MW01260017

UROLOGIC SURGICAL PATHOLOGY

FOURTH EDITION

UROLOGIC SURGICAL PATHOLOGY

FOURTH EDITION

Liang Cheng, MD

Virgil H. Moon Professor of Pathology and Urology
Director of Molecular Diagnostics and Molecular Pathology Laboratory
Chief of Genitourinary Pathology Division
Director, Fellowship in Urologic Pathology
Department of Pathology and Laboratory Medicine
Indiana University School of Medicine
Indianapolis, Indiana, United States

Gregory T. MacLennan, MD

Professor of Pathology, Urology and Oncology
Case Western Reserve University School of Medicine
University Hospitals Cleveland Medical Center
Cleveland, Ohio, United States

David G. Bostwick, MD, MBA

Chief Medical Officer
Bostwick Laboratories, a Division of Poplar Healthcare
Orlando, Florida, United States

ELSEVIER

ELSEVIER

1600 John F. Kennedy Blvd.
Ste 1800
Philadelphia, PA 19103-899

UROLOGIC SURGICAL PATHOLOGY, FOURTH EDITION

ISBN: 978-0-323-54941-7

Copyright © 2020 by Elsevier, Inc. All rights reserved.

Previous editions copyrighted 2014, 2006, 1998

No part of this publication may be reproduced or transmitted in any form or by any means, electronic or mechanical, including photocopying, recording, or any information storage and retrieval system, without permission in writing from the publisher. Details on how to seek permission, further information about the Publisher's permissions policies and our arrangements with organizations such as the Copyright Clearance Center and the Copyright Licensing Agency, can be found at our website: www.elsevier.com/permissions.

This book and the individual contributions contained in it are protected under copyright by the Publisher (other than as may be noted herein).

Notices

Practitioners and researchers must always rely on their own experience and knowledge in evaluating and using any information, methods, compounds or experiments described herein. Because of rapid advances in the medical sciences, in particular, independent verification of diagnoses and drug dosages should be made. To the fullest extent of the law, no responsibility is assumed by Elsevier, authors, editors or contributors for any injury and/or damage to persons or property as a matter of products liability, negligence or otherwise, or from any use or operation of any methods, products, instructions, or ideas contained in the material herein.

Library of Congress Control Number: 2018959513

Content Strategist: Michael Houston
Content Development Manager: Katie De Francesco
Content Development Specialist: Angie Breckon
Publishing Services Manager: Deepthi Unni
Project Manager: Janish Ashwin Paul
Design Direction: Renee Duenow

Printed in Canada

Last digit is the print number: 9 8 7 6 5 4 3 2

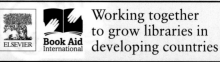

Contributors

Hikmat A. Al-Ahmadie, MD
Associate Attending Pathologist
Memorial Sloan Kettering Cancer Center
New York, New York, United States

Mahul B. Amin, MD
Professor and Chairman
Department of Pathology and Laboratory Medicine
University of Tennessee Health Sciences
Memphis, Tennessee, United States

Md. Shahrier Amin, MD, PhD
Nephropathologist
Arkana Laboratories
Little Rock, Arkansas, United States

Alberto G. Ayala, MD
Professor of Pathology
Weill Medical College of Cornell University
Department of Pathology and Genomic Medicine
Houston Methodist Hospital
Ashbel-Smith Professor Emeritus of Pathology
The University of Texas MD Anderson Cancer Center
Houston, Texas, United States

Stephen M. Bonsib, MD
Nephropathologist
Arkana Laboratories
Little Rock, Arkansas, United States

David G. Bostwick, MD, MBA
Chief Medical Officer
Bostwick Laboratories, a Division of Poplar Healthcare
Orlando, Florida, United States

Liang Cheng, MD
Virgil H. Moon Professor of Pathology and Urology
Director of Molecular Diagnostics and Molecular Pathology
Chief of Genitourinary Pathology Division
Director, Fellowship in Urologic Pathology
Department of Pathology and Laboratory Medicine
Indiana University School of Medicine
Indianapolis, Indiana, United States

Mukul Divatia, MD
Assistant Professor
Department of Pathology and Genomic Medicine
Houston Methodist Hospital
Weill Medical College of Cornell University
Houston, Texas, United States

Eva Compérat, MD
Professor
Service d'Anatomie et Cytologie Pathologiques
Hôpital Tenon and Sorbonne University
Paris, France

Robert E. Emerson, MD
Professor
Department of Pathology and Laboratory Medicine
Indiana University School of Medicine
Director of Anatomic Pathology
Eskenazi Hospital
Indianapolis, Indiana, United States

Pilar González-Peramato, MD, PhD
Associate Professor of Pathology
Department of Pathology
University Autonoma de Madrid
Section of Genitourinary Pathology
Department of Pathology
University Hospital La Paz
Madrid, Spain

Kyu-Rae Kim, MD, PhD
Professor of Pathology
Department of Pathology
The University of Ulsan College of Medicine
Asan Medical Center
Seoul, South Korea

Ernest E. Lack, MD
Senior Consulting Pathologist
Joint Pathology Center
Silver Spring, Maryland, United States

Antonio Lopez-Beltran, MD, PhD
Professor of Anatomic Pathology
Unit of Anatomic Pathology
Department of Surgery
Cordoba University School of Medicine
Cordoba, Spain

Jun Ma, MD
Staff Pathologist
Bostwick Laboratories, a Division of Poplar Healthcare
Orlando, Florida, United States

Gregory T. MacLennan, MD
Professor of Pathology, Urology and Oncology
Case Western Reserve University
University Hospitals Cleveland Medical Center
Cleveland, Ohio, United States

Rodolfo Montironi, MD
Professor of Pathology
Head, Genitourinary Cancer Program
Section of Pathological Anatomy
United Hospitals
Polytechnic University of the Marche Region
Ancona, Italy

Manuel Nistal, MD, PhD
Professor of Histology
Department of Anatomy, Histology and
    Neuroscience
University Autonoma de Madrid
Head of Service
Department of Pathology
University Hospital La Paz
Madrid, Spain

Edina Paal, MD
Assistant Professor
The George Washington University
Staff Pathologist
Pathology and Laboratory Medicine Service
Veterans Administration Medical Center
Washington, DC, United States

Ricardo Paniagua, MD, PhD
Professor of Cell Biology
Department of Biomedicine and Biotechnology
University of Alcalá
Alcalá de Henares
Madrid, Spain

Andrew A. Renshaw, MD
Staff Pathologist
Department of Pathology
Baptist Hospital of Miami and Miami Cancer Institute
Miami, Florida, United States

Victor E. Reuter, MD
Professor of Pathology
Weil Medical College of Cornell University
Attending Pathologist and Vice Chair
Memorial Sloan Kettering Cancer Center
New York, New York, United States

Jae Y. Ro, MD, PhD
Director of Surgical Pathology
Department of Pathology and Genomic Medicine
Houston Methodist Hospital
Weill Medical College of Cornell University
Adjunct Professor
The University of Texas MD Anderson Cancer Center
Houston, Texas, United States

Thomas M. Ulbright, MD
Lawrence M. Roth Emeritus Professor of Pathology
Department of Pathology and Laboratory Medicine
Indiana University School of Medicine
Indianapolis, Indiana, United States

Robert H. Young, MD
Robert E. Scully Professor of Pathology
Harvard Medical School
Pathologist, James Homer Wright Pathology Laboratories
Massachusetts General Hospital
Boston, Massachusetts, United States

Preface to the Fourth Edition

It is our great privilege to present the fourth edition of *Urologic Surgical Pathology*. As our understanding of urologic diseases continues to rapidly evolve and advance, this newest edition has been substantially revised and incorporates the most current knowledge, understanding, and terminology in the field of genitourinary pathology. As with previous editions, the fourth edition is authored by leading contemporary international experts and serves as an evidence- and criterion-based reference that encompasses the present scope of our specialty. The emphasis remains on the practical aspects of diagnostic pathology with detailed discussions of the clinical and histopathologic components across the continuum of urologic disease processes. Additionally, there is added focus on novel diagnostic biomarkers, newly characterized histologic variants, and recent advances within the understanding of cancer genomics. The text's framework also incorporates the most recently published TNM staging classifications (2017 revision) by the American Joint Committee on Cancer (AJCC) and the 2016 World Health Organization (WHO) Classification of Tumours of the Urinary System and Male Genital Organs.

This work is designed to provide contemporary, comprehensive, and evidence-based information not only for pathologists, but also for urologists, medical oncologists, and other healthcare professionals involved in patient care. In today's era of precision medicine, effective patient care is a collaborative effort requiring medical professionals of various specialties to synthesize new pathologic discoveries toward translational clinicopathologic correlations at the patient's bedside. With this in mind, the fourth edition of *Urologic Surgical Pathology* highlights the burgeoning role that molecular pathology has secured within modern health care, particularly in the management of urologic malignancy. The reader will subsequently appreciate the increased emphasis placed on discussions of new molecular genetic discoveries and their applications within tumor diagnosis, classification, and practical utility in personalized patient care.

We are grateful to our contributing authors for sharing their knowledge and experience with our readers. We extend utmost thanks to both Fredrik H. Skarstedt from the Multimedia Education Division of the Department of Pathology at Indiana University, who edited the digital images for this book, and Tracey Bender, who provided outstanding editorial assistance. We also thank the dedicated and talented staff at Elsevier, especially Angie Breckon and Michael Houston, who have given invaluable support throughout the development and production of this book. Finally, we are incredibly grateful to our colleagues and readers for their continued support in our efforts to produce the most comprehensive and up-to-date reference for the study and understanding of urologic disease. We hope that the fourth edition of *Urologic Surgical Pathology* becomes a valuable resource for all of our readers.

Liang Cheng
Gregory T. MacLennan
David G. Bostwick

January 2019

Contents

1

Nonneoplastic Diseases of the Kidney

MD. SHAHRIER AMIN AND STEPHEN M. BONSIB

"Study with me, then, a few things in the spirit of truth alone so we may establish the manner of Nature's operation. For this essay which I plan, will shed light upon the structure of the kidney. Do not stop to question whether these ideas are new or old, but ask, more properly, whether they harmonize with Nature. I never reached my idea of the structure of the kidney by the aid of books, but by the long and varied use of the microscope. I have gotten the rest by the deductions of reason, slowly, and with an open mind, as is my custom."

—Marcello Malpighi, 1666

CHAPTER OUTLINE

Introduction

In keeping with the spirit of Marcello Malpighi, this chapter also aspires to reveal "the manner of Nature's operation" as it affects the kidney.[1] However, unlike Malpighi, today's knowledge draws extensively on the labors, discoveries, and insights of investigators of the past centuries.

Knowledge of the normal structure and function of the kidney has been acquired over centuries of scholarly effort. We have come a long way since Aristotle taught that urine was formed by the bladder and that kidneys were present "not of actual necessity, but as matters of greater finish and perfection."[1] Reference to the excretory functions of the bladders and kidneys can be found in early Indian Ayurveda, Chinese, or Egyptian literature.[2-4] Some of the earliest scientifically valid experimental methods are described in *The Canon of Medicine* by the famous Persian Muslim physician Abu Ali Sina, also known as "Avicenna."[5-13] He meticulously described the layers of the bladder and its two-stage function, the intramural ureter and antireflux mechanisms, and scientifically classified urethral and bladder diseases, notably calculi. The foundation of modern urology was established in the sixteenth century by Leonardo da Vinci and Vesalius, who provided the first accurate and detailed drawings of the female and male genitourinary tracts (Fig. 1.1).[14,15] More than 300 years passed before William Bowman, in 1842, coupled intravascular dye injection with microscopic examination to demonstrate the structural organization of the nephron and its vascular supply (Fig. 1.2).[16,17] Bowman's

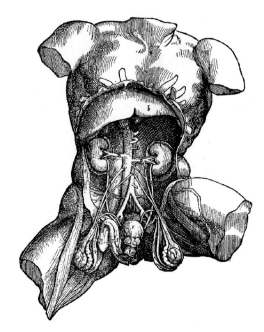

Fig. 1.1 Vesalius's anatomic illustration of the male genitourinary tract published in 1543. Note that the left kidney is incorrectly placed lower than the right. (From Murphy LJT, ed. The history of urology. Springfield, Ill: Charles C Thomas, 1972; with permission.)

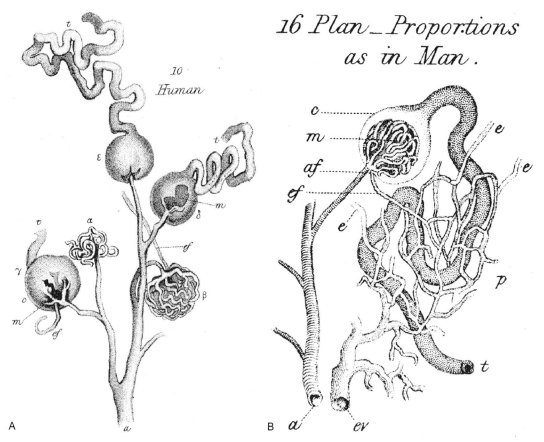

Fig. 1.2 William Bowman's illustration of the vascular supply to glomeruli and the relationship of the efferent arteriole to the convoluted tubules (A and B). (From Bowman W. On the structure and use of the malpighian bodies of the kidney, with observations on the circulation through that gland. Philos Trans R Soc Lond Biol 1842;132:57; with permission.)

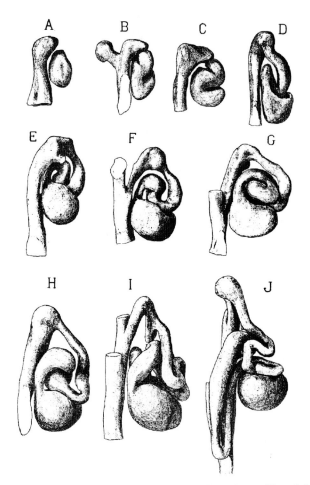

Fig. 1.3 Wax model serial reconstruction of nephron differentiation by Huber. (From Huber GC. On the development and shape of uriniferous tubules of certain of the higher mammals. Am J Anat 1905;4:29; with permission.)

observations provided morphologic support for Malpighi's seventeenth-century speculation of a filtration function for the malpighian body (the glomerulus).[1,18] Sixty years later the embryologic development of the nephron was demonstrated by Huber in a thin-section serial reconstruction study of embryos (Fig. 1.3).[19] Huber's observations were refined and elegantly illustrated by Brödel in Kelly and Burnam's *Diseases of the kidneys, ureters and bladder* published in 1914.[20] Potter and Osathanondh validated the findings in a series of microdissection studies of developing kidneys, which were published in the 1960s.[21-26]

The ultrastructural features and immunohistochemical profiles of the normal kidney and of many diseases were elucidated in the 1970s and 1980s after refinement of the percutaneous biopsy technique and advances in morphologic analyses. Since 1990 there has been an explosion of new information about the genetic basis of normal and abnormal renal development, and about numerous disease processes.[27-34]

Embryologic Development and Normal Structure

This chapter begins with a brief review of the embryology and normal gross and microscopic structure of the kidney. For more in-depth coverage of these topics, several excellent resources are available.[27-34]

The development of the urinary and genital tracts is closely related (Fig. 1.4). These tracts both develop from paired longitudinal

cords of tissue lateral to the aorta that are known as the intermediate mesoderm.[26,27,33] From the portion caudal to the seventh somite, known as the nephrogenic mesoderm (or nephrogenic cord), three nephronic structures develop in quick succession: the pronephros, the mesonephros, and the metanephros. Although the pronephros and the mesonephros are transient organs, they are crucial for the proper development of both the urinary and the reproductive tracts.

Pronephros

The first embryologic derivative of the nephrogenic cord is the pronephros, a structure functional only in the lowest forms of fish. It arises from the most cranial portion of the nephrogenic cord during the third week of gestation (1.7 mm stage; 7th to 14th somite stage). Approximately seven pairs of tubules form, only to regress 2 weeks later (Figs. 1.4 and 1.5). The pronephros is important because the pronephric tubules grow caudally and fuse with the next pronephric unit, which gives rise to the pronephric duct. The pronephric duct is the only remnant of the pronephros, and henceforth is called the mesonephric duct.

Mesonephros

The mesonephros develops from the dorsolumbar segments of the nephrogenic cord from day 24 of gestation. Cells of the mesonephric duct proliferate caudally (Fig. 1.4) and begin to form the mesonephric kidney during the fourth week of gestation (4 mm; 26th to 28th somite stage). The mesonephros is a highly differentiated structure and is the functional kidney of higher fishes and amphibians.

The mesonephric kidney consists of approximately 40 pairs of nephrons. The cranial nephrons sequentially regress while caudal nephrons form, with 7 to 15 nephrons functional at all times (Figs. 1.4 and Fig. 1.5). The nephrons are induced in a fashion analogous to their metanephric counterparts.

A fully developed mesonephric nephron consists of a glomerulus connected to the mesonephric duct by a convoluted proximal and distal tubule (Figs. 1.6A and 1.7A). The glomerulus is vascularized by capillaries that branch from small arterioles originating from the aorta, and its efferent arteriole empties into the posterior cardinal vein. The glomerulus appears to filter plasma. Its proximal tubule possesses a brush border; the proximal and distal tubules appear capable of nutrient resorption, as well as concentration and dilution of urine. The tubules connect with the mesonephric duct, which extends distally to connect to the cloaca at about 4 weeks postconception. The mesonephric kidney remains functional until the end of the fourth month of gestation.

Portions of the mesonephric kidney can be easily identified in small embryos (1 to 3 cm), which are occasionally encountered in surgical specimens such as those from ectopic pregnancies. In the male, some of the caudal mesonephric tubules develop into the efferent ducts of the epididymis, while the mesonephric duct becomes the epididymis, the seminal vesicle, and ejaculatory duct. In the female, the entire mesonephros degenerates during the end of the first trimester; however, vestigial structures such as the epoophoron, paroophoron, and Gartner duct, as well as mesonephric remnants, can occasionally be seen in surgical specimens from the ovary and fallopian tubes.

Metanephros

The metanephric kidney is the product of a complex orchestration of embryologic processes. Although discussed separately, it must be

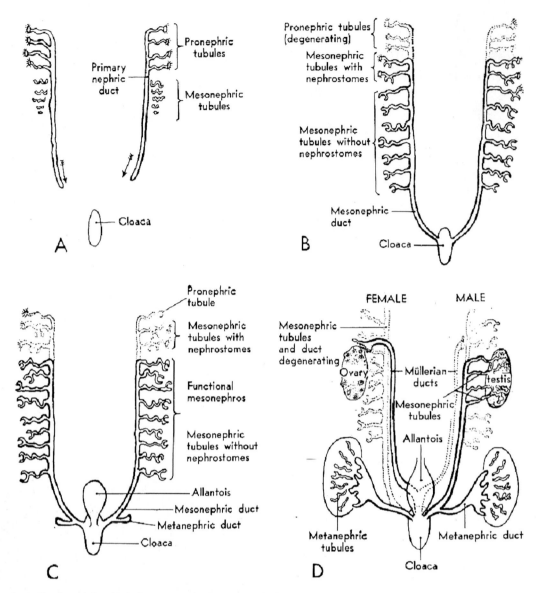

Fig. 1.4 Diagram illustrating the relationship between reproductive tract and urinary tract development. (From Patton BM. Human embryology. New York: McGraw Hill, 1968; with permission.)

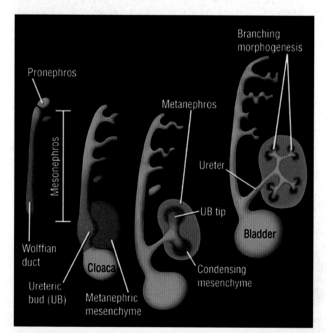

appreciated that while the collecting system and renal pyramids are forming there is simultaneous induction of thousands of nephrons, and neurovascular and lymphatic components ramify in a carefully organized architecture throughout the cortex.

The formation of the adult metanephric kidney begins during the fourth to sixth weeks of gestation (4 to 5 mm), after the mesonephric duct has established communication with the urogenital sinus (Fig. 1.5). A diverticulum, known as the ureteric (or ampullary) bud, forms on its posterior medial aspect (Figs. 1.4 and Fig. 1.5) and then establishes contact with the sacral portion of the nephrogenic mesoderm, the nephrogenic blastema. A complex

Fig. 1.5 Early morphogenesis of the kidney. The pronephros and mesonephros begin to develop at 3 and 3.5 weeks, respectively, but gradually regress. The metanephros forms in the metanephric mesenchyme at the distal end of the mesonephros, after the mesonephric duct has established connection with the urogenital sinus, usually after 4 weeks of gestation. It is then invaded by the ureteric bud, which undergoes branching to form the collecting system while the overlying condensing mesenchyme forms the nephrons.

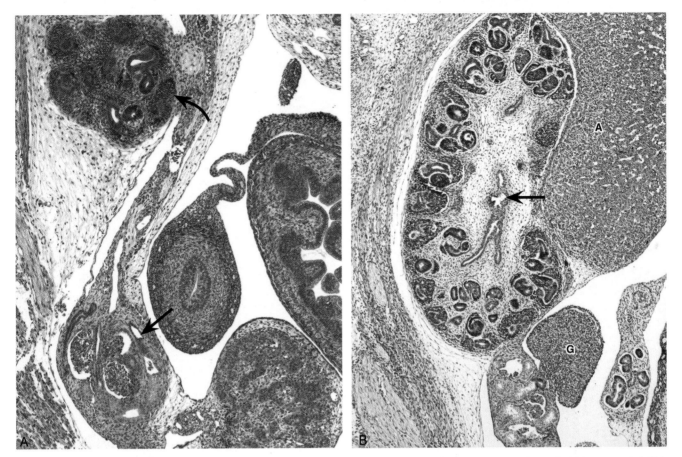

Fig. 1.6 (A) An embryo of 7 weeks of gestation showing initial induction of the metanephric kidney (*curved arrow*) and glomeruli of the mesonephric kidney (*arrow*). (B) Embryo 12 weeks of gestation showing a metanephric kidney with a rudimentary collecting system (*arrow*) and active nephrogenesis. The adrenal gland (*A*), gonad (*G*), and mesonephric kidney are also visible.

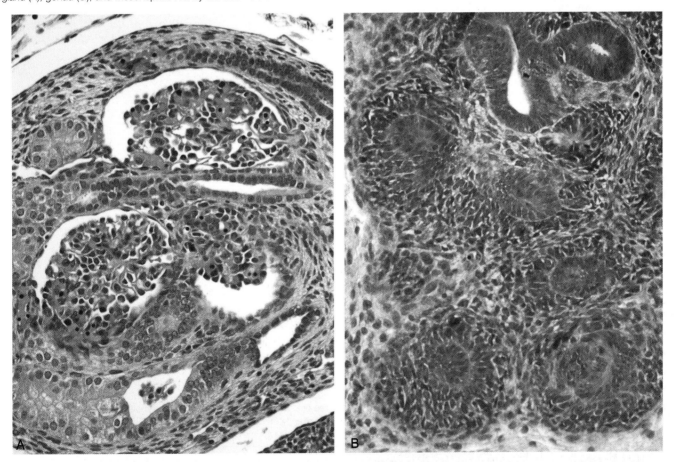

Fig. 1.7 (A) A portion of the mesonephric kidney (from Fig. 1.6A) showing well-developed glomeruli and tubules. (B) Metanephric kidney (from Fig. 1.6A) beginning to form and showing condensations of cells destined to form a nephron.

reciprocal inductive process results in dichotomous ureteric bud branching and nephron induction that eventually culminate in the adult metanephric kidney. The metanephros is therefore a product of two embryonic derivatives; the nephrons are of blastemal origin, whereas the ureter, pelvis, calyces, and cortical and medullary collecting ducts are derived from the ureteric bud.

On contact with metanephric blastema the ureteric bud undergoes a rapid sequence of dichotomous branching and fusion, forming the renal collecting system by the 14th week (Figs. 1.8 and 1.9). The initial two branches form the renal pelvis, the third to sixth branches form the major and minor calyces, and the sixth to eleventh branches form the papillary ducts (Fig. 1.9). Because ureteric bud branching is more rapid in the upper and lower poles, the calyces and papillae in those regions are more numerous.

While the collecting system is forming, nephron induction has already begun (Figs. 1.6B, 1.7B, 1.8, 1.10, and 1.11). The kidneys have moved into the flanks because of a combination of migration out of the pelvis and rapid caudal growth of the embryo (Fig. 1.12). The kidney also has rotated from its original position with the pelvis anterior, to its final position with the pelvis medial.[20] By week 13 or 14, the minor calyces and renal pyramids are well formed and

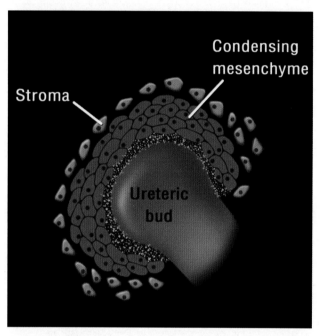

Fig. 1.8 Invasion of the ureteric bud into the mesenchyme results in condensation of the mesenchyme around the ureteric bud tip. (From Jain S. "Normal kidney development." In "Diagnostic pathology: kidney diseases" by Colvin RB and Chang A, pages 36–45. Philadelphia: Elsevier, 2016; with permission.)

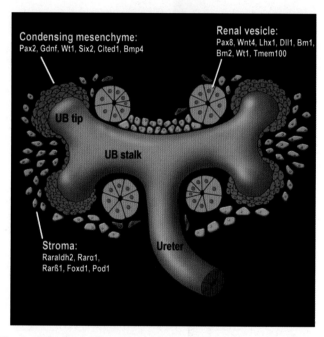

Fig. 1.10 Reciprocal interactions between the ureteric bud, condensing mesenchyme, and stroma involve cross talk between cells with involvement of many genes and their products, some of which are highlighted in this figure. (From Jain S. "Normal kidney development." In "Diagnostic pathology: kidney diseases" by Colvin RB and Chang A, pages 36–45. Philadelphia: Elsevier, 2016; with permission.)

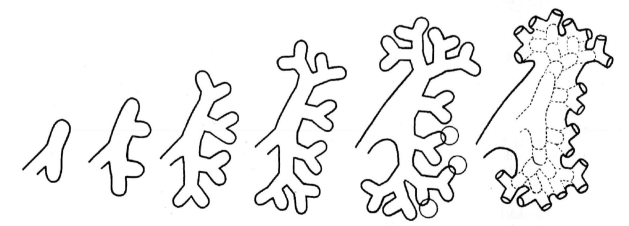

Fig. 1.9 Development of the renal pelvis. Diagram showing branches of the ureteral bud. *Circles* indicate possible locations of minor calyces at level of third-, fourth-, or fifth-generation branches. The figure at the right indicates ureteral bud branches that may dilate to form the renal pelvis. (From Osathanondth V, Potter EL. Development of the human kidney as shown by microdissection III. Formation and interrelationship of collecting tubules and nephrons. Arch Pathol 1963;76:61. Copyright © 1963. American Medical Association. All rights reserved.)

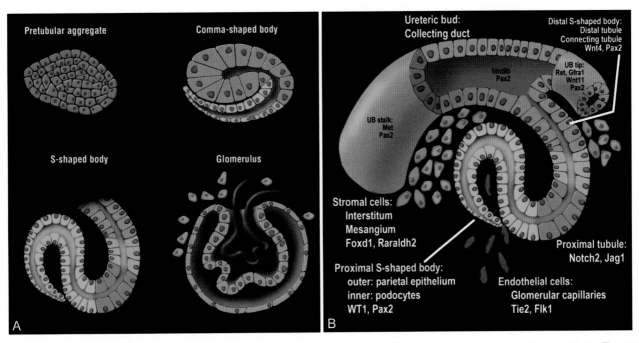

Fig. 1.11 (A) Schematic showing how the pretubular aggregate differentiates to form successively the comma shaped body and S-shaped body. The proximal portion becomes the tubules, and the distal portion forms the glomerular epithelial cells. (B) Endothelial cells invade the cleft of the S-shaped body and form the glomerular tuft. Some of the involved genes are also shown. (From Jain S. "Normal kidney development." In "Diagnostic pathology: kidney diseases" by Colvin RB and Chang A, pages 36–45. Philadelphia: Elsevier, 2016; with permission.)

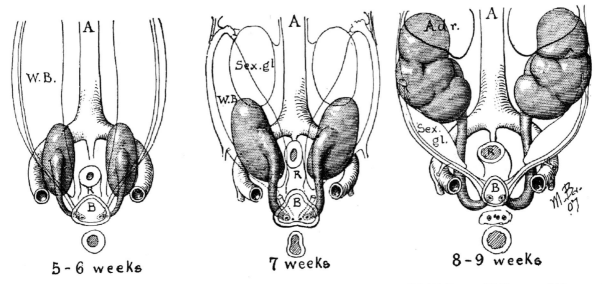

Fig. 1.12 A 1907 diagram by Max Brödel showing the ascent and medial rotation of the kidney. (From Kelly HA, Burnam CF. Diseases of kidneys, ureters and bladder. New York: Appleton, Century Crofts, 1914; with permission.)

the lobar architecture can be appreciated grossly (Figs. 1.13 through 1.15). At this time, the cortex contains several generations of nephrons, and the lateral portions of adjacent lobes begin to merge to form the columns of Bertin.

By weeks 20 to 22 the renal lobes are well formed, and the kidney is a miniature of the adult kidney (Fig. 1.15). The ureteric bud has ceased branching, but the branches continue to lengthen. As they lengthen they induce arcades of four to seven nephrons, which are connected to the collecting duct by a connecting tubule (Fig. 1.16). Additional groups of three to seven nephrons then

form, each attached directly to a collecting duct without a connecting tubule. Therefore each cortical collecting duct will have 10 to 14 generations of nephrons attached, with the most recently formed and least mature nephrons located beneath the renal capsule.

Nephron Differentiation

The formation of individual nephrons begins as early as 7 weeks of gestation and results in a limited degree of "renal function" by

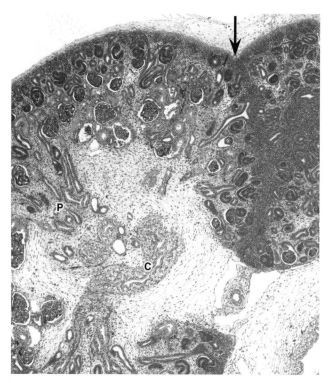

Fig. 1.13 Kidney from a 13-week fetus (compare with Fig. 1.14) showing a renal lobe with a pyramid (*P*) and the collecting system (*C*). Fusion of adjacent lobes forms columns of Bertin (*arrow*).

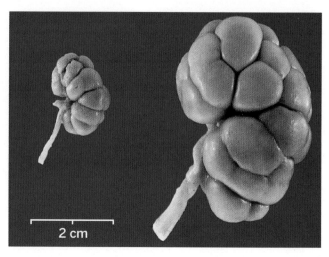

Fig. 1.15 A 22-week fetal kidney (*left*) and a 40-week term kidney (*right*) showing distinct fetal lobes.

9 weeks. In the subcapsular nephrogenic zone of any immature kidney (Fig. 1.17) the sequence of nephron induction can be observed in its various stages of completion. The historic wax models and illustrations made by Huber (Fig. 1.18), the drawing by Brödel (Figs. 1.3 and 1.14), and the illustrations by Dressler and Jain (Figs. 1.5, 1.8, 1.10, and 1.11) provide a three-dimensional

perspective useful in understanding the cellular events during renal development as demonstrated in Fig. 1.17.[26,28]

An individual nephron begins to form when the metanephric blastema aggregates adjacent to the ureteric bud to form a hollow vesicle (Fig. 1.10). The molecular basis for this event is complex and involves the coordinated induction of numerous genes that encode for growth factors, adhesion molecules, matrix components, and other regulatory proteins (Table 1.1 and Figs. 1.10 and 1.11). The cells within the vesicle grow differentially, first forming a comma-shaped aggregate of cells that then elongate and eventually develop two indentations creating an S-shaped structure (Fig. 1.11). The distal portions of the S-shaped body (segments attached to the ureteric bud) are destined to become the proximal and distal tubules (Fig. 1.11). They form tubular structures and establish communication with the collecting duct. The proximal part of the S-shaped body (segment away from the

Fig. 1.14 Microdissected 13-week kidney showing the collecting system, renal pyramids, and several generations of glomeruli. Most of the tubules have been removed. (From Osathanondth V, Potter EL. Development of the human kidney as shown by microdissection III. Formation and interrelationship of collecting tubules and nephrons. Arch Pathol 1963;76:61. Copyright © 1963. American Medical Association. All rights reserved.)

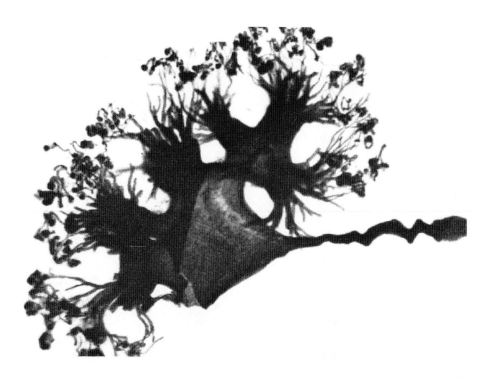

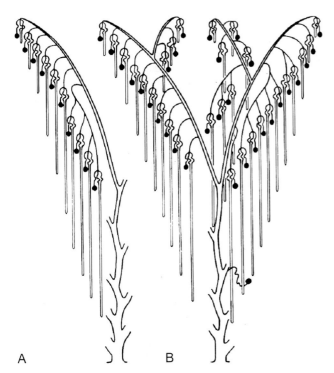

Fig. 1.16 Kidney showing arrangement of nephrons at birth. (A) Usual pattern. (B) Possible variations. (From Osathanondth V, Potter EL. Development of the human kidney as shown by microdissection III. Formation and interrelationship of collecting tubules and nephrons. Arch Pathol 1963; 76:61. Copyright © 1963. American Medical Association. All rights reserved.)

ureteric bud) gradually broadens and separates into two cell layers: the outer layer becomes the parietal epithelium of the Bowman capsule, whereas the inner layer becomes the visceral epithelium (podocytes). Endothelial cells migrate into the indentation in the proximal part and eventually form a podocyte-invested and vascularized glomerular tuft within Bowman capsule.

Cells of the upper layer continue to proliferate to form a connecting duct and the distal convoluted tubule, whereas cells of the middle limb produce the proximal convoluted tubule and the limb

of Henle. Finally, the limb of Henle grows down along the collecting duct to form the medullary rays. Nephrogenesis is usually complete by 32 to 36 weeks of gestation. Maturation occurs beyond this period and continues until adulthood, with resulting renal enlargement that reflects tubular elongation and cellular enlargement of the tubular portions of the nephron. There appears to be some correlation (Table 1.2) between fetal gestational age and layers/rows of mature glomeruli, which can be useful in forensic assessment or to correlate with development in other organs.

Gross Anatomy

The kidneys are paired retroperitoneal organs that normally extend from the 12th thoracic vertebra to the 3rd lumbar vertebra. The upper poles are tilted slightly toward the midline, and the right kidney is slightly lower and shorter than the left kidney. The average adult kidney is 11 to 12 cm long, 5 to 7 cm wide, and 2.5 to 3 cm thick, and it weighs 125 to 170 g in men and 115 to 155 g in women.[20,27,31,33,34] The combined mass of the kidneys correlates with body surface area, whereas age, sex, and race have relatively less influence.[35] Its volume can increase or decrease by 15% to 40% with major fluctuations in blood pressure (BP), hydration, or interstitial expansion by edema.

The posterior surfaces are flatter than the anterior, and the medial surface is concave with a 3-cm slitlike space called the *hilum*. The hilum is the vestibule through which the collecting system, nerves, arteries, veins, and lymphatics pass. In the adult, these structures are invested by fat within the renal sinus and are usually arranged from anterior to posterior as artery and vein and ureter.

The subcapsular surface of the renal cortex may be smooth and featureless, or may show grooves corresponding to the individual renal lobes (Fig. 1.19). The persistence of distinct fetal lobes is common and is a normal anatomic variant. In some kidneys, three zones are created by two shallow superficial grooves that radiate from the hilum to the lateral border (Fig. 1.20). The three regions define the upper pole, middle zone, and lower pole, and usually reflect regions drained by the three lobar veins.

The normal adult kidney has a minimum of 10 to 14 lobes, each composed of a central conical medullary pyramid surrounded by a

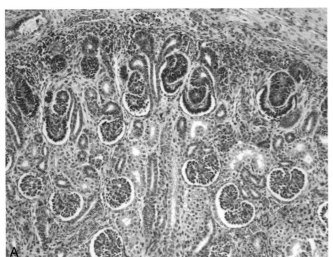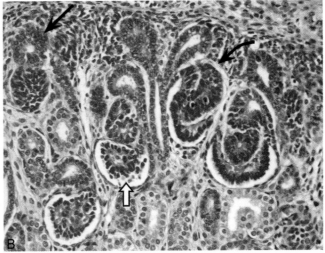

Fig. 1.17 (A) Nephrogenic zone of a 14-week kidney. (B) Notice the ampullary bud and hollow vesicles (*arrow*), early S-phase (*curved arrow*), primitive glomerular tuft (*open arrow*), and increasingly mature glomeruli.

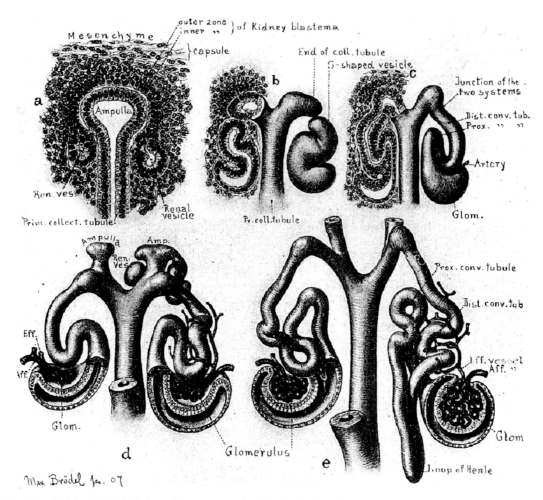

Fig. 1.18 1907 illustration by Max Brödel that shows the sequence of nephron induction. (From Kelly HA, Burnam CF. Diseases of kidneys, ureters and bladder. New York: Appleton, Century Crofts, 1914; with permission.)

TABLE 1.1	Expression of Selected Genes and Proteins Involved in the Development of the Kidneys			
Name	**Role in Development**	**Effect of Mutations**	**Expression in Normal Kidney**	**Comment**
PAX2 (paired box 2)	Acts as a survival signal in ureteric bud/collecting duct lineage	Renal agenesis in null mutant; large gene deletions implicated in 3% of cases of renal-coloboma syndrome[582]	Intermediate mesoderm, nephric duct, mesonephros, ureteric bud, induced metanephric mesenchyme	Nuclear stain; can be used to confirm renal, Müllerian, or Wolffian duct origin of cells
N-myc (avian myelocytomatosis viral oncogene homologue)	Differentiation and organogenesis	Hypoplastic mesonephros, decreased ureteric bud tips and nephrons, renal hypoplasia	Induced metanephric mesenchyme	Amplification (>10 copies) associated with poor prognosis in neuroblastoma
HNF1B (hepatocyte nuclear factor 1β)	Maintains differentiated state of renal epithelia	Null mutants do not survive; renal cysts, single kidneys, renal hypoplasia, electrolyte abnormalities	All tubular epithelia and collecting ducts	Renal tubules become cystic if HNF1B is mutated
WT1 (Wilms tumor 1)	Transcription factor	Renal agenesis in null mutant; proteinuria in heterozygous mice; disturbed podocyte differentiation, glomerulosclerosis	Intermediate mesoderm, mesonephros, uninduced and induced metanephric mesenchyme, comma- and S-shaped bodies; restricted to podocytes in adult kidney	Marker in tumors

Name	Role in Development	Effect of Mutations	Expression in Normal Kidney	Comment
FOXD1 (forkhead box D1)	Expressed in interstitial progenitor cells in the cortex and medulla	Fused kidneys	FOXD1 + progenitors form stroma that becomes vascular smooth muscle, juxtaglomerular cells, mesangial cells, pericytes, and resident fibroblasts	Marker of interstitial progenitor cells that form renal stroma
RARα/RARβ2 (retinoic acid receptor)	Ureteric bud branching, stroma signaling	Kidney and ureter malformations	RARα: ureteric bud, metanephric mesenchyme, stroma RARβ: stroma only	Marker in tumors
GDNF (glial cell line–derived neurotrophic factor)	Growth factor	Ureteric bud fails to form or has abnormal branching; renal hypoplasia or agenesis	Intermediate mesoderm, mesonephros, induced metanephric mesenchyme, pretubular aggregate	
Angiotensinogen	Renin substrate	Hypoplastic papillae, hydronephrosis, thickened blood vessels, hypotension	Ureteric bud, stroma, glomeruli, proximal tubules	
Angiotensin receptor types 1a and 1b	Angiotensin receptor	Hypoplastic papillae, hydronephrosis, thickened blood vessels, hypotension	Ureteric bud, stroma, proximal tubules	
Angiotensin receptor type 2	Angiotensin receptor	Duplicated collecting system, hydronephrotic upper pole	Stroma adjacent to ureteric bud stalk	
Fibroblast growth factor	Growth factor	Increased apoptosis, truncated nephrons, renal hypoplasia	Pretubular aggregates, vesicles, tubule progenitors	
Platelet-derived growth factor (PDGF) receptor b	Growth factor (PDGF) receptor	Dilated glomerular capillaries with no mesangial cells	Glomerular mesangial cells	
Vascular endothelial growth factor	Growth factor	Small glomeruli, lack capillary loops, few endothelial cells	S-shaped body, podocytes, collecting ducts	
Laminin α5	Basement membrane protein	Abnormal glomeruli with displaced endothelial and mesangial cells, and clustered podocytes	Basement membrane of ureteric bud, developing tubules, and glomeruli	
Laminin β2	Basement membrane protein	Absence of podocyte foot processes, proteinuria	Glomerular basement membrane	Nephrotic syndrome
Laminin α3β2	Transmembrane adhesion receptor	Dilated and fewer capillary loops; loss of podocyte foot processes, dual GBMs	Ureteric bud, collecting ducts, podocytes	
Nephrin	Transmembrane protein	Foot process effacement, absence of filtration slit diaphragm, proteinuria	Podocyte filtration slit diaphragm	Congenital nephrotic syndrome of the Finnish type
PKD1 and PKD2 (polycystin 1 and 2)	Transmembrane proteins	Metanephric cysts in null mutants; postnatal PKD in heterozygous mice	Developing nephron segments and collecting ducts	Mutated in autosomal dominant PKD
UP II and III (Uroplakin)	Transmembrane proteins	Hydronephrosis; vesicoureteric reflux (UPII); ureteric obstruction (UPIII)	Superficial umbrella cells of urothelium	

GBM, Glomerular basement membrane; *PKD*, polycystic kidney disease.

cap of cortex (Fig. 1.21). Often there are six lobes in the upper pole and four lobes each in the middle zone and lower pole. However, substantial variability occurs both in the number of lobes in the adult kidney and in their visibility when the renal capsule is removed.

The renal parenchyma consists of the cortex and the medulla, which are grossly quite distinct (Fig. 1.21). The renal cortex is the nephron-containing parenchyma. It forms a 1.0-cm layer between the renal capsule and medulla (also known as the renal pyramids) and extends down between the renal pyramids forming the columns of Bertin. The midplane of a column of Bertin is the line of fusion of two renal lobes. The renal medulla is divided into an outer medulla and the inner medulla or papilla (Fig. 1.21). The outer medulla is further divided into an outer stripe and an inner stripe. Each segment of the renal medulla is defined by its unique tubular components, as discussed later. The outer medulla receives input from nephrons in the overlying cortex and nephrons in the adjacent half of a column of Bertin. The papilla protrudes into a minor calyx. Its tip has 20 to 70 openings of the papillary collecting ducts (Bellini ducts).

The arterial supply to the kidney follows a general overall blueprint, and knowledge of its details is useful when evaluating lesions in a kidney affected by vascular abnormalities.[36-38] In 1901, Brödel first appreciated the distinctive renovascular segmentation of the kidney.[38] The nomenclature used here was established by Graves in 1954.[37]

The main renal artery arises from the aorta and divides into an anterior and a posterior division, and five segmental arteries are usually derived from these two divisions (Figs. 1.20 and 1.22). The anterior division supplies most of the kidney and often divides into four segmental arteries: the apical, upper, middle, and lower segmental branches. The apical and lower segmental arteries supply

TABLE 1.2	Correlation of Fetal Gestational Age and Glomerular Development	
Gestational Age (weeks)	Rows of Glomeruli in Cortex From Medulla to Capsule	Number of Mature Glomerular Layers
16-23	3	–
24	3-5	4.3 ± 0.8
25	4-6	4.6 ± 0.7
26	5-7	–
27	6-8	6.1 ± 1.1
28	7-9	6.0 ± 1.2
29	8-10	6.3 ± 1.3
30	9-11	–
31	10-12	7.1 ± 0.9
32	11-13	–
33	12-13	7.7 ± 0.8
34	12-14	–
35-42	12-14	7.6 ± 0.4 to 8.6 ± 1.3
Newborn to adult	12-14	–
	Cortex between columns of Bertin	Radial counts; excludes columns of Bertin

From Jain S. Normal kidney development. In: Diagnostic pathology: kidney diseases. Philadelphia: Elsevier, 2016 (with permission).

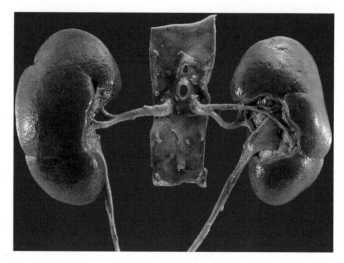

Fig. 1.20 Kidneys showing two grooves defining the renal poles. In each kidney an anterior and posterior division of the renal artery is visible. The left kidney (*right side*) is incompletely rotated.

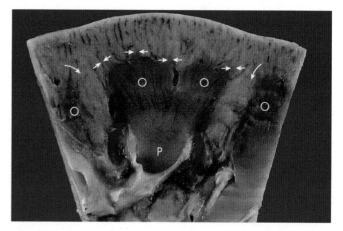

Fig. 1.21 This renal lobe shows the cortical medullary rays. The columns of Bertin invest the outer medulla (*O*), whereas the papilla (*P*) or inner medulla is nestled within a minor calyx.

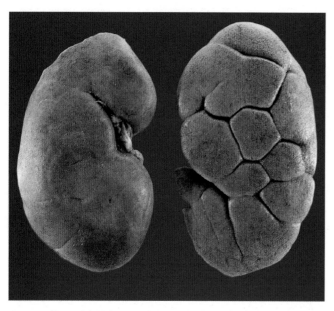

Fig. 1.19 Two adult kidneys with capsules removed showing subtle fetal lobation (*left*) and prominent fetal lobation (*right*).

the anterior and posterior aspects of the upper and lower poles, respectively (Fig. 1.22). In 20% to 30% of kidneys, one or both arteries will arise separately from the aorta to form supernumerary arteries (also known as aberrant, accessory, or polar arteries). The posterior division becomes the posterior segmental artery. It passes behind the pelvis and supplies the middle two-thirds of the posterior surface. The five segmental arteries and all their branches are end arteries with no collateral blood flow. Thus occlusion of a segmental artery or any of its subsequent branches results in infarction of the zone of parenchyma it supplies.[36]

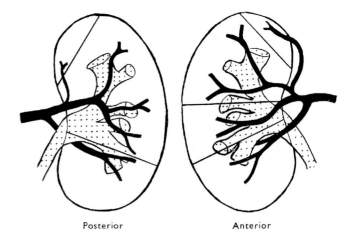

Posterior　　　　　　　Anterior

Fig. 1.22 A diagram of the most common arterial pattern of the kidney showing the main renal artery, anterior and posterior divisions, and the segmental, interlobar, and arcuate arteries. (From Graves FT. The anatomy of the intrarenal arteries and its application to segmental resection of the kidney. Br J Surg 1954;42:133; with permission.)

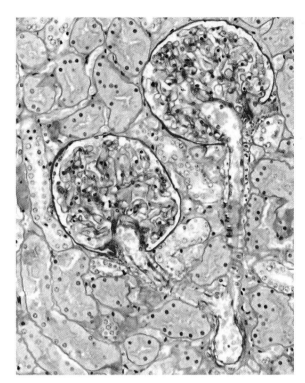

Fig. 1.23 The interlobular artery supplies arterioles to glomeruli (periodic acid–Schiff stain).

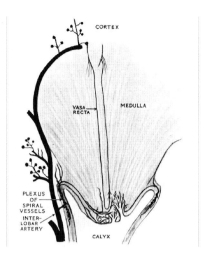

Fig. 1.24 Diagram of the dual blood supply to the papillae. (From Baker SB. The blood supply to the renal papillae. Br J Urol 1959;31:57; with permission.)

Microscopic Anatomy

The cortex is organized into two regions: the cortical labyrinth and the medullary rays (Fig. 1.25). The labyrinth contains glomeruli, proximal and distal convoluted tubules, connecting tubules, and the initial portion of the collecting ducts, as well as interlobular vessels, arterioles, capillaries, and lymphatics. The principal components of the labyrinth are the proximal tubules. In the normal cortex, the tubules are closely packed with closely apposed basement membranes (Figs. 1.23 and 1.25). The interstitial space is scant. It contains the peritubular capillary plexus and inconspicuous numbers of interstitial fibroblasts and reticulum cells. A medullary ray consists of collecting ducts and the proximal and distal straight tubules that course down into and back up from the medulla. The nephrons that empty into the collecting ducts of a single medullary ray comprise a renal lobule, the functional unit of the kidney.

The medulla is divided into an outer medulla, composed of an outer stripe and an inner stripe, and the inner medulla or papilla. Each zone contains specific tubular segments arranged in an

From segmental arteries, the interlobar arteries, arcuate arteries, interlobular arteries, and arterioles are sequentially derived. A segmental artery branches within the renal sinus and creates several interlobar arteries. An interlobar artery enters the parenchyma in a column of Bertin between two renal pyramids (i.e., at the junction of two lobes) and forms a splay of six to eight arcuate arteries. The arcuate arteries course along the corticomedullary junction and terminate at the midpoint of a renal lobe. At perpendicular or slightly oblique angles, the interlobular arteries arise from an arcuate artery and may branch as they pass through the cortex toward the renal capsule. The interlobular arteries course between medullary rays and are encircled by tiers of five to six glomeruli, which they supply with afferent arterioles (Fig. 1.23). The glomerular efferent arteriole forms a portal system of capillaries, which supply the adjacent tubules that arise from more than one glomerulus (Fig. 1.2B).

The renal medulla has a dual blood supply.[39,40] Its principal blood supply arises from the efferent arterioles of the juxtamedullary glomeruli, which course directly into the medulla to form the vasa recta (Fig. 1.24). In addition, as an interlobar artery courses along a minor calyx it gives rise to several spiral arteries, which supply capillaries to the papillary tip. These capillaries anastomose freely with capillaries from the opposite side and form a plexus around the ducts of Bellini.

The interlobular, arcuate, and interlobar veins parallel the arteries. Unlike the arcuate arteries, the arcuate veins have abundant anastomoses. They combine to form three large segmental veins that drain the three poles of the kidney.[31,40,41] The veins lie anterior to the pelvis and unite to form the main renal vein.

The lymphatic drainage is a dual system.[31,41] The major lymphatic drainage follows the blood vessels from parenchyma to the renal sinus, to the hilum, and terminates in lateral aortocaval lymph nodes. In addition, minor capsular lymphatic drainage from the superficial cortex courses into the capsule and then around to the hilum to join the major lymphatic flow.

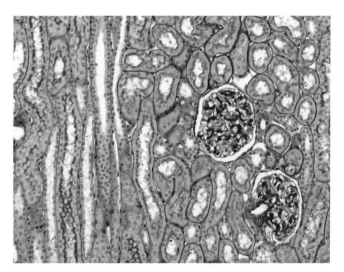

Fig. 1.25 Renal cortex sectioned perpendicular to the renal capsule that shows a medullary ray (*left side*) and the cortical labyrinth with two glomeruli (*right side*) (periodic acid–Schiff stain).

elaborate architecture to create the countercurrent concentration system. The outer stripe contains the straight portions of the proximal tubule, thick ascending limb of loop of Henle and collecting ducts. The inner stripe contains the thin descending and thick ascending limbs of loops of Henle and collecting ducts. The inner medulla contains the thin descending and ascending limbs of loops of Henle and collecting ducts of Bellini. For further details of the microscopic anatomy of the medulla, or for the ultrastructural features of all nephron components, several excellent resources are available.[27,31,41]

Parenchymal Maldevelopment and Cystic Kidney Diseases

"The more complicated an organ in its development, the more subject it is to maldevelopment, and in this respect the kidney outranks most other organs."[33]

—**Edith Potter**

Developmental anomalies and cystic kidney diseases occur in approximately 10% of the population.[27,42-45] They encompass a vast number of complex entities that may be limited to the kidney or part of a multiorgan malformation syndrome. These diseases may be sporadic, hereditary and syndromic, or acquired, and they include several that are associated with a neoplastic diathesis. Enormous progress has been made in unraveling the pathogenesis of many entities with delineation of their genetic and molecular basis. This knowledge has minimized the validity of the simplistic anatomic contribution of urinary tract obstruction popular for so many years by placing it within a larger paradigm of sequential genetic and molecular misadventures that culminate in the malformed kidney and urinary tract.[27,46-56]

These diseases can be separated into two large categories based on pathogenesis. A heterogeneous group of diseases results from mutation of one or more key master genes crucial for proper development of the kidneys and lower urinary tract. Collectively, these are referred to as congenital anomalies of the kidneys and urinary tract (CAKUT). These lesions may be sporadic or hereditary and syndromic. They are common and very important because they account for up to 50% of cases of renal failure in children (Table 1.3).

A second category encompasses a "family" of cystic kidney diseases, the ciliopathies, which result from mutation of genes that

---

TABLE 1.3   **Classification of Cystic Kidney Diseases and Congenital Anomalies of the Kidney and Urinary Tract**

I. Polycystic kidney diseases

A. Autosomal recessive polycystic kidney disease
   Classic in neonates and infants
   Childhood with hepatic fibrosis
B. Autosomal dominant polycystic kidney disease
   Classic adult form
   Early-onset childhood form
C. Glomerulocystic kidney
   Primary GCKD
      Sporadic GCKD
      Familial GCKD
      Hereditary GCKD associated with *UROM* or *HNF1B* mutations
   Secondary glomerular diseases in which glomerular may be present
      Associated with ADPKD/ARPKD/TSC
      Syndromic nonhereditary glomerulocystic kidney
      Ischemic glomerular atrophy
      Renal dysplasia
D. Acquired cystic kidney disease

II. Congenital anomalies of the kidney and urinary tract (CAKUT)

A. Renal agenesis and dysplasia
   Agenesis
      Sporadic: unilateral or bilateral
      Syndromic
      Nonsyndromic multiple malformation syndromes
   Renal dysplasias
      Sporadic: unilateral or bilateral
      Syndromic
      Nonsyndromic multiple malformation syndromes
   Hereditary adysplasia
B. Renal hypoplasias
   Simple hypoplasia: unilateral or bilateral
   Oligomeganephronic hypoplasia
   Cortical hypoplasia (reduced nephron generations)
   Reduced nephron numbers (premature and low birth weight risk for hypertension)
C. Abnormalities in form, position, and number
   Rotation anomaly
   Renal ectopias

Renal fusions
Supernumerary kidney
In combination with A, B, or D
D. Ureteral and urethral abnormalities
   Ureteropelvic junction obstruction
   Ureteral duplication/bifid ureter
   Vesicoureteral reflux
   Primary megaureter
   Ureteral ectopia
   Posterior urethral valves
   In combination with A, B, or C

III. Tubulointerstitial syndromes that may be cystic

A. Nephronophthisis
B. Autosomal dominant tubulointerstitial disease
   UROM kidney disease
   REN kidney disease
   HNF1B kidney disease
   MUC1 kidney disease
C. Renal tubular dysgenesis
D. Bardet-Biedel syndromes

IV. Cystic neoplasms and neoplastic cysts

A. Mixed epithelial and stromal tumor family (includes cystic nephroma)
B. Cystic partially differentiated nephroblastoma
C. Multilocular cystic renal cell carcinoma of low malignant potential
D. Tubulocystic renal cell carcinoma
E. von Hippel–Lindau disease
F. Lymphangioma/lymphangiectasia

V. Miscellaneous cysts

A. Simple cortical cysts
B. Medullary sponge kidney
C. Localized cystic kidney disease

ACE, Angiotensin-converting enzyme; *ADPKD*, autosomal dominant polycystic kidney disease; *ARPKD*, autosomal recessive polycystic kidney disease; *GCKD*, glomerulocystic kidney disease; *HNF1B*, hepatocyte nuclear factor 1β; *MUC1*, mucin-1; *REN*, renin; *TSC*, tuberous sclerosis complex; *UROM*, uromodulin.

TABLE 1.4 The Ciliopathies

Autosomal dominant

Autosomal dominant polycystic kidney disease
Von Hippel–Lindau disease
Uromodulin-associated kidney diseases (medullary cystic kidney disease
    type II, familial juvenile hyperuremic nephropathy, glomerulocystic
    kidney disease)

Autosomal recessive

Autosomal recessive polycystic kidney disease
Nephronophthisis (with or without renal-retinal dysplasia, Joubert
    syndrome, or Senior-Loken syndrome)
Bardet-Biedl syndrome
Meckel-Gruber syndrome
Orofacial-digital syndrome
Jeune syndrome

encode for certain proteins crucial to the formation and function of the primary cilium of renal tubular cells. Most renal tubular cells have a single primary cilium, a slender organelle that originates from the basal body and extends from the apical surface of tubular cells. It is a structure long regarded as vestigial, but it is now apparent that the primary cilium has critical sensory and cell signaling functions that affect cell proliferation, polarity, and differentiation. The ciliopathies are hereditary diseases. Several have associated liver diseases that include bile duct cysts and bile duct plate malformations that may lead to congenital hepatic fibrosis.[55] The ciliopathies include one of the most common genetic diseases, autosomal dominant polycystic kidney disease (ADPKD), as well as numerous other uncommon syndromic disorders. The members of this family of diseases are listed in Table 1.4. However, this list is likely not complete because new entities are regularly added.

Finally, there are miscellaneous other cystic kidney diseases of uncertain pathogenesis. These include the common simple cortical cyst, the uncommon isolated polycystic kidney disease that resembles ADPKD, and acquired cystic kidney disease, which is of great importance because of its neoplastic diathesis.

Construction of a classification system designed to logically organize this vast compendium of developmental and cystic diseases is challenging. Many schemas have been proposed.[57,58] The ideal scheme would account for morphologic features, their clinical importance, and their pathogenesis. Although knowledge of the embryologic development of the kidney provides a tempting basis for explaining departures from the normal renal development, it must be accepted that little experimental evidence exists to defend such conjectures.

Classification of developmental anomalies and cystic kidney diseases based on their underlying genetic defects will likely gradually replace current schemes. However, even with a more thorough understanding of the genetic basis of these diseases, organizing these entities will remain difficult. For instance, CAKUT lesions may affect a single kidney–lower urinary tract unit with a completely normal contralateral kidney. Conversely, CAKUT lesions may show distinctly different types of anomalies that affect each kidney–lower urinary tract unit. Finally, the spectrum of CAKUT diseases may arise in both syndromic and nonsyndromic contexts. Similarly, although the diseases associated with mutation of ciliary proteins are all hereditary, the inheritance can be dominant or recessive. In addition, the renal diseases encountered in the ciliopathies range from cystic diseases that arise in normally formed kidneys, to cystic kidney disease resulting from

metanephric maldevelopment identical to several CAKUT abnormalities, to chronic progressive tubulointerstitial diseases that may or may not form cysts. Another complicating factor is the polygenetic nature of many disorders, in which the variable presence of, or accumulation of, multiple minor genetic defects affects susceptibility and influences the nature of the malformation expressed. This conundrum of developmental misadventures prompted Edith Potter to offer the comment quoted earlier. The classification scheme offered in this chapter is more of a tabulation of entities based on a selected major anatomic feature that is the avenue through which pathologists encounter these entities (Table 1.5).

Abnormalities in Form and Position

It is useful to group abnormalities of form and position because they often occur in combination. For instance, fused kidneys are always ectopic, and most ectopic or fused kidneys also are

TABLE 1.5 Parenchymal Maldevelopment and Cystic Kidney Disease

Abnormalities in form and position

Rotation anomaly
Ectopia
Fusion

Abnormalities of mass and number

Supernumerary kidney
Renal hypoplasia
    Simple hypoplasia
    Oligomeganephronia
    Cortical hypoplasia
    Segmental hypoplasia (Ask-Upmark kidney)
Renal agenesis
    Unilateral renal agenesis
    Bilateral renal agenesis (Potter syndrome)
    Syndromic and hereditary renal agenesis

Renal dysplasia

Multicystic and aplastic dysplasia
Segmented dysplasia
Dysplasia associated with lower tract obstruction
Dysplasia associated with hereditary syndromes
Hereditary renal dysplasia and urogenital dysplasia

Polycystic kidney disease

Autosomal recessive polycystic kidney disease
Autosomal dominant polycystic kidney disease

Cysts (without dysplasia) in hereditary syndromes

Nephronophthisis
Medullary cystic disease
Von Hippel–Lindau disease
Tuberous sclerosis
Glomerulocystic kidney

Miscellaneous

Renal tubular dysgenesis
Acquired cystic kidney disease
Localized cystic kidney disease
Medullary sponge kidney
Simple cortical cyst
Pyelocaliceal ectasia and diverticula

abnormally rotated. Each anomaly may occur in isolation or may represent one component of a more serious complex of malformations affecting other urologic sites or other organ systems. Each may be completely innocent and asymptomatic; however, if urinary tract symptoms develop, they invariably result from impaired urinary drainage, which may cause hydronephrosis or pain, and may be complicated by infection or nephrolithiasis.

Rotation Anomaly

During ascent of the kidney to a lumbar location, the renal pelvis rotates 90 degrees from an anterior to a medial position (Fig. 1.12). Failure of the pelvis to assume a medial orientation, reverse rotation, and overrotation to a posterior or even lateral location comprises a spectrum of orientation abnormalities known as rotation anomalies.[59] Some degree of malrotation occurs in 1:400 to 1:1000 individuals. The most common rotation anomaly is nonrotation or incomplete medial rotation resulting in an anterior location of the pelvis and ureter (Figs. 1.20 and 1.26). This may occur as an isolated abnormality in an otherwise normal kidney. It always accompanies renal ectopia or renal fusion. Ureteropelvic obstruction may on occasion result from a crossing vessel (Fig. 1.26). Excess rotation and reverse rotation with the pelvis posterior or lateral are rare.

Renal Ectopia

Failure of the kidney to assume its proper location in the renal fossa is known as renal ectopia.[60-63] The several varieties are named according to location (Table 1.6). Renal ectopia should be distinguished from renal ptosis in which a normally situated kidney shifts

TABLE 1.6	Types of Renal Ectopia

Pelvic: opposite sacrum
Iliac: opposite sacral prominence
Abdominal: above iliac crest
Cephaloid: subdiaphragmatic
Thoracic: supradiaphragmatic
Crossed: contralateral
    With fusion (90%)
    Without fusion (10%)
    Solitary crossed (rare)
    Bilateral crossed (rarest)

to a lower position. The origin of the renal artery from a normal aortic location identifies a lower-situated kidney as ptotic rather than ectopic. The incidence of ectopia at autopsy ranges from 1:660 to 1:1200. Renal ectopia is bilateral in 10% of cases.

The three most common forms of renal ectopia are pelvic, iliac, and abdominal, all of which are inferiorly located. The kidney may be nonreniform in shape, its pelvis and ureter are anterior (nonrotated), and the ureter is short and usually placed in the bladder, but it may have a high insertion on the pelvis that leads to obstruction. The vascular supply is influenced by the final location of the kidney, arising from the aorta or from the common iliac, internal or external iliac, or inferior mesenteric arteries (Fig. 1.27). The contralateral kidney may be normal or occasionally may be absent or even dysplastic. Other anomalies of urologic organs and cardiovascular, skeletal, and gastrointestinal systems are frequent in both sexes.

Cephaloid ectopia is usually associated with an omphalocele. The kidney appears to continue its ascent when the abdominal organs herniate into the omphalocele sac. The ureter and pelvis are typically normal. Thoracic ectopia is rare and usually involves the left kidney. The kidney resides in an extrapleural location in the

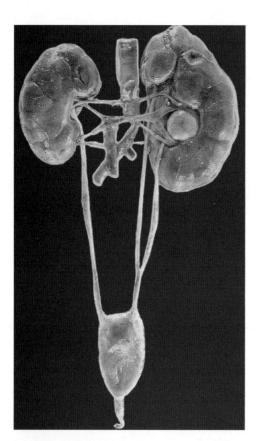

Fig. 1.26 A duplex left kidney with a bifid ureter and a nonrotated (anterior) lower pelvis. An inferior supernumerary artery and a normal vein cross the ureter, with resulting ureteropelvic junction obstruction.

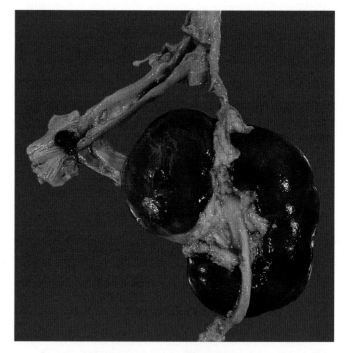

Fig. 1.27 A hypertrophic ectopic pelvic kidney from an asymptomatic patient with unilateral agenesis. Notice the anterior ureter and the vascular supply derived from the iliac vessels.

posterior mediastinum. The diaphragm must be intact to distinguish this anomaly from herniation of the kidney and possibly other abdominal organs into the thorax secondary to diaphragmatic hernia. The lower lobe of the lung may be hypoplastic, but other anomalies are not present. Thoracic ectopia is usually asymptomatic, with a normal ureter and pelvis.

In crossed ectopia the kidney is situated opposite the side of insertion of its ureter in the trigone. Four combinations are possible (Table 1.6). In 90% of cases there is also fusion to the other kidney. In crossed fused ectopia the kidneys may assume a variety of shapes and positions giving rise to six "types": inferior, superior, lump, sigmoid, disk, and L-shaped. The kidneys function normally and their ureters are normally located within the bladder, but their pelves are nonrotated. Extrarenal anomalies (genital, skeletal, and anorectal) occur in 20% to 25% of patients.

Renal Fusion

Horseshoe kidney is the most common form of renal fusion.[64-66] It is the midline fusion of two distinct renal masses, each with its own ureter and pelvis (Figs. 1.28 and 1.29). Horseshoe kidney is relatively common (1:400 to 1:2000) with a 2:1 male predominance. Horseshoe kidney is commonly seen as part of other anomalies such as trisomy 18 (25%), caudal dysplasia syndrome, and Zellweger syndrome.[67] The fusion is typically at the lower poles but can vary greatly in the quantity of fused parenchyma. A horseshoe kidney is ectopic and usually situated anterior to the aorta and vena cava. Occasionally the fusion is posterior to the vena cava or

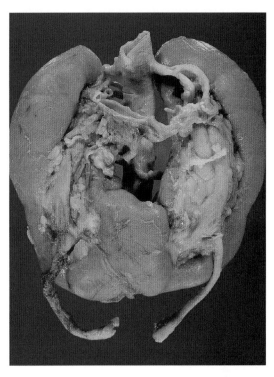

Fig. 1.29 Horseshoe kidney as an incidental autopsy finding in an adult.

posterior to both the aorta and vena cava. The ureters and pelves are always anterior. This placement, coupled with commonly encountered high insertion of the ureter on the pelvis, can result in obstruction (Fig. 1.28). Approximately 30% of patients also have other anomalies of the urinary tract, central nervous system, heart, gastrointestinal tract, or skeletal system.

Abnormalities in Mass and Number

The following group of anomalies is much less common than those described in the preceding section. Hypoplasia is usually bilateral, whereas supernumerary kidney is usually unilateral, and neither is hereditary. The renal parenchyma in each is normally formed. In contrast, renal agenesis can be either unilateral or bilateral, and may be hereditary.

Supernumerary Kidney

A supernumerary or duplicated kidney is one of the rarest disorders.[68,69] It has been defined as "a free accessory organ that is a distinct, encapsulated, large or small parenchymatous mass topographically related to the usual kidney by a loose, cellular attachment at most and often by no attachment whatsoever."[68] It may be located below (most common), above, or adjacent to the kidney and is rarely bilateral. It is connected to the lower urinary tract by either a bifid ureter or its own separate ureter (Fig. 1.30). In half of the reported cases, complications have developed related to obstruction and infection.

Hypoplasia

Hypoplasia refers to a small (<50% of normal) but otherwise normally developed kidney.[70] By definition, nephron formation is normal, albeit deficient, in quantity, and dysplastic elements (metanephric dysgenesis) are absent. There are four types of hypoplasia (Table 1.7).

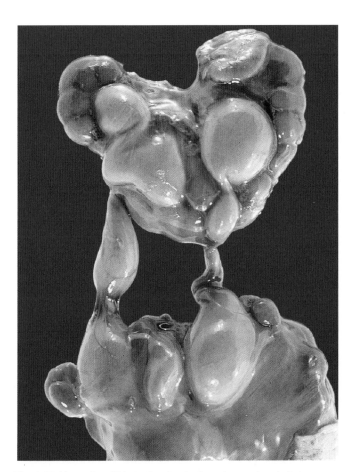

Fig. 1.28 Horseshoe kidney showing hydroureteronephrosis from a neonate with trisomy 18 and multiple congenital anomalies.

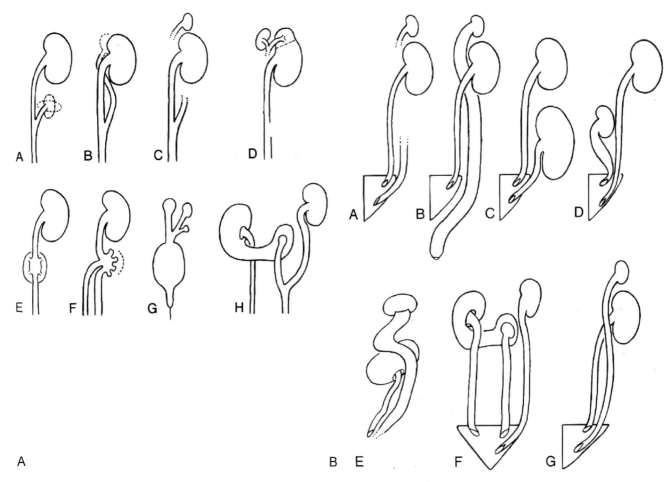

Fig. 1.30 Morphologic variants of supernumerary kidneys with bifid ureters (A) and separate ureters (B). (From N'Guessan G, Stephens FD. Supernumerary kidney. J Urol 1983;130:651; with permission.)

TABLE 1.7	Types of Renal Hypoplasia

Simple hypoplasia
Oligomeganephronia
Cortical hypoplasia
Segmental hypoplasia/Ask-Upmark kidney

Simple Hypoplasia

Simple hypoplasia is a rare, usually bilateral, and often nonhereditary disease in which the small size of the kidney usually reflects a marked reduction in the number of renal lobes.[70] Frequently only one to five lobes are present (Fig. 1.31). Dysplastic elements, by definition, are absent. When the condition is unilateral, the contralateral kidney may be hypertrophied. When it is bilateral, the small kidneys may eventually fail to provide renal function with body growth, and renal failure and nephron sclerosis may develop, the onset of which is determined by the degree of hypoplasia.

Oligomeganephronia

Oligomeganephronia may be the most common form of renal hypoplasia. It is a bilateral, nonhereditary disorder.[71-76] Most cases are sporadic; however, few associations have been described with mutations in transcription factors involved in renal development including PAX2, HNF1B, and SIX.[77-79] The kidneys are small because of a reduction in the number of renal lobes and the number of nephrons within each lobe. Microscopically, the nephrons present are tremendously enlarged (Fig. 1.32). Glomerular and tubular volumes have been measured to be 12 times and 17 times normal, respectively.

Children with oligomeganephronia present with a concentration defect causing polyuria, polydipsia, and salt wasting, resembling patients with nephronophthisis. Renal insufficiency and proteinuria gradually develop with body growth as progressive glomerular and tubulointerstitial scarring occur. The absence of a family history of renal disease, the presence of proteinuria, and imaging studies revealing symmetrically small noncystic kidneys usually permit separation from nephronophthisis.

Cortical Hypoplasia

Cortical hypoplasia is a type of hypoplasia not generally recognized; it does not appear in standard texts of urologic pathology. Examples of cortical hypoplasia, however, are amply demonstrated in the *Atlas of Medical Renal Pathology* by Bonsib.[70] *Cortical hypoplasia* refers to a reduction in the number of nephron generations that results in cortical thinning, reduction in overall renal size, and, if severe, a clinically significant reduction in nephron endowment, a major risk factor for hypertension and renal insufficiency.[80-82] The "normal" number of generations ranges from 10 to 14, although rarely are more than 9 to 10 generations evident even in a well-oriented section. Determination of nephron generations is best performed with a nephrectomy specimen with sections

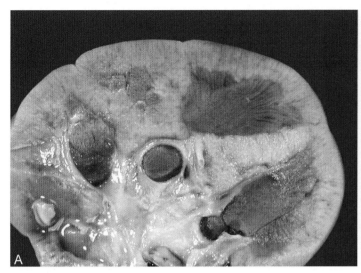
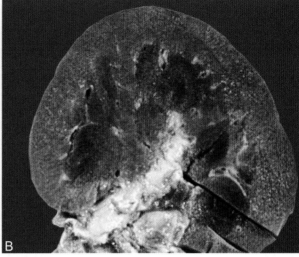

Fig. 1.31 (A) This 3-cm hypoplastic kidney was from a 2-year-old child with a contralateral duplex kidney. It appears to have only five lobes. (B) This 5.5-cm hypoplastic kidney was from an adult with a 13.5-cm hypertrophic contralateral kidney.

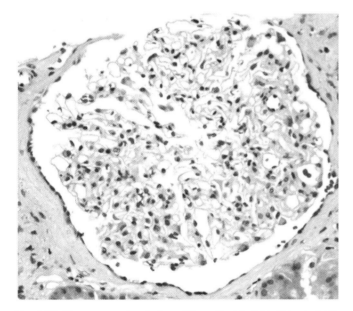

Fig. 1.32 Oligomeganephronia in a 22-month-old child. This markedly enlarged glomerulus is twice the normal diameter. Notice the numerous capillary loops, far more than in a normal glomerulus.

oriented along medullary rays. Nephron generation counting is admittedly imprecise. However, if there is a 50% reduction in nephron generations, that is, four to five generations in a properly oriented section, then the reliability of this assessment is reasonable (Fig. 1.33). This form of hypoplasia may coexist with other forms of hypoplasia, especially Ask-Upmark segmental hypoplasia.

Segmental Hypoplasia (Ask-Upmark Kidney)

Segmental hypoplasia may manifest in neonates or adults and is often associated with hypertension.[83-87] There is widespread agreement that vesicoureteral reflux is the fundamental injury. Some investigators regard it as an acquired lesion because its evolution over time has been radiographically documented in a few cases. Others agree with reflux-related injury but believe that most cases are developmental in origin secondary to in utero reflux that

damages the developing renal lobe. That this condition often manifests in neonates and children supports a developmental basis. Furthermore, it is associated with renal vascular anomalies in 40% of cases and may be coexistent with lobes that show cortical hypoplasia. Segmental hypoplasia is defined as a small kidney with a deep cortical groove and dilatation of adjacent calyx (Fig. 1.34A). Microscopic features include sharply delineated cortical lesions (Fig. 1.34B). The cortex contains few tubules, with no or only rare glomeruli. There is little or no inflammation, nor is glomerulosclerosis or tubular atrophy present to indicate a regressive lesion. Finally, the kidney should have no evidence of metanephric dysgenesis. The medulla is characteristically absent. If present it may be rudimentary or flattened, with no loops of Henle, and may contain a distinctive cellular interstitial mesenchymal tissue not present in the normal renal pyramid.

Renal Agenesis

Absence of the kidney and its corresponding ureter is known as renal agenesis (Table 1.8).[88-94] The corresponding bladder hemitrigone is also absent because it represents the distal continuation of the ureteral smooth muscle (Fig. 1.35).[90] Failure to identify a kidney in a child or an adult does not prove congenital absence of the kidney because cystic dysplastic kidneys identified in newborns have been shown radiographically to regress further over time and may become undetectable.[95]

Unilateral Renal Agenesis

In unilateral renal agenesis the contralateral kidney may be hypertrophic up to twice the normal size. The overall renal function may be normal, and the condition may be entirely asymptomatic (Fig. 1.27). Several genetic and environmental factors have been associated with an increased risk, such as African American race, maternal diabetes mellitus, and maternal age younger than 18 years.[93] In up to 70% of patients, renal agenesis is associated with additional anomalies, most often affecting the genital tract.[90,91,93-97] This presumably reflects a common abnormality affecting development of both the mesonephric duct– and Müllerian duct–derived structures. Female genital anomalies include absence of the ipsilateral fallopian tube, uterine horn, and proximal vagina or uterine didelphia or vaginal septum. Male

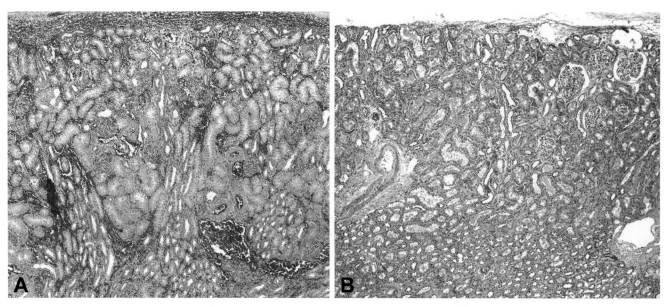

Fig. 1.33 (A) Cortical hypoplasia in a newborn kidney. Two medullary rays are visible. The renal medulla is at the bottom, and the renal capsule is at the top. Only three or four nephron generations are present. (B) This is an adult kidney with cortical hypoplasia. The medulla is at the bottom, and the renal capsule is at the top. Only two or three nephron generations are present.

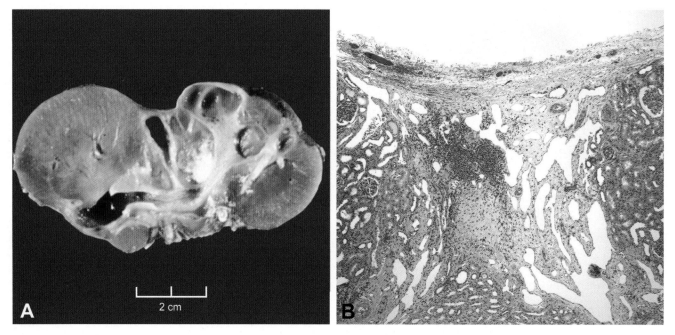

Fig. 1.34 (A) This is a bivalved Ask-Upmark segmental hypoplasia kidney showing the deep linear groove with approximation of the renal capsule and a dilated calyx. (B) The cortical groove in the Ask-Upmark kidney shows an abruptly delineated lesion with dilated veins and complete absence of normal nephrons and atrophic nephrons. (A, Courtesy of The Jay Bernstein, M.D. Consultative Collection, Nephropath, Little Rock, AR.)

genital anomalies may include absence of the ipsilateral epididymis, vas deferens, or seminal vesicle, or a seminal vesicle cyst may be encountered. Identification of a patient with a unilateral genital anomaly or renal agenesis should therefore prompt evaluation of the other organ system.

Bilateral Renal Agenesis (Potter Syndrome)
Bilateral renal agenesis is a uniformly fatal disorder known as Potter syndrome (Fig. 1.36). Both ureters are also absent, so the bladder

has no ureteral orifices.[89] Approximately 40% of affected fetuses are stillbirths, and those born alive die of pulmonary failure within 48 hours. Mothers present with severe oligohydramnios because fetal urine normally accounts for most of the amniotic fluid in the second half of gestation. Oligohydramnios impairs pulmonary development that results in pulmonary hypoplasia and produces a variety of distinctive gross features known as the Potter phenotype or oligohydramnios phenotype (Table 1.9).[98-100] Figs. 1.37 and 1.38 demonstrate some of the characteristic facial and placental

TABLE 1.8	Renal Agenesis

Sporadic forms of renal agenesis

Unilateral renal agenesis
Bilateral renal agenesis (Potter syndrome)

Syndromic and hereditary renal agenesis

Chromosomal anomalies (trisomy 13 and 18)
VATER association
Müllerian aplasia syndrome (MURCS syndrome)
Sirenomelia (caudal regression syndrome)
Cloacal exstrophy
Fraser syndrome
Williams syndrome
Multiple malformation syndromes, not otherwise specified
Hereditary renal adysplasia

MURCS, Müllerian duct aplasia or hypoplasia, unilateral renal agenesis, and cervicothoracic somite dysplasia; *VATER,* vertebral defects, imperforate anus, tracheoesophageal fistula, radial and renal dysplasia.

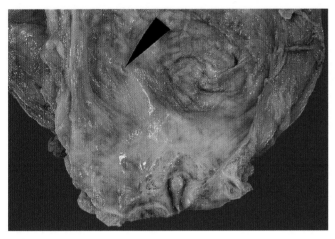

Fig. 1.35 This bladder has an absent left hemitrigone in an adult with a sporadic form of unilateral renal agenesis. The right hemitrigone with its ureteral orifice is indicated by an *arrowhead.*

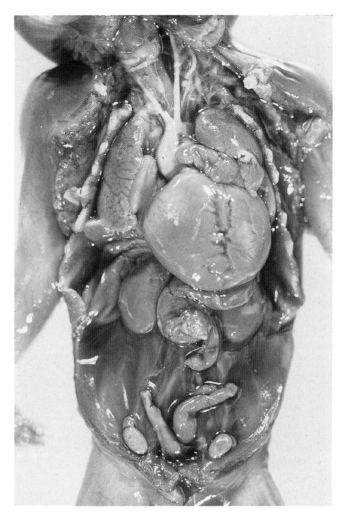

Fig. 1.36 This is the third consecutive fetus affected with bilateral renal-ureteral agenesis in a family with familial renal adysplasia. The small and large bowels have been removed to reveal the adrenal glands. Both kidneys are absent.

TABLE 1.9	Oligohydramnios Phenotype

Potter facies
Increased interocular distance
Broad, flattened nose
Prominent inner canthic folds (sweeping downward and laterally)
Receding chin
Large, low-set ears with little cartilage
Positional deformities (flexion of hips and knees, clubbed feet)
Dry skin
Hypoplastic lungs
Small bladder with absent trigone
Placenta: amnion nodosum

findings. Some urologists refer to any fetus born with the oligohydramnios phenotype as having Potter syndrome, rather than reserving the term for the entity of bilateral renal-ureteral agenesis as initially described. This can be confusing because oligohydramnios has other causes (Table 1.10).[98]

Syndromic Renal Agenesis

Many syndromes are characterized by absence of one kidney or, rarely, both kidneys as a component of a constellation of congenital anomalies.[101-105] The list includes chromosomal anomalies, several malformation syndromes, and multiple malformation events affecting the gastrointestinal, cardiac, central nervous system, or skeletal system that do not conform to a specific syndrome. Finally, renal agenesis may also occur in a familial disorder with renal dysplasia (see Hereditary Renal Adysplasia section later in this chapter).[106-109] In each disorder, identification of extrarenal components and a detailed family history are essential for proper classification and appropriate genetic counseling. The extrarenal anomalies are responsible for many complications and for the lethal nature of many of the syndromes.

Renal Dysplasia

A dysplastic kidney is a metanephric structure with aberrant nephronic differentiation.[27,42-45,110-116] The term *dysplasia* is used in a developmental sense and does not connote any relationship with neoplasia. Dysplastic kidneys should not be confused with hypoplastic kidneys, which are small but have normal nephron

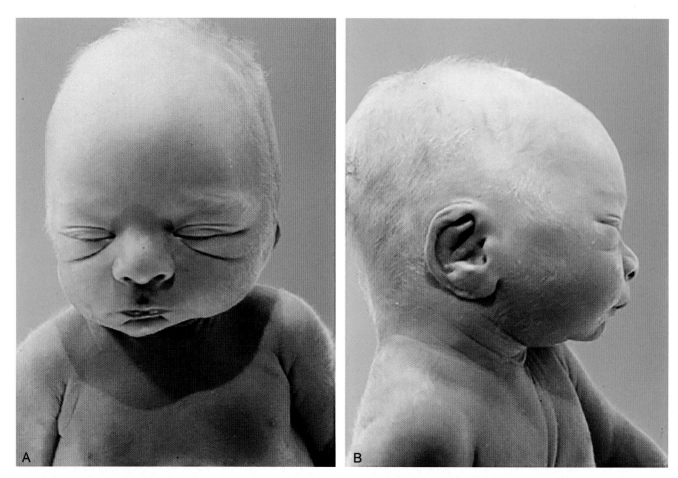

Fig. 1.37 An infant born with oligohydramnios and the characteristic Potter facies in anterior (A) and lateral (B) views.

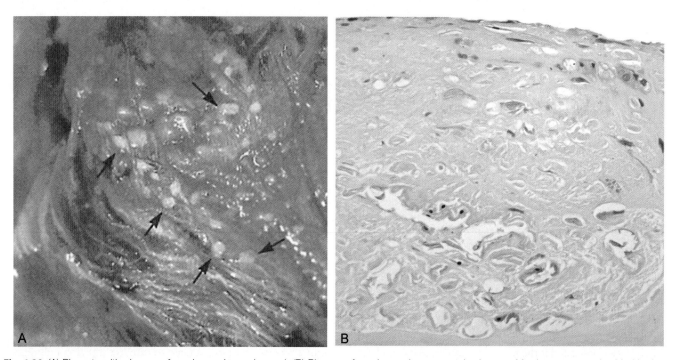

Fig. 1.38 (A) Placenta with plaques of amnion nodosum (*arrows*). (B) Plaques of amnion nodosum contain clumps of fetal squames embedded in dense collagen.

TABLE 1.10	Causes of Oligohydramnios

Major causes

Potter syndrome (bilateral renal agenesis)
Bilateral renal dysplasia
Distal (complete) urinary tract obstruction

Rare causes

Autosomal recessive polycystic kidney disease
Glomerulocystic kidney disease
Renal tubular dysgenesis
Chronic amniotic fluid leak
In utero acute renal failure
Idiopathic conditions

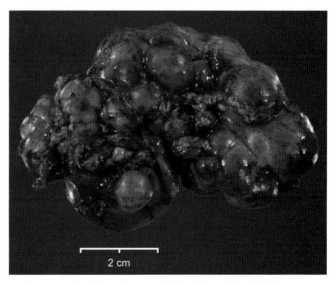

Fig. 1.40 This is the external appearance of a typical multicystic dysplastic kidney. It is markedly enlarged and diffusely cystic with cysts of variable size.

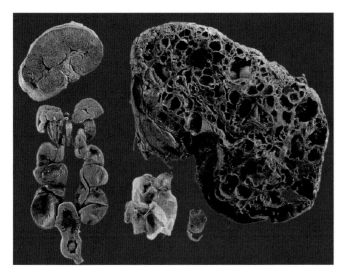

Fig. 1.39 Autosomal recessive polycystic kidney (*upper left*), autosomal dominant polycystic kidney (upper right), and three forms of renal dysplasia: aplastic dysplasia from a 35-year-old patient, multicystic dysplasia from a neonate, and bilateral dysplasia associated with lower tract obstruction (*lower left*).

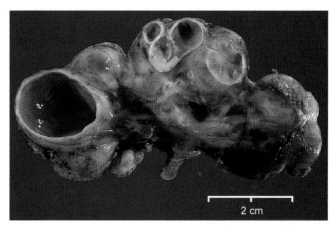

Fig. 1.41 Transverse section of a typical multicystic dysplastic kidney. There is no discernible normal architecture, and no corticomedullary junction or collecting system is seen. The parenchyma is composed solely of cysts and nondescript connective tissue.

development, or with polycystic kidney diseases, which although cystic do not contain dysplastic elements. Dysplastic kidneys are, by definition, maldeveloped (Figs. 1.39 to 1.41). They are usually not reniform, can vary greatly in size and appearance, and occur in several patterns: unilateral, bilateral, or confined to the upper pole of a duplex kidney (Table 1.11). Approximately 90% of cases have a ureteral abnormality or are associated with distal obstruction resulting in ureteral stenosis or dilation and megacystis or bladder hypertrophy. Renal dysplasia most commonly is sporadic, but it may be familial, part of a multiple malformation complex, or a component of a hereditary malformation syndrome (Table 1.12). Table 1.13 and Fig. 1.39 compare the major anatomic and clinical features of renal dysplasias with the autosomal recessive polycystic kidney disease (ARPKD) and ADPKD discussed in the following sections.

Dysplastic kidneys vary tremendously in gross appearance, ranging from the large multicystic kidney to the small aplastic kidney (Fig. 1.39).[70] The typical multicystic kidney is composed entirely of variably sized cysts and is the most common cause of a unilateral renal mass in a child (Fig. 1.40). The cysts contain serous fluid. Typically, there is no corticomedullary differentiation, and a

TABLE 1.11	Renal Dysplasias: Gross Variations and Clinical Associations

Multicystic and aplastic dysplasia
Segmental dysplasia
Dysplasia associated with lower urinary tract obstruction
Dysplasia associated with malformation syndromes
Hereditary adysplasia and urogenital adysplasia

collecting system is often absent (Fig. 1.41). The typical aplastic dysplasia is tiny and contains no cysts or only microscopic cysts (Fig. 1.39). Corticomedullary differentiation and a collecting system are again absent. The multicystic and aplastic dysplasias represent extremes of a morphologic continuum differing only in the extent of cyst formation. Intermediate forms commonly occur. Most often renal dysplasia is a unilateral process, and the

TABLE 1.12	Multiple Malformation Syndromes in Which Renal Dysplasia May Occur

Common occurrence

VATER (VACTERL) association
MURC syndrome
Prune-belly syndrome
Caudal regression syndrome
Cloacal exstrophy
Urogenital sinus syndrome
Urorectal septum syndrome sequence
Meckel-Gruber syndrome[a]
Dandy-Walker syndrome[a]
Short rib–polydactyly syndrome[a]
Elejalde syndrome

Occasional occurrence

Trisomy C
Trisomy 13
Trisomy 18
Persisting mesonephric duct syndrome
Zellweger syndrome[a]
Jeune syndrome[a]
Smith-Lemli-Opitz syndrome[a]
Beckwith-Wiedemann syndrome[a]
Laurence-Moon-Bardet-Biedl syndrome[a]

MURC, Müllerian duct aplasia or hypoplasia, unilateral renal agenesis, and cervicothoracic somite dysplasia; *VACTERL*, vertebral, anal, cardiac, tracheal, esophageal, renal, limb; *VATER*, vertebral defects, imperforate anus, tracheoesophageal fistula, radial and renal dysplasia.
[a]Autosomal recessive inheritance.

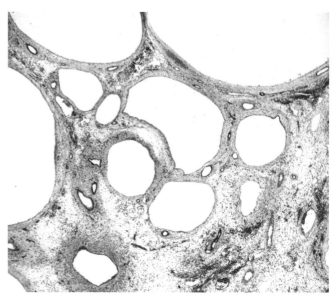

Fig. 1.42 Dysplastic kidney composed of cysts, dysplastic ducts, and a few primitive tubules.

contralateral kidney is normal or larger than normal. When multicystic dysplasia or aplastic dysplasia is bilateral, the neonate presents with a Potter phenotype and dies of pulmonary hypoplasia.

The histologic appearance of a dysplastic kidney can also be quite varied.[106-109,111,113-115] The kidney may be composed entirely of large cysts with little or no metanephric tissue represented (Fig. 1.42). The cysts are of variable size and usually lined by flat-

TABLE 1.13	Comparison of Renal Agenesis, Hypoplasia, and Dysplasia		
	Agenesis/Aplasia	**Hypoplasia**	**Dysplasia**
Definition	Agenesis: no kidneys Aplasia: rudimentary kidneys	Small, architecturally normal kidneys, weight <50% expected; decreased number of nephrons (<2 SD normal)	Architecturally abnormal kidney with immature nephrons
Incidence	Unilateral: 1:1000 Bilateral: 1:10,000	Unilateral: 1:1000 Bilateral: 1:4000	Unilateral: 1:7500 Bilateral: 1:7500
Etiology	Defect in formation of Wolffian duct and/or ureteric bud	Slow induction or incorrect position of ureteric bud, decreased branching	Defective branching
Clinical presentation	Unilateral: M = F; may be asymptomatic, risk of FSGS Bilateral: M > F; perinatal death	May be asymptomatic (if unilateral) or symptomatic: • Failure to thrive • Hypertension • Salt wasting • Excessive thirst	May be asymptomatic (if unilateral) or symptomatic: • Failure to thrive • Hypertension • Salt wasting • Excessive thirst
Radiologic features	Absent kidney	Small kidney	Small kidney with noncommunicating hypoechogenic cysts
Gross appearance	No kidneys Earlobe-shaped, elongated adrenals	Small kidneys Decreased number of pyramids	Nonreniform, multicystic mass Small, normal, or large size
Microscopic features	Normal or compensatory hypertrophy in unilateral agenesis	• Normal organization • Large nephrons in oligomeganephronia	• Disorganized parenchyma • Immature glomeruli and tubules • Smooth muscle collarettes • Metaplastic cartilage (30%)

F, Female; *FSGS*, focal segmental glomerulosclerosis; *M*, male; *SD*, standard deviation.

tened cells. Immature or dysplastic ducts are commonly present. They are lined with columnar epithelium and surrounded by collars of spindle cells that express estrogen receptor and/or progesterone receptor (Fig. 1.43). Immature-appearing cartilage may be also present but is far less frequent than dysplastic ducts (Figs. 1.43B and 1.44A). The dysplastic ducts are thought to originate from the ampullary bud, whereas the immature cartilage is regarded as blastemal derived.[107] Immature tubules and aberrantly formed glomeruli may be present, or relatively normal-appearing tubules and well-formed glomeruli may be present but not sufficiently organized to contribute appreciably to renal function (Fig. 1.44).

Occasionally an infant presents with renal insufficiency and small reniform kidneys with normal ureters and pelves. Simple hypoplasia may be suspected, but biopsy reveals an admixture of normal nephrons and aberrantly formed nephrons with microcysts and cartilage or dysplastic ducts. The renal prognosis is bleak, and the infant usually develops progressive renal failure with further growth.[110]

Segmental forms of dysplasia occur in kidneys with duplication of the collecting system (duplex kidney).[93,101] Usually the duplication is complete with two separate ureters. The upper pole moiety is affected, and histologic examination shows the same range of aberrant nephrogenesis encountered in aplastic and multicystic dysplasia (Fig. 1.45). The upper pole ureter is usually ectopic, in a more cranial or caudal location relative to the normally situated lower pole ureter. The incidence and severity of dysplasia increase with the severity of the ectopia.[106,109]

Bilateral renal dysplasia can be associated with distal obstruction resulting from urethral stenosis, posterior urethral valves, or

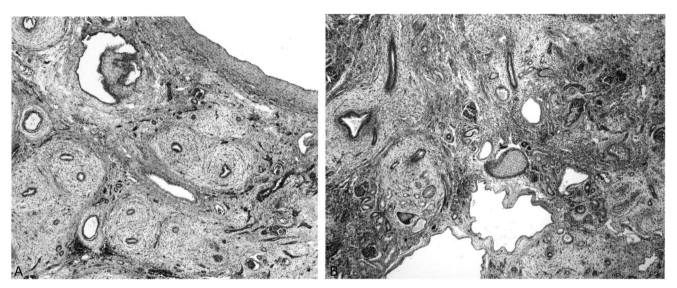

Fig. 1.43 (A) This dysplastic kidney contains large cysts and numerous dysplastic tubules with collarettes of spindle cells. (B) This dysplastic kidney contains numerous dysplastic tubules with collarettes of spindle cells and an island of immature cartilage in the center.

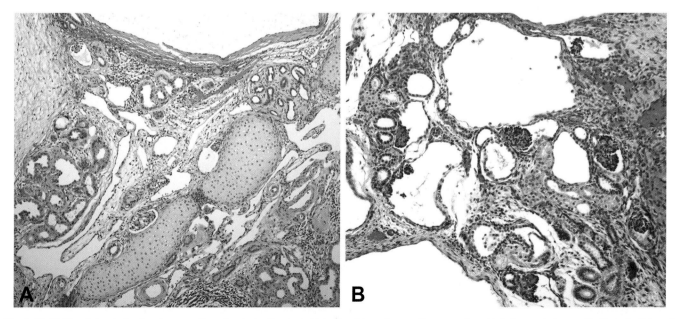

Fig. 1.44 (A) Renal dysplasia showing a portion of a cyst with several islands of immature cartilage, scattered tubules, and abnormally formed glomeruli. (B) This dysplastic kidney has microcysts (at least one is a glomerular cyst), small tubules, and atubular glomeruli.

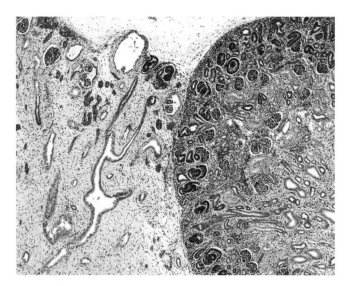

Fig. 1.45 Segmental form of renal dysplasia in a fetal duplex kidney. To the left is the dysplastic upper pole. To the right is the normally developing lower pole.

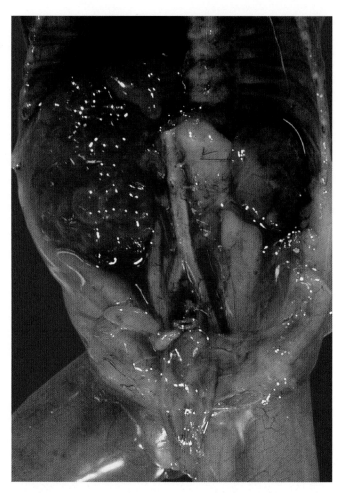

Fig. 1.47 Hereditary renal adysplasia with unilateral multicystic dysplasia and contralateral renal agenesis shown in situ.

bladder neck obstruction. This form of dysplasia may have a distinctive gross appearance. The kidneys are typically reniform, and they may be large or small, but they often show corticomedullary differentiation. The bladder is either hypertrophic or greatly dilated, and the ureters are dilated and tortuous (Figs. 1.39 and 1.46A). There may be a severe degree of dysplasia with scant nephronic elements (Fig. 1.46B) or only a peripheral zone of dysplastic elements with normal deeper nephrons.

Renal dysplasia may develop in many multiple malformation syndromes, chromosomal anomalies, and hereditary malformation syndromes (Table 1.12).[70] When multiple malformations are encountered in a pediatric autopsy, it is important to obtain tissue for karyotype or genetic analysis, and to meticulously document all anomalies. Consultation with specialists in pediatrics and genetics is advisable to provide the proper classification of the disease so that appropriate family counseling can be provided.

The major features of renal aplasia, hypoplasia, and dysplasia are compared in Table 1.13. Multicystic dysplasia, aplastic dysplasia, and renal agenesis are the most severe forms of metanephric maldevelopment. When they are not associated with extrarenal anomalies of a multiple malformation syndrome, they usually are sporadic events with low risk of a subsequently affected sibling. Rarely, however, renal agenesis or renal dysplasia, either unilateral or bilateral (Figs. 1.39 and 1.47), or combined agenesis and dysplasia may be familial (usually autosomal dominant). This is

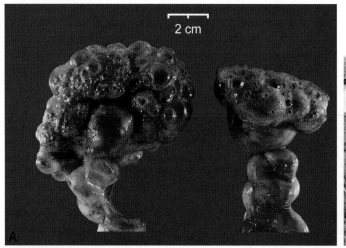

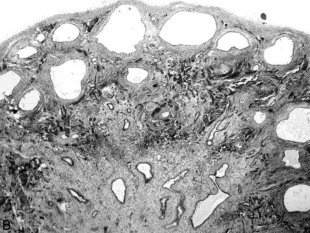

Fig. 1.46 (A) Renal dysplasia associated with urinary tract obstruction. These small kidneys have numerous small cysts and markedly dilated ureters. (B) Cortical medullary development is present, but few differentiated nephron elements.

known as hereditary renal adysplasia.[101-105] There also may be concomitant malformation of Müllerian structures, a condition referred to as hereditary urogenital adysplasia.[87] Unfortunately, neither syndrome can be anticipated until a second family member is identified with either agenesis or dysplasia.

Polycystic Kidney Disease

Autosomal Recessive Polycystic Kidney Disease

Autosomal recessive polycystic kidney is a rare disorder that occurs in 1 in 20,000 to 50,000 births (Table 1.14). In ARPKD, parents lack the disease and 25% of siblings are affected.[117-124] It is associated with mutations of the polycystic kidney and hepatic disease 1 (*PKHD1*) gene, on chromosome 6p12.[117-126] The product of this gene, fibrocystin/polyductin, localizes to the primary cilium and centrosome of renal tubule epithelial cells. Organogenesis in ARPKD appears normal based on microdissection studies of severe neonatal forms.[33] The primary lesion is fusiform ectasia of cortical and medullary collecting ducts, eventually leading to renal failure in severely affected cases. The renal lesion is accompanied by a bile duct plate malformation that develops into congenital hepatic fibrosis in surviving older patients.

Recessive polycystic kidney disease was originally believed to be an invariably lethal neonatal disorder. Observation of some patients who survived into childhood prompted Blyth and Ockenden to propose a classification of patients into perinatal, neonatal, infantile, and juvenile forms.[119] These forms vary in the degree of cyst formation. Although conceptually useful, it is often difficult to place a patient into a given category. More than 100 mutations of the *PKHD1* gene have been identified that account for the clinical spectrum.[118,120,123] The most severe neonatal cases manifest with pulmonary hypoplasia secondary to the massive renal enlargement that compromises pulmonary development. It appears that as the extent of cyst formation decreases, the child has better pulmonary development and a greater likelihood of survival. Unfortunately, with increasing duration of survival there is worsening of the liver disease that may culminate in congenital hepatic fibrosis.[55,127] If one examines the kidneys of children with congenital hepatic fibrosis, two-thirds have a concentrating defect and have some degree of medullary cyst formation, findings indicating that ARPKD and congenital hepatic fibrosis are different manifestations of a single entity.

Most cases of ARPKD result in stillbirth, early neonatal death, or end-stage kidney disease by age 20 years. Affected neonates have massively enlarged and diffusely cystic kidneys that produce abdominal distention and compress thoracic organs (Fig. 1.48A). The lungs cannot develop normally, and death results from pulmonary hypoplasia. Despite the impressive cyst formation, the kidneys may be functional. If they are nonfunctional, oligohydramnios and a Potter phenotype may develop.

In severe cases, the cysts extend throughout the cortex and medulla in a distinctive radiating pattern imparting a spongy quality (Fig. 1.48B). Histologically, the cysts consist of dilated collecting ducts lined with uniform cuboidal cells (Figs. 1.49 and 1.50). The nephrons between the collecting ducts appear normal.

The liver in patients dying in the neonatal period shows portal bile duct proliferation that assumes a distinctive dilated and irregular branched pattern of anastomosing channels at the periphery of portal triads (Fig. 1.51). There is an increase in the size of portal areas with increased fibrous tissue. In older patients, congenital hepatic fibrosis develops, resulting in portal hypertension and hepatosplenomegaly.

In less severely affected kidneys of older children the appearance is variable, and the diagnosis may be less obvious. The kidneys are smaller, and the cysts are fewer. Medullary cysts are always present and tend to be elongated. Cortical cysts if present are often rounded and variably distributed (Fig. 1.52). The parenchyma adjacent to the cysts eventually develops atrophic changes with tubulointerstitial scarring and glomerulosclerosis. These features may create a resemblance to ADPKD. The presence of the liver lesion of congenital hepatic fibrosis therefore is a useful diagnostic feature. However, many diseases may be associated with renal cysts and liver disease, and awareness of additional anomalies is required for proper classification (Table 1.15).[55,114]

Autosomal Dominant Polycystic Kidney Disease

ADPKD is the most common cystic kidney disease and the most common genetically transmitted renal disease.[128-136] It occurs with an estimated frequency of between 1:500 and 1:1000 (Table 1.14). It is the fourth leading cause of end-stage renal disease, and affected patients comprise 5% to 10% of patients treated with dialysis. Although patients vary greatly in the age of onset of symptoms, most present in their third to fifth decade of life. Penetrance is nearly 100% if the individual survives to 80 years. Approximately 25% of affected patients lack a family history and presumably represent a new mutation. The disease results from mutations of *PKD1* and *PKD2* that localize to chromosome 16 in 90% of patients and to chromosome 4 in 10%, respectively. The gene product of *PKD1* is polycystin-1, a transmembrane glycoprotein involved in cell signaling. *PKD2* encodes for polycystin-2, a member of the transient receptor potential channel superfamily of nonselective cation channels.

Patients with ADPKD present with a variety of symptoms, most referable to the urinary tract. Chronic flank pain is the most common and correlates with renal weight and cyst size greater than 3 cm. Acute flank pain often reflects hemorrhage into a cyst. Hematuria is the second most common symptom. This may be gross, resulting in clot formation and urinary tract obstruction. Hypertension often develops early in the disease, and activation of the renin-angiotensin system secondary to intrarenal vascular occlusion by expanding cysts has been implicated. Urinary tract infection develops in 50% to 75% of patients and affects women more often than men. The infection may be confined to the collecting system or a cyst, or it may involve the parenchyma. Perinephric extension with abscess is a serious complication with a 60% mortality rate. Urate or calcium oxalate nephrolithiasis develops in 10% of patients. Extrarenal complications related to

TABLE 1.14	Comparison of Major Cystic Kidney Diseases		
	Dysplasia	ARPKD	ADPKD
Incidence	1:1000-2000	1:50,000	1:500-1000
Bilateral	+/−	+	+
Segmental	+/−	−	−
Ureter abnormal	+	−	−
Reniform shape	+/−	+	+
Uniform cysts	−	+	−
Liver abnormal	+/−	+	+
Other malformations	+/−	−	−

ADPKD, Autosomal dominant polycystic kidney disease; *ARPKD*, autosomal recessive polycystic kidney disease.

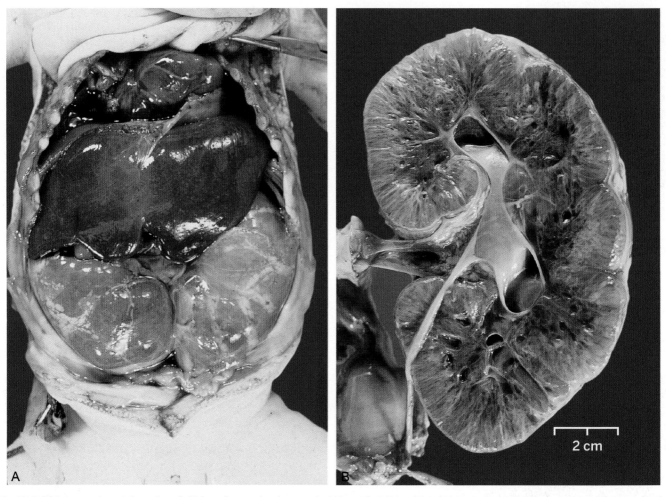

Fig. 1.48 (A) Autosomal recessive polycystic kidney disease showing massive kidneys that distend the abdomen, elevate the diaphragm, and compromise the thoracic cavity. (B) The bivalved kidney has a reniform shape and a normal collecting system. The cortex and medulla contain diffuse, relatively uniform cysts.

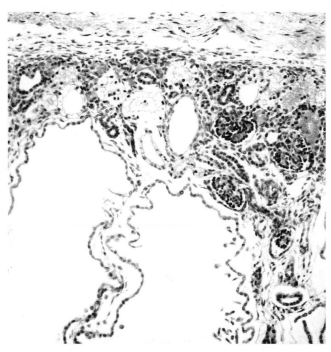

Fig. 1.49 The cortical cysts in autosomal recessive polycystic kidney disease are elongated and lined by cuboidal epithelium. Normally formed nephron elements are between the cysts.

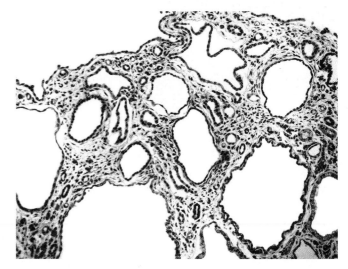

Fig. 1.50 The medullary cysts in autosomal recessive polycystic kidney disease are also lined with uniform cuboidal epithelium.

hypertension and berry aneurysms develop in 5% to 15%. Infection and cardiovascular disease represent the most common causes of death.[135,137]

Early in the disease (Fig. 1.53), the kidney may appear nearly normal with only scattered cysts in the cortex and medulla, and

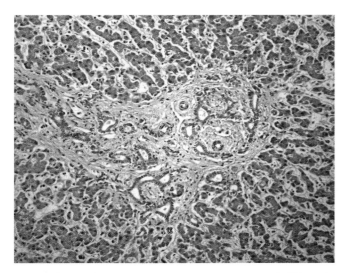

Fig. 1.51 The liver in perinatal autosomal recessive polycystic kidney disease showing the irregular branched architecture of the portal bile ducts and portal fibrosis.

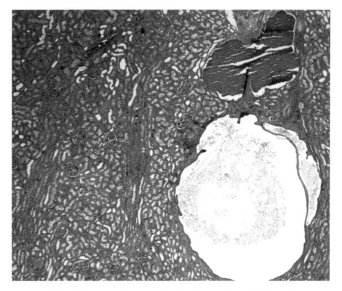

Fig. 1.53 Infantile onset of autosomal dominant polycystic kidney disease at age 7 years with a largely intact cortex and several cysts.

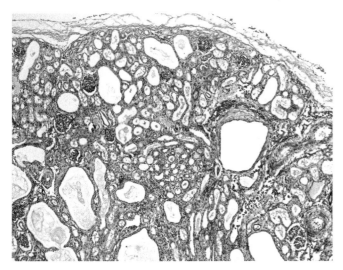

Fig. 1.52 This is an example of the infantile form of autosomal recessive polycystic kidney disease in a 4-year-old child. Collecting duct ectasia is less prominent. Interstitial fibrosis is developing.

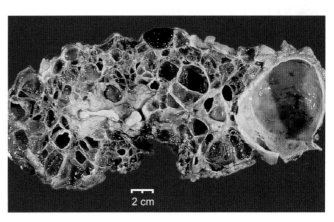

Fig. 1.54 Transverse section of an advanced-stage autosomal dominant polycystic kidney disease kidney. Both the cortex and the medulla are replaced by cysts.

TABLE 1.15	Cystic Renal Disease Associated with Congenital Hepatic Fibrosis or Biliary Cysts

Autosomal recessive polycystic kidney disease
Autosomal dominant polycystic kidney disease
Nephronophthisis
Joubert syndrome
Bardet-Biedl syndrome
Meckel-Gruber syndrome[a]
Oral-facial digital syndrome
Glomerulocystic kidney disease
Zellweger syndrome[a]
Ivemark syndrome[a]
Chondrodysplastic syndromes[a]
Trisomy C[a]
Trisomy D[a]

[a]Additional malformations are present.

normal intervening parenchyma. The cysts initially are small and develop in only about 1% of nephrons. Microdissection studies have shown that the cysts develop in all segments of the nephron.[132] Scanning electron microscopy and immunohistochemistry of cyst lining cells have confirmed these observations.[138]

As the disease progresses, the cysts grow in size and number, with resulting massive renal enlargement (Fig. 1.54). The cysts range in size from a few millimeters to several centimeters, and cyst contents vary from transparent to opaque to hemorrhagic fluid. Most cysts are lined with a single layer of flattened to cuboidal epithelium (Fig. 1.55). Hyperplastic foci or polyp formation are detectable in some cysts (Fig. 1.56).[139,140] The cyst contents may be proteinaceous or include red cells or calcific deposits. The intervening parenchyma shows interstitial fibrosis with a lymphoid infiltrate, tubular atrophy, and glomerular and vascular sclerosis. Despite the cystic transformation, the kidneys retain a reniform shape and preserve their collecting systems.

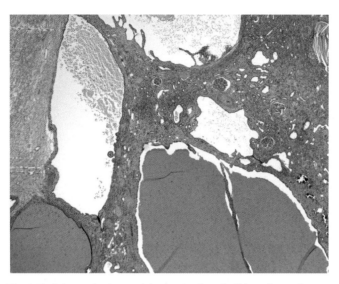

Fig. 1.55 Advanced autosomal dominant polycystic kidney disease from an adult with chronic renal failure shows severe interstitial scarring with calcifications and cysts that contain proteinaceous fluid.

Cystic Diseases (Without Dysplasia) in Hereditary Syndromes

Nephronophthisis

Nephronophthisis is an autosomal recessive tubulointerstitial nephropathy in which cysts often develop. It inevitably leads to end-stage kidney disease.[53,141-146] The first description of nephronophthisis was by Smith and Graham in 1945, who used the term *medullary cystic disease* to highlight the grossly visible medullary cysts.[141] Fanconi, in 1951, coined the term *juvenile familial nephronophthisis* in reference to its histologic outcome; *nephronophthisis* is Greek for "disintegration of nephrons." Most reports of nephronophthisis that appeared before the 1990s combined the

two entities into the *medullary cystic disease/juvenile nephronophthisis complex* because of their morphologic similarities, a practice no longer appropriate considering differences in genetics and pathogenesis. Nephronophthisis is autosomal recessive and a ciliopathy, whereas medullary cystic kidney disease, now referred to as autosomal dominant tubulointerstitial disease (ADTID), is autosomal dominant and is not a ciliopathy as discussed later.[141,143-157]

There are three clinical phenotypes of nephronophthisis that are distinguished by age of onset: infantile, juvenile, and adolescent forms. Affected individuals present with polyuria and polydipsia resulting from salt wasting, a concentration defect, anemia disproportionately severe for the level of renal insufficiency, and growth retardation. Although fundamentally a tubulointerstitial disease, 15% of patients have extrarenal components: retinal dystrophy (Senior-Loken syndrome), oculomotor apraxia (Cogan syndrome), situs inversus (infantile nephronophthisis), and rarely, congenital hepatic fibrosis.[53,141-146,149]

Twenty mutated genes have been identified in nephronophthisis that encode for proteins expressed in the primary cilium, centrosome, and cell junctions of renal epithelial cells. These mutations, however, account for only 30% of nephronophthisis cases. Most mutations are responsible for some of the juvenile and adolescent forms, whereas *NPHP2* and occasionally *NPHP3* mutations are responsible for the infantile form. The juvenile and adolescent forms cannot be histologically distinguished. However, the infantile form has several distinctive features.

The kidneys in nephronophthisis are normally developed at birth. Cyst formation occurs in approximately 70% of patients but is usually delayed until advanced or end-stage disease develops. Sequential imaging shows that most patients lack cysts at presentation but many subsequently develop cysts, and that cyst frequency and size increase over time. Therefore early in the disease no cysts may be detectable to assist in the diagnosis.

Kidney size in the juvenile and adolescent forms is usually normal or smaller than normal. When cysts develop, they congregate at the corticomedullary junction and may range from 1 to several

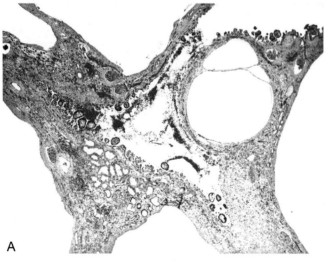

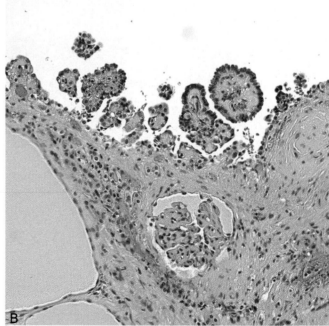

Fig. 1.56 Papillary tufts lining a cyst in autosomal dominant polycystic kidney disease (A and B).

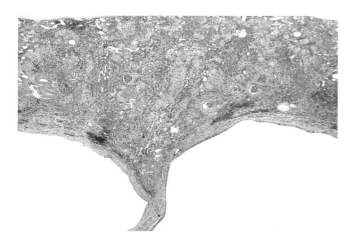

Fig. 1.57 Whole-mount kidney in nephronophthisis showing outer medullary cysts. The cortex has advanced scarring and scattered small cysts in the deep cortex. *(Courtesy of The Jay Bernstein, M.D. Consultative Collection.)*

centimeters in diameter (Fig. 1.57). In the infantile form the kidneys may be larger than normal because cyst formation occurs earlier in the disease, before contraction from tubulointerstitial scarring. If cysts develop they may involve the medulla but generally are cortical in location.

The primary histologic findings in nephronophthisis are nonspecific, so complete laboratory and clinical data are necessary. The juvenile and adolescent forms show a radial distribution of cortical injury with atrophic zones that alternate with zones of normal or hypertrophied tubules largely localized to medullary rays (Fig. 1.58A). Before end-stage renal disease the tubulointerstitial injury exceeds the extent of glomerulosclerosis, thus implicating a primary tubulointerstitial process (Fig. 1.58A). The tubules have an irregular profile sometimes described as figure-eight or T-shaped because of the tubule diverticula, particularly numerous in the limbs of Henle. Many small "cysts" are not true cysts but are localized segments of tubular dilatation with patent afferent and efferent tubule connections.[155]

The irregularly shaped atrophic tubules show prominent multilayering of their tubular basement membranes, or the tubule basement membranes may range from thick and irregular, to thin and attenuated, to segmental absence of basement membrane (Fig. 1.58B). Dense interstitial fibrosis is present often with a prominent lymphoid cell infiltrate. Periglomerular fibrosis is a common finding, as it is in other chronic inflammatory interstitial diseases. As the tubulointerstitial disease progresses, glomeruli undergo sclerosis. Advanced cases show marked fibrointimal thickening of arteries and medial hypertrophy.

Medullary cysts, when present, arise from the loops of Henle and collecting ducts. The cyst cell lining is variable. A cuboidal cell lining is present in small cysts, but large cysts may have a flattened, nondescript cell lining surrounded by a rim of dense fibrous tissue. Medullary inflammation is not usually present.

In the infantile form of nephronophthisis the cysts affect tubules, predominantly distal tubules and collecting ducts, in the form of tubular dilation or ectasia (Fig. 1.59). Macrocystic dilation of tubules occurs and may be visible grossly. The ectatic and grossly cystic tubules are lined by cuboidal to columnar epithelium typical of distal tubules and collecting ducts. The tubules between the cysts may be normal or atrophic. Atrophic tubules are small and lined by inconspicuous cuboidal epithelium with thin tubular basement membranes that lack the irregular basement membrane multilayering of the juvenile and adolescence forms. Glomeruli may develop microcysts in which the Bowman capsule is enlarged two to three times normal. Although mild interstitial inflammation occurs, it is usually less than in the juvenile and adolescent forms.

Autosomal Dominant Tubulointerstitial Disease

ADTID, previously referred to as medullary cystic kidney disease (MCKD), is like nephronophthisis, a chronic progressive tubulointerstitial disease in which cysts may develop. It is a rare disease primarily of adults, but the age of onset overlaps with older patients with nephronophthisis.[151,158-169] There are four known causes of ADTID due to mutation of uromodulin (UROM; Tamm-Horsfall glycoprotein), mucin 1 (MUC1; epithelial membrane antigen), renin (REN), and hepatocyte nuclear factor 1β (HNF1B;

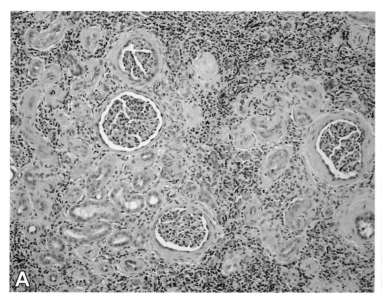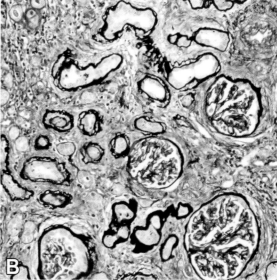

Fig. 1.58 (A) Nephronophthisis showing a chronic interstitial nephritis. Although there is periglomerular fibrosis the glomeruli otherwise are intact, associated with severe chronic tubulointerstitial injury. (B) The atrophic tubules typically show basement membrane multilayering (Jones methenamine silver stain). *(A and B, Courtesy of The Jay Bernstein, M.D. Consultative Collection.)*

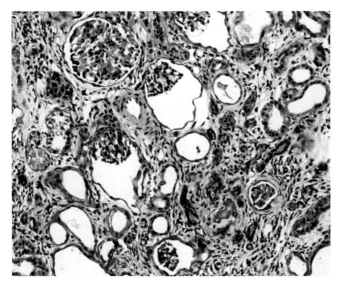

Fig. 1.59 This infantile form of nephronophthisis also shows chronic interstitial nephritis. Glomerular microcysts are visible, and the atrophic tubules lack basement membrane multilayering (periodic acid–Schiff stain.) *(Courtesy of The Jay Bernstein, M.D. Consultative Collection.)*

Table 1.16). One or more additional mutations remain to be identified. The recommended terminology for these diseases is UROM kidney disease, MUC1 kidney disease, REN kidney disease, and HNF1B kidney disease.

Most patients present in the third to fourth decade of life with polyuria and polydipsia as a result of salt wasting and a concentration defect (Table 1.16). They progress to end-stage disease, usually by the fourth to seventh decade, although the rate of progression varies within and between affected families. Hyperuricemia and gout are common, especially in UROM and REN kidney disease. REN kidney disease patients have anemia refractory to treatment, hyperkalemia, and often low BP.

The kidneys in ADTID may be enlarged if cysts are prominent. Although medullary cysts are common, they are usually present in small numbers and develop late in the disease. Within a family not all affected individuals have cysts. The cysts congregate at the corticomedullary junction and can be several centimeters (Fig. 1.60A). Microscopically, all four ADTIDs show a nonspecific chronic interstitial nephritis with tubular atrophy, interstitial fibrosis, and periglomerular fibrosis similar to nephronophthisis. If cysts are present, they are lined with a flattened to cuboidal epithelium. UROM kidney disease contains uromodulin intracellular aggregates in thick ascending limb of Henle cells (Fig. 1.60B). REN kidney disease shows reduced to absent renin staining in cells of the juxtaglomerular apparatus. MUC1 and HNF1B kidney disease have no defining histologic findings. However, patients with HNF1B kidney disease often have congenital anomalies of the kidney and/or lower urinary tract.[78,170]

Von Hippel–Lindau disease

Von Hippel–Lindau disease is an uncommon autosomal dominant disorder due to germline mutation of the *VHL* gene in which renal and extrarenal cysts and neoplasms develop.[171] The extrarenal manifestations include retinal, cerebellar, and spinal hemangioblastomas, pheochromocytoma, epididymal and pancreatic cysts, and cystadenomas. The renal manifestations consist of multiple and bilateral cysts that develop in 75% of patients, and renal cell carcinomas, often bilateral and multicentric, that develop in approximately 50% of patients (Fig. 1.61).[172-176] The mutant *VHL* gene has been localized to chromosome 3p25, adjacent to the gene implicated in development of sporadic clear cell renal cell carcinoma.[172,174,175]

The renal cysts are lined with glycogen-rich cells like those of grade 1 to 2 clear cell renal cell carcinoma (Fig. 1.62).[173,176-178] These range from a benign-appearing lining of one to two cell layers of clear cells to multiple layers of cells. The broad spectrum of neoplastic proliferative lesions ranges from cysts with papillary tufts of mildly atypical cells, to cysts with solid mural nodules of clear cell renal cell carcinoma, to markedly cystic clear cell renal cell carcinoma. This morphologic spectrum represents a challenge in the classification of lesions in biopsy and nephrectomy material. Despite awareness of the high frequency of renal cell carcinoma in this syndrome, metastatic renal cell carcinoma remains the leading cause of death.

Tuberous Sclerosis

Tuberous sclerosis complex (TSC) is an autosomal dominant disorder characterized by mental retardation, epilepsy, angiofibromas, cardiac rhabdomyomas, renal angiomyolipomas, renal cell carcinomas and renal cysts.[179-184] Two genes have been identified that cause TSC, *TSC1* and *TSC2*, mapped to chromosomes 9 and 13 that encode for hamartin and tuberin, respectively. The latter locus is within a few nucleotides of the *PKD1* locus. Although renal cysts are uncommon and usually not extensive, some individuals, usually children, have dual mutations involving *TSC2* and *PKD1*. They develop a diffuse cystic kidney disease with numerous large cortical and medullary cysts that resemble autosomal dominant polycystic disease; this disorder is known as the *TSC2/PKD1* contiguous gene syndrome.

TABLE 1.16	Autosomal Dominant Tubulointerstitial Diseases: Comparison of Major Clinical and Pathologic Features					
Mutation	Onset/ESRD (years)	Laboratory/Clinical Results	Extrarenal Disease	Biopsy	Renal Cysts	Other Pathology
UROM	20-70/avg. 54	Gout, conc. defect	None	CTIN	40%	UROM inclusions
MUC1	20-70/avg. 40	Gout, conc. defect	None	CTIN	12%-17%	None
REN	Childhood/30-40	Gout, conc. defect, ↓ BP, anemia, ↑ K	None	CTIN	None	↓ Renin in JGA
HNF1B	24/Adulthood	Gout, conc. defect, DM, ↓ Mg	Pancreas hypoplasia/agenesis	CTIN	60%-80%	CAKUT

avg., Average; *BP*, blood pressure; *CAKUT*, congenital anomalies of the kidney and urinary tract; *Conc*, concentrating; *CTIN*, chronic tubulointerstitial nephritis; *DM*, diabetes mellitus; *ESRD*, end-stage renal disease; *HNF1B*, hepatocyte nuclear factor 1β; *JGA*, juxtaglomerular apparatus; *K*, potassium; *Mg*, magnesium; *MUC1*, mucin-1; *REN*, renin; *UROM*, uromodulin.

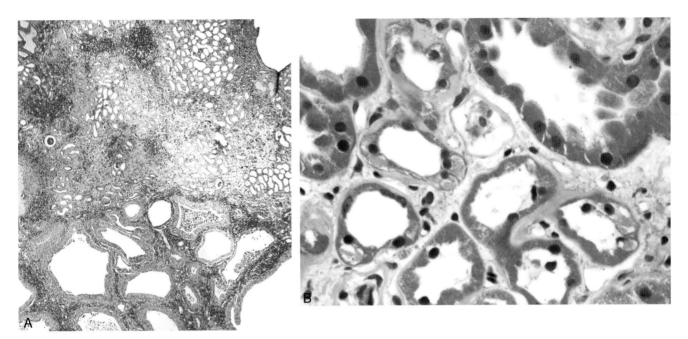

Fig. 1.60 (A) Medullary cystic disease showing cysts along the outer medulla and advanced cortical scarring. *(Courtesy of The Jay Bernstein, M.D. Consultative Collection.)* (B) This is UROM (uromodulin) kidney disease. Trichrome stain nicely demonstrated the intracellular aggregates of retained uromodulin (Tamm-Horsfall protein).

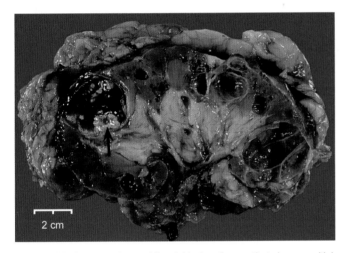

Fig. 1.61 Nephrectomy in von Hippel–Lindau disease that shows multiple cysts. One cyst contains a mural nodule *(arrow)* of renal cell carcinoma.

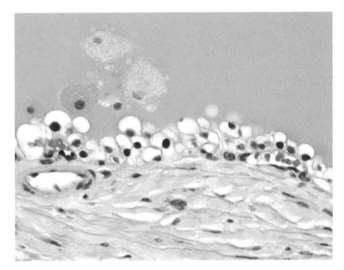

Fig. 1.62 Cyst in von Hippel–Lindau disease is lined with low nuclear grade clear cells.

Many tubules and cysts in tuberous sclerosis are distinctive and provide diagnostic specificity in the recognition of this disorder.[143,153] The cysts are lined with large eosinophilic cells with large hyperchromatic nuclei (Fig. 1.63). The cyst lining cells may form papillary or polyploid masses, and may show occasional mitotic activity. Renal cell carcinomas of several types also develop in TSC but are far less frequent than in von Hippel–Lindau disease.[185]

Glomerulocystic Kidneys

A glomerulocystic kidney (GCK) is defined as the presence of glomerular cysts in more than 5% of glomeruli in the absence of another cystic kidney disease. A GCK may be primary or secondary. *Glomerulocystic kidney disease* is used in reference to the primary forms that include a sporadic form, a familial form, and forms caused by mutations of UROM and HNF1B (Table 1.3). Secondary forms of glomerular cysts occur in many unrelated disorders such as ADPKD, ARPKD, TSC, a variety of syndromes, ischemic glomeruli, and renal dysplasias.[186-191] In these diseases, glomerular cysts may be present, but glomerular cysts are not definitional of the entity.

A glomerular cyst is defined as cystic dilation of Bowman capsule to two to three times normal. The glomerular tuft itself may be normal or abnormally formed. In most cases of GCK the glomerular cysts are widespread and affect far more than 5% of glomeruli (Fig. 1.64). The Bowman capsule dilation in some cases of GCK may be massive, sufficient to result in a grossly cystic kidney. In other cases the kidneys may be small and hypoplastic.

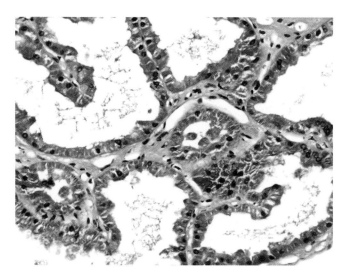

Fig. 1.63 The cysts, as well as scattered individual tubules in noncystic kidneys, in tuberous sclerosis are often lined by large cells with densely eosinophilic cytoplasm and prominent nuclei. *(Courtesy of The Jay Bernstein, M.D. Consultative Collection.)*

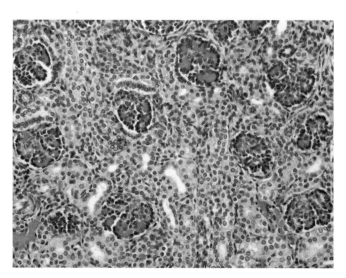

Fig. 1.65 Congenital renal tubular dysgenesis manifesting with oliguric acute renal failure. No normal proximal tubules are present. All cortical tubules resemble distal tubules and are lined by small cuboidal cells without interstitial expansion.

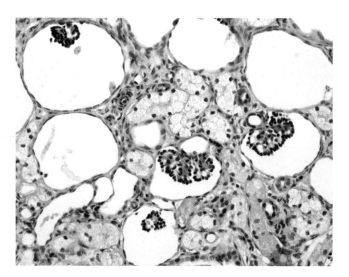

Fig. 1.64 Glomerulocystic kidney disease showing microcysts principally involving Bowman capsules.

Miscellaneous Diseases

Renal Tubular Dysgenesis

Failure of proximal tubule differentiation is known as renal tubular dysgenesis.[192-201] It results in neonatal renal failure with the oligohydramnios sequence, a Potter syndrome phenotype, and death from pulmonary hypoplasia. Renal tubular dysgenesis may be primary or secondary. Primary renal tubular dysgenesis is an autosomal recessive disorder due to mutation of one of the renin-angiotensin system genes. Secondary causes include monochorionic twins with twin–twin transfusions in which only the donor twin is affected, congenital renal artery stenosis, major cardiac malformations, and as a complication of maternal use of angiotensin-converting enzyme inhibitors (can be associated with hypocalvaria).[172]

The kidneys are usually grossly normal, although they may be decreased in weight. The glomeruli are close together because of the lack of the normally voluminous proximal tubule cells. The intervening tubules resemble distal tubules. The cells and tubular

profiles are small (Fig. 1.65). The tubule cells demonstrate distal tubule and collecting duct phenotype by immunohistochemistry and lectin staining. Ultrastructural studies show an undifferentiated phenotype. The cells lack a microvillous brush border and contain scant organelles.

Acquired Cystic Kidney Disease

Acquired cystic kidney disease refers to the development of multiple and bilateral renal cysts in patients whose chronic renal failure cannot be attributed to a hereditary cystic disease. Although identified as long ago as 1847 by Simon, in 1977 Dunnill revived interest in this phenomenon when in an autopsy study of hemodialysis patients he not only observed a high prevalence of renal cysts, but also found renal tumors in 20% of the patients.[202,203] One patient had died of metastatic renal cell carcinoma. The development of both cysts and tumors appears to be related to the uremic state because it is independent of the type of dialysis and the cause of the original renal disease.[204-215]

Acquired cystic kidney disease is bilateral and asymptomatic in its early stages. Cysts are present in 8% of patients at the time dialysis is initiated and increase in incidence, number, and size proportional to the duration of dialysis. After 3 to 5 years of dialysis, cysts have developed in approximately 50% of patients, whereas by 10 years, almost 90% of patients have cysts.[216] The complications of acquired cystic kidney disease include intrarenal and retroperitoneal hemorrhage, cyst infection, and renal cell carcinoma, which may account for 3% to 4% of all deaths.[211-215] All of the major types of renal cell carcinoma can develop in the setting of acquired cystic kidney disease. However, one tumor, acquired cystic kidney disease–associated renal cell carcinoma, appears to be the most common cancer. This tumor has a distinctive morphology and a feature unique among renal cell carcinomas: the frequent presence of calcium oxalate crystals. Although improvement in the cystic disease occurs in many patients after successful renal transplantation, the influence of transplantation on neoplastic complications remains unclear. As the number of patients receiving dialysis increases and their survival rates improve, the occurrence of cystic disease and neoplastic complications can also be expected to increase.

The cysts initially form in the proximal tubules of kidneys with end-stage disease. Most cysts are less than 0.5 cm in diameter, but 2- to 3-cm cysts can develop. Initially the cysts are cortical, but in advanced cases medullary cysts form and the entire kidney may be replaced by cysts and resemble a smaller version of ADPKD (Fig. 1.66). The cysts are lined with flattened, cuboidal, or columnar epithelium and may contain a proteinaceous to hemorrhagic fluid. Foci of epithelial hyperplasia are common in the cysts and tubules. Papillary adenomas are also commonly present.

Localized Cystic Kidney Disease

Localized cystic kidney disease is an uncommon cystic kidney disease that histologically resembles ADPKD. It is not a genetic disease and lacks the progressive renal failure and extrarenal complications of ADPKD.[58,217-220] The affected kidney is usually partially involved but may be diffusely cystic (Fig. 1.67). The contralateral kidney should be noncystic. When the kidney is partially involved, it has a tight collection of variably sized cysts with thin cyst septa. The lesion is surrounded by normal kidney. The cystic lesion invariably involves the medulla but may extend into the cortex. The cysts contain serous fluid and are lined by a low cuboidal to flattened epithelium. Excision and follow-up may be required to establish the diagnosis and exclude a cystic neoplasm.

Medullary Sponge Kidney

Medullary sponge kidney is a cystic renal malformation in which there is ectasia of the papillary collecting ducts of one or more renal pyramids associated with nephrocalcinosis and nephrolithiasis (Fig. 1.68).[221,222] Medullary sponge kidney is usually bilateral and is more common in male patients. It is usually detected radiographically in adults evaluated for nephrolithiasis. The kidneys are not enlarged, and renal function is normal, although a concentrating defect may be present in more severely affected patients.

Microscopically, the collecting ducts are dilated and lined with cuboidal or flattened epithelium. Intratubular calcifications (microliths) are common. If stones have obstructed the ducts, overlying cortical scarring may be present. Medullary sponge kidney can be most readily distinguished from other diseases with medullary cysts such as ADTID, nephronophthisis (NPHP), and juvenile presentation of ARPKD by the presence of nephrolithiasis and nephrocalcinosis on imaging studies.

Simple Cortical Cyst

Simple cortical cysts are the most common cystic renal lesions.[223,224] They are rare before the age of 40 years. Therefore any cyst in a child or young adult, especially if bilateral, can be an important clue to the presence of a cystic kidney disease. Simple cysts increase in frequency with advancing age. In older patients the cysts may be multiple and large, and typically are exophytic (Fig. 1.69). The cysts are lined with a flattened layer of cells or lack

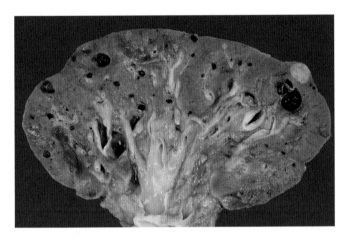

Fig. 1.66 Acquired cystic disease of the kidney. There are multiple cysts in both cortex and medulla. Although this is a mild or early example with abundant noncystic parenchyma, notice the small neoplasm to the upper right. Several smaller tumors are also present elsewhere.

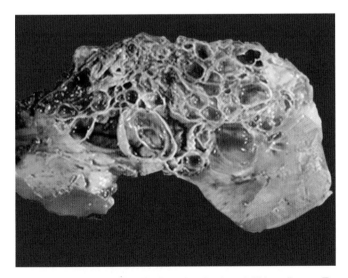

Fig. 1.67 This is an example of isolated/localized cystic kidney disease. The central portion of the kidney is replaced by a diffusely cystic lesion that on imaging studies would likely be regarded as a cystic neoplasm such as a cystic nephroma. (Courtesy of The Jay Bernstein, M.D. Consultative Collection.)

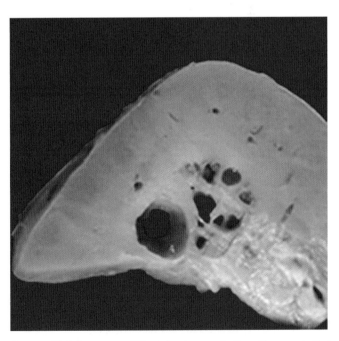

Fig. 1.68 Medullary sponge kidney showing a collection of large cysts that replace the distal renal medulla. These represent prominent ectasia of the distal collecting ducts. (Courtesy of The Jay Bernstein, M.D. Consultative Collection.)

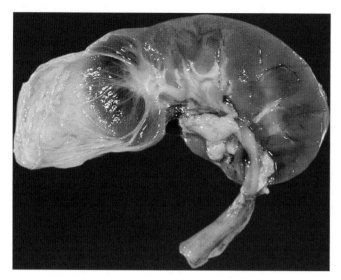

Fig. 1.69 A large, simple cortical cyst found incidentally at autopsy. Notice its thin translucent wall.

TABLE 1.17	Vascular Diseases of the Kidney

Hypertension-associated renal disease
    Benign nephrosclerosis
    Malignant nephrosclerosis
Thrombotic microangiopathy
Renal artery stenosis
    Atherosclerosis
    Fibromuscular dysplasia
Renal artery dissection
Renal artery aneurysm
Arteriovenous malformation and fistula
Renal emboli and infarcts
Renal cortical necrosis
Renal papillary necrosis
Renal cholesterol microembolism syndrome
Renal artery thrombosis
Renal vein and renal venous thrombosis
Bartter syndrome
Vasculitis

an epithelial lining. The cyst wall may occasionally calcify, a radiographic finding mimicking infection or malignancy.

Hydrocalyx, Megacalycosis, and Calyceal Diverticulum

Several lesions—hydrocalyx, megacalycosis, and calyceal diverticulum—have in common a cavity lined with urothelium that communicates with the collecting system and are associated with recurrent infections and nephrolithiasis.[225-227] In hydrocalyx there is caliectasis secondary to infundibular stenosis. The stenosis may be congenital or the sequela of inflammation. By contrast, in megacalycosis obstruction is not evident. In both lesions the renal pyramid is flattened or concave, and in cases complicated by infection, parenchymal inflammation and scarring may be present. In calyceal diverticulum the cavity communicates with a minor calyx via a narrow isthmus, and no obstruction is present. The upper pole calyx is involved in 54% of cases. Parenchymal inflammation and scarring usually are absent unless the case is complicated by infection.

Vascular Diseases

Hypertension-Associated Renal Disease

Vascular disease in its various forms is the most common cause of renal injury encountered at autopsy because of the high incidence of atherosclerosis and hypertension (Table 1.17 and Fig. 1.70).[228-230] A connection between hypertension and renal and cardiovascular diseases has been recognized for more than 100 years.[228-236] Hypertension-associated renal disease was first separated from other forms of renal disease in 1914 by Volhard and Fahr, who first recognized the existence of two forms.[237] The most common form, which they called *benign nephrosclerosis*, occurred in older individuals who had mild hypertension and little renal impairment. The second form, which Volhard and Fahr called *malignant nephrosclerosis*, occurred in younger patients with severe hypertension and renal failure.[237] Although most patients (90% to 95%) with hypertension have idiopathic disease, numerous secondary causes can produce either benign or malignant nephrosclerosis (Table 1.18).

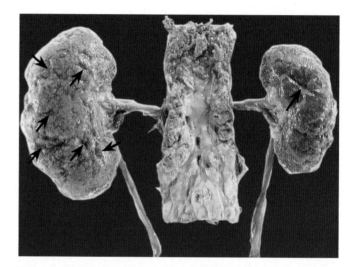

Fig. 1.70 Complicated atherosclerotic vascular disease showing arterial nephrosclerosis, small atheroembolic infarcts (*arrows*), and an atrophic right kidney from renal artery stenosis.

Benign Nephrosclerosis

Benign (or essential) hypertension is an asymptomatic disorder that affects approximately 50 million people in the United States.[228-230] The pathogenesis of essential hypertension is presumed to be multifactorial, involving genetic, epigenetic, environmental, and immune mechanisms. Heritability of BP is estimated to be 31% to 68%, but genome-wide association and linkage studies to date were able to identify only factors with small effects on BP or those that impart increased predisposition to hypertension in certain ethnic groups. Interestingly most monogenic forms of hypertension are related to defects in renal sodium handling (Table 1.19). Unfortunately, in most patients the cause of hypertension remains enigmatic. Hypertension is often first diagnosed around age 45 to 54 years, but there has been an increasing incidence of early-onset hypertension.[238-241] If unchecked, hypertension places the patient at risk not only for complications related to atherosclerotic vascular

TABLE 1.18	Types and Causes of Hypertension

Primary

Benign (essential) hypertension
Malignant hypertension

Secondary

Renal artery stenosis
Acute glomerulonephritis
Chronic renal diseases
Neoplasms
   Renin-producing tumors
   Adrenal cortical tumors
   Pheochromocytoma
Endocrine abnormalities
   Thyrotoxicosis
   Adrenal cortical hyperplasia
   Hyperparathyroidism
   Oral contraceptives
Neurogenic
Miscellaneous vascular
   Preeclampsia
   Thrombotic microangiopathy
   Vasculitis
   Coarctation of aorta

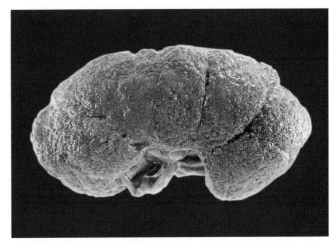

Fig. 1.71 Granular subcapsular surface of benign hypertension-associated arterial nephrosclerosis.

TABLE 1.19	Examples of Monogenic Forms of Hypertension
	Causative Gene/Mutation
Liddle syndrome	Epithelial sodium channel
Gordon syndrome (pseudohypoaldosteronism type II)	Thiazide-sensitive sodium chloride cotransporter
Geller syndrome	Mineralocorticoid receptor
Glucocorticoid remediable hyperaldosteronism	11-α-hydroxylase, aldosterone synthase
Syndrome of apparent mineral corticoid excess	11-α-hydroxysteroid dehydrogenase
Congenital adrenal hyperplasia	11-α-hydroxylase or 17-β-hydroxylase

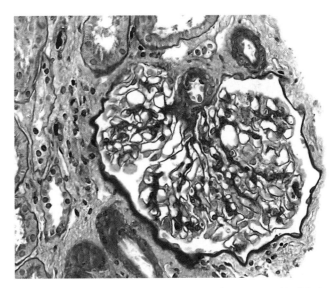

Fig. 1.72 Arteriolar hyalinosis in hypertension. In contrast with diabetes, hyalinosis in hypertension is often limited to the afferent arteriole (periodic acid–Schiff stain).

disease such as renal insufficiency, congestive heart failure, coronary artery disease, and stroke, but also other diseases such as diabetes mellitus.[242,243] Although benign hypertension will not cause renal failure in most patients, it is sufficiently prevalent to account for approximately 15% to 30% of patients with end-stage renal disease.

In benign nephrosclerosis the kidneys are symmetrically reduced in size and weigh between 60 and 100 g. They have granular subcapsular surfaces and cortical thinning, the extent of which is influenced by the severity and duration of the hypertension (Fig. 1.71).[231-233] Microscopically, arteries of interlobar size or greater show fibrous intimal thickening with reduplication or fragmentation of the elastic lamina and smooth muscle hyperplasia. In contrast with atherosclerotic disease, lipid and calcification are not usually present. The afferent arteriolar media shows thickening by hyaline material (Fig. 1.72). Hyaline deposition also occurs in diabetes mellitus but tends to affect both afferent and efferent arterioles, and develops to a mild degree in the absence of hypertension in individuals who are older than 60 years. Hyaline arteriolar

thickening may be encountered in young adults, in whom it is associated with early-onset coronary artery disease. The grossly visible subcapsular granularity corresponds to shallow subcapsular scars that contain sclerotic glomeruli, atrophic tubules, and thick-walled hyalinized or hyperplastic arterioles (Fig. 1.73).

Malignant Nephrosclerosis

Malignant nephrosclerosis develops as a consequence of malignant hypertension.[244,245] Malignant hypertension usually arises in a patient with preexisting benign hypertension, but it may develop as a de novo disorder. Patients present with headache, dizziness, and impaired vision. Their diastolic BP exceeds 120 to 140 mm Hg. Retinal hemorrhages, exudates, and papilledema are present. Hematuria, proteinuria, and microangiopathic hemolytic anemia develop. Without treatment, the patient will experience renal failure and may die suddenly of heart failure, myocardial infarction, or cerebral hemorrhage.

The kidney in malignant nephrosclerosis often has petechial subcapsular hemorrhages or a mottled red and yellow cortex if

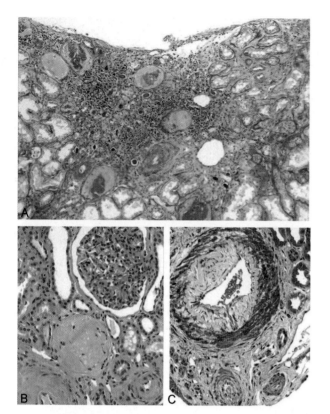

Fig. 1.73 (A) The shallow subcapsular scars contain sclerotic glomeruli and atrophic tubules and thickened arterioles (periodic acid–Schiff [PAS] stain). (B) Glomerular injury in hypertension showing an obsolescent solidified glomerulus (PAS stain). (C) Fibrointimal thickening of an arcuate artery.

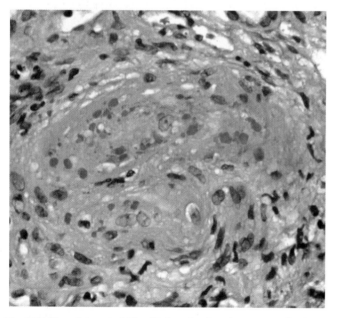

Fig. 1.74 Necrotizing arteriolitis with thrombosis and extravasated red cells in malignant hypertension.

infarcts are present. Microscopically, a range of lesions are encountered depending on whether the lesions are acute or chronic.

Acute thrombotic microangiopathy develops in the acute phase of malignant hypertension (Fig. 1.74). The glomeruli show capillary loop thrombosis and mesangiolysis reflecting necrosis of

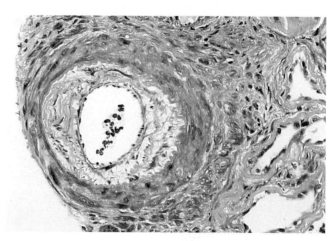

Fig. 1.75 Mucoid intimal edema in an artery in malignant hypertension (trichrome stain).

endothelial and mesangial cells, and may develop segmental capillary loop necrosis with crescent formation. In arterioles, necrosis of endothelium and medial smooth muscle cells results in luminal thrombosis and red blood cell fragmentation and extravasation into the media. The interlobular arteries and arcuate arteries show a distinctive mucoid or edematous-appearing intimal thickening and may also contain subendothelial fibrin or intraluminal and fragmented red blood cells (Fig. 1.75). These acute changes may resolve with adequate treatment.

In more protracted cases, chronic or reparative changes are present alone or superimposed on the acute thrombotic microangiopathy. At this stage with basement membrane stains such as periodic acid–Schiff (PAS) or a silver stain, the glomeruli may either show ischemic wrinkling and collapse or capillary loop basement membrane reduplication. The arterioles and arteries show concentric (onion-skin) myointimal proliferation resulting in severe luminal occlusion (Fig. 1.76). Increasing fibrosis of the intima can be noted in untreated cases.

Thrombotic Microangiopathy

Thrombotic microangiopathy may develop in many pathogenically distinct diseases (Table 1.20).[244-252] Patients often present with thrombocytopenia, microangiopathic hemolytic anemia, peripheral blood schistocytes, and elevated lactate dehydrogenase levels. However, in smoldering or indolent cases these findings may be minimally abnormal or absent. The two classic thrombotic microangiopathy syndromes are hemolytic uremic syndrome (HUS) and thrombotic thrombocytopenic purpura.

Hemolytic Uremic Syndrome

HUS is characterized by the presence of renal failure, thrombocytopenia, and microangiopathic hemolytic anemia. HUS (Fig. 1.77) is divided into two major categories: diarrhea-associated HUS (classic HUS) and atypical HUS not associated with diarrhea (aHUS).

Classic HUS is the most common cause of pediatric acute renal failure. It is a food-borne illness usually secondary to verotoxin-producing bacteria, especially *Escherichia coli*. It has a good prognosis with a high rate of recovery.

In contrast, aHUS has a poor prognosis with a high incidence of renal failure and death. It can be seen in both children and adults, and is often the result of a genetic defect or an acquired disorder of one of several alternative complement pathway regulatory proteins.

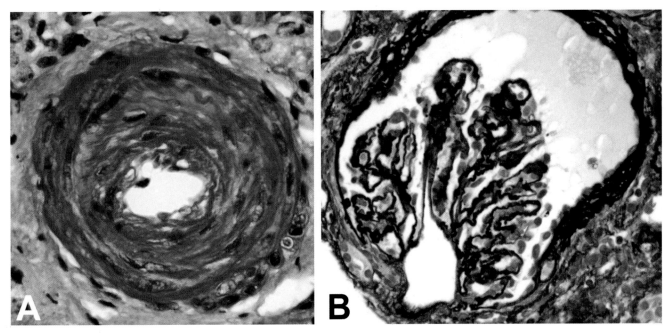

Fig. 1.76 (A) Hyperplastic arteriolitis (periodic acid–Schiff stain). (B) Ischemic capillary loop wrinkling in malignant hypertension (silver stain).

TABLE 1.20   Thrombotic Microangiopathies

Primary thrombotic microangiopathy

Classic hemolytic uremic syndrome
Atypical hemolytic uremic syndrome
Thrombotic thrombocytopenic purpura

Secondary causes of thrombotic microangiopathy

Disseminated intravascular coagulation
Malignant hypertension
Antiphospholipid antibodies
Scleroderma renal crisis
Postpartum hemolytic uremic syndrome
HIV-associated thrombotic microangiopathy
Irradiation-associated thrombotic microangiopathy
Drugs
    Chemotherapeutic agents
    Calcineurin inhibitors
    Cocaine
    Oral contraceptives

HIV, Human immunodeficiency virus.

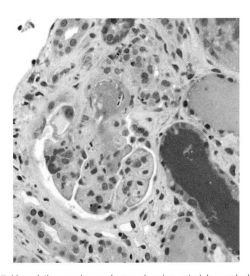

Fig. 1.77 Hemolytic uremic syndrome showing arteriolar and glomerular capillary thrombosis.

Thrombotic Thrombocytopenic Purpura

Thrombotic thrombocytopenic purpura is characterized by neurologic symptoms, thrombocytopenia, microangiopathic hemolytic anemia, fever, and renal failure. It results from von Willebrand factor/ADAMTS13 deficiency. This deficiency may have one of several causes that include a genetic disorder of ADAMTS13, an acquired autoimmune cause, and defective cobalamin metabolism. It has a poor prognosis with a significant risk for renal failure and death.

Microangiopathic vascular changes, with or without obvious thrombosis, can be seen as a primary morphologic finding in a number of diverse conditions (Table 1.20). This list includes malignant hypertension, as discussed earlier. Unfortunately, none of these causative factors have distinguishing morphologic features; therefore clinical information is critical to the diagnosis.

Thrombotic microangiopathies of all causes may have a range of acute and chronic features.

The acute lesions include necrosis of endothelial cells, vascular smooth muscle cells, and/or glomerular mesangial cells leading to microvascular thrombosis of arterioles and small arteries, and glomerular thrombosis and mesangiolysis (Figs. 1.77, 1.78, and 1.79). Red blood cell fragmentation is common. The larger arteries show basophilic mucoid intimal expansion (Fig. 1.75).

The chronic lesions represent repair that leads to vascular occlusion and glomerular capillary loop basement membrane duplication or to ischemic glomerular obsolescence (Fig. 1.79).

Renal Artery Stenosis

In 1934, Goldblatt and associates established a role for decreased renal perfusion in the generation of systemic hypertension by partially occluding one renal artery of a dog, and thus producing

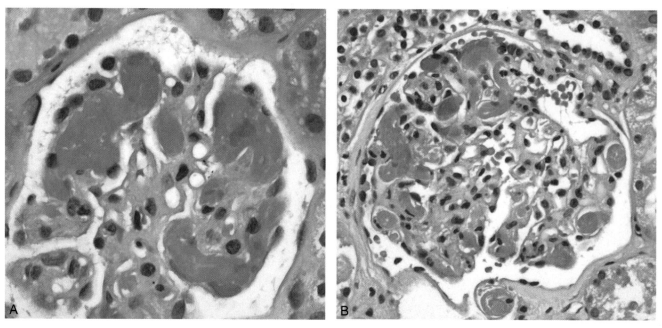

Fig. 1.78 (A) Disseminated intravascular coagulation showing glomerular capillary thrombi. (B) Cyclosporine toxicity showing glomerular capillary loop thrombi in a renal allograft.

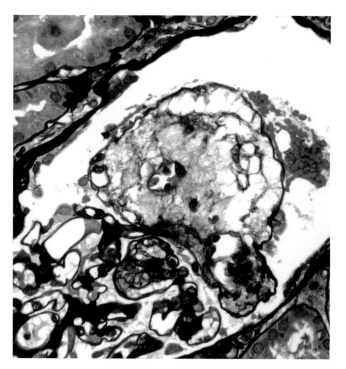

Fig. 1.79 Chronic chemotherapy-related thrombotic microangiopathy showing basement membrane duplication and severe mesangiolysis in a bone marrow transplant recipient (silver stain).

TABLE 1.21	Fibromuscular Dysplasia
Intimal fibroplasia	
Medial fibroplasia	
Medial hyperplasia	
Medial fibroplasia with aneurysms	
Perimedial fibroplasia	
Periarterial fibroplasia	

TABLE 1.22	Causes of Renal Artery Stenosis
Atherosclerosis	
Fibromuscular dysplasia	
Rare other causes	
Renal artery dissection	
Renal artery aneurysm	
Renal artery thrombosis	
Renal artery emboli	
Arteriovenous malformation	
Arteritis	
Radiation injury	
Transplant artery stenosis	
Neurofibromatosis	

hypertension that was reversed after restoration of blood flow.[253] Hypertension resulting from decreased renal perfusion and relieved by restoration of flow is known as renovascular hypertension. Renal artery stenosis is the most common cause.[254,255] The two major causative factors of renal artery stenosis are atherosclerosis (66% of cases) and fibromuscular dysplasia (33% of cases) (Table 1.21).[256-259] The remaining causes of renal artery stenosis, although numerous, comprise less than 1% of cases (Table 1.22).

Atherosclerosis-Related Renal Artery Stenosis

Atherosclerosis is associated with several renal complications and is responsible for 60% to 70% of cases of renal artery stenosis.[259] The disorder has a male predominance. Patients usually present from age 50 to 70 years and have significant atherosclerosis of the aorta and other major arteries that influences the management of the disease and its prognosis. Because atherosclerosis develops over many

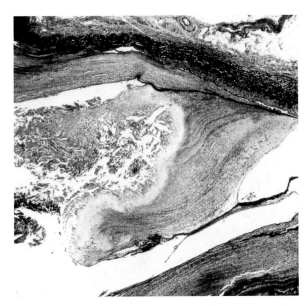

Fig. 1.80 Atherosclerotic renal artery stenosis with a plaque at the renal artery ostium (elastic stain).

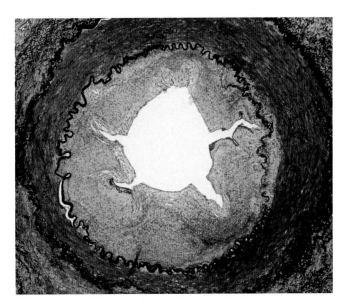

Fig. 1.81 Intimal fibromuscular dysplasia showing fibroblastic intimal thickening and intact internal elastic lamina (Movat elastic stain).

years and is a complication of prolonged essential hypertension, the kidney may exhibit benign nephrosclerosis, or it may contain remote infarcts from aortic atheroemboli (Fig. 1.70). Bilateral disease occurs in 30% of cases and, if severe, causes ischemic chronic renal failure. Revascularization can improve renal function in some patients; however, because these patients have a long history of hypertension, arterial nephrosclerosis is usually implicated in the renal failure, and renal artery stenosis may not be recognized.

The renal artery is occluded by eccentrically thickened intima at its aortic ostium or in its proximal portion (Fig. 1.80). Intimal thickening begins when myointimal cells enter the media and synthesize connective tissue components and mucopolysaccharides.[200,260,261] Lipid and foam cells accumulate, and fibrosis develops. The advanced lesion contains atheromatous material in the form of acingulate (rigid or nonconforming) cholesterol clefts, foamy macrophages, and calcification. It also has irregular duplication of elastica with sclerosis and atrophy of medial smooth muscle.

Fibromuscular Dysplasia

Fibromuscular dysplasia is the second most common cause of renal artery stenosis in adults and is the most common cause in children.[254-258,262-265] It consists of a group of lesions that, despite histologic differences, have a similar clinical presentation and affects women in their second to fourth decade of life. Multifocal stenosis with a string-of-beads appearance, generally involving the distal two-thirds of branches of the renal artery, is the classic radiologic appearance in about 80% of cases. The prognosis for fibromuscular dysplasia is much better than for atherosclerosis-associated renal artery stenosis because the patient is younger, the hypertension is of recent onset, and hypertension and atherosclerosis-related diseases in other sites are absent. There are five subtypes (Table 1.21).

Intimal Fibroplasia

Intimal fibroplasia is a rare (<1% of cases) form of fibromuscular dysplasia. It produces circumferential intimal thickening in a substantial segment of the renal artery and may also extend into its segmental branches. The thickened intima is composed of fibroblastic tissue (Fig. 1.81). It is distinguished from atherosclerotic intimal thickening by the absence of lipids and calcification, and the

presence of an intact internal elastic lamina. It is prone to develop thrombosis and dissection.

Medial Hyperplasia

Medial hyperplasia consists of a localized segment of disorganized medial smooth muscle thickening. Radiographically, it resembles the intimal form and is also prone to develop thrombosis and dissection. The intima is not thickened, and the internal elastic lamina is intact.

Medial Fibroplasia With Aneurysms

Medial fibroplasia with aneurysms is the most frequent and distinctive form of fibromuscular dysplasia. It tends to involve the distal main renal artery and its segmental branches, and is commonly bilateral. It is characterized by ridges of medial thickening without fibrosis alternating with areas of extreme medial thinning and close approximation of the internal and external elastic lamina (Figs. 1.82 and 1.83). These areas of thinning represent the "aneurysms" and result in a characteristic pattern (string of pearls) on angiogram.

Perimedial Fibroplasia

Perimedial fibroplasia is the second most common form of fibromuscular dysplasia. It is characterized by an irregular pattern of fibrosis that replaces the outer one-half to two-thirds of the media by fibrous tissue (Fig. 1.84). It can lead to severe stenosis and the development of thrombosis and renal infarcts.

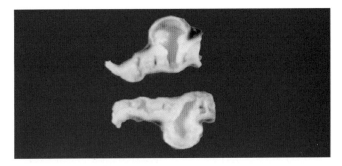

Fig. 1.82 A segment of the main renal artery showing medial fibroplasia complicated by a saccular aneurysm.

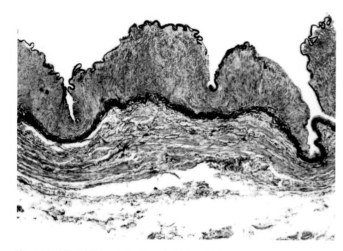

Fig. 1.83 Medial fibroplasia (Movat elastic stain).

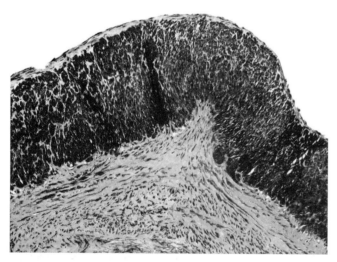

Fig. 1.84 Perimedial fibroplasia (trichrome stain).

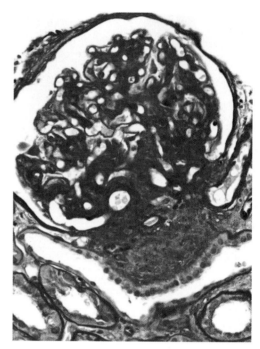

Fig. 1.85 Acute renal artery stenosis in a renal transplant showing prominent enlargement of the juxtaglomerular apparatus.

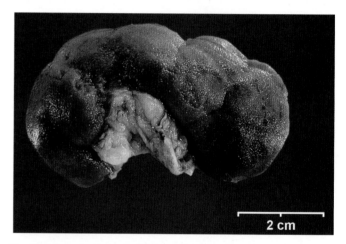

Fig. 1.86 A small, contracted kidney with a smooth surface in chronic renal artery stenosis secondary to fibromuscular dysplasia.

Periarterial Fibroplasia

Periarterial fibroplasia is the rarest form of fibromuscular dysplasia. It consists of dense collagenous tissue that forms within the adventitia and restricts arterial expansion during systole. The collagenous tissue can extend into the adjacent fibrofatty tissue and create a vague similarity to retroperitoneal fibrosis.

Kidney in Renal Artery Stenosis

In renal artery stenosis of recent onset, initial enlargement of the juxtaglomerular apparatus results from an increase in the number of the extraglomerular mesangial cells, or lacis cells (Fig. 1.85). There is metaplasia of smooth muscle cells of the afferent arteriole to form contractile filament–poor renin-synthesizing cells. Distinctive renin protogranules and mature renin granules can be detected in increased quantities in these cells by the Bowie stain, immunocytochemistry, or electron microscopy.

After several weeks of renal artery stenosis the juxtaglomerular apparatus shrinks, again becoming inconspicuous. At this time the parenchyma supplied by the stenotic artery shows a very distinctive alteration. Grossly, uniform cortical thinning (Fig. 1.86) results from diffuse atrophy of tubules that causes close approximation of glomeruli secondary to loss of tubular volume. The glomeruli appear slightly contracted but remain viable. The tubules appear distinctive. They are small and lined by small cuboidal epithelium, and lack tubular basement membrane thickening of typical

atrophic tubules (Fig. 1.87). Furthermore, little interstitial fibrosis separates the tubules. If the main renal artery is the site of stenosis, then the entire kidney becomes small (40 to 70 g) and uniformly contracted with a smooth subcapsular surface. If a segmental artery is stenotic, or conversely, if it is free of stenosis while the main renal artery is stenotic (Figs. 1.88 and 1.89), then a characteristic line of transition from a thinned cortex to a thicker cortex will become grossly apparent. Interestingly the degree of sclerosis and hypertensive changes in the distal arteries in the affected side or segments are often less pronounced because of the protective effects. In contrast the contralateral kidney can often show severe sclerosis in arteries and arterioles and nephrosclerosis.

Renal Artery Dissection

Dissection of the renal artery refers to a disruption of the intima that extends into the media (Figs. 1.90 and 1.91), with creation of a false lumen or a double channel, or results in a complete vascular occlusion causing renal infarction.[263,266-268] Dissection is associated with hypertension, flank pain, and hematuria. The hypertension may not always precede the dissection but is invariably present after the dissection. Renal artery dissection has several causes, with the most common being extension from aortic dissection (Table 1.23). Primary renal artery dissection is rare and, in the past, was usually a complication of preexisting fibromuscular dysplasia. Catheter-related causes are increasing with the more frequent use of that procedure to correct renal artery stenosis.[269] Dissection caused by blunt trauma is rare and is usually the consequence of an automobile accident.

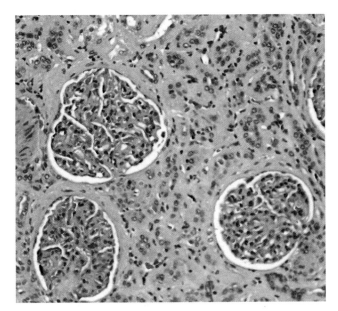

Fig. 1.87 The thin cortex in chronic renal artery stenosis shows diffuse small atrophic tubules and crowding of nonsclerotic glomeruli.

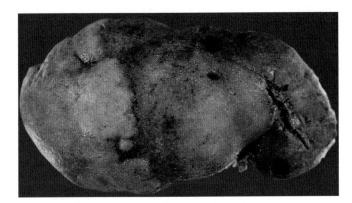

Fig. 1.88 Chronic renal artery stenosis affecting the middle and lower poles. The upper pole was supplied by a patent supernumerary (polar segmental) artery.

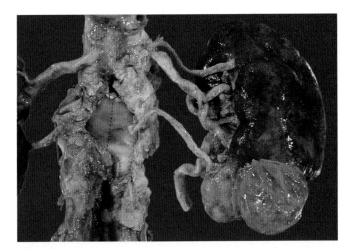

Fig. 1.89 Chronic renal artery stenosis affecting a lower pole accessory artery in a patient with severe aortic atherosclerotic disease. The atrophic pole is also affected by a large simple cortical cyst.

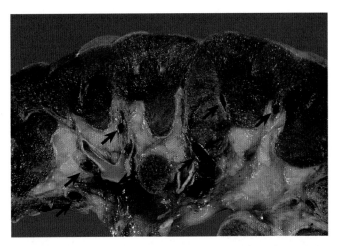

Fig. 1.90 Extensive renal artery dissection (*arrows*) after unsuccessful angioplasty.

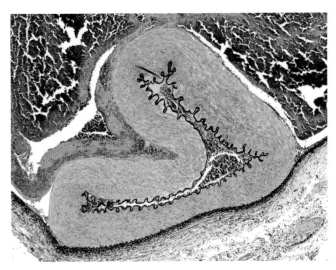

Fig. 1.91 The dissection (from Fig. 1.90) developed at the interface of the media and adventitia (elastic stain).

TABLE 1.23 Causes of Renal Artery Dissection

Extension of aortic dissection
Fibromuscular dysplasia
Blunt abdominal trauma
Catheter injury
Spontaneous or idiopathic conditions

Renal Artery Aneurysm

Aneurysms of the main renal artery or one of its tributaries are rare, found in 0.01% of autopsies.[270-273] They may be classified as true aneurysms, which may be either congenital or acquired, or false aneurysms, which are usually the result of trauma. Most are small and asymptomatic. If a large vessel is involved, renal artery aneurysms may be associated with thrombosis and vascular occlusion leading to infarction or hypertension. Pain is an ominous symptom that usually indicates impending rupture or dissection. The risk for rupture is greatest during pregnancy and parturition, and is usually fatal. Three categories of aneurysms have been identified: saccular, fusiform, and intrarenal. Dissecting aneurysm is not included in this list because aneurysmal enlargement is not a feature of renal arterial dissection.

Saccular Aneurysm

Saccular aneurysms develop in the main renal artery at the bifurcation of the anterior and posterior divisions, or at a branch point of a segmental artery. Although they are frequently calcified or show atherosclerotic changes, they are usually regarded as congenital, and the atherosclerosis is considered a secondary event. They may be small or enlarge to 4 to 5 cm. Especially if noncalcified, the large aneurysms are prone to rupture or may erode into an adjacent vein to produce an arteriovenous fistula.

Fusiform Aneurysm

Fusiform aneurysms usually occur in young patients and represent a poststenotic dilation that develops distal to renal artery stenosis, often secondary to fibromuscular dysplasia. Thrombosis with secondary renal infarction is a serious potential complication.

Intrarenal Aneurysm

Intrarenal aneurysms are usually false aneurysms. They have many causes: trauma (biopsy, surgery), arteritis (polyarteritis nodosa), postinflammatory injury (tuberculosis [TB] or transplant rejection), and neurofibromatosis. Rarely, intrarenal aneurysms may be congenital.

Arteriovenous Malformation and Fistula

Direct communication between renal arteries and veins may be either congenital or acquired.[274-276] Congenital lesions are referred to as arteriovenous malformations, whereas acquired lesions are called *arteriovenous fistulas*. High-output heart failure, hypertension, and hematuria may develop depending on the size of the shunt and location of the lesion. The most common type is an acquired fistula (65% to 75% of cases). It usually has a single point of communication between an artery and a vein. It may have several causes; the most common is iatrogenic (Table 1.24).

Congenital arteriovenous malformations are rare. Most consist of cirsoid arteriovenous communications with multiple points of communication between artery and vein. Most are located within the medulla or in the calyceal or pelvic mucosa and usually cause gross hematuria. Hilar vessels may also be affected. When a single cavernous channel connects an artery with a vein, an abdominal bruit may be heard.

Renal Emboli and Infarcts

Renal artery emboli invariably cause infarction because of the end-artery organization of the renal blood flow.[31,277] If the infarct is small, it may be clinically and functionally asymptomatic. Larger infarcts cause flank pain, hematuria, and hypertension.[278-284] If the infarct is bilateral and widespread, renal insufficiency results. Emboli originate either from the heart in patients with valvular disease or atrial fibrillation, or from the aorta. Aortic atheroemboli are by far the most frequent (Fig. 1.92). If an infected vegetation is responsible, a more complicated picture develops with hematogenous pyelonephritis and microabscesses (Fig. 1.93). Familiarity

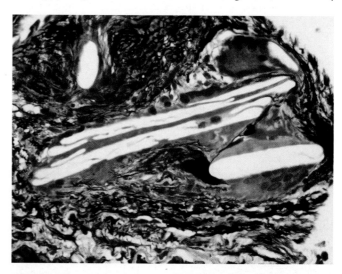

Fig. 1.92 This atheroembolus has elicited a multinucleated giant cell reaction.

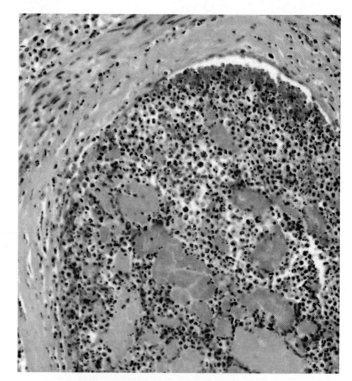

Fig. 1.93 This thromboembolus from a patient with infective endocarditis contains gram-positive cocci and has destroyed a portion of the arterial wall.

TABLE 1.24	Causes of Acquired Arteriovenous Fistula
Surgical injury	
Needle biopsy	
Penetrating injury	
Neoplasia	
Arterial aneurysm erosion	
Inflammation	

TABLE 1.25	Gross Recognition of Occluded Arterial Segment	
Artery	Size of Infarct	Relationship to Lobes
Segmental	4-5 cm	Entire lobe and portion of adjacent lobe
Interlobar	2-3 cm	Columns of Bertin and portion of adjacent lobe
Arcuate	0.5-1.0 cm	1/6-1/8 of a lobe extending to the middle of the lobe
Intralobular	0.1-0.2 cm	Small portion of a lobe

with the arterial supply to the kidney often enables one, on gross examination, to infer the caliber of vessel occluded by the size of infarct and its relationship with the renal lobes (Table 1.25).

The acute infarct shows a sharply demarcated zone of transcortical coagulation necrosis, which will also involve the medulla if an arcuate or larger artery is involved (Figs. 1.94 and 1.95). The margins of the infarct are hemorrhagic and contain many neutrophils and histiocytes. Cholesterol clefts or infected material in the arteries may reveal the source of the embolus (Figs. 1.92 and 1.93).

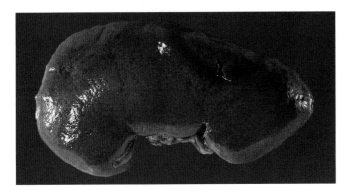

Fig. 1.94 Acute infarct resulting from an interlobar artery occlusion. The acute infarct appears as a circumscribed pale lesion with a hyperemic rim.

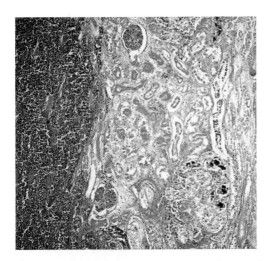

Fig. 1.95 The acute infarct shows coagulation necrosis centrally with a peripheral rim of hemorrhage and acute inflammation.

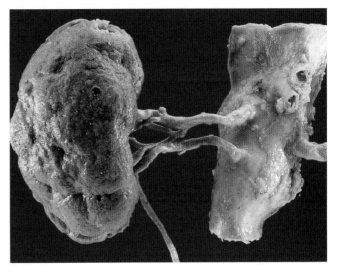

Fig. 1.96 This kidney shows multiple depressed scars resulting from arcuate and interlobular atheroembolic infarcts.

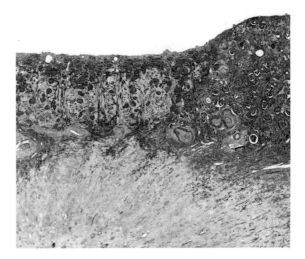

Fig. 1.97 This is a remote cortical infarct from atheroembolic disease. Note the solidified periodic acid–Schiff–positive glomeruli.

Eventually infarcts become depressed cortical scars (Fig. 1.96). Within them, ghostlike remnants of glomeruli and tubules are present (Fig. 1.97). A PAS stain is helpful in determining whether a scar is an infarct or a more chronic form of injury because infarcted glomeruli contain condensed masses of capillary loop basement membranes without the collagenous tissue in Bowman space that forms with other causes of glomerulosclerosis.

Renal Cortical Necrosis

Renal cortical necrosis is a serious bilateral ischemic injury that can complicate a variety of extrarenal diseases.[285-287] Obstetric causes are most frequent (Table 1.26). Patients experience acute renal failure, usually associated with anuria and hematuria, which may be gross. The condition has a high fatality rate related to extrarenal complications. The kidneys develop diffuse or patchy sharply demarcated zones of cortical pallor with hyperemic rims that also involve the columns of Bertin. The renal pyramids and a thin subcapsular rim of cortex are spared. There is coagulation necrosis of the glomeruli and tubules, usually with widespread thrombosis.

TABLE 1.26	Causes of Renal Cortical Necrosis

Obstetric complications
Abruptio placentae
Septic abortion
Intrauterine fetal demise

Infections
Sepsis
Peritonitis

Burns

Gastrointestinal hemorrhage

Transfusion reactions

Toxins

Hemolytic uremic syndrome

Renal Papillary Necrosis

Necrosis of portions of the renal medulla is known as renal papillary necrosis.[288-297] Several diseases are associated with papillary necrosis (Table 1.27). When bilateral and diffuse, renal papillary necrosis manifests as an acute devastating illness with renal failure, fever, chills, flank pain, and hematuria. Alternately, it may be an insidious process that manifests as a urinary concentrating defect or with the gradual development of renal failure. Renal papillary necrosis is always a complication of some other disease process, and most patients have more than one risk factor. In the United States diabetes is the most prevalent underlying disorder.

Because of the strong association with infection, renal papillary necrosis is often included in discussions of pyelonephritis. However, its pathogenesis is ischemia related to the marginal medullary blood supply. This accounts for its association with disorders that compromise medullary blood flow.

Renal papillary necrosis is usually a disease of adults; however, it can also develop in infants. Although the disorder is often referred to in the pediatric literature as renal medullary necrosis, approximately 25% to 30% of patients will also experience development of focal cortical infarcts.[288,292] Infants with renal papillary necrosis are usually younger than 1 month and have perinatal asphyxia or a severe infantile disease associated with vascular collapse and dehydration, such as gastroenteritis.

In the 1950s and 1960s renal papillary necrosis became a serious problem, particularly in Australia and in Scandinavian countries, where analgesic combinations were in widespread use.[291,294-297] Analgesic nephropathy, as it came to be known, rapidly became the leading cause of chronic renal failure and renal papillary

TABLE 1.27	Causes of Renal Papillary Necrosis

Diabetes mellitus
Urinary tract obstruction
Acute pyelonephritis
Analgesic abuse
Sickle cell disease
Hypoxia
Dehydration
Combination of these factors = 55%

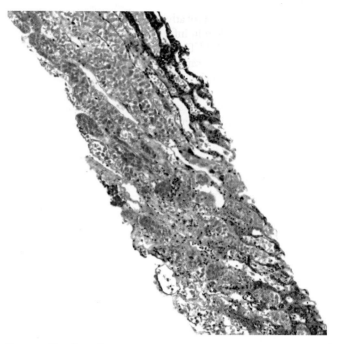

Fig. 1.98 Renal papillary necrosis in a patient with diabetes. The renal medulla shows coagulation necrosis with a peripheral rim of acute inflammation.

necrosis in those regions (see Analgesic Nephropathy section later in this chapter).

In renal papillary necrosis the necrosis usually does not involve the entire medulla. The papillary tip is most vulnerable, whereas the outer medulla is often preserved. A medullary form and a papillary form have been described. In the medullary form the calyceal spiral arteries are patent and peripheral, or fornical portions of the pyramid are intact with the central portions necrotic (Fig. 1.98). In the papillary form the necrosis is more extensive, and the entire papilla or inner medulla is necrotic (Fig. 1.99). In both forms the necrosis is of a coagulation type, in keeping with its ischemic etiology.

Renal Cholesterol Microembolism Syndrome

Atherosclerotic vascular disease may affect the kidneys in several fashions. In 1965 Richards and colleagues distinguished embolic

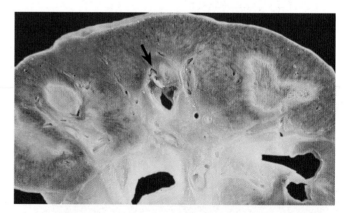

Fig. 1.99 This kidney shows diffuse papillary necrosis in a patient with diabetes. The renal papilla in the center has completely sloughed.

complications of fragments of atherosclerotic plaques that occluded large arteries and resulted in infarcts from microemboli of cholesterol crystals.[278-284,298-300] This syndrome usually develops after a vascular procedure such as catheterization or aneurysm surgery, but occasionally arises spontaneously. Emboli shower the microvasculature of multiple organs including kidneys, skin, brain, and gastrointestinal tract, and produce a systemic disease resembling systemic vasculitis with abdominal pain, acute onset of hypertension, livedo reticularis, and neurologic symptoms. In the initial reports of microembolic disease that appeared in the 1960s to 1980s, the fatality rate was very high. More recently, patients with milder forms have been identified, and these patients may completely or partially recover renal function.

Cholesterol microembolization is associated with several potentially confusing laboratory findings. Cholesterol microembolization is frequently associated with eosinophilia in 15% to 80% of cases. In a given patient, eosinophilia may be impressive, with absolute eosinophil counts reported as high as 19,700/mm^3. Eosinophiluria is infrequent. Less commonly encountered but potentially more confusing are hypocomplementemia, thrombocytopenia, and proteinuria that may be in the nephrotic range.

Not every biopsy sample with a cholesterol crystal should elicit alarm. Asymptomatic cholesterol embolization has been identified at autopsy in 4% of patients with aortic atherosclerotic disease, a finding attesting that cholesterol embolization can be clinically insignificant. When multiple emboli are noted on biopsy, concern escalates because the percentage of kidney examined in a single biopsy is minute. Many thousands of emboli may have been delivered to the kidneys for every crystal noted in a biopsy (Fig. 1.100). If the patient presents with impaired renal function and no other cause is identified, implicating cholesterol embolization as a cause of the renal failure becomes unavoidable. Autopsy studies have demonstrated that fresh or recent cholesterol crystals are intraluminal without a cellular reaction. Within days macrophages appear followed by a fibroblastic reaction. Eventually endothelial cell and

collagen investment incorporates the crystals into the wall or provokes further fibroblastic reaction with luminal obliteration. Correlation of the clinical event that may have caused cholesterol embolization with the foregoing features may assist interpretation of finding crystals in a renal biopsy.

Renal Artery Thrombosis

Thrombosis of the renal artery is an uncommon event that usually follows a traumatic injury to the renal artery or to the aorta (Table 1.28).[301] Renovascular hypertension and renal infarction are the major complications.

Renal Vein Thrombosis

In the past renal vein thrombosis was believed to cause nephrotic syndrome.[302-304] With the increased use of renal biopsy and advances in understanding of the physiologic consequences of nephrotic syndrome, it is now clear that renal vein thrombosis is a complication of the hypercoagulable state that develops in patients with nephrotic syndrome. Patients with renal vein thrombosis present with flank pain or tenderness and hematuria, and often have hypertension. Renal failure and pulmonary emboli are serious complications. Although renal vein thrombosis has no pathognomonic histologic findings, interstitial edema and marginating neutrophils

TABLE 1.28   Causes of Renal Artery Thrombosis

Umbilical artery catheters in neonates
Blunt abdominal trauma
Intraaortic balloons in adults
Renal transplantation
Electrical injury

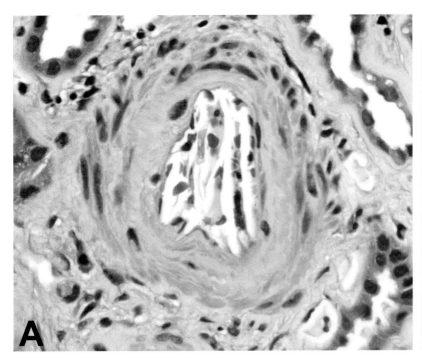
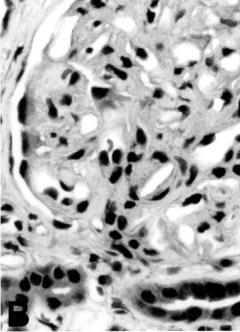

Fig. 1.100 Renal cholesterol microembolism syndrome with cholesterol emboli in an arteriole (A) and in the glomerular hilum (B).

within dilated glomerular capillaries have been described in acute cases. Organizing thrombi are seen in veins at autopsy.

Renal venous thrombosis differs from renal vein thrombosis in that smaller intrarenal vessels are affected, such as interlobular and arcuate veins, rather than the main renal vein.[305-307] Infants are usually affected, and the condition is associated with serious illnesses such as diarrhea, congenital heart disease, maternal diabetes mellitus, seizures, and birth trauma. Hemorrhagic cortical infarcts may develop if the thrombosis is sufficiently widespread to interfere with collateral blood flow.

Bartter syndrome

Bartter syndrome is characterized by hyperplasia of the juxtaglomerular apparatus, hyperaldosteronism, and hypokalemic alkalosis.[308-312] It is caused by mutations of several Cl channels (types I to IV) or a calcium-sensing receptor (type V). The mutations affect function of the channels in the thick ascending limb of loop of Henle, leading to decreased NaCl reabsorbtion. The resultant electrolyte and water depletion causes persistent activation of the renin-angiotensin-aldosterone system. Despite the impressive enlargement of the juxtaglomerular apparatus and hyperreninemia, both renal artery stenosis and systemic hypertension are absent. This syndrome is most commonly identified in children and, in many cases, appears to be familial, with autosomal recessive inheritance.

Vasculitis

Vasculitis comprises a large and heterogeneous group of disorders that have in common inflammatory injury to vascular structures.[313] The first major account of vasculitis dates to the 1866 description of periarteritis (polyarteritis) nodosa by Küssmaul and Maier (Fig. 1.101).[314] The seriousness of systemic vasculitis with major visceral involvement was graphically captured in their report. They stated, "He was one of those patients for whom one could make the prognosis even before making the diagnosis, he gave the impression of being one whose days were numbered."[314]

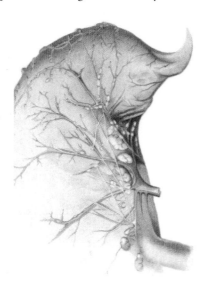

Fig. 1.101 Nodules along renal arteries in polyarteritis nodosa, from the 1866 description by Küssmaul and Maier. (From Küssmaul A, Maier R. Ueber eine bisher niche beschriebene eigenthumliche arteriener-krankung (periarteritis nodosa), die mit morbus Brightii und rapid fortschreitender ailgemeiner muskellahmung. Dtsch Arch Klin Med 1866;1:484; with permission.)

TABLE 1.29	Vasculitis and Anti-Neutrophil Cytoplasmic Antibodies	
ANCA-Positive Vasculitis (% Positive)	**ANCA-Negative Vasculitis**
Wegener granulomatosis (>90%)	Temporal arteritis
Microscopic polyarteritis (>90%)	Takayasu arteritis
Polyarteritis nodosa (30%-50%)	Henoch-Schönlein purpura[a]
Idiopathic crescentic (>90%)	Connective tissue diseases[a]
Kawasaki disease (50%)	Glomerulonephritis
Churg-Strauss syndrome (50%-60%)	Cryoglobulinemia
	Drug reaction[a]
	Infectious arteritis

ANCA, Antineutrophil cytoplasmic antibody.
[a]Rare positive cases.

A major advance in the diagnosis and management of patients with vasculitis was the discovery of a serologic marker for certain forms of vasculitis, the antineutrophil cytoplasmic antibody (ANCA).[315-329] ANCA refers to a family of autoantibodies detectable in the serum of patients with the major forms of systemic vasculitis involving the kidney and in idiopathic (immune complex negative or "pauci-immune") crescentic glomerulonephritis (Table 1.29). These autoantibodies are directed against lysosomal components of neutrophils and monocytes, and can be detected by indirect immunofluorescence on alcohol-fixed neutrophils. Two principal patterns are detected, a cytoplasmic pattern (c-ANCA) and a perinuclear pattern (p-ANCA). The c-ANCA pattern is now known to be due to antiproteinase 3 (PR3) antibodies, whereas p-ANCA pattern is due to antimyeloperoxidase (MPO) antibodies. In about 75% patients, c-ANCA pattern/PR3 autoantibodies correlate with granulomatosis with polyangiitis (GPA, formerly known as Wegener granulomatosis). The p-ANCA pattern/MPO autoantibodies are less specific and seen in about 70% of cases of renal limited pauci-immune crescentic glomerulonephritis and about 40% to 50% of cases of microscopic polyangiitis or eosinophilic GPA (Churg-Strauss syndrome). Thus although the typing of ANCA does not permit a specific diagnosis, the presence of a positive ANCA test result is important because it simplifies the morphologic and clinical differential diagnosis (Table 1.29). ANCA can also be used to monitor response to therapy (insensitive, because of slow decline in titer with remission) and to distinguish a clinical relapse (rising titer) from a therapeutic complication (falling titer).

The kidney is the most commonly affected organ in systemic vasculitis. Either necrotizing and crescentic glomerulonephritis or true arteritis may develop (Fig. 1.102). Crescentic glomerulonephritis is the most common pattern of renal involvement by vasculitis. A crescent forms after necrosis of the glomerular capillary wall. Extravasation of fibrin, protein, and red cells ensues, and epithelial cell proliferation occurs in the area of damage. If healing occurs, a segmental-to-circumferential scar (fibrous crescent) forms, the size of which varies with the size of the initial necrosis. When the percentage of glomeruli affected by necrosis exceeds 50%, patients present with rapidly progressive renal failure. Their urine contains protein, red cells, and often red cell casts.

The process of crescent formation is not specific for vasculitis. Crescents also form in other types of glomerulonephritis. The process is subclassified by the findings on direct immunofluorescence (Table 1.30). Crescentic glomerulonephritis in vasculitis is

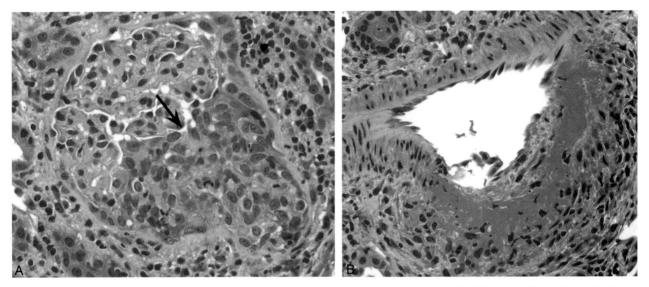

Fig. 1.102 (A) A cellular crescent (*arrow*) in a patient with granulomatosis with angiitis (Wegener granulomatosis). (B) Segmental fibrinoid necrosis of an artery in a patient with microscopic polyangiitis.

TABLE 1.30	Direct Immunofluorescence in Crescentic Glomerulonephritis

Linear immunofluorescence

Goodpasture syndrome
Antiglomerular basement membrane disease

Granular immunofluorescence

Immune complex glomerulonephritis

Pauci-immune/negative immunofluorescence

ANCA-associated crescentic glomerulonephritis
Idiopathic crescentic glomerulonephritis

ANCA, Antineutrophil cytoplasmic antibody.

distinctive because of the absence of appreciable detectable immune reactants by direct immunofluorescence, referred to as pauci-immune crescentic glomerulonephritis. Even though most cases are ANCA-positive, 15% to 20% cases can be negative, although these are also treated the same way as ANCA-positive cases.[330-336]

Necrotizing arteritis and arteriolitis are less common lesions than crescentic glomerulonephritis when vasculitis affects the kidney. They are characterized by fibrinoid necrosis of the vessel wall, karyorrhexis, and a mixed inflammatory cell response rich in neutrophils (Fig. 1.102B). The prominent inflammatory component distinguishes vasculitis from acute thrombotic microangiopathy. Although necrotizing arteritis is most common in microscopic polyangiitis and GPA (Wegener granulomatosis), necrotizing arteritis can develop in other forms of vasculitis. Serologic data and clinical correlation are crucial to proper classification.

Tubulointerstitial Disease

Disorders of tubules and interstitium are discussed together because they rarely occur in isolation. Any alteration in one affects the other. Tubulointerstitial diseases encompass many entities and include the most common causes of acute and chronic renal failure (Table 1.31). Although diverse in etiology, tubulointerstitial diseases have a limited spectrum of histologic abnormalities; therefore clinical information is crucial in establishing the cause of any tubulointerstitial disease. Because the severity of tubulointerstitial alterations correlates with the severity of renal dysfunction, patients with tubulointerstitial disease present with renal insufficiency.

The rate of development of renal insufficiency can be used to separate entities with the greatest potential for recovery of renal function from those in which some irreversible injury is present and likely to persist. Acute tubulointerstitial diseases have a rapid clinical onset, are associated with edema and variable inflammation, and are potentially reversible. The inflammation is usually neutrophilic in infectious causes (pyelonephritis) and is principally lymphocytic, plasmacytic, and histiocytic in allergic and autoimmune forms. Chronic tubulointerstitial diseases have a gradual or insidious onset and are associated with irreversible tubular atrophy and interstitial fibrosis. A lymphocytic infiltrate is also present, even in forms associated with chronic or smoldering infection.

Acute and Chronic Renal Failure

Acute renal failure manifests as a sudden deterioration in renal function usually defined as evolving over 2 days to 2 weeks. Patients experience an increase in serum creatinine of 0.5 to 1.0 mg/dL/day. The urine may contain red blood cells, but red blood cell and white blood cell casts are absent, urinary protein is less than 1 g/day, and the urinary sodium concentration is increased. Many patients also are oliguric (<400 mL urine/day). The rapid evolution of renal failure correlates with the rapid expansion of the interstitial areas by edema. Tubular cell injury and edema, without or with inflammation, are the principal morphologic findings in the two most common causes, acute tubular injury (previously referred to as acute tubular necrosis) and acute tubulointerstitial nephritis, respectively (Tables 1.31 to 1.34).

Chronic renal failure manifests as a gradual decline in renal function usually defined as renal failure evolving over a period of 2 months or longer. There is typically a mononuclear cell interstitial infiltrate. However, the histologic picture is dominated by

TABLE 1.31 Tubulointerstitial Diseases

Acute tubular injury (acute tubular necrosis)

Acute and chronic noninfection-associated tubulointerstitial nephritis

Allergic tubulointerstitial nephritis
Chronic tubulointerstitial nephritis, not otherwise specified
Herbal and slimming agents and aristocholic acid nephropathy
Immunoglobulin G4–related sclerosing tubulointerstitial nephritis
Analgesic nephropathy

Bacterial infection–associated tubulointerstitial nephritis

Acute pyelonephritis
　Ascending
　Hematogenous
　Emphysematous
Chronic pyelonephritis
　Obstructive nephropathy
　Reflux nephropathy

Virus-associated tubulointerstitial nephritis

Granulomatous tubulointerstitial nephritis

Sarcoidosis

Xanthogranulomatous pyelonephritis
Malakoplakia
Tuberculosis
Diverse other granulomatous infection-related diseases, especially fungal

Metabolic abnormalities, heavy metals, and crystal-associated tubulointerstitial diseases

Heavy metals
Nephrocalcinosis
Randall plaque and nephrolithiasis
Oxalosis
Cystinosis
Uric acid nephropathy and gout

Amyloidosis and paraprotein-associated tubulointerstitial disease

Amyloidosis
Light chain cast nephropathy
Immunoglobulin/light chain deposition disease
Light chain crystal tubulopathy
Light chain proximal tubulopathy
Crystal-storing histiocytosis

TABLE 1.32 Causes of Acute Tubular Injury (Necrosis)

Ischemic injury

Nephrotoxic injury

Antibiotics
Radiographic contrast agents
Nonsteroidal antiinflammatory drugs
Chemotherapeutic agents
Cocaine
Organic solvents
Insecticides and herbicides
Heavy metals
Rhabdomyolysis
Hemolysis
Insect stings
Snake bites
Mushroom poisoning

TABLE 1.33 Causes of Acute Interstitial Nephritis

Drug associated

β-Lactam and other antibiotics
Diuretics
Nonsteroidal antiinflammatory drugs
Allopurinol
Rifampicin
Cimetidine
Sulfa drugs
Phenytoin

Connective tissue diseases

Systemic lupus erythematosus
Sjögren syndrome

Transplant rejection

Sarcoidosis

Acute interstitial nephritis–uveitis syndrome

Antitubular basement membrane disease

Bacterial infections

Scarlet fever
Diphtheria
Typhoid fever
Brucellosis
Leptospiral infection
Rickettsia

Viral infection

Cytomegalovirus
Epstein-Barr virus
Polyomavirus
Human immunodeficiency virus
Hantavirus

interstitial fibrosis and tubular atrophy (IFTA). Many of the same agents that cause acute tubular injury or acute interstitial nephritis also produce chronic interstitial nephritis, such as heavy metals, drugs, connective tissue diseases, and sarcoidosis, and many entities cause a mixed pattern of acute and chronic changes. In some patients, no specific cause can be established, and this is called *idiopathic chronic tubulointerstitial nephritis.*

Acute Tubular Injury (Necrosis)

Acute tubular injury is the most common renal parenchymal cause of acute renal failure.[337-347] It usually is divided into ischemic and toxic forms. Ischemic injury is more common. Its causative factor can usually be established because it results from decreased renal perfusion secondary to hemorrhage, hypotension, or dehydration.

TABLE 1.34	Exogenous Causes of Chronic Interstitial Nephritis

Herbal remedies and slimming agents

Drugs
Analgesics
Chemotherapeutic agents
Cyclosporine
Lithium

Heavy metals
Lead
Cadmium

In some patients these features are not observed directly but are inferred based on the clinical setting. The causes of toxic acute tubular injury are diverse (Table 1.32), and they may be difficult to identify because they often develop in the context of therapy for other illnesses or may result from exogenous agents.

For acute tubular injury to result in acute renal failure, it must be diffuse and bilateral. If unilateral or even focal in one kidney, then renal insufficiency will not occur. The renal size and weight are increased as a consequence of interstitial edema. In certain situations, such as older patients with arterial nephrosclerosis with underlying renal atrophy, acute tubular injury may not result in a change in renal size and weight. Grossly the cortex usually is pale and may bulge slightly compared with the medulla. The medulla, particularly the outer medulla, often is congested and dark, secondary to dilation of the vasa recta.

In acute tubular injury, there is interstitial expansion resulting from edema without significant inflammation. If inflammation is present, it consists of a predominantly mononuclear cell infiltrate at the corticomedullary junction or within the vessels in the vasa recta of the outer medulla. The tubules themselves can show two patterns of injury. In the more obvious and severe form, there is extensive coagulative necrosis of tubular cells, particularly of the

proximal tubules, with loss of nuclei (Fig. 1.103A). This form is usually seen at autopsy. In autopsies it must be distinguished from autolysis.[344] Autolytic tubules may be recognized by the tendency of their epithelium to separate from their tubular basement membranes and from each other, with preservation of their nuclei and intact cell membranes (Fig. 1.103B).

The second pattern of acute tubular necrosis is subtler. It is characterized by attenuation or flattening of the tubular epithelium causing luminal enlargement and widely spaced nuclei (Fig. 1.104A and B). At low magnification this imparts a microcystic appearance to the cortex because of single-cell necrosis and sloughing. The remaining cells lose their brush border and spread out to cover the basement membrane. There may be short segments of denuded tubular basement membranes. Mitotic figures may be present but are usually very infrequent. Atypia of the lining epithelia and karyomegaly may be noted in tubular injury because of radiation or certain drugs such as tenofovir (Fig. 1.104C). Distal tubules and collecting ducts may contain granular casts of sloughed cells.

In heavy metal lesions such as those caused by bismuth, cadmium, and lead, proximal tubule intranuclear inclusions may be present. Myeloid bodies detectable by electron microscopy are present in lesions caused by aminoglycoside antibiotics, although their presence does not correlate with toxicity. Pigmented myoglobin casts in distal tubules are found in lesions caused by rhabdomyolysis, often have a distinctive granular morphology, and can easily be confirmed with a myoglobin stain (Fig. 1.105). Extensive intranephron bleeding from a variety of glomerular diseases can also result in acute tubular injury. Red blood cells and red blood cell casts are observed within tubules lined by extremely attenuated epithelium.

Acute Tubulointerstitial Nephritis

Acute tubulointerstitial nephritis is an inflammatory cause of acute renal failure.[347-353] The term *acute* refers to the rapid development of renal failure rather than the character of the infiltrate, which consists of lymphocytes, plasma cells, and histiocytes with scattered eosinophils (Fig. 1.106A). Acute interstitial nephritis represents

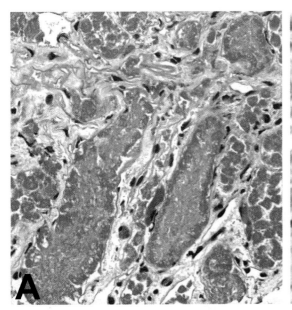 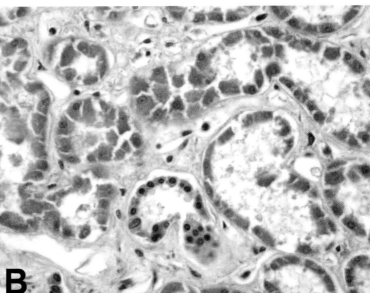

Fig. 1.103 (A) Acute tubular necrosis at autopsy showing coagulation necrosis. (B) Kidney at autopsy showing autolysis. Notice the retention of nuclei and the separation of the epithelial cells from each other and from the tubular basement membrane.

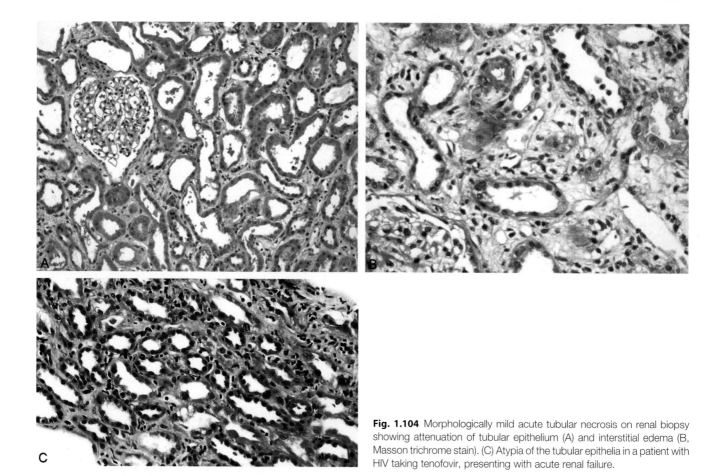

Fig. 1.104 Morphologically mild acute tubular necrosis on renal biopsy showing attenuation of tubular epithelium (A) and interstitial edema (B, Masson trichrome stain). (C) Atypia of the tubular epithelia in a patient with HIV taking tenofovir, presenting with acute renal failure.

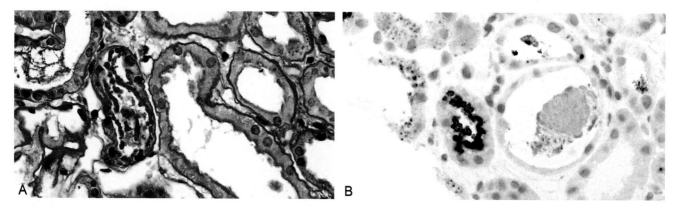

Fig. 1.105 (A) Tubular injury in a patient with rhabdomyolysis and acute renal failure. Note the granular debris in the tubular lumina (periodic acid–Schiff stain). (B) Myoglobin stain is positive in the granular debris.

a hypersensitivity or autoimmune reaction to a variety of stimuli (Table 1.33), and most are T-cell–mediated reactions.

The history and certain laboratory data are required to establish the cause because, except for identifying an infective agent or an antibody-mediated lesion, this condition has no morphologic features to discriminate among the various causative agents. Before the use of antibiotics, acute tubulointerstitial nephritis was usually caused by infections, most often scarlet fever or diphtheria. Today an allergic drug reaction is often the first consideration. The presence of a rash, fever, eosinophilia, or eosinophiluria can corroborate that impression, but often these features are absent. Almost any drug can cause an allergic reaction. Unfortunately the most common cause

of an allergic reaction is ingestion of some commonly prescribed drugs. Frequently the clinician will attribute the allergic reaction to the drug most recently taken. Proteinuria is usually less than 1 g/day, so the presence of significant proteinuria is very useful because it is commonly associated with nonsteroidal antiinflammatory drugs.

Patients often have enlarged, tender kidneys. Morphologically, one sees prominent interstitial expansion with tubular separation by edema and a mixed cell infiltrate consisting of lymphocytes, plasma cells, and monocytes (Fig. 1.106A). Smaller numbers of eosinophils may be present. However, eosinophils are particularly prominent in allergic conditions (Fig. 1.106B). The inflammatory process infiltrates tubule epithelium (tubulitis). The tubule cells may appear

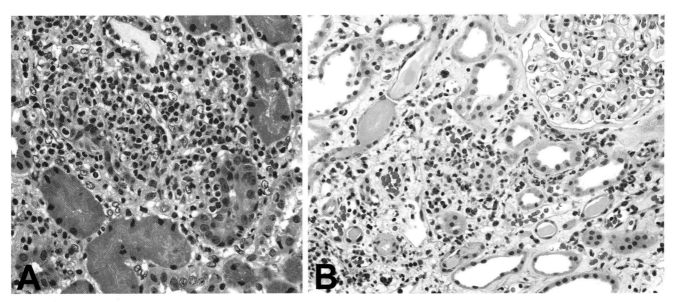

Fig. 1.106 (A) Acute tubulointerstitial nephritis is characterized by a mixed cell interstitial infiltrate with interstitial expansion by edema. Inflammatory cell infiltration of tubules, known as tubulitis, is present. (B) In allergic forms of acute interstitial nephritis secondary to drug reaction, eosinophils may be particularly numerous, as in this case.

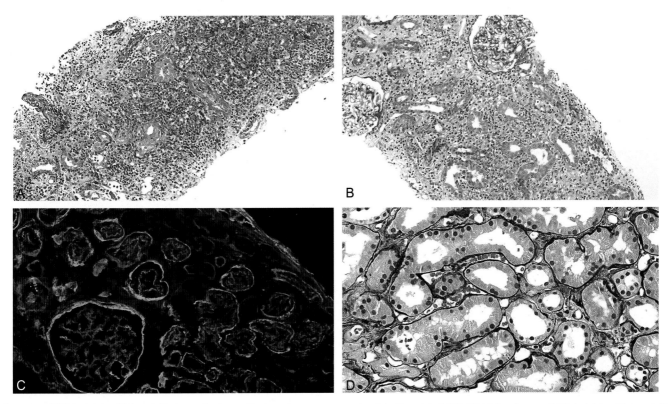

Fig. 1.107 (A) Tubulointerstitial nephritis in a patient recently placed on programmed cell death protein 1 (PD-1) inhibitor therapy. (B) Tubulointerstitial nephritis in a patient with uveitis, suggestive of tubulointerstitial nephritis with uveitis syndrome. (C) Positive immunoglobulin G (IgG) deposits along the tubular basement membranes in a patient with anti–brush border antibodies (IgG immunofluorescence). (D) Relatively thick basement membranes in anti-brush border antibody (same patient as in C) (silver stain).

reactive or may show individual cell necrosis. A mixed inflammatory infiltrate, almost resembling pyelonephritis, is often seen in tubulointerstitial nephritis due to programmed cell death protein 1 (PD-1) inhibitors (Fig. 1.107A). Clinical history of PD-1 inhibitor use is crucial.[354] A history of recent or concomitant uveitis is required in the diagnosis of tubulointerstitial nephritis with uveitis syndrome

(Fig. 1.107B).[351,355,356] In antibody-mediated cases immune complex deposits may be identified within tubular basement membranes or in peritubular capillaries, or a tubular basement membrane reaction can be demonstrated if antitubular basement membrane antibody is present (Fig. 1.107C and D).[357,358] Occasionally, necrotizing vasculitis or granulomas may also develop in allergic reactions.

Herbal Remedies, Slimming Agents and Aristocholic Acid Nephropathy

Many unregulated over-the-counter herbal remedies and slimming agents contain many plant-derived components and assorted chemical additives that may be nephrotoxic.[359-365] Of the many possible ingredients, aristocholic acid is known to be particularly nephrotoxic. However, other components alone or in combination may have similar renal consequences. Patients present with renal failure and low-grade proteinuria. The renal failure is often progressive, and end-stage renal disease may develop within weeks to months of ingestion (Fig. 1.108). Toxicity is usually proportional to the dosage and duration of ingestion.

Immunoglobulin G4–Related Sclerosing Tubulointerstitial Nephritis

Immunoglobulin G4 (IgG4)–related systemic disease is a multiorgan autoimmune disease first identified in the pancreas as autoimmune pancreatitis.[366-370] IgG4-related systemic disease is now known to affect many organs and body sites. Renal involvement may manifest as a discrete mass noted radiologically, or renal failure secondary to sclerosing tubulointerstitial disease. A biopsy will show a lymphoplasmacytic infiltrate associated with dense expansile fibrosis that may have a storiform quality (Fig. 1.109). The interstitium becomes effaced with relative glomerular preservation. The fibrosing process may abruptly transition into normal cortex. Eosinophils and phlebitis may be present. The infiltrate is enriched in IgG4-postive plasma cells, greater than 10 in a high-power field. Immunofluorescence shows tubular basement membrane and interstitial deposits of IgG, C3, κ, and λ. Occasionally, concomitant membranous glomerulonephritis is present, and the patient has heavy proteinuria. Patients often have laboratory abnormalities such as eosinophilia, low complement, and hypergammaglobulinemia with elevation of serum IgG4 levels. A combination of imaging, clinical and laboratory features, and histology is needed to make the diagnosis.

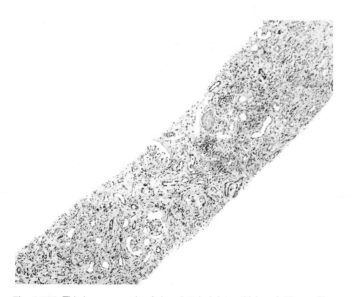

Fig. 1.108 This is an example of chronic tubulointerstitial nephritis, resulting from use of an herbal remedy. It shows glomerular preservation with diffuse tubular atrophy and dense interstitial fibrosis. Mild interstitial inflammation is present consisting chiefly of lymphoid cells.

Analgesic Nephropathy

Analgesic nephropathy is characterized by renal papillary necrosis and cortical chronic interstitial nephritis resulting from the prolonged use (10 to 20 years) of phenacetin-containing compound analgesic preparations.[291,294-297] This association was first recognized following a marked increase in chronic interstitial nephritis and renal papillary necrosis in several geographic regions in Scandinavia and Australia. Originally the chronic interstitial nephritis was recognized; however, Kincaid-Smith demonstrated that papillary necrosis was the primary injury and the cortical scarring was secondary.[291] Analgesic abuse has been implicated as the cause of 80% to 90% of renal papillary necrosis in nondiabetic Australians.[294] In addition to chronic renal disease approximately 34% of patients experienced coronary artery disease and other atherosclerotic complications.[319] Furthermore, 8% of patients experienced development of urothelial carcinoma.

Phenacetin and aspirin combined with caffeine or codeine were the original offending preparations. The substitution of acetaminophen for phenacetin, control over marketing practices, and increasing recognition of the risk factors have substantially lowered the prevalence of analgesic nephropathy. However, a similar chronic renal disease has now been identified by long-term misuse of nonsteroidal antiinflammatory drugs.

The renal lesions of analgesic abuse begin in the inner medulla and have been divided into three stages. The first stage is characterized by a yellowish radiating discoloration of the papillary tip. Microscopically, there is necrosis of the loops of Henle and interstitial cells with thickening and sclerosis of small vessels. In the second stage the process involves the entire inner medulla with widespread necrosis of collecting ducts, loops of Henle, and vasa recta. Interstitial calcification frequently is present.

During the third stage, cortical changes develop after necrosis of the renal pyramid. The cortex overlying the pyramid becomes thin and atrophic, histologically showing a nonspecific chronic interstitial nephritis with tubular atrophy, interstitial fibrosis, and a lymphoid infiltrate. The columns of Bertin may be spared, producing an alternating pattern of atrophy and thickening of the cortex. The necrotic papillae often have been described as darkly colored, and focally may detach and slough. In contrast with other forms of papillary necrosis a neutrophilic response is not evident. A distinctive capillary sclerosis affects the small vessels of the papillary tip and the small mucosal vessels of the renal pelvis, ureter, and bladder characterized by extensive reduplication of the basal lamina best demonstrated by PAS stain.

Bacterial Infection–Associated Tubulointerstitial Disease

Acute Pyelonephritis

Acute pyelonephritis is a bacterial infection of the kidney.[83,371-389] Patients present with fever, leukocytosis, and flank tenderness, and may suffer a variety of complications (Table 1.35). Pyuria and urinary white blood cell casts are usually present. The kidneys may be seeded by organisms via two major pathways: ascending infection and the hematogenous route.

The most common avenue of infection is ascent from a lower urinary tract infection. *E. coli* is the most frequent organism followed by other enteric organisms such as *Proteus*, *Klebsiella*, and *Enterobacter*. In most individuals with bacterial cystitis the infection remains localized to the bladder. In susceptible individuals, vesicoureteral reflux occurs, permitting colonization of the upper

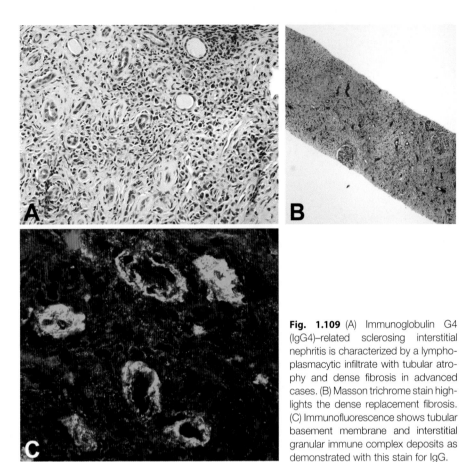

Fig. 1.109 (A) Immunoglobulin G4 (IgG4)–related sclerosing interstitial nephritis is characterized by a lympho-plasmacytic infiltrate with tubular atrophy and dense fibrosis in advanced cases. (B) Masson trichrome stain highlights the dense replacement fibrosis. (C) Immunofluorescence shows tubular basement membrane and interstitial granular immune complex deposits as demonstrated with this stain for IgG.

TABLE 1.35	Complications of Acute Pyelonephritis

Renal abscess
Pyonephrosis
Perinephric abscess
Emphysematous pyelonephritis
Sepsis

tracts.[83,379,380] This most often occurs in children with primary vesicoureteral reflux, a congenital, often hereditary, abnormality of the anatomy of the uretero–vesical junction. Reflux can also develop in nonrefluxing systems if the cystitis is severe or if there is distal obstruction or a neurogenic bladder.

Even with an upper urinary tract infection, parenchymal infection is not inevitable. The organisms must first gain access to the papillary collecting ducts, a process known as intrarenal reflux. The architecture of the renal pyramids influences their susceptibility to intrarenal reflux (see the Reflux Nephropathy [Chronic Nonobstructive Pyelonephritis] section later in this chapter). After initial infection of the pyramids the infection extends up the medullary rays before more generalized cortical spread.

Acute pyelonephritis in surgical and autopsy specimens represents the most severe examples. The collecting system is thickened, and yellow-white suppurative foci or overt abscesses are present in both pyramids and cortex (Fig. 1.110). When the infectious process is early, neutrophils can be seen within the collecting ducts of the cortex and medulla (Fig. 1.111). Bacteria may be present, but this is usually seen only at autopsy in which the postmortem period allows unchecked growth of organisms. Glomeruli may be spared initially, but with increasing severity, generalized parenchymal destruction occurs and may liquefy, resulting in abscess formation.

Hematogenous pyelonephritis usually complicates prolonged sepsis or infectious endocarditis. The kidneys are usually peppered with abscesses, which are more numerous in the cortex than in the medulla (Figs. 1.112 and 1.113). The organisms responsible are more often gram-positive bacteria or fungi.

Pyonephrosis

Pyonephrosis refers to the near-total destruction of an obstructed kidney by acute pyelonephritis. The parenchyma is replaced by suppurative inflammation that transforms the kidney into a large abscess. The patient is typically septic. Urine culture results may be negative because of the urinary tract obstruction.

Perinephric Abscess

A perinephric abscess is the accumulation of infectious material and neutrophils within perinephric fat (Fig. 1.114). It usually originates from rupture of a renal abscess or from pyonephrosis, but it can develop after a surgical procedure such as renal transplantation or surgical treatment of calculi.[385,386] Rarely, it may originate from an infected nidus extrinsic to the kidney, such as the gastrointestinal tract in diverticulitis and Crohn disease, or from bone in osteomyelitis. Either gram-negative or gram-positive organisms can be responsible.

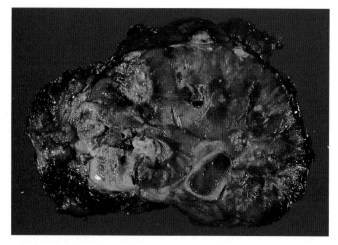

Fig. 1.110 This kidney is affected by ascending acute pyelonephritis complicated by abscess formation. The lower pole (*left*) is most severely involved.

Emphysematous Pyelonephritis

Emphysematous pyelonephritis is an uncommon but potentially life-threatening complication of acute suppurative bacterial (rarely fungal) infection of the kidney.[390-392] In emphysematous pyelonephritis, gas bubbles develop within the renal parenchyma and may extend into perinephric and even retroperitoneal sites. This disorder should be distinguished from emphysematous pyelitis and ureteritis, which are far less dangerous conditions. Approximately 90% of patients with this infection have diabetes mellitus, and urinary tract obstruction is present in approximately 40%. Women

outnumber men by a 2:1 ratio. *E. coli* is the responsible organism in 68% of cases and *Klebsiella* in 9% of cases, with a mixed infection in 19% of cases. No reported cases have been attributed to *Clostridium*.

The kidney of a patient with emphysematous pyelonephritis grossly shows widespread abscesses with papillary necrosis and cortical infarcts. It may have a cystic appearance resulting from gas bubbles. Microscopically, the characteristic feature consists of empty spaces lacking epithelial cell linings and distorting the parenchyma (Fig. 1.115). Adjacent areas show vascular thrombosis, ischemic necrosis, suppurative inflammation, and abscesses.

Chronic Pyelonephritis

Chronic pyelonephritis is a chronic destructive tubulointerstitial disease usually regarded as a sequel of recurrent or persistent episodes of bacterial infection of the kidney. It is responsible for 5% to 15% of cases of end-stage kidney disease. Usually it is subdivided into reflux nephropathy (or chronic nonobstructive pyelonephritis) and obstructive pyelonephritis.

Reflux Nephropathy (Chronic Nonobstructive Pyelonephritis)
In 1960, Hodson and Edwards established a link between nonobstructive chronic pyelonephritis and vesicoureteral reflux.[389] Appreciation of the nearly ubiquitous association between nonobstructive forms of chronic pyelonephritis and vesicoureteral reflux led Bailey, in 1973, to coin the term *reflux nephropathy*.[393-395] Reflux nephropathy appears to be responsible for the majority of pyelonephritic scars.

Vesicoureteral reflux is a congenital disorder in which urine regurgitates from the bladder into a ureter because of inadequate development of its musculature or because the submucosal portion of the ureter is too short. Often it is a familial disorder and usually is

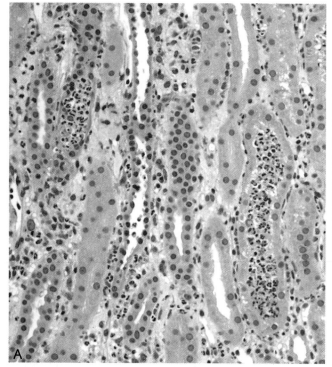

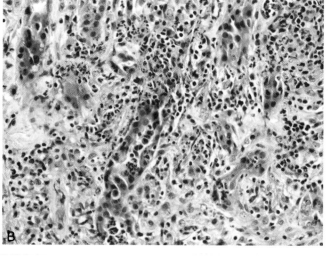

Fig. 1.111 (A) At autopsy, this kidney shows the early phase of ascending acute pyelonephritis. There are numerous neutrophils within the outer medullary collecting ducts. These would have been destined to form urinary white blood cell casts had the patient survived. (B) This shows cortical involvement. Although most neutrophils remain within tubules that will soon be destroyed, interstitial neutrophils are also present.

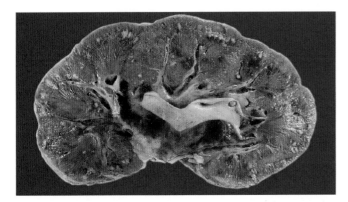

Fig. 1.112 At autopsy, this kidney shows hematogenous pyelonephritis. Notice the miliary pattern of microabscesses. The patient died of sepsis.

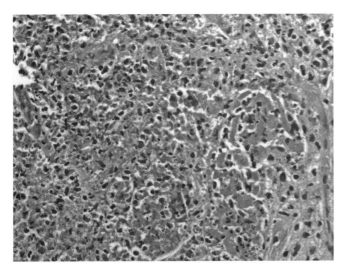

Fig. 1.113 In hematogenous pyelonephritis, multiple discontinuous rounded microabscesses develop. This shows a cortical microabscess with central liquefactive necrosis and acute inflammation.

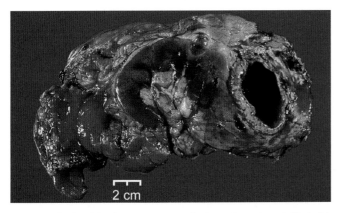

Fig. 1.114 Perinephric abscess can complicate acute pyelonephritis. In this case the intrarenal infection appears to have cleared. However, a perinephric abscess formed that resulted in nephrectomy.

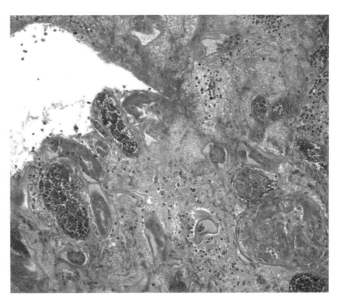

Fig. 1.115 Emphysematous pyelonephritis is a devastating complication of acute pyelonephritis. This kidney shows diffuse coagulation necrosis. Bacterial colonies are present (*blue*). The large clear space represents a gas bubble.

infection. Scars are usually noted only in patients with the most severe degrees of reflux.

Not all patients with urinary tract infections and vesicoureteral reflux experience development of reflux nephropathy. This observation was explained by Ransley and Risdon, who identified two types of renal pyramids, simple and compound (Fig. 1.116).[379] In simple pyramids, Bellini ducts open through a convex papilla at an oblique angle and close with an increase in intrapelvic pressure. However, compound pyramids that drain multiple lobes have concave surfaces and the orifices of Bellini ducts fail to close, resulting in intrarenal reflux. Reflux nephropathy is believed to represent the combined effect of recurrent or persistent vesicoureteral reflux and intrarenal reflux, which permits infection within the urinary tract to gain access to the renal parenchyma. It also is possible that high pressures in the absence of infection may result in similar segmental scarring. Compound papillae are usually located in the polar regions of the kidney, the location of most scars in reflux nephropathy.

The kidneys are small and irregularly contracted, usually weighing from 30 to 50 g. Their capsular surfaces show broad depressed scars, typically in polar regions. On cut surface, scalloping and loss of the renal pyramids beneath the cortical scars result in dilated calyces (Fig. 1.117). The cortex adjacent to the scars may be unaffected or hypertrophic. The pelvicaliceal system and ureter usually are dilated and their walls thickened.

Microscopically, the cortical scars show chronic tubulointerstitial nephritis with a lymphoid interstitial infiltrate (Fig. 1.118). There is extensive tubular atrophy, and tubules frequently contain eosinophilic casts (thyroidization). Periglomerular fibrosis and global glomerular sclerosis also are typical. The vessels show striking intimal sclerosis, a finding not present in the adjacent cortex. The uninvolved cortex may appear essentially normal or show compensatory hypertrophy of nephrons. The collecting system shows chronic pyelitis and ureteritis with lymphoid aggregates or germinal centers in the mucosa.

Some patients experience hypertension, proteinuria, and progressive renal failure. Proteinuria (often in the nephrotic range)

detected after a urinary tract infection at an early age. Although reflux tends to decrease in frequency with increasing age as the submucosal ureteral segment matures or lengthens, the renal scars are already present, possibly developing at the time of the first

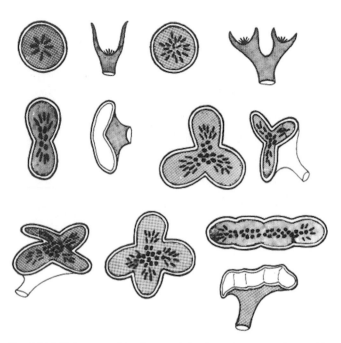

Fig. 1.116 Various possible shapes of simple and compound pyramids. (From Hodson CJ. Reflux nephropathy: a personal historical review. AJR Am J Roentgenol 1981;137:456; with permission).

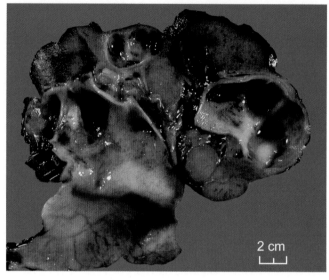

Fig. 1.117 This kidney was damaged by reflux nephropathy. It shows dilated calyces with overlying thin cortices separated by intact lobes of cortex.

is an important finding because it identifies patients at risk for renal failure. The glomerular lesion of focal segmental glomerulosclerosis is responsible for the proteinuria. Unfortunately, correction of the reflux or prevention of recurrent infection does not prevent progression of the glomerular lesion.

Chronic Obstructive Pyelonephritis

In chronic obstructive pyelonephritis, the kidney is damaged by a combination of pressure-related atrophy and bacterial infection. In advanced cases the kidney is hydronephrotic with diffuse calyceal dilation, blunting or effacement of papillae, and cortical thinning. This uniform alteration contrasts with the irregular pattern of

scarring characteristic of reflux nephropathy (Fig. 1.119). Microscopically, the picture is that of diffuse chronic interstitial nephritis with tubular atrophy, interstitial fibrosis, and glomerular sclerosis (Figs. 1.120 and 1.121). Sections including renal pyramids may show mild blunting of papillary tips in mild cases or complete effacement of pyramids in advanced cases.

Viral Infections

Viruses can produce a variety of renal diseases including acute tubulointerstitial nephritis, glomerulonephritis (most common), and arteritis (Table 1.36).[396-414] Direct infection of the kidney with diagnostic findings occurs with cytomegalovirus, adenovirus, and polyomavirus infections. These infections cause typical acute interstitial nephritis in which viral inclusions are visible within the

Fig. 1.118 Reflux nephropathy shows an abrupt delineation of the scarred cortex (*right side*) secondary to reflux, from the normal cortex (*left side*) supplied by a nonrefluxing pyramid (periodic acid–Schiff stain).

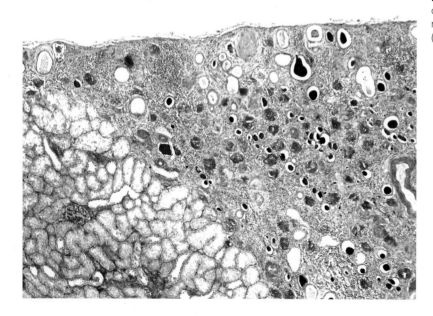

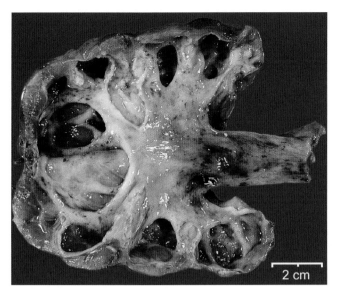

Fig. 1.119 This kidney was damaged by chronic obstruction. It shows diffuse cortical attenuation, effacement of all pyramids, and a dilated collecting system and ureter.

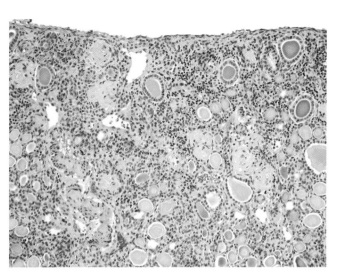

Fig. 1.121 This case of chronic pyelonephritis shows diffuse tubular atrophy and interstitial fibrosis with a modest bland lymphoid infiltrate and thyroidization of the tubules.

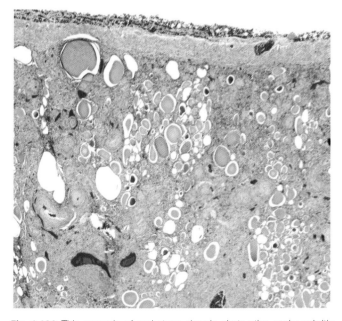

Fig. 1.120 This example of end-stage chronic obstructive pyelonephritis shows thyroidization of tubules, glomerulosclerosis, and secondary occlusive vascular changes.

TABLE 1.36 Viral Renal Diseases

Acute tubulointerstitial nephritis

Cytomegalovirus
Adenovirus
HIV
BK polyomavirus
Hantavirus

Glomerulonephritis

Hepatitis B
Hepatitis C
HIV
Parvovirus B-19
Rare others
   Mumps
   Varicella
   Echovirus
   Cytomegalovirus

Arteritis

Hepatitis B

HIV, Human immunodeficiency virus.

kidney. Polyomavirus and cytomegalovirus produce characteristic large intranuclear inclusions (Figs. 1.122 and 1.123). Adenovirus infection often also results in microabscess formation, as well as smudgy-appearing intranuclear inclusions within tubular cells (Fig. 1.124). Immunostains for adenovirus, polyomavirus, and cytomegalovirus are useful in diagnosis (Figs. 1.122 through Fig. 1.124).

Viral inclusions are not visible in the other viral renal diseases listed in Table 1.36. Many viruses can cause one of several forms of immune complex disease–associated glomerulonephritis. Human immunodeficiency virus (HIV) causes a complex renal disease known as HIV nephropathy. This is characterized by a triad of interstitial nephritis with large tubular casts, glomerulonephritis resulting from a collapsing form of focal-segmental glomerulosclerosis, and numerous endothelial reticulotubular inclusions (Fig. 1.125). Hepatitis C usually associated with cryoglobulins can produce necrotizing arteriolitis or arteritis and proliferative glomerulonephritis with membranoproliferative features. Fibrillary glomerulopathy also appears to be associated with hepatitis C infection (Fig. 1.126).[415-417] Hantavirus (nephropathia epidemica, hemorrhagic fever with renal syndrome) can produce an uncommon rodent-derived, acute, self-limited influenza-like illness with acute tubulointerstitial nephritis.

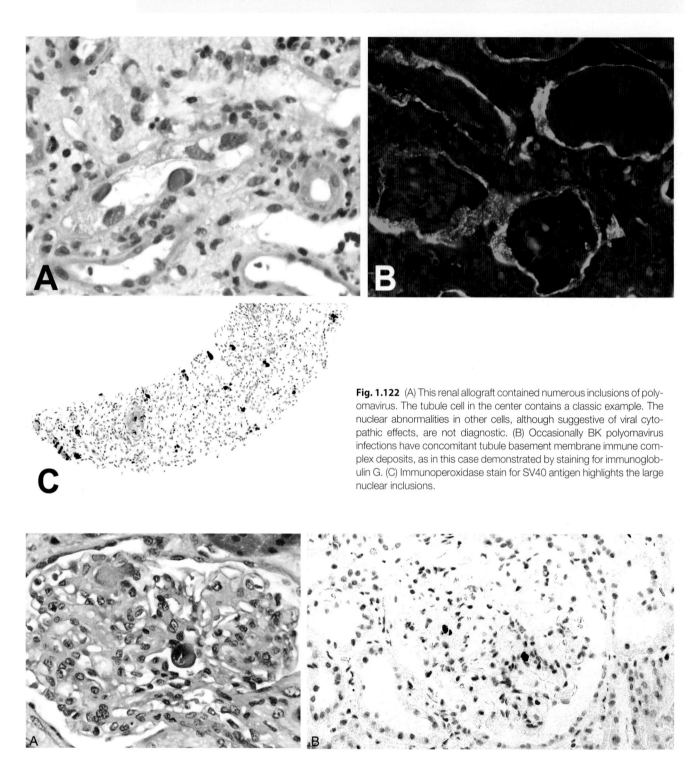

Fig. 1.122 (A) This renal allograft contained numerous inclusions of polyomavirus. The tubule cell in the center contains a classic example. The nuclear abnormalities in other cells, although suggestive of viral cytopathic effects, are not diagnostic. (B) Occasionally BK polyomavirus infections have concomitant tubule basement membrane immune complex deposits, as in this case demonstrated by staining for immunoglobulin G. (C) Immunoperoxidase stain for SV40 antigen highlights the large nuclear inclusions.

Fig. 1.123 (A) Cytomegalovirus can infect tubule cells, endothelial cells, and podocytes. This case contains two infected podocytes. The podocyte in the center has classic intranuclear and cytoplasmic inclusions. (B) Immunostain for cytomegalovirus highlights the inclusions.

Granulomatous Tubulointerstitial Disease

Sarcoidosis

Sarcoidosis is a chronic disease of unknown cause in which multiple organ systems are affected, usually by noncaseating granulomas. Symptomatic renal disease occurs in less than 10% of patients with sarcoidosis.[418-425] The most frequent renal abnormalities result from hypercalcemia, which causes a reduction in glomerular filtration rate, a decrease in concentrating ability, renal tubular acidosis, nephrocalcinosis, or the formation of calcium stones. In addition, granulomatous acute tubulointerstitial nephritis (Fig. 1.127) or chronic tubulointerstitial nephritis may develop.

Xanthogranulomatous Pyelonephritis

Certain granulomatous diseases may affect the kidney and urinary tract (Table 1.37).[418-421,426-431] Most are the result of infections. Xanthogranulomatous pyelonephritis is the inflammatory sequel of chronic suppurative renal infections and usually develops in an

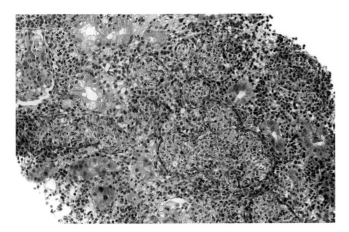

Fig. 1.124 Adenovirus infection shows marked tubulointerstitial nephritis with occasional lymphoepithelial-type lesions.

obstructed kidney in which portions of the renal parenchyma are transformed into a xanthomatous and suppurative inflammatory mass.[418-420,432,433] Although various theories of pathogenesis have been proposed, such as metabolic abnormalities, aberrant immune responses, lower virulence organisms, or ineffective antimicrobial therapy, the most plausible and simplest mechanism is renal outflow obstruction in the presence of a pyogenic infection. This view accommodates the major clinical and pathologic features encountered in most patients. The principal importance of xanthogranulomatous pyelonephritis relates to the difficulty in preoperative diagnosis and its ability clinically, radiographically, and grossly to mimic the destructive growth of a renal neoplasm.

Xanthogranulomatous pyelonephritis begins with suppurative inflammation and edema within the pelvic lamina propria and adjacent sinus fat that result in pelvicaliceal ulceration and fat necrosis. The inflammatory process extends into the medulla, also resulting in necrosis. The cortex, perinephric fat, and even retroperitoneal tissue may eventually be involved. The gross extent of the process has been classified into three "stages": in stage I (nephric stage) the process is confined within the renal capsule, in stage II (perinephric stage) the perinephric fat is involved, and in stage III (paranephric stage) there is extension outside Gerota capsule.

Xanthogranulomatous pyelonephritis may involve all or only portions of the renal parenchyma, thus creating three general patterns: diffuse, segmental, and focal. The diffuse form is most common (Fig. 1.128). It arises in a completely obstructed kidney,

usually because of calculi, often of staghorn form (Fig. 1.129). The kidney is nonfunctional, and nephrectomy is the treatment of choice. Preoperative diagnosis is most accurate in this form. The segmental and focal forms are more difficult to diagnose preoperatively and are more likely to be mistaken for neoplasms. They show the same microscopic features as diffuse xanthogranulomatous pyelonephritis but differ anatomically. Segmental xanthogranulomatous pyelonephritis is polar and is more common in children. The focal (or tumefactive) form is a cortical variant that lacks communication with the pelvis and is not associated with pyelitis or urinary tract obstruction. These two forms are amenable to partial nephrectomy.

The collecting system is thickened by the xanthomatous process, which can involve one or more renal pyramids and extend into the cortex (Fig. 1.128). The xanthogranulomatous nodules show a zonal pattern. A central nidus of necrotic debris and neutrophils is surrounded by the zone of foamy macrophages (Fig. 1.130). The most peripheral tissue shows a fibroblastic response as the host attempts to confine or organize the inflammatory process.

The presence of the xanthogranulomatous mass, coupled with its histologic cellularity, can elicit concern regarding a neoplasm, particularly if a biopsy or frozen section is examined. The foam cells can resemble clear cell renal carcinoma, whereas the fibroblastic response can resemble a spindle cell neoplasm. The bubbly microvesicular fat of the foam cells contrasts with the cleared-out cytoplasm, characteristic of renal carcinoma. Additional features include a lack of cohesive growth on touch preparations and the absence of cytologic atypia or mitoses. Immunohistochemical markers are useful to support the diagnosis: xanthogranulomatous pyelonephritis showing abundance of macrophages (CD68+, CD163+, and cytokeratin-negative), but neoplasms showing staining for epithelial markers (cytokeratin, epithelial membrane antigen [EMA], etc.).

Malakoplakia

Malakoplakia is an uncommon chronic granulomatous disease most frequently observed in the urinary tracts of middle-aged women as a complication of recurrent infections.[426,427,433,434] Bladder involvement is 4 to 10 times as common as upper urinary tract involvement, and renal involvement is rare. Diverse extraurinary tract sites also are rarely affected, a situation often associated with concomitant malignancy. Like nephrogenic adenoma, immunosuppressed patients have been reported to be at greatest risk for development of urinary tract malakoplakia.

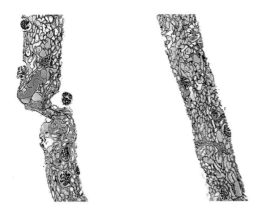
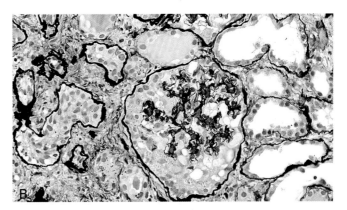

Fig. 1.125 (A) Human immunodeficiency virus (HIV)–associated nephropathy can have a classic triad of collapsing glomerulopathy, tubulointerstitial inflammation, and microcystic tubular dilatation. However, in patients with African American ancestry, these features may also be attributed to inheritance of Apo-L1 risk mutations. (B) Collapsing glomerulopathy in a patient with HIV (silver stain).

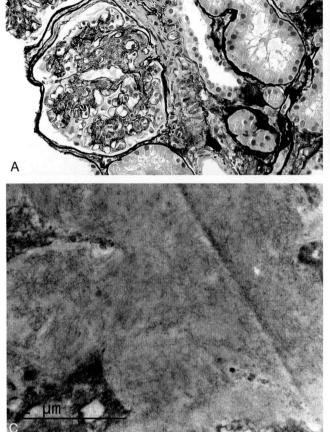

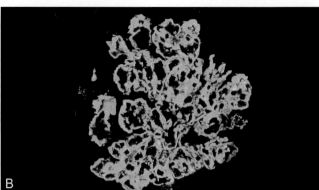

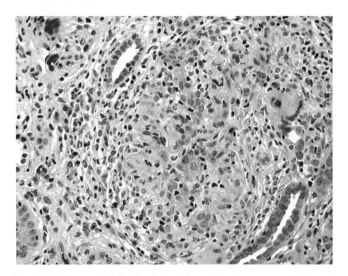

Fig. 1.126 (A) Fibrillary glomerulopathy in a patient with hepatitis C infection. (B) Smudgy deposits of IgG are shown by immunofluorescence study along the glomerular basement membrane. (C) Electron microscopy confirms the fibrillar architecture of the deposits.

Fig. 1.127 The most distinctive, but not the most common, renal findings in sarcoidosis are small, noncaseating granulomas. Multinucleated giant cells may be present, and asteroid and Schaumann bodies are occasionally encountered.

TABLE 1.37	Granulomatous Diseases of the Kidney
Sarcoidosis	
Xanthogranulomatous pyelonephritis	
Malakoplakia	
Mycobacterial infection	
Fungal infection	
Parasitic infection	
Urate nephropathy	
Vasculitis	
Drug hypersensitivity	

bodies) (Fig. 1.131). PAS stain and special stains for calcium or iron enhance the target-like appearance of these cytoplasmic inclusions and indicate their mineralized nature. These inclusions have been shown by a variety of methods to represent incompletely digested bacilli.

Tuberculosis

Genitourinary TB is the second most common extrapulmonary site of infection, accounting for 30% to 40% cases of extrapulmonary TB, second only to lymph node involvement. Urogenital involvement is present in 2% to 20% of patients with pulmonary TB (2% to 10% in developed countries, and 15% to 20% in developing countries).[428,431,435-437] It is principally a disease of young to middle-aged patients, 75% of whom are younger than 50 years. Men are affected more than women (2:1). Most patients have

The typical mucosal lesion of malakoplakia is characterized by a yellow-brown, soft (*malakos*) plaque (*plakos*) that often has a central umbilication. The parenchymal lesions consist of similar soft, yellow-brown nodules. Microscopically, masses of large eosinophilic histiocytes (von Hansemann histiocytes) are present, many of which contain basophilic inclusions (Michaelis-Gutmann

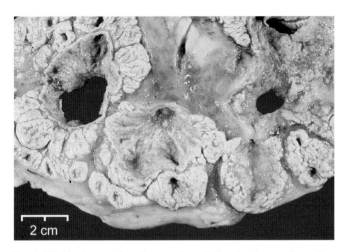

Fig. 1.128 Xanthogranulomatous pyelonephritis showing xanthomatous thickening of the collecting system. There are xanthomatous nodules centered on the pyramids that also involve the cortex.

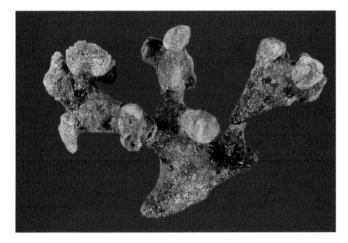

Fig. 1.129 Staghorn calculus from a patient with xanthogranulomatous pyelonephritis. It represents a calcified cast of the pelvis and calyces.

no radiographic or clinical evidence of pulmonary disease at the time the genitourinary tract involvement is identified. Symptoms arise usually when there is bladder impairment. Considering the higher prevalence of cystic kidney disease in TB-endemic areas, there appears to be a yet ambiguous association between TB and cystic kidney disease.[438,439]

In genitourinary TB, the renal parenchyma initially becomes infected by hematogenous dissemination resulting in bilateral development of small cortical neutrophilic microabscesses that gradually evolve into more typical granulomas and may caseate. Although progressive active disease may occur, in most patients the process is arrested. It may reactivate after a long latency period after a perturbation in the immune system. Renal involvement due to retrograde or ascending infection by TB after instillation of bacillus Calmette-Guérin for treatment of superficial bladder cancer or urothelial carcinoma in situ is rare.[435,440]

Medullary involvement results with reactivation. The organisms appear to favor the thin limbs of Henle, where they proliferate and cause destructive granulomatous lesions that caseate and cavitate (Fig. 1.132). Spread to the renal pelvis can produce a tuberculous pyelonephritis that can progress to a pyonephrosis-like lesion, also known as a "cement" or "putty" kidney.[435] Papillary necrosis follows, with seeding of the collecting system and lower urinary tract. Infection in these sites elicits granulomatous and fibrotic sequelae resulting in contraction of the collection system, ureter, and bladder. The patient thus presents with a concentrating defect, dysuria, and hematuria. Cavitary lesions, calyceal deformity, and ureteral strictures are demonstrable by various imaging studies.

Diverse Other Granulomatous Diseases

Granulomatous interstitial disease has been described in a variety of other clinical settings including drugs, infections, and hematologic disease.[429,430,441-446] Acute fungal tubulointerstitial nephritis is usually encountered in immunocompromised or diabetic patients. Antibiotic therapy and urinary tract instrumentation are other major risk factors. As with bacterial infections, the kidney may be seeded by either an ascending or a hematogenous route. *Candida* species and *Torulopsis* are the most common organisms. In patients with acquired immunodeficiency syndrome (AIDS), almost any fungus may be encountered (Fig. 1.133). The kidney

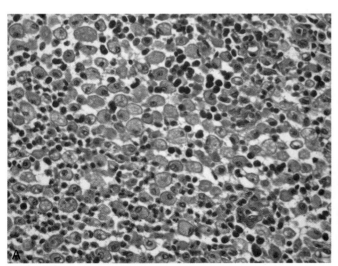
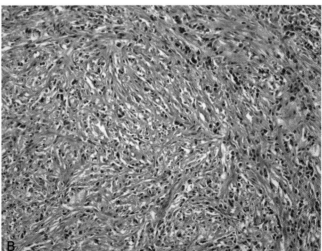

Fig. 1.130 (A) The center of a xanthogranulomatous nodule usually contains neutrophils and cell debris, and is surrounded by foamy macrophages. (B) The peripheral areas show fibrosis, chronic inflammation, and giant cells.

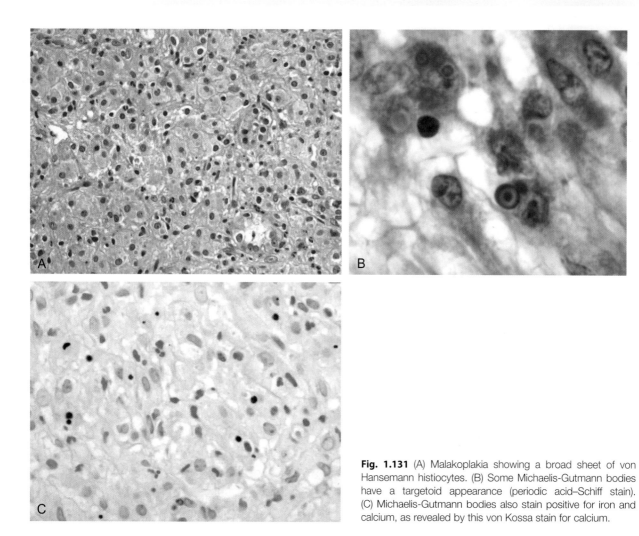

Fig. 1.131 (A) Malakoplakia showing a broad sheet of von Hansemann histiocytes. (B) Some Michaelis-Gutmann bodies have a targetoid appearance (periodic acid–Schiff stain). (C) Michaelis-Gutmann bodies also stain positive for iron and calcium, as revealed by this von Kossa stain for calcium.

Fig. 1.132 (A) This kidney is heavily replaced by caseating tuberculous granulomatous masses. This bears strong resemblance to xanthogranulomatous pyelonephritis. In contrast with xanthogranulomatous pyelonephritis, renal tuberculosis (TB) lower urinary tract involvement results in a contracted renal pelvis and ureter. (B) This is a caseating granuloma from a kidney involved by miliary TB.

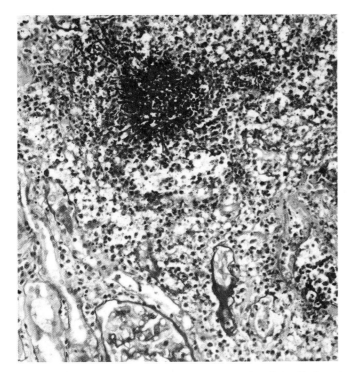

Fig. 1.133 This kidney from an immunosuppressed patient with fungal endocarditis contained numerous fungal microabscesses of hematogenous origin (periodic acid–Schiff stain).

shows a mixed neutrophilic and granulomatous response, and fungal elements are usually demonstrable.

Metabolic Abnormalities, Heavy Metals, and Crystal-Associated Tubulointerstitial Diseases

Heavy Metals

A variety of therapeutic agents and heavy metal exposures can cause the insidious development of chronic interstitial nephritis, and have been associated with increased prevalence of glomerular diseases such as membranous nephropathy.[447-455] The tubulointerstitial scarring is irreversible, but if the toxic injury is recognized early enough and the agent is eliminated, some improvement in renal function is possible. For most agents, no distinctive histologic features develop. In lead and cadmium toxicity, however, intranuclear inclusions in tubule cells may be present, and chronic lead toxicity often manifests with gout and hypertension. Papillary necrosis is the principal underlying lesion in analgesic nephropathy.

A variety of metabolic abnormalities may affect the kidney. The four most important involve calcium, uric acid, oxalate, and cystine. Each can exert its effect by parenchymal mineral deposition or by formation of calculi.

Hypercalcemic Nephropathy

Hypercalcemia can result from many systemic diseases (Table 1.38), and it has several renal consequences.[456-459] The most common renal effects are a decrease in glomerular filtration rate and a decrease in concentrating capacity, which may lead to polyuria and, when severe and prolonged, to volume depletion and acute renal failure.

TABLE 1.38 Major Causes of Hypercalcemia

Primary and secondary hyperparathyroidism
Vitamin D intoxication
Milk-alkali syndrome
Sarcoidosis
Malignant neoplasms
- Small cell carcinoma
- Multiple myeloma
Increased bone turnover
Idiopathic

Hypercalcemia also can have direct morphologic effects: nephrolithiasis, calcium phosphate crystal formation in tubules, and calcium deposition along cortical tubule basement membranes (Fig. 1.134). The pattern of deposition can sometimes be a clue to the type of salt deposited: globular or shell-like calcifications (phosphate type) in hyperphosphatemia and/or hyperphosphaturia, and clumpy or finely granular calcifications (calcium type) in hypercalcemia or hypercalciuria.[460]

Nephrolithiasis

Nephrolithiasis is the commonest urologic condition worldwide, with an estimated prevalence rate of 7.1% in women and 10.6% in men in the United States alone.[459,461-467] The lifetime risk for development of a systematic stone event has continued to increase over the last several decades.[468,469] It is not a single disease but rather a common end point with obstructive complications that may arise within the context of diverse abnormalities of metabolism or renal tubular cell function, or may result from urinary tract diseases such as obstruction or bacterial infections. Nephrolithiasis is a dynamic process. In its early stages, medical therapy can potentially control or prevent its complications by modifying factors that permit crystallization. There are several types of stones, which may be pure or heterogeneous in composition (Table 1.39). Each has multiple causative agents and clinical associations.

Calcium-containing stones are the most common variety and can have a variable composition such as calcium oxalate or calcium

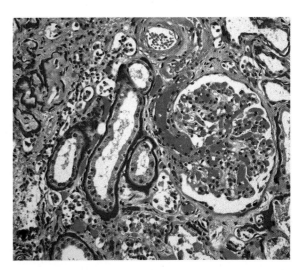

Fig. 1.134 Nephrocalcinosis showing tubule basement membranes encrusted with calcium.

TABLE 1.39	Types of Renal Stones
Calcium phosphate	
Calcium oxalate	
Struvite	
Uric acid	
Cystine	
Matrix stone	

phosphate (hydroxyapatite, carbonate apatite, or brushite). Most patients with calcium oxalate–containing stones do not have an abnormality of oxalate metabolism. Hypercalcuria is the most common underlying metabolic abnormality, encountered in 60% of patients.

Struvite stones (infection or triple-phosphate stones) are a combination of struvite ($MgNH_4PO_4$-$6H_2O$) and carbonate-apatite ($Ca_{10}[PO_4]_6$-CO_3). These form usually in the presence of urea-splitting organisms such as *Proteus*, *Staphylococcus albus*, *Pseudomonas*, and *Klebsiella*; however, recent studies also show significant colonization by nonurea splitting organisms.[470,471] Struvite stones can form very rapidly and cause most staghorn calculi (Fig. 1.129).

Not all stones are heavily mineralized. Matrix stones are composed principally of a glycoprotein matrix with focal calcification.[466,472] Matrix stones form large casts of the collecting system and have a soft yellow to tan gross appearance and a laminated structure histologically. They are often associated with urinary tract infection.

Because nephrolithiasis can result from urinary tract obstruction or cause urinary tract obstruction, affected kidneys may show diverse changes such as hydronephrosis, acute or chronic pyelonephritis, or xanthogranulomatous pyelonephritis. Many also contain small calcified plaques along the papillary tips known as Randall plaques. In the 1950s Randall noted that 20% of patients with stones had 2- to 4-mm submucosal calcified plaques, which he believed represented precursor lesions in stone formation.[462,467] These plaques are derived from interstitial and tubular basement membrane calcification (Fig. 1.135), which in certain patients becomes a nucleation site for stone formation.

Oxalate-Associated Renal Disease

Oxalic acid is the simplest dicarboxylic acid found in nature.[473] It is a major constituent of many plants and a metabolic by-product of endogenous and exogenous compounds. The kidneys may be confronted with an excessive oxalate load in several situations (Table 1.40), and this results in oxalosis and calcium oxalate calculi.[463,473-486] However, most patients with calcium oxalate stones have none of these disorders but rather have abnormalities in calcium metabolism.

Primary hyperoxaluria types I and II are autosomal recessive inborn errors in metabolism that result in excessive production of oxalate.[473,474,480,487-489] Calcium oxalate deposits form in vessels in several extrarenal tissues such as the heart, brain, eye, and bone marrow. Renal tubular oxalosis and calcium oxalate calculi form and result in renal failure at an early age.

Secondary hyperoxaluria and renal oxalosis may result from ethylene glycol (automobile antifreeze) ingestion or from methoxyflurane anesthesia, and may cause acute renal failure with renal tubular oxalosis. In ethylene glycol intoxication, glycol is

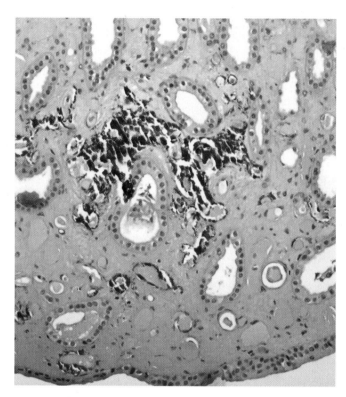

Fig. 1.135 Randall plaque in a papillary tip from a patient with nephrolithiasis. Calcification of thin loops of Henle has extended into the interstitium.

TABLE 1.40	Causes of Hyperoxaluria
Primary hyperoxaluria, types I and II	
Secondary hyperoxaluria	
Ethylene glycol ingestion	
Methoxyflurane anesthesia	
Gastrointestinal disease	
Pancreatobiliary disease	
Chronic renal failure	
Idiopathic conditions	
Small-intestinal and/or gastric bypass	
Oxalate-rich foods	
Vitamin C intoxication	

metabolized to oxalate, which precipitates in the distal tubules and causes obstruction (Fig. 1.136A). Glycol also has a direct toxic effect on tubular epithelium that contributes to the renal injury. The free fluoride in methoxyflurane appears to stimulate excessive oxalate production by the liver and causes a heavy acute oxalate load to the kidney. In renal tubular oxalosis, calcium oxalate crystals are found within both renal tubule lumina and tubule epithelial cells. The crystals are strongly birefringent under polarized light (Fig. 1.136B).

Secondary hyperoxaluria of a more chronic form, leading to stone formation, occurs in patients with small-bowel or pancreatobiliary tract disease (enteric oxalosis), and may be a complication of ingestion of oxalate-rich foods such as star fruit, citrus fruits, grape, rhubarb, among others. Unabsorbed lipids bind intraintestinal calcium and leave insufficient calcium to precipitate the oxalate

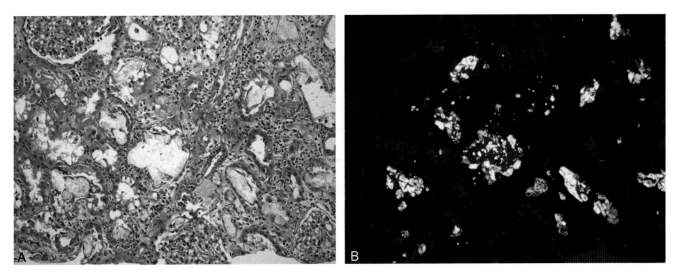

Fig. 1.136 (A) This kidney from a patient with acute renal failure secondary to ethylene glycol ingestion shows extensive calcium oxalate deposition. (B) Calcium oxalate crystals show strong birefringence under polarized light.

within the gut, thus leading to increased oxalate absorption. Finally, it also is common to encounter scattered calcium oxalate crystals within renal tubules at autopsy in patients with chronic renal failure and in the absence of overt renal disease.

Cystinosis

Cystinosis is an autosomal recessive storage disease characterized by impaired transport of the amino acid cystine across lysosomal membranes. The result is the excessive accumulation of cystine in several organs, including the kidney.[490-496] Three forms are recognized: an infantile nephropathic form, an adolescent form, and an adult form. In the infantile nephropathic form, initial tubular dysfunction characterized by Fanconi syndrome progresses to uremia and death by 9 to 10 years of age if untreated. This condition is accompanied by growth retardation, photophobia, and hypothyroidism. Its progress can be arrested by treatment with cysteamine,

which reduces intracellular cystine levels. The adolescent form is rare and slowly progressive, whereas the adult form causes only ocular disease.

In the early phase of nephropathic cystinosis, the kidneys may have enlarged multinucleated podocytes (referred to as polykaryocytosis), and cystine crystals may be visible in macrophages within glomeruli or in interstitial areas. With progression of the disease, chronic tubulointerstitial nephritis develops with tubulointerstitial scarring and clusters of crystal-containing macrophages in the interstitium (Fig. 1.137). Because cystine crystals are birefringent and soluble in water, alcohol fixation and polarization provide optimum demonstration and retention of the crystals.

Uric Acid–Associated Renal Disease

Uric acid is the final degradation product of purine metabolism in humans. It is poorly soluble in plasma. When uric acid causes

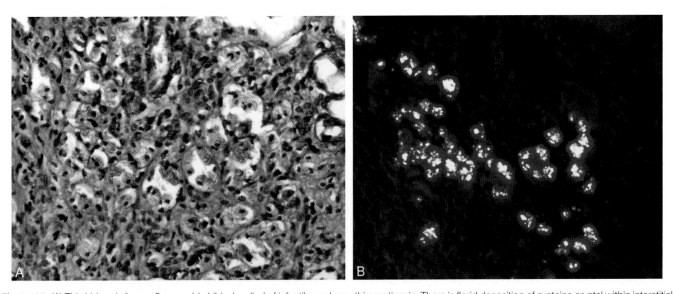

Fig. 1.137 (A) This kidney is from a 6-year-old child who died of infantile nephropathic cystinosis. There is florid deposition of cysteine crystal within interstitial cells. (B) Cystine crystals show strong birefringence under polarization microscopy.

TABLE 1.41	Causes of Hyperuricemia and Gout

Lymphoproliferative disorders
Myeloproliferative disorders
Lead (saturnine gout)
Diuretics
Alcohol
Aspirin
Endocrine dysfunctions
Starvation
Hypoxanthine-guanine phosphoribosyltransferase deficiency
Phosphoribosylpyrophosphate synthetase increased activity

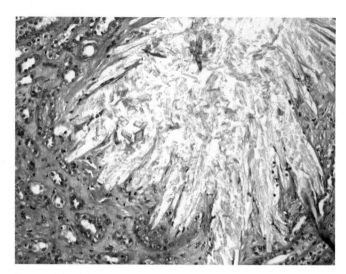

Fig. 1.138 Medullary urate granuloma.

symptoms and is deposited in tissues, the condition is known as gout. Outside the joints, the kidney is the major site of clinically significant disease caused by hyperuricemia. There are multiple causes of uric acid elevation (Table 1.41). The association between serum uric acid levels and chronic renal disease remains controversial, but three forms of the disease—acute uric acid nephropathy, uric acid lithiasis, and chronic gouty nephropathy—are thought to directly contribute to renal dysfunction.[497-501]

In acute uric acid nephropathy, acute renal failure results from intratubular uric acid crystals. It develops as a complication of rapid tumor lysis in lymphoproliferative and myeloproliferative disorders after initiation of chemotherapy. The acidity and concentration in the collecting ducts favor uric acid crystal formation. The renal medulla, particularly the papilla, may have grossly visible yellow streaks. Uric acid crystals are very soluble in water and birefringent. Therefore the histologic demonstration of uric acid crystals requires tissue fixed in absolute alcohol (or the use of touch smears or frozen sections) and viewing under polarized light. Crystals may also form within the collecting system and be detectable in the urine. Hydration, alkalization of urine, and pretreatment with allopurinol have greatly reduced the incidence of crystal formation.

Uric acid stones, which may be composed of pure uric acid, are radiolucent or mixed with calcium oxalate and radiopaque. Uric acid stones develop in 20% of patients with gout. Stones become more prevalent with increased amounts of uric acid excreted. Stone formation can be inhibited by alkalization of the urine and hydration.

Chronic gouty nephropathy develops in patients with sustained hyperuricemia. It is characterized by the interstitial deposition of sodium urate. Urate elicits a mononuclear cell reaction and a giant cell reaction resulting in microtophus formation (Fig. 1.138). These lesions develop mainly within the outer medulla. Small urate granulomas can also be seen in azotemia of other causes and occasionally in otherwise normal kidneys. In patients with renal failure attributed to chronic gout the cortex shows changes of hypertension-associated arterial nephrosclerosis and chronic interstitial nephritis. Tophi usually are not identified.

It was previously believed that primary gout caused renal failure in a substantial number of patients with gout. This concept has been challenged because the gout in many of the patients in older reports was probably secondary, and the renal disease was caused by lead toxicity and underlying diabetes and hypertension. It is now known that chronic lead nephropathy causes clinical gout and hypertension, and produces the same histologic findings previously regarded as typical of chronic gouty nephropathy.

Diabetic Kidney Disease

Diabetes mellitus (both types I and II) remains the major cause of end-stage renal disease. With the increasing prevalence of the metabolic syndrome pandemic worldwide, it is predicted that more than 400 million people will be affected by 2030.[502-509] Although the effects of diabetes are more easily identified in the glomeruli, diabetes affects virtually all compartments of the kidney, including the vasculature and tubulointerstitium. In most patients, renal disease manifests after 10 to 15 years in patients with type 1 diabetes and 5 to 10 years in patients with type 2 diabetes. Prevalence of nephropathy is highest among Native Americans, followed by African Americans, Hispanics, and Caucasians. In contrast, Asians and Hispanics tend to have a higher risk for end-stage renal disease from diabetes compared with other ethnic groups.

In type 1 diabetes, autoimmune destruction of the islets cells due to failure of self-tolerance in T cells leads to insulin deficiency. Either an HLA-DR3 or HLA-DR4 haplotype is present in 90% to 95% of Caucasians with type 1 diabetes. The pathogenesis of type 2 diabetes is multifactorial, with several susceptibility loci identified by genome-wide association studies. Of these, transcription factor 7–like-2 on chromosome 10q shows the strongest association. There is both decreased insulin secretion by beta cells and decreased response of peripheral tissues to insulin. In both types, insulin deficiency and hyperglycemia are the major driving force for the biochemical changes in basement membranes and resultant morphologic alterations.

The morphologic changes in both type 1 and type 2 diabetes are similar. The size of the kidneys depends on duration of disease. In early stages, kidneys are often bilaterally enlarged because of hyperfiltration.[510] However, as disease progresses, there is progressive shrinkage due to atrophy and fibrosis. Consequently end-stage kidneys may be normal or even slightly small in advanced-stage diabetic nephropathy.

In the early stages of diabetes, increased glomerular filtration rate and increased capillary pressure lead to glomerular hypertrophy and increased glomerular filtration area.[511-513] There is diffuse thickening of the glomerular and to a lesser degree of tubular basement membranes due to a combination of factors including cross-linking by advanced glycation end products, increased protein deposition, decreased protein degradation, and trapping of plasma

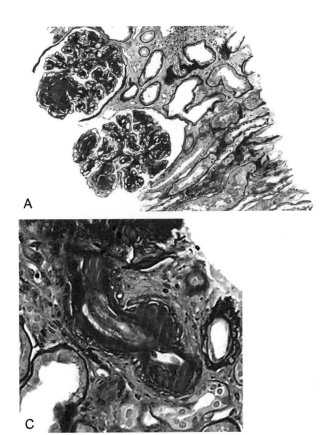

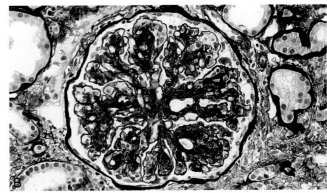

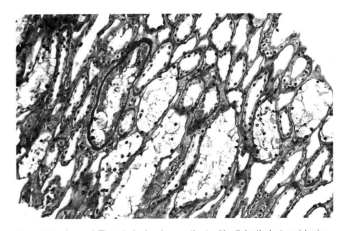

Fig. 1.139 (A) Diabetic nodular glomerulosclerosis showing a Kimmelstiel-Wilson nodule. (B) Thick glomerular and tubular basement membranes in diabetes. (C) Afferent and efferent arteriolar hyalinosis in diabetic nephropathy.

Fig. 1.140 Armani-Ebstein lesion in a patient with diabetic ketoacidosis.

proteins.[514,515] Thickening of the glomerular basement membrane can be seen as early as 2 years after onset of type 1 diabetes. There is concurrent increased deposition of matrix proteins in the mesangium leading to mesangial widening. In approximately 15% to 30% of individuals with long-term diabetes, round to oval lesions form in the mesangial core. These mesangial nodules are typically acellular or paucicellular, although in early stages hypercellularity and mesangiolysis may be noted (Fig. 1.139). They gradually enlarge with progression of disease. Named after Paul Kimmelstiel and Clifford Wilson, who first described these in an autopsy series, these so-called Kimmelstiel-Wilson nodules differ from segmental glomerulosclerosis in that they are often surrounded by patent or aneurysmally dilated capillary lumina.[516] The nodules in diabetes are PAS-positive, argyrophilic on a silver stain, Congo red–negative and blue on trichrome (Fig. 1.139). Interestingly many murine models of diabetes do not show the nodular glomerulosclerosis that is typically seen in human diabetes. There is also extensive deposition of PAS-positive hyaline material in the glomerular capillary loops, Bowman capsule, and both afferent and efferent arterioles (Fig. 1.139). Efferent arteriolar hyalinosis is a typical feature in diabetes. Progressive disease with sclerosis and hyaline deposition ultimately results in obliteration of the capillary lumina, segmental adhesions, ischemia, global glomerulosclerosis, tubular atrophy, and interstitial fibrosis.

In addition to thickening of the tubular basement membranes, protein resorption and lipid droplets are often noted in the tubules. An interesting lesion can be seen in patients who have, or have succumbed to, diabetic ketoacidosis. This so-called Armanni-Ebstein lesion consists of abundant clear vacuoles in a subnuclear location in proximal tubules (Fig. 1.140). Diffuse thickening of the tubular basement membranes is also often prominent in diabetes, and can be seen in both the atrophic and the nonatrophic tubules. A prominent lymphoplasmacytic infiltrate with abundant eosinophils, resembling tubulointerstitial nephritis, is often seen in the atrophic and fibrotic areas in diabetes (Fig. 1.140). Recognizing inflammation due to diabetes from tubulointerstitial inflammation due to other causes is clinically significant. Clinical history, location of the inflammation, and other pertinent features of diabetes are helpful in making this distinction.

Amyloidosis and Paraprotein-Associated Tubulointerstitial Disease

Patients with chronic infections, multiple myeloma, lymphoma, or leukemia frequently develop renal disease either from a direct effect of the neoplasm or mediators of inflammation, or from a therapeutic complication. Either glomerular or tubulointerstitial lesions may develop and result in proteinuria and renal insufficiency (Table 1.42).[517-529]

Amyloidosis

Amyloidosis is a group of protein folding disorders that have in common the tissue deposition of thin (8 to 11 nm) fibrils rich in β-pleated sheet structure as demonstrated by x-ray diffraction. This structure resists proteolysis and leads to perpetuation of the fibrils in tissue. Deposition usually occurs in multiple organs, in diverse combinations, although localized deposits (amyloidomas) or organ-isolated forms also occur. Organ-isolated forms may evolve into a systemic process. Renal involvement usually manifests as nephrotic syndrome with eventual development of renal failure, although occasional cases of interstitial-limited or vascular-limited disease occur. Cardiomyopathy, enteropathies, neuropathies, ocular involvement, and hepatic involvement are other major clinical presentations. Almost any organ or site may be affected. Although renal disease is a poor prognostic finding, cardiac involvement represents the gravest threat to the patient's survival.

Classification of amyloid by its precursor molecules provides an etiopathogenetic correlation and has therapeutic implications (Table 1.43). AA is the most common type of systemic amyloidosis worldwide and in children, whereas AL/AH amyloid is the more common type in the developed nations and elderly.[520] The third most common category is familial amyloid. Several familial forms have been identified: transthyretin, fibrinogen Aα, apolipoprotein AI, apolipoprotein AII, lysozyme, cystatin C, and gelsolin. All are autosomal dominant, and most may involve the kidney. A recently described amyloidogenic protein is LECT2 (leukocyte chemotactic factor 2), that shows strong racial predilection in certain populations including Mexican, Native American, Punjabi, Sudanese, and Egyptian individuals. It tends to present more often with chronic renal failure rather than proteinuria.[530-532]

The kidneys in amyloidosis are often stated to be grossly enlarged. However, the kidneys may initially be normal in size because early involvement affects the glomeruli, which are not appreciably expanded. Conversely, in advanced cases, amyloid deposition may result in renal contraction because tubular atrophy

TABLE 1.42	Renal Lesions Associated with Hematopoietic Neoplasms

Amyloidosis
Immunoglobulin or light chain deposition disease
Light chain cast nephropathy
Light chain proximal tubulopathy
Light chain crystal tubulopathy
Crystal-storing histiocytosis
Nephrocalcinosis
Uric acid nephropathy
Neoplastic infiltration

TABLE 1.43	Amyloidosis Classification	
Clinical Syndrome	Amyloid Protein	Precursor Molecule
Primary, myeloma or lymphoproliferative disease associated	AL	Immunoglobulin light or heavy chain
Secondary, reactive	AA	Serum AA protein
Familial amyloid syndromes	ATTR	Transthyretin
	Afib	Fibrinogen Aα chain
	AApoI	Apolipoprotein AI
	AApoII	Apolipoprotein AII
	AGel	Gelsolin
	ALys	Lysozyme
	ACys	Cystatin C
Leukocyte chemotactic factor 2	ALect2	
Senile cardiac	ATTR	Transthyretin
Familial Mediterranean fever	AA	Serum AA protein
Dialysis associated	Aβ2M	β2-Microglobulin
Medulla limited	AApoIV	Apolipoprotein AIV

accompanies glomerular obliteration, with a consequent decrease in cortical mass. The kidneys may have a pale or sallow gross appearance, with blurring of the delineation of cortex and medulla.

Renal amyloidosis manifests in a variety of tissue deposition patterns, defined by location and appearance of the amyloid fibrils, and somewhat dependent on the type of the amyloidogenic protein. Most types of amyloid characteristically form in the glomerulus, initially expanding the mesangium and forming acellular nodules. Later the capillary loops are involved, leading to glomerular obliteration (Fig. 1.141). This form is referred to as nodular amyloidosis. The deposits have a distinctive homogeneous, eosinophilic, glassy appearance on hematoxylin and eosin staining (Fig. 1.141A). Usually no tissue reaction is observed, but occasionally a giant cell reaction may be seen. The nodular mesangial deposits may resemble the nodular Kimmelstiel-Wilson lesions of diabetic glomerulosclerosis and nodular immunoglobulin deposition disease. However, the amyloid deposits are often pale on PAS stain (Fig. 1.141B), nonargyrophilic by silver stains (Fig. 1.141C), and blue on trichrome (Fig. 1.141D). Interestingly, in some cases of amyloidosis the amyloid fibrils extend through the capillary loop basement membrane in parallel arrays and form long, delicate, spikelike arrangements. This form of amyloid deposition can be seen as spicules in a silver stain (Fig. 1.142) because of peculiar argyrophilia of the amyloid itself or accompanying basement membrane, and is often referred to as spicular amyloid. Patients with this form often demonstrate rapid progression of disease. Confirmation of amyloid requires Congo red stain demonstrating orangeophilia under brightfield examination and apple-green or anomalous birefringence when examined with polarized light (Fig. 1.143). Other histochemical methods that can be used include thioflavin fluorescence, crystal violet, and sulfated Alcian blue. Electron microscopy of amyloid reveals delicate, randomly arrayed fibrils (Fig. 1.144).

Extraglomerular deposition in arterioles and arteries, and deposition in the interstitium of the cortex and medulla occur in advanced cases of amyloidosis (Fig. 1.145A). Interstitial deposition of amyloid is particularly common in the hereditary forms and secondary to LECT2 (Fig. 1.145B).[530,531] Rarely, amyloid deposition is confined to vessels in the kidney and elsewhere, resulting in renovascular hypertension and systemic occlusive vascular disease. This

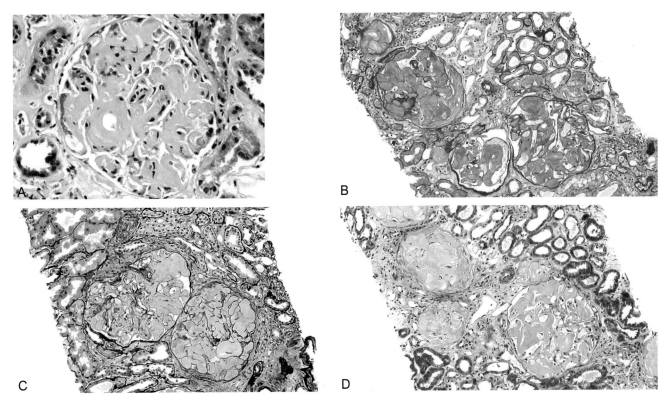

Fig. 1.141 (A) This glomerulus is replaced by homogeneous eosinophilic material characteristic of amyloid (hematoxylin and eosin stain). Amyloid deposits are typically periodic acid–Schiff negative (B), nonargyrophilic with silver stain (C), and stained blue with trichrome stain (D).

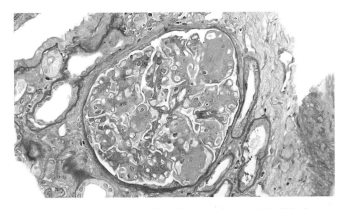

Fig. 1.142 This glomerulus contains silver-negative amyloid within the capillary loop and mesangium, with thin spicular arrays of amyloid extending perpendicular to the capillary loop basement membrane into Bowman space (Jones methenamine silver stain).

form is known as vascular amyloidosis. Medulla predominant deposition is seen in apolipoprotein AIV amyloidosis (Fig. 1.145C and D).[533]

Typing of the amyloidogenic protein is important for the subsequent management of the patient. Immunofluorescence stains for κ and λ light chains and immunoperoxidase stain for AA (Fig. 1.145A), LECT2 (Fig. 1.145B), or TTR protein-derived forms are most commonly used. Mass spectrometry is usually needed when the histochemical stains are negative and for definitive typing of the rare forms of amyloidosis.[532,534,535]

Light Chain Cast Nephropathy

Light chain cast nephropathy ("myeloma kidney") is a disease resulting from acute tubular injury (Fig. 1.146) due to the intratubular formation of large, eosinophilic, PAS-negative, and often cracked or fractured casts composed of a restricted light chain (Fig. 1.147).[521,536] The updated International Myeloma Working Group consensus criteria recognize cast nephropathy as a myeloma-defining condition.[537-539] The casts form in the distal tubules and collecting ducts, and may extend into the adjacent interstitium. They may elicit an inflammatory response that includes neutrophils, histiocytes, and sometimes multinucleated giant cells (Fig. 1.148). Immunohistochemical demonstration of light chain restriction is required for diagnosis (Fig. 1.149).

Immunoglobulin and Light Chain Deposition Disease

Immunoglobulin and light chain deposition disease refers to the deposition of granular paraprotein deposits in glomeruli, tubulointerstitial areas, or both, that causes nephrotic syndrome, Fanconi syndrome, and renal insufficiency (Fig. 1.150). The glomerular lesion resembles amyloid; however, the deposits are granular rather than fibrillar in appearance by electron microscopy

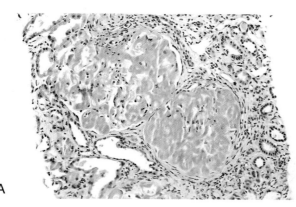

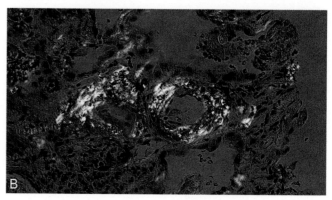

Fig. 1.143 (A) Deposits of amyloid in these glomeruli are highlighted by rosy color with Congo red stain. (B) This artery is involved by amyloid. The diagnostic apple-green birefringence of amyloid is demonstrated on Congo red stain under polarization.

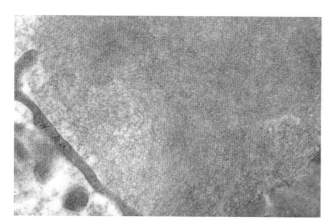

Fig. 1.144 Electron micrograph showing the thin, delicate, randomly arrayed fibrils characteristic of amyloid.

(Fig. 1.151).[540,541] Similar tubulointerstitial deposits form along the outside of the tubular basement membrane, within the interstitium, and in small vessels. Like amyloidosis, systemic involvement also occurs.

Light Chain Proximal Tubulopathy

Light chain proximal tubulopathy is another monoclonal light chain tubular disease. Patients present with proteinuria and renal failure from acute tubular injury.[521,542-545] On immunofluorescence, light chain restriction is noted within the proximal tubule cytoplasm, where lysosomal granules are filled with a single light chain (Fig. 1.152). Most cases are the result of κ light chains. The lesion may be seen alone or in combination with other light chain lesions such as light chain cast nephropathy. Most patients are subsequently shown to have multiple myeloma.

Light Chain Crystal Tubulopathy

In this type of light chain disease, the light chain crystals are located within the tubular epithelium.[542-545] The tubular lumina are empty. Patients present with renal failure and often have Fanconi syndrome. Although the crystals are abundant, the histologic findings may be subtle. This problem can be compounded because the crystals may not stain by immunofluorescence. However, antigenic

sites are more readily available to light chain antisera with pronase digestion, as noted earlier (Fig. 1.153).

Crystal-Storing Histiocytosis

Crystal-storing histiocytosis is another rare form of light chain crystal deposition.[546] In this disease the crystals are located within infiltrating histiocytes rather than in the cells of the nephron (Fig. 1.154). As in light chain crystal tubulopathy, the antigenicity of the crystals may be impaired in frozen tissue, thus necessitating pronase digestion to demonstrate light chain restriction.

Monoclonal Gammopathy of Renal Significance

Although the term *monoclonal gammopathy of renal significance* may encompass all entities with a monoclonal gammopathy resulting in renal dysfunction, the term is recently being used to characterize cases where any of the specific entities, as described earlier, cannot be identified as a reason for the renal disease.[547,548] Possible mechanisms include tubulointerstitial inflammation or direct injury from the light chains. However, it is still used as a waste basket where the mechanism for renal disease in a patient with underlying lymphoproliferative disease cannot be well characterized.

Renal Transplantation

Renal allograft biopsy evaluation is a mainstay in the management of renal transplant dysfunction.[549] Biopsy findings have been shown to change the clinical diagnosis in 27% to 46% patients, and therapy in approximately 59%, with no diminishing value in the last 20 years.[550] The recommendations regarding biopsy of a transplanted kidney are varied and often institution dependent. Although some centers perform "protocol" biopsies at predetermined intervals, in most institutions declining renal function is the major indication for an allograft biopsy. In addition to evaluating for possible rejection, numerous other potential causes of allograft dysfunction must also be considered when reviewing a biopsy. Many diseases tend to recur in the transplanted kidney, and many conditions do not manifest before a certain time interval (Fig. 1.155); thus knowledge of other clinical parameters including allograft age is crucial. The list also includes identification of transplant surgery–associated injury, therapy-associated injury,

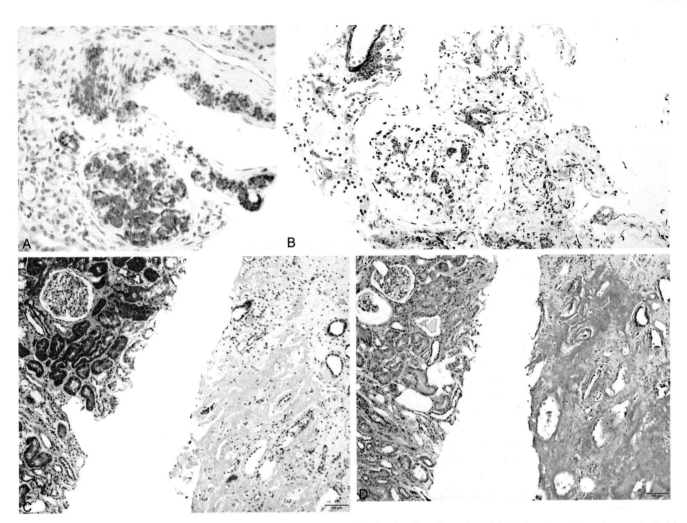

Fig. 1.145 (A) This kidney is from a patient with AA-associated amyloidosis. Notice the deposition of amyloid in the glomerulus, artery, and arteriole (immunoperoxidase stain for AA protein). (B) Positive stain for LECT2 in a Hispanic patient. (C) Hematoxylin and eosin stain showing glassy, homogeneous deposits in the medulla only (on the right) in a case of apolipoprotein AIV amyloidosis. (D) Congo red stain highlighting the amyloid deposits in the medulla.

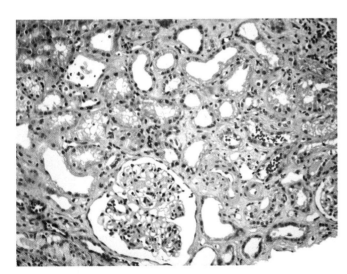

Fig. 1.146 Light chain cast nephropathy causes diffuse acute tubular injury.

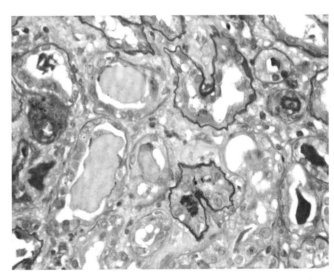

Fig. 1.147 Monoclonal light chain casts are invariably periodic acid–Schiff (PAS) stain–negative. In contrast, the usual protein casts stain strongly on PAS stain; note PAS-positive protein casts on the right side.

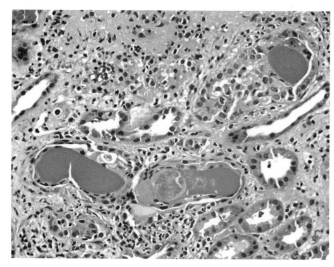

Fig. 1.148 The casts of light chain cast nephropathy often, but not always, elicit a cellular reaction. In this example there is a mononuclear cell and multinuclear giant cell reaction to the casts.

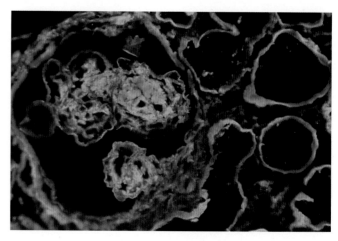

Fig. 1.150 Direct immunofluorescence showing λ light chain deposition along tubular and glomerular capillary basement membranes and within the mesangium. Staining for κ light chain is negative.

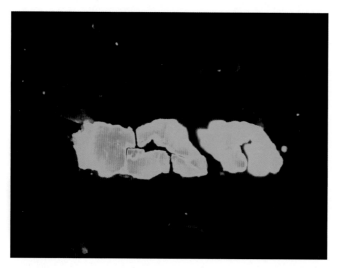

Fig. 1.149 Direct immunofluorescence showing light chain restriction. There is intense staining for κ light chain within this cast. The λ light chain stain was negative.

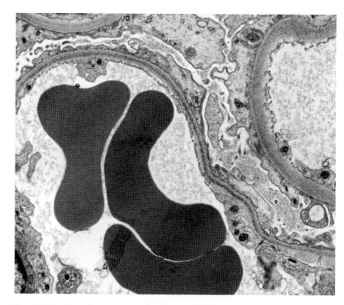

Fig. 1.151 Granular paraprotein deposits of λ light chains along the inner aspect of a capillary loop basement membrane.

immunosuppression-associated complications, and the entire spectrum of diseases that can affect a native kidney.

Evaluation of Preimplantation/Procurement and Zero-Hour Implantation Biopsy

Most institutions perform preimplantation biopsy to assess suitability of a kidney for transplantation, usually from a deceased donor, to identify active renal disease or to evaluate the clinical significance of incidentally identified neoplasms. Zero-hour implantation biopsies are useful to provide an insight into the condition of the kidney for future comparative analysis. An abnormal finding in the preimplantation biopsy is the largest reason for discard of donor organs, leading to 37% to 43% of kidney discards.[550-552] Proper evaluation of such biopsies is crucial to avoid unnecessary organ discards. Evaluation is often limited to frozen sections of a subcapsular wedge. Awareness of the pitfalls of a frozen section is important when

evaluating these biopsies, which is often performed by the surgical/urologic pathologist. Conventional frozen sections have prominent artificial interstitial spaces that can be mistaken for fibrosis or edema. Even though thrombi or crescents can be identified, glomerular cellularity cannot be reliably assessed. Evaluation of at least 25 glomeruli, from as deep in the cortex as feasible, should be performed. Scarred areas with clusters of sclerotic glomeruli, as often present in a subcapsular sample, should be excluded from the overall estimate of percent sclerosis and mentioned separately. No study has yet established an absolute threshold for glomerulosclerosis, fibrosis, and arteriosclerosis, beyond which a donor kidney cannot be used.[550] Individual case-by-case judgment should be used when deciding whether to use a particular kidney in a particular recipient, because studies have shown that even marginal donor organs may be beneficial for some recipients, especially in "old for old" or dual-organ transplantation programs.[550]

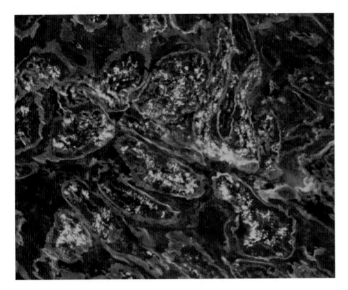

Fig. 1.152 In light chain proximal tubulopathy, there are numerous light chain–restricted protein droplets within the proximal tubule cells. This is the stain for κ light chain. The λ light chain stain was negative.

Evaluation of a Transplant Biopsy

A kidney biopsy is the gold standard for evaluation of renal dysfunction posttransplantation. The Banff classification is the most widely used system for reporting of a transplant biopsy. It is a working classification that is continuously refined and updated, and provides information on the type of rejection, the intensity of rejection, and the presence of chronic changes.[31,553-572] The Banff Diagnostic Scoring System was originally formulated in the early 1990s. It has undergone a series of revisions and updates.

Tables 1.44 through 1.60 show the revised classification with updated recommendations and respective grading of components. Interstitial inflammation and tubulitis are the hallmarks of T-cell–mediated rejection (TCMR). The key components of acute antibody-mediated rejection (ABMR) include glomerulitis, peritubular capillaritis, and C4d staining of peritubular capillaries. Endotheliitis or intimal arteritis per se can be a component of T-cell or ABMR, or an isolated finding (so-called isolated v-lesion). When seen in the context of TCMR, presence of arteritis is used to upgrade the class of rejection from I to II or III, depending on severity. Additional scores are also provided for indices of chronic rejection such as transplant glomerulopathy, and other chronic changes including arterial fibrointimal thickening, arteriolar hyalinosis, tubular atrophy, and interstitial fibrosis. For those interested in greater detail, the original Banff reports and several excellent book chapters on the topic are cited in the References.[31,550,553-575]

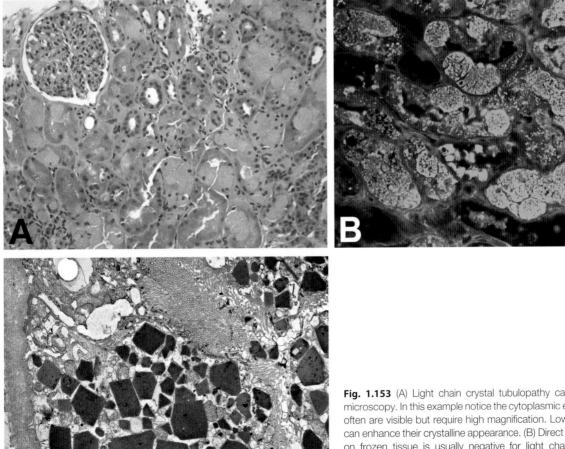

Fig. 1.153 (A) Light chain crystal tubulopathy can be subtle by light microscopy. In this example notice the cytoplasmic enlargement. Crystals often are visible but require high magnification. Lowering the condenser can enhance their crystalline appearance. (B) Direct immunofluorescence on frozen tissue is usually negative for light chains. Use of paraffin-embedded tissue can show light chain restriction because of pronase predigestion. (C) The light chain crystals have a sharp, angulated appearance on electron microscopy.

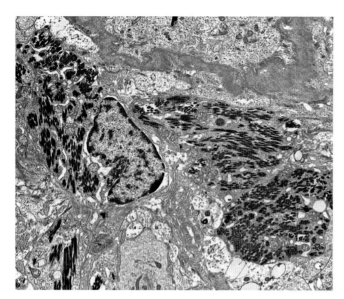

Fig. 1.154 This example of crystal-storing histiocytosis shows interstitial histiocytes filled with light chain crystals (electron microscopy).

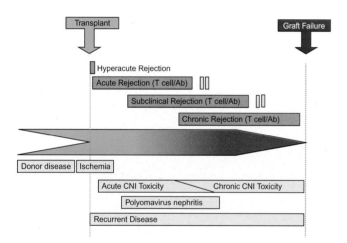

Fig. 1.155 Timeline of events after a renal transplant. Ab, antibody; CNI, calcineurin inhibitor.

Antibody-Mediated Rejection

ABMR has both acute and chronic forms. It can happen both early posttransplantation in a presensitized patient and late posttransplantation because of preexisting or de novo donor-specific antibodies (DSAs). The term *chronic* in the context of ABMR is not related to a certain time posttransplantation and rather indicates morphologic changes of remodeling seen in the allograft because of antibody-mediated injury. C4d is often detected in peritubular capillaries and arterioles, regarded as evidence of a preexisting antibody event (immunoglobulins are not detected), and neutrophils or mononuclear inflammatory cells are usually present within glomerular tufts and dilated peritubular capillaries (Fig. 1.156A-D). However, even moderate inflammation in the microcirculation can be associated with the development of overt transplant glomerulopathy in the presence of DSA and in C4d-negative cases.[576] Positive staining for C4d is therefore no longer required for the diagnosis of ABMR according to the updated Banff classification.[574] Acute ABMR clinically resembles acute cellular rejection but is more resistant to immunosuppressive reversal. The morphologic pattern of injury is variable and ranges from acute tubular injury to thrombotic microangiopathy to arterial fibrinoid necrosis or transmural inflammation (Table 1.44). In chronic active ABMR, one sees manifestations of protracted endothelial injury including glomerular basement membrane duplication (so-called chronic transplant glomerulopathy) (Figs. 1.156A and 1.157A), multilayering of peritubular capillary basement membranes (Fig. 1.157B; electron microscopy finding), fibrointimal thickening of arteries, or interstitial fibrosis/tubular atrophy. Intimal arteritis is thought to be seen in both ABMR and TCMR.

T-Cell–Mediated Rejection

Acute TCMR (previously also known as type 1 cellular or interstitial rejection) usually develops in the first few weeks to months after transplantation. A predominance of T lymphocytes with lesser numbers of monocytes is observed. Eosinophils and plasma cells are present in modest numbers, but they may on occasion be numerous. Acute TCMR is separated into three types of rejection. Type I rejection is most common. Its hallmark is interstitial inflammation associated with infiltration of tubular epithelium by mononuclear cells, known as tubulitis (Fig. 1.158). Tubulitis is best recognized with the aid of a basement membrane stain such as PAS (Fig. 1.158B) or silver stain. Edema and tubular epithelial and tubular basement membrane damage are also present.

Type II rejection is a more serious form of rejection, less responsive to immunosuppressive treatment. It is characterized by endothelial cell enlargement with subendothelial mononuclear cells, known as endovasculitis or endotheliitis (Fig. 1.159A). Fibrin may be observed but is not required for the diagnosis. Endothelial cell necrosis can develop with thrombosis. Glomeruli can also be involved in acute rejection, known as acute transplant glomerulopathy. This is characterized by mononuclear cell accumulation within glomerular capillary loops and mesangium. The hypercellular appearance of glomeruli resembles proliferative glomerulonephritis that can develop in allografts as a recurrent or de novo condition. If glomerular hypercellularity is associated with changes of type I rejection, or especially type II rejection, recurrent or de novo glomerulonephritis is unlikely. Immunofluorescence and electron microscopy may be required, however, to exclude the presence of immune deposits in certain cases. Type III rejection is uncommon and is characterized by transmural inflammation (Fig. 1.159B) or fibrinoid necrosis.

Chronic active TCMR, as introduced in the Banff 2017 classification, is thought to be a manifestation of chronic underimmunosuppression.[572] It shows inflammation (ti score 2 or 3) in areas of fibrosis and atrophy, amounting to more than 25% of the sampled cortex (i-IFTA score 2 or 3), with foci of moderate (t2) or severe (t3) tubulitis involving one or more tubules, but not including severely atrophic tubules. In chronic transplant arteriopathy, there is marked fibrointimal thickening of arteries, usually interlobular or arcuate (Fig. 1.160). Mild intimal inflammation may be present, and foam cells and fibrin may be observed. Within the thickened intima, smooth muscle proliferation resembles a new media.

Calcineurin Inhibitor Nephrotoxicity

Calcineurin inhibitors (cyclosporine and FK506) have effects on several cell types in the kidney and produce a variety of acute and

TABLE 1.44 Banff Classification of Renal Allograft Diagnostic Scoring

Category I. Normal biopsy or nonspecific changes

Category II. Antibody-mediated changes

A. Active ABMR (all three criteria must be present for diagnosis):
1. Histologic evidence of acute tissue injury, including one or more of the following:
   - Microvascular inflammation (g > 0 and/or ptc > 0), in the absence of recurrent or de novo glomerulonephritis (in the presence of acute TCMR, borderline infiltrate, or infection, ptc ≥ 1 alone is not sufficient and g must be[1]
   - Intimal or transmural arteritis (v > 0)
   - Acute thrombotic microangiopathy, in the absence of any other cause
   - Acute tubular injury, in the absence of any other apparent cause
2. Evidence of current/recent antibody interaction with vascular endothelium, including at least one of the following:
   - Linear C4d staining in peritubular capillaries (C4d2 or C4d3 by IF on frozen sections, or C4d > 0 by IHC on paraffin sections)
   - At least moderate microvascular inflammation ([g + ptc] ≥ 2)
   - Increased expression of gene transcripts in the biopsy tissue indicative of endothelial injury, if thoroughly validated
3. Serologic evidence of DSAs (HLA or other antigens): C4d staining or expression of validated transcripts/classifiers as noted earlier in criterion 2 may substitute for DSAs; however, thorough DSA testing, including testing for non-HLA antibodies if HLA antibody testing is negative, is strongly advised whenever criteria 1 and 2 are met
B. Chronic, active ABMR (all three criteria must be present for diagnosis):
1. Morphologic evidence of chronic tissue injury, including one or more of the following:
   - Transplant glomerulopathy (cg > 0), if no evidence of chronic thrombotic microangiopathy or chronic recurrent/de novo glomerulonephritis; includes changes evident by EM alone (cg1a)
   - Severe peritubular capillary basement membrane multilayering (requires EM)
   - Arterial intimal fibrosis of new onset, excluding other causes; leukocytes within the sclerotic intima favor chronic ABMR, if there is no history of prior TCMR, but are not required
2. Same as criterion 2 for active ABMR
3. Same as criterion 3 for active ABMR
C. C4d staining without evidence of rejection (all four criteria must be present for diagnosis):
1. Linear C4d staining in peritubular capillaries (C4d2 or C4d3 by IF on frozen sections, or C4d > 0 by IHC on paraffin sections)
2. Criterion 1 for active or chronic, active ABMR not met
3. No molecular evidence for ABMR as in criterion 2 for active and chronic active ABMR
4. No acute or chronic active TCMR, or borderline changes

Category III. Borderline changes/suspicious for acute T-cell–mediated rejection

1. Foci of tubulitis (t > 0) with minor interstitial inflammation (i0, or i1) or, moderate to severe interstitial inflammation (i2, or i3) with mild tubulitis (t1)
2. No intimal arteritis

Category IV. T-cell-mediated rejection

A. Acute TCMR
   Grade Ia—significant interstitial inflammation and moderate tubulitis (i2, or i3 and t2)
   Grade Ib—significant interstitial inflammation and severe tubulitis (i2, or i3 and t3)
   Grade IIa—mild-to-moderate intimal arteritis (v1), with or without interstitial inflammation and tubulitis
   Grade IIb—severe intimal arteritis (v2) involving >25% of luminal area, with or without interstitial inflammation and tubulitis
   Grade III—transmural arteritis and/or arterial fibrinoid change and necrosis of medial smooth muscle cells with accompanying lymphocytic inflammation (v3)
B. Chronic active TCMR
   Grade Ia—significant interstitial inflammation in areas of fibrosis and atrophy (i-IFTA ≥ 2 and ti ≥ 2) and moderate tubulitis (t2)
   Grade Ib—significant interstitial inflammation in areas of fibrosis and atrophy (i-IFTA ≥ 2 and ti ≥ 2) and severe tubulitis (t3)
   Grade IIa—chronic allograft arteriopathy (arterial intimal fibrosis with mononuclear cell infiltration in fibrosis and formation of neointima)

Category V. Interstitial fibrosis and tubular atrophy, no specific etiology

A. Mild: <25% cortical area
B. Moderate: 26%-50% cortical area
C. Severe: >50% cortical area

Category VI. Other non–rejection-associated injuries and complications

A. Acute tubular injury
B. Drug toxicities
   1. Calcineurin inhibitor toxicities
   2. mTOR inhibitor toxicities
   3. Antiviral tubular toxicities
   4. Drug-associated acute tubulointerstitial nephritis
C. Infections
   1. BK polyomavirus
   2. Cytomegalovirus
   3. Adenovirus
D. De novo and recurrent diseases
E. Allograft rupture
F. Posttransplant lymphoproliferative disorders
   1. Epstein-Barr virus–related
   2. Not Epstein-Barr virus–related
G. Pyelonephritis
H. Drug-induced interstitial nephritis

ABMR, antibody-mediated rejection; *DSA,* donor-specific antibody; *EM,* electron microscopy; *HLA,* human leukocyte antigen; *IF,* immunofluorescence; *IHC,* immunohistochemistry; *mTOR,* mammalian target of rapamycin; *t,* tubulitis; *TCMR,* T-cell–mediated rejection.

chronic lesions (Table 1.58).[577-581] However, the most common manifestation of nephrotoxicity is an absence of morphologic findings. Renal failure results from arteriolar vasoconstriction with a reversible decrease in the glomerular filtration rate. This form of toxicity is implicated when urinary tract obstruction has been clinically excluded and the biopsy shows no signs of rejection, acute tubular necrosis, or any lesion described in the following paragraphs.

Two nephrotoxic lesions affect arterioles and glomeruli. Acute thrombotic microangiopathy with glomerular and/or arteriolar thrombi may develop, usually in the initial weeks to months after transplantation. A second chronic hyaline arteriopathy may develop, in which hyaline deposits replace smooth muscle cells (Fig. 1.161), preferentially along the outer aspect of the arteriole. The external location of hyaline distinguishes this lesion from hypertension and diabetic arteriolar hyalinosis, in which the deposits form along the inner aspect of the arteriole.

A distinctive tubular lesion of acute reversible nephrotoxicity is isometric vacuolization. The tubular epithelial cell cytoplasm

TABLE 1.45 Tubulitis (t)[a] Score

t 0   None
t 1   Foci with 1-4 cells/tubular cross section or 10 tubular cells
t 2   Foci with 4-10 cells/tubular cross section or 10 tubular cells
t 3   Foci with >10 cells/tubular cross section or 10 tubular cells
      Or, 2 foci of tubular basement membrane destruction and t2 and
      i2 or i3

[a]Mononuclear cells inside of tubular basement membrane; severely atrophic tubules should not be scored. A severely atrophic tubule is defined as one with each of the following three features: a diameter <25% of that of unaffected or minimally affected tubules on the biopsy; an undifferentiated-appearing, cuboidal, or flattened epithelium; and pronounced wrinkling and/or thickening of the tubular basement membrane.

TABLE 1.46 Interstitial Inflammation (i)[a] Score

i 0   <10% of cortex
i 1   10%-25% of cortex
i 2   26%-50% of cortex
i 3   >50% of cortex

[a]Excluding the subcapsular zone and fibrotic areas.

TABLE 1.47 Intimal Arteritis (v)[a] Score

v 0   No intimal arteritis/arteriolitis
v 1   Intimal arteritis/arteriolitis <25% lumen (minimum 1 cell, 1 artery/
      arteriole)
v 2   Intimal arteritis/arteriolitis >25% lumen
v 3   Transmural arteritis and/or arterial fibrinoid change and medial
      smooth muscle necrosis with lymphocytic infiltrate in vessel

[a]Mononuclear cells beneath endothelium or within media. "v" lesions are scored only in arteries having a continuous media with two or more smooth muscle layers.

TABLE 1.48 Glomerulitis (g)[a] Score

g 0   No glomerulitis
g 1   Glomerulitis in <25% of glomeruli
g 2   Segmental or global glomerulitis in 25%-75% of glomeruli
g 3   Glomerulitis (mostly global) in >75% of glomeruli

[a]Complete or partial occlusion of more than one glomerular capillary by leukocyte infiltration and endothelial cell enlargement.

TABLE 1.49 Peritubular Capillaritis (ptc)[a] Score

ptc 0   At least 1 leukocyte in <10% of cortical PTCs and/or maximum
        number of leukocytes <3
ptc 1   At least 1 leukocyte cell in ≥10% of cortical PTCs with 3 or 4
        leukocytes in most severely involved PTC
ptc 2   At least 1 leukocyte in ≥10% of cortical PTCs with 5-10
        leukocytes in most severely involved PTC
ptc 3   At least 1 leukocyte in ≥10% of cortical PTCs with >10
        leukocytes in most severely involved PTC

[a]Recommended to comment on the composition (mononuclear cells versus neutrophils) and extent (focal, ≤50% versus diffuse, >50%) of peritubular capillaritis.

TABLE 1.50 Transplant Glomerulopathy (cg) Score

cg 0   No GBM double contours by light microscopy or EM
cg 1a   No GBM double contours by light microscopy, but GBM double
        contours (incomplete or circumferential) in at least three
        glomerular capillaries by EM with associated endothelial
        swelling and/or subendothelial electron lucent widening
cg 1b   ≥1 glomerular capillaries with GBM double contours in >1
        nonsclerotic glomerulus by light microscopy; EM confirmation
        is recommended if EM is available
cg 2   Double contours affecting 26%-50% of peripheral capillary loops
        in the most affected of nonsclerotic glomeruli
cg 3   Double contours affecting >50% of peripheral capillary loops in
        the most affected of nonsclerotic glomeruli

EM, Electron microscopy; *GBM*, glomerular basement membrane.

TABLE 1.51 Arteriolar Hyalinosis (ah) Score

ah 0   No PAS-positive hyaline thickening
ah 1   Mild-to-moderate PAS-positive hyaline thickening in at least one
       arteriole
ah 2   Moderate-to-severe PAS-positive hyaline thickening in more than
       one arteriole
ah 3   Severe PAS-positive hyaline thickening in many arterioles

PAS, Periodic acid–Schiff.

TABLE 1.52   Vascular Fibrous Intimal Thickening (cv)[a] Score

cv 0	No chronic vascular changes
cv 1	Vascular narrowing of up to 25% luminal area by fibrointimal thickening of arteries +/− breach of internal elastic lamina or presence of foam cells or occasional mononuclear cells
cv 2	Increased severity of changes described earlier with 26%-50% narrowing of vascular luminal area
cv 3	Severe vascular changes with >50% narrowing of vascular luminal area

[a]In the most severely affected vessel. Note whether lesions characteristic of chronic rejection (breaks in the elastica, inflammatory cells in fibrosis, formation of neointima) are seen.

TABLE 1.53   Interstitial Fibrosis (ci) Score

ci 0	Interstitial fibrosis in up to 5% of cortical area
ci 1	Mild—interstitial fibrosis in 6%-25% of cortical area
ci 2	Moderate—interstitial fibrosis in 26%-50% of cortical area
ci 3	Severe—interstitial fibrosis in >50% of cortical area

TABLE 1.54   Tubular Atrophy (ct) Score

ct 0	No tubular atrophy
ct 1	Tubular atrophy in up to 25% of the cortical tubules
ct 2	Tubular atrophy involving 26%-50% of the area of cortical tubules
ct 3	Tubular atrophy involving >50% of the area of cortical tubules

TABLE 1.55   Total Inflammation (ti) Score

ti 0	No or trivial interstitial inflammation (<10% of parenchyma)
ti 1	10%-25% of parenchyma inflamed
ti 2	26%-50% of parenchyma inflamed
ti 3	>50% of parenchyma inflamed

TABLE 1.56   Mesangial Matrix (mm)[a] Score

mm 0	No mesangial matrix increase
mm 1	Up to 25% of nonsclerotic glomeruli affected (at least moderate matrix increase)
mm 2	26%-50% of nonsclerotic glomeruli affected (at least moderate matrix increase)
mm 3	>50% of nonsclerotic glomeruli affected (at least moderate matrix increase)

[a]The threshold criterion for the moderately increased mesangial matrix (mm) is the expanded mesangial interspace between adjacent capillaries. If the width of interspace exceeds two mesangial cells on the average in at least two glomerular lobules, the mm is moderately increased.

TABLE 1.57   C4d Score[a]

C4d 0	0%
C4d 1	Minimal C4d staining (>0 but <10% of PTCs)
C4d 2	Focal C4d staining (10%-50% of PTCs)
C4d 3	Diffuse C4d staining (>50% of PTCs)

[a]Percentage (%) of peritubular capillaries (PTCs) with C4d scored in at least five high-power fields. It should be mentioned whether scoring is done by immunofluorescence on frozen sections or by immunohistochemistry on paraffin-embedded sections. A score of C4d2 or C4d3 on frozen sections and C4d > 0 on paraffin-embedded sections is considered positive.

TABLE 1.58   Peritubular Capillaropathy Score by Electron Microscopy

Mild	≤3 circumferential layers in 3 PTCs
Moderate	4-6 circumferential layers in 1 or 2 PTCs
Severe	1 PTC with ≥7 layers and at least 2 with ≥5 layers

TABLE 1.59   Quantitative Criteria for Inflammation in Areas of Interstitial Fibrosis and Tubular Atrophy (i-IFTA) Score

i-IFTA0	No inflammation or <10% of scarred cortical parenchyma
i-IFTA1	Inflammation in 10%-25% of scarred cortical parenchyma
i-IFTA2	Inflammation in 26%-50% of scarred cortical parenchyma
i-IFTA3	Inflammation in >50% of scarred cortical parenchyma

TABLE 1.60   Calcineurin Inhibitor Nephrotoxicity

Normal histology
Thrombotic microangiopathy
Hyaline arteriopathy
Tubular isometric vacuolization
Interstitial fibrosis

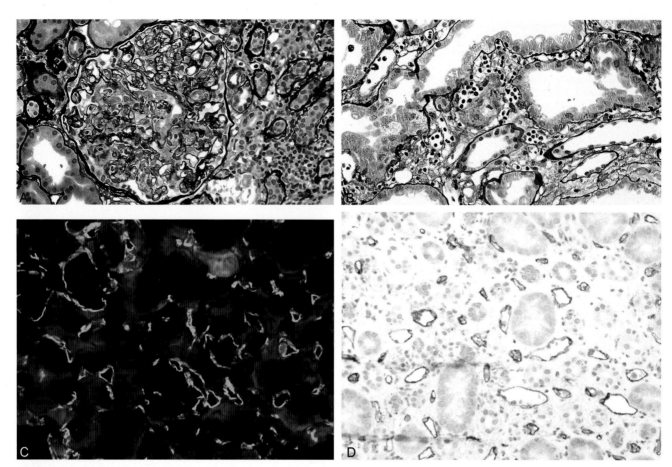

Fig. 1.156 Features commonly seen in antibody-mediated rejection. (A) Glomerulitis and glomerular basement double contours. (B) Peritubular capillaritis showing dilated peritubular capillaries with mononuclear inflammatory cells (silver stain). (C) C4d immunofluorescence stain with strong circumferential staining in the peritubular capillaries. (D) Immunoperoxidase stain for C4d with strong circumferential staining in the peritubular capillaries.

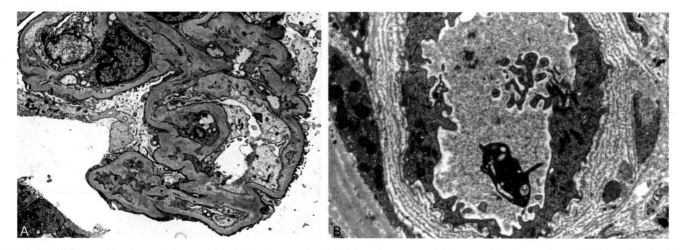

Fig. 1.157 (A) Glomerulitis, glomerular basement double contours, and endothelial swelling are seen in this case with advanced transplant glomerulopathy. (B) This peritubular capillary has prominent multilayering of its basement membrane (electron microscopy).

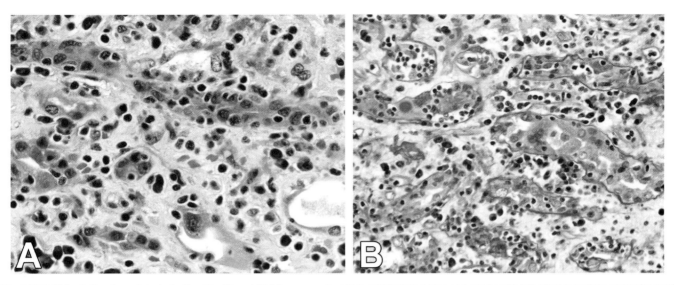

Fig. 1.158 (A) Acute T-cell–mediated rejection, Banff type I. Visible are prominent interstitial inflammation and edema with inflammatory cells involving the renal tubules. (B) Periodic acid–Schiff stain highlights the tubulitis showing numerous lymphoid cells with small, dark nuclei located inside the tubular basement membranes.

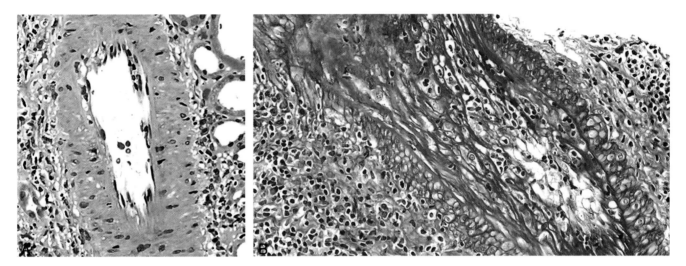

Fig. 1.159 Endotheliitis and transmural vasculitis can be a component of both T-cell– or antibody-mediated rejection. (A) Endotheliitis in a case with acute T-cell–mediated rejection; this case was categorized as Banff type IIa. The endothelial cells are enlarged, and subendothelial mononuclear cells are present. (B) Transmural arteritis in a case with severe T-cell– and antibody-mediated rejection.

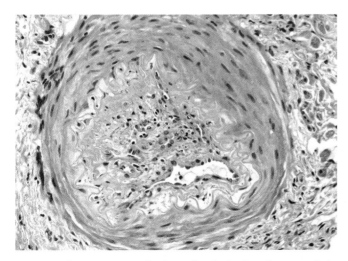

Fig. 1.160 Chronic active antibody-mediated rejection. Severe occlusive fibrointimal thickening is present.

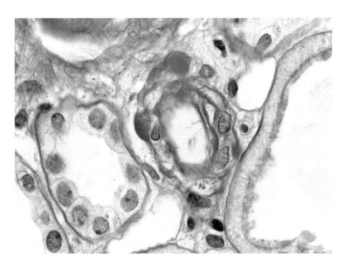

Fig. 1.161 Cyclosporine-associated hyaline arteriopathy. Periodic acid–Schiff–positive hyaline globules are located on the outer aspect of this arteriole.

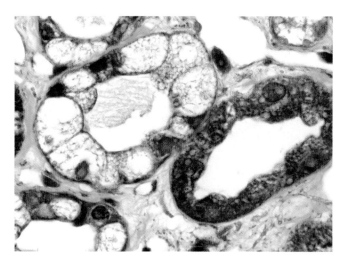

Fig. 1.162 Cyclosporine-associated isometric tubular epithelial cell vacuolization (trichrome stain).

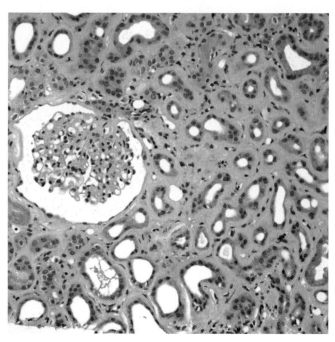

Fig. 1.163 Cyclosporine-associated diffuse interstitial fibrosis.

contains numerous small vacuoles that impart a foamy appearance and represent dilated smooth endoplasmic reticulum (Fig. 1.162). A second chronic irreversible lesion of nephrotoxicity is interstitial fibrosis with tubular atrophy (Fig. 1.163). It usually appears months to years after transplantation. When cyclosporine was first introduced, however, interstitial fibrosis was observed to develop rapidly when large loading doses were administered in the context of acute tubular necrosis.

References are available at expertconsult.com

2

Neoplasms of the Kidney

GREGORY T. MACLENNAN AND LIANG CHENG

CHAPTER OUTLINE

The first renal neoplasm was reported nearly 200 years ago.[1,2] In 1953, about eight renal tumors were described in a well-known textbook on surgical pathology.[3] As a consequence of the contributions of numerous investigators over many decades, the most recent World Health Organization (WHO) classification of renal neoplasms includes about 50 well-defined and distinctive renal tumors, as well as various miscellaneous and metastatic tumors.[4] In addition, a number of emerging or provisional new entities are under active investigation and may be included in future classifications. In this chapter, we examine these diverse and fascinating neoplasms.

Renal Cell Carcinomas

General Considerations

Incidence

Excluding cancer of the renal pelvis and ureter, kidney cancer is the seventh most common malignancy worldwide, accounting for 3.3% of all newly diagnosed cancers in 2012.[5-8] In 2018, nearly 65,340 new cases were reported, with ~14,970 related deaths in the United States.[9] At diagnosis, 25% to 30% of patients had metastatic cancer.[10] Highest incidences were in the Czech Republic, Lithuania, Slovakia, and Northern America, and lowest rates were in Middle, Western, and Sub-Saharan Africa. Mortality rates were higher in more developed regions than in less developed regions.[6,11-13]

Epidemiology

Renal cell carcinoma (RCC) afflicts males approximately twice as often as females, and is most commonly diagnosed in patients in their early sixties.[5,11-13] The risk for development of RCC is two to three times higher in individuals who have a first-degree relative with RCC.[14] Approximately 2% to 4% of cases of RCC are associated with several distinctive hereditary cancer syndromes that will be discussed in this chapter under the appropriate headings; the remainder are considered sporadic.

Recognized risk factors for renal cancer include cigarette smoking, obesity, and hypertension.[15] Cigarette smoking has consistently been shown to be a causal risk factor for RCC. The risk increases with consumption level and gradually decreases after years of cessation.[16] There is strong epidemiologic support for a causal association between trichloroethylene exposure and kidney cancer.[17] Overweight and obesity are estimated to contribute to the development of more than 40% of renal cancers in the United States and more than 30% in Europe, possibly mediated by insulin resistance and chronic hyperinsulinemia, increased bioavailability of steroid hormones, and localized inflammation.[18,19] Although the role of hypertension in the development of RCC is difficult to assess, the bulk of epidemiologic evidence implicates it as a causal risk factor.[20,21] Long-term renal dialysis exposes patients to a considerably higher average annual incidence of RCC than the general population.[22] The major risk factor in such patients appears to be the presence of acquired cystic kidney disease (ACKD).[23]

Hereditary Aspects of Renal Cell Neoplasia

Hereditary renal tumors comprise single neoplasms or a constellation of tumor types in more than one first-degree or second-degree family member that are inherited through the passage of germline mutations, each of which is specific for a hereditary renal tumor syndrome.[24] Bilaterality, multifocality, and early age of onset are typical of hereditary renal tumors. It is estimated that between 2% and 4% of renal cell neoplasms arise based on an underlying hereditary abnormality. Well-characterized examples include the following occurrences: clear cell renal cell carcinoma (CCRCC) in von Hippel–Lindau (VHL) syndrome and constitutional chromosome 3 translocations syndrome; papillary renal cell carcinoma (PRCC) in hereditary PRCC syndrome, hereditary leiomyomatosis and renal cell carcinoma (HLRCC) syndrome (non-PRCC1 only), familial papillary thyroid carcinoma syndrome, hyperthyroidism-jaw tumor syndrome, and Birt-Hogg-Dubé syndrome; oncocytoma in hyperthyroidism-jaw tumor syndrome; and chromophobe RCC and hybrid chromophobe oncocytoma in Birt-Hogg-Dubé syndrome. A meta-analysis of reported cases in 1998 failed to establish a link between tuberous sclerosis complex (TSC) and renal cell neoplasms, but more recent reports indicate that the incidence of RCC in patients with TSC is 2% to 4% higher than its incidence in the general population.[25-31] Although patients with autosomal dominant polycystic kidney disease appear to have a higher incidence of renal cortical adenoma than the general population, there is no convincing evidence that patients with this condition have a higher risk for development of RCC than the general population.[32-34]

Grading Renal Cell Carcinoma

It has been a long-held tenet that cytologic grading is important in predicting the biologic behavior of RCC.[35-53] Several grading systems proposed in the last 50 years have fallen into disuse because they lacked sufficient validation or applicability to the currently accepted classification of RCC.[35,37,39,52,54-56] In an ideal grading system, significant outcome differences should be demonstrable between patients with different tumor grades, both univariate and after adjusting for important clinical and pathologic features. Until recently, the most widely used grading system was the one proposed by Fuhrman et al.[37] The validation, reproducibility, and interpretation of the Fuhrman system drew substantial criticism, and consequently the four-tiered WHO/International Society of Urologic Pathology (ISUP) grading system has been recommended for use in grading CCRCC and PRCC, cancers for which there is sufficient outcome data to allow the system to be used for predicting prognosis.[2,57,58] Nucleolar prominence defines grades 1 to 3 (Fig. 2.1 through 2.3). Pronounced nuclear pleomorphism, tumor giant cells, and rhabdoid or sarcomatoid changes are all features of grade 4 tumors (Fig. 2.4 through 2.6). These grades are assigned based on these criteria within the single

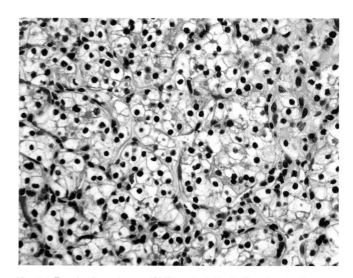

Fig. 2.1 Renal cell carcinoma, ISUP grade 1. Nucleoli are inconspicuous or absent at 400× magnification.

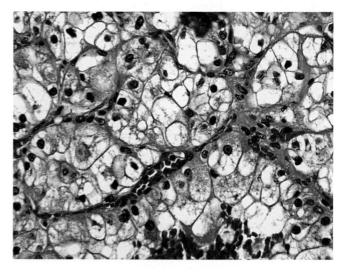

Fig. 2.2 Renal cell carcinoma, ISUP grade 2. Nucleoli are distinctly visible at 400× magnification, but inconspicuous or invisible at 100× magnification.

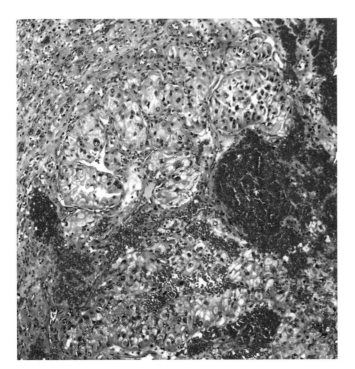

Fig. 2.3 Renal cell carcinoma, ISUP grade 3. Nucleoli are distinctly visible at 100× magnification.

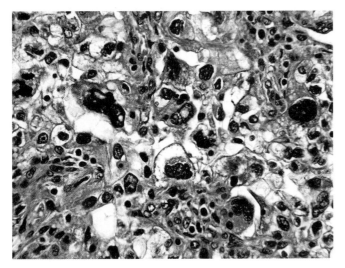

Fig. 2.4 Renal cell carcinoma, ISUP grade 4. Tumor giant cells are present, and extreme nuclear pleomorphism is evident.

high-power field (hpf) showing the highest nucleolar grade or greatest degree of nuclear pleomorphism (Table 2.1). The WHO/ISUP grading system is not applicable for predicting outcome for other types of RCC due to a current paucity of outcome data for those tumors.

Analysis of the utility of the WHO/ISUP system continues. One group of investigators did not find a statistically significant difference in outcome between patients with ISUP grade 1 or 2 and ISUP grade 3 tumors, perhaps, in part, because their dataset did not include cases of multilocular cystic renal neoplasm of low malignant potential (MCRNLMP) or cases of clear cell PRCC (CCPRCC).[59] In contrast, others have found clear separation of

cancer-free survival curves between the four grades of the WHO/ISUP system, and once again found evidence of its superiority over the now-abandoned Fuhrman grading system.[60]

There has been some interest in further refining the accepted WHO/ISUP grading system by amalgamating defined grades with the presence or absence of tumor necrosis (defined as homogeneous clusters and sheets of dead cells, or coalescing groups of cells forming a coagulum, containing nuclear and cytoplasmic debris). Two studies furnished evidence that combining these parameters for cases of CCRCC provides additional prognostic information compared with the use of WHO/ISUP nucleolar grade alone.[59,61]

Staging Renal Cell Carcinoma

Tumor stage reflects the extent of anatomic spread and involvement of disease and is considered to be the most important factor in predicting the clinical behavior and outcome of RCC.[62] Staging systems for RCC have been in use for nearly 50 years and have been continually updated and improved. Since undergoing simplifications and refinements in 1992, the tumor, nodes, and metastasis (TNM) staging system has become the predominant staging system for RCC.[63] In 2017, the eighth edition of the *AJCC Cancer Staging Manual* was published.[64] Staging parameters for carcinomas arising in the kidney are provided, and definitions for primary tumor (T), regional lymph nodes (N), and distant metastasis (M) are given (Table 2.2). T1 and T2 tumors are localized to the kidney and are defined by their greatest dimensions. T1 tumors are ≤7 cm and are subclassified as T1a (≤4 cm) or T1b (>4 cm but ≤7 cm). T2 tumors are more than 7 cm and are subclassified as T2a (>7 cm but ≤10 cm) or T2b (>10 cm). T3 tumors extend beyond the renal parenchyma to involve major veins (renal vein or segmental branches, or vena cava), the pelvicaliceal system (Fig. 2.7), or perinephric tissues, but do not involve the ipsilateral adrenal and do not extend beyond Gerota fascia. T3a tumors conform to this description but do not extend into the vena cava. T3b tumors extend into vena cava below the diaphragm (Fig. 2.8), and T3c tumors extend into vena cava above the diaphragm. T4 tumors invade the ipsilateral adrenal gland directly or invade beyond Gerota fascia (Fig. 2.9). Lymph nodes submitted and uninvolved by tumor define N0; node involvement is staged N1. NX denotes absence of lymph nodes in the surgical specimen. Stage M1 denotes known distant metastases (Figs. 2.10 and 2.11); M0 denotes absence of known distant metastases.

Clear Cell Renal Cell Carcinoma

CCRCC accounts for 60% to 70% of all cases of RCC.[56,65] It is believed to arise in epithelial cells lining the proximal tubule.[66,67] Although patients in all age groups are at risk for its occurrence, the great majority develop in patients older than 40 years, and the majority are males, with a ratio of approximately 1.5:1.[68,69]

More than 90% of cases of CCRCC have characteristic cytogenetic abnormalities that involve loss of genetic material from the short arm of chromosome 3 (3p) and mutations in the VHL gene.[70-76] The VHL gene, which is located at 3p25–26 and functions as a tumor suppressor gene, was identified through studies of patients with VHL disease, and subsequent investigations implied the presence of one or more additional genes near this site.[72,76-78] The VHL gene in CCRCC is typically found to be inactivated by a combination of allelic deletion and either mutation or, less often, hypermethylation.[79,80] Loss of the VHL protein function contributes to tumor initiation, progression, and metastasis.[61] It is suspected that other genes on 3p may act as tumor suppressors and

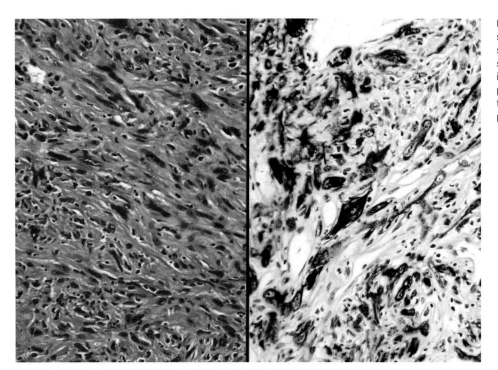

Fig. 2.5 Renal cell carcinoma, ISUP grade 4, sarcomatoid differentiation. There is no consensus regarding the precise definition of sarcomatoid renal cell carcinoma. In this instance, the tumor cells are spindled and pleomorphic, and reminiscent of undifferentiated sarcoma. Tumor cells show strongly positive immunostaining for keratin CAM5.2.

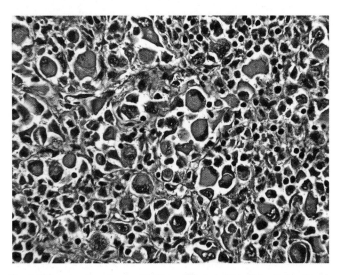

Fig. 2.6 Renal cell carcinoma, ISUP grade 4, rhabdoid differentiation. Tumor cells resemble rhabdomyoblasts Tumor cells are slightly discohesive, with central eosinophilic intracytoplasmic inclusions and large eccentric and irregular nuclei, some of which have prominent nucleoli.

TABLE 2.1	International Society of Urologic Pathology Grading for Clear Cell and Papillary Renal Cell Carcinoma

1. Nucleoli are inconspicuous or absent at 400 × magnification.
2. Nucleoli are distinctly visible at 400 × magnification, but inconspicuous or invisible at 100 × magnification.
3. Nucleoli are distinctly visible at 100 × magnification.
4. Tumor exhibits the presence of tumor giant cells and/or extreme nuclear pleomorphism and/or sarcomatoid differentiation and/or rhabdoid differentiation.

Adapted from Delahunt B, et al. The International Society of Urologic Pathology (ISUP) grading system for renal cell carcinoma and other prognostic parameters. Am J Surg Pathol 2013;37:1490-1504.

may be involved in the development of CCRCC, particularly 3p14.2 deletions, possibly resulting in inactivation of the FHIT gene, as well as another tumor suppressor gene at 3p12.[81] A continuous deletion from 3p14.2–p25, including the FHIT and VHL genes, can be identified in up to 96% of cases.[82] The 3p locus harbors at least four other CCRCC tumor suppressor genes: KD-M6A, KDM5C, SETD2, and PBRM1. After the initiating event involving the 3p gene, additional genetic alterations occur in clonal tumor cell populations as tumor progression occurs and metastatic capability increases. Consequently, these additional genetic abnormalities, when detectable, are often associated with higher histologic grade, higher pathologic stage, and an adverse prognosis. The genetic abnormalities associated with these effects are losses on chromosome 14q, loss of 4p, loss of 9p, and loss-of-function mutations in the *BAP1* gene.[83-86]

There are several familial settings in which CCRCC may arise, the commonest of which is VHL disease. This condition affects 1 in every 36,000 births. It is an autosomal dominant disease associated with the development of retinal angioma, cerebellar and spinal angioma and hemangioblastoma, bilateral multifocal pheochromocytoma, papillary cystadenoma of the epididymis, pancreatic cyst and malignant neuroendocrine tumor, inner ear endolymphatic sac tumor, and renal cyst. In addition, 35% to 45% of affected patients with VHL experience development of bilateral multifocal CCRCC. An average VHL kidney may harbor as many as 1100 cysts and 600 microscopic CCRCCs.[87] Onset of renal carcinoma in patients with VHL is often early; clinically evident renal cancer has been reported in adolescence, and the mean age at diagnosis is 39 years. Historically, without treatment, up to 40% of patients with VHL died of advanced renal carcinoma. In VHL disease, patients are born with a germline defect in one of the two alleles of the VHL gene, located on chromosome 3p925–26,

TABLE 2.2	American Joint Committee on Cancer 2017 TNM Staging of Carcinomas Arising in the Kidney (8th Edition)

Definition of primary tumor (T)

TX Primary tumor cannot be assessed
T0 No evidence of primary tumor
T1 Tumor ≤7 cm in greatest dimension, limited to the kidney
    T1a Tumor ≤4 cm in greatest dimension, limited to the kidney
    T1b Tumor >4 cm but ≤7 cm in greatest dimension, limited to the kidney
T2 Tumor >7 cm in greatest dimension, limited to the kidney
    T2a Tumor >7 cm but ≤10 cm in greatest dimension, limited to the kidney
    T2b Tumor >10 cm, limited to the kidney
T3 Tumor extends into major veins or perinephric tissues, but not into the ipsilateral adrenal gland and not beyond Gerota fascia
    T3a Tumor extends into the renal vein or its segmental branches, or invades the pelvicaliceal system, or invades perirenal and/or renal sinus fat, but not beyond Gerota fascia
    T3b Tumor extends into the vena cava below the diaphragm
    T3c Tumor extends into the vena cava above the diaphragm or invades the wall of the vena cava
T4 Tumor invades beyond Gerota fascia (including contiguous extension into the ipsilateral adrenal gland)

Definition of regional lymph node (N)

NX Regional lymph nodes cannot be assessed
N0 No regional lymph node metastasis
N1 Metastasis in regional lymph node(s)

Definition of distant metastasis (M)

M0 No distant metastasis
M1 Distant metastasis

American Joint Committee on Cancer (AJCC) Prognostic Stage Groups

When T is…	And N is…	And M is…	Stage group is:
T1	N0	M0	I
T1	N1	M0	III
T2	N0	M0	II
T2	N1	M0	III
T3	N0	M0	III
T3	N1	M0	III
T4	Any N	M0	IV
Any T	Any N	M1	IV

Used with permission of the American College of Surgeons, Chicago, Illinois. The original source for this information is the AJCC Cancer Staging Manual, Eighth Edition (2017) published by Springer International Publishing.

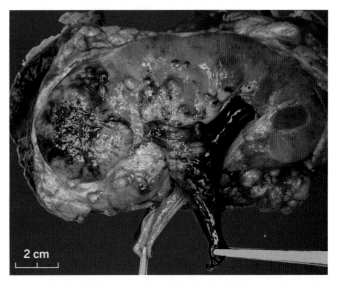

Fig. 2.7 Sarcomatoid clear cell carcinoma extending into renal collecting system. The tumor also had extended into renal vein and inferior vena cava.

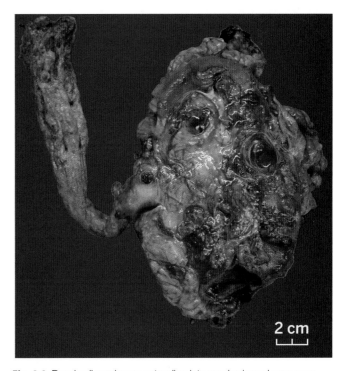

Fig. 2.8 Renal cell carcinoma extending into renal vein and vena cava.

which functions as a tumor suppressor. Loss of the second allele results in clinical disease expression.[87] Additional heritable settings in which CCRCC may develop include Cowden syndrome, Birt-Hogg-Dubé syndrome, families segregating constitutional chromosome 3 translocations, tuberous sclerosis, and families with succinate dehydrogenase B (*SDHB*) deficiency germline mutations.[88,89]

Grossly, CCRCC ranges from a few millimeters to very large, weighing several kilograms; the average size is about 7 cm. It is usually unilateral and unicentric; bilaterality or multicentricity are features of hereditary CCRCC. It commonly forms a bosselated mass that protrudes from the cortical surface (Fig. 2.12). The cut surface is at least in part a characteristic bright golden yellow color, owing to

the abundance of cholesterol, phospholipids, and neutral lipids within the tumor cells. The cut surface is typically variegated with areas of gray-white fibrosis and recent or old hemorrhage. It usually has an expansile pushing growth pattern and is well demarcated from the adjacent normal kidney by a fibrous pseudocapsule of varying thickness; in some cases it may appear to infiltrate the adjacent renal parenchyma (Fig. 2.13). Areas of cystic change and calcification are commonly found, particularly within areas of necrosis.

Microscopically, CCRCC displays a variety of architectural patterns. Tumor cells are arranged most often in sheets, compact nests, alveolar, acinar, and microcystic or macrocystic structures, separated by an abundance of thin-walled blood vessels (Fig. 2.14). Tubular structures are variable in size. Microcysts contain extravasated red blood cells or eosinophilic fluid.

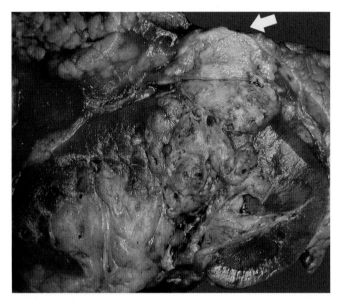

Fig. 2.9 Renal cell carcinoma extending into cortical fat and involving inked Gerota fascia (*arrow*).

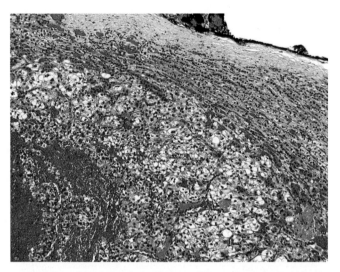

Fig. 2.10 Metastatic renal cell carcinoma. Clear cell renal cell carcinoma involves the adrenal in a radical nephrectomy specimen, not by direct extension.

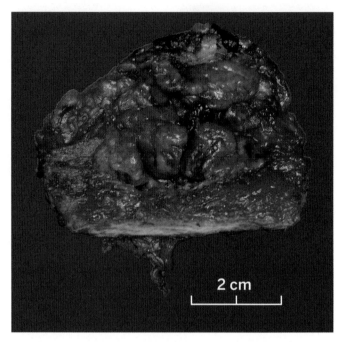

Fig. 2.11 Renal cell carcinoma metastatic to a rib. Tumor was excised because clinically it was a solitary metastasis.

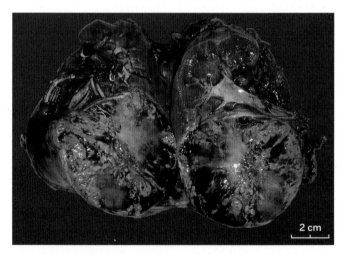

Fig. 2.12 Renal cell carcinoma. Bosselated, well-circumscribed, low-grade clear cell renal cell carcinoma, bright golden yellow with extensive hemorrhage and fibrosis.

Infrequently, small papillary structures lined by clear cells may be present focally but account for an insignificant proportion of the overall architecture.

The classic cell of CCRCC has distinct cell membranes and optically clear cytoplasm due to loss of cytoplasmic lipids and glycogen during histologic processing. Some cases of CCRCC display varying numbers of cells with granular eosinophilic cytoplasm; such cells are more often seen in high-grade cancer or near areas of hemorrhage or necrosis. The nuclei of CCRCC show considerable variation in size, shape, and nucleolar prominence, as discussed in the earlier Grading Renal Cell Carcinoma section, and these features are assessed when assigning a nuclear grade to an individual tumor (Figs. 2.1 through 2.6).

Numerous uncommon histologic variations have been described in CCRCC including heterotopic bone formation (Fig. 2.15), intracellular and extracellular hyaline globules, basophilic cytoplasmic inclusions, abundant multinucleated giant cells, sarcoid-like granulomas, myospherulosis, and lymphomatoid features.[90-98] The significance of these rare findings is unknown.

Immunohistochemically, CCRCC typically shows positive immunostaining for vimentin, CAM5.2, AE1/AE3, RCC-Ma, CD10, PAX2, PAX8, and carbonic anhydrase-IX (CA-IX) (Table 2.3). Immunostains for 34E1β2, cytokeratin 7 (CK7), CK20, mucin 1 (MUC1), parvalbumin, α-methylacyl–coenzyme A racemase (AMACR), kidney-specific cadherin, and CD117 are negative in most cases.[99-114]

Pathologic stage most accurately predicts the prognosis for patients with CCRCC.[53,115,116] Prognosis for tumors within the same stage is further definable by tumor grade, the presence or absence of tumor necrosis, and the presence or absence of

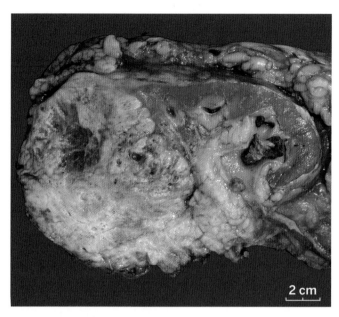

Fig. 2.13 Renal cell carcinoma. High-grade clear cell renal cell carcinoma, not sharply circumscribed, extensively involving renal sinus and perirenal fat, as well as Gerota fascia.

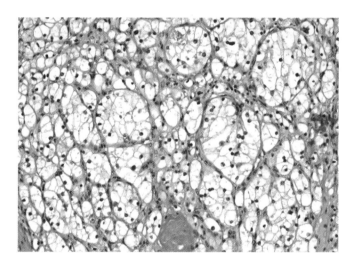

Fig. 2.14 Renal cell carcinoma. Clear cell renal cell carcinoma composed of nests of cells with clear cytoplasm, surrounded by abundant thin-walled blood vessels.

sarcomatoid or rhabdoid differentiation. Grade and tumor necrosis were discussed in the earlier section Grading Renal Cell Carcinoma. Progressively higher tumor grades are associated with progressively worsening prognosis. Tumor necrosis accounting for more than 10% of the total tumor volume is associated with a less favorable outcome. Sarcomatoid differentiation is seen in 5% to 8% of cases of CCRCC.[117] Rhabdoid differentiation is seen in 3% to 7% of RCC overall and is most frequently associated with CCRCC.[117,118] The presence of either sarcomatoid or rhabdoid differentiation worsens the prognosis. Patients whose tumors exhibit sarcomatoid change have a 5-year survival rate of 15% to 22%; for those whose tumors exhibit rhabdoid differentiation, the median survival is 8 to 31 months.[117]

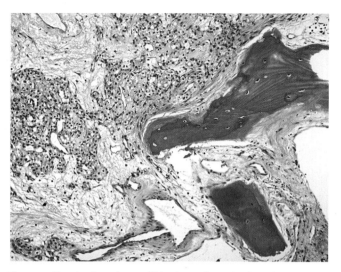

Fig. 2.15 Renal cell carcinoma. This clear cell renal cell carcinoma shows heterotopic bone formation.

Multilocular Cystic Renal Neoplasm of Low Malignant Potential

MCRNLMP is an uncommon renal tumor that was described as an entity distinguishable from conventional CCRCC in 1991.[119] By definition it has a fibrous pseudocapsule, and is composed entirely of cysts and septa with no expansile solid nodules; the septa should contain aggregates of epithelial cells with clear cytoplasm that are indistinguishable from the tumor cells that compose grade 1 RCC.[4] It accounts for less than 1% of all renal tumors and has a male-to-female ratio of approximately 2:1.[120-124] Age range is 20 to 76 years; most patients are in their fifties or sixties, and females tend to present at a younger age than males.

Although most patients are asymptomatic, and their tumors are discovered incidentally, a minority have either a palpable mass, gross hematuria, abdominal or back discomfort, or rarely, systemic symptoms. Laboratory findings may include anemia and microhematuria, but most patients have no laboratory abnormalities. Imaging studies usually reveal a complex cystic mass that may have focal calcification.

Grossly, MCRNLMP ranges from 0.5 to 13.0 cm in greatest dimension. It is typically a unilateral and solitary well-circumscribed mass composed entirely of cysts, separated from adjacent renal parenchyma by a fibrous wall; however, it can be multifocal, as well as bilateral (Fig. 2.16).[124] The cysts are of variable size and contain clear or hemorrhagic fluid. The septa between cysts are thin. Necrosis is absent, and there are no grossly visible nodules expanding the septa, a feature that differentiates this tumor from extensively cystic CCRCC.[125]

Microscopically, the cysts are lined by epithelial cells, usually as a single layer, but occasionally multilayered, and occasionally forming minute papillary structures; some cysts lack any lining cells (Fig. 2.17). The lining cells have variable amounts of cytoplasm that may be clear or lightly eosinophilic; however, the cytologic characteristics of the lining epithelial cells do not constitute part of the criteria for defining MCRNLMP, because renal cystic lesions of many types may sometimes be lined by epithelium with clear cells.[120] The septa consist of fibrous tissue. More than 20% of tumors show calcifications within the septa, and metaplastic bone formation is sometimes observed. Within the septa in all cases there are clusters of epithelial cells with clear cytoplasm (Fig. 2.18).

TABLE 2.3   Selected Immunohistochemical Stainings in Renal Epithelial Neoplasms

	PAX8	CD10	CA-IX	RCC-Ma	Melanocytic markers[a]	Vimentin	CK7	CK20	P63	HMWCK	CD117 (c-kit)	AMACR	GATA3
Clear cell RCC	+	+	+	+	-	+	-	-	-	-	-	-/+	-
Papillary RCC	+	+	+/-	+	-	+	+[b]	-	-	-	-	+	-
Clear cell papillary RCC	+	-[c]	+ (cuplike)	+/-	-	+	+	-	-	+/-	-	-	-
Chromophobe RCC	+	-/+	-	+/-	-	-	+	-	-	-	+	-	+/-
Oncocytoma	+	-/+	-	-	-	-	Focal[d]	-	-	-	+	-/+	-
Angiomyolipoma	-	-	-/+	-	+	-/+	-	-	-	-	-	-	-
ESC RCC	+	-/+	-/+	NA	-	+	-/+	+	-	-	-	-/+	-
Collecting duct carcinoma	+	-	-/+	-	-	+	+/-	-	-/+	+	-	-	-
Tubulocystic carcinoma	+	+	+/-	+	-	+/-	-/+	-	-	-	-	+/-	-
Translocation RCC	+	+/-	-/+	+/-	+/-	+	-	-	-	-	-	+/-	-
MTSCC	+	-/+	-/+	+/-	-	+	+	-	-	-/+	-	+/-	-
UCUUT	-/+[e]	-/+	-/+	-	-	+/-	+	+	+	+	-/+	-/+	+

+, usually positive; -, usually negative; +/-, frequently positive; -/+, occasionally positive; *AMACR*, alpha-methylacyl-CoA racemase (P504S); *CA-IX*, carbonic anhydrase 9; *CK7*, cytokeratin 7; *CK20*, cytokeratin 20; *ESC RCC*, eosinophilic solid and cystic renal cell carcinoma; *HMWCK*, high molecular weight cytokeratin 34βE12; *MTSCC*, mucinous tubular and spindle cell carcinoma; *NA*, not available; *PAX8*, paired box 8 transcription factor; *RCC*, renal cell carcinoma; *RCC-Ma*, renal cell carcinoma marker; *UCUUT*, urothelial carcinoma of the upper urinary tract.
[a]Melanocytic makers include HMB45, Melan-A/Mart-1, tyrosinase A, and microphthalmia-associated transcription factor (*MITF*).
[b]CK7 may be negative in type II papillary RCC.
[c]CD10 can be focally positive in the cyst lining cells of clear cell papillary RCC.
[d]In contrast with diffuse and strong immunoreactivity for CK7 in chromophobe renal cell carcinoma, oncocytoma typically shows scattered focal positivity for CK7(<5% of tumor cells staining).
[e]Approximately 20% to 30% of UCUUTs showed positive staining for PAX8.

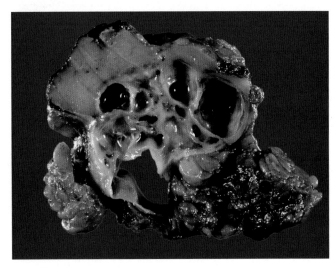

Fig. 2.16 Multilocular cystic renal neoplasm of low malignant potential. This small renal neoplasm is composed entirely of variably sized cysts.

Ploidy studies reveal diploid DNA content in more than 90% of cases.[121] Electron microscopy in one case revealed apical microvilli and other ultrastructural features in the tumor cells that were similar to those seen in conventional CCRCC of the kidney.[120] VHL gene mutations are identifiable in about 25% in MCRNLMP, and there is no difference in the status of chromosome 3p deletion between low-grade CCRCC and MCRNLMP, supporting the concept that MCRNLMP is a subtype of CCRCC.[126,127] Tumor cells of MCRNLMP are strongly immunoreactive for PAX8 and CA-IX.[128]

Only rare cases have shown extension beyond the kidney into the perirenal fat.[121,124] The proper diagnosis hinges on strict adherence to the diagnostic criteria for this entity. There are no reports of recurrence or metastasis of MCRNLMP.[53,120-124] Surgical resection is indicated to exclude extensively cystic RCC.

Papillary Renal Cell Carcinoma

PRCC, the second most common type of RCC, accounts for up to 18.5% of all renal epithelial neoplasms.[53,129-131] Most cases occur sporadically, but some develop in members of families with hereditary PRCC, an inherited renal cancer characterized by mutations in the *MET* oncogene at 7q31 and by a predisposition to development of multiple bilateral papillary renal tumors.[132-137]

The mean age of patients with PRCC ranges from 52 to 66 years, and males are affected slightly more than twice as often as females (2.4:1 male-to-female ratio).[129,138,139] Currently only 5% to 10% of patients diagnosed with PRCC present with flank pain, hematuria, or abdominal mass; discovery is predominantly incidental by various radiologic studies. About 30% of PRCC contain foci of calcification; furthermore, PRCC tends to appear

These cells resemble the cyst lining cells, usually have small, dark nuclei, and do not form expansile nodules; this is a critical feature that distinguishes MCRNLMP from extensively cystic CCRCC (Figs. 2.19 and 2.20).[125] They are often difficult to distinguish from histiocytes or from lymphocytes with surrounding retraction artifact. In difficult cases, the epithelial nature of the tumor cell clusters can be confirmed by their immunoreactivity to antibodies against CK and epithelial membrane antigen (EMA); immunostains for histiocytic markers are negative.[120]

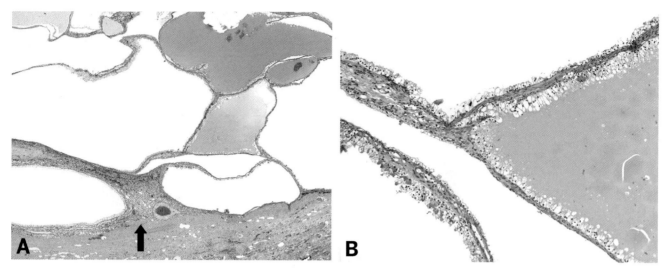

Fig. 2.17 Multilocular cystic renal neoplasm of low malignant potential (A and B). Tumor consists of cysts separated by delicate septa. *Arrow* points to aggregate of neoplastic clear cells.

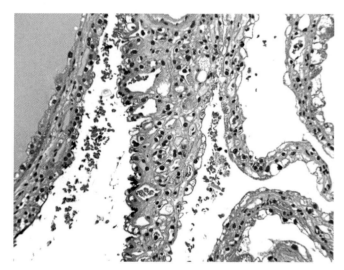

Fig. 2.18 Multilocular cystic renal neoplasm of low malignant potential. The delicate septa are lined by clear cells, and clear cells are present within the septa, but are not forming expansile nodules.

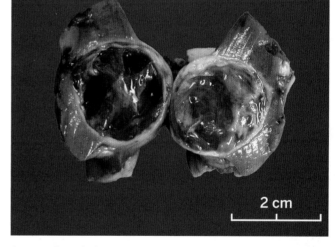

Fig. 2.19 Extensively cystic clear cell renal cell carcinoma. Grossly the differential diagnosis in this case included multilocular cystic renal neoplasm of low malignant potential; however, mural thickening is evident in the cystic portion on the right, and expansile tumor is demonstrated microscopically in Fig. 2.20.

hypovascular on radiologic studies because of spontaneous ischemic necrosis. PRCC is also more likely to be multifocal (8% of cases) and necrotic (46%) than other common RCC subtypes, as well as being overrepresented in end-stage renal disease.[53,140] When multiple papillary tumors are found in patients without a family history of renal tumors, each papillary tumor arises independently; multifocality is not the result of intrarenal metastasis.[141,142] In patients with hereditary papillary renal cancer, it has been estimated that each kidney may harbor as many as 3400 separate microscopic papillary tumors.[133]

Grossly, PRCC is typically well circumscribed, and up to 90% of cases are confined to the renal parenchyma.[53] Multifocality may be grossly evident, particularly in cases of hereditary PRCC (Figs. 2.21 and 2.22).[132,133] A thick, fibrous pseudocapsule is present in up to two-thirds of cases (Fig. 2.23).[138,139,143] The degree of pseudocapsule formation often parallels the extent of hemorrhage and necrosis in the tumor. The cut surface varies from light gray-tan to golden yellow to red-brown, depending on the

preponderance of macrophages in the stroma and the degree of remote hemorrhage and hemosiderin accumulation (Figs. 2.24 and 2.25).

Microscopically, PRCC is composed of varying proportions of papillary and tubular structures and, in some instances, contains cysts with papillary excrescences or with tumor infiltrating the cyst wall (Fig. 2.26).[139] Papillae are lined by a single layer of tumor cells that may sometimes appear pseudostratified.[139,144] The stalks of the papillary structures contain fibrovascular cores and are commonly infiltrated by variable numbers of macrophages; the prevalence of macrophages has no apparent correlation with the extent of accompanying hemorrhage or necrosis. The architectural arrangement of the papillary stalks varies. They may form exquisite and readily recognizable papillae. Compact and tight packing in some tumors results in a solid appearance (Fig. 2.27). In some tumors, the papillae are arranged in long parallel arrays, creating a trabecular appearance (Fig. 2.28).[138]

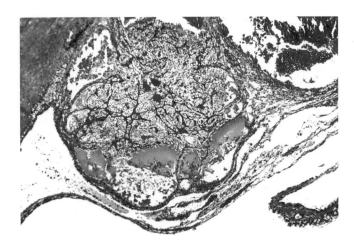

Fig. 2.20 Extensively cystic clear cell renal cell carcinoma (CCRCC). The expansile nodule of CCRCC excludes a diagnosis of multilocular cystic renal neoplasm of low malignant potential.

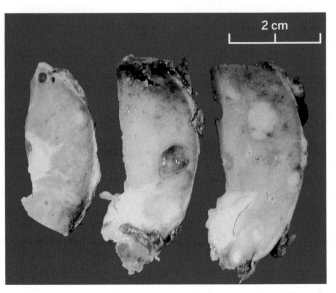

Fig. 2.22 Papillary renal cell carcinoma. Multiple tumors are evident. This was a well-documented case of hereditary papillary renal carcinoma.

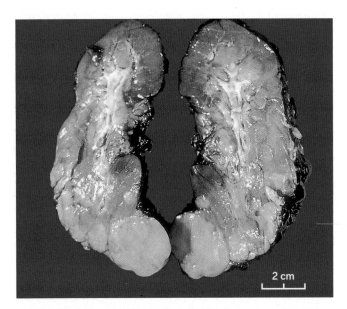

Fig. 2.21 Papillary renal cell carcinoma. Multiple tumors are evident. There was no family history of renal neoplasms.

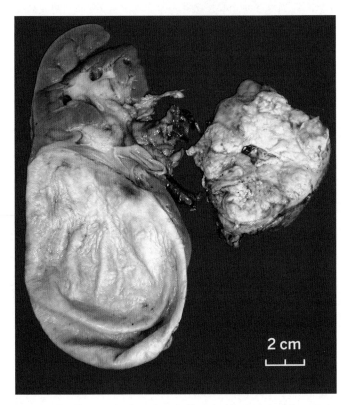

Fig. 2.23 Papillary renal cell carcinoma. Grossly this tumor had the appearance of a thick-walled cyst filled with liquefied bloody material; a sarcomatoid papillary renal carcinoma in the wall had already metastasized to form a large hilar mass.

Infrequently, PRCC exhibits solid areas composed of spindle cells with low-grade nuclear features, admixed with variable amounts of tumor with tubular or papillary architecture.[145,146] In one series of such cases, all were confirmed to be PRCC by molecular studies.[145] It is important to distinguish these tumors from mucinous tubular and spindle cell carcinoma, and to recognize that the low-grade spindle cell proliferations do not represent sarcomatoid change.

For more than two decades, morphologic heterogeneity in histologic grade and cytoplasmic quality (eosinophilic or basophilic) has been recognized in PRCC.[138] Based on studies of morphology, immunohistochemical staining, growth kinetics, clinicopathologic staging parameters, and patient survival data, it was proposed that PRCC could be subclassified into two morphologic variants, which have been designated types 1 and 2 (PRCC1 and PRCC2, respectively).[144,147,148] Notably, both types exhibit tumor-associated acute and chronic inflammation, extensive necrosis,

evidence of recent hemorrhage, psammoma bodies, cholesterol clefts, foreign-body-type giant cells, and areas of dystrophic calcification.[144,147] However, beyond that, there are a number of substantial differences.

PRCC1 is composed of papillae covered by a single or double layer of small epithelial cells of low nuclear grade, bearing small round to ovoid nuclei with inconspicuous nucleoli, and possessing minimal pale or clear cytoplasm (Fig. 2.29). Tubular structures in

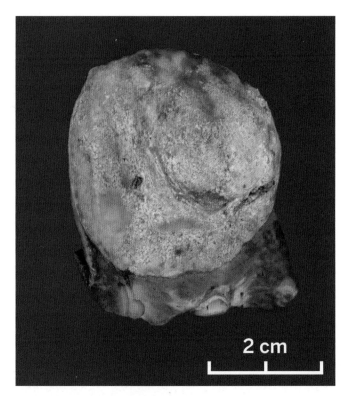

Fig. 2.24 Papillary renal cell carcinoma. Tumor is well circumscribed. The yellow color reflects an abundance of stromal macrophages.

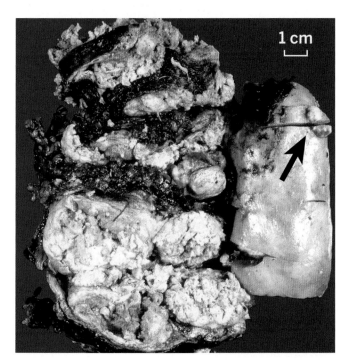

Fig. 2.25 Papillary renal cell carcinoma. The small cortical nodule (*arrow*) was a papillary renal cell carcinoma that had metastasized to form a large hilar mass.

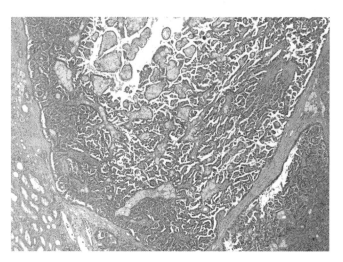

Fig. 2.26 Papillary renal cell carcinoma. This low-power view demonstrates the papillary architecture. Abundant stromal macrophages are evident.

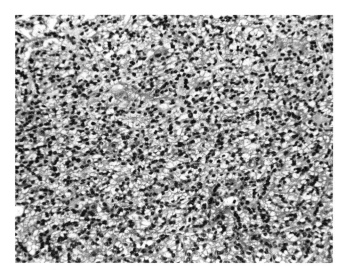

Fig. 2.27 Papillary renal cell carcinoma. In the solid variant, papillae may not be readily evident.

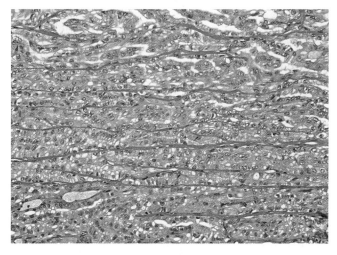

Fig. 2.28 Papillary renal cell carcinoma. Papillary structures are compactly packed into long parallel arrays.

these neoplasms have similar lining cells. The papillae of PRCC1 are usually thin, delicate, and often short, and frequently show expansion by edema fluid.[144,147] The short complex papillae may impart a glomeruloid appearance. Aggregates of foamy macrophages are commonly noted within the papillary cores or

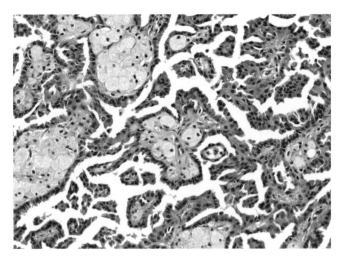

Fig. 2.29 Papillary renal cell carcinoma. In this type 1 tumor the papillae are delicate and are lined by cells with small, dark nuclei and scant cytoplasm. Abundant stromal macrophages are present.

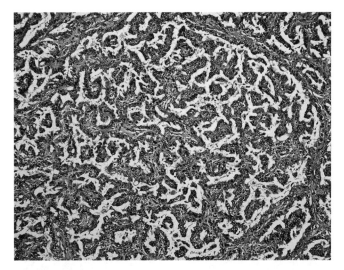

Fig. 2.30 Papillary renal cell carcinoma (PRCC). This section is from a case of familial PRCC. The epithelial cells are small and of low nucleolar grade. Cytoplasm is minimal and eosinophilic. Papillae are thin, delicate, and short.

within sheets of tumor cells. PRCC1 tumor morphology is characteristic of papillary neoplasms that occur in hereditary PRCC (Fig. 2.30).[136]

PRCC2 tends to be larger than PRCC1 (mean diameters, 6 cm for PRCC1 and 9.5 cm for PRCC2) and is of significantly higher nucleolar grade.[144,147] Tumor cells in PRCC2 exhibit large and spherical nuclei, prominent nucleoli, and varying degrees of nuclear pseudostratification. The cytoplasm is abundant and typically eosinophilic (Fig. 2.31). The fibrovascular cores of the majority of PRCC2 tumors tend to be dense and fibrous rather than thin and delicate, and edema and glomeruloid bodies are less prevalent than in PRCC1 tumors. Macrophages, rather than populating the papillae, are more likely to be found near areas of necrosis.

The histologic distinctions noted earlier have been augmented by molecular analysis. PRCC1 exhibits loss of Y chromosome and gains in chromosomes 7, 17, 16, and 20.[149] Activation of the MET pathway is a feature of up to 80% of PRCC1 tumors.[150,151] PRCC2 tumors exhibit a heterogeneous array of chromosomal gains and losses, involving chromosomes 1, 3, 4, 5, 6, 8q, 9, 14, and 15.[150-154]

PRCC2 tumors are more often associated with aggressive clinicopathologic parameters than PRCC1 tumors, including higher TNM stage, larger tumor size, and an overall worse prognosis.[147,148,155] The worsened prognosis for PRCC2 tumors was evident in some studies on univariate analysis, but in other studies the statistical significance of specific tumor subtype was not maintained on multivariate survival analysis when adjusting for grade and stage.[147,148,152,155-157]

Immunohistochemically, PRCCs often expresses AE1/AE3, CK7, CAM5.2, EMA, 34βE12, AMACR, CA-IX, RCC marker (RCC-Ma), CD10, and vimentin (Table 2.3). PRCC1 tumors are more likely than PRCC2 to express CK7 (Fig. 2.32).

The practicality of subtyping PRCC is complicated by the fact that a clearcut distinction may be difficult in some cases.[154,158] In various studies, the proportion of PRCC1 tumors varies between 32% and 70%, and conversely the percentage of PRCC2 tumors ranges from 30% to 68%.[144,148,152,159] Specifically some papillary tumors exhibit nuclear features typical of PRCC1 but cytoplasmic features typical of PRCC2, and some are composed of mixtures of cells of generally low nuclear grade but with substantial variations in cytoplasmic characteristics.[154,158] In short, it seems clear that a

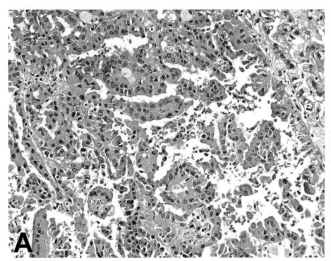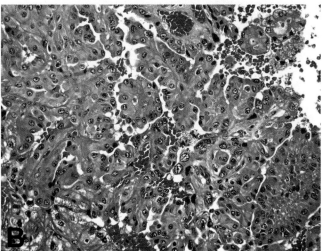

Fig. 2.31 Papillary renal cell carcinoma (A and B). In this type 2 tumor the papillae are thicker and are lined by cells with large irregular nuclei and abundant eosinophilic cytoplasm.

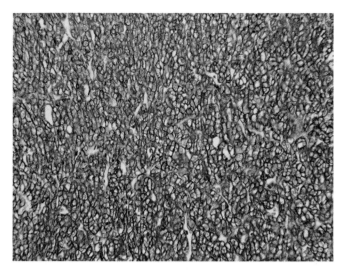

Fig. 2.32 Papillary renal cell carcinoma. Diffuse strongly positive cytokeratin 7 immunostaining is evident in this solid variant of papillary renal carcinoma.

the PRCC, not otherwise specified, category have been developed, indicating that 45% to 47% of PRCCs fall into this category.[150,160] Furthermore, an oncocytic low-grade variant of PRCC has been identified, composed predominantly of tumor cells with oncocytic cytoplasm and round, nonoverlapping low-grade nuclei with inconspicuous nucleoli, and a linear arrangement toward cell apices (Fig. 2.33).[161,162] These tumors resemble PRCC1 molecularly, with similar gains of chromosomes 7 and 17, and clinically, exhibiting indolent behavior, and they have a good prognosis.[160,162,163]

Alternative classifications and suggested classifications of PRCC have been published recently. Based on comprehensive molecular characterization of 161 PRCCs, the Cancer Genome Atlas (TCGA) Research Network showed that PRCC1 and PRCC2 are different types of renal cancer. PRCC1 is associated with MET alterations. Multiple molecular clusters were described within the PRCC2 group. PRCC2 tumors were characterized by CDKN2A silencing, SETD2 mutations, transcription factor E3 (TFE3) fusions, and increased expression of the NRF2-antioxidant response element pathway. A CpG island methylator phenotype was observed in a distinct subgroup of PRCC2 that was characterized by poor survival and mutation of the gene-encoding fumarate hydratase (FH).[151] Disregarding the fact that the TCGA study included tumors that were not conventional PRCCs (specifically translocation carcinomas and FH-deficient carcinomas were included in the study and the report), it seems clear that PRCC2,

number of PRCC cases do not meet the well-accepted histologic criteria for either PRCC1 or PRCC2, and such tumors have been variously designated as mixed, unclassified, overlapping, or not otherwise specified.[151,154,160] Strict histologic criteria for assignment to

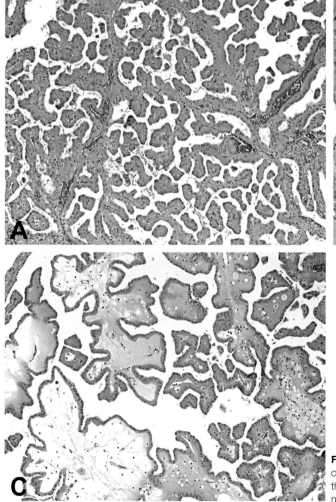

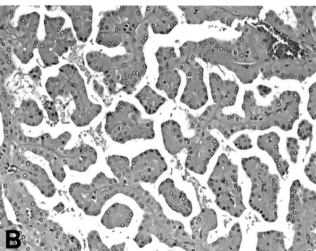

Fig. 2.33 Papillary renal cell carcinoma, oncocytic variant (A to C). Tumor cells have relatively abundant cytoplasm and round nonoverlapping nuclei that are arranged linearly toward the cell apices and bear inconspicuous nucleoli (A to C).

rather than being homogeneous, represents a heterogeneous group of tumors that requires further study.

A recent study using several immunohistochemical stains (CA9, GATA3, and ABCC2), microRNA (miRNA) expression, and copy number variation analysis provided evidence in support of subclassifying PRCC into four subtypes, designated PRCC1, PRCC2, and two new subtypes, PRCC3 and PRCC4/OLG (the latter representing the oncocytic low-grade variant of PRCC noted earlier). PRCC1, PRCC2, and PRCC3 each have unique staining signatures. The PRCC subtypes have different clinical characteristics, justifying their proper stratification.[156]

Compared with other common types of RCC, the cancer-specific survival rates at 5 years after surgery for a large series of patients with CCRCC, PRCC, and chromophobe RCC were 72%, 91%, and 88%, respectively.[164] PRCC has a more favorable outcome than collecting duct carcinoma and HLRCC-RCC.[165,166] Patients with PRCC1 tumors have significantly longer survival than those with PRCC2, but the difference is better related to the stage and grade at presentation than the actual tumor type.[160] ISUP nucleolar grading has been validated for use in pathologic descriptions of PRCC. Sarcomatoid and rhabdoid change are included in ISUP grading as grade 4; grade 4 tumors are associated with decreased survival.

Hereditary Leiomyomatosis and Renal Cell Carcinoma–Associated Renal Cell Carcinoma

Germline mutations of the FH gene at chromosome 1q42 is the underlying genetic abnormality in an inherited autosomal dominant disorder known as HLRCC syndrome. Biallelic inactivation of the gene in FH-mutated cells results in accumulation of fumarate, which reacts spontaneously, via protein succination, with the cysteine sulfhydryl group of proteins to form *S*-2(2-succino)-cysteine (2SC).

These accumulations modulate the activity of various transcription factors, notably HIF1A, NRF2, and AMPK, resulting in increased proliferation and resistance to apoptosis.[167-169]

Cutaneous leiomyomas occur in 76% of family members overall (Fig. 2.34), and uterine leiomyomas arise in 100% of female members. In addition, about 20% to 30% of family members develop a distinctive type of aggressive RCC that is already metastatic in 50% of cases when first diagnosed.[166,170-173]

Renal tumors are, with rare exceptions, unilateral and solitary, rather than multiple and bilateral, as observed in other familial RCC syndromes, and typically there is little in the history of patients with these seemingly sporadic tumors to suggest a familial tendency. Patients with HLRCC renal tumors tend to present at a relatively young age (mean, 36 years), but 25% of patients are older than 50 years at diagnosis.[166] Tumors range in size from 2.3 to 20 cm. Some are cortical, some are medullary, and some involve both regions. The degree of tumor circumscription is widely variable. Cystic or multicystic change is noted infrequently.[165] Histologically, tumors exhibit a wide range of architectural patterns. Intracystic papillary, tubulopapillary, and tubulocystic patterns are most prevalent and characteristic of FH-deficient RCC.[165] Other architectural patterns include papillary, tubular, solid, and cystic elements; collecting duct carcinoma-like areas with infiltrating tubules, nests, and single cells surrounded by desmoplastic stroma; and sarcomatoid change.[166,169,174] The morphologic hallmark of these tumors is the presence of a characteristic large nucleus with a very prominent inclusion-like orangiophilic or eosinophilic nucleolus, surrounded by a clear halo (Fig. 2.35). However, this feature is often not uniformly present throughout the tumor.[169]

An early study of 2SC immunostaining detected positivity for 2SC in various HLRCC-related tumors, but not in normal tissues or a variety of non-HLRCC-related tumors, and predicted genetic

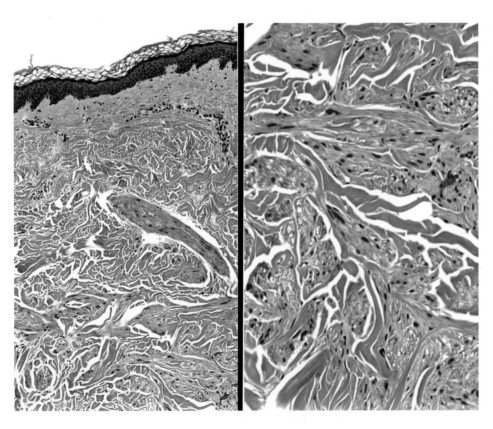

Fig. 2.34 Hereditary leiomyomatosis and renal cell cancer (HLRCC) syndrome. Male patient, aged 48 years, with a history of metastatic renal cell carcinoma, was seen in a dermatology clinic regarding multiple red-brown firm dermal nodules. All six of his female siblings had undergone hysterectomy for leiomyomas. Sections shown here illustrate a dermal leiomyoma. Findings were regarded as probable evidence for HLRCC syndrome. (Courtesy John Miedler, MD.)

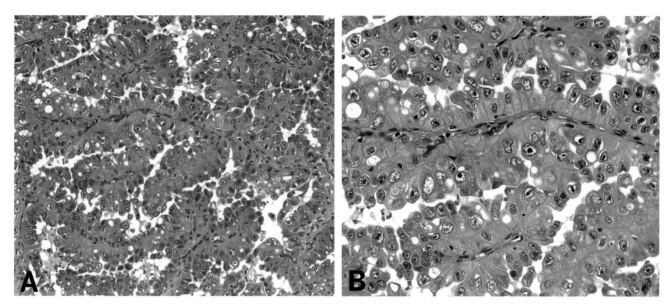

Fig. 2.35 Hereditary leiomyomatosis and renal cell cancer (HLRCC) syndrome. Section from the renal cancer of the patient described in Fig. 2.34 shows a papillary carcinoma, similar to conventional type 2 papillary renal cell carcinoma (A). However, many of the large nuclei exhibit very prominent inclusion-like orangiophilic or eosinophilic nucleoli, surrounded by a clear halo (B).

alterations of the FH gene in patients referred for genetic testing.[175] Subsequently, it was found that all confirmed HLRCC tumors demonstrate diffuse and strong nuclear and cytoplasmic 2SC immunostaining, a finding not present in a wide range of other renal carcinoma types. In addition, positive nuclear and cytoplasmic 2SC staining correlated well with the presence of FH germline mutation. Somatic inactivation of the remaining FH allele is found in HLRCC renal cancers, consistent with the role of FH as a tumor-suppressor gene. Its loss of function in the tumor cells corresponded to strong 2SC staining, whereas adjacent renal parenchyma maintained a wild-type allele and did not show 2SC immunoreactivity.[169]

After reports of loss of FH immunostaining in HLRCC-associated tumors, a study was conducted to ascertain the status of 2SC and FH immunostaining in many high-grade unclassified RCC, unclassified RCC with papillary pattern, and PRCC2.[176-179] One-fifth of renal cancers initially diagnosed as "unclassified RCC, high grade" or "unclassified RCC with papillary pattern" were found to have deficient FH immunostaining, almost invariably accompanied by FH mutations, as well as strong 2SC immunoreactivity. A small minority (0.5%) of tumors previously diagnosed as PRCC and 3% of tumors previously diagnosed as PRCC2 showed FH deficiency by immunostaining and FH mutations.[179] Furthermore, the FH-deficient RCC exhibited considerable clinicopathologic similarities with well-documented cases of HLRCC-associated RCC. Further testing confirmed an association with HLRCC syndrome in about one-third of patients with FH-deficient RCC in this study.[179] Evaluation of both FH and 2SC immunostaining status appears to be warranted in cases exhibiting the morphologic and clinical features noted earlier.

As noted later in the Tubulocystic Renal Cell Carcinoma section, about 50% of poorly differentiated renal carcinomas with areas resembling classic tubulocystic carcinoma exhibit loss of FH immunoreactivity and positive 2SC immunostaining.[180] The term *FH-deficient RCC* has been proposed provisionally for tumors with a combination of suggestive morphology and immunophenotype but where genetic confirmation is unavailable at the time of diagnosis.[180]

HLRCC-RCC is a lethal disease with rapid aggressive growth and early metastasis even when the tumor is small.[166] The majority of patients present with advanced stage disease and succumb to their cancers. Consequently, recognition of the characteristic features of this tumor are important not only in managing the affected patient but in counseling and follow-up of family members. Aggressive excision of even small tumors in syndromic patients is warranted.

Chromophobe Renal Cell Carcinoma

Chromophobe cells were first described in chemically induced renal tumors in rats.[181] Chromophobe RCC was first reported in 1985; its name was derived from the morphologic similarity between the predominant tumor cells in the human tumor to those comprising the experimentally produced rat kidney tumor.[182] Subsequently, the eosinophilic variant was described in 1988.[183]

Genomic studies indicate that chromophobe RCC arises from cells of the distal nephron.[184] Most cases arise sporadically. Some are associated with an folliculin (FLCN) germline mutation in the autosomal dominant cancer predisposition Birt-Hogg-Dubé syndrome, characterized by hair follicle fibrofolliculomas (mainly on the face and neck) and a predisposition to development of bilateral multifocal renal tumors, as well as pulmonary cysts, that can give rise to spontaneous pneumothorax.[185] Chromophobe RCC comprises approximately 34% of the renal neoplasms that occur in patients with this syndrome; the remaining neoplasms include oncocytoma (7%), CCRCC (9%), and tumors with features that resemble a mixture of oncocytoma and chromophobe carcinoma (50%). Another hereditary predisposition to development of chromophobe RCC results from a germline mutation of PTEN in Cowden syndrome.[186]

Chromophobe RCC accounts for 4.9% of surgically excised renal epithelial neoplasms. It comprises a higher proportion of renal cancers in the Middle East. Patients range in age from childhood to extreme old age, with a slight male preponderance.[131,187-192] The majority of cases are found incidentally. Symptomatic patients typically report flank pain or gross hematuria; rarely a mass is palpable, or weight loss has occurred. Paraneoplastic symptoms are generally absent. Radiologically, there are no features that reliably distinguish chromophobe RCC from other renal epithelial neoplasms (see later Oncocytoma section with respect to [99m] Tc-sestamibi single-photon emission computed tomography/computed tomography [SPECT/CT] scanning).

Sporadic chromophobe RCC is typically solitary, with rare exceptions. Tumors are well circumscribed and vary widely in size, from 1.5 to 25 cm in diameter; mean diameter ranges from 6.9 to 8.5 cm.[131,187-189,191,192] The cut surface is usually solid, homogeneous, and light brown or beige; less often the tumor is mahogany brown, gray-tan, light pink, or yellow-white (Figs. 2.36 and 2.37). A minority show hemorrhage or necrosis, and these features, when present, are limited in extent. An area of central scarring is infrequently present.

Microscopically, the tumor cells of chromophobe RCC are typically arranged in solid sheets; in some cases, areas of tubulocystic architecture are present.[182] Tumors are intersected randomly by delicate to broad fibrous septa and blood vessels that are predominantly of medium caliber, in contrast with the small sinusoidal vessels that are seen in CCRCC (Fig. 2.38).[193,194]

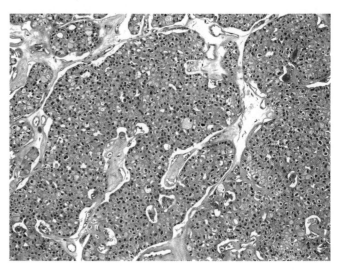

Fig. 2.38 Chromophobe renal cell carcinoma. Sheets of tumor cells are intersected by delicate to broad fibrous septa.

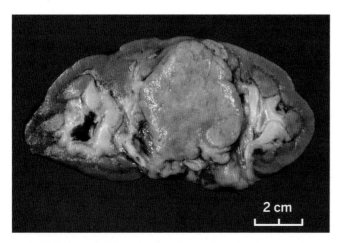

Fig. 2.36 Chromophobe renal cell carcinoma. This classic type of chromophobe carcinoma is tan and well circumscribed.

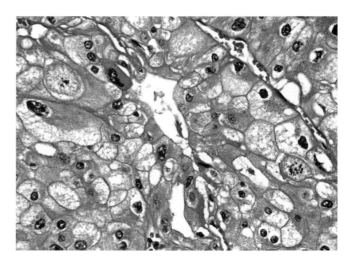

Fig. 2.39 Chromophobe renal cell carcinoma. Numerous chromophobe cells have abundant flocculent cytoplasm and sharply outlined plantlike cell membranes.

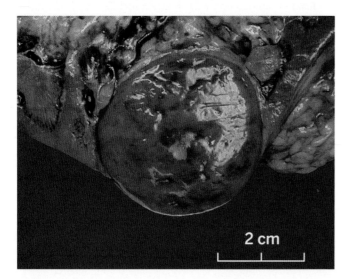

Fig. 2.37 Chromophobe renal cell carcinoma. This eosinophilic type of chromophobe carcinoma is mahogany and well circumscribed.

Two types of tumor cells may be present in varying proportions. One type, the chromophobe cell, is a large polygonal cell with abundant, almost transparent and slightly flocculent cytoplasm and prominent, often "plantlike" cell membranes (Fig. 2.39). The chromophobe cells are frequently found adjacent to vascular channels. Usually they are admixed with a second population of smaller cells with less abundant cytoplasm that is granular and eosinophilic (Fig. 2.40). This combination of cell types characterizes the "typical" variant of chromophobe RCC.[182] The nuclei of both cell types are typically hyperchromatic with irregular wrinkled nuclear contours; binucleation is common. Perinuclear halos are frequently present in the more eosinophilic cells, and this feature can be of considerable diagnostic importance.

A variant of chromophobe RCC that is virtually entirely composed of intensively eosinophilic cells with prominent cell membranes has been designated as the eosinophilic variant of this neoplasm (Figs. 2.41 and 2.42).[183] In some cases of this variant the problem of making a distinction from oncocytoma is compounded by areas of tumor architecture that entirely mimic that

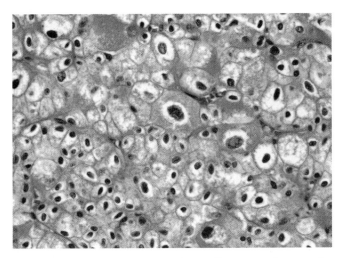

Fig. 2.40 Chromophobe renal cell carcinoma. The tumor cells are smaller, with more densely granular eosinophilic cytoplasm, raisinoid nuclei, and perinuclear halos.

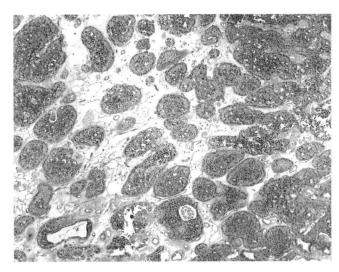

Fig. 2.43 Chromophobe renal cell carcinoma. The compact tumor cell nests in this chromophobe carcinoma mimic the findings in oncocytoma (same patient as in Fig. 2.42).

entity (Fig. 2.43). It may be difficult to distinguish chromophobe RCC, especially the so-called eosinophilic variant of chromophobe RCC, from oncocytoma. Strong diffusely positive tumor cell immunoreactivity for CK7 is supportive of a diagnosis of eosinophilic variant of chromophobe RCC (see later Oncocytoma section) (Fig. 2.44). Hale's colloidal iron stainings are positive in chromophobe RCC and negative in oncocytoma.

Sarcomatoid transformation, a feature common to other types of RCC, may be found in up to 9% of cases, and in certain geographic locations, it may be unusually prevalent (Fig. 2.45).[195-198] Rare cases with osteosarcoma-like differentiation, rhabdoid differentiation, or extensive calcification and ossification have been reported.[101,199,200] The ISUP has recommended that chromophobe RCC should not be graded.[117]

Some renal neoplasms exhibit mixed morphologies, with elements suggestive of oncocytoma and chromophobe RCC in the same tumor, and have been referred to as hybrid oncocytic/chromophobe tumors.[201-203] Such tumors arise in several distinct

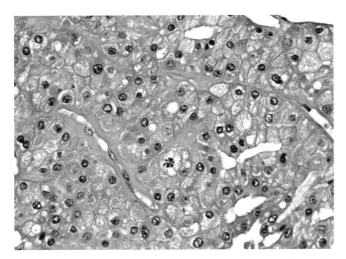

Fig. 2.41 Chromophobe renal cell carcinoma. This eosinophilic variant closely mimicked oncocytoma, but mitotic figures were readily evident in parts of the tumor.

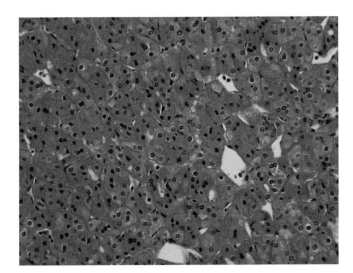

Fig. 2.42 Chromophobe renal cell carcinoma. This eosinophilic variant closely mimicked oncocytoma, but it showed strong and diffusely positive immunostaining for cytokeratin 7.

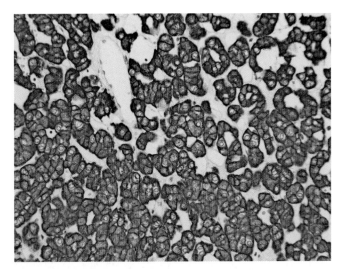

Fig. 2.44 Chromophobe renal cell carcinoma. Typically chromophobe carcinoma shows strongly and diffusely positive immunostaining for cytokeratin 7.

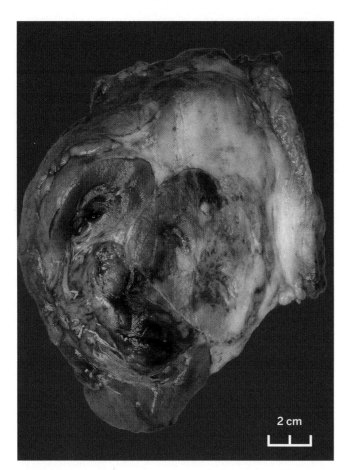

Fig. 2.45 Chromophobe renal cell carcinoma. Sarcomatoid differentiation was evident in this large chromophobe carcinoma. The patient died of cancer less than 3 months after nephrectomy.

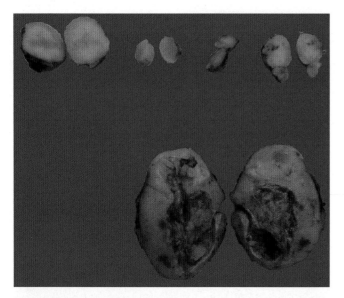

Fig. 2.46 Birt-hogg-dubé oncocytic tumors. Female, aged 29 years, who had eight oncocytic tumors removed from her left kidney at age 26 years, underwent excision of five additional oncocytic tumors from her right kidney, shown here. (Image courtesy Bhunesh Maheshwari, MD.)

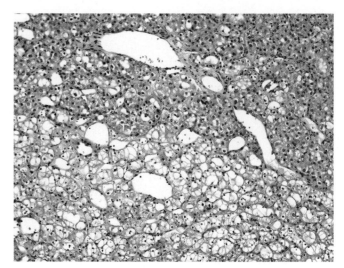

Fig. 2.47 Hybrid oncocytic chromophobe tumor. Section from a renal neoplasm in a patient with Birt-Hogg-Dubé syndrome shows an admixture of eosinophilic cells with round nuclei resembling oncocytes and cells with clear or lightly eosinophilic cytoplasm and prominent nuclear membranes, reminiscent of chromophobe renal cell carcinoma.

settings: as tumors present in cases of renal oncocytosis, as tumors arising in patients with Birt-Hogg-Dubé syndrome (Fig. 2.46), and as sporadic tumors.[204-206] Descriptions of hybrid oncocytic/chromophobe tumors vary somewhat with the setting in which they arise, but a common theme is the admixture of tumor cells resembling typical oncocytoma with tumor cells resembling chromophobe RCC, either gradually transitioning from one morphology to another, or as fairly distinctly separate tumor cell clusters adjacent to one another, or intimately admixed with one another (Fig. 2.47). Remarkably, despite somewhat overlapping morphologies, tumors from all three groups have different molecular genetic makeups, and their molecular signatures are different from those of oncocytoma and chromophobe RCC.[203,206,207] The precise nature of these tumors awaits further elucidation. Available data on follow-up of patients with hybrid oncocytic/chromophobe tumors indicate that tumors in all three groups exhibit indolent behavior.

Ultrastructurally, chromophobe cells contain numerous round, ovoid, or elongate microvesicles ranging from 150 to 300 nm in diameter, scant numbers of small mitochondria with tubulovesicular cristae, and rare glycogen particles.[183,208] The nature and origin of the microvesicles are unknown; it is postulated that they are derived from mitochondria.[182] Eosinophilic cells have fewer microvesicles and more abundant mitochondria with tubulovesicular or lamellar cristae.[183,199]

The genetic abnormality most consistently observed in chromophobe RCC has been loss of one copy of the entire chromosome for most or all of the chromosomes 1, 2, 6, 10, 13, 17, and 21 (in 86% of cases), as well as losses of various other chromosomes (at frequencies varying from 12% to 58% of cases).[183,184,209-225] Chromosomal losses result in a hypodiploid DNA index.[111,113,188] Sarcomatoid chromophobe RCC frequently has multiple gains (polysomy) of chromosomes 1, 2, 6, 10, and 17; distant metastases in cases of metastatic chromophobe RCC show the same genetic patterns, usually chromosomal losses (monosomy), as are found in the primary tumors.[223] About one-half of cases of the eosinophilic variant of chromophobe RCC do not share the same chromosomal abnormalities as the classic type.[184]

Chromophobe RCC virtually always shows positive immunohistochemical staining for PAX8, CD117 (ckit), pancytokeratin, EMA, and parvalbumin, and negative immunostaining for vimentin, CK20, and AMACR (Table 2.3).[99-101,108,112,113,226,227] Hale colloidal iron stainings are positive in chromophobe RCC. The use of immunostaining in distinguishing chromophobe RCC from oncocytoma is discussed in the Oncocytoma section. The most useful staining is CK7. CK7 are typically diffusely positive in chromophobe RCC, in contrast with oncocytomas, which usually show focal scattered stainings (<5% of tumor areas). Oncocytoma is negative for Hale colloidal iron stainings.

Genetic analysis allows separation of these entities based on the finding that oncocytomas do not demonstrate combined losses of heterozygosity at chromosomes 1, 2, 6, 10, 13, 17, and 21, characteristic of chromophobe RCC.[228] Fluorescence in situ hybridization (FISH) studies indicate that detection of losses of chromosomes 2, 6, 10, or 17 effectively excludes the diagnosis of oncocytoma and supports the diagnosis of chromophobe RCC.[209]

A more recent study demonstrated that approximately 70% of chromophobe RCCs carry either a hemizygous deletion of RB1 or ERBB4, and no oncocytomas showed the deletions of these genes.[229] The combined use of RB1 and ERBB4 FISH to detect deletion of these genes may offer a highly sensitive and specific assay to distinguish chromophobe RCC from oncocytoma.[229]

The prognosis for chromophobe RCC has been shown in a number of large series to be significantly better than for CCRCC, and there is no significant difference in outcome between the typical and the eosinophilic variants of chromophobe RCC.[53,131,189] Stage at presentation with chromophobe RCC is usually significantly lower than with CCRCC. Only 4% of patients with chromophobe RCC present with metastases, compared with 27% of patients with CCRCC. The cancer-specific survival rate for chromophobe RCC at 5 years after nephrectomy is about 90%.[53] Adverse risk factors for survival include histologic tumor necrosis and sarcomatoid change. Metastatic chromophobe RCCs have been found to be enriched for TP53 mutations, PTEN mutations, and imbalanced chromosome duplications (duplication of three or more chromosomes).[230] Median cancer-specific survival for patients with metastatic chromophobe RCC is 0.6 year, similar to the prognosis for patients with other types of metastatic RCC.

Collecting Duct Carcinoma

A formal description of collecting duct carcinoma was first published in 1986.[231] This neoplasm arises in the principal cells of the collecting ducts of Bellini. It accounts for less than 1% of renal malignancies. Patients range in age from 13 to 87 years of age, with a mean age of 55 years. Collecting duct carcinoma occurs more commonly in males, with a male-to-female ratio of at least 2:1.[165,232,233] Although up to 25% of cases are discovered incidentally, the majority of patients present with symptoms, including abdominal or flank pain and hematuria. Less common symptoms include weight loss, fatigue, fever, musculoskeletal pain, anorexia, and gastrointestinal disturbances, and rarely the presenting symptoms are those of metastatic cancer.[232,234,235] Imaging studies usually demonstrate a predominantly solid mass consistent with renal carcinoma.[232,236,237] Urine cytology is positive for malignant cells in a small percentage of cases.[233,238,239] Bone metastases, which may be present at the time of diagnosis, are often osteoblastic.

Small collecting duct carcinomas are usually located centrally and may be localized to a medullary pyramid. However, collecting ducts extend from the medulla to the cortex, and therefore

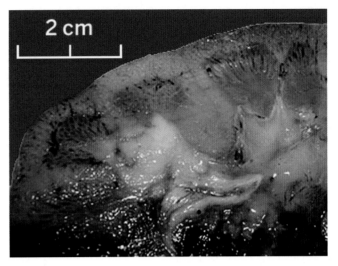

Fig. 2.48 Collecting duct carcinoma. A gray-white tumor with ill-defined borders occupies a medullary pyramid. (Courtesy Rodolfo Montironi, MD.)

collecting duct carcinoma can originate anywhere in the parenchyma, and identification of the site of origin may not be possible, particularly in large tumors. Tumors range from 1 to 16 cm in greatest dimension.[232,233] The cut surface of collecting duct carcinoma is usually gray-white and firm, and areas of necrosis may be evident (Fig. 2.48). Tumor borders are irregular and indistinct. Intrarenal metastases may be evident as satellite tumor nodules. Tumor involvement of the adrenal gland, perirenal fat, renal sinus fat, renal pelvis, Gerota fascia, renal vein, or regional lymph nodes is grossly evident in most cases.

Microscopically, collecting duct carcinoma has an ill-defined border, with extensive infiltration of adjacent parenchyma and frequently an interstitial growth pattern with preservation of glomeruli.[165] Usually there is an acute and chronic inflammatory cell infiltrate at the interface between tumor and normal parenchyma (Figs. 2.49 and 2.50). Pronounced stromal desmoplasia is a constant feature (Fig. 2.50). A variety of growth patterns may coexist within a given tumor. Tumors may grow in solid sheets/cords/nests, form tubulopapillary structures, or infiltrate desmoplastic stroma as small to medium-sized elongated tubules, but do not

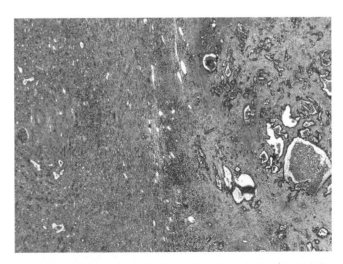

Fig. 2.49 Collecting duct carcinoma. At low power, tumor demonstrates complex tubulopapillary architecture and a pronounced inflammatory reaction at the interface between tumor and normal kidney.

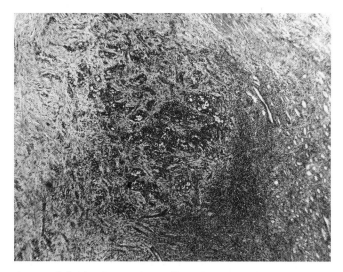

Fig. 2.50 Collecting duct carcinoma. Tumor is composed of tubulopapillary structures in a background of pronounced stromal desmoplasia; there is an intense inflammatory reaction at the interface between tumor and normal kidney.

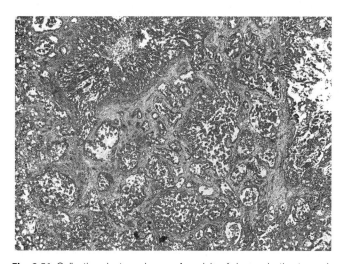

Fig. 2.51 Collecting duct carcinoma. A nodule of desmoplastic stroma is infiltrated by a tumor with predominantly papillary architecture.

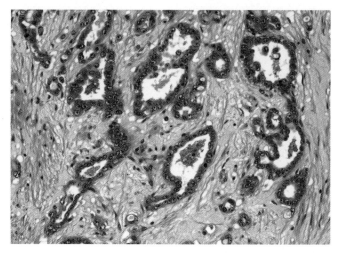

Fig. 2.52 Collecting duct carcinoma. Tumor cells lining the malignant tubules are of high nuclear grade.

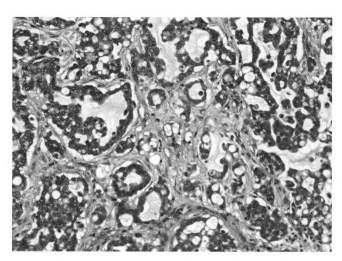

Fig. 2.53 Collecting duct carcinoma. Wispy mucin can be seen in the tubules.

exhibit the type of tubulocystic architecture that typifies tubulocystic carcinoma.[165] The presence of multiple nodules of desmoplastic stroma infiltrated by papillary tumor is a feature somewhat distinctive for collecting duct carcinoma (Fig. 2.51).[165] Some tumors have microcysts with intracystic papillary proliferations of high-grade carcinoma. Some tumors show intratubular extension with microscopic subcapsular deposits distant from the main tumor. The epithelium lining native ducts adjacent to or distant from the main tumor mass may show marked cytologic atypia or frank carcinoma in situ. Tumor cells are almost always of high nuclear grade, with nuclear pleomorphism and prominent nucleoli and varying amounts of eosinophilic cytoplasm (Fig. 2.52). Cells lining luminal structures may display a hobnail appearance, a finding that is not typical of other types of RCC. Small vessel invasion is common, and renal vein involvement is evident in about 20% to 44% of cases.[165,232] The incidence of sarcomatoid change varies from 16% to 36%.[198,240,241]

Mucin is often demonstrable by mucicarmine, Alcian blue, or undigested periodic acid–Schiff stains, within the tumor

cell cytoplasm, at the luminal borders, or extracellularly (Fig. 2.53).[231,242,243]

A diagnosis of collecting duct carcinoma is challenging, in that several other entities enter the differential (Table 2.4). Metastatic adenocarcinoma must be excluded on clinical grounds. High-grade urothelial carcinoma must be excluded by generous sampling of the pelvicaliceal system. An immunohistochemical panel of PAX8,

TABLE 2.4	Diagnostic Criteria for Collecting Duct Carcinoma

1. Medullary involvement
2. Predominantly tubular morphology
3. Desmoplastic stromal reaction
4. Cytologically high grade
5. Infiltrative growth pattern
6. Absence of other renal cell carcinoma subtypes or urothelial carcinoma

Adapted from Moch H, Humphrey PA, Ulbright TM, Reuter VE, eds. *WHO Classification of Tumors of the Urinary System and Male Genital Organs.* Lyon: IARC; 2016:31-32.

p63, and GATA3 may assist: tumors that are GATA3[+] or p63[+] and PAX8[-] are more likely urothelial, whereas collecting duct carcinoma is likely to be PAX8[+], p63[-], and GATA3[-] (Table 2.3). [244,245] Unfortunately, PAX8 has also been noted in urothelial carcinomas of the renal pelvis. [246] Tumors expressing both PAX8 and S100 protein are highly likely to be of renal origin, and use of this panel may assist in excluding urothelial carcinoma. [165] In confirming a diagnosis of collecting duct carcinoma, renal medullary carcinoma (RMC) must be considered and excluded. This issue is addressed later in the Renal Medullary Carcinoma section. Finally, recent experience with aggressive high-grade renal cancers has shown that as many as 25% previously diagnosed as collecting duct carcinoma are in fact examples of FH-deficient RCC. [165] These tumors are addressed more fully in the Hereditary Leiomyomatosis and Renal Cell Carcinoma–Associated Renal Cell Carcinoma section. Consequently, immunostains for FH and 2SC should be performed on tumors suspected of being collecting duct carcinoma, complemented as needed by molecular genetic testing for FH mutations. In short, a diagnosis of collecting duct carcinoma is most confidently rendered after exclusion of metastatic adenocarcinoma, urothelial carcinoma of the pelvicaliceal system, RMC, and FH-deficient RCC. [165]

The reported molecular changes in collecting duct carcinoma are markedly variable and limited, and no distinctive molecular mechanism or pathway has been proposed for collecting duct carcinoma. [247]

The prognosis for collecting duct carcinoma is poor. Tumor stage is often advanced at the time of presentation; in one series 91% were pT3 or pT4 when initially diagnosed. [165] Nearly 50% of patients have nodal or distant metastases at the time of initial diagnosis. [165,232,233] Lung, bone, and brain are common sites of metastasis. [165] Approximately two-thirds of patients with collecting duct carcinoma die of cancer within 2 years, and mortality rates as high as 83% have been reported by some investigators. [234]

Renal Medullary Carcinoma

First reported in 1995, RMC is an uncommon, highly aggressive renal malignancy. [248] It is believed to arise in the terminal collecting ducts and their adjacent papillary epithelium. [165,248-252] Its occurrence is very strongly associated with sickle cell hemoglobinopathies, so it has been postulated that the earlier-noted epithelium suffers chronic ischemic damage related to sickling erythrocytes, and that RMC originates in a setting of chronic regenerative proliferation of this damaged epithelium. The majority of affected patients have been African Americans with sickle cell trait (HbAS) or hemoglobin SC disease (HbSC), but it has also been reported in a patient with sickle cell disease (HbSS). [247,249,253]

Most reported patients with RMC are in their second and third decades of life (range, 5 to 58 years); mean age at diagnosis is approximately 20 years. The male-to-female ratio is at least 2:1, and for reasons that are inapparent, about 75% of tumors occur on the right and 25% occur on the left. [254] The patients are most commonly of African ancestry, but individuals of Central and South American and Mediterranean ancestry are also at risk for RMC. In reported cases in which sickle cell status was known, 87% had sickle cell trait (HbAS), 9% had hemoglobin SC disease (HbSC), and 4% had sickle cell disease (HbSS).

Abdominal or flank pain (52%), gross hematuria (52%), and weight loss (23%) are the most common presenting symptoms. [254] Fever, nausea, and vomiting are also common, and about 10% of patients have a palpable abdominal mass. [248,249,252,253,255]

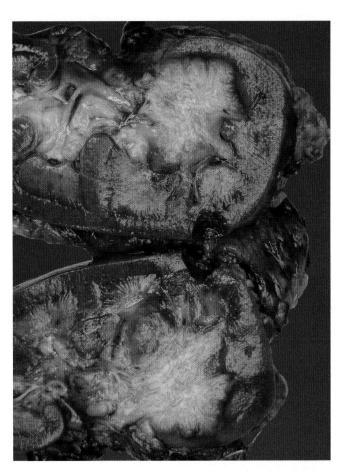

Fig. 2.54 Renal medullary carcinoma. Medullary-based tumor in a 34-year-old African American woman with sickle cell trait, presenting with hematuria.

Duration of symptoms before diagnosis ranges from 2 days to 60 weeks, but the median is relatively short (8 weeks).

Grossly, these tumors typically occupy the renal medulla and are poorly circumscribed, lobulated, firm to rubbery, tan to gray, with varying degrees of hemorrhage and necrosis (Fig. 2.54). They range in size from 1.8 to 13 cm in greatest dimension, with a mean of 7 cm. [249,256,257] Satellite nodules are commonly present, as is extension into the perinephric and sinus fat. Microscopically, they demonstrate a variety of morphologic patterns. The most characteristic finding is a reticular or microcystic growth pattern that resembles yolk sac tumor of the testis. Sievelike/cribriform growth patterns are also commonly noted. Other common patterns include tubule formation and growth in solid sheets, cords, or nests. Tumor cells are typically pleomorphic, with large nuclei, prominent nucleoli, and varying amounts of eosinophilic cytoplasm. Tumor cells may have a squamoid or rhabdoid appearance, particularly in areas of sheetlike growth. Abundant neutrophils may be noted within the tumor, and there is often an intense inflammatory response at the interface between tumor and the adjacent renal parenchyma (Fig. 2.55). The tumor incites a prominent desmoplastic stromal reaction. Varying degrees of mucin production are evident in most RMCs (Fig. 2.56). In most histologic sections, sickled erythrocytes are identified (Fig. 2.57).

Tumor cells in all cases show positive immunostaining for PAX8. Loss of expression of SMARCB1 (INI1), a nuclear transcription regulator encoded on chromosome 22, is considered to be a necessary criterion for a diagnosis of RMC (Fig. 2.58). [165] This is due to loss of heterozygosity or hemizygous deletions

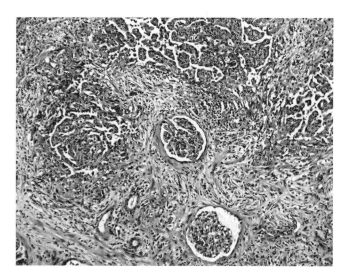

Fig. 2.55 Renal medullary carcinoma. Tumor freely infiltrates renal interstitium and shows complex tubulopapillary architecture. The stroma shows prominent desmoplasia.

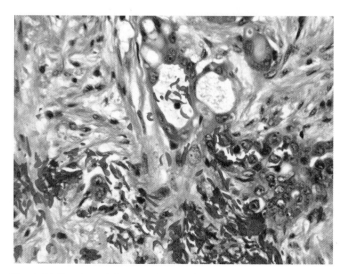

Fig. 2.57 Renal medullary carcinoma. Sickled erythrocytes are readily apparent.

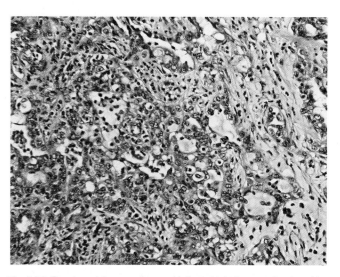

Fig. 2.56 Renal medullary carcinoma. Malignant tubules contain wispy blue mucin. A substantial infiltrate of neutrophils is present.

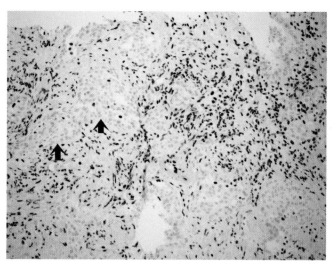

Fig. 2.58 Renal medullary carcinoma. In a core biopsy specimen, tumor cells (*arrows*) exhibit loss of INI1 immunostaining. Background nonneoplastic cells show normal (positive) immunostaining.

at the SMARCB1 locus, and in rare instances, loss of chromosome 22.[258] In one study, inactivation of the *SMARCB1* gene was shown to be due to interchromosomal balanced translocations.[259] In the same study, whole exome sequencing showed that RMC has no other recurrent genetic alterations and an overall stable genome, underscoring the oncogenic potency of *SMARCB1* inactivation.[259] Between 40% and 70% of RMCs show positive immunostaining for OCT3/4 (also known as POU5F1).[165,260] Variable degrees of positive immunostaining are noted for AE1/AE3 and CAM5.2, CK7, CK20, polyclonal carcinoembryonic antigen (CEA), *Ulex europaeus* agglutinin (UEA-1), and EMA.[247,249,250,255,261]

In view of the fact that 95% of patients with RMC have metastatic cancer at the time of diagnosis or shortly thereafter, it is not surprising that the prognosis for this neoplasm is poor.[254] Common sites of metastasis are lymph nodes, lung, liver, and adrenals. Long-term disease-free survival is rare; survival ranges from 2 to 68 weeks,

with a mean survival duration of 19 weeks.[247,256,257] Survival is somewhat longer overall in patients given adjuvant therapy, but is usually limited in duration, and even in cases of prolonged remission, recurrence and death are the usual outcome.[262,263]

There is some overlap in the clinical and pathologic features of collecting duct carcinoma and RMC, prompting speculation that RMC is a subtype of collecting duct carcinoma.[247,264] Some investigators have adopted the stance that loss of SMARCB1 immunostaining and documentation of hemoglobinopathy by history and appropriate laboratory studies, and evidence of diffuse sickling within the tumor stroma as well as blood vessels, are of paramount importance in making a diagnosis of RMC.[165] The rare tumors that exhibit RMC-like histology, SMARCB1-deficient immunophenotype, and aggressive clinical features but arising in patients in whom sickle cell trait or disease has been rigorously excluded are designated as RCC, unclassified, with medullary phenotype.[4,165]

MiT Family Translocation Renal Cell Carcinoma

Tumors in this class of RCCs are characterized by gene fusions involving *TFE3* or *TFEB*, two members of the MiT family of transcription factors.[265] Translocation renal cell carcinomas (TRCCs) that are associated with Xp11 translocations harbor gene fusions involving *TFE3*, and those with t(6;11) translocation harbor a *MALAT1-TFEB* gene fusion. The t(6;11) TRCCs are less common than Xp11 TRCCs.

Although the majority of patients with TRCC are younger than 50 years, patients up to 79 years of age have been reported.[266-270] Translocation carcinoma occurs with approximately equal frequency in males and females, and in some patients its development has been associated with prior chemotherapy treatment.[271-274] About one-half of patients present with abdominal or flank pain or hematuria; some tumors are detected as a palpable mass, and some are found incidentally.

Renal carcinoma accounts for less than 5% of pediatric renal neoplasms. Half or more of pediatric RCCs are translocation RCCs.[275,276] Translocation carcinoma accounts for between 1% and 4% of adult RCCs.[276-279]

Xp11 Translocation Renal Cell Carcinoma

TFE3 rearranged tumors involve the Xp11.2 gene locus and fall into one of three general categories: Xp11 TRCCs, melanocytic Xp11 TRCCs, and Xp11 PEComas.[280-283]

Xp11 TRCCs are defined by a variety of chromosome translocations, all of which involve a breakpoint at Xp11.2, and all of which result in the fusion of any one of multiple translocation partners with the TFE3 transcription factor gene at this locus, triggering oncogenic activation of the TFE3 transcription factor.[266,271,276] Known TFE3 fusion partners include *ASPSCR1 (ASPL)*, *PRCC*, *SFPQ1 (PSF)*, *NONO*, *CLTC*, *PARP14*, *LUC7L3*, *DVL2*, and *KHSRP*.[281] Of these the most common are the *ASPSCR1-TFE3* (also known as *ASPL-TFE3*) TRCC that results from a t(X;17)(p11;q25) translocation and the *PRCC-TFE3* TRCC, resulting from a t(X;1)(p11;q21) translocation.[268,284]

PRCC-TFE3 TRCC is typically yellow or gray, ranges in size from 3 to 14 cm in diameter, and has a fibrous pseudocapsule that has varying degrees of calcification in the majority of cases, sometimes substantial enough to impart an egg shell–like consistency (Fig. 2.59).[268] It is composed of tumor cells in papillary formations

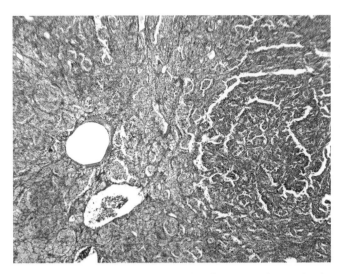

Fig. 2.60 Translocation carcinoma. PRCC-TFE3 renal carcinoma showing compact nested and papillary architecture at low power.

and in nests surrounded by thin-walled capillary vessels (Figs. 2.60 and 2.61). The tumor cell nests are usually solid, but may be centrally discohesive, imparting an alveolar appearance, and some nests have central lumina; fresh blood in these lumina imparts a "bloody-gland" appearance typical of conventional CCRCC. The extent of the papillary component is variable; it may be the predominant pattern, or it may account for less than 10% of the tumor. Foam cells are evident in the minority of papillae. Psammoma bodies are often present and, although usually rare and isolated, may be abundant in some tumors. Transitions between areas of nested and papillary architecture are usually sharply demarcated. Tumor cells are uniformly polygonal, with sharply defined cell borders and with abundant cytoplasm that varies from clear and finely granular to distinctly eosinophilic. Proportions of clear and eosinophilic cells vary from tumor to tumor. Nuclei appear rounded at low power, but appear wrinkled and irregular at high power; nuclear grade is 2 or 3 in most cases. Areas of necrosis are seen in the majority of cases, but mitotic activity is very limited.

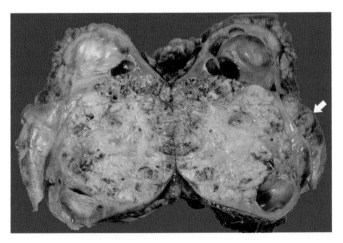

Fig. 2.59 Translocation carcinoma in a 42-year-old woman. Tumor extended into renal pelvis (*arrow* at right), as well as renal vein and vena cava.

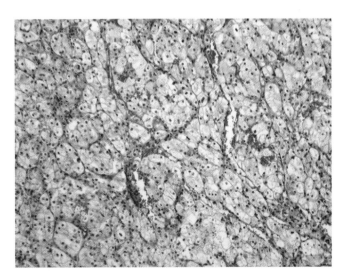

Fig. 2.61 Translocation carcinoma. PRCC-TFE3 renal carcinoma at high power showing clear to faintly eosinophilic cytoplasm and sharply defined cell borders.

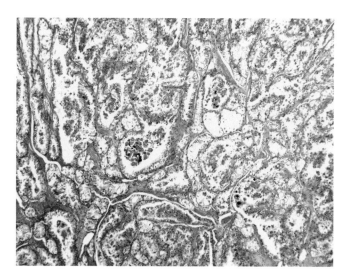

Fig. 2.62 Translocation carcinoma. ASPL-TFE3 renal carcinoma at low power showing nested to pseudopapillary architecture and numerous psammomatous calcifications.

ASPSCR1-TFE3 TRCC is usually well circumscribed but unencapsulated.[284] It displays nested and pseudopapillary growth patterns and psammomatous calcifications (Fig. 2.62). Papillary structures lack foam cells and intracytoplasmic hemosiderin.[285] Tumor cells are epithelioid, with well-defined cell borders and voluminous cytoplasm that is predominantly clear, but may also be finely granular, eosinophilic, or densely granular (Fig. 2.63). Nuclei have vesicular chromatin and a single prominent nucleolus.

Rare examples of melanotic Xp11 translocation renal cancers have been reported in recent years.[280,281,286,287] These tumors are composed of solid sheets and nests of polygonal epithelioid cells with clear to finely granular cytoplasm, containing variable amounts of finely brown pigment confirmed to be melanin by histochemical stains (Fig. 2.64). Tumor cells show patchy immunoreactivity for melanoma antigens but negative immunostaining for keratins, PAX-8, and PAX-2.[281]

Immunohistochemically, MiT family RCCs consistently express PAX-8, but they underexpress epithelial immunohistochemical

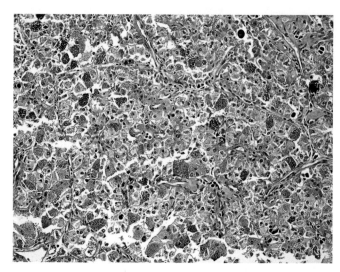

Fig. 2.64 Melanotic translocation carcinoma. Section from a 4-cm renal mass in a 14-year-old girl consists of polygonal epithelioid cells with fairly distinct cell borders and abundant clear to finely granular cytoplasm. Many cells contain brown-pigmented cytoplasmic granules. Tumor cells showed strongly positive immunostaining for transcription factor E3 and HMB45, and negative immunostaining for AE1/AE3, epithelial membrane antigen, Melan A, microphthalmia transcription factor, and S100 protein.

markers. Only about one-half of these tumors show positive staining for various cytokeratins or EMA, and the staining is often weak and/or focal.[288,289] Only about 60% of Xp11 TRCCs express cathepsin K, and they only infrequently express melanocytic markers.[290-292]

Although TFE3 immunostaining to detect the C-terminal portion of TFE3 is the most distinctive, sensitive, and specific immunohistochemical marker for Xp11 TRCCs, reliability of this stain has proven to be challenging because of fixation issues. A TFE3 break-apart FISH probe can be used to confirm the diagnosis (Fig. 2.65).[269,293–295]

The number of patients with documented follow-up after treatment for the various types of translocation carcinoma is

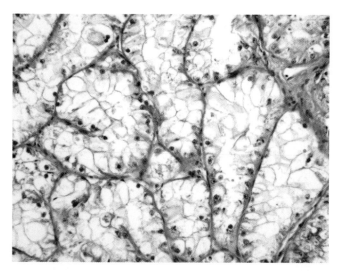

Fig. 2.63 Translocation carcinoma. ASPL-TFE3 renal carcinoma at higher power showing cells with voluminous clear cytoplasm and vesicular nuclei with prominent nucleoli.

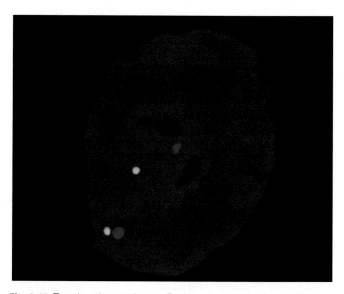

Fig. 2.65 Translocation carcinoma. Positive transcription factor E3 fluorescence in situ hybridization (FISH) result from a female patient. The break-apart FISH assay showed a fused or closely approximated green-red signal pair (representing the uninvolved X chromosome) and another pair of split signals.

limited.[268,272,277-279,284,285,296,297] Regarding TFE3 TRCCs, there are notable clinical differences between *PRCC-TFE3* TRCC and *ASPSCR1-TFE3* TRCC.[296] TFE3 TRCC patients who present with distant metastases usually have *ASPSCR1-TFE3* TRCC and usually die of cancer or exhibit disease progression. More than two-thirds of *ASPSCR1-TFE3* TRCCs have metastatic cancer in regional lymph nodes; despite this, in the absence of concurrent distant metastases, the great majority of these patients achieve long-term freedom from disease. Only about one-third of *PRCC-TFE3* TRCCs have positive nodes at presentation. However, *PRCC-TFE3* TRCC occasionally recurs as late as 20 to 30 years after surgery, requiring long-term follow-up.[266,268,296] The specific type of TFE3 TRCC appears to have no significant impact on outcome; only older age or advanced stage at presentation are predictive of death from cancer.[296] Overall, cancer-specific survival for patients with TFE3-rearranged RCC is similar to the survival of patients with conventional CCRCC, but worse than the survival of patients with PRCC.[277]

t(6;11) Translocation Renal Cell Carcinoma

Only about 50 cases of t(6;11) TRCC have been reported. It is characterized by a t(6,11)(p21;q12) translocation that results in fusion of the 5′ portion of the *Alpha* gene with the transcription factor gene *TFEB* at 6p21.[270,288,298-303]

Patients with t(6;11) TRCC range in age from 3 to 68 years, with a mean and median age of about 33 to 34 years.[288] About one-half of patients report abdominal pain or hematuria, and the rest are asymptomatic.

Macroscopically, tumors are solid but often contain cysts, which rarely may be very large.[288] Tumors are usually confined within a pseudocapsule, and range from 2 to 12 cm in greatest dimension (mean diameter, 7 cm). They typically display a homogeneous tan-yellow-brown color, without evidence of necrosis.

Microscopically, tumors demonstrate a solid, nested pattern of growth, characteristically with entrapment of single native renal tubules at their periphery, and distinctively biphasic cell populations. The predominant cell type is epithelioid, with well-defined borders, abundant clear, finely granular, or eosinophilic cytoplasm, and rounded or vesicular nuclei that have prominent nucleoli evident at low magnification and mild nuclear membrane irregularities at high power.

In the majority of cases, there is a second cell population comprising 5% to 30% of the tumor and consisting of smaller cells with denser chromatin, usually clustered around nodules of hyaline basement membrane material; these nodules have been described by some as "pseudorosettes" (Fig. 2.66). Less commonly, tumors contain areas resembling epithelioid angiomyolipoma, chromophobe carcinoma, or CCRCC with cystic change.[270] Mitotic figures are inapparent. Abortive papillae, brown pigmentations, psammomatous calcifications, and well-formed tubules are seen in a minority of cases.

The t(6;11) TRCCs consistently express the cysteine protease cathepsin K and melanocytic markers Melan A and HMB45. They also express the KP1 clone of CD68, but do not express the PG-M1 clone of CD68.[297] This can be used to distinguish them from pure epithelioid angiomyolipomas (AML), which express both the KP1 and the PG-M1 clones of CD68, as well as cathepsin and melanocytic markers.[297] Although positive nuclear immunostaining is highly specific for t(6;11) TRCCs, a transcription factor EB (TFEB) break-apart FISH assay in formalin-fixed paraffin-embedded tissue is preferable as a diagnostic marker.[270,300,302]

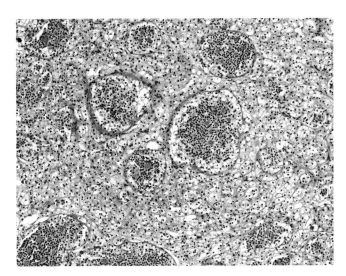

Fig. 2.66 The t(6:11) renal cell carcinoma: transcription factor EB gene (*TFEB*) rearranged renal cell carcinoma. Two cell populations are evident: some with abundant clear cytoplasm and a second cell population consisting of smaller cells with denser chromatin, clustered around nodules of hyaline basement membrane material, forming "pseudorosettes."

The t(6;11) TRCCs are generally confined within an intact pseudocapsule and usually present at stage pT1 or pT2.[300] Of about 50 reported t(6;11) TRCCs, 11 patients were known to have metastatic cancer and of these, 4 were known to have died.[297]

Succinic Dehydrogenase–Deficient Renal Cell Carcinoma

A subset of tumors occurs in the setting of germline mutations of SDHA, SDHB, SDHC, SDHD, and SDHAF2. These include pheochromocytomas/paragangliomas, gastrointestinal stromal tumors, RCC, and pituitary adenomas. Tumors associated with germline mutations of SDHB, SDHC, SDHD, and SDHAF2 show loss of immunostaining for SDHB, but retain positive staining for SDHA, whereas tumors associated with SDHA mutation show loss of immunostaining for SDHB, but also show loss of staining for SDHA. In 2010, a morphologically unique renal tumor occurring in a patient with a germline mutation and somatic loss of the wild-type SDHB allele was reported.[304] In 2011, it was reported that renal carcinomas related to SDH mutation could be identified by loss of immunohistochemical staining for SDHB, and later that year it was reported that SDH-deficient RCC had distinctive morphologic features that could prompt immunohistochemical staining for SDHB, with the premise that loss of staining could prompt definitive genetic testing.[305,306] In recent years, more than 60 renal neoplasms arising in the setting of germline SDH mutation have been reported, with mutation frequencies approximately as follows: SDHB, 81%; SDHC, 9%; SDHD, 5%; and SDHA, 5%.[305,307-309] The molecular abnormality that defines SDH-deficient RCC is double-hit inactivation of one of the SDH genes, and this is an event that occurs only rarely, if ever, in the absence of a germline mutation.[305,307] With this in mind, all patients with SDH-deficient RCC should be offered genetic testing, and surveillance for other SDH-deficient neoplasms (e.g., paraganglioma, pituitary adenoma, SDH-deficient gastrointestinal stromal tumor) should be initiated.

SDH-deficient RCC is estimated to account for about 0.05% to 0.2% of renal neoplasms.[305] Vague flank pain is noted in some instances, but many are found incidentally. Mean age at presentation is 37 years (range, 14 to 76 years), and there is a male predominance of nearly 2:1.[305,307] The tumors are typically well circumscribed, 2 to 20 cm in diameter, with a tan to red-brown cut surface, and sometimes with a cystic component. Tumors are expansile with a lobulated or pushing border and infrequently are separated from the adjacent normal kidney by a pseudocapsule. At the interface between tumor and normal kidney, tumors may surround benign elements from the adjacent kidney. Microcysts and macrocysts are commonly noted, usually containing pale eosinophilic fluid (Fig. 2.67).[305] Stromal myxoid change or hyalinization is seen in some tumors. Tumors are composed of cuboidal to ovoid cells with round nuclei. Nucleolar prominence consistent with ISUP nucleolar grade 2 is seen in the majority, but some exhibit grade 3 nucleoli, and sarcomatoid change consistent with ISUP grade 4 is noted in some cases. Cell borders may be indistinct (Fig. 2.68). The cytoplasm is eosinophilic or flocculent and may appear bubbly, but not truly oncocytic. A distinctive finding is the presence of cytoplasmic vacuoles and inclusion-like spaces,

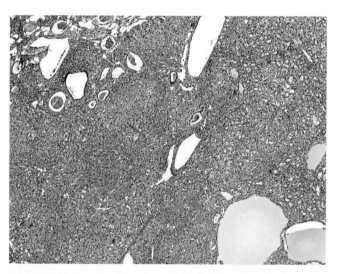

Fig. 2.67 Succinate dehydrogenase–deficient renal cell carcinoma. Tumor infiltrates and surrounds native renal elements at the interface between tumor and normal kidney; microcysts are present.

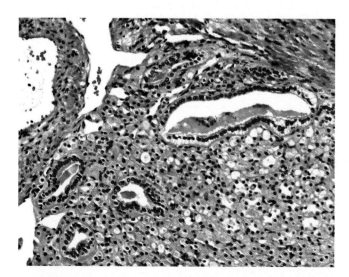

Fig. 2.68 Succinate dehydrogenase–deficient renal cell carcinoma. Tumor cells have small, round, low-grade nuclei. Cytoplasm is pale, eosinophilic, finely granular, or flocculent.

containing either pale eosinophilic fluid or flocculent material.[305] True coagulative necrosis is seen in some tumors, usually in nucleolar/nuclear grade 3 or 4 tumors. Tumor cells show positive immunostaining for PAX8 and kidney-specific cadherin, but absence of immunostaining for SDHB.[305,307] Other immunostains are not helpful in establishing the diagnosis. Notably, immunostains for CD117, RCC-Ma, and CA-IX are negative, and keratin markers are frequently negative.[307]

Patients whose SDH-deficient RCCs are uniformly low grade and lack coagulative necrosis have about a 90% likelihood of a good outcome.[305,307] Tumors that exhibit coagulative necrosis, grade 3 nucleoli, or sarcomatoid change have a guarded prognosis, with metastasis in up to 70% of cases.[305] Cases in which metastatic cancer appeared 16 to 30 years after tumor excision may represent metastasis of an unsampled metachronous tumor in the opposite kidney.[305,307]

Mucinous Tubular and Spindle Cell Carcinoma

Five examples of mucinous tubular and spindle cell carcinoma were first reported in 1997 by MacLennan and colleagues under the name of "low-grade collecting duct carcinoma." Four similar cases were reported in 2001, described as "low-grade myxoid renal epithelial neoplasms," and five more patients with similar tumors in 2002 as "low-grade tubular-mucinous renal neoplasms."[310–312] The tumor occurs predominantly in females, with a 1:3 male-to-female ratio. Patients range in age from 13 to 82 years, with a mean age of 58 years. Although some tumors are symptomatic, the majority are discovered incidentally.

Tumors range in diameter from 2.2 to 12 cm, averaging 6 to 7 cm. Tumors are sharply circumscribed, gray-white, tan, or yellow, sometimes with minimal hemorrhage or necrosis (Fig. 2.69). Classic tumors are composed of tightly packed, small elongated tubules separated by abundant basophilic extracellular mucin, sometimes with a "bubbly" myxoid consistency (Figs. 2.70 and 2.71).[310-312] Focally, aggregates of spindled cells may be present (Fig. 2.72).[313,314] The mucin stains strongly with Alcian blue at pH 2.5 (Fig. 2.73). Tubules are lined by uniform low cuboidal cells with scant cytoplasm and round nuclei of low nuclear grade with absent or inconspicuous nucleoli. Mitotic figures are rare.

The spectrum of acceptable histologic findings in mucinous tubular and spindle cell carcinoma has expanded with increasing recognition of this tumor, to include cases with relative paucity of mucinous matrix, aggregates of foamy macrophages, papillations or small components of well-formed papillae, focal clear cell change in tubular cells, focal necrosis, oncocytic tubules, numerous small vacuoles, psammomatous calcification, or heterotopic bone formation (Figs. 2.74 and 2.75).[315] Rarely the spindle cell component rivals or even exceeds the tubular component (Figs. 2.76 through 2.79). Furthermore, there is increasing recognition that high nuclear grade, areas of coagulative tumor necrosis, sarcomatoid change, and aggressive biologic behavior can be encountered in a small subset of these tumors.[316-319] Tumor cells have a complex and markedly variable immunophenotype, but are typically immunoreactive for CK7, AMACR, and PAX8 (Table 2.3).[320-322]

Despite morphologic similarities to PRCC in some cases, the gains of chromosomes 7 and 17 and loss of Y chromosome that are characteristic of PRCC are not seen in mucinous tubular and spindle cell carcinoma.[323] Alterations in the Hippo pathway are present in mucinous tubular and spindle cell carcinoma but are not seen in PRCC.[324] Cytogenetic analyses and comparative

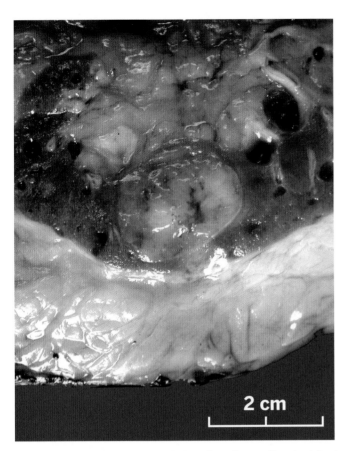

Fig. 2.69 Mucinous tubular and spindle cell carcinoma. Sharply defined gray-white neoplasm with a slightly bulging glistening cut surface.

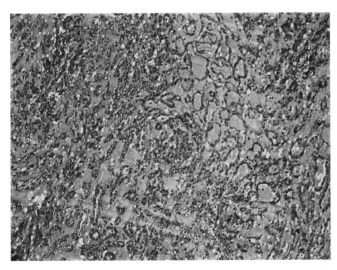

Fig. 2.70 Mucinous tubular and spindle cell carcinoma. Abundant mucin fills and separates variably sized tubular structures.

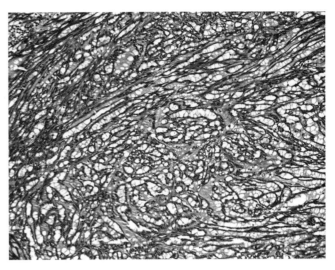

Fig. 2.71 Mucinous tubular and spindle cell carcinoma. Round and closely packed elongated tubular structures filled and separated by "bubbly" mucin.

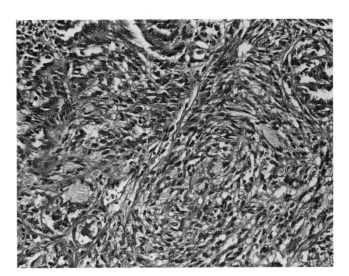

Fig. 2.72 Mucinous tubular and spindle cell carcinoma. Aggregates of spindle cells are present.

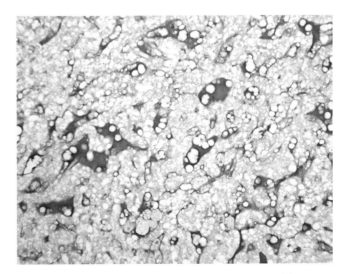

Fig. 2.73 Mucinous tubular and spindle cell carcinoma. The tumor-associated mucin shows positive staining with Alcian blue.

genomic hybridization studies have revealed multiple genetic alterations that include losses of chromosome 1, 4, 6, 8, 9, 13, 14, 15, 18, and 22.[312,314,325-327]

These tumors are generally of low pathologic stage at the time of excision, and most tumors with classic histologic findings behave in an indolent fashion. However, high nuclear grade and sarcomatoid change in isolated cases have been associated with fatal outcomes.[316,328,329]

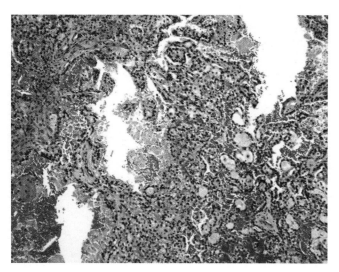

Fig. 2.74 Mucinous tubular and spindle cell carcinoma. In this example, small papillary structures were focally present.

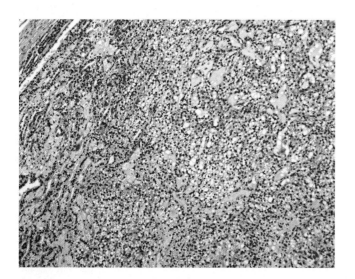

Fig. 2.75 Mucinous tubular and spindle cell carcinoma. In this variant case, mucin-filled tubules are at upper right, abundant macrophages are at upper left, and centrally the cells have clear cell morphology.

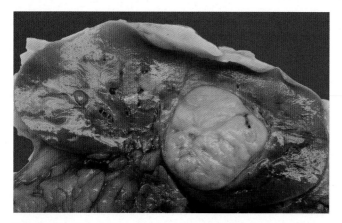

Fig. 2.76 Spindle cell–predominant mucinous tubular and spindle cell carcinoma. Tumor is sharply circumscribed and lacks hemorrhage or necrosis.

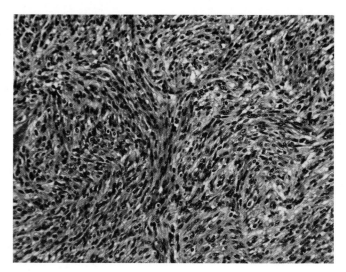

Fig. 2.77 Spindle cell–predominant mucinous tubular and spindle cell carcinoma. More than 95% of the tumor was composed of bland uniform spindle cells. Areas of tubule formation were widely scattered and inconspicuous. Spindle cells showed diffuse strongly positive immunostaining for keratin CAM5.2.

Tubulocystic Renal Cell Carcinoma

Tubulocystic renal cell carcinoma is a rare distinctive neoplasm; examples of it were presented at a meeting of the United States and Canadian Academy of Pathology and described in abstract form in 1994, and several illustrations of the gross and microscopic appearance of these neoplasms were presented in the AFIP Atlas of Tumor Pathology, Series III, in 1994.[330,331] Details of the clinical and pathologic details of eight examples of this neoplasm were first reported in 1997 by MacLennan and colleagues.[310,332] It was emphasized that although the neoplasm had some features suggestive of collecting duct origin, it was distinctly different from classic collecting duct carcinoma in many ways. Because these tumors were clearly composed of tubules and ductlike structures, showed areas of hobnail change, and had immunohistochemical characteristics similar to those of classic collecting duct carcinoma (i.e., positivity for 34βE12 and UEA-1), it was hypothesized that they were of collecting duct origin and that they represented the low-grade end of a spectrum of findings in collecting duct carcinoma, hence the term *low-grade collecting duct carcinoma.*[310] Subsequently, the clinical and pathologic features of additional examples of similar tumors were reported, and the name of the lesion was changed to tubulocystic carcinoma.[333]

Close to 100 cases of this neoplasm have been reported, with a strong male preponderance ($\geq$7:1).[334-338] Tubulocystic carcinoma of the kidney is a well-circumscribed tumor that ranges in size from 0.7 to 17 cm, is often grossly cystic, and lacks hemorrhage or necrosis; some show a "bubble-wrap" appearance of the cut surface (Fig. 2.80). The microscopic appearance at very low power is reminiscent of a spiderweb or lace doily (Fig. 2.81). The tumor is composed of tubules and cystic structures of markedly variable size, separated by septa that are commonly delicate and "spiderweb-like," or by fibrotic septa of variable thickness (Fig. 2.82). Tubules are lined by a single layer of low cuboidal epithelial cells with modest to abundant amounts of eosinophilic cytoplasm, commonly with areas of hobnail appearance (Fig. 2.83). Nuclei are round, with evenly dispersed chromatin, and have readily evident nucleoli in some cases. Nuclear grade is 1 or 2 in all instances. No necrosis is present, and mitotic activity is extremely limited.[310,333]

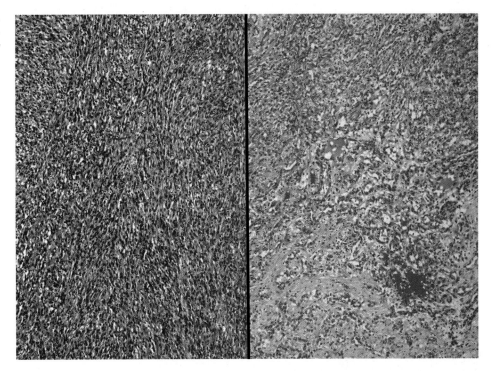

Fig. 2.78 Spindle cell–predominant mucinous tubular and spindle cell carcinoma. Spindle cell component is on the left, and tubular component is on the right.

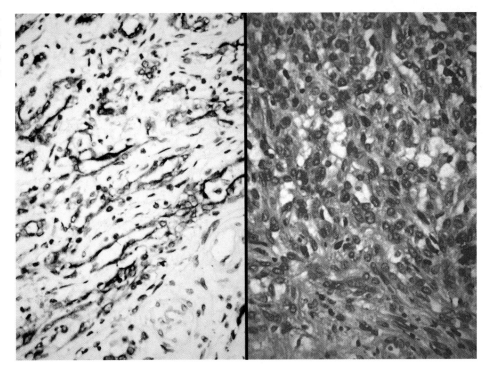

Fig. 2.79 Spindle cell–predominant mucinous tubular and spindle cell carcinoma. Cells lining the scant tubules showed positive immunostaining for keratin AE1/AE3. The tubules contained scant mucin, which is highlighted by Alcian blue stain.

Immunohistochemically, tumor cells in classic cases of pure tubulocystic carcinoma show strong and diffuse labeling for PAX8, with frequent AMACR expression (Table 2.3). The minority show focal immunoreactivity for CA-IX and patchy reactivity with antibody against CK7 (in 30% to 40% of cells).[337]

Molecular studies in classic cases of pure tubulocystic carcinoma show no gains of chromosomes 7 or 17, and no TFE3 translocation by FISH.[337] Other investigators have noted disomy of chromosome 7 in the majority, loss of Y chromosome in one case, and polysomy or gain of chromosome 17 in 50% of their classic cases.[338] Gene expression profiling demonstrates that the molecular signature of tubulocystic carcinoma is distinct from those of papillary, clear cell, and chromophobe carcinomas.[336] Tubulocystic carcinoma and collecting duct carcinoma are unrelated from a molecular perspective.[339]

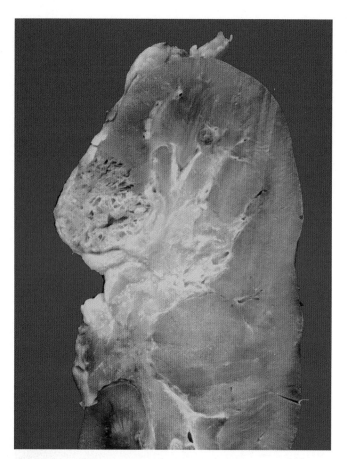

Fig. 2.80 Tubulocystic carcinoma. Tumor is composed of myriad small cysts. Some examples have a "bubble-wrap" appearance on sectioning.

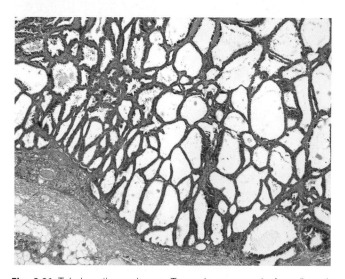

Fig. 2.81 Tubulocystic carcinoma. Tumor is composed of small cystic spaces separated by delicate septa, with a "spider web" or "lace doily" appearance.

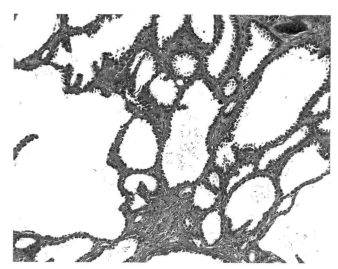

Fig. 2.82 Tubulocystic carcinoma. Delicate septa lined by eosinophilic cells with "hobnail" appearance.

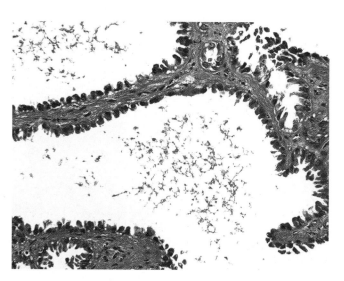

Fig. 2.83 Tubulocystic carcinoma. At high power the hobnail cells have small, dark nuclei; nucleoli are absent or inconspicuous.

Stage and nuclear grade are typically low, and biologic activity is indolent, with a potential for metastasis that is less than 10%.[310] Staging data and available follow-up in currently reported patients showed that one patient had lymph node metastases when first diagnosed, but was alive without disease at follow-up, another

had a local recurrence, one patient experienced bone metastases, and a fourth developed both bone and liver metastases and died of cancer.[310,333-336]

The diagnosis of tubulocystic carcinoma should be restricted to tumors with the classic histologic features.[201] Some investigators have proposed a close relationship between tubulocystic carcinoma and PRCC, based on evaluation of tumors with papillary components admixed with areas resembling tubulocystic architecture.[335,340] Some have noted morphologic similarities between tubulocystic carcinoma and t(6,11) TRCC, and others have reported tumors with poorly differentiated solid and papillary components admixed with areas resembling tubulocystic architecture.[180,338,341,342] Poorly differentiated high-grade renal carcinomas that have areas closely resembling tubulocystic carcinoma have been shown in many instances to be examples of FH-deficient RCC.[180] Cases of tubulocystic carcinoma with purely classic morphology are distinctive and lack the full spectrum of genetic and immunohistochemical features that are classically seen in PRCC.[336-338]

Acquired Cystic Disease–Associated Renal Cell Carcinoma

The incidence of ACKD in the dialysis population is proportional to dialysis interval, with close to 100% of patients affected by 10 years of dialysis.[343] Patients with ACKD are especially prone to the development of carcinoma, with an incidence rate of 3% to 7% and a risk that increases with the duration of dialysis, approaching 100 times that of the general population.[344,345] The biologic basis for increased renal carcinogenesis in end-stage renal disease is undefined. Depressed immunity, excessive free radical production related to inflammation, impaired antioxidant defenses, and deposition of oxalate crystals have been postulated.

The RCCs that arise most commonly in a setting of ACKD are, in descending order of frequency, acquired cystic disease–associated RCC (ACD-RCC) (36%), CCPRCC (23%), CCRCC (18%), PRCC (15%), and chromophobe RCC (5%).[344] Of these tumors, only ACD-RCC, by definition, occurs only in patients with ACKD. The earliest report of RCC with abundant oxalate crystals appeared in 1998.[346] The characteristics of ACD-RCC were subsequently described more fully in large series of cases in 2005 and 2006.[344,347] Patients with ACD-RCC tend to be relatively young and predominantly male. Tumors are identified primarily through routine screening protocols, although some present with microscopic hematuria or flank pain.

Grossly, ACD-RCCs range from 1 to 8 cm, and are often multifocal and bilateral (Fig. 2.84). More than 50% of cases are multifocal, and more than 20% are bilateral.[201,344] Tumors are generally well circumscribed. Foci of hemorrhage and necrosis are common, and some have focally calcified capsules. Many appear to have arisen in cysts. Histologically the tumor architecture demonstrates various combinations of solid sheetlike, papillary, acinar, and cribriform and tubulocystic patterns. The tumor cells are typically large with abundant granular eosinophilic cytoplasm and large round to oval, mildly irregular nuclei with prominent nucleoli.[344,346,347] About 80% of these tumors show abundant intratumoral calcium oxalate crystals within luminal structures and in the stroma (Figs. 2.85 and 2.86). The crystals are not associated with fibrosis, necrosis, increased mitoses, or inflammation. Intratumoral calcium oxalate deposition is a feature that appears to be restricted to tumors arising in a background of ACKD.

Studies indicate that ACD-RCC arises from cells of the proximal nephron.[348] Tumor cells show positive immunostaining for CD10, RCC-Ma, and often for AMACR.[347,349] Tumor cells typically show no immunostaining for CK7.[344,349] Gains in chromosomes 3, 7, 16, and 17 and the sex chromosomes are noted with high frequency in ACD-RCC.[348,350,351]

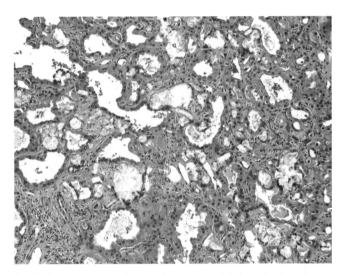

Fig. 2.85 Acquired cystic kidney disease–associated renal cell carcinoma. This carcinoma exhibits tubulocystic architecture and abundant calcium oxalate crystals.

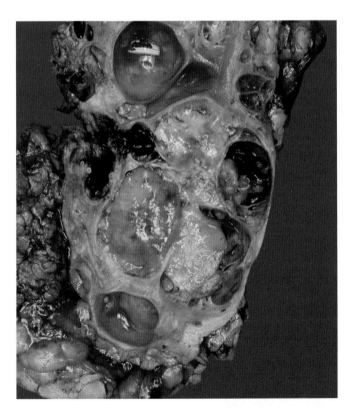

Fig. 2.84 Acquired cystic kidney disease–associated renal cell carcinoma. A solid and cystic neoplasm is present in a background of extensive cystic change in this patient with a long-standing history of dialysis for renal failure.

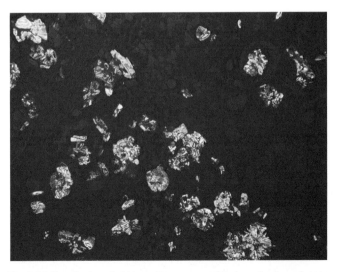

Fig. 2.86 Acquired cystic kidney disease–associated renal cell carcinoma. Abundant oxalate crystals are demonstrable under polarized light, a unique property of this neoplasm.

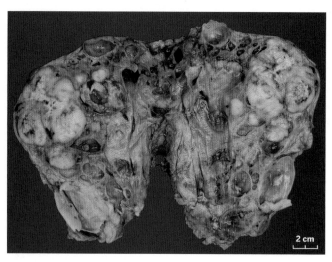

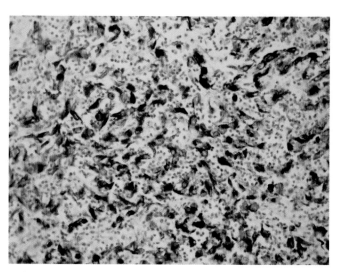

Fig. 2.87 Acquired cystic kidney disease–associated renal cell carcinoma with sarcomatoid features. A large multinodular and partially necrotic tumor is present in a background of acquired cystic kidney disease. This dialysis-treated patient had bilateral sarcomatoid carcinoma. Patient died of cancer less than 6 months after bilateral nephrectomy.

Fig. 2.89 Acquired cystic kidney disease–associated renal cell carcinoma with sarcomatoid features. The spindle cell component of the tumor shown in Fig. 2.88 showed strong immunoreactivity for CAM5.2.

The prognosis for ACD-RCC is generally favorable, because it tends to have an indolent behavior, and constant medical surveillance of dialysis patients facilitates diagnosis at an early stage. However, when sarcomatoid or rhabdoid morphology is identified, it often portends a poor outcome (Figs. 2.87 through 2.89).[344,352]

Clear Cell Papillary Renal Cell Carcinoma

Although originally described as one of two unique tumors typically arising in end-stage renal disease, with and without acquired cystic change, it is now known that the majority of CCPRCCs arise sporadically, accounting for up to 4.3% of resected kidney tumors, occurring about equally in males and females, and comprising the fourth most common renal tumor.[344,350,353-361] Patients range in age from 18 to 88 years, with a mean age of ~60 years.[358] In one series, there was a propensity for occurrence in African American patients.[362]

Grossly, CCPRCC is typically small, with a mean diameter of 2.0 cm, but varies in size between 0.2 and 9 cm. Tumors are well circumscribed, often cystic, with a thin, fibrous capsule and without hemorrhage or necrosis (Fig. 2.90), and may be multiple or bilateral.[358,363,364] Necrosis and hemorrhage are absent. Cyst formation is nearly universal and is extensive in about one-third of tumors. Solid areas appear white-tan to pale yellow.

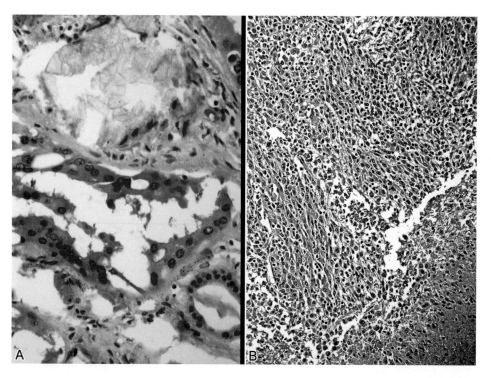

Fig. 2.88 Acquired cystic kidney disease–associated renal cell carcinoma with sarcomatoid features. (A) Typical acquired cystic kidney disease–associated renal cell carcinoma is present in a section from the tumor shown in Fig. 2.87. (B) In the same kidney was a spindle cell neoplasm with abundant mitotic activity and extensive necrosis.

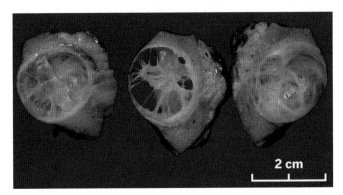

Fig. 2.90 Clear cell papillary renal cell carcinoma. The tumor is sharply circumscribed and extensively cystic, but nodules of solid tumor are readily visible.

Histologically, papillary architecture is usually limited to focal branching or small blunt papillae; extensively branched papillae are uncommon (Fig. 2.91). Most tumors exhibit areas of a dense, compact arrangement of tubular structures, similar to CCRCC. A distinctive finding is the presence of cells with nuclei aligned at the apical end of the cells, similar to early secretory phase endometrium (Fig. 2.92). Most cells lining the papillary and tubular structures exhibit clear cytoplasm and a low nucleolar grade. Necrosis is absent.

A small subset of tumors (previously designated renal angiomyoadenomatous tumors) show similar cytologic findings but with "collapsed" acini, variable tubular/acinar architecture, and prominent components of fibrous or smooth muscle stroma.[353,355,365,366]

Immunohistochemically, tumor cells show positive immunostaining for CK7 and CA-IX (Table 2.3) and negative immunostaining for AMACR and CD10. Positive immunostaining for 34βE12 is noted in more than 90% of cases.[367]

In contrast with conventional CCRCC and PRCC, CCPRCC lacks the VHL 3p25 deletion and also lacks VHL gene mutations, VHL promoter hypermethylation, trisomies of chromosomes 7

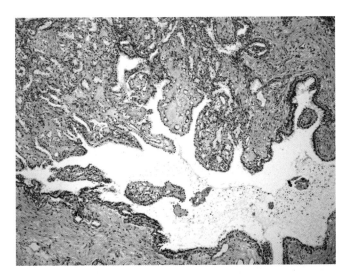

Fig. 2.91 Clear cell papillary renal cell carcinoma. At low power the cystic nature of the tumor is evident. Tumor exhibits papillary architecture, but the papillae are relatively small and blunt, with limited branching. Even at low power, it is evident that most tumor cells have clear cytoplasm.

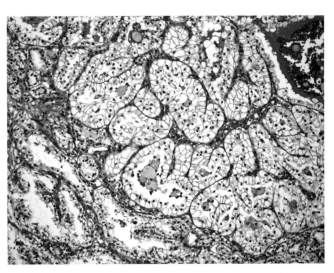

Fig. 2.92 Clear cell papillary renal cell carcinoma. A typical finding is the presence of areas of a densely and compactly arranged tubular structures, lined by cells with clear cytoplasm, whose nuclei are of low nuclear grade and are arranged at the apical end of the cells, similar to early secretory phase endometrium.

and 17, and loss Y chromosome, although low copy number gains of chromosomes 7 and 17 have been reported in a small number of cases.[358,361] No mutations of *KRAS*, *NRAS*, *BRAF*, *PIK3CA*, *ALK*, *ERBB2*, *DDR2*, *MAP2K1*, *RET*, or *EGFR* genes were detected in a recent study.[368] Currently no specific characteristic genetic abnormality has been found.

Although the differential diagnosis for CCPRCC is broad, the morphologic distinction between CCPRCC and conventional CCRCC presents the greatest challenge.[360,369] Immunopositivity for CK7 does not exclude CCRCC. Discordant immunoprofiles, such as immunopositivity for CD10 or AMACR, or an immunoprofile that fits neither CCPRCC nor CCRCC, are best regarded as a reason to avoid making a diagnosis of CCPRCC.[360,369] Similarly, tumors with solid growth or large nested areas resembling CCRCC are best not diagnosed as CCPRCC, nor may it be prudent to make a definitive diagnosis of CCPRCC on limited material.[369]

Rare cases of CCPRCC have been reported to arise in patients with VHL disease.[355] Studies of a number of CCPRCC-like tumors occurring in patients with VHL disease showed that they usually lack the characteristic immunohistochemical profile of sporadic CCPRCC, and FISH analysis of chromosomes 3p, 7, and 17 supported a molecular pathogenesis more similar to that of CCRCC than of CCPRCC.[359,370]

More than 90% of CCPRCCs are stage pT1 at presentation.[353,358,360,361] A single patient with sarcomatoid change in a CCPRCC had a fatal outcome.[361] Of several hundred reported cases of conventional CCPRCC, no patient has reportedly died of or suffered recurrence of this neoplasm, leading some to propose that CCPRCC be renamed "clear cell papillary neoplasm of low malignant potential."[361]

Renal Cell Carcinoma, Unclassified

Renal cell carcinoma, unclassified is a diagnostic category for the designation of RCCs that have histologic features that do not resemble those of any of the well-characterized RCC subtypes, accounting for 0.7% to 5.7% of RCC cases.[4] Examples of tumors that are appropriately assigned to this category are tumors that are composites of recognized types, tumors composed of unrecognizable cell types, tumors with mucin production, and renal carcinomas with entirely sarcomatoid morphology, lacking recognizable epithelial elements (Fig. 2.93).[371] Low- or high-grade unclassifiable oncocytic neoplasms were also included in this category.[4]

Reported age at presentation ranges from 21 to 91 years.[372-378] There is a general tendency for such tumors to be large, at an advanced stage at presentation, and to exhibit histologic features that correlate with poor outcome, such as high nuclear grade, tumor necrosis, and microvascular invasion.[371,374-376] The limited data available suggest that unclassified RCC have marked genetic instability; in one study, 40 mutated genes were identified in the tissues of unclassified RCC compared with a number of normal renal tissue samples.[377] In another study of 62 unclassified RCC, molecular analysis revealed that about 75% of cases fell into one of several subsets of abnormalities of variable prognostic significance, raising the possibility that molecular analysis of these enigmatic tumors may have diagnostic and therapeutic implications.[379]

Unclassified RCC is a histologically and clinically heterogeneous category of tumors whose prognosis seems to be linked to the same clinical and pathologic findings that influence outcome in conventional renal cancers.[371,375,376] One study compared unclassified RCC with a 4:1 matched group of patients with CCRCC, with respect to year of surgery, symptoms at presentation, tumor size, stage, regional lymph node involvement, metastases, grade, coagulative tumor necrosis, and sarcomatoid change, and found no statistically significant differences in outcome after adjusting for these features in a matched analysis.[376] Other investigators have reported that unclassified RCC tend to behave more aggressively than conventional renal carcinomas of the same stage and grade.[374,375]

Emerging or Provisional Renal Cell Carcinomas

Oncocytic Renal Cell Carcinoma Occurring After Neuroblastoma

Secondary malignant neoplasms develop in approximately 13% of children treated for cancer.[380] More than 30 cases of RCC arising in children who survived neuroblastoma in childhood have been reported in the last 40 years.[68,381-395] Although the great majority were exposed to chemotherapy or radiation therapy, at least two never had either exposure, raising the possibility that the cause of such cancers may lie in an underlying genetic relationship or susceptibility.[391,393,396] The tumors reported include CCRCC, PRCC, MiT family RCC, hybrid oncocytic-chromophobe tumor, and SDHB-deficient RCC, as well as a unique oncocytic RCC that is rare but is included in the category of emerging/provisional RCC.[391,392,395]

The interval between a diagnosis of neuroblastoma and of oncocytic RCC postneuroblastoma ranges from 3 to 38 years, and age at diagnosis of oncocytic RCC postneuroblastoma ranges from 8 to 40 years.[395] Tumors form expansile masses, composed microscopically of cells arranged in solid sheets intersected by cystic areas, nests, papillary structures, or forming tubules (Fig. 2.94).[391,392,395] Occasional psammoma bodies are present. Tumor cells have sharply defined cell membranes and abundant eosinophilic granular cytoplasm, giving them an "oncocytoid" appearance. Cells with

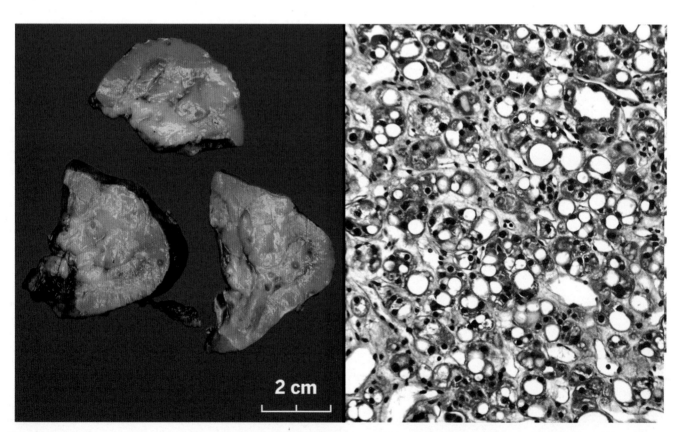

2 cm

Fig. 2.93 Renal cell carcinoma, unclassified. (Left) This unusual carcinoma had a fatty appearance, grossly suggestive of angiomyolipoma. (Right) The tumor was composed of epithelial cells with extensively vacuolated cytoplasm. Tumor cells showed positive immunostaining for AE1/AE3 and CAM5.2 and no immunoreactivity for cytokeratin 7, HMB45, Melan A, S100 protein, 34βE12, or *Ulex europaeus*.

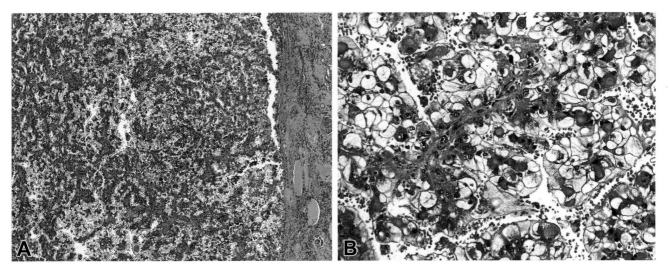

Fig. 2.94 Oncocytic renal cell carcinoma occurring after neuroblastoma. (A) Tumor is solid and expansile; this example has prominent papillary architecture. (B) Tumor cells have sharply defined cell membranes and abundant eosinophilic granular cytoplasm. Nuclei are irregular, and many have prominent nucleoli.

abundant reticular cytoplasm may be present, with some morphologic resemblance to chromophobe cells (Fig. 2.94). Tumor cell nuclei are medium sized and irregular, and many bear prominent nucleoli. Only occasional mitotic figures are observed. The tubular and solid architecture with varying cyst formation, cyst lining cells with a hobnail appearance and eosinophilic to flocculent cytoplasm, and variably sized cytoplasmic granules are similar to the findings in a recently described but not fully characterized renal carcinoma, eosinophilic solid and cystic RCC. There are insufficient data regarding molecular features and outcome for these tumors.

Eosinophilic Solid and Cystic Renal Cell Carcinoma

More than 50 cases of this rare tumor have been well studied and reported.[378,397-401] Although it was initially identified in patients with TSC, it is now known to occur sporadically as well (Fig. 2.95).[29,30,402,403] The earliest reported patients were all women with a mean age of about 55 years (range, 31 to 79), but in a more recently reported series of cases, this tumor has been identified in males as well as females, and in younger patients as well (median age, 27 years; range, 14 to 35 years).[29,30,378,397-403] The majority of eosinophilic solid and cystic renal cell carcinomas are single, but multifocality and bilaterality have been reported.[378] Grossly they are tan or yellow-gray and most often solid and cystic grossly, although about 25% are entirely solid. They range from 1.5 to 13.5 cm in greatest dimension (median, 3.8 cm). With rare exceptions, they present at stage pT1 or pT2.

Microscopically, they are arranged in solid nests or sheets, always with interspersed aggregates of lymphocytes and histiocytes, and with psammoma bodies in about 50% of tumors (Fig. 2.95). All tumors harbor variably sized macrocysts and microcysts; cells lining the cysts often exhibit a prominent hobnail appearance. Tumors are composed of cells with voluminous eosinophilic cytoplasm and round to oval nuclei, with focally prominent nucleoli. Multinucleated tumor cells are common. Intracytoplasmic vacuoles may be present. A unique and striking feature is the presence of cytoplasmic "stippling" by eosinophilic or basophilic amorphous granular structures of variable size and prominence.

Immunohistochemically, tumor cells are always PAX-8+ and CK8/18+. Distinctively, about 75% of these tumors express CK20, and 75% do not express CK7, so the majority have a CK20+/CK7− phenotype. About 75% of tumors express keratin AE1/AE3, AMACR (patchy), and CD10 (patchy). Importantly, these tumors express the following markers only rarely (CD117; CK5/6) or never (melanocytic markers). SDHA and SDHB staining, as well as FH staining, is retained, and MiT family translocations are not present.

A recurring set of genomic alterations has been identified: copy number gains in 16p, 7p, 13q, and 19p; copy number losses in Xp11.2 and 22q; and a variety of losses of heterozygosity.

Initially it was believed that eosinophilic solid and cystic RCC was an indolent tumor. With increasing awareness of this tumor, currently two patients are known to have developed metastases (an incidence rate of about 3% in known cases).[378,400]

Thyroid-like Follicular Carcinoma of the Kidney

The first reports of a primary renal neoplasm bearing a striking resemblance to follicular carcinoma of the thyroid appeared in 2006 and 2009.[404,405] To date 39 cases have been reported. In all cases, no evidence of thyroid cancer was discovered, concurrently or subsequently. About 70% are found incidentally; the remainder experience hematuria or flank or abdominal pain.[406] Patients range in age from 19 to 83 years (median, 35 years; mean, 43 years), and male-to-female ratio is nearly 1:2. Tumors are brown, tan-yellow, or gray; range in size from 1.1 to 1.3 cm; and are typically well circumscribed, often with a pseudocapsule. Cysts and areas of hemorrhage or necrosis are noted in about 50% of cases. Gross or microscopic extension into perinephric tissues is noted in 13% of cases, but extension into renal pelvis or renal vein has not been noted.[406] Microscopically, tumors exhibit a striking resemblance to thyroid tissue or thyroid neoplasia with follicular architecture, being composed of variably sized follicles with inspissated colloid-like material in the follicular lumina (Fig. 2.96).[406] The follicles are lined by cuboidal or flattened epithelial cells with uniform nuclei of modest size. About 20% of cases have microcalcifications. Exclusion of metastatic thyroid carcinoma or ovarian struma ovarii is necessary. In this regard immunostains for thyroglobulin and TTF1 have been uniformly negative in reported cases.[406] About 10% of patients have metastases at presentation or have them later; lymph nodes, lung, and skull are favored sites. The carcinoma has not resulted in patient death in any case.[406]

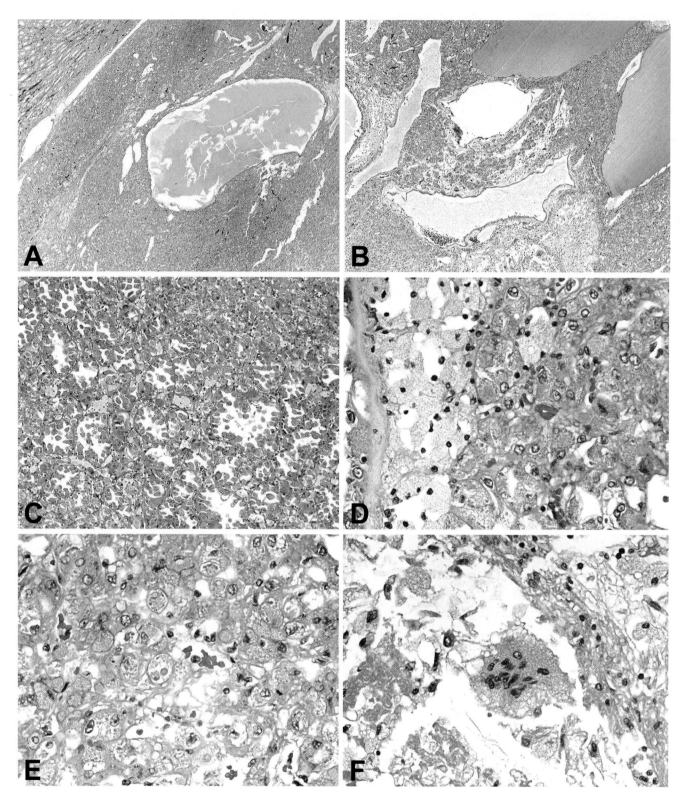

Fig. 2.95 Eosinophilic solid and cystic renal cell carcinoma. (A) At low power, tumor shows solid architecture, with a large cyst. (B) Cysts of variable size are separated by septa composed of tumor cells. (C) Microcysts are lined by cells with prominent hobnail morphology. (D) Tumor cells have voluminous eosinophilic cytoplasm. Nuclei are round to oval, and some have prominent nucleoli. (E) Cytoplasm of some tumor cells is stippled by basophilic amorphous granular structures. (F) Scattered multinucleated tumor giant cells are present.

ALK Rearrangement–Associated Renal Cell Carcinoma

There are recent reports of about 10 cases of RCC characterized by translocations resulting in fusion of a variety of genes with the anaplastic lymphoma kinase (*ALK*) gene, occurring in children with sickle cell trait and adults without sickle cell trait.[407-413] In children with VCL-ALK gene fusions the tumors are medullary based, have prominent lymphoplasmacytic infiltrates, and are composed of discohesive polygonal or spindle-shaped cells with prominent

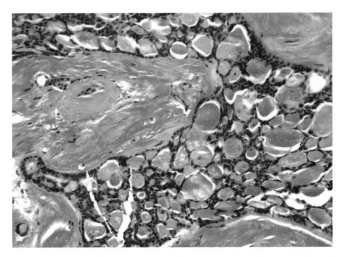

Fig. 2.96 Thyroid follicular carcinoma–like carcinoma. This unusual renal neoplasm is remarkably reminiscent of a thyroid follicular neoplasm, set in a diffusely hyalinized fibrotic background.

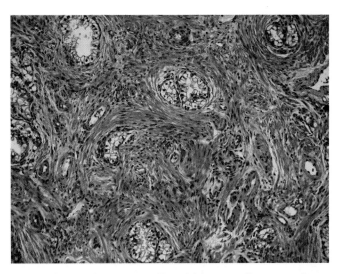

Fig. 2.97 Renal cell carcinoma with angioleiomyoma-like stroma. Stroma exhibits a smooth muscle–like appearance and separates the neoplastic epithelial glandular structures, many of which are rimmed by a prominent layer of endothelial cells that mimic a myoepithelial cell layer.

cytoplasmic vacuoles that can be highlighted with EMA immunostaining. Focal membranous immunostaining for ALK protein is noted, INI1 protein is intact, and *ALK* gene rearrangements are found on molecular studies. In adults the VCL gene is not the fusion partner. Morphologic similarities in adult cases include heterogeneous solid architecture, eosinophilic cells, mucinous cytoplasmic elements, rhabdoid cells, and intracytoplasmic lumina.[413] In some adults the tumors have behaved in an indolent manner, but in others, the tumors proved fatal within 4 years.[407,408] Detection of the ALK rearrangement can be of critical importance in the management of a patient with metastatic cancer.

Renal Cell Carcinoma With Angioleiomyoma-like Stroma

A small group of renal epithelial neoplasms exhibit clear cell cytologic features and angioleiomyoma or leiomyoma-like stromal smooth muscle proliferation.[365,414-417] The precise nature of these tumors, and their relationship with CCRCC or CCPRCC, if any, remains under investigation. Evaluation of several such tumors has disclosed no chromosome 3p or VHL alterations, and no trisomy of 7 or 17.[414,415]

Males and females are about equally affected, with a median age of 66 years.[415] Tumors range in size from 1.0 to 3.5 cm. Tumors are pink-tan or whitish, rather than having the variegated often hemorrhagic golden-yellow cut surface seen in conventional CCRCC. Microscopically, the stroma contains areas with a smooth muscle–like appearance, interspersed with stromal hyalinization and edema. Slitlike vascular spaces dispersed in the smooth muscle stroma are always seen (similar to the solid pattern of angioleiomyoma) and in some tumors the stroma also contains vascular channels with thicker, muscular walls, similar to the venous pattern of angioleiomyoma.[415] The smooth muscle proliferation often entraps adjacent nonneoplastic renal tubules and commonly extends into adjacent fat. The tumor epithelium forms glandular structures distributed in the smooth muscle proliferation and rimmed by a prominent layer of endothelial cells that mimics a basal cell or myoepithelial cell layer (Fig. 2.97). The cytoplasm of the epithelial cells is abundant and varies from clear to pale, flocculent or eosinophilic. Nuclear grade varies between 2 and 3.[415]

The epithelium is immunoreactive for CA-IX, CD10, vimentin, CK7, 34βE12, and PAX8, but not for AMACR. The stroma

is immunoreactive for caldesmon, desmin, and smooth muscle actin. Neither component is immunoreactive for HMB45, Melan A, cathepsin K, or TFE3 protein.[415] This tumor seems clearly unrelated to CCRCC. Although some of its features overlap with those of CCPRCC, it differs from that entity by its prominent smooth muscle component, relative paucity of cyst formation, higher nuclear grade, increased prominence of CD10 labeling, and absence of a "secretory cell" pattern.[415] The tumors with the earlier-noted features described in the literature have demonstrated no evidence of malignant behavior.[365,414-417]

Benign Epithelial Neoplasms

Papillary Adenoma

Renal papillary adenoma is defined as an unencapsulated renal neoplasm with papillary or tubular architecture, composed of cells of low ISUP nucleolar grade and measuring ≤15 mm in greatest dimension.[4] Before 2015, the upper limit of size acceptable for a diagnosis of papillary adenoma was ≤5 mm. The size cutoff was increased in 2015, based on analyses of the malignant potential of small renal masses. Evidence indicates that for each 1-cm increase in tumor size, the incidence of synchronous metastases increases 22%. Combined experience in nephrectomies performed at Mayo Clinic and Memorial Sloan-Kettering Cancer Center demonstrated that of 519 renal tumors less than 2 cm in diameter, none had synchronous metastases and none developed asynchronous metastases after surgical excision of the primary tumor. Similar findings were reported from Fox Chase Cancer Center.[418-420]

Autopsy studies of small renal cortical tumors have shown that papillary adenomas are quite frequent, being present in 21% of patients overall, and their frequency increases linearly with age, being found in 10% of patients aged 21 to 40 years and in 40% of those aged 70 to 90 years.[421,422] They are frequently observed in patients undergoing chronic dialysis, occurring in 33% of patients with ACKD.[423] They are commonly found in nephrectomy specimens from patients with hereditary PRCC.[133] They are more commonly found in nephrectomy specimens bearing PRCC than in normal kidneys.[424,425]

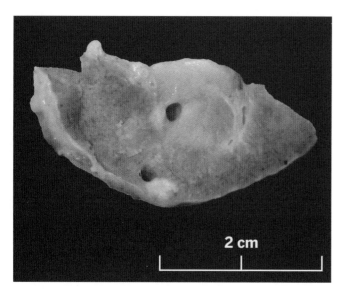

Fig. 2.98 Papillary adenoma. Circumscribed oval nodule just below the capsule, approximately 3 mm in diameter.

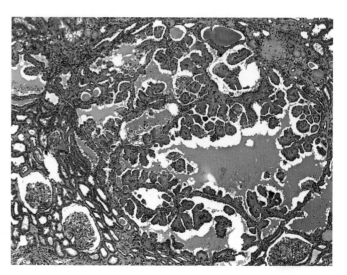

Fig. 2.100 Papillary adenoma. This small, completely circumscribed papillary adenoma exhibits the features typical of the oncocytic variant of papillary renal cell carcinoma.

Papillary adenoma is visible in the renal parenchyma, often just below the renal capsule, as one or more well-circumscribed gray-white to tan nodules (Fig. 2.98), varying in shape from conical to roughly spherical. Although most are solitary, in some patients they are multiple and bilateral, and in rare cases innumerable; this latter condition has been termed *renal adenomatosis*.[426-428] Most have a seamless interface with the adjacent renal parenchyma, but a thin, fibrous pseudocapsule is apparent in some. Tumor architecture may be papillary, tubular, or tubulopapillary. In most, the tumor cells resemble those of PRCC1, bearing nuclei that are round to oval and occasionally grooved, with stippled to clumped chromatin and inconspicuous nucleoli, lacking mitotic activity, and accompanied by scant cytoplasm that varies from pale to eosinophilic to basophilic (Fig. 2.99).[144,429] Much less frequently, tumor cells possess abundant eosinophilic cytoplasm (Fig. 2.100). Psammoma bodies and foamy macrophages are frequently present.[430]

Immunohistochemically, the majority of cases of papillary adenoma show positive staining for EMA, CAM5.2, 34E1β2, and AMACR.[108,424,431,432] Papillary adenomas typically exhibit loss of the Y chromosome and a combined trisomy of 7 and 17.[149,433]

Oncocytoma

Renal oncocytoma was first well categorized in 1976 as a benign and relatively common neoplasm distinctly separable from RCC.[434] It is believed to arise from the intercalated cells of renal collecting tubules and accounts for 5% to 7% of surgically resected nonurothelial renal neoplasms.[434-438]

Patients range in age from 10 to 94 years old (median, 62 years), and the majority are males, with a 1.7:1 male-to-female ratio.[56,421,422,437-440] Approximately 75% of patients are asymptomatic at the time of diagnosis, their tumor discovered incidentally during investigation of nonrenal complaints. In some patients the diagnosis is prompted by the discovery of a palpable mass; in others the lesion is identified during investigation of hypertension, hematuria, or flank or abdominal pain. Radiologic findings are too nonspecific to discriminate between oncocytoma and renal carcinoma, with the result that oncocytoma generally is managed by surgical excision.[441,442] (99m)Tc-sestamibi SPECT/CT scanning has shown some promise in distinguishing oncocytoma and hybrid oncocytic tumors from RCC, but sensitivity (87.5%) and specificity (95.2%) need further refinement.[443]

Grossly, oncocytoma is typically solid, ranging from 0.3 to 26 cm in greatest dimension, with reported mean size ranging from 4.8 to 8.1 cm. It is commonly mahogany brown and less often tan to pale yellow, and well circumscribed, with varying degrees of encapsulation (Fig. 2.101). An area of central scarring is often present (in up to 33%, particularly in larger tumors); other gross findings may include recent hemorrhage (up to 20%) and, rarely, foci of cystic degeneration.[439,444-449] Gross extension of tumor into perirenal fat and rarely into large blood vessels is sometimes evident. Multiplicity is common; up to 13% of oncocytomas are multifocal, and up to 13% are bilateral (Fig. 2.102).[446-448,450] Other benign renal neoplasms are often present, including papillary adenoma and AML, and concurrent RCC has been observed in up to 32% of cases.

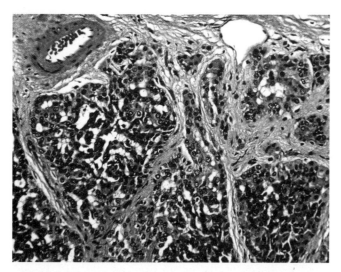

Fig. 2.99 Papillary adenoma. This example exhibits tubulopapillary architecture. Lesional cells are small, with scant cytoplasm and small, dark nuclei that lack nucleoli.

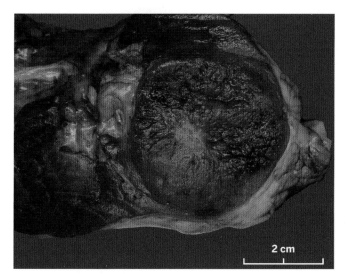

Fig. 2.101 Renal oncocytoma. Tumor is circumscribed, mahogany brown, and slightly hemorrhagic, with a central stellate scar.

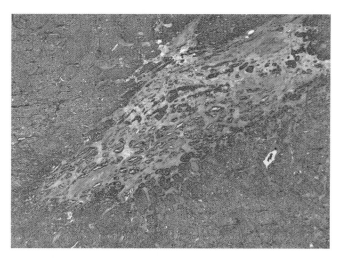

Fig. 2.103 Renal oncocytoma. Low-power view of an area of scarring demonstrates organoid architecture and the disposition of cell nests in a hyalinized hypocellular stroma.

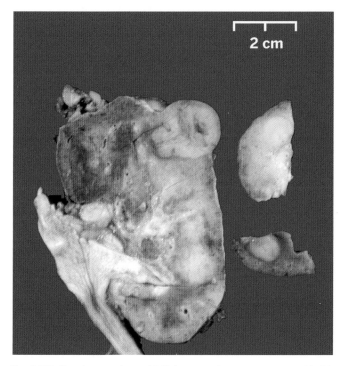

Fig. 2.102 Renal oncocytoma. Multiple oncocytomas were present in this nephrectomy specimen.

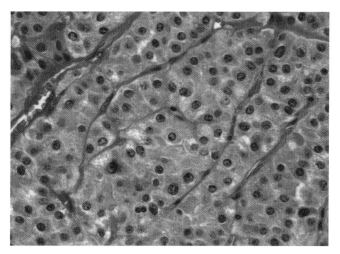

Fig. 2.104 Renal oncocytoma. Typical oncocytic cells with abundant, densely granular eosinophilic cytoplasm and uniform, round nuclei with inconspicuous nucleoli.

Microscopically, the areas of scarring are represented by hypocellular hyalinized or myxoid stroma (Fig. 2.103). The classic appearance of oncocytoma is that of a tumor composed predominantly of round to polygonal cells with densely granular eosinophilic cytoplasm, round uniform nuclei with smoothly dispersed chromatin, and a central nucleolus (Fig. 2.104).[439,445-447] Scattered binucleated cells are often present.[451] A minor component of cells with scant granular cytoplasm, dark hyperchromatic nuclei, and a high nuclear-to-cytoplasmic ratio may be present. Cells with enhanced amounts of cytoplasm and pronounced nuclear atypia are often present, but the nuclear atypia in such cells is usually degenerative, the nuclei have poorly preserved smudgy chromatin

patterns, and there are often associated intracytoplasmic inclusions (Fig. 2.105).[445,452] The degree of nuclear abnormality is reminiscent of that observed in benign endocrine tumors in other organs (e.g., endocrine "anaplasia"). Mitotic figures are only rarely identified. Tumor architecture may be nested, organoid (classic), tubulocystic, or mixed. In the classic pattern, tumor cells form nests, islands, organoid clusters, cords, trabeculae, or confluent solid sheets of cells lacking stroma. The tubulocystic pattern exhibits variably sized luminal structures lined by cells indistinguishable from those of the classic pattern (Fig. 2.106). The mixed pattern includes both organoid and tubulocystic components. Findings observed in some tumors include focal papillary structures projecting into dilated luminal structures, stromal calcifications, and osseous and myeloid metaplasia.

The neoplasm that is most difficult to distinguish from oncocytoma is the eosinophilic variant of chromophobe RCC, and the distinction is obviously of considerable importance, because one entity is benign and the other is malignant. Findings that are considered impermissible for a diagnosis of oncocytoma include

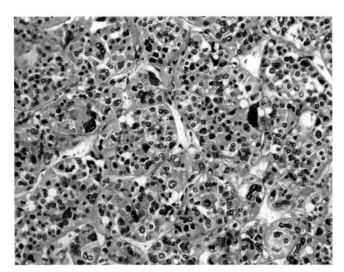

Fig. 2.105 Renal oncocytoma. Compact nests of cells, some of which show pronounced nuclear pleomorphism and hyperchromasia.

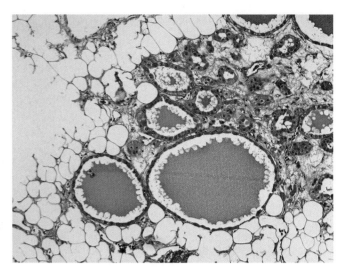

Fig. 2.107 Renal oncocytoma. This otherwise typical oncocytoma showed areas of extension into perirenal fat.

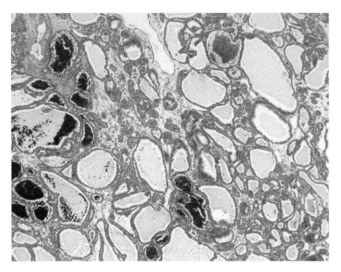

Fig. 2.106 Renal oncocytoma. This tumor was remarkable by the degree of cystic change that was present; otherwise it was entirely compatible with oncocytoma.

diagnosis acceptability were recorded: invasion of perinephric fat, 59% (Fig. 2.107); invasion of sinus fat, 53%; and invasion of renal vein or a vein branch, 35%. Invasion of medium and large renal vessels, including grossly visible tumor in the renal vein, is identified in about 1.5% of otherwise typical oncocytomas.[455] Cumulative data from several investigators indicate that vascular invasion is consistent with a diagnosis of oncocytoma, provided the morphologic features of the tumor are classic (Figs. 2.108 and 2.109).[446,447,452,453,455] Although definitive assessment of these features is facilitated by adequate tumor sampling, two-thirds of respondents indicated willingness to issue an outright diagnosis of oncocytoma on a needle biopsy specimen.[454]

Use of immunostains to make the earlier distinction has been evaluated extensively. Currently the stain reported to be used most widely by experienced renal pathologists is CK7.[454] The great majority (82%) regarded positivity of less than 5% of tumor cells as supportive of a diagnosis of oncocytoma (Fig. 2.110), and 100% of respondents regarded diffuse CK7 positivity as supportive of a diagnosis of chromophobe RCC (Figs. 2.43 and 2.44). A large number of immunohistochemical stains has been evaluated

areas of clear cell or spindle cell carcinoma, prominent papillary architecture, macroscopic or conspicuous microscopic necrosis, and atypical mitotic figure. Certain morphologic findings, when noted in tumors otherwise compatible with oncocytoma, raise concern for malignancy.[445-447,453,454] Recently a group of experienced renal pathologists were queried regarding their level of acceptance of these features in the spectrum of diagnosis of oncocytoma.[454] Regarding mitotic activity, 82% considered identification of a single mitotic figure still compatible with a diagnosis of oncocytoma, but more than one was considered worrisome by 59% and incompatible with oncocytoma diagnosis by 35%. Intranuclear pseudoinclusions were considered acceptable by more than one-half unless this was a widespread finding. More than one-half considered absence of separate round nests, with a mainly solid, compact growth pattern or trabecular nests, worrisome for carcinoma. About 75% regarded small clusters of cells with clear cytoplasm embedded in hyalinized stroma, minute papillary projections into dilated tubules, as compatible with oncocytoma. The following features and the corresponding acceptance rates for oncocytoma

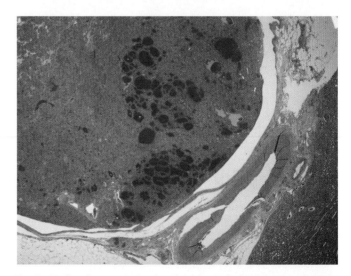

Fig. 2.108 Renal oncocytoma. An otherwise typical oncocytoma (see also Fig. 2.109) was noted to have tumor within a large renal vein.

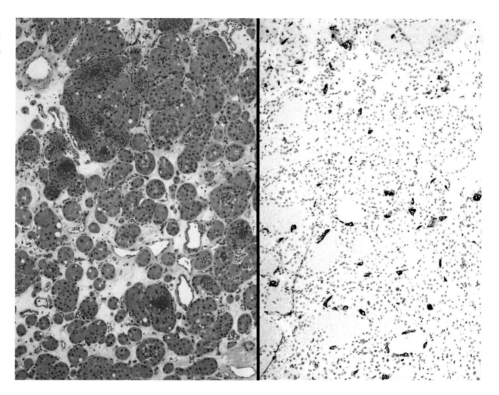

Fig. 2.109 Renal oncocytoma. The morphology and immunostaining pattern with cytokeratin 7 are typical for oncocytoma (same case as shown in Fig. 2.108).

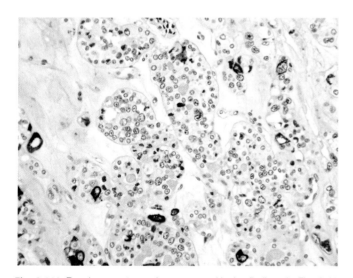

Fig. 2.110 Renal oncocytoma. In contrast with the findings in Fig. 2.44, oncocytoma typically exhibits only scattered cells with positive immunostaining for cytokeratin 7.

and shown to be insufficiently specific as single markers for distinguishing between oncocytoma and chromophobe RCC, including EMA, vimentin, parvalbumin, antimitochondrial antibody (113-1), caveolin-1, CD117, vinculin, peanut agglutinin antigen, UEA-1, cytokeratin KL1, S100 protein, lysozyme, E-cadherin, MIB1, cyclin D1, epithelial cell adhesion molecule, CK7, RON protooncogene, ankyrin-repeated protein with a proline-rich region, CD63, vimentin 3, amylase α-1A, and MOC31.[99,100,109,112,192,193,223,226,227,456-469]

Several panels of immunohistochemical markers have been proposed for making this distinction, and none has gained widespread clinical use (Table 2.3).[470-473] Distinction of oncocytoma and

chromophobe RCC from RCC subtypes (CCRCC and PRCC) that sometimes exhibit prominent eosinophilic cytoplasm can be facilitated by stains for CD117 and vimentin, because the former two frequently show positive staining for CD117 and negative staining for vimentin, and the latter two have the opposite immunoprofile (Table 2.3).

Diffuse reticular cytoplasmic colloidal iron staining is a classic finding in chromophobe RCC. Positive staining is also noted in 11% of oncocytomas, usually in a luminal distribution. Many laboratories find this to be a technically difficult stain for routine use.[456,474] Because of an overlap in ultrastructural findings between the two entities, electron microscopy cannot be relied on to make the distinction in all cases.[208,475,476]

From a molecular perspective, oncocytoma tends to fall into one of three categories: those with no identifiable clonal cytogenetic alterations, those that show losses of a sex chromosome and chromosome 1, and those that exhibit structural rearrangements involving chromosome region 11q12~q13.[477-482] Partial or complete loss of chromosome 14 is another frequently reported abnormality.[483-485] In general, loss of chromosome 1 or a diploid karyotype in a tumor with appropriate morphologic and immunohistochemical findings is supportive of a diagnosis of oncocytoma.[486]

Bilaterality and multifocality are relatively common in oncocytoma. Extreme examples of multifocality, variably termed *oncocytosis* or *oncocytomatosis*, often involving both kidneys, have been reported.[202,204,205,487-489] The number of oncocytomas present in such cases may be impossible to determine, and rarely such cases are associated with renal failure.[205,490,491] Typically, at least one dominant tumor is present, usually oncocytoma, and less frequently chromophobe RCC, accompanied by innumerable other oncocytic nodules. Other findings in these cases include diffuse oncocytic change in nonneoplastic tubules, benign oncocytic cortical cysts, and an "interstitial pattern" characterized by diffuse intermingling of oncocytic tubules and cell clusters with the normal renal interstitium. In some cases "hybrid tumors" are present, with mixed histologic features of both oncocytoma and chromophobe RCC.

Renal oncocytoma is considered to be benign, because follow-up of large numbers of patients with renal oncocytoma has disclosed no examples of patient deaths attributable to metastases.[439,444-449] Nonetheless, several experienced renal pathologists report having seen tumors that closely mimicked an oncocytoma, yet which metastasized, emphasizing the difficulty of accurately diagnosing oncocytoma in every case.[454] When borderline features hamper the distinction between oncocytoma and chromophobe RCC, the great majority of experienced renal pathologists are willing to use terminology that does not definitively label the tumor as benign or malignant.[454]

Metanephric Tumors

Metanephric Adenoma

The clinical and pathologic features of this tumor were delineated between 1980 and 1995.[249,492-497] For some time it was postulated that metanephric adenoma might represent the differentiated end of the Wilms tumor spectrum, because it closely resembles differentiated epithelial nephroblastoma and consistently expresses WT1 protein immunoreactivity.[498,499] Recently, it has been shown that mutations in the *BRAF* gene (specifically V600E) are detectable in more than 90% of metanephric adenomas in adults and children.[500-502] This mutation has not been found in sequencing analyses of Wilms tumor, suggesting that metanephric adenoma and Wilms tumor do not share a common molecular pathogenesis, unless one postulates that small subsets of Wilms tumors either have BRAF mutation from the outset or acquire such a mutation during their evolution, resulting in a nonproliferative state and terminal differentiation to a metanephric adenoma.[502,503] Documentation of the presence of BRAF V600E mutations in all members of the metanephric tumor family (metanephric adenoma, metanephric adenofibroma, and metanephric stromal tumor) suggests that a clonal event occurs that affects primordial renal cells before the mesenchymal-to-epithelial transition of primitive metanephric mesenchymal cells.[504,505]

The majority of patients with metanephric adenoma are female, with a male-to-female ratio of ~1:2.[249,497,498,506] BRAF-mutated metanephric adenomas tend to be more frequently associated with female gender and older age, whereas a strong male predominance has been noted in those that are BRAF wild-type.[507] Although most patients are in their fifth or sixth decade of life, the reported age range for metanephric adenoma is 15 months to 83 years.[249,496,497] In the majority of cases the tumor produces no symptoms and is discovered incidentally, but some patients present with flank or abdominal pain, intermittent fever, or hematuria, and some are found to have a palpable abdominal mass or polycythemia.

Metanephric adenoma ranges from 0.3 to 20 cm in greatest dimension, with a mean of 5.5 cm.[249,508] It is typically unilateral and rarely multifocal. The majority are either unencapsulated or have only a limited and discontinuous pseudocapsule. Tumors are tan to gray to yellow, and soft to firm (Fig. 2.111). Although most are solid, some have areas of hemorrhage, necrosis, and cystic degeneration. Calcification within the solid areas or within the walls of cystic structures is common. Infrequently, coexistent RCC is present.[249,509,510]

Microscopically, metanephric adenoma may appear solid at low power, but on closer inspection it is composed of very small acini

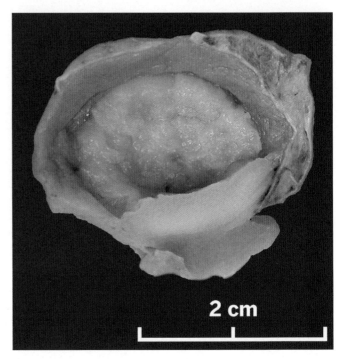

Fig. 2.111 Metanephric adenoma. Light tan, well-circumscribed, but unencapsulated tumor in a kidney from a 48-year-old woman.

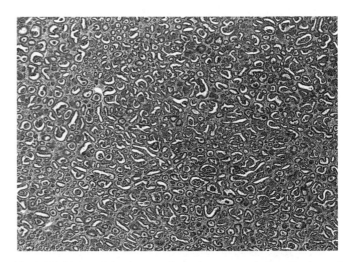

Fig. 2.112 Metanephric adenoma. Tumor is composed of small embryonal epithelial cells forming densely packed tubules, set in a very limited hyalinized paucicellular stroma. Numerous "glomeruloid bodies" are present.

separated by acellular stroma consisting only of edema fluid or a smoothly hyalinized matrix (Fig. 2.112). The degree of acinar crowding is variable. Extensive replacement of tumor by hyalinized scar is observed in about one-third of cases. In some, tumor cells are arranged to form nests and tubules. In about one-half of cases, papillary structures are noted, consisting of polypoid fronds or short papillary infoldings within tubular or cystic spaces, producing a glomeruloid appearance. Less commonly, tumor cells form solid aggregates that resemble blastemal nodules of Wilms tumor, and infrequently microcysts are present, lined by flattened tumor cells like those noted elsewhere in the tumor. The great majority of tumors display calcification, either in the form of calcific deposits and foci of dystrophic calcification within areas of stromal

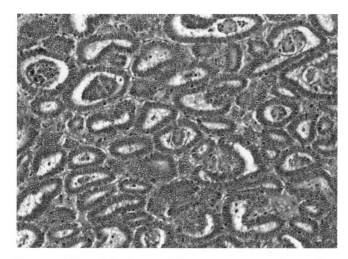

Fig. 2.113 Metanephric adenoma. At higher power, tumor cells are uniform, with evenly dispersed chromatin and scant cytoplasm, lacking nucleoli and mitotic activity.

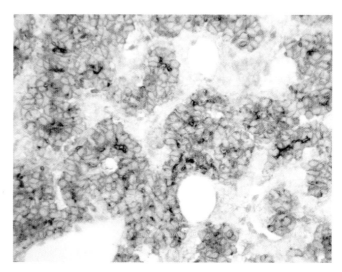

Fig. 2.115 Metanephric adenoma. Tumor cells show positive immunostaining for CD57.

hyalinization and scarring, or as psammoma bodies associated with papillary structures.

Tumor cells of metanephric adenoma possess little cytoplasm, which is usually pink or clear (Fig. 2.113). Nuclei are slightly bigger than lymphocytes, irregularly rounded or ovoid, sometimes displaying a central fold. Nuclear chromatin is delicate, nucleoli are absent or inconspicuous, and mitotic figures are rare or absent.

The main differential diagnostic considerations for metanephric adenoma are epithelial-predominant Wilms tumor in children and the solid variant of PRCC in adults. Metanephric adenoma is typically immunopositive for WT1 and CD57, and immunonegative for AMACR and CK7, an immunoprofile that is the exact opposite to that of PRCC (Figs. 2.114 and 2.115). Metanephric adenoma and WT share immunopositivity for WT1 and immunonegativity for AMACR and CK7, but are distinguishable by positive staining for CD57 in metanephric adenoma and negative immunostaining for this marker in Wilms tumor (Table 2.5).[498,511] Positive VE1 immunostaining is exhibited by 80% of BRAF-mutated metanephric adenomas.[507] Cadherin 17 has been reported to be

TABLE 2.5 Immunohistochemical Profiles of Metanephric Adenoma, Wilms Tumor, and Papillary Renal Cell Carcinoma (Including Solid Variant)

	CK7	CD57	AMACR	WT1	BRAF
Metanephric adenoma	-	+	-	+	+
Wilms tumor	-	-	-	+	-
PRCC	+	-	+	-	-

AMACR, α-Methylacyl–coenzyme A racemase; CK, cytokeratin; PRCC, papillary renal cell carcinoma.

expressed in 81% of metanephric adenomas, whereas PRCC and epithelial-predominant Wilms tumors show no immunoreactivity for this marker.[512] FISH analysis has shown that the gains of chromosomes 7 and 17, and losses of Y that are typical of PRCC are not found in metanephric adenoma.[506]

Metanephric adenoma, with rare exception, has shown benign biologic behavior. In one case a nephrectomy specimen that harbored metanephric adenoma also had demonstrable regional lymph node metastases. Possibly the underlying neoplasm in this case was a Wilms tumor that metastasized and subsequently matured into a metanephric adenoma through acquisition of a BRAF mutation.[499,502]

Metanephric Adenofibroma

Metanephric adenofibroma, a rare biphasic renal neoplasm with epithelial and stromal components, was first described in 1992.[513] It is now recognized that the epithelial component is indistinguishable from metanephric adenoma, and that the stromal component, in addition to being distinct from congenital mesoblastic nephroma (CMN), is morphologically identical to the metanephric stromal tumor.[499,514,515] As noted earlier in the Metanephric Adenoma section, BRAF V600E mutation has been identified in both the epithelial and stromal components of metanephric adenofibroma.[502,516] Most metanephric adenofibromas arise in young people. Patients range in age from 5 months to

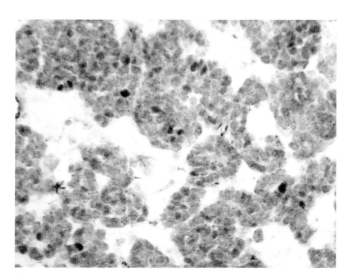

Fig. 2.114 Metanephric adenoma. Tumor cells show positive immunostaining for WT1.

36 years, with a median age of about 7 years and a male-to-female ratio of 2:1.[515]

Metanephric adenofibroma is typically solitary, centered in the renal medulla, and sometimes grossly papillary, occasionally protruding into the renal pelvis.[515] Tumor borders are indistinct. Tumors range from 1.8 to 11 cm, with a median size of 3.85 cm. Most are yellow-tan and partially cystic.

Microscopically, there is marked variability in the relative proportions of stromal and epithelial components. All tumors have the same stromal component, indistinguishable from metanephric stromal tumor, but there is variability in the epithelial component. Tumors with usual histology have epithelial components that are identical to those of metanephric adenoma, lacking mitotic activity. In some instances, the epithelial component shows increased mitotic activity (>5 mitoses/20 hpf). Metanephric adenofibroma has rarely been part of a composite tumor in association with Wilms tumor or RCC.[515,517] In one instance, the RCC component metastasized, with a fatal outcome.[517] Conventional metanephric adenofibroma is regarded as a benign tumor.[499]

Metanephric Stromal Tumor

After recognition of a distinctive and unique biphasic renal neoplasm, metanephric adenofibroma, it was recognized that a separate subset of renal neoplasms consisted entirely of stromal elements identical to the stromal component of metanephric adenofibroma.[513] This subset was designated metanephric stromal tumor.[518,519] The putative pathogenesis of the members of the metanephric tumor family is described in the Metanephric Adenoma section.

Most patients are children, ranging from a few days old to 15 years, with a mean age of 2 years.[520,521] A single adult patient has been reported.[499] The majority are detected as a palpable abdominal mass, and about 20% have hematuria. Less common manifestations of tumor include hypertension, flank pain, or tumor rupture.[520,522] Some are found incidentally.

Metanephric stromal tumor is typically a tan lobulated partially cystic fibrous tumor with a mean diameter of 5 cm. It is often centered in the renal medulla and is usually unifocal, but about one-sixth of cases are multifocal.[520] Mean diameter is 5 cm. It is unencapsulated and has a scalloped border that, on close inspection, subtly infiltrates the adjacent normal parenchyma.

Microscopically, it is composed of spindled and stellate cells with thin hyperchromatic nuclei and indistinct cytoplasmic extensions (Fig. 2.116).[499] Scattered epithelioid stromal cells may be noted. Metanephric stromal tumor tends to surround native renal tubules and blood vessels, forming concentric "onion-skin" rings or collarettes around these structures in a myxoid background (Fig. 2.117). Geographic differences in the degree of cellularity versus the degree of myxoid change produce a vaguely nodular variation in tumor cellularity at low power. In most tumors, angiodysplasia is evident within entrapped arterioles, manifested by epithelioid transformation of medial smooth muscle cells and myxoid change. Juxtaglomerular cell hyperplasia within entrapped glomeruli is observed in 25% of cases, a feature that may be responsible for hypertension with hyperreninism (Fig. 2.118). Heterologous stromal differentiation results in the presence of glia or cartilage in 20% of cases; the association of glial elements with metaplastic embryonal epithelium produces "glial–epithelial complexes."

Immunohistochemically, tumor cells of metanephric stromal tumor show patchy reactivity for CD34 and no immunostaining for cytokeratins, S100 protein, or desmin.[438] Areas with glial

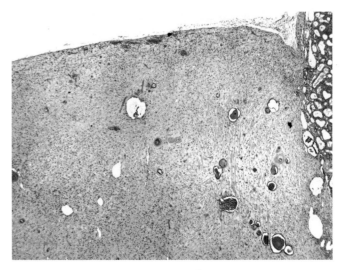

Fig. 2.116 Metanephric stromal tumor. Spindle cell neoplasm entraps native renal elements and subtly infiltrates at its interface with adjacent kidney.

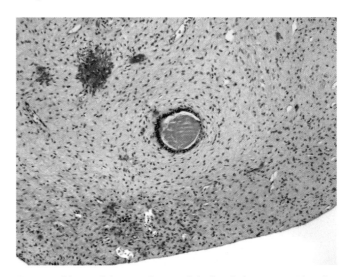

Fig. 2.117 Metanephric stromal tumor. Spindle cells form concentric collarettes that encircle a native tubule ("onion-skinning").

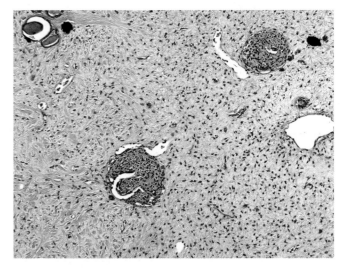

Fig. 2.118 Metanephric stromal tumor. Entrapped glomerulus demonstrates juxtaglomerular cell hyperplasia.

differentiation show positive immunostaining for S100 protein and glial fibrillary acidic protein. The distinction of metanephric stromal tumor from other pediatric renal tumors with purely stromal morphology has been aided by the application of studies for BRAF exon 15 mutations. Recently, it has been found that BRAF exon 15 mutations (specifically V600E) are demonstrable in about 70% of metanephric stromal tumors, providing evidence that metanephric stromal tumor is linked with metanephric adenoma and metanephric adenofibroma, which also exhibit these mutations in both their epithelial and stromal components.[504,505] It is known that other pediatric renal tumors with purely stromal morphology, specifically CMN, clear cell sarcoma of kidney (CCSK), some stromal-predominant Wilms tumors, ossifying renal tumor of infancy (ORTI), and rhabdoid tumor, do not exhibit BRAF exon 15 mutations, a finding that could be useful in distinguishing among these neoplasms in limited tissue samples of such tumors.[504] Metanephric stromal tumor is considered benign, lacking the capacity to metastasize. A single case of local recurrence after surgery has been reported.[523]

Nephroblastic and Cystic Tumors That Occur Mainly in Children

Nephrogenic Rests

Nephrogenic rests are regarded as precursor lesions of nephroblastoma (Wilms tumor). There are two distinct categories of nephrogenic rest: perilobar nephrogenic rests (PLNRs) and intralobar nephrogenic rests (ILNRs).[524,525] They represent abnormal persistence in the kidney of embryonal cells or their derivatives, past 36 weeks of gestation into postnatal life. They are defined as "foci of abnormally persistent nephrogenic cells, retaining cells that can be induced to form a Wilms tumor."[524,526] They are found in less than 1% of infants during routine autopsy examination and are only rarely of intralobar type in this setting.[524-528] In contrast, nephrogenic rests have been identified in 42% of patients with nephroblastoma (Wilms tumor): 20% PLNRs, 18% ILNRs, and 4% PLNRs and ILNRs.[529] They are found in 28% of patients with unifocal tumors, and in more than 90% of those with multifocal disease.[529] They are found in virtually all patients with bilateral nephroblastoma, suggesting germline changes in these individuals that predispose them to development of nephroblastoma.[530] About 5% to 10% of patients with nephroblastoma have bilateral abnormalities: bilateral nephroblastoma, bilateral nephrogenic rests, or unilateral nephroblastoma with contralateral nephrogenic rests.[531]

PLNRs are strictly confined to the periphery of the renal lobe. They are composed of blastema, embryonal epithelial cells, and scant stroma; have an ovoid shape and a subcapsular location; and are sharply demarcated from the adjacent renal parenchyma. Dormant or incipient rests show no features of involution or proliferation. Nephrogenic rests may undergo maturation, sclerosis, involution, obsolescence, and eventual disappearance.[524,525] PLNRs that exhibit focal or diffuse overgrowth of blastemal or embryonal epithelial cell types are designated "hyperplastic rests." In extreme cases when one or occasionally both kidneys are involved by a more or less continuous subcapsular band of nephrogenic rests, the condition is designated "diffuse hyperplastic perilobar nephroblastomatosis" (Figs. 2.119 and 2.120).[532] The blastema and embryonal epithelium that comprise hyperplastic PLNRs show marked proliferative changes including abundant

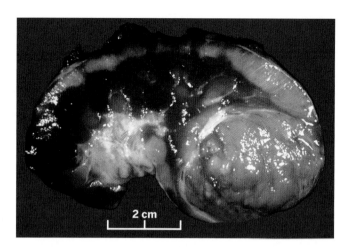

Fig. 2.119 Nephrogenic rests. Diffuse hyperplastic perilobar nephroblastomatosis: a more or less continuous subcapsular band of nephrogenic rests, associated with a Wilms tumor after preoperative chemotherapy; patient had bilateral Wilms tumors.

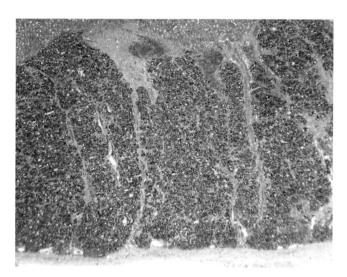

Fig. 2.120 Nephrogenic rests. Diffuse hyperplastic perilobar nephroblastomatosis after preoperative chemotherapy; patient had bilateral Wilms tumors.

mitotic activity and prominent nucleoli. Hyperplastic PLNRs interface directly with adjacent normal renal tissue and lack the pseudocapsule that characterizes nephroblastoma. Furthermore, hyperplastic PLNRs remain subcapsular and tend to be ovoid, in contrast with the spherical expansile growth seen in nephroblastoma. The distinction between the two entities may be virtually impossible on a limited biopsy specimen. PLNR rarely progress to malignancy, but the presence of PLNRs in a kidney removed for nephroblastoma, especially in a patient younger than 12 months, puts the child at an increased risk for development of nephroblastoma in the opposite kidney.[533]

ILNRs can be located anywhere in the renal lobe and may also be identified in the renal sinus and the walls of the pelvicaliceal system. They are composed of multiple cell types including abundant immature or mature stroma, and lie between normal nephrons, forming an indistinct interdigitating interface with the adjacent normal tissue (Figs. 2.121 and

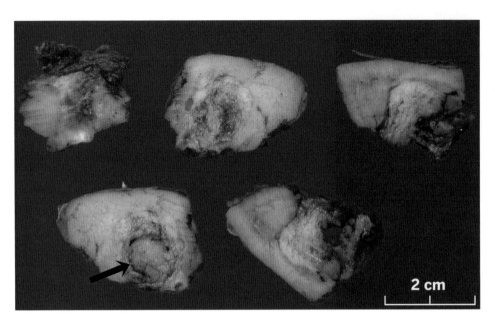

Fig. 2.121 Intralobar nephrogenic rests (ILNRs). Patient was carefully monitored after previous treatment for contralateral nephroblastoma and a new lesion developed, which was excised by partial nephrectomy. Most of the lesion consisted of ILNRs, but the yellowish nodule indicated by the *arrow* was a nephroblastoma.

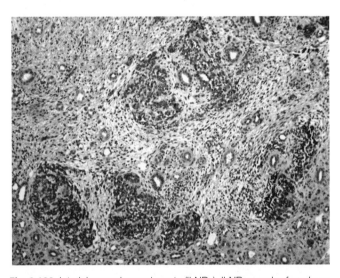

Fig. 2.122 Intralobar nephrogenic rests (ILNRs). ILNRs may be found anywhere in the renal lobe, in the renal sinus, and even in the walls of the pelvicaliceal system. They lie between normal nephrons. Composed of blastema and immature tubules, they form an indistinct interdigitating interface with the adjacent normal tissue.

TABLE 2.6	Relative Frequencies of Pediatric Renal Neoplasms

Neoplasm	Approximate Frequency
Nephroblastoma (not anaplastic)	75%-80%
Nephroblastoma (anaplastic)	5%-8%
Congenital mesoblastic nephroma	4%
Clear cell sarcoma of kidney	3%-4%
Rhabdoid tumor	2%
Renal cell carcinoma	3%-4%
Miscellaneous pediatric renal neoplasms: Ewing sarcoma, synovial sarcoma, angiomyolipoma, lymphoma, and other rare neoplasms	1%-2%

Adapted from Moch H, Humphrey PA, Ulbright TM, Reuter VE, eds. WHO Classification of Tumors of the Urinary System and Male Genital Organs. Lyon: IARC; 2016.

2.122). Like PLNRs, ILNRs may be dormant, obsolescent, or hyperplastic. Overgrowth in ILNRs is usually triphasic, involving stromal prominence, and often with heterologous elements. ILNRs progress to nephroblastoma significantly more often than do PLNRs and are associated more commonly with WT1 mutations and congenital syndromes.

Patients with diffuse hyperplastic nephroblastomatosis are commonly treated with chemotherapy, because the risk for development of multiple nephroblastoma, as well as anaplastic nephroblastomas, is exceptionally high; furthermore, the gradually increasing burden of cumulative neoplasia can degrade renal function. Obviously, such patients require close monitoring and surgical intervention if tumor response is inadequate.[534]

Nephroblastoma (Wilms Tumor)

Nephroblastoma is a malignant neoplasm that is believed to arise from a precursor cell capable of generating the entire kidney, such as the cells of the intermediate mesoderm from which both the metanephric mesenchyme and the ureteric bud are derived.[535] This may explain the variable histologic features of mesenchymal to epithelial differentiation seen in nephroblastoma.[535] Nephroblastoma accounts for about 5% to 6% of all pediatric cancers and comprises approximately 80% to 85% of all pediatric kidney tumors (Table 2.6).[4] It is the second most common intraabdominal cancer of childhood and the fifth most common pediatric cancer overall.[536] In the United States, ~650 new cases of nephroblastoma are diagnosed each year, representing ~8 new cases per million children younger than 15 years.[536] Nearly 50% of nephroblastomas are seen in children younger than 3 years old, 90% occur in children younger than 6 years old, and 98% occur in children younger than 10 years old, with a peak incidence at age 2 to 3 years.[530,537-539] Nephroblastoma occurs slightly more often in females than in males, particularly when it is bilateral.[540] Synchronous or metachronous bilateral involvement occurs in 5% to 10% of patients.[541,542] The risk of its occurrence is lowest among Asians, higher in whites, and highest among African Americans.[543-545] Patients with horseshoe kidneys have a twofold risk for development of nephroblastoma compared with the general population.[546-549] Although nephroblastoma is considered relatively rare in adolescents and adults, the numbers of reported cases have been sufficient for the development of useful treatment protocols.[550,551]

About 10% of nephroblastomas occur in a setting of one of several well-recognized syndromes, manifesting clinical and biologic features that suggest an influence of predisposing germline mutations.[552] Congenital anomalies such as aniridia and genitourinary anomalies accompany nephroblastoma in 1% and 3% of cases, respectively, and about 4% of cases are accompanied by somatic overgrowth syndromes. Approximately 2% of nephroblastoma patients have a family history.[553]

The best known genetic underpinnings of nephroblastoma involve aberrations of WT1, abnormalities of 11p15 methylation, and Wnt-activating mutations involving CTNNB1 and AMER1. In recent years, additional novel mutations have been identified involving miRNA-processing genes *DROSHA*, *DGCR8*, and *DICER1*; renal developmental genes *SIX1* and *SIX2*; and *MYCN*.[554] Many more driver mutations have been identified; nonetheless, recurrent driver mutations have not been identified in most nephroblastomas. It appears likely that many different genetic changes converge on a limited number of developmental pathways, resulting in oncogenesis. One pathway is regulated by miRNA biogenesis, promoting a progenitor state, and another is transcriptional elongation that prevents normal induction.[554]

The best-characterized genetic changes in nephroblastoma involve losses of chromosomal material on the short arm of chromosome 11. The Wilms tumor gene (*WT1*) is located on chromosome 11p13.[555,556] The *WT1* gene is altered by germline heterozygous deletions in the WAGR (Wilms tumor, anirida, genitourinary anomalies, and intellectual disability [formerly referred to as mental retardation]) syndrome, involving loss of most or all of the 11p13 band, and imparting a 30% chance of developing nephroblastoma, and by germline point mutations that impart a 90% risk of developing nephroblastoma in the Denys-Drash syndrome (Wilms tumor, pseudohermaphroditism, and nephropathy). The *WT1* gene is mutated in about 20% of nephroblastomas unassociated with clinical syndromes.[555-557] Another important nephroblastoma locus is located at 11p15, and multiple different mutations at this site are associated with the Beckwith-Wiedemann syndrome (macroglossia, macrosomia, hypoglycemia, visceromegaly, and omphalocele).[558] Additional nephroblastoma loci have been identified at 16q and distal chromosome 1p.[536] About one-third of nephroblastomas can be shown to have somatic deletions involving the *WTX* gene on the X chromosome.[559]

The most common presenting sign of nephroblastoma is a palpable smooth, nontender abdominal mass, detected by a parent during bathing or clothing an otherwise healthy child. Microscopic and occasionally gross hematuria is observed in 20% to 25% of patients; hypertension in 20%; anorexia, fever, and weight loss in 10%; and flank pain or hematuria after trauma in 10%.[560,561] Anemia, polycythemia caused by erythropoietin production by the tumor, free rupture into the peritoneal cavity, and symptoms related to tumor extension into the great vessels (varicocele, hepatomegaly, ascites, congestive heart failure, or sudden death caused

by tumor embolism) are rarely reported presentations.[560,561] Although radiologic techniques may not specifically distinguish nephroblastoma from other pediatric renal neoplasms, such imaging modalities are helpful in staging the neoplasm; furthermore, demonstration of bilaterality or multifocality is unusual in pediatric renal tumors other than nephroblastoma.[561,562]

Most nephroblastomas are solitary and unilateral (Fig. 2.123); however, multifocal tumors in a single kidney are found in 7% of cases (Fig. 2.124), and in 5% of cases, bilateral primary tumors are

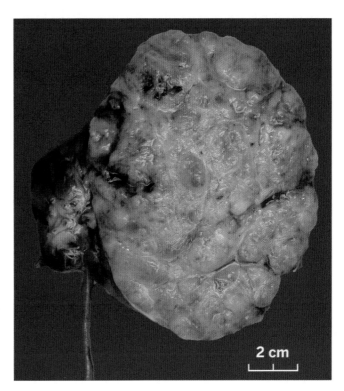

Fig. 2.123 Wilms tumor. This well-circumscribed tumor has a bulging cut surface and a thin fibrous pseudocapsule.

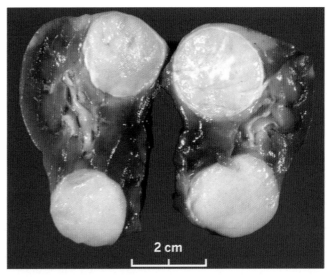

Fig. 2.124 Wilms tumor. Multifocal tumors are present in a single kidney, a finding noted in 7% of cases.

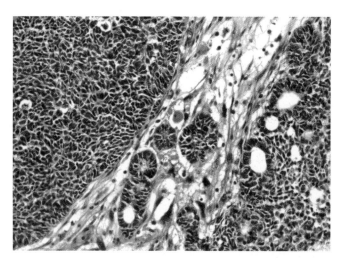

Fig. 2.125 Wilms tumor. Three histologic components are typically present: blastema, epithelium-forming tubules, and stroma.

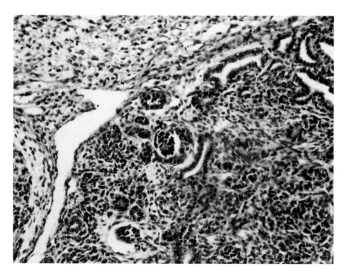

Fig. 2.126 Wilms tumor. Blastema, tubules, and a glomerular structure lacking capillaries are noted.

noted.[533,561,563] Grossly, nephroblastomas are usually sharply circumscribed and confined within a fibrous pseudocapsule, with a wide size range, and weighing up to 6 kg. Their color varies from pale gray to tan, and consistency varies from soft to firm, depending on the content of mature stromal elements.[564,565] Some tumors are extensively cystic; rarely protrusion of the tumor into the renal pelvis results in a "botryoid" appearance.[566,567]

Histologically, most nephroblastomas are triphasic, containing elements of blastema, epithelium, and stroma in varying proportions; however, biphasic and monophasic nephroblastomas also occur (Fig. 2.125). Each cell or tissue type can exhibit a variable degree of differentiation.

Blastema consists of cells that are small, round, densely packed and overlapping, with minimal cytoplasm and little evidence of differentiation. Their nuclei are round or polygonal, relatively uniform in size, with evenly dispersed chromatin and small nucleoli. Abundant mitotic figures are usually present. Blastema exhibits several different growth patterns—diffuse, nodular, and serpentine and basaloid—and these are often admixed within a given tumor. The diffuse pattern is characterized by lack of circumscription at the periphery of the tumor, accompanied by extensive invasion of adjacent soft tissues. Nodular and serpentine patterns show sharply defined round or undulating cords or nests of blastemal cells in a myxoid or fibromyxoid stroma, and if a distinctive layer of epithelial cells is arrayed at the periphery of these cell groups, the pattern is designated as basaloid.[552,564,565]

The epithelial component, present in most nephroblastomas, is characterized by tubular and occasionally glomeruloid structures that recapitulate the developmental stages of metanephric tubules. The tubules range from primitive rosette-like structures virtually indistinguishable from similar structures seen in neuroblastomas to easily recognizable tubular structures with small lumina. Glomerular structures, reminiscent of those seen in normal kidneys but usually lacking capillaries, are seen in some tumors (Fig. 2.126). An appearance of epithelial maturation may be evident, particularly after therapy; foci of readily recognizable squamous, mucinous, or even ciliated epithelium may be present.[552,564,565]

The stromal component exhibits considerable diversity in its relative abundance and patterns of differentiation. Most often it comprises spindle cells in a myxoid background, resembling embryonal mesenchyme. Skeletal muscle with varying degrees of differentiation is the most commonly observed heterologous stromal component. Other differentiation patterns seen in the stromal component of nephroblastoma include smooth muscle, fibrous tissue, cartilage, bone, adipose tissue, and glial and mature ganglion cells.

In the absence of unfavorable histology, most nephroblastomas are highly responsive to chemotherapy. Unfavorable histology is characterized by the presence of nuclear anaplasia, and less commonly by the secondary development of a high-grade sarcoma or carcinoma within a nephroblastoma.[565,568-572] Nuclear anaplasia denotes nuclear hyperchromasia and gigantism with multipolar mitotic figure (Fig. 2.127). It is the cytologic manifestation of extreme polyploidy of tumor cells and is associated with multiple chromosomal rearrangements.[573,574] It can be found in 5% to 8% of nephroblastomas overall; it is rare in tumors from patients younger than 2 years old, but its incidence gradually increases to 13% in tumors from patients 5 years of age or older. The definition of anaplasia requires that the nucleus must be hyperchromatic and that all its major dimensions must be at least three times larger than those

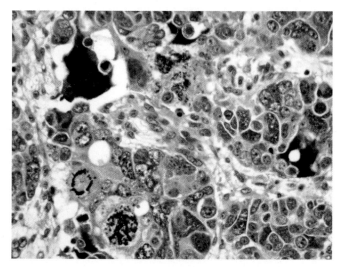

Fig. 2.127 Wilms tumor with nuclear anaplasia: nuclear hyperchromasia and gigantism with multipolar mitotic figure.

TABLE 2.7 Definition of Focal Versus Diffuse Anaplasia

Focal anaplasia

- Clearly defined anaplasia within the primary tumor, and must be circumscribed[a]
- Anaplasia confined to the renal parenchyma
- Anaplasia not present within vascular spaces
- No severe nuclear pleomorphism or hyperchromasia (so-called severe nuclear unrest) in nonanaplastic tumor

Diffuse anaplasia

- Nonlocalized (multifocal) anaplasia
- Anaplasia beyond the tumor capsule
- Anaplastic cells in intrarenal or extrarenal vessels, renal sinus, extracapsular invasive sites, or metastatic deposits
- Anaplasia that is focal, but with nuclear atypia approaching the criteria for anaplasia (so-called unrest nuclear change) present elsewhere in the tumor
- Anaplasia not clearly delimited from nonanaplastic tumor
- Anaplasia present in a biopsy or other incomplete tumor sample
- Anaplasia not meeting criteria for focal anaplasia

[a]The tumor's perimeter must be completely examined, which may require mapping of anaplastic foci that extend to the edge of tissue sections.

Adapted from Moch H, Humphrey PA, Ulbright TM, Reuter VE, eds. WHO Classification of Tumors of the Urinary System and Male Genital Organs. Lyon: IARC; 2016.

of neighboring nonanaplastic nuclei. Each component of the abnormal metaphase of the multipolar polyploid mitotic figure must be as large as, or larger than, a normal metaphase.[564,565]

Anaplasia may be either focal or diffuse (Table 2.7).[4] Focal anaplasia is defined as anaplastic changes confined to sharply restricted foci within the primary tumor sample. The focus must be circumscribed, and its perimeter completely examined, and there must be no severe nuclear pleomorphism or hyperchromasia in nonanaplastic tumor. Focal anaplasia portends a prognosis between that of tumors with favorable histology and tumors with diffuse anaplasia.[573,575] Diffuse anaplasia is defined as follows: multifocal anaplasia; focal anaplasia associated with severe nuclear pleomorphism or hyperchromasia in nonanaplastic tumor; anaplasia identified outside the primary tumor or not clearly delimited from nonanaplastic tumor; or anaplastic cells in intrarenal or extrarenal vessels, renal sinus, extracapsular invasive sites or metastases, or in a biopsy or other incomplete specimen.[573]

Anaplasia is significant because its presence implies increased tumor aggressiveness and portends resistance to chemotherapy.[570,572,576,577] Mutations of the TP53 gene are known to be associated with anaplasia in nephroblastomas, but not in more than 60% of anaplastic tumors, and TP53 mutations have also been recorded in nonanaplastic tumors.[565,578-583] It has been suggested that TP53 positivity in the absence of anaplasia may represent progression events with strong intratumor heterogeneity that are closely linked but not limited, to anaplasia.[584] The presence of *TP53* mutations within tissue containing diffuse anaplasia confers an increased risk for tumor recurrence and death compared with tumors that lack *TP53* abnormalities.[585]

Immunohistochemistry has not been of substantial utility in the pathologic evaluation of nephroblastoma. Nuclear immunostaining for WT1 can be demonstrated in the blastemal and epithelial components of nephroblastoma, but this finding is nonspecific, having been demonstrated in other tumors including desmoplastic small round cell tumor, leukemia, and various carcinomas.[552,565,586,587]

Therapeutic protocols for treatment of nephroblastoma have been developed by the Children's Oncology Group (COG) and the International Society of Pediatric Oncology, and the staging systems used by these groups are similar, but not identical, reflecting the fact that the COG advocates primary resection of the tumor, followed by therapy determined by stage and histologic findings, whereas the International Society of Pediatric Oncology advocates preoperative chemotherapy (with or without initial biopsy) and sometimes radiotherapy, followed by nephrectomy. Outcomes for both sets of protocols are similar; each reports long-term survival rates of approximately 90%.[585,588,589] Prognostic factors used to generate current COG treatment protocols include stage, histology, patient age, tumor weight, completeness of lung nodule response, and loss of heterozygosity at chromosomes 1p and 16q.[575]

The staging system used for nephroblastoma in North America is that of the COG (Table 2.8).[4] This takes into account penetration of the renal capsule, involvement of renal sinus vessels, surgical margins, regional lymph nodes, distant metastases, and bilaterality at presentation.

Nephroblastomas have limited and usually predictable local and metastatic growth patterns. They extend locally into perirenal soft tissues, renal vein, and vena cava (Fig. 2.128). Metastases are most common to regional lymph nodes, lungs, and liver.[590,591] Bone and brain metastases are exceptional.

Cystic Partially Differentiated Nephroblastoma

Cystic partially differentiated nephroblastoma is a multilocular cystic Wilms tumor that is composed entirely of cysts separated by delicate septa; within the septa are small foci of blastema, primitive

TABLE 2.8 Children's Oncology Group Staging System for Renal Tumors

Stage	Definition
I	Tumor limited to the kidney, resected completely, renal capsule intact. The following are accepted: minimal infiltration of renal sinus soft tissues without sinus vessel involvement; protrusion into pelvicaliceal system without infiltration of pelvic/ureteral wall; tumor presence within intrarenal vessels
II	Tumor penetrates renal capsule, extends beyond kidney, but is resected completely; includes tumors infiltrating renal sinus soft tissues more than minimally, and sinus vessels, as well as tumors infiltrating adjacent organs or vena cava, but completely resected
III	Gross or microscopic residual but confined to the abdomen; includes the following: gross or microscopic resection margin positivity; tumor in abdominal lymph nodes; peritoneal involvement by tumor growth; peritoneal contamination by tumor spillage before or during surgery; residual tumor in abdomen; tumor removed piecemeal; tumor underwent biopsy (including fine-needle aspiration) before preoperative chemotherapy
IV	Hematogenous metastasis or lymph node metastasis outside the abdominopelvic region
V	Bilateral renal involvement at diagnosis; tumor in each kidney substaged separately

Adapted from Moch H, Humphrey PA, Ulbright TM, Reuter VE, eds. *WHO Classification of Tumors of the Urinary System and Male Genital Organs*. Lyon: IARC, 2016.

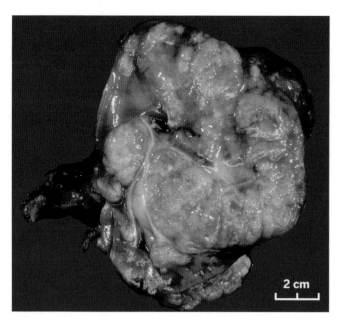

Fig. 2.128 Wilms tumor. This tumor involved the soft tissues of the renal sinus and extended into the renal vein.

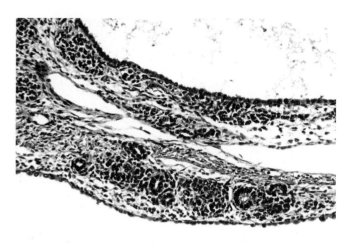

Fig. 2.130 Cystic partially differentiated nephroblastoma. The delicate septa contain blastema and immature tubules.

or immature epithelium, and immature-appearing stromal cells.[592,593] Virtually all such tumors are identified in children younger than 24 months old, and males are affected about twice as often as females.[120]

Cystic partially differentiated nephroblastomas are typically well circumscribed and clearly demarcated from the adjacent normal kidney. They range up to 18 cm in diameter, are entirely composed of cysts of variable size, and entirely lack expansile nodules of tumor (Fig. 2.129).[120] The cysts are lined by flat, cuboidal, or hobnail cells; sometimes no lining epithelium is evident.[593] The septa exhibit variable cellularity and contain blastema, nephroblastomatous epithelial elements in the form of luminal structures

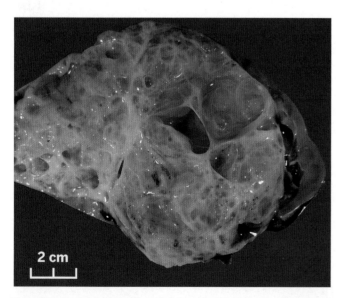

Fig. 2.129 Cystic partially differentiated nephroblastoma. Tumor is entirely composed of cysts of variable size and entirely lacks expansile nodules of tumor.

resembling tubules and ill-formed papillary structures resembling immature glomeruli, and undifferentiated and differentiated mesenchymal elements, most often in the form of skeletal muscle and myxoid mesenchyme, and less often cartilage and fat (Fig. 2.130). Septal elements may form microscopic papillary infoldings within the cysts; in the papulonodular variant they may form grossly evident polyps protruding into cystic spaces.[594]

Cystic partially differentiated nephroblastoma is distinct from pediatric cystic nephroma.[595] Complete surgical excision cures cystic partially differentiated nephroblastoma.[594,596,597] Recurrence may occur in the event of incomplete surgical resection.[596]

Pediatric Cystic Nephroma

Pediatric cystic nephroma is a multilocular cystic neoplasm that occurs in children younger than 24 months and is more common in boys than in girls.[595,598,599] When diagnosed, most are quite large, with a mean diameter of 9 cm. It consists exclusively of cysts entirely lacking any solid component (Fig. 2.131).

The cysts are of variable size and are lined by flattened, cuboidal, or hobnail epithelium. They are separated by fibrous septa that contain cellular aggregates and well-differentiated tubules. Conspicuously and diagnostically absent, in contrast with the findings in the septa of cystic partially differentiated nephroblastoma, are nephroblastomatous epithelial elements, islands of blastema, or undifferentiated or differentiated mesenchymal elements such as cartilage, fat, or skeletal muscle (Fig. 2.132).

Most pediatric cystic nephromas can be shown to have DICER1 mutations.[595,599] These mutations are not found in cystic partially differentiated nephroblastoma and only rarely are detectable in adult cystic nephroma.[595,599]

Germline DICER1 mutations are known to occur, and children in families who carry these mutations are at risk for development of pediatric cystic nephroma (sometimes bilateral) or pleuropulmonary blastoma.[600-602] Germline mutations of this sort are not identified in children with nephroblastoma.[601] Most anaplastic sarcomas of the kidney also have DICER1 mutations, and it is postulated by some investigators that these rare pediatric renal cancers may represent a progression from pediatric cystic nephroma.[595,603,604]

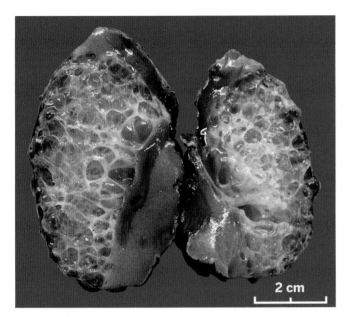

Fig. 2.131 Pediatric cystic nephroma. Entirely cystic renal tumor, lacking tumor nodules, in a young man.

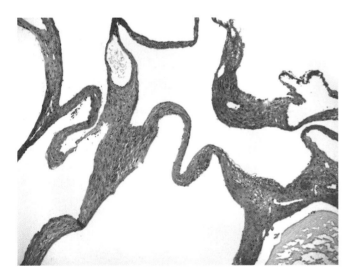

Fig. 2.132 Pediatric cystic nephroma. The septa throughout the tumor lacked elements of nephroblastoma.

Mesenchymal Tumors

Mesenchymal Tumors That Occur Mainly in Children

Clear Cell Sarcoma

The existence of a pediatric renal sarcoma with a propensity to metastasize to bone was reported in 1970 and further delineated in 1978 in three separate reports under three different names, of which "clear cell sarcoma" eventually became the accepted term for this neoplasm.[568,605-607] Evidence suggests that CCSK arises from a mesodermal cell type that retains the capacity to initiate differentiation toward both nephrons and stroma, but remains locked in a primitive state.[608] CCSK accounts for approximately 3% of all

pediatric renal neoplasms and is seen in patients ranging from 2 months to 14 years old; approximately 50% of patients are in their second or third year of life, and mean age at diagnosis is 3 years.[609-611] Male patients outnumber females by a ratio of 2:1. CCSK is neither familial nor associated with renal dysplasia or any known syndrome. The great majority (>90%) of CCSKs harbor internal tandem duplications in the last exon of the *BCOR* (Bcl6 interacting corepressor) gene; it is thought that this gene in CCSK regulates gene transcription through an epigenetic silencing mechanism.[612] In a little less than 10% of cases, a t(10;17)(q22; p13) translocation is demonstrable, resulting in a YWHAE-NUTM2 B/E gene fusion.[613-615] These two genetic changes in CCSK are very likely mutually exclusive.[616] A small subset of CCSK cases harbor neither alteration.[616] Some evidence suggests that there may be links between CCSK and bone/soft tissue sarcomas that harbor BCOR-CCNB3 and other gene fusions.[616]

Most CCSKs are large, unicentric masses that greatly distort or nearly efface the native kidney (Fig. 2.133). Tumors are well circumscribed and sharply demarcated from the adjacent kidney. Apparent origin in the renal medulla is noted in some cases.[519] Tumors range in size from 2.3 to 24 cm in diameter (mean, 11.3 cm). Cut surfaces are generally gray-tan, soft, and mucoid, and cysts are noted in most, sometimes representing the dominant gross finding. Hemorrhage and small foci of necrosis are commonly observed, and extension of tumor into the renal vein is present in 5% of cases. Lymph node metastases are present in approximately 30% of patients at the time of diagnosis.

Microscopically, tumor cells are separated by regularly spaced fibrovascular septa coursing through the tumor, frequently creating vascular arcades that divide the tumor cells into cords or columns 4 to 10 cells in width.[519,617] The width of the fibrovascular septa varies considerably, from thin "chicken-wire" capillaries to capillaries

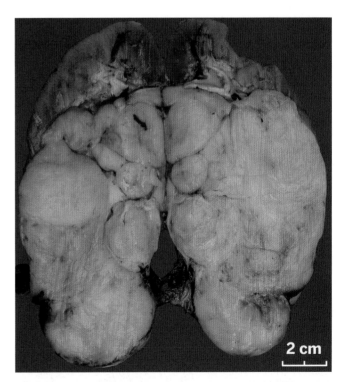

Fig. 2.133 Clear cell sarcoma of kidney. This large, well-circumscribed and sharply demarcated, bulky, bulging unicentric tumor with a soft gray-tan cut surface extensively effaces the native kidney. Necrosis and hemorrhage are not prominent.

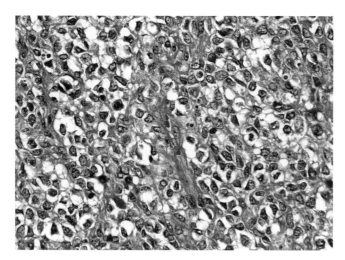

Fig. 2.134 Clear cell sarcoma of kidney. Tumor cells are plump, ovoid, and spindled, with uniform round or oval nuclei, separated by optically clear extracellular mucopolysaccharide matrix material, imparting a clear cell appearance.

surrounded by sheaths of spindle cells in a collagenous matrix. In classic cases, the tumor cells within the cords are plump and ovoid or spindled, with fairly uniform nuclei that are round to oval and often vesicular, with finely dispersed chromatin, inconspicuous nucleoli, and infrequent mitotic figure. Tumor cells are separated by optically clear material, which consists of extracellular mucopolysaccharide matrix, imparting a clear cell appearance (Fig. 2.134). Tubules and glomeruli are typically entrapped at the periphery of the tumor, and cystic dilation of these tubules may simulate cystic nephroma.

Although about 90% of CCSKs exhibit classic microscopic findings, the majority show one of several variant patterns, creating some extraordinarily difficult diagnostic challenges. In the myxoid pattern, cord cells are separated by pools of amphophilic mucinous material. In the sclerosing pattern, osteoid-like material compresses residual cord cells. In the cellular pattern, small nodules of overlapping cord cells may simulate blastemal condensations of Wilms tumor. Both epithelioid patterns, acinar and trabecular, mimic the tubules of Wilms tumor and carcinoma, respectively. The palisading pattern simulates the Verocay bodies of schwannoma, the storiform pattern resembles fibrohistiocytic neoplasms, and the purely spindle cell variant is difficult to distinguish from monophasic synovial sarcoma and cellular CMN. Anaplasia, defined by the same criteria used in Wilms tumor, is noted in about 3% of cases.[439]

Immunohistochemically, the cord cells of CCSK often show positive staining for vimentin, SATB2, cyclin D1, and BCL2.[609,616,618] Immunostains for CD34, S100 protein, desmin, CD99, CK, and EMA are uniformly negative.[611]

With current therapeutic regimes that include radiotherapy and multiagent chemotherapy, 5-year event-free survival rate is 75% to 85%, and 5-year overall survival rate is 85% to 90%.[619] Relapse occurs in about 15% of patients and is most common in younger patients and in those with advanced stage disease. When relapse occurs it is generally within 4 years of treatment, although later relapses occasionally occur; the brain is the most common site of metastasis, likely because of a blood–brain barrier to effective chemotherapy, followed by lung and bone.[619]

Rhabdoid Tumor

Rhabdoid tumor of the kidney (RTK) was first described in 1978.[568] It accounts for about 2% of malignant renal tumors in children.[4,609,620] Although the component cells resemble rhabdomyoblasts, the tumor does not exhibit muscle differentiation. The cell of origin of RTK is not known. The occurrence is limited to patients younger than 5 years; more than 80% occur in children younger than 2 years, and median age is 1 year.

In approximately 15% of RTK cases, a brain tumor, most often located in the midline cerebellum, is present simultaneously or becomes apparent a short time later.[621] Most associated brain tumors resemble medulloblastoma, primitive neuroectodermal tumor, or atypical teratoid/rhabdoid tumor, and have been shown to be second primaries rather than metastases from RTK.[609,622-625] The molecular hallmark of RTK is biallelic inactivation of the HSNF5/INI1 tumor suppressor gene located on the long arm of chromosome 22, a finding that is shared by rhabdoid tumors occurring in the soft tissue, brain, and other tissue sites.[626]

RTK is usually unicentric and unilateral.[622] Most weigh less than 500 g. It is typically bulging, soft, and pale, sometimes with hemorrhage or necrosis, and with an ill-defined interface with the adjacent normal kidney (Fig. 2.135).[621,622] Satellite tumor nodules may be evident.[609]

Microscopically, RTK is composed of monotonous sheets of loosely cohesive cells with distinct cell borders. The tumor cells are large and polygonal, and characteristically show vesicular nuclei, single cherry-red nucleoli of variable prominence, and juxtanuclear, globular, eosinophilic cytoplasmic inclusions, which are ultrastructurally whorled intermediate filaments. Not all tumor cells contain cytoplasmic inclusions, and cells with such cytoplasmic inclusions tend to be clustered rather than diffusely distributed (Figs. 2.136 and 2.137). Rhabdoid tumor demonstrates aggressive infiltration of adjacent renal parenchyma, and extensive vascular invasion is common.[609,622,627]

Immunohistochemically, tumor cells of RTK most consistently show positive staining for vimentin and focal but intense staining for EMA. Expression of other markers, including cytokeratin, neuron-specific enolase, S100 protein, CD99, desmin, and Leu 7, is inconsistent. Immunostaining for INI1 is uniformly negative

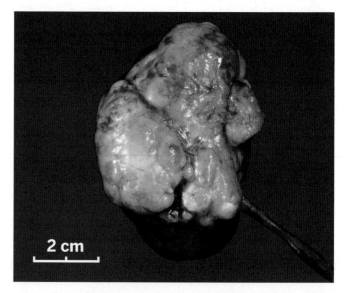

Fig. 2.135 Rhabdoid tumor of kidney. Tumor is bulging and soft, and pale, with an ill-defined interface with adjacent normal kidney.

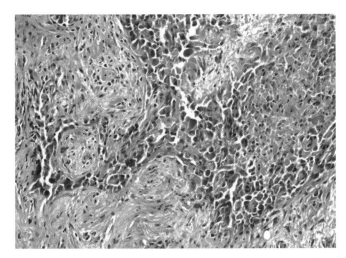

Fig. 2.136 Rhabdoid tumor of kidney. Tumor is composed of sheets of large polygonal, loosely cohesive cells with eccentric nuclei; tumor necrosis is evident.

An abdominal mass is the presenting concern in 76% of patients. In utero detection by ultrasound occurs in up to 16% of cases, and some cases have been associated with polyhydramnios, hydrops fetalis, and premature delivery.[169,631-633] Reported tumor-associated biochemical abnormalities include hypercalcemia and hyperreninemia; in all cases tumor removal has eliminated these biochemical abnormalities.[169,634,635]

CMN is typically unilateral and solitary. It varies from 0.8 to 14 cm in greatest dimension, with a mean of 6.2 cm. Most tumors involve the renal sinus.[609,622] CMN is classified into three subtypes with the following approximate frequencies: classic (39%), cellular (42%), and mixed (10%); subtype was not specified in about 9% of reported cases.[169,636] Classic CMN is typically firm and may exhibit a whorled and myomatous texture. Its interface with the adjacent normal kidney is not sharply demarcated (Fig. 2.138). Cellular CMN is more often bulging and soft, with areas of hemorrhage, necrosis, and cystic degeneration, and its interface with the adjacent normal kidney is more sharply delineated (Fig. 2.139).[609,622,629,637,638] Microscopically, classic CMN is

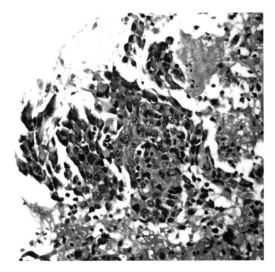

Fig. 2.137 Rhabdoid tumor of kidney. The tumor cells are large and polygonal, with vesicular nuclei that contain nucleoli of variable prominence. Mitotic figures and necrosis are readily apparent. Many tumor cells exhibit juxtanuclear, globular, eosinophilic cytoplasmic inclusions, composed ultrastructurally of whorled intermediate filaments.

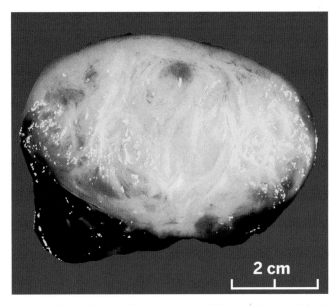

Fig. 2.138 Congenital mesoblastic nephroma. This example was of classic type; it has a whorled and myomatous-appearing cut surface.

in RTK but is retained in virtually all tumors that enter the differential diagnosis. Gene expression profile analysis, used in conjunction with traditional diagnostic tools, has recently been shown to be a powerful tool for separating RTK from Wilms tumor, CCSK, and CMN.[620]

RTK is aggressive and lethal. In most cases disease stage is advanced at presentation. Thus far no satisfactory treatment for children with RTK has been reported; 5-year survival rates range from 10% to 23%.[609,628]

Congenital Mesoblastic Nephroma

CMN was first recognized in 1967.[629] It occurs in approximately 1 in 500,000 infants, and accounts for about 4% of pediatric renal tumors.[630] Male-to-female ratio is 1.5:1. It is the most common renal neoplasm diagnosed in the first month of life, and virtually all cases have occurred in children younger than 30 months.[609]

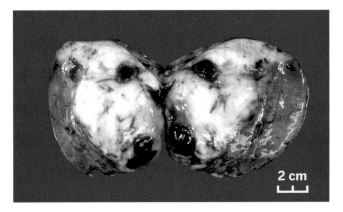

Fig. 2.139 Congenital mesoblastic nephroma. This cellular mesoblastic nephroma has a bulging cut surface and areas of hemorrhage and cystic degeneration.

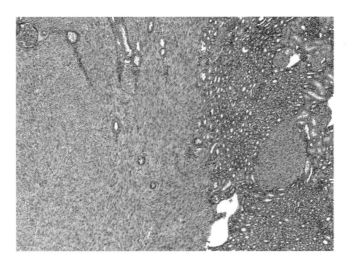

Fig. 2.140 Congenital mesoblastic nephroma. This classic type of mesoblastic nephroma is composed of bland spindle cells that infiltrate between and around adjacent native renal structures.

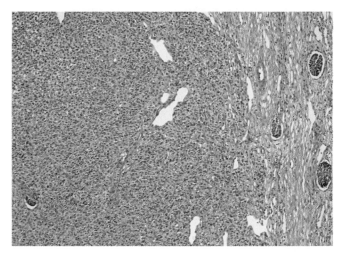

Fig. 2.142 Congenital mesoblastic nephroma. This cellular type of mesoblastic nephroma is densely cellular, with an expansile pushing border where it meets normal kidney.

composed of bland fibroblastic/myofibroblastic cells arranged in fascicles, with only rare mitotic figure and no necrosis. It is indistinguishable from infantile fibromatosis. It subtly infiltrates adjacent tissues, surrounding islands of native kidney at the interface between tumor and normal renal parenchyma (Figs. 2.140 and 2.141).[609,622] Long, narrow tongues of tumor typically extend into perirenal soft tissue, particularly in the renal hilum.

Cellular CMN is microscopically indistinguishable from infantile fibrosarcoma.[609,622] It is expansile, with a "pushing" but unencapsulated border at its interface with normal kidney (Fig. 2.142). It is more densely cellular than the classic variant, and its architecture is more sheetlike than fascicular. It is composed of monomorphic sheets of closely packed small cells with vesicular nuclei and minimal cytoplasm, which may impart a small blue cell appearance (Fig. 2.143). Tumor cells may become plump and elongated with slight to moderate nuclear pleomorphism. The presence of tumor cells with prominent nuclei, in a background of necrosis, may raise concern for rhabdoid tumor. Mitotic figure and necrosis are readily apparent. Mixed CMN is composed of classic and cellular elements

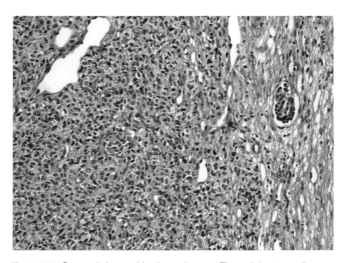

Fig. 2.143 Congenital mesoblastic nephroma. The cellular type of mesoblastic nephroma is composed of monomorphic sheets of closely packed small cells with vesicular nuclei and minimal cytoplasm.

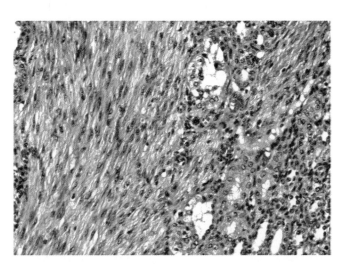

Fig. 2.141 Congenital mesoblastic nephroma. This classic type of mesoblastic nephroma is composed of spindle cells that lack cytologic atypia or mitotic activity.

in variable proportions; the classic variant is often seen at the periphery of a centrally expansile nodule of cellular CMN.

Tumor cells of both variants of CMN show positive immunostaining for vimentin. They often show positive immunostaining for actin and rarely for desmin. They show no immunostaining for cytokeratins, CD34, BCL2, or WT1.[618,622] Ultrastructurally, tumor cells of CMN have features of fibroblasts or myofibroblasts.

All cases of cellular CMN are associated with a specific translocation, t(12;15)(p13;q25), resulting in ETV6-NTRK3 fusion. This rearrangement is identical to that seen in infantile fibrosarcoma but is not found in classic CMN.[639,640] Cellular CMN appears to represent congenital infantile fibrosarcoma arising in the kidney.[609,640,641] There is lack of uniformity in detection of the ETV6-NTRK3 fusion gene in cases of mixed CMN.[641] A variant fusion (EML4-NTRK3) has been reported in cellular CMN, emphasizing that expanding the scope of genetic testing in these cases may be warranted at times.[636]

Cumulative data indicate that 96% of patients with CMN survive.[642] Relapse occurs in about 4% of patients, and more than one-half of patients with relapse achieve a second complete remission. Of the 4% of patients who die, about 2% die of cancer and 2% die of surgical or chemotherapy-related issues.[642]

Ossifying Renal Tumor of Infancy

ORTI was first described in 1980, and so far only about two dozen cases have been reported.[643-645] ORTI is clinically, radiologically, and morphologically distinct from all other pediatric renal tumors. Most patients are males. Patients range in age from 6 days to 2.5 years at the time of diagnosis. Most present with gross hematuria; rarely a mass is palpable. Radiologic studies disclose upper collecting system abnormalities such as dilatation, distortion, filling defects or obstructions, associated with punctate calcifications or a calcified mass within the collecting system. The renal contour is not distorted.[644–646]

At operation a polypoid neoplasm is noted to be attached to the renal medulla, growing exophytically into the pelvicaliceal system, and sometimes reminiscent of a staghorn calculus. In one reported case, two neoplasms were observed.[644] Although the largest ORTI measured 6.5 cm, most are 2 to 3 cm in diameter. ORTI is typically firm to hard, sometimes compressing adjacent renal tissue.[644,645] On sectioning, ORTI is usually pink-white or tan-white and solid, rarely with small cysts.

Microscopically, ORTI appears to originate in the papilla of the medullary pyramids. It is composed of a central partially calcified osteoid matrix surrounded by two populations of cells: an epithelioid component of osteoblast-like cells and a blastemal-like component of round, oval, or spindle cells. Osteoblast-like cells are generally positive immunohistochemically for EMA and vimentin, and variably positive for cytokeratins, whereas the blastemal-like cells are negative for EMA and cytokeratins, and variably positive for vimentin.[646] The precise histogenesis of the tumor is unknown. No cases of ORTI have been associated with Wilms tumor, but some investigators have speculated that it may be derived from ILNR; in support of that, in three recent cases the blastemal-like cells showed strongly positive immunostaining for WT1.[646,647] A recent study of five cases has shown that clonal trisomy 4 may be considered to be a characteristic finding in this tumor.[647,648] ORTI is regarded as a benign tumor, and conservative surgical excision is recommended when possible; nonetheless, the majority of patients have been treated by total nephrectomy.[644]

Mesenchymal Tumors That Occur Mainly in Adults

Leiomyosarcoma

Leiomyosarcoma, a malignant neoplasm demonstrating smooth muscle differentiation, is the most common primary renal sarcoma, accounting for <0.2% of all primary renal malignancies, but comprising 50% to 60% of primary renal sarcomas.[649-654] Slightly more than 100 cases have been reported. Nearly all occur in adults, with a mean age of about 58 years, and with no striking gender difference.[652] Renal leiomyosarcoma may arise from the renal parenchyma, renal capsule, main renal vein, or smooth muscle of the renal pelvis, and rarely, in a background of renal AML (Fig. 2.144); only about 30% are intrarenal.[651,653,655-657] Presenting symptoms may include hematuria, flank pain, fever, or symptoms related to metastases; in some patients a mass is palpable.[649,652,658-661]

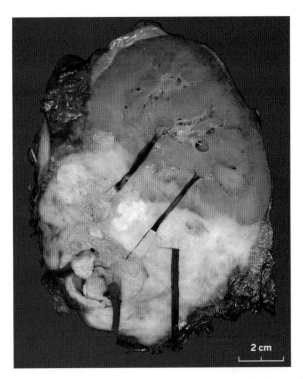

Fig. 2.144 Leiomyosarcoma of kidney. This tumor arose in a background of renal angiomyolipoma; it diffusely infiltrates normal kidney and surrounding soft tissues, with abundant necrosis.

Tumors are solid and can measure up to 23 cm, with a mean tumor diameter of 13 cm.[651] Necrosis is seen in up to 90% of cases, and cystic degeneration may be apparent.[652] Tumors are generally well circumscribed and may appear encapsulated.[652,660,661] They are typically gray-white and soft to firm; some have a whorled cut surface.

The microscopic features of renal leiomyosarcoma are like those of leiomyosarcoma in other sites, composed of spindled, nontapered eosinophilic cells with blunt-ended nuclei, having a fascicular, plexiform, or haphazard architecture (Figs. 2.145 and 2.146). Nuclear pleomorphism is evident in a variable proportion of cases. Mitotic rates are remarkably variable, with a mean of 10.6 per 10 hpf. Myxoid change, usually focal, but sometimes extensive, is frequently observed. Microscopic vascular invasion is commonly noted.

Immunohistochemically, tumor cells typically, although not uniformly, show positive staining for smooth muscle actin, desmin, vimentin, calponin, and h-caldesmon (Fig. 2.147). Immunostains for cytokeratin (Oscar), myogenin, CD117, CD34, HMB45, Melan A, and S100 protein are negative.[652,654]

Leiomyosarcoma must be distinguished from sarcomatoid RCC or urothelial carcinoma, AML, and leiomyoma. The distinction from sarcomatoid carcinoma requires extensive tumor sampling and is aided by use of the immunostains noted earlier. In the distinction of leiomyoma from leiomyosarcoma, tumors exhibiting necrosis, nuclear pleomorphism, and more than rare mitotic figures are considered malignant.[654] AML typically expresses melanocytic markers and cathepsin K, markers that are usually absent in leiomyosarcoma.[652] It should be noted, however, that leiomyosarcoma can rarely arise in a background of AML.[662]

The prognosis for renal leiomyosarcoma is generally poor; 3-year survival rate was 20% and median survival period was

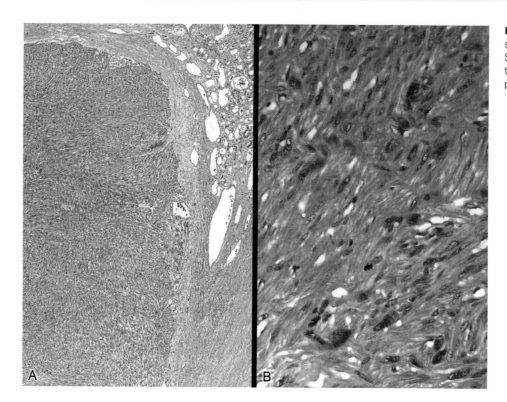

Fig. 2.145 Renal leiomyosarcoma. Expansile tumor with a thick fibrous capsule (A). Spindle cell tumor with haphazard architecture, blunt-ended nuclei, nuclear pleomorphism, and mitotic activity (B).

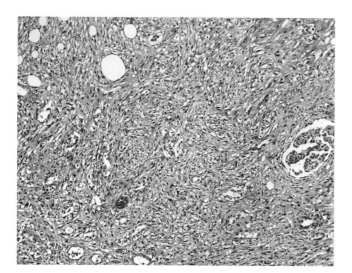

Fig. 2.146 Leiomyosarcoma of kidney arising in angiomyolipoma (same patient as in Fig. 2.144). This spindle cell neoplasm diffusely infiltrates the native kidney. Adipose cells of underlying angiomyolipoma are visible at the upper left.

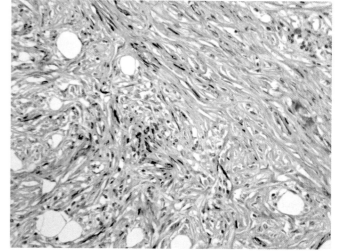

Fig. 2.147 Leiomyosarcoma of kidney arising in angiomyolipoma (same patient as in Fig. 2.144). Spindled tumor cells show positive immunostaining for smooth muscle actin.

18 months in one large series.[651] Most tumors are French Federation of Cancer Centers grade 2 or 3.[654] It is notable that patients with low-grade leiomyosarcoma have a relatively favorable prognosis; those with high-grade tumors fare poorly.[652,661]

Angiosarcoma

Only 2% of all soft tissue sarcomas are angiosarcomas, and less than 5% of angiosarcomas arise in the genitourinary tract.[663] Slightly more than 60 cases of renal angiosarcoma have been reported. Most patients are men between 50 and 69 years old (mean age,

61 years; range, 24 to 95 years).[664] There are no known causative predisposing factors. In one remarkable instance, two brothers developed renal angiosarcoma.[665]

Patients present with hematuria, weight loss, flank pain, hematuria, or symptoms related to metastatic cancer.[663,665-669] Tumors vary in size, measuring up to 23 cm. They have ill-defined borders, are hemorrhagic, yellow to gray-tan, soft, sometimes necrotic, and locally infiltrative.

Microscopically, renal angiosarcoma is similar to angiosarcoma in other sites, exhibiting vasoformative architecture with channels

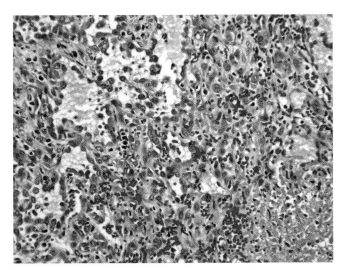

Fig. 2.148 Renal angiosarcoma. This tumor from a 48-year-old man shows vasoformative architecture with channels resembling vascular spaces and sinusoids containing red blood cells, lined by pleomorphic epithelioid and spindle cells.

resembling vascular spaces and sinusoids containing red blood cells, lined by pleomorphic epithelioid cells, as well as areas that are more solid, composed of plump atypical spindle cells with eosinophilic cytoplasm, pleomorphic nuclei, and frequent mitotic figures (Fig. 2.148).[663,665,667-669] Tumor cells show positive immunostaining for CD31, CD34, ERG, FLI1, and factor VIII-RA.

The prognosis for renal angiosarcoma is poor.[663,665-669] Survival is rare and has been noted predominantly in patients whose tumors were less than 5 cm in diameter.[664] About 75% of patients have metastatic cancer at the time of diagnosis or experience metastases shortly thereafter. Mean survival time after diagnosis is 7.7 months.

Rhabdomyosarcoma

Rhabdomyosarcoma is a malignant neoplasm composed of cells with varying degrees of skeletal muscle differentiation. The literature contains fewer than 20 well-documented cases of primary renal rhabdomyosarcoma.[670-673] The majority have arisen in children. Tumors are often large but circumscribed, gray-white and nodular, with necrosis, cystic degeneration, and gross findings indicative of advanced disease stage.

The diagnosis requires absence of sarcoma elsewhere, gross appearance indicative of origin within the kidney rather than spread from a retroperitoneal primary, and extensive tumor sampling to exclude nephroblastoma in children and sarcomatoid carcinoma in adults. The histologic findings and immunoprofile are the same as in rhabdomyosarcomas at other sites (Fig. 2.149). In children, embryonal rhabdomyosarcoma is the commonest subtype, whereas those arising in adults are more likely to be of pleomorphic type. The prognosis for this aggressive cancer is poor.

Osteosarcoma

There are fewer than 30 reported cases of primary renal osteosarcoma.[674-680] Patients are in their fifth to ninth decade of life, and present with abdominal or flank pain, weight loss, or hematuria; the male-to-female ratio is about 2:1.[679] In about one-half of patients, an abdominal mass is palpable. Intratumoral calcifications are typically evident radiologically, may mimic nephrolithiasis, and may create a "sunburst" appearance in the kidney on CT scanning.[58]

Tumors may be as large as 28 cm.[677] Most are locally infiltrative high-stage cancers; 92% present at stage pT3–4 with metastases at diagnosis or soon after.[679] Tumors are described as friable, brown or gray-pink or gray-white, with hemorrhage, necrosis, and bony hard areas.[674,676,677] Microscopically, the tumors are composed of pleomorphic polygonal to spindled cells with associated fibrous stroma and osteoid formation, as well as osteoclastic giant cells. The osteoid shows lacelike ossification. Abundant mitotic activity

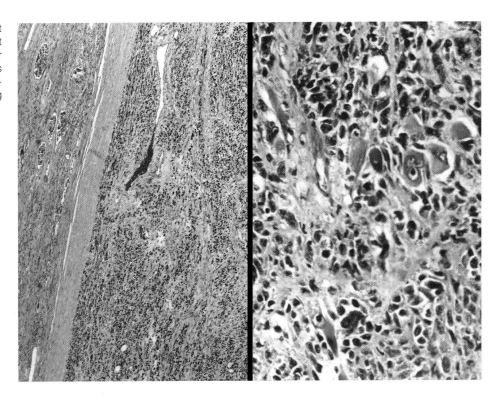

Fig. 2.149 Renal rhabdomyosarcoma. At low power, on left, the appearance is that of a small round blue cell tumor. At higher magnification, on right, small round blue cells are intermingled with cells resembling rhabdomyoblasts and others resembling strap cells.

is usually noted, and atypical cartilage formation may be focally present.

The overall prognosis for renal osteosarcoma is poor. Mean survival is 15 months, and most patients die of cancer within a few months of diagnosis.[679-684] Long-term survival is rare and is associated with low pT stage.[674,679]

Synovial Sarcoma

Synovial sarcoma is a malignant mesenchymal neoplasm capable in some instances of exhibiting epithelial differentiation. Its morphology may be one of three types: monophasic, composed entirely of spindle cells; biphasic, composed of spindle cells and a population of cells with epithelial differentiation; or poorly differentiated. Its defining characteristic is a t(X;18) chromosome translocation [t(X:18)(p11.2/q11.2)], which results in fusion between the SYT gene on chromosome 18 (SS18) and a member of the SSX gene family (SSX1, SSX2, SSX4, or SS18L) on the X chromosome. The most common of these fusions is SS18-SSX2. More than 80 cases of renal synovial sarcoma have been reported to date.[685-693]

Renal synovial sarcoma affects males and females about equally, occurring predominantly in young to middle-aged adults (median age, ~37 years) and infrequently in older adults. Tumors are typically large, ranging from 5 to 20 cm in diameter, with a soft or rubbery consistency, and variegated cut surfaces (Fig. 2.150). Hemorrhage and necrosis are usually evident, and most exhibit smooth-walled cysts. Extension into large vessels is noted in some cases.[685,686]

Of reported cases, 81% were monophasic, 13% were biphasic, and 6% were poorly differentiated.[692,693] Microscopically, renal synovial sarcoma is composed of monomorphic plump spindle cells growing in solid sheets or in short intersecting fascicles that typically infiltrate the adjacent normal renal parenchyma, encircling normal structures (Figs. 2.151 and 2.152). Necrosis is present and is often extensive. The spindle cells in most instances are nonpleomorphic, with ovoid nuclei and indistinct cell borders. However, examples of this tumor with extensive rhabdoid morphology

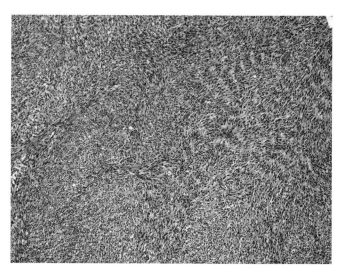

Fig. 2.151 Renal synovial sarcoma, monomorphic. Section from tumor in Fig. 2.150. Tumor cells showed positive immunostaining for TLE1 and bcl2, weak staining for CD99, and negative staining for keratin markers, smooth muscle markers, HMB45, WT1, and PAX8.

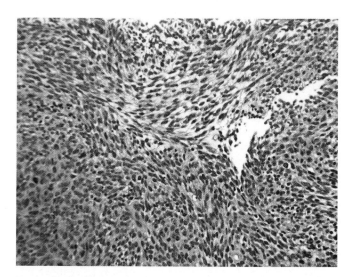

Fig. 2.152 Renal synovial sarcoma, monomorphic. Section from tumor in Fig. 2.150. FISH analysis of the tumor was positive for SS18(SYT) gene rearrangement.

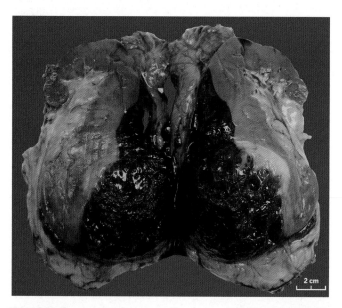

Fig. 2.150 Renal synovial sarcoma. Renal mass in a 29-year-old woman who experienced an abrupt onset of flank pain. Computed tomographic scan showed a perirenal hematoma, with suspicion for an associated neoplasm. (Image courtesy Liwei Jia, MD.)

have been identified, emphasizing that synovial sarcoma needs to be considered part of the differential of mesenchymal kidney tumors with prominent rhabdoid features.[688] Mitotic figures are abundant. Areas of dense cellularity often alternate with hypocellular myxoid, edematous, or sclerotic areas. Cysts of variable size are present, lined by mitotically inactive hobnail epithelium with abundant eosinophilic cytoplasm; the cysts are regarded as entrapped and cystically dilated native renal tubules (Fig. 2.153).[685,686]

Immunohistochemically, tumor cells consistently show positive nuclear immunostaining for TLE1 and cytoplasmic staining for BCL2, but no immunoreactivity for S100 protein, CD34, desmin, or muscle-specific actin. Scattered positive immunostaining for keratin markers is seen in about 50% of cases.[685-688,692]

Outcome data for renal synovial sarcoma are somewhat limited, but available statistics indicate that metastases are present at the

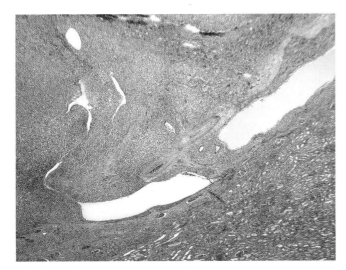

Fig. 2.153 Synovial sarcoma of kidney. Sheets of monomorphic spindle cells surround cysts that are probably trapped and cystically dilated native renal tubules.

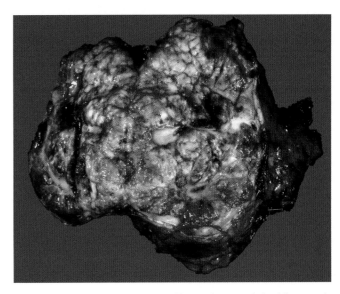

Fig. 2.154 Ewing sarcoma of kidney. Tumor almost entirely obliterates the native kidney.

time of diagnosis or develop later in at least 40% of patients, and that metastasis usually indicates a very poor prognosis, with a median survival of 6 months.[685-693]

Ewing Sarcoma

Peripheral neuroectodermal tumor and Ewing sarcoma are small, round cell sarcomas that are members of a common histologic spectrum known as the Ewing family of tumors.[694] Members of this family share a balanced translocation [t(11;22) (q24;q12)] that encodes an oncogenic fusion protein and transcription factor, EWS/FLI. This tumor-specific chimeric fusion retains an element of EWS, a member of the TET family of microRNA (mRNA)-binding proteins, and an element of FLI, a member of the ETS family of transcription factors. Other translocation fusions belonging to the TET/ETS family also occur in Ewing sarcoma.[695,696] The specific gene fusion does not affect prognosis.[697] Although extraskeletal Ewing sarcoma most commonly arises in deep soft tissues of the extremities, more than 120 cases of primary Ewing sarcoma of the kidney (ESK) have been reported.[698-718] The cell of origin for ESK is not known. Studies suggest that it is derived from a mesenchymal stem or progenitor cell, rather than from a type of neural crest cell.[719]

The age range for patients with ESK is 3 to 78 years old, with a median age of ~27 years and a slight male preponderance.[718] Patients present with abdominal pain, hematuria, a palpable mass, and sometimes with constitutional symptoms.

Tumors are typically large (>10 cm in many instances), poorly circumscribed gray-tan to white tumors that extensively obliterate the native renal parenchyma (Fig. 2.154).[710] Hemorrhage, necrosis, and renal vein invasion are common gross findings. ESK falls into a category of small, round, blue cell tumors of the kidney, including blastemal Wilms tumor, small cell neuroendocrine carcinoma, rhabdomyosarcoma, synovial sarcoma, CIC-DUX4 and BCOR-CCNB3 translocated sarcomas, lymphoma, and poorly differentiated RCC; hence its diagnosis is especially challenging.

Microscopically, ESK consists of sheets of monotonous polygonal cells with high nuclear-to-cytoplasmic ratios, arranged in a vaguely lobular pattern (Fig. 2.155). Cell overlapping is not prominent. Nuclei are round and hyperchromatic, with dispersed

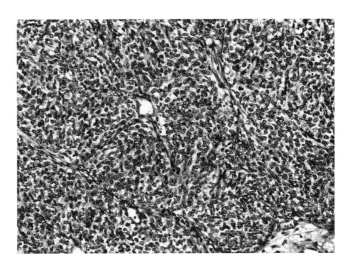

Fig. 2.155 Ewing sarcoma of kidney. Sheets of monotonous polygonal cells with high nuclear-to-cytoplasmic ratios are arranged in a vaguely lobular pattern. Nuclei are round and hyperchromatic, with dispersed chromatin and absent or inconspicuous nucleoli.

chromatin and absent or inconspicuous nucleoli. Mitotic figures are readily apparent and may be numerous. In well-preserved specimens, cells may show a small amount of clear cytoplasm, corresponding to the presence of intracytoplasmic glycogen. Tumor cells infiltrate adjacent renal parenchyma as broad sheets or finger-like projections. Pseudorosette formation may be noted (Fig. 2.156). Immunohistochemically, ESK shows positive immunostaining with the following frequencies: CD99, almost 100%; vimentin and S100 protein, 52% to 70%; NSE and synaptophysin, 48% to 95%; FLI1 protein, 71% to 84%; cytokeratin or desmin, rarely. None of the immunohistochemical markers are specific for the diagnosis.[718] Neurosecretory granules may be evident ultrastructurally.

Because the morphology and immunoprofile of ESK overlap with several other tumors as noted earlier, confirmation of the diagnosis by molecular studies is necessary. Reciprocal translocations

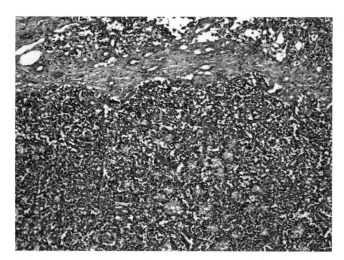

Fig. 2.156 Ewing sarcoma of kidney. An area of rosette formation is demonstrated.

between chromosomes 11 and 22 involving bands q24 (containing the *FLI1* gene locus) and q12 (containing the *EWS* gene locus) are found in 85% to 95% of ESKs; hence demonstration of the EWS/FLI1 fusion transcript by cytogenetic or polymerase chain reaction assays can assist in confirming the diagnosis, but bearing in mind that translocation partners other than FLI1, such as the ERG locus and other rare partners, are also found in ESK, and the EWS gene rearrangement can be found in CCSK, neuroblastoma, and desmoplastic small, round cell tumor as well. Break-apart FISH probes that demonstrate displacement of the ESWR1 locus are useful adjunctive tests. False-negative molecular tests can result from sampling errors or variant fusions. In short, an accurate diagnosis of ESK requires correlation of all available clinical, morphologic, immunohistochemical, and molecular genetic data.[718]

The prognosis for renal peripheral primitive neuroectodermal tumor is guarded. Nearly one-half of patients have metastatic cancer at the time of presentation, and less than 40% of patients with metastases at presentation survive 4 years.[712,717,718] In a recent analysis of 40 patients with ESK, 57% were free of disease during 5 to 58 months of follow-up, but 43% died of their disease.[712]

Angiomyolipoma

AML is a member of the PEComa family. Neoplasms in this family are composed of perivascular epithelioid cells (PECs), an enigmatic cell type that lacks an established nonneoplastic counterpart, and typically occupies a perivascular location. There is experimental evidence supporting the premise that the progenitor of renal AML is the lymphatic endothelial cell.[720] Lymphatic endothelial cell marker D2-40 reportedly highlights endothelial-lined spaces with rounded, elongated, irregular shapes, or complex sinusoidal or labyrinth-like formations.[721] PECs coexpress contractile proteins (predominantly α-smooth muscle actin and calponin); melanocytic markers including microphthalmia-associated transcription factor (MITF), HMB45, HMSA1, and Melan A/MART1; and cathepsin K, PNL2, estrogen receptor (ER), and progesterone receptor (PR). A small subset of PEComa neoplasms harbor TFE3 gene fusions, demonstrable not only by strong nuclear immunohistochemical staining for TFE3, but also by a break-apart FISH assay.[722] PECs are capable of exhibiting a variety of morphologic and immunophenotypical appearances: spindle shapes resembling smooth muscle, expressing actin more strongly than

HMB45; epithelioid shapes expressing HMB45 and little, if any, expression of actin; or they may develop vacuolization to the extent of resembling an adipocyte. Members of the PEComa family include AML, clear cell "sugar" tumor of the lung and extrapulmonary sites, lymphangioleiomyomatosis, clear cell myomelanocytic tumor of the falciform ligament/ligamentum teres, and rare clear cell tumors in other anatomic sites. Renal PEComa tumors encountered in surgical pathology practice include classic AML, epithelioid AML, and AML with epithelial cysts.[723]

The term *angiomyolipoma* came into popular use in 1951, although its existence had been documented many decades before that.[724] Initially regarded as a hamartoma, it is now known to be a neoplasm.[713,725-728] The development of PEComa neoplasms, such as AML, is related to the genetic alteration that is seen in patients with and without the clinical criteria necessary for a diagnosis of TSC, and the association between AML and TSC has been known for a long time.[649,729,730] TSC is an autosomal dominant genetic disorder characterized by seizures, mental retardation, autism, and the development of diverse tumors in multiple sites, including AML, subependymal giant cell tumor, cutaneous angiofibroma, cardiac rhabdomyoma, lymphangioleiomyomas, and pulmonary multifocal micronodular hyperplasia.[723,731-733] TSC results from inactivating heterozygous or mosaic mutations in either TSC1 (9q34) (21% of cases) or TSC2 (16p13.3) (79% of cases).[732,734,735] Proteins that are encoded by the TSC1 and TSC2 genes form a complex (TSC1/TSC2) that acts as a negative regulator of mammalian target of rapamycin complex 1 (mTORC1). Hyperactivation of mTORC1 occurs when the TSC1/TSC2 complex is disrupted, resulting in unregulated protein translation and cell growth.[694,736,737] AMLs that arise in patients with TSC occur because of biallelic inaction of either TSC2 or TSC1, and arise in both males and females equally in the third and fourth decades of life (Fig. 2.150). Sporadic, non–TSC-associated renal AMLs arise nearly exclusively in association with mutations in TSC2 and develop in the fourth through sixth decades of life, predominantly in females.[723,738,739]

AMLs account for about 1% of surgically removed renal tumors; of these, four to five times as many sporadic AMLs are removed in comparison with AMLs removed from patients with TSC, and four times as many are removed from females as from males, possibly because of hormonal influences on tumor growth in females.[649,740-743]

AML occurs in patients of all ages.[740] Many AMLs, particularly those less than 4 cm in diameter, produce no symptoms and are found incidentally or during screening in patients with tuberous sclerosis.[744] However, more than 80% of AMLs that exceed 4 cm in diameter are associated with symptoms or signs, which include acute or chronic abdominal or flank pain, hematuria, nausea, vomiting, and fever. An abdominal or flank mass is often present, and some patients have associated hypertension. More than one-half of tumors more than 4 cm in diameter are associated with some degree of bleeding, which may be sufficient to result in hypovolemic shock.[742,744] Rupture of renal AML during pregnancy is a well-recognized complication.[745,746]

Renal AML can be accurately diagnosed in most cases using ultrasound or CT scanning, because of their fat content.[747,748] Exceptions to this include AMLs that are almost entirely composed of smooth muscle components, AMLs with extensive intratumoral bleeding, and rare renal malignancies that contain fat, mimicking AMLs.[749-753]

Classic AML is the commonest renal mesenchymal tumor; may be situated in the renal cortex, medulla, or capsule; and may be

Fig. 2.157 Renal angiomyolipoma. Multiple tumors were resected from a 19-year-old woman with tuberous sclerosis.

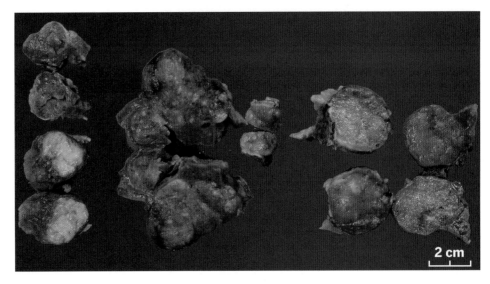

solitary or multiple (Fig. 2.157). Most surgically excised specimens are greater than 4 cm in diameter and can be as large as 30 cm in greatest dimension.[754] Most are smoothly rounded or ovoid and circumscribed, but not encapsulated. They compress and distort the adjacent renal parenchyma but do not infiltrate it. Extension into the perirenal fat is often seen, and rarely AML infiltrates adjacent structures to an extent that makes it unresectable (Fig. 2.151).[649,747] There are about two dozen reports of AML that extended into the renal vein or vena cava, in one instance even extending as far as the right atrium.[740] Tumors vary from pink-tan or gray to yellow, depending on the relative contents of smooth muscle and fat.

Microscopically, the interface between AML and the adjacent renal parenchyma is sharp, with minimal intermingling of tumor and native renal tubules. Although all AMLs are composed of smooth muscle, fat, and abnormal blood vessels, the relative proportions of these elements vary from tumor to tumor and even within different regions of the same tumor. Aggregates of thick-walled artery-like blood vessels are admixed with large mature fat cells and smooth muscle cells (Fig. 2.158). The blood vessels typically are devoid of elastica.[755] The smooth muscle cells show some degree of pleomorphism; some are spindled cells resembling normal smooth muscle, and some are rounded epithelioid cells.[740] Although smooth muscle cell nuclei are usually small and regular, lacking mitotic activity, focal areas of marked nuclear atypia may be present, with occasional mitotic figure. The smooth muscle cells typically form a collar around the adventitia of the abnormal blood vessels and may exhibit a perpendicular orientation in relation to it, creating a "hair on end" appearance (Fig. 2.159).[747] Hemorrhage and areas of necrosis are commonly seen.

AML with epithelial cysts is characterized by the presence of prominent intratumoral cysts of variable size (Fig. 2.160). Usually there is one large cyst; this may be accompanied by smaller cysts.[756,757] The cysts represent entrapped and cystically dilated native renal tubules; they are lined by cuboidal to hobnail cells. Beneath the cyst epithelium is a compact cellular "cambium-like" layer of stromal cells likely representing Müllerian differentiation of PEC. AML with epithelial cysts typically have a component of muscle-predominant AML. Prominent curvilinear and branching lymphatic spaces are evident within the smooth muscle, most

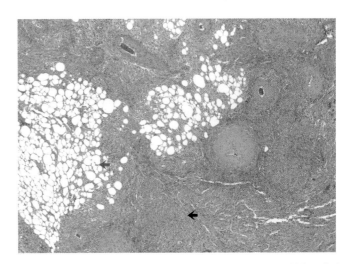

Fig. 2.158 Renal angiomyolipoma. Tumor is composed of thick-walled artery-like blood vessels (*green arrow*), admixed with large mature fat cells (*red arrow*), and smooth muscle cells (*black arrow*).

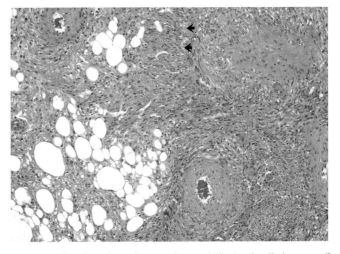

Fig. 2.159 Renal angiomyolipoma. *Arrows* indicate the "hair on end" appearance of smooth muscle cells adjacent to blood vessels.

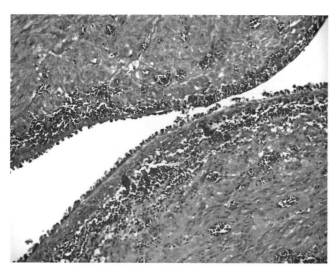

Fig. 2.160 Renal angiomyolipoma with epithelial cysts. This otherwise typical angiomyolipoma containing a cyst lined by cuboidal to hobnail cells, representing an entrapped and cystically dilated native renal tubule.

prominently in the subepithelial myomatous layer. The mesenchymal cells show positive immunostaining for melanocytic markers, cathepsin K, CD10, ER, and PR.

As noted in the introduction, the spindled and epithelioid smooth muscle cells of classic AML are typically immunoreactive to antibodies against MITF, Melan A, HMB45, smooth muscle actin, and calponin (Fig. 2.161).[758,759] Cathepsin K is highly expressed in the entire spectrum of PEC lesions of the kidney.[760,761] PNL2, a sensitive and specific biomarker for melanoma, has been shown to have high sensitivity and specificity for AML. It does not stain other renal neoplasms, with the exception of melanocytic Xp11.2 translocation RCC.[762] Positive staining for CD68, S100 protein, desmin, ER, and PR is seen in some AMLs, but none shows immunoreactivity for epithelial markers (Fig. 2.154).[763-767]

AML in regional lymph nodes in nephrectomy specimens containing AML is regarded as an expression of multicentricity of disease rather than metastasis.[740,768-772] Renal AML has also

been reported to coexist with AML in the perirenal fat, the opposite kidney, the adrenal, the liver, the lung, and the spleen.[740,773]

Although classic AML is regarded as a benign neoplasm, it can be associated with a variety of adverse outcomes. Rupture with massive blood loss can lead to fatal consequences.[740,773] Renal disease, comprising confluent, multiple bilateral AML and renal cysts, causes renal insufficiency in approximately 15% of patients with tuberous sclerosis and is the second most common cause of death in such patients after central nervous system causes, and the most common cause of death in such patients older than 30 years.[738,740] As noted previously, AML has infrequently been reported to infiltrate local structures to an extent that precluded surgical excision and ultimately caused death.[774,775] Two cases of sarcoma arising in AML have been documented.[662,776] AML can exist concurrently with RCC, which is most often of clear cell type and less frequently of chromophobe cell type.[738,777,778]

Studies of large series of patients and observations of the behavior of AML followed radiologically over periods of many years have allowed various management regimens to be proposed.[649,738,742-744,774,779] However, details of management algorithms are beyond the scope of this chapter.

Epithelioid Angiomyolipoma

The existence of AML with epithelioid elements was recognized gradually over a period of years beginning in the late 1980s.[26,113,780-783] Currently the designation of epithelioid AML requires that this variant of AML must be composed of at least 80% epithelioid cells.[784,785] The realization that such tumors could exhibit malignant behavior also evolved gradually.[662,776,782,786-789]

Males and females are equally affected, and the mean age at diagnosis is 50 years (range 30 to 80 years). Like classic AML, epithelioid AML occurs sporadically, as well as in patients with tuberous sclerosis. Loss of heterozygosity of the *TSC2* gene has been reported in epithelioid AML.[782] Because very little fat is present in most epithelioid AMLs, they mimic carcinoma radiologically. Tumors tend to be large, gray-tan, white, or brown (Fig. 2.162). Hemorrhage is common, and necrosis may be present and sometimes extensive. Gross involvement of perirenal fat, renal veins, or vena cava by tumor may be apparent.

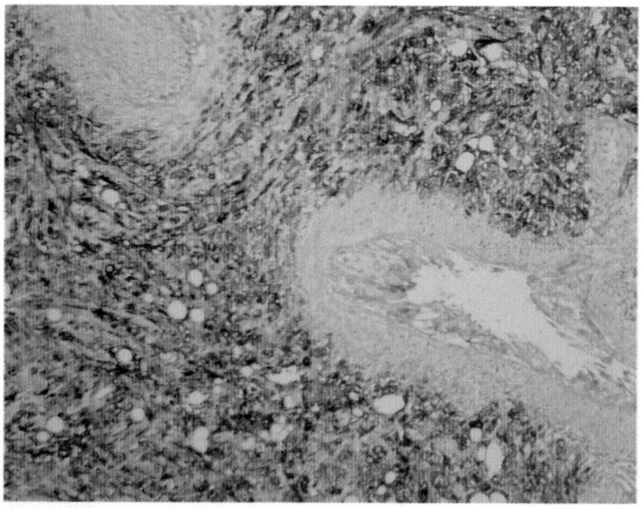

Fig. 2.161 Renal angiomyolipoma. Tumor cells show positive immunostaining for Melan A.

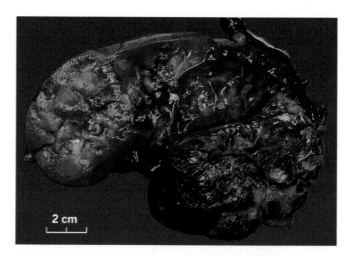

Fig. 2.162 Renal epithelioid angiomyolipoma. Woman, aged 74 years, who had a needle biopsy of a renal mass that was diagnosed as angiomyolipoma mainly composed of epithelioid cells. Imaging 2 years later disclosed a dramatic increase in size, prompting radical nephrectomy.

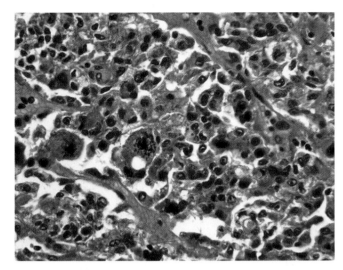

Fig. 2.163 Renal epithelioid angiomyolipoma. Tumor with a "carcinoma-like pattern." Thin vascular septa separate compartmentalized sheets of round to polygonal epithelioid cells with abundant eosinophilic cytoplasm, vesicular nuclei with prominent nucleoli, and abundant highly atypical mitotic figure.

Histologically, epithelioid AMLs tend to exhibit two different growth patterns. In the "carcinoma-like" pattern, tumor cells are arranged in cohesive nests, broad alveoli, and compartmentalized sheets separated by thin vascular-rich septa (Fig. 2.163).[723] Tumor cells are large and polygonal, somewhat discohesive, and have dense, deeply eosinophilic cytoplasm and atypical nuclei with prominent nucleoli, and sometimes intranuclear inclusions.[723] Some tumors with this architecture exhibit two or more mitotic figures per 50 hpf, but most have none or only one mitotic figure per 50 hpf. Necrosis and hemorrhage may be present. Another common morphology in epithelioid AML is described as

"epithelioid and plump spindled cells with diffuse growth" (Fig. 2.164).[723] In these tumors, noncompartmentalized epithelioid and spindled cells grow diffusely in densely packed sheets. The epithelioid cells are smaller and more uniform than in the carcinoma-like tumors and have clear to granular feathery eosinophilic cytoplasm. Their nuclei lack significant atypia but have vesicular chromatin and prominent nucleoli. Intranuclear inclusions and mitotic figures are absent or rare. Multinucleated giant cells may be seen in either growth pattern.[723,781,782,786,789,790] Vascular invasion and extension into perirenal soft tissues may be seen in some cases. Components of classic AML may be apparent.[740,781-783] Some tumors are partially or predominantly composed of cells with clear cytoplasm, sometimes with patchy dark-brown melanin pigment, and, rarely, the degree of pigmentation may be quite striking.[791-794]

Immunohistochemically, epithelioid AML expresses melanocytic markers (HMB45, HMB50, MITF, and MART1/Melan A), as well as smooth muscle markers (smooth muscle actin and muscle-specific actin) (Fig. 2.165).[113,781,782,795,796]

Although it is universally agreed that epithelioid AMLs have malignant potential, the magnitude of that potential has been the subject of much debate, likely because of wide variability of the nature of the patient cohorts reported by various investigators and the definitions used to define the reported tumors as epithelioid AML.[784,785,797,798] Somewhat dire outcomes have been reported in series that very likely include a large number of consultation cases and therefore may reflect a nonstandard experience.[784,798] Tumors harboring epithelioid components with substantial cytologic atypia, defined as atypical polygonal cells with abundant cytoplasm, vesicular nuclei, prominent nucleoli, and nuclear size more than two times the size of adjacent nuclei, have been designated "epithelioid AML with atypia."[798] About 25% of patients whose tumors fall into this category experienced adverse events including recurrence, distant metastasis, and in some instances, cancer-related death.[798] Histologic features most often

Fig. 2.164 Renal epithelioid angiomyolipoma. Sections from the tumor shown in Fig. 2.162. Another common tumor morphology in epithelioid angiomyolipoma, distinct from the "carcinoma-like" pattern shown in Fig. 2.163. On the left the cells are epithelioid, with abundant finely granular, flocculent, or denser eosinophilic cytoplasm. Nuclei are round, with vesicular chromatin and prominent nucleoli. Other portions of this tumor were dominated by plump spindle cells, as shown on the right. Mitotic figures are absent.

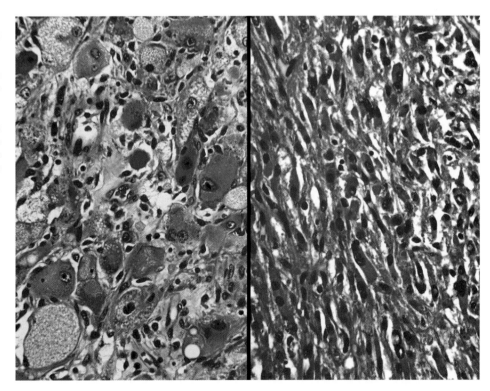

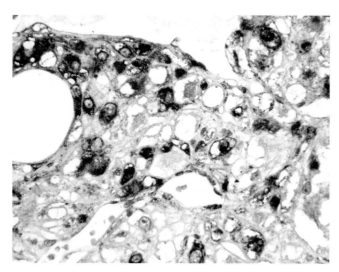

Fig. 2.165 Renal epithelioid angiomyolipoma. Tumor cells show positive immunostaining for HMB45.

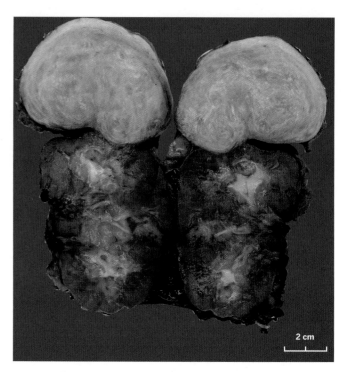

Fig. 2.166 Renal leiomyoma. This renal tumor was discovered incidentally in a 78-year-old woman, mimicking renal cell carcinoma radiologically and clinically. (Image courtesy Akisha Glasgow, MD.)

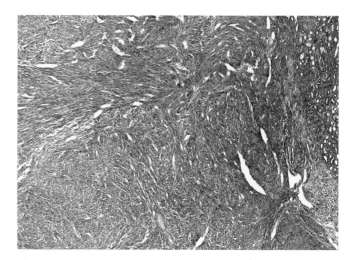

Fig. 2.167 Renal leiomyoma. Tumor is composed of spindle cells arranged in small intersecting fascicles, typical of smooth muscle.

associated with malignant behavior include nuclear atypia in ≥70% of the epithelioid cells, mitotic count ≥2 per 10 hpf, presence of atypical mitotic figure and necrosis. Tumors with fewer than three of these features tend to have a benign course, whereas three or four of these features predict an aggressive course.[798] In a series of epithelioid AMLs entirely composed of epithelioid elements ("pure" [monotypic] epithelioid PEComa neoplasms), 17% suffered recurrence postsurgery, metastases were present initially or developed later in nearly one-half of patients, and cancer-related death occurred in one-third of patients in whom follow-up could be obtained.[784] In this study, adverse prognostic factors included extrarenal tumor extension, renal vein extension, and carcinoma-like histologic growth pattern.

Conversely, in two large series of consecutively resected AMLs, epithelioid morphology accounting for as little as 10% of the tumor comprised only 8% of the cases, and in the other, tumors with at least 80% epithelioid morphology comprised only 4.6% of the cohort. No adverse events were recorded in the first series, and in the second series, only 1 of 20 patients with epithelioid AMLs experienced development of distant metastases.[785,798] Putting this in perspective, although some epithelioid AMLs, when defined as those that have ≥80% epithelioid morphology, can exhibit malignant behavior in the form of local recurrence or distant metastasis, the proportion of AMLs that comprise this category is probably less than 5% overall.[785]

Leiomyoma

Leiomyoma is a benign neoplasm with smooth muscle differentiation. Those arising in the kidney are exceptionally uncommon; fewer than 50 well-documented cases have been reported.[654,799,800] Leiomyoma may arise in the renal capsule, cortical vascular smooth muscle, or smooth muscle of the renal pelvis.[801] It occurs almost exclusively in adult females, with mean age ranging from 58 to 63 years. Although the great majority of cases are detected incidentally, some have been associated with gross hematuria or abdominal pain.

Tumors range from 0.3 to 20 cm in greatest dimension, with a mean diameter of 3 to 4 cm. Renal leiomyoma is typically firm, bulging, and well circumscribed, with a gray-white whorled fibrous or trabeculated cut surface (Fig. 2.166). Microscopically, it is composed of long fascicles of elongated, fusiform cells with scant to moderate eosinophilic cytoplasm, elongated "cigar-shaped" blunt-ended nuclei with fine chromatin and inconspicuous nucleoli, arranged in nodules of intersecting fascicles separated by variable amounts of stroma (Fig. 2.167).[800] Stromal hyalinization and sclerosis are common and may be extensive. Thick vessels, like those seen in uterine leiomyomas, are sometimes present. Nuclear atypia, necrosis, vacuolated cytoplasm, and lipid-containing cells are absent, and mitotic figures are rare to absent.[654,799,800]

Immunohistochemically, tumor cells exhibit a low Ki67 proliferation rate, positive staining for all smooth muscle markers, and positive immunostaining for ER/PR/WT1 in nearly all instances (Fig. 2.168). Immunostains for HMB45, Melan

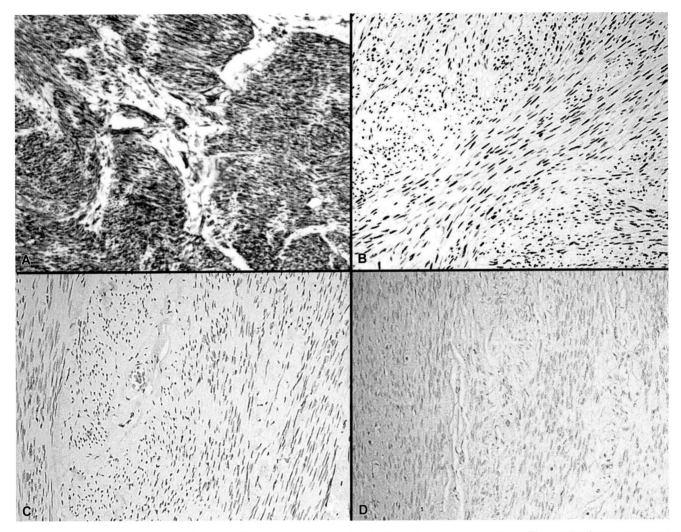

Fig. 2.168 Renal leiomyoma. Tumor cells showed positive immunostaining for desmin (A) and for progesterone receptor (B), as well as for estrogen receptor and smooth muscle actin (not shown). Immunostains for HMB45 (C) and cathepsin K (D) were negative, as were immunostains for Melan A and S100 protein (not shown). (Images courtesy Akisha Glasgow, MD.)

A/MART1, and cathepsin K are negative.[654,800] The lack of immunoreactivity for HMB45 and cathepsin K is regarded as very helpful in distinguishing renal leiomyoma from lipid-poor renal AML, because the latter will commonly express one or both of these markers.[800]

Hemangioma

More than 200 cases of renal hemangioma have been reported. Some cases occur sporadically, and some present in a background of other vascular disorders such as Klippel-Trenaunay syndrome, Sturge-Weber syndrome, or systemic angiomatosis. Although the age spectrum of patients with renal hemangioma is broad, ranging from infancy to old age, the majority are young to middle-aged adults. The cardinal manifestation of renal hemangioma is hematuria, but some patients present with abdominal or flank pain; the tumor is discovered incidentally in some, and in small children a palpable mass may draw attention to the lesion. Most renal hemangiomas are small, 1 to 2 cm in greatest dimension, but may be as large as 18 cm. They are most often located in the renal pelvis or renal pyramids, but may also be found in the renal cortex, the renal capsule, or within peripelvic blood vessels or soft tissues (Fig. 2.169).[802-810]

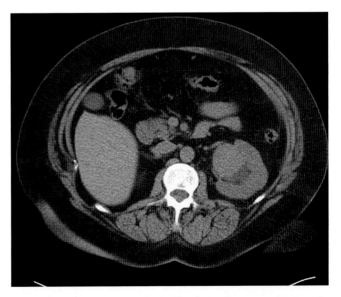

Fig. 2.169 Renal hilar hemangioma. On computed tomography scan, the lesion occupying the hilum of the right kidney was indistinguishable from a malignancy.

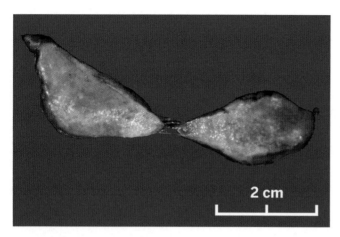

Fig. 2.170 Renal hilar hemangioma. Same patient as shown in Fig. 2.169. At surgery, this soft, uniformly tan-red lesion was loosely attached to large vessels in the renal hilum but was not an intrinsic part of the kidney.

Grossly, renal hemangioma may be difficult to visualize, appearing as a small, mulberry-like lesion or a small red streak. Larger lesions exhibit varying degrees of circumscription and often appear red or gray-tan and spongy (Fig. 2.170).

Microscopically, renal hemangioma is composed of irregular, blood-filled, vascular spaces lined by a single layer of endothelial cells that lack mitotic activity and nuclear pleomorphism (Fig. 2.171). Both cavernous and capillary hemangiomas have been reported. A variant, anastomosing hemangioma, can raise concern for angiosarcoma.[811] This highly vascular neoplasm may mimic splenorenal fusion, grossly and microscopically (Fig. 2.172).[610] More renal than nonrenal cases of this entity have been reported, and some of the renal cases are associated with extramedullary hematopoiesis.[610] It consists of anastomosing sinusoidal capillary-sized vessels with scattered hobnail endothelial cells within a framework of nonendothelial supporting cells; the vessels may appear "sievelike" (Fig. 2.173). The endothelial cells have a consistent immunophenotype expressing positivity for CD31, CD34, factor VIII-Ra, and FLI1, and negativity for GLUT1, D2-40, CD8, and HHV8.[610] Although the microscopic

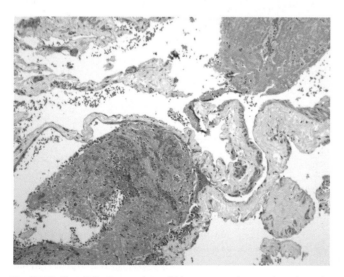

Fig. 2.171 Renal hilar hemangioma. This cavernous hemangioma/vascular malformation has thick- and thin-walled blood vessels.

appearance of the tumor may resemble splenic parenchyma, the immunophenotype of the vascular endothelial cells (CD34⁺ and CD8⁻) is precisely the opposite of that of splenic red pulp sinusoidal tissue, which is CD34⁻ and CD8⁺ (Figs. 2.174 and 2.175).[610] In contrast with angiosarcoma, necrosis and diffuse infiltration are absent, the vessels lack significant endothelial nuclear atypia and pleomorphism, and mitotic figures are rare or absent. Some benign renal vascular lesions represent arteriovenous malformations rather than hemangiomas; they are composed of an admixture of abnormally arranged thick- and thin-walled vessels, resembling malformed veins, venules, arteries, and arterioles, with or without associated thrombosis.[669]

Lymphangioma

Renal lymphangioma, also designated peripyelic–pericalyceal lymphangiectasis, is a rare cystic renal lesion that is regarded as a developmental malformation resulting from failure of developing lymphatic tissue to establish normal communication with the remainder of the lymphatic system.[807,812-814] Fewer than 50 cases have been reported. The great majority of lymphangiomas occur in the head and neck and axillary regions; other sites include the retroperitoneum, mediastinum, mesentery, omentum, colon, and pelvis.[815]

Renal lymphangioma has been reported in neonates, infants, children, and adults.[807,812] Approximately two-thirds occur in adults. The lesion may involve one or both kidneys in localized or diffuse distribution, and rarely may be restricted to the lymphatics of the renal capsule, either unilaterally or bilaterally.[812,816] Some cases manifest as abdominal masses in children, some are found incidentally, some present with renin-dependent hypertension, and some present with hematuria or pain related to renal obstruction.[813,815-819]

Renal lymphangioma is typically a well-encapsulated multicystic mass; the cut surface is composed of innumerable fluid-filled cysts ranging from 0.1 to 2.0 cm, often mimicking polycystic kidney disease or a multilocular renal cyst (Fig. 2.176).

Microscopically, the cysts are lined by flattened endothelial cells and are separated by a variable amount of stroma that may contain smooth muscle, glomeruli, tubules, lymphoid infiltrates, and blood vessels (Fig. 2.177).[807,817] The nature of the endothelial cells lining the cysts can be ascertained, if necessary, by appropriate immunostains.

Renal lymphangioma is benign. However, once discovered, it is usually excised surgically because the radiologic differential may include cystic RCC in adults, or cystic variant of Wilms tumor, clear cell sarcoma, or rhabdoid tumor in children.[815,817]

Hemangioblastoma

Fewer than 20 cases of sporadic renal hemangioblastoma, a benign tumor arising in the absence of VHL disease and lacking evidence of VHL gene mutation, have been reported.[820-824] Males and females are equally affected, and mean age is 50 years, with a range of 16 to 71 years. Tumors range in diameter from 1.2 to 6.8 cm; they are well circumscribed, gray-white, yellow, or brownish, but lack the golden yellow appearance often seen in CCRCC.[824] Microscopically, the tumor is composed of polygonal epithelioid stromal cells with pale to eosinophilic cytoplasm, arranged in sheets and sometimes lobulated nodules, intersected by an abundant arborizing capillary network (Fig. 2.178). Cytoplasmic vacuolization is common, to the extent that some cells may resemble lipoblasts; others may have a rhabdoid appearance. Intracytoplasmic

Fig. 2.172 The dark beefy-red color, due to its content of erythrocytes, mimics the appearance of splenorenal fusion.

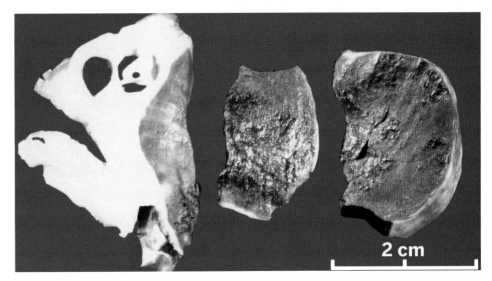

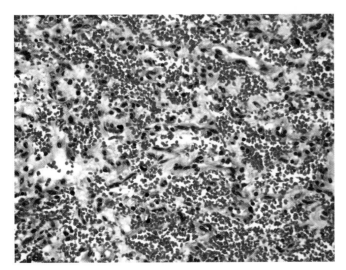

Fig. 2.173 Renal anastomosing hemangioma. Tumor is composed of capillary-sized anastomosing sinusoidal-like spaces, lined by a single file of endothelial cells lacking significant cytologic atypia or mitotic activity.

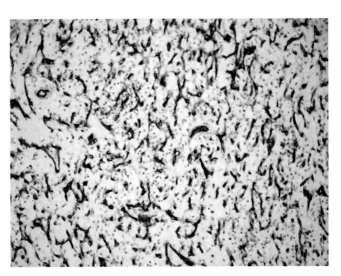

Fig. 2.174 Renal anastomosing hemangioma. Immunostain with CD34 sharply highlights the complex anastomosing architecture of the tumor. Endothelial cells of this tumor uniformly express CD31, factor VIII, and FLI1. Expression of CD34 by the sinusoidal endothelium of splenic red pulp is usually weak or absent.

hyaline globules and intranuclear cytoplasmic pseudoinclusions may be present, as well as scattered psammoma-like calcifications.[823,824] Nuclei are mainly cytologically bland, but scattered bizarre nuclei may be noted. Mitotic figures are absent or rare, and necrosis and hemorrhage are not seen. Tumor cells show positive immunostaining for α-inhibin, NSE, S100 protein, GLUT1, and vimentin, as well as positive nuclear staining for PAX8 (Fig. 2.179). Immunomarkers for cytokeratins are usually negative, as are markers of neuroendocrine, endothelial, mesothelial, melanocytic, and muscle differentiation.

Distinction of this tumor from CCRCC, epithelioid AML, and translocation-associated RCC is challenging. Tumor cells radiating from the walls of hemangiopericytoma-like blood vessels, scattered psammoma-like calcifications, and intranuclear cytoplasmic invaginations may give a clue to the correct diagnosis and may prompt immunohistochemical studies that will aid in separating it from its mimics.[823] Because it is benign, the distinction is clearly important.

Juxtaglomerular Cell Tumor

Juxtaglomerular cell tumor was first described in 1967.[825] It is a renal neoplasm that arises from specialized smooth muscle cells present in the glomerular afferent arteriole of the juxtaglomerular apparatus. Approximately 100 cases of juxtaglomerular cell tumor have been reported, more often in women than in men (1.9:1 ratio).[826-828] Patients range from 6 to 69 years of age, but the majority of patients are in their twenties and thirties, with a mean age of 27 years. Clinical findings often facilitate an accurate preoperative diagnosis. Almost all patients have hypertension that is difficult to control. In the rare instances in which the tumor produces an inactive form of renin, the patient's blood pressure may be normal.[829] Other symptoms reported include pain, headache, polyuria, nocturia, dizziness, and vomiting. Other typical clinical findings include high serum renin levels, elevated serum aldosterone, and hypokalemia.

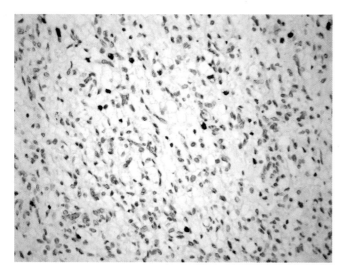

Fig. 2.175 Renal anastomosing hemangioma. Immunostain for CD8 highlights background lymphocytes but is not expressed by the vascular endothelial cells. This is the most compelling distinction of this tumor from splenorenal fusion. The sinusoidal endothelial cells of splenic red pulp show strong and diffusely positive immunostaining for CD8; no other endothelium within the body expresses this antigen, and its function on these cells is unknown.

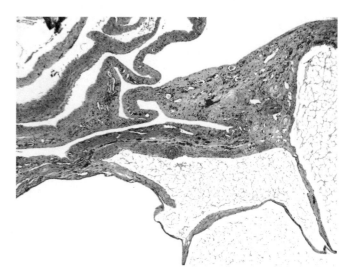

Fig. 2.177 Renal lymphangioma. Lymphangioma consists of numerous thin-walled cysts separated by delicate fibrous septa. The cysts are lined by flattened endothelial cells and are separated by septal structures that may contain normal renal structures such as glomeruli, tubules, and blood vessels.

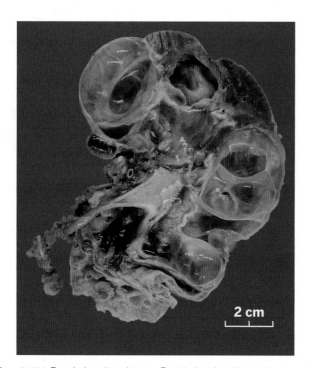

Fig. 2.176 Renal lymphangioma. Renal lymphangioma is a well-encapsulated multicystic mass that may be unilateral or bilateral, localized or diffuse. The cut surface is composed of innumerable fluid-filled cysts ranging from 0.1 to 2.0 cm in diameter, mimicking polycystic kidney disease or a multilocular renal cyst.

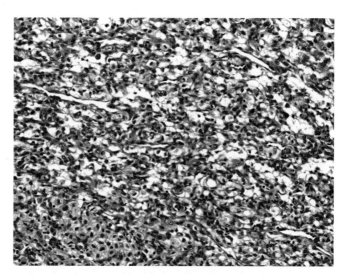

Fig. 2.178 Renal hemangioblastoma. The stromal cells of hemangioblastoma contain numerous lipid vacuoles, imparting a clear cell appearance. The tumor is traversed by numerous arborizing thin-walled blood vessels. Distinction from clear cell renal cell carcinoma is challenging.

Grossly, juxtaglomerular cell tumor is usually well circumscribed by a fibrous capsule of variable thickness.[826] It is typically 2 to 4 cm in diameter, but can be as large as 9 cm.[830] It has a yellow to gray-tan and often hemorrhagic cut surface (Fig. 2.180). Microscopically, it is composed of polygonal to round to elongated, spindle-shaped cells (Figs. 2.181 and 2.182). Cells tend to have slightly eosinophilic cytoplasm and centrally located nuclei. Most

cases show some degree of nuclear atypia. Mitotic figures are usually absent. Cell borders may be well defined or ill-defined. Cellular arrangement also varies; the cells may be arranged in irregular trabeculae, papilla, organoid patterns, or solid compact sheets.[826,831] The background stroma may be scant, abundant and hyalinized, or edematous, imparting a microcystic appearance. Abundant thin-walled vessels are usually present, and most tumors demonstrate thick-walled vessels, sometimes in clusters or branching (Fig. 2.182).[826,832]

Because of the varied histologic appearance, immunohistochemical staining of tumors suspected to be juxtaglomerular cell tumor can be helpful in confirming the diagnosis and in differentiating it from other renal neoplasms.[826] Juxtaglomerular cell tumor shows positive immunostaining for actin, CD34, and CD117, and negative immunostaining for cytokeratins, desmin,

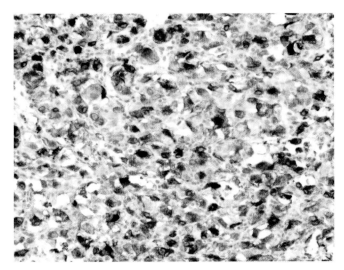

Fig. 2.179 Renal hemangioblastoma. Tumor cells show positive nuclear immunostaining for α-inhibin. Distinction of this tumor from clear cell renal cell carcinoma (RCC), epithelioid angiomyolipoma, and translocation-associated RCC is challenging and requires a battery of immunostains.

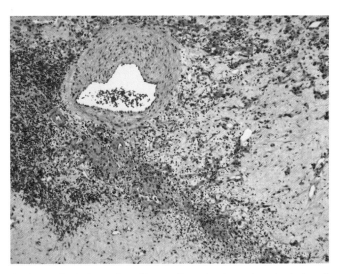

Fig. 2.181 Juxtaglomerular cell tumor. Round, polygonal, and spindle cells are present in a myxoid background, with scattered inflammatory infiltrate and thick-walled blood vessels.

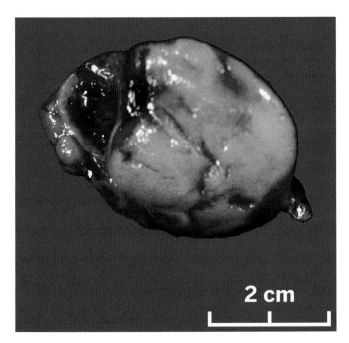

Fig. 2.180 Juxtaglomerular cell tumor. This small, hemorrhagic, yellow tumor has a bulging cut surface.

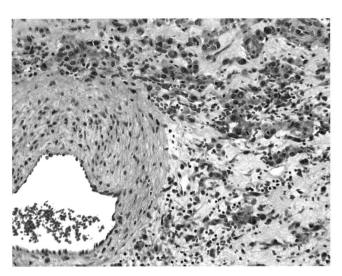

Fig. 2.182 Juxtaglomerular cell tumor. This is a higher-power view of findings shown in Fig. 2.181.

studies suggest that the oncogene(s) or tumor suppressor gene(s) responsible for the pathogenesis of juxtaglomerular cell tumor may be localized on chromosomes 4 and 10, or chromosomes 9 and 11, respectively.[827,828]

Surgical removal of the tumor usually normalizes the patient's blood pressure and relieves other symptoms. These tumors are almost exclusively benign, although there has been one documented case of juxtaglomerular cell tumor that metastasized to the lung.[825,826,829-835]

Renomedullary Interstitial Cell Tumor

Renomedullary interstitial cell tumor is a benign lesion derived from renomedullary interstitial cells, which synthesize several vasoactive agents, such as prostaglandin, that exert antihypertensive effects. Absence of known clinical correlations, such as heart weight or hypertension, and demonstrable clonality in some cases, favor the premise that it is a benign neoplasm.[836] It is typically a small spherical or ovoid tumor in the renal medulla, found incidentally in nearly one-half of patients in their teens and older, with a slight

S100 protein, HMB45, chromogranin, and synaptophysin.[826,832,833] Tumors that may be confused with juxtaglomerular cell tumor include RCC, AML, and glomus tumor. Immunohistochemical staining is helpful in that RCC stains positive for cytokeratins, and AML stains positive for HMB45; these stains are negative in juxtaglomerular cell tumor. Immunohistochemical staining does not differentiate juxtaglomerular cell tumor from glomus tumor because both tumors arise from smooth muscle cells and stain positive for actin and CD34. However, electron microscopy of juxtaglomerular cell tumor reveals both rhomboid-shaped renin protogranules and smooth muscle microfilaments, findings that are unique to this neoplasm and that account for its characterization as a tumor derived from "myoendocrine cells." Genetic

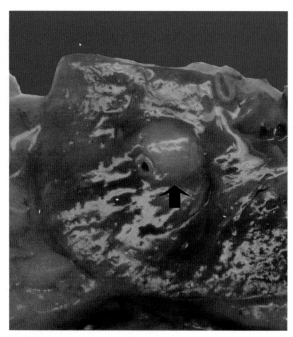

Fig. 2.183 Renomedullary interstitial cell tumor. This small pale inconspicuous nodule (*arrow*) was noted near the tip of a renal papilla in a radical nephrectomy specimen. (Courtesy Wei Chen, MD.)

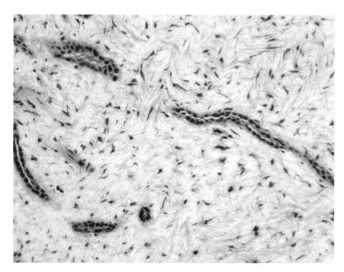

Fig. 2.185 Renomedullary interstitial cell tumor. This is a higher-power view of findings described in Fig. 2.184.

female predilection.[421,422] It is bilateral in ~50 of cases and multiple in more than 50 of cases.[421,422,790,807,836] Most are 0.1 to 0.6 cm in diameter (Fig. 2.183). Rarely, it is large enough to obstruct renal pelvic outflow and cause pain, and with the use of increasingly sensitive radiologic studies, asymptomatic lesions indistinguishable from malignancy are discovered incidentally, requiring surgical excision.[837,838]

Microscopically, it is composed of small spindle or stellate cells set in a background of loose, faintly basophilic stroma containing interlacing bundles of delicate fibers (Figs. 2.184 and 2.185).[836] A number of changes seem to coincide with advancing patient age. Tumors tend to be larger, the stroma becomes less cellular and begins to exhibit deposition of ropey eosinophilic amorphous material that is composed of collagen type III, the tumor border changes from being ill-defined to well circumscribed, and entrapped renal medullary tubules, which are present in about 85% of tumors overall, become marginated at the tumor periphery or obliterated entirely.[836]

Schwannoma

Only about two dozen cases of renal schwannoma have been reported.[839-847] Patients range from 24 to 89 years of age (average, 59 years), without apparent gender predilection. The tumor may arise in the renal parenchyma or the renal capsule, but is often centrally located, impinging on renal pelvis or hilar soft tissues. Some are discovered incidentally; in some cases, nonspecific symptoms such as malaise, fever, weight loss, or abdominal discomfort are reported, or an abdominal mass is palpable.

Grossly, renal schwannoma ranges from 4 to 16 cm in greatest dimension (mean, 9.7 cm). It is typically tan to yellow, well circumscribed, and sometimes multinodular.[843,844]

Microscopically, renal schwannoma is composed of bland uniform spindle cells with wavy nuclei and is sharply circumscribed with a dense fibrous capsule (Figs. 2.186 and 2.187). Classic

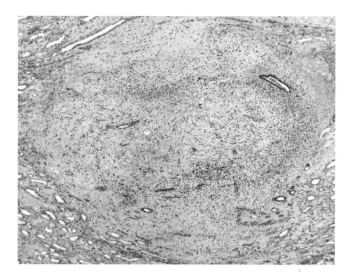

Fig. 2.184 Renomedullary interstitial cell tumor. Tumor is composed of small stellate cells in a background of loose faintly basophilic stroma containing interlacing bundles of delicate fibers.

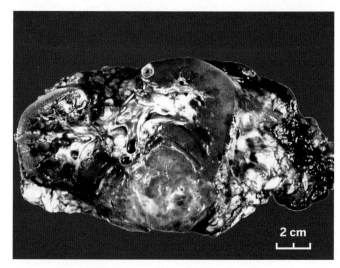

Fig. 2.186 Renal schwannoma. This well-circumscribed tumor is from a young female patient.

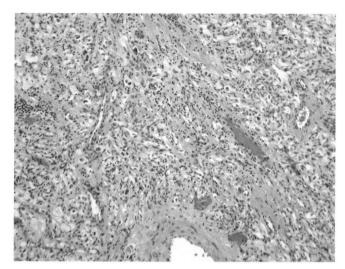

Fig. 2.187 Renal schwannoma. Although not showing classic findings, this lesion was regarded as most consistent with schwannoma, based primarily on its immunoprofile (the only significant immunostaining was strong diffuse positivity for S100 protein).

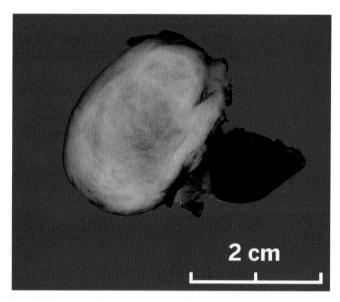

Fig. 2.188 Renal solitary fibrous tumor. Renal solitary fibrous tumor is typically a well-circumscribed, pseudoencapsulated, lobulated, rubbery, or firm mass with a homogeneous gray or tan-white whorled cut surface, usually without necrosis, cyst formation, or hemorrhage.

schwannoma exhibits variable cellularity, with cellular Antoni A areas alternating with hypocellular Antoni B areas, nuclear palisading, and Verocay body formation.[840-842,844] Cellular schwannoma shows fascicular growth and relatively uniform cellularity, cystic change with macrophage aggregates and relative paucity of palisading, Verocay bodies, and Antoni A and Antoni B areas. Numerous thick-walled hyalinized blood vessels are present in either type of schwannoma. Mitotic figures and necrosis are absent. Tumor cells show strong and uniformly positive immunostaining for S100 protein, and no immunoreactivity to antibodies against cytokeratin, CD34, CD57, smooth muscle actin, or desmin.

Renal schwannoma is benign, but in rare instances undergoes malignant transformation in the form of angiosarcoma or malignant peripheral nerve sheath tumor.[847]

Solitary Fibrous Tumor

Solitary fibrous tumor is a spindle cell neoplasm that was first described in 1931. Although it is most often found in the pleura, it also occurs in a variety of extrapleural sites, including the kidney.[848-853] About 40 cases of renal solitary fibrous tumor have been reported.[854-856] It has been postulated that solitary fibrous tumor is a neoplasm of fibroblast/primitive mesenchymal cells with features of multidirectional differentiation.[857] More than one-half of patients are more than 40 years old (range 28 to 83 years; average age, 52 years), and the male-to-female ratio is approximately equal.[851,853] Symptoms include flank or abdominal pain or hematuria; some patients are asymptomatic, and in others, a mass is palpable.[848-853]

Renal solitary fibrous tumor ranges from 2 to 25 cm, with a mean of 8.75 cm; in one patient, bilateral lesions were present.[851,853] It is typically well circumscribed and pseudoencapsulated, lobulated, rubbery, or firm, and has a homogeneous gray or tan-white whorled cut surface (Fig. 2.188). In most cases, necrosis, cyst formation, and hemorrhage are absent. Microscopically, solitary fibrous tumor is composed of a proliferation of spindle cells arranged in a patternless architecture, with areas of alternating hypocellularity and hypercellularity separated from one another by thick bands of hyalinized collagen and branching

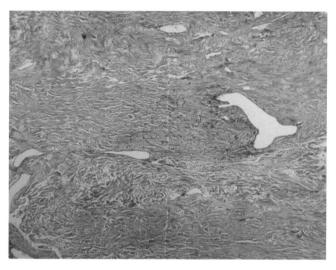

Fig. 2.189 Renal solitary fibrous tumor. Region of hypocellularity, composed mainly of hyalinized collagen, and containing branching hemangiopericytoma-like blood vessels.

hemangiopericytoma-like blood vessels (Figs. 2.189 and 2.190). Tumor cells have scant and indistinct cytoplasm, and elongate nuclei with finely dispersed chromatin and only occasional nucleoli. Criteria for malignancy include more than 4 mitotic figures per 10 hpf, with or without necrosis, hypercellularity, cytologic atypia, or infiltrative growth patterns.[848-854]

Tumor cells typically show positive immunostaining for CD34, and most also show positive staining for CD99 and BCL2. Nuclear STAT6 expression is a highly sensitive and almost perfectly specific immunohistochemical marker for solitary fibrous tumor (Fig. 2.191).[858] By FISH analysis, NAB2-STAT6 gene fusion is demonstrable in two-thirds of cases, but the gene fusion is not uniformly related to STAT6 immunoreactivity, nor does the fusion correlate with malignant-appearing histologic findings or clinical outcome, although available data are limited to date.[854]

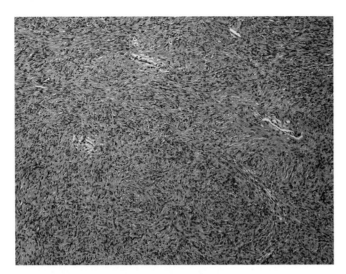

Fig. 2.190 Renal solitary fibrous tumor. Region of hypercellularity, composed of spindle cells arranged in a patternless architecture.

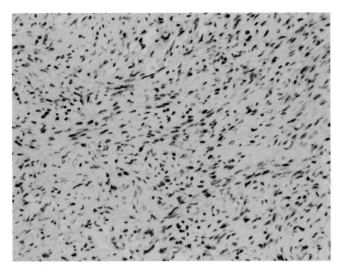

Fig. 2.191 Renal solitary fibrous tumor. Nuclear STAT6 expression strongly supports the diagnosis.

The differential diagnosis of renal solitary fibrous tumor includes a broad spectrum of epithelial and mesenchymal neoplasms. There are no distinctive ultrastructural findings that aid in the diagnosis of solitary fibrous tumor. The combination of immunopositivity for STAT6, CD34, BCL2, and CD99, and the absence of expression of α-smooth muscle actin, S100 protein, CD31, and CD117 are helpful in distinguishing solitary fibrous tumor from lesions such as monophasic synovial sarcoma, leiomyoma, low-grade leiomyosarcoma, and schwannoma.[849,859] About 10% to 15% of renal solitary fibrous tumors exhibit aggressive biologic behavior in the form of local recurrence or distant metastasis, and long-term follow-up of affected patients is recommended.[855]

Mixed Epithelial and Stromal Tumor Family

Adult Cystic Nephroma

Adult cystic nephroma, first described in 1892, is a benign renal neoplasm composed entirely of epithelial-lined cysts separated by septa of variable thickness, but usually less than 2 mm thick, and lacking an expansile solid component.[860] Because it has clinical and morphologic features that overlap with those of mixed epithelial and stromal tumor (MEST), it has been hypothesized that the two entities are closely related, if not the same.[861-866] Consequently, adult cystic nephroma is classified within the spectrum of the MEST family.[201]

Cystic nephroma in adults is seen mainly in females (1:8 male-to-female ratio). The peak incidence is between ages 50 and 60 years. Median age in women and men is 55 and 44 years, respectively; it is rare before age 30 years.[866] Although it may present as a painless abdominal mass, with flank or abdominal pain, or hematuria, most are discovered incidentally.[862,867,868] Tumors are well circumscribed, always unilateral, commonly but not always separated from the adjacent renal parenchyma by a fibrous pseudocapsule, and range in size from 1.4 to 22 cm, with an average diameter of approximately 7 cm. They tend to be larger in women than in men (Fig. 2.192).[866] Most tumors involve the renal cortex, but rarely tumors may be predominantly intrapelvic.[866,869] They are composed of multilocular cysts of varying sizes, filled with serous fluid (Fig. 2.193). The cysts are lined by epithelium that is flattened, hobnail, or cuboidal in appearance; in one-third of cases, cysts are focally lined by clear cells with apical eosinophilic granules (Fig. 2.194). Mitotic figures are absent.[120,861,866] Calcifications, often linear and thin, are seen in about 50% of cases. The septal stroma shows a variety of appearances. It may be hypercellular, collagenized and hypocellular, edematous and hypocellular, or hypercellular with wavy spindle cells.[866] Hypercellularity is often noted adjacent to cysts (Figs. 2.195 and 2.196). Hypocellularity and collagenization tend to be noted in larger tumors and in older women, whereas hypercellularity and wavy spindle cell stroma tend to be found in younger women and in smaller tumors.[866] In about one-third of cases, nodules of hyalinized stroma with an appearance somewhat reminiscent of ovarian corpora albicantia are present. Inconspicuous embedded epithelial elements occupy the stroma in about 40% of cases. These may consist of a few cells with no lumen, tiny cysts with pinpoint lumens, or slightly larger readily identified small cysts.[866] It is hypothesized that the epithelial component of adult cystic nephroma arises from a stromal–epithelial transition that continues throughout the life of the tumor.[866]

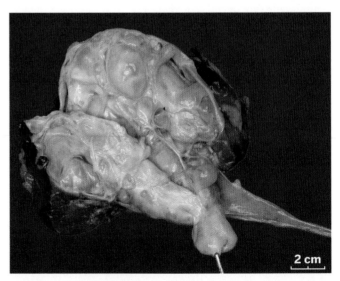

Fig. 2.192 Cystic nephroma. Tumor extends into the renal pelvis.

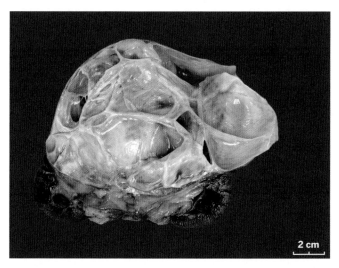

Fig. 2.193 Cystic nephroma. Tumor is composed of multilocular cysts of varying sizes, separated by thin delicate septa, and containing serous fluid. No solid tumor nodules are visible.

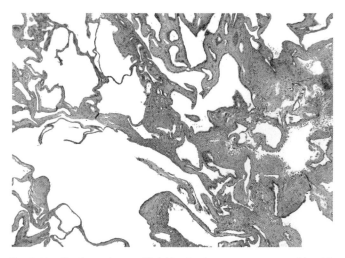

Fig. 2.194 Cystic nephroma. Variably sized cysts are separated by thin septa that correspond to the outline of the cysts; expansile nodules are absent. Septal stroma is composed of spindle cells in a collagenous background.

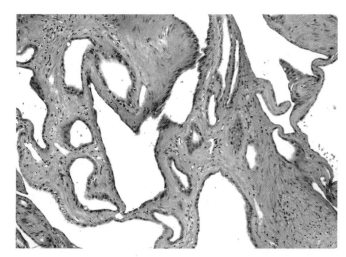

Fig. 2.195 Cystic nephroma. The lining epithelium is flattened or cuboidal.

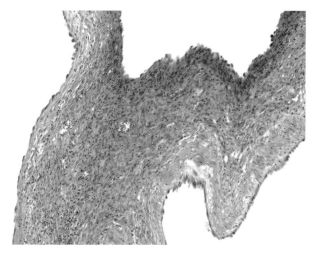

Fig. 2.196 Cystic nephroma with hypercellular stroma.

The lining epithelium of cysts expresses PAX8 in all cases, GATA3 in about one-third of cases, and CD10 in slightly less than one-third of cases. These cells do not express ER or PR.[866] Stromal cells express smooth muscle actin in all cases, and PR and CD10 in 80% to 85% of cases. The following markers are expressed in 40% to 60% of cases: desmin, caldesmon, ER, inhibin, and CD34.[866] The following markers are not expressed in stromal cells: S100 protein, Melan A, cathepsin K, PAX8, or GATA3.[866]

Adult cystic nephroma is regarded as a benign neoplasm and cured by adequate surgical excision. Recurrence has been attributed to incomplete resection.[870] However, there are a number of reports of sarcoma arising in a background of cystic nephroma in adults, at least three of which have had a fatal outcome (Figs. 2.197 through 2.199).[867,871]

Adult cystic nephroma is clinically, morphologically, immunohistochemically, and genetically distinct from the entity known as pediatric cystic nephroma.[120,599] The adult tumor occurs predominantly in middle-aged females; the pediatric tumor occurs predominantly in young boys.[120] The adult tumors commonly have an element of wavy, ropy collagen that is not seen in the pediatric cases.[599] The majority of adult tumors show at least focal

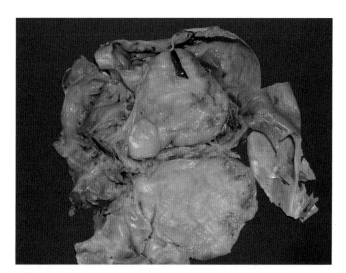

Fig. 2.197 Cystic nephroma with superimposed sarcoma. A sarcoma has developed with a solid fleshy cut surface. (Courtesy John Kunkel, MD.)

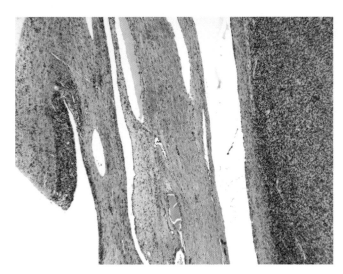

Fig. 2.198 Cystic nephroma with superimposed sarcoma. Typical cystic nephroma is seen, coexisting with sarcoma component in the same image.

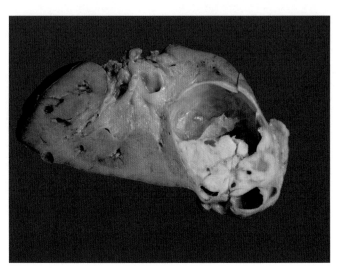

Fig. 2.200 Mixed epithelial and stromal tumor. Tumor is variably solid and cystic. (Image courtesy Rodolfo Montironi, MD.)

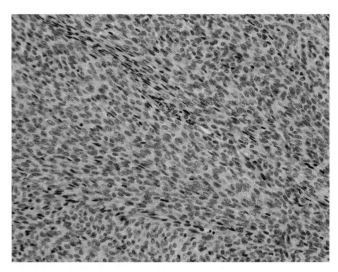

Fig. 2.199 Cystic nephroma with superimposed sarcoma. Final diagnosis was sarcoma, not otherwise specified, based on inconclusive immunohistochemical and molecular studies.

immunostaining for inhibin; this is not seen in pediatric cases.[599] Whereas the great majority of pediatric cystic nephromas harbor DICER1 mutations, this has been found in only one adult cystic nephroma.[595,598,599]

Mixed Epithelial and Stromal Tumor

MEST of the kidney is a biphasic neoplasm composed of epithelial and stromal components. There is compelling evidence that both the stromal and the epithelial elements arise from a common progenitor cell that possesses capacity for dual differentiation; in short, that both elements are clonal and neoplastic.[872] After being reported under a variety of other names since 1973, it received its current appellation in 1998.[873-880] Along with cystic nephroma, it is classified as a member of the MEST family. Its relationship to cystic nephroma was discussed in the beginning of the Adult Cystic

Nephroma section. It occurs predominantly in middle-aged women, is usually, but not always, benign, and is composed of a variety of epithelial elements set in stroma with variable morphology.[862-864,881-884] The majority of patients with MEST of the kidney are female, with a 7:1 predominance and a mean age of about 50 years. Male patients tend to be older, with a median age of 71 years.[883] Some patients present with hematuria or flank pain, and some tumors are discovered incidentally.

Grossly, MEST tumor is typically single, unilateral, and circumscribed, and most are 4 to 6 cm in diameter (range 0.3 to 17.5 cm).[881-883] Some protrude into the collecting system.[879] Tumors are variably solid and cystic; the cysts may be clustered or dispersed, and the solid areas may be firm and rubbery, or fleshy (Fig. 2.200). Some are invested with a pseudocapsule, but in most cases, spindle cells simply infiltrate the adjacent renal parenchyma. The epithelial and stromal elements exhibit remarkable variability and complexity (Fig. 2.201). The stromal component is the predominant constituent of these tumors.[883] The stromal spindle cells may have hyperchromatic nuclei with scant cytoplasm; may have vesicular nuclei and more cytoplasm; may have elongated nuclei; or may appear plump, with abundant cytoplasm.[883] The spindle cell component typically varies considerably in cellularity and often shows condensation around cystic areas (Fig. 2.202). It may be hypocellular with extensive collagenization or with myxoid change; it may be cellular and arranged in fascicles resembling smooth muscle or in a woven pattern resembling ovarian stroma (Fig. 2.203); it may be densely cellular and arranged in patterns resembling fibrosarcoma or synovial sarcoma; or it may show alternating zones of hypocellularity and hypercellularity with fibrocytic cells in a keloid-like background resembling solitary fibrous tumor. Smooth muscle stroma is present in two-thirds of cases, and fat is present in one-third of cases (Fig. 2.204).[883] Vascular stromal components may include thick-walled blood vessels, artery-like and lymphatic-like structures surrounded by hypocellular fibrous stroma, and vessels in various stages of sclerosis, resembling a corpus albicans of the ovary when sclerosis is advanced.[883] The epithelial component may be represented by tiny crowded glands, branching ducts, small round glands lined by tall cuboidal cells, luminal structures resembling thyroid follicles, spatulate papillae, aggregated luminal structures resembling nephrogenic adenoma, or complex papillae. Cells

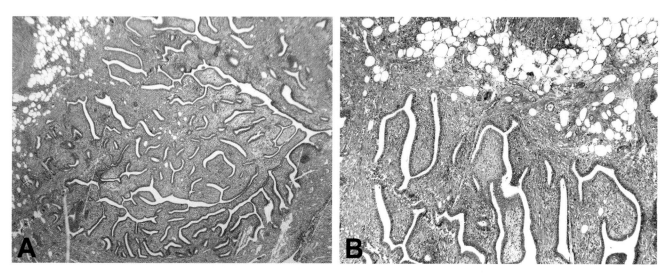

Fig. 2.201 Mixed epithelial and stromal tumor. Complex branching architecture and broad papillae; stromal component includes smooth muscle (A), fat (B), and fibrous tissue.

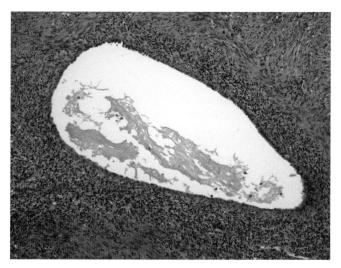

Fig. 2.202 Mixed epithelial and stromal tumor. Condensation of spindle cell component around cystic areas is apparent.

lining the glands or cysts are commonly flat, cuboidal, or hobnail type. Less common luminal cell types include urothelium, ciliated cells, clear cells with or without subnuclear vacuoles, oxyphilic epithelium, columnar with stratified nuclei, and mucinous goblet cells.[883] No significant cytologic atypia or mitotic activity is evident within either the spindle cell or the epithelial components.[416,812,880-883,885-887]

Immunohistochemically, the spindle cells in 90% or more of cases show immunoreactivity to the following antibodies: smooth muscle actin, desmin, caldesmon, ER, PR, and CD10. CD34 and WT1 are expressed in less than 50% of cases. The epithelial elements show uniformly positive immunostaining for keratin markers and PAX8, and for GATA3 in a little more than 50% of cases. ER, PR, and CD10 markers are expressed by epithelial cells in about 10% of cases. All tumors are negative for inhibin, SF1, HMB45, Melan A, and cathepsin K.[883]

Although MEST was initially considered benign, increasingly there are reports of such tumors showing malignant transformation of either the stromal or epithelial components, or of both, and in two cases, the patients succumbed to the renal cancer.[872,888-895]

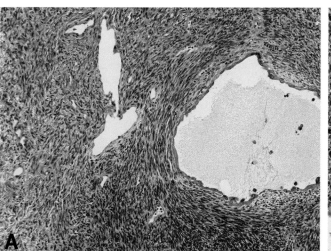

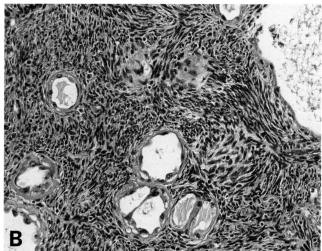

Fig. 2.203 Mixed epithelial and stromal tumor (A and B). Biphasic tumor is composed of smooth muscle, fat, and fibrous elements admixed with complex epithelial-lined structures.

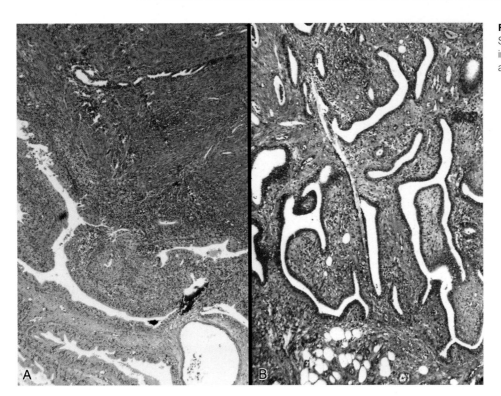

Fig. 2.204 Mixed epithelial and stromal tumor. Stromal cell nuclei are very closely packed, imparting an ovarian stroma–like appearance (A and B).

Malignancies have been in the form of undifferentiated sarcoma, carcinosarcoma, undifferentiated large cell–type carcinoma, sarcoma with heterologous features, mucinous borderline tumor, and endometrioid adenocarcinoma.

Neuroendocrine Tumors

Well-Differentiated Neuroendocrine Tumor

Primary renal well-differentiated neuroendocrine tumor, a low-grade malignancy with neuroendocrine differentiation, is uncommon. It is frequently associated with other renal abnormalities including horseshoe kidney (18%), renal teratoma (14%), and polycystic kidney disease (2%).[896-905] A recently reported case was found incidentally in association with multiple bilateral CCPRCCs.[906] More than 80 cases have been reported; average age at diagnosis is 49 (range 12 to 78) years. Almost 30% of cases are discovered incidentally; presenting symptoms in the other 70% include abdominal or flank pain, hematuria, constipation, fever, weight loss, and testicular pain. Neuroendocrine syndromes occur in about 12% of patients, and a mass is palpable in 27%.[907,908] Renal well-differentiated neuroendocrine tumor is typically hypovascular or avascular on radiologic studies, and frequently displays intratumoral calcification.[909] Somatostatin receptor scintigraphy can be helpful in preoperative and postoperative assessment of disease status.[910]

Tumors range from 1.5 to 30 cm in greatest dimension, with a mean of 8.4 cm. They are yellow-white to red-tan, and although most are solid, about one-third are partially or predominantly cystic (Fig. 2.205A). About one-half are confined to the renal parenchyma, one-third involve perirenal fat, and renal vein involvement occurs in slightly more than 10% of cases. Histologically, renal well-differentiated neuroendocrine tumor shows findings typical of this tumor arising in other body sites. Most tumors have a mixed growth pattern, with cells arranged in a trabecular pattern, solid nests, acinar structures, or insular, tubular, or rosette-like structures (Fig. 2.205B). Mitotic activity is limited.[900]

The immunoprofile of renal well-differentiated neuroendocrine tumor is similar to that of well-differentiated neuroendocrine tumor occurring elsewhere, with positive immunostaining for synaptophysin, chromogranin, neuron-specific enolase, and cytokeratin in a high percentage of cases.[911] It is notable that renal well-differentiated neuroendocrine tumor often shows positive immunostaining for prostatic acid phosphatase.[912] Cytogenetically, numerical or structural aberrations of chromosomes 3 and 13 have been noted.[913,914] Loss of heterozygosity at the D3F15S2 locus of 3p21 in one case suggested the possibility of a common genetic event in the genesis of renal well-differentiated neuroendocrine tumor and conventional RCC.

Metastases are present at the time of diagnosis or appear within 7 years of follow-up in 50% of patients. Metastases are more common in patients older than 40 years and are more often seen in association with tumors that are solid, larger than 4 cm, outside the renal capsule, or that have a mitotic rate higher than 1 per 10 hpf. The mortality rate is less than 10%, indicating that the disease is relatively indolent, and that resection of positive lymph nodes can be curative.[900]

Large Cell Neuroendocrine Carcinoma

Primary large cell neuroendocrine carcinoma of the kidney is exceptionally rare. The lone well-described case had a solid cut surface with necrosis grossly and a solid growth pattern with large-zone necrosis.[905] Tumor cells were large, with a low nuclear-to-cytoplasmic ratio, vesicular chromatin, and prominent nucleoli. Mitotic activity was brisk (50 per 10 hpf). Tumor cells were diffusely and strongly positive for synaptophysin, but negative for vimentin, CD10, and EMA. At presentation the tumor was at an advanced stage, and the patient died of local tumor progression 2 months after the initial diagnosis.[905]

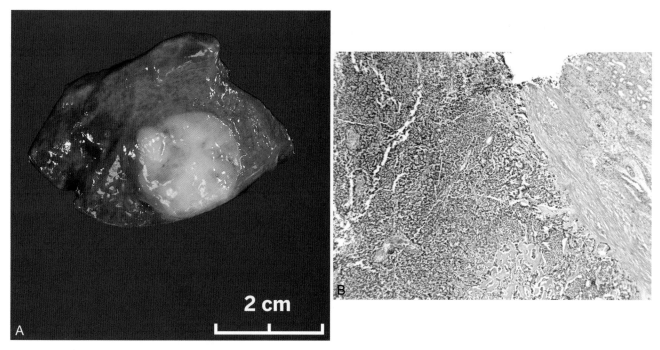

Fig. 2.205 Well-differentiated neuroendocrine tumor of kidney, found incidentally at autopsy. Well-circumscribed tumor is confined to renal parenchyma (A). Tumor cells are arrayed in ribbons, cords, and solid sheets (B).

Small Cell Neuroendocrine Carcinoma

Many reported cases of primary renal small cell carcinoma probably originate in the urothelium of the renal pelvis or calyces, judging from their reported locations, and from the fact that many reported cases were admixed with components of urothelial carcinoma, squamous cell carcinoma, and adenocarcinoma, similar to small cell carcinomas that arise in the urothelium of the urinary bladder.[905,915-921] Fewer than 30 well-documented cases of pure small cell carcinoma of the kidney have been reported.[905,920,922-927]

Patients range in age from 37 to 83 years, with a mean of 59 years. Symptoms include hematuria, back or abdominal pain, fatigue and other constitutional symptoms, and nonspecific gastro-intestinal complaints. Most tumors range between 10 and 18.5 cm in greatest dimension, frequently obliterating large portions of the native kidney.[922,923,925]

Tumors are typically solid, poorly circumscribed, gray-yellow, and extensively necrotic and hemorrhagic (Fig. 2.206). Tumor stage at the time of nephrectomy is often advanced, with involvement of perirenal structures, renal vein, and regional lymph nodes.[922,923,926] Histologic, immunohistochemical, and ultrastructural findings are similar to those of small cell carcinoma in more conventional locations (Figs. 2.207 and 2.208).[922,923,925,926]

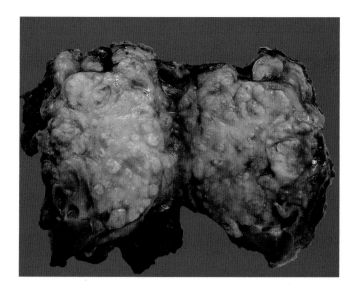

Fig. 2.206 Small cell neuroendocrine carcinoma of kidney. The tumor arose in a 73-year-old woman who had never used tobacco products. It extended into the renal vein and vena cava, and mimicked renal cell carcinoma clinically and radiologically. (Image courtesy Mohadese Behtaj, MD.)

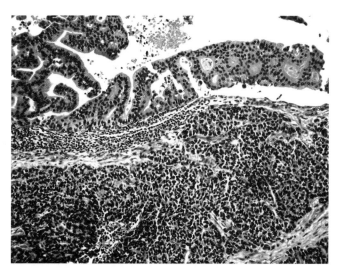

Fig. 2.207 Small cell neuroendocrine carcinoma of kidney. More than 99% of the tumor consisted of typical small cell carcinoma. However, several sections that included renal pelvic epithelium demonstrated the presence of urothelial carcinoma, which overlies the small cell carcinoma in this image.

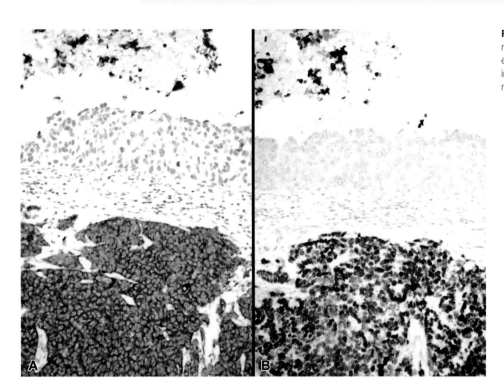

Fig. 2.208 Small cell neuroendocrine carcinoma of kidney. The small cell carcinoma expressed synaptophysin (A) and TTF1 (B), in contrast with the overlying urothelial carcinoma, which expressed neither.

Although some patients have had a favorable outcome, the prognosis for most patients with renal small cell carcinoma is poor, possibly because of a propensity for occult metastases at the time of presentation.[920,923,925] Median survival is less than 1 year, regardless of the therapeutic regimen used; survival is prolonged by platinum-based chemotherapy.[918]

Paraganglioma

There are fewer than a dozen well-documented cases of renal paraganglioma. In a large series of 710 patients with pheochromocytoma or paraganglioma, only 2 cases were primary renal paragangliomas.[906] Tumors have been detected through evaluation of a palpable abdominal mass, microhematuria, recurrent flank pain, and hypertension. Distinction of intrarenal from capsular lesions is difficult and probably irrelevant, because these tumors are radiologically indeterminate for renal malignancy and are removed on that basis.

The tumors range from 1.6 to 18 cm in greatest dimension.[906,928-934] Some are predominantly solid with yellow-brown or gray-pink cut surfaces, and others have been predominantly cystic, either unilocular or multilocular, containing hemorrhagic or thick dark-brown fluid. Histologically, most have had the classic "Zellballen" morphology, being composed of organoid clusters of cells surrounded by delicate fibrovascular stroma and sustentacular cells. Some tumors include sheets of large polygonal cells with eccentric nuclei having coarse chromatin and prominent nucleoli. Tumor cells show positive immunostaining for vimentin, neuron-specific enolase, chromogranin, and synaptophysin, and are negative or show only focally positive staining for cytokeratins. Sustentacular cells show positive immunostaining for S100 protein.

Prognosis for renal paraganglioma is difficult to ascertain because, in most reported cases, follow-up has been short. In one remarkable case, lung metastases developed 13 years after the original nephrectomy.[928] A patient with a 13.2-cm primary renal paraganglioma was alive at last follow-up 24 months after diagnosis, but with widespread metastases.[906]

Miscellaneous Tumors

Renal Hematopoietic Neoplasms

Lymphoma

Lymphoma involves the genitourinary system more frequently than any other solid organ system.[935] Involvement of the kidneys by lymphoma is not infrequent and occurs in several patterns, including secondary, primary, posttransplant, and renal intravascular lymphomatosis.[936] Risk factors for renal lymphoma include status post renal transplantation and acquired immunodeficiency syndrome.[936-941]

Renal involvement during the course of systemic lymphoma defines secondary renal lymphoma and is the most common setting for renal lymphoma. Imaging studies at the time of presentation disclose renal involvement in 3% to 8% of patients with systemic lymphoma, and autopsy evidence of renal involvement has been reported in 34% to 62% of patients dying of lymphoma.[936,942] When renal involvement is noted at autopsy, it is bilateral in 75% of cases. Despite its frequency, the great majority of patients with secondary renal lymphoma do not experience symptoms or clinical findings relative to it.[943]

Primary renal lymphoma is rare; it accounts for 0.7% of all extranodal lymphomas in North America and 0.1% in Japan.[944] Only about 50 cases are reported in the literature.[945] It is defined as lymphoma that presents initially with signs and symptoms related to the kidneys, and by all diagnostic criteria is initially limited to one or both kidneys; about 10% to 20% of cases are bilateral.[946] Symptoms and signs include flank or abdominal pain or mass, weight loss, fever, malaise, night sweats, hematuria, pyuria, proteinuria, hypertension, and azotemia. Nearly all patients tend to fall into one of two clinical scenarios: those with renal masses mimicking RCC, and those who present with acute renal failure associated with massive bilateral renal infiltration by lymphoma.[935,936,941-944,947-962] In those with renal masses, clinical and radiologic features that suggest renal lymphoma include multifocal lesions, bilateral lesions, predominantly perirenal plaques, extrarenal extension of tumor, and very prominent hilar adenopathy—all features that are not typical of other renal neoplasms including RCC.[936,963] A confounding feature of some lymphomas, however, is tumor extension into the renal vein, and in some cases the vena cava, a radiologic feature typical of RCC.

Posttransplant lymphoproliferative disorder is a nodal or extranodal lymphoid proliferation that follows solid organ or bone marrow transplantation. It is a consequence of therapeutic suppression of T-cell function, which facilitates infection of B lymphocytes by Epstein-Barr virus, resulting in B-cell proliferations that range from benign reactive polyclonal proliferations to monoclonal proliferations (lymphoma).[936] Although the majority of solid organ transplantation–related lymphoproliferative disorders are of recipient origin, some reported examples of renal lesions have been documented to be of donor origin.[937-940]

Renal intravascular lymphomatosis is a component of angiotrophic large cell lymphoma wherein the renal involvement is characterized by extensive infiltration of glomerular and peritubular capillaries by lymphoma cells.[964,965]

Lymphoma in kidneys resected with a presumptive diagnosis of renal carcinoma show single or multiple tumor nodules that are variably described as friable, soft and fleshy, or firm or rock hard.[941-943,948,949,966] The nodules are typically pale tan, pink, or gray-white, with varying degrees of necrosis or hemorrhage (Fig. 2.209). Tumors often obliterate substantial portions of the renal parenchyma, with varying degrees of circumscription. Involvement of perirenal soft tissues and infiltration of the adrenal or renal hilar vessels are common findings. Nephrectomy is not

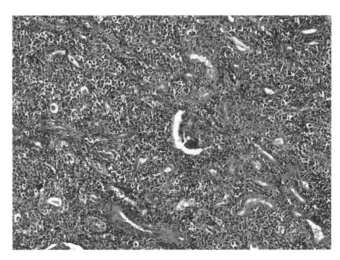

Fig. 2.210 Renal lymphoma. Sheets of monotonous lymphoma cells infiltrate between native renal tubules and glomeruli.

usually done in cases presenting with acute renal failure and diffuse bilateral renal enlargement; in these cases the diagnosis is made by percutaneous needle biopsy.[936,943,944,953-962] The kidneys may appear grossly normal in cases of renal intravascular lymphomatosis.[964]

In nephrectomy specimens, lymphoma obliterates the underlying parenchyma except at the interface between tumor and normal kidney, where the lymphoma cells infiltrate in an interstitial pattern, sparing tubules and glomeruli.[943] This interstitial infiltrative pattern is also seen in needle biopsy specimens (Fig. 2.210).[953-955,958-960,962] Virtually all histologic lymphoma subtypes may be encountered. Diffuse large B-cell lymphoma and its variants are the most commonly encountered primary renal lymphomas; fewer than six cases have been T-cell lymphomas.[945,967]

Renal lymphoma arising in a background of systemic lymphoma has a poor prognosis. The prognosis for primary renal lymphoma is guarded and difficult to quantify due to the lack of long-term follow-up in many of the cases, but there are many reports of complete remission, although reported follow-up periods are often short.[935,941,945,954-956,961,966] Some patients with renal lymphoma die of complications of therapy.[947,953,958] Detection of extrarenal disease after an initial diagnosis of primary renal lymphoma portends a poor outcome in some instances, but successful treatment of such relapses, with prolonged remissions, has been reported.[942,943,947,949,951,957,962]

Plasmacytoma

About 25 cases of primary renal plasmacytoma have been reported, and 20% involved patients with a prior history of plasma cell dyscrasia.[649,968-975] The majority of reported cases have been in patients without a history or clinical evidence of plasma cell neoplasm elsewhere, and the kidneys were resected with a clinical diagnosis of RCC.[975] The great majority of patients are male; patients range in age from 22 to 64 years of age, although most are in their fifties and sixties. Some are noted to have an abdominal mass, some present with hematuria, and in some cases the renal lesion is found incidentally.

Tumors range from 3 to 21 cm in greatest dimension. They are often noted to obliterate large portions of the renal parenchyma and to involve perirenal fat and regional lymph nodes.[968,970,971] Tumors are described as soft or firm and light gray or tan, with small foci of hemorrhage.[969,971,973] Microscopically, tumors are

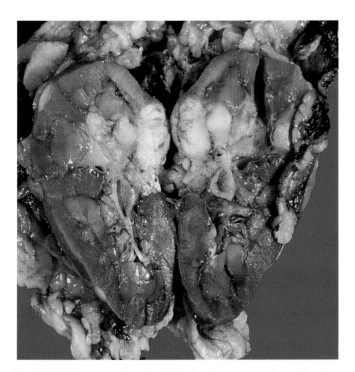

Fig. 2.209 Primary renal lymphoma. Nephrectomy was performed because of a radiologically indeterminate mass. Lesion was diffuse large B-cell, non-Hodgkin lymphoma. Complete staging was negative. Patient was in complete remission 18 months after chemotherapy.

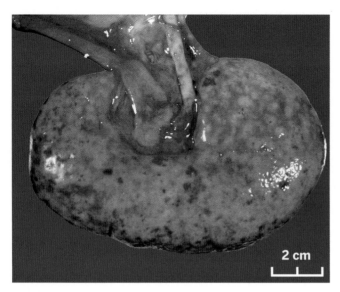

Fig. 2.211 Leukemia involving kidney. Autopsy specimen from a patient recorded as dying of eosinophilic leukemia. Kidney appears swollen, hyperemic, and ecchymotic.

composed of sheets of plasma cells with varying degrees of cytologic atypia and mitotic activity.

Prognosis for primary renal plasmacytoma is difficult to quantify due to its rarity. The overall prognosis for extramedullary plasmacytoma is generally favorable, but local recurrence (30%) and development of systemic disease (40%) make the prognosis guarded.[975]

Leukemia

Myeloid sarcoma is a neoplastic mass formed by proliferating myeloblasts or immature myeloid cells occurring in an extramedullary site. It may arise in a setting of myelodysplastic syndrome, myeloproliferative disorder, or acute myeloid leukemia.[976] Most cases of myeloid sarcoma are identified at autopsy in patients dying of myeloid leukemia, occurring with a frequency of 3% to 7% of such cases (Fig. 2.211).[977] The frequency of documented renal involvement by myeloid sarcoma in autopsy series varies considerably, but with rare exceptions; in most instances, no clinical manifestations of renal involvement are apparent ante mortem.

Rarely myeloid sarcoma occurs de novo as a forerunner of acute myeloid leukemia in patients without leukemia.[976,978,979] Patients may have no renal symptoms or may have flank pain. Renal involvement usually takes the form of diffuse enlargement; in one case the kidney was noted to have an ill-defined green lesion at autopsy, and in another case the kidney was diffusely infiltrated by a grayish tumor. Microscopically, renal tissue shows dense interstitial infiltration by immature granulocytic cells. The frequency of tumor cell positivity for the following histochemical and immunohistochemical stains is as follows: myeloperoxidase, 92%; CD43, 91%; CD34, 44%; CD117, 42%; CD68, 61%; lysozyme, 10%; CD99, 78%; and naphthol ASD-chloroacetate esterase, 55%.[980]

Germ Cell Tumors

There are fewer than a dozen well-documented cases of intrarenal teratoma.[901,902,981-989] In some reports the precise relationship between the tumor and the renal capsule has been difficult to ascertain, and a large proportion of reported cases may represent Wilms tumor with teratoid features. Although most have occurred in children younger than 7 years, several have been encountered in adults.

Tumors may be single or multiple. Associated anomalies have included renal dysplasia and horseshoe kidney. One case was associated with an ipsilateral malignant neuroepithelial tumor of the adrenal gland, and several had elements of carcinoid tumor.[986] A single case of intrarenal mixed germ cell tumor, composed of yolk sac tumor and teratoma, has been reported.[990] The morphology of the reported tumors has been similar to that noted in more conventional sites.

Reported cases of choriocarcinoma metastatic to the kidney are more common than those deemed to have arisen in the kidney.[991,992] Regarding those reported to be renal primaries, it is difficult to exclude the possibility that some originate from spontaneous regression of postgestational choriocarcinoma, a clinically occult "burnt-out" testicular primary, or from urothelial carcinoma of the renal pelvis.[993,994] The morphology of such tumors is indistinguishable from that of their gonadal or uterine counterparts.

Metastatic Tumors

Cancer metastatic to the kidney from other sites is commonly observed at autopsy of patients who died of cancer, occurring in up to 7.2% of cases.[995,996] Occasionally symptoms related to the renal metastasis are the initial manifestations of disease.[997] The commonest primary sites are the lung, breast, melanoma of skin, opposite kidney, gastrointestinal tract, ovary, and testis.[998] In patients with a history of malignancy, renal metastases outnumber RCC by a ratio of about 4:1; a new renal lesion in a patient with advanced incurable cancer is more likely a metastasis than a new primary.[999] However, when a renal mass is found concurrently with another nonrenal malignancy, it is a renal primary nearly as often as it is a metastasis from the other malignancy.[1000] Most metastases are multiple, bilateral, well-defined nodules; some are single and poorly circumscribed (Figs. 2.212 and 2.213). In some cases, metastases are confined to the glomeruli, and rarely this may result in renal insufficiency (Fig. 2.214).[1001,1002] It is notable that RCC is the malignant neoplasm most receptive of tumor-to-tumor metastasis; in this circumstance, lung cancer is the tumor most likely to metastasize to RCC.[1003]

References are available at expertconsult.com

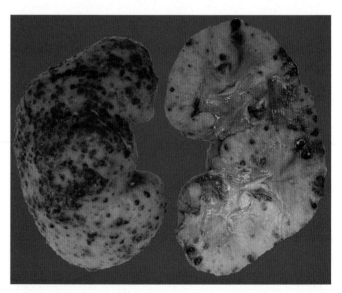

Fig. 2.212 Metastasis to kidney. Specimen shows innumerable metastases of melanoma.

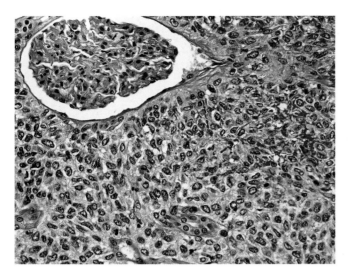

Fig. 2.213 Metastasis to kidney. Section from the kidney shown in Fig. 2.212 shows a glomerulus surrounded by melanoma in the renal parenchyma.

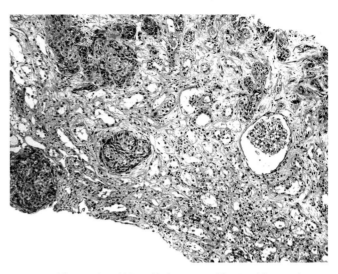

Fig. 2.214 Metastasis to kidney. Patient was a 68-year-old man who presented with hematuria and renal failure. Clinical diagnosis was acute glomerulonephritis until needle biopsy disclosed the presence of extensive glomerular involvement by metastatic non–small cell lung carcinoma.

3

Renal Pelvis and Ureter

EVA COMPERAT, STEPHEN M. BONSIB AND LIANG CHENG

CHAPTER OUTLINE

The renal pelvis and ureter are muscular conduits lined by urothelium that function to propel urine from the renal calyceal system to the urinary bladder.[1] The ureter and renal pelvis are affected by developmental, reactive, and neoplastic disorders. The developmental disorders are a group of closely related entities that include abnormalities in ureteral number, ureteral location, and structure and function of pelvic and ureteral muscularis propria. The mucosa is the site of major reactive and neoplastic disorders.[1]

Development

The ureter and renal pelvis develop from the ampullary bud, which arises from the distal mesonephric duct during the fourth week of development.[2] Contact of the ampullary bud with metanephric blastema induces nephrogenesis. During the months that follow, the ampullary bud elongates and branches dichotomously in parallel with development of the nephrons to create the adult metanephric kidney with its renal pelvis and ureter.[3] As the ureter elongates, there is a period of luminal obliteration followed by recanalization in the fifth week. Recanalization begins in the middle of the ureter and extends proximally and distally with the ureteropelvic and ureterovesical junctions, which are the last segments to recanalize.[4]

The mesonephric duct distal to the ampullary bud (the common nephric duct) is incorporated into the developing urogenital sinus, whereas the ureteral orifice migrates to the trigone of the urinary bladder.[2] The common nephric duct forms the trigone and contributes to the prostatic urethra in the male. Concomitant development of the male and female reproductive tracts from the mesonephric (wolffian) and Müllerian ducts, respectively, and division of the cloaca into bladder and hindgut occur nearby as the ureter and kidney develop. Thus multiple malformations in these areas often occur together.[3]

Anatomy

The lumen of the renal pelvis and ureter is lined by the urothelium, which rests on a basement membrane over a lamina propria composed of highly vascular loose connective tissue (Fig. 3.1A). The urothelium is composed of three to five layers of cells in the pelvis and four to seven layers of cells in the ureter (Fig. 3.1B).[1,4] The pelvis and ureter have a continuous muscular wall that originates in the fornices of the minor calyces as small interlacing fascicles of smooth muscle cells.[5] These take on a spiral architecture in the pelvis and ureter that is necessary for effective peristalsis.[5] The muscularis propria is not divided into distinct layers. Near the bladder, the ureter acquires an external sheath from the detrusor muscle, and the muscle fascicles become oriented longitudinally.[5] The longitudinal fibers continue through the wall of the bladder and into the submucosa, where they spread about the ureteral orifice to contribute to the trigone muscle. Ultimately they terminate near the bladder neck in the female and at the verumontanum in the male.

Peristalsis is initiated by "pacemaker" cells in the renal pelvic muscle near the calyces. These generate electrical impulses that propagate from cell to cell through gap junctions. Effective peristalsis requires both continuity of gap junctions and appropriate quantity and organization of muscle fascicles.[6] As discussed later, disruption of this pattern, even focally, may cause ureteral incompetence or functional obstruction.[3,5]

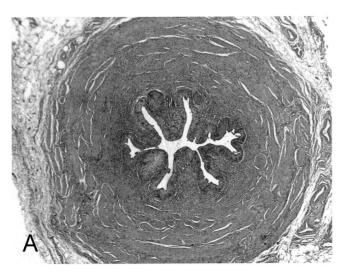 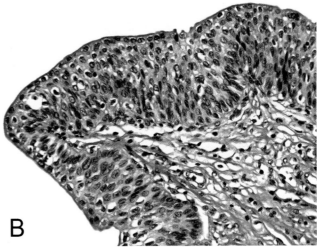

Fig. 3.1 Adult ureter. (A) Cross section showing adventitia, muscularis propria, and irregular contour of relaxed mucosa. (B) The mucosa consists of a few layers of urothelial cells overlying loose connective tissue. No muscularis mucosa is visible.

Congenital Malformations

Genitourinary tract malformations occur in 10% of the population and are the most common group of congenital anomalies (Fig. 3.2).[7] Some, such as bifid ureters, are clinically insignificant.[8] Others are associated with ureteral incompetence or obstruction, with increased risk for renal damage or renal dysplasia.[4] Some are components of multiple malformation syndromes (e.g., VATER [vertebrae, anus, trachea, esophagus, renal] association or prune belly syndrome), are associated with chromosomal abnormalities (e.g., trisomy syndromes), or have a familial predisposition.[9,10] Congenital malformations of the ureters frequently occur together (Table 3.1).

Patients with ureteropelvic anomalies usually present with symptoms of ureteral or pelvic distention, such as flank pain or mass, or with complications such as infection, calculi, or renal insufficiency. Magnetic resonance imaging is the examination of reference.[11] Most such lesions encountered in surgical pathology consist of intrinsic structural defects of the muscularis, usually involving the ends of the ureters, the last segments to recanalize during embryogenesis. These malformations are congenital and

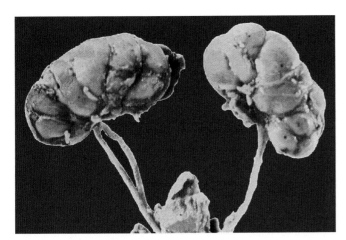

Fig. 3.2 Bifid ureter joining to form a single ureter above the bladder.

of developmental origin, but patients may present at any age from newborn to adulthood. Surgical therapy usually consists of excision of the abnormal segment to preserve renal function. The pathologist should define the anatomic basis of the functional deficit, which usually consists of a distinct but localized defect in smooth muscle quantity or organization (Table 3.2).[12] Recognition of these lesions requires an appreciation of the normal muscle pattern, and their histologic demonstration requires well-oriented sections in which the pattern of the muscle fascicles is highlighted by a trichrome stain. For most lesions, longitudinal orientation of the specimen best shows the deviation from the normal muscle pattern. Primary megaureter (discussed later) is an exception in which cross sections optimally display the predominance of circular fibers and thickening of the periureteral sheath.[13]

Abnormalities in Number or Location of Ureters

Ureteral agenesis, ureteral duplication, and ureteral ectopia are a group of related malformations resulting from defective formation of the ampullary bud.[2] Isolated failure of bud formation causes ureteral agenesis with absence of the ipsilateral hemitrigone and kidney.[2] Another cause of agenesis of the ureter and kidney is wolffian duct failure, which is often associated with genital tract malformations (e.g., absent testis or unicornuate uterus).[2,7] Unilateral agenesis of the kidney and ureter is associated with additional urologic malformations in 20% to 40% of patients.[14,15] Bilateral renal agenesis (Potter syndrome) is lethal because of associated pulmonary hypoplasia; treatment possibilities exist but introduce ethical problems.[16]

Bifid ureter and duplex ureter, the most common (0.8% of all autopsies) ureteral anomalies, result from premature branching of the ampullary bud or development of two separate ampullary buds.[17] Premature branching results in two separate renal pelves and proximal ureters that join to form a single ureter at some point above the bladder (Fig. 3.3). Duplex ureters (Fig. 3.3) have two separate ureteral orifices in the bladder.[18] The ureter from the lower pole usually has its orifice normally situated on the trigone or displaced laterally. The orifice of the ureter from the upper pole can be normally placed, but displacement toward the bladder neck or to an extravesical location is more common.[19] Ureteral ectopia

TABLE 3.1   Common Associations Among Ureteral Anomalies

Ureteral Anomaly	Bifid/Duplex	Ectopia	Reflux	Obstruction of Ureteropelvic Junction	Ureterocele	Dysplasia
Bifid/duplex		+	+	+	+	+
Ectopia	+		+	+	+	+
Reflux	+	+		+	+	+
Obstruction of ureteropelvic junction	+	+	+		+	+
Ureterocele	+	+	+	+		+
Diverticulum	-	+	+	-	-	+
Primary megaureter	-	-	-	-	-	+

TABLE 3.2   Ureteral Muscle Findings in Ureteral Anomalies

Ureteral Anomalies	Muscle Normal	Muscle Deficient	Muscle Dysplastic	Longitudinal Fiber Predominance	Circular Fiber Predominance	Sheath Thick
Refluxing megaureter	+	+	+	-	-	-
Obstruction of ureteropelvic junction	+	+	+	+	-	-
Primary megaureter	-	-	+	-	+	+
Ureterocele	+	+	+	-	-	-
Paraureteral diverticulum	+	+	+	-	-	-

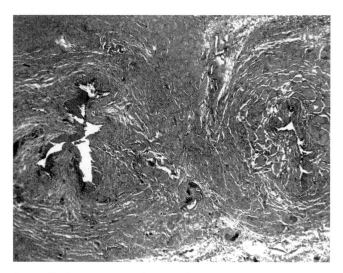

Fig. 3.3 Duplex ureter near point of confluence.

results from abnormally high or low origin of the ampullary bud from the mesonephric duct. Eighty percent of ureteral orifice ectopia is associated with the ureter from the upper pole of a duplicated system.[3,4] The ectopic ureteral orifice may be intravesical (lateral or caudal to the normal site) or extravesical in the urethra, vestibule, or genitalia. Symptoms are influenced by gender and the site of the ureteral orifice, and may consist of urethral dribbling, vaginal "discharge," epididymoorchitis, or pyelonephritis if reflux or obstruction are present.[20] The greater the degree of ectopia in a lateral or extravesical location, the more likely it is that the corresponding renal unit will be dysplastic. The resected specimen thus may include a segmental or complete nephrectomy for dysplasia or pyelonephritis, or a distal ureter excised for reflux, obstruction, or ureterocele.[7,8]

Refluxing Megaureter

Reflux from the bladder is the most common ureteral problem requiring surgical intervention. Patients usually present in early childhood with urinary tract infections and often already have renal scars (reflux nephropathy).[21] Reflux may be unilateral or bilateral, and in about one-third of cases, the patients' siblings have similar urologic abnormalities.[22] Vesicoureteral reflux is caused by incompetence of the ureterovesical junction. There is a 2:1 predominance of females over males, possibly resulting from the additional mechanical support provided to the bladder by the prostate and seminal vesicles.[23]

The affected ureters have abnormally short submucosal segments or deficiency of longitudinal fibers in the intramural segment, or both. Short submucosal segments are apparent to the urologist but difficult to demonstrate histologically. Deficiency of longitudinal fibers can be identified in longitudinal sections of the intramural segment and may appear to the urologist as an abnormally thin and translucent segment of distal ureter (Fig. 3.4). Excision of the defective distal ureteral segment and reimplantation of the ureter is usually curative.[21]

Ureteropelvic Junction Obstruction

Ureteropelvic junction obstruction is the most common cause of ureteral obstruction and may present at any age. When occurring in childhood, it is frequently bilateral (16%), associated with other urologic malformations (15% to 20%), predominantly on the left side, and predominantly in boys; urinary tract infections are frequent. In contrast, cases presenting in adulthood are most often

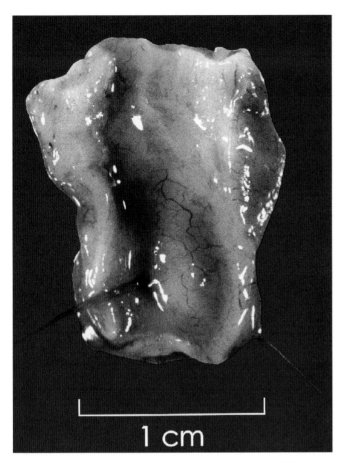

Fig. 3.4 Longitudinal section showing mucosal aspect of distal ureter in reflux. Note the thin wall.

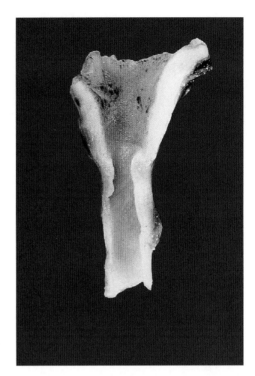

Fig. 3.5 Funnel-shaped zone of ureteropelvic junction obstruction.

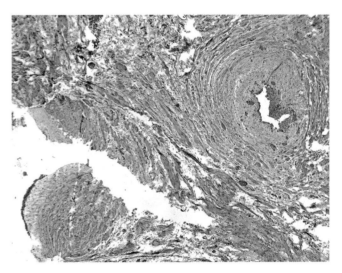

Fig. 3.6 Ureteropelvic junction obstruction.

unilateral and occur in women. Treatment usually includes laparoscopic or robotic surgery.[24] The two most common causes are defects in the muscularis (75%) and renal nonrotation associated with polar vessels (6% to 24%).[25]

The obstructed ureteropelvic junction is characteristically funnel shaped (Fig. 3.5). It may have a grossly visible area of thin muscle, a valvelike intraluminal protrusion of edematous mucosa or muscularis, or may be stenotic.

The histologic appearance is varied. There may be segmental smooth muscle attenuation, often with a predominance of longitudinal fibers, diffuse lack of fascicular organization of pelvic muscles (i.e., dysplastic; see Ureteral Dysplasia section later in this chapter), segmental absence of smooth muscle, or stenotic lumen with normal muscle (Fig. 3.6). "Valves" or "pleats" have also been described that probably result from herniation at the site of muscle abnormality.[26]

Renal polar blood vessels are common anatomic variants of the renal vasculature that usually do not obstruct the ureter because of the medial origin at the renal hilum. In congenitally nonrotated kidneys the pelvis is anterior, and polar vessels may cause significant ureteral obstruction.

Primary Megaureter

Primary megaureter is a nonrefluxing form of ureteral dilation. The gross appearance is distinctive (Fig. 3.7), consisting of narrow and straight ureters immediately above the bladder that merge with segments that are fusiform and markedly dilated. This fusiform dilation differs from the tortuous appearance of ureteral dilation secondary to reflux or obstruction. In 80% of cases, there is functional obstruction at the level of the narrow segment that must be excised.[27] In cross section the narrow segment shows predominance of circular fibers, hypoplasia, and fibrosis of the smooth muscle, or thickening of the periureteral sheath (Fig. 3.8). The only abnormality of the dilated segment is smooth muscle hypertrophy. In the other 20% of cases the narrow segment of ureter has normal muscle, and the dilated segment above it has an almost complete absence of muscle.[28] This has been referred to as dysplastic ureters (see Ureteral Dysplasia section later in this chapter) and is commonly associated with dysplastic kidney.[7,29] However, this terminology may be misleading because there is no relationship with dysplastic (preneoplastic) urothelium.

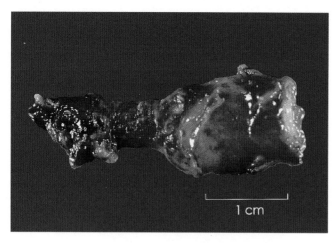

Fig. 3.7 Primary megaureter with abrupt dilation at the superior end.

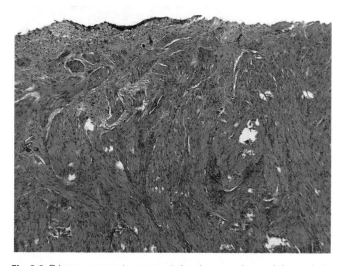

Fig. 3.8 Primary megaureter segment showing smooth muscle hyperplasia.

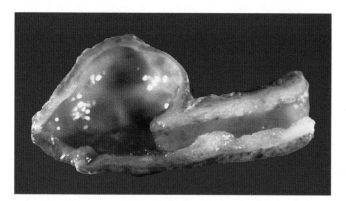

Fig. 3.9 Ureterocele of upper pole ureter. Orifice is near bladder neck.

Ureterocele

Ureterocele consists of congenital dilation of the distal ureter within the bladder (Fig. 3.9). It may balloon into the bladder and occasionally protrudes into the urethra.[30] Most ureteroceles occur in the upper pole ureter of a duplicated system in which the ureter usually passes dorsal to the lower pole ureter. Its dilated

portion may undermine and distort the trigone, often resulting in obstruction or reflux of the normally situated lower pole ureter or, if the ureterocele is large, the contralateral ureter as well. Ureterocele rarely affects a single ureter.[31]

Microscopically, the muscle of the wall of ureterocele varies from hypertrophic to atrophic or absent (Fig. 3.10).[5] Consistent with the usual ectopic location of the ureteral orifice associated with duplex kidneys, 70% of cases have segmental dysplasia of the upper pole of the kidney.[28]

Paraureteral Diverticulum

Herniation of the urinary bladder involving the distal ureter is called *paraureteral diverticulum*. It is usually congenital and detected in childhood, but may result from urethral or bladder neck obstruction at any age.[32] Vesicoureteral reflux is commonly associated with paraureteral diverticulum. The location of the ureteral orifice within the diverticulum correlates with the risk for renal dysplasia (Fig. 3.11). When the ureter opens into the dome

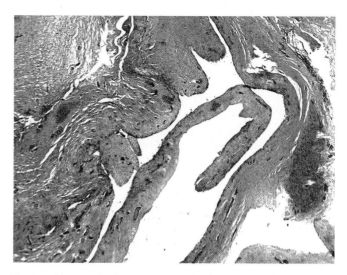

Fig. 3.10 Ureterocele showing thinning or lacking muscle in its wall.

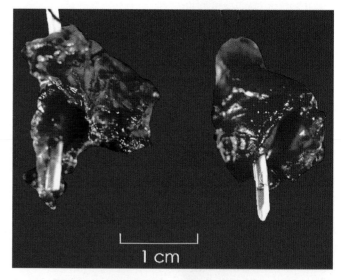

Fig. 3.11 Bilateral paraureteral diverticula. Probes indicate ureteral orifices at the mouth of each diverticulum.

of the diverticulum (a form of lateral ectopia) rather than near its orifice, the likelihood of renal dysplasia is great. There are few histologic studies of diverticula, but deficient ureteral muscle and sheath development have been reported.[33]

Ureteral Dysplasia

Ureteral dysplasia refers to ureters composed of infrequent smooth muscle cells lacking organization and failing to form fascicles. It is unrelated to urothelial dysplasia. Tokunaka et al. showed that involved muscle cells possess thin actin filaments but lack thick myosin filaments essential for normal contractility.[28] Recognition of ureteral dysplasia is important because of the strong association with ipsilateral renal dysplasia (56% to 70% of cases).

Dysplastic ureters vary in appearance from atresia to dilation (Fig. 3.12), and may have an anomalous location. Recognition of the dysplastic nature is not possible on gross examination, because ureters with normal muscle fascicle formation may have a similar appearance.[34]

Nonneoplastic Proliferative, Metaplastic, and Inflammatory Lesions

Nonneoplastic lesions of the ureter share similarities with those in the bladder, although inverted lesions may be more common in the ureter.[35]

Hyperplasia, von Brunn Nests, and Ureteropyelitis Cystica and Glandularis

The most common nonneoplastic urothelial proliferative lesions are simple hyperplasia, von Brunn nests, and ureteropyelitis cystica

and glandularis.[6,7] Simple hyperplasia consists of an increase in the number of layers of urothelial cells without cytologic atypia that commonly accompanies inflammation and neoplasia. von Brunn nests are small, cohesive aggregates of normal urothelial cells within the lamina propria (Fig. 3.13). They are most common in the trigone of the bladder but are also found in 10% of normal ureters at autopsy.[7] When von Brunn nests have central lumens lined by urothelium or columnar cells, they are referred to as ureteritis or pyelitis cystica and ureteritis or pyelitis glandularis (Fig. 3.14), respectively. These changes are common in patients with stone disease.[1] Although usually microscopic, ureteritis and pyelitis cystica may rarely produce grossly visible fluid-filled cysts that elevate the urothelium (Fig. 3.15).[1]

Squamous and Glandular Metaplasia

Squamous metaplasia is the most common form of urothelial metaplasia.[1,36,37] It may be nonkeratinizing or keratinizing (Fig. 3.16), with or without atypia. When squamous metaplasia is encountered in the renal pelvis and ureter, it is often keratinizing. The keratin may be so copious that squames are seen in the urine or collect in the pelvis, forming a mass.[38,39] Keratinizing squamous metaplasia

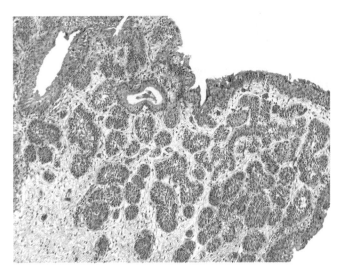

Fig. 3.13 von Brunn nests of the ureter.

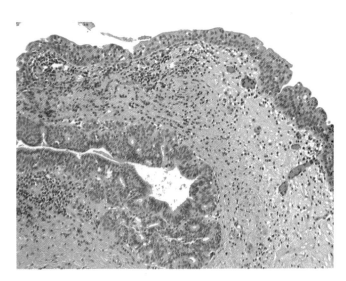

Fig. 3.14 Ureteritis glandularis.

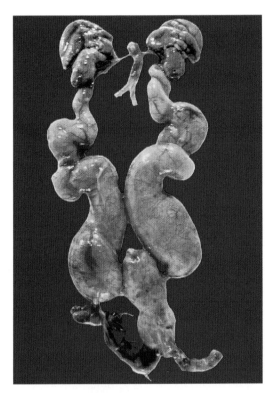

Fig. 3.12 Dysplastic megaureter associated with bilateral renal dysplasia.

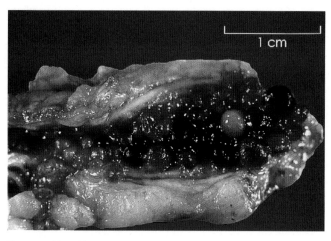

Fig. 3.15 Ureteritis cystica with cobblestone appearance of vesicles protruding into the ureteral lumen.

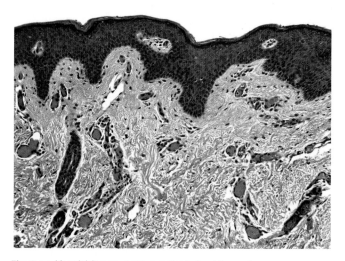

Fig. 3.16 Keratinizing squamous metaplasia of the ureter.

is usually the result of chronic irritation. Conditions such as chronic infection, indwelling catheters, and calculi are present in 60% to 70% of patients. Keratinizing squamous metaplasia may coexist with squamous cell carcinoma and urothelial carcinoma.[40]

Mucinous (glandular, enteric, intestinal, colonic) metaplasia indicates the presence of colonic-type mucinous epithelium, often containing enterochromaffin cells.[41] Intestinal metaplasia of the renal pelvis and ureter is rare, and most cases coexist with adenocarcinoma.[42,43]

Nephrogenic Adenoma

Nephrogenic adenoma is rare in the upper urinary tract, often appearing as an exophytic lesion that may cystoscopically mimic urothelial carcinoma.[44] Microscopically, it consists of a benign papillary and tubular proliferation lined by cuboidal or hobnail epithelium.[45] Nephrogenic adenoma is discussed in detail in Chapter 5.

Reactive Changes (Reactive Atypia)

Reactive changes may affect the urothelium and mimic urothelial carcinoma in situ. In the bladder this is a well-known phenomenon,

whereas it is less common in the upper urinary tract. Its etiology may be inflammatory or idiopathic, and similar alterations may be produced by irradiation and catheterization.[46,47] The resultant striking cytologic atypia characteristically affects superficial cells, which can be enlarged. The cells have low nuclear/cytoplasmic ratios, nuclear or cytoplasmic vacuoles, and smudged chromatin; intraepithelial abscess formation has been described.[37,48] The mixture of normal urothelial cells with occasional large atypical cells is distinctive. Reactive atypia may be encountered in the urothelium of patients who have vesicoureteral reflux.[49] Contrary to the bladder, instillations normally do not interfere with the urothelium, so changes may not be seen. These aspects can be very difficult to analyze in urinary cytology.[48,50]

Malakoplakia

Malakoplakia is an uncommon chronic granulomatous disease that occurs most frequently in the urinary tract of middle-aged women as a complication of recurrent infection.[51,52] Bladder involvement is 4 to 10 times more common than that of the renal pelvis and ureter.[1,37] Nevertheless, malakoplakia has become a rare finding with improved treatment of urinary tract infections.[53]

The typical lesion is a yellow-brown soft ("malakos") plaque ("plakos") (Fig. 3.17) that often has central umbilication. Microscopically, masses of large eosinophilic histiocytes (von Hansemann histiocytes) are present, many of which contain basophilic inclusions (Michaelis–Gutmann bodies; Fig. 3.17). Periodic acid–Schiff stain and special stains for calcium and iron enhance the targetoid appearance of these cytoplasmic inclusions and indicate their mineralized nature.[1,37] Malakoplakia is discussed in detail in Chapter 5.

Endometriosis

Endometriosis is defined by the presence of endometrial tissue beyond the confines of the uterine cavity. It affects approximately 10% to 20% of premenopausal women.[54] However, only 1% to 2% of all cases involve the urinary tract. *Ureteral* endometriosis is especially rare.[54] Antonelli et al. reported the largest series of ureteral endometriosis (19 cases), of which 4 cases (21%) had coexisting bladder endometriosis.[55] Presenting symptoms include flank pain, gross hematuria, dysuria, uremia, and pelvic mass. Approximately 50% of cases are asymptomatic. The lesion is similar in appearance to those in other organ sites, consisting of benign endometrial glands and stroma (Fig. 3.18). It may also present as a polypoid lesion. Malignant transformation of ureteral endometriosis is exceptional.[56]

Retroperitoneal Fibrosis

Retroperitoneal fibrosis is a proliferative process of inflammation and fibrosis occurring in elderly men that may encase affected structures, with the ureters frequently exhibiting medial deviation on intravenous pyelography.[57] It may be primary and idiopathic, although a variety of secondary causes have been identified, including iatrogenic (drugs, surgery, irradiation), inflammatory (vasculitis, aneurysms, diverticulitis, inflammatory bowel disease), and neoplastic (sclerosing lymphoma, urothelial carcinoma) disorders. Regardless of etiology, the typical histology is a prominent mixed inflammatory cell infiltrate with fibroplasia and edema (Fig. 3.19).[57] The major challenge is to identify those secondary causes that merit different therapy. Idiopathic retroperitoneal

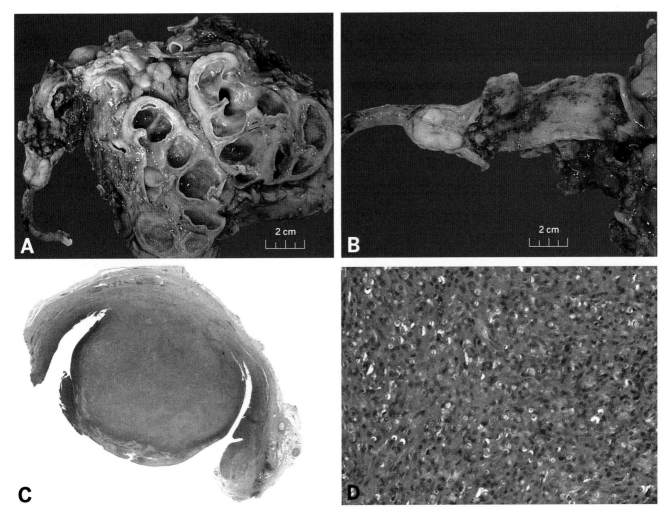

Fig. 3.17 Malakoplakia (A) Malakoplakia involving both kidney and ureter. (B) Malakoplakia involving the ureter. Malakoplakia has a yellowish appearance. (C) Malakoplakia of the ureter. Whole-mount view. (D) Malakoplakia is characterized by granulomatous inflammation, composed of numerous macrophages with target or "owl-eye"-shaped intracytoplasmic basophilic inclusions (Michaelis-Gutmann bodies).

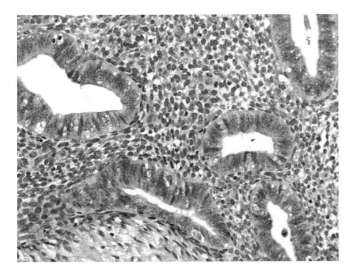

Fig. 3.18 Endometriosis of the ureter.

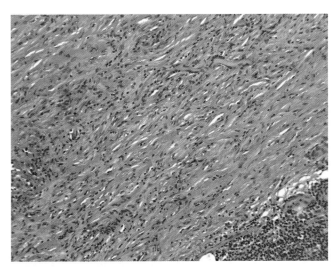

Fig. 3.19 Retroperitoneal fibrosis.

fibrosis has been linked to the immunoglobulin G4 (IgG4)-driven autoimmune process.[58] IgG4-related sclerosing disease is a recently recognized entity and encompasses many organ systems with multiple organ involvement. Recent data indicate that a significant proportion of idiopathic retroperitoneal fibrosis cases in females are associated with clonal expansion of fibroblasts.[59]

Neoplasms

Neoplasms of the ureter and pelvis represent less than 10% of upper tract tumors in adults; renal cell carcinoma comprises most of the remaining cases.[35,60-62] Pyelocaliceal tumors are approximately twice as common as ureteral tumors.[61] Ninety-five percent are epithelial, and 80% are malignant. Of the malignant neoplasms, urothelial carcinoma and primary nonurothelial carcinoma account for 90% and 1.9%, respectively.[61,63]

Benign Epithelial Neoplasms

Inverted Papilloma

Inverted papilloma is a benign urothelial tumor that occurs less commonly in the renal pelvis and ureter than in the urinary bladder.[64] It is almost twice as common in the ureter as in the renal pelvis.[65] Men predominate (male/female ratio = 9:1), with a mean age at presentation of about 65 years.[65] In the upper tract, it may be symptomatic, presenting with hematuria, or it may be found incidentally on radiologic examinations performed for reasons unassociated with inverted papilloma. Inverted papilloma may be multiple and associated with urothelial carcinoma at other sites. Grossly, it may form a mass mimicking carcinoma (Fig. 3.20). The tumor consists of trabeculae of histologically typical urothelium (see Chapter 6).[1,37] Rarely, urothelial carcinoma may arise within inverted papilloma of the ureter, which is the major differential diagnosis.[66]

Urothelial Papilloma

Urothelial papilloma consists of a small (several millimeters or less), delicate papillary structure most often found incidentally. Biopsies of this structure are only rarely performed because of a tendency for urologists to fulgurate this small, clinically innocent-appearing lesion. Microscopically, it consists of thin, delicate fibrovascular fronds invested by epithelium of normal thickness that lacks atypia. By definition, there is no extension into the lamina propria.[1] No recent literature is available for the upper urinary tract.

Malignant Epithelial Neoplasms

Urothelial Dysplasia and Carcinoma In Situ

In keeping with the concept of the urothelium of the renal pelvis, ureter, and bladder as a single anatomic unit affected by similar neoplastic influences, the same relationships between dysplasia and cancer shown for bladder cancer apply in the upper tract. The mucosa adjacent to invasive pelvic and ureteral tumors is abnormal (dysplasia or carcinoma in situ) in 95% of specimens. Patients presenting with concomitant carcinoma in situ have a worse outcome than those who present with pure/primary carcinoma in situ, suggesting a need to differentiate these two entities in the treatment decision process.[62,67] Grossly, the mucosa appears normal or erythematous (Fig. 3.21). The histologic criteria are identical to those described in Chapter 6 (Fig. 3.22). There is an excellent prognosis for upper tract carcinoma in situ treated with radical nephroureterectomy or bacillus Calmette–Guérin.[68-71]

Urothelial Carcinoma

Urothelial carcinoma of the upper tract is epidemiologically similar to that of the bladder. The incidence and prevalence of upper urinary tract urothelial carcinoma is not well defined, because they are usually combined with other forms of neoplams.[72,73] Pyelocaliceal tumors are approximately twice as common as ureteral tumors. There is a male predominance (male/female ratio = 3:1), and it is most common in older individuals aged 70 to 90 years.[74] Hematuria is the principal symptom, but flank pain also is frequent.[61] Upper tract involvement likely represents 5% to 10% of cases of urothelial carcinoma, with an estimated annual incidence in Western countries of almost 2 cases per 100,000 inhabitants.[61,72,73,75]

Cigarette smoking, industrial carcinogens, and chronic irritation (stones and infection) are risk factors.[61,69,76] Phenacetin abuse

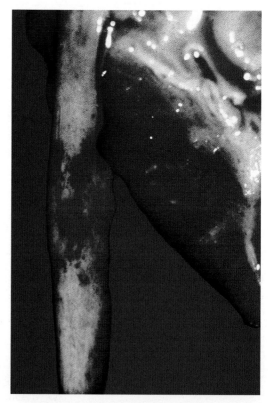

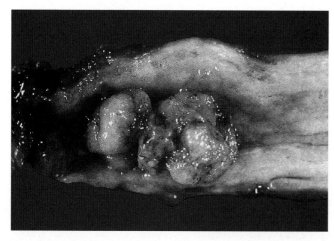

Fig. 3.20 Inverted papilloma of the ureter.

Fig. 3.21 Red patches of urothelial carcinoma in situ of the ureter.

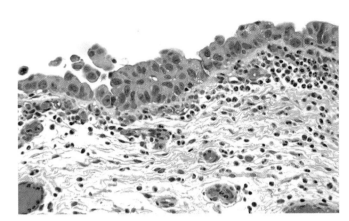

Fig. 3.22 Urothelial carcinoma in situ of the ureter.

is the most important causative factor in some populations, accounting for nearly 25% of renal pelvic tumors and more than 10% of ureteral tumors. Balkan nephropathy and exposure to thorium-containing radiologic contrast material are risk factors for upper tract carcinoma, but not for bladder involvement.[61,77-79] Advanced age, race (black non-Hispanic patients), obesity (body mass index ≥30), Eastern Cooperative Oncology Performance Status (≥1), smoking history, the presence of hydronephrosis, and systemic symptoms are associated with worse prognosis.[74,78,80]

The right and left sides are equally affected, and approximately 2% to 8% of cases are bilateral. Multifocality is a significant problem for patients with upper tract tumors.[61,72,81] There is no survival difference between patients with unilateral or synchronous bilateral upper urinary tract cancers in some studies.[82] However, patients with bilateral subsequent (metachronous) upper tract tumors have a shorter survival.[82-84] More recent studies indicate tumor multifocality is a poor prognostic factor.[83,85]

Ureteral carcinoma seems to have a worse prognosis than renal pelvic involvement, perhaps because the former is usually more invasive. In a report limited to upper urinary tract cancer, muscular invasion was found in the ureter and renal pelvis in 78% and 38%, respectively. Ureteral carcinoma tends to have higher grade and stage than in the bladder.[61,68,80]

In the ureter the most common location of tumor is the distal segment.[86,87] Due to the high rate of recurrence (more than 15%) in the ureter distal to the resected tumor, nephroureterectomy with resection of a cuff of urinary bladder is the operation of choice.[88]

Recurrence in the bladder occurs in 22% to 47% of cases of upper tract urothelial carcinoma. Patients may also have urothelial carcinoma in the contralateral upper tract (2% to 6%).[89,90] In 9% to 17% of cases, concurrent bladder carcinoma is present, and nearly 50% of patients with upper tract cancer subsequently experience bladder involvement.[78,89,91-93] In contrast, the incidence of upper urinary tract tumors is low (0.7% to 4%) among patients with primary bladder cancer.[85]

Patients with multiple bladder tumors are at high risk for development of upper tract cancer. The location of bladder involvement is also important; those with cancer in the trigone are at approximately sixfold higher risk for a synchronous tumor in the upper tract.[91,92] Patients with synchronous or prior history of bladder carcinoma have worse prognosis than those patients without bladder involvement.[81,83,92]

Comparison of upper tract and bladder cancer revealed that the former was more likely to have advanced tumor stage, higher grade, lymphovascular invasion, and lymph node metastasis. Among patients with non–muscle-invasive urothelial carcinoma, those with bladder involvement were more likely to experience higher recurrence and lower cancer-specific survival rates than those with renal pelvicalyceal tumor, but not ureteral tumor.[94] Patients with stage Ta bladder cancer with two or more recurrences are also at high risk for development of upper urinary tumor.[95] In pT2 and pT3 tumors, there was no difference in outcome between the three tumor locations (urinary bladder, ureteral, and renal pelvicalyceal). In pT4 tumors, patients with ureteral and pelvicalyceal tumors were more likely to experience recurrence and mortality than those with bladder involvement. However, an earlier study of 425 patients did not show outcome difference between different locations.[94]

Overall, 60% of cases of upper tract carcinoma are invasive at diagnosis compared with 15% to 25% of bladder tumors.[61,74] In patients who had undergone nephroureterectomy for upper tract carcinoma, pathologic stage was an independent predictor of cancer-specific survival.[78,96]

The gross appearance is similar to that in the bladder (Fig. 3.23), except that large papillary tumors frequently fill the ureters and cause obstruction, resulting in hydronephrosis (Fig. 3.24). Large tumors of the pelvis may extensively invade the renal parenchyma in an ill-defined infiltrative manner (Fig. 3.25), and may extend into paracortical fat, eliciting a

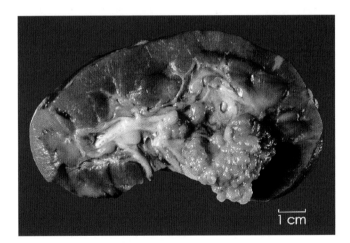

Fig. 3.23 Papillary urothelial carcinoma of the renal pelvis.

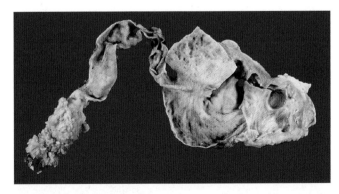

Fig. 3.24 Papillary urothelial carcinoma of the ureter causing hydronephrosis.

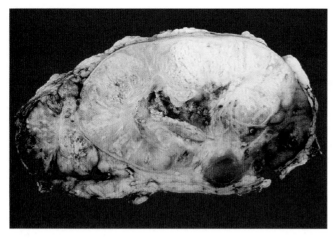

Fig. 3.25 Infiltrative urothelial carcinoma of the pelvis replacing most of the kidney.

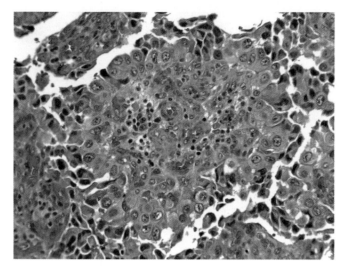

Fig. 3.28 Noninvasive papillary urothelial carcinoma, high grade (grade 3 of 3).

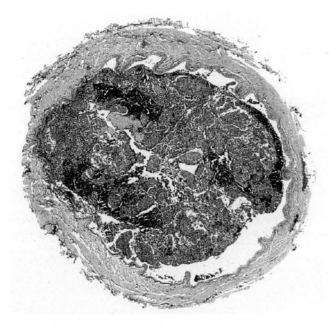

Fig. 3.26 Papillary urothelial carcinoma filling the lumen of the ureter.

scirrhous response. In large tumors, little evidence may remain of mucosal origin in the pelvis, and extensive histologic sampling is required. Gross fat extension or invasion into renal parenchyma should be documented.[97,98]

Grade and stage are the most important prognostic factors in urothelial carcinoma of the upper tract.[35,61,77] The grading scheme is identical to that applied in the bladder (see detailed discussion in Chapter 5) (Figs. 3.26 through 3.28). Both 1973 and 1998 International Society of Urologic Pathology/2004 World Health Organization (WHO) grading systems have been used in recent years. The WHO 2016 recommends the distinction of low and high grades in an effort to standardize terminology and definitions, eliminates ambiguity in diagnostic categories in the WHO 1973 system, and better defines the high-risk group.[36,99] The American Joint Committee on Cancer recommends low grade and high grade, and in squamous cell and adenocarcinoma, GX, G1–3 (Table 3.3).[77]

Histopathology of urothelial carcinoma of the renal pelvis and ureter (Fig. 3.29) has the same spectrum as urothelial carcinoma of the urinary bladder, including squamous and glandular differentiation, and sarcomatoid (Fig. 3.30), lymphoepithelioma-like,

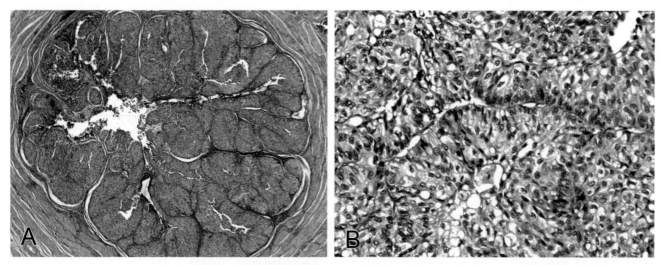

Fig. 3.27 Noninvasive papillary urothelial carcinoma, low grade (grade 2 of 3) (A and B).

TABLE 3.3 — The 2017 American Joint Committee on Cancer TNM Staging for Carcinoma of the Renal Pelvis and Ureter[77]

Primary tumor (T)

TX	Primary tumor cannot be assessed
T0	No evidence of primary tumor
Ta	Papillary noninvasive carcinoma
Tis	Carcinoma in situ
T1	Tumor invades the subepithelial connective tissue
T2	Tumor invades the muscularis
T3	(For renal pelvis only) tumor invades beyond muscularis into peripelvic fat or the renal parenchyma T3 (For ureter only) tumor invades beyond muscularis into periureteric fat
T4	Tumor invades adjacent organs or through the kidney into the perirenal fat

Regional lymph nodes (N)[a]

NX	Regional lymph nodes cannot be assessed
N0	No regional lymph node metastasis
N1	Metastasis in a single lymph node ≤2 cm in greatest dimension
N2	Metastasis in a single lymph node >2 cm or multiple lymph nodes

Distant metastasis (M)

M0	No distant metastasis
M1	Distant metastasis

[a]Laterality does not affect the N classification.
Used with permission of the American College of Surgeons, Chicago, Illinois. The original source for this information is the AJCC Cancer Staging Manual, Eighth Edition (2017) published by Springer International Publishing.

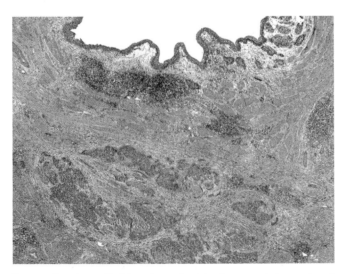

Fig. 3.29 Invasive urothelial carcinoma involving the muscularis propria wall.

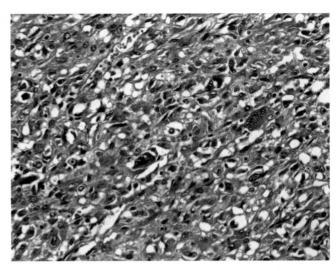

Fig. 3.30 Sarcomatoid urothelial carcinoma of the ureter.

plasmacytoid, micropapillary, inverted, microcystic, and small cell variants. Approximately 25% harbor histologic variants, and some of these are associated with worse prognosis (see Chapter 6).[100-102] Rare variants, including those with trophoblastic differentiation and osteoclast-type giant cells, have also been reported.[103-106] For some entities, immunohistochemical studies may be of diagnostic help.

In addition to grade and stage, other histologic factors are prognostically important, including concomitant carcinoma in situ, sessile tumor growth pattern, tumor size, tumor necrosis, lymphovascular invasion, lymph node involvement, tumor architecture, positive surgical margins, and histologic variants. Extranodal extension is an independent predictor of poor clinical outcome in patients with upper tract urothelial carcinoma with lymph node metastasis.[36,61,107,108]

Immunophenotypically, upper tract urothelial carcinoma is similar to its counterpart in bladder, staining for GATA3, S-100P, uroplakin III, thrombomodulin, cytokeratins 7 and 20, p63, and high-molecular-weight cytokeratin.[109] PAX2 and PAX8, nephric cell lineage transcription factors that play key roles in renal organogenesis, are often expressed in upper tract urothelial carcinoma, but are usually nonreactive in bladder urothelial carcinomas.[110]

Cytology for detection or surveillance in the upper urinary tract is challenging, with sensitivity and specificity of 54% and 56%, respectively.[48,50,111] Patients with clinical low-grade tumors on biopsy run the risk of upgrading, particularly with positive urine cytology. The predictive value of biopsy can be improved by extensive ureteroscopic sampling.[112] Fluorescence in situ hybridization analysis of chromosomes 3, 7, 9, and 17 abnormalities provides superior sensitivity compared with cytology for the detection of upper urinary tract urothelial carcinoma while maintaining a similar specificity.[113]

Genetic factors play a role in carcinogenesis of upper tract urothelial carcinoma. The risk is significantly increased in patients with family history of hereditary nonpolyposis colon cancer (Lynch syndrome), with upper tract tumors developing at a younger age and more likely in the ureter, with an almost equal gender ratio.[114-116] Although some believe these tumors have high-grade potential, similar to that in the general population, others report that patients with microsatellite instability (MSI) more often have low-grade, low-stage cancer with an inverted growth pattern and good prognosis.[117,118] Another group found no pathologic difference in invasion depth or growth type, but noted higher grade than with non MSI-H tumors.[119] When cancer arises in the upper tract, it is more common in the ureter among patients with Lynch syndrome than the general population (51% versus 45%, respectively), and the likelihood is greater for high-grade tumor (88% and 74%, respectively).[118,120] High incidence of MSI (21%) was initially reported in sporadic tumors of the upper tract,[121] although others reported a lower incidence (7%).[86,122] High MSI was associated with better prognosis.[119,123] These tumors often display

TABLE 3.4	Four Clusters of Gene Expression[126]			
Subtypes of UUT-UC	Cluster 1	Cluster 2	Cluster 3	Cluster 4
Mutation	No PIK3CA mutation	100% FGFR3 mutations	100% FGFR3 mutations; 71% PIK3CA mutations; no TP53 mutations	No PIK3CA mutation; 62% KMT2D mutations; 50% TP53 mutations
Tobacco history	Nonsmokers		High tobacco use	High tobacco use
Grade	High grade	Enriched low grade		High grade
Stage	NMIUC	NMIUC		MIUC
Recurrence	High recurrence	No bladder recurrence	Bladder recurrence	Carcinoma in situ
Survival	Favorable survival			Short survival

MIUC, Muscle-invasive urothelial carcinoma; *NMIUC*, non-muscle-invasive urothelial carcinoma; *UUT-UC*, upper urinary tract-urothelial carcinoma.
From Moss TJ, Qi Y, Xi L, et al. Comprehensive genomic characterization of upper tract urothelial carcinoma. *Eur Urol* 2017;72:641-649.

inflammation, suggesting likely response to immune checkpoint inhibitors, similar to bladder cancer.[121] Patients identified as high risk for Lynch syndrome should undergo DNA sequencing for patient and family counseling.[118] Screening of patients with Lynch syndrome is important to predict development of new primary tumors.[116]

Cytogenetic studies of sporadic tumors show that genetic changes in upper tract urothelial carcinoma are similar to those in the urinary bladder.[124] Promoter hypermethylation was an independent predictor of progression-free survival in patients with upper tract urothelial carcinomas.[125] Nevertheless, important differences exist between sporadic and inherited forms.[124,126]

Different molecular subgroups in bladder and upper urinary tract cancers have been described. Several pathways other than MMR (mismatch repair) are differentially deregulated, including TP53 signaling and level of genomic instability. Higher rate of TP53 mutations and related pathways lead to important genomic instability, alterations of copy numbers, and dysfunction of the cell cycle and apoptosis. FGFR3 (fibroblast growth factor receptor 3) is commonly mutated in high-grade tumors, with higher rates than in the bladder. Up to 60% of high-grade tumors display FGFR3 mutations. Four major different tumor clusters with different outcomes have been identified (Table 3.4).[126]

Squamous Cell Carcinoma

Approximately 10% of renal pelvic tumors are squamous cell carcinoma, with a lower percentage of cases of ureteral involvement.[40,100] Calculi, horseshoe kidney, and chronic infection are risk factors.[127] The relationship with squamous metaplasia is controversial, perhaps owing to the rarity of squamous cell carcinoma of the upper urinary tract. Epstein-Barr virus infection is not implicated.[128] The most common presenting symptoms are flank pain and gross hematuria.

Most squamous cell carcinomas of the renal pelvis and ureters are high stage; extensive infiltration of the renal parenchyma is common (Fig. 3.31), and survival at 5 years is rare.[63] The histopathology of this tumor is similar to squamous cell carcinoma in the bladder. This tumor should be distinguished from metastatic squamous cell carcinoma, which usually is straightforward when clinical and pathologic features are considered.

Adenocarcinoma

Primary adenocarcinoma of the upper tract is rare, and reports consist of single cases or small series of cases (Fig. 3.32). Most occur in adults, but rare pediatric cases have been described.[129] Calculi, chronic inflammation, and infection appear to be predisposing

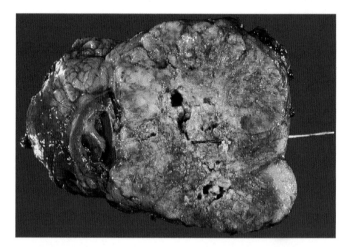

Fig. 3.31 Squamous cell carcinoma of the renal pelvis. the probe indicates the course of the ureter.

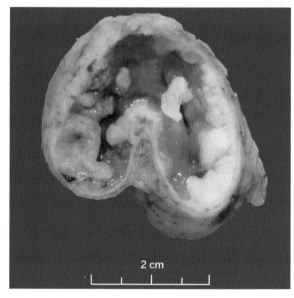

Fig. 3.32 Mucinous adenocarcinoma of the renal pelvis.

conditions.[101] Most patients present with advanced cancer, similar to those with squamous cell carcinoma, and have a poor prognosis. Intestinal metaplasia and villous adenoma may be precursors based on common coexistence, and noninvasive carcinoma is sometimes

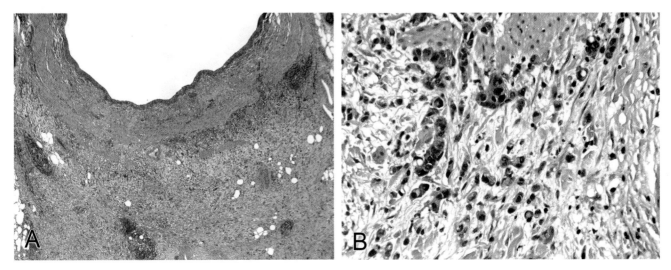

Fig. 3.33 Mucinous adenocarcinoma of the ureter infiltrating the lamina propria (A and B). The tumor cells display signet ring cell features.

found in the adjacent mucosa.[130] Variants of adenocarcinoma have been described, and the prognostic significance of subclassification is uncertain. The prognosis is generally poor.[63] Papillary architecture and resemblance to mucinous adenocarcinoma of the colon (Fig. 3.33) are common.

Metastases

Neoplastic involvement of ureters may occur by direct local extension or metastasis.[131] Contiguous ureteral involvement is more frequent and is usually caused by carcinoma of the cervix, prostate, or bladder. Metastatic involvement is less common, and breast and colon are the most common sites of primaries. Ureteral involvement is rarely the initial manifestation. When distant metastasis occurs, the lung is the most common site of metastasis for patients with urothelial carcinoma of upper tract.[132]

Mesenchymal Neoplasms

Mesenchymal neoplasms are uncommon in the ureter and pelvis. Fibroepithelial polyp is most common, followed by benign and malignant smooth muscle tumors. A variety of additional tumors have been reported as single cases including hemangioma, neurofibroma, and malignant schwannoma.

Fibroepithelial Polyp

Fibroepithelial polyp is more common in the ureters and renal pelvis than in the bladder. It is an uncommon benign mesenchymal tumor of the renal pelvis and ureter. Approximately 70% of patients are male, and it occurs at all ages from infancy to old age (mean, approximately 40 years).[133] Fibroepithelial polyp is the most common benign polypoid lesion of the ureter in children. Colicky flank pain and hematuria are the most common symptoms. The cause is uncertain.[134]

Grossly, fibroepithelial polyp consists of single or multiple slender smooth-surfaced vermiform polyps that usually arise from a common base. The ureteropelvic junction is a common site, and the polyp may cause obstruction at that narrow point. Rarely, it is bilateral. Microscopically, the polyp is covered by normal urothelium, which may be focally eroded. The core of the polyp is composed of loose edematous and vascular stroma with few inflammatory cells (Fig. 3.34).[1]

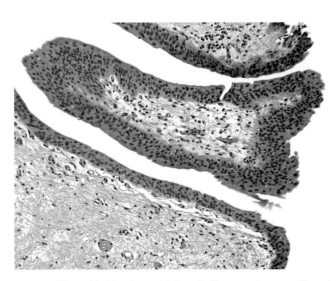

Fig. 3.34 Fibroepithelial polyp consisting of a fibrovascular core with scattered inflammatory cells and a covering of normal urothelium.

Leiomyoma and Leiomyosarcoma

Smooth muscle tumors of the ureter and pelvis are much rarer than those of the kidney, and patients have an approximately equal frequency of benign and malignant tumors. Patients present with hematuria, pain, or mass, findings indistinguishable from those of urothelial neoplasms.[135,136] Grossly, small tumors may form polypoid masses (Fig. 3.35), whereas larger tumors are often infiltrative. Histologically, they resemble their counterparts elsewhere.[1]

Hemangioma

Hemangioma of the ureter and renal pelvis is an uncommon polypoid tumor (Fig. 3.36) consisting of hypervascular fibrous stroma covered by normal urothelium. Occurring in children and adults, this lesion may be multiple and frequently causes obstruction.[137]

Other Tumors

Other sarcomas, such as osteogenic sarcoma, extraosseous Ewing sarcoma, liposarcoma, rhabdomyosarcoma, and malignant schwannoma are rare. Malignant melanoma may arise in the mucosa of the

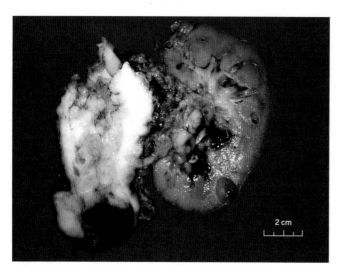

Fig. 3.35 Leiomyosarcoma of ureter, gross appearance.

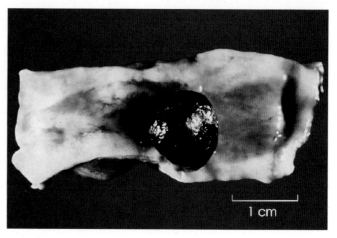

Fig. 3.36 Hemangioma of the ureter.

renal pelvis. Carcinosarcoma, combining squamous or urothelial carcinoma with heterologous sarcoma, such as osteogenic sarcoma, chondrosarcoma, or rhabdomyosarcoma, is rare. Choriocarcinomatous differentiation may be seen in coexisting urothelial carcinoma. Pure choriocarcinoma of the renal pelvis has been reported. Inflammatory myofibroblastic tumor involving the ureter is rare (see

detailed discussion in Chapters 5 and 6). Obstruction caused by secondary infiltration by malignant lymphoma occurs in approximately 16% of cases of disseminated lymphoma.[101,103-106,129]

References are available at expertconsult.com

4

Fine Needle Aspiration of the Kidney

ANDREW A. RENSHAW

CHAPTER OUTLINE

Introduction

Fine needle aspiration (FNA) of the kidney is a useful technique for diagnosing a specific subset of renal lesions.[1-5] Most renal lesions in adults are either benign cysts (based on their radiographic appearance) that can be left alone or are sufficiently worrisome that resection is indicated regardless of the results of FNA. It is estimated that only 10% to 30% of all renal masses are candidates for FNA.[6,7]

Until recently, renal FNA in the pediatric population was contradicted because aspiration of a suspected Wilms tumor, the most common renal tumor in children, resulted in clinical "upstaging." This has been changed and has resulted in an increase in the use of FNA in pediatric patients in some centers. Interpretation of these specimens is challenging, and it is discussed more fully in the Fine Needle Aspiration in Pediatric Patients "section at the end of" this chapter.[8-10]

Both FNA and core needle biopsy can be performed. Immunohistochemistry and genetic studies can be done on both types of specimens.[11,12] Although each technique has its own advantages and disadvantages, the combination of FNA and core needle biopsy has the highest yield.[13-19] However, in some cases an aspirator may be willing to do an FNA but unwilling to do a core needle biopsy because of the risk for hemorrhage. Thus the ability to interpret FNA material remains an important skill. Because the interpretation of core biopsies is similar to that of routine histologic assessment, which is discussed in more detail in other chapters of this textbook, this chapter will focus on interpretation of FNA specimens. Regardless of the biopsy method, accurate identification of some unusual subtypes of renal cell carcinoma (RCC) may depend on both adequate sampling and ancillary studies, and these may not always be available.[20] As a result, accurate subtyping of some unusual types of RCC may not always be possible with either FNA or core needle biopsy.

Background to Renal Fine Needle Aspiration

Indications

FNA has several indications. First, FNA can provide a diagnosis in a patient who is not a candidate for resection. This includes patients whose primary tumor is high stage, patients with presumptive metastatic disease, or patients who are not medically able to undergo resection. In addition, many urologists will consider following rather than resecting benign lesions such as oncocytoma, and this is a relatively common indication for FNA. Second, FNA has traditionally been used to evaluate patients with radiographically indeterminate lesions, usually cysts. However, the utility of the technique in this setting is quite limited; see the section on renal cysts. Finally, although the ultimate decision to perform a partial rather than total nephrectomy is a surgical one, the results of FNA can be useful in triaging these patients. Candidates for partial nephrectomy include patients with small lesions, young patients, and patients who are at risk for multiple and bilateral lesions, such as patients with von Hippel–Lindau syndrome.[21] More and more patients are potential candidates for partial nephrectomy, in part because higher-resolution imaging techniques can identify smaller lesions than in the past. FNA can provide a specific or differential diagnosis in most of these patients. Finally, in the patient with focal bacterial pyelonephritis or a renal abscess, needle placement permits both diagnosis and therapeutic drainage.

Specimen Collection and Preparation

Virtually all renal aspirations are performed percutaneously by radiologists using ultrasound, computed tomography, or magnetic resonance imaging.[22-24] Rarely a surgeon might obtain an FNA intraoperatively. Most of the literature is on alcohol-fixed specimens prepared with either Papanicolaou (Pap) or hematoxylin and eosin stains, or air-dried Giemsa-stained material. Cell blocks can be particularly helpful for identifying papillae and other architectural features, and many lesions are best diagnosed with immunohistochemical support (e.g., angiomyolipoma). Genetic studies can be useful, and sometimes necessary, in subtyping RCCs.[25-28] Fluorescence in situ hybridization can be performed on unstained cytospins, monolayers, smears, and cell block sections.[12,29]

Complications

The complications of renal FNA include hemorrhage, pneumothorax, infection, arteriovenous fistula, and urinoma. All are uncommon. Morbidity, mortality, and needle track cancer seeding are rare in the modern era with the use of smaller (less than 18 gauge) needles.[18,30]

Accuracy

Based on historical studies, renal FNA accurately distinguishes benign from malignant lesions in 73% to 94% of cases; correct subclassification of RCC is achieved in 74% to 80% of cases, and up to 90% for the most common subtypes of RCC using routine cytology.[14,15,31-53] More recent studies show that accuracy can be increased up to 99% on core biopsy material for the most common subtypes of RCC by using immunohistochemistry for carbonic anhydrase IX, CD117, α-methylacyl-coenzyme A racemase, cytokeratin (CK) 7, and CD10.[46] Other panels have also been shown to be of value.[51] To date, subtyping RCC is generally not necessary for the treatment of most patients, although it may provide prognostic information. As therapies other than surgery continue to improve, this may not remain true, especially if some of these therapies prove subtype specific. As noted earlier, recognition of the common subtypes is highly reliable. The recognition of unusual RCC subtypes on limited material without adequate ancillary studies may be impossible, and this may drive the need for the development of more thorough sampling protocols. Unfortunately, no specific immunohistochemical stain exists for oncocytoma, making this a diagnosis of exclusion, and perhaps less reliable than a diagnosis of RCC.[51]

Renal FNA is performed infrequently, and many cytopathologists may not have much experience evaluating these specimens. False-positive results have occurred when xanthogranulomatous pyelonephritis, angiomyolipoma, benign hepatocytes, benign

tubular cells, glomeruli, and benign adrenal cortical cells have been misinterpreted as RCC.[18] In the past, interpretation of renal FNA has been one of the poorest performers on survey material, with a false-positive rate of 30.4% and a false-negative rate of 13.9%.[54] Many of these errors relate to misinterpretation of normal elements as tumor. Recent surveys have shown improved performance.

Cellularity is important to consider when interpreting a kidney FNA; rare atypical cells are common in many benign lesions. Hypocellular kidney aspirates therefore should *never* be diagnosed as positive.

Adequacy

Up to 30% of renal aspirates are nondiagnostic (inadequate); repeat aspiration is helpful in approximately half of cases.[31,32,35,37-40,44] Most inadequate specimens are related to technical failure to obtain adequate diagnostic material.[55] Although specific adequacy criteria are not well defined, awareness of the radiographic appearance of the lesion is important. For example, an aspirate composed exclusively of macrophages from a known Bosniak category 1 lesion (see later discussion of cysts for definition) being drained for symptomatic relief is both adequate and diagnostic (benign); in contrast, the same aspirate from a solid Bosniak category 2 or 3 lesion is neither adequate nor diagnostic, and is best reported as "nondiagnostic" rather than negative.

Normal Elements

Normal elements are commonly present in renal FNA.

Glomeruli

Glomeruli (Fig. 4.1) are highly cellular globular structures that may mimic the papillae that are seen in papillary RCC, especially at low power. In contrast with papillary RCC, however, endothelial cells lining the capillary loops can be seen at the extreme edge of many glomeruli. In RCC the neoplastic cells may be at the edge of a large cluster, but the cytoplasm of the cell almost always extends even more peripherally than the nucleus, and the nucleus is rounder than that of an endothelial cell.

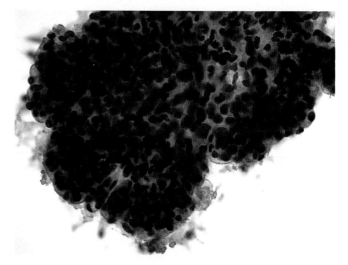

Fig. 4.1 Glomeruli appear as rounded masses that superficially resemble papillae. At the top, the capillary loops and flattened endothelial cells are visible at the periphery. Hematoxylin and eosin stain, original magnification ×400.

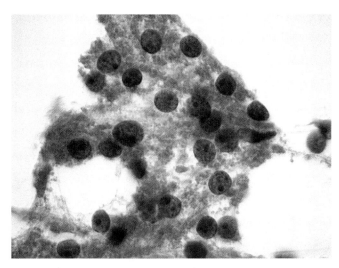

Fig. 4.2 Proximal tubular cells. The cells have abundant granular cytoplasm and disrupted cell membrane with overflowing granules. Hematoxylin and eosin stain, original magnification ×1000.

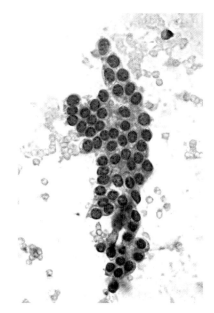

Fig. 4.3 Distal tubular cells. The cells have scant clear cytoplasm and round nuclei with small nucleoli. Papanicolaou stain, original magnification ×1000.

Proximal Tubular Cells

Proximal tubular cells (Fig. 4.2) consist of single cells with round bland nuclei, small but easily seen nucleoli, and abundant, granular cytoplasm. These normal cells are often ripped from their tubules, and as a result, the cell membrane is usually torn and the granules often appear to be spilling out of the cells. Less commonly, entire tubules may be aspirated, resulting in small round to elongate nests of cells. These cells are similar, if not identical, to those seen in aspirates from oncocytoma and some cases of papillary and chromophobe RCC. However, FNAs of tumors are typically quite cellular. Papillary tumors have papillae that are best seen on cell block preparations. Chromophobe RCC tumor cells are often binucleate; there is variation in cell and nuclear size and shape. The cell borders of the tumor cells are usually well defined because these cells are only loosely cohesive and relatively easily removed from the tumor, and chromophobe RCC rarely produces round nests of cells.

Distal Tubular Cells

Distal tubular cells (Fig. 4.3) are small, single or cohesive cells in sheets of up to about 20 cells, with scant clear to slightly granular cytoplasm and small, round nuclei with or without very small nucleoli. Cell membranes are usually intact, but may be difficult to see because the cytoplasm is scant. What little cytoplasm that is present is clear to minimally granulated, but should not be vacuolated.[56] These cells are identical to those seen in either low-grade clear cell or papillary RCC. However, aspirates of tumors should be more cellular, both tumors may have intracytoplasmic hemosiderin, and papillary RCC may form papillae and spherules.

Benign Lesions

Oncocytoma

Oncocytoma comprises 3% to 5% of all renal tumors and is benign, although rare metastases have been reported (see Chapter 2 for additional discussion of the metastatic potential of oncocytoma).[57-63] The tumor cells have abundant granular cytoplasm and uniform round nuclei, with variably prominent nucleoli, and in many cases salt-and-pepper type chromatin.[64] Occasional large bizarre nuclei

may be present (similar to "endocrine atypia"), but mitotic figures are absent or rare. The arrangement of the neoplastic cells in rounded nests is distinctive and stands in contrast with the trabeculae (ribbons) of chromophobe RCC.[65] In addition, although the classic gross description of this tumor as a mahogany brown lesion with a central scar continues to be perpetuated in most textbooks, a more accurate description is a well-circumscribed lesion that is exactly the same color as the adjacent cortex, which is mahogany brown if the kidney is removed without draining the blood first or more pale gray or tan if the kidney has been drained before resection.

Cytologically, the cells of oncocytoma are easily dissociated and aspirates are typically highly cellular. The specimens are composed of numerous single cells and loosely cohesive small clusters of up to about 10 cells, with abundant, eosinophilic, granular cytoplasm, well-defined cell membranes, frequent binucleation, and round nuclei with small but distinct nucleoli, and in many but not all cases, salt-and-pepper chromatin (Fig. 4.4).[66-70] Although atypia can be present in oncocytoma, it is of a specific type. In general this is "endocrine" atypia and consists of nuclei with marked size variation and relatively dark chromatin without prominent nucleoli.[68] This is in marked contrast with the prominent nucleoli and fine chromatin of most RCCs. Although hyaline globules have been reported in oncocytomas, they are not specific.[71,72]

The differential diagnosis includes normal proximal tubules, clear cell RCC, chromophobe RCC, papillary RCC, and hepatocytes. The cells of proximal tubules are identical, but aspirates are scant and the cell membranes are rarely intact. Even though oncocytoma may have cohesive cells, it rarely forms the rounded nests that one sees in normal proximal tubules. Instead the clusters of cells are more loosely cohesive and irregular. Although clear cell RCC is always listed in the differential diagnosis of oncocytoma, this is usually easy to resolve. The aspirates of clear cell RCC are more cohesive, have fewer single cells, more nuclear atypia, and less uniformly granular cytoplasm. Although some clear cell tumors may have abundant granular cytoplasm, most are higher-grade tumors. In addition, clear cell RCC is CD117⁻, whereas oncocytoma is CD117⁺. In contrast, chromophobe RCC may be extremely difficult to distinguish from

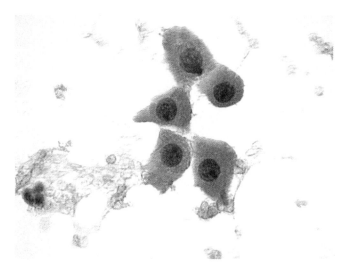

Fig. 4.4 Oncocytoma. The cells are single, small, and uniform with abundant granular cytoplasm and round nuclei with small nucleoli and intact cell membranes. Hematoxylin and eosin stain, original magnification ×1000.

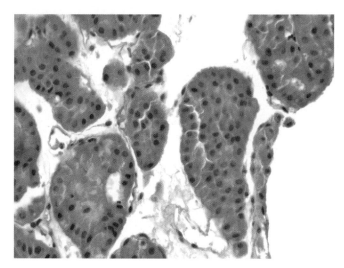

Fig. 4.5 Oncocytoma on core biopsy. The architecture of small nests is extremely helpful in confirming the diagnosis. Hematoxylin and eosin stain, original magnification ×200.

oncocytoma, but in general has less uniformly granular cytoplasm and often more nuclear outline irregularity; nucleoli are rare and the chromatin is finer (although it may be either light or dark). Chromophobe tumors show diffuse cytoplasmic positivity with Hale colloidal iron staining, a finding that supports the diagnosis. However, oncocytoma usually shows focal to moderate membranous staining with Hale colloidal iron stain, which can be difficult to interpret. Both tumors are CD117⁺. Chromophobe RCC is reported to be more diffusely positive for CK7, CK20, and PAX8 than oncocytoma, but reactivity is often patchy in both tumors.

Rare low-grade papillary tumors can have cells that are identical to those seen in oncocytoma, but the papillary architecture is diagnostic, and these tumors should be diffusely CK7⁺. As in clear cell tumors, most papillary tumors with granular cytoplasm are higher-grade tumors that are not typically in the differential with oncocytoma. Inadvertent sampling of the liver can superficially resemble oncocytoma because hepatocytes have abundant granular cytoplasm. However, hepatocytes are usually aspirated in groups as well as singly, may contain bile, and have more variation in the size of the cells and their nuclei.

It is currently controversial whether oncocytoma should be diagnosed on FNA alone. There is no specific immunohistochemical marker for oncocytoma, and currently the diagnosis of oncocytoma on aspirate material alone is a diagnosis of exclusion.[73] Individual cells in both clear cell and papillary tumors can be identical to those seen in oncocytoma, and chromophobe RCC can strongly resemble oncocytoma even on resection. Hybrid tumors that have features of both chromophobe RCC and oncocytoma have been described, both sporadically and in association with Birt-Hogg-Dube syndrome.[73] In general the best diagnosis for these lesions is oncocytic neoplasm with a differential diagnosis of oncocytoma versus RCC, including chromophobe RCC. If a definitive diagnosis is mandatory, a core needle biopsy (Fig. 4.5) exhibiting the nested architecture may assist in distinguishing the lesion from chromophobe RCC. However, it is often possible to satisfy the clinical needs of the patient without making a definitive diagnosis. For example, in an elderly patient with multiple comorbidities and a relatively limited life expectancy, a diagnosis of favor oncocytoma is often enough for the urologist to forgo excision and likely represents the best clinical care.

Papillary Adenoma

Papillary adenoma (renal cortical adenoma) is histologically, immunohistochemically, and cytogenetically indistinguishable from low-grade papillary RCC except by size.[74,75] Renal adenoma is defined as a small lesion less than 1.5 cm in diameter.[76] Aspirates from adenoma, like those from papillary RCC (see later), are cellular, with bland cells forming tubules spherules and true papillae. Cytologic atypia may be minimal, and the diagnosis often relies on the presence of abundant cellularity and distinct architectural pattern. Both adenoma and papillary RCC are CK7⁺, in contrast with clear cell RCC, which may be composed of similar cells (although it does not form distinct architectural patterns).

Many adenomas are too small to be identified radiologically or aspirated, but larger adenomas may undergo a biopsy. Therefore when diagnosing a papillary lesion in the kidney, ideally one should know its size. If one has an aspirate from a small lesion, or does not know how big the lesion is, the best diagnosis is low-grade papillary neoplasm, adenoma versus carcinoma. Regardless of the final diagnosis, when diagnosed on cytologic material, both lesions are candidates for resection, because adenomas may grow beyond 1.5 cm.

Angiomyolipoma

Angiomyolipomas occur in two distinct clinical settings.[77-79] Approximately half occur in young adults with tuberous sclerosis, in whom the tumors are usually multiple and bilateral. The remaining cases occur in young and middle-aged women without any known clinical syndromes, and angiomyolipoma is usually solitary in these patients. These lesions can bleed spontaneously, and those larger than 5 cm are often resected to circumvent catastrophic hemorrhage. The tumor is composed of three elements in varying proportions: blood vessels, mature fat, and an atypical smooth muscle/perivascular cell that is reactive for various melanocytic markers such as HMB45 and Melan A.

FNAs of typical lesions with abundant adipose tissue are easy to diagnose, but these tumors are rarely aspirated because they can be diagnosed by identifying the fat radiographically.[80-90] Rarely a case with abundant adipose tissue is aspirated to rule out a liposarcoma, but most FNAs from angiomyolipoma are from those with little adipose tissue.[91] In general, the vessels are too large to be aspirated, although rarely large intact vessels are identified. As a result, the predominant cells in most aspirates are the atypical smooth muscle/perivascular cells, and these can be very challenging to interpret (Fig. 4.6). The aspirates are generally paucicellular and on low power consist of relatively large groups of elongate and round cells that resemble abnormal stroma (Fig. 4.7). The cells are very cohesive, and single cells are rare. In comparison with the cellular groups of RCC, these groups are less dense and have more cytoplasm. On higher power, the cells consist predominantly of atypical smooth muscle/perivascular cells that can be elongate (Fig. 4.8) or round (Fig. 4.9), bland, or markedly atypical. The cytoplasm is often stringy or crystalline rather than granular or vacuolated, but this may be difficult to appreciate in most specimens. Infrequent, relatively large clear vacuoles are also present, perhaps representing fat (Fig. 4.10). The atypia is characterized by markedly enlarged, darkly hyperchromatic, generally round nuclei (Fig. 4.11). In contrast with atypia seen in most FNAs from clear cell RCC, the chromatin is usually much darker, nucleoli are absent, and the

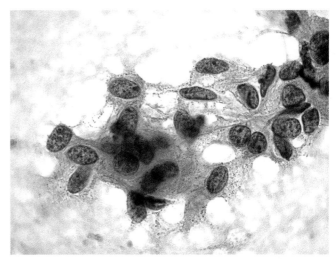

Fig. 4.8 Angiomyolipoma. Some cells are elongated. Hematoxylin and eosin stain, original magnification ×1000.

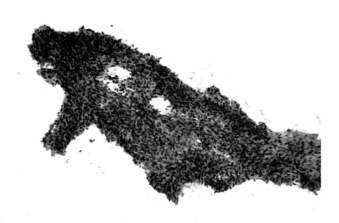

Fig. 4.6 Angiomyolipoma. Often all that is seen is a tight clump of atypical spindle cells that is hard to see through. Hematoxylin and eosin, original magnification ×200.

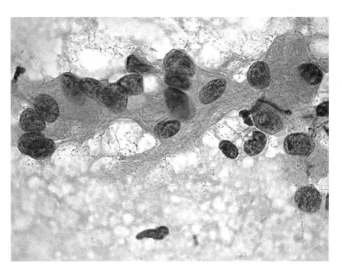

Fig. 4.9 Angiomyolipoma. Some cells are round, but the cytoplasm is still stringy rather than vacuolated. Hematoxylin and eosin stain, original magnification ×1000.

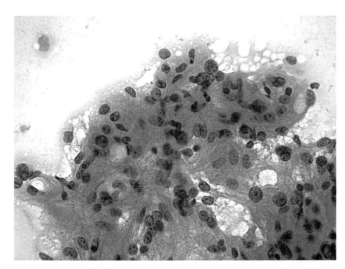

Fig. 4.7 Angiomyolipoma. On low power, there are cohesive clusters of epithelioid and spindle cells with abundant stringy cytoplasm. Hematoxylin and eosin stain, original magnification ×200.

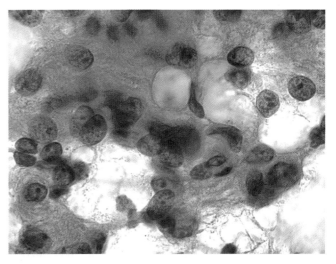

Fig. 4.10 Angiomyolipoma. Large vacuoles possibly representing fat are present, but the cytoplasm remains stringy or crystalline rather than vacuolated. Hematoxylin and eosin stain, original magnification ×1000.

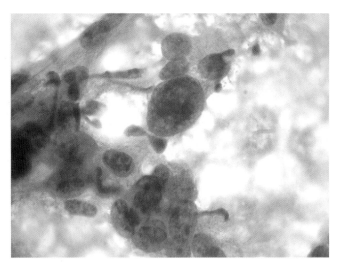

Fig. 4.11 Angiomyolipoma. The atypia consists most often of single markedly enlarged and round nuclei with dark hyperchromatic chromatin and no nucleolus. Hematoxylin and eosin stain, original magnification ×1000.

strikingly atypical cells tend to be surrounded by less atypical cells. However, the atypia in some angiomyolipomas can be both quite marked and varied, and virtually any pattern may be seen in such cases. Immunoreactivity for melanocyte markers can be extremely helpful whenever the diagnosis of a renal aspirate is not clear, especially when the aspirate appears to consist only of stromal elements.

Several lesions fall in the differential diagnosis. When atypical smooth muscle/perivascular cells are round, they can resemble clear cell RCC.[32,90,92] Often the nuclei will have more granular and dark chromatin and lack the prominent nucleoli of clear cell RCC. In addition, the quality of the cytoplasm is different, consisting of stringy or granular material with rare larger clear vacuoles, rather than the mixture of clear and granular material. Staining with epithelial membrane antigen (EMA), keratin, and melanocyte markers is advisable in any pleomorphic round cell aspirate. When the cells are elongated, the foremost differential diagnosis is sarcoma or sarcomatoid RCC.[93] Immunohistochemistry is the best way to distinguish these lesions.

Notably, aspirates and biopsies from angiomyolipoma are often scant and difficult to interpret, being composed of stroma and rare spindle-shaped cells that may resemble fibroblasts. Nevertheless, these difficult and otherwise nondiagnostic aspirates or biopsies often contain cells that stain with melanocyte markers, facilitating a definitive diagnosis. Thus it is prudent to obtain immunostains on any atypical or paucicellular spindle cell or epithelioid cell renal lesion.

Metanephric Adenoma

Metanephric adenoma is another benign lesion in which metastases have been reported (see Chapter 2 for additional discussion of the metastatic potential of metanephric adenoma).[94-98] It typically occurs in women in their fifth decade of life, and is composed of tubules and papillae forming "glomeruloid bodies" lined by uniformly bland cells with occasional psammoma bodies. The tumor is WT1+, EMA−, and has a normal karyotype, which can be helpful in distinguishing it from RCC. The cytologic features consist of small, short papillae and loose sheets of cells and individual cells that have been pulled out of the papillae, with scant cytoplasm, round nuclei, fine even chromatin, and rare small nucleoli.[99,100] The chromatin resembles that seen in papillary carcinoma of the thyroid.

The differential diagnosis includes Wilms tumor, low-grade papillary RCC, and metastatic malignancy. It may not be possible to distinguish metanephric adenoma from Wilms tumor (also WT1+, EMA variable) in which only the epithelial elements have been sampled, although it is helpful to remember that Wilms tumor is composed of larger cells with more hyperchromasia and mitoses.[95] Low-grade papillary RCC also has very similar features, but the tumor cells have more cytoplasm, are WT1−, and are uniformly EMA+.[75,95] Finally, like metanephric adenoma, metastases often have a very high nuclear/cytoplasmic (N/C) ratio, but metastases should never be diagnosed in the absence of a clinical history and are typically EMA+.

Cystic Nephroma/Mixed Epithelial and Stromal Tumor

Cystic nephroma/mixed epithelial and stromal tumor (MEST) is a benign cystic neoplasm that can mimic RCC radiographically and typically presents as an isolated mass. It is composed of stroma and small cysts lined by atypical epithelium.[79] FNAs are usually misdiagnosed as either RCC, angiomyolipoma, or sarcoma because they contain markedly atypical round cells or, less commonly, spindle cells.[41,101,102] The round cells are typically single and contain clear to vacuolated cytoplasm, nuclear membrane irregularity, and prominent nucleoli (Fig. 4.12).[103,104] The spindle cells are large, pleomorphic, and admixed with cells with intracytoplasmic vacuoles simulating fat.[105] Without a cell block or a core biopsy to show the characteristic arrangement of cysts and cellular stroma, most aspirates consisting of scant atypical round cells with clear cytoplasm cannot be reliably distinguished from clear cell RCC. Nevertheless, these specimens are almost always hypocellular and consist of single cells without large groups. Diagnosing these scant specimens as atypical or suspicious rather than positive for malignancy is the best way to avoid misdiagnosis.

Renal Abscess

Focal bacterial pyelonephritis and a renal abscess can appear mass-like radiologically.[6,106] Aspirates contain necrotic material, numerous neutrophils, and rare atypical cells that are easily confused with

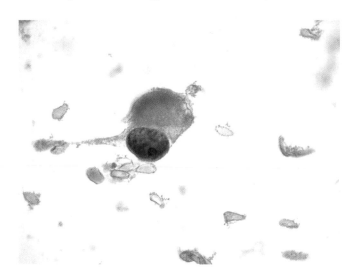

Fig. 4.12 Cystic nephroma/mixed epithelial and stromal tumor. Aspirates most often contain round cells with marked atypia that may not be distinguishable from renal cell carcinoma. Most aspirates, however, are scant. Hematoxylin and eosin stain, original magnification ×1000.

those of clear cell RCC. The atypical cells are few, however, and in the context of abundant acute inflammation should not be reported as positive for malignancy. Tuberculosis and malakoplakia have also been described in the kidney.[107,108]

Xanthogranulomatous Pyelonephritis

Xanthogranulomatous pyelonephritis is a reactive process that can present as a mass lesion that mimics RCC.[40] The lesion is composed of histiocytes and multinucleated giant cells. The histiocytes may be grouped and resemble clear cell RCC (Fig. 4.13), but in general the histiocytes have more "dirty" cytoplasm, have smaller microvesicles in their cytoplasm, lack nuclear atypia, and most often have a bean-shaped nucleus rather than the round nucleus typical of RCC. In addition, histiocytes are positive for CD68 and negative for keratin and EMA.

Renal Infarct

Rarely, renal infarcts may have a radiographic appearance suspicious for malignancy.[109] Specimens are hypocellular and composed of necrotic material that may contain rare atypical cells resembling those of clear cell RCC. As in other settings, scant specimens with rare atypical cells should not be diagnosed as malignant.

Renal Cysts

Renal cysts are common; 70% to 85% of all renal lesions are cysts, and 50% of men older than 50 years have at least one.[110,111] The majority of these are benign, acquired, and solitary; only 1% to 4% are cystic RCC, most often multilocular clear cell RCC, although conventional clear cell and papillary RCC also occur.[79,112-118] The prognosis of a patient with a cystic RCC is generally excellent, but metastases can occur in patients with clear cell RCC, and resection, either by partial or radical nephrectomy, is indicated.[119-121]

Aspirates of cystic renal masses are problematic because they have relatively low sensitivity. Indeed, in patients with cystic RCC, FNA is much more likely to yield a false-negative diagnosis than a true positive result.

Cysts are classified according to the Bosniak system.[122-127] Most lesions are category 1 (benign) and receive no further evaluation. Category 4 lesions are worrisome enough that they are usually resected. Categories 2 and 3 are indeterminate; 5% to 57% of indeterminate cysts are malignant, and these are the lesions that might be selected for FNA.

It is difficult to determine the exact sensitivity of FNA for Bosniak category 2 or 3 lesions. Most literature on FNA of cystic lesions predates computed tomography and magnetic resonance imaging, and includes a high preponderance of both category 1 and 4 lesions.[38,106,111,114,115,128-130] In general, 9% to 37% of FNAs of *all* RCCs, most of which are solid, are nondiagnostic.[32,34,38,41,49,131,132] Most RCCs interpreted as negative on FNA have a cystic component.[49] In addition, most radiographically suspicious cysts prove to be RCC.[32,34,41] In the largest series of cystic RCC (11 cases), only 2 cases had atypical cells on cytologic examination, and repeat aspirates in both patients were negative.[133]

Based on these data, the sensitivity of renal FNA for Bosniak category 2 or 3 lesions is likely no more than 10% to 20%. In patients for whom a positive or suspicious diagnosis can be rendered, renal FNA is of value, but this represents a minority of patients. Most patients with Bosniak category 2 or 3 lesions will have a negative aspirate. Because the risk for malignancy is 5% to 57% before the FNA, a negative result does not change the patient's pretest probability of malignancy.

How should these aspirates be interpreted? Some urologists aspirate benign Bosniak category 1 cysts for symptomatic relief. In this setting, one should take a very conservative approach, and any diagnosis other than benign/nondiagnostic would be extraordinary and demand clinical correlation concerning the imaging characteristics. For Bosniak category 2 or 3 cases, most often one sees proteinaceous debris and macrophages. These should be signed out as nondiagnostic. Occasionally a few small epithelial cells are identified with no significant atypia. Most of these are single cells or very small groups of large but bland cells (most often cyst lining cells [Fig. 4.14]), and can be signed out as negative with a note stating either that RCC cannot be ruled out or clinical correlation is necessary to ensure the sample is representative of any underlying lesion. In some cases, these rare epithelial cells will show either nuclear or cytoplasmic atypia (Fig. 4.15). Nuclear atypia consists of nuclear enlargement with or without prominent nucleoli or nuclear outline irregularity. Cytoplasmic atypia consists of any clearing of the cytoplasm, a finding that is distinctly uncommon in normal renal epithelial

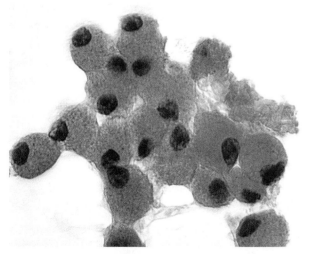

Fig. 4.13 Xanthogranulomatous pyelonephritis. When histiocytes cluster together they can resemble renal cell carcinoma. Hematoxylin and eosin stain, original magnification ×1000.

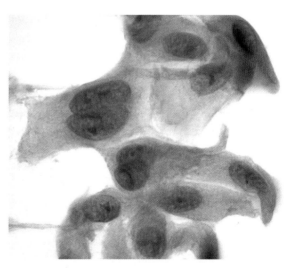

Fig. 4.14 Cyst lining cells, benign cyst. The cells are elongated and appear to be streaming. Hematoxylin and eosin stain, original magnification ×1000.

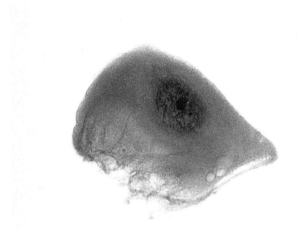

Fig. 4.15 Atypical cyst lining cells, benign cyst. The cell is single and has a prominent nucleolus. The cell could represent either renal cell carcinoma or cystic nephroma, and should be diagnosed as either atypical or suspicious. However, in comparison with both of those entities, the cytoplasm is harder, more opaque, and less vacuolated. Hematoxylin and eosin stain, original magnification ×1000.

cells, although it can be seen in atypical cyst lining cells. In either case the aspirate should be diagnosed as suspicious for malignancy, knowing that some of these will turn out to be reactive cyst lining cells, but this is all the atypia that is likely to be seen in a cystic RCC. Unless the case is very cellular, one should never diagnose these lesions as positive for malignancy.

Acquired Cystic Disease and Adult Polycystic Disease

Patients with acquired cystic disease secondary to renal failure often experience development of multiple cysts, and 9% have RCCs, which are often multifocal and papillary.[134-137] Similarly, patients with adult polycystic kidney disease, an autosomal dominant disease, are also at an increased risk for RCC, which is typically papillary and may be multifocal. In both settings, however, these patients routinely experience papillary hyperplasia within the cysts, and distinction between this hyperplasia and carcinoma is not always possible on FNA.[138] In contrast with most nonneoplastic cysts, cohesive groups of cells rather than single cells may be aspirated. Fortunately the underlying disease is almost always known in these patients, and the best response is simply to avoid aspiration. However, when faced with an aspirate from a patient with a disease that contains atypical cells, cellularity is the best diagnostic clue. Abundantly cellular aspirates should be diagnosed as positive; all other aspirates should be diagnosed as either atypical or suspicious.

Malignant Lesions

Renal Cell Carcinoma

The most common tumor of the kidney is RCC. These tumors have been graded in the past using the Fuhrman system, although the International Society of Urologic Pathology system is now recommended.[64,139] There is good cytologic and histologic correlation in Fuhrman grading, and one would expect the same with the International Society of Urologic Pathology system.[140-142] RCC is classified histologically according to the most recent World Health Organization (WHO) classification system.[76] Histologic typing of the common subtypes on aspiration material is well correlated with resection.[49,84] Data for more recently described and less common subtypes are limited and may be less reliable, because these subtypes are less commonly recognized on resection and may require both more extensive sampling and ancillary studies for accurate diagnosis.

Clear Cell Renal Cell Carcinoma

Clear cell or conventional RCC comprises 75% of all RCCs. Genetic analysis shows frequent deletions of chromosome 3p, the site of the *VHL* gene.[143-146] The cytology of these tumors can be divided into three overlapping patterns, depending on grade and whether the cells are easily spread out on the slide. In the first and classic pattern most often seen with higher-grade tumors, the aspirate is highly cellular, with large groups and isolated cells containing abundant cytoplasm, low N/C ratio, and centrally located round to slightly irregular nuclei with prominent nucleoli (Fig. 4.16).[38,40,56,147] The nuclei may be eccentric and are

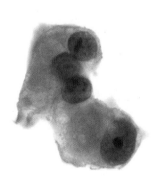

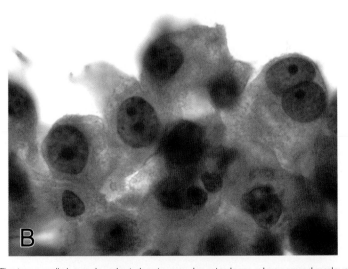

Fig. 4.16 Clear cell renal cell carcinoma, classic cytology, high-grade tumor. The tumor cells have abundant clear to granular cytoplasm, a large round nucleus that is eccentrically placed, and prominent nucleolus (A and B). Hematoxylin and eosin stain, original magnification ×1000.

occasionally so eccentrically placed that they appear to be partially extruded. The cytoplasm is translucent and vacuolated, and often the vacuoles are peripherally placed while the remaining cytoplasm is centrally placed. This combination of eccentric round nuclei with centrally placed cytoplasm mimics the cytology of plasma cells, and these cells have been described as plasmacytoid. Higher-grade tumors have more isolated cells and less cytoplasmic vacuolization. Occasionally clear cell tumors, usually high-grade ones, will have neutrophils within their cytoplasm. Such a finding is relatively specific for the clear cell subtype, although uncommon.

The second pattern is that seen in very low-grade tumors. In this setting the cells are quite bland and closely resemble normal distal tubular cells (Fig. 4.17). Generally the cells are in small flat sheets. The best way to distinguish these cells from normal cells is by the cellularity, although some low-grade tumors may not produce very

cellular aspirates. In a minority of low-grade clear cell tumors, a scant amount of intracytoplasmic hemosiderin will also be present; although helpful, this finding is more common in papillary tumors.[148] However, in general, these tumors are very difficult to diagnose on direct smears, but relatively easy to diagnose on cell block material.

The third pattern occurs in both low- and high-grade tumors. In this pattern the tumor cells are difficult to aspirate because the neoplastic cells are tightly adherent to the fibrous stroma. The aspirate consists of fragments of highly cellular fibrous tissue, and one must go to high power and diligently screen the edge of the tissue to identify the neoplastic cells lining the fibrous tissue (Fig. 4.18). The tumor cells are best identified based on their clear cytoplasm and location lining the fibrous stroma. As with the second pattern, although the direct smears of such cases are extremely difficult, cell

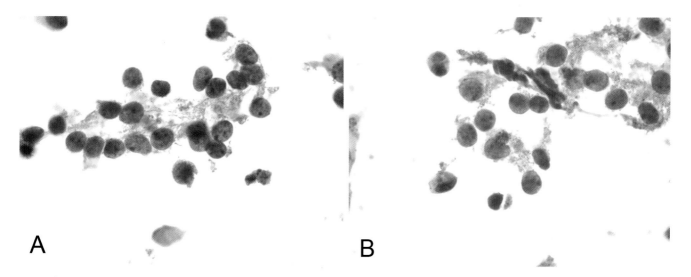

Fig. 4.17 Clear cell renal cell carcinoma, low grade. The cells are small with scant cytoplasm and minimal atypia. The cells resemble distal tubular cells (A). Some clear cell tumors have a scant amount of hemosiderin in a perinuclear location, which is quite characteristic (B). However, intracytoplasmic hemosiderin is much more common in papillary tumors. Abundant cellularity may be the best clue that this is a tumor rather than distal tubules. Hematoxylin and eosin stain, original magnification ×1000 (A and B).

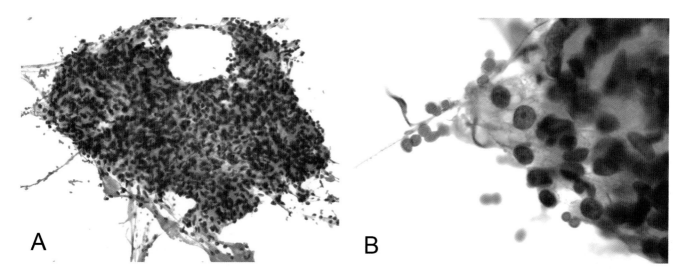

Fig. 4.18 Clear cell renal cell carcinoma. The cells are tightly cohesive and present as highly cellular chunks of tissue (A). In cases like this, diligent screening around the edge of the cluster can reveal identifiable neoplastic cells (B). Hematoxylin and eosin stain, original magnification ×1000.

blocks are much easier to interpret. In some cases an EMA stain can be helpful in distinguishing the tumor cells from macrophages.

The differential diagnosis includes benign tubular cells, macrophages, adrenal cortical cells, hepatocytes, cystic nephroma/MEST, cystic renal disease, and other types of RCC. Aspirates of tubular cells are typically scant and rarely contain large groups. The cells do not have vacuolated cytoplasm and do not contain hemosiderin. Macrophages rarely produce large groups of cells, do not have an extruded nucleus, are more uniformly microvacuolated, have "dirty cytoplasm," kidney bean-shaped rather than round nuclei, and lack atypia. Adrenal cortical cells are more uniform, have smaller vacuoles, and routinely have their cytoplasm stripped so one typically sees bare nuclei in a background of proteinaceous debris (Fig. 4.19). Hepatocytes are also more uniformly granular, may contain bile, and have round nuclei of various sizes that are almost always centrally placed (Fig. 4.20). Cystic nephroma/MEST may have individual cells that are virtually identical to clear cell RCC and may be markedly atypical. In general,

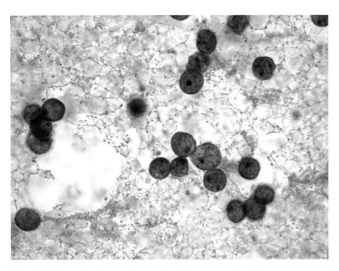

Fig. 4.19 Adrenal cortical cells consist of bare, round nuclei in a background of granular debris representing stripped cytoplasm. Hematoxylin and eosin stain, original magnification ×1000.

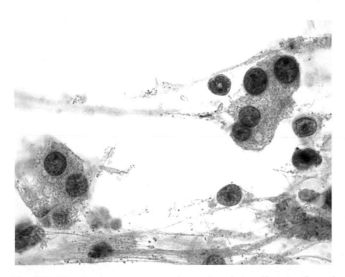

Fig. 4.20 Hepatocytes are common in renal aspirates. Hematoxylin and eosin stain, original magnification ×1000.

however, these aspirates are scant and should be diagnosed as atypical or suspicious rather than positive. Cystic renal disease, including acquired cystic disease and adult polycystic renal disease, can also have cells that are virtually identical to those seen in clear cell RCC, but the cellularity is also low.

Papillary Renal Cell Carcinoma

Papillary RCC is defined histologically as a tumor with at least 50% true papillae (although in some cases these may be so closely packed that they appear solid.[75] Papillary RCC represents between 7% and 15% of all RCCs.[75,149,150] This subtype of RCC is associated with trisomies of chromosomes 7, 16, and 17, renal cortical adenomas, and multifocality.[74,151-154] Larger papillary RCCs may be cystic and necrotic. Patients with low-grade/low-stage papillary RCC have an excellent prognosis, whereas those with high-grade/high-stage have a poor prognosis.[152,155] Papillary RCC is immunoreactive for EMA, low-molecular-weight keratins, and CK7 and negative for high-molecular-weight keratin 34βE12 and WT1.[75,156]

Like clear cell RCC, FNAs of papillary RCC exhibit several overlapping patterns. The most common pattern is seen in low-grade tumors.[157-160] These tumors can only be recognized by their architectural appearance because they lack virtually any cytologic atypia and the cells are identical to those of distal tubules with scant clear cytoplasm. Architecturally, papillae are often recognized at low power, but more commonly one sees spherules, tubules, or rosettes that lack fibrovascular cores (Fig. 4.21) or cellular swirls.[161,162] In the vast majority of such tumors, the lesional cells have clear cytoplasm, although infrequently the tumor cells of low-grade papillary tumors have abundant granular cytoplasm (Fig. 4.22).[163] Cytologically the cells are identical to those seen in oncocytoma, but the papillary architecture assists in making the correct diagnosis. More commonly, tumors with abundant granular cytoplasm are higher grade and have relatively prominent nucleoli (Fig. 4.23). In some of these tumors, there are true papillae with fibrovascular cores distended with macrophages. This feature is especially well appreciated on cell block material. In general the cells in tumors with this appearance have more granular cytoplasm and resemble proximal tubular cells more than distal tubular cells. In some cases, there is abundant intracytoplasmic hemosiderin, much more than that which is occasionally seen in FNAs of clear cell RCC. This is strongly suggestive of a papillary tumor. Psammoma bodies are rare but helpful when present. High-grade tumors tend to resemble high-grade clear cell tumors and have very large round nuclei, prominent nucleoli, and most often have relatively abundant granular cytoplasm.

The differential diagnosis includes renal cortical adenoma, distal tubular cells, proximal tubular cells, oncocytoma, other types of RCC, and cystic renal disease. Low-grade tumors can be distinguished from distal tubular cells by their increased cellularity and their architecture including papillae, spherules, rosettes, and swirls. Renal cortical adenomas are identical to papillary tumors but are <1.5 cm in diameter. Rare low-grade tumors are cytologically identical to oncocytoma, but the papillary architecture helps make the distinction. Most papillary tumors with abundant granular cytoplasm are high grade, and the large nuclear size and prominent nucleoli are the best distinguishing features. However, distinguishing these high-grade tumors from clear cell RCC can be extremely difficult, although reactivity for CK7 may be helpful.[49] Cystic renal disease, including acquired cystic disease and adult polycystic renal disease, can also have cells that are virtually identical to those seen in papillary RCC, but the cellularity is typically low.

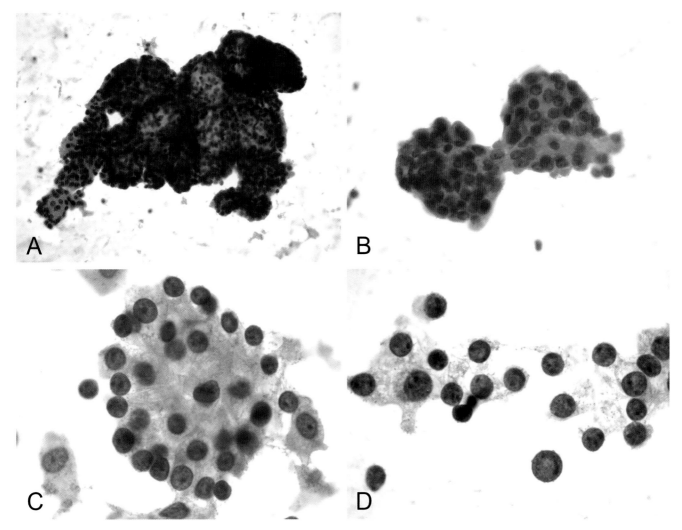

Fig. 4.21 Papillary renal cell carcinoma, low grade. Classic features include papillae (A), spherules (B), and rosettes (C). Cytologic atypia is minimal (D). Hematoxylin and eosin staining, original magnification ×200 (A); ×400 (B); ×1000 (C and D).

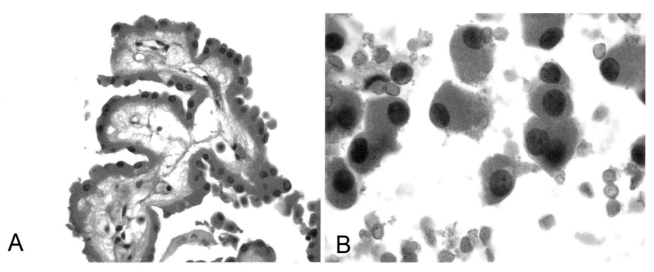

Fig. 4.22 Papillary renal cell carcinoma, low grade, with granular cytoplasm. Such tumors are rare. The papillae are diagnostic (A). See Chapter 2 for additional discussion of oncocytic low-grade variant of papillary renal cell carcinoma. If only individual cells are seen (B), the tumor cannot be distinguished from onco-cytoma. Hematoxylin and eosin stain, original magnification ×400 (A); ×1000 (B).

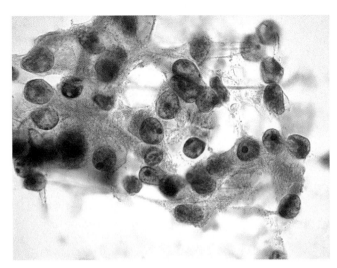

Fig. 4.23 Papillary renal cell carcinoma. Tumors with abundant granular cytoplasm are typically higher grade and may strongly resemble clear cell tumors. Hematoxylin and eosin stain, original magnification ×1000.

Chromophobe Renal Cell Carcinoma

Chromophobe RCC comprises 3% to 5% of all RCCs and is associated with numerous chromosomal monosomies.[153,164-169] Patients have an excellent prognosis.[169-172] The cytoplasm stains diffusely positive with Hale colloidal iron stain.[173]

Most aspirates are very cellular, consisting of tumor cell groups and isolated tumor cells that are generally less cohesive than the cells aspirated from clear cell RCC (Figs. 4.24 and 4.25).[174-177] The cells of chromophobe RCC may have a "koilocytic" appearance as a result of their cytoplasmic and nuclear features, resembling koilocytes seen in Pap smears. These consist of very large cells with prominent cell membranes and abundant fluffy cytoplasm, which is granular but not uniformly so. There may be perinuclear clearing of the cytoplasm. Binucleation is common. Although some nuclei can be very round and bland, in general the nuclei of chromophobe carcinoma have markedly irregular outlines, fine chromatin that can be either very light or dark and hyperchromatic, and marked size variation. Prominent nucleoli are uncommon. These nuclear features are distinctly different from those of most other RCCs. Eosinophilic variants have more granular cytoplasm, whereas typical variants have more clear cytoplasm. The cells stain diffusely positive in a cytoplasmic pattern with Hale colloidal iron stain.

The differential diagnosis depends on whether the tumor is a typical or eosinophilic variant. The typical variant resembles clear cell tumors, whereas the eosinophilic variant resembles oncocytoma. Unlike clear cell tumors, chromophobe RCC has more variation in cell and nuclear size, finer (and often darker) chromatin without nucleoli, and much more irregular nuclear outlines, including grooves. Clear cell tumors are CD117⁻, whereas chromophobe tumors are CD117⁺. In contrast with oncocytoma, chromophobe RCC has more nuclear size variation and nuclear outline irregularity, but some cases may be impossible to distinguish with cytology alone (Fig. 4.26). Diffuse cytoplasmic staining with Hale colloidal iron is diagnostic of chromophobe RCC, but oncocytoma can have significant cell membrane staining. Nevertheless, in the setting of diffuse Hale colloidal iron staining the diagnosis is relatively straightforward. Both tumors are CD117⁺. Chromophobe tumors are more often diffusely positive for both CK7 and CK20 than oncocytoma, but patchy staining is not uncommon in both tumors.

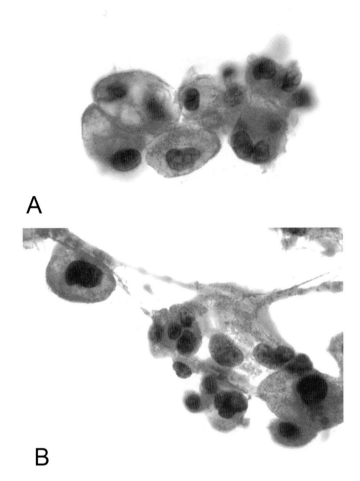

A

B

Fig. 4.24 Chromophobe renal cell carcinoma. Typical (A) and eosinophilic (B) variants. The cells have a "koilocytic" appearance with prominent cell membranes and central cytoplasmic clearing. Hematoxylin and eosin staining, original magnification ×1000.

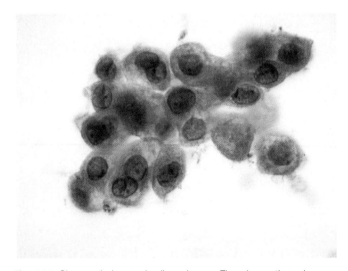

Fig. 4.25 Chromophobe renal cell carcinoma. Fine chromatin and numerous nuclear grooves. The koilocytic appearance is present in some cells. Hematoxylin and eosin stain, original magnification ×1000.

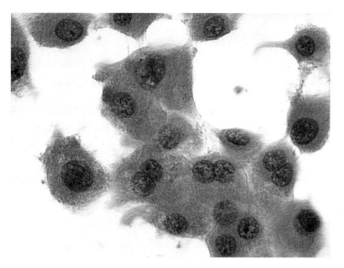

Fig. 4.26 Chromophobe renal cell carcinoma. Areas like this may be difficult to distinguish from oncocytoma. Hematoxylin and eosin stain, original magnification ×1000.

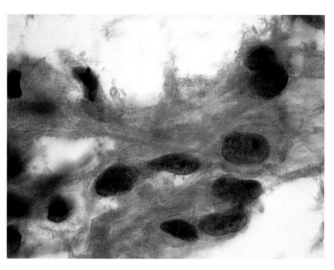

Fig. 4.28 Sarcomatoid renal cell carcinoma. Occasionally the spindle cells appear cohesive. Hematoxylin and eosin stain, original magnification ×1000.

Sarcomatoid Renal Cell Carcinoma

Sarcomatoid RCC comprises about 3% of all RCCs. Many of these tumors cannot be resected at presentation and are thus potential candidates for FNA.[178,179] Nevertheless, increasing numbers of these tumors are identified at lower stage because of advanced imaging methods, and these patients may have a better prognosis. The tumors, by definition, must have at least a small component of spindle cells (Figs. 4.27 and 4.28).[147,180] The tumor may also have an identifiable epithelioid cell component. If this is lacking, then the tumor must be keratin- or EMA-positive to confirm this diagnosis.

The cytologic diagnosis and the differential diagnosis are strongly dependent on sampling. Most aspirates are highly cellular and easily diagnosed as a high-grade tumor. To make the diagnosis of sarcomatoid RCC, a spindle cell component must be identified, although this component is often less spindled on cytology than it is in histology. If only the spindle cell area is sampled, sarcoma or angiomyolipoma would be the most common alternative diagnoses. If only the epithelioid area is sampled, clear cell RCC would be the most likely alternative diagnosis. Immunohistochemical evaluation is generally necessary to confirm this diagnosis.

Collecting Duct Carcinoma

This is a rare tumor that is poorly defined, but characterized by a medullary location, tubulopapillary histology, high-grade cytology, and prominent desmoplasia.[181-192] It may be confused with other tumors, especially renal medullary carcinoma and papillary RCC.[183,186,188,193-195] Characteristically, it is immunoreactive for high-molecular-weight cytokeratin 34βE12.[181,187]

Although there are numerous case reports of the cytology of this tumor, given the uncertainty of the diagnostic criteria, it is not clear whether the histologic diagnosis in many of these cases is correct. Nevertheless, the features most commonly described include large hyperchromatic nuclei and scant cytoplasm, which resemble metastatic cancer.[196-200] The differential includes metastatic disease, urothelial carcinoma, and RCC, not otherwise specified.

Translocation-Associated Renal Cell Carcinomas [TFE3-Associated Tumors, Including the MiT Family, Xp11, and t[6,11]]

Translocation-associated RCC was described in 1999 as a distinct histologic lesion that occurs primarily in children.[201] Subsequent genetic studies confirmed the histologic features, identified cases in adults, and showed a strong association with translocations on chromosome X involving the *TFE3* gene.[202,203] Several distinct cytogenetic rearrangements have since been described, and an association with different histologic and clinical features has been proposed. Histologically the tumor most commonly has a mixed nested and papillary architecture made up of cells with abundant voluminous cytoplasm and frequent calcifications; however, as more genetic variants are recognized, the spectrum of histologic features has expanded.[201] The diagnosis is confirmed by demonstrating immunoreactivity for TFE3 and relatively scant staining for EMA and keratin. Cytologic preparations reveal cells with abundant clear and granular cytoplasm, and most cases will resemble clear cell or, less likely, papillary RCC.[204-206] A strong clinical suspicion (young patient) and immunocytochemistry (lack or only focal reactivity for EMA and keratin, and subsequent confirmation with TFE3) or molecular studies are necessary to diagnose this tumor on cytology.

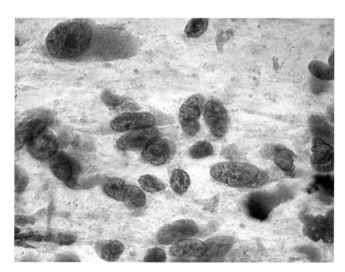

Fig. 4.27 Sarcomatoid renal cell carcinoma. Most often, isolated spindle cells are mixed with rounder cells. Hematoxylin and eosin stain, original magnification ×1000.

Mucinous Tubular and Spindle Cell Carcinoma

Mucinous tubular and spindle cell carcinoma is a rare tumor that thus far has had an excellent prognosis.[207] Tumors are composed of a mixture of tubular and spindle cells, often in a mucoid matrix. Tumor cells are reactive for EMA, α-methylacyl-coenzyme A racemase, and CK7.[208] Chromosomal losses have been reported.[208] Cytologically, aspirates consist of aggregates of relatively uniform oval to spindle cells with abundant myxoid matrix.[208-210] The myxoid matrix is relatively unique to this tumor, although it may be seen in metastatic cancer such as adenoid cystic carcinoma. In the absence of this matrix the tumor may be confused with a low-grade clear cell or papillary RCC, or a sarcomatoid RCC. Papillary RCC is also CK7+ but typically displays spherules, rosettes, or swirls. Sarcomatoid RCC is typically higher grade.

Clear Cell Papillary Renal Cell Carcinoma

Clear cell papillary RCC is an uncommon subtype of RCC that has features of both clear cell and papillary RCC but has an extremely indolent course. Although the cytologic features (including papillae, some with vascular cores, columnar cells, and fine chromatin) of the tumors have been described, the distinction from other subtypes of RCC relies on its characteristic immunohistochemical pattern (CD117− and CK7+ and carbonic anhydrase IX-positive).[211]

Other Subtypes of Renal Cell Carcinoma

A wide variety of additional less common subtypes of RCC have been accepted in the most recent WHO classification but have not been described on cytologic material.[76] A partial list of these include ALK-translocation RCC, succinate dehydrogenase B deficiency–associated RCC, and hereditary leiomyoma and RCC syndrome. Many of these tumors require thorough sampling and additional ancillary studies, including both immunocytochemistry and molecular analysis, for diagnosis. Although most of these tumors likely can be identified as RCC on adequate cytologic material, whether these rare subtypes can be routinely identified in cytologic specimens is not yet known.

Metastases

Metastases to the kidney are present in 7% of all cancer patients at autopsy, but most are clinically silent.[212] It is extremely uncommon for a metastasis to the kidney to be the initial manifestation of malignancy. Most "metastases" without a known primary probably represent unusual primary renal tumor.[213]

The lung is the most common primary site, although metastases can arise from any site (Fig. 4.29). Many cases have dark nuclei and irregular nuclear outlines, but some metastatic lung cancers have abundant clear cytoplasm and prominent nucleoli, and thus mimic high-grade clear cell RCC.[34,38,49,214-216] Knowledge of the clinical history and judicious application of immunocytochemistry is necessary to diagnose a metastatic cancer. Adenocarcinoma of the lung is often positive for TTF1 and Napsin A, whereas squamous cell carcinoma is positive for p40 and p63. All of these markers are negative in RCC. The distinction from typical variants of RCC is usually not difficult, particularly with immunocytochemistry, because RCC is often positive for CD10, PAX2, and PAX8. A variety of rare primary renal tumors, however, including collecting duct carcinoma, mucin-positive RCC, small cell carcinoma of the kidney, and primary lymphoma of the kidney, are impossible to distinguish from metastatic tumor by cytomorphology alone.[217-220] In addition, primary urothelial carcinoma should also be distinguished from metastatic cancer.

Urothelial Carcinoma

Urothelial carcinoma that arises in the renal collecting system is treated differently (nephroureterectomy) than RCC (nephrectomy), making its distinction important on cytology specimens.

Cytologically, low- and high-grade urothelial tumors have different appearances.[34,36,38,221] Low-grade tumors are characteristically composed of sheets and papillae of cells with moderate amounts of opaque cytoplasm without vacuolization, containing large hyperchromatic nuclei with granular chromatin. In some cases, cells with long cytoplasmic tails that narrow in the middle and then widen at the end and become flattened are present (Fig. 4.30). These cells, termed *cercariform cells*, are characteristic of urothelial carcinoma, and when present in large numbers can

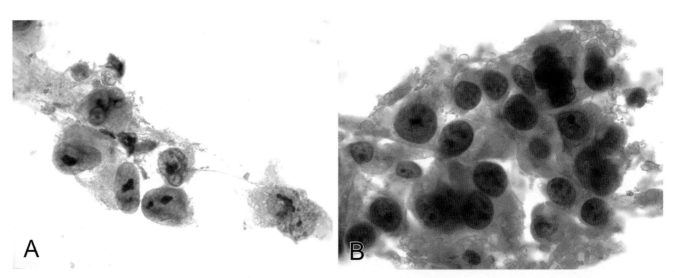

Fig. 4.29 Metastases. Most metastases have relatively high N/C ratios and granular chromatin. These two examples from lung (A) and melanoma (B) could easily be confused with a primary renal cell carcinoma. History and immunohistochemistry are essential. Hematoxylin and eosin stain, original magnification ×1000.

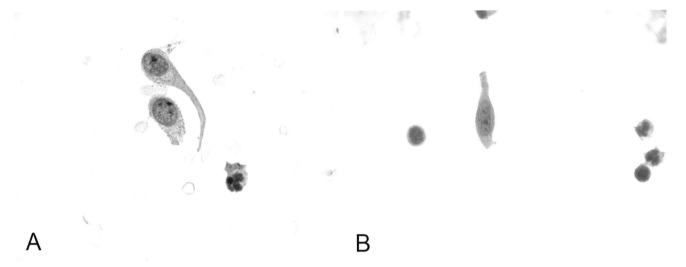

Fig. 4.30 Urothelial carcinoma. These cercariform cells have a long, flat tail that is highly characteristic of urothelial carcinoma. Hematoxylin and eosin stain, original magnification ×1000 (A and B).

be helpful in distinguishing this tumor from renal cortical neoplasms.[222-224]

Typically, high-grade tumors present as isolated cells and small clusters with scant cytoplasm that may contain vacuoles, high N/C ratios, dense hyperchromatic chromatin, and irregular nuclei (Fig. 4.31). Cercariform cells may also be present. These cases are usually easy to distinguish from RCC. In difficult cases, immunohistochemical studies can be helpful, because urothelial carcinomas are usually positive for GATA3 and negative for PAX8, an immunoprofile not characteristic of renal cell neoplasms. Distinction between urothelial tumor and metastatic cancer can be very difficult on cytology alone, but consideration of clinical history, judicious use of immunohistochemistry, and identification of cercariform cells may be of value in making the distinction.

Other Rare Tumors

The cytology of a variety of less common tumors has also been described in the literature. These tumors include low-grade myxoid renal epithelial neoplasm, primitive neuroectodermal tumor, synovial sarcoma, solitary fibrous tumor, mesoblastic nephroma in an adult, low-grade fibromyxoid sarcoma, acute leukemia, renal lymphoma, renal medullary carcinoma, Wilms tumor in adults, neuroblastoma, desmoplastic small round cell tumor, angiosarcoma, and intravascular papillary endothelial hyperplasia.[225-242]

Future Trends

Fine Needle Aspiration in Pediatric Patients

Until recently, FNAs of tumors in children were uncommon, because the most common tumor in this age group (Wilms tumor) was upstaged by the aspiration itself. Currently, aspiration no longer automatically upstages a tumor, and aspirates in this group of patients are becoming more common. Accuracy rates as high as 90% have been described.[243,244] Nevertheless, aspirates in these patients can be quite challenging.[9] Although Wilms tumor is the most common tumor, there are several other tumors, including metanephric adenoma, which can mimic the epithelial component, and cellular mesoblastic nephroma, which can mimic the stromal component of Wilms tumor.[245-247] In addition, tumors such as clear cell sarcoma of the kidney and rhabdoid tumor have protean histologic and cytologic appearances.[248-251] For example, clear cell sarcoma of the kidney has myxoid, sclerosing, cellular, epithelioid, spindled, and palisading histologic appearances, only some of which have been described in cytologic preparations.[8,79,246,248,249] Rhabdoid tumor can present as single cells or groups of cells that can be spindled, round, rhabdoid, or epithelioid.[250,251] Both clear cell sarcoma and rhabdoid tumor of the kidney have been misdiagnosed in large series of pediatric renal FNAs, and awareness of the variety of appearances of these tumors is the best defense against misdiagnosis.[244] Other uncommon neoplasms that are sometimes aspirated in children include Ewing sarcoma/PNET, adrenocortical carcinoma, extramedullary hematopoiesis, synovial sarcoma, rhabdomyosarcoma, and neuroblastoma.[226-228,230,239,252-255] Immunohistochemistry and genetic studies are often of value in this setting.

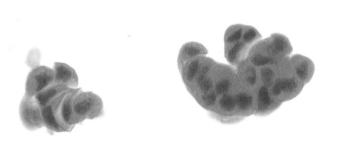

Fig. 4.31 Urothelial carcinoma, high grade. The hyperchromatic and markedly angulated nuclei are easily distinguished from renal cell carcinoma. A metastasis may be difficult to rule out. Hematoxylin and eosin stain, original magnification ×1000.

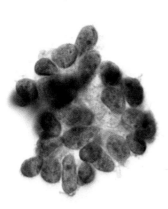

Fig. 4.32 Wilms tumor, epithelial type. A rosette is shown. The cytology of the cells is like that of metanephric adenoma with scant cytoplasm and fine even chromatin. Hematoxylin and eosin stain, original magnification ×1000.

The cytology of Wilms tumor has been well described (Fig. 4.32).[10,243] Most of these aspirates contain either biphasic or triphasic components, facilitating the diagnosis. Atypia (anaplasia) can be diagnosed on aspirate material as well. However, some triphasic tumors show only blastema on aspiration because of sampling error. These aspirates can be difficult to distinguish from other round cell tumors of childhood that rarely present in the kidney. Immunohistochemistry and genetic studies can be of help in some cases. Aspirates that are predominantly epithelial may be difficult to distinguish from metanephric adenoma.[246,256]

Renal Mass Ablation

Since the 1990's, radiologists have used a variety of methods, including chemicals, heat, and radiofrequency, to destroy renal masses in situ without resection.[257] The procedure has been shown to be safe, and many of these patients remain disease free after the procedure. However, recurrences do occur, particularly after ablation of larger lesions.[258] Renal FNA with immediate assessment has been shown to be an accurate method of diagnosing these lesions.[259] Unfortunately, many patients who undergo the procedure do not have material taken for pathologic diagnosis. The lack of pathologic material is a hindrance in the event of tumor recurrence or metastasis. Although immediate evaluation of cytology before ablation is not always necessary, cytologists should continue to encourage radiologists to at least attempt to obtain some material from the lesion for diagnosis to facilitate subsequent therapy in the event of an adverse outcome.

Conclusions

FNA of renal lesions can be helpful in the appropriate clinical setting. Routine diagnosis of metastatic cancer, primary RCC, and a wide variety of benign and malignant lesions is possible. The diagnosis of oncocytoma and many of the less common subtypes of RCC remains a challenge that often requires both adequate sampling and additional ancillary studies. The development of adjuvant therapies for RCC, some of which may be type specific, is likely to make cytologic diagnosis more common, more useful, and more challenging.

References are available at expertconsult.com

5
Nonneoplastic Disorders of the Urinary Bladder

ANTONIO LOPEZ-BELTRAN AND ROBERT H. YOUNG

CHAPTER OUTLINE

Embryology and Anatomy

Embryology

The common excretory ducts (the dilated segments of the mesonephric ducts distal to the ureteral buds) become absorbed into the urogenital sinus after the fourth week of gestation. Their epithelium merges toward the midline and forms a triangular patch that will become the trigone of the urinary bladder. The ends of the developing ureters implant there. The anterior abdominal wall closes with the caudal migration of the cloacal membrane, and during this process mesenchyme is induced to form the anterior wall of the bladder. During the seventh week of gestation, the urorectal septum of the cloaca fuses with the proctodeum, separating the rectum from the parts of the urogenital sinus that will form the dome and posterior wall of the bladder. Thus most of the bladder is derived from the rostral part of the urogenital sinus.[1]

In early embryogenesis the allantois projects outward from the yolk sac into the body stalk, which later forms the umbilical cord. The allantois originates from the part of the yolk sac that gives rise to the cloaca. As the urinary bladder forms, the allantois remains connected to its apex. The urachus (from the Greek o' o'υραχυς, plural urachi) is the intraabdominal structure that connects the apex of the bladder to the umbilicus and contains the allantois. The urachus grows with the embryo to maintain its bridge between the dome of the bladder and the body stalk. By the sixth month of gestation, the urachus has become a cordlike structure little more than 1 mm in diameter between the umbilicus and the dome of the bladder. At birth the dome of the bladder is near the umbilicus, the urachus is 2 to 3 mm long, the adjacent umbilical arteries are 5 to 7 mm in diameter, and the umbilical vein is 10 mm in diameter. Superiorly the urachus usually divides into three bands of fibrous tissue. The middle band passes through the abdominal wall into the umbilical cord, where it disperses into fine strands. The other two bands attach to the adventitia of the umbilical arteries.

Gross Anatomy

The bladder is located within the pelvis minor, beneath the peritoneum. When it fills, it expands into the abdomen and may reach the level of the umbilicus. In children younger than 6 years, the empty bladder is partially in the abdomen. Between age 6 years and puberty, the bladder descends to its adult position. At the bladder neck, the bladder is fixed in place by the pubovesical ligaments in the female and the puboprostatic ligaments in the male. The rest of the bladder is loosely contained by the pelvic fat and fibrous tissue and is free to expand as the need arises. The empty bladder has roughly the shape of an inverted pyramid. The superior surface, the dome, is covered by peritoneum. The most anterior and superior point, the apex, is the usual point of insertion of the median umbilical ligament and the urachus. The posterior surface faces posteriorly and inferiorly, forming the base of the bladder. Between it and the rectum are the uterine cervix and the superior end of the vagina in females, and the lower vasa deferentia and seminal vesicles in the male. On either side the lateral surfaces are in contact with the fascia of the levator ani muscles.

The trigone lies at the base of the bladder and borders the posterior side of the bladder neck.[2] At the lateral points of the trigone the ureters empty into the bladder cavity through the ureteral orifices.[3] The muscle of the trigone is derived from the detrusor muscle of the bladder and the muscle of the ureters.[4] Within the wall of the bladder the ureters are surrounded by sheaths of muscle and fibrous tissue known as Waldeyer sheath.[5] The ureters pass obliquely through the wall of the bladder in such a way that when the bladder fills, the pressure compresses and closes the ureters, preventing reflux.[6,7] The region where the walls of the bladder converge and connect with the urethra is the neck of the bladder.[8] In this area muscle fibers from the detrusor muscle, the muscle of the trigone, and the muscle of the urethra merge.[4] The internal sphincter is in the bladder neck and consists principally of fibers from the detrusor muscle.[9]

The urachus lies in the space of Retzius anterior to the peritoneum and surrounded anteriorly and posteriorly by the umbilicovesical fascia. On either side of it lie the umbilical arteries, which are enveloped in the umbilicovesical fascia. Caudally the layers of the umbilicovesical fascia spread over the dome of the bladder. This space is pyramidal and separated from the peritoneum and other structures by fascial planes. After birth the apex of the bladder

descends and draws the urachus with it, bringing along the obliterated umbilical arteries. Within the umbilical fascial tunnel, the adventitia of the umbilical arteries is teased out into fibrous strands, referred to as the *plexus of Luschka.*

Hammond et al. recognized four anatomic variants of the urachus (Fig. 5.1).[10] Type I consists of a well-formed urachus that extends from the bladder to the umbilicus, distinct from the umbilical arteries. In type II the urachus is joined with one of the umbilical arteries, and these continue jointly to the umbilicus. In type III the urachus and both umbilical arteries join and continue to the umbilicus as the ligamentum commune. Type IV consists of a short tubular urachus that terminates before fusing with either of the umbilical arteries. Hammond et al. found urachi of type I urachus in almost 33% of adults, type II in 20%, type III in 20%, and type IV in 25%.[10] Blichert-Toft et al. found a different distribution of the types in a study of 81 specimens: 9% type I, 12% type II, 25% type III, and 54% type IV.[11] In adults the urachus outside the bladder wall is usually 5 to 5.5 cm long and at its junction with the bladder is 4 to 8 mm broad, tapering to approximately 2 mm at the umbilical end. Pathologically and clinically, it is convenient to divide the urachus into supravesical, intramuscular, and intramucosal segments (Fig. 5.2).

The urinary bladder is supplied by two pairs of vessels, the superior and inferior vesical arteries, branches from the internal iliac arteries.[12,13] The lymphatics of the anterior and posterior bladder walls drain through the internal and middle chains of the external iliac lymph nodes, and those of the trigone drain to both the external iliac nodes and the hypogastric nodes.[14]

Histology

The bladder is lined by a specialized epithelium variously referred to as *urothelium* for its adaptation to the urinary environment or

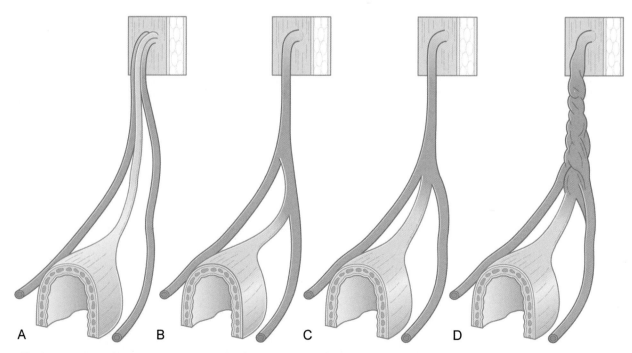

Fig. 5.1 The four common variants of urachal anatomy. Type I: the urachus extends to the umbilicus (fetal type). Type II: the urachus joins one of the umbilical arteries. Type III: the urachus and umbilical arteries merge and continue to the umbilicus. Type IV: the urachus and umbilical arteries form a complex of fine strands, the plexus of Luschka.

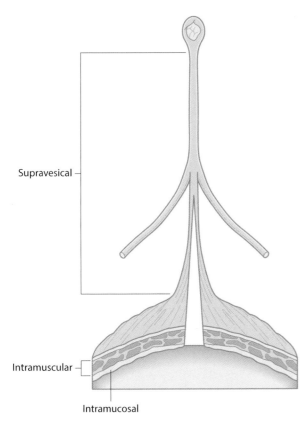

Fig. 5.2 The urachus is composed of intramucosal, intramuscular, and supravesical segments.

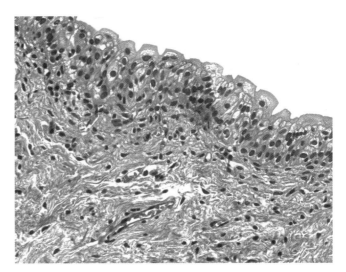

Fig. 5.3 Umbrella cells have voluminous cytoplasm and large nuclei with inconspicuous nucleoli.

transitional cells after the anal transition zone, a vestige of the cloaca, or because of its morphology, which early microscopists perceived as transitional between squamous and glandular. The designation *urothelium* is preferred here for its reflection of the function of these cells. The urothelial lining of the human urinary tract is composed of three to six layers of cells. The apparent number of layers varies with the degree of distention or stretching at the time of fixation. There are two subtypes of urothelial cells: the umbrella cells, which cover the surface and are in direct contact with urine, and the underlying cells, which comprise the other layers.

The umbrella cells (also referred to as superficial cells) are the largest cells of the urothelium (Fig. 5.3) and have eosinophilic cytoplasm, which may contain small amounts of mucin. Their nuclei are large and often somewhat irregular with condensed hyperchromatic chromatin and inconspicuous nucleoli. Superficial (umbrella) cells are frequently binucleated and occasionally multinucleated. Ultrastructurally, umbrella cells have asymmetric cell membranes with a thick outer layer, an irregular angular surface resulting from insertion of stiff segments of membrane, and a variety of intercellular connections.[15,16] These specializations enable the umbrella cells to cope with the rigors of the urinary environment and maintain the blood–urine barrier as the bladder expands and contracts.[15] Superficial umbrella cells express uroplakins, GATA3, and CK20 on immunohistochemistry (Fig. 5.4).[17]

The urothelial cells of the other layers are smaller and more uniform than the umbrella cells, with pale cytoplasm.[18] The nuclei are central, predominantly oval, and, in the deeper layers, oriented perpendicular to the basement membrane.[19] Often there is a noticeable nuclear groove. The chromatin is very fine and evenly dispersed, and nucleoli are small and inconspicuous. Mitotic figures are uncommon, and DNA replication studies reveal that the urothelium is renewed approximately once a year. The epithelial cells of the basal layer express BCL2, whereas the intermediate cells express RB1 and PTEN at varying intensities. The basal layer of urothelium rests on a basement membrane, which can be highlighted with immunohistochemistry for laminin and type IV collagen. Beneath the basement membrane is the lamina propria, a zone of loose connective tissue that contains delicate vessels and thin, delicate bundles of smooth muscle fibers referred to as the

Fig. 5.4 Umbrella cells with characteristic immunohistochemical expression of CK20.

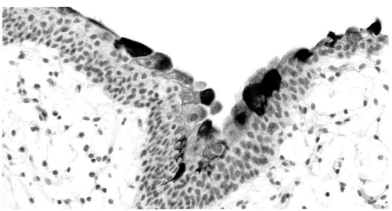

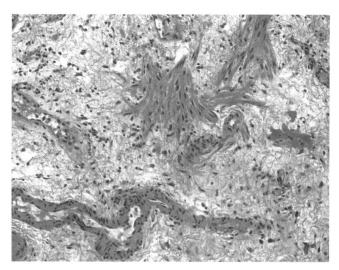

Fig. 5.5 Smooth muscle in lamina propria is arranged in small irregular bundles.

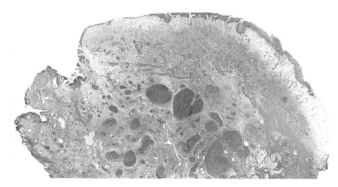

Fig. 5.6 Bladder wall seen after transurethral resection. Beneath the epithelium, there is edematous lamina propria with muscularis mucosae. The connective tissue beneath the muscularis mucosae contains an arcade of larger vessels.

muscularis mucosae (Fig. 5.5). The muscularis mucosae of the bladder is variable, ranging from an essentially complete layer, analogous to that seen in the colon, to a sparse and incomplete array of smooth muscle fibers.[20-24] In the bladder dome and trigone, the muscularis mucosae may become hypertrophic/hyperplastic, resulting in compact bundles of smooth muscle separated by stroma. In cases of bladder outlet obstruction (prostatic hyperplasia) the muscularis mucosae may become hyperplastic (compensatory hyperplasia) and disorganized with fibers splayed in different directions. The connective tissue beneath the muscularis mucosae contains an arcade of larger vessels (Fig. 5.6). The lamina propria is usually thinner in the bladder neck and trigone. Beneath this is the *muscularis propria*, composed of large bundles of muscle fibers with a scant amount of loose connective tissue. The arrangement of muscle bundles varies in pattern and thickness at different locations in the bladder. Distinct layers, analogous to those of the bowel, are seen only in the area of the internal sphincter. In the bladder neck and superior urethral regions the muscle bundles are more uniform and densely packed than seen elsewhere. In the trigone the muscularis propria is located very superficially. Also, the interface between the muscularis propria and the perivesical soft tissue is often irregular, a finding that may cause difficulties in assessing microscopic invasion for staging purposes.[25] A number of immunohistochemical stains have been applied in an attempt to differentiate muscularis mucosae from muscularis propria. Smoothelin, desmin, and vimentin have been reported to be differentially expressed in both. However, contradictory reports with overlapping results are on record. None is currently recommended in practice.[26] Normal adipose tissue is present within the lamina propria and through all layers in the bladder wall.

Histologically, urachal remnants typically consist of a central lumen lined by epithelium and surrounded by a narrow zone of dense connective tissue, then bundles of smooth muscle fibers, and finally a connective tissue adventitia (Fig. 5.7).[27] Such tubular remnants are present in about 33% of adults.[28] Schubert et al. classified intramural urachal remnants into three groups, ranging from simple tubular structures to more complex canals (Figs. 5.8 and 5.9).[28]

The mucosal segment of the urachus may consist of a papilla, a small opening flush with the surface, a wide diverticular opening, or may be absent (Figs. 5.10 and 5.11). Hammond et al. found a mucosal opening in 10% of specimens.[10] Blichert-Toft et al. found that the epithelial component was present in more than 50% of supravesical segments of the type I variant but was often absent or limited to the segment immediately above the bladder in type IV.[11] Urothelium is the most common lining, present in more than 66% of intramural remnants.[28] The remaining intramural remnants are lined by columnar cells that occasionally may be mucus-secreting.[29] Rarely, remnants are lined by flattened epithelium, and some cases may not show covering epithelium.

Fig. 5.7 The structure of the urachus in cross section.

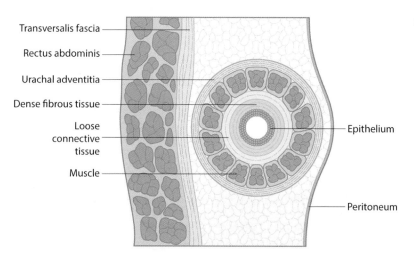

Transversalis fascia

Rectus abdominis

Urachal adventitia

Dense fibrous tissue

Loose connective tissue

Muscle

Epithelium

Peritoneum

Fig. 5.8 Variation in the course and structure of the urachus. Type I is a simple canal with a smooth course. Type II has saccular dilations. Type III is more complex with dilations, outpouchings, and an irregular course.

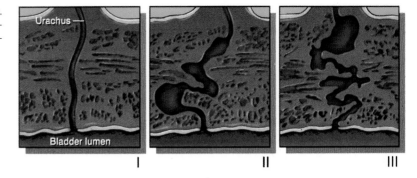

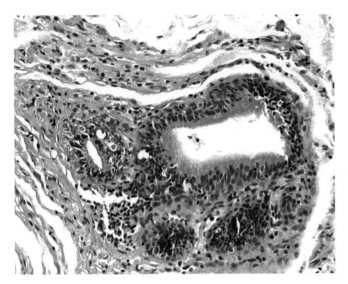

Fig. 5.9 A complex of urachal channels with focal dilation in the supravesical segment.

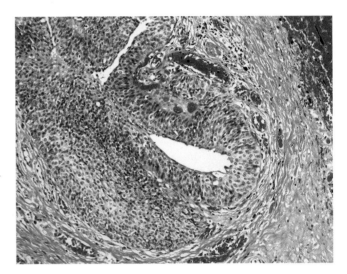

Fig. 5.11 Type A intramucosal urachus ending in a papilla.

Fig. 5.10 The intramucosal urachus varies from (A) lumen terminating in a papilla, (B) a patent lumen smoothly continuous with bladder mucosa, (C) smooth bladder mucosa closing the urachal lumen, (D) to dimpled bladder mucosa covering the urachal lumen.

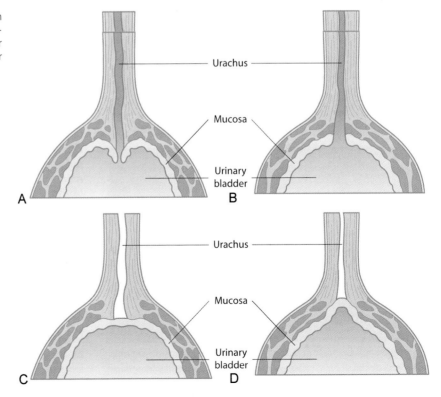

Epithelial Abnormalities

von Brunn Nests

Well-circumscribed nests of urothelial cells in the lamina propria, von Brunn nests, arise by a process of budding from the overlying epithelium or by migration and may or may not be attached to the epithelium.[30-36] Autopsy studies reveal von Brunn nests in 85% to 95% of bladders, most commonly in the trigone.[31,33,34,37] Previously some considered these nests to be related to inflammation or a precursor of carcinoma, but neither view is currently accepted. Today they are viewed as normal features of the bladder mucosa.

Histologically, von Brunn nests are rounded, well-circumscribed groups of urothelial cells in the lamina propria, usually close to the urothelium but occasionally appreciably deep (Fig. 5.12). Central lumina are often present within florid von Brunn nests, sometimes with cystic dilatation. Their regular shape and orderly spatial arrangement contrast with the features of rare carcinomas with a nested pattern that are occasionally confused with von Brunn nests. In contrast, small, crowded nests with variable spacing and an infiltrative base characterize the nested variant of urothelial carcinoma.[35,38-40] The nuclei of the cells in von Brunn nests lack significant atypia. Reactive and metaplastic changes in the surface urothelium may also occur in von Brunn nests. Urothelial carcinoma in situ may extend into von Brunn nests and should not be mistaken for invasion of the lamina propria. When von Brunn nests are numerous, closely packed, and hyperplastic, the distinction from inverted papilloma may be difficult and arbitrary. Rarely, florid epithelial proliferations may occur in cases of von Brunn nests, like those seen in the setting of radiation or chemotherapy (see later discussion).

Cystitis Glandularis and Intestinal Metaplasia

The existence of the typical and mucinous forms of cystitis glandularis have been recognized for many years, leading, however, to somewhat confusing terminology. The more common form can be referred to as *typical* or *conventional type* of cystitis glandularis, and the second form as the *intestinal type*.[41] Cystitis glandularis of intestinal type is currently designated *intestinal metaplasia*.[42-55] Molecular and immunohistochemical evidence of divergent pathways of histogenesis for these two metaplastic processes have been reported.[56,57] Although the two lesions may coexist, one may predominate or be present exclusively.

Cystitis Glandularis and Cystitis Cystica

The term *cystitis glandularis* refers to a lesion that evolves from and merges imperceptibly with von Brunn nests.[35,41,42,58-65] Cystitis glandularis is so common that it may be considered a normal feature of the vesical mucosa. Autopsy studies reveal its presence in up to 71% of bladders, most commonly in the trigone.[37] Most foci of cystitis glandularis are microscopic. However, it occasionally forms irregular, rounded, or nodular elevations of the mucosa.[66] Exceptionally it forms larger polypoid lesions that may be mistaken for a neoplasm before microscopic examination.[67-70] Microscopically, cystitis glandularis is composed of glands in the lamina propria that are lined by cuboidal to columnar cells surrounded by one or more layers of urothelial cells (Fig. 5.13). Similar epithelium may also be present on the mucosal surface. The glands of cystitis glandularis may be dilated. Although the lining cells are sometimes characterized as mucinous, they usually do not appear overtly mucinous in sections stained with hematoxylin and eosin, and mucin stains are often negative or weakly positive.[41] Cystitis cystica consists of von Brunn nests in which the central cells have degenerated to form small cystic cavities.[14,33,71-74] Albeit somewhat less common than von Brunn nests and cystitis glandularis, cystitis cystica is present in up to 60% of bladders.[34] It is most common in adults but also occurs in children. At cystoscopy, its cystic nature is usually apparent.[73] Grossly, the lesions appear as translucent, submucosal cysts that are pearly-white to yellow-brown (Fig. 5.14).[66] Most are less than 5 mm in diameter, but rare examples measuring a few centimeters in diameter have been reported.[72] The cysts contain clear yellow fluid. Microscopically, the cysts are lined by urothelium or cuboidal epithelium (Fig. 5.15) and filled with eosinophilic fluid in which a few inflammatory cells are often present. Cystitis cystica et glandularis need to be differentiated occasionally from a microcystic variant of urothelial carcinoma. The presence of at least focal cellular atypia and invading nests deeper in the bladder wall would favor carcinoma.[75] Recent TERT mutation analysis studies support cystitis glandularis as a benign reactive process.[76]

Cystitis glandularis and cystitis cystica are interrelated lesions in which cystitis cystica would be the end of spectrum with higher level of anomalies (Fig. 5.16). In line with this thought, both lesions are frequently reported with the single term of cystitis glandularis et cystica. Cystitis glandularis and cystitis cystica have

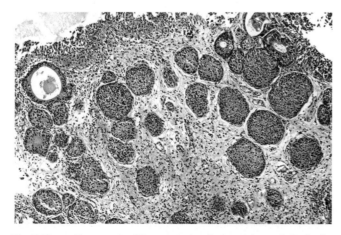

Fig. 5.12 von Brunn nests at the mucosal surface and deeper in the lamina propria. Note the smooth round contours of the nests.

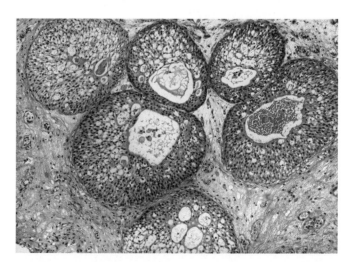

Fig. 5.13 Cystitis glandularis of the typical/conventional type. The lining cells are columnar, goblet cells are not present, and mucus is absent or inconspicuous.

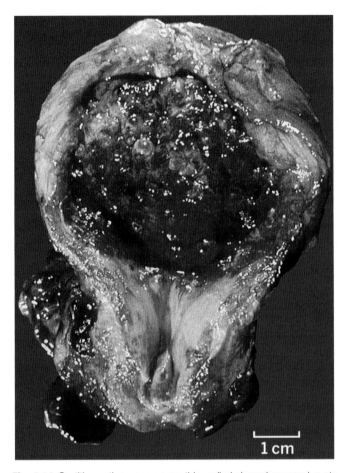

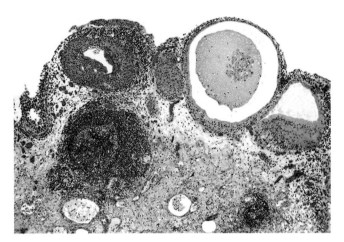

Fig. 5.16 Cystitis glandularis and cystitis cystica may frequently be seen together and are part of the so-called proliferative cystitis in urologic literature.

Fig. 5.14 Cystitis cystica appears as thin-walled domed mucosal cysts or blebs.

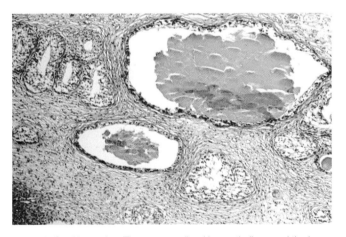

Fig. 5.15 Cystitis cystica. The cysts are lined by urothelium, and the lumen contains proteinaceous fluid.

characteristic immunostaining with CK7, similar to normal urothelium, and lack expression of CDX2 and CK20, markers associated with intestinal differentiation.[57,75]

Intestinal Metaplasia (Cystitis Glandularis, Intestinal Type)

Intestinal metaplasia may be extensive, affecting both the lamina propria and the mucosa.[41,70,77,78] The lining cells in intestinal metaplasia are tall and columnar with obvious mucin production.

In such cases, goblet cells are often present, and the glands closely resemble colonic glands. Rarely, Paneth cells and argentaffin-, argyrophil-, or chromogranin A–positive cells are present.[42,43,56,59,77] Biopsies from such areas closely resemble colonic mucosa, with tubular glands and numerous goblet cells (Fig. 5.17). The mucin produced by these cells is of the colonic type.[79,80] These lesions have characteristic immunostaining with CDX2 and CK20, and lack the expression of CK7. In some cases the cells also stain immunohistochemically with antibodies to prostate-specific antigen (PSA) and prostatic acid phosphatase (PAP).[81,82]

Rarely, colonic epithelium may be present in the bladder as a developmental abnormality.[83] Diffuse forms of *intestinal metaplasia* usually occur in chronically irritated bladders such as those of paraplegics or in patients with stones or long-term catheterization (Fig. 5.18).

Intestinal metaplasia usually poses no diagnostic problem, but occasional cases are difficult to distinguish from adenocarcinoma, in particular florid extensive forms and cases showing a variable degree of dysplasia (Fig. 5.19).[35,46,64,84,85] Rare cases of intestinal metaplasia may coexist with mucin extravasation into the stroma, a finding not to be misdiagnosed as adenocarcinoma (Fig. 5.20). Mitosis and cellular atypia are found only rarely in intestinal metaplasia. Intestinal metaplasia is typically confined to the lamina propria, with only rare cases extending superficially to the muscularis propria. Exceptionally, isolated glands of intestinal metaplasia may show moderate dysplasia in an analogous fashion to what is seen in colonic adenoma; the significance of this finding is uncertain. Nonetheless, suggested treatment is complete resection of the bladder lesion with close follow-up of the patient. It seems to be judicious to report these cases as intestinal metaplasia with adenomatous change, stating the level of dysplasia as a note. An irregular haphazard arrangement of glands in the lamina propria or deeper in the bladder wall with high degree of cytologic atypia should raise the suspicion of adenocarcinoma.

For many years there has been debate regarding the malignant potential of intestinal metaplasia. Sporadic reports describing the occurrence of adenocarcinoma in a background of longstanding intestinal metaplasia have led to speculation that intestinal metaplasia is a premalignant lesion.[42-55,86] In support of this a recent study reported levels of telomere shortening in intestinal metaplasia

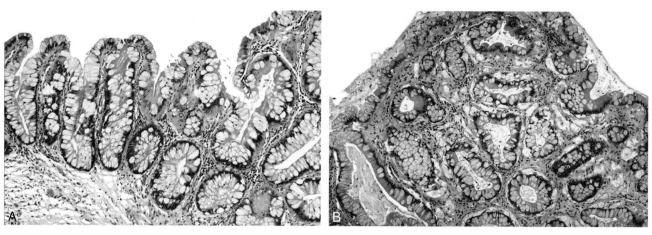

Fig. 5.17 (A) Cystitis glandularis, intestinal type. There are spaced tubular glands lined by goblet cells. The surface epithelium is also mucinous. (B) Cystitis glandularis, intestinal type. The glands closely resemble colonic glands.

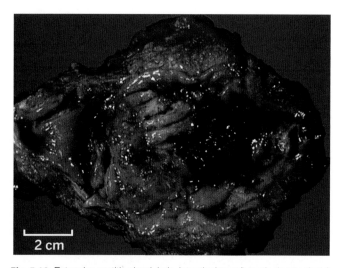

Fig. 5.18 Extensive cystitis glandularis, intestinal type (intestinal metaplasia). Large and small foci of glistening red mucosa mimic a bladder tumor.

consistent with a premalignant nature of this lesion.[54] In contrast, no instances of bladder adenocarcinoma were identified in a study of 53 patients with intestinal metaplasia followed for more than 10 years, suggesting that intestinal metaplasia is not a strong risk factor for cancer.[86]

Squamous Metaplasia

Metaplastic squamous epithelium is common in patients with severe chronic cystitis such as nonfunctioning bladders or schistosomiasis.[87-95] It is about four times more common in women than men. Squamous metaplasia may occur anywhere in the bladder but is most frequent on the anterior wall. Areas of metaplasia often are white or gray-white (Fig. 5.21) and may blend into the surrounding mucosa or be sharply demarcated.[87,89] Abundantly keratinizing lesions may have a bulky irregular appearance similar to carcinoma.[96,97] Histologically, the lesions show squamous epithelium of variable thickness, often covered by a layer of keratin (Figs. 5.22 and 5.23). In most cases there is no nuclear atypia, but changes as severe as those of carcinoma in situ are occasionally seen and should raise the possibility of invasive carcinoma elsewhere in the specimen or in nearby mucosa.

Keratinizing squamous metaplasia (leukoplakia) appears to be a significant risk factor for the development of carcinoma of the urinary mucosa.[98-101] A Mayo Clinic study of 78 patients with keratinizing squamous metaplasia found that 22% had synchronous carcinoma and another 20% later had carcinoma (the mean interval was 11 years).[102] Similar findings were reported by Khan et al. with a longer duration of follow-up.[103] Most were squamous cell carcinoma. Where schistosomiasis is endemic, squamous metaplasia commonly precedes squamous cell carcinoma.[104,105]

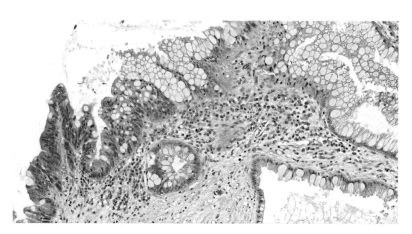

Fig. 5.19 Occasionally intestinal metaplasia shows a variable degree of focal cellular dysplasia (*left*) similar to adenomatous change seen in the colon.

Fig. 5.20 Occasionally intestinal metaplasia may be associated with extensive mucin extravasation.

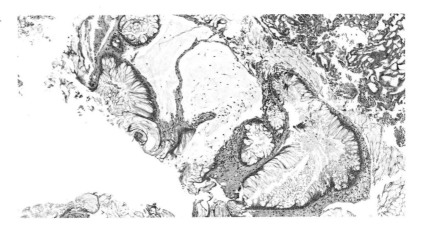

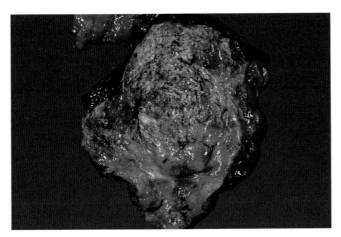

Fig. 5.21 Keratinizing squamous metaplasia is gray with flecks of light-colored keratin.

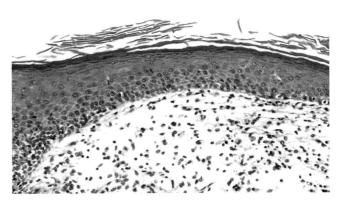

Fig. 5.23 Keratinizing squamous metaplasia with parakeratosis.

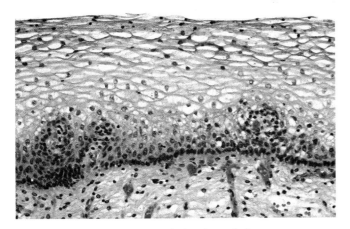

Fig. 5.22 Squamous metaplasia replacing the urothelium.

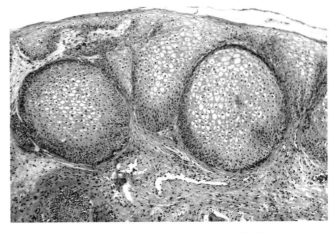

Fig. 5.24 Nonkeratinizing glycogenated squamous epithelium.

Nonkeratinizing glycogenated squamous epithelium, resembling vaginal epithelium (Fig. 5.24), is present in the trigone and bladder neck in up to 86% of women of reproductive age and in almost 75% of postmenopausal women.[106-111] This normal finding should not be diagnosed as squamous metaplasia. Cystoscopically, these areas are pale gray-white with irregular borders, often with a surrounding zone of erythema. The clinical association of this cystoscopic finding with symptoms of urgency and frequency has been called *pseudomembranous trigonitis.* This type of squamous epithelium is rare in men but has been reported in patients receiving estrogen therapy for adenocarcinoma of the prostate.[108,112]

Verrucous squamous hyperplasia is a form of squamous metaplasia recently described to occur in the bladder, and consists of spiking or church spirelike squamous hyperplasia. The lesion presents with marked hyperkeratosis and elongation of the rete pegs.

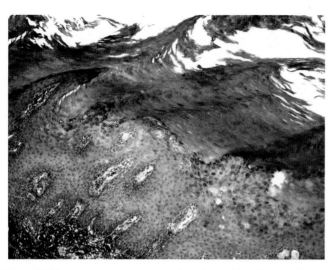

Fig. 5.25 Verrucous squamous hyperplasia is considered a premalignant lesion of squamous cell carcinoma when present in the bladder. This case was found adjacent to a verrucous squamous cell carcinoma.

Occasional signs of maturation, such as focal granular cell layer, may be seen. It is considered a premalignant lesion with potential to evolve into verrucous or other forms of squamous cell carcinoma (Fig. 5.25).[103]

Nephrogenic Adenoma

First described as a hamartoma in 1949 by Davis, the name *nephrogenic adenoma* was given a year later by Friedman and Kuhlenbeck in a report of eight cases.[113,114] They chose this name because, in its most common form, the tumor is composed of small tubules resembling renal tubules.[115-121] The terms *nephrogenic metaplasia* and *adenomatous metaplasia* are preferred by some.[118,122,123] More than 75% of reported cases have involved the bladder, but lesions in the urethra, ureter, and rarely the renal pelvis have also been reported.[119] Recent evidence in renal transplant patients suggests that nephrogenic adenoma is derived from tubular renal cells and is not a metaplastic proliferation of the urothelium as has long been thought.[124] Molecular evidence suggests that clear cell adenocarcinoma of the bladder may rarely arise from nephrogenic adenoma.[125]

Approximately 90% of patients with nephrogenic adenoma are adults, and there is a male predominance of 2:1. In children, it is more common in girls than in boys.[126,127] Nephrogenic adenoma is frequently found after genitourinary surgery (61% of cases) or associated with calculi (14% of cases), trauma (9% of cases), and cystitis.[119] Renal transplant recipients comprise about 8% of patients.[119,128] Reports of hematuria, dysuria, and frequency are common, but the association with other lesions makes it difficult to categorically attribute any of these symptoms to nephrogenic adenoma.

Approximately 56% are papillary, 34% sessile, and 10% polypoid. It is rare on the anterior wall of the bladder, but nearly evenly distributed over the rest of the mucosa.[119] About two-thirds are smaller than 1 cm in diameter, most being incidentally discovered microscopic lesions. Approximately 25% are from 1 to 4 cm in diameter, and only 10% are larger. In less than 20% of cases, there are multiple lesions, which rarely include diffuse involvement of the bladder.

Microscopically, nephrogenic adenoma displays tubular, cystic, polypoid, papillary, flat, fibromyxoid, and diffuse patterns.[129-132] The most common architecture is tubular (present in 96% of cases). The tubules are typically small, round structures lined by cuboidal epithelium (Fig. 5.26), but occasionally are elongated and solid. Sometimes they are surrounded by a prominent basement membrane. Cystic dilatation of the tubules is common (Fig. 5.27) (present in 72% of cases) and may predominate. Tubules and cysts often contain eosinophilic or basophilic secretions, which may react with mucicarmine (present in 25% of cases). Polypoid and papillary structures (Fig. 5.28) are present in 65% of cases. Edematous polyps are more common than delicate papillae, which are present in only 10% of cases. Focal solid growth (Fig. 5.29) is uncommon. Rarely, a fibromyxoid stroma is present (Figs. 5.30 through 5.32).

Most tubules, cysts, and papillae have cuboidal to low columnar epithelium with scant cytoplasm, but epithelium with abundant clear cytoplasm is seen in up to 40% of cases. Hobnail cells (Fig. 5.26B) focally line the tubules and cysts in 70% of cases, and rarely they predominate.[129] Larger cysts may be lined by flat epithelial cells. Glycogen is present in some cells in 10% to 15% of cases.[133] The nuclei are regular and round, and atypia is rare, usually appearing degenerative.[129,134] Mitotic figures are absent or rare. Nephrogenic adenoma is often associated with chronic

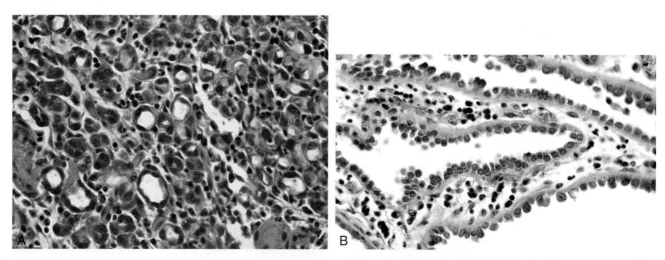

Fig. 5.26 (A) Tubules of nephrogenic adenoma lined by cuboidal epithelium resembling renal medullary tubules. (B) Tubules of nephrogenic adenoma lined by hobnail cells.

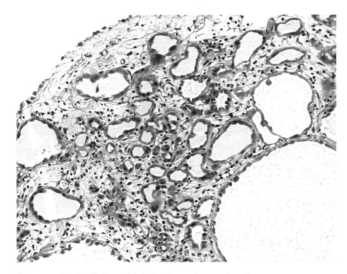

Fig. 5.27 Cystic dilation of tubules in nephrogenic adenoma.

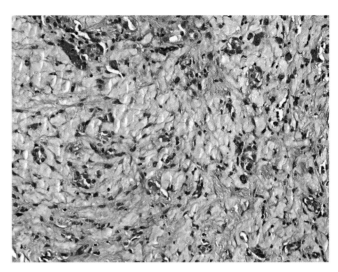

Fig. 5.30 Fibromyxoid nephrogenic adenoma with small tubules embedded in a myxoid background stroma.

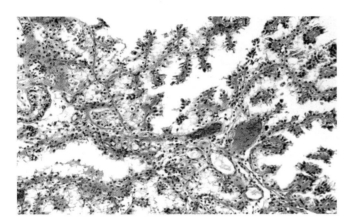

Fig. 5.28 Papillary nephrogenic adenoma. The papillae are covered by a single layer of cuboidal cells.

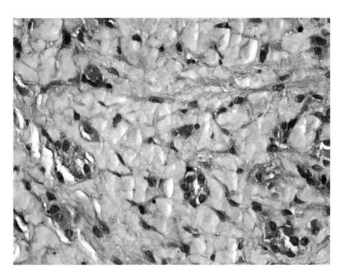

Fig. 5.31 Magnified view of case depicted in Fig. 5.30.

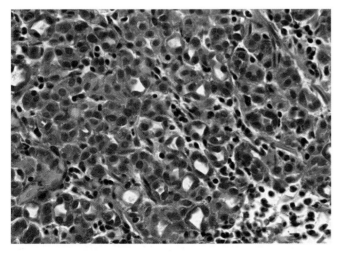

Fig. 5.29 Diffuse or solid pattern of nephrogenic adenoma. The cells have abundant eosinophilic cytoplasm.

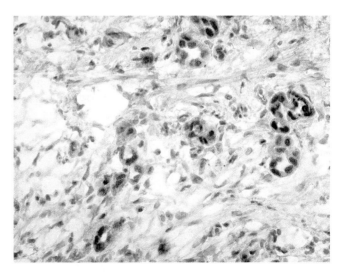

Fig. 5.32 Positive PAX8 stainings in fibromyxoid nephrogenic adenoma.

cystitis, which may obscure it. Rarely, it is associated with stromal calcification, squamous metaplasia, or cystitis glandularis.[115,135]

Nephrogenic adenoma has a number of features that may cause confusion with bladder carcinoma.[130] Tiny mucin-filled tubules apparently lined by a single cell with a compressed nucleus may resemble signet ring cells. The irregular disposition of the tubules may simulate invasive adenocarcinoma, especially when they are among the fibers of the muscularis mucosae. Hobnail cells may suggest clear cell adenocarcinoma, which shares architectural features of tubular, cystic, and papillary structures with nephrogenic adenoma (see Chapter 6). Clinical and pathologic features that help to distinguish nephrogenic adenoma from clear cell adenocarcinoma are listed in Table 5.1.

In a few cases of nephrogenic adenoma, papillae are the predominant feature (Fig. 5.33); cytologic atypia may be present (Figs. 5.34 and 5.35) and may cause confusion with other papillary lesions, such as urothelial carcinoma and papillary cystitis. Recognition of the cuboidal epithelium covering the papillae of nephrogenic adenoma differentiates it from these lesions, which are covered by urothelium.

Nephrogenic adenoma may be confused with prostate adenocarcinoma because of immunoreactivity for racemase (P504S) and negative reactivity for basal cell–specific cytokeratin (34βE12) and p63.[136] However, negative reactivity for PSA and PAP differentiates

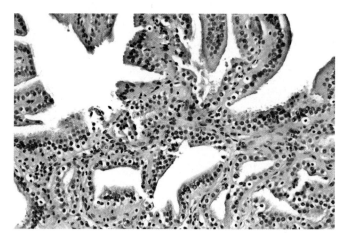

Fig. 5.33 Nephrogenic adenoma with predominance of the papillary component.

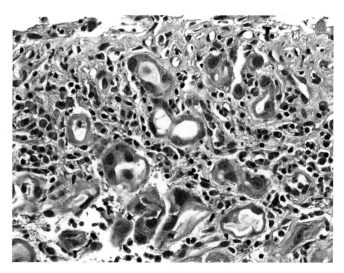

Fig. 5.34 Cytologic atypia in nephrogenic adenoma.

TABLE 5.1	Features Distinguishing Nephrogenic Adenoma From Clear Cell Adenocarcinoma (*See Also Chapter 6*)	
Feature	Nephrogenic Adenoma	Clear Cell Adenocarcinoma
Gender predominance	Male	Female
Age	33% <30 years	All >43 years
Associated genitourinary conditions	Very common	Absent
Size	Usually small	Often large
Solid growth pattern	Rare	Common
Clear cells	Uncommon	Common
Glycogen in cytoplasm	Rare	Common and abundant
Hobnail cells	Common	Common
Necrosis	Absent	Often present (53%)
Luminal mucin	Common	Common
Nuclear atypia and mitotic figures	Rare	Common
Prostate-specific antigen	Negative	Negative
34βE12	Positive	Positive (occasionally negative)
CK7	Positive	Positive
CK20	Negative	Positive
EMA	Positive	Positive
AMACR (P504S)	Often positive	Often positive
PAX2	Positive	Positive
PAX8	Positive	Positive
Ki67-MIB1 labeling index (clone Ki67)	<5%	Often >15%
p53	Occasional focal positive	Positive

AMACR, alpha-methylacyl-CoA racemase; EMA, epithelial membrane antigen

nephrogenic adenoma from prostate adenocarcinoma.[137-139] S100A1 is also a useful marker to distinguish nephrogenic adenoma from prostatic adenocarcinoma.[140] Immunohistochemical staining for nuclear transcription factors for renal development, PAX2 and PAX8, is useful for differentiating nephrogenic adenoma from prostate adenocarcinoma, benign urothelium, and papillary urothelial carcinoma.[141-146] Focal GATA3 positivity has rarely been observed in nephrogenic adenoma. Pathologic features that favor clear cell adenocarcinoma over nephrogenic adenoma include the predominance of clear cells, severe cytologic atypia, high mitotic rate, the presence of tumor necrosis, high Ki67 count, and strong reactivity for p53.[147]

Papillary Hyperplasia

The urothelial mucosa overlying inflammatory or neoplastic processes may occasionally have a papillary appearance on microscopic examination. In some cases, discovery of the bladder lesion precedes identification of the underlying condition, and in these cases the bladder lesion is referred to as a *herald lesion*.[148] The term *papillary hyperplasia* is used when papillae are not seen grossly or at cystoscopy.[66] Most often the underlying lesion originates in the prostate, female genital tract, or colon.[148,149] When associated

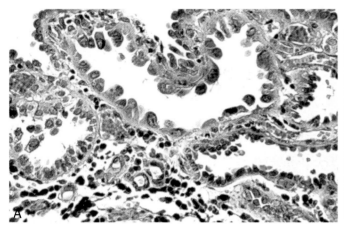
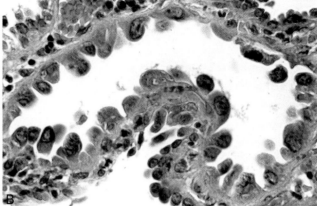

Fig. 5.35 Cytologic atypia in nephrogenic adenoma (A and B).

with prostatic disease, the papillary lesions are found in the trigone in the midline; those associated with uterine disease are found in the midline above the trigone. When associated with intestinal disease, the bladder lesions are often on the left and posterior. In this context, papillary hyperplasia is seen as a nonspecific reactive process. This reactive hyperplasia should be distinguished from the papillary urothelial hyperplasia that is seen as the earliest manifestation of papillary carcinoma, a lesion renamed by the current World Health Organization classification of the tumors of the urinary tract as urothelial proliferation of uncertain malignant potential.[150]

Inflammation and Infection

Nonspecific Cystitis

Polypoid and Papillary Cystitis

Polypoid and papillary cystitis result from inflammation and edema in the lamina propria leading to papillary and polypoid mucosal lesions.[151-156] The term *papillary cystitis* is used for finger-like papillae (Figs. 5.36 and 5.37) lined by reactive urothelium and *polypoid cystitis* for broad-based edematous lesions (Figs. 5.38 and 5.39). The latter are more common. Chronic inflammation in the lamina propria and dilated blood vessels are prominent and diagnostically helpful features of both papillary and polypoid cystitis. Depending on the degree of edema of the lamina propria, there is a continuous morphologic spectrum from papillary cystitis to polypoid cystitis to *bullous cystitis* (Fig. 5.39). In papillary and polypoid cystitis the lesion is taller than it is wide, whereas in bullous cystitis the opposite applies. There may be associated metaplastic changes in the epithelium covering or adjacent to the lesion.

In the clinical settings of indwelling catheter and vesical fistula, the surgical pathologist should be alert to the possibility that an exophytic bladder lesion may be inflammatory.[157] Polypoid cystitis is present in up to 80% of patients with indwelling catheters.[154] Although most lesions are microscopic in size, polypoid or bullous lesions up to 5 mm in diameter (mostly in the dome or on the posterior wall) are found in about 33% of cases. Prolonged catheterization may induce widespread polypoid and bullous cystitis. Most lesions disappear within 6 months of removal of the irritant.[153]

Vesical fistulae, whether resulting from intestinal diverticulitis, Crohn disease, colorectal cancer (Fig. 5.40), or appendicitis, are often associated with polypoid cystitis and, less commonly, with

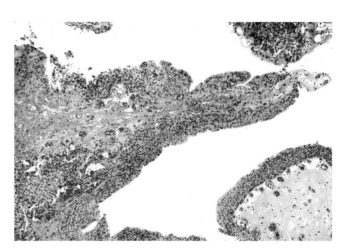

Fig. 5.36 Papillary cystitis with finger-like fronds covered by a few layers of urothelium.

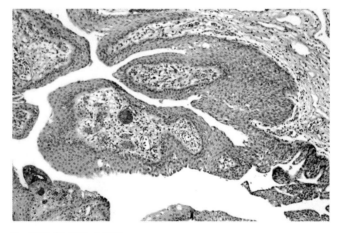

Fig. 5.37 Papillary cystitis.

papillary cystitis.[158-164] Fistulae between the urinary bladder and the alimentary tract are about three times more common in men than in women.[160,165] Pneumaturia and fecaluria are typical symptoms.[160] In about 50% of cases, indications of extravesical disease are initially absent, making the diagnosis more difficult. Patients may present with frequency, urgency, and dysuria. Cystoscopically, the appearance often suggests bladder carcinoma.[153]

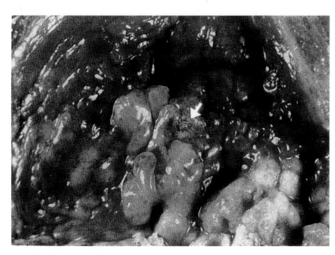

Fig. 5.38 Polypoid cystitis. *Arrow* shows biopsy site.

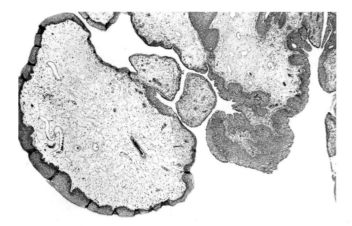

Fig. 5.39 Polypoid cystitis.

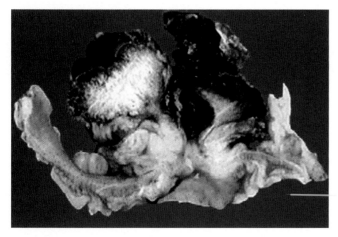

Fig. 5.40 Colovesical fistula secondary to adenocarcinoma of colon. The dimpled outlet in the bladder mucosa (*top*) connects with the colon (*bottom*).

Papillary and polypoid cystitis must be distinguished from papillary urothelial carcinoma. Grossly and microscopically, the fronds of polypoid cystitis are much broader than those of most papillary carcinomas. The delicate papillae of papillary cystitis more closely resemble those of carcinoma. Branching is much less prominent in

papillary cystitis than in papillary carcinoma. In papillary cystitis the epithelium may be hyperplastic, but usually not to the degree seen in carcinoma. Umbrella cells are more often present in papillary cystitis than in carcinoma.

Follicular Cystitis

Follicular cystitis occurs in up to 40% of patients with bladder cancer and 35% of those with urinary tract infection.[166,167] Grossly, the mucosa is erythematous with pink, white, or gray nodules (Fig. 5.41).[168-171] Microscopically, the nodules consist of lymphoid follicles in the lamina propria, usually with germinal centers (Fig. 5.42). Malignant lymphoma is the most important differential diagnostic consideration, particularly in biopsies. The criteria used to distinguish lymphoma from chronic inflammation at other sites apply here.[172]

Giant Cell Cystitis

Atypical mesenchymal cells with enlarged, hyperchromatic, or multiple nuclei are frequently seen in the lamina propria of the bladder. Wells found them in 33% of cases of cystitis at autopsy and coined the term *giant cell cystitis.* Such cells are common in

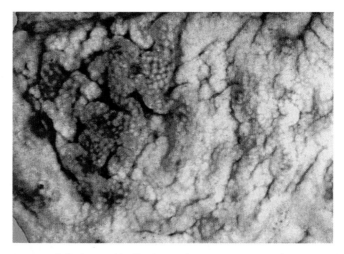

Fig. 5.41 Follicular cystitis. The lymphoid aggregates are visible as small domed lesions on the mucosal surface.

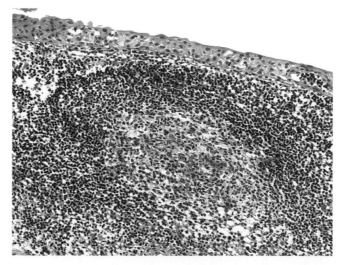

Fig. 5.42 Follicular cystitis. The lamina propria contains a lymphoid follicle.

bladder biopsies including those without other evidence of cystitis.[173] Histologically, the cells often have bipolar or multipolar tapering eosinophilic cytoplasmic processes (Fig. 5.43). The nuclei are often irregular in size and shape and hyperchromatic. Mitotic figures are absent or rare. If present in large numbers, these cells may suggest pseudoneoplastic lesions such as postoperative spindle cell nodule and neoplasms such as sarcomatoid urothelial carcinoma or sarcoma. Similar cells may be seen in the lamina propria after radiation therapy and anticancer chemotherapy.[174-177]

Hemorrhagic Cystitis

Cystitis with a predominantly hemorrhagic clinical presentation (Fig. 5.44) may be caused by chemical toxins, radiation, viral infection, or may be idiopathic. Chemical causes include drugs (such as cyclophosphamide, busulfan, and thiotepa), derivatives of aniline and toluidine (such as dyes and insecticides), and a host of other compounds.[178,179] Radiation and chemotherapy for cancer account for most cases.

Since its introduction in the late 1950s, cyclophosphamide has been recognized as a potent bladder toxin associated with hemorrhagic cystitis.[176,180,181] Hemorrhage may be severe, and early experience reported mortality of nearly 4%.[181,182] Hemorrhage

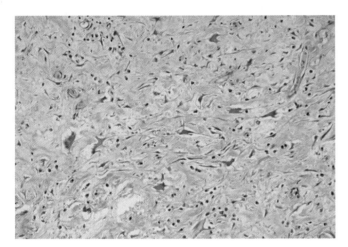

Fig. 5.43 Giant cell cystitis. The lamina propria contains large stromal cells, some with elongated cytoplasmic processes and some that are multinucleated.

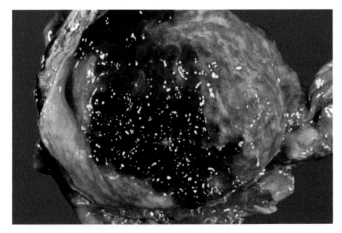

Fig. 5.44 Hemorrhagic cystitis.

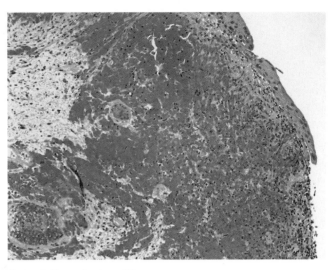

Fig. 5.45 Hemorrhagic cystitis.

usually begins during or shortly after treatment. Within 4 hours the mucosa is edematous and congested (Fig. 5.45), and the epithelium shows changes like those seen in the irradiated bladder, including nuclear pleomorphism and variable cell size. As the bladder heals the urothelium becomes hyperplastic and may form papillae. High doses of cyclophosphamide and repeated exposure may lead to irreversible fibrosis and a small contracted bladder.[174] Epithelial and mesenchymal neoplasms may arise in the bladder after cyclophosphamide therapy.[183-185]

Special Types of Cystitis

Interstitial Cystitis (Bladder Pain Syndrome)

Interstitial cystitis has also been referred to as *Hunner ulcer*, but that term is used less frequently today because it has been recognized that ulcers are not always present. The term *interstitial cystitis* was introduced by Skene in 1887, and Nitze described most of the characteristic features before the work by Hunner in 1914.[186–188] Interstitial cystitis poses diagnostic problems for both pathologists and urologists. The pathologic features are not specific, and the pathologist must correlate them with the clinical and cystoscopic features.

At least 90% of patients with interstitial cystitis are women, and it is seen most often in middle and old age.[189-200] Patients report marked frequency, urgency, and pain when the bladder becomes full and when it is emptied.[201] The urine is sterile. Cystoscopy may reveal small foci of hemorrhage (glomerulations), hemorrhagic spots that ooze blood, and linear cracks in the mucosa.[201,202] Occasionally there are ulcers with radiating scars. Ulcers and scars are more frequent in older patients with long-standing cystitis.[203] In advanced cases the wall of the bladder becomes fibrotic and contracted, resulting in very low bladder capacity (Fig. 5.46). Interstitial cystitis most often affects the dome and posterior and lateral walls.

Biopsy specimens from patients with interstitial cystitis have a variety of appearances. When present, ulcers are often wedge shaped, and the urothelium is either absent or mixed with a surface exudate of fibrin, erythrocytes, and inflammatory cells (Fig. 5.47). The ulcers usually extend deep into the lamina propria, which is edematous and congested. The muscularis propria may also be edematous or fibrotic. Generally, there is a dense infiltrate of lymphocytes and plasma cells. When ulcers are not present, the changes are less striking. Small mucosal ruptures, edema of the

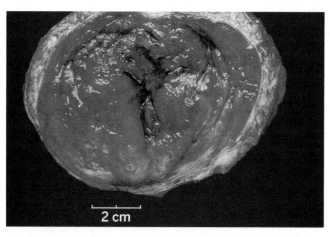

Fig. 5.46 Chronic interstitial cystitis. The mucosa is punctuated by depressed scars, and the wall is thick and rigid.

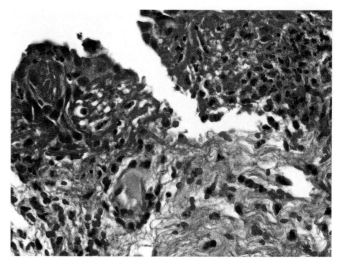

Fig. 5.48 Bladder mucosa rupture in interstitial cystitis.

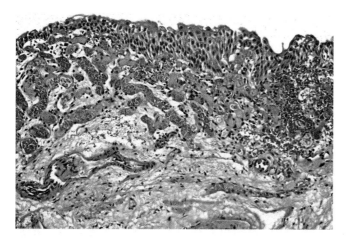

Fig. 5.47 The lamina propria is prominently vascular in interstitial cystitis.

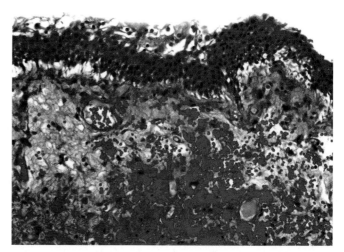

Fig. 5.49 Glomerulation seen in interstitial cystitis.

lamina propria, and foci of hemorrhage in the lamina propria are usually present and correspond to the glomerulations seen at cystoscopy (Figs. 5.48 and 5.49).

Mast cells are often seen in the mucosa, lamina propria, and muscularis propria in interstitial cystitis.[204] Their significance has been debated since Simmons and Bunce first reported an increase in mast cells in interstitial cystitis in 1958.[205] Kastrup et al. concluded that more than 20 mast cells/mm^2 in the muscularis propria was strongly suggestive of interstitial cystitis, and Larsen et al. found that 28 mast cells/mm^2 was the upper limit for normal bladders.[206,207] Johansson and Fall found an average of 164 mast cells/mm^2 in the lamina propria of patients with ulcers, 93/mm^2 in those without, and 88/mm^2 in a control group.[203] The difficulty of counting mast cells and the lack of consensus on what is "normal" are evident. Conditions of tissue fixation also affect the count. Thus the histologic features of interstitial cystitis are not pathognomonic and, therefore, the main indication of bladder biopsy in these patients is to exclude urothelial carcinoma in situ, a condition that may present with symptoms that overlap with those of interstitial cystitis.

The extensive urothelial denudation that often occurs with carcinoma in situ may result in an appearance of ulceration, inflammation, and vascular congestion closely resembling that seen in interstitial cystitis. When urothelium is absent or scant in a biopsy,

multiple sections should be obtained to look for foci of atypical cells. Tamm-Horsfall protein is deposited in the epithelium and submucosa in patients with interstitial cystitis, indicating a barrier defect in this disease. When other conditions are excluded, often the pathologist can report only that the pathologic findings are consistent with interstitial cystitis.

Eosinophilic Cystitis

Bladder inflammation with a striking infiltrate of eosinophils is known to have associations with allergic diseases and with invasive urothelial carcinoma. In some cases, there is simply a history of transurethral resection or biopsy. In other cases, no inciting factor can be identified.[208-211]

Eosinophilic cystitis associated with allergic disease is rare, and most cases have involved patients with asthma or eosinophilic gastroenteritis.[212,213] Rarely, eosinophilic cystitis is associated with parasitic infection.[214,215] Patients range in age from newborn to elderly, and more than 33% are children. The ratio of females to males is 2:1. The usual symptoms are dysuria, frequency, and hematuria. At cystoscopy, there often are polypoid lesions resembling those of polypoid cystitis, and in children sarcoma botryoides may come to mind. Nodular and sessile lesions and ulcers also are seen. Occasionally, the lesions mimic carcinoma.[216,217] Histologically, the lamina propria is edematous, containing a mixed inflammatory infiltrate in which eosinophils are prominent (Fig. 5.50). Occasionally, edema causes ureteral obstruction and upper tract complications, but most patients respond to nonspecific medical treatment including antihistamines, nonsteroidal antiinflammatory agents, and steroids. However, the disease tends to be persistent or recurrent, so long-term follow-up is recommended.[218,219]

Patients with no history of allergy are typically older men with various urologic diseases, such as prostatic hyperplasia and carcinoma of the bladder.[220] Many patients have a history of transurethral resection or biopsy, and eosinophilic cystitis may be a reaction to bladder injury. Inflammation with prominent eosinophils is also commonly seen at the periphery of invasive carcinoma in cystectomy specimens.

Postsurgical Necrobiotic Granulomas

After transurethral surgery using diathermic cautery, the bladder may contain necrotizing palisading granulomas.[221-223] Similar lesions have been reported subsequent to laser surgery.[224] Postsurgical granulomas are found in approximately 10% of cases, and the frequency increases with the number of operations. Typically, these granulomas have elongated linear or serpiginous outlines. Their centers contain acellular, finely granular eosinophilic material in which flecks of brown debris are often present (Fig. 5.51). Around the necrotic areas is a band of histiocytes arranged radially like the stakes of a palisade fence. Epithelioid histiocytes and foreign body giant cells also are commonly present. Surrounding this layer is dense chronic inflammation in which eosinophils may be numerous. Eventually the granulomas are replaced by fibrous scars, sometimes with dystrophic calcification.

Bacillus Calmette–Guérin Granulomas

Since 1976, urothelial carcinoma in situ has been treated with intravesical instillation of the mycobacterium bacillus Calmette–Guérin.[225] This therapy often produces remission but is not usually curative.[226,227] A profound inflammatory reaction ensues after instillation with the result that the urothelium is lost and the lamina propria develops dense chronic inflammatory infiltrates among which are interspersed small granulomas composed of epithelioid histiocytes and multinucleated giant cells (Fig. 5.52).[228-233] These granulomas are usually round or ovoid lesions in the superficial lamina propria and lack necrosis. Acid-fast stains only rarely

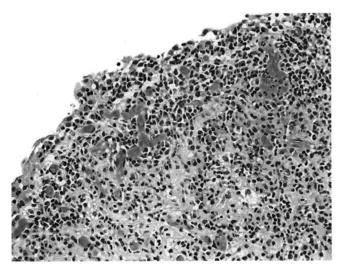

Fig. 5.50 In eosinophilic cystitis, the lamina propria contains sheets of eosinophils.

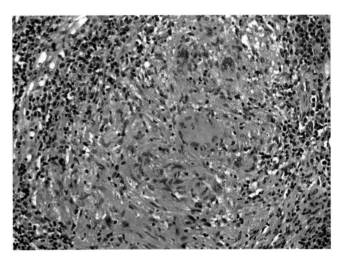

Fig. 5.52 Granuloma of bacillus Calmette–Guérin.

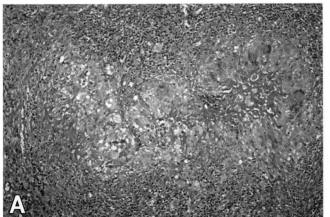
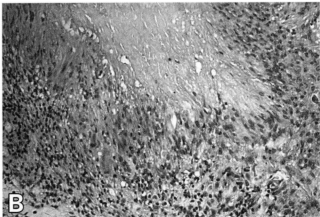

Fig. 5.51 (A) Postoperative granuloma with amorphous debris. (B) Postoperative granuloma with strands of coagulated tissue in the center and a palisade of histiocytes surrounding the necrotic material.

demonstrate organisms. Granulomatous inflammatory changes may also be seen in urine cytology specimens.[234,235] Rarely, nephrogenic adenoma may arise after therapy with bacillus Calmette–Guérin.[236]

Other Noninfectious Granulomas

After herniorrhaphy, suture granuloma may produce an inflammatory mass in or near the bladder.[237-243] Usually the herniorrhaphy wound has been infected. Because of the long interval between herniorrhaphy and bladder symptoms (up to 11 years), the clinical diagnosis is often of bladder neoplasm. Microscopic examination shows a predominantly inflammatory process with foreign body giant cells and fibrosis around fragments of suture.

Rarely, diffuse infiltrates of histiocytes without the features specific for malakoplakia may form nodules in the bladder, and this has been termed xanthogranulomatous cystitis.[244] Xanthogranulomatous cystitis has been described in association with benign and malignant bladder neoplasms, as well as nonneoplastic conditions such as urachal diverticula or infections. Fewer than one dozen cases have been reported.[244-254] Collections of foamy histiocytes may also be found in the lamina propria in patients with disorders of lipid metabolism (Fig. 5.53), but also may be seen along the papillary cores of some urothelial carcinomas, and have been called xanthoma of the bladder.[253,255,256] Granulomatous inflammation of the bladder has also been reported in association with granulomatous disease of childhood, rheumatoid arthritis, infarcted leiomyoma, and fistulae of Crohn disease.[257-260] Sarcoidosis rarely affects the bladder.[261]

Radiation Cystitis

Radiation frequently induces a variety of abnormalities in the bladder.[262-265] At 3 to 6 weeks after treatment, there is acute cystitis with loss of the urothelium and congestion and edema in the lamina propria.[266] The remaining urothelial cells show varying degrees of nuclear atypicality. Features of radiation injury in the urothelium include vacuoles in the cytoplasm and nuclei, karyorrhexis, and a normal nuclear–cytoplasmic ratio. In the stroma, marked edema and telangiectasis are common. Blood vessels also undergo hyalinization and thrombosis. The lamina propria usually contains atypical spindle cells like those of giant cell cystitis (Fig. 5.54).

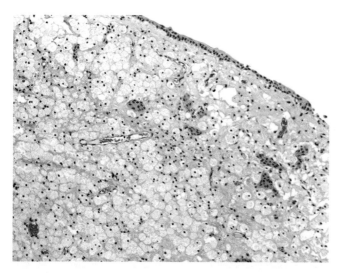

Fig. 5.53 Xanthoma of the bladder occupying lamina propria.

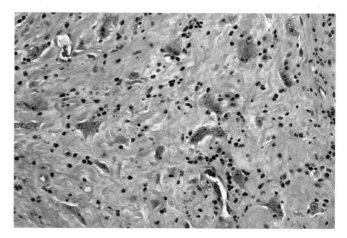

Fig. 5.54 Radiation cystitis with atypical stromal cells.

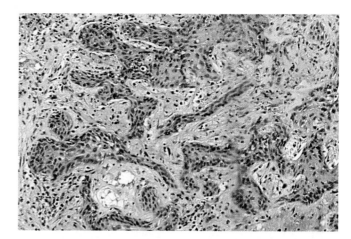

Fig. 5.55 Florid epithelial proliferations (pseudocarcinomatous hyperplasia) after radiation therapy.

Later, ulcers and fibrosis and contraction of the bladder wall and stricture of the ureters may occur.[266,267]

Florid epithelial proliferations (also reported as pseudocarcinomatous hyperplasia) that can simulate carcinoma have been seen (Figs. 5.55 and 5.56).[262-264,266-270] The individual urothelial cells may have an eosinophilic cytoplasm with somewhat "squamoid" appearance.[271] Attention to the reactive nature of the background and patient's clinical history is crucial to avoid a misdiagnosis of carcinoma.

Reaction to Chemotherapy

Urothelial carcinoma in situ is commonly treated with intravesical topical chemotherapy. The most frequently used agents are the alkylating agents triethylenethiophosphoramide (thiotepa) and mitomycin C. These drugs induce denudation of the bladder mucosa in 37% of biopsies.[177] The remaining epithelium often shows nuclear changes, such as pleomorphism and hyperchromasia with frequent cytoplasmic eosinophilia, which may be mistaken for residual carcinoma in situ (Figs. 5.57 and 5.58).[272]

Pseudocarcinomatous lesions like those seen in radiation cystitis have been seen in patients who have been treated with chemotherapy.[262,270,271,273]

Fig. 5.56 Florid epithelial proliferations (pseudocarcinomatous hyperplasia) seen in a patient with a history of radiation therapy for prostate cancer. Notice cytoplasmic eosinophilia with squamoid appearance and moderate nuclear atypia.

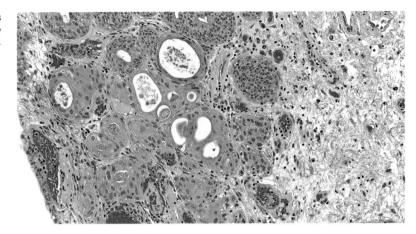

and diphtheroids are implicated. A predisposition to bacterial cystitis is associated with structural factors including exstrophy, urethral malformations, fistulae with other pelvic organs, diverticula, calculi, and foreign bodies. Urinary stasis and alkalinity also promote infection. Systemic illnesses such as diabetes mellitus, chronic renal disease, and immunosuppression are predisposing conditions. Most pathogens gain access to the bladder by ascending the urethra. Mycobacteria are an exception and usually descend from the upper tract in the urine.

Early in bacterial infection, the appearance of the mucosa ranges from moderately erythematous to deeply hemorrhagic; these changes may be diffuse or focal. In addition to the classic symptoms of dysuria, urgency, and frequency, hematuria may result from leakage of erythrocytes through the mucosa. Later, a gray fibrinous membrane may cover the mucosal surface. With progression, a thin purulent exudate may adhere to the surface, creating a suppurative or exudative cystitis. Edema may thicken the vesical wall, and in chronic infections, fibrosis may thicken and stiffen the wall and the mucosa may be ulcerated (Fig. 5.59).

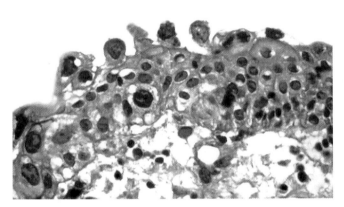

Fig. 5.57 Epithelial atypia and sloughing associated with intravesical thiotepa.

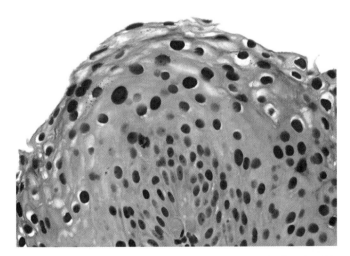

Fig. 5.58 Epithelial atypia associated with intravenous cyclophosphamide.

Infectious Cystitis

Bacterial Cystitis

Bacterial infection is the most common cause of cystitis and is usually caused by coliform organisms such as *Escherichia coli*, *Klebsiella pneumoniae*, and *Streptococcus faecalis*. Less commonly, *Proteus vulgaris*, *Pseudomonas pyocyanea*, *Neisseria gonorrhea*, *Salmonella typhi*,

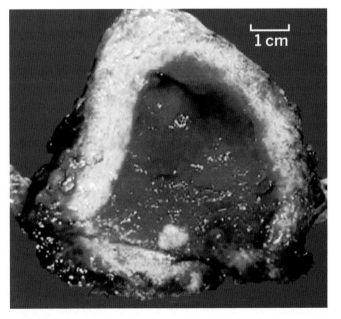

Fig. 5.59 Bladder of a patient with spinal cord injury with chronic and acute cystitis.

Microscopically, the urothelium may be hyperplastic or metaplastic. Ulceration may be extensive, and the surface of the ulcer may be covered by a fibrinous exudate in which neutrophils are mixed with bacterial colonies. Early in the infection, edema is often the predominant finding. Initially, leukocytes are not numerous, but as the infection progresses, they become prominent in the lamina propria. In severe cases, suppuration is followed by abscess formation, which may involve the entire thickness of the bladder wall. When the inflammatory reaction is less intense and more indolent, the process may be characterized as subacute. In such cases the mucosa is usually denuded, the lamina propria is edematous, and eosinophils may be prominent.

In chronic cystitis, the urothelium may be hyperplastic, thin, or denuded, and ulceration may occur. The urothelium may display reactive atypia. Granulation tissue may replace parts of the lamina propria and muscularis propria, eventually becoming densely fibrotic.

Gangrene

Gangrene may arise as a consequence of circulatory compromise, debilitating systemic illness (e.g., uncontrolled diabetes mellitus or carcinoma), vascular insufficiency, or instillation of corrosive chemicals.[274-278] Gangrene usually begins in the mucosa, and the necrotic tissue is sloughed to expose deeper structures (Fig. 5.60). Occasionally the muscularis propria is deeply penetrated and gangrene extends to the serosa. Deposition of mineral salts from the urine may give the sloughed material a gritty texture.

Encrusted Cystitis

When urea-splitting bacteria alkalinize the urine and inorganic salts are deposited in a damaged mucosa (Fig. 5.61), the term *encrusted cystitis* is applied.[279-286] Encrusted cystitis is most common in women and may occur in association with conditions in which inflammation or trauma damages the mucosa. In recent years, an increasing number of cases of encrusted cystitis have been diagnosed, especially in immunosuppressed patients such as renal transplant recipients. Numerous species of bacteria have been demonstrated in this infection, but *Corynebacterium* group D2 (*Corynebacterium urealyticum*) is currently isolated in most cases.[287-289] Urine culture in selective media and prolonged incubation are necessary to isolate *Corynebacterium urealyticum*.[290]

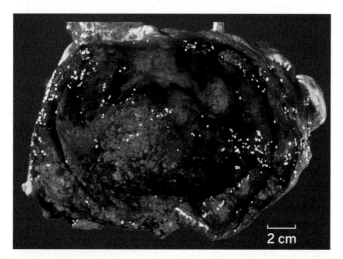

Fig. 5.60 Gangrenous cystitis from a patient with *Klebsiella* sepsis. The mucosa is diffusely necrotic.

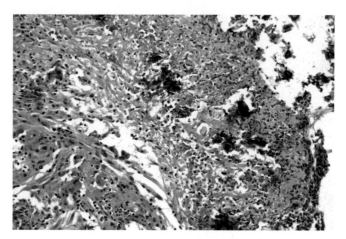

Fig. 5.61 Encrusted cystitis with deposits of calcium salts.

Patients report longstanding dysuria, frequency, and sometimes hematuria. The urine contains gritty material, blood, mucus, and pus. When the salts are rich in calcium, the deposits may be visible on radiographs.[285,291] Cystoscopically, the lesions are usually multiple and have a gritty appearance. Rarely, the entire mucosa is involved. Histologically, the lesions are covered with a shaggy coat of fibrin mixed with calcified necrotic debris and inflammatory cells. The underlying tissue may be quite inflamed early in the course of the disease, but later, inflammatory cells become scant and the lamina propria becomes fibrotic. Mineral salts may also be deposited on the surface of urothelial carcinoma, particularly in areas of necrosis or fulguration.[291] Treatment is based on adapted antibiotic therapy, acidification of urine, and excision of calcified plaques. The consequences of treatment failure are serious and can result in graft nephrectomy in kidney transplant recipients.[289]

Emphysematous Cystitis

In some cases of cystitis, gas-filled blebs are seen on cystoscopy or at gross examination, a condition termed *emphysematous cystitis*.[292-301] Emphysematous cystitis is more common in women than men. Approximately half of the patients have diabetes, usually also with bacterial infections with *E. coli* or *Aerobacter aerogenes*.[302] Less frequently, the infection is fungal.[297,301] Other predisposing conditions include cystoscopy, trauma, fistula, and urinary stasis. The blebs range from 0.5 to 3 mm in diameter and may be present throughout the mucosa. Histologically, the blebs are cavities lined by flattened cells and surrounded by thin septa in the lamina propria. Occasionally they extend into the muscularis propria.

Other Rare Lesions

Rare cases of Langerhans cell histiocytosis, crystal storing histiocytosis, and mesonephric rests or hyperplasia of the mesonephric remnants involving the bladder have been reported.[303]

Urachal Abscess

Most bacterial infections of the urachus are associated with a urachal malformation or cyst.[304-306] Many of these develop into abscesses (Fig. 5.62) that may drain into the bladder or through the umbilicus. Rupture into the peritoneal cavity can cause severe peritonitis, a serious complication. When the abscess is large and associated with much inflammation and fibrosis in surrounding tissues, it may be difficult or impossible to determine precisely the

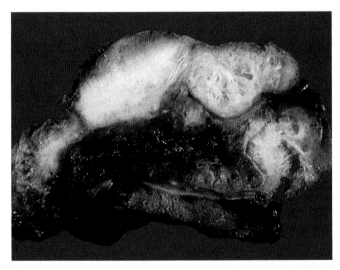

Fig. 5.62 Urachal abscess. *Arrow* indicates outlet of urachus in the bladder mucosa.

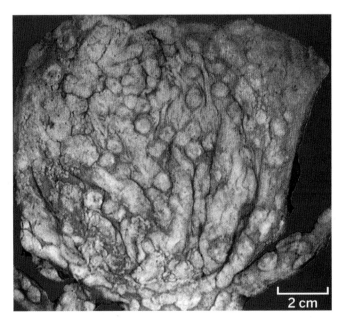

Fig. 5.63 Malakoplakia of the bladder and ureters.

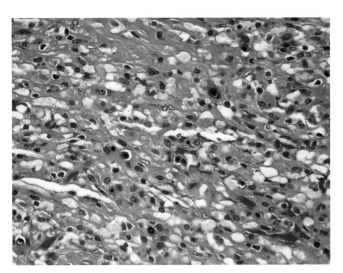

Fig. 5.64 Malakoplakia.

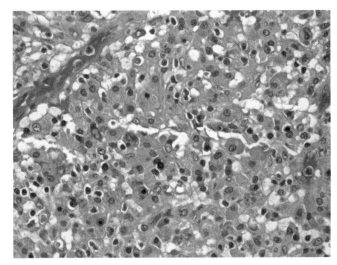

Fig. 5.65 Malakoplakia. Note von Hansemann cells in the lamina propria.

nature of the underlying urachal abnormality. The combination of antibiotic therapy with surgical excision of the urachal malformation and abscess is usually curative.[307] On rare occasions, urachal abscess may be caused by tuberculous, echinococcal, or actinomycotic infections.[27]

Malakoplakia

First described in 1902 and 1903 by Michaelis and Gutmann and by von Hansemann, respectively, malakoplakia occurs most frequently in the urinary bladder, where it is visible as yellow-white soft raised plaques on the mucosal surface.[308–310] It was this appearance, combined with a reluctance to speculate on the pathogenesis of the disorder, that prompted von Hansemann to combine the Greek roots for plaque (*plakos*) and soft (*malakos*) to coin the term *malakoplakia*.[311] Urinary tract malakoplakia primarily affects women (more than 75% of cases) and has a peak incidence in the fifth decade of life.[311,312] It occasionally occurs in children.[313] Malakoplakia is an uncommon granulomatous process that results from impairment of the capacity of mononuclear cells to kill phagocytosed bacteria.[314,315] It is usually associated with infection by coliform organisms. Most patients present with the usual symptoms of urinary tract infection, including hematuria. *E. coli* is most frequently cultured from the urine, but *P. vulgaris*, *A. aerogenes*, *K. pneumoniae*, and α-hemolytic streptococci have also been isolated. Despite this, bacteria have rarely been identified within the lesions of malakoplakia without the use of transmission electron microscopy.[316,317]

Grossly, the lesions are usually multiple, soft yellow or yellow-brown plaques (Fig. 5.63). Often there is a central dimple and a rim of congestion about the plaque. Lesions larger than 2 cm are unusual. In some cases the lesions are nodular, but rarely large and polypoid.

Microscopically, there is an accumulation of histiocytes with granular eosinophilic cytoplasm (von Hansemann histiocytes) in the superficial lamina propria beneath the urothelium, which is usually intact (Fig. 5.64). The histiocytes contain the characteristic intracytoplasmic inclusions known as Michaelis–Gutmann bodies. These are typically spherical, 5 to 8 μm, concentrically laminated bodies with a bull's-eye appearance (Fig. 5.65). Often they are basophilic but also may be pale and difficult to see. They always

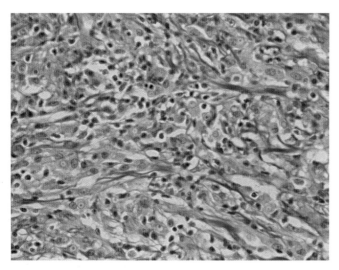

Fig. 5.66 Malakoplakia. The von Kossa stain for calcium highlights the Michaelis–Gutmann bodies.

contain calcium and sometimes iron salts so the von Kossa (Fig. 5.66) and Perl Prussian blue stains highlight them. They also react with the periodic acid–Schiff stain, but so does the cytoplasm of the von Hansemann histiocytes (Fig. 5.67), so this technique is less helpful than staining for calcium. Early in the disease, Michaelis–Gutmann bodies may be scant and very difficult to appreciate in sections stained with hematoxylin and eosin. Thus when there is an infiltrate of histiocytes in the bladder, a section should be stained for calcium to find inapparent Michaelis–Gutmann bodies. These bodies are required for the diagnosis, so it is possible that there is an early prediagnostic phase of the disease in which there is insufficient calcification to make them detectable. In some cases, there is abundant granulation tissue, extensive fibrosis, or a dense infiltrate of acute and chronic inflammatory cells that may obscure the von Hansemann histiocytes and Michaelis–Gutmann bodies. Late in the disease, there may be extensive fibrosis and few Michaelis–Gutmann bodies.

Ultrastructural and immunohistochemical studies have shown that the cytoplasm of von Hansemann histiocytes contains many phagolysosomes in which there are fragments of bacterial cell walls.[318] It appears that Michaelis–Gutmann bodies form when the phagolysosomes fuse and calcium is transported across the

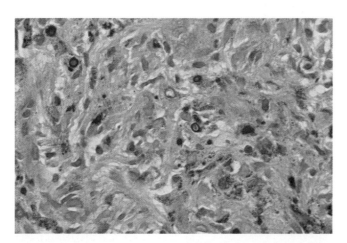

Fig. 5.67 Malakoplakia. The von Hansemann histiocytes react with the periodic acid–Schiff stain.

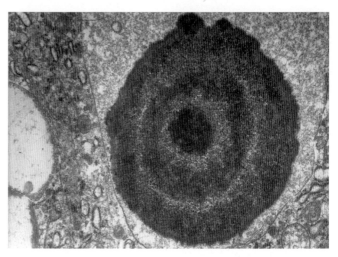

Fig. 5.68 Ultrastructural appearance of a Michaelis–Gutmann body.

phagolysosomal membranes and forms hydroxyapatite crystals with phosphate from the bacterial cell walls. The bodies enlarge over time, producing the typical laminated structure. Ultrastructurally, Michaelis–Gutmann bodies range from 5 to 10 μm in diameter (Fig. 5.68).[319] At the center is a dense crystalline core surrounded by a homogeneous zone that is not crystalline but rather granular or composed of myelin figures.

Tuberculous Cystitis

Tuberculous cystitis is almost always caused by *Mycobacterium tuberculosis*; *Mycobacterium bovis* accounts for only about 3% of cases.[320–322] Tuberculous cystitis is almost always secondary to renal tuberculosis from which organisms in infected urine implant in the bladder. In one study, 66% of patients with surgically treated renal tuberculosis had vesical tuberculosis.[323] Some cases occurring in men appear to be secondary to genital infection, and spread of the infection is directly along the mucosa. Frequency, urgency, hematuria, and dysuria are common symptoms.

Early in the infection the lesions are in the region of the ureteral orifices and consist of marked mucosal congestion, sometimes with edema. These lesions may progress to form 1- to 3-mm tubercles, or may ulcerate and become covered by friable necrotic material. Initially the tubercles are sharply circumscribed, firm, and solid. As they enlarge, they coalesce and ulcerate.

The tuberculous granuloma in which central caseous necrosis is surrounded by multinucleated giant cells, plasma cells, and lymphocytes is the characteristic histologic lesion. Acid-fast or auramine-rhodamine–stained sections will usually disclose mycobacteria.

Chronic tuberculous cystitis may result in a small, scarred, low-capacity bladder. The ureteral orifices may be distorted and obstructed, causing hydronephrosis and hydroureter. Rarely the infection penetrates the wall of the bladder, causing peritonitis or a fistula.

Fungal and Actinomycotic Cystitis

Fungal cystitis is uncommon and most often is caused by *Candida albicans*.[324-326] Infection may ascend the urethra or may be hematogenous. Ascending infection is usually limited to the trigone. Most candidal cystitis cases occur in debilitated patients or those receiving antibiotic therapy. Many patients have diabetes, and most are women. Nocturia, constant pain, and marked frequency are typical symptoms. The urine is usually turbid and bloody.

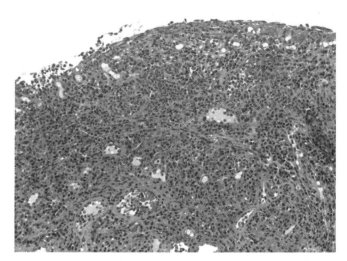

Fig. 5.69 Candidal cystitis. Fungus is present in the inflammatory exudate and debris.

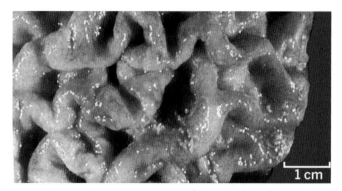

Fig. 5.70 Condyloma of the bladder with prominent folds.

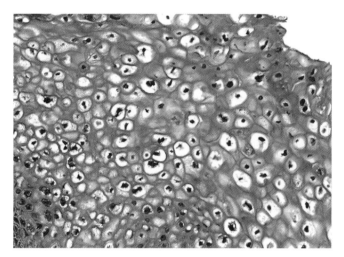

Fig. 5.71 Koilocytes in the condyloma of the bladder.

The lesions are typically slightly raised, sharply demarcated white plaques with irregular shapes. Occasionally a fungus ball may form in the lumen of the bladder. Microscopically, there is ulceration and inflammation of the lamina propria. The typical hyphae and budding yeast forms may be seen in routine sections (Fig. 5.69) or with periodic acid–Schiff or Gomori methenamine silver stains.

Rare cases of fungal cystitis caused by *Aspergillus* species and other fungi have been reported.[325,327]

Vesical actinomycosis is rare in the general population but complicates actinomycosis of the ovary or fallopian tube in about 10% of cases.[328] Symptoms are nonspecific. Microscopically, the bladder wall is focally or diffusely thickened, and there is often continuity with the lesions in adjacent organs. The infection may form a mass simulating a neoplasm. The mucosa may be edematous or ulcerated, and if the infection is transmural, a fistula may form. Microscopically, there is abundant granulation tissue within which are small abscesses containing colonies of *Actinomyces* (sulfur granules).

Viral Cystitis

Human Papillomavirus

A few dozen cases of condyloma acuminatum of the bladder have been reported.[329-337] There is a male predominance of approximately 2:1. Patients range in age from early adulthood to old age, but most are younger than 50 years. Most patients, many of whom are immunocompromised, have had condylomata of the urethra, vulva, vagina, anus, or perineum, but some have had condylomata only in the bladder. In some immunocompromised patients the lesions have been particularly difficult to eradicate and may rarely progress to invasive disease.[338,339]

Cystoscopy usually shows a solitary lesion in the bladder neck or trigone. These appear papillary, and the clinical differential diagnosis includes papillary carcinoma and other papillary lesions of the vesical mucosa. Alternatively the mucosa may have prominent folds and scattered white flecks (Fig. 5.70).[331]

Microscopically, the lesions show the characteristic features of condylomata including koilocytotic cells with abundant clear cytoplasm (Fig. 5.71) and wrinkled hyperchromatic nuclei. These features distinguish the lesions from the rare squamous papilloma and papillary squamous cell carcinoma of the bladder.

Other Viruses

Adenovirus is recognized as an important cause of hemorrhagic cystitis, especially in children.[340] Otherwise healthy children may be affected, as well as children after bone marrow transplantation. Adenovirus types 11 and 21 are most frequently identified.[341-345] Papovavirus also causes hemorrhagic cystitis in children and adults.[346] Herpes simplex type 2 has caused hemorrhagic cystitis in a few patients, and herpes zoster has also caused cystitis.[347,348] Cytomegalovirus also is sometimes seen in the bladder, particularly in immunosuppressed patients.[349] BK virus infection has been seen in association with posttransplant urothelial carcinoma.[350,351] Polyomavirus infection of the urothelium may mimic urothelial carcinoma in situ (Fig. 5.72).

Schistosomiasis

Schistosomiasis is the fourth most prevalent disease in the world and the leading cause of hematuria.[352] In humans the trematode *Schistosoma hematobium* commonly resides in the paravesical veins and causes urinary schistosomiasis, which also is known as *bilharziasis*.[353,354] The adult forms of these flat worms are dioecious, living as pairs in veins, with the male surrounding the female. Estimates of adult life spans vary from 2 to 20 years, and each pair can produce up to 200 eggs per day. In endemic areas, children have the highest incidence of infection, but it is adults who suffer the severe effects of chronic infection.

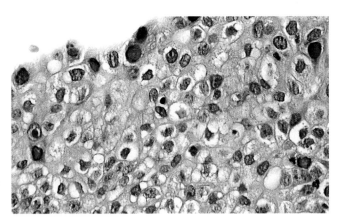

Fig. 5.72 Polyoma virus infection in the urothelium in a patient with kidney transplantation. Notice characteristic nuclear inclusion in urothelial cells.

Schistosomiasis has various clinical manifestations, but the underlying process begins with the deposition of eggs in small veins and venules. Subsequently the eggs may pass into the lumina of hollow organs, such as the bladder, or become trapped in the walls of viscera, where they produce a granulomatous response and may be destroyed or calcified. Alternatively, they may enter the circulation from the small veins and embolize other sites. For unknown reasons the predominant site for oviposition by *S. hematobium* is the venous systems of the lower urinary tract. *S. hematobium* deposits eggs in clusters, causing a patchy distribution of lesions.[355] The eggs are not acid-fast in histologic sections, whereas those of other common human schistosomes, *S. mansoni, S. intercalatum,* and *S. japonicum,* are acid-fast. *S. mattheei,* which usually infects animals but may cause urinary schistosomiasis in humans, also is not acid-fast. In humans the eggs of *S. hematobium* are intermediate in size between those of *S. mansoni* and *S. japonicum.*

Schistosomiasis may be categorized as active or inactive. The active form is characterized by the presence of active pairs of flatworms depositing eggs, which elicit a strong granulomatous response (Fig. 5.73). Polypoid inflammatory masses may obstruct the ureters or the bladder outlet.[355] The number of ova in the urine correlates with the burden of eggs in the bladder wall, and the active stage is most readily diagnosed by examination of the urine. The inactive form occurs after the worms have died and there are no viable eggs in urine or tissue. However, eggs remain in the tissue, and high concentrations of calcified eggs may be detected

radiographically. Evaluation of the quantity of ova in tissue requires special digestion techniques.[356-359] In the inactive phase the patient is not infectious.

The principal nonneoplastic manifestations of schistosomiasis in the bladder are polyps and ulcers. In most cases the trigone and ureteral orifices are the sites of the lesions, which may lead to bladder neck obstruction.[300,360] The deposits of ova are heaviest in the submucosa.[95] During active disease, heavy burdens of eggs produce multiple large inflammatory polyps, which may obstruct the ureteral orifices and may bleed sufficiently to cause anemia or clot retention.[361-363] Obstruction may lead to stone formation in the kidneys, ureters, and bladder.[364,365] In inactive schistosomiasis the polyps are fibrocalcific. In a small percentage of cases the polyps are composed of hyperplastic epithelium that appears more villous than polypoid. The inflammation in the bladder also gives rise to polypoid cystitis, biopsy specimens of which may not contain any eggs. In the early active stage, ulcers rarely form when a necrotic polyp detaches. Ulcers are more common in the chronic stage, when large numbers of eggs (more than 250,000/g of bladder tissue) are present. These constantly painful ulcers are often in the posterior bladder wall of young adults and have stellate or ovoid contours.[366] Metaplastic changes, including keratinizing squamous metaplasia and intestinal metaplasia, are also common.[352] The bladder mucosa may also contain raised granules known as *bilharzial tubercles.*[367] These may calcify to form the classic sandy patches. Neoplastic complications of schistosomiasis are discussed in Chapter 6.

Calculi

Bladder stones are most common in men with bladder outlet obstruction (Fig. 5.74) and in children in underdeveloped countries. Most are free in the bladder, but occasionally calculi form about a suture after surgery (Fig. 5.75).[368] The symptoms are similar to those of bladder outlet obstruction, and include hesitancy, frequency, and nocturia. Other symptoms include hematuria, dysuria, and suprapubic pain radiating down the penis. Radiography or cystoscopy is usually diagnostic of bladder calculus. Because bladder stones may be composed of radiolucent uric acid, cystoscopy is the most definitive diagnostic procedure.

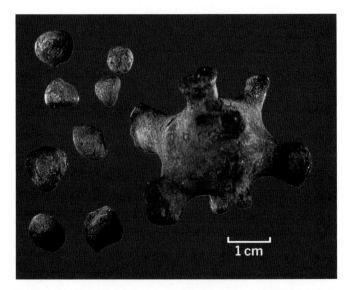

Fig. 5.74 Bladder calculi from a man with obstructive prostatic hyperplasia.

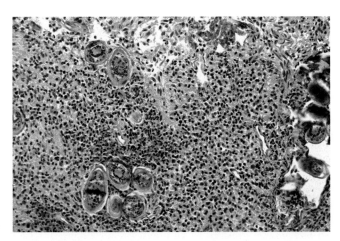

Fig. 5.73 Schistosomiasis, active form with numerous ova.

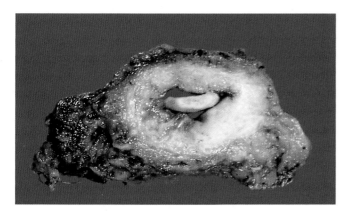

Fig. 5.75 Free calculus in the bladder of a patient with invasive bladder carcinoma.

Bladder calculi were common in children in Europe before 1800 and remain relatively common in some parts of Asia and the Middle East. Most patients are boys younger than 10 years, and the stones are composed of calcium oxalate and ammonium acid urate. Patients usually do not have renal stones. A diet low in protein and minerals, along with low fluid intake, seem to be factors that promote stone formation in these children. In North America and Europe, only 2% to 3% of patients with bladder calculi are children. Most of these patients also have renal or ureteral calculi, and their stones are composed of calcium oxalate, calcium phosphate, or a mixture of the two. Although most of these children have bacterial infections, the causative organisms do not often produce urease. Children with a history of multiple urologic procedures are more likely to have struvite stones and infections with *Proteus* species.

Polyps and Other Mass Lesions

Ectopic Prostate

Polyps composed of prostatic epithelium resembling those more commonly seen in the prostatic urethra rarely occur in the bladder.[369-373] Reported cases have occurred in men from 20 to 67 years of age, and hematuria has been the most consistent symptom. About two-thirds of the lesions arise in the trigone, and the architecture varies from papillary to polypoid. The stroma contains prostatic glands, and the surface is covered by columnar epithelium or urothelium (Fig. 5.76). Immunohistochemistry for PSA, prostate-specific membrane antigen (PSMA), and PAP confirms the prostatic

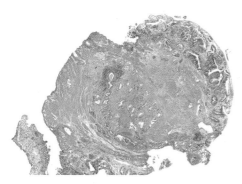

Fig. 5.76 Ectopic prostate tissue (prostate-type polyp) in the bladder.

character of the glands and columnar cells. Prostatic hyperplasia may also expand into the bladder lumen as a polypoid mass.[374-376]

Other Polyps

Fibroepithelial polyps of the bladder are rare and resemble their more common counterpart in the ureter.[377-380] They are distinguished from polypoid cystitis by being solitary, with a more fibrous core and a paucity of inflammatory cells. Rare cases of collagen polyps (collagenoma) resulting from the accumulation of injected collagen in the bladder to control stress incontinence have been reported.[381]

Hamartoma

Hamartoma of the bladder is a rare (fewer than a dozen reported cases) polypoid mass (Fig. 5.77) composed of epithelial elements resembling von Brunn nests, cystitis glandularis, or cystitis cystica distributed irregularly in a stroma that may be muscular, fibrous, or edematous.[382-386] Occasional cases have intestinal metaplasia of the glands, small tubules resembling renal tubules, or markedly cellular stroma.

Amyloidosis

More than 100 cases of primary amyloidosis of the bladder have been reported.[387-398] The lesions appear throughout adulthood and are equally common in both sexes. In most cases, the deposits are limited to the bladder, but in some the ureters and urethra have also been involved. Hematuria is almost always the presenting symptom.[399] On cystoscopy the lesions range from sessile and ulcerated to nodular or polypoid, and are often mistaken for carcinoma.[121] In about 25% of cases, there are multiple lesions. In the Mayo Clinic series of 31 cases of primary amyloidosis of the bladder, 24 patients had immunoglobulin light chain and 3 had transthyretin-related amyloid. Although local recurrences were common, none of the patients experienced systemic amyloidosis.[400] Histologically, the amyloid deposits are predominantly in the lamina propria and muscularis propria (Fig. 5.78). Vascular involvement is less prominent. A foreign body giant cell reaction may be present adjacent to the deposits, and rarely the deposits become calcified. Congo red or thioflavin T stains bladder amyloid, which is most frequently AL type (immunoglobulin light chain).

Secondary involvement of the bladder is rare in systemic amyloidosis.[401] Reported cases are associated with rheumatoid arthritis,

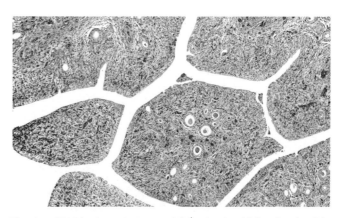

Fig. 5.77 Bladder hamartoma consisting of polypoid fronds of cellular stroma containing small tubular structures lined by epithelium.

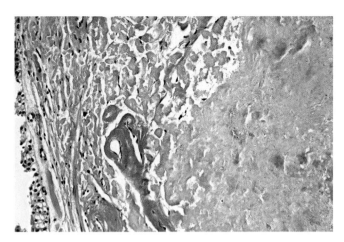

Fig. 5.78 Amyloid fills the lamina propria in this biopsy specimen.

Crohn disease, ankylosing spondylitis, myeloma, and familial Mediterranean fever. Hematuria is universal and often very severe.[399,401] Although primary localized amyloidosis often presents with hematuria, it is generally much less severe than that associated with secondary amyloidosis. Cystoscopically, there is diffuse erythema, sometimes with petechiae or necrosis. Histologically, the amyloid is mainly in the blood vessels; occasionally there are lesser deposits in the lamina propria.

Proteinoma (Tamm-Horsfall Protein Deposits)

Tamm-Horsfall protein (uromodulin) may accumulate in the bladder, where it produces a tumor-like proteinoma, with waxy eosinophilic extracellular material or homogeneous eosinophilic flecks in areas of fibrinous exudate. It has no clinical significance (Fig. 5.79). Rare cases may simulate neoplasia mainly when occurring in the upper urinary tract.[402]

Fallopian Tube Prolapse

In one instance, portions of fallopian tube prolapsed into a vesical fistula that developed after surgery, mimicking a bladder neoplasm endoscopically.[403]

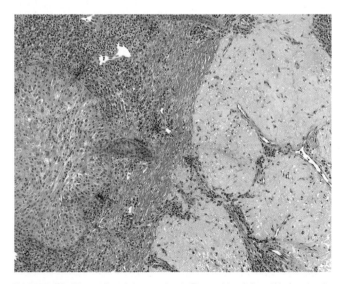

Fig. 5.79 Bladder wall proteinoma due to Tamm-Horsfall protein (uromodulin) deposit in the context of severe chronic cystitis.

Postoperative Spindle Cell Nodule

The term *postoperative spindle cell nodule* was coined by Proppe et al. in 1984 for a proliferative spindle cell lesion occurring in the lower urinary tract and female genital tract within 120 days of surgery at the site where the lesions arise. Subsequently, others have reported identical lesions.[404–408] At cystoscopy the bladder lesions are nodular (Fig. 5.80) and described as a "heaped-up tumor" and a "friable vegetant mass." The possibility of confusion with malignancy is heightened by the microscopic examination, which shows interlacing fascicles (Fig. 5.81) of mitotically active spindle cells (Fig. 5.82) resembling leiomyosarcoma or some other spindle cell sarcoma. Other histologic features include delicate vasculature, scattered inflammatory cells, small foci of hemorrhage, edema, and focal myxoid change. Although there may be many mitotic figures, the nuclei usually show little pleomorphism or hyperchromasia.

The original and subsequent reports have shown that postoperative spindle cell nodules are benign reactive proliferations that resolve spontaneously or with medical therapy and must be distinguished from sarcoma. Well-differentiated leiomyosarcoma is the most important consideration in this differential diagnosis. This

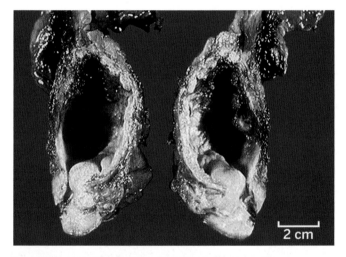

Fig. 5.80 Postoperative spindle cell nodule in bladder neck.

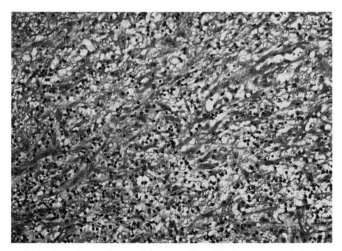

Fig. 5.81 Postoperative spindle cell nodule composed of cellular bundles of spindle cells.

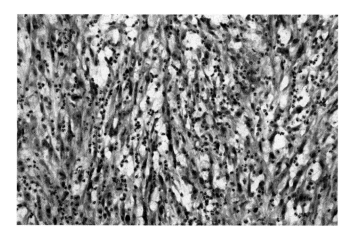

Fig. 5.82 Postoperative spindle cell nodule with mitotic figure.

distinction may be very difficult because both postoperative spindle cell nodule and well-differentiated leiomyosarcoma have similarly bland nuclei, may infiltrate the muscularis propria, and have similar numbers of mitotic figures. The prominent array of delicate blood vessels seen in many postoperative spindle cell nodules is not a common feature of leiomyosarcoma. Myxoid change may be seen in both and is not helpful unless extensive, a finding more common in leiomyosarcoma. The clinical history of recent surgery at the site powerfully suggests postoperative spindle cell nodule. In these cases, follow-up with cystoscopy and additional biopsies are warranted. The proliferating cells are immunoreactive for AE1/AE3, CAM5.2, and vimentin in some cases.[409]

Inflammatory Myofibroblastic Tumor (Pseudosarcomatous Fibromyxoid Tumor; Inflammatory Pseudotumor)

Patients without a history of recent surgery may also have benign proliferative spindle cell lesions that mimic sarcoma.[410] A variety of terms have been applied to these, but inflammatory myofibroblastic tumor is emerging as the preferred term.[35,264,408,411-421] Most patients range in age from 20 to 50 years, and there appears to be a slight predominance of women. Gross hematuria is the most common presenting symptom.

Grossly, the lesions have ranged from pedunculated masses protruding into the bladder cavity (Fig. 5.83) to small nodules or ulcers in the mucosa. Usually the lesions are solitary, 2- to 5-cm polyps with broad bases. Some lesions are sessile and deeply infiltrate the muscularis propria (Fig. 5.84). The cut surface may be gelatinous or mucoid.

Histologically, inflammatory myofibroblastic tumor is typically composed of spindle cells arranged in a widely spaced, haphazard pattern in a myxoid matrix containing a prominent network of small blood vessels (Fig. 5.85).[417] A second pattern that is sometimes seen is more cellular with spindle cells arranged in fascicles with variable amounts of collagen between them (Fig. 5.86). In both patterns the spindle cells are similar with long bipolar eosinophilic or amphophilic cytoplasmic processes. In the myxoid pattern, stellate and polygonal cells are also present. The nuclei are large and occasionally multiple. In most cases there are fewer than two mitotic figures per 10 high-power fields, but occasional cases have more.[417] The myxoid pattern (Fig. 5.87) usually contains a sparse inflammatory infiltrate, whereas in the second pattern, lymphocytes and plasma cells may be prominent. An example of the

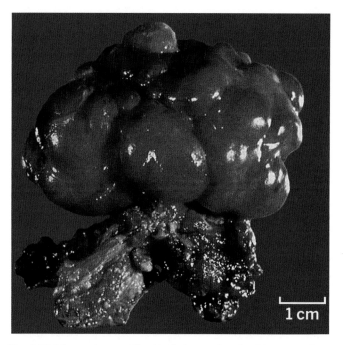

Fig. 5.83 Inflammatory myofibroblastic tumor. A polypoid mass projects into the bladder lumen.

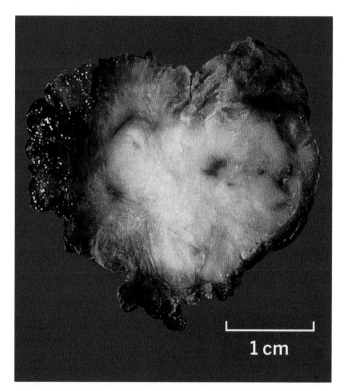

Fig. 5.84 Inflammatory myofibroblastic tumor. The cut surface shows involvement of the full thickness of the bladder wall.

second pattern has been reported as a plasma cell granuloma.[422] Eosinophils are often common in both patterns. Infiltration of the muscularis propria is common, and the process may extend into perivesical fat. Anaplastic lymphoma kinase 1 (ALK1) staining is often positive in these tumors (Fig. 5.88).

The main differential diagnostic consideration for inflammatory myofibroblastic tumor is malignancy, particularly myxoid

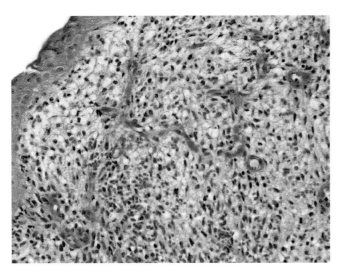

Fig. 5.85 Inflammatory myofibroblastic tumor showing delicate blood vessels in a background of spindle cells.

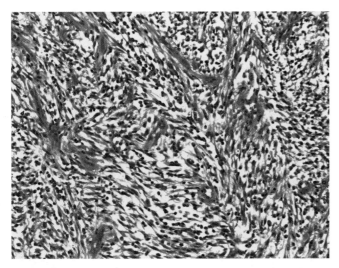

Fig. 5.86 Inflammatory myofibroblastic tumor composed of fascicles of spindle cells.

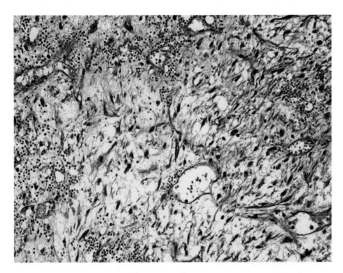

Fig. 5.87 Inflammatory myofibroblastic tumor with myxoid areas.

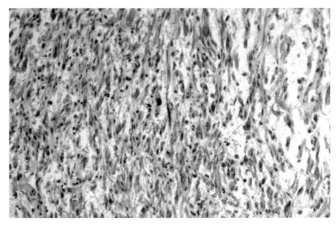

Fig. 5.88 ALK1 staining.

sarcomatoid carcinoma and other sarcomas including myxoid leiomyosarcoma.[35,408,421,423] Inflammation and vascularity are more prominent in inflammatory myofibroblastic tumor than in leiomyosarcoma, and the cellularity is more variable, although a destructively infiltrative margin favors leiomyosarcoma. Inflammatory myofibroblastic tumor also may invade the muscularis propria. The most reliable criteria to separate sarcoma from inflammatory myofibroblastic tumor are nuclear atypia and the presence of necrosis at the tumor–detrusor muscle interface in muscle-invasive cases.[419] Sarcoma also shows less prominent microvasculature, less variable cellularity, consistently less than one mitotic figure per 10 high-power fields, and predominant acute inflammation without plasma cells.[417,419,424] Immunohistochemical evidence of smooth muscle actin, desmin, and other muscle-specific differentiation favors leiomyosarcoma, but this is not absolutely reliable. Immunohistochemically, the spindle cells of the inflammatory myofibroblastic tumor are strongly positive for vimentin, variable for smooth muscle actin, and focally for cytokeratin (Fig. 5.89).[408,425-427] Fluorescence in situ hybridization, with translocation of the *ALK* gene or cytoplasmic immunohistochemical staining for cytoplasmic ALK protein, is present in 40% to 89% of inflammatory myofibroblastic tumors.[408,425,428-431] To date, ALK1 staining or translocation of the *ALK1* gene has not been identified in any case of bladder leiomyosarcoma or rhabdomyosarcoma. However, spindle cell lesions in sites other than the urinary bladder may display *ALK1*

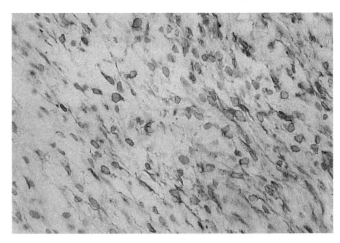

Fig. 5.89 Cytokeratin immunoreactivity in inflammatory myofibroblastic Tumor.

expression, which has been reported in 40% of inflammatory myo-fibroblastic tumors, 19% of rhabdomyosarcomas, and 10% of leiomyosarcomas at other sites (see Chapter 6). The expression of GATA3, as well as high-molecular-weight cytokeratins, CK5/6 and p63, favors sarcomatoid carcinoma, whereas immunoreactivity for smooth muscle actin and desmin with overall absence of other markers would suggest leiomyosarcoma in the proper clinical context.[17,409]

Müllerian Lesions

Endometriosis

The bladder is the most common site of urinary tract involvement in endometriosis, but only about 1% of women with endometriosis have bladder involvement.[35,64,432-440] As many as 50% of these patients have a history of pelvic surgery, and approximately 12% lack evidence of endometriosis at any other site. The average age is approximately 35 years. Frequency, dysuria, and hematuria are the most common symptoms, but more than 50% of patients have no vesical symptoms. Endometriosis of the muscularis propria may give symptoms similar to those of interstitial cystitis.[441] There is a palpable suprapubic mass in almost 50% of cases, and this may undergo catamenial enlargement. Rarely, endometriosis has been reported in postmenopausal women treated with estrogen and in men treated with estrogen for prostate cancer.[442-447] At cystoscopy the lesions usually appear as congested, edematous mucosal elevations overlying blue, blue-black, or red-brown cysts. Grossly, a hemorrhagic ill-defined mass may project into the bladder lumen (Fig. 5.90). The overlying urothelium may be intact or eroded. If the lesions are limited to the muscularis propria (Fig. 5.91) or serosa, the mucosa may be normal. Fibrosis and hyperplastic muscle around the lesions may thicken the bladder wall. Microscopically, the lesions resemble endometriosis as seen elsewhere. In some cases not all of the glands are surrounded by endometrial stroma, and in some foci, stroma is absent.[433] Positivity immunohistochemistry for estrogen receptors (ER), progesterone receptors (PR), CK7, and CA125 in the epithelial component, with CD10 expression in the stromal component, is characteristic of endometriosis.[438] A case of malignant transformation of endometriosis of bladder has been reported.[448]

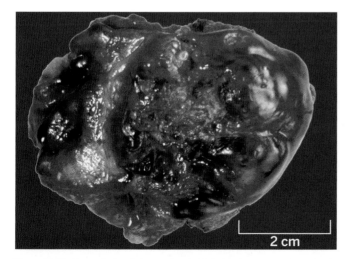

Fig. 5.90 Endometriosis. A hemorrhagic ill-defined mass projects in the bladder lumen.

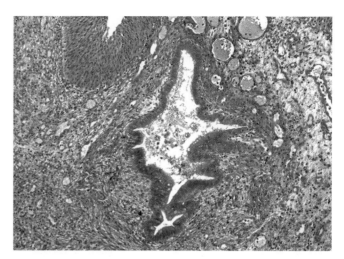

Fig. 5.91 Endometriosis. Endometrioid glands surrounded by endometrial stroma.

Endocervicosis

Endocervicosis of the bladder is less common than endometriosis.[35,64,350,449,450] Patients typically present in their fourth and fifth decades with symptoms such as suprapubic pain, dysuria, frequency, or hematuria and may have catamenial exacerbation of symptoms. They often have a history of cesarean section. Most lesions are in the muscularis propria, but the mucosa (Fig. 5.92A) and adventitia also may be involved. In endocervicosis, there is a haphazard proliferation of irregularly shaped mucinous glands in the bladder wall (Fig. 5.92B). The epithelium lining the glands consists of a single layer of columnar cells with abundant pale cytoplasm that reacts with periodic acid–Schiff and mucicarmine stains.[451] Ciliated cells often are interspersed among the mucinous cells. When the glands are dilated, the epithelium is cuboidal or flattened. The glandular lumina usually contain mucus. Ruptured glands with extravasated mucus and a stromal reaction may be seen. The most common of the benign Müllerian glandular lesions in women, endosalpingiosis, is, enigmatically, the one least often seen in the bladder. Indeed it has only recently been described.[452] Vesical endosalpingiosis consists of numerous tubal-type glands (Fig. 5.93A) lined at least focally by ciliated cells (Fig. 5.93B). The Müllerian epithelium may replace the urothelium of the mucosa and cover polypoid intraluminal projections (Fig. 5.94). In some cases a mixture of several different types of Müllerian epithelium is present, and the term *müllerianosis* may be appropriate.[35,452,453] CDX2⁻/ER⁺ is the typical immunohistochemistry panel in endocervicosis. This might also be useful in differentiating endocervicosis from intestinal metaplasia (CDX2⁺/ER⁻) in small bladder biopsies.

Müllerian Cyst

In men, Müllerian duct cysts usually lie between the bladder and rectum, and may involve the posterior wall of the bladder.[454-456] Patients usually present with irritative bladder symptoms, and clinical evaluation reveals a midline supraprostatic mass. Grossly, the cyst is unilocular or multilocular and filled with clear or hemorrhagic fluid. Microscopically, the cyst lining is often lost throughout much of its area, but a layer of Müllerian epithelium can usually be found at least focally. In contrast with seminal vesicle cysts, spermatozoa are absent from Müllerian duct cysts.

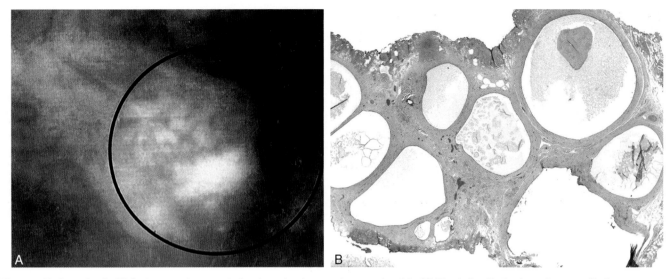

Fig. 5.92 Endocervicosis. (A) Cystoscopy shows vesical endocervicosis as a submucosal nodule. (B) Glands lined by benign columnar epithelium are present in the muscularis propria.

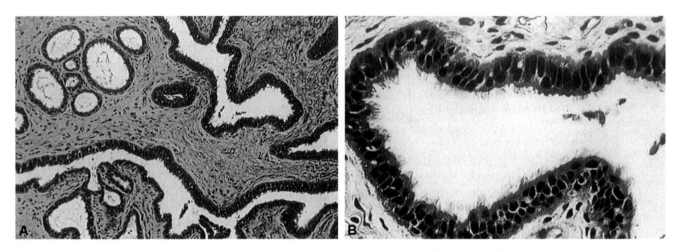

Fig. 5.93 Endosalpingiosis. (A) Glands, some of them branching, are lined by tubal-type epithelium. (B) Higher magnification demonstrates cilia on the surfaces of the epithelial cells.

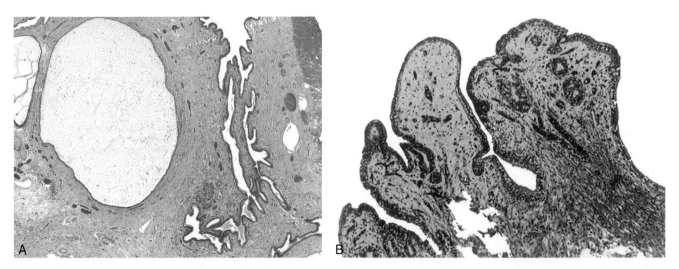

Fig. 5.94 Müllerianosis. (A) The lesion is designated müllerianosis when both endocervicosis and endometriosis are present. (B) Polyps lined by Müllerian epithelium protrude into the bladder lumen. Epithelia of endocervical, endometrial, and tubal types were present in this case.

Müllerian sinus lined by mucus-secreting epithelium connecting the posterolateral wall of the bladder with the broad ligament is a rare lesion.[457]

Malformations

Agenesis

Agenesis of the bladder is rare, and only a few dozen cases have been recorded, almost all of them in girls.[458-463] Agenesis results from failure of separation of the ureters from the wolffian ducts. In this situation the ureters enter the Müllerian tract or posterior urethra. Alternatively the urorectal septum fails to form and the cloaca remains. Usually there is ureteral obstruction with megaureter and hydronephrosis. When development of the distal ureters fails, the trigone of the bladder does not develop. Vesical agenesis is strongly associated with sirenomelia, a syndrome characterized by fusion of the lower extremities and other anomalies. Most such cases have no ureters, lending support to the concept that vesical agenesis is related to failure of ureteral development.

Exstrophy

Exstrophy (incomplete closure) of the bladder and its associated malformations have long been recognized, and the 1855 description and review by Duncan can hardly be improved on today.[464] Exstrophy is more common than agenesis and occurs in approximately 1 of 10,000 to 40,000 live births.[465] Although there is little risk (1%) to siblings of patients with exstrophy, among offspring of parents with exstrophy the rate is 1 in 70 live births.[466,467] Exstrophy occurs in two variants, bladder exstrophy and cloacal exstrophy. The latter is much less common than the former (1 in 200,000 live births).[468]

Exstrophy results from perforation of an abnormally developed cloacal membrane. In normal development the ingrowth of mesenchyme between the ectodermal and endodermal layers of the cloacal membrane permits fusion of the midline structures below the umbilicus and closure of the abdominal wall. Downward growth of the urorectal septum divides the cloaca into the bladder anteriorly and the rectum posteriorly. The urorectal septum joins the cloacal membrane in the perineum before perforating it to produce the anal and urogenital openings. Before perforation, the genital tubercles migrate medially and fuse in the midline. Defective development of the cloacal membrane with premature perforation results in a variety of abnormalities, including superior vesical fissure, bladder exstrophy, and cloacal exstrophy.[469]

Bladder exstrophy is five to seven times more common in boys than in girls.[470] It is often accompanied by other malformations such as epispadias, intestinal malformations, and defects of spinal closure. Genital malformations are the rule, with epispadias in 86% of boys and unfused labia in 71% of girls.[471] Epispadias is so often associated with exstrophy that the two are sometimes called the exstrophy–epispadias complex.[467] Spina bifida is present in 18% of cases.[471]

Bladder exstrophy is a true malformation rather than an arrest of development.[472] In exstrophy the urinary tract is open to the body wall from the urethral meatus to the umbilicus.[469] The mucosa of the bladder and urethra is fused to the adjacent skin, and the urethra and bladder are foreshortened. The ureters end in a widened trigone and are prone to reflux after surgical closure. The pubic symphysis is widely open (3 to 10 cm).[469] The rectus muscles

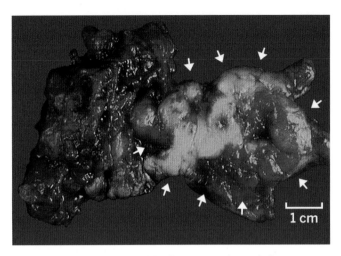

Fig. 5.95 Exstrophy of the bladder. The mucosa (*arrows*) shows congestion, edema, and fibrosis.

are widely separated, and umbilical and inguinal hernias are common. At birth the exstrophic bladder mucosa is usually smooth and has a normal appearance. This condition is short-lived, and trauma and infection quickly produce ulcers and inflammation (Fig. 5.95). The anus is often anteriorly displaced, and there may be rectal prolapse. In girls the Müllerian system shows variable duplication and failure of closure.[473] In boys the penis is short, with a dorsal chordee. Incomplete variants of this constellation of anatomic lesions are rare.[474]

Histologically, the mucosa often shows acute and chronic inflammation with ulceration and metaplastic changes at the time of surgical closure.[475-477] Squamous and intestinal metaplasia are absent or slight at birth and become extensive and profound with time.[478] After closure the mucosa often remains inflamed and squamous metaplasia is common, although changes such as cystitis cystica and glandularis diminish.[475]

Without surgery, more than 66% of patients with bladder exstrophy die by age 20 years.[470] Early surgical intervention, with or without urinary diversion, is successful in many cases, allowing preservation of renal function, urinary continence, and eliminating urinary infections in more than 50% of patients.[479,480] The chronic inflammation and metaplasia of untreated exstrophy predispose the patient to carcinoma, particularly adenocarcinoma.[470] Surgical reconstruction prevents this, and exstrophy-associated carcinoma has become rare.[481]

Cloacal exstrophy is a complex malformation that also is known as *exstrophia splanchnia*, which conveys the extensiveness of the defects.[482] Typically, the lower abdominal wall consists of a large area of exposed mucosa, above which is usually an omphalocele. At the center of the area of mucosa is a patch of intestinal mucosa with one to four orifices. The most superior orifice connects to the ileum, and the lowest connects to a short segment of colon that ends blindly. The other orifices are appendices. The anus is imperforate. Lateral to the intestinal mucosa is exstrophic bladder mucosa containing the ureteral orifices and occasionally the vasa deferentia and vagina. Patches of bladder mucosa may join above or below the intestinal mucosa, or may encircle it. The testes are undescended, and the external genitalia are absent or malformed. Double penis is common in boys.[483] The pubic symphysis is diastatic, and vertebral abnormalities are common. Abnormalities of other organ systems are rare. Cloacal exstrophy was invariably fatal four decades ago, but modern surgical techniques have greatly improved patient outcome, and the survival rate is now almost 50%.[468]

Duplication and Septation of the Bladder

The complete form of duplication is rare and consists of two fully formed urinary bladders with complete mucosal and muscular elements.[484,485] Each unit receives the ureter from its side and drains into a duplicate urethra.[486] In the great majority of cases, this anomaly is accompanied by either diphallus or duplication of the uterus and vagina. In almost 50% of cases, the hindgut is duplicated and the lumbar vertebrae may also be duplicated.[487]

In partial duplication the bladder is divided either sagittally or coronally by a complete wall, and each side is connected to the ureter from the kidney on its side.[484,485,488] Partial duplication differs from complete duplication in that the two units usually communicate and drain into a common urethra. Partial duplication is even rarer than complete duplication.

In septation of the urinary bladder, a septum composed of mucosa, with or without muscularis, partitions the bladder in either the sagittal plane or the coronal plane.[484,488] The partition may be complete or incomplete. When the septum is in the sagittal plane, the ureter from each side connects with its respective chamber. Because there is a single bladder neck and urethra, complete septation is associated with dysplasia and obstruction of one side.[489] If the partition is incomplete, drainage may be normal. Hourglass bladder is an allied condition in which the bladder narrows near its middle, giving it the shape of an hourglass.[490,491]

Urachal Cysts and Persistence

Completely patent urachus is a dramatic lesion in which urine flows from the umbilicus or stump of the umbilical cord. This abnormality is uncommon, with fewer than 300 reported cases.[221,492] The ratio of males to females is approximately 2:1. Most patients with patent urachus have no other developmental abnormality, although Lattimer found that 50% of patients with prune belly syndrome (congenital deficiency of the abdominal musculature) had patent urachus. In most cases, patent urachus does not appear to result from increased intravesical pressure.[493] Schreck and Campbell found that only two of eight children with patent urachus had urinary outlet obstruction.[494] Embryologically, the sequence of development indicates that the urachus is normally already closed before the development of other structures can lead to increased pressure, which might keep it open. The concept that increased pressure later in development might lead to the reopening of the urachus after normal closure was refuted by Begg's anatomic studies.[495]

Incompletely patent urachus is classified by Vaughan as umbilicourachal sinus, vesicourachal sinus or diverticulum, and the blind variant in which the urachus is closed at both ends but remains open centrally (Fig. 5.96).[496] Later, Hinman added alternating urachal sinus to the classification to account for individuals without a history of umbilical urinary drainage in whom urachal infections drained both into the bladder and from the umbilicus.[497] Alternating urachal sinus should be distinguished from completely patent urachus, in which the lumen is patent from bladder to umbilicus at birth. Hinman concluded that, in patients with alternating urachal sinus, the lumen is a potential space in which accumulating epithelial cellular debris becomes a focus for infection.[497] Rarely stones form within urachal malformations. These may be urinary in origin, similar in composition to other urinary calculi,

or may be of different origin, in which case they are usually small and yellow-brown or brown.

Urachal cysts are found at any point in the urachus (Fig. 5.97) and range from small lesions found incidentally (Figs. 5.98 and 5.99) to immense masses containing as much as 50 L of fluid.[498] Small cysts are usually lined by urothelium or cuboidal epithelium (Fig. 5.100), but columnar epithelium may be present. The lining of large cysts is usually flattened. Calcification may be present.

Diverticulum

Diverticulum of the bladder (Fig. 5.101) is a common clinical problem that infrequently requires surgical treatment. The cause of bladder diverticulum is generally attributed to increased luminal pressure, although some lesions in children are attributable to localized deficiency of the muscularis propria and others to syndromes such as Ehlers–Danlos syndrome.[499-507] Diverticula are common in children with Menkes syndrome (kinky hair syndrome).[508] They are found in patients of all ages, but most often in men older than 50 years with outflow obstruction caused by prostatic hyperplasia, suggesting that they are caused by increased pressure.[499,505,509-513] Diverticula are most common in the vicinity of the ureteral orifices. At this site, diverticula can cause ureteral obstruction or reflux and predispose the patient to infection. Although most diverticula are small and asymptomatic, large ones may rival or exceed the volume of the bladder and be associated with infection and stone formation.[499] Less than 10% of diverticula develop neoplasms, most of which are urothelial carcinoma, rarely osteosarcoma.[514-518]

The excised specimen usually includes a small orifice connecting the bladder and the diverticulum.[513] The passage between the two consists of a narrow intramural neck in the inner layer of the muscularis propria, and the wall of the diverticulum may contain attenuated muscle fibers from the outer layer in patients without a history of chronic inflammation. In patients with a history of chronic inflammation, the muscle fibers often are absent, having been replaced by fibrous tissue. Consequently, cancers involving a bladder diverticulum cannot be assigned a pT2 stage.[519] Squamous metaplasia also is seen in association with chronic inflammation.[519]

Other Congenital Malformations and Anomalies

A congenital fistula between the bladder and the anterior abdominal wall may form a superior or inferior vesical fissure and is considered a less severe form of exstrophy than typical exstrophy. Noncongenital fistulas are common samples seen in uropathology practice.

Congenital prepubic sinus is a midline sinus from the skin immediately superior to the pubis that may communicate with the anterior bladder wall. Microscopically, the sinus tract is lined by urothelium and surrounded by a smooth muscle sheath. The sinus is considered a urethral duplication rather than a variant of exstrophy. Trigonal cyst is a developmental anomaly located at or near the trigone that is lined by normal-looking urothelium. An enlarged bladder (megacystis) may result from any distal anatomic obstruction, often at the bladder neck or urethral valves, or as a manifestation of a syndrome complex such as the prune belly syndrome, a rare birth defect also characterized by bilateral cryptorchidism, other urologic malformations, and absence of the abdominal wall musculature. Megacystis is one component of the syndrome of megacystis-microcolon-intestinal hypoperistalsis.

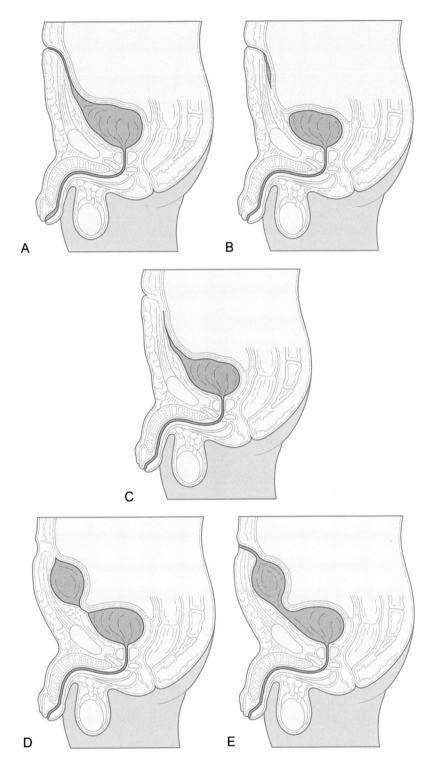

Fig. 5.96 Types of persistent or patent urachus. (A) Complete patency. (B) Umbilicourachal sinus. (C) Vesicourachal sinus. (D) Blindly patent urachus. (E) Alternating urachal sinus.

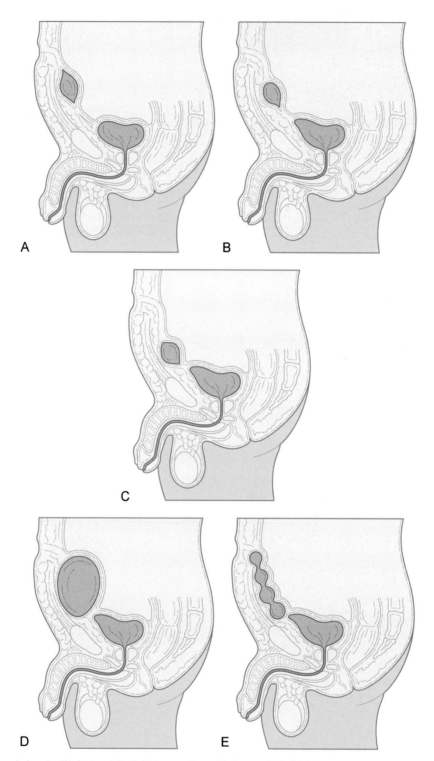

Fig. 5.97 Classification of urachal cysts. (A) Juxtaumbilical. (B) Intermediate. (C) Juxtavesical. (D) Giant cyst. (E) Multiple cysts.

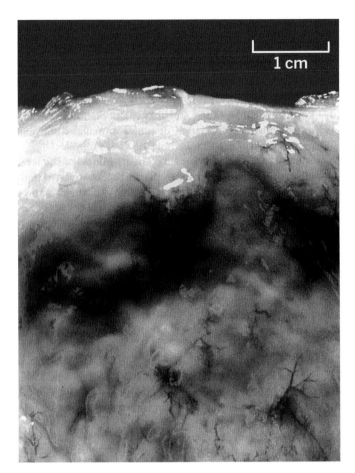

Fig. 5.98 Small urachal cyst found as a submucosal nodule in the bladder dome.

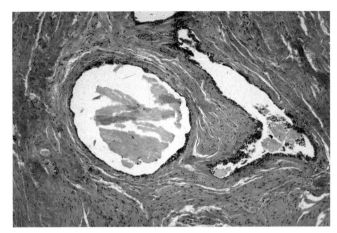

Fig. 5.100 Multilocular urachal cyst lined by cuboidal and atrophic epithelium.

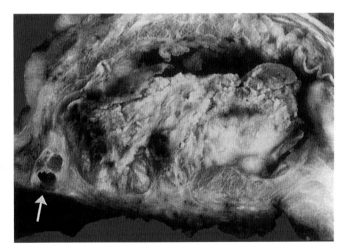

Fig. 5.99 Urachal cyst (*arrow*). An incidental finding in a radical cystoprostatectomy specimen.

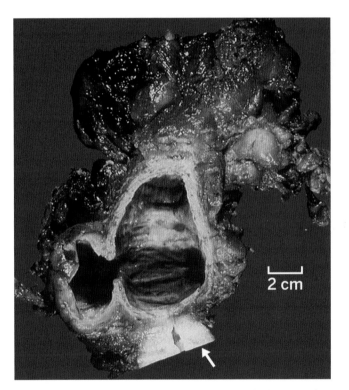

Fig. 5.101 Bladder diverticulum (*arrow* indicates hyperplastic prostate).

Congenital bladder neck obstruction (Marion disease) is an obstructive condition due to dyssynergic voiding that results in bladder dysfunction and various side effects that can stem from inefficient bladder emptying. It can occur in males of all ages, including children. It can be readily and accurately diagnosed with the appropriate video-urodynamic studies. Histologically, there is concentric fibromuscular hypertrophy and elastosis of the bladder neck and secondary detrusor muscle hypertrophy, often with chronic inflammation of the bladder mucosa.

References are available at expertconsult.com

6

Neoplasms of the Urinary Bladder

LIANG CHENG, ANTONIO LOPEZ-BELTRAN, GREGORY T. MACLENNAN, RODOLFO MONTIRONI AND DAVID G. BOSTWICK

CHAPTER OUTLINE

Carcinoma of the urinary bladder is the fourth most common malignancy in men, accounting for an estimated 60,490 new cases and 12,240 cancer deaths in the United States in 2018.[1,2] Significant progress has been made in the diagnosis and treatment of bladder cancer.[3-5] Bladder cancer is morphologically heterogeneous; more than 90% of bladder cancer cases are urothelial (transitional cell) carcinoma, whereas primary squamous cell carcinoma, adenocarcinoma, small cell carcinoma, and other tumors are less common.[1] The classification system of urinary bladder neoplasia used in this chapter has been modified according to the 2016 World Health Organization (WHO) classification of tumors of the urinary system.[6]

Benign Urothelial Neoplasms

Urothelial Papilloma and Diffuse Papillomatosis

Urothelial papilloma is a benign exophytic urothelial neoplasm that typically occurs in patients younger than 50 years.[7] The male-to-female ratio is 2:1. The most common symptom is hematuria.[7] Most tumors are located near the ureteric orifices. Urothelial papilloma may recur, but recurrent papilloma does not progress.[7-9]

The diagnostic criteria for urothelial papilloma in the 2016 WHO classification are identical to those defined in the 1973 WHO classification.[6,10] Using the restrictive diagnostic criteria recommended by the WHO, urothelial papilloma represents less than 1% of papillary urothelial neoplasms.[7,11-14] Urothelial papilloma is composed of a delicate fibrovascular core covered by cytologically and architecturally normal urothelium with no more than seven layers of cells (Fig. 6.1). The superficial cells are often prominent and may have vacuolization of the cytoplasm, eosinophilic syncytial or apocrine-like morphology, or may demonstrate mucinous metaplasia. Mitotic figures are absent to rare and, if present, are in the basal cell layer. The stroma may show edema or inflammatory cells. Rare cases show dilated lymphatics within the fibrovascular fronds. Occasionally, foamy histiocytes accumulate within the fibrovascular stalks. Secondary budding of small fronds from larger simple primary papillary fronds is commonly observed.

Papilloma is a diploid tumor with a low proliferation rate, undetectable or very limited p53 accumulation, and frequent fibroblast growth factor receptor 3 (FGFR3) mutation (75% of cases).[15] Cytokeratin (CK) 20 expression is limited to the superficial (umbrella) cells.[14,16] Telomerase reverse transcriptase (TERT) promoter mutations are present in 46% of urothelial papilloma cases.[17]

The designation of diffuse papillomatosis is applicable when the mucosa is extensively involved by multiple small delicate papillary processes, creating a velvety cystoscopic appearance.[12,14,18] These papillary structures are covered by normal urothelium with no cytologic atypia (Fig. 6.2). The malignant potential of this lesion is uncertain.

Inverted Papilloma

Inverted papilloma is usually found in males in the sixth or seventh decade of life.[19-28] The male-to-female ratio is 7:1.[19] Hematuria and obstructive symptoms are the most common symptoms at presentation. The majority of inverted papillomas develop in the region of the trigone and bladder neck (Fig. 6.3). Some cases may be multifocal.[19,29] The incidence of multiplicity ranges from 1.3% to 4.4%.[19,21] A significant number of patients have a history of smoking, suggesting a possible link between tobacco use and inverted papilloma.[19] Human papillomavirus (HPV) infection is not a causative agent of urothelial inverted papilloma.[30]

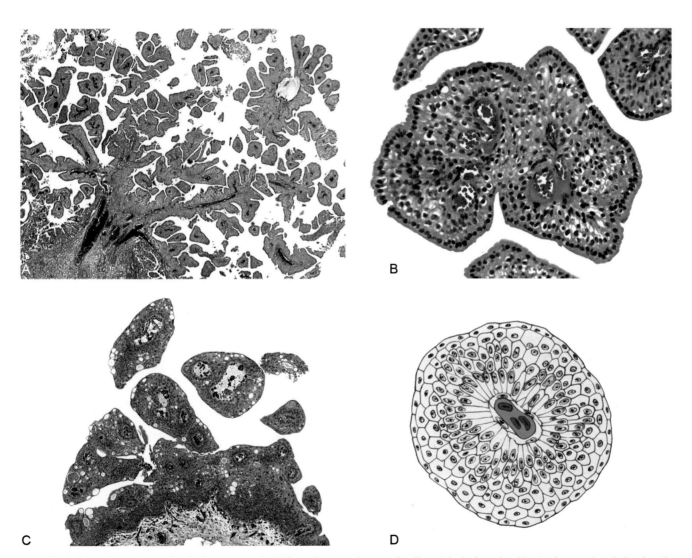

Fig. 6.1 Urothelial papilloma is a papillary lesion composed of delicate fibrovascular cores lined by cytologically and architecturally normal urothelium less than seven cell layers thick. (A) Low-power view of urothelial papilloma. (B) High-power view of the same tumor as in (A). (C) Another example of urothelial papilloma. (D) Schematic diagram of urothelial papilloma. (From Cheng L, Darson M, Cheville JC, et al. Urothelial papilloma of the bladder: clinical and biological implications. *Cancer* 1999;86:2098–2101, with permission.)

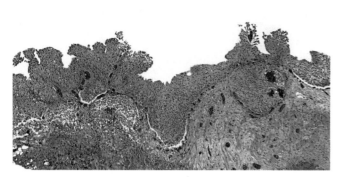

Fig. 6.2 Diffuse papillomatosis. Multiple papillary excrescences are present in the mucosa. Cytologically, the lining cells are normal.

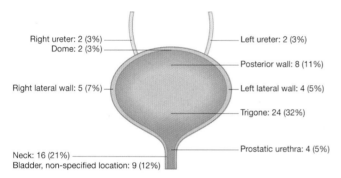

Right ureter: 2 (3%)
Dome: 2 (3%)
Left ureter: 2 (3%)
Posterior wall: 8 (11%)
Right lateral wall: 5 (7%)
Left lateral wall: 4 (5%)
Trigone: 24 (32%)
Neck: 16 (21%)
Prostatic urethra: 4 (5%)
Bladder, non-specified location: 9 (12%)

Fig. 6.3 Distribution of inverted papillomas in the urinary tract. (From Sung MT, MacLennan GT, Lopez-Beltran A, et al. Natural history of urothelial inverted papilloma. *Cancer* 2006;107:2622–2262, with permission.)

Histologically, inverted papilloma shows an inverted growth pattern, usually composed of anastomosing islands and trabeculae of histologically and cytologically normal urothelial cells invaginating from the surface urothelium into the subjacent lamina propria but not into the muscularis propria (Fig. 6.4). Although the term *inverted papilloma* was initially introduced in 1963 by Potts and Hirst to describe this architecturally distinctive urothelial neoplasm, the Viennese urologist Paschkis had previously reported four morphologically identical urothelial tumors in 1927 under the name of *adenomatoid polyp*.[31,32] Kunze et al. proposed the subdivision of inverted papilloma into two morphologically distinct variants, trabecular and glandular.[20] By their criteria the trabecular variant is composed of anastomosing cords and trabeculae of urothelial cells invaginating the lamina propria at various angles. These invaginating structures demonstrate mature urothelium centrally, with darker and palisading basal cells peripherally, usually surrounded by fibrotic stroma without marked inflammation. The glandular variant is composed of nests of urothelium with either pseudoglandular spaces lined by mature urothelium or even true glandular elements, containing mucicarminophilic secretions and mucous-secreting cells. The glandular variant, as proposed by these investigators, has considerable morphologic overlap with florid cystitis glandularis and is not widely accepted as a diagnostic entity.

Within the spectrum of findings in inverted papilloma, vacuolization and foamy xanthomatous cytoplasmic changes may be seen. These "clear cells" may be concentrated within distinct regions of the tumor, but more frequently are diffusely intermingled with usual inverted papilloma cells. Foci of nonkeratinizing squamous metaplasia and neuroendocrine differentiation have been reported.[29] Mitotic figures are either absent or rare. Some cases may demonstrate focal minor cytologic atypia that is likely degenerative in nature and has no clinical significance.[33] Inverted papilloma may coexist with carcinoma, and it is most important to differentiate inverted papilloma from urothelial carcinoma with inverted growth pattern. Such distinction may be difficult, especially in limited biopsy specimens or when interpretation is confounded by crush artifact.[33] Inverted papilloma usually exhibits orderly maturation of invaginated trabeculae and cords, composed of spindling and peripherally palisading cells. In contrast, urothelial carcinoma with an inverted growth pattern often has thick and irregular tumor columns with transition to more solid nests. In addition, the presence of an exophytic papillary component and unequivocal tumor invasion in the lamina propria or muscularis propria justifies a diagnosis of inverted urothelial carcinoma.

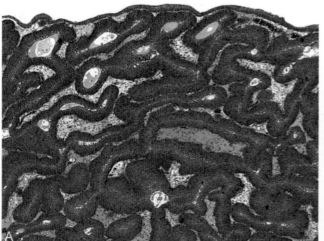
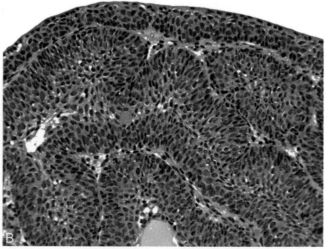

Fig. 6.4 Inverted urothelial papilloma. (A) The low magnification demonstrates a distinct downward growth pattern of a typical inverted papilloma composed of intact surface-lining urothelium and underlying thin anastomosing trabeculae of urothelium in the lamina propria. (B) At higher magnification the trabeculae are lined by uniform urothelial cells without cytologic atypia.

Marked cytologic atypia, including nuclear pleomorphism, nucleolar prominence, and abundant mitotic activity, further supports a diagnosis of malignancy.

Several investigators have voiced concern regarding the malignant potential of inverted papilloma based on the subsequent development of urothelial carcinoma, but most patients with this complication have a history of a prior or concurrent urothelial carcinoma.[23,34-37] In a large series of 75 patients, all but 1 patient had an uneventful course without either tumor recurrence or progression to urothelial malignancy during a mean follow-up of 68 months.[19] Consequently, transurethral resection of inverted papilloma is adequate treatment, and surveillance protocols as rigorous as those used in the management of urothelial carcinoma seem unnecessary for this benign entity.

It has been well documented by the finding of nonrandom inactivation of X chromosomes that inverted papilloma is a clonal neoplasm that arises from a single progenitor cell. Sung and colleagues studied the status of loss of heterozygosity (LOH) in inverted papilloma using microsatellite markers that are commonly altered in urothelial carcinoma.[38] The incidence rate of LOH in inverted papilloma is low (8% to 10%) and contrasts with the high frequency of LOH (29% to 80%) in urothelial carcinoma and papillary urothelial neoplasm of low malignant potential (PUNLMP).[39-46] The low frequency of allelic loss in inverted papilloma is similar to that of normal urothelium.[47] Lott and et al. evaluated mutations of *FGFR3* and *TP53* genes by DNA sequencing in 20 cases of inverted papilloma of the urinary tract.[48] Point mutations of the FGFR3 gene were identified in 45% (9/20) of inverted papillomas, with four cases exhibiting mutations at multiple exons. Seven cases had exon 7 mutations of the *FGFR3* gene, containing R248C, S249T, L259L, P260P, and V266M. Two cases had exon 10 and 15 mutations, including A366D, H412H, E627D, D641N, and H643D; five cases had N653H. The most frequent mutation of the *FGFR3* gene was identified at R248C. None of the inverted papillomas exhibited mutations in TP53.

Telomere shortening using fluorescence in situ hybridization (FISH) analysis is seen in about 70% of urothelial carcinomas with inverted growth, but in only 9% of inverted papillomas.[49] Telomere FISH analysis is useful to separate these two entities in selected challenging cases.[49] A recent TERT promoter mutation status study reported 15% mutation in inverted papilloma compared with 58% in urothelial carcinoma with inverted growth, suggesting that there is a subpopulation of inverted papilloma that shares a carcinogenetic pathway with urothelial carcinoma with inverted growth and conventional urothelial carcinomas.[50]

The markedly reduced frequency of LOH, the absence of *TP53* mutations, the absence of telomere shortening, and the pattern of *FGFR3* mutations in inverted papilloma compared with that of urothelial carcinoma suggest that inverted papilloma does not harbor the key genetic abnormalities that predispose to the development of urothelial carcinoma and may indicate that these entities arise through separate and distinct pathogenetic mechanisms.[24-26,48]

Squamous Papilloma

Squamous papilloma is a rare benign neoplasm; it may represent the squamous counterpart of urothelial papilloma.[51] It is unrelated to HPV infection, usually occurs in elderly women, and follows a benign clinical course.[51] Histologically, it is composed of papillary cores with overlying benign squamous epithelium

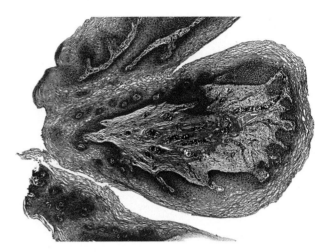

Fig. 6.5 Squamous cell papilloma of the urinary bladder. (From Cheng L, Leibovich BC, Cheville JC, et al. Squamous papilloma of the urinary tract is unrelated to condyloma acuminata. *Cancer* 2000;88:1679–1686, with permission.)

(Fig. 6.5). These tumors are diploid with undetectable or very limited nuclear p53 accumulation. Some demonstrate immunohistochemical expression of epidermal growth factor receptor (EGFR) protein.[52]

Urothelial Proliferation of Uncertain Malignant Potential

Papillary Urothelial Hyperplasia/Urothelial Proliferation of Uncertain Malignant Potential

In the 2016 WHO classification of tumors of the urinary tract, the term *urothelial proliferation of uncertain malignant potential* (UPUMP) was recommended for lesions previously known as papillary urothelial hyperplasia and flat urothelial hyperplasia.[6] It also recognized that some may actually represent a "shoulder" lesion of previously resected urothelial papillary tumor.

UPUMP typically occurs in patients with either a prior or concurrent low-grade papillary urothelial neoplasia.[53] Most patients are men with a mean age of 67 years. These lesions are characterized by undulating folds of urothelium that lack cytologic atypia and fibrovascular cores (Fig. 6.6).[37,53-55] Cytologically, the cells in UPUMP lack atypia and maintain nuclear polarity. There may be increased vascularity in the stroma at the base of the papillary folds.

Recent data suggest that papillary hyperplasia may be a precursor to low-grade papillary neoplasms.[37,53-55] These lesions may also evolve into a high-grade noninvasive (Ta) papillary urothelial carcinoma. Swierczynski and Epstein reported 15 cases of papillary urothelial hyperplasia with varying degrees of atypia ranging from dysplasia to flat carcinoma in situ (atypical papillary urothelial hyperplasia).[56] On follow-up examination, most of these patients had experienced high-grade urothelial neoplasms. These cases may be viewed as urothelial carcinoma in situ or dysplasia with early papillary formation.

Flat Urothelial Hyperplasia/Urothelial Proliferation of Uncertain Malignant Potential

The term *urothelial proliferation of uncertain malignant potential* (UPUMP), recently introduced in the 2016 WHO classification

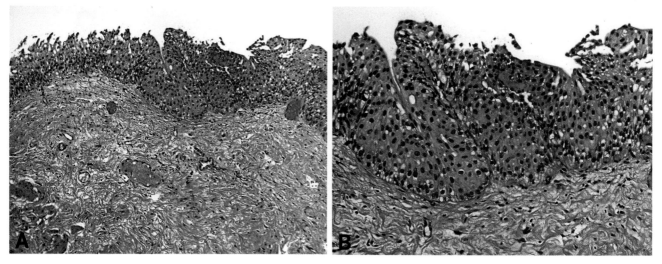

Fig. 6.6 Papillary urothelial hyperplasia (urothelial proliferation of uncertain malignant potential; A and B).

of urinary tract tumors, is meant to include flat urothelial hyperplasia in addition to papillary hyperplasia (see earlier discussion), but in practice we recommend that the term *flat urothelial hyperplasia* be used.

Normal urothelium is a multilayered epithelium composed of basal, intermediate, and superficial cells (Fig. 6.7). The number of cell layers (usually less than seven) may vary because of tangential sectioning.[57] Urothelial hyperplasia is characterized by markedly thickened mucosa with an increase in the number of cell layers, usually ≥10 (Fig. 6.8). However, it is not necessary to count the number of cell layers for the diagnosis. The cells in urothelial hyperplasia do not show any significant cytologic abnormalities, although slight nuclear enlargement may be focally present. Morphologic evidence of maturation from base to surface is generally evident. Urothelial compression artifact or tangential sectioning of mucosa with pseudopapillary growth (lacking a true vascular core) may resemble flat urothelial hyperplasia.

Flat urothelial hyperplasia has been observed in association with a variety of conditions including inflammatory disorders, urolithiasis, papillary urothelial hyperplasia, dysplasia, carcinoma in situ,

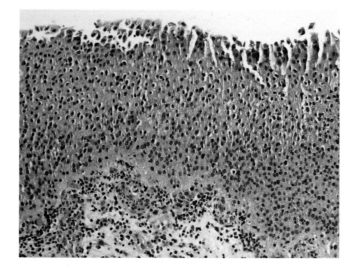

Fig. 6.8 Flat urothelial hyperplasia (urothelial proliferation of uncertain malignant potential).

and low-grade papillary tumors.[58] When seen as an isolated phenomenon, there is no evidence to suggest that primary urothelial hyperplasia has a premalignant potential. However, molecular analyses showing chromosome 9q deletions and mutations in the *FGFR3* gene in both urothelial hyperplasia and low-grade papillary neoplasia suggest that this lesion may be clonally related to the papillary tumors in patients with bladder cancer.[16,59,60] Flat urothelial hyperplasia has been considered by some authors to be the source of papillary neoplasia, usually associated with low-grade tumors.[61]

Flat Intraepithelial Lesions

The classification of nonpapillary (flat) intraepithelial lesions and conditions of the urothelium has evolved over the years and was redefined at the International Consultation on the Diagnosis of Noninvasive Urothelial Neoplasms held in Ancona (Italy, 2001) (Table 6.1).[58] This classification includes epithelial abnormalities (reactive urothelial atypia and flat urothelial hyperplasia), presumed preneoplastic lesions and conditions (keratinizing

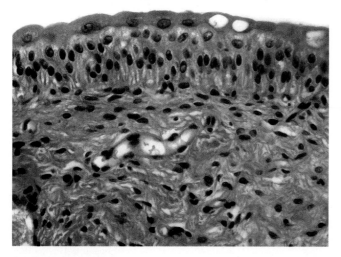

Fig. 6.7 Normal urothelium.

TABLE 6.1	Classification of Flat Urothelial Lesions of the Urinary Bladder Based on the Ancona International Consultation

Flat urothelial hyperplasia
Reactive urothelial atypia
Presumed preneoplastic lesions and conditions
  Keratinizing squamous metaplasia
  Intestinal metaplasia
  Malignancy-associated cellular changes
Preneoplastic lesions
  Dysplasia
Neoplastic noninvasive lesion
  Urothelial carcinoma in situ

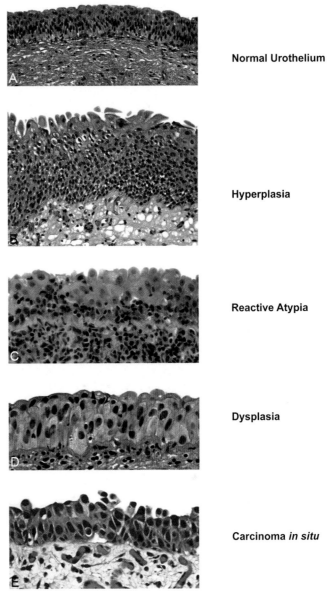

Normal Urothelium

Hyperplasia

Reactive Atypia

Dysplasia

Carcinoma *in situ*

Fig. 6.9 Flat intraepithelial lesions. (A) Normal urothelium. (B) Urothelial (simple) hyperplasia. (C) Reactive atypia. (D) Urothelial dysplasia. (E) Urothelial carcinoma in situ.

squamous and glandular metaplasia and malignancy-associated cellular changes), as well as preneoplastic (dysplasia) and neoplastic noninvasive (carcinoma in situ) lesions (Fig. 6.9).[57,58] Each of these lesions is defined with strict morphologic criteria to provide more accurate information to urologists in managing patients (Table 6.2).

Great advances have been made in the molecular genetic and biomarker characterization of bladder cancer in recent years.[15,41,44,46,62-81] Malignancy-associated cellular change is a recently introduced concept, encompassing urothelial abnormalities in bladders harboring neoplasia that are not evident by routine light microscopy but are demonstrable by chromatin analysis or genetic studies.[58,82-84] The clinical relevance of malignancy-associated cellular changes remains to be established, but these parameters may be important in evaluating the status of residual urothelium after surgical bladder tumor resections.[83] Recent studies have shown that 50% of the histologically normal urothelium adjacent to superficial urothelial carcinoma harbors genetic anomalies on chromosome 9, similar to the anomalies found in the coexisting carcinoma. In addition, nondiploid nuclear DNA histograms occur in 4% to 54% of histologically normal urothelium adjacent to bladder tumors.[82] These genetic alterations suggest a neoplastic potential for flat urothelial lesions, regardless of whether cytologic atypia is present.

Urothelial Reactive Atypia

Urothelial abnormalities whose architectural and cytologic changes are of lesser degree than those of dysplasia have often been termed *atypia*.[58] The term *atypia* is, by its very nature, nonspecific. The intraobserver and interobserver variations in recognition and interpretation of *urothelial atypia* are substantial. Nevertheless, the term *atypia* is still in use at many institutions. Two similar categories of atypia have been recently recognized, namely reactive atypia and atypia of unknown significance.[85] Both of them are placed among the "benign" urothelial abnormalities.[58]

Reactive Atypia

Reactive atypia is characterized by mild nuclear abnormalities occurring in acutely or chronically inflamed urothelium. In most cases there is a history of cystitis, instrumentation, infection, stones, or previous therapy.[57] The epithelium may or may not be thickened in reactive atypia. The cells are often larger than normal, with more abundant cytoplasm than normal urothelial cells

(Fig. 6.10). These features occasionally impart a squamoid appearance. Nuclei are uniformly enlarged, vesicular, and may have prominent, usually centrally located nucleoli. Mitotic figures may be frequent but always occur in the lower epithelial layers (Table 6.2). Inflammatory cells occupying the lamina propria and infiltrating into the urothelium are invariably present. CK20, CD44, p53, and p16 immunohistochemical stains may be particularly useful from a differential diagnosis perspective (Table 6.3) (see Urothelial Dysplasia section).[86-90]

Atypia of Unknown Significance

The term *atypia of unknown significance* was introduced by the International Society of Urological Pathology (ISUP) consensus group to describe lesions in which the pathologist was uncertain whether the changes were reactive or preneoplastic.[85] Atypia of

TABLE 6.2   Comparison of Flat Intraepithelial Lesions of the Urinary Bladder

Features	Reactive Atypia	Hyperplasia	Dysplasia	Carcinoma In Situ
Cell layers	Variable	>7 cells	Variable	Variable
Polarization	Slightly abnormal	Normal	Slightly abnormal	Abnormal
Cytoplasm	Vacuolated	Homogeneous	Homogeneous	Homogeneous
Nuclear-to-cytoplasmic ratio	Normal or slightly increased	Normal or slightly increased	Slightly increased	Increased
Nuclei				
Anisonucleosis	Normal	Normal	Mild	Moderate to severe
Borders	Regular/smooth	Regular/smooth	Notches/creases	Pleomorphic
Chromatin	Fine/dusty	Fine	Slight hyperchromasia	Coarse/hyperchromatic
Chromatin distribution	Even	Even	Even	Uneven
Nucleoli	Large	Small/absent	Small/absent	Large/prominent
Mitotic figures	Variable	Absent	Rare	Often
Denudation	Variable	No	No	Variable
CK20	Surface	Surface	Variable	Variable
Stromal microvascular proliferation	Variable	Variable	Less prominent	Often prominent

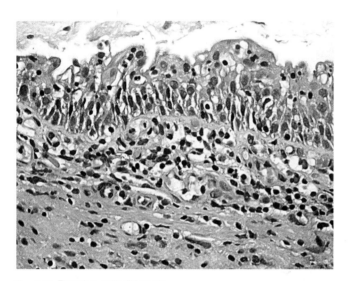

Fig. 6.10 Reactive urothelial atypia.

unknown significance is characterized by nuclear changes similar to those seen in reactive atypia. However, the degree of nuclear pleomorphism and hyperchromasia is greater than in reactive atypia, and dysplasia cannot be ruled out. Inflammation in the lamina propria with urothelial infiltration is often present. However, the cellular changes seem to be disproportionate to the degree of inflammation. Atypia of unknown significance is often seen in patients with a previous diagnosis of urothelial neoplasia. Progression to urothelial carcinoma has not been documented.[57] No

evidence currently supports a premalignant nature of such lesions. The clinical outcome of patients with atypia of unknown significance is identical to that of patients with reactive atypia.[57] The utility of creating this diagnostic category has been questioned, and the use of the designation "atypia of unknown significance" is discouraged.[86-91]

Therapy-Induced Changes in the Urothelium and Mimics of Urothelial Flat Neoplasia

Antineoplastic agents used in the bladder or systemically, such as thiotepa (triethylenethiophosphoramide), mitomycin C, cyclophosphamide, bacillus Calmette–Guérin (BCG), and radiation therapy, produce urothelial changes that can mimic cancer histologically.[90,92] Pathologists must be aware of the diagnostic pitfalls and exercise caution when evaluating urothelial atypia after treatment with chemotherapy or irradiation.[58,89,93-95] In most cases, knowledge of the prior treatment is crucial to correctly diagnosing the epithelial and stromal changes present. If the distinction between treatment-induced atypia and dysplasia/carcinoma in situ is uncertain, a conservative approach with repeat cystoscopy and biopsy is indicated, preferably after the inflammation has subsided.

Cyclophosphamide therapy may induce stromal fibrosis, vascular intimal thickening, mural fibrin deposition in vessels, and vascular ectasia.[94] It also induces epithelial necrosis followed by rapid atypical regeneration. Treatment-induced urothelial atypia may mimic dysplasia or carcinoma in situ (Fig. 6.11). The metabolic effects of cyclophosphamide including arrest of cell and nuclear division produce binucleated and multinucleated cells, often with

TABLE 6.3   Immunohistochemical Features of Flat Intraepithelial Lesions of the Urinary Bladder

Conditions	CK20	CD44	p53	p16
Normal	Limited to umbrella cells	Limited to basal cells	Often negative	Absent
Flat urothelial hyperplasia	Limited to umbrella cells	Limited to basal cells	May be positive	Unknown
Reactive atypia	Limited to umbrella cells	Increased reactivity in all cell layers	May be positive	Absent
Atypia of unknown significance	Limited to umbrella cells	Increased reactivity in all cell layers	May be positive	Unknown
Dysplasia	Deep layers	Absent	Often positive	Often positive
Urothelial carcinoma in situ	Full-thickness expression	Absent	Positive	Positive

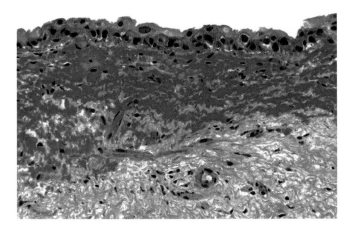

Fig. 6.11 Cyclophosphamide (Cytoxan)-induced changes include urothelial atypia and hemorrhagic cystitis.

large, bizarre nuclei resembling radiation injury changes that can be mistaken for malignancy. Cyclophosphamide may also induce reactivation of polyomavirus infection (BK virus), causing marked nuclear atypia in the surface urothelium. In rare cases, BK virus infection mimics flat intraepithelial lesions in immunocompromised patients.

In BCG-treated bladders, it is important to keep in mind that residual carcinoma in situ might only be present in von Brunn nests. Loss of intercellular cohesion in carcinoma in situ may result in the so-called denuding cystitis or in residual neoplastic cells loosely attached to the surface ("clinging" pattern). Also of importance are the reactive changes associated with BCG therapy, which include both acute and chronic inflammation. There may also be a pattern of reactive epithelial atypia and granulomatous reaction deep in the bladder wall.[94,95]

Mitomycin C and thiotepa, when used as topical chemotherapeutic agents in the bladder, produce identical histologic changes. These include exfoliation, epithelial denudation, multinucleation, cytoplasmic vacuolization, and the appearance of bizarre, nonmalignant nuclei in the superficial layer of the urothelium. A marked necroinflammatory process follows administration of topical mitomycin C. There is a histiocytic response extending deep into the bladder wall. Mitomycin C may also initiate eosinophilic cystitis, a useful clue for the surgical pathologist when evaluating small bladder biopsies in this setting. These agents are not metabolic inhibitors of DNA replication, and thus do not produce full-thickness urothelial atypia, as is seen after cyclophosphamide therapy. Patients receiving ketamine may present reactive urothelial changes that can mimic urothelial carcinoma in situ.[96]

Radiation therapy produces a variety of bladder lesions associated with a progression of pathologic findings. The earliest change, usually seen after 3 to 6 weeks, consists of acute cystitis with desquamation of urothelial cells and hyperemia with edema of the lamina propria. The urothelium shows varying degrees of atypia, including cytoplasmic and nuclear vacuolization, karyorrhexis, stromal hyalinization, thrombosis of blood vessels, and mesenchymal cell atypia similar to that seen in giant cell cystitis.[94] Enlarged nuclei may have large nucleoli, but degenerative nuclear features are usually present. Surface ulceration with fibrin deposition, or a reactive, tumor-like epithelial proliferation associated with fibrosis of the lamina propria or muscularis propria, arteriolar mural thickening and hyalinization, and atypical and sometimes multinucleated stromal cells are features seen in late cases of radiation cystitis, usually becoming evident months or years after radiation therapy. An important long-term effect of radiotherapy is the development of de novo radiation-induced bladder cancer, which usually is a urothelial carcinoma but occasionally is a squamous cell neoplasm. Rare examples of sarcomatoid carcinoma (or carcinosarcoma) and sarcoma of the urinary bladder have been reported.[58,94,95,97-99]

Several inflammatory conditions of the urinary bladder, some related to treatment, may cause urothelial atypia leading to overdiagnosis of dysplasia and carcinoma in situ. In addition, the damaged mucosa may become ulcerated, with adjacent atypical regenerating urothelium showing pseudocarcinomatous hyperplasia (Fig. 6.12).[58,95,100,101] This change is more common after ulceration related to radiation therapy.[90,91]

Urothelial Dysplasia

Urothelial dysplasia is defined as abnormal urothelium with cytologic and architectural changes that do not meet all the criteria for an unequivocal diagnosis of urothelial carcinoma in situ

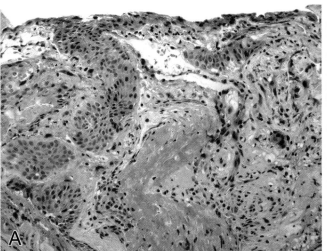
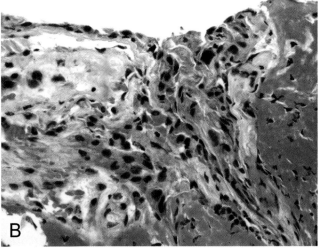

Fig. 6.12 Pseudocarcinomatous urothelial hyperplasia (A and B).

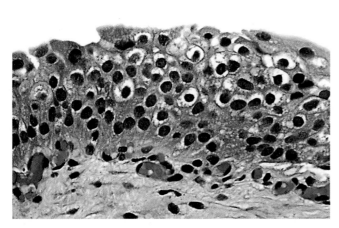

Fig. 6.13 Urothelial dysplasia. Dysplastic urothelium shows variability in nuclear size and shape, increase in nuclear-to-cytoplasmic ratio, and loss of cellular polarity. Cytoplasmic clearing is common. The superficial umbrella cell layer is intact. The degree of cytologic atypia is insufficient for an unequivocal diagnosis of carcinoma in situ.

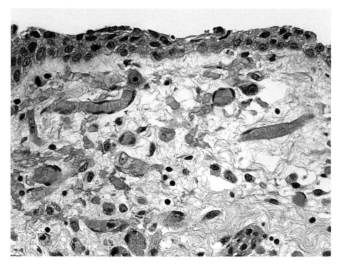

Fig. 6.15 Urothelial dysplasia.

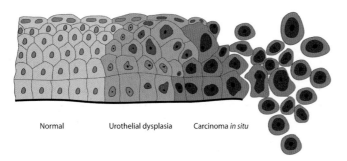

Normal   Urothelial dysplasia   Carcinoma *in situ*

Fig. 6.14 Morphologic continuum from normal urothelium through dysplasia to carcinoma in situ and invasion. The dysplastic urothelium shows loss of orderly maturation and cellular polarity. The progression from dysplasia to carcinoma in situ is characterized by the increasing nuclear-to-cytoplasmic ratio, nuclear hyperchromasia, and nuclear and nucleolar enlargement. The superficial umbrella cell layer is often absent in urothelial carcinoma in situ, but its loss is not a prerequisite for the diagnosis. Urothelial carcinoma in situ often progresses to invasive cancer.

(Fig. 6.13).[57,58,102,103] The overall appearance is that of the urothelium in low-grade papillary urothelial carcinoma. The cytologic abnormalities in urothelial dysplasia, characterized by cellular crowding, loss of orderly maturation, and loss of cellular polarity, are not present in the full thickness of the urothelium (Fig. 6.14). Occasionally there may be an increased number of cell layers. The superficial umbrella cells are usually present. Most cellular abnormalities in dysplasia are restricted to the basal and intermediate cell layers. Individual dysplastic cells show enlarged nuclei and nucleoli with irregular contours and coarsening of the chromatin. Multiple nucleoli and nuclear overlapping may be seen. The cells often show cytoplasmic clearing. Mitotic figures, when present, are generally basally located. The transition from normal to abnormal urothelium is subtle, and nondysplastic urothelial cells are often dispersed among the dysplastic cells.

The diagnosis of urothelial dysplasia can be made in cases in which the urothelium demonstrates significant cytologic atypia that cannot be attributed to inflammation or a reparative process and yet lacks the full complement of cytologic abnormalities that characterize carcinoma in situ (Fig. 6.15). Nuclear and

architectural features are the primary criteria for distinguishing dysplasia from reactive atypia and urothelial carcinoma in situ. Aberrant CK20 expression in urothelial cells plus overexpression of p53 and Ki67 are indicators of dysplastic change in urothelial mucosa (Table 6.3).[103-108] Molecular markers may be helpful in the differential diagnosis. CK20 immunostaining is limited to the superficial cell layers in normal urothelium; in contrast, it is usually present in the superficial and intermediate cell layers of dysplastic urothelium.[104,109] CD44 may be of particular value in the distinction between urothelial dysplasia and reactive atypia.[105,110] Positive CD44 immunostaining is observed only in the basal cells in normal urothelium and is either absent entirely or present only in scattered cells in urothelial dysplasia, whereas full-thickness positive membranous CD44 staining is typical of reactive urothelium.[110] Dysplastic cells show increased p53 expression, whereas p53 nuclear accumulation is predominantly undetectable or only weakly evident in the basal and parabasal cells in reactive urothelium. Alterations of p53 and allelic losses, particularly in chromosome 9, may occur in dysplasia.[60] p16 has been reported as variably positive in urothelial dysplasia and negative to weak or patchy in reactive urothelium.[106,111]

It has proven difficult to create standardized nomenclature for intraurothelial cytologic abnormalities. Consequently, grading of urothelial dysplasia is not currently recommended. The use of the term *atypia* as a synonym for urothelial dysplasia is discouraged. Intraurothelial cytologic abnormalities that cannot be attributed to a reactive or reparative process and yet lack sufficient abnormalities to be diagnosed as carcinoma in situ should be diagnosed as urothelial dysplasia without qualifiers.

Primary Dysplasia

Primary dysplasia occurs in the absence of other urothelial tumors. Its prevalence in the general population is unknown due to lack of large-scale screening studies. In an autopsy series of 313 patients without gross lesions, urothelial dysplasia was present in 6.8% of males and 5.7% of females.[112] Only a few studies provide clinical information on patients with primary dysplasia.[57,102,113,114] These patients are predominantly middle-aged men with irritative symptoms with or without hematuria. The lesion has a predilection for posterior wall location.[102] Dysplasia is not cystoscopically visible, although occasionally the urothelium may appear raised and irregular or mildly erythematous. It is estimated that de novo (primary) dysplasia progresses to bladder neoplasia in 14% to 19% of cases.[57,102,113,114] Using modern criteria for urothelial dysplasia, Cheng et al. found a 19% progression rate in 36 patients with isolated urothelial dysplasia during a mean follow-up of 8.2 years.[102] A similar progression rate (15%) was found in a different cohort of patients.[57]

Secondary Dysplasia

Secondary dysplasia is seen in patients with a history of bladder neoplasia. The incidence of dysplasia in patients with established bladder neoplasia varies from 22% to 86% and approaches 100% in patients with invasive carcinoma.[58,115-120] As many as 24% of random biopsies from patients with stage Ta and T1 carcinomas show epithelial abnormalities that include dysplasia and carcinoma in situ.[121] The presence of urothelial dysplasia indicates urothelial instability and is a harbinger of recurrence and progression.[82,120,122-128] Recurrence rate was 73% of patients with superficial neoplasia and concomitant dysplasia compared with 43% without coexisting dysplasia.[121] Of the 30% of patients with superficial urothelial carcinoma who experienced muscle invasive cancer within 5 years after the initial diagnosis, most had dysplasia or carcinoma in situ adjacent to the primary tumor.[122] Of the patients with dysplasia elsewhere in the bladder mucosa, 36% eventually had muscle-invasive tumors, whereas only 7% of patients with normal urothelium in adjacent biopsies subsequently had muscle-invasive cancer.

Urothelial Carcinoma In Situ (High-Grade Intraurothelial Neoplasia)

Urothelial carcinoma in situ is a flat, noninvasive lesion in which the urothelium is entirely composed of cytologically malignant cells. Melamed et al. first described the natural history of urothelial carcinoma in situ and found that 9 of 25 patients (36%) experienced development of invasive carcinoma within 5 years after the initial diagnosis.[129] In Cheng et al.'s study of 138 patients with urothelial carcinoma in situ in the absence of invasive cancer, the ages at diagnosis ranged from 32 to 90 years (mean, 66 years).[130] The male-to-female ratio in patients with carcinoma in situ is approximately 7:1. Clinical presentations include gross and microscopic hematuria, irritative symptoms (dysuria, pain, frequency), nocturia, and sterile pyuria. Approximately 25% of patients are asymptomatic. Carcinoma in situ usually is multifocal, with a predilection for the trigone, lateral wall, and dome of the bladder. Cystoscopically, it may appear as erythematous velvety or granular patches, although it may also be visually undetectable. Erythematous changes are often apparent at gross examination (Fig. 6.16).

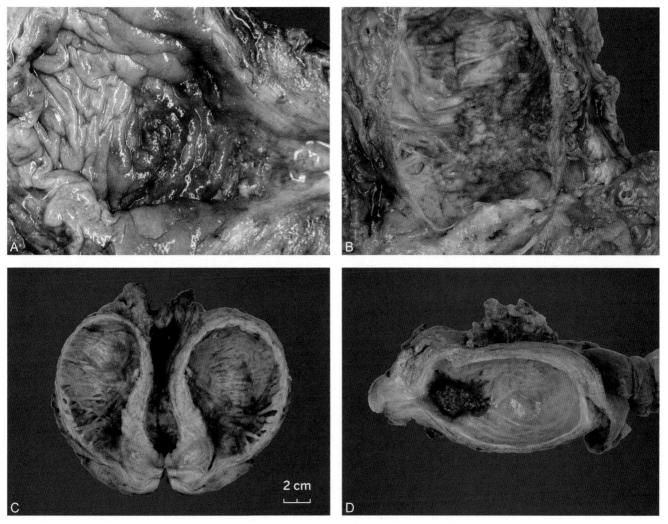

Fig. 6.16 Gross appearance of urothelial carcinoma in situ (A to D). Erythematous changes are common.

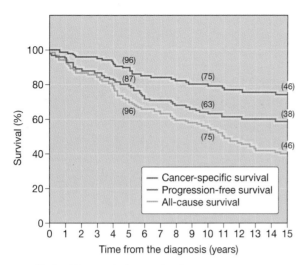

Fig. 6.17 Kaplan-Meier survival curves for 138 patients with primary urothelial carcinoma in situ of the bladder. No patients had invasive urothelial carcinoma at the time of diagnosis. The numbers in parentheses represent the number of patients under observation at 5, 10, and 15 years. Progression was defined as development of invasive carcinoma, distant metastasis, or death from bladder cancer. (From Cheng L, Cheville JC, Neumann RM, et al. Survival of patients with carcinoma in situ of the urinary bladder. *Cancer* 1999;85:2469–2474, with permission.)

De novo or isolated carcinoma in situ (often referred to as primary carcinoma in situ) accounts for 1% to 3% of bladder neoplasms.[14,58,130-135] Clinical presentation often closely mimics that of interstitial cystitis. Urothelial carcinoma in situ is often multifocal. Mapping studies of cystectomy specimens show extensive carcinoma in situ, with involvement of the prostatic urethra and the ureter in as many as 67% and 57% of cases, respectively.[136-142] Urothelial carcinoma in situ has a high likelihood of progressing to invasive carcinoma if left untreated.[130] The mean interval between a diagnosis of carcinoma in situ and the detection of cancer progression is 5 years. The actuarial progression-free survival, cancer-specific survival, and all-cause survival rates are 63%, 79%, and 55%, respectively, at 10 years and 59%, 74%, and 40%, respectively, at 15 years (Fig. 6.17).[130] Factors predictive of progression include multifocality, coexistent bladder neoplasia, DNA aneuploidy, CCND3 gene amplification, prostatic urethral involvement, and recurrence after treatment.[13,14,58,63,84,130,143-145]

Urothelial carcinoma in situ is often associated with invasive carcinoma elsewhere in the bladder (referred to as *secondary carcinoma in situ*).[146] The frequency of carcinoma in situ increases with the grade and stage of the associated urothelial neoplasm. Patients with coexisting invasive urothelial carcinoma have a greater risk for cancer progression and cancer-specific death than patients with primary carcinoma in situ.[58]

Microscopic Pathology

Urothelial carcinoma in situ is characterized by flat, disordered proliferation of urothelial cells with marked cytologic abnormalities (Fig. 6.18). The morphologic diagnosis of carcinoma in situ requires severe cytologic atypia (anaplasia).[14,58,130] Full-thickness change is not required, which may range from one cell layer to the thickness of hyperplasia (greater than seven cells). Superficial (umbrella) cells may or may not be present. Marked disorganization of cells is characteristic, with loss of cellular polarity and decreased cellular cohesiveness. The tumor cells tend to be large

and pleomorphic, with moderate to abundant cytoplasm. Nevertheless, the cells of carcinoma in situ are sometimes small with a high nuclear-to-cytoplasmic ratio. The chromatin tends to be coarse and clumped. Nucleoli may be multiple, and they are large and prominent in at least some of the cells. Mitotic figures, which are often atypical, are seen in the uppermost layers of the urothelium. The adjacent mucosa often contains lesser degrees of cytologic abnormality. Tissue edema, vascular ectasia, and proliferation of small capillaries are frequently observed in the lamina propria (Fig. 6.18).

An immunohistochemical panel, consisting of CK20, CD44, p53, and Ki67, may be helpful in differential diagnosis.[58,104,105,147-151] Carcinoma in situ shows intense CK20 and p53 positivity in most malignant cells. Increased Ki67 labeling is noted in carcinoma in situ, but this can be seen also in reactive atypia of the urothelium, thus limiting its usefulness in practice. The neoplastic cells are uniformly negative for CD44 immunostaining.[147] In contrast, CK20 staining shows patchy cytoplasmic immunoreactivity only in the superficial umbrella cell layer, and CD44 stains only the basal cells in the adjacent normal urothelium. p16 and racemase have been reported as variably positive in urothelial carcinoma in situ and negative to weak and focal in reactive urothelium.[91,106,111]

Histologic Variants of Carcinoma In Situ

Several morphologic variants and growth patterns of carcinoma in situ have been recognized over the years (Figs. 6.19 to 6.21; Table 6.4). Variations in subtype of urothelial carcinoma in situ do not alter patient prognosis. Although it is not necessary to mention these specific growth patterns or morphologic variants in the surgical pathology report, awareness of the histologic diversity of carcinoma in situ may aid in the diagnosis of this therapeutically and biologically important lesion.[58,152] These lesions may be associated with microinvasion, sometimes clinically unsuspected and histologically subtle.

Large Cell Carcinoma In Situ

Large cell carcinoma in situ constitutes the most common morphologic form of this entity. Cytologic findings include nuclear pleomorphism, variably abundant cytoplasm, and anaplastic nuclear features (Fig. 6.19A). In rare cases large cell carcinoma in situ may have minor nuclear pleomorphism but still exhibit architectural disarray. Rare cases may focally exhibit high pleomorphism with bizarre giant cells.

Small Cell Carcinoma In Situ

The small cell pattern refers to the size of the cells and may or may not coexist with small cell carcinoma (Fig. 6.19B); it is unrelated to neuroendocrine differentiation of carcinoma in situ. In such cases the pleomorphism is usually minimal, the cytoplasm is scant, and the nuclei are enlarged and hyperchromatic, with coarse unevenly distributed chromatin. The scattered prominent nucleoli are distorted and angulated. Recognition of the small cell pattern of carcinoma in situ is important to avoid misdiagnosis of basal cell hyperplasia, which has been observed in patients treated with BCG, and show a small cell pattern but lack nuclear atypia or loss of polarity.

Denuding and "Clinging Pattern" Carcinoma In Situ

In some cases the neoplastic urothelial cells are strikingly discohesive and undergo extensive exfoliation, with the result that biopsies

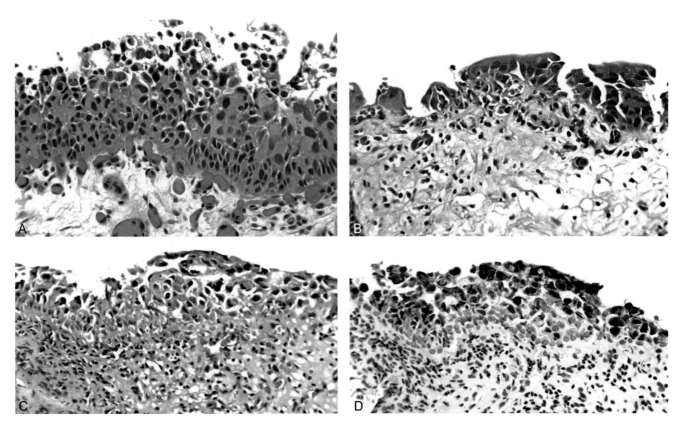

Fig. 6.18 Urothelial carcinoma in situ displaying disordered proliferation of malignant urothelial cells that demonstrate a high nuclear-to-cytoplasmic ratio, nuclear pleomorphism, irregular nuclear contours, coarsely granular chromatin, and prominent nucleoli. Loss of cellular polarity and cell cohesion are seen in urothelial carcinoma in situ (A to C). Vascular proliferation is often prominent in the underlying stroma. Full-thickness involvement is not required for the diagnosis of urothelial carcinoma in situ. The superficial umbrella cell layer may still be present. (D) Aberrant expression of cytokeratin 20 is observed.

may show only a few residual carcinoma cells on the surface ("clinging carcinoma in situ") or no recognizable epithelial cells on the surface, a condition referred to as "denuding cystitis" (Fig. 6.19C and D).[153] In the clinging pattern of carcinoma in situ, there is a patchy, usually single layer of atypical cells. In mucosal biopsies entirely lacking surface epithelium, carcinoma in situ may be present only in von Brunn nests. A careful search for carcinoma in situ in deeper sections or in other submitted biopsy fragments is important, and a recommendation for evaluation of urine cytology for carcinoma cells is warranted.

Pagetoid and Undermining (Lepidic) Carcinoma In Situ

Another pattern of carcinoma in situ, also referred to as cancerization of the urothelium, shows either pagetoid spread (clusters or isolated single cells) (Fig. 6.20A to C) or undermining or overriding of the normal urothelium (lepidic growth) (Fig. 6.20D). Carcinoma in situ exhibiting pagetoid growth is characterized by large single cells or small clusters of cells within otherwise normal urothelium of ureter, urethra, prostatic ducts, or in areas of squamous metaplasia. Individual cells showing pagetoid spread have enlarged nuclei with coarse chromatin; frequently the cytoplasm is clear.

Pagetoid growth patterns can be found in up to 15% of carcinoma in situ cases.[58] Most patients are male and their ages range from 31 to 78 years (mean, 64 years). Pagetoid carcinoma in situ is usually a focal lesion and is easily overlooked. It occurs in a clinical and histologic setting of conventional carcinoma in situ with coexisting invasive urothelial carcinoma, and such patients essentially

have the same progression and survival rates as patients without pagetoid changes. In cases with extensive urothelial denudation, pagetoid carcinoma in situ may be focally present in adjacent otherwise normal-looking urothelium, thus alerting the surgical pathologist to search for additional carcinoma in situ elsewhere in the bladder.

Because primary extramammary Paget disease of the external genitalia and of the anal canal may extend to the bladder, and conversely, some cases of pagetoid carcinoma in situ of the bladder may extend to the urethra, ureter, and external genitalia, differentiating between these two entities represents an important diagnostic and therapeutic challenge. A panel of immunostains, including CK7, CK20, and thrombomodulin, may assist in differentiating pagetoid urothelial carcinoma in situ from extramammary Paget disease, which is known to be CK7+ and CK20-.[58]

Carcinoma In Situ With Squamous or Glandular Differentiation

Rare cases of carcinoma in situ may exhibit squamous differentiation characterized by intercellular bridges. Carcinoma in situ with squamous features is most often observed in association with urothelial carcinoma showing extensive squamous differentiation elsewhere in the bladder (Fig. 6.21A). A much less frequently encountered pattern is carcinoma in situ with morphologic and immunohistochemical evidence of glandular differentiation (Fig. 6.21B). Some authors refer to this as adenocarcinoma in situ; such lesions may show papillary, cribriform, or flat morphology. Carcinoma in situ involving von Brunn nests

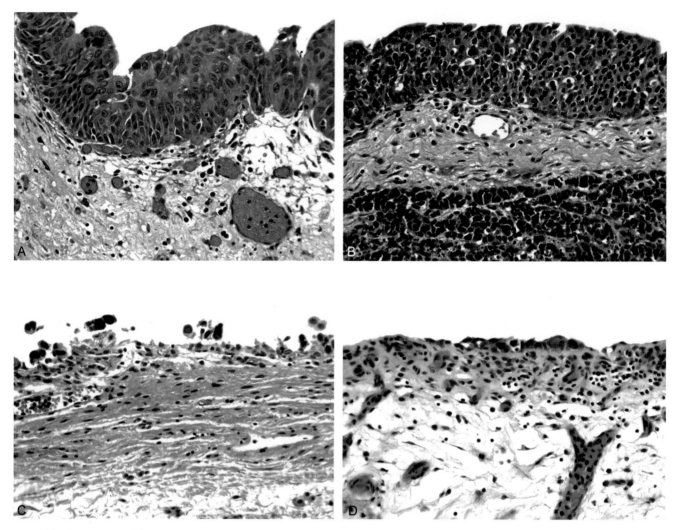

Fig. 6.19 Histologic variants of urothelial carcinoma in situ. (A) Large cell carcinoma in situ. (B) Small cell carcinoma in situ. Small cell carcinoma is present in the lamina propria. (C) "Clinging" carcinoma in situ. (D) Denuding carcinoma in situ. The urothelium is partially denuded; residual carcinoma in situ cells are present in the remainder of the urothelium.

(Fig. 6.22), cystitis glandularis, or cystitis cystica may be difficult to distinguish from adenocarcinoma in situ in the absence of concurrent invasive adenocarcinoma. A recent report based on 25 cases of urothelial carcinoma in situ with glandular differentiation showed high Ki67 index and p53 accumulation, high nuclear and cytoplasmic p16 expression, and diffuse PTEN expression, a phenotype that also characterized concurrent conventional carcinoma in situ.[154] MUC5A, MUC2, CK20, and HER2 were positive in all 25 cases of urothelial carcinoma in situ with glandular differentiation, and CDX2 was present in 19 cases; MUC1, CK7, or 34βE12 was focally present in 21, 19, and 18 cases, respectively. The authors concluded that urothelial carcinoma in situ with glandular differentiation is a variant of carcinoma in situ that follows the natural history of conventional urothelial carcinoma in situ. The immunophenotype suggests urothelial origin with the expression of MUC5A and CDX2 as signature for glandular differentiation.[154]

Carcinoma In Situ With Micropapillary Pattern

On rare occasions, urothelial carcinoma in situ may have a micropapillary architecture, characterized by a flat surface with micropapillae (pseudopapillae without vascular cores) lined by markedly atypical cells (Fig. 6.23). This morphology is seen in the context of conventional urothelial carcinoma and seems to be unrelated to invasive micropapillary urothelial carcinoma.[155]

Carcinoma In Situ With Microinvasion

Carcinoma in situ with microinvasion was initially defined by Farrow and Utz as invasion into the lamina propria to a depth ≤5 mm from the basement membrane.[156] At a recent consensus it was suggested that cases with more than 20 cells measured from the stroma-epithelial interface should be classified as fully invasive.[58] Microinvasion appears as direct extension in cords (tentacular), single cells, or single cells and clusters of cells (Fig. 6.24). The clusters of cells may have retraction artifact that mimics vascular invasion. Stromal response may be present, but in most cases it is absent. In cases with a prominent stromal inflammatory response the invasive neoplastic cells may be interspersed among lymphocytes, making them inconspicuous. In these circumstances, immunohistochemical staining with antibodies against CKs, such as AE1/AE3, highlights the invading cells.[157]

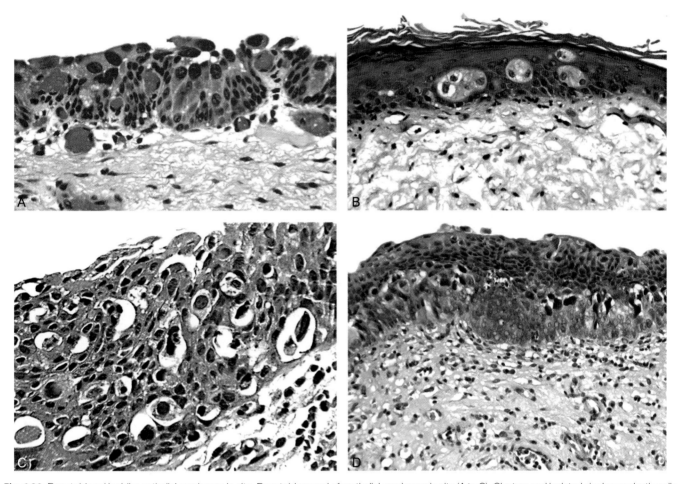

Fig. 6.20 Pagetoid and lepidic urothelial carcinoma in situ. Pagetoid spread of urothelial carcinoma in situ (A to C). Clusters and isolated single neoplastic cells (B and C) are present in the urothelium. (D) Urothelial carcinoma in situ also may display an undermining or lepidic growth pattern.

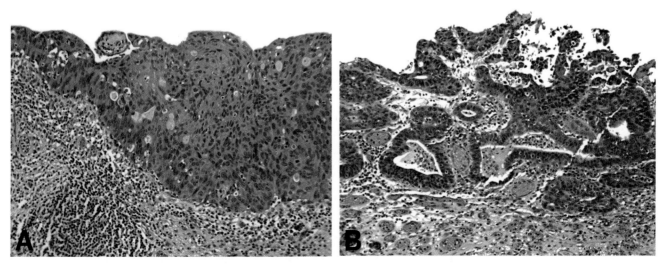

Fig. 6.21 Urothelial carcinoma in situ may show squamous (A) or glandular differentiation (B).

TABLE 6.4	Morphologic Patterns of Urothelial Carcinoma in situ

Large cell carcinoma in situ
Small cell carcinoma in situ
Denuding and "clinging pattern" carcinoma in situ
Pagetoid and undermining (lepidic) carcinoma in situ
Carcinoma in situ with squamous or glandular differentiation
Carcinoma in situ with microinvasion
Carcinoma in situ with micropapillary pattern

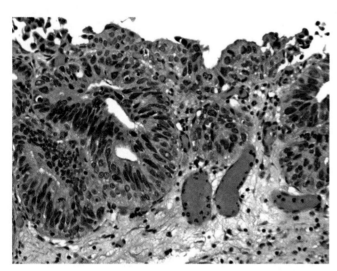

Fig. 6.22 Urothelial carcinoma in situ involving von Brunn nest may be misdiagnosed as adenocarcinoma in situ.

Urothelial Carcinoma

General Features

Epidemiology and Risk Factors

Bladder cancer is the seventh most common cancer worldwide, accounting for an estimated 330,380 new cases globally in 2012.[158] There are significant variations in incidence, morbidity,

recurrence, progression, and mortality rates of bladder cancer in different countries and ethnicity groups.[144,159-165] African American men have a much lower incidence of bladder cancer, but their mortality rates are similar to Caucasians.[144,166-169] Bladder cancer occurs two to five times more frequently in men than in women. This has been attributed to different smoking and occupational exposure between men and women.[144,166-168]

Multiple risk factors have been linked to bladder cancer. Exogenous factors, such as tobacco smoking, occupational risk, and lifestyle exposure to carcinogens, all play important roles. Smokers have two to four times the risk for urothelial cancer as the general population, and heavy smokers have five times the risk.[167] It is estimated that 20 years of smoking is needed for development of bladder cancer, and the probability of this event is directly correlated with the lifetime number of cigarettes consumed. The relative risk for active smokers experiencing development of bladder cancer compared with never smokers is 3:1 and for previous smokers is 1.9:1. Although the exact mechanism by which tobacco causes bladder cancer is not known, many known carcinogens in cigarette smoke, such as acrolein, 4-amino-biphenyl, arylamine, and oxygen free radicals, have been implicated. Furthermore, increased duration, intensity of tobacco consumption, and degree of inhalation significantly contribute to cancer development. The beneficial effects of smoking cessation, in contrast, include an almost immediate decline in risk for bladder cancer. Continued smokers have a worse recurrence-free survival than those who quit at the time of diagnosis.[144,170] Ex-smokers and current smokers also have a significantly shorter recurrence-free survival after treatment for bladder cancer.[171]

Occupational exposure to aniline dyes and aromatic amines such as 2-naphthylamine and benzidine is the second most prevalent risk factor for bladder cancer. Benzidine, the most carcinogenic aromatic amine, is used in dye production and as a hardener in the rubber industry.[170] The degree of carcinogenesis caused by occupational exposure varies with the degree of industrialization, but in heavily industrialized nations, occupational exposure may account for up to one-fourth of all urothelial cancers. The latency period between exposure and tumor development is usually prolonged.[144] Occupational bladder cancer has also been observed in gas workers, painters, and hairdressers. Nutrition may also play a role. Vitamin A supplementation apparently reduces the risk for

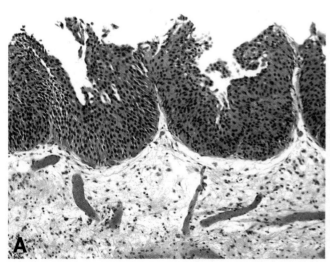
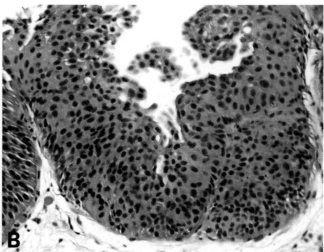

Fig. 6.23 Urothelial carcinoma in situ with micropapillary pattern (A and B).

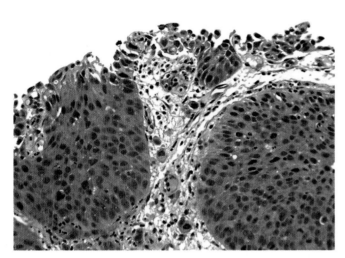

Fig. 6.24 Urothelial carcinoma in situ with microinvasion is characterized by individual single cells in the stroma. The adjacent von Brunn nests are also involved by carcinoma in situ.

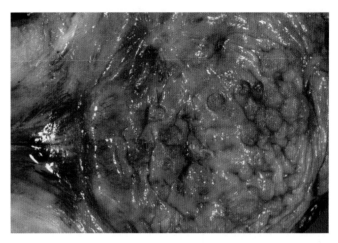

Fig. 6.25 Gross appearance of multifocal urothelial carcinoma. The papillary architecture of these tumors is apparent.

bladder cancer, whereas fried food and fat ingestion increases the risk. A high fluid intake reduced the risk for bladder cancer in one study, but this remains controversial. Epidemiologic studies in Taiwan and Chile have shown an increased risk for urothelial cancer in people whose drinking water has a high content of arsenic. Other water contaminants with putative toxic effects on urothelium are also being actively investigated.[144]

Additional factors implicated in the development and progression of bladder cancer include analgesic use, urinary tract infections (bacterial, parasitic, fungal, or viral), urinary lithiasis, pelvic radiation, and chemotherapeutic agents such as cyclophosphamide.[172] Although caffeine ingestion has been implicated as a risk factor for bladder cancer, risk estimates for this association decrease after controlling for concomitant tobacco use. Similarly, saccharin-containing artificial sweeteners have induced bladder neoplasia in rats, but human epidemiologic studies have failed to establish this relationship in humans. There is a relationship between the parasite *Bilharzia* (schistosomiasis) and squamous cell cancer in the bladder, more frequently seen in the Middle East, where waterborne flatworms are endemic.[144]

Signs and Symptoms

The majority of patients with bladder cancer present with hematuria. Approximately 20% of patients being evaluated for gross hematuria will subsequently be diagnosed with bladder cancer. Similarly, of patients presenting with microscopic hematuria, up to 10% will be diagnosed with bladder cancer. A significant proportion of patients also have irritative voiding symptoms including urgency, frequency, and dysuria; their symptoms are mistakenly attributed to urinary tract infection.

The initial evaluation and management for patients with suspected bladder cancer involve cystoscopic evaluation of the bladder and prostatic urethra for mucosal lesions. Small lesions and flat lesions worrisome for carcinoma in situ can be sampled with cold-cup biopsy forceps, whereas larger suspicious lesions are resected transurethrally as completely as possible. Transurethral resections and biopsies should include muscularis propria if possible.[173] Tumor recurrence is a significant risk factor for cancer progression.[174-177] New guidelines of the International Consultation on Urological Diseases were recently published.[178-183] Advances in

multiparametric magnetic resonance imaging are likely to change the clinical approach to bladder cancer diagnosis in years to come.

Field Cancerization and Tumor Multicentricity

Development of multifocal tumors in the same patient, either synchronous or metachronous, is a common characteristic of urothelial malignancy (Fig. 6.25).[44,65,66,76,78,81,102,142,184-187] Multiple coexisting tumors have often arisen before clinical symptoms are apparent. The separate tumors may or may not share a similar histology. Two theories have been proposed to explain the frequency of urothelial tumor multifocality. The monoclonal theory suggests that the multiple tumors arise from a single transformed cell that proliferates and spreads throughout the urothelium either by intraluminal implantation or by intraepithelial migration. The field effect theory explains tumor multifocality as a development secondary to field cancerization effect. Chemical carcinogens cause independent transforming genetic alterations at different sites in the urothelial lining, leading to multiple genetically unrelated tumors.

The issue of monoclonal versus oligoclonal origin of multifocal urothelial carcinomas is clinically important for understanding patterns of early tumor development when planning treatment and surgical strategies, and when molecular diagnostic techniques are used in the detection of recurrent or residual disease.[43,44,63,65,66,71,102,144,188] The cause of multifocality also influences test design for genetic detection of recurrent or residual tumor cells in posttreatment urine samples. No consensus currently exists concerning which theory is most important in the development of multifocal urothelial carcinoma. Many studies have suggested a monoclonal origin for multifocal urothelial carcinoma, but other studies have shown an independent origin for some multicentric urothelial tumors using similar methods.[59,60,189-205] A recent study suggests that both field cancerization and monoclonal tumor spread may coexist in the same patient.[44] Molecular evidence supporting an oligoclonal origin for multifocal urothelial carcinomas in the majority of cases was found, consistent with the field cancerization theory for multicentric urothelial carcinogenesis.

Field cancerization, which is an important cause of multicentric squamous cell carcinomas of the head and neck, postulates that

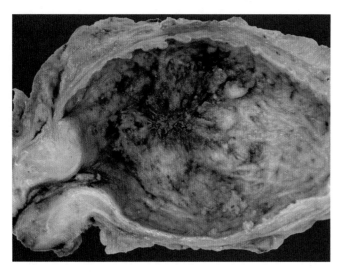

Fig. 6.26 Multifocal bladder cancer. Urothelial carcinoma in situ is often associated with invasive urothelial carcinoma.

multifocal urothelial carcinomas arise in the same way.[71] In the field cancerization process, simultaneous or sequential tumors result from numerous independent mutational events at different sites in the urothelial tract. These independent transformations are a consequence of external cancer-causing influences. In support of the field effect theory is the frequent finding of genetic instability in normal-appearing bladder mucosa in patients with bladder cancer in the adjacent urothelium.[47,206] Premalignant changes, such as dysplasia or carcinoma in situ, often are found in urothelial mucosa away from an invasive bladder cancer (Fig. 6.26). Many genetic comparisons and mapping of atypia in cystectomy specimens have emphasized the role of oligoclonality and field cancerization in the development of multifocal urothelial tumors, especially in early-stage disease. Because the monoclonal and oligoclonal theories to explain urothelial tumor multifocality are not mutually exclusive, various theories have been proposed to combine the two mechanisms. It has been suggested that oligoclonality is more common in early lesions with progression to higher stages leading to the overgrowth of one clone and pseudomonoclonality.[199,207] Thus early or preneoplastic lesions may arise independently with a specific clone undergoing malignant transformation, which subsequently spreads through the urothelium by either an intraluminal or intraepithelial dissemination. Whereas tumor multifocality seems to be an oligoclonal phenomenon in the majority of cases, there is undeniable support for the monoclonal hypothesis in some cases.[44]

Molecular Taxonomy

Recent studies have sought to better define the molecular characteristics of urothelial carcinoma using broad-based genomic and transcriptomic approaches to differentiate distinct molecular classes of urothelial carcinoma.[208-211] Historically, a dual-pathway model was developed in which noninvasive lesions (low-grade papillary Ta) are associated with frequent HRAS and FGFR3 alterations, and frequent TP53 and RB alterations characterize high-grade urothelial carcinomas. The findings in more recent studies suggest that this model may somewhat oversimplify the genomic complexity of urothelial cancer. Based on complex gene expression studies, the number of bladder cancer subtypes has been reappraised. One group of investigators identified five categories of tumors that demonstrated differential expression of CK, FGFR3 mutational status, cell adhesion gene profiles, and cell-cycle regulator gene profiles.[212,213] These five categories include the so-called urobasal A, urobasal B, genomically unstable, squamous cell carcinoma–like, and infiltrated. Three major subtypes—urobasal, genomically unstable, and squamous cell carcinoma–like—can also be distinguished based on immunohistochemical profile, enabling identification of such cases in daily pathology practice.[212,213]

A simplified classification system was recently published that divides urothelial carcinoma into "luminal" and "basal-like" categories. Whereas *luminal (CK20+, GATA3+)* carcinomas expressed genes frequently associated with superficial umbrella cells and appeared similar to superficial papillary tumors, *basal-like (CK5/6+, CD44+, CK20−)* carcinomas expressed genes more characteristic of urothelial basal cells and also had a significantly worse prognosis but may be more responsive to neoadjuvant chemotherapy. In addition to the luminal and basal-like tumors, some classification systems have identified a third group of tumors, "p53-like," which are associated with resistance to neoadjuvant chemotherapy.[214]

Immune Checkpoint Inhibitor Therapy

Immunotherapeutic strategies to target the programmed cell death-1/ programmed cell death-1 ligand (PD-1/PD-L1) axis represent a breakthrough in the treatment of bladder cancer.[215-219] These agents act on T-cell–inhibitory pathways, unleashing profound antitumor effects. Drug options for patients with bladder cancer now include atezolizumab, pembrolizumab, nivolumab, durvalumab, and avelumab. The suggested cutoffs for evaluating available immunohistochemical markers associated with a specific drug are summarized in Table 6.5.

Histologic Grading

Histologic Grading According to the 1973 World Health Organization Classification

Histologic grading is one of the most important prognostic factors in bladder cancer.[1,220-222] The first widely accepted grading system for papillary urothelial neoplasms was the 1973 WHO classification system, which divided urothelial tumors into four categories: papilloma, grade 1 carcinoma, grade 2 carcinoma, and grade 3 carcinoma.[10] Histologic grading is based on the degree of cellular anaplasia, with grade 1 tumors having the least degree of anaplasia compatible with a diagnosis of malignancy, grade 3 tumors having the most severe degree of anaplasia, and grade 2 tumors having an intermediate degree of cellular anaplasia (Fig. 6.27). Anaplasia is further defined by the authors of the 1973 WHO classification as increased cellularity, nuclear crowding, disturbed cellular polarity, failure of differentiation from the base to the surface, nuclear polymorphism, irregular cell size, variations in nuclear shape and chromatin pattern, displaced or abnormal mitotic figures, and giant cells.[10]

The 1973 WHO histologic grading of bladder cancer is one of most successful grading systems among all organ sites and has been validated since its introduction three decades ago.[222-225] The 1973 WHO grading system has been accepted by pathologists, urologists, oncologists, and cancer registrars in the United States and elsewhere. An enormous amount of data have been accumulated using this system in studies of the morphologic properties, clinical behavior, treatment, and follow-up of urothelial tumors. Because of its relative simplicity and its well-documented powerful

TABLE 6.5	Comparison of Programmed Cell Death-1 Ligand Immunostainings in Selected Anti–Programmed Cell Death-1/Anti–Programmed Cell Death-1 Ligand Agents						
Characteristics	Durvalumab	Atezolizumab		Nivolumab		Pembrolizumab	Avelumab
Manufacturer	MedImmune/ AstraZeneca	Genetech/Roche		Bristol-Meyers Squibb		Merck	Merck/ Pfizer
Target	PD-L1	PD-L1		PD-1		PD-1	PD-L1
PD-L1 assay	Ventana SP263	Ventana SP142		Dako 28-8		Dako 22C3	Dako 73-10
Cell types scored for urothelial carcinoma	TIC and TC	TIC		TC		TC and TIC	TC
No. of lines of therapy	≥1	≥2	1 (cisplatin ineligible)	≥2	≥2	2	1 (cisplatin ineligible)	≥2
PD-L1 cutoffs							
High/positive	≥25% TC or TIC	≥5% TIC	≥5% TIC	≥1% TC	≥1%, ≥5% TC	≥10% CPS	≥10% CPS	≥5% TC
Low/negative	<25% TC and TIC	<1% TIC	<1% TIC	<1% TC	<1% TC	Not available	<10% CPS	No visible staining

CPS, Combined positive score (tumor and immune cell PD-L1 expression); PD-1, programmed cell death-1; PD-L1, programmed cell death-1 ligand; TC, tumor cells; TIC, tumor-infiltrating immune cells.

predictive value, it has been well accepted by urologists and used globally for several decades in making clinical decisions for management of patients with urothelial cancer.

A recent systematic review surveyed 3593 published articles and compared the prognostic performance and reproducibility of the 1973 WHO and 2004/2016 WHO grading systems.[226] They found that higher tumor grade in both classifications was associated with higher disease progression and recurrence rates. Progression rates in grade 1 patients were similar to those in low-grade patients. However, the 1973 system identifies more aggressive tumors. Reproducibility of the 2004/2016 system was marginally better than that of the 1973 system. The authors could not confirm that the 2004/2016 classification outperforms the 1973 classification in prediction of recurrence and progression.[226]

The European Association of Urology (EAU) guidelines on non–muscle-invasive urothelial carcinoma of the bladder recommend the use of both 1973 and 2004/2016 WHO classifications (Table 6.6) (see further discussion later in this chapter).[177]

Grade 1 Urothelial Carcinoma

Grade 1 papillary carcinoma consists of an orderly arrangement of normal urothelial cells lining delicate papillae with minimal architectural abnormality and minimal nuclear atypia (Fig. 6.27A and B). Nuclear grooves are usually present. There may be some complexity and fusion of the papillae, but this is usually not prominent. The urothelium is often thickened to more than seven cell layers. The urothelium displays normal maturation and cohesiveness, with an intact superficial cell layer. The nuclei tend to be uniform in shape and spacing, although there may be some enlargement and elongation. The chromatin texture is finely granular, without significant nucleolar enlargement. Mitotic figures are rare or absent, and basally located. Grade 1 tumor should be distinguished from urothelial papilloma, which is a benign lesion (Table 6.7).

Grade 1 carcinoma appears to have a predilection for the ureteric orifices. In one study, 69% of grade 1 urothelial carcinomas were centered near a ureteric orifice, but the remainder was seen in all other portions of the bladder. Patients with grade 1 carcinoma are at increased risk for local recurrence, progression, and dying of bladder cancer. Significant levels of morbidity and mortality are associated with grade 1 urothelial carcinoma of the bladder if patients are followed for a sufficient interval.[227-240] With 20 years of follow-up, Holmang et al. found that 14% of patients with noninvasive grade 1 urothelial carcinoma (pTa G1) died of bladder cancer.[229] In a recent review of 152 patients with stage Ta grade 1 urothelial carcinoma, Leblanc et al. found that 83 patients (55%) had tumor recurrence, including 37% with cancer progression.[231] Patients who remained tumor-free for 1 year still had a 43% chance of late recurrence. In Greene et al.'s study of 100 patients with grade 1 cancer, 10 patients (10%) died of bladder cancer after more than 15 years; of the 73 patients who had recurrences, 22% were of higher grade than the original tumor.[241] The mean interval from diagnosis to the development of invasive cancer was 8 years. Jordan et al. studied 91 patients with grade 1 papillary urothelial tumors and found that 40% had recurrence.[239] Twenty percent of patients with recurrences had high-grade (grade 3) cancer, and four patients (4%) died of bladder cancer.[239] Long-term follow-up is recommended for patients with grade 1 papillary urothelial carcinoma.

Grade 2 Urothelial Carcinoma

Grade 2 carcinoma represents a broad group of tumors encompassing a spectrum of cytologic atypia and some variability in the relative proportions of cells with atypical features (Fig. 6.27C and D). Grade 2 carcinomas retain some of the orderly architectural appearance and maturation of grade 1 carcinoma but display at least focal moderate variation in orderliness, nuclear appearance, and chromatin texture, apparent at low magnification. Cytologic abnormalities are invariably present in grade 2 carcinoma, with moderate nuclear crowding, moderate loss of cell polarity, moderate nuclear hyperchromasia, moderate anisonucleosis, and mild nucleolar enlargement. Mitotic figures are usually limited to the lower half of the urothelium, but this is an inconstant feature. Superficial cells are usually present, and the urothelial cells are predominantly cohesive, although variation in cohesion may be present. Some tumors may be extremely orderly, reminiscent of grade 1 carcinoma, with only a small focus of obvious disorder or irregularity. These are considered grade 2 cancer, recognizing that tumor grade is based on the highest level of abnormality present.

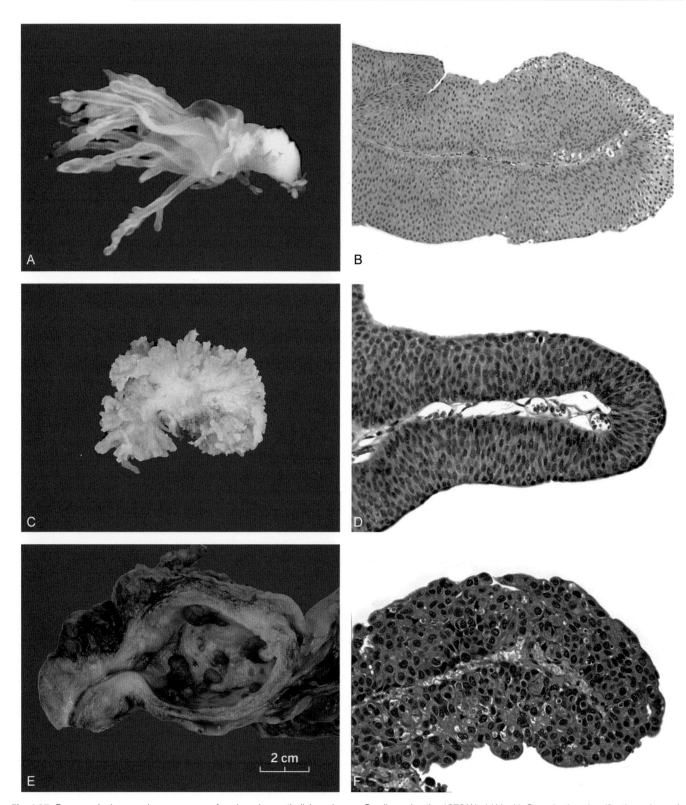

Fig. 6.27 Gross and microscopic appearance of noninvasive urothelial carcinoma. Grading using the 1973 World Health Organization classification scheme is recommended. Grade 1 urothelial carcinoma (A and B). Grade 2 urothelial carcinoma (C and D). Grade 3 urothelial carcinoma (E and F).

The prognosis for patients with grade 2 urothelial carcinoma is significantly worse than for those with lower-grade papillary cancer. Recurrence risk for patients with noninvasive grade 2 cancer is 45% to 67%.[13,14,242] Invasion occurs in up to 20%, and cancer-specific death is expected in 13% to 20% after surgical treatment.[13,14,242] Patients with grade 2 cancer and lamina propria invasion are at even greater risk, with recurrences in 67% to 80% of cases, the development of muscle-invasive cancer in 21% to 49%, and cancer-specific death in 17% to 51% of those treated surgically.[13,14,242] Some authors consider both nuclear

TABLE 6.6

Risk Group Stratification for Non–Muscle-Invasive Urothelial Carcinoma of the Bladder[177]

Risk Grouping	Criteria
Low-risk tumors	Primary, solitary, Ta, LG/G1, <3 cm, no CIS
Intermediate-risk tumors	All tumors not defined in the two adjacent categories (between the category of low and high risk)
High-risk tumors	Any of the following: • T1 tumor • HG/G3 tumor • Carcinoma in situ • Multiple and recurrent and large (>3 cm) Ta G1G2 tumors[a]

HG, high grade; *LG*, low grade.
[a]All conditions must be present at this point.

TABLE 6.7

Diagnostic Features of Urothelial Papilloma and Grade 1 (Low-Grade) Noninvasive Papillary Urothelial Carcinoma

Characteristics	Urothelial Papilloma	Grade 1 (Low-Grade) Urothelial Carcinoma
Age	Younger	Older
Sex (male:female)	2:1	3:1
Size	Small, usually <2 cm	Typically, larger than papilloma
Microscopic findings		
Well-formed papillae	Present	Present, rarely fused
Thickness of urothelium	≤7 layers	>7 layers
Superficial umbrella cells	Present	Usually present
Cytology	Minimal or absent	Mild
Nuclear enlargement	Rare or none	None or slightly enlarged
Nuclear hyperchromasia	Rare or none	Slight or minimal
Chromatin	Fine	Fine, slightly granular
Nucleolar enlargement	Absent	Absent or inconspicuous
Nuclear pleomorphism	Absent	Absent
Mitotic figures	None	Rare or basal location
Stromal invasion	Absent	Rare

Grade 1 (low-grade) urothelial carcinoma in the newly proposed grading system corresponds to those previously classified as "papillary urothelial neoplasm of low malignant potential" (PUNLMP) in the 2004 World Health Organization and International Society of Urological Pathology classification system.
Modified from Cheng L, MacLennan GT, Lopez-Beltran A. Histologic grading of urothelial carcinoma: a reappraisal. *Hum Pathol* 2012;43:2097–2108.

pleomorphism and mitotic count as criteria for subdividing grade 2 urothelial cancer (grades 2A and 2B), and they have been successful in identifying groups of cancers with different outcomes.[222,243-246] However, subclassification of grade 2 urothelial carcinoma is not recommended because of significant interobserver variability.

Grade 3 Urothelial Carcinoma

Grade 3 carcinoma displays the most extreme nuclear abnormality of any papillary urothelial cancer, similar to changes observed in urothelial carcinoma in situ (Fig. 6.27E and F). The obvious urothelial disorder and loss of polarity are present at scanning magnification. The superficial cell layer is partially or completely absent with grade 3 carcinoma, accompanied by prominent cellular discohesion. There is obvious loss of normal architecture, cell polarity, and frequent atypical mitotic figures. Cellular anaplasia, characteristic of grade 3 carcinoma, is defined as increased cellularity, nuclear crowding, random cellular polarity, absence of normal mucosal differentiation, nuclear pleomorphism, irregularity in cell size, variation in nuclear shape, capricious chromatin pattern, increased frequency of mitotic figures, and occasional neoplastic giant cells.[10]

Recurrence risk for patients with noninvasive grade 3 cancer is 65% to 85%, with invasion occurring in 20% to 52% and cancer-specific death in up to 35% after surgical treatment.[13,247] Of surgically treated patients with grade 3 cancer and lamina propria invasion, 46% to 71% experience recurrences, 24% to 48% have muscle-invasive cancer, and 25% to 71% suffer cancer-specific death, emphasizing the need for aggressive treatment of these patients.[14,242,248]

Histologic Grading According to the 2004/2016 World Health Organization Classification

The first widely accepted grading system for papillary urothelial neoplasms was the 1973 WHO classification system.[10] In 1998 a revised system of classifying noninvasive papillary urothelial neoplasms of the urinary bladder was proposed by the ISUP (Table 6.8).[249] This system was formally adopted by the WHO in 1999 and was published in *Pathology and Genetics of Tumors of the Urinary System and Male Genital Organs* (3rd and 4th editions), which is part of a series of WHO "Blue Books" for the classification of tumors.[250] This system separates noninvasive papillary urothelial neoplasms into four categories, designated papilloma, PUNLMP, low-grade carcinoma, and high-grade carcinoma (Fig. 6.28; Table 6.8).[6]

Papillary Urothelial Neoplasm of Low Malignant Potential

A PUNLMP is a low-grade urothelial tumor with a papillary architecture and a purported low incidence of recurrence and progression.[46,223-225,248,251-258] This lesion is histologically defined by the 2004/2016 WHO classification system as a papillary urothelial tumor, which resembles the exophytic urothelial papilloma but with increased cellular proliferation exceeding the thickness of normal urothelium (Fig. 6.28A). All such tumors would have been considered grade 1 urothelial carcinomas by the 1973 WHO grading system. Cytologic atypia is minimal or absent, and architectural abnormalities are minimal with preserved polarity. Mitotic figures are infrequent and usually limited to the basal layer. Clinically, these tumors show a male predominance (3:1) and occur at a mean age of 65 years.[259] They are most commonly identified during investigation of gross or microscopic hematuria. Cystoscopically, these lesions are typically 1 to 2 cm in greatest dimension and located on the lateral wall of the bladder or near the ureteric orifices.[259] They have been described as having a "seaweed in the ocean" appearance.

Several studies have shown that the 2004 WHO classification can differentiate noninvasive papillary urothelial tumors into prognostic groups.[248] When applied to transurethral resection of bladder tumor specimens, this classification system predicted the

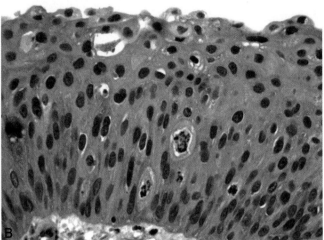

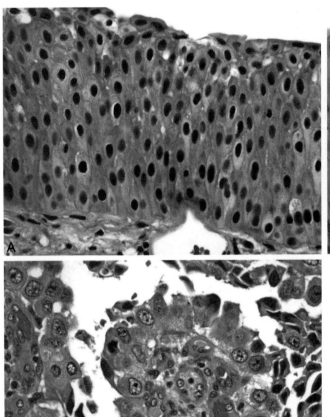

Fig. 6.28 Histologic grading of urothelial tumors using the 2004 World Health Organization (WHO) grading system. (A) Papillary urothelial neoplasm of low malignant potential, formerly 1973 WHO grade 1 urothelial carcinoma. (B) Low-grade urothelial carcinoma, formerly 1973 WHO grade 2 urothelial carcinoma. (C) High-grade urothelial carcinoma, formerly 1973 WHO grade 3 urothelial carcinoma.

TABLE 6.8 Grading of Urothelial Carcinoma of the Urinary Bladder: Comparison of Different Grading Systems

1973 WHO	1998 WHO/ISUP	1999 WHO	2016 WHO	Current Proposal
Papilloma	Papilloma	Papilloma	Papilloma	Papilloma
Grade 1	PUNLMP	PUNLMP	PUNLMP	Grade 1 (low grade)
Grade 2	Low grade	Grade 1	Low grade	Grade 2 (low grade)
		Grade 2		Grade 3 (high grade)
Grade 3	High grade	Grade 3	High grade	Grade 4 (high grade)

ISUP, International Society of Urological Pathology; *PUNLMP,* papillary urothelial neoplasm of low malignant potential; *WHO,* World Health Organization.

All grading schemes have substantial interobserver and intraobserver variabilities. Exact correlation does not exist among the grading systems. Some 1973 WHO grade 2 tumors are "low grade," and some are classified as "high grade." The 1998 WHO/International Society of Urological Pathology system is the same as the 2004 WHO system.

Modified from Cheng L, MacLennan GT, Lopez-Beltran A. Histologic grading of urothelial carcinoma: a reappraisal. *Hum Pathol* 2012;43:2097–2108.

pathologic stage in the corresponding cystectomy.[259] However, the published recurrence and progression rates are variable.[223,224,260-262] A recent meta-analysis suggests that both 1973 and 2004 WHO grading systems predict progression and recurrence. They also conclude that the 1973 WHO grading system identifies more aggressive tumors.[226] These results may argue in favor of reporting both grading systems in daily practice.[220]

In a series of 112 patients diagnosed with PUNLMP, with up to 35 years of follow-up (median, >12 years), tumor recurrence was observed in 29% of patients. Seventy-five percent of patients with tumor recurrence had a higher tumor grade (i.e., low-grade or high-grade urothelial carcinoma according to the 2004/2016 WHO classification). The overall disease progression rate in these patients with PUNLMP was 4%.[259] With a median follow-up of 56 months, the 1973 WHO grade 1 tumors had a progression rate of 11%, whereas the 2004/2016 WHO PUNLMP tumors had a progression rate of 8%.[263] The tumor recurrence rate after PUNLMP resection was reported to be 35% in the study by Holmang et al. and 47% in the study by Pich et al.[262,264] These authors concluded that PUNLMP and low-grade carcinoma have similar risks for progression. More recently Pan et al. showed recurrence and progression rates were 18% and 2%, respectively, for PUNLMP.[258] Also, in a study of 53 PUNLMP tumors with a mean follow-up period of 11.7 years, Fujii et al. reported a recurrence rate of 60%, with 34% progressing to low-grade carcinoma and 8% progressing to invasive carcinoma (stage T1).[260] Taken together, these data indicate that patients with PUNLMP do not have a benign neoplasm, but instead have a significant risk for tumor recurrence and disease progression. PUNLMP is not substantially different from noninvasive Ta grade 1 carcinoma as defined by 1973 WHO criteria; long-term clinical follow-up is recommended for these patients.[223,224] A recent study reported that TERT promoter mutations are present in 43% of PUNLMP cases.[17]

Despite provision of detailed histologic criteria for the diagnostic categories in the 2004/2016 WHO system, improvement in intraobserver and interobserver variability compared with the 1973 WHO system was limited.[223,224,265-268] In fact, Mikuz demonstrated that interobserver agreement was higher using the 1973 WHO classification than when using either the 2004/2016 WHO or 1999 WHO/ISUP systems.[269] In a study by Yorukoglu et al. the intraobserver and interobserver reproducibility of both the 2004/2016 WHO and the 1973 WHO systems were evaluated by assigning six urologic pathologists to the task of independently reviewing 30 slides of noninvasive papillary urothelial tumors in a study set.[267] They found no statistical difference between the reproducibility achieved with either system; the new system failed to improve reproducibility.[267] There was agreement for PUNLMP in only 48% of cases, and reproducibility was lower for low-grade tumors in both the 2004/2016 WHO and the 1973 WHO systems.[267] Murphy et al. recorded a 50% discrepancy rate among pathologists attempting to distinguish between PUNLMP and low-grade papillary urothelial carcinoma after a period of structured pathologist education.[266]

Low-Grade Urothelial Carcinoma

A low-grade papillary urothelial carcinoma shows fronds with recognizable variation in architecture and cytology.[248,270-272] The tumor shows slender papillae with frequent branching and variation in nuclear polarity; nuclei show enlargement and irregularity; chromatin is vesicular, and nucleoli are often present (Fig. 6.28B). Mitotic figures may occur at any level in low-grade papillary urothelial carcinoma. Such cases would have been considered as grade 1 or 2 in the 1973 WHO classification scheme. Altered expression of CK20, CD44, p53, and p63 is frequent. Some tumors are diploid, but many are aneuploidy. FGFR3 mutations are seen with about the same frequency as in PUNLMP.[46,78,248,270,273] The male-to-female ratio is 2.9:1, and the mean age is 70 years (range, 28 to 90 years). Most patients present with hematuria and have a single tumor in the posterior or lateral bladder wall. However, 22% of patients with low-grade papillary urothelial carcinoma have two or more tumors. Tumor recurrence, stage progression, and tumor-related mortality rates are 50%, 10%, and 5%, respectively. Stage progression may be as high as 13% as reported in one series.[248]

Pellucchi et al. were able to further stratify 2004/2016 WHO low-grade urothelial carcinomas into two separate risk groups using the 1973 WHO grading scheme.[274] According to the 1973 WHO grading system, 87 low-grade (2004/2016 WHO) tumors (32%) were classified as 1973 WHO grade 1 tumors, and 183 low-grade (2004/2016 WHO) tumors (68%) were classified as 1973 WHO grade 2 tumors among 270 consecutive patients with a first episode of low-grade pTa bladder cancer at transurethral resection of the bladder between 2004/2016 and 2008. Five-year recurrence-free survival rate was 49% for the low-grade population and 62% and 40% for the

1973 WHO grade 1 and 2 groups, respectively.[274] In a recent analysis of 348 patients the authors found that the 1973 WHO grading system is more suitable than the 2004/2016 WHO grading system for predicting prognosis in non–muscle-invasive bladder cancer.[275]

Low-grade invasive urothelial carcinomas have been reported recently.[276,277] In a series of 23 cases, 5 (23%) experienced high-grade invasive urothelial carcinoma and 2 experienced metastatic disesae.[276]

High-Grade Urothelial Carcinoma

In high-grade papillary urothelial carcinoma the cells lining papillary fronds show obvious disordered arrangement with cytologic atypia (Fig. 6.28C). All tumors classified as grade 3 in the 1973 WHO scheme, as well as some tumors assigned grade 2 in that classification, would be considered high-grade carcinomas in the 2004/2016 WHO classification. The papillae are frequently fused. Both architectural and cytologic abnormalities are recognizable at scanning power.[248] The nuclei are pleomorphic with prominent nucleoli and altered polarity. Mitotic figures are frequent. The thickness of the urothelium varies considerably. Carcinoma in situ is frequently evident in the adjacent mucosa. Changes in CK20, p53, and p63 expression, as well as aneuploidy, are more frequent than in low-grade lesions. Molecular alterations in these tumors include overexpression of p53, HER2, or EGFR and loss of p21Waf1 or p27kip1 as seen with invasive cancers. Genetically, high-grade noninvasive lesions (pTa G3) resemble invasive tumors.[248,270] A comparative genomic hybridization-based study showed deletions at 2q, 5q, 10q, and 18q, as well as gains at 5p and 20q.[278] Hematuria is common, and the endoscopic appearance varies from papillary to nodular or solid. There may be single or multiple tumors. Stage progression and death due to disease are observed in as many as 65% of patients.[270] In a recent analysis of 85 patients with Ta high-grade urothelial carcinoma, recurrence and tumor progression rates were 37% and 40%, respectively.[279]

Histologic Grading of Urothelial Carcinoma: The Four-Tier Proposal

A four-tier grading categorization of urothelial carcinomas was proposed in 2012.[220] In this system noninvasive papillary urothelial carcinomas are separated into four categories: grade 1 urothelial carcinoma (low grade), grade 2 urothelial carcinoma (low grade), grade 3 urothelial carcinoma (high grade), and grade 4 urothelial carcinoma (high grade) (Table 6.9; Figs. 6.29 and 6.30). PUNLMP is classified as "grade 1 urothelial carcinoma (low grade)" in the four-tier grading scheme. Urothelial papilloma remains as a benign urothelial tumor following identical diagnostic criteria and terminology to those defined in the 1973 and 2004/2016 WHO classifications.[10,270]

Grade 1 Urothelial Carcinoma (Low Grade)

The diagnostic criteria are identical to those defined in the 1998 WHO/ISUP and 2004/2016 WHO classifications for PUNLMP (Fig. 6.30A). We propose to change the terminology of PUNLMP to "grade 1 urothelial carcinoma (low grade)." In these tumors, cytologic atypia is minimal or absent, and architectural abnormalities are slight with preserved polarity. Mitotic figures are infrequent and usually limited to the basal layer. Grade 1 tumor should be distinguished from urothelial papilloma, which is a benign lesion without invasive potential or risk for progression. The key difference between papilloma and grade 1 urothelial

TABLE 6.9	Diagnostic Criteria for the Newly Proposed Grading System of Urothelial Carcinoma of the Bladder			
Features	Grade 1 (Low Grade)	Grade 2 (Low Grade)	Grade 3 (High Grade)	Grade 4 (High Grade)
Increased cell layers (>7)	Yes	Variable	Variable	Variable, usually <7 layers
Superficial umbrella cells	Present	Often present	Usually absent	Usually absent
Polarity/overall architecture	Normal	Mildly distorted	Moderately distorted	Severely distorted
Discohesiveness	Normal	Normal	Mild to moderate	Severe
Clear cytoplasm	May be present	May be present	Usually absent	Usually absent
Nuclear size	Normal or slightly increased	Mildly increased	Moderately increased	Markedly increased
Nuclear pleomorphism	Uniform, slightly elongated to oval	Mild, round to oval with slight variation in shape and contour	Moderate	Marked
Nuclear polarization	Normal to slightly abnormal	Abnormal	Abnormal	Absent
Nuclear hyperchromasia	Slight or minimal	Mild	Moderate	Severe
Nuclear grooves	Present	Present	Absent	Absent
Nucleoli	Absent or inconspicuous	Inconspicuous	Enlarged, often prominent	Multiple prominent nucleoli
Mitotic figures	None/rare, basal location	May be present, at any level	Often present	Prominent and frequent, atypical forms
Stromal invasion	Rare	Uncommon	May be present	Often present

In the current proposal, grade 1 (low-grade) tumors are classified as "papillary urothelial neoplasm of low malignant potential" (PUNLMP) in the 2004 World Health Organization (WHO) classification system; grade 2 (low-grade) tumors are classified as "low grade urothelial carcinoma" (2004 WHO/International Society of Urological Pathology [ISUP]); grade 3 (high-grade) and grade 4 (high-grade) tumors are both classified as "high-grade urothelial carcinoma" (2004 WHO/ISUP).

Modified from Cheng L, MacLennan GT, Lopez-Beltran A. Histologic grading of urothelial carcinoma: a reappraisal. *Hum Pathol* 2012;43:2097–2108.

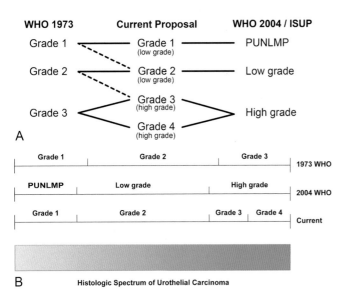

Fig. 6.29 Comparisons of different grading systems. (A) The 1973 World Health Organization (WHO) grade 1 carcinomas are reassigned, some to the papillary urothelial neoplasm of low malignant potential (PUNLMP) category and some to the low-grade carcinoma category in the 2004 WHO classification. Similarly, 1973 WHO grade 2 carcinomas are reassigned, some to the low-grade carcinoma category and others to the high-grade carcinoma category. All 1973 WHO tumors are assigned to the high-grade carcinoma category. In the current proposal, PUNLMP has been reassigned as grade 1 carcinoma, 2004 low-grade urothelial carcinoma has been reassigned as grade 2 urothelial carcinoma, and 2004 high-grade urothelial carcinoma has been divided into grade 3 and 4 urothelial carcinomas (all high grade). Grade 4 urothelial carcinomas are more commonly associated with invasion. (B) Urothelial carcinomas encompass a continuous spectrum of diseases with various biologic behavior and morphologic manifestations. Defining exact cutoff for each disease category can be challenging. *ISUP,* International Society of Urological Pathology.

carcinoma (low grade) is the number of epithelial layers covering the papillae (Table 6.9).

Grade 2 Urothelial Carcinoma (Low Grade)

The diagnostic criteria are identical to those defined in the 1998 WHO/ISUP and 2004/2016 WHO classifications for low-grade urothelial carcinomas (Fig. 6.30B). These tumors are characterized by an overall orderly appearance, but with areas of variation in architectural and cytologic features recognizable at scanning power (Table 6.9). They are differentiated from grade 1 urothelial carcinoma (low grade) by the presence of easily recognizable cytologic atypia including variation of polarity and nuclear size, shape, and chromatin texture. Mitotic figures are infrequent and may be seen at any level of the urothelium.

Grade 3 Urothelial Carcinoma (High Grade)

Grade 3 urothelial carcinomas (high grade) display an intermediate degree of architectural and cytologic abnormality between grade 2 urothelial carcinomas (low grade) and grade 4 urothelial carcinomas (high grade) (Fig. 6.30C). Architectural disorder in these tumors is obvious, with branching and bridging of papillary projections. Nevertheless, a certain degree of polarity and nuclear uniformity are still discernible. Severe anaplasia is not seen in these tumors. All grade 3 urothelial carcinomas would be classified as high-grade urothelial carcinoma using the 2004/2016 WHO classification scheme.

Grade 4 Urothelial Carcinoma (High Grade)

Cases with severe nuclear anaplasia are considered grade 4 urothelial carcinoma in the current proposal. These tumors present an overall impression of complete architectural disorder with absence of polarity, loss of superficial umbrella cells, and marked variation of all nuclear parameters (Table 6.9). Numerous irregularly distributed mitotic figures are frequently noted. Severe cytologic atypia is

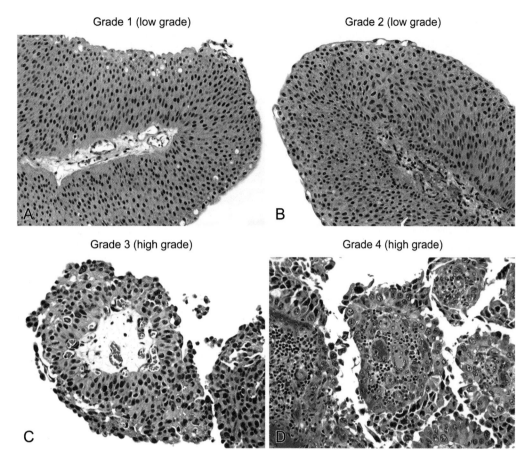

Fig. 6.30 Histologic grading of urothelial carcinoma, new proposal. (A) Grade 1 urothelial carcinoma (low grade), previously "papillary urothelial neoplasm of low malignant potential" (PUNLMP). (B) Grade 2 urothelial carcinoma (low grade), previously low-grade urothelial carcinoma (2004 World Health Organization [WHO] classification) (hematoxylin and eosin stain, original magnification ×200.) (C) Grade 3 urothelial carcinoma (high grade), previously high-grade urothelial carcinoma (2004 WHO classification) (hematoxylin and eosin stain, original magnification ×200). (D) Grade 4 urothelial carcinoma (high grade), previously high-grade urothelial carcinoma (2004 WHO classification). (From Cheng L, MacLennan GT, Lopez-Beltran A. Histologic grading of urothelial carcinoma: a reappraisal. Hum Pathol 2012;43:2097-2108, with permission.)

usually uniformly present in all fields or all histologic sections examined (Fig. 6.30D). Unlike grade 1 or grade 2 urothelial carcinoma (low grade), these tumors often have less than seven layers in thickness. Cellular discohesiveness is remarkable. These cases are typically associated with stromal invasion and advanced stage bladder cancer.

Unusually aggressive variants of urothelial carcinoma, including nested variant, micropapillary variant, plasmacytoid variant, sarcomatoid carcinoma, small cell carcinoma, undifferentiated carcinoma, and giant cell carcinoma, should also be graded as grade 4 tumors.[220]

Other Proposals for Bladder Cancer Grading and Tumor Heterogeneity

The ANCONA 2001 Refinement of the 1973 World Health Organization Classification

To improve understanding and to standardize use of the 1973 WHO classification, an expanded and refined contemporary description of the scheme was presented in 2001. This proposal is known as the Ancona refinement of the 1973 WHO grading system.[10,14,242] This effort was inspired by discussions during the international consensus meeting on bladder cancer held in Ancona, Italy, in 2001. It was proposed that urothelial tumors be divided into two main groups based on growth pattern: flat and papillary.

Flat tumors form a morphologic continuum whose classification includes reactive changes, dysplasia, and carcinoma in situ (see previous discussion). Papillary tumors include papilloma, grade 1 papillary carcinoma, grade 2 papillary carcinoma, and grade 3 papillary carcinoma. The diagnostic criteria for each of these categories were refined and optimized for reproducibility.[14,242] The use of terms that had been recently introduced for new urothelial neoplasia grading schemes, including *low malignant potential* and *atypia of uncertain clinical significance*, was discouraged. Grading of bladder cancer should be based on the highest level of abnormality noted. No formal recommendation has been previously made regarding the amount or extent of a higher grade needed for upgrading, but the Ancona refinement requires at least one high-power field (40× objective magnification with 20× ocular magnification).[14,242]

The 1999 World Health Organization Grading Proposal

The publication of the 1999 WHO blue book introduced a grading scheme.[250] This new classification retained the three-tiered numbering system (grade 1, grade 2, and grade 3 carcinomas). However, tumors formerly classified as 1973 WHO grade 1 were subdivided into PUNLMP and grade 1 tumors (Table 6.8). In the 1999 WHO classification, which differed from the 1998 WHO/ISUP and 1973 WHO classifications, papillary tumors of the

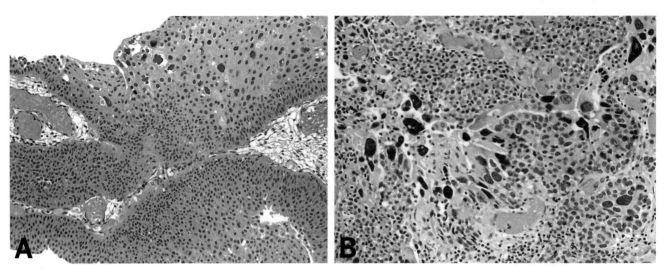

Fig. 6.31 Cancer heterogeneity of urothelial carcinoma (A and B). The same tumor may have areas with different histologic grades.

urinary bladder were subclassified as papilloma, PUNLMP, grade 1, grade 2, and grade 3. The definition of papilloma remains the same in all new grading systems and is defined as a papillary tumor with a delicate fibrovascular stroma lined by cytologically and architecturally normal urothelium without increased cellularity or mitotic figures.[7]

Tumor Heterogeneity: Implications for Grading

Papillary urothelial neoplasms encompass a spectrum of morphologic findings including tumors that behave aggressively and tumors that are biologically benign. Attempting to differentiate biologic behavior based solely on subtle histopathologic criteria is fraught with difficulties and perils, especially considering the significant interobserver variability that has been documented in numerous studies with all classification schemes.[266-269] The 2004/2016 WHO/ISUP system provides clearly defined histologic criteria for each of its diagnostic categories; however, urothelial neoplasms frequently demonstrate features of more than one grade (Fig. 6.31). The grading of papillary urothelial tumors is typically based on the worst grade present. However, cancer heterogeneity could have a significant impact on patient outcome. Cheng et al. examined 164 patients with stage Ta urothelial tumors and found that approximately one-third of tumors had morphologic tumor heterogeneity consistent with more than one histologic grade.[221] They graded both the primary and secondary patterns of tumor growth by the 2004/2016 WHO/ISUP criteria with PUNLMP, low-grade carcinoma, and high-grade carcinoma patterns receiving scores of 1, 2, and 3, respectively. Each tumor was then evaluated by a combined scoring system on a scale of 2 to 6. With a median follow-up of 9.2 years, the prognosis of patients with a combined score of 6 (the entire tumor consisting of high-grade carcinoma) is considerably worse than those with a combined score of 5 (a tumor consisting of low- and high-grade carcinoma) (26% versus 68% 10-year progression-free survival; $P = 0.02$).[221] The significant survival difference (42%) between score 5 and score 6 groups may suffice to warrant different management strategies in appropriate settings. Subsequent studies have also suggested that combined scoring systems may be useful in the grading of bladder tumors.[280] Grading should take cancer heterogeneity into consideration, because prognostic accuracy was increased when the combined primary and secondary grades were applied.[221] This finding (two-numbered grading system) was recently validated.[281,282]

Neither the 2004/2016 WHO/ISUP system nor the 1973 WHO system takes tumor heterogeneity into account; however, the 1973 WHO system does allow a greater amount of diagnostic flexibility in that tumors are frequently classified as grade 1 to 2 or grade 2 to 3. This added flexibility may give a more accurate representation of the tumor histology than attempting to force a lesion into a single diagnostic category. It appears that prognostic accuracy is improved when heterogeneity is considered.[221] Future investigations are needed to fully address the impact of tumor heterogeneity on clinical outcome.

Staging of Invasive Bladder Cancer

General Features of Invasive Urothelial Carcinoma

At gross examination, most tumors present as a single, solid, polypoid mass with or without ulceration, and may also appear sessile and extensively infiltrate the bladder wall (Fig. 6.32). Histologically, the neoplastic cells invade the bladder wall as nests, cords, trabeculae, small clusters, or single cells that are often separated by a desmoplastic stroma. The tumor sometimes grows in a more diffuse, sheetlike pattern, but even in these cases, focal nests and clusters are generally present. The cells show moderate to abundant amphophilic or eosinophilic cytoplasm and large hyperchromatic nuclei. In larger nests, palisading of nuclei may be seen at the edges of the nests. The nuclei are typically pleomorphic and have irregular contours with angular profiles. Nuclear grooves may be identified in some cells. Nucleoli are highly variable in number and appearance. Some cells contain single or multiple small nucleoli, and others have large eosinophilic nucleoli. Foci of marked pleomorphism may be seen, with bizarre and multinuclear tumor cells present. Mitotic figures are common, including many abnormal forms. Invasive tumors are most commonly high grade, usually showing marked anaplasia with focal giant cell formation.[220,283]

Pathologic stage is most critical for assessing patient prognosis.[283] The 2017 TNM (tumor, lymph node, and metastasis) staging information should be provided in the pathology report (Figs. 6.33 and 6.34; Table 6.10).[284]

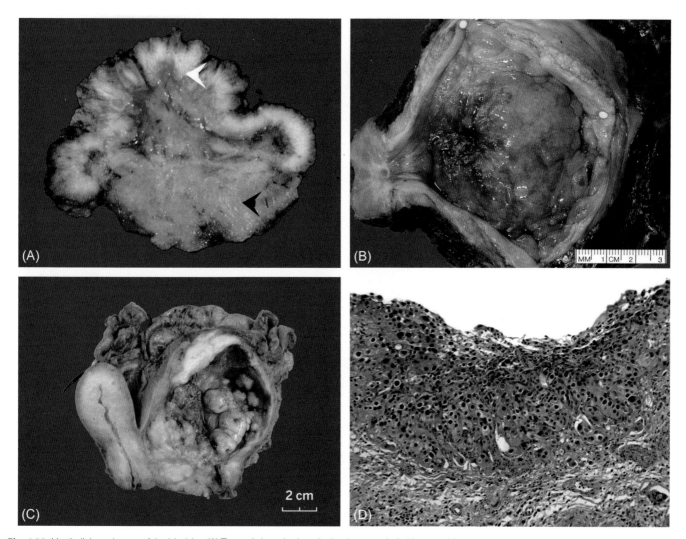

Fig. 6.32 Urothelial carcinoma of the bladder. (A) Tumor is invasive into the lamina propria (*white arrow*) but does not involve muscularis propria (*black arrow*). (B) Urothelial carcinoma often coexists with urothelial carcinoma in situ, which was present in the areas of widespread mucosal erythema. (C) Invasion into an adjacent organ (uterine cervix) is evident grossly. (D) The mucosal surface of invasive cancer is often denuded or ulcerated, with a ragged appearance.

Stage pT1 Tumor

Infiltrating urothelial carcinoma is defined by the WHO as a urothelial tumor that invades beyond the basement membrane.[285] The 2017 TNM staging system defines pT1 tumors of the bladder as those invading the lamina propria, but not the muscularis propria.[284] The recognition of lamina propria invasion by urothelial carcinoma is one of the most challenging fields in surgical pathology, and the pathologist should follow strict criteria in its assessment (Table 6.11; Fig. 6.35).[1,157,286]

Histologic Grade

Although invasion is not necessarily an unexpected finding in low-grade tumors, it is much more commonly encountered in high-grade lesions, reaching 70% to 96% in some series (Fig. 6.35A).[157] In addition, histologic grade at transurethral resection has been correlated with pathologic stage at cystectomy.[287]

Stroma-Epithelial Interface

Tangentially sectioned, densely packed, noninvasive papillary tumors exhibit a stroma–epithelial interface that is smooth and regular. In instances of true invasion, one is likely to see variably sized and irregularly shaped nests or individual tumor cells insinuating through the stroma (Fig. 6.35B and C). When the specimen includes tangential sections through noninvasive tumor or when urothelial carcinoma involves von Brunn nests, the basement membrane preserves a regular contour, whereas it is frequently absent or disrupted in cases of true invasion. The smoothness of the stroma-epithelial interface may be assessed on hematoxylin and eosin stains. In some cases, however, additional findings may be helpful; for example, there is a parallel array of thin-walled vessels that evenly line the basement membrane of noninvasive nests. These are absent in patients with invasive tumors.

Invading Epithelium

The invasive front of the neoplasm may show one of several features. Most commonly, tumors invade the underlying stroma as single cells or irregularly shaped nests of tumor cells (Fig. 6.35). Sometimes tentacular or finger-like extensions can be seen arising from the base of the papillary tumor. Frequently the invading nests appear cytologically different from cells at the base of the

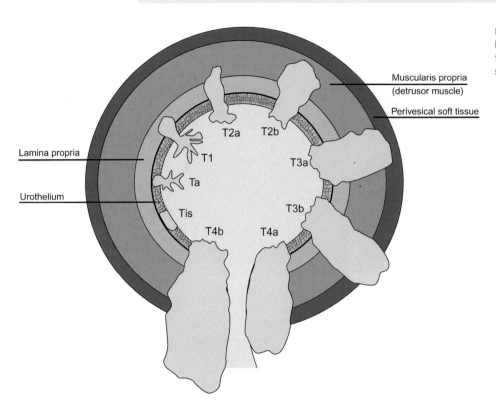

Fig. 6.33 Schematic diagram of staging of bladder carcinoma according to the 2016 tumor, lymph node, and metastasis (TNM) staging system.

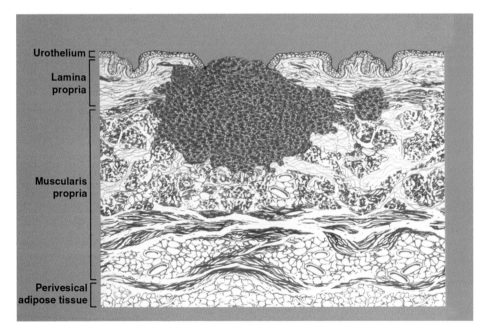

Fig. 6.34 The bladder is organized into the urothelium, lamina propria, muscularis propria, and perivesical adipose tissue. Adipose tissue can be present in the lamina propria or muscularis propria layer. Current staging system for bladder cancer is based on the depth of invasion. A tumor invading into muscular propria (detrusor muscle) is illustrated. (From Cheng L, Neumann RM, Scherer BG, et al. Tumor size predicts the survival of patients with pathologic stage T2 bladder carcinoma: a critical evaluation of the depth of muscle invasion. *Cancer* 1999;85:2638–2647, with permission.)

noninvasive component. Invasive tumor cells often have more abundant cytoplasm and a higher degree of nuclear pleomorphism. In some cases, particularly in microinvasive disease, the invasive tumor cells may acquire abundant eosinophilic cytoplasm. At low- to medium-power magnification, these microinvasive cells seem to be more differentiated than the overlying noninvasive disease, a feature known as paradoxical differentiation (Fig. 6.35D and E).

Stromal Response

The stromal response to invading carcinoma is not always uniformly present in invasive urothelial carcinoma, and the diagnosis of invasion may rely on identification of the typical characteristics of the invading epithelium. The stromal reaction in the lamina propria associated with invasive tumor may be inflammatory, myxoid, or fibrous (Fig. 6.36). Assessment of differences in stromal growth pattern provides an important diagnostic clue.[288] Although the

TABLE 6.10	Tumor Node Metastasis (TNM) Classification of Bladder Cancer

Primary tumor (T)[a]

TX	Primary tumor cannot be assessed
T0	No evidence of primary tumor
Ta	Noninvasive papillary carcinoma
Tis	Carcinoma in situ
T1	Tumor invades subepithelial connective tissue (lamina propria)
T2	Tumor invades muscularis propria
T2a	Tumor invades superficial muscularis propria (inner half)
T2b	Tumor invades deep muscularis propria (outer half)
T3	Tumor invades perivesical tissue
T3a	Microscopically
T3b	Macroscopically (extravesical mass)
T4	Tumor invades any of the following: prostatic stroma, uterus, vagina, pelvic wall, and abdominal wall
T4a	Tumor invades prostatic stroma* or uterus or vagina
T4b	Tumor invades pelvic wall or abdominal wall

*Subepithelial invasion of prostatic urethra does not constitute T4 staging status.

The suffix "m" should be added to the appropriate T category to indicate multiple tumors. The suffix "is" may be added to any T to indicate the presence of associated carcinoma in situ.

Regional lymph nodes (N)

NX	Regional lymph nodes cannot be assessed
N0	No regional lymph node metastasis
N1	Single regional lymph node metastasis in the true pelvis (perivesical, obturator, internal and external iliac, or sacral lymph node)
N2	Multiple regional lymph node metastasis in the true pelvis (perivesical, obturator, internal and external iliac, or sacral lymph node)
N3	Lymph node metastasis to the common iliac lymph nodes

Distant metastasis (M)

M0	No distant metastasis
M1	Distant metastasis
M1a	Distant metastasis limited to lymph nodes beyond the common illiacs
M1b	Non–lymph node distant metastases

Used with permission of the American College of Surgeons, Chicago, Illinois. The original source for this information is the AJCC Cancer Staging Manual, Eighth Edition (2017) published by Springer International Publishing.

[a]TNM descriptors: For identification of special cases of TNM or pTNM classifications, the "m" suffix and "y" and "r" prefixes are used. The "m" suffix indicates the presence of multiple primary tumors in a single site and is recorded in parentheses: pT(m)NM. The "y" prefix indicates those cases in which classification is performed during or after initial multimodality therapy. The "r" prefix indicates a recurrent tumor when staged after a documented disease-free interval and is identified by the "r" prefix: rTNM.

TABLE 6.11	Histologic Features that are Useful for the Diagnosis of Stromal Invasion

Histologic grade

- Invasive cells are usually higher nuclear grade

Invading epithelium

- Irregularly shaped nests
- Single-cell infiltration
- Irregular or absent basement membrane
- Tentacular finger-like projections
- Paradoxical differentiation
- Angiolymphatic invasion

Stromal response

- Desmoplasia or fibrotic stroma
- Retraction artifact
- Inflammation
- Myxoid stroma
- Pseudosarcomatous stroma

Modified from Lopez-Beltran A, Cheng L. Stage pT1 bladder carcinoma: diagnostic criteria, pitfalls and prognostic significance. *Pathology* 2003;35:484–491.

majority of bladder tumors with unquestionable lamina propria invasion exhibit some sort of stromal reaction, microinvasive disease usually does not, making its identification even more difficult. In some cases, retraction artifact around superficially invasive individual tumor cells may mimic angiolymphatic invasion. Often this finding is focal and may itself be one of the early signs of invasion into the lamina propria.

Lamina propria invasion may elicit a brisk inflammatory response. Numerous inflammatory cells in the lamina propria often obscure the interface between epithelium and stroma (Fig. 6.37). This makes small nest or single-cell invasion difficult to recognize. CK immunostaining is useful in difficult cases.

Invasive urothelial carcinoma may have a cellular stroma with spindled fibroblasts and variable collagenization, or a hypocellular stroma with myxoid background. Rarely the tumor induces an exuberant proliferation of fibroblasts, which may display alarming cellular atypia similar to giant cell cystitis. This feature, although a helpful clue to invasion, should not be mistaken for the spindle cell component of sarcomatoid urothelial carcinoma. Immunostains for CK are helpful in difficult cases, although some myofibroblasts may also be positive for keratin.[289] The proliferating stroma is usually nonexpansile, being limited to areas around the neoplasm, and is composed of cells that have a degenerate or smudged appearance.

Diagnostic Pitfalls

Transurethral resection specimens are excised in a piecemeal fashion. Submitted tissue fragments are of variable shape and size, and are difficult, if not impossible, to orient properly (Table 6.12). Furthermore, due to their complex architecture, papillary tumors are inevitably tangentially sectioned in multiple planes, resulting in the presence of isolated nests of noninvasive tumor cells within connective tissue. Smooth, round, and regular contours favor tangential sectioning, whereas irregular, jagged nests with haphazard arrangement favor stromal invasion. Papillary tumors may show variable and often brisk inflammation at the tumor-stromal interface. This may obscure isolated cells or small nests of invasive tumor. Diagnosis of invasion in some of these cases can be facilitated by immunohistochemical study with anti-CK antibodies. Thermal injury or cautery artifact produces severely distorted morphology, rendering accurate diagnosis of invasion difficult. Tumor cells involving von Brunn nests may also mimic lamina propria invasion. This is especially problematic when von Brunn nests are prominent or when they have been distorted by inflammatory or cautery artifact.

Substaging of pT1 Tumors

The recurrence and progression rates for pT1 tumors are highly variable.[146,157,159,286,290-298] A need exists for an accurate, easy-to-use, reproducible substaging system to stratify pT1 patients into different prognostic groups.[283] Several studies have explored the utility of evaluating the spatial relationship of invasive tumor to the muscularis mucosae for subclassification of pT1 tumor.[157,299-306]

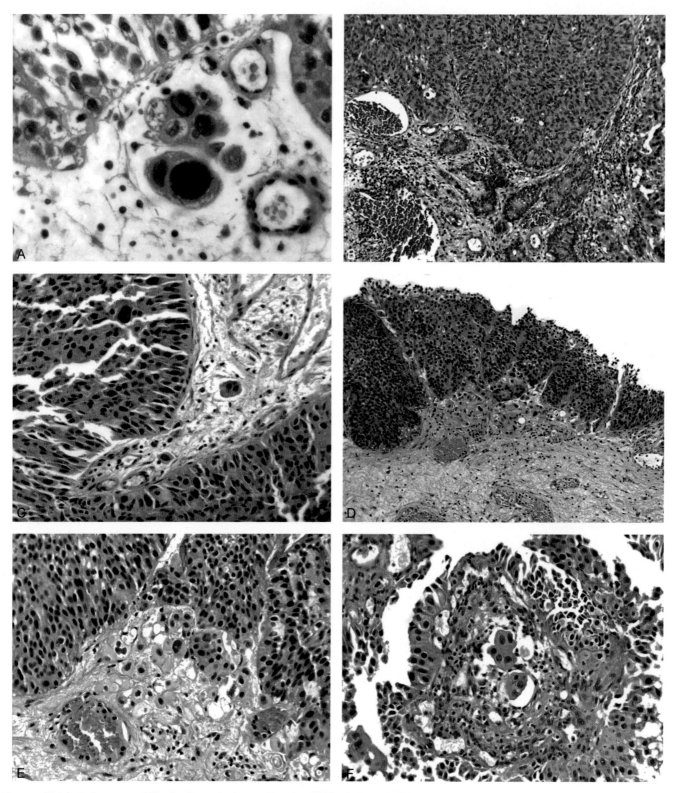

Fig. 6.35 Histologic features useful for the diagnosis of stromal invasion. (A) Histologic grade. (B) Irregular contour of invading fronts. (C) Single individual cells. Paradoxical differentiation (D and E). Invading tumor cells may have more eosinophilic cytoplasm than overlying noninvading tumor cells. (F) Retraction artifact is most useful in the diagnosis of stalk invasion in the papillae.

Muscularis mucosae consist of thin and wavy fascicles of smooth muscle frequently associated with large, thin-walled blood vessels. Muscularis mucosae can be identified in 15% to 83% of biopsy specimens (Fig. 6.38); however, 6% of radical resection specimens do not have discernible muscularis mucosae.[157,159,292,299-304,307-310] Thus the "large" vessels have been used as a surrogate marker of muscularis mucosae in all published studies that have proposed T1 substaging based on muscularis

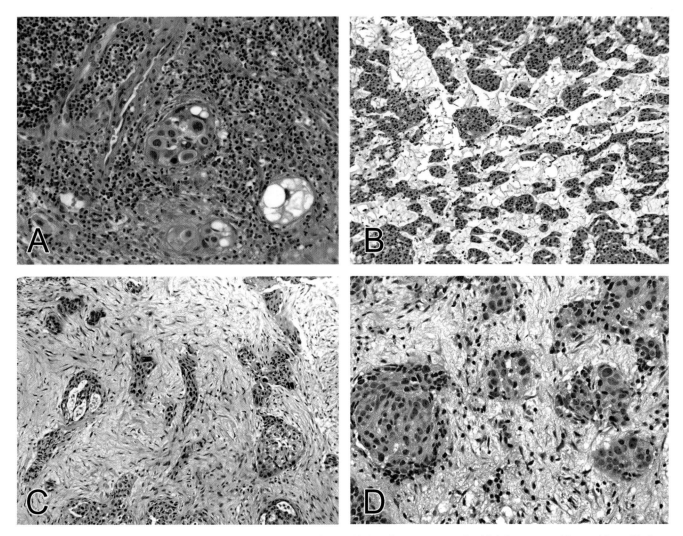

Fig. 6.36 Diagnosis of stage T1 bladder cancer. The stroma associated with invasive cancer may be (A) inflammatory, (B) myxoid, or (C) fibrous. (D) Hypocellular stroma with myxoid background.

mucosae invasion. For example, Angulo et al. were able to identify muscularis mucosae in 39% of their cases, and they used the blood vessel landmark in another 26%.[299] Thus in 35% of their cases substaging could not be performed because neither muscularis mucosae nor large vessels could be found. Platz et al. identified muscularis mucosae in only 33% of their cases and found no significant prognostic value in substaging pT1 cancer using the level of muscularis mucosae invasion.[303] These problems have raised concerns about the practicality and validity of substaging pT1 disease based on assessment of muscularis mucosae invasion, and currently this practice is not universally advocated.[249] Nonetheless, pathologists should provide assessment of lamina propria invasion depth or extent of disease when possible.

Cheng et al. proposed a system for substaging pT1 tumors based on the ocular micrometer measurement of tumor invasion into the subepithelial connective tissue (Fig. 6.39).[159,286,292] Using an ocular micrometer to measure the depth of invasion from the mucosal basement membrane, they found a significant correlation between depth of invasion in the transurethral resection specimens and final pathologic stage at cystectomy.[286,311] A depth of invasion of 1.5 mm predicted an advanced stage of disease at cystectomy with a sensitivity of 81%, a specificity of 83%, and positive and negative predictive values of 95% and 56%, respectively. The same

investigators subsequently applied the same criteria to a group of 83 consecutive patients diagnosed with pT1 bladder cancer. When depth of tumor invasion was greater than 1.5 mm, 5-year survival was 67%, whereas with a depth of invasion less than 1.5 mm, the 5-year survival rate was 93%.[159]

Modifications of Cheng's criteria for pT1 substaging, as well as other proposals for T1 substaging, have recently been reported.[312-315] In one study substaging was performed using 0.5, 1.0, and 1.5 mm as thresholds to distinguish extensive from focal invasion. No prognostic differences were found between Ta and T1 low-grade papillary urothelial carcinomas. T1 >1-mm high-grade papillary urothelial carcinomas were associated with significantly greater risks for recurrence, progression, cancer-specific mortality, and all-cause mortality compared with T1 ≤1-mm and Ta tumors. Therefore the authors recommended using a 1.0-mm cutoff in pT1 substaging.[312] Substaging pT1 bladder cancer by measurement of the size of infiltrating tumor area by high-power fields may improve risk stratification.[315] Others have subclassified the patterns of pT1 tumor invasion into three categories: focal invasion confined to the papillary stalk, focal invasion of the tumor base, or extensive invasion of the tumor base.[316] None of the patients with stalk-only invasion progressed, whereas progression rates were 31% and 76%, respectively, for those patients with focal base invasion

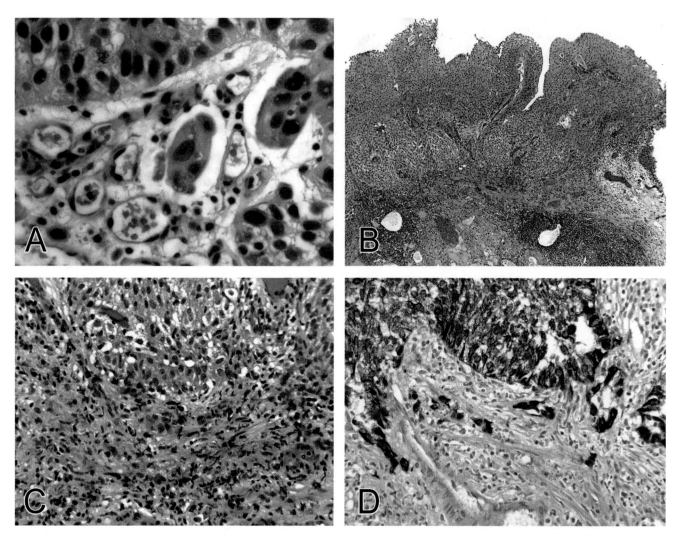

Fig. 6.37 Diagnosis of stage T1 bladder cancer. (A) Retraction artifact around superficially invasive individual tumor cells may mimic angiolymphatic invasion. Invasive tumor also may show variable and often brisk inflammation at the tumor-stromal interface (B and C). (D) Immunostaining with anticytokeratin antibodies (AE1/AE3) is useful for identification of individual tumor cells.

TABLE 6.12	Pitfalls in the Diagnosis of Stage pT1 Urothelial Carcinoma

Tangential sectioning and poor orientation
Obscuring inflammation
Thermal injury
Urothelial carcinoma in situ involving von Brunn nests
Muscle invasion indeterminate for type of muscle (muscularis propria versus muscularis mucosae)
Variants of urothelial carcinoma with deceptively bland cytology
Pseudoinvasive nests of benign proliferative urothelial lesions

and extensive base invasion.[316] The recently released American Joint Committee on Cancer (AJCC) cancer staging manual strongly recommends subclassification of pT1 bladder cancer in the reporting, although the exact criteria whereby such subclassification is to be accomplished were not specified.[284]

Substaging of pT1 bladder tumors may also be facilitated by CK immunohistochemistry, especially in difficult cases where specimen orientation and tissue artifacts hinder accurate assessment.[157,288,317,318] The fact that some myofibroblasts in lamina propria may also be positive for keratin represents a potential pitfall with clinical relevance.[289]

Occasionally, muscularis mucosae bundles are difficult to differentiate from muscularis propria, particularly when muscularis mucosae bundles are hypertrophic. In these cases, smoothelin, a recently identified biomarker that facilitates distinguishing muscularis mucosae from muscularis propria, may be helpful. Muscularis propria typically displays intense and strong smoothelin staining, in contrast with muscularis mucosae, which has weak or negative smoothelin staining.[319-321]

Stage pT2 Tumor

The 2017 AJCC and Union for International Cancer Control bladder cancer TNM staging systems subclassify pT2 tumors into two categories: cancer invading less than one-half of the depth of muscular propria (pT2a) and cancer invading more than one-half of the depth of muscularis propria (Fig. 6.40A and B).[284] The clinical utility of substaging of pT2 tumors has been questioned.[159,283,322-326]

The subdivision of the T2 category is based on the work by Jewett and Strong in 1952.[327] In a study of 18 patients with

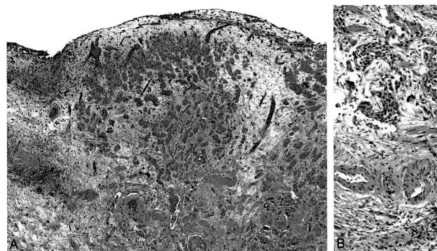

Fig. 6.38 Muscularis mucosae is not uniformly present in the lamina propria (A and B). Substaging of pT1 cancer based on muscularis mucosae invasion is not recommended.

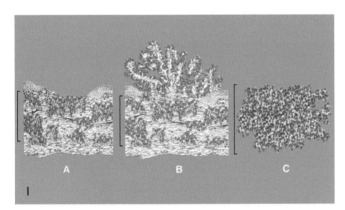

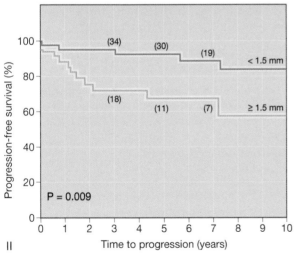

Fig. 6.39 Substaging of pT1 bladder cancer based on the depth of invasion. The depth of stromal invasion in transurethral resection or biopsy specimens is measured from the basement membrane of the bladder mucosa to the deepest invasive cancer cells using ocular micrometer (*top panel, A and B*). When tissue fragments contained cancer without intervening stroma or the specimens were not oriented, the depth of invasion was measured from the shortest distance to avoid overestimation of the depth of invasion (*top panel, C*). Cancer progression-free survival according to the level of depth of invasion (1.5 mm) in the transurethral resection specimens (*bottom panel*). Numbers in parentheses represent the number of patients

muscle-invasive carcinoma (5 T2a cases and 13 T2b cases), they found that 80% of this small series of patients with stage T2a bladder carcinoma patients survived, whereas only 8% of those with stage T2b survived. Data accumulated in the 46 years since this original publication of a series of only 18 patients do not support the subdivision of T2 by depth of muscularis propria invasion.[324,328-356] Jewett stated in 1978 that "it seems probable that our arbitrary dividing line drawn 30 years ago at the halfway level to separate B1 from B2 tumors was too superficial."[357]

Cheng et al. found that tumor size, rather than the depth of invasion, was predictive of distant metastasis-free and cancer-specific survival in patients with muscularis propria invasion.[159] Ten-year distant metastasis-free and cancer-specific survival rates were 100% and 94%, respectively, for patients with cancer <3 cm, and 68% and 73%, respectively, for patients with cancer ≥3 cm in the largest tumor dimension.[159] In a recent study of 311 patients with pT2 bladder cancer, Yu et al. found no significant difference in clinical outcome between pT2a and pT2b cancers after controlling for lymph node status.[324] Ten-year recurrence-free survival rates were 84% and 72%, respectively, for pT2a and pT2b lymph node–negative bladder cancers. Among patients with lymph node–positive bladder cancer, 10-year recurrence-free survival rate was 50% for pT2a carcinoma and 48% for pT2b carcinoma.[324]

Jimenez et al. introduced a morphologic classification of invasive bladder tumors distinguishing three patterns of growth (nodular, trabecular, and infiltrative).[358] Tumors with an infiltrative growth pattern are associated with a worse prognosis than tumor displaying a noninfiltrative (nodular or trabecular) growth pattern.

under observation at 3, 5, and 7 years. Progression was defined as the development of muscle-invasive or more advanced stage carcinoma, distant metastasis, or death from bladder cancer. (From Cheng L, Weaver AL, Neumann RM, et al. Substaging of T1 bladder carcinoma based on the depth of invasion as measured by micrometer: a new proposal. *Cancer* 1999;86:1035–1043; and Cheng L, Neumann RM, Weaver AL, et al. Predicting cancer progression in patients with stage T1 bladder carcinoma. *J Clin Oncol* 1999;17:3182–3187, with permission.)

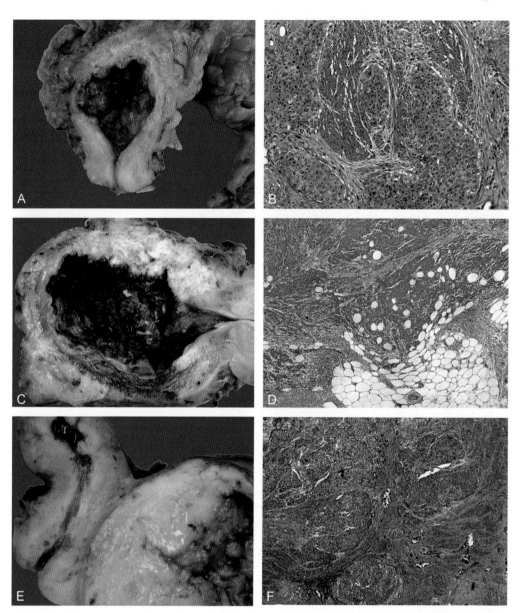

Fig. 6.40 Invasive urothelial carcinoma. pT2 urothelial carcinoma with muscularis propria invasion (A and B). pT3 urothelial carcinoma with invasion into perivesicular adipose tissue (C and D). Extensive urothelial carcinoma in situ is also present (C). pT4 cancer with invasion into adjacent uterine wall (E and F).

Stage pT3 Tumor

Stage pT3 bladder carcinoma is defined as tumor invading into perivesical soft tissue (Fig. 6.40C and D). The subdivision of pT3 tumors into T3a (tumors with microscopic extravesical tumor extension) and pT3b (tumors with gross extravesical extension) is also of questionable utility.[359-362] Quck et al. examined 236 patients with pT3 tumors.[360] With a median follow-up of 8.9 years, no difference in recurrence or survival was found between patients with pT3a and pT3b tumors. Lymph node and surgical margin status were the only factors that significantly impacted patient prognosis in this study.

Currently there is no reliable method to predict extravesical extension (pT3) from transurethral resection or biopsy specimens. The presence of fat invasion in transurethral resection or biopsy specimens does not constitute a pT3 cancer. Cheng and his colleagues analyzed 90 patients with bladder cancer diagnosed with invasive bladder cancer at transurethral resection.[311] The depth

of invasion was measured from the transurethral resection specimens by ocular micrometer. All patients were treated by radical cystectomy. Median interval from transurethral resection to cystectomy was 44 days. Extravesical extension ($\geq$T3) at cystectomy was present in 39 patients (43%). The authors found that the depth of invasion was associated with final pathologic stage (Spearman correlation $r = 0.58$; $P < 0.001$).[311] The overall accuracy of the depth of invasion for the prediction of extravesical extension, measured by the area under the receiver operating characteristic curve, was 0.81 (standard error, 0.045). The mean depth of invasion among patients with extravesical extension at cystectomy was 4.0 mm, compared with 2.2 mm for those without extravesical extension. Based on a 4.0-mm cutpoint, the sensitivity, specificity, positive predictive value, and negative predictive value for extravesical extension were 54%, 90%, 81%, and 72%, respectively. Among patients with depth of invasion greater than 4 mm in biopsies, 100% had advanced-stage ($\geq$pT2) bladder cancer; 81%

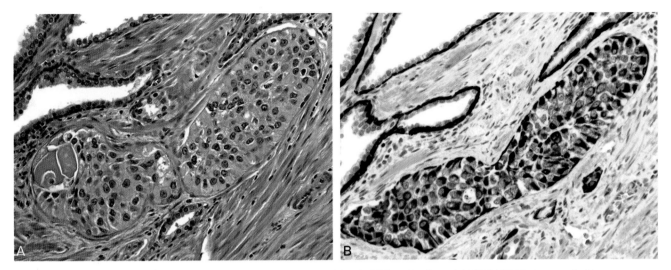

Fig. 6.41 pT4 bladder cancer with invasion into the prostate (A). Immunostaining for high-molecular-weight CK highlights tumor cells (B).

had pT3 or pT4 bladder cancer. The authors concluded that patients with bladder cancer depth of invasion greater than 4 mm in the transurethral resection specimens, measured by micrometer, are likely to have extravesical extension, and more aggressive treatment should be considered.[311]

Stage pT4 Tumor

Stage pT4 bladder cancer is defined as tumor invading into adjacent organs or structures including the uterus (Fig. 6.40E and F), vagina, prostatic stroma (Fig. 6.41), pelvic wall, or abdominal wall. In the 2017 AJCC and Union for International Cancer Control bladder cancer TNM staging guidelines, pT4a includes invasion of prostatic stroma, uterus, or vagina, and pT4b indicates pelvic or abdominal wall invasion.[284]

In men, T4 cancer is defined as prostatic stromal invasion by direct extension from a primary bladder tumor in the bladder. Prostatic stomal invasion by urothelial cancers involving the prostatic urethra does not constitute T4 cancer. Esrig et al. studied 143 bladder cancers with prostatic involvement, dividing them into two groups: group 1 penetrated the full thickness of the bladder wall to involve the prostate, and group 2 involved the prostate by extension from the prostatic urethra.[363] Five-year overall survival rates were 21% and 55% for group 1 and 2 patients, respectively. Among group 2 patients, the presence of prostatic stromal invasion was associated with a worse prognosis than for patients in whom urothelial cancer was confined to the urethral mucosa only.[363] Similarly, Pagano et al. found that 5-year survival rate was only 7% among group 1 patients, compared with 46% among group 2 patients.[364] In group 2 cases, all patients with only urethral mucosal involvement were alive and free of disease at 5 years, compared with 40% to 50% survival among patients with prostatic stromal invasion. In a detailed mapping study of 214 radical cystoprostatectomy specimens, Shen et al. found the presence of prostatic involvement and levels of involvement are significant prognostic factors in patients with bladder cancer.[365] About 26% of the invasive bladder cancer in the prostate resulted from direct prostatic infiltration from the primary bladder tumor in the bladder, and in the remaining 72% of cases the prostate was infiltrated by urothelial carcinoma arising in the prostatic urethra.[365]

In men, direct perivesical tumor extension involving the seminal vesicles was associated with poor prognosis similar to that of

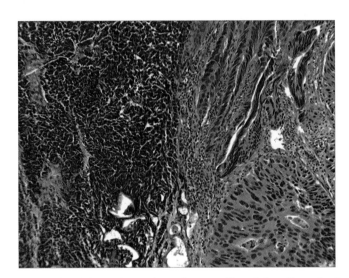

Fig. 6.42 Urothelial carcinoma shows divergent differentiation with small cell carcinoma (*left*) and adenocarcinoma component (*top right*).

pT4b bladder cancer.[366,367] Five-year overall survival rate for these patients was only 10%, similar to pT4b cancer (7%). The 5-year overall survival rate for patients with prostatic stromal involvement was 38%.[366] However, the prognostic significance of seminal vesicle invasion via intraepithelial extension from the prostate is less certain and should be reported separately.[368]

Reyes et al. recently described six women with urothelial carcinoma involving gynecologic organs.[369] The first site of involvement was usually the vagina, and vaginal bleeding was the main presenting symptom. Immunohistochemistry revealed strong CK7 and focal to diffuse strong CK20 positivity in all patients, as well as at least focal p16 positivity in five patients.[370] HPV in situ hybridization was negative in all patients.

Histologic Variants of Urothelial Carcinoma

Urothelial carcinoma has a propensity for divergent differentiation.[3,69,259] Virtually the entire spectrum of bladder cancer variants described next may be seen in variable proportions in otherwise conventional urothelial carcinoma (Fig. 6.42). The clinical outcome of some variants differs from conventional urothelial carcinoma. Therefore recognition of these variants is important (Tables 6.13 to 6.16). The recently published 2016 WHO Classification of Tumors of the Urinary System and Male Genital Organs presents refined criteria of pathologic features useful in establishing the correct diagnosis, and updates terminology and molecular characteristics of these important subtypes of bladder cancer.[6] Histologic variants not included in the current WHO classification of tumors of the urinary tract and relevant growth variation patterns of urothelial carcinoma are also briefly discussed here.

TABLE 6.13 **Histologic Variants of Infiltrating Urothelial Carcinoma According to the 2016 World Health Organization Classification of Tumors of the Urinary Tract**

Urothelial carcinoma with divergent differentiation
    With squamous cell differentiation
    With glandular differentiation
    With trophoblastic differentiation
    Other (small cell carcinoma, germ cell differentiation, other)
Micropapillary urothelial carcinoma
Plasmacytoid urothelial carcinoma
Nested urothelial carcinoma (including large nested variant)
Microcystic urothelial carcinoma
Lymphoepithelioma-like urothelial carcinoma
Lipid-rich urothelial carcinoma
Clear cell (glycogen-rich) urothelial carcinoma
Sarcomatoid urothelial carcinoma
Giant cell urothelial carcinoma
Poorly differentiated urothelial tumors
    Osteoclast-rich undifferentiated carcinoma

TABLE 6.14 **Histologic Variations and Variants of Urothelial Carcinoma not Included in the Current World Health Organization Classification of Tumors of the Urinary Tract**

Urothelial carcinoma, inverted growth (inverted papilloma-like)
Pseudoangiosarcomatous (pseudoangiosarcoma-like) urothelial carcinoma
Urothelial carcinoma with chordoid features
Urothelial carcinoma with syncytiotrophoblastic giant cells
Urothelial carcinoma with acinar/tubular differentiation
Urothelial carcinoma with chordoid
Undifferentiated carcinoma
    Undifferentiated carcinoma, not otherwise specified
    Undifferentiated carcinoma with rhabdoid features
    Giant cell undifferentiated carcinoma
    Osteoclast-rich undifferentiated carcinoma
Urothelial carcinoma with unusual stromal reactions
    Pseudosarcomatous stroma
    Stromal osseous metaplasia
    Stromal cartilaginous metaplasia
    Osteoclast-type giant cells
    Prominent lymphoid infiltrate
Urothelial carcinoma in augmentation cystoplasty
Urothelial carcinoma in children and young adults
Urothelial carcinoma in bladder diverticulum

Urothelial Carcinoma With Divergent Differentiation

The most common urothelial carcinoma variant is known as urothelial carcinoma with divergent differentiation, which may include squamous, glandular, neuroendocrine, and/or trophoblastic elements. Typically, divergent differentiation occurs in a background of conventional urothelial carcinoma.

Approximately 20% of urothelial carcinomas contain areas of squamous or glandular differentiation (Fig. 6.43). Urothelial carcinomas with squamous and/or glandular differentiation tend to be more biologically aggressive and are more likely to have extravesical tumors and node-positive disease.[341,342] Squamous differentiation, defined by the presence of intercellular bridges or keratinization, occurs in 21% of urothelial carcinomas of the bladder (Fig. 6.43A and B).[343-346] It frequently increases with grade and stage. Detailed histologic maps of urothelial carcinoma with squamous differentiation have shown wide variation in the proportion of the squamous component. Some cases have urothelial carcinoma in situ as the only urothelial component. Cases with areas of squamous differentiation may have a less favorable response to therapy than pure urothelial carcinoma.[344,345,347,348] Of 91 patients with metastatic carcinoma, 83% with mixed adenocarcinoma and 46% with mixed squamous cell carcinoma experienced disease progression despite intense chemotherapy, whereas the carcinoma progressed in less than 30% of patients with pure urothelial histology.[349] Low-grade urothelial carcinoma with focal squamous differentiation has a higher recurrence rate than pure low-grade urothelial carcinoma. Tumors with any identifiable urothelial element are classified as urothelial carcinoma with squamous differentiation, and an estimate of the percentage of squamous component should be provided. CK14, L1 antigen, and caveolin-1 have been reported as immunohistochemical markers of squamous differentiation in urothelial carcinoma.[350,351] Urothelial carcinoma with prominent squamous differentiation in the setting of neurogenic bladder has been linked to HPV infection, although sporadic urothelial carcinoma with squamous differentiation is not related to HPV infection.[352,353]

Immunostaining with squamous differentiation biomarkers is useful in differential diagnosis.[371-373] Urothelial carcinoma with squamous differentiation may express urothelial (S100P, 83%; GATA3, 35%; uroplakin 3, 13%) and squamous-associated markers CK14 (87%) and desmoglein 3 (70%).[372]

Glandular differentiation is less common than squamous differentiation and may be present in about 6% of urothelial carcinomas of the bladder (Fig. 6.43C and D).[374-376] Glandular differentiation is defined by the presence of true glandular spaces within the tumor. These may be tubular or enteric glands with mucin secretion. A colloid-mucinous pattern characterized by nests of cells "floating" in extracellular mucin, occasionally with signet ring cells, may be present. Cytoplasmic mucin-containing cells are present in 14% to 63% of typical urothelial carcinoma and are not considered to represent glandular differentiation. The diagnosis of adenocarcinoma is reserved for pure tumors. A tumor with mixed glandular and urothelial differentiation is classified as urothelial carcinoma with glandular differentiation, and an estimate of the percentage of glandular component should be provided. A form of glandular differentiation with villous-like appearance has been described as associated with papillary urothelial carcinoma.[377]

The expression of MUC5AC-apomucin may be useful as an immunohistochemical marker of glandular differentiation in urothelial carcinomas.[378,379] A panel of immunohistochemical markers including cadherin-17, GATA3, and β-catenin is useful in distinguishing primary urinary bladder adenocarcinoma and

TABLE 6.15 — Diverse Morphologic Manifestations and Pitfalls in the Diagnosis of Urothelial Carcinoma Variants

Variants of Urothelial Carcinoma	Main Differential Diagnosis
Urothelial carcinoma with squamous and/or glandular differentiation	Squamous cell carcinoma, adenocarcinoma
Urothelial carcinoma, nested variant	von Brunn nest hyperplasia, cystitis glandularis, nephrogenic adenoma, paraganglioma, carcinoid, prostatic adenocarcinoma
Urothelial carcinoma, inverted variant	Inverted papilloma
Urothelial carcinoma, micropapillary variant	Adenocarcinoma, metastasis from other sites including serous carcinoma of the ovary
Urothelial carcinoma, microcystic variant	Cystitis cystica and cystitis glandularis, endocervicosis, nephrogenic adenoma, adenocarcinoma
Lymphoepithelioma-like (urothelial) carcinoma	Urothelial carcinoma with prominent lymphoid infiltrate, lymphoma (MALTOMA type), chronic cystitis
Urothelial carcinoma, plasmacytoid variant	Plasmacytoma, melanoma
Urothelial carcinoma, clear cell (glycogen-rich) variant	Clear cell carcinomas from kidney and other sites, clear cell adenocarcinoma
Urothelial carcinoma, lipid cell variant	Carcinosarcoma/sarcomatoid carcinoma with heterologous elements (liposarcoma), signet ring cell adenocarcinoma
Urothelial carcinoma with syncytiotrophoblastic giant cells	Choriocarcinoma, sarcomatoid carcinoma
Large cell undifferentiated carcinoma	Metastasis from other sites (lung)
Urothelial carcinoma with rhabdoid feature	Plasmacytoma, melanoma, inflammatory myofibroblastic tumor, metastasis from other sites
Urothelial carcinoma with pseudosarcomatous stroma	Sarcomatoid carcinoma
Urothelial carcinoma with stromal osseous or cartilaginous metaplasia	Sarcomatoid carcinoma with heterologous elements
Urothelial carcinoma with osteoclast-type giant cells	Reactive granulomatous lesion, giant cell carcinoma
Urothelial carcinoma with prominent lymphoid infiltrate	Lymphoma, lymphoepithelioma-like carcinoma
Rare urothelial carcinomas with discohesive, acinar differentiation or endometrioid-like morphologies	Lobular carcinoma of breast, endometrial carcinoma, prostatic adenocarcinoma

TABLE 6.16 — Variants of Urothelial Carcinoma and their Potential Clinical Significance by Pathologic Category

Variant Type	Differential Diagnosis and Molecular Alteration
Urothelial carcinoma with divergent differentiation	
With squamous cell differentiation	Primary or secondary squamous cell carcinoma. Common basal molecular classification; most unrelated to HPV
With glandular differentiation	Primary or secondary adenocarcinoma
	Unknown
With trophoblastic differentiation	Trophoblastic cells present in urothelial carcinoma; choriocarcinoma either primary or secondary; β-human chorionic gonadotropin (serum/tissue) in 30% of high-stage urothelial carcinoma
	True choriocarcinoma either primary or secondary shows high copy number of isochromosome 12p
Urothelial carcinoma with deceptively benign features	
Nested urothelial carcinoma (including large nested)	Von Brunn hyperplasia, nephrogenic adenoma
	TERT promoter mutation
Microcystic urothelial carcinoma	Cystitis cystica, cystitis glandularis, adenocarcinoma
	TERT promoter mutation
Differential diagnosis with metastases to the bladder	
Micropapillary urothelial carcinoma	Serous carcinoma of the ovary; micropapillary carcinomas from other sites; micropapillary morphology in carcinoma in situ or in NMIBC carcinoma seems less aggressive than invasive micropapillary carcinoma
	Variable HER2 (ERBB2) gene amplifications or mutations; basal molecular classification in 50% of cases
Plasmacytoid/signet ring cell/diffuse urothelial carcinoma	Plasmacytoma; lymphoma; metastases from adenocarcinoma of stomach (poorly cohesive/diffuse); plasmacytoid morphology in carcinoma in situ or in NMIBC carcinoma seems less aggressive than invasive plasmacytoid carcinoma; CDH1 loss (mutation or methylation) in >80% of cases; E-cadherin loss in >70% of cases
Sarcomatoid urothelial carcinoma (carcinosarcoma)	Inflammatory myofibroblastic tumor (inflammatory pseudotumor); metastatic sarcomatoid carcinoma; sarcoma either primary or metastatic
	Altered EMT protein expression by immunohistochemistry
Giant cell urothelial carcinoma	Highly bizarre pleomorphic tumor giant cells similar to giant cell carcinoma of lung
	Unknown
Clear cell (glycogen-rich) urothelial carcinoma	Clear cell carcinomas from kidney or gynecologic organs; other
	Similar to conventional urothelial carcinoma
Urothelial carcinoma, lipid cell variant	Liposarcoma; carcinosarcoma (heterologous sarcomatoid carcinoma)
	Similar to conventional urothelial carcinoma
Poorly differentiated tumors (undifferentiated carcinoma not otherwise specified, osteoclast-rich undifferentiated carcinoma, other)	Large cell carcinoma of lung; giant cell tumor of bone
	Unknown
Marked immune cell response	
Lymphoepithelioma-like urothelial carcinoma	Metastases from other sites; may be missed in small biopsies because of marked inflammatory background
	Mostly unrelated to Epstein-Barr virus

NMIBC, Non–muscle-invasive urothelial carcinoma; TERT, telomerase reverse transcriptase.

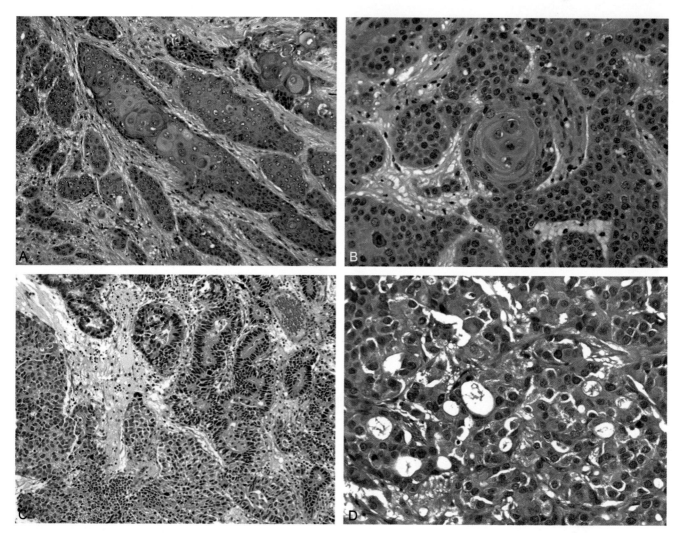

Fig. 6.43 Urothelial carcinoma with mixed differentiation. Squamous differentiation (A and B). Glandular differentiation (C and D). (D) Mucin secretion is noted in the luminal space of glandular differentiation.

TABLE 6.17	General Immunohistochemical Features Helpful in Resolving the Differential Diagnosis of Urinary Bladder Glandular Malignancies			
Tumors	**Cadherin-17**	**GATA3 (Nuclear)**	**β-Catenin**	**p63**
Primary urinary bladder adenocarcinoma	Positive	Negative	Usually membranous	Negative
Urothelial carcinoma with glandular differentiation	Negative	Sometimes positive (urothelial > glandular)	Usually membranous for both urothelial and glandular components	Urothelial carcinoma component usually positive; glandular component negative
Secondary involvement of bladder by colorectal adenocarcinoma	Positive	Negative	Usually nuclear	Negative
Primary colorectal adenocarcinoma	Positive	Negative	Usually nuclear	Negative

urothelial carcinoma with glandular differentiation from secondary colorectal adenocarcinoma (Table 6.17).[380] The typical immunohistochemical profile of primary adenocarcinoma of the urinary bladder is as follows: cadherin-17+, GATA3–, and β-catenin membranous and cytoplasmic positive. Cadherin-17 is a relatively specific and sensitive marker in diagnosing primary adenocarcinoma of the urinary bladder, distinguishing it from urothelial carcinoma with glandular differentiation. However, it does not distinguish primary adenocarcinoma of the urinary bladder from secondary

involvement by colorectal adenocarcinoma, in which case β-catenin is the most useful marker. Although GATA3, when positive, supports a diagnosis of urothelial carcinoma with glandular differentiation, nuclear expression is present only in a minority of cases.[380]

When adenocarcinoma is present in association with urothelial carcinoma, even focally, it portends a poor prognosis. Glandular differentiation is an important finding and usually dictates more aggressive therapy (see later in this chapter).

Different lines of germ cell differentiation, including trophoblastic differentiation, in an otherwise conventional urothelial carcinoma may rarely be seen as a form of divergent differentiation (see further discussion later in this chapter).

Some urothelial carcinomas may present components of small cell carcinoma, which mimics its pulmonary counterpart, coexisting with conventional urothelial carcinoma, squamous carcinoma, adenocarcinoma, or sarcomatoid carcinoma.[381] Any amount of small cell carcinoma should be reported because it is relevant in prognosis and therapeutic approach, as noted later in the Neural and Neuroendocrine Tumors section.[382,383]

Micropapillary Urothelial Carcinoma

Micropapillary carcinoma is a distinct variant of urothelial carcinoma that resembles papillary serous carcinoma of the ovary (Fig. 6.44).[155,376,384-395] The first description of micropapillary carcinoma included 18 patients whose ages ranged from 47 to 81 years (mean, 67 years), with a male-to-female ratio of 5:1.[376,386,387,391] The most common presenting symptom is hematuria.

Micropapillary carcinoma is accompanied by noninvasive papillary or invasive urothelial carcinoma in 80% of reported cases. The presence of a micropapillary component at the surface in bladder biopsy specimens is an unfavorable prognostic feature. In such cases, deeper biopsies may prove useful, because muscle invasion is a significant concern in these cases.[376,387] Micropapillary carcinoma is composed of infiltrating, slender, delicate filiform processes or small, tight papillary tumor cell clusters that lie within lacunae that resemble lymphovascular spaces; however, no lining endothelial cells are demonstrable by immunohistochemistry in these small lacunar spaces.[391,392]

Interobserver reproducibility for the diagnosis of invasive micropapillary carcinoma was moderate (κ, 0.54).[396] Although the diagnosis among the classic cases was relatively uniform (93% agreement), the classification in the subset of invasive urothelial carcinomas with extensive retraction and varying sized tumor nests was more variable. Multiple nests within the same lacunar space had the highest association with a diagnosis of classic invasive micropapillary carcinoma.[396]

Twenty-five percent of cases show glandular differentiation, and some authors consider it a variant of adenocarcinoma. Psammoma bodies are infrequent. True vascular and lymphatic invasion is commonly demonstrable, and most cases show invasion of the muscularis propria or deeper.[397] Metastases are common at the time of initial diagnosis.[387] The main differential consideration is metastatic serous micropapillary ovarian carcinoma in women or mesothelioma in either gender.

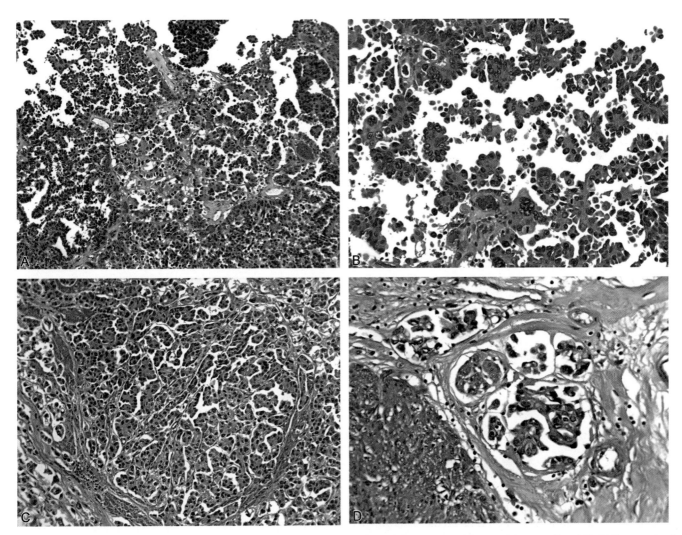

Fig. 6.44 Urothelial carcinoma, micropapillary variant. Surface component resembling papillary serous carcinoma of the ovary (A and B). (C) Tumor extends into muscularis propria. (D) Infiltrating tumor may form tight clusters of micropapillary aggregates within lacunae.

Expression of keratins by tumor cells of micropapillary carcinoma is similar to that of typical urothelial carcinoma, but micropapillary carcinomas are much more likely to express CA125, suggesting that the micropapillary phenotype is a form of glandular differentiation.[398] Micropapillary carcinoma also shows positive immunostaining for epithelial membrane antigen (EMA), CK7, CK20, Leu-M1 (CD15), and FOXA1.[388,399] MUC1 expression is seen in the stroma-facing aspect of the tumor cell groups, indicating a reversal of the normal cell orientation in these tumors.[400] Forty-two percent of micropapillary variant urothelial carcinomas harbor *HER2* gene ammplification.[401]

Carcinomas with micropapillary histology have also been reported in the lung, breast, pancreas, colorectum, and salivary glands. Clinical correlation is usually required, but the possibility of a bladder primary may be suggested if there is no obvious primary tumor at another anatomic site. Identification of an admixed urothelial carcinoma of more typical morphology or immunohistochemical support (CK7, CK20, and uroplakin 3 positivity) would be helpful.[402]

Recent molecular data suggest that most micropapillary carcinomas belong to a molecular subtype of urothelial carcinoma, the so-called luminal urothelial carcinoma subtype, rather than being a discrete pathologic identity.[403] This luminal subtype appears as a dominant trait, such that even urothelial carcinomas with small components of micropapillary growth belong to this category. Luminal tumors may have wild-type p53 and can be resistant to current chemotherapy regimens.[403]

Micropapillary carcinoma should be considered a variant of urothelial carcinoma with a poor prognosis. In one study 62% of patients with invasive micropapillary carcinoma had lymph node metastases, and 85% of patients died of cancer at a mean interval from the diagnosis of 6.2 months.[388] Another study by the MD Anderson Cancer Center suggested that high-grade stage pT1 urothelial carcinomas have a high frequency of micropapillary carcinoma (so-called superficial micropapillary carcinoma), and that patients in this category should be offered aggressive therapy instead of intravesical immunotherapy to improve long-term survival.[389,390] Samaratunga and Khoo found that the prognosis is related to the proportion and location of the micropapillary component.[398] Cases with a moderate or extensive micropapillary component are at high risk for having an advanced stage at presentation. Cases with less than 10% micropapillary component and a surface micropapillary component have a high chance of detection at an early stage.

Plasmacytoid Urothelial Carcinoma

Zukerberg et al. described bladder carcinoma in two patients that diffusely permeated the bladder wall and was composed of cells with a monotonous appearance mimicking lymphoma.[404] Approximately one-third of the patients presented with intraperitoneal disease spread, and 20% had subsequent metastasis involving serosal surfaces.[405] The tumor cells were medium size, with eosinophilic cytoplasm and eccentric nuclei producing a plasmacytoid appearance (Fig. 6.45).[405-412] The epithelial nature of the malignancy

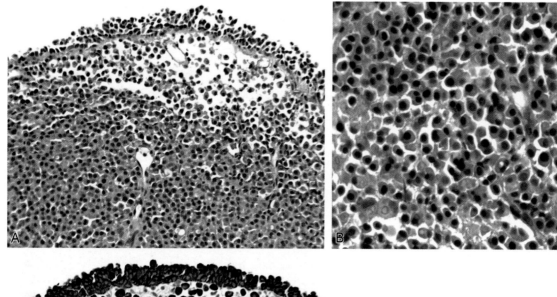

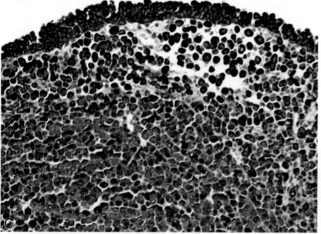

Fig. 6.45 Urothelial carcinoma, plasmacytoid variant. The tumor cells have an eccentric nucleus and eosinophilic cytoplasm reminiscent of plasma cells (A and B). (C) CK stain is strongly positive in tumor cells.

was confirmed by immunohistochemistry.[413] The differential diagnostic considerations include lymphoid reaction, lymphoma, multiple myeloma, urothelial carcinoma with rhabdoid feature, signet ring cell adenocarcinoma, paraganglioma, neuroendocrine carcinoma, melanoma, and rhabdomyosarcoma. Identification of an epithelial component by immunohistochemistry confirms the diagnosis.

A series report of 11 cases showed that the plasmacytoid component comprised greater than 50% of the tumor in eight cases, with two additional cases showing pure plasmacytoid carcinoma.[406] All patients had advanced-stage cancer (>pT3), and 73% had lymph node metastases. On follow-up, 82% of patients died of disease from 2 to 11 months, and two patients were alive with disease at 8 and 16 months.[406]

The architectural pattern of the tumor varied from solid expansile nests with discohesive cells to mixed solid and alveolar growth; a streaking discohesive architecture was additionally present in two cases (18%).[406] Rarely a myxoid pattern can be present. Histologically, the individual tumor cells had an eccentrically placed nucleus and abundant eosinophilic cytoplasm reminiscent of plasma cells. Most neoplastic cells had nuclei of low-to-intermediate nuclear grade with occasional nuclear pleomorphism. In addition to the plasmacytoid morphology, several single cells with cytoplasmic vacuoles, with or without mucin, which impart a signet ring cell appearance, are typically present. These tumors are not associated with any extracellular mucin production, a useful parameter to differentiate plasmacytoid carcinoma from adenocarcinoma with signet ring cells, which is typically associated with extracellular mucin. Some of these tumors have been previously designated as lobular-like carcinoma because of morphologic reminiscence of this subtype to lobular breast carcinoma.

Immunohistochemical staining demonstrated that both plasmacytoid and associated conventional urothelial carcinoma were positive for CK7, CK20, AE1/AE3, and EMA; CD138 (marker of plasma cells) was often positive.[406]

Loss of E-cadherin, encoded by the *CDH1* gene, has recently been described in a large cohort of patients with plasmacytoid urothelial carcinoma and may account for the marked discohesion of these malignant cells.[414] Loss of E-cadherin protein by immunohistochemistry may be seen in about 70% of plasmacytoid carcinomas in contrast with only 11% of conventional urothelial carcinomas. CDH1 mutations have been described in 87% of plasmacytoid carcinomas, whereas no CDH1 mutations were seen in conventional urothelial carcinomas.[415] Some cases show CDH1 methylation instead of mutation.[415]

Nested Urothelial Carcinoma

The nested variant of urothelial carcinoma is an aggressive neoplasm with fewer than 50 reported cases.[376] There is a marked male predominance, and in early studies, 70% of patients died 4 to 40 months after diagnosis despite therapy.[416,417] This rare pattern of urothelial carcinoma was first described as a tumor with a "deceptively benign" appearance that closely resembles von Brunn nests infiltrating the lamina propria (Fig. 6.46).[416-419] Nuclei generally show little or no atypia, but invariably the tumor contains foci of unequivocal cancer with cells exhibiting enlarged nucleoli and coarse nuclear chromatin. Anaplastic features are often more apparent in the deeper aspects of the cancer.[420] The architectural pattern of nested carcinoma component ranged from a predominantly disorderly proliferation of discrete, small, variably sized nests to tubular growth pattern with focal random nuclear atypia centered within the base of the tumor.

The definition of nested urothelial carcinoma has been expanded to include other tumors showing deceptively benign histology, such as large nested variant urothelial carcinoma. Larger infiltrative nests may be present in variable proportions. A component of conventional urothelial carcinoma is frequently present.

The differential diagnosis of the nested variant of urothelial carcinoma includes lesions and tumors with nested-like morphology as prominent von Brunn nests, cystitis cystica, cystitis glandularis, inverted papilloma, nephrogenic metaplasia, carcinoid tumor, paraganglionic tissue, and paraganglioma (Table 6.18).[376,416,420,421] The occurrence of a large nested variant of urothelial carcinoma (Fig. 6.47) further emphasizes the importance of recognizing these diverse morphologic manifestations.[421,422]

The immunohistochemical features of the nested variant of urothelial carcinoma are similar to those of aggressive urothelial carcinomas of the usual type, with frequent loss of p27 and a high MIB1 (Ki67) labeling index.[423] In the differential diagnosis between florid von Brunn nests and the nested variant of urothelial carcinoma, CK20 immunohistochemical evaluation does not

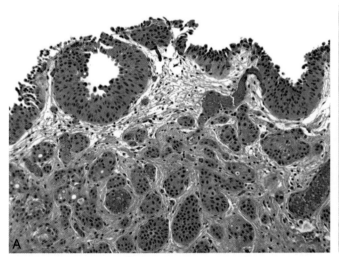
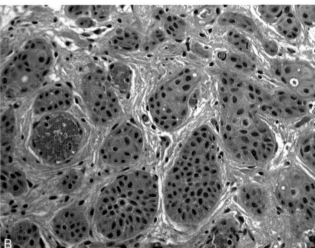

Fig. 6.46 Urothelial carcinoma, nested variant. (A) Tumor invades into the lamina propria. (B) The cells are relatively uniform without significant cytologic atypia. The key differential diagnostic consideration is von Brunn nest hyperplasia.

TABLE 6.18 Key Features in the Differential Diagnosis of the Nested Variant of Urothelial Carcinoma

Conditions	Lumen Formation	Marked Cytologic Atypia in Deeper Portion	Infiltrative Base	Muscle Invasion	Immunohistochemistry
Nested variant urothelial carcinoma	Present, variable	Present, frequent	Present, frequent	Present, frequent	Low p27^{kip1}, high MIB1 (Ki67) proliferation index
Florid von Brunn nests	Present, variable	Absent	Absent	Absent	Variable
Nephrogenic metaplasia	Present	Absent	Present, frequent	Present, rare	Variable, PAX8$^+$ and AMACR$^+$
Cystitis cystica, cystitis glandularis	Present	Absent	Absent	Absent	Variable
Paraganglionic tissue and paraganglioma	Absent, associated prominent vascular network	Absent	Absent	Present	Neuroendocrine markers positive

AMACR, α-Methylacyl-coenzyme A racemase (P504S).

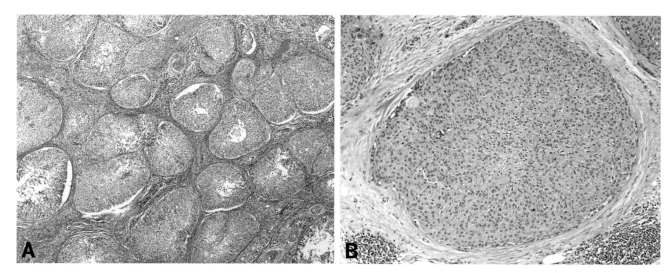

Fig. 6.47 Large urothelial carcinoma, nested variant (A and B).

appear to be useful, but significantly greater MIB1 and p53 expressions are seen in nested-variant urothelial carcinoma compared with florid von Brunn nests, with MIB1 expression in more than 7% of lesional cells and p53 expression in more than 3% of lesional cells seen only in carcinoma.[424] Most nested tumor cells are also positive for high-molecular-weight CK, CK7, p63, and variably CK20. Nested urothelial carcinoma may be distinguished from benign mimickers by the presence of the TERT promoter mutation associated with the tumor cells.[17,425]

The outcome for nested urothelial carcinoma, seen either in pure form or with a component of usual urothelial carcinoma, has generally been regarded as poor. However, in a recent study, nested urothelial carcinoma appears to be similar in immunohistochemical features and clinical outcomes to conventional urothelial carcinoma, with no difference in recurrence rate or survival when surgically treated.[426]

Microcystic Urothelial Carcinoma

Microcystic urothelial carcinoma is a variant of invasive urothelial carcinoma with a deceptively benign appearance, exhibiting microcysts, macrocysts, or tubular structures, with cysts ranging from microscopic to 2 cm in diameter (Fig. 6.48).[427,428] The cysts are round to oval and of varying sizes; the periphery of large cysts

was frequently punctuated by many smaller cysts. The cysts and tubules may be empty, contain necrotic debris, or be filled with mucin demonstrable by periodic acid–Schiff (PAS) stain after diastase predigestion. The cysts are lined by urothelial, low columnar cells or by a single layer of flattened epithelium of low to intermediate nuclear grade. Focal high-grade conventional urothelial carcinoma is present in about 40% of cases. There are no survival differences for microcystic carcinoma compared with conventional urothelial carcinoma.[429]

This variant of urothelial carcinoma may be confused with benign proliferations such as florid polypoid cystitis cystica and glandularis and nephrogenic metaplasia.[428] This pattern should be separated from the nested variant of urothelial carcinoma with tubular differentiation.[376]

Rarely, microcystic variant may simulate Gleason 3 + 3 prostatic adenocarcinoma but can be distinguished from it by negative prostate markers (prostate-specific antigen [PSA], NKX3.1) and positive urothelial markers (CK7, CK20, thrombomodulin, p63, GATA3, or S100P). Microcystic urothelial carcinoma appears to be similar in immunohistochemical features to conventional urothelial carcinoma. Microcystic urothelial carcinoma may be distinguished from benign mimickers by the presence of TERT promoter mutation associated with the tumor.

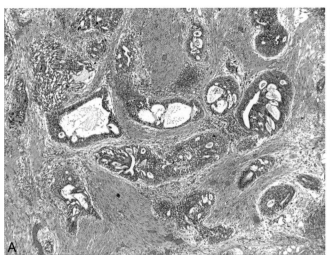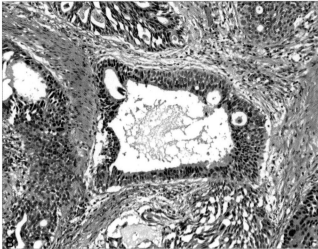

Fig. 6.48 Urothelial carcinoma, microcystic variant (A and B).

Lymphoepithelioma-like Urothelial Carcinoma

Carcinoma that histologically resembles lymphoepithelioma of the nasopharynx has been described in the urinary bladder, with fewer than 100 cases reported.[376,407,427,430-433] It is more common in men than in women (3:1 ratio) and tends to occur in late adulthood (range, 52 to 81 years; mean, 69 years). Most patients present with hematuria. The tumor is solitary and usually involves the dome, posterior wall, or trigone, often with a sessile growth pattern. Histologically, it may be pure or mixed with typical urothelial carcinoma, the latter being focal and inconspicuous in some instances. Glandular and squamous differentiation may be seen. The epithelial component is composed of nests, sheets, and cords of undifferentiated cells with large pleomorphic nuclei and prominent nucleoli (Fig. 6.49).[376,407] The cytoplasmic borders are poorly defined, imparting a syncytial appearance. The background consists of a prominent lymphoid stroma that includes T and B lymphocytes, plasma cells, histiocytes, and occasional neutrophils or eosinophils with a predominant population of CD3+ T lymphocytes. Neither Epstein-Barr virus nor HPV infection has been identified in lymphoepithelioma-like carcinoma of the bladder.[430,434,435] Immunohistochemistry reveals CK immunoreactivity (CK AE1/AE3 and CK7) in the malignant cells, confirming their epithelial nature; the tumor cells are also reactive for GATA3 and S100P but are rarely positive for CK20.

Lymphoepithelioma-like carcinomas of the urinary bladder have common urothelial genetic alterations detected by UroVysion and frequent p53 accumulations supporting a similar pathogenesis to conventional urothelial carcinoma.[430] The major differential diagnostic considerations are poorly differentiated urothelial carcinoma with lymphoid inflammatory response, poorly differentiated squamous cell carcinoma, and lymphoma. Lymphoepithelioma-like bladder carcinoma has been found to be responsive to chemotherapy if the tumor is encountered in its pure form. Although most reported cases occurring in the urinary bladder are associated with a relatively favorable prognosis when pure or predominant, when lymphoepithelioma-like carcinoma is only focally present in an otherwise typical urothelial carcinoma, the prognosis is the same as that of patients with conventional urothelial carcinoma of the same grade and stage.

Lipid-Rich Urothelial Carcinoma

Lipid cell variant is a rare neoplasm defined as a urothelial carcinoma that exhibits transition to a cell type resembling signet ring lipoblasts (Fig. 6.50). A report based on 27 patients showed that the lipid cell component varied from 10% to 50% of the tumor specimen.[420] Pathologic stage at diagnosis was Ta (n = 1), T1 (n = 2), T2, (at least n = 7), T3a (n = 4), T3b (n = 8), and T4a (n = 5). Sixteen of the patients died of disease at 16 to 58 months (mean, 33 months).[436]

The architectural pattern of the tumor varies from solid expansile to infiltrative nests. The large epithelial tumor cells have an eccentrically placed nucleus and abundant vacuolated cytoplasm resembling signet ring lipoblasts. Mucin stains are negative in all cases. Most neoplastic cells have nuclei of intermediate nuclear grade with occasional nuclear pleomorphism.

Immunohistochemical staining demonstrates that the lipid cell component is positive for CK7, CK20, CAM5.2, high-molecular-weight CK (34βE12), AE1/AE3, EMA, and thrombomodulin; vimentin and S100P were negative. LOH analysis results are the same for the lipid variant and concurrent conventional urothelial carcinoma.[436]

Electron microcopy analysis of two cases confirmed the presence of lipid in tumor cells. In limited samples, lipid cell variant urothelial carcinoma may be misdiagnosed as liposarcoma, sarcomatoid carcinoma (carcinosarcoma) with a liposarcomatous component, or signet ring cell carcinoma. The finding of lipid-containing cells immunoreactive for epithelial markers can be useful in this setting.[436]

Clear Cell (Glycogen-Rich) Urothelial Carcinoma

Up to two-thirds of urothelial carcinoma cases have foci of clear cell change resulting from abundant glycogen.[376,437,438] The glycogen-rich clear cell "variant" of urothelial carcinoma, recently described, appears to represent the extreme end of the morphologic spectrum. It consists predominantly or exclusively of cells with abundant clear cytoplasm (Fig. 6.51). Tumor cells show positive immunostaining for CK7, GATA3, S100P, and p40; some cases may express desmoglein 3, which suggests squamous differentiation.[439] Recognition of this pattern avoids confusion with clear cell adenocarcinoma of the bladder and metastatic clear cell carcinoma

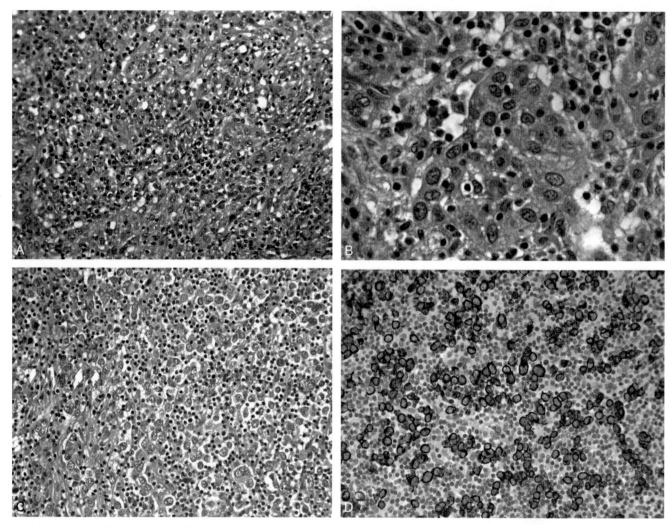

Fig. 6.49 Lymphoepithelioma-like (urothelial) carcinoma. Infiltrating tumor shows typical syncytial arrangement of the cells in an inflammatory background with abundant eosinophils (A to C). (D) The tumor cells display strong immunoreactivity to antibodies against AE1/AE3.

from the kidney or prostate. Immunohistochemical markers of prostate and kidney lineage are not expressed in clear cell (glycogen-rich) urothelial carcinoma. Cytoplasmic clearing as a result of thermal artifact in transurethral resections should not be mistaken for this variant of bladder cancer.[437,438]

Sarcomatoid Urothelial Carcinoma

The term *sarcomatoid variant of urothelial carcinoma* should be used for any biphasic malignant neoplasm that exhibits morphologic or immunohistochemical evidence of both epithelial and mesenchymal differentiation (Fig. 6.52). The presence or absence of heterologous elements should be recorded in the report (see Sarcomatoid Carcinoma section).

Giant Cell Urothelial Carcinoma

Giant cell carcinoma is a rare form of bladder cancer recognized by the current WHO classification of urologic tumors.[6] It is an aggressive variant of urothelial carcinoma associated with poor prognosis that presents at an advanced stage.[440,441] It may represent an extreme form of dedifferentiation in bladder carcinoma.[442]

A study based on eight cases showed that the pleomorphic giant cell component varied from 20% to 100% of the tumor specimen;

in two cases the giant cell component composed greater than 50% of the tumor, with one case showing pure pleomorphic giant cell carcinoma.[440] The architectural pattern of the tumor varied from infiltrating pleomorphic tumor with bizarre giant cells to solid expansile nests with discohesive growth pattern; a hypocellular desmoplastic stromal response was present in two cases (25%) with giant single cells in sclerotic stroma.[440]

Histologically, giant bizarre anaplastic cells with frequent typical or atypical mitotic figures are present in all cases (Fig. 6.53).[440] Seven mixed cases had concurrent conventional high-grade urothelial carcinoma; two cases presented features of micropapillary or lymphoepithelioma-like urothelial carcinoma. Variably sized intracytoplasmic vacuoles were present in two cases. All patients had advanced-stage cancer (>pT3), and six (75%) had lymph node metastases. Immunohistochemical staining demonstrated that both pleomorphic giant cell and associated conventional urothelial carcinoma were positive for CK7, CAM5.2, AE1/AE3, and EMA; p63, thrombomodulin, and uroplakin 3 were positive in six, three, and two cases, respectively. On follow-up, five patients died of disease from 6 to 17 months and two patients were alive with metastases at 11 and 19 months. One patient had no evidence of disease at 74 months.[440]

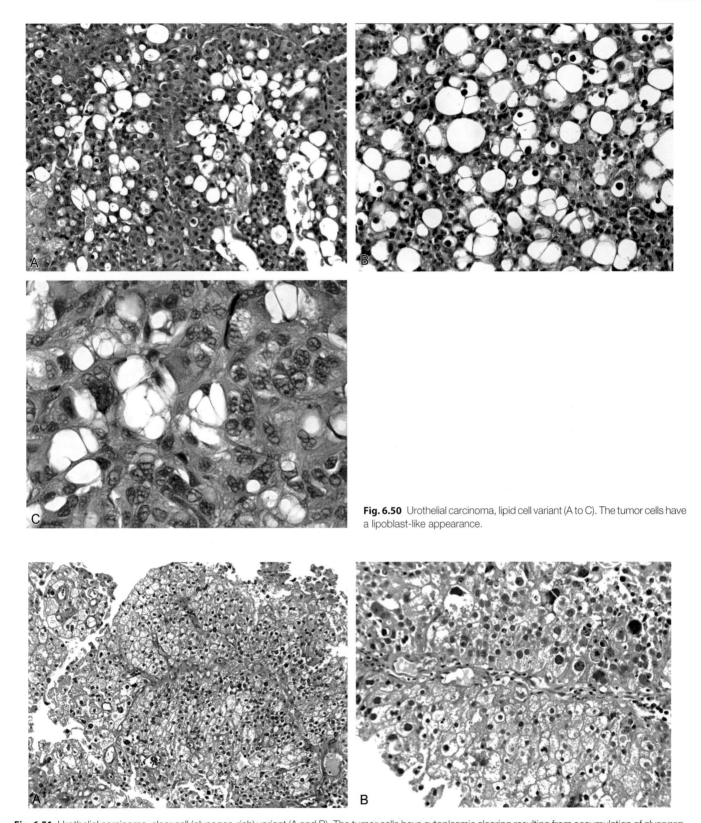

Fig. 6.50 Urothelial carcinoma, lipid cell variant (A to C). The tumor cells have a lipoblast-like appearance.

Fig. 6.51 Urothelial carcinoma, clear cell (glycogen-rich) variant (A and B). The tumor cells have cytoplasmic clearing resulting from accumulation of glycogen.

The main differential diagnosis includes giant cell carcinoma primary in the lung or other anatomic sites, but this distinction can be made only on clinical grounds. The tumor giant cells display CK and vimentin immunoreactivity. Bladder tumors with giant cells associated with β-human chorionic gonadotropin (β-hCG) production, osteoclast-type giant cells, and sarcomatoid carcinoma with occasional pleomorphic giant cells should enter the differential diagnosis. In limited samples, giant cell carcinoma may be misdiagnosed as sarcoma, a pitfall of paramount importance for its clinical management.

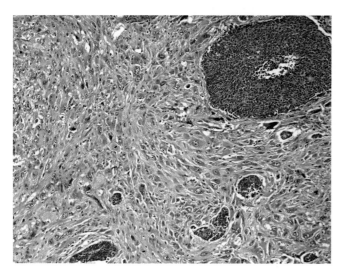

Fig. 6.52 Sarcomatoid urothelial carcinoma. Note the abrupt transition between sarcomatoid and urothelial carcinoma.

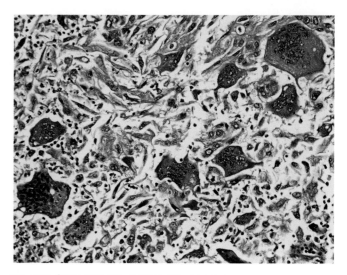

Fig. 6.54 Osteoclast-rich undifferentiated carcinoma.

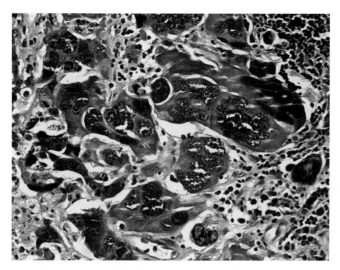

Fig. 6.53 Giant cell urothelial carcinoma.

Poorly Differentiated Tumors (Including Those With Osteoclast-like Giant Cells)

Poorly differentiated tumors is a newly included category in the current WHO classification of urinary tract tumors.[6] Poorly differentiated tumors span a spectrum that includes tumors with mixed morphologies including tumors such as small cell undifferentiated carcinoma, sarcomatoid carcinoma, giant cell carcinoma (see earlier discussion), undifferentiated carcinoma not otherwise specified (see further discussion later in this chapter), and the so-called osteoclast-rich undifferentiated carcinoma.[6,443,444] The poorly differentiated urothelial tumors may be associated with conventional urothelial carcinoma or other forms of divergent differentiation, including glandular, trophoblastic, or squamous differentiation, or with combinations of poorly differentiated patterns. Limited reported data portend poor outcomes for this category of poorly differentiated urothelial tumor with multiple histologic patterns at time of first diagnosis.[6,443,444]

A rare pattern of poorly differentiated tumors seen in the bladder includes the so-called osteoclast-rich undifferentiated carcinoma, a pattern including giant cell tumors or osteoclastoma-like giant cell tumors of the pancreas, gallbladder, liver, breast, salivary gland, thyroid, skin, lung, intestines, larynx, and female genital tract. Fewer than 20 tumors with similar histologic findings have been reported in the bladder, most as case reports.[445-447] In a series of six patients, four of five with follow-up died of disease, three with documented metastasis.[444] A large majority of patients reported in case reports who had adequate follow-up also had documented metastatic cancer or died of cancer. These tumors should be distinguished from urothelial carcinoma with syncytiotrophoblastic giant cells and urothelial carcinoma with osteoclast-type giant cell reaction of the stroma.

Osteoclast-rich undifferentiated carcinoma is composed of mononuclear cells (frequently positive for epithelial markers), osteoclast-like giant cells (positive CD68, CD51, and CD54), and recognizable usual urothelial neoplasia (carcinoma in situ, papillary, or invasive carcinoma) in varying proportions (Fig. 6.54).[444] Some areas may have a histologic appearance like that of giant cell tumors of bone, whereas other areas may show single cells or aggregates of mononuclear cells with a spectrum of atypia, including marked pleomorphism, distinct from the nuclei of the osteoclast-like giant cells. These mononuclear cells may stain for pan-CK, EMA, CAM5.2, and CK7, and rarely for S100P, actin, desmin, and p53. Although these tumors have several histologic features of their skeletal counterparts, including areas with blood-filled cysts mimicking aneurysmal bone cyst, it is believed that they represent true undifferentiated carcinomas because of CK positivity, concurrent presence of high-grade urothelial neoplasia, matched p53 positivity in mononuclear cells and urothelial tumor cells, and the poor prognosis of tumors with this histology.[444]

See further discussion in Undifferentiated Carcinoma (Including Those With Rhabdoid Features) section.

Other Aspects and Variants of Urothelial Carcinoma Not Included in the Current World Health Organization Classification

Other aspects and variants of urothelial carcinoma not included or not sufficiently covered in the current WHO classification of tumors of the urinary tract are discussed here (Table 6.14).

Urothelial Carcinoma, Inverted Growth
(Inverted Papilloma-like)

The inverted variant also has been referred to as urothelial carcinoma with endophytic (inverted papilloma-like) growth and as inverted urothelial carcinoma (Fig. 6.55). The potential for misinterpretation of urothelial carcinoma with inverted growth as benign inverted papilloma is high.[33,376,448-451] The inverted variant of urothelial carcinoma demonstrates significant nuclear pleomorphism, architectural abnormality, and increased mitotic activity. In most cases the surface of the neoplasm shows similar abnormalities and is readily recognized as typical urothelial carcinoma (Fig. 6.55). An exophytic papillary or invasive component is often associated with the inverted element.[33,449] However, in cases of inverted papilloma fragmented during transurethral resection, a pseudoexophytic pattern may result. Large papillary tumors with prominent endophytic growth may appear to "invade" the lamina propria with a pushing border. Unless this pattern is accompanied by true destructive stromal invasion, the likelihood of metastasis is minimal because the basement membrane is not truly breached. One proposal suggests grading these tumors following the same criteria as conventional urothelial carcinoma.[33,376]

Inverted papillomas of the urinary bladder and urothelial carcinomas with an inverted growth pattern may be distinguished using a combination of morphologic, immunohistochemical, and molecular genetic assessments (Table 6.19).[33] Whereas inverted papillomas usually do not demonstrate immunoreactivity for Ki67, p53, or CK20, urothelial carcinomas with inverted growth pattern frequently express one or more of these biomarkers. Similarly, inverted papillomas do not show the molecular features of urothelial carcinoma, whereas inverted pattern urothelial carcinomas often demonstrated genetic alterations that are commonly seen in bladder cancer.[33,452]

Telomere shortening using FISH analysis is a feature seen in about 70% of urothelial carcinoma with inverted growth but in only 9% of inverted papilloma, a finding that can be useful to separate these two entities in difficult cases.[50] A recent TERT promoter mutation status study reported 15% mutation in inverted papilloma compared with 58% in urothelial carcinoma with inverted growth. These studies suggest that there is a subpopulation of inverted papilloma that shares a carcinogenetic pathway with urothelial carcinoma with inverted growth and conventional urothelial carcinomas.[49,50]

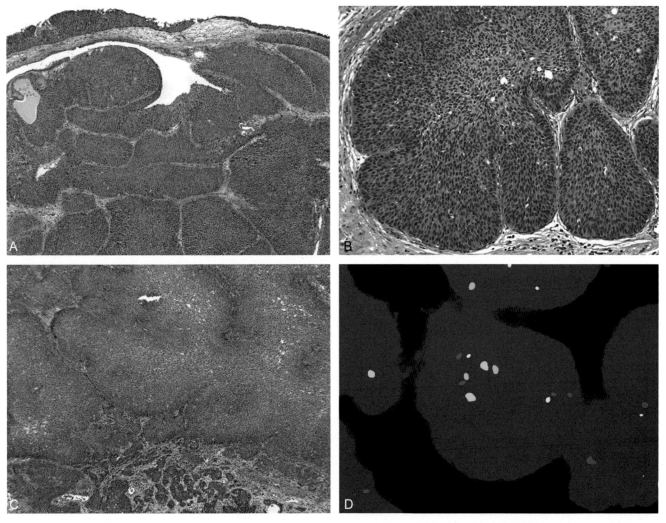

Fig. 6.55 Urothelial carcinoma, inverted variant. Thick columns and cords of neoplastic cells of irregular width and areas of solid growth are seen (A and B). (C) Stromal invasion is obvious. (D) Multicolor interphase fluorescence in situ hybridization using the UroVysion probes is useful in difficult cases. The cancer cell showed four copies of chromosome 3 (*red*) and two copies each of chromosomes 7 (*green*), 17 (*aqua*), and p16 gene (*gold*).

TABLE 6.19 Differences Between Urothelial Carcinoma with Inverted Growth and Inverted Papilloma

Characteristics	Urothelial Carcinoma, Inverted Growth	Inverted Papilloma
Surface	Variable, usually exophytic papillary lesion present	Smooth, dome shaped, usually intact cytologically unremarkable surface urothelium
Growth pattern	Endophytic, thick trabeculae, circumscription variable	Endophytic, sharply delineated, anastomosing cords and trabeculae
Cytologic features	Cytologic atypia is invariably present, mitotic figures often present, less maturation or palisading	Orderly polarized cells, some spindling and palisading at periphery, absence of necrosis and diffuse severe cytologic atypia; mitotic figures absent or rare
Biologic potential	Recurrences and progression may occur	Benign, no recurrences when completely resected[a]
Ki67 labeling index	Variable with grade; usually high p53	Low
UroVysion FISH	Positive	Negative
TP53 mutation	Frequent	Absent
Telomere length	Shortened	Normal
FGFR3 mutation	Frequent	Frequent (45%)
TERT promoter mutation	Often present	Rare

FGFR3, Fibroblast growth factor receptor 3; *FISH,* fluorescence in situ hybridization; *TERT,* telomerase reverse transcriptase.
[a]Rare recurrences related to incomplete surgical excision.

Pseudoangiosarcomatous (Pseudoangiosarcoma-like) Urothelial Carcinoma

The pseudoangiosarcomatous pattern recently described in bladder cancer is unique for its striking morphologic resemblance to angiosarcoma. Reported patients were males ranging in age from 47 to 87 years, and all had high-stage cancers at cystectomy. Follow-up data available in six cases revealed a poor outcome with an overall median survival of 8.5 months.[453]

Histologically, the pseudoangiosarcomatous carcinomas were characterized by tumor cell discohesion and lysis that created pseudolumina formations surrounded by attached residual tumor cells (Fig. 6.56). Detached degenerating tumor cells variably admixed with inflammatory cells were common in the false lumina. Partially intact urothelial carcinoma nests contained irregular or cleftlike spaces and disintegrating tumor cells with stretched intercellular bridges. The tumor was commonly associated with a dense collagenous matrix, often surrounding the lytic nests. Similar tumor cell discohesion and breakdown were observed in three tumors with foci of squamous cell differentiation, distinguished by the presence of dyskeratosis and keratin formation.

Other associated nonpseudoangiosarcomatous carcinoma components included conventional urothelial carcinoma, squamous differentiation, sarcomatoid spindle cell carcinoma, small cell carcinoma, micropapillary carcinoma, and glandular differentiation.

Pseudoangiosarcomatous urothelial carcinomas were all diffusely CK7+, most were GATA3+, and none expressed vascular-associated markers.

Urothelial Carcinoma With Chordoid Features

These cases were initially described as urothelial carcinoma with chordoid features, characterized by prominent cellular cording and associated myxoid stromal matrix, a pattern closely resembling that of extraskeletal myxoid chondrosarcoma (Fig. 6.57).[454] Urothelial carcinoma with chordoid features is a morphologic pattern of urothelial carcinoma that may potentially mimic a spectrum of primary vesical and nonvesical neoplasms with myxoid or mucinous components. These carcinomas maintain an immunophenotype characteristic of urothelial carcinoma and usually manifest with high-stage disease.[454]

In the study by Cox et al. of 12 patients (8 male and 4 female), the patients' ages ranged from 50 to 85 years (mean, 68 years).[454] The specimens consisted of five cystectomies, six transurethral resections, and one anterior exenteration with right nephroureterectomy. Morphologically, each patient had at least focal areas in which acellular myxoid stroma was associated with the carcinoma cells. When well developed, the neoplastic cells had scant eosinophilic cytoplasm and were arranged into cords closely mimicking extraskeletal myxoid chondrosarcoma, chordoma, mixed tumor and myoepithelioma of soft tissue, and yolk sac tumor. The

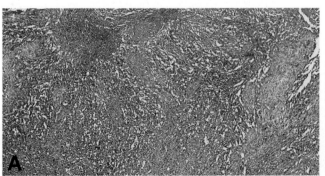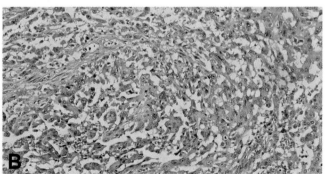

Fig. 6.56 Pseudoangiosarcomatous urothelial carcinoma (A and B).

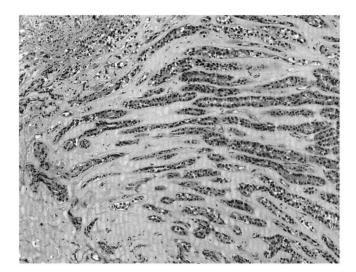

Fig. 6.57 Urothelial carcinoma with chordoid features.

percentage of tumor with a chordoid appearance ranged from 5% to 95% (mean, 39%; median, 25%). No conventional sarcomatous differentiation, no intracytoplasmic mucin, and no glandular formation were present in any patient. All 12 patients had foci of typical urothelial carcinoma present at least focally, and a gradual transition to the chordoid pattern was commonly seen.[454]

Immunophenotypically, these tumors show strong immunoreactivity for p63 (nuclear) and CK 34βE12 (cytoplasmic). Immunostains for CK20, calponin, glial fibrillary acidic protein, oncofetal protein glypican-3, and Brachyury were negative in the seven cases studied, whereas S100P had focal staining (<5%) in one case. The myxoid stromal component was diffusely colloidal iron and Alcian blue positive. PAS was negative in all eight cases, whereas mucicarmine was only focally positive in two of eight cases. Most cases were high stage (pT4, 5; pT3, 4; pT2, 2; and pT1, 1), and six of eight cases (75%) with nodal sampling had metastatic disease. In one case the lymph node metastasis had areas with chordoid morphology. Nine of 12 patients had available follow-up: 2 were dead of disease (1 and 10 months); 4 were alive with disease (5 to 8 months), with distant metastasis in 3; and 3 had no evidence of disease at last follow-up (2 to 120 months).[455]

Urothelial Carcinoma With Syncytiotrophoblastic Giant Cells

Urothelial carcinoma with syncytiotrophoblastic giant cells or trophoblastic differentiation is not uncommon. Small clusters of syncytiotrophoblastic giant cells may be present in typical urothelial carcinomas and should not be confused with choriocarcinoma (see further discussion later in this chapter). These cells can produce substantial amounts of immunoreactive β-hCG, indicative of syncytiotrophoblastic differentiation (Fig. 6.58).[376,456,457] The number of β-hCG–immunoreactive cells is inversely associated with cancer grade.[458,459] Secretion of β-hCG into the serum may be associated with a poor response to radiation therapy.[457,460,461]

β-hCG expression in poorly differentiated urothelial carcinoma without overt syncytiotrophoblastic differentiation probably represents a metaplastic phenomenon.[462] A definitive diagnosis of primary choriocarcinoma of the bladder requires a high copy number of chromosome 12p or the presence of isochromosome 12p, as seen by FISH, thus supporting germ cell differentiation.[463] It seems likely that many, if not all, reported cases of "primary choriocarcinoma of the bladder" represent urothelial carcinoma with syncytiotrophoblasts.[427,456,460]

Urothelial Carcinoma With Acinar/Tubular Differentiation

Urothelial carcinoma with acinar/tubular type differentiation is uncommon (Fig. 6.59). Although a prominent acinar or tubular component may accompany a nested carcinoma, some urothelial carcinomas may have an almost exclusive component of acini or small- to medium-sized tubules that may be misdiagnosed as nephrogenic adenoma or cystitis glandularis.[418,464,465] The differential diagnosis with an extension of a prostatic carcinoma is also a consideration but easily handled by immunohistochemistry (PSA and prostatic-specific acid phosphatase are positive in prostate cancer; CK20, high-molecular-weight CK, and p63 are positive in the majority of urothelial carcinomas).[464]

Undifferentiated Carcinoma (Including Those With Rhabdoid Features)

The newly proposed category of "poorly differentiated tumors" in the 2016 WHO classification is confusing. We suggest that these tumors should be put in the category of "undifferentiated

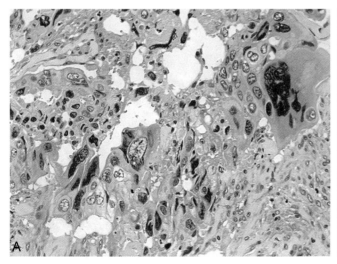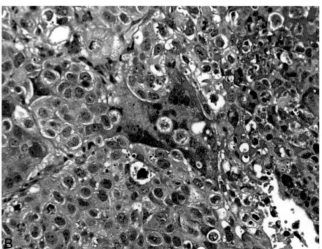

Fig. 6.58 Urothelial carcinoma with syncytiotrophoblastic giant cells (A and B).

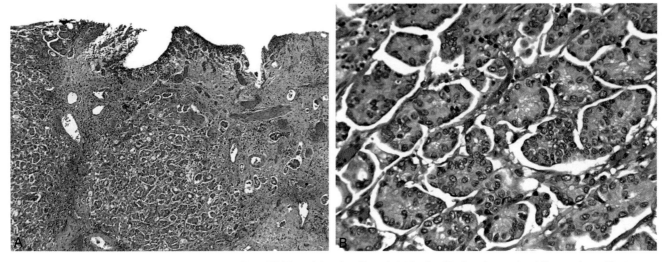

Fig. 6.59 Urothelial carcinoma with acinar differentiation (A and B). The acini are lined by cuboidal cells with abundant eosinophilic cytoplasm. The tumor may mimic prostatic adenocarcinoma.

carcinoma," which can be further subclassified as follows: (1) undifferentiated carcinoma, not otherwise specified; (2) undifferentiated carcinoma with rhabdoid features; (3) giant cell undifferentiated carcinoma; and (4) osteoclast-rich undifferentiated carcinoma (Table 6.14).

Undifferentiated carcinoma of the urinary bladder is an aggressive variant of urothelial carcinoma that manifests at an advanced stage with poor prognosis (see also previous discussion of "poorly differentiated tumors"). Such cancers are composed of cells whose cytologic and architectural findings display no recognizable form of differentiation. These tumors do not conform to urothelial, squamous, adenocarcinoma, or any other recognized category of bladder carcinoma. They are rare and, if present in a metastatic site, the histology would not suggest urothelial primary.

A series of eight such cases was reported by Lopez-Beltran et al.[443] The tumors were composed of sheets of large polygonal or round cells with moderate to abundant cytoplasm and distinct cell borders (Fig. 6.60). The large cell undifferentiated component varied from 90% to 100% of the tumor specimen, with five patients showing pure tumors. The architectural pattern of the tumor varied from infiltrating tumor to solid expansile nests with focal (<5%) discohesive growth pattern in two patients. All patients had advanced-stage cancer (≥pT3), and seven (88%) had lymph node metastases. Six patients died of disease at 5 to 26 months, and two patients were alive with metastases at 6 and 14 months.

Positive immunohistochemical staining for AE1/AE3, CK7, CAM5.2, CK20, thrombomodulin, and uroplakin 3 has been demonstrated in large cell undifferentiated cases. Other immunohistochemical markers performed in the differential diagnosis context included α-fetoprotein, β-hCG, PSA, vimentin, synaptophysin, and chromogranin, and all were negative. Ki67 and p53 labeling indices ranged from 50% to 90% and 40% to 90%, respectively.

A variety of tumors with rhabdoid differentiation has been described in the literature in different organ sites. Few cases have been described in the urinary tract.[466-469] This morphologic pattern is better considered within the spectrum of undifferentiated carcinoma of the bladder.[470] These tumors are highly aggressive: 50% of patients die of bladder cancer shortly after the diagnosis.[471] In most cases the rhabdoid component was admixed with other components, including conventional urothelial carcinoma, sarcomatoid carcinoma, and/or small cell carcinoma. Rhabdoid cells have abundant eosinophilic cytoplasm, vesicular nuclei, and prominent nucleoli (Fig. 6.61); they show positive immunostaining for CK markers (EMA, CAM5.2, and AE1/AE3). These tumors are characterized by (SMARCB1) INI1 negativity because of loss of the SWI/SNF chromatin remodeling complex.[470]

Urothelial Carcinoma With Unusual Stromal Reactions

Infiltrating urothelial carcinoma may be associated with a variety of stromal reactions. A pseudosarcomatous stroma (Fig. 6.62A) may be present that rarely displays sufficient cellularity, cytologic atypia, spindle cell proliferation, or myxoid appearance to raise serious concern about sarcomatoid carcinoma.[445-447] The stromal cells in these circumstances are invariably CK⁻ or only focally positive. Tumor-associated osseous (Fig. 6.62B) or chondroid metaplasia is present in some cases of urothelial carcinoma and its metastases. This stromal reaction may be difficult to differentiate from osteosarcoma or chondrosarcoma.[472-474] The metaplastic bone or

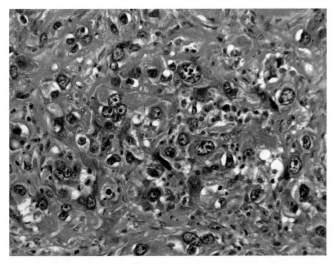

Fig. 6.60 Undifferentiated carcinoma.

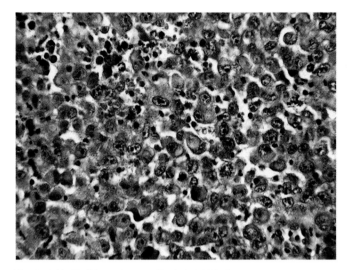

Fig. 6.61 Urothelial carcinoma with rhabdoid features.

cartilage is histologically benign. Zukerberg et al. described the presence of osteoclast-like giant cells in two cases of invasive high-grade urothelial carcinoma.[447] The giant cells had abundant eosinophilic cytoplasm and numerous small, round, regular nuclei

(Fig. 6.62C). These giant cells displayed immunoreactivity for vimentin and CD68 but not for epithelial markers.[445] The presence of osteoclast-like giant cells does not appear to influence prognosis.[376] An inflammatory cell response in the stroma adjacent to invasive tumors is relatively common.[475] This response usually takes the form of a lymphocytic infiltrate with a variable admixture of plasma cells (Fig. 6.62D).[476] Generally this cellular reaction is mild to moderate, but occasionally it may be intense. Sometimes a neutrophilic response is observed, with or without extensive eosinophilic infiltration. Evidence suggests that carcinomas occurring in the absence of a cellular immune response are likely to behave more aggressively.[476] One study reported intense inflammation in bladder carcinoma was indicative of a good prognosis.[477] Exclusion of lymphoepithelioma-like carcinoma of the urinary bladder is important when extensive inflammation in the stroma is present.[376,427]

Urothelial Carcinoma in Augmentation Cystoplasties and Neurogenic Bladder

Primary or recurrent urinary bladder cancers, including carcinoma in situ, may rarely occur in these settings. Early lesions might be difficult to diagnose due to the lack of anatomic landmarks and the frequently associated inflammatory and reactive changes.

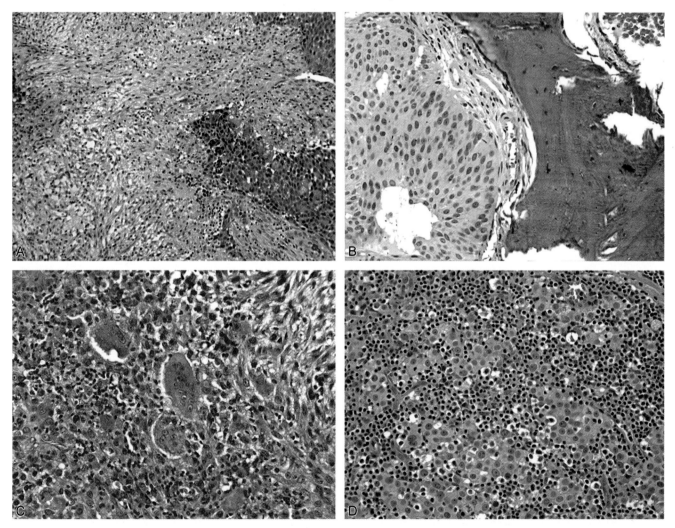

Fig. 6.62 Urothelial carcinoma with prominent stromal reaction. (A) Pseudosarcomatous stroma. (B) Osteoid formation. (C) Osteoclast-type giant cells. (D) Lymphoid-rich stroma.

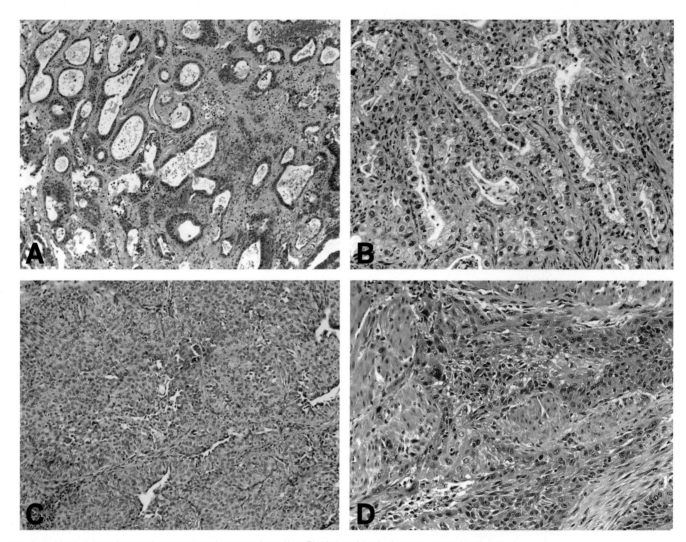

Fig. 6.63 Urothelial carcinoma after augmentation cystoplasty (A to D). Various histologic patterns can be observed.

Aggressive biologic behavior in tumors arising in augmentation cystoplasties has been observed (Fig. 6.63).[478]

In neuropathic bladder, most pathologic findings are related to the high frequency of bladder infections; therefore cystitis may be seen in these patients. Additional changes may be seen related to long-term catheter drainage. Keratinizing squamous metaplasia is an important premalignant lesion predisposing to development of squamous cell carcinoma, a tumor than can be seen in these patients.

Urothelial Carcinoma in Children and Young Adults

Urothelial neoplasms in children and young adult patients are rare and historically are noted to have a lower rate of recurrence and progression than those of older patients. Because of their rarity, data regarding clinical, pathologic, and molecular abnormalities in these tumors are limited.[160]

Reported cases include low-grade papillary urothelial carcinoma, high-grade papillary urothelial carcinoma, urothelial papilloma, and PUNLMP (Fig. 6.64).

Mutations of the *FGFR3* and *TP53* genes are rare or absent in urothelial neoplasms of young patients. In contrast, chromosomal abnormalities detected by UroVysion FISH are usually present in patients older than 19 to 20 years, a finding in support of the

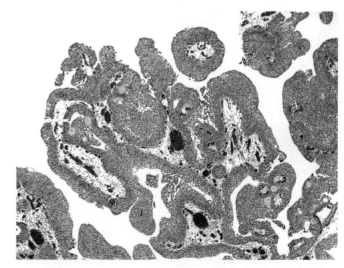

Fig. 6.64 Urothelial carcinoma in children (noninvasive low-grade papillary urothelial carcinoma).

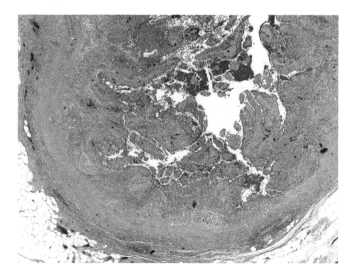

Fig. 6.65 Urothelial carcinoma in bladder diverticulum.

recently proposed hypothesis that an age of 19 to 20 years separates distinct molecular pathways of urothelial carcinogenesis.[479]

Urothelial Carcinoma in Bladder Diverticulum

These tumors occur in 0.8% to 14.3% of all bladder diverticula and constitute about 1% of bladder neoplasms. Most neoplasms seen in diverticula are solitary. Although most tumors found in diverticula are urothelial carcinomas of variable grade and invasiveness, rare cases of adenocarcinoma, carcinosarcoma, small cell carcinoma, squamous cell carcinoma, or undifferentiated carcinoma have been reported (Fig. 6.65).[480] No pT2 stage can be assigned in diverticula because of lack of detrusor muscle layer.[481]

Specimen Handling and Reporting

Appropriate assessment and reporting of pathologic findings in cases of urothelial malignancy assist the urologist with management of the patient (Tables 6.20 and 6.21).[1,181,283,287,482-488] The most common bladder specimens are endoscopic biopsies and transurethral resections, both of which contain subepithelial tissue of varying depth.[221,482] Other specimens include cystectomy (partial or total), cystoprostatectomy, pelvic exenteration (en bloc resection), and diverticula resections. Surgical excision of urachal adenocarcinoma usually includes the bladder dome, urachus, and umbilicus.

A bladder biopsy can provide information that helps assess risk factors for recurrence, progression, and response to treatment. Small, noninvasive papillary neoplasms are often excised by biopsy using cold-cup forceps, diathermy forceps, or a small diathermy loop.[482] To avoid tissue distortion, these specimens should be transferred to fixative with minimal handling. Larger neoplasms are often sampled by transurethral resection using a diathermy loop that produces strips of tissue 6 mm in diameter and of variable length. Additional resection of the bladder base after a previous transurethral resection may provide additional information for assessment of tumor staging. Hyperemic or velvety areas of urothelium are typically sampled to exclude carcinoma in situ; random biopsies are commonly taken from macroscopically normal urothelium distant from the tumor site to determine the extent of involvement.[489,490] Some urologists also submit biopsy specimens of the urethra, particularly in patients with high-grade papillary urothelial carcinoma or carcinoma in situ.

The pathology report should include clinically relevant historical information, as well as clinically useful macroscopic and microscopic information.[221,485] Reporting of bladder cancer should include information related to: (1) specimen type, (2) tumor site and size, (3) histologic type, (4) associated epithelial lesions, (5) histologic grade, (6) tumor configuration, (7) adequacy of material for determining T category, (8) pathologic staging, and (9) additional pathologic findings.

Muscularis mucosae is often present in the lamina propria and consists of thin and wavy fascicles of smooth muscle, which are frequently associated with large-caliber blood vessels.[288,299,491] Muscularis mucosae invasion (pT1) should not be mistaken for muscularis propria invasion (pT2), and it is unacceptable to simply state in the pathology report that smooth muscle invasion is present.[299] The presence or absence of muscularis propria (detrusor muscle) should also be mentioned in the pathology report as an indication of the adequacy of resection.[157,492,493]

An additional feature of importance in bladder tumor evaluation is the presence of blood vessel or lymphatic channel invasion (Fig. 6.66).[181,361,485,494-507] Identifying vascular or lymphatic invasion is sometimes difficult, because lymphovascular spaces may easily be confused with artifactual clefting around nests of invasive carcinoma. In suspicious cases, blood vessels can be highlighted by immunohistochemical staining for CD31 or CD34. The presence of vascular or lymphatic invasion, and whether immunohistochemical stains assisted in identifying this finding, should be included in the report.

The presence of associated urothelial carcinoma in situ should also be reported in cases of bladder carcinoma, because patients with associated carcinoma in situ are at much greater risk for tumor recurrence and disease progression.

Tumor involving the resection margin in partial or complete cystectomy specimens is assumed to correspond to residual tumor in the patient. Positive margins should be classified as macroscopic or microscopic according to the findings at the specimen inked surfaces.[508] The resection margin status should be carefully specified. Statements about deep soft tissue margins should specify whether peritoneal surfaces are involved by tumor. In cases of urachal adenocarcinoma in which partial cystectomy with excision of the urachal tract and umbilicus is performed, the margins of the urachal tract (i.e., the soft tissue surrounding the urachus and the skin around the umbilical margin) should be specified.

Glandular Neoplasms

Villous Adenoma

Villous adenoma is an uncommon benign glandular epithelial neoplasm with exophytic growth that is often associated with urachal adenocarcinoma (Fig. 6.67).[509,510] Patients often present with hematuria or irritative symptoms. Mucinuria may be present in rare cases. There is no apparent gender predominance. The tumor usually occurs in elderly patients (mean age, 65 years; range, 23 to 94 years) with a predilection for the urachus, dome, and trigone of the urinary bladder. Its cystoscopic appearance is that of an exophytic tumor. Histologically, villous adenoma of the bladder is identical to villous adenoma of the colon, with columnar mucin-filled goblet cells lining delicate fibrovascular stalks (Fig. 6.68). Nuclear findings include pseudostratification, crowding, occasional prominent nucleoli, and hyperchromasia, as in the colon. Villous adenomas of the bladder show positive immunostaining for CK20 (100% of cases), CK7 (56%), and carcinoembryonic

TABLE 6.20 **Reporting of Cystectomy Specimens**

Gross findings

Fresh or fixed specimen

Nature of the specimen: partial cystectomy, radical cystectomy, cystoprosta-tectomy, pelvic exenteration

Three-dimensional measurements of recognizable anatomic structures and of tumors or other recognizable lesions

Site of involvement (such as trigone, right or left lateral wall, anterior or posterior wall, dome)

Tumor focality

Growth pattern (papillary, flat, ulcerated, solid/nodular, infiltrative, indeterminate)

Gross assessment of invasion (into lamina propria or muscularis propria)

Gross extravesical soft tissue extension

Gross invasion into adjacent organs, such as prostate, ureter, urethra, uterus, vagina, pelvic and abdominal wall

Gross assessment of margin status, including perivesical soft tissue and peritoneal surface

Lymph nodes

Location and the number of lymph nodes sampled

Report the presence or absence of extranodal extension

Report if the lymph nodes are bisected or completely embedded

Report if the lymph nodes are grossly involved by cancer

Microscopic findings

Anatomic location of the tumor

Histologic diagnosis

Tumor size and multifocality

Histologic grade (we recommend using both 1973 and 2016 WHO grading systems)

Pattern of invasion (nodular, trabecular, or infiltrative)

Extent of invasion (pathologic staging)

No invasion (pTa or pTis)

Invasion into the lamina propria (pT1)

Invasion into inner (pT2a) or outer half of muscularis propria (pT2b)

Invasion into perivesical soft tissue (pT3)

Surgical margins

Ureteral margin

Urethral margins

Perivesical soft tissue margin

Pelvic soft tissue margin (for pelvic exenteration specimens)

Presence or absence of lymphovascular invasion

Other intraepithelial abnormalities

Presence or absence of dysplasia and carcinoma in situ in adjacent mucosa, including pagetoid spread of carcinoma in situ

Location and multifocality

Other findings such as intestinal metaplasia, squamous metaplasia, thera-peutic treatment effects, etc.

Extent of tumor invasion into adjacent organs

Prostate

Involvement of the prostatic urethra with or without stromal invasion

Involvement of prostatic ducts/acini without stromal invasion

Prostatic stromal invasion

Direct extension into the prostate from carcinoma through the bladder neck

Direct extravesical extension into the prostatic parenchyma

Seminal vesicle invasion through intraprostatic epithelium or by direct perivesical extension

Ureter and urethra

Report any dysplastic/neoplastic change of the mucosa, including pagetoid spread of carcinoma in situ

Report invasion into adjacent lamina propria or muscularis propria

Seminal vesicles

Report spread of carcinoma in these organs either through epithelium or by direct extension of an infiltrative carcinoma

Vagina/uterus

Report direct extension or metastases to either organ

Rectum, pelvic and abdominal wall

Report direct extension or metastases

Lymph node status

Report the number of lymph nodes sampled

Report the presence or absence of metastases

If metastases are present, state the following in the report:

The number of positive nodes

The diameter of the largest metastasis

The presence or absence of extranodal extension

Final pathologic staging (using the 2017 American Joint Committee on Cancer TNM staging)

Response to preoperative treatments (complete response, incomplete response, or no response)

Results of ancillary studies (if performed)

Correlation with frozen section diagnosis (if performed)

---

antigen (89%). Acid mucin is demonstrable in 78% of cases with Alcian blue PAS stain.[509] Patients with an isolated villous adenoma have an excellent prognosis, but progression to adenocarcinoma appears to occur in 21% to 33% of cases.

The differential diagnosis includes adenocarcinoma of blad-der.[509] Villous adenomas of the bladder may coexist with in situ and invasive adenocarcinoma. On limited sampling there may be only changes of villous adenoma. Therefore the entire specimen should be processed to exclude invasive disease.

Clear Cell Carcinoma (Tumors of Müllerian Type)

Clear cell carcinoma is a rare variant of urinary bladder carci-noma that morphologically resembles its counterpart in the female genital tract. In the 2016 WHO classification, clear cell carcinoma is included in a category of tumors of müllerian type, which also includes endometrioid carcinoma of müllerian origin.[6]

A rare case of müllerian adenosarcoma of the urinary bladder has been recently described, adding a new entity to the spectrum of tumors of müllerian type.[511]

Patients with clear cell carcinoma of the bladder are typically females who present with hematuria or dysuria. Occasionally, clear cell adenocarcinoma has been associated with endometriosis or müllerianosis; occurrence in a bladder diverticulum has been reported. Tumors are typically exophytic, nodular, or sessile in appearance (Fig. 6.69). Clear cell carcinomas may infiltrate the bladder wall and metastasize to lymph nodes and distant organs in a pattern similar to other types of bladder cancer.

Clear cell carcinoma exhibits a distinctive histologic appearance, with a variety of architectural patterns, forming tubulocystic or papillary structures, or growing in diffuse solid sheets. The tubules vary in size and may contain either basophilic or eosinophilic secre-tions. The papillae are generally small, and their fibrovascular cores may be extensively hyalinized. The tumor cells range from flat to cuboidal to columnar, and they may have either clear or eosino-philic cytoplasm. The cytoplasm often contains glycogen. Hobnail cells are frequently seen. Cytologic atypia is usually moderate to severe, and high mitotic counts are frequently observed. In some cases clear cell carcinoma is associated with urothelial carcinoma, and rarely with adenocarcinoma not otherwise specified.[512]

TABLE 6.21 Reporting of Bladder Biopsy and Transurethral Resection Specimens

Gross findings

Cold-cup biopsy

The estimated number of tissue fragments, aggregate dimensions
The presence or absence of papillary growth
All tissue fragments should be submitted

Transurethral resection of the bladder

The estimated number of tissue fragments, aggregate dimensions
Total weight of resected tissue fragments
The proportion of tissue embedded, if not completely embedded[a]

Microscopic findings

General assessment

Epithelial surface (intact, ulcerated, denuded)
Presence or absence of muscularis propria (detrusor muscle)
Comment on cautery artifact if it compromises evaluation

Tumor assessment

Anatomic location (if available)
Histologic diagnosis
    Specify invasive or noninvasive urothelial carcinoma
Histologic grade (we recommend to use both 1973 and 2016 World Health
    Organization grading systems)
Overall architecture (e.g., papillary, flat, ulcerated, solid, or nodular)
Pattern of invasion (nodular, trabecular, or infiltrative)
Presence or absence of lymphovascular invasion
Extent of invasion (specify whether stromal invasion is present and the level
    of invasion)
Invasion into lamina propria
    Extent and/or depth of invasion should be provided
    Reporting of muscularis mucosae invasion is optional because mus-
        cularis mucosae is not uniformly present in the biopsy specimens
Invasion into muscularis propria (detrusor muscle)
    T2 substaging (pT2a versus T2b) cannot be performed on biopsy
        specimens
Statements of tumor stage should be provided (e.g., at least T1, or T2)
    Comment that accurate staging may require complete resection of the
        tumor
    T2 substaging (pT2a versus T2b) cannot be performed on biopsy
        specimens
    Fat invasion in biopsy is not necessarily indicative of extravesical
        invasion (pT3) because fat can be present throughout the bladder
        wall
Findings in the adjacent mucosa
    Presence or absence of dysplasia, carcinoma in situ
    Other findings: intestinal metaplasia, cystitis glandularis, keratinizing
        squamous metaplasia, etc.

[a]We recommend that a minimum of 10 cassettes be submitted for initial evaluation. If lamina propria invasion is identified, the entire specimen may be submitted to rule out muscularis propria invasion and to further assess the extent of invasion.

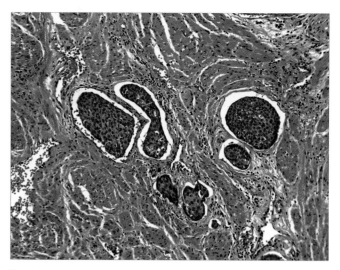

Fig. 6.66 Lymphovascular invasion by an invasive urothelial carcinoma.

strong p53 staining and MIB1 counts of greater than 32 per 200 cells in clear cell adenocarcinoma.[515] However, p53 nuclear accumulation (up to 20%), increased MIB1 labeling index (up to 5%), and aneuploid DNA patterns have been observed in atypical nephrogenic metaplasia.[514] All cases of atypical nephrogenic metaplasia display positive immunoreactivity for high-molecular-weight CK (34βE12), CK7, and EMA.[514] In contrast with atypical nephrogenic metaplasia, clear cell carcinomas will typically display greater cytologic atypia, a significant mitotic rate, and necrosis.[515] Clear cell adenocarcinoma of the urinary tract is positive for both CK7 and CK20.[516] Positive α-methylacyl-coenzyme A racemase (P504S; AMACR) and PAX8 immunoreactivity for both clear cell adenocarcinoma and nephrogenic adenoma has been noted.[516-522] CD10 is focally positive in clear cell adenocarcinoma.[516]

The other differential diagnostic considerations include clear cell variant of urothelial carcinoma, metastatic clear cell renal carcinoma, cervical or vaginal clear cell adenocarcinoma, and, in males, prostatic adenocarcinoma secondarily involving the bladder. In addition to the immunostaining characteristics noted previously, clear cell carcinoma may show positive staining for carcinoembryonic antigen and LeuM1, but is negative for estrogen and progesterone receptors, and these stains may be helpful in the differential diagnosis.

Adenocarcinoma

Adenocarcinoma is defined as a malignant neoplasm derived from the urothelium showing histologically pure glandular phenotype.[6] It accounts for 0.5% to 2% of all malignant bladder tumors. Adenocarcinoma of the urinary bladder occurs more commonly in males than in females, with a peak incidence in the sixth decade of life.[523] Patients typically present with hematuria. Two major categories have been recognized: those arising in the bladder proper and those arising from urachal remnants. Approximately one-third arise in the urachus.[524] Molecular evidence suggests that intestinal metaplasia is a putative precursor for adenocarcinoma.[525]

Adenocarcinoma of the bladder may show a variety of histologic growth patterns: (1) enteric (colonic) type; (2) mucinous (colloid) type; (3) signet ring cell type; (4) hepatoid type; (5) mixed forms; and (6) adenocarcinoma, not otherwise specified (Fig. 6.70; Table 6.24). However, the 2016 WHO classification divides adenocarcinoma into the following categories: enteric type; mucinous type; mixed type (tumors with mixture of the enteric and mucinous patterns); and adenocarcinoma, not otherwise specified (tumors do not resemble a specific type).[6]

Tumor cells are positive for CA125, suggestive of müllerian origin, but CA125 staining may also be seen in urothelial carcinoma and carcinoma from a variety of other sites, so this finding does not prove müllerian origin (Table 6.22).[437,513] These tumors are typically positive for CK7 with variable CK20 staining.[437] Stains for PSA and prostate-specific acid phosphatase are negative.[513] The main differential diagnostic consideration for clear cell carcinoma is nephrogenic metaplasia (nephrogenic adenoma) (Table 6.23).[514] Several immunohistochemical stains have been evaluated for utility in making this distinction, but only p53 and MIB1 appear useful, with at most focal p53 staining and MIB1 counts of less than 14 per 200 cells in nephrogenic adenoma, and

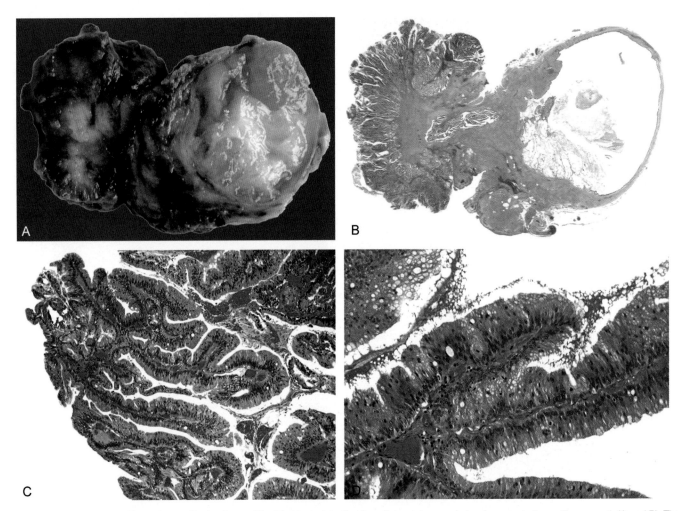

Fig. 6.67 Villous adenoma. Tumor located in the dome of the bladder, originating from the urachus, and showing exophytic papillary growth (A and B). The tumor has long papillary fronds lined by intestinal-type columnar epithelium with scattered goblet cells (C and D).

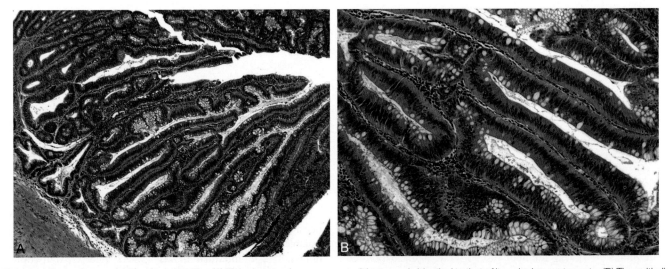

Fig. 6.68 Villous adenoma of the urinary bladder. (A) The microscopic appearance of the tumor is identical to that of its colonic counterparts. (B) The epithelial cells display nuclear stratification, nuclear crowding, nuclear hyperchromasia, and occasional prominent nucleoli.

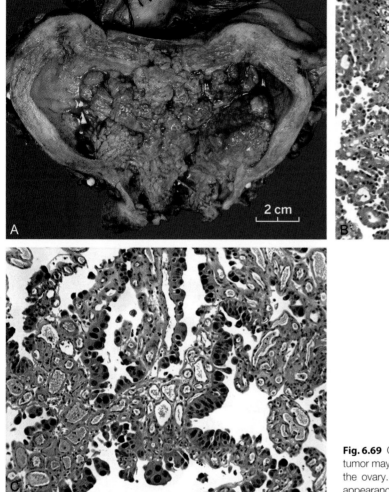
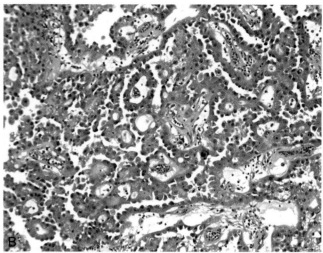

Fig. 6.69 Clear cell carcinoma. (A) Gross appearance at cystectomy. (B) The tumor may display various growth patterns similar to clear cell carcinoma of the ovary. (C) The tubules are lined by columnar cells with a "hobnail" appearance.

TABLE 6.22 Typical Staining Patterns of Primary and Secondary Adenocarcinomas of the Bladder

	34βE12	CK7	CK20	CEA	PSA	PSAP	CDX2	Villin	CA-125	Vimentin	PAX8
Primary bladder adenocarcinoma	+	+/-	+/-	+	-	+/-	+	+/-	+/-	-	-
Clear cell carcinoma		+	+/-		-	-			+		+
Prostatic adenocarcinoma	-	-	+/-	+/-	+	+	-	-	-	-	-
Seminal vesicle adenocarcinoma	+	-							+		+
Renal cell carcinoma	-	-	-	-		-	-	-	-	+	+
Colorectal adenocarcinoma	-	-	+	+	-	-	+	+	+/-	-	-
Endometrial adenocarcinoma	+	-	-	-		+/-			+	+	+

+, Usually positive; *+/-*, variable staining; *-*, usually negative; *34βE12*, high-molecular-weight CK34 E12; *CEA*, carcinoembryonic antigen; *CK*, cytokeratin; *PSA*, prostate-specific antigen; *PSAP*, prostate-specific acid phosphatase.

The enteric type closely resembles adenocarcinoma of the colon.[523] The not otherwise specified type consists of adenocarcinoma with a nonspecific glandular growth pattern. Tumors that show abundant mucin and tumor cell clusters apparently floating in mucin are classified as mucinous (colloid) type. The signet ring cell variant may be diffuse or mixed and may have a monocytoid or plasmacytoid phenotype. Pure signet ring cell carcinoma carries the worst prognosis among different histologic types of adenocarcinoma. It is not uncommon to find a mixture of these growth patterns. The grading system for adenocarcinoma of the bladder is based on degree of glandular differentiation and nuclear pleomorphism, categorized as well, moderately, and poorly differentiated.[1,512]

The reported immunohistochemical profile of bladder adenocarcinoma is variable but generally resembles that of colonic adenocarcinoma (Table 6.22).[105,147,373,380,526] CK7 positivity is variable, whereas CK20 is positive in most bladder adenocarcinomas.[523] The "intestinal marker" CDX2, a nuclear transcription factor, may be misleading in this situation because primary bladder adenocarcinomas are virtually always also CDX2+.[527] It is notable

TABLE 6.23 Differential Diagnosis of Atypical Nephrogenic Metaplasia and Clear Cell Carcinoma[a]

Characteristics	Nephrogenic Adenoma	Clear Cell Carcinoma
Sex	Male predominance (male-to-female ratio, 3:1)	Female predominance (male-to-female ratio, 1:2)
Mean age	62 years	58 years
Clinical presentation	Hematuria and voiding symptoms	Hematuria and voiding symptoms
Biologic behavior	Benign	Aggressive
Location	No apparent predilection	Predilection for urethra
Size	Small	Large
Microscopic Findings		
Necrosis	Absent	Often present (53%)
Mitotic figures	Absent or inconspicuous	Easily identifiable
Stromal edema	Common	Uncommon
Luminal mucin	Common	Common
Clear cell change	May be seen	Common
Hobnail cells	Common	Common
Infiltrative growth	Usually absent	Present
Psammoma bodies	Absent	May be seen
Inflammation	Invariably present	May be present
Cytologic atypia		
Nuclear enlargement	Present	Present
Nuclear hyperchromasia	Present	Present
Prominent nucleoli	Present	Present
Nuclear pleomorphism	Minimal	Present
Immunostaining		
Prostate-specific antigen	Negative	Negative
34βE12	Positive	Positive (occasionally negative)
CK7	Positive	Positive
CK20	Negative	Positive
Epithelial membrane antigen	Positive	Positive
AMACR (P504S)	Often positive	Often positive
PAX2	Positive	Positive
PAX8	Positive	Positive
MIB (Ki67) labeling index	<5%	Often >15%
p53	Occasional focal positive	Positive
DNA ploidy	Aneuploid pattern may be seen	Unknown

34βE12, High-molecular-weight CK; *AMACR*, α-methylacyl-coenzyme A racemase (P504S); *CK*, cytokeratin.
[a]Nuclear pleomorphism is more pronounced in clear cell adenocarcinoma.

TABLE 6.24 Histologic Variants of Adenocarcinoma of the Urinary Bladder[a]

Enteric (colonic type) adenocarcinoma
Mucinous or colloid adenocarcinoma
Signet ring cell adenocarcinoma
Hepatoid adenocarcinoma
Mixed adenocarcinoma
Adenocarcinoma, not otherwise specified

[a]Clear cell carcinoma is included in a category of tumors of müllerian type in the 2016 World Health Organization classification.

that CDX2 positivity has been observed in 2% of urothelial carcinomas in a tissue microarray study; consequently, CDX2 immunostaining cannot be used to exclude a urothelial primary in cases of metastatic carcinoma of uncertain origin.[528] Areas of intestinal metaplasia in the bladder also routinely stain positive for CDX2.[105,529] Villin, an actin-binding protein found in epithelial cells with a brush border, is positive in colon adenocarcinoma and bladder adenocarcinomas of enteric type but not in urothelial carcinomas with glandular differentiation.[530] Nuclear β-catenin staining is seen in 81% of colorectal carcinomas involving the bladder, whereas staining restricted to the cytoplasm is typical of primary bladder adenocarcinoma.[380,512,531] A small subset of primary bladder adenocarcinomas may harbor KRAS mutation; therefore KRAS mutation is not helpful in the differential diagnosis between bladder and colonic adenocarcinoma.[532]

Hepatoid Adenocarcinoma

Primary hepatoid adenocarcinoma of the bladder is rare, with only three well-illustrated case reports.[533] The pathologic diagnosis is based on a combination of histologic features resembling hepatocellular carcinoma and positive immunostaining for α-fetoprotein. The tumor occurs in elderly men and is biologically aggressive. Lymph node metastases are common.[533] The histogenesis is uncertain. Tumors are composed of polygonal cells with abundant granular eosinophilic cytoplasm, vesicular nuclei, and prominent nucleoli, arranged in nests and trabecular structures; the overall appearance is reminiscent of hepatocellular carcinoma (Fig. 6.71). Occasionally, hyaline globules and bile production are seen. Immunoreactivity for α-fetoprotein, CAM5.2, α1-antitrypsin, albumin, hepatocyte paraffin-1, EMA, and a striking

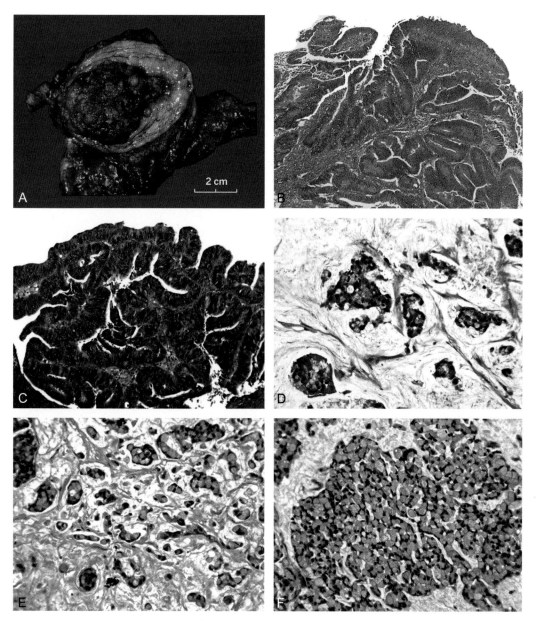

Fig. 6.70 Adenocarcinoma. (A) Gross appearance. (B) Adenocarcinoma, not otherwise specified. (C) Enteric type, resembling typical colonic adenocarcinoma. (D) Colloid (mucinous) type. Malignant cells float in a pool of mucin. (E and F) Signet ring cell type. Mucin pool formation is common (F).

canalicular pattern with polyclonal anticarcinoembryonic antigen staining all indicate hepatocellular differentiation.[533] The hepatic nature of the cells was further confirmed by the demonstration of albumin gene messenger RNA (mRNA) by nonisotopic in situ hybridization.[533]

Urachal Adenocarcinoma

Urachal adenocarcinoma is far less common than nonurachal adenocarcinoma of the bladder.[534-540] Urachal adenocarcinomas arise from the urachus, the fibrous remnant from the embryonic allantoic stalk connecting the umbilicus to the bladder (Fig. 6.72). Urachal remnants are reported to occur most frequently in the bladder dome or posterior wall. Most cases of urachal adenocarcinoma occur in the fifth and sixth decades of life, which is about 10 years younger than those patients with nonurachal bladder adenocarcinoma. This tumor occurs slightly more often in men than in

women.[535,536] Presenting signs and symptoms may include a suprapubic mass, mucinuria, or irritative symptoms.[541]

Urachal carcinoma usually involves the muscular wall of the bladder dome, and it may or may not destroy the overlying mucosa (Fig. 6.73). The mass may be relatively small and discrete, but in some cases it forms a large mass invading the retropubic space of Retzius and may extend as far as the anterior abdominal wall. Mucinous lesions tend to calcify, and these calcifications on plain x-ray films of the abdomen may be the initial clinical manifestation.[535] The mucosa of the urinary bladder remains intact in early stages of the disease, but it eventually becomes ulcerated as the tumor extends toward the bladder cavity. The cut surface of this tumor exhibits a glistening, light tan appearance, reflecting its mucinous contents. A specific staging system for this neoplasm has been proposed. Histologically, urachal adenocarcinomas are subdivided into mucinous, enteric, not otherwise specified, signet

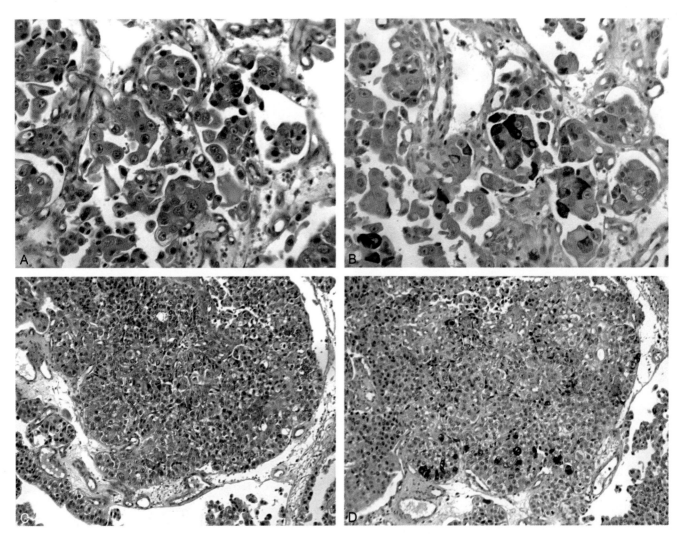

Fig. 6.71 Hepatoid adenocarcinoma (A to D). Trabecular (A) and solid growth (C) patterns. Immunostains for α-fetoprotein are positive (B and D).

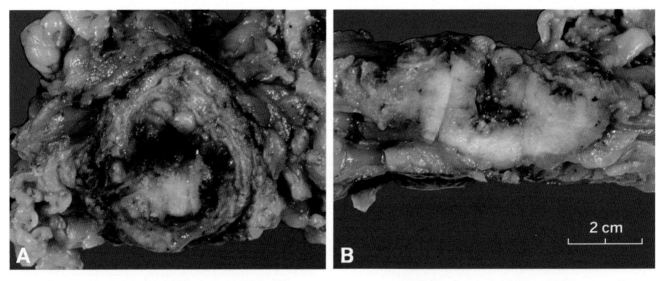

Fig. 6.72 Gross appearance of urachal adenocarcinoma (A and B).

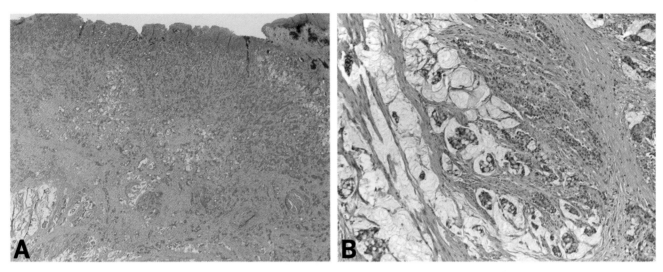

Fig. 6.73 Urachal adenocarcinoma (A and B). The tumor invades into the muscularis propria wall and bladder mucosa.

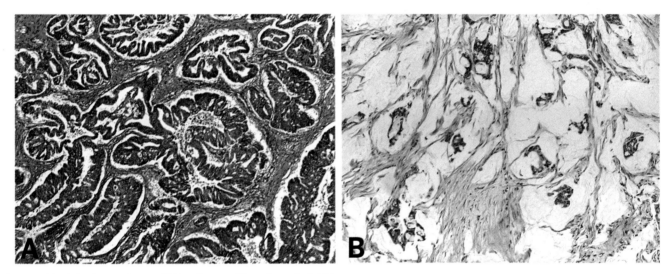

Fig. 6.74 Urachal adenocarcinoma. (A) Enteric type; (B) mucinous (colloid) type.

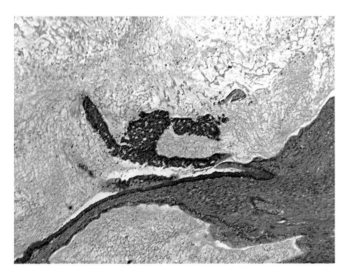

Fig. 6.75 Mucinous cystadenocarcinoma of the urachus.

ring cell, and mixed types; these subtypes are like those of adenocarcinoma of the urinary bladder (Fig. 6.74).

Mucinous cystadenocarcinoma has a prominent cystic component and is within the spectrum of mucinous cystadenoma and mucinous cystic tumor of low malignant potential, homologous to ovarian mucinous tumors (Fig. 6.75). Cyst walls lined by a single layer of mucinous columnar cells with no cytologic atypia define the morphologic signature of mucinous cystadenoma. Epithelial abnormalities range from low-grade cytologic atypia to intraepithelial carcinoma in mucinous cystic tumor of low malignant potential. Intraepithelial carcinomatous change is characterized by severe atypia, abundant mitotic activity, and complex architecture. Mucinous cystadenocarcinoma may present with microinvasion (<2 mm comprising <5% of the tumor) or as frankly invasive neoplasm.[541]

Specific criteria to classify a tumor as urachal in origin were initially established by Wheeler and Hill in 1954 and consisted of the following: (1) tumor in the dome of the bladder; (2) absence of cystitis cystica and cystitis glandularis; (3) invasion of muscle or deeper structures and either intact or ulcerated epithelium; (4) presence of urachal remnants; (5) presence of a suprapubic mass; (6) a sharp demarcation between the tumor and the normal surface epithelium; and (7) tumor growth in the bladder wall, extending into the space of Retzius.[542] These rather restrictive criteria were modified by Johnson et al., who proposed the following criteria: (1) tumor in the bladder dome; (2) a sharp demarcation between the tumor and the surface epithelium; and (3) exclusion of primary adenocarcinoma located elsewhere that has spread secondarily to the bladder.[825] According to Johnson's criteria, urachal adenocarcinoma may be associated with areas of cystitis cystica and cystitis glandularis in the adjacent or distant bladder mucosa if they show no dysplastic intestinal metaplasia (adenomatous change). Although urachal adenocarcinoma may arise from villous adenoma of the urachus, intestinal metaplasia of the urachal epithelium is believed to be the factor predisposing to malignant transformation at this site.[512]

Whenever urachal adenocarcinoma or primary adenocarcinoma of the bladder is considered, direct extension or metastasis from colorectal carcinoma must be excluded. Management of urachal adenocarcinoma consists of partial or radical cystectomy, including resection of the umbilicus. Recurrences are common, however, especially when a partial cystectomy is done. It is important to distinguish between urachal and nonurachal adenocarcinomas for treatment purposes. Resection of urachal adenocarcinoma must include removal of the entire urachal remnant.

Nonurachal bladder adenocarcinomas show positive immunostaining with carcinoembryonic antigen in 67% of cases and Leu-M1 (CD15) in 73% of cases, whereas urachal adenocarcinomas consistently stain with both.[105,543]

A recent study including 34 urachal adenocarcinoma and 6 secondary adenocarcinomas concluded that using β-catenin (frequently membranocytoplasmic β-catenin staining) and CK7 (positive in 50% of urachal adenocarcinomas) may have value in differentiating urachal adenocarcinoma of enteric morphology from colonic adenocarcinoma.[537]

Squamous Cell Neoplasms

Squamous Papilloma

Refer to earlier discussion in the Benign Urothelial Neoplasms section.

Squamous Cell Carcinoma In Situ

Only a few reports on squamous cell carcinoma in situ of the bladder are available. Histologically, it is identical to squamous cell carcinoma in situ found in other organ sites (Fig. 6.76). This finding is often associated with subsequent or concurrent invasive urothelial carcinoma with squamous differentiation. In a report of 11 patients, 1 patient had no evidence of disease at 8 months, 1 had residual squamous cell carcinoma in situ at 10 months, 1 had high-grade urothelial carcinoma (not otherwise specified) at rebiopsy after 6 months, 3 patients were noted to have invasive squamous cell carcinoma at intervals of 2, 3, and 4 months,

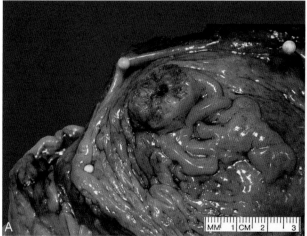

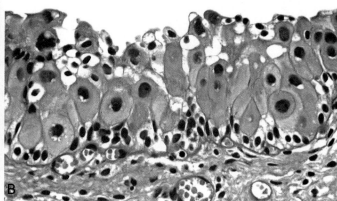

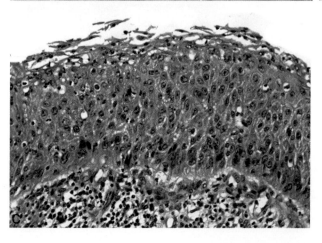

Fig. 6.76 Invasive squamous cell carcinoma. (A) Gross appearance of nodular elevated invasive squamous cell carcinoma, surrounded by extensive areas of dysplastic squamous epithelium. Cytologic atypia in squamous cell dysplasia (B) is less severe than in squamous cell carcinoma in situ (C).

respectively, and 1 was found to have invasive urothelial carcinoma with squamous features in the cystectomy specimen at 12 months.[52] Wide-range HPV DNA signal was detected in one case. Enhanced expression of EGFR in these bladder squamous lesions suggests a possible therapeutic target in cases that are difficult to manage clinically.[52]

A closely related squamous lesion designated "verrucous squamous hyperplasia" has been described as a possible precursor of verrucous or other types of squamous carcinoma; therefore it should be followed and treated accordingly.[544]

Squamous Cell Carcinoma

Squamous cell carcinoma is defined as a malignant neoplasm derived from the urothelium that shows a pure squamous cell phenotype (Fig. 6.77).[544-548] When urothelial elements (either urothelial carcinoma in situ or any conventional urothelial carcinoma component) are present, the tumor should be classified as urothelial carcinoma with squamous differentiation. Risk factors associated with the development of squamous cell carcinoma include tobacco smoking, chronic nonspecific urinary tract infections, and schistosomiasis.[549-555] Keratinizing squamous metaplasia may be present in the adjacent epithelium in cases of squamous cell carcinoma of the bladder, and frequently displays the full spectrum of dysplastic lesions or carcinoma in situ.[545] Invasive squamous cell carcinoma of the bladder displays a range of differentiation, from well differentiated to poorly differentiated, with a histologic spectrum that can vary from well-defined islands of squamous cells with keratinization, prominent intercellular bridges, and minimal nuclear pleomorphism to tumors exhibiting marked nuclear pleomorphism and only focal evidence of squamous differentiation. Histologic grading

is based on the amount of keratinization and the degree of nuclear pleomorphism using a three-tiered system (grades 1, 2, and 3).[546,556] Several morphologic variants of squamous cell carcinoma, including verrucous, basaloid, and clear cell pattern, have been recognized. A rare case of NUT (nuclear protein in testis gene) undifferentiated carcinoma with an extensive squamous cell component has been reported.[557] Immunohistochemically, most squamous cell carcinomas of the bladder are positive for MAC387, CK7, p63, p40, CK14, and desmoglein 3, and usually negative for GATA3 and uroplakins 2 and 3.

Schistosoma-Associated Squamous Cell Carcinoma

Schistosomiasis is known to be associated with squamous cell carcinoma of the bladder (Fig. 6.78A and B). Tumors arising in this setting are typically large, often filling the bladder lumen, and frequently polypoid or solid with visible necrosis and keratin debris; others are ulcerated infiltrating tumors. Histologically, the presence of keratinizing squamous metaplasia in the adjacent flat epithelium is relatively constant and may be associated with dysplasia or carcinoma in situ. The prevalence of associated squamous metaplasia in cases of squamous cell carcinoma of the bladder ranges from 17% to 60% and is widely variable according to geographic location of the patient population. Similar to non–Schistosoma-associated squamous cell carcinoma, these tumors range from well to poorly differentiated, but most commonly are well differentiated with prominent keratinization and intercellular bridge formation with minimal nuclear pleomorphism. Pathologic stage and lymph node status are significant prognostic and predictive factors, and pathologic grade according to the degree of keratinization and the degree of nuclear pleomorphism is also considered an important prognostic indicator. Radical surgical excision currently is

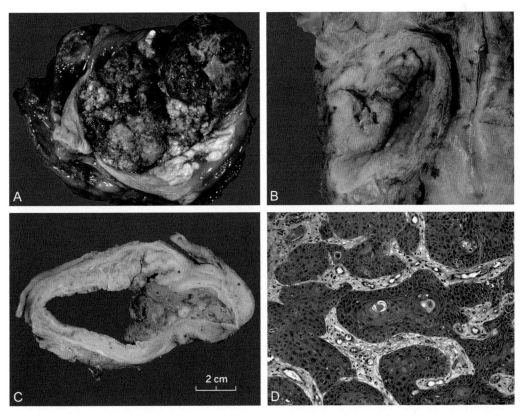

Fig. 6.77 Squamous cell carcinoma of the urinary bladder. Tumors are often bulky and exophytic (A to C). (D) Keratin pearl formation is typical of squamous cell carcinoma.

the most widely used treatment option; neoadjuvant radiation has been reported to improve survival in aggressive tumors.

Verrucous Squamous Cell Carcinoma

Verrucous carcinoma is an uncommon variant of squamous cell carcinoma that accounts for 3% to 5% of squamous bladder cancers. It occurs most often in patients with schistosomiasis but has also been reported in patients from nonendemic areas.[51] This tumor grossly appears as a "warty" mass. Histologically, it shows epithelial acanthosis and papillomatosis, minimal nuclear and architectural atypia, and rounded, pushing deep borders (Fig. 6.78C and D; Table 6.25). Cases of squamous carcinoma with verrucous features but which additionally have an infiltrative component have been described. It is recommended by the 2004/2016 WHO classification to diagnose such cases not as verrucous carcinoma but as regular squamous cell carcinoma.

Verrucous carcinoma in the bladder is associated with minimal risk for progression regardless of whether associated with schistosomiasis. A link to HPV infection has not been established.[51] p16 expression in squamous cell carcinoma is unrelated to HPV infection in these tumors.[558]

Basaloid Squamous Cell Carcinoma

A single case of basaloid squamous cell carcinoma of the urinary bladder has been reported.[559] The patient had a long-standing history of recurrent urinary tract infections. Grossly, it was a sessile multilobulated tan-brown mass involving the posterior wall of the bladder. Architecturally the tumor was characterized by small nests of basaloid cells with minimal cytoplasm arranged with peripheral palisading (Fig. 6.78E and F). Cytologically, the tumor cells had a high nuclear-to-cytoplasmic ratio with dense hyperchromatic nuclei. Central necrosis of the larger nests and

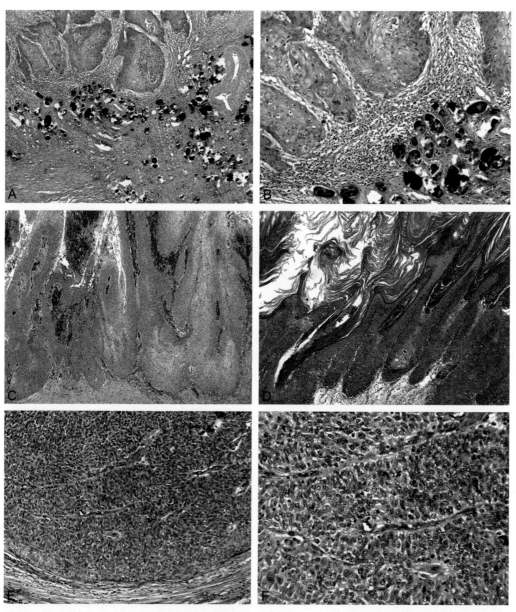

Fig. 6.78 Variants of squamous cell carcinoma. *Schistosoma*-associated squamous cell carcinoma (A and B). Numerous schistosomal eggs are seen. Verrucous squamous cell carcinoma (C and D). The tumor forms broad endophytic fronds of squamous epithelium with pushing growth pattern at its base. Basaloid squamous cell carcinoma (E and F). The tumor is characterized by nests and trabeculae of basaloid cells with minimal cytoplasm.

TABLE 6.25	Differential Diagnosis of Squamous Papilloma, Condyloma Acuminatum, and Verrucous Squamous Cell Carcinoma of the Urinary Bladder		
	Squamous Papilloma	Condyloma Acuminatum	Verrucous Squamous Cell Carcinoma
Age (years)	62 (range, 32-82)	40 (range, 17-76)	66 (range, 43-83)
Sex (male:female)	1:6	1:1.6	1.2:1
Clinical history	Nonspecific	External genitalia condyloma or history of immunosuppression	Nonspecific
Clinical presentation	Irritative symptoms	Irritative symptoms	Irritative symptoms
Biologic behavior	Rarely recurs	Aggressive	Aggressive
Location	No predilection	No predilection	No predilection
Extent	Small, solitary	Multiple, extensive	Diffuse, extensive
Histologic changes			
Architecture	Papillary	Papillary	Expansive and endophytic
Pushing margin	Absent	Absent	Present
Cytologic atypia	Usually not seen or mild	Usually not seen or mild	May be present
Stromal invasion	Absent	Absent	Present
p53 alteration	+/-	+	+
Human papilloma virus detection	-	+	-
DNA ploidy	Diploid	Aneuploid	Aneuploid

+, Usually positive; +/-, variable staining; -, usually negative.

pseudoglandular arrangement of the small nests was focally present. The tumor stroma was desmoplastic. Mitotic figures and apoptotic bodies were frequent. The reported case also had microscopic foci of urothelial cell carcinoma with squamous differentiation. Squamous metaplasia was present elsewhere in the bladder in addition to dysplasia and squamous cell carcinoma in situ. This tumor is probably best categorized as urothelial carcinoma with squamous cell differentiation (basaloid type).

Neural and Neuroendocrine Tumors

Small Cell Carcinoma

Epidemiology and Clinical Features

Small cell carcinoma is a malignant neuroendocrine neoplasm of the urothelium that histologically mimics its pulmonary counterpart.[560] It is a rare malignancy that accounts for less than 1% of urinary bladder cancers.[560-579] The demographic and clinical features of small cell carcinoma of the urinary bladder are similar to those of conventional urothelial carcinoma.[382,383] The majority of patients are male, and most patients are in the sixth to seventh decades of life. The mean age at the time of diagnosis is 66 years, ranging from 36 to 85 years, with a male predominance (male-to-female ratio is 3:1).[560] Most patients have a history of cigarette smoking. There is no link between small cell carcinoma of the urinary bladder and HPV infection.[580] Clinical presentations include site-specific and systemic symptoms. Site-specific symptoms are like those of urothelial carcinoma. Clinical presentations include hematuria, irritative symptoms such as dysuria, nocturia, frequency, urinary obstructive symptoms, or localized abdominal/pelvic pain.[560] Systemic symptoms are nonspecific and include anorexia and weight loss. Occasionally, patients have paraneoplastic syndromes with hypercalcemia, hypophosphatemia, or ectopic secretion of adrenocorticotropic hormone.[370,561,568,581]

Staging, Treatment, and Outcome

Most patients with small cell carcinoma of the urinary bladder have advanced stage when first diagnosed, typically with muscularis propria invasion or extravesical extension. A significant proportion of patients also present initially with metastatic cancer including metastases to regional lymph nodes, bone, liver, or lung.[560] Therefore careful and accurate pathologic and clinical staging are necessary to guide further therapy. The overall prognosis for small cell carcinoma of the urinary bladder is poor, with a median survival time of 1 to 2 years, although a few patients have had long-term survival (Fig. 6.79).[560] In Cheng et al.'s report of 64 cases, the cancer-specific survival rate at 5 years was 16%, consistent with the 14% rate reported by Choong et al. from the Mayo Clinic.[560,568] The overall median survival was 1.7 years.[568] Cytotoxic chemotherapy plays a major therapeutic role in the treatment of limited- and advanced-stage small cell carcinoma of the urinary bladder. Chemotherapy is usually combined with other therapeutic modalities such as radiation therapy or surgical resection. Neoadjuvant therapy appears to improve survival.[579] Because of the rarity of small cell carcinoma of the urinary bladder, it is difficult to conduct clinical trials. Therefore the treatment of small cell carcinoma of the urinary bladder will continue to mirror that of small cell lung cancer. Improvement in survival may depend on the identification of new molecular markers for early diagnosis and the development of novel targeted therapies.[41,574,582-586]

Histogenesis and Genetics

Several hypotheses have been proposed to explain the histogenesis of small cell carcinoma of the urinary bladder. One theory, the stem cell theory, is that small cell carcinoma originates from multipotential, undifferentiated stem cells. This is supported by the observation that small cell carcinoma frequently coexists with other histologic types of bladder carcinoma.[566,571,587] Another theory is that small cell carcinoma originates from neuroendocrine cells in normal or metaplastic urothelium. It is speculated that Kulchitsky-type neuroendocrine stem cells may exist within the urothelium and may give rise to neuroendocrine tumors.[588,589] Others have suggested that small cell carcinoma of the bladder may be derived from a poorly defined population of submucosal cells of neural crest origin, the same cells from which paragangliomas and neurofibromas arise in the urinary bladder.[590,591]

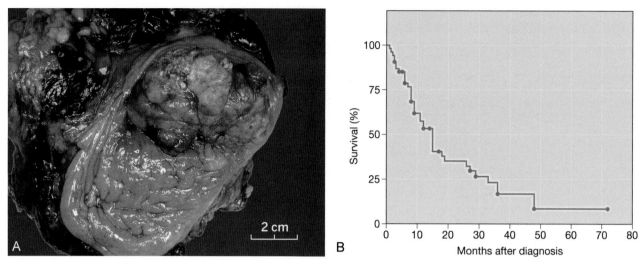

Fig. 6.79 Small cell carcinoma of the urinary bladder. (A) The gross appearance of small cell carcinoma is not different from that of typical urothelial carcinoma. (B) Kaplan-Meier survival curve for patients with small cell carcinoma of the urinary bladder. The prognosis is extremely poor. (From Cheng L, Pan CX, Yang XJ, et al. Small cell carcinoma of the urinary bladder: a clinicopathological analysis of 64 patients. *Cancer* 2004;101:957–962, with permission.)

Molecular data indicate that both urothelial and small cell carcinomas originate from the same stem cell in the urothelium.[41]

At the molecular level, small cell carcinoma of the urinary bladder demonstrates chromosomal aberrations that are commonly seen in small cell lung cancer.[573,574,582,584] Loss of 4q, 5q, 10q, and 13q is common in small cell carcinoma of the urinary bladder.[592] Cheng et al. identified allelic loss at 3p25 to 3p26, 9p21, 9q32 to 9q33, and 17p13 and nonrandom inactivation of X chromosome in a large series of small cell carcinomas of the urinary bladder.[41] Homozygous deletion of p16 and gain or high level of amplification at 1p22 to 1p32, 3q26.3, 8q24, 12q14 to 12q21, and 5q, 6p, 8q, and 20q, chromosomes 1 to 3, 5 to 7, 9, 11, and 18 have also been found.[592,593,594] Some of these regions contain oncogenes. For example, 8q24 includes the oncogene *MYC*, which is found to be highly amplified in small cell carcinoma of the urinary bladder.

Small cell carcinoma of the urinary bladder also shares some of the aberrant signaling pathways seen in small cell lung cancer. For instance, an autocrine loop through the c-kit (CD117)/stem cell factor pathway has been frequently identified in small cell lung cancer.[595,596] It is well known that CD117, a transmembrane receptor tyrosine kinase involved in many physiologic and pathologic processes including hematopoiesis and carcinogenesis, is a target of the tyrosine kinase inhibitor imatinib. CD117 expression can be detected in up to 40% of small cell carcinoma of the urinary bladder.[574] TERT promoter mutation is more commonly seen in small cell carcinomas of the bladder.[597]

Pathology

Most tumors appear as a single large, solid, polypoid mass (Fig. 6.79), but may also appear sessile and ulcerated, and extensively infiltrate the bladder wall. The lateral walls and dome of the bladder are the most frequent topographies, but rare cases may arise in a bladder diverticulum.[584-586,598] Histologically, small cell carcinoma of the urinary bladder consists of sheets or nests of small- or intermediate-size cells with nuclear molding, scant cytoplasm, inconspicuous nucleoli, and evenly dispersed finely stippled chromatin (Fig. 6.80A to D). Mitotic figures are readily evident and may be frequent.[560] There may be extensive nuclear disruption, which can make diagnosis difficult in biopsy specimens. Punctate or geographic necrosis is common, and DNA encrustation of blood vessel walls (Azzopardi phenomenon) may be

noted.[566,570] Occasionally, tumor rosettes are present. Vascular invasion is invariably present.[560,599] In most cases extensive tumor infiltration of detrusor muscle is evident.

Coexisting nonsmall cell carcinoma components, in the form of carcinoma in situ, conventional urothelial carcinoma, adenocarcinoma, squamous cell carcinoma, or sarcomatoid carcinoma, are present in 12% to 61% of cases.[560] In a largest series reported by Cheng et al., 20 cases (32%) were pure small cell carcinoma, and 44 cases (68%) consisted of small cell carcinoma admixed with other histologic types (urothelial carcinoma in 35 cases, adenocarcinoma in 4 cases, sarcomatoid urothelial carcinoma in 2 cases, and both adenocarcinoma and urothelial carcinoma in 3 cases).[560] In another series only 12% of cases were pure small cell carcinoma, whereas a mixture of small cell and urothelial carcinoma was noted in 36 cases (70%), a mixture of small cell carcinoma and adenocarcinoma was present in 4 cases (8%), and a mixture of small cell carcinoma and squamous cell carcinoma was present in 5 cases (10%).[562]

Ultrastructurally, tumor cell nuclei are irregular with coarse chromatin. Cytoplasm is scant with sparse organelles including polyribosomes, short segments of rough endoplasmic reticulum, mitochondria, and occasional Golgi complexes. A finding of diagnostic importance is the presence of membrane-limited, rounded dense core granules ranging from 150 to 250 nm in diameter, which have been observed in almost all cases examined.[566,570] Tonofilaments and dendrite-like processes are also present in the some of the cases.

Immunohistochemistry

The immunohistochemical profile of small cell carcinoma of the urinary bladder has been extensively investigated.[105,373,562,566,567,574,585,586,600-602] It typically exhibits both epithelial and neuroendocrine differentiation. However, the diagnosis of small cell carcinoma can be made on the typical morphologic features alone, even if neuroendocrine differentiation cannot be demonstrated. Markers that have been helpful in confirming neuroendocrine differentiation in small cell carcinoma include neuron-specific enolase, chromogranin, synaptophysin, Leu 7, protein gene product 9.5, serotonin, and vasoactive intestinal peptide. Neuroendocrine differentiation has been demonstrated in 30% to 100% cases of small cell carcinoma by various markers in different studies. Chromogranin A appears to be a relatively

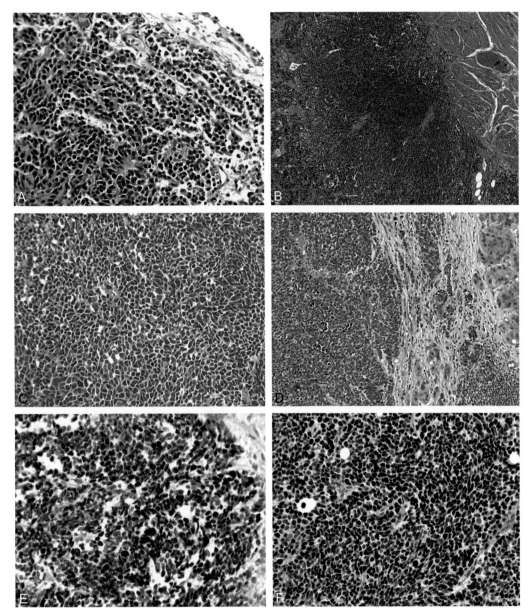

Fig. 6.80 Small cell carcinoma of the urinary bladder. Tumors are composed of sheets and cords of small cells with scant cytoplasm and hyperchromatic nuclei with nuclear crowding and overlapping (A to C). These tumors typically present with high stage with invasion into muscularis propria, as evident in (B). (D) Coexisting urothelial carcinoma component is often present. (E) Immunostain for p53 is diffusely positive. (F) These tumors often show positive immunostaining for thyroid transcription factor-1.

insensitive marker, demonstrable immunohistochemically in only one-third of cases.

Positive immunostaining for CK7 has been observed in about 60% of cases.[566,567,569,601,603] GATA3, CK20, and uroplakins 2 and 3 immunostains are negative in small cell carcinoma of the urinary bladder.[576,601,604,605] Strong and focally intense cytoplasmic dotlike CAM5.2 reactivity is reported in about two-thirds of cases studied.[562,600] Positive immunostaining for CK 34βE12 has been observed in 40% of cases, and positive EMA immunostaining in about 78% of cases.[566,567,576] p53 is overexpressed in 52% of cases (Fig. 6.80E).[586] Reported frequencies of Ki67 expression have varied from 15% to 80%.[576,604]

CD44v6 may be useful in distinguishing poorly differentiated urothelial carcinoma from small cell carcinoma. CD44, a member of a family of transmembrane glycoproteins, mediates cell-cell and cell-matrix adhesion, the latter by serving as a receptor for hyaluronate binding. CD44v6 splice variant is an isoform conferring metastatic potential and has been correlated with aggressive behavior in some cancers. CD44v6 immunoreactivity is demonstrable in 60% of cases of urothelial carcinoma, compared with only 7% positivity in small cell carcinoma.[606,607]

Thyroid transcription factor 1 (TTF1) is a nuclear transcriptional factor protein that is expressed in thyroid and lung epithelium. TTF1 is a reliable marker for distinguishing primary adenocarcinomas of the lung from adenocarcinomas of extrapulmonary origin, and for distinguishing pulmonary small cell carcinoma from Merkel cell carcinoma. Jones et al. showed that approximately 40% of cases of small cell carcinoma of the urinary bladder had positive TTF1 staining (Fig. 6.80F).[601] Therefore TTF1 immunostaining cannot reliably distinguish between a lung or a urinary bladder primary in cases of metastatic small cell carcinoma of uncertain primary location. In general, small cell carcinoma metastatic to the urinary bladder can only be distinguished from a bladder primary by knowledge of the clinical setting.[601]

Differential Diagnosis

The main differential diagnoses include metastasis of small cell carcinoma from another site, lymphoma, lymphoepithelioma-like carcinoma, plasmacytoid carcinoma, and poorly differentiated urothelial carcinoma.[560] Immunohistochemical studies can be quite helpful in distinguishing these entities in difficult cases. Small cell carcinoma can occasionally mimic malignant lymphoma when the tumor cells of small cell carcinoma appear to grow in a discohesive pattern, a finding that may result from artifacts produced by fixation and specimen processing. Lymphoma shows positive immunostaining for leukocyte common antigen and negative immunostaining for keratin and neuroendocrine markers that typically are positive in small cell carcinoma. Plasmacytoid carcinoma, poorly differentiated urothelial carcinoma, and squamous cell carcinoma do not express neuroendocrine markers such as synaptophysin or chromogranin, as small cell carcinoma does. Large cell neuroendocrine carcinoma is morphologically characterized by large tumor cells with low nuclear-to-cytoplasmic ratios, coarse chromatin, and frequent nucleoli and high mitotic activity with areas of necrosis; confirmation of its true nature requires positive immunostaining with appropriate neuroendocrine markers.

Distinction between small cell carcinoma of the prostate and urinary bladder may be challenging, especially in small biopsy specimens without associated prostatic adenocarcinoma or urothelial carcinoma.[608] Recently gene fusions between *ETS* genes, particularly *TMPRSS2* and *ERG*, have been identified as a frequent event in prostate cancer. Thus molecular methods may be helpful in determining the primary site of small cell carcinoma. In a recent study of 30 cases of prostatic small cell carcinoma and 25 cases of bladder small cell carcinoma, Williamson et al. found *TMPRSS2-ERG* gene fusion in 47% (14/30) of prostatic small cell carcinoma.[608] Small cell carcinomas of the bladder were negative for *TMPRSS2-ERG* gene fusion. The presence of *TMPRSS2-ERG* gene fusion in small cell carcinoma established prostatic origin.[608]

Large Cell Neuroendocrine Carcinoma

Large cell neuroendocrine carcinoma is a poorly differentiated and high-grade neuroendocrine tumor (Fig. 6.81), morphologically identical to its counterpart in the lung. Primary large cell neuroendocrine carcinomas of the urinary bladder are rare, and experience with these tumors is limited to a few anecdotal case reports.[609-612] The age at diagnosis ranges from 32 to 82 years. These tumors are either pure or can be associated with other components such as

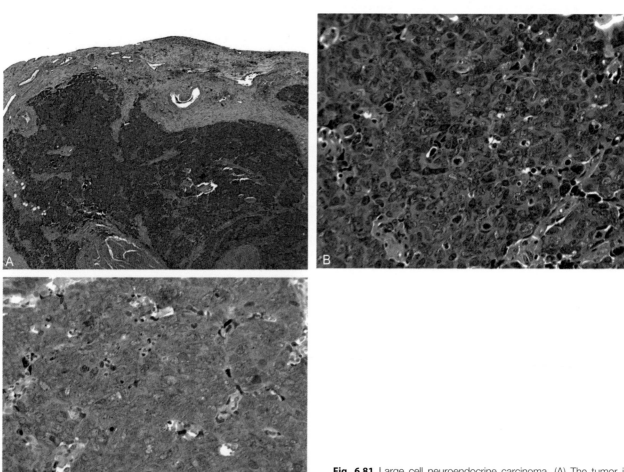

Fig. 6.81 Large cell neuroendocrine carcinoma. (A) The tumor is highly aggressive, with invasion into muscularis propria. (B) Tumor forms solid sheets composed of cells with large hyperchromatic nuclei and amphophilic cytoplasm. (C) Immunostain for synaptophysin is positive.

typical urothelial carcinoma, squamous cell carcinoma, adenocarcinoma or sarcomatoid carcinoma. Immunohistochemically, the tumor cells frequently show immunoreactivity to chromogranin A, CD56, neuron-specific enolase, and synaptophysin. In addition to neuroendocrine markers the tumor cells typically show positive immunostaining for CAM5.2, AE1/AE3, and EMA and may show focal positivity for vimentin.[602] In situ hybridization for the detection of Epstein-Barr virus in one reported case was negative. These tumors are aggressive and tend to metastasize systemically despite aggressive adjuvant therapy. Metastasis from a lung primary should be considered before diagnosing a primary bladder large cell neuroendocrine carcinoma.

Well-Differentiated Neuroendocrine Tumor (Carcinoid)

Well-differentiated neuroendocrine tumor is a potentially malignant neuroendocrine neoplasm of the bladder. Fewer than two dozen cases of carcinoid tumors of the urinary bladder have been reported, usually occurring in elderly patients (age range, 29 to 75 years), with a slight male predominance.[588,601,613-622] Hematuria is common, but irritative voiding symptoms may be the first symptom. Association with carcinoid syndrome has not been reported. Most tumors are submucosal with a predilection for the trigone. They range in size from 0.3 to 3.0 cm. Well-differentiated neuroendocrine tumors are often polypoid at cystoscopy. Their coexistence with other bladder tumors, such as inverted papilloma and adenocarcinoma, has been reported.

Well-differentiated neuroendocrine tumors of the bladder are histologically like their counterparts in other organ sites. The tumor cells have abundant amphophilic cytoplasm and are arranged in an insular, acinar, trabecular, or pseudoglandular pattern with a delicate vascular stroma. An organoid growth pattern, resembling paraganglioma, is sometimes seen. Tumor cell nuclei have finely stippled chromatin and inconspicuous nucleoli. Mitotic figures are infrequent, and tumor necrosis is absent. Tumor cells show immunoreactivity for neuroendocrine markers (neuron-specific enolase, chromogranin, serotonin, and synaptophysin), as well as AE1/AE3. Differential diagnostic considerations include paraganglioma, nested variant of urothelial carcinoma, and metastatic prostate carcinoma. About 25% of patients have or experience development of regional lymph node or distant metastasis, but the majority is cured by excision.

Paraganglioma

Clinical Features

Primary paraganglioma of the bladder occurs infrequently. The largest series, which included 16 patients followed for a mean of 6.3 years, was reported by Cheng et al.[590] Females are more likely to experience bladder paraganglioma, the male-to-female ratio is 1:3. The tumor tends to occur in young patients (mean age, 45 years), and symptoms are present in more than 80% of cases. Presenting symptoms include hematuria; hypertension, which may be exacerbated during voiding; and other symptoms of catecholamine excess.[623-643] At cystoscopic examination, small (<3 cm), dome-shaped nodules covered by normal mucosa are found in the trigone, dome, or lateral wall (Fig. 6.82).

In contrast with extraadrenal paragangliomas at other sites, of which approximately 10% exhibit malignant behavior, the frequency of malignancy in bladder paragangliomas is about 20%.[590] No reliable histologic criteria exist to distinguish malignant from benign neoplasms.[628,631,642,644-646] The findings of nuclear pleomorphism, mitotic figures, and necrosis are not a reliable predictor of clinical outcome in patients with paraganglioma of the urinary bladder.[627,631] Malignancy in these tumors can only be confirmed by the occurrence of regional or distant metastases. No metastases or tumor recurrences have been observed in patients whose tumors were confined within the bladder wall.[590]

Histogenesis

The origin of paraganglioma of the bladder is uncertain. It is thought to arise from embryonic rests of chromaffin cells in the sympathetic plexus of the detrusor muscle.[590] It is postulated that small nests of paraganglionic tissue may persist along the aortic axis and in the pelvic regions, and these remnants of paraganglionic tissue may migrate into the urinary bladder wall during fetal development.[647-650] In an autopsy study of 409 patients, Honma identified paraganglia of the urinary bladder in 52% of the cases examined and found that paraganglia were present throughout different layers of the bladder wall, with a predilection for the anterior and posterior walls.[651] The trigone of the bladder was the least common location of paraganglia. In Cheng et al.'s study, the majority of tumors (94%) involved the muscularis propria of the bladder wall, with a predilection for the posterior and lateral walls.[590] A significant number of patients (37%) also had extravesical extension or pelvic involvement. These findings support the hypothesis that paraganglioma of the bladder originates from paraganglionic cells that migrated into the bladder wall.[647] The high prevalence of paraganglionic cells within the muscular wall (63% of all paraganglia of the bladder) is consistent with the frequent occurrence of paraganglioma in this location.[651]

Genetics

Genomic analyses have identified germline mutations responsible for sporadic as well as familial paraganglioma syndromes.[652-659] The susceptibility genes include *SDHB*, *SDHC*, and *SDHD*. Succinate dehydrogenase (SDH), which consists of four polypeptides [SDHA, SDHB(1p36), SDHC(1q21), and SDHD(11q23)], is the major mitochondrial enzyme linking the aerobic respiratory chain and the Krebs cycle, which oxidizes succinate to fumarate.[652,654] The SDH genes are tumor suppressor genes, the inactivation of which is involved in the hypoxia-angiogenic pathway activating the transcription factor hypoxia-inducible factor (HIF).[652] Non-sense and missense mutations, insertions, and small and large deletions have been reported in the *SDH* genes of patients with pheochromocytoma or paraganglioma. These mutations are generally seen in younger patients. *SDHD* mutations have been identified in patients with pheochromocytoma or functional paraganglioma. Patients with these mutations usually have a paternal family history of disease due to maternal imprinting. *SDHB* gene mutations are usually associated with abdominal paragangliomas and are often identified in patients with no family history of the disease. The *SDHB* gene mutation is associated with a high risk for malignancy.[652]

HIF dysregulation is also linked to inactivation of the *VHL* tumor suppressor gene (3p25 to 3p–26), which is seen in von Hippel–Lindau disease. Pheochromocytomas or paragangliomas may be seen in this disease.[660] Other autosomal dominant diseases associated with pheochromocytomas/paragangliomas include multiple endocrine neoplasia type 2 (caused by mutation of the *RET* proto-oncogene) and neurofibromatosis type 1 (caused by a mutation in *NF1*, a tumor suppressor gene). Genetic aberrations at other loci

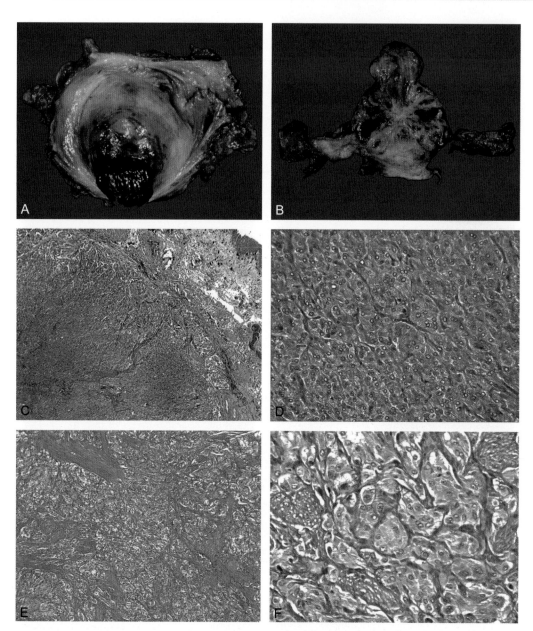

Fig. 6.82 Paraganglioma (pheochromocytoma) of the urinary bladder. Gross appearance (A and B). The tumor is composed of large polygonal cells with eosinophilic granular cytoplasm and central vesicular nuclei (C and D). (E) Tumor invades into the muscularis propria. (F) A Zellballen growth pattern is characteristic of paraganglioma. (A and B, From Cheng L, Leibovich B, Cheville J, et al. Paraganglioma of the urinary bladder: can biologic potential be predicted? *Cancer* 2000;88:844–852, with permission.)

(2q and 16p) have also been recently found to be associated with familial pheochromocytoma.[661] Similarly, Lemeta et al. found abnormalities in tumor suppressor genes located at 6q23 to 6q24, which may play a role in the tumorigenesis of pheochromocytomas.[662]

Pathology

Histologically, bladder paraganglioma is similar to its counterparts in other body sites; most are covered by normal urothelium (Fig. 6.82).[590] The tumor consists of round or polygonal epithelioid cells with abundant eosinophilic or granular cytoplasm. Tumor cell nuclei are centrally located and are vesicular with finely granular chromatin. The cells are arranged in discrete nests (Zellballen), with intervening vascular septa. Sustentacular cells may be present. Mitotic figures, necrosis, and vascular invasion are usually absent.[590]

Immunohistochemistry

Paraganglioma typically demonstrates immunoreactivity with neuroendocrine markers such as chromogranin, synaptophysin, and neuron-specific enolase.[590] The sustentacular cells exhibit immunostaining for S100P. Tumor cells are usually immunoreactive for GATA3, but usually show no immunoreactivity for CK7, CK20, or AE1/AE3.[652]

Differential Diagnosis

The differential diagnosis for paraganglioma includes granular cell tumor, nested variant of urothelial carcinoma, metastatic large cell neuroendocrine carcinoma, or malignant melanoma.[416,417,419,590,663,664] Granular cell tumor has abundant eosinophilic granular cytoplasm, shows strongly positive immunostaining for S100P, and lacks the Zellballen growth pattern, the fine vascular stroma, chromogranin immunoreactivity, and sustentacular cell S100P immunostaining.[665-669] The nested variant of urothelial carcinoma also lacks a fine vascular network and is immunohistochemically negative for S100P and chromogranin. Metastatic large cell neuroendocrine carcinoma is characterized by necrosis, abundant mitotic activity, and cellular anaplasia. Although it is immunoreactive for neuroendocrine markers similar to paraganglioma, it is also immunoreactive for CK and negative for sustentacular cell S100P immunoreactivity. History is important in differentiating paraganglioma from metastatic carcinoid. Carcinoid tumor is negative for sustentacular cell S100P immunoreactivity. Malignant melanoma must be considered in the differential diagnosis because paraganglioma may contain melanin pigment.

Neurofibroma

Neurofibroma of the urinary bladder is rare. Most of these lesions occur in the setting of neurofibromatosis type 1 rather than as isolated lesions.[591] Classically, neurofibromas of the urinary bladder occur in young patients with a slight male predominance. The average age at diagnosis is 17 years. Presenting symptoms include hematuria, irritative symptoms, and pelvic mass. Neurofibroma is a benign, probably neoplastic tumor of various nerve sheath cells including Schwann cells, perineurium-like cells, fibroblasts, and intermediate type cells.[670] The histologic findings are the same as in neurofibromas of other organs; tumors are composed of a hypocellular proliferation of spindle cells, loosely arranged into fascicles with scattered "shredded carrot" bundles of collagen (Fig. 6.83).[591,671] Individual cells have wavy, bland nuclei. In a

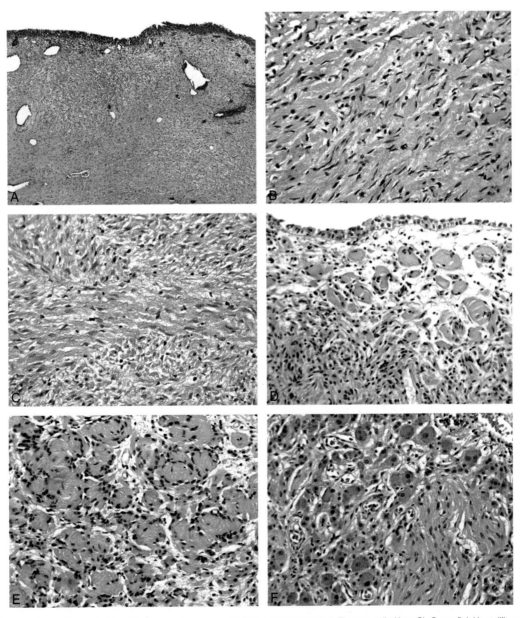

Fig. 6.83 Neurofibroma of the urinary bladder. The tumor shows a proliferation of uniform neurofibroma cells (A to C). Superficial bandlike subepithelial pseudomeissnerian corpuscles are prominent (D and E). (F) Ganglion cells may be involved by neurofibroma.

recent series by Cheng et al., three of four bladder neurofibromas were transmural with both diffuse and plexiform growth patterns.[591] Another case had only diffuse pattern with submucosal involvement and subepithelial pseudomeissnerian corpuscles on biopsy. Areas of diffuse involvement were hypocellular with small- to medium-size spindle cells with ovoid to elongate nuclei in a collagenized matrix. A few mast cells were present. Immunohistochemical staining was reactive in all cases for S100P, as well as type IV collagen.[591] Three were positive for neurofilament protein in axons. A recent report indicates that bladder neurofibromas do not express ALK1 (anaplastic lymphoma kinase 1) protein. The differential diagnosis of bladder neurofibroma includes other spindle cell tumors such as leiomyoma, postoperative spindle cell nodule (PSCN), inflammatory pseudotumor, low-grade leiomyosarcoma, other nerve sheet tumors, and rarely rhabdomyosarcoma.[591]

Schwannoma

Schwannoma of the urinary bladder is derived from Schwann cells in nerve sheaths. It occurs in both men and women, and is often associated with von Recklinghausen disease.[672] The age at presentation ranges from the fourth to sixth decade of life.[672,673] The presenting symptoms include bladder pressure, suprapubic pain, back pain, urgency, and frequency. No recurrences have been reported during follow-up periods of 1 to 3 years after surgical resection.[672,673]

Grossly, the tumor appears as a circumscribed mass, often arising from the lateral wall, beneath a normal mucosa. It may or may not extend into the perivesical fat. Histologically, schwannoma consists of spindle cells with uniform round to oval nuclei arranged in a palisading or organoid pattern. There is no nuclear pleomorphism and mitotic figures are infrequent.[672,673] Tumor cells show positive immunostaining for S100P, neuron-specific enolase, and vimentin. Immunostains for myoglobin, factor VIII, keratins, actin (HHF-35), and desmin are negative.[672,673]

Primitive Neuroectodermal Tumor

Primary primitive neuroectodermal tumor (PNET) of the bladder is a rare and aggressive neoplasm.[674] Morphologically, it is a small, round, blue cell tumor that is often associated with extensive areas of necrosis (Fig. 6.84). Tumor cells show strong expression of CD99, vimentin, and CD117, and focal reactivity to CK and S100P. Ultrastructural study reveals sparse neurosecretory granules.[674] Molecular genetic analysis supports the diagnosis of PNET by showing the EWS/FLI1 fusion transcript type 2 by reverse transcriptase-polymerase chain reaction and *EWS* gene rearrangement by FISH. A patient treated with imatinib after systemic chemotherapy and radical surgery remained alive after 6 years of follow-up.[674]

Malignant Peripheral Nerve Sheath Tumor

Malignant peripheral nerve sheath tumor (MPNST) is rare in the urinary bladder. Only a few cases have been documented, predominantly in patients younger than 40 years.[675] Some have arisen in the setting of neurofibromatosis type 1, possibly originating in neurofibromas of autonomic nerve plexuses in the bladder wall. MPNST is typically a highly malignant and rapidly growing tumor. Patients present with hematuria, and a suprapubic mass is sometimes noted.[676] The lesion has been seen arising from the trigone, as well as from the lateral and posterior walls of the bladder. It may form multiple large nodules with surface ulceration and areas of necrosis. The tumor may infiltrate the entire thickness of the bladder wall, involving perivesical soft tissues or pelvic peritoneum. Distant metastases may be present at diagnosis. Prognosis is generally poor, with local recurrence or distant metastases often evident within 2 months of initial surgical resection.

Histologically, MPNST is a poorly differentiated tumor that grows in sheets and nodules consisting of interlacing fascicles of malignant spindle cells.[675] The tumor cells are pleomorphic, with variable amounts of eosinophilic cytoplasm.[676] Most have a single nucleus, but multinucleated tumor cells may be present. Nuclei are round to oval with prominent irregular eosinophilic nucleoli or elongated and tapered with marked atypia. Mitotic activity may be moderate. An extensive infiltrate of acute and chronic inflammatory cells, including eosinophils, may be present. An epithelioid variant, as well as a variant with rhabdomyoblastic differentiation (malignant triton tumor), has been described.[676]

Immunohistochemical stains can help with the identification of this tumor, which typically shows positive immunostaining for S100P and vimentin, and focally positive staining for neuron-specific enolase. It usually does not stain for EMA, AE1/AE3,

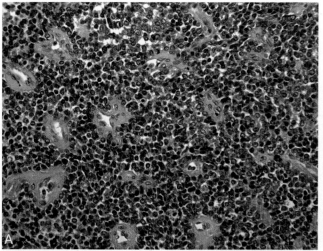
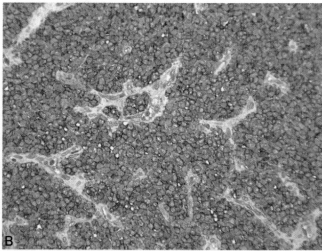

Fig. 6.84 Primitive neuroectodermal tumor of the urinary bladder. (A) The tumor is highly cellular and consists of small, round blue cells in sheets surrounded by fibrovascular stroma. Pseudorosette formation is apparent. (B) The tumor is immunoreactive for CD99.

muscle-specific actin, desmin, myoglobin, CK, chromogranin, or neurofilament.[675,676] In one case rhabdomyoblastic differentiation with focal immunostaining for myoglobin was identified in a tumor that arose in an infant with neurofibromatosis type 1.[677]

The differential diagnosis of this tumor includes epithelioid sarcoma, undifferentiated carcinoma, melanoma, epithelioid angiosarcoma, rhabdoid tumor, carcinosarcoma, and epithelioid leiomyosarcoma. Immunoreactivity to HMB45 or Melan-A, or strong, diffuse S100P immunoreactivity would favor melanoma. Carcinosarcoma would show evidence of epithelial differentiation with immunoreactivity for CK and EMA. Unlike epithelioid sarcoma, tumor cells of MPNST are immunoreactive for S100P, focally immunoreactive for neuron-specific enolase, and are not immunoreactive for EMA or CK. Immunohistochemistry can also be used to help rule out endothelial, muscular, and neuroendocrine differentiation, as well as anaplastic lymphoma.

Sarcomatoid Carcinoma

Definition and Terminology

The term *sarcomatoid carcinoma* applies when a malignant neoplasm exhibits morphologic or immunohistochemical evidence of both epithelial and mesenchymal differentiation.[80] Heterologous elements may be present and should be acknowledged in the pathology report.[678] There is considerable confusion and disagreement in the literature regarding nomenclature and histogenesis of these tumors. Molecular data and morphologic evidence support the hypothesis that sarcomatoid carcinoma is a common final pathway of all forms of epithelial bladder tumors (Fig. 6.85).[69,80] Sarcomatoid transformation has been observed in various epithelial tumors of the urinary bladder including conventional urothelial carcinoma, small cell carcinoma, adenocarcinoma, squamous cell carcinoma, and large cell neuroendocrine carcinoma.

Various terms have been used for these neoplasms including carcinosarcoma, sarcomatoid carcinoma, pseudosarcomatous transitional cell carcinoma, malignant mesodermal mixed tumor, spindle cell carcinoma, giant cell carcinoma, and malignant teratoma. In some reports both carcinosarcoma and sarcomatoid carcinoma are included under the term *sarcomatoid carcinoma*. In other reports they are regarded as separate entities. There is widespread consensus that the most appropriate term for all of these neoplasms is *sarcomatoid carcinoma*.[679] The term *sarcomatoid carcinoma* is preferred for the majority of cases in which there is a spindle cell

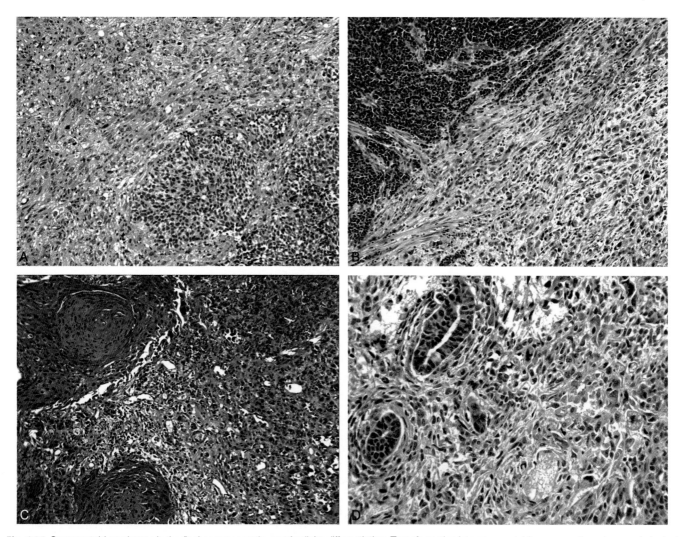

Fig. 6.85 Sarcomatoid carcinoma is the final common pathway of cellular differentiation. Transformation into sarcomatoid component can be seen in typical urothelial carcinoma (A), small cell carcinoma (B), squamous cell carcinoma (C), and adenocarcinoma (D).

component with positive vimentin staining. Some may use the term *carcinosarcoma* for cases with identifiable heterologous elements on hematoxylin and eosin–stained sections or positive staining for markers of specific mesenchymal differentiation. Both diagnostic categories appear to be variations of the same neoplastic transformation process and have the same clinical features and prognosis.

Clinical Features

Sarcomatoid carcinoma represents approximately 0.3% of bladder carcinomas. The most frequent presenting symptoms are hematuria, dysuria, nocturia, acute urinary retention, and lower abdominal pain.[80] The mean patient age is 66 years (range, 50 to 77 years).[97,680-682] In some patients there is a history of exposure to cyclophosphamide therapy or carcinoma treated by radiation.[680,681] The presence of specific types of differentiation of the spindle cell component does not influence the prognosis, but sarcomatoid carcinoma is usually high grade, biologically aggressive, and associated with a poor prognosis.[97,682] Pathologic stage is the best predictor of survival in sarcomatoid carcinoma.[80]

Histogenesis and Genetics

Recent molecular studies strongly argue for a monoclonal origin of both the epithelial and mesenchymal components in sarcomatoid carcinoma and carcinosarcoma. These two categories have similar clinical characteristics including patient age, gender presentation, and outcome. An analysis of 30 sarcomatoid urothelial carcinomas for X chromosome inactivation status, as well as LOH, has shed light on the pathogenesis of this tumor. Results of this study found identical patterns of allelic loss in the carcinomatous and sarcomatous components, and identified four of six polymorphic microsatellite markers where genetic alterations occur frequently in urothelial carcinomas, including D8S261 (86%), D9S177 (75%), IFNA (57%), and D11S569 (78%) loci.[69] Furthermore, discordant allelic loss of microsatellite markers was also found at the various sites as the bladder tumors underwent malignant progression leading to genetic divergence of high-grade anaplastic malignancies after the initial neoplastic transformation. In addition, the study found the same pattern of nonrandom X chromosome inactivation in both carcinomatous and sarcomatous components in five of eight female patients.[69] The identical X-chromosome inactivation and significant concordance of LOH support the contention that both carcinomatous and sarcomatous tumor components arise from a monoclonal primordial cell. Clonal divergence may occur during tumor progression and lead to differentiation into mesenchymal and epithelial phenotypes.[76,79-81]

Markers representative of epithelial-mesenchymal transition, including vimentin, FoxC2, SNAIL, and ZEB1, are often overexpressed in sarcomatoid urothelial carcinoma.[683] A concurrent loss of E-cadherin and elevated N-cadherin expressions is also evident in most cases. A recent report found TERT promoter mutations in 35% of sarcomatoid carcinomas. All patients with TERT mutation died of cancer within 2 years after surgery.[684]

Pathology

The gross appearance is characteristically "sarcoma-like," with a dull gray fleshy cut surface and infiltrative margins. The tumors are often polypoid and tend to form large intraluminal masses (Fig. 6.86). Microscopically, sarcomatoid carcinoma is composed of a urothelial, glandular, or small cell epithelial component showing variable degrees of differentiation (Fig. 6.87).[678] Carcinoma in situ is present in 30% of cases and occasionally is the only apparent epithelial component. A small subset of sarcomatoid

carcinomas may have a prominent myxoid stroma. The mesenchymal component most frequently observed is an undifferentiated high-grade spindle cell neoplasm. The most common heterologous element is osteosarcoma, followed by chondrosarcoma, rhabdomyosarcoma, leiomyosarcoma, liposarcoma, angiosarcoma, or multiple types of mesenchymal differentiation (Fig. 6.88).

Differential Diagnosis and Immunohistochemistry

Sarcomatoid carcinoma is characterized by strong staining with CK (AE1/AE3, CAM5.2) and/or EMA with coexpression of vimentin in the majority of cases (Fig. 6.62; Tables 6.26 and 6.27).[97,105,441,680,682,685-688] In contrast with smooth muscle neoplasms, actin and desmin are typically negative. However, sarcomatoid carcinomas with heterologous differentiation may rarely be encountered, and in this situation expression of other mesenchymal markers, such as actin, desmin, or S100P, may be observed.[689,690]

Sarcomatoid carcinoma of the urinary bladder is usually biphasic, composed of both epithelial and mesenchymal elements. In cases exclusively composed of spindle cells, the main differential diagnostic consideration is sarcoma, particularly leiomyosarcoma. In view of the rarity of primary bladder sarcoma, any malignant spindle cell tumor in the urinary bladder in an adult can be considered sarcomatoid carcinoma until proved otherwise. CK immunostaining may be helpful in this setting. One should also bear in mind that focal CK immunoreactivity may be seen in smooth muscle tumors and pseudosarcomatous myofibroblastic proliferations. Smooth muscle tumors are additionally immunoreactive for desmin and vimentin, even when they express CK antigens.[678,679]

Sarcomatoid carcinoma with prominent myxoid and sclerosing stroma may be mistaken for pseudosarcomatous myofibroblastic tumor, PSCN, or urothelial carcinoma with pseudosarcomatous stroma.[686-688] The presence of slitlike vessels and the absence of mitotic figures and significant cytologic atypia favor the diagnosis of benign lesion.

Soft Tissue Tumors

Pure sarcomas of the urinary bladder are rare and have been described only in small series and isolated case reports.[691,692] Myofibroblastic proliferations, including pseudosarcomatous myofibroblastic tumor and PSCN, still invoke a degree of uncertainty for classification and differential diagnosis. Other rare benign lesions of the bladder include leiomyoma, hemangioma, and neurofibroma. Other examples of benign soft tissue tumors are rarely described.[691-693] Differentiation of benign lesions from malignant lesions is critical to avoid overly aggressive therapy. Malignant mesenchymal tumors of the urinary bladder include leiomyosarcoma, rhabdomyosarcoma, angiosarcoma, and undifferentiated pleomorphic sarcoma (UPS). Recognizing these spindle cell lesions and differentiating them from sarcomatoid carcinoma is important because these two diagnostic categories have differing therapeutic and prognostic implications.[691,692,694]

Myofibroblastic Proliferations and Benign Soft Tissue Tumors

Inflammatory Myofibroblastic Tumor

Inflammatory myofibroblastic tumor of the bladder is a controversial entity and has had many designations including inflammatory pseudotumor, inflammatory pseudosarcomatous fibromyxoid tumor, nodular fasciitis, pseudosarcomatous myofibroblastic

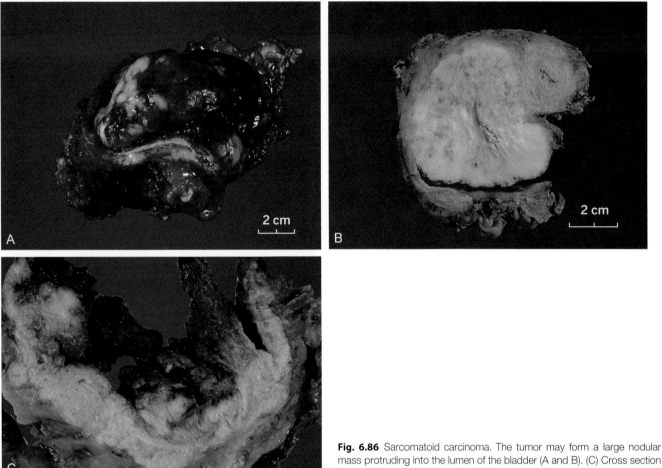

Fig. 6.86 Sarcomatoid carcinoma. The tumor may form a large nodular mass protruding into the lumen of the bladder (A and B). (C) Cross section shows diffusely infiltrative growth.

proliferation, and fibromyxoid pseudotumor.[686,695-719] It was initially described as a lesion showing spindle cells in a myxoid stroma with scattered chronic inflammatory cells.[720] The most frequent presenting symptom is hematuria; other symptoms include irritative or obstructive voiding symptoms, abdominal pain, or the discovery of a mass lesion. Rarely, constitutional symptoms, including fever and weight loss, have been reported, possibly because of the release of cytokines. Grossly, the lesion is either a polypoid mass or a submucosal nodule. The tumor may or may not cause surface ulceration, and the cut surface is often pale, firm, and glistening. Histologically, there is a proliferation of spindle cells with elongated eosinophilic cytoplasmic processes in a loose edematous or myxoid background (Figs. 6.89 and 6.90; Tables 6.26 and 6.27). The nuclei may be large with occasional atypia.[701,718,721] Single, prominent nucleoli may be present. Occasional mitotic figures are seen, none of which is atypical. The mitotic rates vary from 0 to 20 mitoses per 10 high-power fields.[711,716,717] Inflammation, usually chronic and consisting of a lymphoplasmacytic infiltrate, is invariably seen. Some lesions have infiltrates of eosinophils or neutrophils, which may be focally prominent. Extravasated red blood cells may be present. Three histologic patterns have been recognized, the most common of which is the "nodular fasciitis-like" pattern with myxoid, vascular, and inflammatory areas.[699,711] A second pattern, designated "fibrous histiocytoma-like," has a more compact spindle cell proliferation and scattered lymphocytes, plasma cells, or eosinophils. The third pattern, designated "scar or

desmoid-like," has dense collagen with fewer spindled and inflammatory cells (Fig. 6.90). Infiltration into the muscularis propria or even perivesical involvement may be seen. Typically, the lesion occurs in patients ranging in age from 9 to 42 years, with a female predominance. The tumor size ranges from 1.5 to 13 cm. Follow-up data have revealed no evidence of metastases, but the lesion may recur after surgery.[701,718,719]

There is some lack of consistency in the reported immunoprofile, with the result that the utility of immunostaining in separating this lesion from other spindle cell lesions of the bladder is limited. Immunoreactivity for actin and vimentin is usually present but may be focal.[686-688] p53 staining is weak or absent in inflammatory myofibroblastic tumor and PSCN, but strongly and diffusely positive in rhabdomyosarcoma, leiomyosarcoma, and sarcomatoid carcinoma.[702,715] Pan-CK reactivity, which may be patchy, is seen in many cases of inflammatory myofibroblastic tumor. Nevertheless, CK may be seen in other nonepithelial tumors such as leiomyosarcoma.[716,717] Actin immunoreactivity may not help differentiate benign tumors from malignant tumors because α-smooth muscle actin is positive in 43% of sarcomas, in 63% of inflammatory myofibroblastic tumor, and in an intermediate percentage of PSCN. Rhabdomyosarcoma rarely expresses smooth muscle actin, but leiomyosarcoma often does. Iczkowski et al. found 3 of 11 inflammatory myofibroblastic tumors, 2 of 3 PSCNs, and 0 of 8 sarcomas were reactive for desmin, but this marker may be present in leiomyosarcoma at other sites.[715]

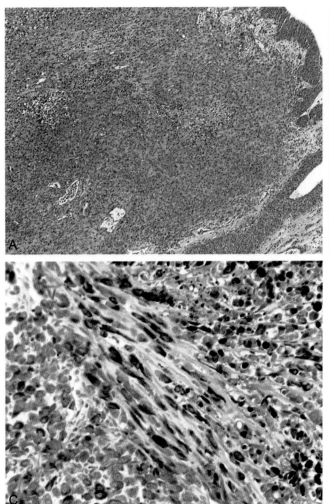
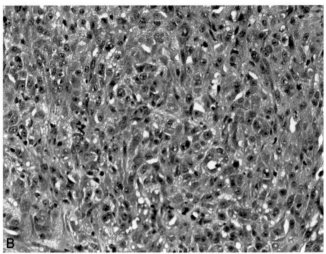

Fig. 6.87 Sarcomatoid carcinoma. Inflammatory cells are invariably present in sarcomatoid carcinoma (A and B). Sarcomatoid urothelial carcinoma should be distinguished from other benign and malignant spindle cell tumors. (C) Strong and diffuse immunoreactivity for CK AE1/AE3 confirms the epithelial nature of the tumor.

Inflammatory myofibroblastic tumor shows variable staining for EMA.[701,718] Inflammatory myofibroblastic tumor is negative for myoglobin, whereas rhabdomyosarcoma is usually positive for skeletal muscle markers such as myogenin or MyoD1. Strong coexpression of smooth muscle actin and CK is characteristic of vesical myofibroblasts and thus should characterize inflammatory myofibroblastic tumor.[712]

The main differential diagnoses include PSCN, embryonal rhabdomyosarcoma, leiomyosarcoma, and sarcomatoid carcinoma.[80,160,465,686-688,692,701,702,715,718,719,722-727] PSCN reportedly is more likely to have eosinophils.[716,717] Inflammatory myofibroblastic tumor may be confused with myxoid leiomyosarcoma because both may have a myxoid stroma. Morphologically, leiomyosarcoma is more uniform in its cellularity and exhibits more cytologic atypia. Inflammatory myofibroblastic tumor, in contrast, has a more prominent network of small blood vessels and a more extensive inflammatory infiltrate. Inflammatory myofibroblastic tumor may have necrosis at the site of surface ulceration and it may infiltrate into the detrusor muscle, but it typically does not exhibit deep necrosis as may be seen in a sarcoma. However, in a recent series by Harik et al., 32% of inflammatory myofibroblastic tumor cases showed necrosis in the deep bladder wall, two of which were extensively necrotic.[697] Recently, positive cytoplasmic immunostaining for ALK1 has been identified in up to 89% of inflammatory myofibroblastic tumors in the

bladder.[702,715,721,728-730] The ALK1 staining was confirmed by FISH to mRNA from a fusion gene resulting from translocation of the *ALK* gene on chromosome 2p23 to the clathrin heavy chain region on chromosome 17q23.[695,721,728] It has been suggested that *ALK* cases are less likely to recur. Neither ALK1 staining nor translocation of the *ALK1* gene has been identified in any case of bladder leiomyosarcoma or rhabdomyosarcoma. However, spindle cell lesions in sites other than the urinary bladder may display ALK1 expression, which has been reported in 40% of inflammatory myofibroblastic tumors, 19% of rhabdomyosarcomas, and 10% of leiomyosarcomas at other sites.[686-688,719,728-730] The ALK translocated inflammatory myofibroblastic tumor has shown sustained response to the ALK inhibitor crizotinib.[731]

Harik et al. proposed that inflammatory myofibroblastic tumor occurring in the adult bladder and PSCN should be combined into a diagnostic category designated *pseudosarcomatous myofibroblastic proliferations*.[697] These investigators further suggested that evidence is sufficient to distinguish pseudosarcomatous myofibroblastic proliferations of the bladder from inflammatory myofibroblastic tumor of childhood. The latter is often associated with systemic findings, such as fever, weight loss, and laboratory abnormalities, including anemia, thrombocytosis, and polyclonal hypergammaglobulinemia.

Given the marked histologic and immunohistochemical overlap between inflammatory myofibroblastic tumor, leiomyosarcoma, and sarcomatoid carcinoma and the relevant clinical implication

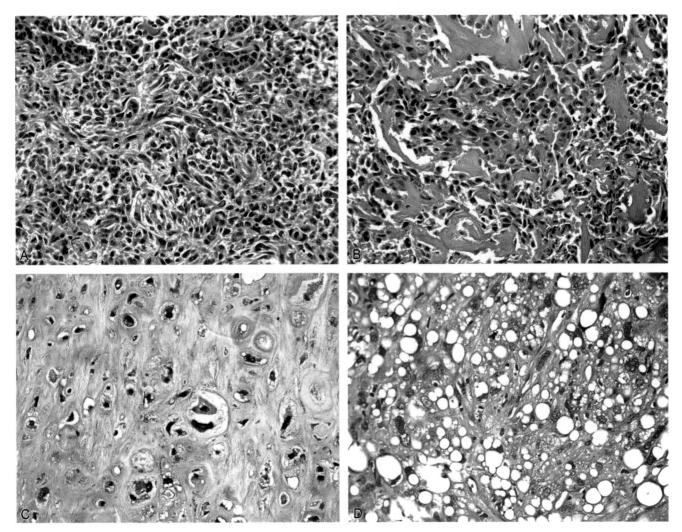

Fig. 6.88 Sarcomatoid carcinoma. (A) Typical sarcomatoid carcinoma is composed of malignant spindle cells with significant cytologic atypia and frequent mitotic figures. Heterologous differentiation, including (B) osteosarcoma, (C) chondrosarcoma, and (D) liposarcoma, may be seen.

TABLE 6.26	Differential Features of Selected Soft Tissue Tumors of the Urinary Bladder						
	Cytologic Atypia	Mitotic Figures	Atypical Mitotic Figures	Tumor Necrosis	Inflammation	Invasion of Muscle	Other Features
Sarcomatoid carcinoma	Present	Present	Present	Present	Often present	May be present	Concomitant carcinoma
Inflammatory myofibroblastic tumor	Minimal	Few	Absent	Surface only	Often prominent	May be present	Delicate capillaries
Leiomyoma	Minimal	Rare	Absent	Absent	Absent	Absent	Well circumscribed
Leiomyosarcoma	Present	Present	Present	Present	Sparse	Present	Uniform appearance
Undifferentiated pleomorphic sarcoma	Present	Present	Present	Present	Present	Present	Multinucleated cells
Neurofibroma	Varies	Absent	Absent	Absent	Sparse	Absent	Strands of collagen
Postoperative spindle cell nodule	Minimal	Variable	Absent	Absent	Present	Absent	Delicate capillaries
Rhabdomyosarcoma	Present	Present	Present	Varies	Absent	May be present	Cambium layer in embryonal RMS, alveolar appearance
Angiosarcoma	Present	Present	Present	May be present	Present	May be present	Anastomosing vessels

TABLE 6.27 Immunohistochemistry in the Differential Diagnosis of Spindle Cell Lesions of the Urinary Bladder

	Sarcomatoid Carcinoma	Inflammatory Myofibroblastic Tumor	Leiomyosarcoma	Leiomyoma	Undifferentiated Pleomorphic Sarcoma	Neurofibroma	Postoperative Spindle Cell Nodule	Rhabdomyosarcoma
ALK1		Pos				Rare pos	Neg	
α_1-Antichymotrypsin					Pos			
CD68					Pos			
Cytokeratin	Pos	Neg/Pos	Neg/Pos		Neg/Pos	Neg	Neg/Pos	Neg/Pos
Desmin	Neg/Pos	Neg/Pos	Pos	Pos	Neg/Pos		Neg/Pos	Pos
Epithelial membrane antigen	Pos	Neg/Pos	Neg			Neg	Neg	Neg
h-Caldesmon			Pos	Pos	Neg			Neg
Muscle-specific actin	Neg/Pos	Pos	Pos	Pos	Neg/Pos		Pos	Pos
MYOD1			Neg		Neg			Pos
Myogenin			Neg		Neg			Pos
Myoglobin								Neg/Pos
Neuron-specific enolase		Neg						Neg/Pos
Smooth muscle actin	Neg/Pos	Pos	Pos	Pos	Neg/Pos		Neg/Pos	Neg/Pos
S100P		Neg	Neg		Neg	Pos		Neg
Vimentin	Neg/Pos	Pos	Pos	Pos	Pos		Pos	Pos
CD31					Neg			
CD34			Neg/Pos		Neg			Neg

ALK, Anaplastic lymphoma kinase; *Neg*, negative; *Neg/Pos*, variable staining; *Pos*, positive.

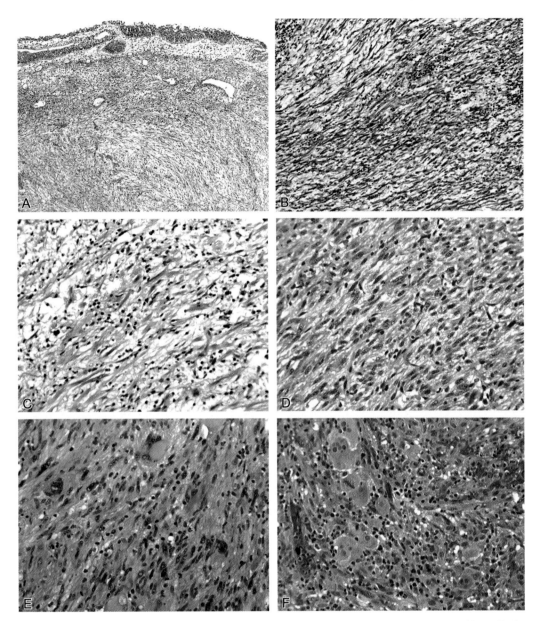

Fig. 6.89 Inflammatory myofibroblastic tumor. The tumor is composed of spindle cells in an edematous stroma (A to C). Scattered acute and chronic inflammatory cells are typically seen in this lesion. (D) The lesion may appear hypercellular. Multinucleated giant cells and mitotic figures may be present (E and F).

of such overlap, a panel of antibodies, including GATA3, CK AE1/AE3, desmin, smooth muscle actin, ALK, high-molecular-weight CK, p63/p40, and CK5/6, may be used in the diagnostic workup (Table 6.24). Positivity for GATA3, CK AE1/AE3, high-molecular-weight CK, p63, and CK5/6 favors sarcomatoid carcinoma. Positivity for smooth muscle actin and desmin with overall absence of all other markers favor leiomyosarcoma. Inflammatory myofibroblastic tumor is likely to express ALK by immunohistochemistry or may be more accurately diagnosed by use of a FISH test.[732]

Postoperative Spindle Cell Nodule

PSCN may be seen in both genders months after surgical instrumentation or resection.[697,702,714,715,733,734] They are characterized by nodules up to 4 cm occurring in the lower genital tract and lower urinary tract.[733] Patients range in age from 29 to 79 years

and typically present with hematuria or obstructive voiding symptoms. Some PSCNs are found incidentally by CT scan or at cystoscopy.[701,718] Microscopically, the tumors are uniform and composed of intersecting fascicles of plump spindle cells with delicate vessels, focal hyalinization, and moderate collagen deposition (Fig. 6.91). The spindle cells have abundant, tapering, eosinophilic cytoplasm. The nuclei vary only slightly in size, and there is no cytologic atypia. There are numerous mitotic figures, ranging from 1 to 25 per 10 high-power fields, none of which is abnormal.[686-688,719] All lesions have ulceration with acute inflammatory cells in the ulcer bed, as well as scattered chronic inflammatory cells in deeper areas. The tumor has infiltrating margins with smooth muscle destruction. Moderate edema and small foci of hemorrhage may be identified. No recurrences or metastases have been reported, but bladder wall eosinophilia may be prominent after resection of the lesion.[733] The proliferating cells are

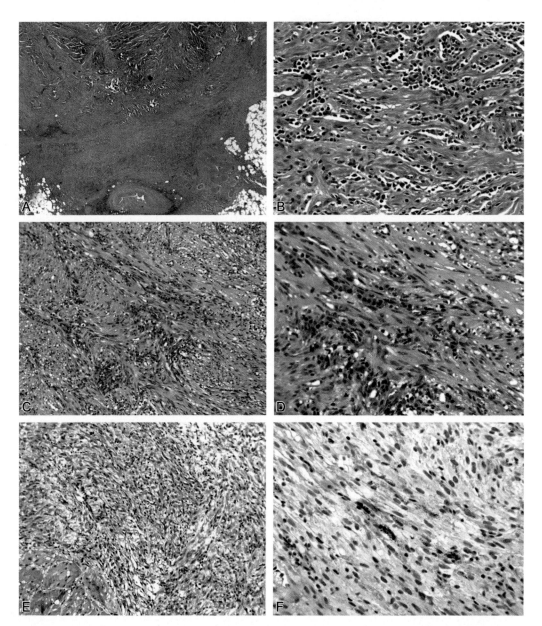

Fig. 6.90 Inflammatory myofibroblastic tumor. End stage of sclerotic and fibrotic variant (A to D). Inflammatory background is almost always present. (E) The lesion may extend into muscle. (F) Immunostaining for ALK1 is useful in confirming the diagnosis.

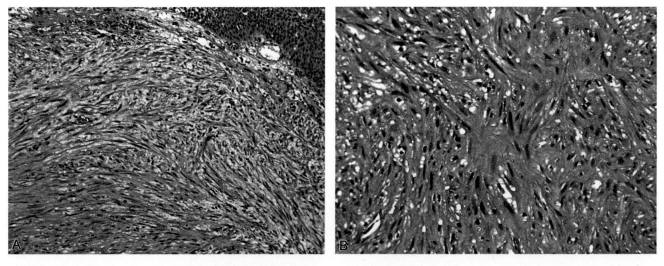

Fig. 6.91 Postoperative spindle cell nodule (A and B). Inflammatory cells are invariably present.

immunoreactive for AE1/AE3, CAM5.2, and vimentin in some cases, similar to the findings in inflammatory myofibroblastic tumor. Some cases exhibit only immunoreactivity for vimentin.[719]

The differential diagnoses for PSCN include sarcomatoid carcinoma, myxoid leiomyosarcoma, rhabdomyosarcoma, and UPS/malignant fibrous histiocytoma (see Inflammatory Myofibroblastic Tumor section for discussion).[711,721] Findings that are helpful in distinguishing PSCN from sarcoma include the lack of necrosis or myxoid degeneration, lack of nuclear atypia, and predominance of chronic over acute inflammation.[702,715] p53 immunostaining may be helpful in distinguishing these lesions, being noted only rarely in PSCN, but showing strong and diffuse staining in malignant lesions.

Leiomyoma

Although rare, leiomyoma is the most common benign neoplasm of the bladder.[693,694,735,736] A review by Goluboff et al. of 37 cases reported that 59% occurred in the third through sixth decades of life with an average patient age of 44 years.[693,736] Leiomyoma of the bladder is more common in women, with a male-to-female ratio of 1:3. About 19% of patients are asymptomatic; others present with obstructive voiding symptoms (49%), irritative symptoms (38%), hematuria (11%), or flank pain (13%). Leiomyomas are most often endovesical, followed by extravesical or intramural.[693] Grossly, the tumors are small, well-circumscribed white nodules without necrosis, ranging from 1.6 to 5.8 cm (Fig. 6.92). Microscopically, leiomyoma consists of intersecting fascicles of smooth muscle cells with moderate to abundant eosinophilic cytoplasm.[736] Cellularity is usually limited, and myxoid change is absent in most cases. The nuclei are oval to cigar-shaped, centrally located, and blunt-ended, and lack significant nuclear atypia, mitotic activity, and necrosis. Examples of angioleiomyoma have been reported. Leiomyoma is immunoreactive for smooth muscle actin, desmin, and vimentin. Some may express CD34, but most are negative for CK and S100P. Excision is usually curative.

Hemangioma

Cheng et al. reported the findings in 19 patients with bladder hemangioma.[737] In this series the mean age at diagnosis was 58 years, whereas in previous reports, hemangiomas occurred in all age groups but predominantly in patients younger than 30 years. Male-to-female ratio is 3.7:1.[737] The usual presenting symptom is gross hematuria, but other complaints may include irritative voiding symptoms and abdominal pain. Endoscopically, a sessile blue raised mass may be seen. The lesion is usually small (median, 0.7 cm). Hemangiomas are most often found on the posterior and lateral walls of the bladder. The histologic findings in bladder hemangioma are the same as those noted in other sites. Cavernous hemangioma is the most common type reported in the bladder, but capillary or arteriovenous types may infrequently be seen (Fig. 6.93). Effective conservative treatment consists of biopsy with or without fulguration. After such treatment, none of the 19 patients reported by Cheng et al. had recurrence (mean follow-up, 6.9 years).[737] The differential diagnosis for bladder hemangioma includes angiosarcoma and Kaposi sarcoma, both of which exhibit more cytologic atypia. Exuberant granulation tissue contains prominent inflammation, which is not a feature of hemangioma. Multiple hemangiomas may be associated with syndromes predisposing to their development, including Klippel-Trenaunay-Weber and Sturge-Weber syndromes.[737]

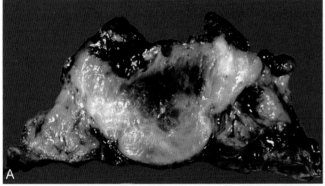

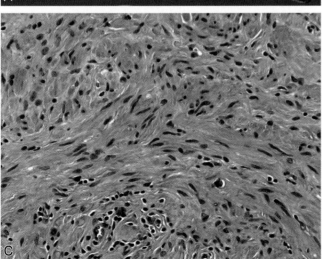

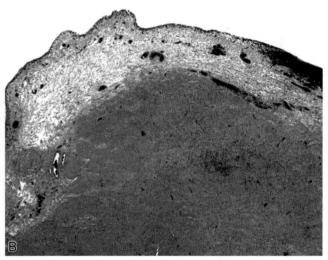

Fig. 6.92 Leiomyoma of the urinary bladder. (A) The tumor is well circumscribed with central hemorrhagic areas. The tumor is composed of intersecting fascicles of benign smooth muscle cells with eosinophilic cytoplasm and cigar-shaped blunt-ended nuclei (B and C).

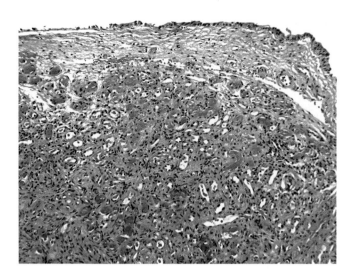

Fig. 6.93 Hemangioma of the urinary bladder, capillary type.

Granular Cell Tumor

Granular cell tumor is rarely seen in the urinary bladder, but reported cases have occurred in adult patients 23 to 70 years of age.[665-669,738] There is no gender predilection.[668] They are usually solitary, well circumscribed, and vary in size up to 12 cm. Histologically, the cells have abundant granular eosinophilic cytoplasm and vesicular nuclei. S100P is invariably expressed in the tumor cells. A congenital granular cell tumor of the gingiva with systemic involvement including urinary bladder has been reported. To date, only one malignant granular cell tumor of the bladder has been described.[738]

Solitary Fibrous Tumors

Solitary fibrous tumor of the urinary bladder occurs in older patients who present with pain or hematuria. Two of the seven reported cases were incidental findings in one study.[739] The tumor is typically a polypoid submucosal mass. Histopathologic features include spindle cells arranged haphazardly in a variably collagenous stroma (Fig. 6.94). Dilated vessels reminiscent of hemangiopericytoma are present.[740] All solitary fibrous tumors of the bladder have had a benign course, although the number of cases is small, and

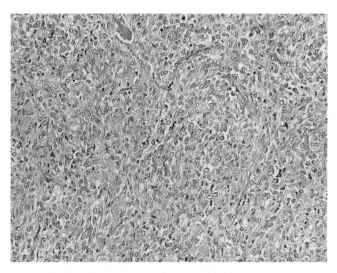

Fig. 6.94 Solitary fibrous tumor of the urinary bladder.

follow-up has been short term in several cases. The proliferating cells typically show CD34 and bcl-2 immunoreactivity. In a recent report of 11 cases of solitary fibrous tumors of the genitourinary tract, these tumors tended to behave aggressively.[741] The *NAB2-STAT6* gene fusion was identified in 64% of cases using a breakapart FISH probe cocktail. However, the *NAB2-STAT6* fusion status was not useful in discriminating between low-risk and high-risk tumors.[741]

Perivascular Epithelioid Cell Tumor

Perivascular epithelioid cell tumors (PEComa) are low-grade mesenchymal tumors composed of histologically and immunohistochemically distinctive perivascular cells.[742-746] The PEComa family consists of entities such as angiomyolipoma, clear cell ("sugar") tumor of the lung, and lymphangioleiomyoma. PEComa have alternatively been termed *clear cell myomelanocytic tumors*.[747] These tumors characteristically exhibit an epithelioid morphology arranged radially around blood vessels and a more spindled morphology distant from the blood vessels, and coexpress muscle and melanocytic immunohistochemical markers (Fig. 6.95). Only a few well-documented examples of this tumor arising primarily in the bladder have been reported.[742,747-750] Patients with the PEComa of the bladder often present with dysuria and hematuria. The mean age at diagnosis is approximately 36 years.

Sukov et al. reported three cases of bladder PEComa.[750] One case showed principally a spindle cell pattern, the second case had principally epithelioid morphology, and the third case demonstrated a mixed pattern. In another report the tumor was described as being composed of epithelioid and occasionally spindled cells, containing abundant cytoplasm that varied from clear to granular and eosinophilic.[748] Nuclei were round and generally uniform; inconspicuous nucleoli and nuclear inclusions were observed. Mitotic figures were rare to absent, and necrosis was not seen.[748] Another tumor exhibited perivascularly arranged cells with granular eosinophilic cytoplasm, round to oval vesicular nuclei, and prominent nucleoli. Focal cytologic atypia and few mitotic figures were identified.[749] Both of these tumors demonstrated intracytoplasmic glycogen in some tumor cells by PAS staining with and without diastase digestion.[748,749] The other tumor, which was designated as a clear cell myomelanocytic tumor, had clear to eosinophilic, epithelioid, and spindle cells arranged in fascicles or packets with delicate vascular stoma among the nests.[747] Interestingly, a normal counterpart to the perivascular epithelioid cell has not been identified in the urinary bladder.

PEComa demonstrate divergent immunoreactivity.[373,742,745,750] Tumor cells may show immunoreactivity to antibodies against melanocytic markers such as HMB45, Melan-A, tyrosinase, and microphthalmia transcription factor, as well as weakly positive immunostaining for myoid markers including smooth muscle actin, smooth muscle myosin heavy chain, desmin, calponin, and CD117. The vasculature is highlighted by reticulin and CD31. The tumor cells typically show no immunostaining for S100P, AE1/AE3, myoglobin, synaptophysin, or chromogranin. Immunoreactivity for vimentin is usually inconspicuous. Interestingly, PEComa are thought to be capable of modulating their immunophenotype according to morphology. For example, a PEComa with prominent spindle cell morphology expresses smooth muscle actin more strongly than HMB45. In contrast, a purely epithelioid PEComa displays HMB45 immunoreactivity and only focal actin positivity. PEComa with spindle cell morphology may display immunoreactivity for progesterone receptors, suggesting a role for this hormone in morphologic and immunophenotypic modulation.

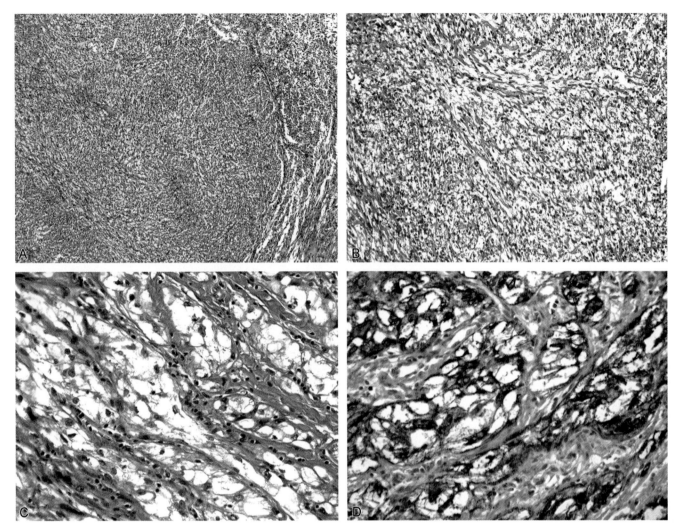

Fig. 6.95 Perivascular epithelioid cell tumor (PEComa) of the urinary bladder. PEComa of the urinary bladder consists of a proliferation of epithelioid cells with fascicular arrangement of cells (A to C). (D) Cells have abundant clear cytoplasm and are HMB-45 immunoreactive.

Pan et al. performed comparative genomic hybridization studies of nine PEComa cases, including one from the urinary bladder.[751,752] All exhibited gross chromosomal aberrations. Frequent imbalances included losses on chromosome 19 (eight cases), 16p (six cases), 17p (six cases), 1p (five cases), and 18p (four cases). Gains were seen on chromosome X (six cases), 12q (six cases), 3q (five cases), 5q (four cases), and 2q (four cases). The single bladder tumor exhibited chromosomal gains at 3p12, 10p15, 12p11.2-p12, and 12q21, and chromosomal loss at 19q13.1. Chromosomal gain on 12q13 to 12q21 has been identified in different types of sarcomas. Although not identified in the bladder PEComa, deletions in chromosome 16p, where the TSC2 gene is located, were frequently identified in such tumors at other sites. These recurrent chromosomal aberrations provide evidence that the PEComa is a distinctive tumor entity at any anatomic location. Recent study suggested that progenitor of renal angiomyolipoma is the lymphatic endothelial cell.[753]

Although PEComa are by far the most common urinary bladder neoplasms in adults, a wide spectrum of soft tissue lesions can occur in the bladder, sometimes creating the false impression of an aggressive urothelial malignancy due to extravesical growth.

In particular, PEComa may generate a broad differential diagnosis at the histopathologic level because of its biphasic light microscopic and immunohistochemical features.[695,724,742,745,750,754,755] Tumors included in the differential diagnoses of PEComa include leiomyoma, leiomyosarcoma, paraganglioma, melanoma, clear cell sarcoma of soft parts, epithelioid sarcoma, PSCN, inflammatory myofibroblastic tumor, sarcomatoid carcinoma, and metastatic carcinoma. Smooth muscle tumor cells are typically more eosinophilic and are not arranged in packets; similarly, they do not typically express melanocytic markers. Primary malignant melanoma is rare in the bladder. It typically develops from the urothelium, is often focally melanotic, and does not demonstrate immunoreactivity for actin. The mixture of spindled and epithelioid morphology in PEComa may also raise consideration of metastatic malignant melanoma, especially in combination with the expression of melanocytic markers. However, in contrast with melanoma, expression of S100P is seen in only a subset of PEComa. Although rare, extragastrointestinal stromal tumor may also show mixed epithelioid and spindled features. Clear cell melanoma is similar to clear cell sarcoma of soft parts. It shares some overlapping histologic features with PEComa, but the thin vascular stroma among tumor nests

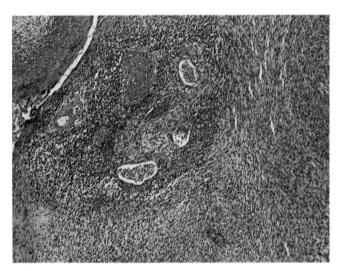

Fig. 6.96 Malignant perivascular epithelioid cell tumor (PEComa) of the urinary bladder.

seen in PEComa is not seen in clear cell sarcoma of soft parts, which instead has nests separated by collagenous avascular stroma. Whereas clear cell sarcoma of soft parts is immunoreactive for HMB45 and S100, it is negative for actin. PSCN and inflammatory myofibroblastic tumor, as well as sarcomatoid carcinoma, can be excluded by reference to their characteristic histologic and immunohistochemical features.[695,742,755]

All reported cases of bladder PEComa have demonstrated indolent biologic behavior, but such tumors occurring at other sites have, in rare instances, behaved in a malignant fashion.[748] We have also seen a case of PEComa that behaved in a malignant fashion (Fig. 6.96).[756] Of the reported cases, no patient had evidence of recurrence at 4 and 6 years.[747,748] Recently, criteria for prediction of malignant behavior in PEComa in general (of all organ sites) have been proposed, including two or more of the following: size greater than 5 cm, infiltrative growth, high cellularity, high nuclear grade, necrosis, vascular invasion, and mitotic rate ≥ 1 per 50 high-power fields. Tumors with only nuclear pleomorphism ("symplastic" features) or size greater than 5 cm are classified as having uncertain malignant potential.[724,742,745,750]

Malignant Soft Tissue Tumors

Leiomyosarcoma

Leiomyosarcoma is the most common malignant mesenchymal tumor of the urinary bladder in adults.[691,692,736,757-759] It is rare, but it has been reported in patients ranging from 15 to 75 years of age; most patients are in the sixth to eighth decade of life. There is male predominance. Some leiomyosarcomas develop several years after the administration of cyclophosphamide. Acrolein, a degradation product of cyclophosphamide, is thought to be the causative agent.[757,759] Patients present with gross hematuria, obstructive voiding symptoms, dysuria, or abdominal mass. Most often the tumor is in the dome of the bladder and less frequently in the lateral walls. Grossly, the tumor is large, unencapsulated, often polypoid with surface ulceration, and exhibits invasive growth involving all layers of the bladder (Fig. 6.97).[759] The cut surface is usually firm or fleshy with a fibrous or myxoid appearance. Some are hemorrhagic, with varying degrees of necrosis. Histologically, interlacing bundles and fascicles of elongated

eosinophilic cytoplasmic processes and spindled to elongated hyperchromatic nuclei are common. High-grade lesions have significant nuclear pleomorphism with hyperchromasia and irregular nuclear membranes. Pleomorphic, vesicular nuclei with macronucleoli and frequent bizarre mitotic figures interspersed with some multinucleate giant cells characterize high-grade lesions. The pleomorphism of high-grade leiomyosarcoma is usually identifiable at low power, along with tumor cell necrosis, increased mitotic activity, and infiltration of the muscularis propria. Grading influences prognosis and is based on the degree of cytologic atypia and mitotic activity. Low-grade leiomyosarcoma has fewer than five mitoses per high-power fields, mild to moderate cytologic atypia, minimal necrosis, and an infiltrative margin.[759] High-grade leiomyosarcoma has more than five mitoses per high-power fields, moderate to marked cytologic atypia, and may show abundant necrosis.

Several morphologic variants including myxoid and epithelioid types have been described. Myxoid leiomyosarcoma may contain moderate numbers of thin-walled blood vessels, and epithelioid leiomyosarcoma has rounded tumor cells, which occasionally exhibit clear and vacuolated cytoplasm.

Immunohistochemically, leiomyosarcomas usually stain positively for vimentin, with variable staining for smooth muscle actin (43% to 100%) and desmin (0% to 60%) (Tables 6.26 and 6.27). Infrequently, they show positive immunostaining with epithelial markers including CK (CAM5.2, AE1/AE3) (10%) and EMA (5%). ALK1 immunostain is usually negative.

Leiomyosarcoma must be differentiated from several other tumors including leiomyoma, sarcomatoid carcinoma, rhabdomyosarcoma, postoperative spindle cell tumor, and pseudosarcomatous myofibroblastic proliferations. Sarcomatoid carcinoma can be recognized if one is aware of a history of a high-grade urothelial carcinoma or of concurrent urothelial in situ or invasive carcinoma. Therefore extensive tissue sampling is recommended before rendering a diagnosis of leiomyosarcoma in the bladder. Sarcomatoid carcinoma is typically immunopositive for low-molecular-weight CK and EMA, and is usually immunonegative for myogenous markers such as desmin and smooth muscle actin, although in rare cases with muscle differentiation, these markers may be diffusely positive.[759] Even though leiomyosarcomas may show CK immunoreactivity, the staining is usually focal and weak. Another differential consideration, rhabdomyosarcoma, may have a myxoid appearance, but this tumor is rare in adults. Features of rhabdomyosarcoma include the presence of cross striations or a cambium layer, as well as positive staining for myogenin. Caldesmon is usually positive in leiomyosarcoma but is usually negative in inflammatory myofibroblastic tumor and rhabdomyosarcoma.[760]

Rhabdomyosarcoma

Rhabdomyosarcoma is infrequently seen in the urinary bladder, and the great majority occur during childhood and adolescence.[670,712,761-768] Only a few cases of bladder rhabdomyosarcoma in adults have been reported.[762] Rhabdomyosarcoma is the most frequent malignant tumor of the bladder in children. There is a slight male predominance. Children with neurofibromatosis type 1 have an increased prevalence of rhabdomyosarcoma with a predominance of bladder or prostate primaries. Although the prognosis in adults is generally poor, significant advances in the treatment of childhood rhabdomyosarcoma have been made, resulting in improved survival with preservation of bladder function. Patients with rhabdomyosarcoma classically present with hematuria; some have obstructive voiding symptoms, and in some

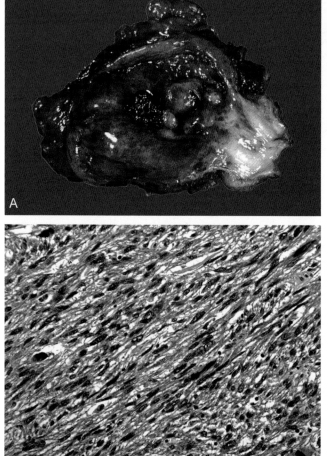

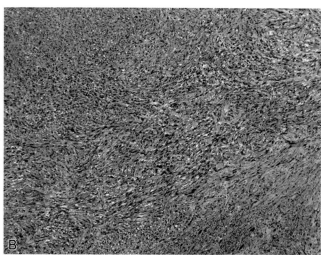

Fig. 6.97 Leiomyosarcoma of the urinary bladder. (A) The tumor is bulky, polypoid, hemorrhagic, and necrotic. It is composed of interwoven fascicles of spindle cells with nuclear pleomorphism, hyperchromasia, and atypical mitotic figures (B and C).

cases an abdominal mass is evident.[769] The most frequent site of involvement is adjacent to the trigone, a feature that essentially precludes the option of partial cystectomy.

Several histologic variants of rhabdomyosarcoma are seen in the bladder, with embryonal type, including the botryoid subtype, being the most common.[761] Grossly, rhabdomyosarcoma, including the sarcoma botryoid variant, appears as a polypoid gelatinous and lobulated mass protruding into bladder lumen with variable hemorrhage and necrosis. The shiny, lobulated, grapelike appearance of the most common type of bladder sarcoma in children is the source of the name *sarcoma botryoid*. Most tumors have a superficial covering epithelium. The botryoid subtype of embryonal rhabdomyosarcoma demonstrates a "cambium" layer, or condensed layer of small, round rhabdomyoblasts under the intact epithelium (Fig. 6.98). The main tumor mass in botryoid rhabdomyosarcoma may be a paucicellular myxoid tumor. These hypocellular areas may be admixed with more cellular areas, especially where the tumor infiltrates deeply into the muscle wall. Histologically, well-differentiated tumor cells (rhabdomyoblasts) have hyperchromatic small nuclei. The cells are small and elongated with frequent cross striations.[761] Less differentiated rhabdomyoblasts have medium or large, irregularly shaped hyperchromatic nuclei with a small rim of cytoplasm and a high mitotic rate. Often, atypical mitotic figures and bizarre cells are seen.[762] A rare variant reported to occur in the bladder is alveolar rhabdomyosarcoma. This sarcoma has closely packed alveolar spaces separated by thin fibrovascular septa lined by a single layer of cuboidal hyperchromatic tumor cells. The polygonal cells lining the fibrovascular septa have a hobnail appearance, with nuclei projecting away from the basement membrane. Tumor cells floating in the alveolar spaces have been described. The solid type of alveolar rhabdomyosarcoma grows in confluent sheets, but the cells are similar to those of the classic pattern.[761] Mixed alveolar and embryonal types occur, and their biologic behavior is similar to that of pure alveolar rhabdomyosarcoma. The botryoid subtype, which tends not to infiltrate deeply into the muscle, is associated with an overall excellent prognosis. Deeply infiltrating embryonal rhabdomyosarcoma and alveolar rhabdomyosarcoma, in contrast, often portend a poor prognosis even with modern multimodality therapy. Immunohistochemical stains of rhabdomyosarcoma usually show positivity for desmin, MyoD1, or myogenin. Also, muscle-specific actin, myoglobin, and myosin may be positive. Rhabdomyoblasts may stain for neuron-specific enolase and infrequently for CK. The alveolar variant has been reported to stain focally with S100. The differential diagnosis of bladder rhabdomyosarcoma includes pseudosarcomatous myofibroblastic tumor, leiomyosarcoma, and neurofibroma and sarcomatoid carcinoma. These tumors can often be distinguished on morphologic grounds.[762] Immunohistochemistry often will point toward skeletal muscle differentiation.

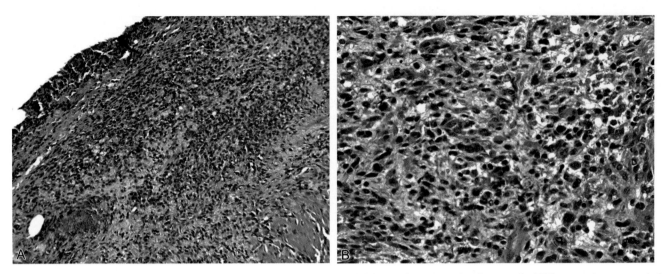

Fig. 6.98 Rhabdomyosarcoma of the urinary bladder. (A) Intact urothelium with underlying cambium layer of malignant cells. (B) The tumor is composed of a mixture of small round to spindle-shaped cells, strap cells, and rhabdomyoblasts, with abundant eosinophilic cytoplasm.

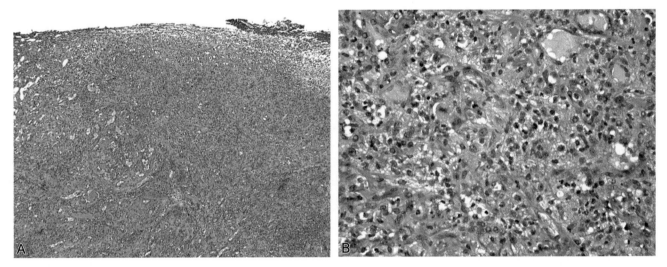

Fig. 6.99 Angiosarcoma of the urinary bladder. (A) The surface epithelium is partially denuded. (B) The tumor is composed of anastomosing vascular channels lined by malignant endothelial cells.

Angiosarcoma

Angiosarcoma of the bladder, which arises from blood vessel endothelium, is rare and carries a poor prognosis.[770-774] Seventy percent of patients die within 2 years of diagnosis. Angiosarcoma can arise in any part of the bladder. The age at presentation ranges from 38 to 85 years.[770] There is a male predominance. The development of angiosarcoma has been linked to certain environmental exposures including vinyl chloride, arsenic, and therapeutic irradiation. All cases have presented with hematuria. Other reported symptoms include flank or groin pain and dysuria. The disease has often extended locally beyond the bladder or metastasized at time of presentation. Frequent sites of metastasis are lung and liver.[770] Histologically, angiosarcoma of the bladder is composed of anastomosing vascular channels lined by atypical endothelial cells (Fig. 6.99). The endothelial cells often are pleomorphic with large hyperchromatic nuclei, prominent nucleoli, and abundant mitotic figures. The vascular lining cells may protrude into the lumen imparting a hobnail appearance. There may be no intervening stroma. The vascular channels range in size from small capillaries to sinusoidal

spaces. A solid growth pattern of monomorphic epithelioid cells with vesicular chromatin and moderate eosinophilic cytoplasm arranged in sheets and nests has been described. Infiltration into the deep muscle layer may be present with either vascular or solid growth patterns. Immunohistochemically, angiosarcoma stains positively for vimentin, CD31, CD34, and ERG. The only reported epithelioid angiosarcoma of the bladder was negative for CK. The differential diagnosis for angiosarcoma of the bladder is hemangioma, which is usually small and lacks cytologic atypia, anastomosing channels, and solid areas. Kaposi sarcoma may be seen in the urinary bladder, especially in immunocompromised patients. The differential diagnosis also includes high-grade urothelial carcinoma.[770]

Undifferentiated Pleomorphic Sarcoma

Primary UPS (previously designated as "malignant fibrous histiocytoma") of the bladder is rare.[270,694,775] It occurs most commonly in men from 45 to 79 years of age, with gross hematuria at time of presentation. The tumor is often large at presentation and involves

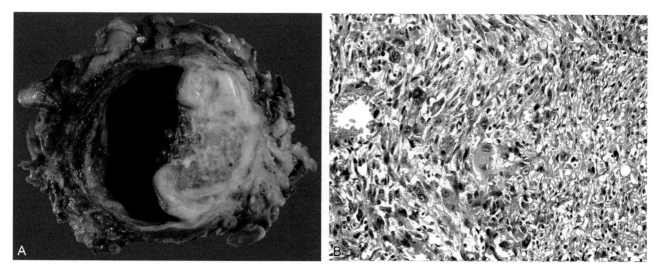

Fig. 6.100 Undifferentiated pleomorphic sarcoma of the urinary bladder. (A) The tumor is fleshy and necrotic, partially filling the lumen. (B) Spindled and pleomorphic cells with nuclear hyperchromasia, admixed with occasional giant cells, are arranged in a storiform and fascicular pattern.

all layers of the bladder wall (Fig. 6.100). The overlying urothelium may be either normal or ulcerated. Four morphologic variants are recognized: myxoid, inflammatory, storiform-fascicular, and pleomorphic types. Histologically, these tumors are composed of spindled or polygonal cells with variably sized oval to round nuclei. The nuclei have coarse chromatin and prominent nucleoli. Mitotic activity is usually moderate to high. Multinucleated giant cells are scattered throughout. Inflammatory-type UPS is characterized by an abundance of inflammatory cells, especially neutrophils infiltrating between fascicles of tumor cells.

Immunohistochemical stains can help differentiate UPS from other spindle cell neoplasms in the bladder. Typically, UPS is nonreactive for CK. It is often reactive for vimentin and α_1-antichymotrypsin and focally reactive for CD68. Some tumors have stained strongly for neuron-specific enolase and S100P.

Several tumors are included in the differential diagnosis of UPS. Sarcomatoid carcinoma of the bladder may have a similar appearance, but an epithelial component immunoreactive to CK and EMA is usually identifiable in sarcomatoid carcinoma. Differentiating UPS from pseudosarcomatous myofibroblastic tumor or PSCN may be difficult. Mixed acute and chronic inflammatory cells and a history of a surgical procedure favors PSCN.

UPS of the bladder is a highly aggressive tumor with a high local recurrence rate and frequent metastasis. Treatment usually is surgical with postoperative chemotherapy and radiation, but no therapy has yet been successful at prolonging survival.

Osteosarcoma

Defined as a malignant tumor showing osteoid production, osteosarcoma of the urinary bladder occurs in male patients 60 to 65 years of age.[776-779] Some have a history of radiation therapy for urothelial carcinoma. Most osteosarcomas arise in the trigone region. Hematuria, dysuria, urinary frequency, and recurrent urinary tract infections are the most common presenting symptoms. Osteosarcoma of the urinary bladder presents as a solitary, large, polypoid, gritty, often deeply invasive, variably hemorrhagic mass. Histologically, tumors are composed of cytologically malignant cells surrounding variably calcified, woven bone lamellae (Fig. 6.101). Foci of chondrosarcomatous differentiation or spindle cell areas may also be observed. The cytologic atypia differentiates

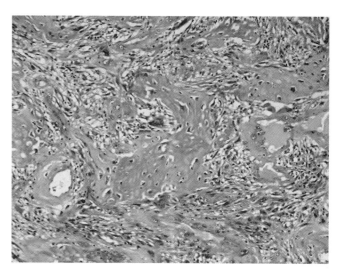

Fig. 6.101 Osteosarcoma of the urinary bladder.

osteosarcoma from stromal osseous metaplasia occurring in some urothelial carcinomas. A recognizable malignant epithelial component is diagnostic of sarcomatoid carcinoma even when osteoid is present. Urothelial sarcomatoid carcinoma is the most important differential diagnostic consideration for osteosarcoma of the bladder. Osteosarcoma of the urinary tract is an aggressive tumor associated with a poor prognosis. Most patients have advanced stage at presentation and die of disease within 6 months, often with lung metastases. The stage of the disease at time of diagnosis is the best predictor of survival.

Other Rare Soft Tissue Tumors Arising in the Bladder

Other malignant mesenchymal neoplasms such as MPNST, liposarcoma, chondrosarcoma, hemangiopericytoma, and Kaposi sarcoma may rarely involve the bladder.[691,692] The diagnosis requires that bladder involvement by direct extension from another site be excluded. In the case of primary chondrosarcoma of the bladder, sarcomatoid carcinoma must be excluded. A rare case of osteoclast-like giant cell tumor of the urinary bladder has been reported in a 73-year-old woman who had recurrence (Fig. 6.102).[780] The tumor

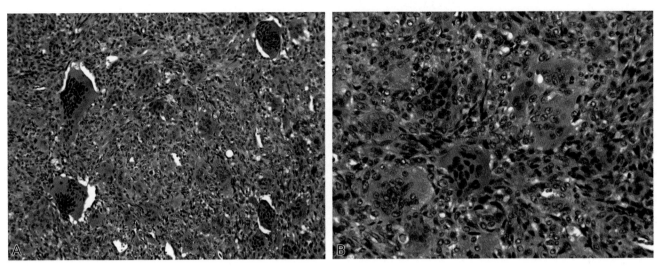

Fig. 6.102 Osteoclast-like giant cell tumor of the urinary bladder (A and B). Numerous osteoclast-like giant cells are seen. This rare tumor histologically resembles its counterpart in the bone and should not be confused with giant cell carcinoma (which falls into the morphologic spectrum of large cell undifferentiated carcinoma). Immunohistochemical stains for CK were negative (not shown).

is morphologically identical to those seen at osseous sites. Immunostaining for CK is negative. A single case report on alveolar soft part sarcoma arising in the bladder has been reported.[781] The tumor showed strong nuclear immunoreactivity for TFE3.

Miscellaneous Tumors

Malignant Melanoma

Malignant melanoma may occur in the urinary bladder as a primary or metastatic tumor. Melanoma primary in the bladder has been reported in fewer than 20 patients.[782,783] All have been adults, with men and women being equally affected. Gross hematuria is the most frequent presenting symptom, but some patients with bladder melanoma have presented with symptomatic metastases. Metastatic melanoma in the bladder is much more common than melanoma primary in the bladder. The generally accepted criteria for determining that melanoma is primary in the bladder are lack of a cutaneous lesion history, failure to find a regressed melanoma of the skin with a Woods lamp examination, failure to find a different visceral primary, and pattern of spread consistent with bladder primary. Almost all the tumors have appeared darkly pigmented at cystoscopy and on gross pathologic examination (Fig. 6.103). Their sizes range from less than 1 to 8 cm. Histologically, the tumors show classic features of malignant melanoma: pleomorphic nuclei, spindle and polygonal cytoplasmic contours, and intracytoplasmic melanin pigment. Pigment production is variable and may be absent. One example of clear cell melanoma has been reported. A few of the tumors are associated with melanosis of the vesical epithelium. One malignant melanoma arose in a bladder diverticulum.

Immunohistochemical procedures have shown positive reactions with antibodies to S100P and with HMB45 or Melan-A, or SOX10. Two-thirds of the patients have died of metastatic melanoma within 3 years of diagnosis. Follow-up of those alive at the time of other reports has been less than 2 years.

Germ Cell Tumors

Several germ cell neoplasms may arise rarely in the bladder, including dermoid cyst, teratoma, seminoma, choriocarcinoma, and yolk sac tumor (Fig. 6.104).[457,458,461,462,775,784-794] Rare cases of teratoma arising in the bladder have been described in both adults and children. Dermoid cyst typically occurs in women between 30 and 49 years of age who present with nonspecific bladder symptoms. Typical histologic features include calcifications and structures consistent with hair and teeth.

Pure choriocarcinoma of the bladder is exceedingly rare and is associated with an aggressive clinical course.[463] Patients usually have symptoms typical of other bladder cancers, including hematuria, dysuria, and frequency. Some male patients may have gynecomastia. Increased urinary levels of β-hCG may be present. Diagnostic features include syncytiotrophoblastic giant cells and cytotrophoblast cells that display β-hCG and glypican 3 immunoreactivity (Fig. 6.105). Choriocarcinoma should not be confused with urothelial carcinoma with syncytiotrophoblastic giant cells (see previous discussion). FISH analysis for isochromosome 12p is diagnostic for germ cell tumors and should be considered before rendering the diagnosis of choriocarcinoma of the bladder. Previously reported cases probably represent urothelial carcinoma with trophoblastic differentiation, rather than true primary choriocarcinoma of the bladder.

The origin of germ cell tumor of the urinary bladder is uncertain. The germinal rests from the urogenital ridge and totipotential cells from the primitive ridge may remain at the urogenital ridge during development of the gonads and undergo subsequent retrodifferentiation into pure germ cell tumor manifestation. In the setting of mixed choriocarcinoma and urothelial carcinoma the choriocarcinoma likely represents a metaplastic variant of urothelial carcinoma. These cases should be classified as urothelial carcinoma with mixed differentiation (trophoblastic differentiation), not true germ cell tumor.

Hematologic Malignancies

Malignant lymphoma may occur in the urinary bladder as a primary lesion or as part of a systemic disease.[795-801] Lymphomas constitute less than 1% of bladder neoplasms. Secondary involvement of the bladder is common (12% to 20%) in advanced stage systemic lymphoma. Bladder lymphomas may form solitary (70%) or multiple (20%) masses at cystoscopy. Occasionally there may be diffuse thickening (10%) of the bladder wall. Ulceration is rare (<20%) in primary lesions but common in secondary lesions.

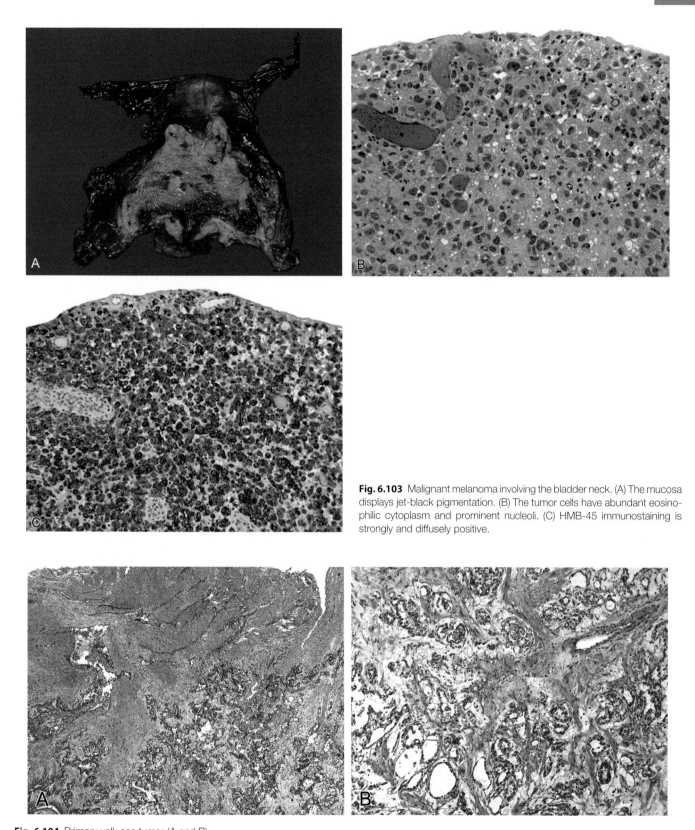

Fig. 6.103 Malignant melanoma involving the bladder neck. (A) The mucosa displays jet-black pigmentation. (B) The tumor cells have abundant eosinophilic cytoplasm and prominent nucleoli. (C) HMB-45 immunostaining is strongly and diffusely positive.

Fig. 6.104 Primary yolk sac tumor (A and B).

Frankly hemorrhagic changes of the mucosa have been observed. The cause of bladder lymphoma remains unclear. Schistosomiasis is associated with a T-cell lymphoma of the bladder. Papillary urothelial tumors may present simultaneously with bladder lymphoma, either primary or secondary. Primary marginal zone B-cell lymphoma of mucosa-associated lymphoid tissue of the bladder

has an excellent prognosis after therapy (Fig. 6.106).[801] Lymphoepithelial lesions may be seen and should not be confused with lymphoepithelioma-like carcinoma or lymphoid-rich variant urothelial carcinoma. Other types of primary bladder lymphoma such as Burkitt lymphoma, T-cell lymphoma, Hodgkin lymphoma, and plasmacytoma are rare. Among secondary bladder

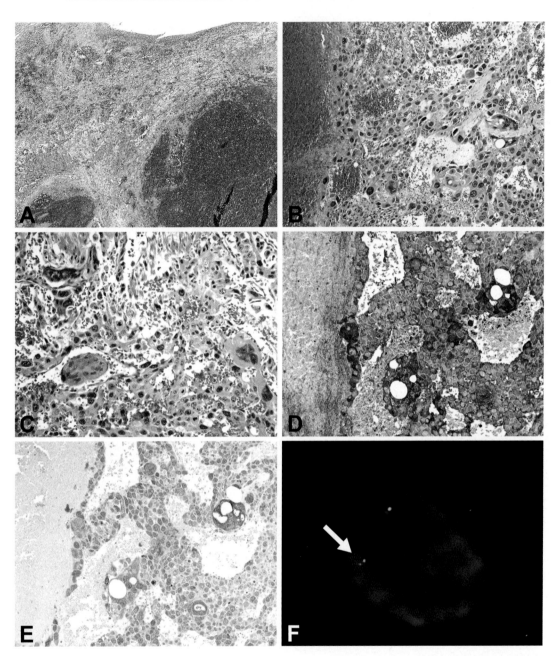

Fig. 6.105 Primary choriocarcinoma of the urinary bladder. Morphologic appearance of bladder choriocarcinoma is identical to those seen in the testis (A to C). (D) β-Human chorionic gonadotropin immunostaining is diffusely positive. (E) Glypican 3 staining is also positive in tumor cells. (F) The *arrow* points to the presence of isochromosome 12p, a genetic hallmark of germ cell tumor.

lymphomas, diffuse large B-cell lymphoma is the single most frequent histologic subtype, followed by follicular, small cell, low-grade mucosa-associated lymphoid tissue, mantle cell, Burkitt, and Hodgkin lymphoma. Involvement of the urinary bladder by acute myeloid leukemia (granulocytic sarcoma or myeloid sarcoma) is rare, and relevant clinical data and high index of suspicion are critical to avoid misdiagnosis (Fig. 6.107).[802-804]

Metastatic Tumors and Secondary Extension

The urinary bladder is secondarily involved by a wide spectrum of malignancies. The most common primary sites and their relative frequencies include colon (Fig. 6.108) (21%), prostate

(Fig. 6.109) (19%), rectum (12%), and cervix (11%).[805] Most tumors from these sites involve the bladder by direct extension. The most common distant sites of origin of tumors metastatic to the bladder and their relative frequencies are stomach (4.3%), skin (3.9%), lung (2.8%), and breast (2.5%). Secondary tumor deposits are almost always solitary (96.7%), and 54% of these are in the bladder neck or trigone. More than one-half of secondary tumors are adenocarcinomas. In terms of differential diagnosis, few secondary tumors have distinctive histologic features, making it difficult to make the appropriate diagnosis. Hence knowledge of the history and clinical setting are particularly important in these cases. Immunohistochemistry is useful for distinguishing primary tumors of the urinary bladder from metastases or direct extension from other sites.[105,806]

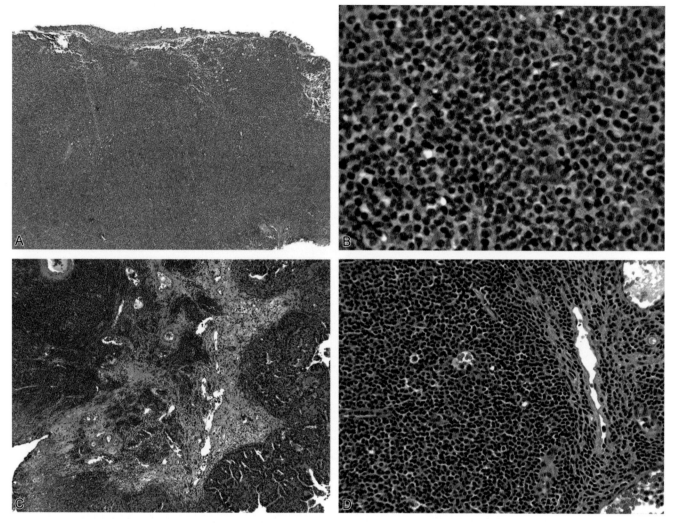

Fig. 6.106 Lymphoma involving the urinary bladder. Primary marginal zone B-cell lymphoma of mucosa-associated lymphoid tissue (A and B). The surface epithelium is largely intact. The tumor is composed of diffuse sheets of small- to medium-size lymphoid cells with pale cytoplasm. A case of coexisting small lymphocytic lymphoma and transitional cell (urothelial) carcinoma (C and D).

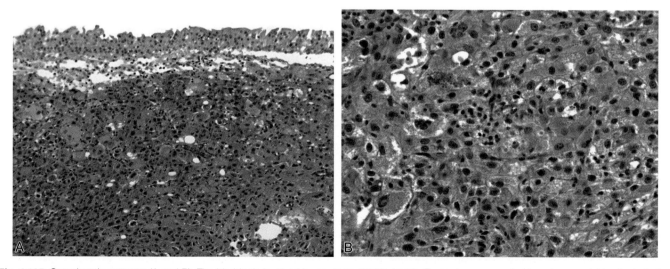

Fig. 6.107 Granulocytic sarcoma (A and B). The bladder is involved by acute myeloid leukemia. Tumor is composed of immature myeloid cells, including promyelocytes and myeloblasts.

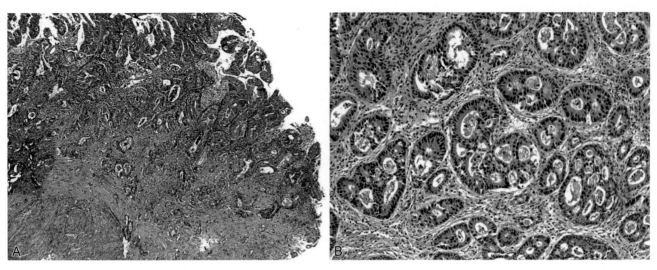

Fig. 6.108 Metastatic colonic adenocarcinoma involving the urinary bladder (A and B).

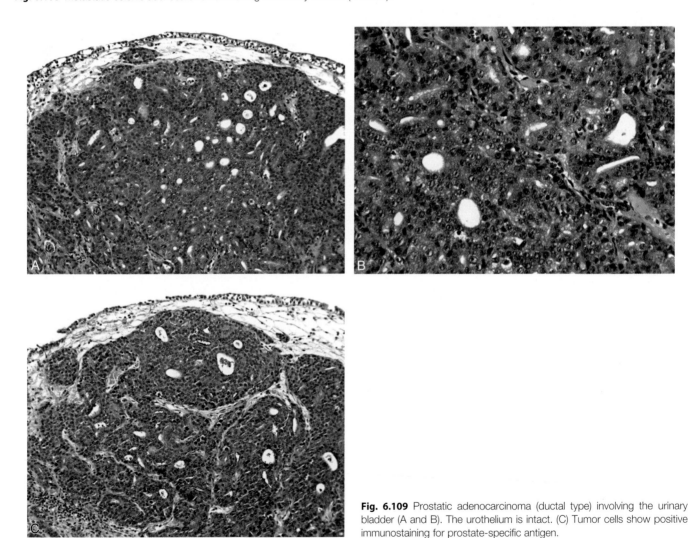

Fig. 6.109 Prostatic adenocarcinoma (ductal type) involving the urinary bladder (A and B). The urothelium is intact. (C) Tumor cells show positive immunostaining for prostate-specific antigen.

Prostatic adenocarcinomas invading the bladder are typically positive for PSA and prostate-specific acid phosphatase. Androgen receptor and PSMA are less specific for prostate lineage determination. The two markers that are more sensitive than PSA and are just as specific are NKX3.1 and P501S (prostein). GATA3 is probably the best marker for urothelial origin and is strongly and diffusely positive in more than 50% of cells in urothelial carcinoma. Rare prostate carcinoma cases can be focally and weakly positive for GATA3. It should be noted that prostatic basal cells often stain for GATA3.

Colorectal adenocarcinoma may infiltrate the bladder directly or as discontinuous metastasis. Intestinal markers such as CDX2 and villin may be expressed also by bladder tumors and therefore are of limited value. As mentioned earlier in this chapter, diffuse nuclear β-catenin expression is highly suggestive of colon primary. Nuclear positivity is rare and focal in primary bladder adenocarcinoma. Most bladder adenocarcinomas express CK7 and CK20, in contrast with colon adenocarcinoma, which is often CK7⁻ and CK20⁺.

Metastatic Urothelial Carcinoma

When urothelial carcinoma presents at other sites, recognition of urothelial origin may be difficult, particularly because squamous and glandular differentiation are common in high-grade urothelial carcinoma (Fig. 6.110).[371,380] Differential CK expression may be of value in the confirmation of metastatic urothelial carcinoma.[373,807-812] Urothelial carcinomas are usually positive for high-molecular-weight CK (34βE12), thrombomodulin, p63, p40, GATA3, uroplakins 2 and 3, and S100P. Expression of the combination of thrombomodulin, high-molecular-weight CK (34βE12), and CK20 is strongly suggestive of urothelial origin in the setting of metastatic carcinoma of unknown primary, whereas the expression of two of these three is still suggestive, albeit more weakly.[811] Expression of uroplakins 2 and 3 is highly specific for tumors of urothelial origin.[811,813-815] GATA3 and S100P are other biomarkers that are helpful for establishing urothelial origin.[816-820]

Ovarian Brenner tumors, which histologically resemble urothelial neoplasms, may stain with uroplakin 3 and therefore may be included as a possible alternate primary site for uroplakin 3⁺ metastatic carcinomas in female patients.[813,815] Some immunophenotypic differences between Brenner tumors and urothelial carcinomas of the bladder do exist. Urothelial carcinomas are frequently positive for thrombomodulin and CK20, whereas Brenner tumors typically do not stain with these antibodies.[821] Ovarian transitional cell carcinomas rarely (6%) express uroplakin 3 and typically have a uroplakin 3⁻/CK20⁻/WT1⁺ phenotype in contrast with the uroplakin 3⁺ phenotype observed in 82% of Brenner tumors.[815] In fact the differences in staining with uroplakin 3 and other markers suggest that Brenner tumors are the only true urothelial neoplasms of the ovary, with ovarian transitional cell carcinomas representing a pattern of poorly differentiated adenocarcinoma.[822,823] Both benign and malignant Brenner tumors lack TERT promoter mutations, commonly seen in urothelial carcinoma.[824]

References are available at expertconsult.com

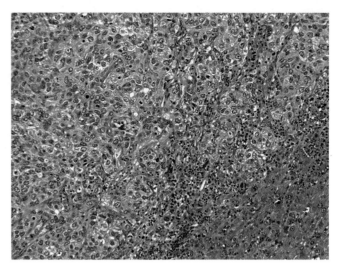

Fig. 6.110 Metastatic urothelial carcinoma involving the liver.

7

Urine Cytology

DAVID G. BOSTWICK

CHAPTER OUTLINE

Introduction

Examination of urine is one of the oldest medical tests, used by Samarians, Babylonians, Egyptians, Indians, and Greeks in their traditional medicine. It was not until after Papanicolaou and Marshall published the first article in 1945 that urine cytology was used to detect urothelial carcinoma.[1] Subsequently, Koss, Melamed, and colleagues characterized urine cytology and histology in 1960.[2-5] Numerous classification systems have been introduced, and those before 2013 are nicely reviewed by Owens et al.[6]

The greatest contemporary issues with urine cytology are low sensitivity detection of low-grade cancer, poor interobserver agreement (especially with atypia), and lack of standardized diagnostic criteria. Recent efforts described in this chapter offer great promise in resolving these concerns.

This chapter discusses the spectrum of cytologic abnormalities in voided urine samples and washings to allow comparison with biopsy findings described in Chapters 5 and 6, and presents classifications published after the last edition of this text. The clinically significant and common problem of hematuria is also addressed from the perspective of the cytopathologist.

Utility of Urine Cytology

Indications

Cytologic examination of the urine sediment is of value in the diagnosis of a wide variety of benign and malignant diseases of the bladder, urethra, ureter, and kidney.[7-10] The chief indications for the use of cytology in disorders of the urinary tract include:

1. Screening and diagnosis of carcinoma in situ and high-grade carcinoma
2. Follow-up of patients with atypical cytology evaluation or urothelial tumor, regardless of grade
3. Monitoring of patients with urothelial tumor undergoing or after treatment, including active surveillance[8,11,12]
4. Evaluation of hematuria, including separation of kidney (upper tract disease) and nonkidney (lower tract) causes

Sources

The sources of urologic cytology specimens include voided urine, catheterized urine, bladder washing (barbotage), brushing, ureteral and renal pelvic brushing and washing, and neobladder urine from an ileal conduit or colonic pouch.[13,14] Initial morning first-void urine includes exfoliated cells, debris, and impurities that have collected in the urinary tract and urethral opening during the night, and may optimize yield of potential pathogens such as human papillomavirus.[15,16] Ureteral washings and other instrumented specimens require caution because they may produce artifactually clustered urothelium.[17]

The specimen source is critically important for diagnosis. For example, upper urinary tract washings were superior to voided samples in detection of upper tract high-grade carcinoma (90% versus 50% yield, respectively).[18] Similarly, urinary diversion cytology specimens from patients who undergo radical cystectomy are often submitted for screening for recurrent urothelial carcinoma, and those with carcinoma (2% to 6% incidence rate) revealed scant, well-preserved urothelial cells either alone or in clusters with high-grade features, including eccentrically located, enlarged, hyperchromatic nuclei; irregular nuclear borders; and high nuclear-to-cytoplasmic (N/C) ratios, often with an inflammatory background.[19,20] The sensitivity, specificity, positive predictive value, and negative predictive value of cytology for high-grade carcinoma in diversion remnants were 82%, 97%, 75%, and 98%, respectively; 21% of patients with atypia were eventually diagnosed with carcinoma.[21] In another study, bladder washing specimens were more predictive of high-grade cancer than voided urine specimens.[22]

Specimen Adequacy

Adequacy is a reflection of how representative the specimen is based chiefly on cellularity, although the presence of obscuring elements is also important.[23] Regardless of the specimen type (voided urine or instrumented), an unsatisfactory or inadequate specimen is one that is poorly cellular, completely obscured, or predominantly degenerate. Obscuring elements include neutrophils, lubricants, other foreign debris, crystals, bacteria, squames, and spermatozoa. Conversely, according to one group, if there are any atypical cells, regardless of the overall cellularity, this represents a satisfactory specimen.[24] Brief exposure to contrast agents does not influence adequacy; thus, contrast washings of the urinary tract can be sent for cytologic diagnosis if fixed within a short time.[25]

Inadequate voided specimens were defined by Bastacky et al. and the Papanicolaou Society of Cytopathology as those that contained fewer than 15 intermediate or basal urothelial cells, obscuring blood or inflammation, or poor cellular preservation.[26,27] Prather et al. defined adequacy as the presence of a total of 2600 cells or 20 urothelial cells in 10 consecutive high-power fields (hpf) in instrumented urine specimens processed using the ThinPrep method.[28] The Paris System 2013 included a category of unsatisfactory/nondiagnostic, but provided no qualifications for different specimen sources (voided, instrumented) and preparation types.[29]

Adequacy is based on multiple features, including: (1) volume, (2) collection method, (3) processing method, (4) underlying patient condition, (5) operator-dependent factors, and (6) logistic factors. Volume is an important determinant of adequacy of voided urine specimens. Adequacy increased linearly for each increment of urine volume submitted to the laboratory up to 30 mL, after which the correlation was nonlinear, and low-volume specimens were less likely to harbor suspicious or malignant cells.[23] Collection methods are also significantly associated with specimen adequacy and cellularity.[30] Comparison of voided urine and bladder washings revealed concordance in more than 99% of cases, indicating

equivalence of these collection techniques.[31] Conversely, in a series of patients with biopsy-proven low-grade carcinoma on follow-up, 56% of urine cytology specimens demonstrated atypical features, including the presence of tissue fragments, cytoplasmic tails, and eccentric and enlarged nuclei, and these features were significantly more common in washings than in voided urine specimens.[32]

Contemporary processing methods include conventional cytospin, Meiers improved filter method, ThinPrep, and SurePath methods (Table 7.1); direct smear has been largely abandoned. The cytospin method was superior to direct smear, Thin Prep, and SurePath in a comparative study of voided urine specimens; the rate of unsatisfactory preparations was quite low (0.30%), and the overall sensitivity, specificity, and positive and negative predictive values for urothelial carcinoma were 0.72, 0.92, 0.97, and 0.46, respectively.[33] Cytospin was also superior to ThinPrep for evaluation of nuclear detail and background material in specimens with nonurothelial malignancies.[34] Conversely, Kim and Kim found similar sensitivity and specificity for cytospin and ThinPrep in a large series of bladder washings (61% versus 60% and 95% versus 95%, respectively).[35] Metaanalysis showed that there was similar sensitivity with cytospin and liquid-based cytology methods.[36] Using the Paris System 2013, cytospin and ThinPrep had similar sensitivity and specificity for the diagnosis of suspicious or high-grade urothelial carcinoma.[37] The filter method was superior to cytospin by decreasing the number of false-negative cases because of higher cellularity and improved detection of atypical or malignant epithelial cells.[38] ThinPrep increased the number of nonatypical urothelial cell clusters compared with cytospin (13% to 21% versus 7%, respectively).[39]

The patient's underlying condition and his or her indication for cytologic evaluation influences specimen adequacy. Increased cellularity is observed in specimens from patients with cancer, calculi, or infection compared with those with only hematuria or irritative voiding symptoms.[29] Other adequacy factors include level of hydration, micturition before specimen acquisition, the use of diuretics or other medications, the presence of obstructive conditions such as benign prostatic hyperplasia, with consequent reduction of bladder capacity, and medical problems resulting in oliguria.

Operator-dependent factors refer to expertise of the examiner and the potential for human bias and error. Logistic factors that influence adequacy include length of time from collection to processing, container leakage with potential drying artifacts, and many others.

Reporting and Classification

Several reporting and classification systems for urine cytology have been published, each of which has relative strengths and weaknesses. Unlike cervical cytology, there has not been widespread acceptance and use of any single reporting system for urine cytology studies. Thus, terminology and criteria for urine cytology reporting are not uniform among pathologists.[6] The major diagnostic categories that we use at our laboratory are presented in Table 7.2.

Recently two international consensus conferences published their classifications: the Paris System 2013 and the International Consultation on Urologic Disease–European Association of Urology 2015 (Table 7.2). Both were based on expert consensus by small, self-selected academic groups with minimal input from other cytopathologists, urologists, oncologists, or others.

TABLE 7.1	Comparison of Processing Methods of Urine Cytology Processing
Method	**Description**
Cytospin smear (two-step centrifugation/fixation method)	Urine samples are sedimented at 700 *g* for 10 minutes. The supernatant is removed to within approximately 1-2 mL of the cell pellet, and the pellet is then resuspended and rinsed with 10 mL of hypotonic solution (0.075 M potassium chloride) for 10 minutes. The cells are resedimented at 600 *g* for 10 minutes, and the supernatant is removed to within 0.5 mL of the pellet. The pellet is then gently vortexed and resuspended in 10 mL 3:1 methanol/glacial acetic acid fixative. Fixed specimens are left at room temperature for 30 minutes. The urinary cells are then sedimented at 600 *g* for 5 minutes, aspirated, and transferred to a 2-mL microfuge tube. The final cell pellet is left in approximately 100-500 μL of residual methanol/glacial acetic acid fixative, depending on the size of the cell pellet. A total of 10 μL of cell sediment is placed on the slide, and the specimen is allowed to dry.[261]
Meiers improved filter method	Urine samples are fixed in ethanol and drawn up into a 60-mL syringe threaded with a Luer lock tip. An 8.0-μM filter mounted in a filter holder is subsequently attached to the syringe tip. The urine sample is then pushed gently through the filter until complete. The membrane filter is placed on a positively charged glass slide. Gauze is placed over the membrane and slight pressure applied with the palm of the hand to transfer the cell filtrate. The cell filtrate is placed on a slide in a manner similar to Cytospin. The membrane is discarded and the filter holder was deposited in a 10% bleach solution overnight until next use.[261]
ThinPrep (Hologic, Bedford, MA)	ThinPrep test is performed with a proprietary automated liquid-based monolayer cell preparation system. Urine samples are immersed in a buffered preservative solution, transferred to a bowl, and a cylinder with a filtration membrane is then placed in the bowl to ensure that the cells are homogeneously distributed. Using negative pressure, the erythrocytes and mucus penetrate the filtration membrane, leaving only the filtration membranes for the diagnostic procedure. This maneuver is repeated until an appropriate number of cells (2000-50,000) is collected. Thereafter the cylinder is removed from the bowl; cells left on the filtration membrane are attached to the slide and then fixed in 95% alcohol.
SurePath (BD Diagnostics, Burlington, NC)	The SurePath test is performed with a proprietary liquid-based monolayer cell preparation system density gradient-based cell enrichment. Urine samples are immersed in ethanolic preservative solution and a device is placed into the vial to ensure that cells are homogenously distributed. A polysaccharide-based density gradient reagent is used to filter debris, centrifuged, resuspended, and centrifuged again. The PrepStain processor creates and stains the slides.

It should be noted that evidence-based guidelines have supplanted such expert panels and simple consensus conference-based conclusions, and are now considered to be the contemporary standard for defining the practice of medicine; thus it is surprising that these recent efforts failed to abide by even the most basic tenets of evidence-based medicine, instead resorting to "biology by democracy." All proper methods of systematic review and guideline generation share certain core concepts, including careful selection of the guideline topic, thorough structured review of the evidence with grading and synthesis, creation of recommendations, consultation and peer review, dissemination and implementation, revision, and updating. According to the U.S. Agency for Healthcare Research and Quality, three key principles are required for successful conduct of systematic reviews: (1) the review must be relevant and timely, focusing on the most important issues and the optimal time to initiate a review; (2) the review must be objective and scientifically rigorous, free from conflicts of interest; and (3) the review must include public participation and transparency to ensure confidence and credibility, and provide for accountability.[40] Thus the recent cytopathology consensus statements should be considered below the standards of current practice of evidence-based medicine. Nonetheless, any efforts to create standardized terminology are laudable and generate renewed interest in refinement of diagnostic criteria, continuing the work of the Papanicolaou Society at creation of uniformity in cytopathology practice.[27]

In Paris System 2013, the recommended diagnostic words are also problematic. The words "negative for high-grade urothelial carcinoma" on a report could easily be mistyped or misinterpreted by the transcriptionist, cytopathologist, or urologist if the word *negative* is overlooked while the word *carcinoma* registers,

potentially resulting in serious consequences for the patient. Reasonable alternatives include "negative for high-grade malignancy," "negative for high-grade neoplasia," and "no definite evidence of malignancy."

The Paris System 2013

The Paris System 2013 focused chiefly on accuracy of identification of high-grade carcinoma, requiring five criteria for a definitive diagnosis: at least 5 malignant cells (10 cells for upper tract cancer), elevated N/C ratio (≥ 0.7), markedly atypical nuclear borders, moderate to severe hyperchromasia, and coarse chromatin (Tables 7.2 and 7.3). However, malignant specimens often contain degenerative changes, and this may limit the number of diagnostic cells; consequently, about half of positive cases failed to fulfill this criterion in a report from Johns Hopkins University.[41] Furthermore less than 20% of cells present in positive specimens fulfilled all five of the criteria. The second most restrictive criterion, N/C ratio ≥ 0.7, was present in only 78% of positive specimens. Nonetheless, the Paris System 2013 upgraded about 40% of indeterminate specimens and did not change the frequency of diagnosis of high-grade carcinoma.[41]

N/C ratio is a critical component of the Paris System, but just how reliable is it? Hang et al. confirmed the importance of the ≥ 0.5 cut point for the diagnosis of atypical urothelial cells using digital image analysis; receiver operating characteristic analysis demonstrated that the maximum N/C ratio alone was highly predictive of high-grade carcinoma on follow-up (area under the curve [AUC], 79%), with a sensitivity of 73% and a specificity of 85%.[42] However, visual quantitation of N/C ratio showed only a fair

TABLE 7.2   Comparison of Cytologic Diagnostic Categories in Urine Sediment

Bostwick Laboratories System (2018)[a]	Paris System for Reporting Urine Cytology (2013)[24]	International Consultation on Urologic Disease–European Association of Urology (2015)[262,b]	Recommended Diagnostic Response[c]
Nondiagnostic	Nondiagnostic	Nondiagnostic	Repeat within 3 months
Negative	Negative for high-grade urothelial carcinoma	Negative for epithelial cell abnormality	Clinical follow-up as needed
Atypical	Atypical urothelial cells	Atypical urothelial cells of undetermined significance	Clinical follow-up; consider ancillary tests
Suspicious	Low-grade urothelial neoplasm[d]	Low-grade urothelial carcinoma	Cystoscopy and biopsy
	Suspicious for high-grade urothelial carcinoma	Atypical urothelial cells, cannot rule out high-grade urothelial carcinoma	Cystoscopy and biopsy
Malignant cells present	High-grade urothelial carcinoma	High-grade urothelial carcinoma	Cystoscopy and biopsy
Other (specify)	Others: primary and secondary malignancies and miscellaneous lesions	Other (specify)	Cystoscopy and biopsy, depending on specificity of findings

[a]Expanded terminology: These are the templated words that appear on the Bostwick Laboratories' reports.
Nontumor-associated cytology:
- Normal cells/negative for malignant cells
- Inflammatory changes: specific type or nonspecific

Tumor-associated cytology:
- Rare single cells and clusters of mildly to moderately atypical urothelial cells; this may represent a reactive process, but neoplasm should be considered; clinical correlation is indicated
- Rare highly atypical urothelial cells suspicious for neoplasm; reactive process cannot be excluded; repeat study and/or further investigation may be of value
- Severely atypical urothelial cells highly suspicious for neoplasm; clinical correlation is recommended
- Malignant cells present most suggestive of urothelial carcinoma
- Malignant cells present (specify squamous cell carcinoma, adenocarcinoma, prostatic adenocarcinoma, renal cell carcinoma, other)
- Malignant cells present, not otherwise specified

[b]Modified from Amin et al.[262]
[c]Modified from Barkan et al.[24]
[d]In the Paris System, the presence of fibrovascular cores is rare and is the only instance in which the diagnosis of low-grade urothelial neoplasm in instrumented urine can be made. Low-grade urothelial neoplasm should be used sparingly and in conjunction with the negative category to clarify the absence of high-grade carcinoma in the Paris System. In the Bostwick Laboratories classification, the presence of fibrovascular cores is considered suspicious.

TABLE 7.3   Comparison of Morphologic Criteria of Abnormal Cells in the Paris System 2013 for Reporting Urinary Cytology Category

Category	Nuclear-to-Cytoplasmic Ratio (Feature 1)	Nuclear Chromasia (Feature 2)	Chromatinic Rim/Nuclear Membrane (Feature 3)	Chromatin Quality (Feature 4)	Mandatory (Major) Features	Minor Features
Atypical urothelial cells[a]	>0.5	Similar to umbrella cells or dark/very dark[a]	Fine and even or uneven shape and thickness[a]	Finely granular or coarsely clumped[a]	1	2-4 (one of the features) 2-4 noted with footnote "a" must be second features identified in the cells of interest in addition to 1
Suspicious[b] and high-grade urothelial carcinoma[b]	>0.7	Very dark	Uneven shape and thickness	Coarsely clumped	1, 2	3, 4 (at least one of the above must be a third feature identified)

[a]Only one minor feature required.
[b]Only difference is the cellular quantity: suspicious, very few cells; high-grade carcinoma, 5-10 cells or more.
Modified from Barkan GA, Wojcik EM, Nayar R, et al. The Paris System for reporting urinary cytology: the quest to develop a standardized terminology. *Acta Cytol* 2016;60:185-97.

correlation with actual N/C ratio, with correlation decreasing with increasing N/C ratio.[43] In the critical range, N/C ratio of 0.5 to 0.7, interobserver correlation (75%), and correlation with true N/C ratio (53%) may be insufficiently accurate for precise category assignment in the Paris System.

Compared with previous classification systems, the Paris System 2013 resulted in a great increase in the rate of "atypical" cases while improving sensitivity but lowering specificity. Granados et al.

found that the incidence of "atypical" increased from 3% to 24% in benign cases, from 2.5% to 25% in low-grade carcinoma, and from 6.6% to 16% in high-grade carcinoma.[39] The false-positive rate (abnormal cytology in negative or low-grade carcinoma cases) increased from 11% to 34%. Sensitivity was higher (63% versus 49%) at the expense of lower specificity (73% versus 91%). The agreement between prior classification and Paris System 2013 was moderate for negative and high-grade carcinoma cases (κ = 0.42 and 0.56, respectively) and weak for low-grade tumors (κ = 0.35). Conversely, Hassan et al. found fewer cases were diagnosed as "atypical" with the Paris System compared with their original diagnoses (26% versus 39%), whereas the correlation of "atypical" with subsequent high-grade cancer increased from 33% to 53%.[44] The new system also resulted in a higher number of low-grade carcinomas diagnosed as "negative" (40%) rather than "atypical" (22%). In another study, 70% of cases of "atypical" cases were reclassified by Paris System 2013 as "negative"; however, 18% of these were found to have high-grade cancer.[45] The sensitivity and specificity of fluorescence in situ hybridization (FISH) with Paris System 2013 were 86% and 33%, respectively, in the "atypical" group and 63% and 100%, respectively, in the "negative" group.

The category of "atypical urothelial cells" no longer includes cellular changes attributed to the BK polyomavirus cytopathic effect, according to the Paris System 2013. Reclassification of such cases as "negative" decreased the rate of "atypical" from 25% to 21%, although the high rate of subsequent "high-grade cancer" among nonsurveillance patients suggested that the reclassification may be "inappropriate."[46]

In Paris System 2013, nonatypical urothelial cell groups are classified as "negative for high-grade carcinoma" except in cases that display fibrovascular cores that are now diagnosed as "low-grade urothelial neoplasm." However, because of the correlation of nonatypical urothelial cells with high-grade carcinoma (high specificity and negative predictive value [87.1% and 94%, respectively]) despite low sensitivity (30.4%), Granados et al. concluded that the presence of nonatypical urothelial cell clusters in voided urine (even without fibrovascular cores) should not be diagnosed as "negative."[39]

The predictive values of "suspicious" and "high-grade carcinoma" diagnoses were unchanged (94% each) after reclassification with Paris System 2013 despite the new exclusion criterion of cellular degeneration for "suspicious."[44] Joudi et al.[22] found that "high-grade carcinoma" with the Paris System 2013 yielded a higher predictive value for carcinoma than the cytologic diagnosis of "suspicious" (79% versus 55%, respectively), similar to results with the Bostwick Laboratories Classification (74% versus 54%, respectively).[22,47]

Addition of anisonucleosis and India ink nuclei (but not tumor diathesis, ragged edge of urothelial cells, apoptotic bodies, or pleomorphism) significantly improved the predictive accuracy of the Paris System 2013 according to Suh et al.[48] With their modification the reporting rate of "atypical" decreased from 25% in their original system to 15% in Paris System 2013 and 11% in Suh's proposed modification; likewise, sensitivity increased from 59% to 71% and 90.0%, respectively.[48]

Interobserver agreement with the Paris System 2013 was adequate for the category of "negative for high-grade carcinoma," but not for the other categories, with mean absolute agreement of 65% and a mean expected agreement of 44%; the mean chance-corrected agreement (κ) was only 0.32.[49] Approximately 15% of disagreements were classified as high clinical impact. The authors concluded that this low level of diagnostic precision may negatively impact the applicability of Paris System 2013 for widespread clinical application.

Normal Components of the Urinary Sediment

The most common cellular elements are benign superficial urothelial cells, followed by intermediate and basal urothelial cells that are more commonly observed in instrumented specimens. Superficial squamous cells from the female genital tract often outnumber urothelial cells. Benign glandular cells (from cystitis glandularis), squamous cells originating in squamous metaplasia of urothelium or external genital tract skin, and, rarely, benign seminal vesical cells also fall into this category. Clusters or fragments of urothelial cells that may be seen in both instrumented and noninstrumented urine specimens should be classified as "negative" unless the cytomorphology of the cells forming the group fulfills the criteria for "atypical." Similarly, changes associated with urolithiasis, treatment-related changes, and polyomavirus cytopathic changes should all be classified as "negative," according to Paris System 2013.

Urothelial cells are the most variably sized cells in the urinary sediment, ranging from 20 μm in diameter for intermediate and basal cells up to 100 μm for typical "umbrella" or superficial cells. Urothelial cells typically have single round to oval nuclei with abundant, homogenous, predominately basophilic cytoplasm. Cells from the basal urothelium are smaller, round, and display well-defined thickened cytoplasmic membranes. Chromocenters and multiple eosinophilic micronucleoli may be prominent, especially in cases with accompanying inflammation.

Fragments of urothelial cells are commonly found in catheterized specimens, as well as bladder washes; however, it is abnormal to see urothelial fragments in spontaneously voided urine, and their presence may be associated with papilloma or low-grade urothelial cancer. Occasionally large urothelial fragments may display cytoplasmic vacuoles containing neutrophils. Multinucleation, nuclear enlargement, and hyperchromasia can be found in inflammatory processes within the lower urinary tract.

Superficial (Umbrella) Cells

Regardless of the type of sample and collection technique used, superficial urothelial cells are a common component of the urine sediment. These cells have one or more nuclei that are large, measuring up to 3 μm in diameter, comparable with superficial squamous cells (Fig. 7.1A).[8] Binucleate and multinucleate cells are common. Such cells are often larger than the mononucleate superficial cells, and their nuclei are somewhat smaller. Large multinucleate superficial cells are by far the most striking component of the urinary sediment, particularly in washings or brushings of the bladder or ureter. Multinucleate superficial cells are particularly large and may be mistaken for giant cells. A potential error in diagnosis is misinterpretation of large superficial cells as macrophages or tumor cells. The DNA content of superficial cells may be polypoid.[50,51]

The chromatinic rim of the nucleus is thick and sharply demarcated. The chromatin is finely granular, often with a "salt and pepper" appearance, and may contain one or more prominent chromocenters. The structure of the nucleus is better preserved in bladder washings than in voided urine. In women there may be a sex chromatin body attached to the nuclear membrane. The cytoplasm of these cells is usually basophilic, often finely granular, and sometimes vacuolated. The cell border is convex (luminal) and concave (deep).

Cells Originating From the Deeper Layers of the Urothelium

All other urothelial cells are smaller than the superficial cells, and often exfoliate in clusters, particularly in instrumented specimens. Single small urothelial cells are observed in voided urine. Clusters

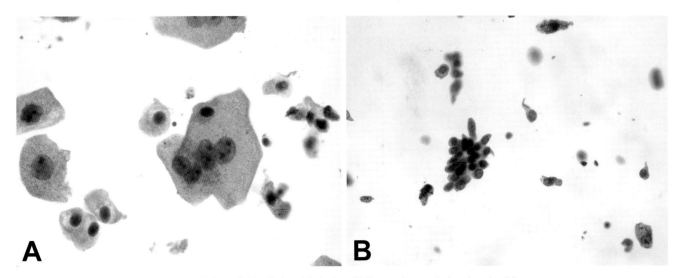

Fig. 7.1 Normal superficial (umbrella) cells. (A) Superficial cells in voided urine. (B) Deeper layer cells (parabasal cells).

of urothelial cells may be tightly packed and assume spherical "pseudopapillary" configurations with sharp borders. Such clusters are often misinterpreted as low-grade papillary carcinoma.[52,53] When deep (basal) cells are removed by instrument, they often appear in loose clusters. These cells are polygonal or elongate, sometimes columnar, and almost always display cytoplasmic extensions in contact with other cells. The amount of basophilic cytoplasm in such cells depends on the layer of origin and is more abundant in cells derived from upper layers. Single cells resemble parabasal squamous cells in size and configuration. These cells are often spherical or round, particularly in voided urine, but may also show cytoplasmic extensions.[8] The nuclei of the smaller urothelial cells are approximately the same size, measuring about 2 to 5 μm in diameter (Fig. 7.1B). They are usually finely granular and benign appearing, containing one or rarely two small chromocenters. In voided urine the nuclei may be pale or opaque and occasionally somewhat darker.

Columnar Cells

Columnar urothelial cells are common, particularly in specimens obtained by instrumentation.[54] Columnar cells often derive from cystitis cystica or the urethra. They can be single or in small groups, often with a tail by which they are attached to the basement membrane (Fig. 7.2).

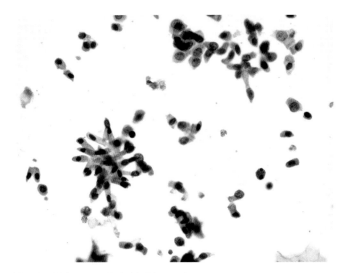

Fig. 7.2 Columnar cells in bladder wash.

Mucus-Containing Epithelial Cells

Occasionally urine specimens contain mucus-secreting columnar epithelial cells with peripheral nuclei and distended clear cytoplasm. These cells may be ciliated. Such cells often derive from cystitis cystica or cystitis glandularis but may represent cells from urachal remnant, nephrogenic metaplasia, or Müllerian rest (endometriosis or endocervicosis).

Squamous Cells

Squamous cells of varying size and degrees of maturation are common in urine sediment, particularly in voided specimens (Fig. 7.3). Such cells are more abundant in female than male patients.[8] In

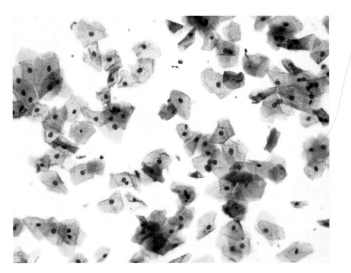

Fig. 7.3 Squamous cells in the urine.

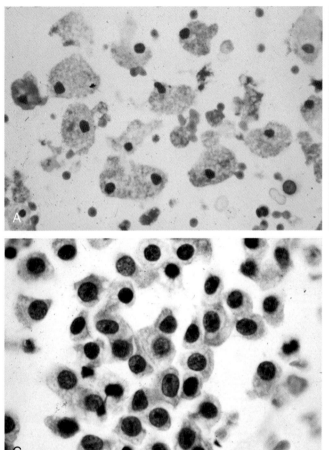

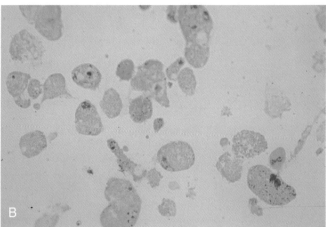

Fig. 7.4 (A) Proximal and distal convoluted cells from the nephron. (B) Necrotic proximal and distal convoluted cells. (C) Collecting duct cells.

women these cells originate in the urethral squamous epithelium and in the trigone of the urinary bladder, and are often glycogenated. Voided urine sediment may also contain squamous cells derived from the vulva, vagina, or uterine cervix. In men the origin of the squamous cells is the terminal portion of the urethra or, in rare cases, vaginal type of squamous metaplasia with bladder origin. Among the benign squamous cells, there may be superficial cells, intermediate cells, and small parabasal cells. Navicular cells are intermediate squamous cells with abundant cytoplasmic glycogen content and peripheral nuclei; these cells stain yellow with Papanicolaou stain. Such cells may be observed during pregnancy, early menopause, and sometimes in women or men receiving hormonal therapy (androgen deprivation therapy for prostate cancer). Squamous cells may also be anucleate and fully keratinized. In such cases these should be reported, because the presence of such "ghost" cells may be of considerable significance, representing leukoplakia or squamous cell carcinoma of the bladder.[7]

Renal Epithelial Cells

Cells derived from renal tubules sometimes appear in the urine sediment. These cells are small and usually poorly preserved, with pyknotic, hyperchromatic, condensed, spherical nuclei, and granular eosinophilic cytoplasm. Occasionally the tubular cells form small clusters or casts. The significance of tubular cells in urine sediment remains uncertain. In patients after kidney transplant the presence of renal tubular cells may indicate rejection of the allograft.[55]

Convoluted Tubular Cells

Cells from the convoluted tubular epithelium are the largest cells in the nephron, present at the entrance to the Bowman capsule and extending to the beginning of the loop of Henle. These cells are rarely seen in healthy individuals but are shed in large numbers in cases of renal toxicity and renal ischemia caused by a wide variety of drugs, heavy metals, immunosuppressant, and other toxins.

Proximal tubular cells in urine are easily identified by their large size (20 to 60 μm in diameter); irregular, elongate, or cigar-like appearance; and coarsely granular basophilic cytoplasm (Fig. 7.4A). Cytoplasmic borders are indistinct and may be ragged or torn. The granular cytoplasm contains large numbers of mitochondria by ultrastructure. Nuclei are slightly larger than erythrocytes and may occasionally be multinucleate. Interestingly, proximal and distal tubular cells appear singly, never in fragments or clusters. These cells are often mistaken for granular casts in unstained bright-field microscopy. Proximal and distal renal tubular cells slough from their basement membranes and can be found in urine as intact preserved cells or as "ghost" or necrotic forms that retain their size and cytoplasmic characteristics (Fig. 7.4B).

Collecting Duct Cells

Renal tubular cells lining the proximal and distal collecting ducts are small (12 to 18 μm in diameter), and each contains a single slightly eccentric nucleus with coarse and evenly distributed chromatin. There may be an occasional prominent nucleolus, because these cells may be reactive, but they are never multinucleate. The cytoplasm is polygonal to columnar, finely granular, and uniform basophilic, with distinct borders (Fig. 7.4C). Vacuolization may occasionally be seen, especially in reactive states. The cells may phagocytize castlike material, crystals, and pigments.

Collecting duct cells in urine may be present in very low numbers in normal individuals, but are significant when found with renal casts or as fragments. An abnormal number (greater than one per hpf) may be found in a wide variety of clinical conditions, including shock, trauma, burn, and exposure to toxins; also, an increased number of cells in renal transplant patients heralds clinical rejection up to 48 hours early.[56]

Renal epithelial cell fragments in urine indicate a severe form of renal tubular injury ("ischemic necrosis") and are exclusively from the collecting duct. This reflects loss of blood flow (ischemic injury) to the renal tubules and subsequent sloughing of entire segments or portions of the renal tubules with regeneration of lost epithelium, a process similar to repair in cervical smears. There are five types of fragments, and these are classified according to morphology: (1) spindle fragments; (2) fragments attached to or surrounding cast material; (3) pavement or "en face" fragments; (4) fragments with reactive cellular or noncellular inclusions (castlike, crystal, or pigmented [bile] inclusions); and (5) cylindrical, tubelike fragments.

Other Benign Cells

Occasionally cells of prostatic and seminal vesicle (Fig. 7.5) origin may be present in the urinary sediment. Such cells accompany spermatozoa and are common after prostatic massage.[57,58] Erythrocytes are a frequent component of the urinary sediment, particularly in patients with clinical evidence of hematuria (see later).[7]

Inflammatory Cells

Macrophages are often observed in inflammatory reactions of the urinary tract. The cells may be mononucleate or multinucleate and contain fine cytoplasmic vacuoles, sometimes with phagocytic debris. Normal urine sediment contains very few lymphocytes or neutrophils. The presence of large numbers of such cells may precede clinical evidence of inflammation. For example, when there were more than 12.5 white blood cells/μL by image analysis, sensitivity and specificity for predicting *Chlamydia* infection were 87% and 89%, respectively, in first voided urines in men at high risk.[59]

Noncellular Components of the Urinary Sediment

In addition to viral inclusions, a variety of intracellular and extracellular findings may be diagnostically valuable in the urine sediment.

Pigment and Pigmented Cells

Numerous normal and pathologic processes result in extracellular pigmented material in the urine and pigmented cells (Table 7.4).[60]

Cytoplasmic Eosinophilic Inclusions (Melamed-Wolinska Bodies)

Nonspecific cytoplasmic inclusions may appear as products of degenerating cells in multiple body fluids and can be seen with careful examination in 43% of urine samples.[61] There is no relationship with any disease. The round, opaque bodies are 12 to 15 μm in diameter, and may be single or multiple, with eosinophilia standing in contrast with the pale-staining urothelial cytoplasm. Nuclei are usually degenerate, with hyperchromasia, karyorrhexis, or pyknosis, but may also be intact.

Nonspecific cytoplasmic eosinophilic inclusions should be distinguished from acid-fast–positive nuclear inclusions in renal tubular cells associated with lead poisoning, as well as nonspecific acid-fast–negative red nuclear inclusions of uncertain significance in older women.[62,63]

Crystals

Polygonal transparent crystalline precipitates of urates are common in voided urine. Their presence results from changes in the acidity of urine after collection but has no diagnostic significance. Crystals derived from true uric acid are rare, and other crystals are rarely of diagnostic value.[64] Voided urine and occasional specimens obtained by instrumentation may contain contaminants and renal casts. For a complete review, refer to other texts.

Casts and Other Findings Attributable to Renal Diseases in Urine

Renal casts are observed in urine sediment in patients with glomerular and renal parenchymal diseases. Casts are composed of Tamm-Horsfall protein and originate in the distal tubules and collecting ducts. In healthy individuals hyaline and rare granular casts may

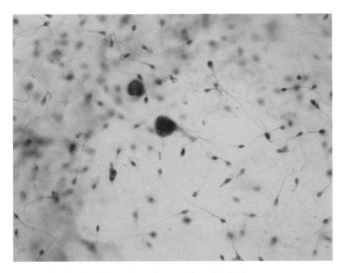

Fig. 7.5 Seminal vesicle cells and sperm in voided urine.

TABLE 7.4	Pigmented Cells in Urine: Differential Diagnosis
Finding	**Description**
Lipofuscin pigment	Granular yellow-brown pigment scattered around nuclei, often obscured by degenerative changes
Hemosiderin	Coarse golden-brown, brown, or black pigment usually in the cytoplasm of macrophages or rarely in urothelium; often observed in the setting of injury, blood transfusions, calculi, or foreign bodies; may be mistaken for melanin
Melanin	Dusty brown pigment found in melanosis, nevi, or melanoma; the greatest difficulty is when melanin pigment is associated with atypical urothelial cells; distinguishing urothelial cells from melanoma cells may require biopsy; with uncertainty, biopsy is indicated

occasionally appear because of dehydration, fever, exercise, and other factors; these casts are considered physiologic. Conversely, nonphysiologic casts made of abnormal urine protein and those that contain cells of various types are easily identified. The type of cells contained within the cast matrix, the width of the casts, and the number of casts is indicative of the severity of the underlying disease. The presence of abnormal amounts of protein, blood, leukocytes, nitrites, and bilirubin all correlate with the type of cast.

"Round cells" are recently described cells in patients with end-stage renal failure that appear to be predictive of early hemodialysis.[65] They are distinct from known cells in sediment and are similar to proximal convoluted tubule-derived cells based on morphology and molecular marker expression (GGT1, but not podocalyxin). These cells also express PAX2, Wilms tumor 1 (WT1), OSR1, and SIX2. The number of round cells correlates with the severity of chronic kidney disease.

The severity of lupus nephritis correlates strongly with voided urine cytology findings, including erythrocytes (isomorphic and dysmorphic), acanthocytes, and leukocytes (0.65 for each); classification tree has an accuracy rate of 84.3%.[66]

Dysmorphic red blood cells may be indicative of urologic or glomerular diseases (see later).

Diagnostic Criteria

Infections

Bacteria

A wide variety of bacteria may affect the epithelium of the urinary tract. Most are coliforms and other gram-negative rods. Cystitis may be acute or chronic. Acute cystitis is usually associated with symptoms that rarely require confirmatory tissue biopsy or cytologic examination. The sediment may contain numerous exfoliated urothelial cells, necrotic material, and inflammatory cells, with a predominance of neutrophils (Fig. 7.6A to C). Marked necrosis and inflammation may also occur in the presence of necrotic tumors, particularly high-grade urothelial carcinoma and squamous cell carcinoma.

The sediment in chronic cystitis usually contains a background of chronic inflammation with macrophages and erythrocytes.[7] Urothelial cells may be abundant and poorly preserved, occasionally forming small clusters. The cytoplasm in these cells tends to be granular and vacuolated; when the cells are degenerate, the cytoplasm contains spherical eosinophilic inclusions (Melamed-Wolinska bodies) (Fig. 7.7).[67] There may be slight nuclear

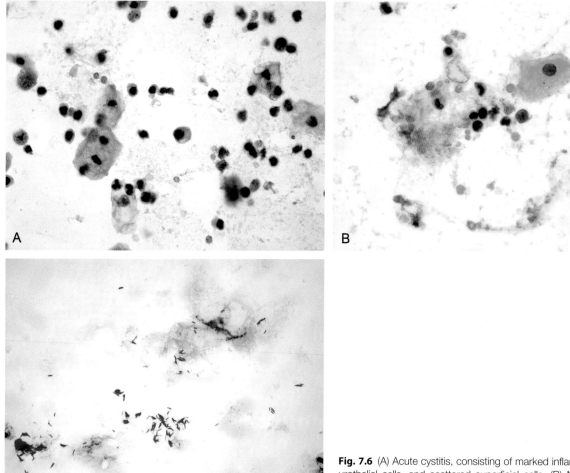

Fig. 7.6 (A) Acute cystitis, consisting of marked inflammation, degenerate urothelial cells, and scattered superficial cells. (B) Necrosis and macrophages in tuberculosis of bladder. (C) Acid-fast bacilli in urine (Ziehl-Neelsen stain).

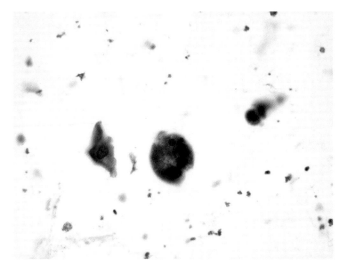

Fig. 7.7 Degenerate urothelial cells with cytoplasmic inclusions (Melamed-wolinska bodies).

enlargement and hyperchromasia, but the contours of the nuclei are usually regular and the chromatin texture is finely granular without the coarse granularity of cancer cells. There may be necrosis of urothelial cells, with nuclear pyknosis and marked cytoplasmic vacuolization. In ulcerative cystitis, large sheets of urothelial cells may exfoliate.

Interstitial cystitis, a form of chronic cystitis associated with chronic inflammation, displays nonspecific cytologic changes.[8] Eosinophilic cystitis has a predominance of eosinophils, a pattern that may be seen in patients with allergic disorders, previous biopsies, or after mitomycin C treatment.[68]

Tuberculous cystitis may be observed in patients with AIDS and those receiving treatment for urothelial carcinoma with bacillus Calmette–Guérin (BCG). In such patients the urine has inflammatory cells, necrosis (Fig. 7.6B), and rarely contains fragments of tubercles consisting of clusters of elongate carrot-shaped epithelioid cells, sometimes accompanied by multinucleated Langhans-type giant cells, and reactive atypia of urothelial cells.[69-71] Ziehl-Neelsen staining may reveal acid-fast bacilli

(Fig. 7.6C). The sediment occasionally contains "decoy" cells with glassy hyperchromatic nuclei.[70] Similar findings may occur in patients with tuberculosis of the bladder.

Fungi

Fungi occasionally affect the lower urinary tract, particularly the urinary bladder, and *Candida albicans* is the most common, usually seen in pregnant women, diabetics, and those with impaired immunity such as patients with AIDS, those undergoing chemotherapy for cancer, and bone marrow transplant recipients. In the sediment the fungi may appear as yeast forms, with small oval bodies, or pseudohyphae, with oblong branching nonencapsulated filaments (Fig. 7.8A and B). Other fungi are uncommon, including *Blastomyces dermatitidis*, *Aspergillus*, and *mucormycosis*. A fungus of the species *Alternaria* is a common laboratory contaminant.[8]

Viruses

Several important viruses cause significant morphologic changes in the urothelial cells, many of which may be confused with malignancy. The dominant feature of viral infection is the formation of nuclear and cytoplasmic inclusions (Table 7.5).

Herpes simplex is an obligate intracellular virus, and florid infection with permissive replication of the virus causes abnormalities in urothelial cells that are readily recognized. In the early stages of viral replication the nuclei of infected cells appear hazy with a ground-glass appearance. Multinucleation is commonly observed in such cells. Multiple nuclei are often densely packed, with nuclear molding and tightly fitting contoured nuclei (Fig. 7.9). In later stages of infection the viral particles concentrate in the center of the nuclei, forming bright eosinophilic inclusions with a narrow clear zone or halo at the periphery. Infected cells may contain single or multiple nuclei.[8,64]

Cytomegalovirus is usually seen in newborn infants with impaired immunity. The infection is common in adults with AIDS. The characteristic changes are readily recognized in the sediment, including large cells with prominent basophilic nuclear inclusions surrounded by an abundant peripheral clear zone (Fig. 7.10). There is a distinct outer band of condensed nuclear chromatin.

Polyomavirus infection is widespread, according to serologic studies of adults. The BK polyomavirus may cause hemorrhagic cystitis in patients with allogeneic hematopoietic stem cell

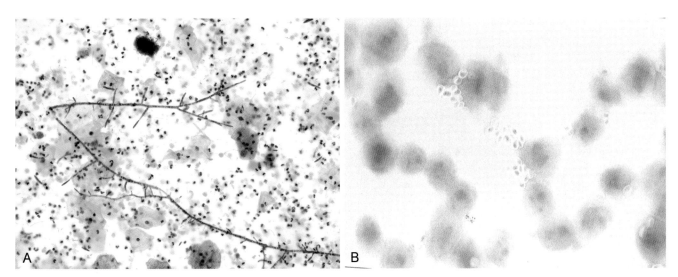

Fig. 7.8 *Candida albicans* in the urinary sediment. (A) Distinctive branching fungal hyphae are abundant in this routine specimen. (B) Note the small oval bodies that stand in contrast with the urothelial cells.

TABLE 7.5 Characteristic Cytologic Changes Associated with Viruses

Cytomegalovirus
- Enlarged cells
- High N/C ratio
- Basophilic intranuclear inclusion with "owl's-eye" appearance; occasionally small, dark intracytoplasmic inclusions

Herpesvirus
- Enlarged, multinucleated cells with "ground-glass" chromatin
- High N/C ratio
- Opaque, structureless chromatin
- Eosinophilic intranuclear inclusion

Polyomavirus
- Enlarged cells
- High N/C ratio
- Opaque, structure-less chromatin, chromatinic membrane is common
- Nuclei stain with a magenta hue
- Intranuclear inclusion fills almost the entire nuclear area

Papillomavirus
- Perinuclear clear cytoplasmic zones (koilocytosis)
- Nuclear enlargement and homogeneous hyperchromasia

N/C, Nuclear-to-cytoplasmic.

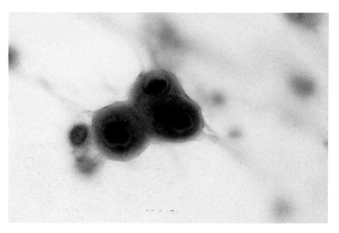

Fig. 7.10 Cytomegalovirus infection.

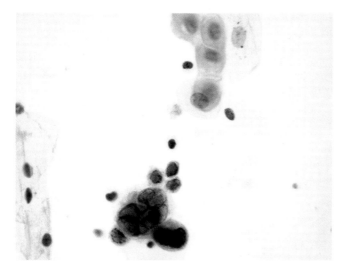

Fig. 7.9 Herpes infection.

transplant and virus-associated nephritis in patients with renal transplant. The occult virus can become activated and recognized in voided urine sediment. Polyomavirus plays a major role in urine cytology because it produces cell abnormalities that may be readily confused with cancer; these cells are also known as "decoy" cells (Fig. 7.11A).[72] In permissive infections, the virus produces large homogeneous basophilic nuclear inclusions that occupy almost the entire volume of the nuclei with only a thin chromatinic rim.[73,74] The background usually contains abundant inflammatory and cellular debris. Infected cells are often enlarged and usually contain a single nucleus, but binucleation and occasional large multinucleated cells may be seen.[75] Elongate cells are referred to

as "comet" cells. Nonspecific eosinophilic inclusions (Melamed-Wolinska bodies) may be present in the cytoplasm.[67] Late infections may contain pale-staining degenerated inclusion-bearing cells in cases in which the virus may be detected in voided urine.[76] When the inclusions regress, the chromatin acquires a distinctive, coarsely clumped appearance. Clearance of decoy cells from urine is closely related to histologic remission of polyomavirus nephropathy.[77] The cytologic picture in some cases may be quite dramatic and has led to misdiagnosis of carcinoma.[78] Decoy cells do not exhibit aneuploidy by FISH, and acid hematoxylin stain appeared to be superior to Papanicolaou stain in identifying and confirming the presence of infection (Fig. 7.11B).[79] Decoy cells occurred in 14% of samples from patients with histologically proven viral nephropathy, with a sensitivity of 67%, specificity of 89%, positive predictive value of 12%, and negative predictive value of 99%.[80] Quantification of decoy cells improved the positive predictive value to 32% (threshold 10 ≥ cells). Immunohistochemical staining of urinary exfoliated cells for SV40T improved sensitivity to 86% for detecting atypical or degenerate infected cells (specificity of 93% and positive predictive value of 33%).

More than 70 types of human papillomavirus have been identified, and types 6 and 11 are associated with condyloma acuminatum. Condyloma may also appear in the urethra and invariably induces koilocytosis. Urothelial carcinoma exhibits a low incidence of human papillomavirus types 16 and 18 infection (Fig. 7.12).[81]

Trematodes and Other Parasites

The most common urine parasite is *Schistosoma haematobium* (Bilharzia). There are two important cytologic manifestations of infection with *S. haematobium*: recognition of the ova and the malignant tumors that may be associated with it.[68] The ova are elongate structures with a thick transparent capsule and a sword-shaped protrusion known as the terminal spine located at the narrow end of the ovum. Fresh or calcified ova may be readily recognized in the sediment. The embryonal form of the parasite, known as miracidium, is released in human stool and urine, retaining the shape of the ovum with its terminal spine. Other common intestinal parasites that affect the bladder include *Ascaris lumbricoides*, *Enterobius vermicularis*, and agents of filariasis. *Trichomonas vaginalis* is a sexually transmitted parasite that is rarely found in urine (0.1% incidence), appearing as round to oval organisms with eccentric nuclei and cytoplasmic granules; acute inflammation is usually present.[82] Hassan et al. described microfilariae of *Wuchereria bancrofti* in an 18-year-old boy in India who presented with chylous hematuria.[273]

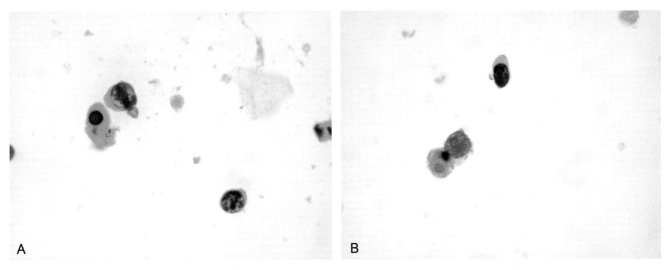

Fig. 7.11 Decoy cells in polyomavirus infection. (A) These may be mistaken for malignant cells. (B) Nuclear details of polyomavirus infection (acid hematoxylin stain).

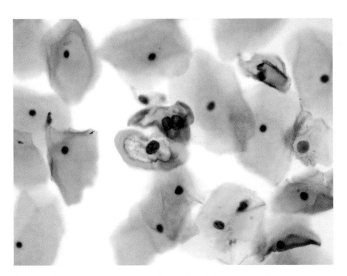

Fig. 7.12 Koilocytes (Human papillomavirus infection) in urine.

TABLE 7.6	Differential Diagnosis of Urothelial Atypia Found in Urinary Sediment

Urinary tract conditions
    Urethral catheterization
    Urinary calculi
    Chronic cystitis and cystitis glandularis
    Polyoma (BK) virus infection[a]
    Cellular changes resulting from radiation therapy and chemotherapy
    Reactive and/or hyperplastic urothelium (e.g., cystitis, inflammation, etc.)
    Papillary urothelial tumor of low malignant potential and low-grade urothelial carcinoma
Renal parenchymal conditions
    Acute tubular necrosis
    Papillary necrosis
    Renal infarction
    Acute allograft rejection with ischemic necrosis

[a]Not considered within the category of "atypical" in Paris System 2013 (categorized as "negative").

Reactive Cytologic Changes

Numerous reactive changes involving the urothelium may be misinterpreted as "atypical" or "suspicious/malignant" (Table 7.6).

Lithiasis

About 40% of patients with calculi have abnormal cytologic findings in voided urine.[52] These patients have numerous large, smooth-bordered clusters of benign urothelial cells with an abundance of superficial cells (Fig. 7.13A). These changes may overlap with the spectrum of findings with low-grade urothelial carcinoma, but the cells tend to cluster, with fewer single cells.[52] Calculi are abrasive to the mucosa when present in the renal pelvis, ureter, or urinary bladder, and the resultant cytologic specimens closely resemble the effects of instrumentation. Significant atypia of urothelial cells due to lithiasis is uncommon, and the clusters have smooth borders (Fig. 7.13B and C).[8] Nonetheless, lithiasis remains a major diagnostic pitfall in urine cytology interpretation.

Drug Effects

Intravesically administered agents and drugs, including BCG (see earlier Bacteria section), mitomycin C, and thiotepa, are commonly used for treatment of primary and recurrent bladder tumors (Figs. 7.14A and B and 7.15). They may induce cell enlargement, cytoplasmic vacuolization, and other reactive changes, including nuclear enlargement of cells, wrinkled nuclear membranes, mild hyperchromasia, pleomorphism, abnormal nuclear morphology, disordered orientation of the urothelium, and eosinophilic inflammation.[83] Intravesical chemotherapy can contribute to false-positive results in urine cytology.[84]

Systemically administered drugs, such as the alkylating agents cyclophosphamide and busulfan, have a marked effect on the urothelium, inducing significant cytologic abnormalities (Fig. 7.16A to C). These drugs may cause changes that include bizarre urothelial cells with marked nuclear and nucleolar enlargement, mimicking poorly differentiated carcinoma.[8,85,86] Large doses of cyclophosphamide have been shown to induce urothelial carcinoma, leiomyosarcoma, and carcinosarcoma.[87,88]

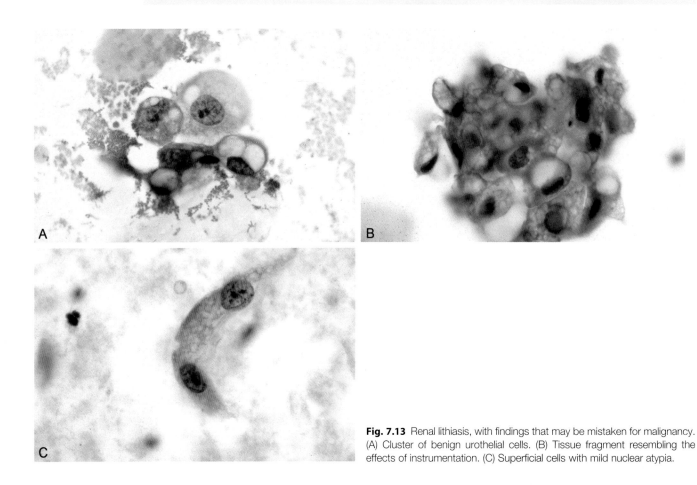

Fig. 7.13 Renal lithiasis, with findings that may be mistaken for malignancy. (A) Cluster of benign urothelial cells. (B) Tissue fragment resembling the effects of instrumentation. (C) Superficial cells with mild nuclear atypia.

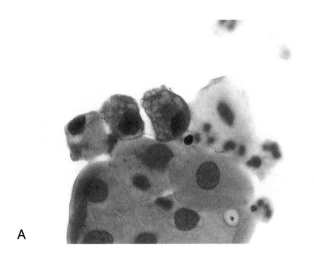
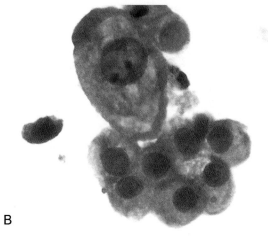

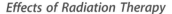

Fig. 7.14 Mitomycin C changes in the urine mimicking malignancy (A and B).

Effects of Radiation Therapy

Radiation therapy typically induces marked cell enlargement, with bizarre cell shapes and vacuolated nuclei, polychromatic cytoplasm, and sometimes multiple nucleoli (Fig. 7.17A and B). These findings may persist for years after treatment.[8] Clinical history is essential for diagnosis.

Degenerative Changes

Degenerating cells with pyknotic, crenated nuclei are often a source of concern in urine cytology caused by inflammation, stone, and

trauma, among others. Although these changes mimic malignancy, the chromatin is usually smudged and degenerated (Fig. 7.18), in contrast with the cancerous cells in which the chromatin is crisp and distinct. Such changes are occasionally observed in polyomavirus infection.[76]

Instrumentation Atypia

Large numbers of superficial cells and intermediate cells can be seen in catheterized urine, bladder washings, and brushings (Fig. 7.19A). Small pseudopapillae, cellular enlargement, and

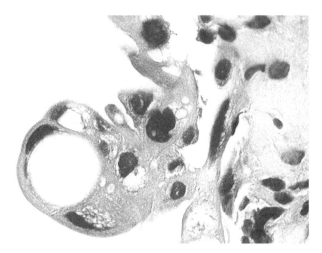

Fig. 7.15 Thiotepa-induced changes, including urothelial detachment with nuclear atypia and cytoplasmic vacuolization.

pleomorphism with large nucleoli can be intimidating features (Fig. 7.19B), but careful examination of the entire sample may be helpful for distinguishing reactive changes from malignancy (Tables 7.6 and 7.7).

Laser-Induced Changes and Other Ablation Changes

Marked cellular spindling is common in post-laser coagulation of the bladder. The spindled cells occur singly, in loose clusters, and in lamellar stacks, and have elongate nuclei with dense chromatin and bipolar cytoplasm (Fig. 7.20). Cytologic interpretation should not be undertaken during the immediate posttreatment period.[89]

Irreversible electroporation, an apoptosis-inducing ablation method used for small renal masses, preserves the urinary collecting system with unaltered normal morphology, temporarily inducing degeneration with vacuolization of detached urothelial cells.[90]

Electromotive drug administration and chemohyperthermia represent minimally invasive methods of intravesical instillation of therapeutic agents such as mitomycin C. In "negative" or "atypical" voided urines, these treatments induce a unique characteristic pattern of increased cellularity with enlarged nuclear size, irregular nuclear membranes, and altered N/C; hyperchromasia and irregular nuclear chromatin are rarely observed.[91]

Electromagnetic and electrohydraulic extracorporeal shockwave lithotripsy for treatment of calculi causes a transient (4 to 10 days) increase (≥10-fold) in red blood cells and epithelial cells that is not observed in basal cells or myocytes.[92,93]

Neobladder and Ileal Conduit Urine

The urine is dominated by degenerated glandular cells. Nuclei are usually dense and hyperchromatic due to degeneration. Urothelial cells are usually sparse or absent. Eosinophilic cytoplasmic inclusions (Melamed-Wolinska bodies) are common (Fig. 7.21A and B). Debris, cytoplasmic fragments, granular deposits, bacteria, occasional inflammatory cells, red blood cells, and small intestinal cells are seen in the background.[94,95] Vegetable cells in urines from Bricker ileal conduit originate from the ostomy adhesive.[96] Fresh specimens should be examined; urine from the collection bag is unsatisfactory for cytologic examination.

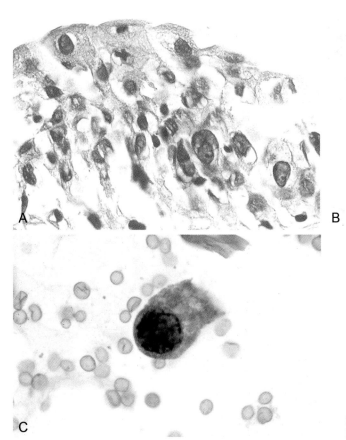

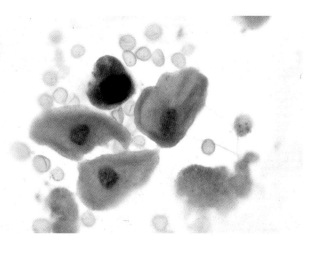

Fig. 7.16 Cyclophosphamide changes. Atypical urothelial cells with large hyperchromatic nuclei that may be mistaken for malignant cells (A to C).

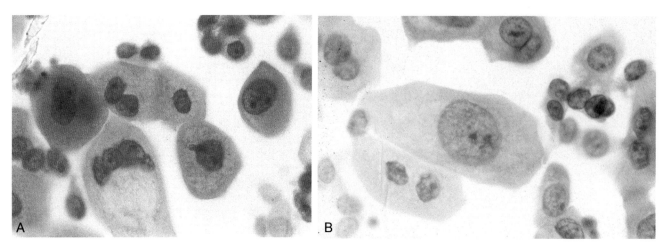

Fig. 7.17 Radiation changes (A and B). Note bizarre enlarged urothelial cells with numerous vacuolations.

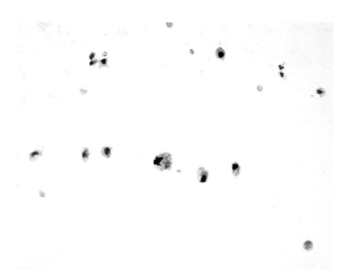

Fig. 7.18 Crenated (Degenerating) cells.

Urine Cytology in Renal Transplant Recipients

Urine cytology is an effective screening method for monitoring patients with renal transplant, with high sensitivity and high negative predictive value, and can be routinely used in follow-up.[97] The epithelial cells of collecting tubules are well preserved. The cells that appear in urine specimens have scant vacuolated cytoplasm with spherical and somewhat opaque nuclei. A feature of impending rejection is the presence of numerous T lymphocytes and erythrocytes in the urine. The erythrocytes have a thick outer border and clear center suggestive of renal origin. In rejection, tissue fragments may be present, including necrotic renal tubules and hyaline casts.[55]

Other Benign Conditions

A wide variety of benign conditions induce unique findings in the urine. Partial or complete keratinization of the squamous epithelium, referred to clinically as leukoplakia, often replaces the urothelium, resulting in a cystoscopic gray-white appearance of the mucosa. In the urinary sediment, anucleated keratinized cells,

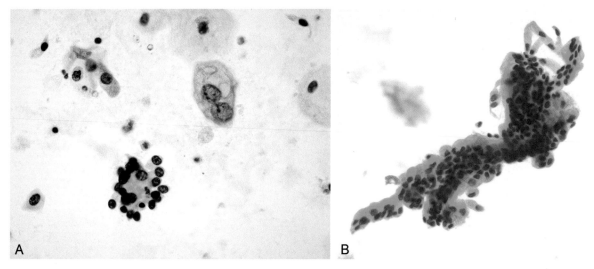

Fig. 7.19 Instrumentation atypia. (A) Ureteric wash with mild increase in nuclear-to-cytoplasmic ratio and prominent nucleoli. (B) Cluster of cells (pseudopapillae) with slightly irregular outline and normal nuclear membrane (bladder wash sample).

TABLE 7.7	Features of Reactive Changes and Urothelial Carcinoma (World Health Organization 1973 Classification)		
Feature	Reactive Changes	Grade 1 Carcinoma	Grades 2 and 3 Carcinoma and Carcinoma In Situ
Cell arrangements	Pseudopapillae	Papillae and tight clusters	Single cells and loose clusters
Cell configuration	Flat groups	Papillary	Variable
Size	Enlarged, pleomorphic	Slightly enlarged, uniform	Markedly enlarged, pleomorphic
Numbers	Few cells	Few groups	Variable
Cytoplasm	Vacuolated	Homogeneous	Variable, vacuolated
Nucleus	Central, uniform	Eccentric, enlarged	Eccentric, pleomorphic
Nuclear-to-cytoplasmic ratio	Normal to slightly increased	Increased	Moderate to markedly increased
Size	Slightly enlarged	Enlarged	Enlarged
Border	Smooth, thick	Slightly irregular, one or two notches, thin	Moderate to markedly irregular, thin
Chromatin	Fine, evenly distributed	Granular, evenly distributed	Coarse, unevenly distributed
Nucleoli	Often large	Small, absent	Large, variable
DNA content	Diploid	Usually diploid	Aneuploid

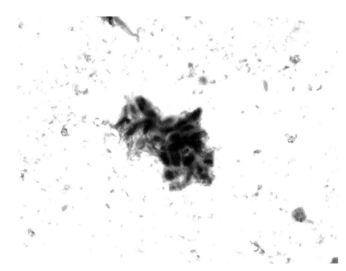

Fig. 7.20 Laser-induced changes.

so-called ghost cells, may be present. When these cells are present, one should exclude the possibility of squamous cell carcinoma.[7,8] Cystitis glandularis may shed ciliated mucus-containing epithelial cells that contain peripheral nuclei and clear cytoplasm. Such cells may be mistaken for adenocarcinoma. Endometriosis of the bladder may result in urine shedding of diagnostic glandular and spindle cells.[98] Large numbers of macrophages may be present in urine samples in patients with malakoplakia, but the release of such inflammatory cells usually occurs after biopsy and is detected in the urine stream (Fig. 7.22A). The spherical, intracytoplasmic, eosinophilic, or calcified Michaelis-Guttmann bodies associated with malakoplakia in the cytoplasm of the macrophages are usually readily identified (Fig. 7.22B). Urinary mulberry cells indicate Fabry disease, a lysosomal storage disorder caused by a deficiency of α-galactosidase A.[99]

Benign Tumors and Tumor-like Processes

There are no cell changes that are characteristic of inverted papilloma (Fig. 7.23A and B) or nephrogenic adenoma, and cytologic

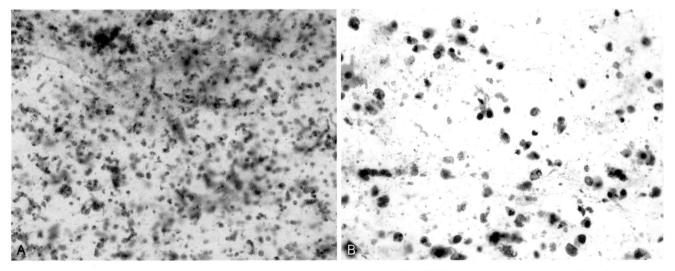

Fig. 7.21 Ileal conduit urine. (A) Cellular sample with many degenerating cells (low magnification). (B) Columnar cells, degenerating cells, red blood cells, and melamed-wolinska bodies.

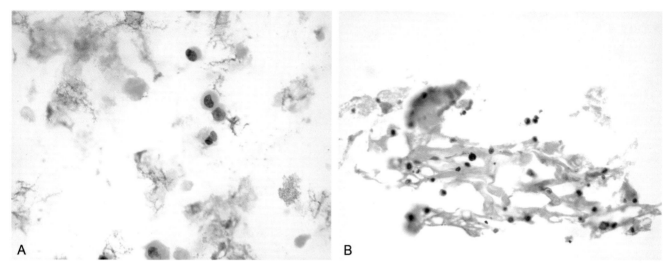

Fig. 7.22 (A) Macrophages and debris in malakoplakia. (B) Michaelis-gutmann bodies (von kossa stain).

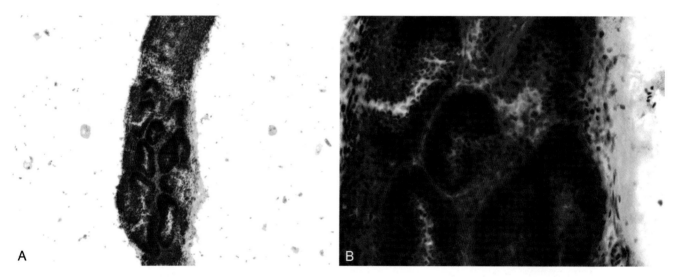

Fig. 7.23 Inverted papilloma in bladder wash. (A) Low magnification. (B) High magnification.

findings from these processes and other benign processes may be difficult to differentiate.[100] Paraganglioma presents with tumor nests composed of epithelioid cells with fine chromatin and moderate cytoplasm admixed with occasional spindle sustentacular cells. Single cells are discohesive and large with moderate cytoplasm and inconspicuous nucleoli.[101]

Condyloma acuminatum of the urinary bladder is uncommon and may be associated with condyloma of the urethra or external genitalia. Koilocytosis is characterized by squamous cells with large hyperchromatic nuclei and perinuclear clear zones or halos. These changes result from infection by human papillomavirus types 6 and 11. The presence of koilocytes in voided urine sediment in males often indicates a lesion in the bladder or urethra (Fig. 7.12). In women, such cells may also indicate contamination from the lower genital tract. Occasionally koilocytes may mimic squamous cell carcinoma.

Endometrial-type glandular cells in urine sediment have been reported in women with endometriosis.[102]

Fragments of benign urachal remnant were found in an unusual voided urine.[103] The specimen was moderately cellular, consisting of sheets, small strips, and clusters of benign-appearing glandular cells with a moderate amount of cytoplasm and smooth round to oval eccentric polarized nuclei, lightly stippled fine chromatin, and inconspicuous nucleoli. There was an absence of mitotic figures, apoptotic bodies, blood, or background inflammation.

Atypical Urothelial Cells

One of the greatest challenges in urine cytology interpretation concerns the category of "atypical." There is a lack of consensus on diagnostic criteria, terminology, clinical significance, and benchmark incidence rate, although all authors agree that the rate should be as low as possible.[104] The incidence of "atypical" is widely variable, with a range of 11% to 33% in large published series with more than 100 patients (Table 7.8). The diagnostic incidence differs according to multiple variables, including patient age, gender, type of cytology specimen (instrumented versus void versus washing), patient selection (hematuria versus urinary tract symptoms versus cancer follow-up), sample processing (routine centrifugation versus liquid-based preparation), and number of cytology

TABLE 7.8 Incidence and Cancer Yield[d] of "Atypical Urine Cytology"[a] and Other Categories

Authors (Date)	Total Cases of Atypical (n)	Atypical Rate (%)	Cases of Atypical with Follow-up Biopsy (n)	Time Interval to Biopsy (months)	Negative	All Atypical, Excluding "Favor Neoplasm" and "Favor High-Grade Carcinoma"	"Suspicious"	"Positive"
Deshpande and McKee (2005)[104]	238	N/A	102	≤12	N/A	23.4	N/A	N/A
Raab et al. (2007)[109]	710	11.1	133	≤14	42	65.4	81.8	79.7
Voss et al. (2008)[263]	b	b	128[b]	≤12	56.9	60.9	73.8	90.7
Brimo et al. (2009)[107]	691	23.2	110	≤12	68.9	78	87	N/A
Siddappa et al. (2012)[250]	464	32.5	464	N/A	N/A	11.5	N/A	N/A
Dimashkieh et al. (2013)[264]	296	16.1	296	≤36	8.3	32.1	N/A	N/A
Bostwick and Hossain (2014)[47]	1074	10.2	1074	≤12	13.5	31.1	54.3	75.1
Muus Ubago et al. (2013)[265]	1320	8.1	N/A	≤138	N/A	21.0[c]	N/A	N/A
Chau et al. (2015)[110]	159	22.8	159	≤24	41.9	61.3	78.3	83.7
Virk et al. (2017)[232]	377	N/A	377	≤12	N/A	16.5	N/A	N/A

The atypical rate may be misleading because many articles reported only cases with matched cytology–histology pairs, and most negative biopsies would be excluded because they do not trigger subsequent biopsy.

N/A, Data not available.

[a]Excludes studies with less than 100 "atypical" cytologies with follow-up biopsy.[45,266-269] Excludes upper tract cases and renal cell carcinoma.[52] Excludes Piaton et al. (2011)[271] and (2014)[270] with an "atypical" rate of 0.8% to 2%.

[b]This study[126] included an additional category of cellular "clusters" that accounted for 579 cases, so the results cannot be directly compared with other studies.

[c]Positive includes 44 cases diagnosed by subsequent positive cytology only (no biopsy) and 17 secondary (nonurothelial) carcinomas.

[d]Cancer yield on biopsy includes suspicious for malignancy and diagnostic of malignancy because both categories require immediate clinical intervention.

specimens obtained.[105] Further, it is compounded by variance in subsequent predictive accuracy of "atypical" for carcinoma. The "atypical" category encompasses findings that may include from low- to intermediate-grade dysplasia (an uncommon histologic finding) (Figs. 7.24 through 7.28) at the low end of the spectrum, although it is difficult, if not impossible, to recognize specific cytologic changes corresponding to histologic low- to intermediate-grade dysplasia.[8,106] High-grade (severe) dysplasia and carcinoma in situ are considered to be equivalent, and the findings in urine may be underinterpreted as "atypical" when they are best classified

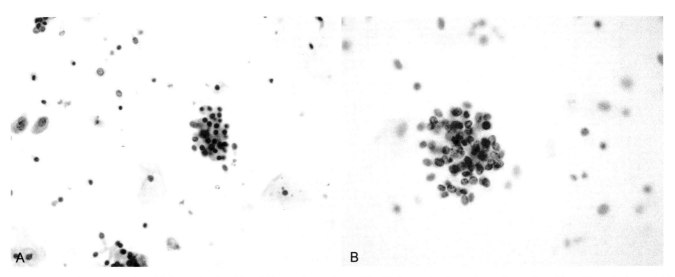

Fig. 7.24 Atypical, favor reactive. (A) Atypical cells with mild hyperchromatic nuclei, slightly overlapping cells, and smooth outlines (Papanicolaou stain). (B) Atypical cells, same case as in (A) with nuclear chromatin details and smooth nuclear membrane (acid hematoxylin stain).

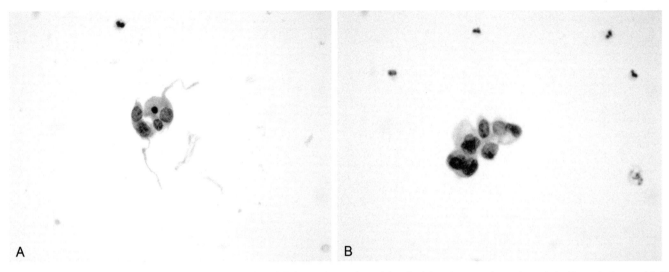

Fig. 7.25 Atypical, uncertain. (A) Groups of atypical cells with mildly hyperchromatic nuclei and mild nuclear membrane irregularity (Papanicolaou stain). (B) Same case as in (A) depicting nuclear details (acid hematoxylin stain).

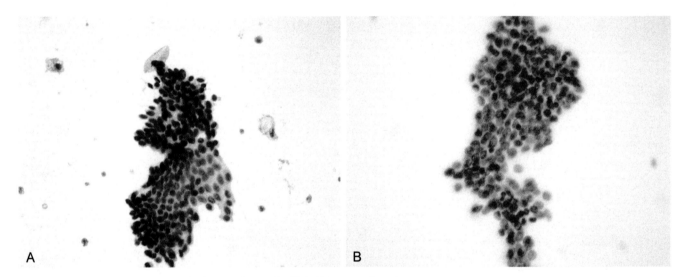

Fig. 7.26 Atypical cells in bladder wash. (A) Papanicolaou stain. (B) Acid hematoxylin stain.

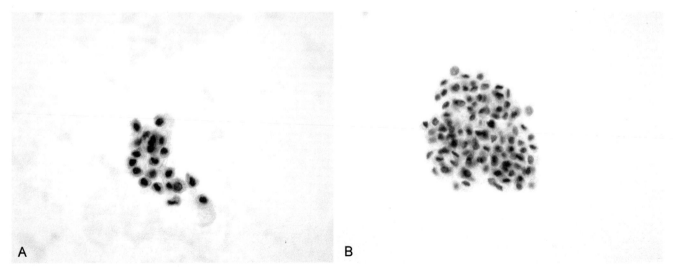

Fig. 7.27 Atypical cells in voided urine. (A) Papanicolaou stain. (B) Acid hematoxylin stain.

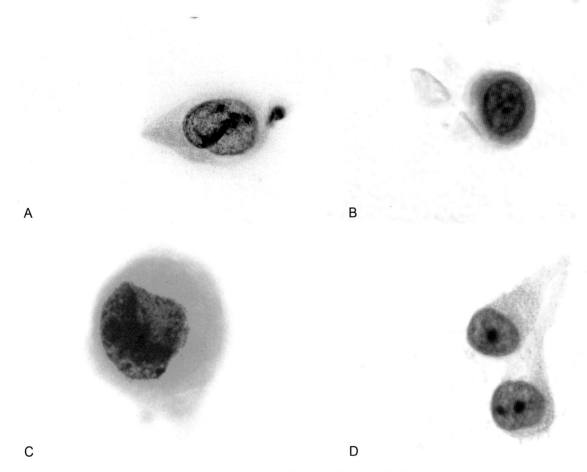

Fig. 7.28 Atypical urothelial cells consistent with dysplasia (A to D). Multiple biopsies of the bladder revealed dysplasia, but no evidence of carcinoma in situ.

as at least "suspicious" and, preferably, "high-grade carcinoma" (see later).

Reported diagnostic criteria for "atypical" usually include specimens in which the N/C ratio is greater than 50%, a criterion adopted by the Paris System 2013 (see earlier).[107,108] Cell clusters are usually classified as "atypical, favor reactive" in combination with smooth uniform nuclear membranes; nucleoli may or may not be enlarged. Deshpande and McKee recognized three groups of urothelial cell clusters: group 1 consisted of flat clusters, group 2 had overlapping clusters with two or more cell layers that may be three-dimensional, and group 3 had overlapping clusters with smooth borders.[104] "Atypical, unclear if reactive or neoplastic" described urothelial cells without degenerate features with irregular intact nuclear membranes, chromatic clumping, or the presence of black structureless nuclei referred to as "India' ink–type nuclei." Degenerate cells (poorly preserved cells) were excluded from classification by some observers, but not others, as were decoy cells of polyomavirus infection.[104,107,108] Increased cellularity, nuclear membrane irregularities, number of "India ink–type nuclei," and number of cell clusters correlated with adverse outcome.[104]

We found that the "atypical" category had significant predictive value for urothelial carcinoma (about 36% overall), especially in patients under active surveillance for recurrent malignancy.[47] Accordingly we believe that it is critical for clinicians to undertake follow-up of these patients. Unfortunately, "atypical" has become a wastebasket category because it is often overused by pathologists,

contributing to complacency and lack of response on the part of many urologists when confronted with this diagnosis. Further, others have suggested that "atypical" is equivalent to "negative," although such studies were based on an insufficient number of cases to reach such a conclusion.[109] Brimo et al. undertook logistic regression and found that "atypical" was not significantly predictive of urothelial carcinoma on follow-up biopsy, but they failed to provide the variables weighed in their multivariate model, so their conclusion cannot be independently confirmed.[107]

Comparison of the two "atypical" categories ("atypical, favor reactive" [see Fig. 7.24A and B] and "atypical, uncertain" [see Fig. 7.25A and B]) revealed similar predictive values for urothelial cancer on subsequent biopsy in our study of more than 9000 consecutive urine cytologies within 12 months (31.1% versus 37.7%), suggesting that this stratification is not very useful clinically, similar to the recommendation of other authors.[107,110] However, some have reported significant stratification of "atypical"; Rosenthal et al. reported predictive values for cancer of 10% and 38% for "atypical, favor reactive" and "atypical, favor high-grade carcinoma," respectively, although they apparently did not recognize the "suspicious" category, lumping those patients into "atypical, favor high-grade carcinoma."[111]

Our rate of atypia (10.2%) was significantly lower than others' (up to 32.5%) (Table 7.8). This difference cannot be attributed to the use of liquid-based cellular enhancement methods, because we used the Meiers improved filter method. Other reports come from academic medical centers with a high level of experience in cytopathology, especially urine cytology, so this is an unlikely source of significant variation. Further, our comparison group did not rely on expert re-review of cases, but rather used the real-life method of reviewing existing diagnoses from reports. Rodgers et al. found that urine cytology was unable to rule out malignancy or exclude patients from further investigation despite ability to confirm the presence of cancer.[112] Interobserver disagreement was "moderate to good" using Kappa statistics, but there were considerable differences in accuracy according to the level of expertise and reporting bias.[113]

It is probable that the improvement in the atypical rate is due to the use of two stains: the acid hematoxylin stain in combination with the Papanicolaou stain. Nuclear details are critical for diagnosis, and the acid hematoxylin provides significant new information beyond that of the routine Papanicolaou stain or routine hematoxylin stain (see later). Examples of atypia in the bladder wash (Fig. 7.26A and B) and atypia in voided urine (Fig. 7.27A and B) are shown to compare Papanicolaou and acid hematoxylin stains.

Suspicious

The reported rate of "suspicious" urine cytology ranges from 1.9% to 28.7%, reflecting variability in definitions and diagnostic cut points.[47,109,114-116] The Paris System 2013 limited this category to "suspicious for high-grade urothelial carcinoma" in recognition of the clinical importance of high sensitivity for detection of high-grade carcinoma at the expense of lower specificity, excluding from consideration suspicion of low-grade carcinoma.[24,39,117] The predictive value of "suspicious" for all grades of cancer before publication of Paris System 2013 varied from 54% to 87% (Table 7.9). Using criteria employed in the Paris System 2013, the predictive value of "suspicious for all cancers" increased to 92%, with high-grade carcinoma found in 79%.[118]

Low-Grade Urothelial Carcinoma

The low-grade urothelial carcinoma category accounts for the urine findings from papillary neoplasm of low malignant potential, World Health Organization (WHO) 1973 grade 1 and 2 carcinomas, low-grade papillary carcinoma, and, likely, papilloma. The diagnosis of low-grade urothelial carcinoma in the WHO 1999 and WHO/International Society of Urologic Pathology 2004

overlaps with WHO 1973 grade 1 and 2 carcinomas, as well as papillary neoplasm of low malignant potential, compounding confusion among pathologists and clinicians (Table 7.10).

It may also be difficult cytologically to separate WHO grade 1 urothelial carcinoma (papillary urothelial neoplasm of low malignant potential) from papilloma in urine cytology specimens.[119,120] The urothelial cell clusters are often arranged in a papillary configuration and are difficult to distinguish from those shed from normal benign urothelium after palpation, instrumentation, or irritation by calculi or inflammation (Figs. 7.29 and 7.30).[52,53] In voided urine, spontaneously shed complex clusters of morphologically benign urothelial cells may be suggestive of a papillary tumor, provided that trauma is excluded clinically. Diagnostic features of WHO grade 1 carcinoma (papillary neoplasm of low malignant potential) include the presence of tumor fragments with connective tissue stalks or central capillary vessels (Tables 7.7 and 7.10).[121] Numerous attempts to define the precise microscopic features of tumor fragments that separate benign urothelial cell clusters from WHO grade 1 carcinoma have met with limited success.[122] Some authors claim that low- to intermediate-grade papillary urothelial tumors shed recognizable cells in the urinary sediment; they note that the characteristic features include increased N/C ratio, enlarged and eccentric nuclei, and inconspicuous nucleoli, features present in 70% of such tumors.[123,124] Mai et al. found that low-grade urothelial carcinoma in urine frequently contained three-dimensional cell clusters with disordered nuclei and cellular dyscohesion, findings that collectively had sensitivity of 70% and specificity of 94%.[125] Scant cellularity was observed in 20% of cases. Others reported correct cytologic diagnosis in 33% of such cases.[122]

Differentiation of WHO grade 1 carcinoma (papillary urothelial neoplasm of low malignant potential) from instrumentation artifact is based on the presence of cell clusters with ragged borders, unlike the smooth borders lined by densely stained cytoplasm at the edge of benign cell clusters.[53] Grade 1 carcinoma can be identified with 45% sensitivity and 98% specificity based on cytologic criteria of increased N/C ratio, irregular nuclear borders, and cytoplasmic homogeneity.[126] In one study, overall observer accuracy was 76%, with a sensitivity of 82% for a definitive negative diagnosis and specificity for a definitive positive diagnosis of 96%.[127] In another study, sensitivity of 90% and specificity of 65% for grade 1 carcinoma was based on the absence of inflammation, the presence of single and

TABLE 7.9	**Incidence and Cancer Yield of "Suspicious"[a] in Recent Reports**				
				Cancer Yield on Biopsy (%)	
Authors (Date)	Cases of Suspicious With Follow-up Biopsy (n)	Incidence of Suspicious (%)	Time Interval to Biopsy (months)	Negative	Suspicious
Voss et al. (2008)[263]	96	4.1	≤12	56.9	73.8
Siddappa et al. (2012)[250,b]	28	2.0	N/A	0	0
Vandenbussche et al. (2013)[272]	62	6.5	36-60	11	89[c]
Bostwick and Hossain (2014)[47]	593	4.1	≤12	16.6	53.6
Piaton et al. (2014)[270]	185	2.0	4-56	N/A	38[c]
Ton Nu et al. (2014)[118]	191	2.5	>6	6.3	93.7
Joudi et al. (2016)[22]	150	N/A	≤6	N/A	55.3

N/A, Data not available.

[a]Suspicious is reported by some as "atypical urothelial cells, cannot exclude high-grade urothelial carcinoma"; the similarity of incidence rates and described criteria suggest that these groups are comparable with "suspicious." The suspicious rate may be misleading because many articles only reported cases with matched cytology–histology pairs, and most negative biopsies would be excluded because they do not trigger subsequent biopsy.

[b]This series included only cases of hematuria.

[c]High-grade carcinoma only (excluded low-grade carcinoma).

TABLE 7.10	Criteria for Cytologic Grading of Urothelial Cancer			
Morphologic Features	Carcinoma In Situ	Grade 1 Carcinoma (Papillary Neoplasm of Low Malignant Potential)	Grade 2 Carcinoma (Low-Grade Urothelial Carcinoma)	Grade 3 Carcinoma (High-Grade Urothelial Carcinoma)
Background	Clean	Clean	Clean	Dirty, tumor diathesis
Cellular arrangement	Numerous single cells, rare fragments	Large fragments of urothelium	Large fragments of urothelium and single cells	Large fragments and numerous single cells
Nuclear features	Syncytia,[a] cannibalism	Slightly enlarged	Nuclear crowding and overlap	Syncytia,[a] cannibalism
Nuclear membrane	Marked membrane irregularity	Regular, round or oval	Minimal membrane irregularity	Marked membrane irregularity
Chromatin	Increased chromatin, coarsely granular, evenly distributed	Finely granular, vesicular	Finely granular, evenly distributed	Increased chromatin, coarsely granular, unevenly distributed
Nucleolus	Rare nucleoli	Occasional micronucleoli	Variable micronucleoli	Macronucleoli
Cytoplasmic features	Variable maturation	Cell maturation present	Moderate degree of maturation	Maturation absent, squamoid and/or glandular features

[a]Loss of cell borders.
Modified from Shenoy UA, Colby TV, Schumann GB. Reliability of urinary cytodiagnosis in urothelial neoplasms. *Cancer* 1985;56:2041-2045.

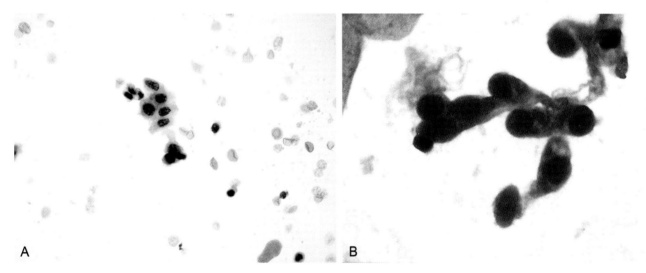

A　　　　B

Fig. 7.29 Examples of grade 1 (of 3) papillary urothelial carcinoma (A and B). In each case the diagnosis was confirmed by biopsy.

overlapping groups of cells with high N/C ratio, hyperchromasia, nuclear grooves and notches, and small nucleoli.[84] A third study showed 26% sensitivity for grade I urothelial carcinoma, and a fourth showed 37% sensitivity (suspicious or malignant diagnoses) and 94% specificity; 48% of these cytology specimens were classified as atypical.[26,128] WHO grade 1 carcinoma is a major source of false-negative results in urine cytology.[84] Chung et al. reported that five distinctive cytologic criteria were helpful in cases in which other conventional criteria for low-grade carcinoma were insufficient for diagnosis (loss of polarity of papillaroid clusters, irregular contours, absence of columnar cells, hobnail features, and hyperchromasia).[129] Stepwise logistic regression analysis revealed that four features distinguished low-grade carcinoma from reactive urothelial cells: increased numbers of monotonous single (nonumbrella) cells, increased N/C ratio, hyperchromasia, and presence of small and large urothelial cells.[130]

The Paris System 2013 recognizes the diagnosis of low-grade urothelial neoplasm (not low-grade carcinoma) based on the

presence of fibrovascular cores in urothelial cell groups and an absence of cytologic atypia.[24] However, in a series of select histologically proven low-grade carcinomas and negative control urines, McCroskey et al. found low sensitivity (21% to 53%) but relatively high specificity (81% to 95%), resulting in poor-to-fair accuracy for the diagnosis of low-grade urothelial carcinoma; overall agreement was fair ($\kappa = 0.30$).[131]

Ancillary techniques (see later) that may be valuable for separating benign and neoplastic urothelial cells include FISH, immunocytochemical tests, and DNA ploidy analysis.[123,132-139] Digital image analysis of voided urine was superior to bladder wash cytology for prediction of tumor recurrence.[140]

High-Grade Carcinoma

"High-grade carcinoma" includes the findings from urothelial carcinoma in situ, characterized by the presence of malignant cells that

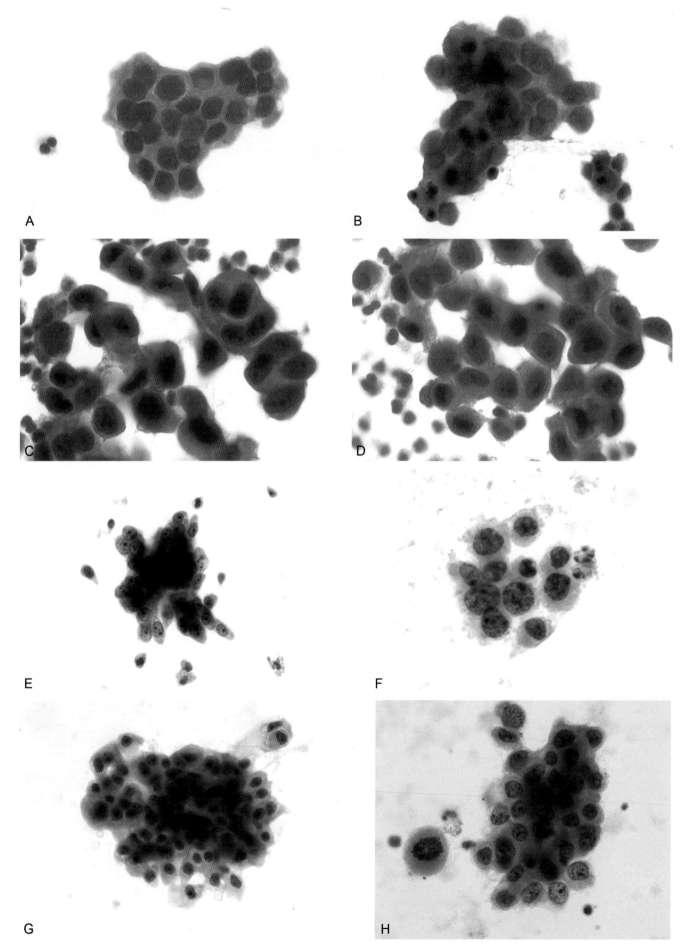

Fig. 7.30 Examples of grade 2 (of 3) papillary urothelial carcinoma (A to H). In each case the diagnosis was confirmed by biopsy.

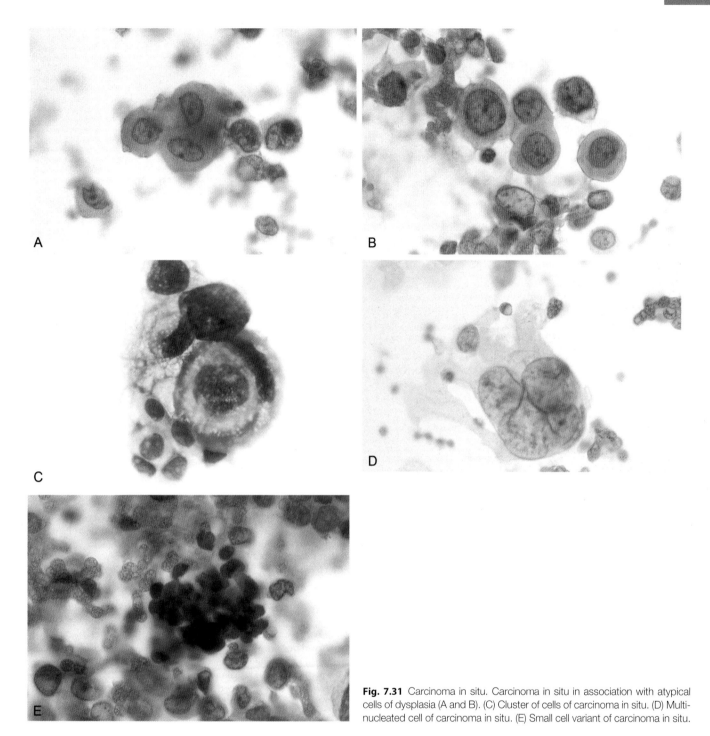

Fig. 7.31 Carcinoma in situ. Carcinoma in situ in association with atypical cells of dysplasia (A and B). (C) Cluster of cells of carcinoma in situ. (D) Multinucleated cell of carcinoma in situ. (E) Small cell variant of carcinoma in situ.

that look like high-grade urothelial carcinoma and are often uniform in size and may be small or large (Fig. 7.31A to E; Table 7.10).[86,141,142] The cells show markedly enlarged nuclei with high N/C ratio, coarse and dark chromatin, and irregular nuclear membranes. Nucleoli may or may not be present. The background is often clean, free of necrotic debris, and lacks inflammation. Occasionally the cells may be heterogeneous and large, particularly after biopsies. When there is prominent inflammation present, it is often prudent not to attempt to separate carcinoma in situ from invasive carcinoma. Microinvasive carcinoma may not be recognizable in cytologic samples, particularly when carcinoma in situ is present. Carcinoma in situ may persist after intravesical therapy such as BCG (Fig. 7.32A and B).

This category also accounts for the urine findings from WHO 1973 grade 2 (intermediate- to high-grade) carcinoma, WHO 1973 grade 3 (high-grade) carcinoma, and carcinoma in situ. It may be difficult to separate grades 2 (Fig. 7.30A to H) and 3 (Fig. 7.33A to F) carcinoma from carcinoma in situ in urine samples (Table 7.10). Unlike benign urothelial cells, these cells have substantial nuclear and cytoplasmic abnormalities. The principal value of urine cytology is the diagnosis and monitoring of high-grade tumors that may not be evident cystoscopically, including carcinoma in situ and occult invasive carcinoma.[142,143]

In voided urine, low-grade and high-grade urothelial carcinoma cells vary in size and shape, and may be small or large. The nuclei are enlarged, with coarsely granular chromatin, hyperchromasia,

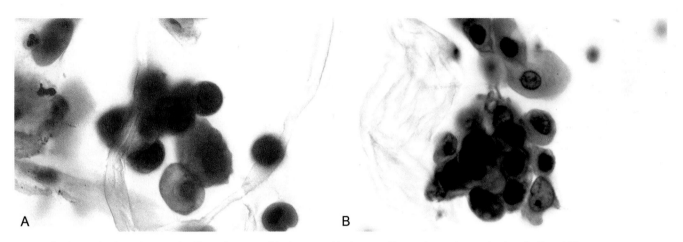

Fig. 7.32 Carcinoma in situ resistant to bacillus calmette–guérin therapy, with clusters of hyperchromatic neoplastic cells (A and B).

abnormal nuclear contours, and prominent nucleoli. Multinucleate cancer cells and mitotic figures are often readily identified.[144]

In washings, urothelial carcinoma may demonstrate a lower degree of nuclear hyperchromasia, perhaps resulting in more prominent large nucleoli. The cells may be poorly preserved, particularly when there is inflammation or necrosis, and a variety of changes may be present, including frayed or vacuolated cytoplasm, nonspecific eosinophilic cytoplasmic inclusions, and pyknotic nuclei. In some high-grade papillary tumors the dominant cytologic finding may be the presence of isolated cancer cells, either singly or in groups of two or three.

Grade 2 carcinoma may present a diagnostic challenge because it is often similar cytologically to grade 1 carcinoma.[8,128,143,145] Fortunately, in most cases, atypical urothelial cells are observed, alerting the clinician of the need for cystoscopic examination. For high-grade urothelial carcinoma, digital image analysis and bladder wash cytology are equally predictive.[140]

Correlation of Urine Cytology and Biopsy Findings (Diagnostic Accuracy)

The diagnostic accuracy of urine cytology is generally high in patients who are symptomatic or being managed after treatment for bladder cancer. However, reported results vary considerably, especially in different patient cohorts. For example, most series of bladder tumors indicate that papilloma and papillary urothelial neoplasm of low malignant potential cannot be reliably diagnosed by urine cytology despite inclusion of several key cytologic findings. Reported sensitivity of urine cytology for grade 1 urothelial carcinoma varied from 26% to 90%.[26,84] The sensitivity increased to 80% for grade 2 and 95% for grade 3.

Carcinoma in situ is usually diagnosed as "suspicious" or "positive" in almost all instances. The overall sensitivity of urine cytology for primary carcinoma of the bladder ranges from 45% to 97%. In a recent report, urine cytology predicted 82% of all recurrent tumors in the bladder.[146] Two major drawbacks of urinary cytology are the high rate of false-positive results in patients receiving intravesical chemotherapy and the high rate of false-negative results in those with grade 1 carcinoma. Scarcity of diagnostic or malignant cells is arguably the greatest single limitation of urine cytology, according to Frost and colleagues.[147] Urine cytology findings, cystoscopy, and possible diagnostic outcomes are summarized in Table 7.11.

False-negative diagnosis of high-grade carcinoma can be attributed to underdiagnosis as "negative," "atypical," or "suspicious"; interestingly, in about 20% of cases, false-negative result was

attributed to overdiagnosis on biopsy of high-grade carcinoma.[148] If poor preservation and obscured samples were considered nondiagnostic, the sensitivity and specificity of cytology for high-grade cancer would be as high as 94% and 71%, respectively.[148]

"Positive" voided urine predicted progression and cancer-specific mortality for non–muscle-invasive carcinoma, independent of and outperforming histologic grade on biopsy.[149] The 5-year cumulative progression and cancer-specific mortality rates for patients with "positive" cytology were 20% and 15%, respectively, compared with 2% and 2%, respectively, for those with "negative" results.

Urine cytology after BCG therapy had sensitivity and specificity of 56% and 56% for cancer recurrence; when combined with cystoscopy, results were 88% and 82%, respectively, obviating the need in many patients for routine biopsy.[150] Urine cytology after radical cystectomy is an early indicator of cancer recurrence, preceding radiographic evidence by a mean of 2.1 years.[151]

Urinary Cells Originating From Other Sites

Prostate

Prostatic adenocarcinoma (Fig. 7.34) may yield cells in voided urine spontaneously or after prostatic massage, particularly when the carcinoma is high grade. Cancer cells in the urine sediment are usually small, often spherical, and columnar, sometimes in small clusters. The cytoplasm is usually basophilic with open vesicular nuclei and prominent nucleoli.

Urethra

Primary cancer of the urethra is rare, and may be urothelial, squamous cell, or adenocarcinoma. Other rare cancers include malignant melanoma and clear cell adenocarcinoma.

Cytologic examination of the urethra after cystectomy for bladder cancer sometimes reveals carcinoma in situ or early invasive carcinoma.[142]

Upper Tract

Urine cytology is usually diagnostic when there is urothelial carcinoma of the renal pelvis and ureter, particularly when the cancers are high grade. With low-grade urothelial malignancies, the same diagnostic problems are encountered as in the bladder. Urine cytology rarely identifies renal cell carcinoma. When malignant cells are present, they are large, with clear or vacuolated cytoplasm and distinct nucleoli.

Among patients with clinical suspicion of upper tract malignancy with positive urine cytology, 42% experienced upper

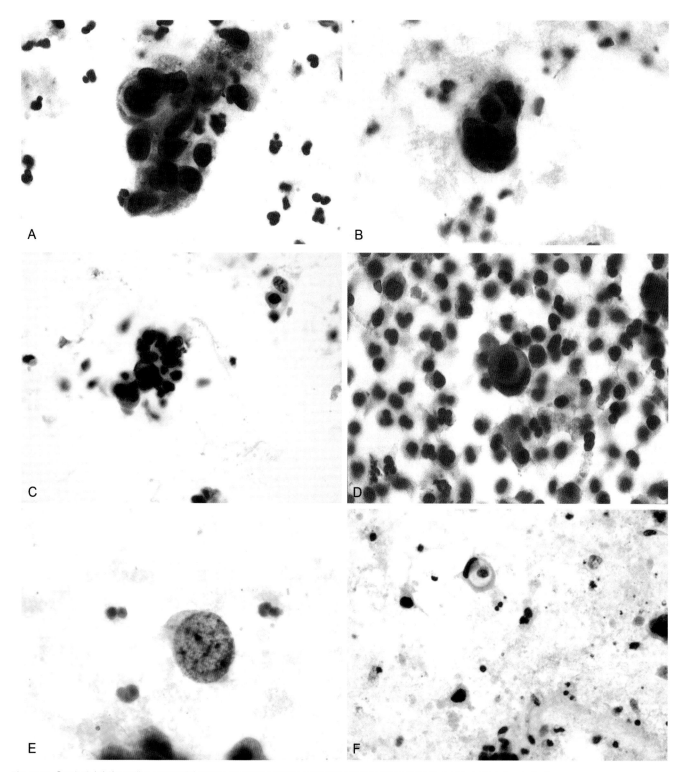

Fig. 7.33 Grade 3 (of 3) papillary urothelial carcinoma with marked cytologic abnormalities (A to F). In (D), note cell cannibalism.

tract cancer and an additional 33% had cancer limited to the bladder.[152] Voided urine, selective urine cytology, ureteral washings, and computed tomography (CT) scan predicted upper tract cancer with a sensitivity and specificity of 63% and 67%, 76% and 73%, 50% and 95%, and 95% and 26%, respectively.[17,153] Patients who had combined abnormal CT and "positive" voided urine had cancer in 83% of cases, whereas 100% of those with combined normal CT and "negative" voided urine (investigated for ongoing symptoms) were

cancer free. FISH hypertetrasomy showed sensitivity and specificity for diagnosis of upper tract carcinoma of 50% and 89%, respectively.[17] Urine cytology alone cannot differentiate upper tract cancer from bladder involvement.

Preoperative "positive" voided urine cytology was predictive of intravesical recurrence after radical nephroureterectomy for upper tract carcinoma. Recurrence-free survival at 1 and 3 years after surgery was 61% and 46% in patients with "positive" urine and 71% and 52% in those with "negative" urine, respectively. Multivariate

TABLE 7.11	Correlation and Outcome in Cytologic and Cystoscopic Findings	
Cytology	Cystoscopy	Outcome
−	−	No tumor
−	+	Low-grade neoplasm
+	+	High-grade cancer, carcinoma in situ
+	−	Carcinoma in situ, upper tract tumor
+ (false-positive result)	−	Chemotherapy, radiation therapy, lithiasis, polyomavirus, cell degeneration (rare) and ileal conduit (rare)

+, Positive; −, negative.

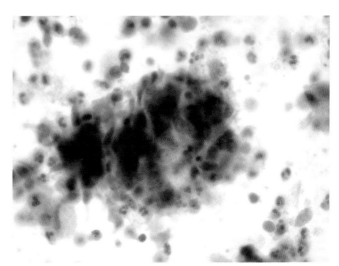

Fig. 7.35 Endometrial carcinoma in urine.

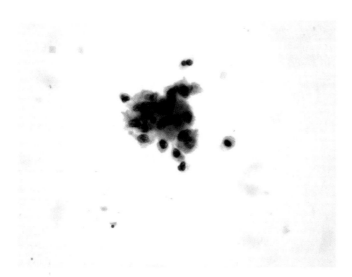

Fig. 7.34 Prostate carcinoma cells in urine.

analysis showed that gender, tumor multifocality in surgical specimens, and "positive" urine cytology were independent risk factors.[154] Ureteral cytology had no additional efficacy beyond voided urine.[155]

Kidney Medulla and Cortex

The strong correlation of chronic kidney disease (58% to 59%) with upper tract urothelial carcinoma, especially among patients receiving dialysis, may result from old age, aristolochic acid nephropathy, and increased risk status after nephroureterectomy, standard treatment for such tumors.[156] Urine cytology is associated with a low detection rate (0.0% to 33.3%) in patients receiving dialysis for all urothelial cancers, especially those with upper tract involvement, because most have anuria.

Renal carcinoma associated with Xp11.2 translocation/TFE3 gene fusions in catheterized urine from the renal pelvis appeared as clusters of cells with abundant clear or eosinophilic granular cytoplasm, large, round nuclei, and prominent nucleoli.[157,158] Papillary clusters containing thin fibrous stroma were occasionally seen. Voided urine showed similar cell clusters but was obscured by degenerative findings. Immunohistochemistry and FISH were useful diagnostic adjuncts.

Secondary Tumors

Numerous secondary malignancies may be observed in the urinary sediment, the most common arising from adjacent or contiguous organs, including the kidney, uterine cervix, endometrium, (Fig. 7.35), ovary, prostate (see earlier), and colon.[34] Clinicopathologic correlation is usually required for diagnosis. Rare cases of carcinoid (low-grade neuroendocrine carcinoma) have been diagnosed by urine cytology.[159] Other rare cancers may be diagnosed by cytology, including bladder and prostatic leiomyosarcoma, primary and secondary lymphoma, mantle cell lymphoma, ALK-negative anaplastic large cell lymphoma, posttransplant lymphoproliferative disorder in patients with renal transplant, melanoma, endometrial adenocarcinoma with squamous differentiation, and choriocarcinoma.[160-168] In many cases urine cytology may not be diagnostic. A recent case of pediatric adrenal neuroblastoma was diagnosed by the presence of highly cellular clusters composed of small, round, atypical cells with scant cytoplasm and high N/C ratio; nuclear molding was also noted.[169] Immunostains were positive for synaptophysin and chromogranin A.

Anticipatory Positive Cytology

Urine-based tests for bladder cancer are frequently apparently falsely positive ("positive" cytology but no clinical or cystoscopic evidence of cancer). However, with further follow-up time, some of these false-positive tests are vindicated as true (anticipatory) positive tests. Among patients with "positive" cytology and initially negative cystoscopy, the hazard ratio of development of a bladder tumor at 1 year was 1.8; 76% of these patients had a tumor within 1 year. Similarly, among patients with a positive FISH and initially negative cystoscopy, the hazard ratio of development of a bladder tumor at 1 year was 1.6; 40% of these patients had a tumor within 1 year.[170] Yafi et al. reported an anticipatory positive rate of 44% after a median time of 15 months.[171]

Other Types of Carcinoma

Squamous Cell Carcinoma

Abnormal squamous cells in the urine may result from squamous metaplasia of the urothelium, cervicovaginal squamous intraepithelial lesion, condyloma acuminatum of the bladder, urothelial carcinoma with squamous differentiation, endometrial adenocarcinoma with squamous differentiation, and squamous cell carcinoma of the urinary tract.[167] Squamous cell carcinoma is common in Africa and the Middle East, particularly in patients infected with

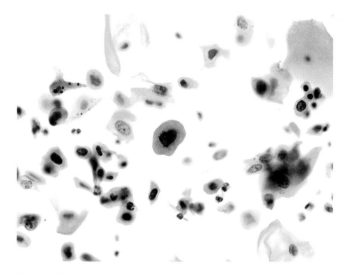

Fig. 7.36 Squamous cell carcinoma in urine.

S. haematobium, but it is relatively uncommon in developed countries, accounting for no more than 3% of bladder tumors.[68] Squamous cell carcinoma has been observed with increasing frequency in long-term survivors with severe spinal cord injury and neurogenic bladder.

Squamous cell carcinoma may display varying degrees of differentiation (Fig. 7.36). In well-differentiated cases, the cytologic findings in voided urine are distinctive, often consisting of keratinized cells with thick, yellow or orange cytoplasm and large, irregular, dark pyknotic nuclei. Squamous pearls, characterized by cell aggregates concentrically arranged around a core of keratin, may be observed.[8] The background often shows evidence of marked necrosis, and ghost cells may be present. A mixture of cancer cells is observed in the urine of the patients with poorly differentiated squamous cell carcinoma, including sharply demarcated cells with eosinophilic cytoplasm and large nuclei.[7,8] Most cases are aneuploid.[172]

Adenocarcinoma

In colonic-type adenocarcinoma of the bladder, the sediment contains columnar cancer cells with large hyperchromatic nuclei and large nucleoli, sometimes in clusters.[173] In poorly differentiated mucus-producing carcinoma, the cancer cells are small, spherical or cuboidal in shape, and contain large hyperchromatic nuclei, often with prominent nucleoli. The cytoplasm is usually basophilic, often scant, and sometimes poorly preserved. When there are large cytoplasmic vacuoles containing mucus, the nuclei may be pushed to the periphery of the cell, features suggestive of or diagnostic of signet ring cell carcinoma.

In clear cell adenocarcinoma the cancer cells are large, with abundant finely vacuolated or granular cytoplasm, open vesicular nuclei, and prominent nucleoli. Such cells usually form round papillary clusters.[7] Most cases are aneuploid.[174]

When numerous mucin-producing goblet cells are present, another consideration is villous adenoma.[175]

Small Cell Undifferentiated Carcinoma (Oat Cell Carcinoma)

In small cell carcinoma, the cancer cells are small and round to oval, about four times the size of lymphocytes, contain compact and finely granular chromatin, often with pyknotic nuclei, high N/C

ratio, and scant basophilic cytoplasm, and are set in a background of inflammatory and necrotic material.[176,177] Nuclear molding may be prominent; nucleoli are not visible. The presence of small clusters of tightly packed tumor cells with nuclear molding is diagnostically helpful.[8] The presence of cell clusters without prominent nucleoli is useful in differentiating these cells from malignant lymphoma; in the latter, cells do not cluster and usually contain small nucleoli. The demonstration of neuroendocrine differentiation in small cell carcinoma may require immunocytologic or ultrastructural studies.[178,179]

Mixed Carcinoma

Urothelial cancer may contain foci with more than one histologic type, including squamous cell carcinoma, adenocarcinoma, and small cell carcinoma. The cytologic findings in such tumors rarely allow the diagnosis of mixed carcinoma. Usually one pattern is dominant, although a mixed population of cancer cells may be observed, including some of the rare variants.

Rare Variants of Urothelial Carcinoma

Signet ring cell, micropapillary, plasmacytoid, urothelial carcinoma with oncocytic features, and sarcomatoid variants have been reported in the cytology literature, mostly as case reports.[180-184] Recognition of variants is critical because many are associated with different clinical outcomes or therapeutic approaches.

Signet ring cell carcinoma consists of scattered malignant epithelial cells displaying distinct cell borders, abundant cytoplasm with single large, discrete mucin vacuoles, and eccentric irregular nuclei with prominent nucleoli.[180] In contrast, metastatic colonic signet ring cell carcinoma displayed predominantly single dispersed malignant cells containing eccentrically placed, oval nuclei with occasional small nucleoli and a moderate amount of vacuolated cytoplasm.

Micropapillary urothelial carcinoma is rarely identified, appearing as numerous small, cohesive groups and single neoplastic cells.[183,185] Pseudopapillae were present in 17 of 20 cases, and in 9 they were a relevant finding; morules were present in 15 cases; isolated microacini were seen in 14 cases; cellular atypia was prominent in 17 cases.[185] In 15 cases a cytologic diagnosis of urothelial carcinoma was made, 1 case was diagnosed as adenocarcinoma, and the remaining 4 cases were considered suspicious of malignancy.

Plasmacytoid carcinoma contains single cells with eosinophilic cytoplasm and characteristic eccentric hyperchromatic nuclei. Immunoreactivity for CD138 is helpful but represents a pitfall because it is also positive in plasma cell dyscrasias.[186]

Urothelial carcinoma with oncocytic features appeared as delicate papillae with cells displaying oncocytic cytoplasm and relatively low N/C ratio; immunostains showed strong p53 immunoreactivity and low Ki-67 labeling.[184]

Major Diagnostic Pitfalls

Most errors in urine cytology are overdiagnosis of benign cellular changes as malignant (Table 7.12). Knowledge of these changes is fundamental to the practice of cytology. The College of American Pathologists Interlaboratory Comparison project of more than 46,000 pathologists found that participants performed well in accurately classifying cases as benign or malignant (overall 92.4% concordance) (Table 7.13).[187] However, the greatest difficulties were with correct identification of adenocarcinoma and squamous cell carcinoma cases, and with overinterpretation of ileal loop and polyomavirus as high-grade carcinoma.[187]

TABLE 7.12	Major Diagnostic Pitfalls in Lower Urinary Tract Cytology

Overdiagnosis of normal and degenerated urothelium as malignant
Overdiagnosis of human polyomavirus infection as malignant
Overdiagnosis of effects of cyclophosphamide as malignant
Underdiagnosis of grade 1 or 2 urothelial carcinoma (papillary urothelial neoplasia of low malignant potential or low-grade urothelial carcinoma) as benign

TABLE 7.13	Concordance with the Urine Cytology Reference Standard in the College of American Pathologists Interlaboratory Comparison Program 2000 to 2010[187,a]

Reference Diagnosis	No. of Responses	Concordance Rate (%)	False Responses (%)
High-grade urothelial carcinoma	71,581	83.8	Atypical urothelial cells (4.1), reactive (3.2), adenocarcinoma (3.1), negative for malignancy (1.3), squamous cell carcinoma (1.1), polyomavirus (0.9), inflammation (0.7), and other (1.8)
Negative for malignancy	2852	73.9	a
Polyomavirus	3535	71.7	Reactive (6.4), high-grade carcinoma (6.2), and cytomegalovirus/herpes (3.1)
Ileal loop urine	5291	55.8	a
Squamous cell carcinoma	756	49.1	a
Adenocarcinoma	1667	42.9	a
Treatment-related changes	1293	36.3	a

[a]Not provided.

Following is a summary of some of the most vexing problems, which are also described and illustrated elsewhere in this chapter.

Trauma or Instrumentation

The normal urothelium tends to exfoliate in the form of tissue fragments that are round or oval, commonly designated as papillary clusters. Vigorous palpation, catheterization, or any form of instrumentation may result in the formation of such epithelial clusters. When present in large numbers, these clusters may be misinterpreted as carcinoma.[53] Another source of error is the presence of numerous superficial urothelial cells that may be mistaken for cancer because of their variable nuclear features.[86] Careful consideration of chromatin pattern, N/C ratio, and nuclear membrane irregularity should enable differentiation of benign and malignant processes in the vast majority of cases.

Cell Preservation

Cells in voided urine sediment, particularly in the first morning void, are often poorly preserved, compounding the diagnostic difficulty. The diagnosis of cancer in voided urine should be avoided unless the findings are unequivocal.[8]

Human Polyomavirus

Polyomavirus (BK virus) infection creates large intranuclear inclusions that may mimic cancer nuclei. However, the inclusions are homogeneous and lack the coarse chromatin granularity of malignancy. This is an important source of diagnostic errors that can contribute to costly and lengthy patient investigations.[78] Polyomavirus-infected cells and malignant cells may coexist in urine cytology.[188]

Lithiasis

Calculi in the lower urinary tract are abrasive, dislodging epithelial fragments that may be quite large and display papillary appearance mimicking low-grade carcinoma.[52] The presence of numerous superficial cells may also create diagnostic difficulty because of nuclear abnormalities.[8,84,86]

Drugs and Other Therapeutic Procedures

Urothelial cell changes may result from a wide variety of inciting agents, including chemotherapy, radiotherapy, and other interventions. Intravesical chemotherapy is responsible for a high rate of false-positive results.[84] A further source of diagnostic difficulty may be synchronous infection with polyomavirus in patients who are immunocompromised.[8] It should be remembered that urothelial carcinoma or sarcoma may develop in patients who are receiving cyclophosphamide for treatment of lymphoma.[87,88]

Ancillary Studies and Immunocytology

This section is limited to discussion of cell-based assays that may be used in the anatomic pathology/cytology laboratory, including digital image analysis, cytochemical and immunocytochemical stains, and FISH. Excluded are clinical laboratory methods such as metabolomics, microRNA and DNA assays, deep sequencing, and serum-based methods of soluble biomarkers.

Digital Image Analysis and Morphometry

Digital image analysis was superior to flow cytometry for DNA ploidy analysis, with sensitivities of 83% to 91% and 71%, respectively, and was even higher in carcinoma in situ, grade 3 cancer, and stages T2 and T3 cancer (all nearly 100%).[134,189]

Digital image analysis can be combined with flow cytometry to identify subpopulations of urothelial cells. The diagnosis of cancer is strongly suspected in cases with abundant aneuploid cells or 16% or more of measured cells with hyperdiploid DNA (greater than twice the DNA content). A specimen is less likely to be malignant if no aneuploid stemline is detected and fewer than 11% of the cells are hyperdiploid. If 11% to 16% of the cells measured are hyperdiploid and no aneuploid stemline is detected, the samples are considered "suspicious."

Recurrent cancer can be detected with the combination of urine cytology and image analysis.[190,191] Digital image analysis by itself was superior to cytologic examination for prediction of tumor recurrence after negative findings by cystoscopic examination and was equivalent to cytology for detection of high-grade cancer.[140] Muralidaran et al. demonstrated the utility of an artificial neural network for urine cytology diagnosis based on nuclear area, diameter, perimeter, standard deviation of nuclear area, and integrated gray density.[192]

Apoptotic index was found to be diagnostically useful. Excluding ileal conduit specimens, the finding of a high apoptotic index with the presence of pyknosis or karyorrhexis in the urine correlated with high-grade cancer.[193]

Quantitative phase imaging is a new method that measures the nuclear mass and entropy of cells, and showed significant differences between "negative" and "positive."[194] There was a progressive increase in patients with "negative" diagnosis compared with those with "atypical," "suspicious," and "positive" cytologic diagnoses that was predictive of subsequent biopsy results.

Nuclear/nucleolar volume ratio creates an index for discrimination of benign and malignant urothelial cells with sensitivity of 56%, specificity of 89%, positive predictive value of 85%, and negative predictive value of 64% (cut point of 1.5%).[195]

Digital image telepathology is feasible. Specificity and sensitivity regarding categorized diagnoses were 83% to 92% and 85% to 93%, respectively; overall accuracy rate was 88% to 90%.[196] Interobserver agreement was substantial ($\kappa = 0.791$). The lowest rate of concordance was with the identification of benign lesions.

Cytochemical Stains

Acid Hematoxylin Stain

Addition of nuclear staining such as the acid hematoxylin stain to Papanicolaou staining increased sensitivity in one laboratory by about 28% by eliminating background debris and improving detection of mitotic figures and other changes in chromatin that may be obscured.[197] The combination of Papanicolaou staining with nuclear staining and image analysis achieved 90% sensitivity for diagnosis of urothelial carcinoma in one report.[198] DNA ploidy analysis was equivalent with the two methods. Both stains were superior to Papanicolaou stain for examination of nuclear chromatin texture and content. These findings indicate that acid hematoxylin is a satisfactory substitute for Feulgen staining in cytologic preparation for DNA ploidy studies and provides additional technical advantages.

In addition to Papanicolaou stain, we routinely use acid hematoxylin stain for urine cytology. This inexpensive, nontoxic, and easily performed stain enhances nuclear chromatin pattern (surrogate Feulgen stain), removes unwanted background debris, and optimizes cellular adherence to the slide. Acid hematoxylin complements Papanicolaou stain for diagnosis of malignant cells (Fig. 7.37A and B) and is superior to Papanicolaou stain for differentiating "decoy" cells from malignant cells (Fig. 7.38A and B).[79]

Acid hematoxylin stain can also be used for DNA ploidy analysis with the aid of an image analyzer.[199,200] The increased accuracy of diagnosis is cost effective, obviating the need for unnecessary cystoscopies and other invasive and expensive techniques. Acid hematoxylin provided superior cellular yield compared with Feulgen stains, as well as more consistent staining and better preservation of nuclear size (Fig. 7.39A and B).[79]

CellDetect

CellDetect is a unique histochemical panel consisting of a proprietary plant extract and three dyes that enables color discrimination between benign (green) and malignant (red) cells based on specific metabolic alterations exclusive to the latter. It was superior to standard cytology (sensitivity of 94% versus 46%, respectively, and specificity of 89% for both), particularly for sensitivity with low-grade tumors (88% versus 17%, respectively).[201,202]

Immunocytochemical Stains

Telomerase

The ribonucleoprotein telomerase is a reverse transcriptase enzyme that adds repeat sequences to the 3' end of telomeres, a region of repetitive sequences at each end of eukaryotic chromosomes. Telomeres protect the ends of the chromosomes from DNA damage or alteration. Telomerase is active in normal stem cells and most cancer cells but is normally absent from, or at very low levels in, most somatic cells. Expression of the hTERT protein has also been analyzed by immunocytochemistry using anti-hTERT antibodies.

The telomeric repeat amplification protocol polymerase chain reaction assay has been most widely used to assay telomerase activity, but it creates false-positive results in the presence of inflammation and nonbladder epithelial cells. The availability of polyclonal and monoclonal antibodies for nuclear and cytoplasmic hTERT protein expression allows cell-specific microscopic visualization of different cell components in urine and other tissues, minimizing the influence of false-positive results (Fig. 7.40).[203-205] Inflammatory cells serve as internal positive controls.

HER2 and Cytokeratins

Immunocytologic expression of HER and high-molecular-weight cytokeratin in cells from voided urine predicted bladder cancer recurrence.[206] HER was expressed in 7% of cases without recurrence

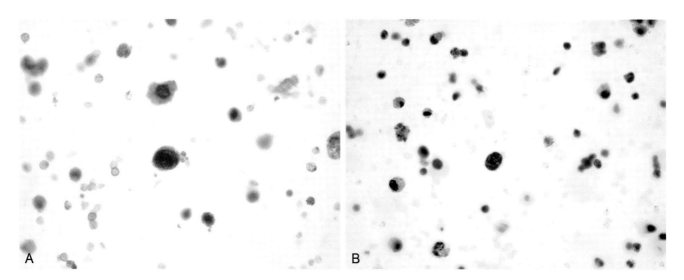

Fig. 7.37 Carcinoma in situ in urine. (A) Papanicolaou stain. (B) Acid hematoxylin stain.

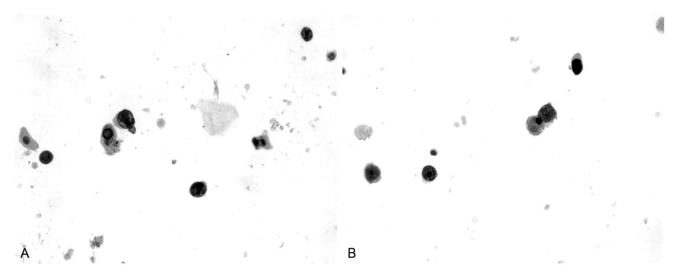

Fig. 7.38 Decoy cells in urine. (A) Papanicolaou stain. (B) Acid hematoxylin stain.

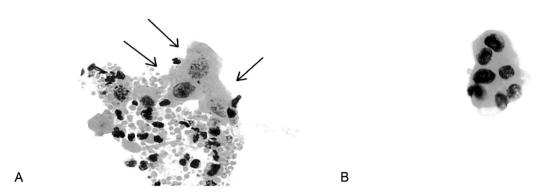

Fig. 7.39 Feulgen stain. (A) Benign urine with stained superficial cell nuclei (*arrows*) with inflammatory cells. Note the detail of the nuclear chromatin, chiseled nuclear membranes (chromatinic rims), and defined small nucleoli. (B) Malignant urothelial cells with densely clumped chromatin, with loss of nuclear detail because of hyperchromasia.

compared with 85% of those with recurrence; results for high-molecular-weight cytokeratin were 43% versus 64%, respectively.[206]

Cytokeratin 20 expression in nonumbrella cells is a robust marker of urothelial carcinoma, and it was confirmatory of low-grade urothelial malignancy in "atypical" voided specimens, as well as excluding cancer in those with reactive changes caused by calculus disease.[207,208] Aberrant staining may be observed in cases of cystitis. The combination of CK20 and p53 immunostaining revealed positivity in 90% of urothelial cancers, 50% of "atypical" cases, and 25% of "negative" cases. Accuracy for cytology versus cytology combined with the two immunostains showed sensitivity of 73% versus 91%, specificity 100% versus 74.3%, positive predictive value 100% versus 89%, and negative predictive value 63% versus 79%.[209] It appears that combined immunocytochemical staining for CK20 and p53 is easy to perform and evaluate, improves sensitivity, helps in establishing the diagnosis of malignancy, and may be of value as a triage tool to select patients who require cystoscopy during clinical follow-up.

Vimentin

Vimentin immunocytochemical staining may be useful as an ancillary method for evaluation of exfoliated atypical reactive/repair renal tubular cells in select urinary specimens. This may avoid unnecessary diagnostic procedures for evaluation of urothelial carcinoma in vimentin-positive cases, suggesting further diagnostic workup for evaluation of renal disease.[210]

ImmunoCyt/uCyt Immunocytology

ImmunoCyt/uCyt consists of a targeted panel of antibodies, including fluorescently labeled M344, LDQ10, 19a211, and glycosylated high-molecular-weight carcinoembryonic antigen. A minimum of 500 epithelial cells is required, and identification of one or more fluorescent cells is positive. Sensitivity is 62% (47% for low-grade and 83% for high-grade cancer); overall specificity was 79%.[211] Metaanalysis revealed that ImmunoCyt had a higher sensitivity (73%) than urine cytology test, but the specificity, positive likelihood ratio (LR), negative LR, diagnostic odds ratio (DOR), AUC, and Q index were lower.[212] The combination of ImmunoCyt and cytology provided sensitivity, specificity, positive LR, negative LR, DOR, AUC, and Q index of 83%, 64%, 2.80, 0.23, 13.50, 0.86, and 0.79, respectively.

ProExC

ProExC is a commercially available immunocytochemical panel biomarker directed against topoisomerase II α and minichromosome maintenance 2 proteins, both of which are involved in DNA replication and overexpressed in dysplastic and malignant tissues. ProExC is positive when nuclear staining identifies at least

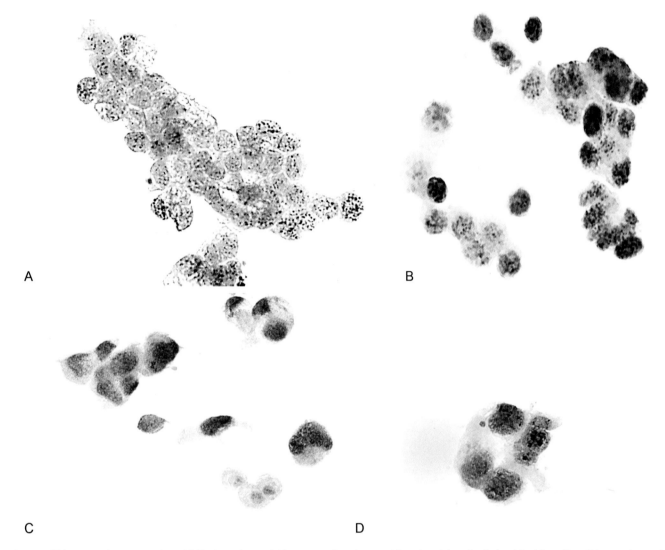

Fig. 7.40 Telomerase Immunocytology. (A) Benign urine nuclei have scant fine dusty staining of nuclei, easily distinguished from (B to D) intense but variable nuclear immunoreactivity in high-grade carcinoma.

one morphologically atypical urothelial cell. Sensitivity and specificity were 85% and 69%, respectively, compared with 85% and 31% for ImmunoCyt, and 93% and 23% for the combination of tests; prediction of high-grade urothelial carcinoma had sensitivity of 92% for ProExC, 86% for ImmunoCyt, and 92% for the combination.[213] ProExC was superior to FISH for prediction of cancer, with sensitivity of 89% and 56%, specificity of 78% and 44%, positive predictive value of 89% and 67%, and negative predictive value of 78% and 33%, respectively.[214]

Other Immunostains

Ubiquilin-2, a ubiquitin-related protein, is expressed in the nuclei of urothelial carcinoma cells, but not benign cells.[215] Overall sensitivity was 88%, specificity was 99%, positive predictive value was 98%, and negative predictive value was 93% for detection of carcinoma.

ERG immunocytochemistry has sensitivity and specificity for prostate cancer in urine of 23% and 100%, respectively; it should be noted that up to half of prostate cancers are ERG$^-$ in prostatic tissues, so the expected sensitivity in urine will be accordingly limited.[216]

WT1 antibody recognizes a podocyte marker that can distinguish normal and nonrenal urinary tract disease from kidney disease.[217] WT1$^+$ cells were found in 50% of voided urine samples,

whereas no positive cells were found in patients with lower urinary tract disease or in healthy volunteers.

Immunostains for p53 or Ki-67 (optimal cutoffs were 5% for p53 and 3% for Ki-67) in combination with cytology increased specificity without penalizing sensitivity for detection of carcinoma; sensitivity and specificity for the detection of all cancers were 86% and 77% for cytology alone, 81% and 93% for cytology and p53, 76% and 88% for cytology and Ki-67, and 69% and 98% for the full combination of cytology, p53, and Ki-67, respectively.[218]

PAX8 is a useful immunostain to diagnose nephrogenic adenoma in voided specimens; however, care must be taken to avoid misinterpretation of positive staining in lymphocyte nuclei.[219]

Epidermal growth factor receptor positivity was an independent risk factor for recurrence after intravesical chemotherapy.[220]

Polyomavirus-infected cells were categorized as SV40$^+$/S100P$^+$ and SV40$^+$/S100P$^-$ by immunostains.[221]

Calreticulin, annexin A2, and annexin A3 were overexpressed in upper tract carcinoma.[222]

In patients with bladder cancer independent of stage, TERT mutations were found in 55%, FGFR3 mutations in 30%, PIK3CA in 14%, and TP53 mutations in 12%, with 70% sensitivity and 97% specificity.[223]

Fluorescence In Situ Hybridization

Multitarget FISH using probes for chromosomes 3, 7, 17, and 9p21 has high sensitivity and specificity for detecting urothelial carcinoma (Fig. 7.41A to E). A positive result is defined as polysomy in four or more cells, which also includes tetrasomy. The sensitivity of FISH for detecting cancer was superior to cytology, despite similar specificity, irrespective of cancer grade and stage: overall, 81% versus 33%; low grade, 76% versus 12%; high grade, 85% versus 50%; nonmuscle invasive, 81% versus 28%; and muscle invasive, 80% versus 45%, respectively.[224] Sensitivity ranged from 55% to 98% and specificity from 55% to 100%. 9p21 loss (>12%) was an independent prognostic factor for recurrence.[225]

About 27% of patients under surveillance for recurrent bladder cancer with no immediate clinical evidence of recurrence had positive FISH, and about 65% of these anticipatory positive patients had recurrent cancer within 29 months.[135,226-231]

FISH may be useful in decreasing the rate of atypia, but it is limited by high false-positive incidence. Carcinoma was diagnosed more frequently in patients with positive than in those with negative FISH results (49% versus 9%, respectively). Sensitivity, specificity, positive predictive value, negative predictive value, and accuracy of FISH were 45%, 82%, 47%, 80%, and 72% for all cancers and 48%, 79%, 28%, 90%, and 74% for high-grade carcinoma, respectively. FISH showed a high false-positive rate (53%)

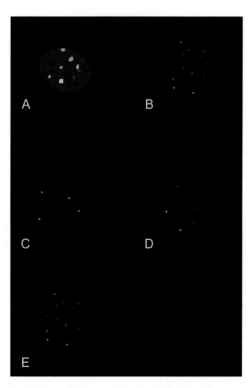

Fig. 7.41 Fluorescence in situ hybridization (FISH) in voided urine cytology. (A) Normal urothelium showing two copies of chromosome 3 (red), two copies of chromosome 7 (green), two copies of chromosome 17 (aqua), and two copies of LSI 9p21 (gold) by FISH. (B) Aneusomic urothelial cell showing five copies of chromosome 3 (red), three copies of chromosome 7 (green), five copies of chromosome 17 (aqua), and no copies of LSI 9p21 (gold) by FISH. (C) Aneusomic urothelial cell showing five copies of chromosome 3 (red), seven copies of chromosome 7 (green), and four copies of chromosome 17 (aqua) by FISH. (D) Aneusomic urothelial cell showing four copies of chromosome 3 (red), two copies of chromosome 7 (green), two copies of chromosome 17 (aqua), and two copies of LSI 9p21 (gold) by FISH. (E) Urothelial carcinoma cell showing gains of chromosomes 3 (red), 7 (green), and 17 (aqua) by FISH.

that remained high even after extended follow-up, arguing against "anticipatory positive" results.[232]

The combination of FISH and cytology, FISH and ImmunoCyt, or cytology and ImmunoCyt all showed negative predictive value of 99% of recurrence in patients with a prior history of high-grade carcinoma.[233]

For upper tract cancer, FISH was superior to voided cytology, with sensitivity of 77% to 84% and specificity of 90% to 95% (64% versus 29% for low-grade urothelial carcinoma and 87% versus 27% for high-grade urothelial carcinoma, respectively).[18,234,235] Comparison revealed that cytology was more suitable for identification of high-grade cancer, FISH was superior for identifying low-grade cancer, and immunostains for p16/Ki-67 were useful for distinguishing high-grade from low-grade cancer.[236]

Alternative evaluation methods may offer superior diagnostic performance compared with the manufacturer's algorithm. Modification of UroVysion scoring criteria with gain of at least one chromosome (3, 7, or 17) or heterozygous or homozygous deletion of 9p21 resulted in moderate increased sensitivity (81%) and only a slight decrease in specificity.[237] In our experience, 9p21 deletion was present in 12% of FISH-positive cases and always occurred with other chromosomal anomalies, rarely if ever a solitary finding.[238] Modification by addition of cytologic prescreening and use of positive results defined as at least one copy number change of a probe target resulted in an increase in sensitivity from to 68% to 81% and a slight decrease in specificity from 84% to 82%.[237] Zellweger et al. found that sensitivity of FISH to predict recurrence was significantly improved by considering specimens with rare (≤10) tetraploid cells as negative, and this observation was later confirmed.[239,240] Zhou and colleagues determined that exclusion of tetrasomy from the polysomy category changed the threshold from 8.5 to 4.5 cells, increased specificity (59% to 79%), but reduced sensitivity (70% to 66%).[241] The introduction of specific cutoffs for tetraploid cells improved specificity.

Molecular grading with FISH increased the accuracy of prediction for both recurrence and progression in patients with intermediate-risk non–muscle-invasive bladder cancer. Low molecular grading was defined as diploid chromosomal pattern or only a loss of p16 or chromosome 3 aneuploidy, and high molecular grading as aneuploidy of chromosome 7 or 17.[242] With median follow-up of 67 months, 57% of tumors were classified as low molecular grading. The 2- and 5-year recurrence-free survival rates were 68% and 49% for low molecular grading, and 47% and 30% for high molecular grading, respectively. The 2- and 5-year progression-free survival rates were 95% and 84% for low molecular grading, and 79% and 58% for high molecular grading tumor patients, respectively. Cancer severity score and molecular grading independently and positively predicted progression in multivariable models.

FISH for AURKA gene copy number in urine yielded a specificity of 79.7% and sensitivity of 79.6%, with an AUC of 0.90.[243]

The Problem of Hematuria

Hematuria is present in about 21% of Americans, including up to 2% of children.[244,245] It is most commonly microscopic, usually discovered incidentally during laboratory studies accompanying physical examination, or gross and typically apparent to patient. Only 1 mL of red blood cells per liter is sufficient to noticeably change the color of urine. Microscopic hematuria is defined as at least three red blood cells per hpf in freshly voided centrifuged urine, preferably documented on three separate occasions.[246] Up to 3% of adults normally excrete small numbers of red blood cells (up to two red blood cells per hpf, or the equivalent of 1000 red blood cells/mL), so it is important in such cases to avoid overdiagnosis. Gross hematuria is the visible discoloration of urine secondary to blood.

Hematuria may be symptomatic or asymptomatic, transient or persistent, but is often accompanied by other physical findings including proteinuria, edema, and hypertension. A thorough history and physical examination is mandatory. Current guidelines around the world recommend against the use of routine urine cytology for evaluation of asymptomatic microscopic hematuria.[247,248] Metaanalysis revealed an overall pooled urinary tract cancer rate for hematuria of 3.3%.[249]

Hematuria may originate anywhere in the urinary tract, from the glomeruli to the distal urethra. Causes of hematuria are numerous and may be benign or malignant (Table 7.14 through Table 7.16). "Atypical urothelial cells" are present in 33% of cases of gross or microscopic hematuria, with 10% of these predictive of carcinoma (3% of all cases of hematuria).[250] The commonest causes of gross hematuria in adults are urinary tract infection (33%), malignancy (23%), and urolithiasis (11%). The most common causes of hematuria in adults are idiopathic (43% of cases of microscopic hematuria) and urinary tract infection (33% of cases of gross hematuria (Table 7.14).[251] Among children the most common causes are idiopathic (80% of cases of microscopic hematuria) and renal disease (34% of cases of gross hematuria).[245] It is critical that the source of persistent hematuria be identified, according to the Best Practice Policy of the American Urologic Association.[251] Such patients should be referred for appropriate urologic workup.

Routine Laboratory Investigation of Hematuria

Routine urinalysis combines the macroscopic reagent strip (dipstick) test with microscopic examination of the sediment to detect disorders of the urinary tract. Dipsticks detect 0.05 to 0.3 mg of

TABLE 7.14	Causes of Hematuria in Children and Adults (%)			
	CHILDREN[245]		ADULTS[251]	
Causes	Microscopic Hematuria	Gross Hematuria	Microscopic Hematuria	Gross Hematuria
Idiopathic	38	80	43	0
Malignancy	0	0	5	23
Calculi	0	1	5	11
Urinary tract infection	0	0	4	33
Renal disease	3	34	2	0
Hypercalciuria	16	22	0	0

TABLE 7.15	Site-Specific Causes of Hematuria

Lower Urinary Tract Bleeding

Tumors (urethra, bladder, prostate, ureters, renal pelvis)
Obstructive uropathy
Benign prostatic hyperplasia
Lithiasis (stones)
Infections (cystitis, prostatitis, schistosomiasis, tuberculosis, condyloma acuminatum)
Coagulopathy
Trauma
Radiation therapy
Instrumentation
Vigorous exercise
Menstrual contamination
Endometriosis

Upper Urinary Tract (Renal) Bleeding

Primary glomerulopathies

Immunoglobulin A nephropathy
Postinfectious glomerulonephritis
Membranoproliferative glomerulonephritis
Focal glomerular sclerosis

Secondary glomerulopathies

Lupus nephritis
Henoch-Schönlein syndrome
Vasculitis (polyarteritis nodosa)
Wegener granulomatosis
Hemolytic-uremic syndrome
Essential mixed cryoglobulinemia
Interstitial nephritis

Familial conditions

Hereditary nephritis (Alport syndrome)
Hemoglobinopathies
Metabolic disorders (hypercalcuria)
Polycystic kidney

Infections

Pyelonephritis (acute or chronic)
Tuberculosis
Cytomegalovirus
Polyomavirus

Nephrolithiasis

Light chain deposition

Diabetic nephropathy

Amyloid

Renal tumors (renal cell carcinoma)

TABLE 7.16 Etiologic Classification of Causes of Hematuria by Ingestion and Pigments

Drugs and Medications	Pigments	Other
Antibiotics	Rhabdomyolysis (myoglobin)	*Diuretics*
Penicillin	Hemoglobin (transfusion reaction)	Thiazides
Cephalosporin		Furosemide
Rifampin	Heme pigment (hemolysis)	Triamterene
Erythromycin		Chlorthalidone
Sulfonamides		
Aminoglycosides		*Other*
Tetracycline		
		Radiocontrast agents
Nonsteroidal antiinflammatory drugs		Cisplatinum
		Heavy metals (gold, cadmium, mercury)
Acetaminophen		Organic solvents
Acetylsalicylic acid		
Naproxen		
Ibuprofen		
Indomethacin		
Phenylbutazone		
Tolmetin		
Mefenamic acid		
Fenoprofen		
Other drugs		
Captopril		
Cimetidine		
Phenobarbital		
Dilantin		
Interferon		
Lithium		

hemoglobin per deciliter of urine. The sensitivity of dipstick examination to detect three or more red blood cells per hpf is around 90%. Myoglobin is also detected by screening reagent strips, so confirmatory testing by an appropriate reagent strip and microscopic examination is necessary. The degree of hematuria bears no relation to the severity of underlying disease and should be considered evidence of disease until proven otherwise.

Dysmorphic Red Blood Cells Indicate Glomerular Disease

Red blood cell morphology is useful for determining the site of origin (glomerular or nonglomerular) of hematuria. Dysmorphic red blood cells are associated with hematuria caused by glomerular injury.[252] Two distinct types of dysmorphic red blood cells have been described: (1) target cells containing a distinct central inclusion of heme pigment surrounded by a clear zone, and (2) cells with multiple cytoplasmic blebs (Fig. 7.42A to D). How dysmorphic red blood cells are formed has not been definitively elucidated, although some suggest that causes include mechanical damage to the red blood cell within the glomerulus followed by osmotic injury sustained during passage through the renal tubules.[253,254] In contrast with dysmorphic red blood cells, isomorphic red blood cells suggest nonglomerular hematuria.

We analyzed 146 patients (Table 7.17) who had diagnostic renal biopsies and prior cytologic examination of urine sediment, including detailed analysis of red blood cell morphology (unpublished

data). Of 108 patients with histologically confirmed glomerulopathy, 67 had dysmorphic red blood cells in urine. One of 38 patients with no glomerulopathy diagnosed at renal biopsy had dysmorphic red blood cells. Using histologically confirmed glomerulopathy as the end point for analysis of dysmorphic red blood cells and glomerulopathy, sensitivity was 70%, specificity was 97%, positive predictive value was 99%, and the negative predictive value was 54%.

Red blood cell morphology alone is not sufficient to categorize patients with hematuria. Although the specificity of dysmorphic red blood cells is high, their absence does not entirely exclude the possibility of glomerulopathy, nor does their presence guarantee renal disease. The evaluation of red cell morphology is most useful when accompanied by evaluation of all components of urine sediment, including urothelial cell morphology, urinalysis with urine chemistry, and serum chemistries.

Studies have evaluated various percentages of dysmorphic red blood cells in patients with known glomerular disease. Increasing the percent required for the diagnosis of glomerular bleeding increases the specificity of the test.[255,256] Among patients exhibiting ≥ 40 dysmorphic red blood cells, 34% had urologic diseases and 29% had glomerular diseases.[257] Urologic diseases included 27% with malignancies and 52% with conditions requiring immediate treatment. For predicting glomerular disease, the presence of proteinuria was more accurate than the number of dysmorphic cells.

Comprehensive Analysis of Urine for Evaluation of Hematuria

Comprehensive quantitative evaluation of the sediment, also known as optimal cytodiagnostic urinalysis, is useful to help discriminate inflammatory, infectious, degenerative, or neoplastic conditions of the kidney and the lower urinary tract, and can often discriminate glomerular and tubular injury.[64,258] This method incorporates routine urinalysis, urine chemistries, and detailed cytologic examination of urothelial and renal cellular elements. Enhanced cytologic preparation improves cell recovery to maximize microscopic visualization and quantitative assessment of dysmorphic and isomorphic red blood cells, inflammatory cells, renal casts, and renal tubular elements. Diagnostic findings are correlated with serum findings, providing the clinician with the full spectrum of chemical and morphologic abnormalities, and allowing triage of patients to the appropriate specialist (e.g., nephrologist, urologist). There are six components in comprehensive analysis of urine for evaluation of hematuria:

1. Patient history
2. Physical examination of the urine sample, including color, character, and specific gravity
3. Chemical examination, consisting of multiparameter reagent dipstick testing and confirmatory tests; albumin, β_2 microglobulin, and protein are reported quantitatively
4. Microscopic urine sediment examination using standardized sediment recovery and high-contrast Papanicolaou stain
5. Quantitative microscopic examination of the sediment entities and 10 specific morphologic categories: background, cellularity, epithelial fragments, inclusion-bearing cells, red blood cells, neutrophils, eosinophils, lymphocytes, renal tubular cells, and casts
6. Diagnostic interpretation

There is a high level of intraobserver and interobserver agreement in determination of origin of renal cells (glomerular, tubular, interstitial, or vascular cells).[258] Similarly, the correlation is high with biopsy findings: 89% correlation in native kidneys and 77% in transplant kidneys. Sensitivity and specificity for glomerular lesions alone in native and transplant kidneys was 91% and

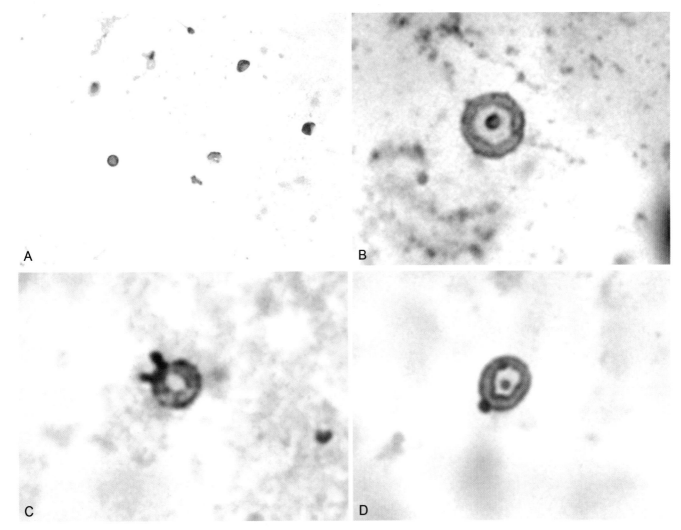

Fig. 7.42 (A) Isomorphic red blood cells. Note the smooth membranes and uniform amount of hemoglobin. Compare with (B), dysmorphic red blood cells, "target cell type." Note the central inclusion of heme pigment. (C) Dysmorphic red blood cells with prominent "blebs" or protrusions of red cell membrane. (D) Dysmorphic red blood cell "target cell type" with cytoplasmic bleb.

TABLE 7.17	Patient Correlation of Urine Red Cell Morphology and Glomerulopathy	
	Glomerulopathy	Negative for Glomerulopathy
Dysmorphic red blood cells (n)	76	1
Isomorphic red blood cells (n)	32	37

85%, respectively. Severity scores showed good correlation between optimal cytodiagnostic urinalysis results and renal biopsy in native and transplanted kidneys, and correlated well with increased creatinine concentration. In cases with biopsy-proven glomerular lesions, more severe changes were found by optimal cytodiagnostic urinalysis when the biopsy showed a proliferative lesion than when only normal glomeruli were found by light microscopy. Optimal cytodiagnostic urinalysis has an advantage over renal biopsy in that it can be repeated as often as necessary, thereby providing data regarding a renal lesion over time.[258]

A study of 201 patients demonstrated that the presence of more than five lymphocytes/hpf correlated with a 4.3 increased odds ratio of acute rejection among patients after antithymocyte globulin induction; the association was lost, however, with alemtuzumab induction. In addition, the study showed that a demonstration of polyomavirus infection was associated with polyomavirus nephropathy.[259]

Data from quantitative measurement of marker proteins (e.g., albumin, transferrin, IgG, α_1-microglobulin, retinol binding protein, α_2-macroglobulin, Bence Jones proteins) have challenged the dominant role of microscopy. Renal biopsy abnormalities were identified in all cases by marker protein excretion, but in only 41% of cases by sediment.[260]

References are available at expertconsult.com

8

Nonneoplastic Diseases of the Prostate

DAVID G. BOSTWICK

CHAPTER OUTLINE

Embryology and Fetal-Prepubertal History

The prostate is derived from the urogenital sinus.[1] During the first 10 weeks of gestation, testosterone from the embryonic testes stimulates ingrowth of epithelial buds into urogenital sinus mesenchyme through a feedback loop.[1] The mesenchyme induces the urogenital sinus epithelium to undergo ductal morphogenesis and differentiation in which the buds grow out into the surrounding mesenchyme and go through the processes of branching morphogenesis, canalization, and cytodifferentiation into basal and luminal cells. This then signals the urogenital mesenchyme to differentiate into smooth muscle cells surrounding the epithelium-lined ducts.[1-3] Concurrently, the seminal vesicles, epididymis, vas deferens, and ejaculatory ducts develop from wolffian (mesonephric) ducts stimulated by fetal testosterone. At 31 to 36 weeks of gestation, the basic structure of the prostate is fully formed. In the fetal prostate, prostatic acini consist of tight aggregates of immature basal cells lining primitive acini, often with

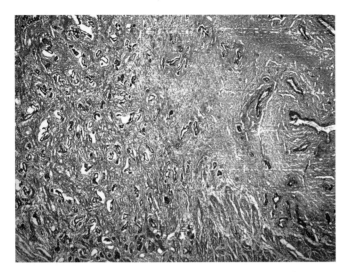

Fig. 8.1 Fetal prostate at 35 weeks with scattered immature glands.

squamous metaplasia of ducts and the urethra (Fig. 8.1). Androgen receptors are required for expression of secretory proteins by the epithelium and for differentiation of the surrounding mesenchyme into smooth muscle (reviewed by Toivanen and Shen).[4]

Immunohistochemical expression of estrogen receptor (ER)-β is evident at 7 weeks throughout the urogenital epithelium, ejaculatory ducts, müllerian ducts, and stroma in all zones, and persists through at least 22 weeks.[5] ER-α is first detectable at 15 weeks of gestation, with minimal staining in the utricle. By 19 weeks, increased expression is present in the luminal cells of the ventral urogenital epithelium, basal cells of the dorsal urogenital epithelium, utricle, distal periurethral ducts, peripheral stroma, and posterior prostatic duct, and this expression becomes more intense in the following weeks.

After birth, the size of the prostate remains stable until 10 to 12 years of age, but duct formation and solid epithelial outgrowth continue.[6-9] During puberty, marked androgen-driven increase in gland size occurs, quickly reaching adult size. By age 20 years, the mean prostate weighs approximately 20 g and remains stable for up to 30 years.[1,7,8]

Developmental anomalies of the prostate are rare and include aplasia, hypoplasia, cystic change, and mesonephric remnants. Aplasia and hypoplasia are associated with androgen deficiency. Cystic change is uncommon and may be congenital or acquired, including utricular and müllerian duct cyst, ejaculatory duct cyst, vas deferens cyst, and seminal vesicle cyst[10-12]; these cysts rarely produce clinical symptoms (Table 8.1).[12-14] Cysts may be also associated with infertility secondary to ejaculatory duct obstruction.[15,16] Mesonephric remnants in the prostate are an unusual mimic of adenocarcinoma that consists of a proliferation of benign acini arranged in lobules or showing infiltrative growth between smooth muscle bundles without stromal desmoplasia (discussed later).[17-21]

Anatomy

The surgical anatomy of the prostate is varied and complex, influencing continence, the spectrum of hyperplastic changes, erectile function, and cancer control.[21]

Zonal Anatomy

The prostate is composed of three zones: the peripheral zone, central zone, and transition zone (Tables 8.2 and 8.3; Fig. 8.2).[1,2,22,23] The peripheral zone contains approximately 70% of the volume of the prostate and is the most common site of prostatic intraepithelial neoplasia (PIN) and carcinoma. Peripheral zone acini are simple, round to oval, and set in a loose stroma of smooth muscle and collagen (Fig. 8.3). Digital rectal examination often includes a description of the left and right "lobes" based on palpation of the median furrow in the midline that divides the peripheral zone into left and right halves.[1,2,22,23]

The central zone is a cone-shaped area that includes the entire base of the prostate and encompasses the ejaculatory ducts; it comprises approximately 25% of the volume of the prostate. A recent report using magnetic resonance imaging (MRI) found that, contrary to McNeal's classical anatomic teachings, the central zone extends below the verumontanum in 95% of men older than 43 years of age, likely because of deformation of the prostate by nodular hyperplasia.[24] Central zone acini are large and complex, with intraluminal ridges, papillary infoldings, and occasional epithelial arches and cribriform glands mimicking PIN (Fig. 8.4).[1,25,26] The ratio of epithelium to stroma is higher in the central zone than in the rest of the prostate, and the stroma is composed of compact interlacing smooth muscle bundles.[1,22]

The transition zone contains the smallest volume of the normal prostate, approximately 5%, but it enlarges together with the anterior fibromuscular stroma to massive size in benign prostatic hyperplasia (BPH) and dwarfs the remainder of the prostate (discussed later). Transition zone glands tend to be simple, small, and round, like those in the peripheral zone, embedded in a compact stroma that forms a distinctive boundary with the loose stroma of the peripheral zone (Fig. 8.5).[1,22,27] The stromal extracellular matrix contains collagen types I, III, IV, and V, fibronectin, laminin, chondroitin sulfate and heparan sulfate proteoglycans, and elastic fibers.[28] The central zone and peripheral zone are often referred to together as the outer prostate or nontransition zone, whereas the transition zone and anterior fibromuscular stroma are often referred to as the inner prostate.[22]

Gene expression differs between the peripheral zone and the transition zone,[29,30] and stromal-epithelial interactions may be responsible for the distinct zonal predilection for select diseases, especially cancer. For example, ERG and ETV1 are upregulated in the glands of the peripheral zone compared with the transition zone; this finding may be important when considering that ERG and ETV1 fusions are found in 80% and 20% of prostate cancers, respectively.[31] Stromal cells from the peripheral zone have a greater capacity to induce development and progression of cancer than those from the transition zone through growth factors regulated by sex hormones.[32]

TABLE 8.1	Prostatic Cysts: Differential Diagnosis		
Type of Cyst	Location	Size	Sperm Within
Prostatic cyst	Lateral	Variable	No
Seminal vesicle cyst	Lateral	Large	Yes
Diverticulum of ejaculatory duct or ampulla	Lateral	Variable	Yes
Müllerian duct cyst	Midline	Large	No

TABLE 8.2 **Zones of the Human Prostate: Histologic Features**

	Central Zone	Transition Zone	Peripheral Zone
Volume of normal prostate (%)	25	5	70
Anatomic landmarks			
Intraprostatic relationships	Ejaculatory ducts	Surrounds proximal prostatic urethra	Distal prostatic urethra
Adjacent structures	Seminal vesicles	Bladder neck	Rectum
Urethral orifices of ducts	Verumontanum; adjacent to ejaculatory ducts	Posterolateral wall of proximal prostatic urethra at its distal end	Posterolateral wall of distal prostatic urethra
Distinctive histologic features			
Epithelium	Complex, large polygonal glands with intraluminal ridges	Simple, small rounded glands	Simple, small rounded glands
Stroma	Compact	Compact	Loose
Biochemical differences			
Production of pepsinogen II	Yes	No	No
Production of tissue plasminogen activator	Yes	No	No
Lectin binding patterns			
LCA, Con-A, WGA, PNA-N, RCA-1	Yes	—	Yes
UEA-1, S-WGA, PNA	Yes	—	No
DBA, SBA, BS-1	No	—	No
Proposed embryonic origin	Wolffian duct	Urogenital sinus	Urogenital sinus

TABLE 8.3 **Zones of the Prostate: Implications for Disease**

	Central Zone	Transition Zone	Peripheral Zone
Tissue sampling techniques			
Transurethral resection	Poor	Good	Poor
Needle biopsy	Variable	Variable	Good
Involvement with pathologic processes			
Atrophy	Infrequent	Variable	Frequent
Nodular hyperplasia	Rare	Frequent	Rare
Prostatitis	Infrequent	Variable	Frequent
Carcinoma (% of prostate cancers)	Infrequent (5)	Frequent (25)	Frequent (70)

common type, the utricle projected out from between the two ejaculatory ducts.[36] The site and shape of the utricular orifice were also diverse; this orifice was most commonly located on the distal three-fourths of the prostatic urethra.

A circumferential sleeve of muscle surrounds the entire urethra. This muscular layer includes a proximal preprostatic smooth muscle sphincter that prevents retrograde ejaculation and a distal sphincter of striated and smooth muscle at the apex that is important in control of micturition.[37]

At the bladder neck, there are three muscle layers: submucosal longitudinal, circular bladder neck, and external longitudinal muscles.[38] Increased prostate volume correlates with an increase in collagen fibers and thinning of muscle in the anterior neck, as well as degeneration of the posterior neck. Nodular hyperplasia increases the amount of fibrosis, with circular muscle fibers becoming thin and fragmented.

Prostatic Urethra, Verumontanum, and Bladder Neck

The urethra serves as a reference landmark for the study of prostatic anatomy (Fig. 8.2).[33] A single 35-degree bend in the center of the prostatic urethra creates proximal and distal segments of nearly equal length. The verumontanum bulges from the posterior wall at the urethral bend and tapers distally to form the crista urethralis. Most prostatic ducts and the ejaculatory ducts empty into the urethra in this part of the middle and distal prostatic urethra, whereas the small periurethral glands of Littre have minute openings throughout the length of the urethra.

Just proximal to the verumontanum is the utricle, a small, 0.5-cm-long epithelium-lined cul-de-sac derived from the urogenital sinus, in contrast with the previous belief that the utricle is a müllerian remnant.[34,35] Careful microdissection study revealed three types of utricle based on the location of its pouch; in the most

Capsule and the Retroprostatic Fascia (Denonvilliers Fascia)

The capsule of the prostate consists of an inner layer of smooth muscle and an outer covering of collagen, with marked variability in the relative amounts in different areas (Fig. 8.6). The collagenous fascia surrounding the prostate is multilayered, consisting of collagen, elastin, and smooth muscle fibers, and may fuse with the muscular capsule depending on location and individual variation.[21]

At the apex, acinar elements may be sparse, and the capsule is ill-defined, composed of a mixture of fibrous connective tissue, smooth muscle, and striated muscle. As a result the prostatic capsule cannot be regarded as a well-defined anatomic structure with constant features, especially at this location.[1,39] In biopsy and surgical specimens the capsule at the apex and bladder base is difficult to identify; consequently, it is often not possible to determine the presence of extraprostatic extension when cancer is present at these sites.[40]

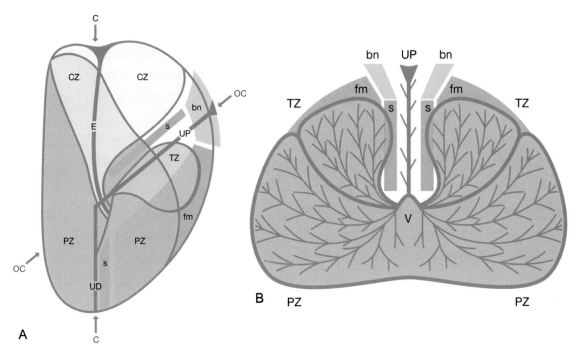

Fig. 8.2 Zonal anatomy of the prostate. (A) Sagittal diagram of the distal prostatic urethral segment (*UD*), proximal urethral segment (*UP*), and ejaculatory ducts (*E*), showing their relationships with a sagittal section of the anteromedial nonglandular tissues (bladder neck [*bn*], anterior fibromuscular stroma [*fm*], prepro-static sphincter [*s*]).[558] These structures are shown in relation to a three-dimensional representation of the glandular prostate (central zone [*CZ*], peripheral zone [*PZ*], transition zone [*TZ*]). The coronal plane (*C*) and the oblique coronal plane (*OC*) are indicated by arrows. (B) Oblique coronal section diagram of the prostate showing location of the PZ and TZ in relation to the UP, verumontanum (*V*), preprostatic sphincter (*s*), bn, and periurethral region with periurethral glands. The branching pattern of the prostatic ducts is indicated; medial TZ ducts penetrate the sphincter.

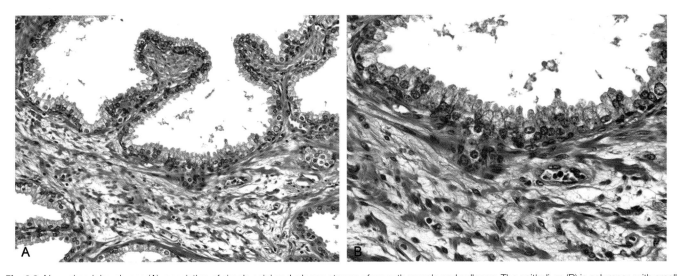

Fig. 8.3 Normal peripheral zone (A), consisting of simple acini and a loose stroma of smooth muscle and collagen. The epithelium (B) is columnar, with small round basal nuclei and an inconspicuous flattened basal cell layer.

At the lateral aspect of the prostate the pelvic fascia and the prostatic capsule are separated by adipose tissue in 52% of cases, but are adherent without fat in the remainder.[41] Anteriorly there is a smooth transition from the capsule to the anterior fibromuscular stroma, but the capsule is recognizable at this location in only 11% of cases. The lateral pelvic fascia connects and fuses with the anterior fibromuscular stroma, and covers the outermost regions of the lateral and anterior surfaces in 85% of cases.[41]

Posteriorly the retroprostatic fascia (Denonvilliers fascia) separate the prostate, seminal vesicles, and bladder from the rectum, with significant interindividual and site-specific variation.[42] The fascial muscular bundles and collagenous fibers posterior to the vas deferens blend with central zone stroma and the ejaculatory duct sheath at the junction of the base of the prostate with the seminal vesicles and vas deferens.[43] The retroprostatic fascia is fused with the capsule at the center of the prostatic posterior aspect in 97% of cases.[41]

Abundant adipose tissue is present around most of the prostate and is a reliable marker of extraprostatic tissue, present on 48% of all prostatic surfaces examined in whole-mount specimens.[44] The

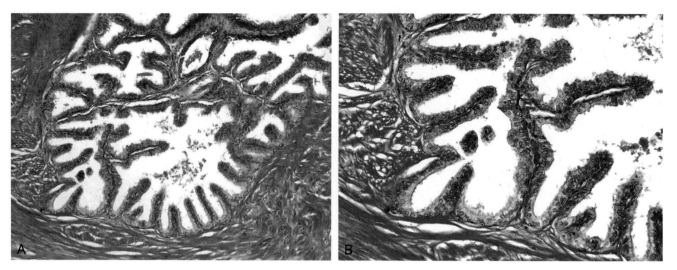

Fig. 8.4 Normal central zone (A), consisting of large acini with complex intraluminal ridges, papillary infoldings, and epithelial arches set in a stroma of compact smooth muscle. The epithelium (B) varies from cuboidal to columnar.

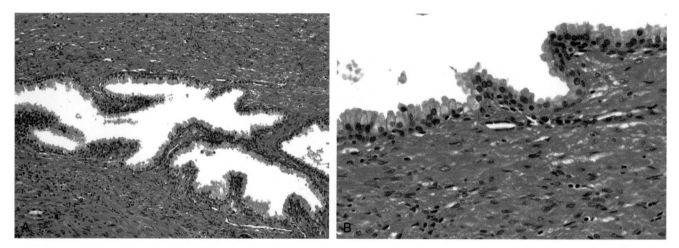

Fig. 8.5 Normal transition zone (A), consisting of simple acini and a compact stroma. The epithelium (B) is cuboidal or low columnar with apical cytoplasmic blebs.

distribution varies among the different surfaces of the prostate, with the anterior, posterior, right, and left surfaces showing 44%, 36%, 59%, and 57% adipose tissue, respectively. Nerve-sparing prostatectomy resulted in slightly less adipose tissue (46%) than did non–nerve-sparing procedures (54%).

Intraprostatic fat is rarely observed and, when present, consists of a small, microscopic focus of a few adipocytes.[45,46] For practical purposes, identification of fat in biopsy specimens is considered sampling of extraprostatic tissue.

Blood Supply

The blood supply of the prostate is furnished by a branch of the internal iliac artery. The most frequent origin is the internal pudendal (56% of cases), followed by the common gluteal-pudendal trunk (28%), the obturator (12%), and the inferior gluteal (4%).[47] Anastomoses are present at the termination of the internal pudendal artery in 24% of cases, with the contralateral arteries in 12%, and to the superior vesical artery in 8%. The two main

arterial pedicles to the prostate from each hemipelvis are the superior and inferior prostatic pedicles. The superior pedicle provides the main arterial supply of the gland and includes branches to both the inferior bladder and the ejaculatory system. The inferior pedicle distributes as a plexus in the apex and anastomoses with the superior pedicle.[48] Prostatic and capsular arteries run along the lateral border of the prostate and serve as a visual landmark in the majority of cases for cavernosal nerve-sparing prostatectomy.[49] Arterial embolization provides symptomatic control in patients with nodular hyperplasia.[48]

Veins drain directly into the prostatic plexus, and an extensive arborizing network is present in the capsule. The venous drainage empties into the internal iliac vein. Lymphatics from the prostate drain mainly into the internal iliac lymph nodes, with lesser drainage into the external iliac and sacral lymph nodes.[1] Antibodies directed against lymphatic vessel endothelial hyaluronan receptor (LYVE1) revealed that lymphatic density was greater in nodular hyperplasia than in carcinoma, whereas microvessel density with anti-CD34 antibodies revealed the opposite.[50]

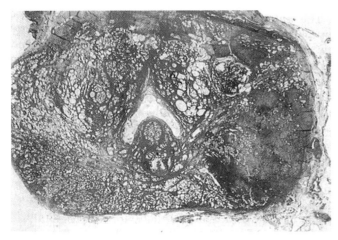

Fig. 8.6 Whole-mount prostate after unilateral nerve-sparing radical prostatectomy (nerves and periprostatic tissue were removed only from the patient's left side adjacent to cancer, which appears on the right side in the image) showing an adherent capsule, extraprostatic fat, and neurovascular bundles on the periphery of the prostate immediately adjacent to a large intraprostatic peripheral zone cancer (*bottom right*). Contrast with the contralateral region (*bottom left*), where there is no bundle (surgical dissection on that side was restricted to the edge of the prostate with capsule without removal of any extraprostatic tissue). This is considered an optimal surgical removal given the size and location of the cancer.

Nerve Supply

The nerve supply of the prostate is furnished by paired neurovascular bundles that run along the posterolateral edge of the prostate from apex to base, embedded between the fascial layers covering the prostate and seminal vesicles.[51] These bundles consist of numerous nerve fibers on a scaffold of veins, arteries, and variable amounts of adipose tissue surrounding almost the entire lateral and posterior surfaces of the prostate. At the apex and the urethra, the neurovascular bundles have two divisions: cavernous nerves (continuation of the anterior and anterolateral fibers around the apex of the prostate on the way to the corpora cavernosa) and corpus spongiosum nerves (continuation of the posterolateral bundles that eventually reach the corpus spongiosum).[52,53] Surgical sparing of these structures during radical prostatectomy preserves sexual

potency.[54] Variation in size and shape of the prostate influences the anatomy of the neurovascular bundles, the urethral sphincter, the dorsal vascular complex, and the pubovesical and puboprostatic ligaments.[55]

Autonomic ganglia are clustered near the neurovascular bundles, with small branching nerve trunks that arborize over the surface of the prostate, penetrate the capsule, and divide to form an extensive network of nerve twigs within the prostate that is often in intimate contact with the walls of ducts and acini.[56] Capsular ganglia are present in 52% of prostates, most frequently at the posterolateral aspect of the base. No obvious differences exist between capsular and periprostatic ganglia.[57] Pacinian corpuscle has also been found in the prostate.[58] The posterior capsule has more nerve fibers than the anterior capsule according to S-100 protein staining.[56]

Caution is warranted in interpretation of perineural space invasion as an absolute criterion for the diagnosis of cancer because this feature can be seen rarely in benign glands (Fig. 8.7).[25,59]

Nerve fiber density is greater in the peripheral zone than in the transition zone, especially in patients with BPH, according to S-100 protein immunohistochemical study.[56] The posterior capsule has significantly more nerve area than the anterior capsule. Innervation appears to decrease with age.

Prostate Sampling Techniques

Needle Biopsy

The introduction of the automatic spring-driven 18-gauge core biopsy gun three decades ago began a new era in the sampling of the prostate for histologic diagnosis (Fig. 8.8). The 18-gauge needle offered important advantages over the older 14-gauge needle. The rate of postbiopsy infection declined from up to 39% to less than 1%, and hemorrhage with urinary clot retention declined from 3% to less than 1%.[60] In recent years the postbiopsy sepsis rate has risen, probably because of increased antibiotic resistance ranging from 3% to 5%.[61,62] The false-negative rate declined from up to 25% to 11%, and the quality of the tissue sample improved, usually with little or no compression artifact at the edges. The main disadvantage of the 18-gauge needle is that it provides less than one-half as much tissue per needle core for pathologic examination

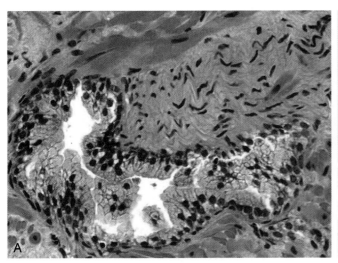
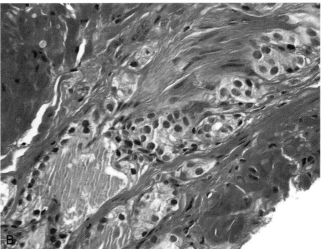

Fig. 8.7 Perineural abutment by benign glands (A and B).

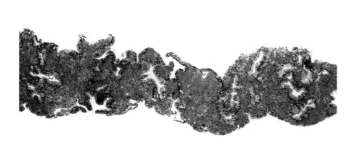

Fig. 8.8 Prostatic needle biopsy core (18 gauge).

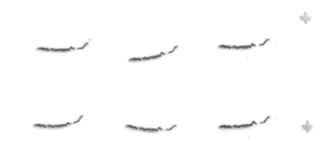

Fig. 8.9 Six sections of a prostate needle biopsy specimen mounted on one slide.

as the traditional 14-gauge biopsy. One report found no difference in cancer yield between 16-gauge and 18-gauge needle biopsies.[63] A recent study found that longer and consistent cores were obtained using novel elongate 15- and 17-gauge biopsy needles that included peripheral and anterior zone tissue sampling in a single core, enhancing determination of cancer location for focal therapy planning.[64]

Current clinical guidelines recommend that extended biopsy schemes with 10 to 12 specimens be obtained.[65] Segregation of specimens into individual vials improves specimen handling, enhancing tissue representation and diagnostic accuracy. Also, focal prostate cancer treatment strategies depend on more precise tumor mapping, requiring even greater tissue sampling.[66] Saturation biopsy using the 18-gauge core biopsy gun significantly increases cancer detection rate over methods with six or fewer cores.[67-70] In recent years the number of positive biopsies with only small foci of cancer has increased because of the success of early detection efforts in identifying smaller tumors at earlier stages. Frequently we encounter small, suspicious foci in biopsies from asymptomatic young men who have no palpable abnormality and only slight elevation of serum prostate-specific antigen (PSA) concentration; this issue is discussed in Chapter 9.

Inking the needle biopsy specimen is useful for identifying tissue cores in paraffin blocks, but this is infrequently performed, although we do this routinely. We found that submission of three cores in a single cassette was equivalent to one core per cassette for cancer detection, despite additional sectioning of the one-biopsy-core-per-cassette blocks.[71] No significant increase occurred in level of detection of atypical small acinar proliferation and adenocarcinoma with greater sampling. Consequently, we now recommend submission of three cores per cassette to minimize labor and cost of processing. However, this recommendation differs from that of the European Society of Uropathology, which prefers separate processing of each core but provides no data to bolster its beliefs.[72]

Laboratories also vary in the number of serial sections obtained from prostate tissue blocks for routine examination. We routinely obtain six sections on each slide from three levels (two sections per level) (Fig. 8.9). A minimum of two slides is prepared: slide 1 for hematoxylin and eosin (H&E) stain, and slide 2 for potential special studies such as immunohistochemistry for keratin 34βE12/p63/racemase/c-myc. In our experience, recutting the block for additional levels is useful in approximately one-half of

cases, because refacing of the block results in further loss of tissue, with usually no more than four additional slides before the specimen is exhausted. Other aspects of tissue processing and handling were recently reviewed.[73]

Fine Needle Aspiration

Fine needle aspiration remains popular for cytologic examination of the prostate in parts of Europe and around the world, but interest in this method in the United States has dropped precipitously because of the ease of acquisition and interpretation of the 18-gauge needle core biopsy.[66] Both techniques have similar sensitivity in the diagnosis of prostatic adenocarcinoma, and both are limited by small sample size; they are best considered complementary techniques.[74,75] Complications of fine needle aspiration occur in less than 2% of patients and are similar to complications of biopsy, including epididymitis, transient hematuria, hemospermia, fever, and sepsis.

Fine needle aspiration produces clusters and small sheets of epithelial cells without stroma (Fig. 8.10).[74] This enrichment for epithelium allows evaluation of single cells and the architectural relationship between cells. Benign and hyperplastic epithelia consist of orderly sheets of cells with distinct margins creating a honeycomb-like pattern. Benign nuclei are uniform with finely granular chromatin and indistinct nucleoli; basal cells are often present at the edge. Carcinoma is distinguished from benign epithelium by increased cellularity, loss of cell adhesion, variation in

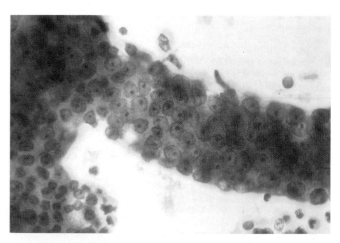

Fig. 8.10 Adenocarcinoma in fine needle aspiration. Note the cohesive cells with prominent nucleolomegaly.

nuclear size and shape, and nucleolar enlargement. Fine needle aspiration is not usually used as a screening test for prostate cancer. However, the specimen obtained from fine needle aspiration can be used for other diagnostic and prognostic testing, such as morphometric analysis, DNA ploidy, cytogenetic studies, and molecular diagnostics.[76-78] Ductal adenocarcinoma may be diagnosed by fine needle aspiration combined with immunohistochemistry.[79]

Imprint cytology of biopsies also relies on the evaluation of single cells and clusters. Compared with histologic findings, imprint cytology had accuracy, sensitivity, specificity, positive predictive value, negative predictive value, false-positive rate, and false-negative rate of 98%, 97%, 98%, 93%, 99%, 2%, and 3%, respectively.[80]

Transurethral Resection

The regions of the prostate sampled by transurethral resection (TURP) and needle biopsy tend to be different.[81,82] TURP specimens usually consist of tissue from the transition zone, urethra, periurethral area, bladder neck, and anterior fibromuscular stroma (Table 8.3). Studies of prostatectomies performed after TURP show that the resection does not usually include tissue from the central or peripheral zone, and not all the transition zone is removed.[83] Most needle biopsy specimens consist only of tissue from the peripheral zone and seldom include the central or transition zones or anterior stroma.

Low-grade adenocarcinoma found incidentally in TURP chips usually has arisen in the transition zone.[84,85] These tumors are frequently small and may be completely resected by TURP. Poorly differentiated adenocarcinoma in TURP chips usually represents part of a larger tumor that has invaded the transition zone from the peripheral zone.[85,86]

The optimal number of chips to submit for histologic evaluation from a TURP specimen remains controversial; some authors advocate complete submission even with large specimens that require many cassettes.[87] The College of American Pathologists recommends a minimum of six cassettes for the first 30 g of tissue and one cassette for every 10 g thereafter.[88]

Tissue Artifacts

Cautery artifact is frequently extensive in TURP specimens and often limits interpretation, particularly at the edge of chips. The epithelium usually shows more damage than the stroma, with separation from the basement membrane, cellular disruption, loss of integrity of nuclear membranes, and homogenization of the chromatin, thus creating featureless, dark nuclei. In severely affected chips, coagulation necrosis is present, including tissue devitalization with loss of cell membranes and indistinct smeared chromatin.[86,89]

Delayed fixation and air drying commonly result in separation of the epithelium and the underlying basement membrane, as well as chromatin smearing and smudging (Fig. 8.11). This artifactual change is more prominent in malignant than benign acini. Cell clusters floating in empty lumina may be mistaken for microvascular invasion.

Degenerating lymphocytes and stromal myocytes may show vacuolization that mimics signet ring cell carcinoma.[89] In difficult cases immunohistochemical stains are useful, with immunoreactivity for leukocyte common antigen in lymphocytes and smooth muscle actin in myocytes; both are negative for keratin AE1/AE3, PSA, and prostatic acid phosphatase (PAP).

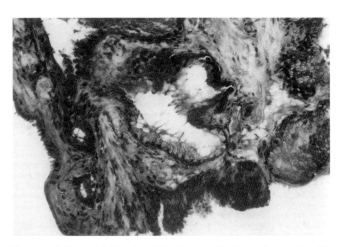

Fig. 8.11 Artifactual drying of prostatic biopsy with chromatin smearing; this specimen is insufficient for diagnosis.

Nonprostatic Tissues in Biopsies

Seminal Vesicle and Ejaculatory Duct Tissue in Biopsies

Up to 20% of prostate biopsy specimens contain fragments of seminal vesicle or ejaculatory duct epithelium, potential sources of diagnostic confusion.[90] The mucosa displays complex papillary folds and irregular convoluted lumina, and the lining consists of a nonciliated pseudostratified tall columnar epithelium. The cells are predominantly secretory, with microvesicular lipid droplets and characteristic age-related refractile golden-brown lipofuscin pigment granules; cytologic atypia is the norm (Figs. 8.12 and 8.13).[91] The muscular wall consists of a thick circumferential coat of smooth muscle.

Cowper Gland Tissue in Biopsies

Cowper glands are small paired bulbomembranous urethral glands that may be mistaken for prostatic carcinoma in biopsies.[92,93] These glands are composed of lobules of closely packed uniform acini lined by cytologically benign cells with abundant apical mucinous cytoplasm (Fig. 8.14). Nuclei are small, solitary, punctate, and basally located, and nucleoli are inconspicuous. Cowper glands are embedded in smooth muscle, thus mimicking the infiltrative pattern of prostatic cancer. Misdiagnosis can be avoided

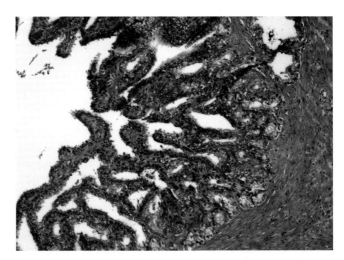

Fig. 8.12 Ejaculatory duct near origin in the seminal vesicles. Note the focal smooth muscle hyperplasia distorting lumen.

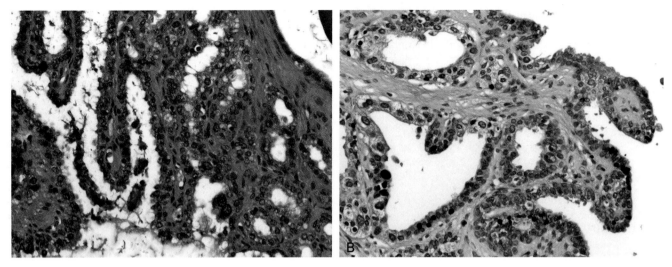

Fig. 8.13 Seminal vesicle (A) and ejaculatory duct (B) showing similar degrees of severe cytologic atypia of epithelium, with occasional bizarre giant cells.

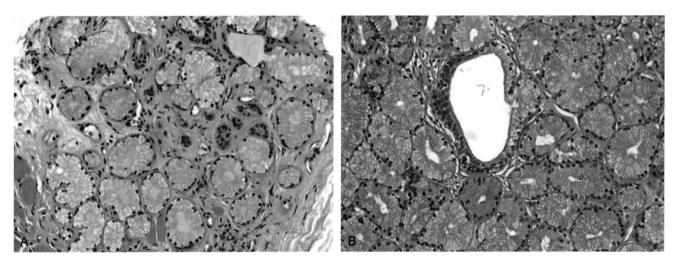

Fig. 8.14 Cowper gland. (A) This lobulated small gland contains multiple small acini with abundant mucinous cytoplasm and small hyperchromatic basal nuclei. (B) These acini surround a central duct.

when samples display immunoreactivity for mucin and smooth muscle actin, and are negative for PSA and PAP.

Disorders of Cowper glands are exceedingly rare. Urethral syringocele is cystic dilatation that may cause voiding dysfunction in children and is not apparently associated with other congenital anomalies.[94] A single case of giant cystadenoma occurred in a 41-year-old man who presented with acute obstruction.[95] Carcinoma is exceedingly rare and is characterized by frank anaplasia of tumor cells.

Rectal Tissue in Biopsies

Rectal tissue is often seen in biopsy specimens of the prostate and may be misinterpreted as benign epithelium or carcinoma when distorted.[96] Immunoreactivity for racemase and negative staining for basal cell–specific antikeratin 34βE12 further confound the diagnostic difficulty, although the combination of PSA and PAP allows accurate differentiation in all cases, when needed. Useful histologic clues to identify rectal mucosa include the presence of detached tissue with an epithelium containing goblet cells, lamina propria and muscularis propria, and abundant inflammatory cells.

Rarely, rectal tissue may contain tubular adenoma, hyperplastic polyp, significant inflammation, or other findings.[97]

Benign Epithelium

The epithelium of the prostate is composed of three principal cell types: secretory luminal cells, basal cells, and neuroendocrine cells. In addition, intermediate cells can be convincingly demonstrated by their unique immunophenotype (keratin phenotype intermediate between basal and luminal cells that coexpresses high levels of keratins 5 and 18 and hepatocyte growth factor receptor c-MET); stem cells are considered a subset of basal cells (see later).[98]

Substantial changes in the epithelium and stroma occur with aging. In addition to emergence of nodular hyperplasia (see later), the volume of glandular lumens in the nonhyperplastic prostate increases, reaching a maximum by the fifth decade.[99] The relative volume of the stroma remains unchanged, but the volume of the epithelium decreases, approximately linearly with age, suggesting that accumulation of fluid develops with aging.

Secretory Luminal Cells

The secretory luminal cells are cuboidal to columnar, with small, round nuclei, punctate or inconspicuous nucleoli, finely granular chromatin, and pale to clear cytoplasm; they account for the bulk (73%) of the epithelium volume.[1,5,22] Despite having the lowest proliferative activity, the terminally differentiated secretory cells produce PSA, PAP, androgen receptors, acidic mucin, and other secretory products. They also express high levels of keratins 8 and 18, but lack keratins 5 and 14, as well as p63.

Basal Cells

The basal cells of the prostate form a flattened, attenuated layer of inconspicuous elongate cells at the periphery of the glands surmounting the basement membrane (Fig. 8.15).[100] These cells possess the highest proliferative activity of the epithelium, albeit low, and a subset is thought to act as stem or "reserve" cells that repopulate the secretory cell layer.[98,100-103] Basal cells retain the ability to undergo metaplasia, including squamous differentiation in the setting of infarction and myoepithelial differentiation in sclerosing adenosis. Epidermal growth factor receptors have been identified in basal cells, but not in secretory cells, a finding suggesting that these cells play a role in growth regulation.[104-106] Basal cells are selectively labeled with antibodies to high-molecular-weight keratins such as clone 34βE12, a property that is exploited immunohistochemically in separating benign acinar processes such as atrophy, which retains a basal cell layer, from cancer, which lacks a basal cell layer. The nuclear protein p63 is another diagnostically useful basal cell marker that consistently decorates nuclei.[107] Basal cell–specific immunohistochemical cocktail (the combination of cytoplasmic antikeratin 34βE12 and nuclear antip63) optimizes the sensitivity of basal cell detection compared with either stain alone.[108,109] Basal cells also express high levels of keratins 5 and 14, in contrast with secretory and intermediate cells, as well as bcl-2, glutathione S-transferase pi, and galactin 3.[110] Basal cells contain little or no PSA, PAP, androgen receptors, keratins 8 or 18, or mucin. The normal prostatic epithelium frequently displays focal basal cell proliferation that is too small to warrant the diagnosis of basal cell hyperplasia. Prostatic basal cells do not normally possess myoepithelial differentiation, unlike basal cells in the breast, salivary glands, pancreas, and other sites, probably because the massive smooth muscle stroma of the prostate propels secretions downstream without need for assistance from basal cells. The basal cell population is heterogeneous in its expression of different combinations of p63, keratin 5, and keratin 14 differentiation markers, and the p63[+]/K5[−]/K14[−] subpopulation is proposed as likely stem cells.[111,112]

Neuroendocrine Cells

Neuroendocrine cells are the least common cell type of the prostatic epithelium, and they are usually not identified in routine H&E-stained sections except for rare cells with large eosinophilic granules.[113,114] Although their function is unknown, neuroendocrine cells probably have an endocrine-paracrine regulatory role in growth and development, similar to neuroendocrine cells in other organs, and contain numerous neuropeptides that modulate cell growth and proliferation.[115,116] Androgen deprivation therapy does not appear to influence the number or distribution of neuroendocrine cells in the normal or neoplastic prostate.[117] These cells coexpress PSA and androgen receptors, a finding suggesting a common cell of origin for epithelial cells and neuroendocrine cells in the prostate.[64,118] Neural crest origin has been shown for at least a subset of these cells.[119]

Recognition that neuroendocrine cells are most numerous near the verumontanum suggests a role in luminal constriction and dilatation. Serotonin and chromogranin are the best immunohistochemical markers in formalin-fixed sections (Figs. 8.16 and 8.17).[115,120-123] African American men have low neuroendocrine cell expression compared with other ethnic groups, and this may play a role in their increased risk for cancer.[124]

Three patterns of neuroendocrine differentiation are seen in human prostatic carcinoma: (1) infrequent small cell neuroendocrine carcinoma, (2) rare carcinoid-like cancer, and (3) conventional prostatic cancer with focal neuroendocrine differentiation (see Chapter 9). Virtually all cases of prostatic adenocarcinoma contain at least a small number of neuroendocrine cells, but special studies such as histochemistry and immunohistochemistry are usually necessary to identify these cells.[123,125-132] Neuroendocrine differentiation typically consists of scattered cells that are inapparent

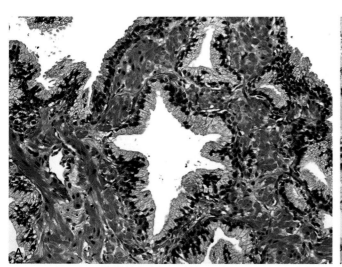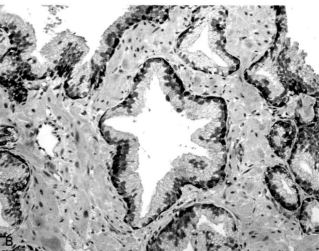

Fig. 8.15 (A) Normal prostatic acinus with prominent basal cell layer resulting from nuclear crowding and hyperchromasia. The basal cell layer is usually inconspicuous. (B) Immunostain for high-molecular-weight keratin and p63 demonstrates a continuous circumferential layer of basal cells.

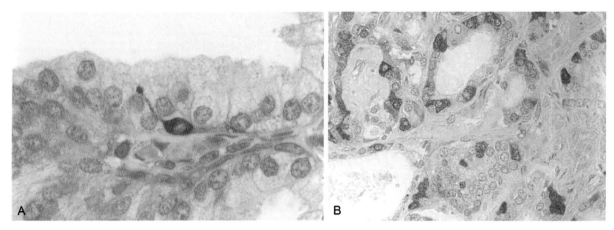

Fig. 8.16 Neuroendocrine cells. (A) When present in normal prostatic epithelium, these cells are infrequent and variable in shape (serotonin immunohistochemical stain). (B) The cells in prostatic adenocarcinoma display dark cytoplasmic reaction product that fills the cytoplasm of scattered cells and obscures the nuclei (chromogranin immunohistochemical stain).

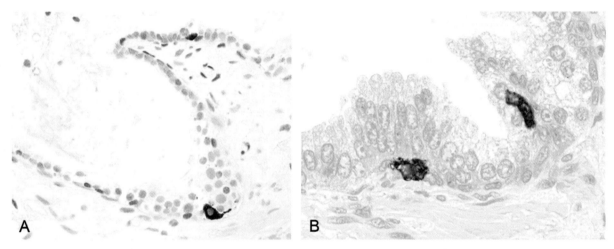

Fig. 8.17 Immunoreactivity of chromogranin A in benign prostatic epithelium (A) and high-grade prostatic intraepithelial neoplasia (B).

by light microscopy but revealed by immunoreactivity for one or more markers. Neuroendocrine cells in prostate cancer are malignant and lack androgen receptor expression.[128,129] These cells have no apparent clinical or prognostic significance in benign epithelium, primary prostatic adenocarcinoma, and lymph node metastases, according to most but not all reports.[130,133]

Stem Cells

Stem cell–derived clonal units found in the normal, atrophic, hyperplastic, and dysplastic epithelium actively replenish the entire epithelium during aging.[134] These deficient areas usually include the basal compartment, a finding indicating the location of stem cells. CD133 has been successfully used as a stem cell marker in both benign and malignant prostate.[135] CD24 is a marker expressed on the basal transit-amplifying cells (transition cells) and may play a role in the differentiation and migration of basal stem cells to the luminal layer.[136] Androgen receptors appear to play a significant regulatory role in maintaining the balance between progenitor basal cells and luminal secretory cells. Androgen receptors are expressed at a low level in basal cells, but they play a suppressive role in the proliferation of the $CK5^+/CK8^+$ progenitor/intermediate cells and a positive (proliferative) role in the $CK5^-/CK8^+$ luminal epithelial cells.[137]

Luminal Products

Intraluminal products of benign prostatic acini may include mucin, degenerating epithelium, crystalloids, proteinaceous debris, prostasomes, corpora amylacea, calculi, and spermatozoa.[138-140]

Prostatic secretions are composed chiefly of simple sugars and are mildly alkaline. The protein content is less than 1%, including proteolytic enzymes, PSA, PAP, β-microseminoprotein, and abundant zinc. In an animal model, luminal secretions increased significantly in the presence of inflammation.[141] Proteinaceous secretions are a frequent nonspecific finding in benign and neoplastic acini (overall 8% incidence rate in one study, with 100% incidence rate in men >70 years of age), and are considered the precursors of corpora amylacea and calculi.[142,143] Dilated acini with thyroid-like secretions are rarely observed in the prostate (Fig. 8.18), reminiscent of the luminal products seen in thyroidization of renal tubules and thyroid-like follicular carcinoma of the kidney; we refer to this as thyroidization of prostatic acini.

Mucin is usually absent in benign acini. Histochemical staining demonstrates neutral mucins (periodic acid–Schiff [PAS] with diastase), whereas neoplastic acini often demonstrate neutral and acidic mucins (Alcian blue–positive [pH 2.5]).[144-147] However, acidic mucin is not specific for cancer because certain benign conditions may also express it, including mucinous metaplasia, sclerosing adenosis, atypical adenomatous hyperplasia (AAH), and

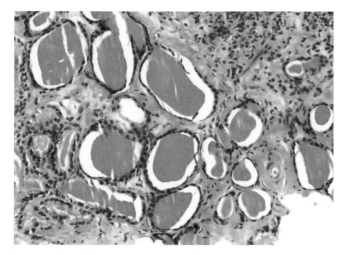

Fig. 8.18 Thyroidization of prostatic acini in association with mild chronic inflammation.

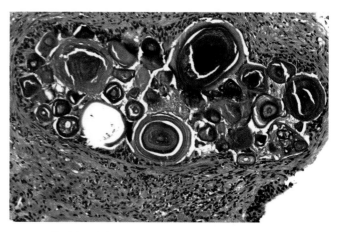

Fig. 8.20 Partially calcified corpora amylacea fill benign prostatic acini.

high-grade PIN. Mucins MUC1, MUC2, MUC4, MUC5AC, and MUC6 are not found in benign epithelium, although conflicting results have been found with MUC1 and MUC4.[148-151] Positive staining for MUC6 in seminal vesicle epithelium may be useful for excluding prostatic origin.[152]

It should be noted that mucin can also be found in the stroma, and raises the following considerations: benign extravasated mucin of unknown origin, stromal Teflon (polytetrafluoroethylene) mimicking mucin (Fig. 8.19; see later), and mucinous adenocarcinoma, in which at least a few cancer cells are invariably found floating in extravasated mucin after careful study.

Corpora amylacea are luminal secretions present in up to 78% of benign acini, but they are observed only rarely in stromal smooth muscle cells and adenocarcinoma (0.4% of needle biopsies with cancer) (Figs. 8.20 and 8.21).[138,153] They vary in size and shape, but most are round (Fig. 8.22). Color ranges from pink-purple to orange, and the presence of concentric laminations and early mineralization is variable. Corpora amylacea result from stasis of prostatic fluid and desquamated epithelial cells, which may further induce deposition of calcium salts leading to calculus formation,

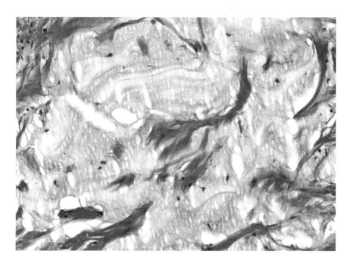

Fig. 8.19 Stromal teflon mimicking extravasated mucin. This may also be mistaken for the extravasated mucin of mucinous adenocarcinoma, but it lacks the diagnostic cancer cells floating in the mucin.

possibly generating a cycle of further irritation, additional blockage, and greater inflammation and mineralization.

Ultrastructurally corpora amylacea are composed of bundles of fibrils and occasional interspersed electron-dense areas.[154] Biochemical analysis and x-ray diffraction reveals that the main constituent is sulfated glycosaminoglycans[155,156]; other components include lactoferrin, calprotectin, myeloperoxidase, and α-defensins, proteins contained in neutrophil granules, thus suggesting a pathogenic role for acute inflammation.[157]

Prostasomes are prostate-derived membranous vesicles that can be isolated from seminal plasma.[158] They have been proposed to perform a variety of functions, including modulation of (immune) cell activity within the female reproductive tract and stimulation of sperm motility and capacitation.[159]

Calculi (microcalcifications), present in 31% to 100% of prostates, are typically found in central large ducts (Fig. 8.23), and are composed predominantly of calcium phosphate in the form of hydroxyapatite.[157,160] One study found calcifications in 89% of prostates, 58% of seminal vesicles, and 17% of ejaculatory ducts.[161] Calcifications occur mainly in benign glands and/or stroma of all zones and the verumontanum, but are most common in the transition zone, often observed in association with inflammation, BPH, and basal cell hyperplasia.[139,162] Whereas luminal microcalcifications are commonly observed in breast cancer, prostatic calculi are rarely seen in malignant acini. Interestingly, stromal microcalcifications are observed in approximately 3% of needle biopsy specimens, invariably in association with chronic inflammation.[163] Gross prostatic calcification, occupying an area of more than 3 cm^2 on a standard x-ray, is rare.[164]

Calcifications are more prevalent in autopsy prostates from African Americans in Washington, DC, than from Africans from West Africa, a finding perhaps reflecting dietary differences.[165] There is a positive correlation of prostatic calcification and age. Calcification is also common in patients with chronic pelvic pain syndrome and is associated with inflammation, bacterial colonization, and symptom duration.[166] Calcific deposits of Mönckeberg medial calcinosis are occasionally observed in arteries and large arterioles in the periprostatic tissue.

Intraprostatic spermatozoa can be identified with Berg stain, present in 26% of prostates at radical prostatectomy, including the peripheral zone (72%), central zone (22%), and transition zone (6%).[167] They are frequently associated with inflammation and atrophy, including postatrophic hyperplasia (PAH).

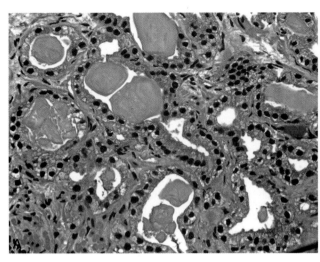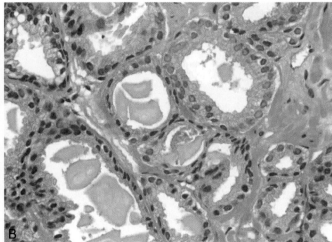

Fig. 8.21 Corpora amylacea in Gleason pattern 3 adenocarcinoma (A and B).

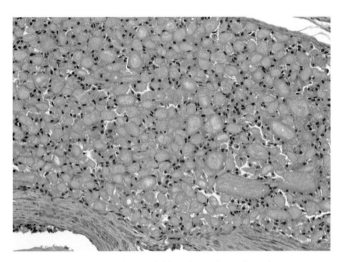

Fig. 8.22 Corpora amylacea mimicking signet ring cell carcinoma.

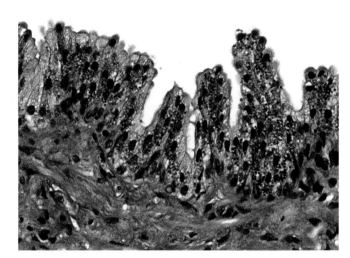

Fig. 8.24 Melanin-like pigment in benign prostatic epithelium.

Pigment

Pigment is occasionally observed in the cytoplasm of the secretory epithelium, including lipofuscin and melanin.[90,168] Lipofuscin granules are golden-brown, gray-brown, or blue by H&E staining (Fig. 8.24), display autofluorescence, and are positive for Fontana-Masson, PAS with diastase, Congo red, Luxol fast blue, and oil red O stains. Similar pigment may be also found in seminal vesicle and ejaculatory duct epithelium, high-grade PIN, and adenocarcinoma. One should avoid misinterpretation of pigmented acini adjacent to carcinoma as evidence of seminal vesicle invasion on needle biopsy. This pigment represents "wear and tear" or "old age" pigment resulting from endogenous cellular by-products.[169] It is present in all zones and is randomly distributed. Less commonly, melanin-like (Fontana-Masson–positive) pigment is found in scattered foci in the normal and hyperplastic epithelium and stroma (Fig. 8.25) (see later Melanosis section).[170]

Immunohistochemistry

The most important immunohistochemical markers in prostate pathology are PSA, PAP, high-molecular-weight keratin 34βE12, p63, racemase (P504S), c-myc, NKX3.1, and ERG. Androgen

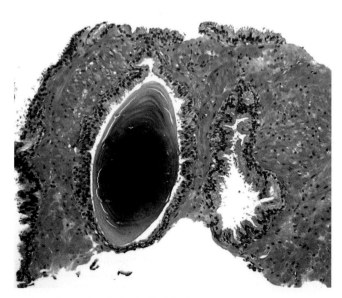

Fig. 8.23 Prostatic calculus in dilated acinus.

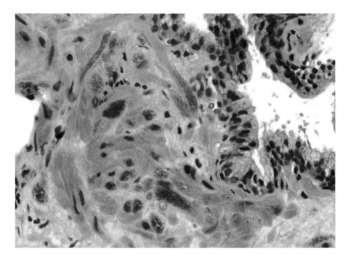

Fig. 8.25 Melanin-like pigment in prostatic stroma (melanosis).

receptor immunostaining has not been used in routine clinical work because of variable results in multiple studies. Standardization of methods of staining and quantitation for all stains is recommended to avoid variable results.[171] These markers are briefly presented here, but they are discussed at length in Chapter 9.

Prostate-Specific Antigen

Immunohistochemical expression of PSA (human glandular kallikrein 3 [hK3]) is useful for distinguishing prostate cancer, especially high-grade cancer, and urothelial carcinoma, colonic carcinoma, granulomatous prostatitis, and lymphoma.[172] PSA also facilitates identification of site of tumor origin in metastatic adenocarcinoma. Table 8.4 lists extraprostatic tissues and tumors that express PSA immunoreactivity.[173-176]

PSA can be detected in frozen sections, paraffin-embedded sections, cell smears, and cytologic preparations of normal and neoplastic epithelium (Fig. 8.26). In the normal and hyperplastic prostate, PSA is uniformly present at the apical portion of the glandular epithelium of secretory cells. The intensity of the staining

TABLE 8.4	Immunoreactivity of Prostate-Specific Antigen in Extraprostatic Tissues and Tumors

Extraprostatic tissues

Urethra: periurethral glands (male and female)
Bladder: cystitis cystica and glandularis
Urachal remnants
Neutrophils
Anus: anal glands (male only)

Extraprostatic tumors

Mature teratoma
Urethra: periurethral gland adenocarcinoma (female)
Bladder: villous adenoma and adenocarcinoma
Penis: extramammary Paget disease
Salivary gland: pleomorphic adenoma (male only)
Salivary gland: carcinoma (male only)

Caveat: In many of these tissues and tumors, staining may be patchy, weak, or equivocal. Many of these reports have not been confirmed or validated. Also, contemporary antibodies to prostate-specific antigen may have different specificity and sensitivity from those used in some of these studies.

decreases in poorly differentiated adenocarcinoma.[173,177] Staining is invariably heterogeneous. Microwave antigen retrieval is usually not necessary, even in tissues that have been immersed in formalin for years. Formalin fixation is optimal for localization of PSA, and variation in staining intensity is only partially the result of fixation and embedding effects.[178] Immunoreactivity is preserved in decalcified specimens and may instead be enhanced.

Prostatic Acid Phosphatase

PAP is a valuable immunohistochemical marker for identifying prostate cancer when it is used in combination with PSA.[179] In the normal and hyperplastic prostate, PAP is uniformly present at the apical portion of the glandular epithelium of secretory cells. There is more intense and uniform staining of low-grade cancer cells, whereas less intense and more variable staining is seen in moderately and poorly differentiated adenocarcinoma. The intensity of PAP immunoreactivity correlates with patient survival, probably because of greater androgen responsiveness in immunoreactive cancers.[180,181] Table 8.5 lists extraprostatic tissues and tumors that express PAP immunoreactivity.[173,174,182,183]

Serum PAP is less useful than PSA because of inherent problems in the accuracy of measurement, including the requirement for special handling related to enzyme instability, diurnal fluctuation, variation in results after prostatic digital examination and biopsy, and cross-reactivity with nonprostatic serum acid phosphatase produced by liver, bone, kidney, and blood cells. Serum PAP has little or no clinical utility.

Keratin 34βE12

Basal cell–specific antikeratin 34βE12 (keratin 903; high-molecular-weight keratin) stains virtually all the normal basal cells; no staining occurs in the secretory and stromal cells. Basal cell layer disruption is present in 56% of cases of high-grade PIN, more commonly in glands adjacent to invasive carcinoma than in distant glands. Loss of more than one-third of the basal cell layer in 52% of foci has been reported in cases of high-grade PIN. Early carcinoma occurs at sites of acinar outpouching and basal cell layer disruption.[26] Prostate cancer cells do not react with this antibody, although it may stain other cancers. Basal cell layer disruption also occurs in inflamed acini, AAH, and PAH.[26,184-187]

Despite the clinical utility of high-molecular-weight keratin, caution is urged in interpretation because of the need to rely on negative results to separate adenocarcinoma from its mimics. Numerous confounding factors can interfere with staining, including poor tissue preservation and fixation, as well as lack of enzyme predigestion.[188]

p63

p63 is the stain of choice for nuclear staining of basal cells and is an excellent complement to high-molecular-weight cytokeratin staining of the cytoplasm (Fig. 8.27).[189] p63 may be more sensitive than 34βE12 in staining benign basal cells, particularly in TURP specimens, and it may offer advantages over 34βE12 in diagnostically challenging cases.[187,190] The immunohistochemical cocktail (34βE12 and p63) increased the sensitivity of basal cell detection and reduced staining variability.[125,191] The p63 gene is also expressed in respiratory epithelia, breast and bronchial myoepithelial cells, cytotrophoblast cells of human placenta, scattered cells of lymph nodes and germinal centers, and squamous cell carcinoma of the lung.[109,192] Quadruple staining with high-molecular-weight cytokeratin, p63, racemase, and c-myc is used by many laboratories for the diagnosis of prostate cancer.[109,187,193]

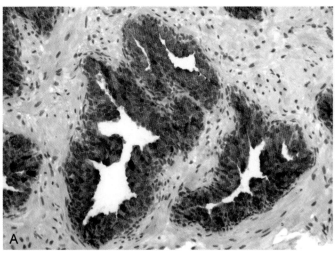
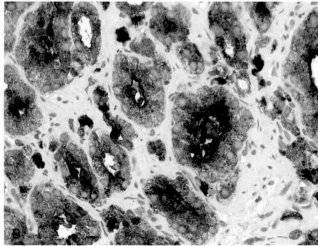

Fig. 8.26 Prostate-specific antigen (PSA) staining. (A) Normal prostate epithelium labeled with PSA antibody. (B) PSA staining in prostate cancer.

TABLE 8.5	Immunoreactivity of Prostatic Acid Phosphatase in Extraprostatic Tissues and Tumors

Extraprostatic cells and tissues

Urethra: periurethral glands (male and female)
Bladder: cystitis cystica and glandularis
Pancreas: islet cells
Kidney: renal tubules
Neutrophils
Colon: neuroendocrine cells
Anus: anal glands (male only)
Stomach: parietal cells
Liver: hepatocytes
Breast: ductal epithelial cells

Extraprostatic tumors

Bladder: adenocarcinoma
Anus: cloacogenic carcinoma
Rectum: carcinoid
Other gastrointestinal carcinoids
Pancreas: islet cell tumor
Mature teratoma
Breast: ductal carcinoma
Salivary gland: pleomorphic adenoma (male only)
Salivary gland: carcinoma (male only)

Caveat: In many of these tissues and tumors, staining may be patchy, weak, or equivocal. Many of these reports have not been confirmed or validated. Also, contemporary antibodies to prostatic acid phosphatase may have different specificity and sensitivity from those used in some of these studies.

p40

In benign tissues p40 displays a remarkably similar pattern of nuclear immunoreactivity as p63, identical in 88% of cases.[194,195] In cancer, cytoplasmic p40 staining is also present in the cytoplasm in 60% of cases, as well as aberrant nuclear staining in 0.6% (compared with 1.4% aberrant staining with p63). If one accounts for the cytoplasmic staining, then p40 staining is more specific than p63.

Racemase

Racemase (α-methylacyl–coenzyme A racemase [P504S]) gene product is an enzyme involved in β-oxidation of branched-chain fatty acids. It is a novel tumor marker for several human cancers and their precursor lesions.[193,196-203] Racemase is expressed in approximately 80% of cases of prostate cancer, but is less intense and more heterogeneous in variants, including atrophic, foamy gland, and pseudohyperplastic cancers (Fig. 8.27; Table 8.6). Positive racemase staining is also found in the majority of cases of high-grade PIN and in 10% to 15% of cases of AAH and occasional benign glands (Fig. 8.27); it is rare in seminal vesicle epithelium.[204-207] The cells of Paneth cell–like change are intensely immunoreactive, but all other benign neuroendocrine cells are negative, whereas malignant neuroendocrine cells are positive.[129,208,209] After radiation therapy, 91% of cancers retain expression, whereas it declines after androgen deprivation therapy.[210,211]

Nephrogenic adenoma is an important mimic of malignancy that is strongly positive for racemase, a result that must be considered in interpretation of small foci in biopsies. Jiang and colleagues found 97% sensitivity and 92% specificity with positive and negative predictive values of 95%.[205]

c-Myc

A compelling need exists for an immunohistochemical stain for cancer nuclei that would provide assistance (the malignant counterpoint to typical benign nuclear staining with p63) in cases in which the cytoplasmic marker racemase staining is marginal or absent.[212] Intense nuclear staining of c-myc is present in luminal secretory cells in 15%, 100%, and 97% of cases of benign tissue, PIN,[213] and cancer, respectively; the mean percentage of c-myc⁺ cells is 0.2% (range, 0% to 5%), 34.4% (range, 10% to 50%), and 32.3% (range, 5% to 70%), respectively. The MYC gene is highly overexpressed in prostate cancer cells, especially in those with negative racemase staining.

Panel of Keratin 34βE12, p63, Racemase, and c-Myc

Cocktail staining of high-molecular-weight cytokeratin, p63, racemase, and c-myc on a single slide is now our standard for the workup of difficult prostate needle biopsies, used in about 15%

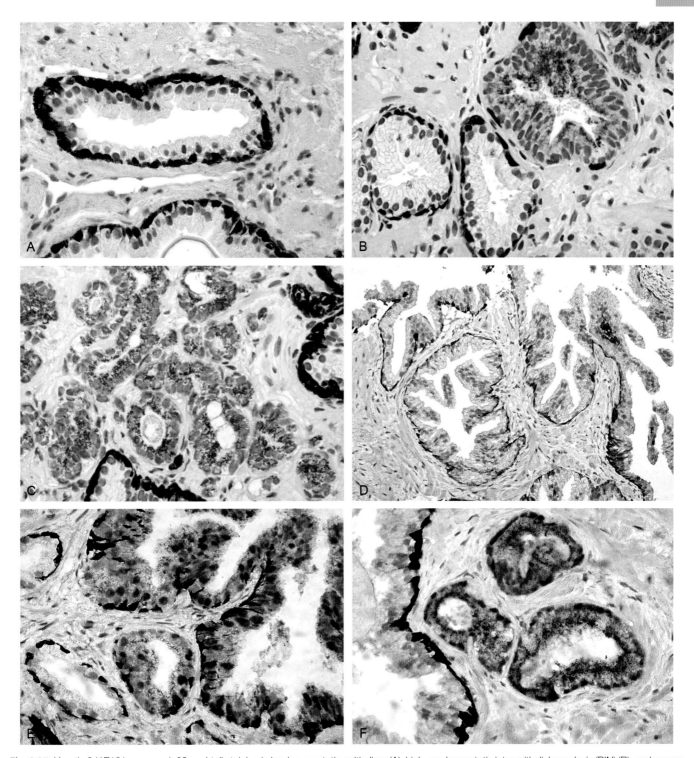

Fig. 8.27 Keratin 34βE12/racemase/p63 cocktail staining in benign prostatic epithelium (A), high-grade prostatic intraepithelial neoplasia (PIN) (B), and cancer (C). Cocktail of keratin 34βE12/p63/racemase/c-myc in benign prostatic epithelium (D), high-grade PIN (E), and cancer (F).

TABLE 8.6	Immunoreactivity of Racemase (α-Methylacyl–Coenzyme a Racemase) in the Benign and Neoplastic Prostate		
	% Immunoreactive Cases (Range)	% Immunoreactive Glands (Range)	Staining Intensity (−, 1+, 2+, 3+)
Benign	8 (0-10)	4.6 (0-24.5)	− ~ 1+
Atypical adenomatous hyperplasia	14 (10-17)	15.1 (1-50)	− ~ 1+
High-grade prostatic intraepithelial neoplasia	88 (80-100)	21.8 (2.7-57.7)	1+ ~ 3+
Cancer	97 (80-100)	35 (6.2-78.2)	2+ ~ 3+

of contemporary cases.[109,187,202] Negative immunohistochemical stain for basal cells is not diagnostic of carcinoma by itself, because occasional benign glands may not show immunoreactivity, so positive markers that are specific for cancer, such as racemase and c-myc, are of great value in confirming malignancy. Positive racemase and c-myc staining converts an atypical diagnosis, based on suspicious histologic features and negative basal cell marker stains, to cancer in up to one-half of cases (Fig. 8.27). Optimizing the staining conditions for cocktail antibodies is important for staining interpretation.

NKX3.1

NKX3.1 expression is the earliest specific marker of the prostatic epithelium during embryogenesis.[4] In neonatal life it is expressed by all epithelial cells, whereas expression in the adult prostate is found in luminal cells, as well as a subpopulation of basal cells. In adults it acts as a tumor suppressor by mediating DNA repair response and interacting with the androgen receptor to ensure accurate transcription, thereby protecting against TMPRSS2-ERG gene fusion.[214]

GATA3

GATA3 immunoreactivity is useful for distinguishing urothelial carcinoma (usually positive) from prostatic adenocarcinoma (negative in 100% of cases, even after radiation therapy).[215] It is expressed in 100% of basal cells in the benign prostate and survives radiation therapy.

ERG

TMPRSS2-ERG, the most common gene fusion in prostate cancer, is associated with expression of a truncated protein product of the oncogene ERG. A novel anti-ERG monoclonal antibody has been characterized, and immunohistochemical ERG expression is highly concordant with the ERG mRNA overexpression (sensitivity, 100%; specificity, 85%).[216] ERG overexpression is the result of TMPRSS2-ERG gene fusion in all cases. ERG protein expression is identified in 52% of cases of high-grade PIN and in 61% of adenocarcinomas on needle biopsies; conversely, only 6% of benign acini adjacent to cancer display weak staining in the secretory cells (Fig. 8.28). No ERG expression is detected in nonprostatic carcinoma, atrophy, and benign and treated tissues of the prostate and seminal vesicles.[217]

Prostate-Specific Membrane Antigen

Prostate-specific membrane antigen (PSMA) is a membrane-bound antigen that is highly specific for benign and malignant prostatic epithelium, although endothelial cells in multiple organs are also immunoreactive. Cytoplasmic epithelial immunoreactivity for PSMA is intense.[218-221] The number of immunoreactive cells increases from benign epithelium to high-grade PIN and prostatic adenocarcinoma. The most extensive and intense staining for PSMA is observed in high-grade carcinoma, with immunoreactivity in virtually every cell in Gleason primary pattern 4 or 5 (Table 8.7).[218] Extraprostatic expression of PSMA is highly restricted other than for vascular staining, and nonprostatic cancer is invariably negative for PSMA, including renal cell carcinoma, urothelial carcinoma, and colonic adenocarcinoma. PSMA immunoreactivity in cancer cells was not predictive of PSA biochemical failure or recurrence in a cohort of organ-confined margin-negative cancers treated by surgery; these findings differ from serum studies in which elevated concentrations of PSMA indicated surgical treatment failure.[221-223] PSMA is expressed in lymph node and bone marrow metastases of prostate cancer (Fig. 8.29), thus underscoring its utility in identifying cancer of an unknown primary

TABLE 8.7	Comparative Immunoreactivity of Prostate-Specific Membrane Antigen and Prostate-Specific Antigen in the Benign and Neoplastic Prostate in 184 Radical Prostatectomies
	% of Immunoreactive Cells + SD (Range)
Prostate-specific membrane antigen	
Benign	69.5 + 17.3 (20-90)
High-grade PIN	77.9 + 13.7 (30-100)
Cancer	80.2 + 13.7 (30-100)
Prostate-specific antigen	
Benign	81.3 + 11.8 (20-90)
High-grade PIN	64.8 + 17.3 (10-90)
Cancer	74.2 + 16.2 (10-90)

PIN, Prostatic intraepithelial neoplasia.

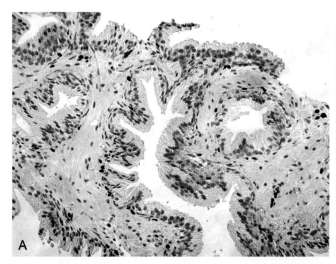 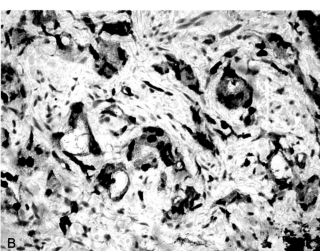

Fig. 8.28 ERG expression (A) in benign prostatic epithelium and (B) cancer.

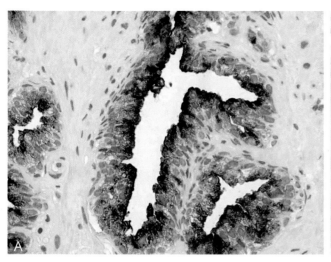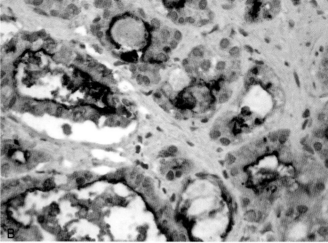

Fig. 8.29 Prostate-specific membrane antigen (PSMA) staining. (A) Normal prostate epithelium labeled with PSMA antibody. (B) PSMA staining in prostate cancer.

site.[219] Serum PSMA is of prognostic significance, especially in the presence of metastases, and correlates well with stage in a screened population. Despite its potential utility, PSMA immunohisto-chemistry is infrequently used in routine practice.

Human Glandular Kallikrein 2

The human kallikrein family consists of three members: hK1, hK2, and hK3 (PSA). The mRNA for hK2 and PSA is located predominantly in prostatic epithelium and is regulated by androgens.[224-226] In addition, hK2 has 78% amino acid homology with hk3 (PSA) and is expressed predominantly in the prostate, a finding suggesting that it may be a clinically useful marker for the diagnosis and monitoring of prostate cancer.[225-228] The intensity and extent of hK2 expression are greater in cancer than in PIN and are greater in PIN than in benign epithelium. Gleason primary grade 4 and 5 cancers express hK2 in almost every cell, whereas heterogeneity of staining is greater in lower grades of cancer.[229] In contrast with hK2, hK3 (PSA) and PAP immunoreactivities are most intense in benign epithelium.[229,230] The number of immunoreactive cells for hK2 and PSA is not predictive of cancer recurrence.[231] Tissue expression of hK2 appears to be regulated independently of PSA and PAP.[232]

Androgen Receptors

Androgen receptors are widely distributed in the nuclei of the basal cell layer, hyperplasia, and localized and metastatic carcinoma.[233] The percentage of cancer cells with androgen receptors is not predictive of time to progression after androgen deprivation therapy.[234] However, greater heterogeneity of receptor immunoreactivity is noted in adenocarcinoma that responds poorly to therapy.[235-237]

Androgen receptor expression in small cell carcinoma appears to predict poor outcome, in contrast with typical adenocarcinoma, which shows no correlation.[238] Androgen receptor gene mutations are present in up to 100% of cases of metastatic hormone-refractory prostate cancer.[239] At present there is no significant role for androgen receptor assays in the diagnosis and treatment of prostate cancer.[240,241]

Other Immunohistochemical Markers

Numerous immunohistochemical markers have been identified in the prostate, and many of these are preferentially found in the basal cell layer (Table 8.8). Basal cells display immunoreactivity at least focally for keratins 5, 10, 11, 13, 14, 16, and 19; of these, only keratin 19 is also found in secretory cells.[192] Keratins found exclusively in the secretory cells include 7, 8, and 18. Expression of S-100A6 (calcyclin), a calcium-binding protein, is restricted in the prostate to the basal cells of benign glands, but not in cancer.[242]

Antioxidant enzyme levels, including glutathione S-transferase, are lower in nodular hyperplasia compared with benign tissue, indicating impairment of oxidation.[243]

MAGI-2 (membrane-associated guanylate kinase, WW and PDZ domain-containing protein 2) expression is significantly higher in adenocarcinoma and high-grade PIN compared with benign tissue.[244]

Benign Stroma

The normal adult prostate stroma consists mainly of smooth muscle cells in combination with myofibroblasts and extracellular matrix. The stroma varies in gene expression according to zone, perhaps because of differences in relative composition, and this may explain differences in origin of nodular hyperplasia and prostate cancer. Stromal cells from the normal peripheral zone lack the capacity to induce epithelial cell growth, whereas the converse is true for hyperplasia-related and cancer-related stroma. The stroma is also affected by aging; inflammatory cells become more abundant, myofibroblasts become senescent and less sensitive to androgens, and the relative proportion of myofibroblasts increases.

Stromal hyaline bodies are small, 15- to 20-μm eosinophilic hyaline bodies occasionally observed within the prostatic stroma, as well as the muscular wall of the seminal vesicles and vas deferens.[245] These round-to-oval structures result from degeneration of smooth muscle actin fibers, and transition forms can be seen. Stromal hyaline bodies stain with Masson trichrome and PAS, but do not stain with phosphotungstic acid–hematoxylin, methyl green pyronine, Feulgen, Alcian blue (pH 2.5), or Congo red stain. Similar inclusions are characteristic of infantile digital fibromatosis and may be seen in phyllodes tumor of the breast.[246]

Telocytes are CD34+ interstitial cells found at the periphery of developing acini in the interacinar stroma and the region surrounding the periductal smooth muscle.[247] They support differentiation of periductal and periacinar muscle and produce networks that

TABLE 8.8	Immunophenotype of Prostatic Basal Cells	
Biomarker	Function	Findings
Proliferating cell nuclear antigen	Cell proliferation marker	Up to 79% of labeled cells are basal cells
MIB1	Cell proliferation marker	Up to 77% of labeled cells are basal cells
Ki67	Cell proliferation marker	Up to 81% of labeled cells are basal cells
Androgen receptors	Nuclear receptors that are necessary for prostatic epithelial growth	Strong immunoreactivity; also present in cancer cells
Prostate-specific antigen	Enzyme that liquefies the seminal coagulum	Present in rare basal cells; mainly in secretory luminal cells
Keratin 8.12	Keratins 13 and 16	Strong immunoreactivity
Keratin 4.62	Keratin 19	Moderate immunoreactivity
Keratin PKK1	Keratins 7, 8, 17, and 18	Moderate immunoreactivity
Keratin 312C8-1	Keratin 14	Strong immunoreactivity
Keratin 34βE12	Keratins 5, 10, and 11	Strong immunoreactivity; most commonly used for diagnostic purposes
p63	A member of the p53 gene family	Strong immunoreactivity; most commonly used for diagnostic purposes
S100A6	Calcium-binding protein	Strong immunoreactivity
EGF receptor	Membrane-bound 170-kDa glycoprotein that mediates the activity of EGF	Strong immunoreactivity; rare in cancer
CuZn-superoxide dismutase	Enzyme that catalyzes superoxide anion radicals	Strong immunoreactivity
Type IV collagenase	Enzyme involved in extracellular matrix degradation	Strong immunoreactivity; decreased in cancer
Type VII collagen	Part of the hemidesmosome complex	Strong immunoreactivity; lost in cancer
Integrins α_1, α_2, α_4, α_6, and α_v; β_1 and β_4	Extracellular matrix adhesion molecules	Strong immunoreactivity; decrease in most with cancer, although α_6 and β_1 are retained
Estrogen receptors	Hormone receptor	Moderate immunoreactivity
bcl-2	Oncoprotein that suppresses apoptosis	Strong immunoreactivity; also found in most cancers
c-erbB2	Oncogene protein in the EGF family	Strong immunoreactivity; also found in most cancers
Glutathione S-transferase gene (GSTP1)	Enzyme that inactivates electrophilic carcinogens	Strong immunoreactivity; rare in cancer
EpCAM	Epithelial cell adhesion molecule	Strong immunoreactivity; absent in cancer
Transforming growth factor-β	Growth factor that regulates cell proliferation and differentiation	Strong immunoreactivity; absent in cancer
Cathepsin B	Enzyme that degrades basement membranes; may be involved in tumor invasion and metastases	Present in many basal cells; rarely in luminal secretory cells; also found in cancer cells
Progesterone receptors	Hormone receptor	Moderate immunoreactivity

EGF, Epidermal growth factor.

separate acinar groups. These cells secrete transforming growth factor (TGF)-β1 and are ER-β^+.

Inflammation

Patchy mild acute and chronic inflammation is present in most adult prostates (77% of biopsies) and probably is a normal finding.[248,249] In healthy men the mean number of intraepithelial lymphocytes per 100 epithelial cells is $\leq$1 lymphocyte, whereas the number in chronic abacterial prostatitis is 8.5 lymphocytes.[250] When the inflammation is severe, extensive, or clinically apparent, the term *prostatitis* is warranted.[251] Prostatitis encompasses a wide spectrum of clinical and pathologic findings, many manifestations of which are rare and poorly understood.[251,252] Stamey considered prostatitis to be a "wastebasket of clinical ignorance" because of significant variation in terminology, diagnostic criteria, and treatment.[253] Up to 25% of men receive a diagnosis of prostatitis in their lifetime, but less than 10% have bacterial infection by culture[254]; this may increase with more sensitive and specific molecular techniques.

Reporting of acute and chronic inflammation in biopsies was routinely included by 56% and 32% of European pathologists, respectively, but only if severe by 39% and 54%, respectively.[255]

Prostatic Immune Response

The immune response in the prostate is primarily cell mediated. Lymphocytes are more numerous in the stroma, and T cells represent more than 90% of the total number of lymphocytes present in both stromal and intraepithelial compartments. Stromal T cells are mainly helper/inducer, whereas intraepithelial T cells are mainly cytotoxic/suppressor cells.[256] This inverted CD4/CD8 ratio in the intraepithelial compartment indicates that cytotoxic/suppressor T cells may represent the first line of defense against luminal foreign agents reaching the prostate through the urethra by retrograde flow. No significant difference exists in the number of lymphocytes (either T or B cells, stromal or intraepithelial) according to the patient age, race, or anatomic zone.[234] These findings indicate that the regulation of lymphocyte function and distribution is tightly controlled, and that there is a constant level of immunosurveillance in the prostate from birth. Increased CD4$^+$ T-lymphocyte infiltration within cancer is stage independent and associated with poor outcome.[257]

Acute Bacterial Prostatitis

Men at high risk for acute prostatitis include those with diabetes, cirrhosis, and suppressed immune systems.[258] The cause is usually

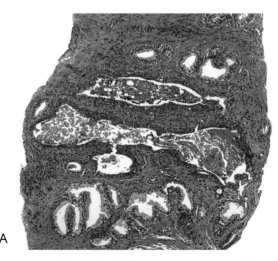
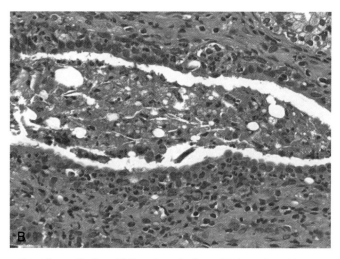

Fig. 8.30 Acute inflammation. (A) Dense acute and chronic inflammation obscures the acinar epithelium. (B) Constipated acinus with circumferential acute and chronic inflammation is evident.

an ascending infection, but bacteria can also be introduced during transrectal biopsy. The prevalence of fluoroquinolone-resistant *Escherichia coli* acute prostatitis was 13% after biopsy in one study.[259] Biopsy-associated acute prostatitis patients are older, have larger prostate volumes, have higher serum PSA concentrations, and show a higher incidence of septicemia and antibiotic-resistant bacteria than those with spontaneous acute prostatitis.[260]

Patients with acute bacterial prostatitis present with sudden onset of fever, chills, irritative voiding symptoms, and pain in the lower back, rectum, and perineum.[252,261] The prostate is swollen, firm, tender, and warm. Microscopically, acute inflammation in the prostate is often intraluminal, with a few scattered neutrophils or aggregates. There are sheets of neutrophils surrounding acini, often with marked tissue destruction and cellular debris (Fig. 8.30). The stroma is edematous and hemorrhagic, and microabscesses may be present. Diagnosis is based on culture of urine and expressed prostatic secretions; biopsy is contraindicated because of the potential for sepsis. Most cases are caused by bacteria responsible for other urinary tract infections, including *Escherichia coli* (80% of infections), other *Enterobacteriaceae* (5% to 10%), and *Pseudomonas, Serratia,* and *Klebsiella* (10% to 15%). Gonococcal prostatitis caused by *Neisseria gonorrhoeae* was common in the preantibiotic era, but it is less common today. Most cases of acute prostatitis respond to antibiotics, although about 10% eventually progress to chronic bacterial prostatitis and another 10% to chronic pelvic pain syndrome.[252,261-263]

Abscess is a rare complication, usually occurring in immunocompromised patients such as those with AIDS. Transrectal ultrasonography is a valuable method for preoperative diagnosis. Many patients with abscesses are treated by TURP and broad-spectrum antibiotics.[264]

Chronic Prostatitis

Chronic bacterial prostatitis is a common cause of relapsing urinary tract infection, and it is often the result of *E. coli*. Lifetime prevalence rate is 2% to 8%.[265] Clinical diagnosis is difficult, often requiring multiple urine cultures obtained after prostatic massage.[252,261,262,266] Treatment is vexing because of the inability of most intravenous antibiotics to enter the prostate and prostatic fluids when the organ is overrun with a chronic inflammatory infiltrate (Fig. 8.31). Prostatic calculi contain bacteria embedded in the

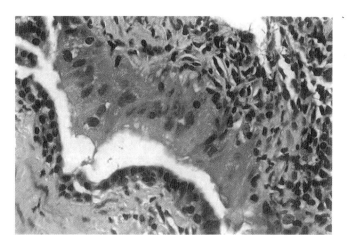

Fig. 8.31 Inflammatory atypia in the setting of chronic inflammation. Note the metaplastic changes adjacent to the inflammation. This was initially misinterpreted as high-grade prostatic intraepithelial neoplasia.

mineral matrix, and this may serve as a nidus of recurrent infection. The secretory products of the inflamed prostate are alkaline, with low levels of zinc, citric acid, spermine, cholesterol, antibacterial factors, and certain enzymes.

Chronic abacterial prostatitis is more common than bacterial prostatitis, and it rarely follows infection elsewhere in the urinary tract. Patients often report painful ejaculation. Results of cultures of urine and expressed prostatic secretions are, by definition, negative. This form of prostatitis has a prolonged indolent course with relapses and remissions.

The causative agent is unknown, but *Chlamydia, Ureaplasma,* and *Trichomonas* have been proposed.[267] Early studies using molecular techniques that do not rely on cultures, including molecular-phylogenetic approaches based on 16S RNA techniques, provided disparate results regarding the contributions of bacterial agents.[268] In patients with nodular hyperplasia and prostatitis, *Trichomonas vaginalis* DNA and antigen were detected in prostate tissue in 25% and 22% of patients, respectively.[269]

No relationship appears to exist between chronic prostatitis and the pathogenesis of BPH.[270,271] Microscopically, several patterns of chronic inflammation have been described including segregated glandular inflammation, periglandular inflammation, diffuse stromal

TABLE 8.9	Histologic Classification of Prostatic Inflammation
Feature	Details
Anatomic location	**Histologic pattern**
Glandular	Inflammatory infiltrates lie within duct/gland epithelium or lumina
Periglandular	Inflammatory infiltrates lie within stroma, are centered around ducts/glands, and approach ducts/glands to within 50 μm
Stromal	Inflammatory infiltrates lie within stroma, but are not centered around ducts/glands, and lie ≥50 μm away
Extent	**Tissue area involved by inflammatory cell infiltrates**
Focal	<10%
Multifocal	10%-50%
Diffuse	>50%
Grade	**Morphologic description (typical inflammatory cell density, cells/mm²)**
1/Mild	Individual inflammatory cells, most of which are separated by distinct intervening spaces (<100)
2/Moderate	Confluent sheets of inflammatory cells with no tissue destruction or lymphoid nodule/follicle formation (100-500)
3/Severe	Confluent sheets of inflammatory cells with tissue destruction or lymphoid nodule/follicle formation (>500)

TABLE 8.10	Etiologic Classification of Granulomatous Prostatitis

I. Idiopathic ("nonspecific")

II. Infectious

  A. Bacterial

    Tuberculosis
    Brucellosis
    Syphilis

  B. Fungal

    Coccidioidomycosis
    Cryptococcosis
    Blastomycosis
    Histoplasmosis
    Paracoccidioidomycosis

  C. Parasite

    Schistosomiasis
    Echinococcosis
    Enterobiasis
    Linguatuliasis

  D. Viral

    Herpes zoster

III. Malakoplakia

IV. Iatrogenic

  A. Postsurgical

  B. Postradiation

  C. Bacillus Calmette-Guérin associated

  D. Teflon associated

V. Systemic granulomatous disease

  A. Allergic ("eosinophilic")

  B. Sarcoidosis

  C. Rheumatoid

  D. Autoimmune/vascular

    Wegener granulomatosis
    Polyarteritis nodosa
    Benign lymphocytic angiitis and granulomatosis
    Churg-Strauss vasculitis
    Immunoglobulin G4–related disease

inflammation, intraepithelial lymphocytes, isolated stromal lymphoid nodules, and single scattered lymphocytes (Fig. 8.31).[272] Total prostatic volume and the aggressiveness of glandular inflammation correlated significantly with serum PSA level in men with nodular hyperplasia.[273] Interstitial infiltration involving T and B lymphocytes with fewer macrophages is a constant finding in early myxoid nodules.[274]

Chronic prostatic inflammation may be classified according to location, extent, and grade (Table 8.9). If more than one grade of inflammation is present for a given anatomic location, the dominant grade and most severe grade are specified (e.g., multifocal mild acinar inflammation, focal mild periacinar inflammation, diffuse mild stromal inflammation, and focal severe stromal inflammation).[275]

Granulomatous Prostatitis

Granulomatous prostatitis comprises a group of morphologically distinct forms of chronic prostatitis, the pathogenesis of which often cannot be determined. Causes include infection, tissue disruption after biopsy, bacillus Calmette-Guérin (BCG) therapy, and others (Table 8.10).[276-279] It accounts for 1.2% of all prostate specimens.[280-282]

Patients range in age from 41 to 75 years, with the majority in the seventh decade of life. Most patients have a prior history of urinary tract infection; cancer is usually suspected clinically. Urinalysis often shows pyuria and hematuria. In one report of 22 cases, serum PSA concentration ranged between 0.9 and 19.2 ng/mL.[281] Hard and fixed nodules were observed on digital rectal examination in 14 cases.

Granulomatous prostatitis is probably caused by blockage of prostatic ducts and stasis of secretions, regardless of cause. The epithelium is destroyed, and cellular debris, bacterial toxins, and prostatic secretions escape into the stroma, including corpora amylacea, sperm, and semen, eliciting an intense localized inflammatory response (Figs. 8.31 to 8.33). This process is similar to intraprostatic sperm granuloma formation. Tissue eosinophilia may be prominent in prostates infested with parasites, systemic allergic or autoimmune disease, iatrogenic post-TURP prostatitis, or nonspecific granulomatous prostatitis. Granulomatous prostatitis may be mistaken for high-grade prostatic adenocarcinoma.[283]

Xanthoma and Xanthogranulomatous Prostatitis

Xanthoma is a rare form of idiopathic granulomatous prostatitis that consists of a localized collection of cholesterol-laden histiocytes; it may also be seen in patients with hyperlipidemia (Fig. 8.34).[284,285] Xanthoma occurs in older men and is usually an incidental finding in patients undergoing TURP or biopsy, although it may appear as a palpable nodule.[286] Serum PSA ranges from 0.5 to 150 ng/mL.[287] Xanthoma usually forms a small, circumscribed, solid nodular pattern, but it may also appear as cords and individual cells infiltrating the prostatic stroma, thus mimicking high-grade prostate carcinoma. Rare cases also contain areas of typical granulomatous prostatitis, and the term

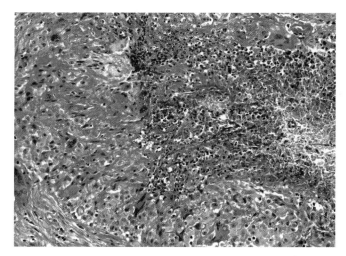

Fig. 8.32 Necrotizing granulomatous prostatitis. The necrosis is surrounded by histiocytes and reactive stroma.

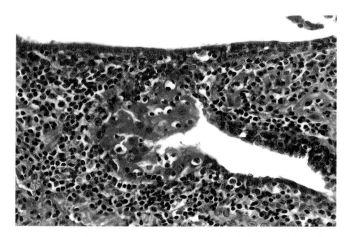

Fig. 8.33 Granulomatous prostatitis with eosinophilic metaplasia of the epithelium.

TABLE 8.11	Clear Cell Proliferations of the Prostate: Differential Diagnosis

Benign

Central zone secretory cells
Atypical adenomatous hyperplasia with clear cell change
Basal cell hyperplasia with clear cell change
Clear cell cribriform hyperplasia
Cowper glands
Mucinous metaplasia
Paraganglia
Storage disease
Stromal nodular hyperplasia with myxoid matrix
Xanthogranulomatous prostatitis
Xanthoma

Malignant

Clear cell adenocarcinoma of the prostate
Transition zone cancer with clear cell pattern
Previous androgen ablation ("nucleolus-poor" clear cell carcinoma)
Mucinous carcinoma
Signet ring cell carcinoma
Epithelioid leiomyoma and leiomyosarcoma
Secondary malignancies
    Clear cell carcinoma of the bladder
    Metastatic renal cell carcinoma, clear cell pattern
    Lymphoma with artifactual signet ring cell–like pattern

xanthogranulomatous prostatitis is appropriate in such cases. One case involved massive enlargement resulting in a 318-g prostate.[288] Distinction from clear cell carcinoma ("hypernephroid" pattern) and foamy gland carcinoma may be difficult, and immunohistochemical stains for PSA, PAP, CAM5.2, and CD68 often assist with this diagnostic concern (Table 8.11).[289]

Idiopathic Granulomatous Prostatitis

Idiopathic (nonspecific) granulomatous prostatitis comprises the majority of cases of granulomatous prostatitis (69%).[279,290] The granulomas are usually noncaseating and associated with

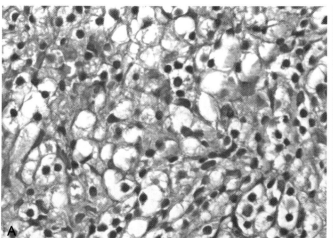
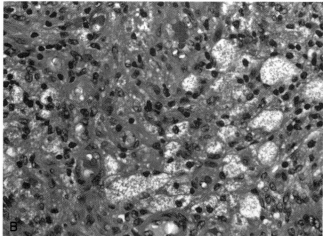

Fig. 8.34 Xanthoma. The needle core (A) contains a collection of cells with clear cytoplasm mimicking signet ring cell carcinoma. The foamy histiocytes (B) have small round to oval hyperchromatic nuclei.

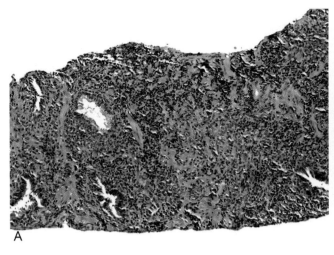
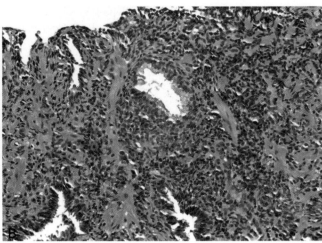
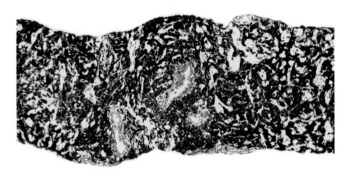

Fig. 8.35 Idiopathic granulomatous prostatitis misinterpreted as poorly differentiated adenocarcinoma. (A) At low magnification, there is a dense cellular infiltrate. (B) At high magnification, there is dense chronic inflammation surrounding benign acini. (C) The inflammatory cells are strongly positive for leukocyte common antigen.

parenchymal loss and marked fibrosis. Classification of eosinophilic and noneosinophilic types is probably of no clinical value. It is important to recognize the wide variety of inciting agents of granulomatous prostatitis and the histologic clues that allow distinction of these different entities, but most cases elude definitive classification (Fig. 8.35). The spectrum of morphologic abnormalities of idiopathic granulomatous prostatitis includes nodular granulomas centered on ducts and acini, central duct and acinar disruption, mixed granulomatous inflammation, and stromal sclerosis. The cellular infiltrate in granulomatous prostatitis is mixed, with epithelioid histiocytes, lymphocytes, neutrophils, eosinophils, plasma cells, and multinucleated giant cells.

Induration may persist on physical examination for years even when the patient has no specific clinical symptoms. Up to 10% of patients with idiopathic granulomatous prostatitis do not respond to conservative management and experience development of severe urethral obstruction that requires TURP. However, TURP is unsuccessful in up to 50% of cases, and some patients require multiple procedures.

Infectious Granulomatous Prostatitis

Infectious granulomatous prostatitis is rare and may be caused by bacteria, fungi, parasites, and viruses. *Mycobacterium tuberculosis* infection of the prostate occurs only after pulmonary infection or miliary dissemination. Small, 1- to 2-mm caseating granulomas coalesce within the prostatic parenchyma and form yellow nodules and streaks. Caseation and cavitation can be extensive and may extend into periprostatic tissues.[291] *Brucellosis* may mimic tuberculosis clinically and pathologically.[292]

Predisposing conditions for fungal infection include immunosuppression, prolonged antibiotic use, diabetes mellitus, malignancy, and an indwelling catheter. Mycotic infections of the prostate such as *Coccidioidomycosis* or *Cryptococcosis* are rare and invariably follow fungemia.[280,293] Most of the deep mycoses induce necrotizing and nonnecrotizing granulomas and fibrosis; *Candida albicans* infection is usually associated with acute inflammation.[280,294]

Granulomas caused by *Schistosoma haematobium* are frequently found in the prostate, bladder, and seminal vesicles in endemic areas such as Egypt. The organisms lodge in vesicular and pelvic venous plexuses as the final habitat. The adult female schistosome migrates into the submucosa of the urinary bladder and prostatic stroma, where she lays eggs that induce granuloma formation and fibrosis. Adenocarcinoma and squamous cell carcinoma of the prostate are rarely associated with *Schistosomiasis*.[295,296]

Malakoplakia

Malakoplakia is a granulomatous disease associated with defective intracellular lysosomal digestion of bacteria. It occasionally occurs in the prostate, where it manifests as a diffuse indurated mass clinically suggestive of carcinoma or occasionally coexisting with cancer.[251,297,298] *E. coli* is commonly isolated from urine cultures.

The prostate is effaced by sheets of macrophages admixed with lymphocytes and plasma cells. Intracellular and extracellular

Michaelis-Gutmann bodies are identified, appearing as sharply demarcated spherical structures with concentric "owl eyes" measuring 5 to 10 μm in diameter. Michaelis-Gutmann bodies represent calcified bacterial debris within phagolysosomes. PAS and von Kossa stains are useful for identifying nonmineralized and mineralized forms, respectively.

Iatrogenic Granulomatous Prostatitis

There are four main causes of iatrogenic granulomatous prostatitis: postsurgical, postradiation, BCG associated, and Teflon associated.

Post-TURP Granulomatous Prostatitis

Post-TURP granulomatous prostatitis may be identified years after surgery as a result of cauterization and surgical disruption of tissues (Figs. 8.36 and 8.37).[299,300] The granulomas are characteristically circumscribed, with central fibrinoid necrosis, an inner rim of palisading macrophages, and an outer rim of T lymphocytes.[301] Multinucleated giant cells are frequently present. The striking histologic resemblance of post-TURP granulomatous prostatitis to

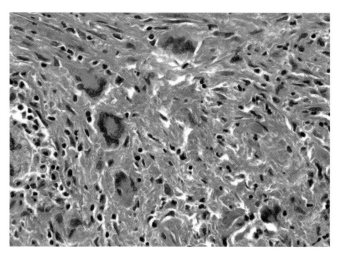

Fig. 8.36 Granulomatous prostatitis after transurethral resection that is characterized by aggregates of multinucleated giant cells.

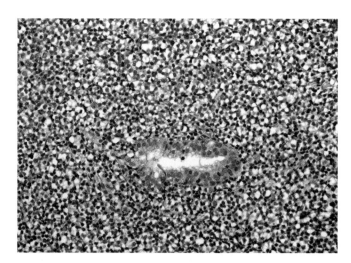

Fig. 8.37 Nonneoplastic focally dense lymphocytic inflammation surrounding benign acinus. This was an incidental finding in a transurethral resection specimen.

rheumatoid nodule suggests hypersensitivity reaction or cell-mediated immune response. Tissue eosinophilia is present in many cases. Treatment is unnecessary.

Postradiation Granulomatous Prostatitis

Although this is an uncommon response to radiation therapy, it should be considered as a possibility in patients with a positive clinical history. There are no unique histologic findings in this form of granulomatous inflammation other than changes of radiation injury in the rest of the prostate.

BCG-Associated Granulomatous Prostatitis

BCG-associated granulomatous prostatitis occurs in virtually all patients treated with intravesicular BCG immunotherapy for superficial urothelial carcinoma of the bladder.[302] Grossly the cut surface of BCG-induced granulomatous prostatitis shows multiple, firm, white nodules or soft, yellow-gray nodules with granular centers, central caseation, and focal cavitation. The granulomas are characteristically discrete, with or without necrosis, and often contain numerous acid-fast bacilli. Smaller granulomas predominantly consist of macrophages and may lack caseating necrosis and giant cells. No therapy is required.

Teflon-Associated Granulomatous Prostatitis

Periurethral and submucosal bladder injections of Teflon were used in the past for treatment of urinary incontinence. This foreign substance may migrate into the prostate and other sites and induce a florid granulomatous response.[303-306] Teflon is basophilic, simulating neoplastic mucin dissecting through the prostatic stroma (Fig. 8.19). Teflon tends to be more basophilic than mucin, and it appears filamentous and birefringent. The adjacent prostatic epithelium is rarely intact, and there are scattered or prominent multinucleated cells and other features of granulomatous prostatitis. Acellular mucin extravasation in the stroma is rare and should be distinguished from extravasated mucin associated with mucin-producing adenocarcinoma by the presence of at least a few cancer cells floating in the mucin.

Systemic Granulomatous Prostatitis

The spectrum of systemic prostatitis is broad and diagnostically vexing because of the rarity of these conditions, especially in the absence of clinical history.

Allergic (Eosinophilic) Granulomatous Prostatitis

Allergic granulomatous prostatitis is a component of Churg-Strauss syndrome.[307] It should be diagnosed only in a patient with a history of asthma or allergy with peripheral eosinophilia and systemic lesions. Histologically there is granulomatous prostatitis with abundant eosinophils, fibrinoid necrosis, and vasculitis (Fig. 8.38).[308] Treatment is with steroids.

Granulomatosis With Polyangiitis and Other Forms of Vasculitis

Prostatic involvement occurs in up to 7.4% of men with granulomatosis with polyangiitis (previously referred to as Wegener granulomatosis) and usually results in urinary obstruction, infection, hematuria, and acute retention; rarely, it may present with abscess.[308,309] The prostate is diffusely enlarged and often indurated. Urinalysis reveals microhematuria, red cell casts, and

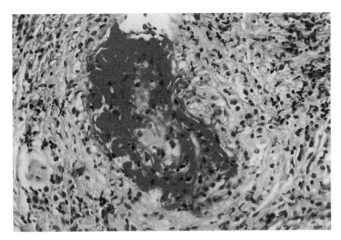

Fig. 8.38 Churg-Strauss vasculitis with fibrin deposition. This prostate biopsy was the first evidence of systemic vasculitis.

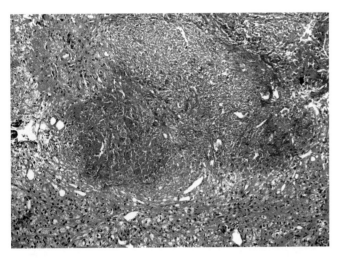

Fig. 8.39 Wegener granulomatosis with serpiginous necrosis rimmed by histiocytes mimicking post–transurethral resection granulomatous prostatitis. This middle-aged man was subsequently found to have lung and kidney involvement.

proteinuria, features indicating renal involvement. The erythrocyte sedimentation rate is frequently elevated. The prostatic urethral mucosa is ragged and friable, and biopsy reveals necrotizing granulomatous inflammation with vasculitis (Fig. 8.39). Stellate and geographic granulomas are present, rimmed by palisading macrophages and occasional multinucleated giant cells. Vasculitis involves small arteries and veins. Results of special stains for organisms are negative. Symptomatic prostatic involvement usually responds to chemotherapy, similar to pulmonary and renal involvement.[310,311] TURP may also be helpful.

Other forms of prostatic vasculitis are also rare and are usually associated with infarct and other forms of prostatitis. Lymphocytic inflammation surrounding small- to intermediate-size blood vessels is present in 93% of infarcts, with a polyarteritis nodosa–like pattern consisting chiefly of T cells.[310] Two cases were reported of antimyeloperoxidase antibody small vessel vasculitis causing prostatic fibrinoid degeneration with and changes involving arterioles.[311,312] Giant cell arteritis also rarely occurs in the prostate, sometimes without systemic involvement.[313]

Autoimmune Prostatitis With Immunoglobulin G4-Related Disease

Immunoglobulin G4 (IgG4)-related disease is a systemic autoimmune fibroinflammatory multiorgan disease, usually involving the pancreas, with occasional involvement of the genitourinary tract, including the kidneys, ureters, testes, and prostate.[314,315] Definitive diagnosis requires three findings: organ swelling, marked elevation of serum IgG4 levels (>135 mg/dL), and positive biopsy findings. Staining for IgG4-immunoreactive plasma cells may offer additional diagnostic support. Characteristic histology includes lymphoplasmacytic inflammation, storiform fibrosis, obliterative phlebitis, and abundant IgG4-immunoreactive plasma cells.

Other Rare Forms of Granulomatous Prostatitis

Other rare forms of granulomatous prostatitis include sarcoidosis, rheumatoid nodule, silicone-induced prostatitis, and systemic vasculitis.[316]

AIDS-Associated Prostatitis

Patients infected with HIV are susceptible to opportunistic infections that may include prostatitis, probably caused by abnormalities of T- and B-lymphocyte function. Infectious prostatitis occurs in 14% of patients with AIDS and in 3% with AIDS-related complex or asymptomatic HIV infection. Prostatitis in these patients may result from a variety of pathogens, including *E. coli, Klebsiella, Enterobacter, Serratia, Pseudomonas, Haemophilus parainfluenzae, Cryptococcus neoformans, M. tuberculosis, Cytomegalovirus, Histoplasma, Candida, Adenovirus,* and *Pneumocystis.*[317-319] Microscopically, organisms can be identified in expressed prostatic secretions, needle biopsy, or prostates at postmortem examination. The prostatic response to infection in patients with AIDS varies from none to necrosis or abscess formation. Patients with AIDS-related prostatitis may be asymptomatic or may present with acute prostatitis, chronic prostatitis, or abscess. Relapses are common despite prolonged antibiotic therapy.

Virus-Associated Prostatitis

Viruses have been occasionally implicated as causative in prostatic inflammation. Cytomegalovirus prostatitis is observed only in immunocompromised patients, with a dense lymphocytic infiltrate punctuated by characteristic inclusions within prostatic secretory cells, endothelial cells of small vessels, and stromal cells.[319,320] Herpes zoster infection may be associated with granulomatous prostatitis. Herpesvirus is present in normal prostates of HIV-infected men, and the expression of viral proteins is associated with increased localized inflammation.[321] Papillomavirus 18 is present in 14% of cases of prostate cancer and 27% of cases of nodular hyperplasia.[322] Zika virus infects, replicates, and produces infectious virus in stromal and epithelial cells in animals, suggesting that its replication may occur in the human prostate, resulting in Zika virus secretion in semen and sexual transmission.[323]

Xenotropic murine leukemia virus–related virus has been dismissed as a potential causative agent in prostatic diseases.[324]

Inflammation After Needle Biopsy

Contemporary transrectal 18-gauge needle biopsy of the prostate induces a predictable inflammatory response along a very narrow linear tract.[60] The biopsy swathe consists of a partially collapsed cavity, often filled with red blood cells, rimmed by mixed acute and chronic inflammation, including lymphocytes, macrophages, and occasional

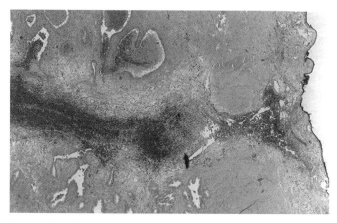

Fig. 8.40 Line of hemorrhage denotes the needle tract beneath the prostatic capsule on the right. This radical prostatectomy specimen was obtained 2 weeks after sextant 18-gauge needle biopsies.

eosinophils (Fig. 8.40). There is a variable amount of hemosiderin pigment, granulation tissue, and fibrosis, usually limited to the edge of the cavity (Fig. 8.41). Venous thrombosis and foreign body giant cell reaction are seen infrequently. Although tumor cells are frequently enmeshed within fibrous connective tissue, they are not seen within the cavity after 18-gauge biopsy.[60] Conversely, tumor is

occasionally identified in the tract after the wider 14-gauge needle biopsy, particularly with perineal biopsy.[325,326]

Biopsy tracts in prostatectomies obtained 4 to 6 weeks after biopsy show fewer red blood cells and less acute inflammation than in those obtained earlier, but no other histologic differences are noted.[60] There is no evidence of the florid granulomatous prostatitis or fibrinoid necrosis that is often seen after TURP. Biopsies involving benign prostatic tissue and cancer are histologically similar.

Inflammation and Nodular Hyperplasia

Inflammation is strongly implicated in the pathogenesis of nodular hyperplasia. An autopsy study of BPH in Caucasian men from Russia and Asian men from Japan revealed similar incidence (70%) of chronic inflammation in both groups.[327]

Patients with inflammation have significantly larger prostates, higher serum PSA concentration, and greater risk for urinary retention, although this last finding has been refuted.[328,329] Expression of proinflammatory cytokines in BPH is elevated; interleukin-6 (IL-6), IL-8, and IL-17 may perpetuate chronic immune response in BPH and induce fibromuscular growth by an autocrine or paracrine loop or by induction of cyclooxygenase-2 expression. Immune reaction may be activated by Toll-like receptor signaling and mediated by macrophages and T cells. Antiinflammatory factors such as macrophage inhibitory cytokine-1 are decreased in symptomatic BPH.[328]

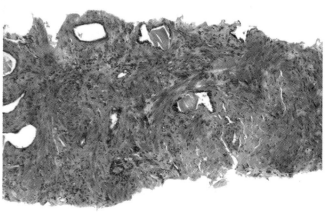

A

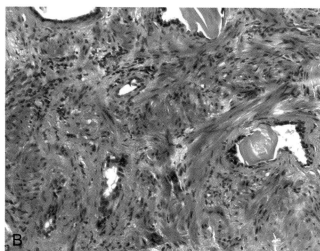

B

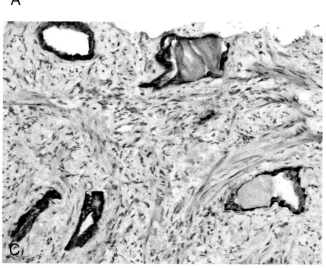

C

Fig. 8.41 Previous biopsy site sampled by second biopsy 3 months later. Note acinar atrophy and distortion with stromal chronic inflammation, features that may be mistaken for carcinoma (A and B). (C) Immunostain panel for keratin 34βE12/p63/racemase reveals intact basal cell layer indicative of benignancy.

Also, the number of high endothelial venule-like vessels correlates positively with the magnitude of chronic inflammation.[330]

Inflammation according to CD45, CD4, and CD68 expression is predictive of progression of BPH.[331] CD4 has the highest risk; men in the highest tertile of moderate/severe inflammation are at twice the risk for progression compared with men in the lower two tertiles combined.

Inflammation and Prostate Cancer

Is inflammation causative of prostate cancer, as it is for other cancers? Inflammation is thought to influence prostate cancer development by relying on immune cells as the primary drivers of this effect.[332] Genomic rearrangements induced by inflammation and oxidative stress are the likely cause of prostate cancer.[333] Metaanalysis showed that use of antiinflammatory drugs such as nonsteroidal antiinflammatory drugs are associated with a decreased risk, although some studies reached an opposite conclusion.[334-337] However, most, but not all, recent clinical studies showed that chronic inflammation is either inversely associated with cancer risk or has no association, arguing against inflammation as causative.[249,338-354] This question remains unresolved.

Atrophy

Atrophy is a common microscopic finding (73% of biopsies), consisting of small, distorted glands with flattened epithelium, hyperchromatic nuclei, and stromal fibrosis.[248] It is usually idiopathic, and prevalence increases with advancing age, particularly in patients who are older than 40 years old. Atrophic changes induced by radiation therapy and androgen deprivation therapy are discussed at the end of this chapter.

Atrophy appears initially as epithelial desquamation resulting from collective detachment and deletion of epithelial cells in response to diverse stimuli.[355] This exposes the luminal side of the basement membrane, activating basal cells to differentiate into intermediate-type cells, which change morphology to cover and remodel the exposed membrane to a new physiologic demand (such as the low androgen environment simulated by surgical or chemical castration) or to support reepithelialization (under normal androgen levels).

Atrophy may be confused with adenocarcinoma because of prominent architectural distortion and cytoplasmic basophilia.[356,357] At high magnification, atrophy usually lacks significant nuclear and nucleolar enlargement except in cases of PAH (discussed later). The nuclear-to-cytoplasmic ratio is high because of scant cytoplasm, and nuclei are dark.

Atrophy usually has regenerative features, particularly in the luminal secretory cells, that account for properties typically associated with high-grade PIN and carcinoma, including immunoreactivity for bcl-2, glutathione S-transferase π, androgen receptors, PSA, PAP, Ki-67, cyclin-dependent kinase inhibitor p15/CDKN2, COX2, and low expression of NKX3.1 protein, versican, and p27.[91,106,358-362] Racemase immunoreactivity is present in up to 31% of foci of atrophy with weak or moderate intensity.[363] However, this marker in isolation is insufficient to distinguish atrophy and the atrophic pattern of adenocarcinoma reliably.[364] Atrophy is enriched by a large number of highly proliferating intermediate cells (phenotypically intermediate between basal cells and secretory cells).[98]

Multiple classifications of atrophy have been proposed (Table 8.12). One classification identified four bins: simple

TABLE 8.12 Proposed Classifications of Atrophy

De Marzo[365]	Billis[366]	Bostwick (this text)
Simple atrophy	Diffuse	Atrophy
Simple atrophy with cyst formation	Focal	Postatrophic hyperplasia
Partial atrophy	Partial	
Postatrophic hyperplasia	Complete	
	Simple	
	Sclerotic	
	Hyperplastic (postatrophic)	
	Combined	

atrophy, simple atrophy with cyst formation, partial atrophy, and PAH (Fig. 8.42).[365] Interobserver agreement was high: median percent agreement for simple was 61%; for simple with cyst formation, it was 100%; for PAH, 88%; and for partial atrophy, 94%; the lower percentage for simple atrophy reflected a propensity to diagnose some cases as simple atrophy with cyst formation.[365] Billis identified six bins: diffuse and focal patterns, with the latter subdivided into partial, complete, or combined, and complete atrophy further subdivided into simple, sclerotic, and hyperplastic (or PAH).[366,367] However, these classifications have no clinical significance, are of questionable pathologic utility, and are not used in practice. The term *partial atrophy* was suggested to describe acini "with relatively scant cytoplasm, yet the glands are not fully atrophic in that they do not appear basophilic at low magnification."[368] We report only two potential diagnoses: atrophy and PAH.

Atrophy may also affect prostatic stromal cells, but the heterogeneity of this compartment masks the changes. In dogs after castration, the number of myocytes and fibroblasts declined, became atrophic and apoptotic, and the atrophic cells were filled with intracellular lipofuscin.[369] The expression of myosin declined, coincident with the increase in TGF-β mRNA level and decline in basic fibroblast growth factor mRNA.

Proliferative changes of the epithelium are linked to carcinogenesis in almost all epithelial malignancies. Proliferative regenerative change in association with inflammation, referred to by some as proliferative inflammatory atrophy, has been postulated to be a premalignant lesion, but this hypothesis has been refuted by most reports (see later). In the original description it included all histopathologic varieties of atrophy, including PAH and simple atrophy. However, this is not a clinicopathologic entity, and it appears to be an inherently redundant name because all patterns of prostatic atrophy have proliferative/regenerative features by definition.[370] Often no inflammation is present, despite claims to the contrary in the original description, so "inflammatory atrophy" is actually a misnomer, and we discourage its use, as well as that of "proliferative inflammatory atrophy."[370] One effort to separate inflammation-associated atrophy and noninflamed atrophy revealed that both were common findings, with a slightly greater incidence of the former in biopsies with cancer.[371,372]

The evidence for and against the linkage between atrophy and high-grade PIN or cancer is presented in Table 8.13. The hypothesis was that cellular injury and regeneration characteristic of proliferative and inflammatory changes in atrophy are induced by

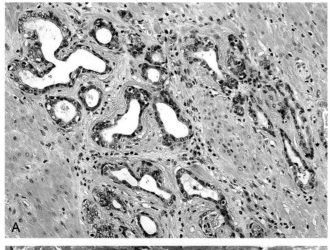

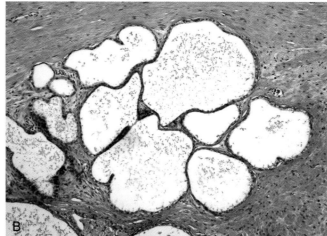

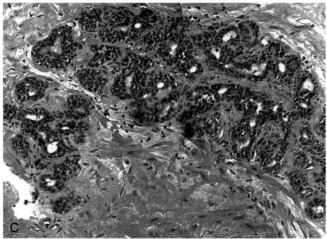

Fig. 8.42 Spectrum of atrophy, including simple atrophy (A), simple atrophy with cyst formation (B), and postatrophic hyperplasia (C).

inflammation and release of reactive oxygen species (oxidative stress) resulting from insult caused by chemicals (e.g., dietary carcinogens), physical factors (e.g., arteriosclerosis-induced ischemia), or bacteria. The regenerating cells are at increased risk for mutation, which also predisposes them to cancerous initiation, promotion, and progression. The clinical implication of this hypothesis is that antiinflammatory drugs could potentially block procarcinogenic inflammatory processes.[373] Despite conflicting views, most reports in recent years have refuted this hypothesis, including level 1 evidence.[346,371,372,374-376] Focal proliferative atrophy lesions are a common finding in biopsy specimens negative for prostate cancer and are not predictive of cancer on follow-up biopsy.[377] At present, proliferative and inflammatory changes in atrophy are best considered to be a rejected hypothesis, because atrophy may occur with or without inflammation or proliferation.[378,379]

Efforts to identify a morphologic continuum between atrophy and high-grade PIN were not convincing, despite claims to the contrary, and this concept has been refuted by most reports. Billis and colleagues found no association of atrophy with high-grade PIN or cancer in autopsy prostates.[380] When atrophy with and without inflammation were considered separately, both lacked topographic association with high-grade PIN or cancer.[381] Iczkowski et al. reported that the cumulative area of atrophy with or without inflammation correlated negatively with that of cancer.[382] Proliferative and inflammatory changes in atrophy were shown in another report to lack a topographic relation to high-grade PIN or cancer.[383] Studying 172 needle biopsy cores with cancer, Billis et al. noted atrophy in 67% of cores, but atrophy without inflammation was a more

common finding (60%) than when inflammation was present (40%).[384] The European Randomized Study of Screening for Prostate Cancer prospectively studied a cohort of 202 random sextant biopsies from men with at least 8 years of follow-up and found atrophy in 94%; extensive atrophy was observed in 5% of biopsies.[385] Similarly, atrophy was detected in 70% (mild, 60%; moderate/marked, 10%) of men between 50 and 75 years old with PSA between 2.5 and 10 ng/mL and a prior negative biopsy in the placebo arm of the REDUCE (Reduction by Dutasteride of Prostate Cancer Events) study of more than 6000 patients.[346] Patients with atrophy were older, had larger prostates, and more acute and chronic prostate inflammation. Baseline atrophy was significantly associated with lower cancer risk compared with absence of atrophy, with an incidence rate of 17% at 2-year biopsy. Only 5% of biopsies had a subsequent diagnosis of cancer, and the authors concluded that atrophy is a common lesion in biopsies and is not associated with a greater risk for high-grade PIN or cancer. Further analysis showed that biopsies with atrophy, chronic inflammation, or both were actually associated with a lower risk for prostate cancer (and lower grade of cancer, when identified) compared with those that contained neither.[386] Other reports have reached a similar conclusion.[353]

What is clear is that any association with cancer requires proliferative changes, and these changes in the setting of atrophy are most often associated with inflammation; atrophy may be an epiphenomenon rather than causative in this setting. Inflammation is often linked with infectious and noninfectious prostatitis, and emerging data suggest a causative role for inflammation (but not necessarily atrophy) in cancer development over time.[374,387,388] Virtually all authors agree

TABLE 8.13 | **Is Atrophy Associated with Prostatic Intraepithelial Neoplasia and Prostate Cancer?**

Evidence supporting the association of atrophy with PIN and prostate cancer

Morphologic similarity to PIN and cancer

Clusters of atypical epithelial cell hyperplasia with nuclear enlargement, hyperchromasia, and prominent nucleoli[475]

Morphologic transition from atrophy to PIN

17%-43% of foci of PIN spatially merged with atrophy

Morphologic transition from atrophy to cancer

Occasional merging of atrophy and cancer without PIN
46% of cancers arise in association with atrophy, often with adjacent PIN

Spatial association with cancer

28% of atrophy (postatrophic hyperplasia) near cancer
43% of atrophy near (<2 mm) cancer
30% of cancers near atrophy
Intermediate cells increased in atrophy
Increased expression of keratin phenotype intermediate between basal and luminal cells (K5 and K18 [K5/18]) and hepatocyte growth factor receptor c-MET

Increased expression of biomarkers compared with otherwise benign epithelium

Increased expression for CK5, GSTP1, c-MET, and CEBPB
Increased nuclear expression of p53 and Ki67 proteins and cytoplasmic expression of Bcl-2, compared with benign nonatrophic epithelium
Increased p53 expression in luminal cells was related to focal infiltration of neutrophils
Tag increased in atrophy and PIN
Increased C/EBPβ and COX2 expression in atrophy, especially those with T-lymphocyte and macrophage inflammation
Increased COX2 expression
Increased cyclin-dependent kinase inhibitor p16
Increased GSTP1 CpG island hypermethylation
Increased GSTA1 and GSTP1

Decreased expression of biomarkers compared with otherwise benign epithelium

NKX3.1 homeobox gene (at 8p21.2) decreased in atrophy and PIN

Evidence arguing against significant association of atrophy with PIN and prostate cancer

Epiphenomenon

Atrophy is present in essentially all adult prostates

Lack of significant nuclear or nucleolar enlargement

No significant cytologic abnormalities

Lack of spatial association with PIN

No topographic or incidental association of atrophy and PIN in autopsy prostates

Lack of spatial association with cancer

No topographic association of atrophy and cancer in biopsies

No transition of atrophy and cancer

Cancer did not merge spatially with atrophy

Lack of association with adverse pathologic findings

No association with cancer grade or stage
Atrophy, chronic inflammation, or both on biopsy were associated with a lower grade of cancer (among those with cancer on biopsy) in a prospective controlled trial[386]

Lack of predictive value for PIN or cancer on subsequent biopsy

Atrophy in an asymptomatic screening population not associated with subsequently greater incidence of PIN or cancer at 8 years
Atrophy in biopsies not predictive of increased risk in follow-up
Atrophy, chronic inflammation, or both on biopsy were associated with a lower risk for prostate cancer in a prospective controlled trial[346]

No increased expression of biomarkers in atrophy compared with PIN and cancer

Myc protein significantly increased in PIN and cancer, but not atrophy
Spermine oxidase increased in PIN and cancer, but not atrophy
TMPRSS2/ERG gene fusion increased in PIN and cancer, but not atrophy

CK, Cytokeratin; *COX2*, cyclooxygenase-2; *GST*, glutathione S-transferase; *PIN*, prostatic intraepithelial neoplasia.
Modified from Bostwick DG, Cheng L. Precursors of prostate cancer. *Histopathology* 2012;60:4–27.

that inflammation-induced oxidative stress is the most plausible explanation for initiation of prostatic carcinogenesis.

Genetic abnormalities in atrophy include loss of 8p22 in 21% of cases and gain of 8p24 in 19%, slightly higher than benign epithelium (16% and 10%, respectively) and lower than in high-grade PIN (25% and 21%, respectively).[389] However, these findings were refuted by another report that found no gains or losses of 8p, 8 centromere, or 8q24 (MYC) in atrophy.[360]

Nonneoplastic Metaplasia

The prostatic epithelium has an interesting but limited repertoire of responses to injury. These responses include a variety of metaplastic and proliferative lesions that may mimic adenocarcinoma (Table 8.14). Metaplasia is a reversible change in which one adult cell type is replaced by another adult cell type.

Squamous Metaplasia

Squamous metaplasia results from a variety of insults to the prostate, including acute inflammation, infarction, radiation therapy,

TABLE 8.14 | **Metaplastic Changes of the Prostate**

Diagnosis	Features
Squamous metaplasia	Intraductal aggregates of flattened cells with eosinophilic cytoplasm, usually at edge of infarcts
Mucinous metaplasia	Mucin-producing columnar or goblet cells in the prostate epithelium or urothelium
Neuroendocrine cells with eosinophilic granules	Isolated cells or small cell clusters with prominent eosinophilic cytoplasmic granules (usually seen as part of tumor)
Urothelial metaplasia	Urothelium within ducts and acini of the prostate; difficult to identify because of variable location of the normal transitional-columnar junction
Nephrogenic adenoma	Inflamed papillary mass of cystic or solid tubules in the urethra; rare; racemase-positive

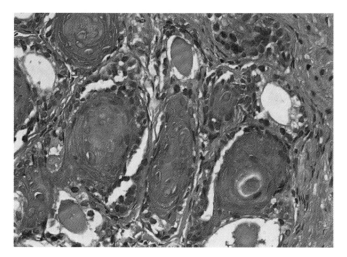

Fig. 8.43 Squamous metaplasia. This syncytial aggregate of basal cells is whorled, with distinct cell borders. Note oval to elongate nuclei with central linear grooves.

and androgen deprivation therapy.[390-392] It commonly involves the urethra in patients with an indwelling catheter. Squamous metaplasia is a specific phenotype in response to estrogen, and ER-α is required to mediate this response.[393] The earliest appearance of ER-α in the fetal prostate at 15 weeks signals the emergence of squamous metaplasia.[5]

Acini may be partially or completely involved by squamous metaplasia. The changes may be focal or diffuse, appearing as intraacinar syncytial aggregates of flattened cells with abundant eosinophilic cytoplasm or cohesive aggregates of glycogen-rich clear cells with shrunken hyperchromatic nuclei (Fig. 8.43). Keratinization is unusual except at the edge of infarcts or areas of acute inflammation.

Mucinous Metaplasia

Mucinous metaplasia refers to clusters of tall columnar cells or goblet cells with cytoplasm filled with blue-gray mucin infrequently observed in the acinar epithelium of all ages (Fig. 8.44).[147,394] This finding is invariably microscopic and can also be seen in the urothelium of large periurethral prostatic ducts, foci of urothelial metaplasia, atrophy, nodular hyperplasia, basal cell hyperplasia, and PAH. The cells contain acid mucin that stains with Mayer mucicarmine,

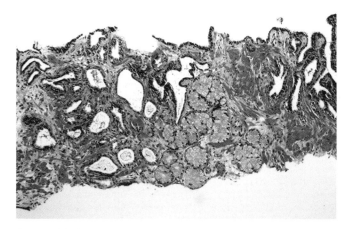

Fig. 8.44 Mucinous metaplasia.

Alcian blue (pH 2.7), and PAS after diastase predigestion; luminal secretions with similar staining are usually present.[395]

The differential diagnosis of mucinous metaplasia includes Cowper glands and adenocarcinoma.[396] Unlike Cowper glands, mucinous metaplasia is usually focal within a small number of acini and lacks complete involvement of a lobular aggregate of acini.[209] The nuclei of the mucinous metaplastic cells are small, dark, and basally situated. No immunoreactivity for PSA and PAP is noted in mucinous metaplasia. An intact basal cell layer can be confirmed by antikeratin 34βE12 or p63 stains.

Neuroendocrine Cells With Eosinophilic Granules (Paneth Cell–like Change)

Neuroendocrine cells with eosinophilic granules (NCEGs) are considered a distinct form of neuroendocrine differentiation in the prostatic epithelium and may represent a normal finding rather than metaplasia.[120,397,398] They account for only a small percentage of cells with neuroendocrine differentiation in benign prostatic acini and adenocarcinoma. Most neuroendocrine cells have small granules that are not apparent on H&E-stained sections. NCEGs are characterized by isolated cells or small groups of cells with prominent eosinophilic cytoplasmic granules, present on routine H&E-stained sections in 10% of serially sectioned radical prostatectomies. It is usually present focally but is occasionally prominent and multifocal. The distribution of cells with NCEGs is always patchy and can be found in usual acinar carcinoma, as well as in cribriform, papillary, and mucinous areas. The nuclei of NCEGs are vesicular with prominent nucleoli, similar to other tumor cells. Luminal mucin is more common in cancer with NCEGs than in cancer without NCEGs. NCEGs invariably display intense cytoplasmic immunoreactivity for chromogranin, neuron-specific enolase, and serotonin.[129] Many of these cells also express PSA and PAP.[399] Lysozyme is negative. NCEGs should be distinguished from another lesion designated eosinophilic metaplasia of the prostate.[400]

NCEGs are not associated with any factors predictive of aggressive behavior of prostate cancer, including tumor stage, serum PSA concentration, or tumor grade, suggesting that this finding does not indicate a poor prognosis.[120,401]

Urothelial Metaplasia

Urothelial metaplasia consists of urothelium within ducts and acini of the prostate proximal to the normal urothelial-columnar junction that apparently arises because of metaplastic change (Fig. 8.45). This junction is variable in location, thus creating difficulty in distinguishing metaplasia from normal urothelium in fragmented specimens such as TURP and needle biopsies. Consequently, the diagnosis of metaplasia for this may be overused. The reported frequency in needle biopsies was 1%.[402]

Microscopically only a few larger ducts or acini are involved in a single focus, but extensive involvement may also be observed. The acini exhibit proliferation of elongate urothelial cells beneath a bland-appearing luminal secretory cell layer.[403] Urothelial metaplasia is benign and is easily distinguished from PIN by its characteristic architectural and cytologic features. Urothelial metaplasia has also been described in phyllodes tumor.[404]

Nephrogenic Metaplasia

Nephrogenic metaplasia (nephrogenic adenoma) most often occurs in adult patients in the urinary bladder, renal pelvis, ureter, and urethra; prostatic urethral involvement is rare, and extension

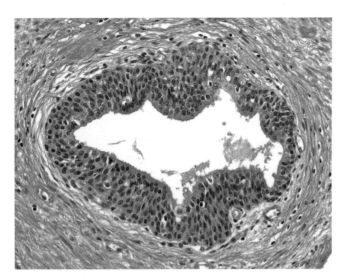

Fig. 8.45 Urothelial metaplasia. This focus of thickened urothelium was found deep within the prostate in a radical prostatectomy specimen. Note the presence of columnar epithelium indicating the junction with the urothelium.

into the parenchyma may create diagnostic confusion with adenocarcinoma (Figs. 8.46 and 8.47). This condition usually follows instrumentation, urethral catheterization, infection, or calculi. Patients present with lower urinary tract symptoms, including hematuria, dysuria, obstruction, and urethral mass.[17,405-408]

Some investigators suggest that nephrogenic metaplasia is neither metaplastic nor neoplastic, but rather represents benign implantation and proliferation of renal tubular cells in the lower urinary tract, similar to implants of endometriosis in the female genital tract and elsewhere. This process of implantation has been confirmed for cases of nephrogenic metaplasia in renal transplant recipients in which the condition is apparently derived from tubular cells of the transplant.[403,408,409] Whether this pathogenetic mechanism applies for nontransplant-associated cases awaits further study, although this hypothesis is gaining popularity. Nephrogenic metaplasia has no apparent association with urothelial metaplasia.

Nephrogenic metaplasia usually appears as an exophytic papillary mass of cystic or solid tubules protruding from the urethral mucosa. Histologic patterns include tubular, tubulocystic, polypoid, papillary, fibromyxoid, and the recently described flat pattern mimicking flat urothelial atypia.[410] The tubules may extend into the underlying prostate as a proliferation of small round-to-oval tubules, sometimes filled with colloid-like material. Occasionally tiny tubules with blue mucin simulate signet ring cells. The lining of nephrogenic metaplasia consists of flattened or simple cuboidal cells, often with a distinctive hobnail appearance. Nuclei display finely granular uniform chromatin with inconspicuous nucleoli; occasional prominent nucleoli are observed. Chronic inflammation and edema of the stroma are noted frequently, but no desmoplasia is present.

The tubules contain scant or moderate mucin that is positive with Alcian blue and PAS stains. The basement membrane appears

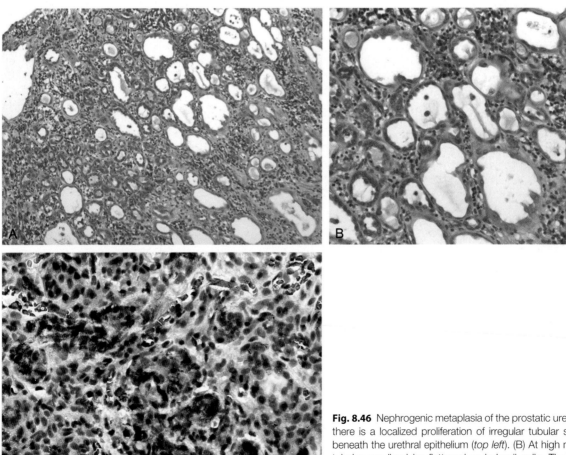

Fig. 8.46 Nephrogenic metaplasia of the prostatic urethra. (A) At low power, there is a localized proliferation of irregular tubular structures immediately beneath the urethral epithelium (*top left*). (B) At high magnification the small tubules are lined by flattened or hobnail cells. The stroma is chronically inflamed. (C) Intense racemase immunoreactivity in nephrogenic metaplasia may contribute to misinterpretation as prostatic adenocarcinoma.

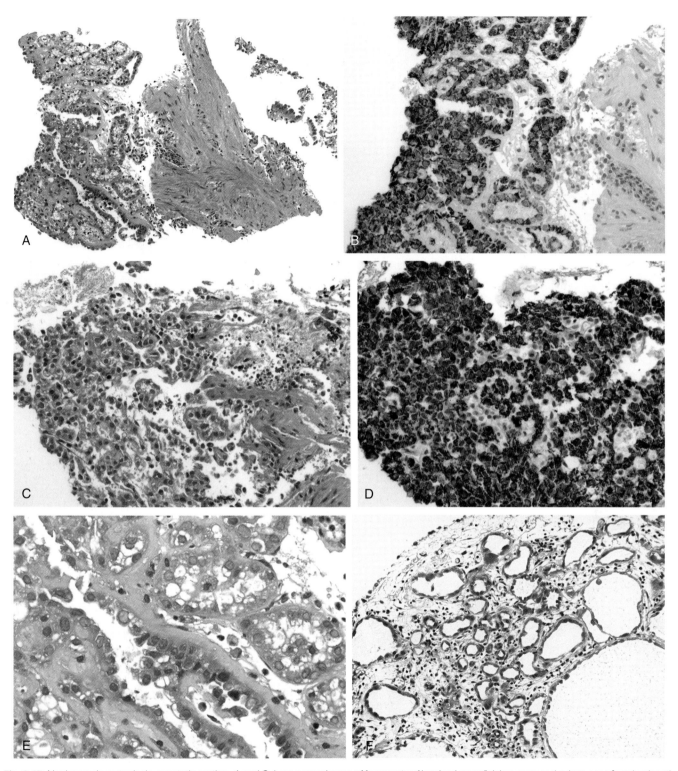

Fig. 8.47 Nephrogenic metaplasia, prostatic urethra. A and C, Low-power image of fragments of involved superficial mucosa and submucosa [predominantly tubular pattern in (A) and mixed solid and tubular pattern in (C)]. Compare with (B) and (D), respectively, showing intense cytoplasmic immunoreactivity for racemase. (E) High magnification showing prominent hobnail cell change, as well as cell vacuolization. (F) Another case with prominent tubular pattern that was misinterpreted initially as adenocarcinoma; note thin overlying urothelium at *top left*.

as a hyaline sheath that is accentuated with PAS stain. Epithelial membrane antigen is consistently expressed in the tubular epithelial cells, and high-molecular-weight keratin 34βE12 and p63 stain many of the basal cells.[402,411] PSA, PAP, p63, and carcinoembryonic antigen (CEA) results are negative. Approximately 58% of nephrogenic metaplasia cases are strongly positive for racemase (Figs. 8.46 and 8.47).[403,406,408] GATA-3 staining is present in 40% of cases.[402] Renal transcription factors PAX2 and PAX8 are also diagnostic markers for nephrogenic metaplasia, thereby underscoring the renal tubular cell implantation hypothesis.[412]

Quinones and colleagues found S-100A1 protein expression in 19 of 20 cases, concluding that a panel composed of PAX8, p63, PSA, S-100A1 protein, and CEA was sensitive and specific in differentiating nephrogenic metaplasia from urothelial and prostatic mimics.[413]

Nephrogenic metaplasia with substantial cytologic atypia (atypical nephrogenic metaplasia) is occasionally encountered and is a benign finding; awareness of the spectrum of cytologic changes within this entity is critical to prevent overdiagnosis of cancer and avoid unnecessary treatment. No direct evidence links atypical nephrogenic metaplasia to cancer.[414]

Hyperplasia and Nodular Hyperplasia

Enlargement of the prostate, also known as nodular hyperplasia or BPH, is the most common clinical ailment of the prostate, although the relationship between histologic findings and severity of symptoms is inexact. It consists of overgrowth of the epithelium and fibromuscular tissue of the transition zone and periurethral area. Symptoms are caused by interference with muscular sphincteric function and by obstruction of urine flow through the prostatic urethra. These symptoms, referred to as lower urinary tract symptoms, include urgency, difficulty in starting urination, diminished stream size and force, increased frequency, incomplete bladder emptying, and nocturia.[415-417]

Other variants, such as basal cell hyperplasia, may harbor microscopic findings that may be misdiagnosed for malignancy.

Nodular Hyperplasia

Development of nodular hyperplasia (BPH, usual acinar and stromal hyperplasia) involves three stages: nodule formation, diffuse enlargement of the transition zone and periurethral tissue, and enlargement of nodules.[418] In men younger than 70 years, diffuse enlargement predominates. In older men, epithelial proliferation and expansile growth of existing nodules predominate, probably because of androgenic and other hormonal stimulation. The proportion of epithelium to stroma increases as symptoms become more severe.[8,419,420]

Grossly, nodular hyperplasia consists of variably sized nodules that are soft or firm, rubbery, and yellow-gray that bulge from the cut surface on transection. If epithelial hyperplasia is present in addition to stromal hyperplasia, the abundant luminal spaces create soft and grossly spongy nodules that ooze a pale-white watery fluid. If the hyperplasia is predominantly fibromuscular, there may be diffuse enlargement or numerous trabeculations without prominent nodularity. Degenerative changes include calcification and infarction. Nodular hyperplasia usually involves the transition zone, but occasionally nodules arise from the periurethral tissue at the bladder neck. Protrusion of bladder neck nodules into the bladder lumen is referred to as median lobe hyperplasia (Fig. 8.48).

Microscopically, nodular hyperplasia is composed of varying proportions of epithelium and stroma (fibrous connective tissue and smooth muscle). The most common types are adenomyofibromatous nodules that contain all elements (Figs. 8.48 and 8.49). The total area, luminal area, and epithelial height of the acini are greater in BPH than in benign epithelium, but the number of acini is similar.[27]

Pure stromal nodule (stromal hyperplasia) is usually microscopic in size and is rarely confused with malignant spindle cell lesion, but it may be confused with leiomyoma. Stromal hyperplasia is well demarcated from the surrounding prostatic tissue, but not encapsulated, characterized by benign-appearing spindle cell proliferation devoid of glandular elements (Fig. 8.50).[421] The spindle cells are arranged in a fasciculated or whorled pattern simulating leiomyoma. It contains small, thick-walled blood vessels embedded in spindle cell proliferation. Myxoid changes may be seen, but nuclear atypia and mitotic figures are not features of usual stromal hyperplasia. The distinction between stromal nodule and leiomyoma is arbitrary; leiomyoma is defined as a lesion greater than 1 cm in diameter that is usually encapsulated. There are four types of pure stromal nodules: (1) immature mesenchymal (5% of stromal nodules); (2) fibroblastic (50%); (3) fibromuscular (36%); and (4) smooth muscular (10%) types.[422] As nodules mature from

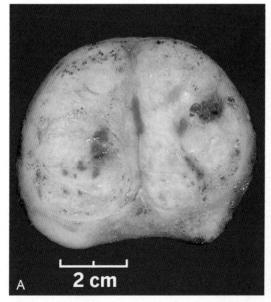
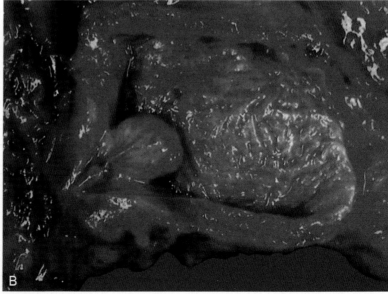

Fig. 8.48 Nodular hyperplasia, gross appearance. (A) Transverse section of the prostate shows massive nodular hyperplasia with small foci of hemorrhagic infarction. A focus of adenocarcinoma forms an ill-defined mass in the peripheral zone at the lower right of the specimen. (B) Hyperplasia of the median lobe of the prostate has created an exophytic mass that protrudes into the bladder.

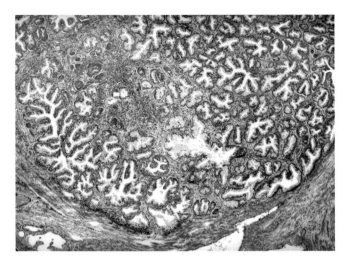

Fig. 8.49 Mixed epithelial-stromal nodule of nodular hyperplasia. Note the dilated peripheral sinus that forms the boundary of the nodule with the transition zone stroma. This sinus often goes in and out of the plane of section and may appear incomplete.

immature mesenchymal to smooth muscular type, there is an increase in expression of all growth factors (vascular endothelial growth factor [VEGF], insulin-like growth factor 1 [IGF1], fibroblast growth factor [FGF], TGF-ss), as well as CD44 and androgen receptors; S-100 protein, c-KIT, and ERs are not expressed.[422]

The diagnosis of nodular hyperplasia is often used by pathologists in needle biopsy specimens when only normal benign peripheral zone tissue is present. The transition zone is infrequently sampled by needle biopsies unless the urologist specifically targets this area or massive hyperplasia compresses the peripheral zone. We require the presence of at least part of a nodule for the diagnosis of nodular hyperplasia in needle biopsies, a very uncommon finding. Narrow 18-gauge needle biopsies virtually never contain the entire nodule unless it is very small and fortuitously sampled. Casual use of the term *nodular hyperplasia* for benign prostatic tissue may mislead the urologist into believing that a palpable nodule or hypoechoic focus of concern has been sampled and histologically evaluated; it is of clinical value for the pathologist to correlate the light microscopic findings with the clinical impression.[423] Variants of hyperplasia are compared in Table 8.15.

Vascular insufficiency probably accounts for infarction of hyperplastic nodules, seen in up to 20% of resected cases. The center of the nodule undergoes hemorrhagic necrosis, often with reactive changes in the residual epithelium at the periphery, including squamous metaplasia and urothelial metaplasia.

Nodular hyperplasia is not a precursor of cancer, but several similarities exist.[424] Both display a parallel increase in prevalence with the patient's age according to autopsy studies, although cancer lags by 15 to 20 years. Both require androgens for growth and development, and both may respond to androgen deprivation treatment. Inflammation is commonly found in both, thus suggesting a potential causative link.[425] Most cancers arise in patients with concomitant nodular hyperplasia, and cancer is found incidentally in a significant number (10%) of TURP specimens. Nodular hyperplasia may be related to cancer arising in the transition zone, perhaps in association with certain forms of hyperplasia.[424,426]

The pathogenesis of nodular hyperplasia is still poorly understood, but many hypotheses have been considered. It is possible that nodular hyperplasia has no single mechanism, but rather represents a synergistic effect of multiple events within biologic communication systems (neural, endocrine, and immune systems) during aging.[143] The increased density of immune cells, predominantly CD3+ T cells, in nodular hyperplasia suggests that the initial response to cellular damage is mediated by cell-mediated immunity.[427] Patients with nodular hyperplasia have defective one-way valves in the vertically oriented internal spermatic veins that result in elevated hydrostatic pressure (sixfold greater than normal) in the venous drainage of the male reproductive system.[428] The elevated pressure propagates to all interconnected vessels and leads to a unique biologic phenomenon: venous blood flows in retrograde fashion from the high-pressure testicular venous drainage system to the low-pressure drainage system of the prostate (law of communicating vessels).[428] Selective venous occlusion provided symptomatic improvement for patients with hyperplasia. There is an increased number of neuroendocrine cells in small adenomas, and the number of cells decreases as nodules enlarge, suggesting a role at inception of nodular hyperplasia.[429,430]

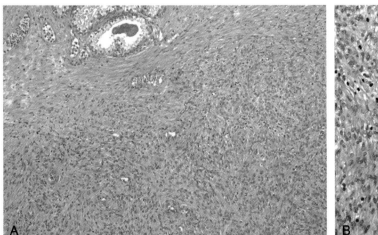
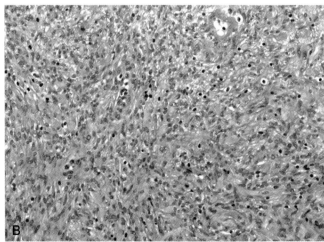

Fig. 8.50 Pure stromal nodule of nodular hyperplasia. (A) This circumscribed nodule is uniform and circumscribed. (B) The nodule consists of stromal fibroblasts with scattered lymphocytes.

TABLE 8.15 | Histopathologic Spectrum of Hyperplasia (Excluding Benign Prostatic Hyperplasia)

Variant	Microscopic Features	Usual Location
Postatrophic hyperplasia	Atrophic acini with epithelial proliferative changes; easily mistaken for adenocarcinoma due to architectural distortion	All zones
Stromal hyperplasia with atypia	Stromal nodules in the setting of cellularity and nuclear atypia	Transition zone
Basal cell hyperplasia	Proliferation of basal cells two or more cells in thickness; may have prominent nucleoli (atypical basal cell hyperplasia) or form a nodule (basal cell adenoma)	Transition zone
Cribriform hyperplasia	Acini with distinctive cribriform pattern, often with clear cytoplasm; easily mistaken for proliferative acini of the central zone	Transition zone
Atypical adenomatous hyperplasia	Localized proliferation of small acini in association with benign prostatic hyperplasia nodule, which architecturally mimics adenocarcinoma but lacks cytologic features of malignancy	Transition zone
Sclerosing adenosis	Circumscribed proliferation of small acini in a dense spindle cell stroma without significant atypia; usually solitary and microscopic	Transition zone
Verumontanum mucosal gland hyperplasia	Small benign acinar proliferation in the verumontanum	Verumontanum
Hyperplasia of mesonephric remnants	Rare benign lobular proliferation of acini with colloid-like material in the lumina; may mimic nephrogenic metaplasia focally; acini do not apparently express prostate-specific antigen or prostatic acid phosphatase	All zones (rare)
Pseudoangiomatous hyperplasia	Proliferation of slitlike spaces with only mild cytologic atypia	Peripheral zone

Postatrophic Hyperplasia

Clusters of atrophic prostatic acini that display proliferative epithelial changes are referred to as PAH (postinflammatory hyperplasia, postsclerotic hyperplasia) (Fig. 8.51).[185,431] It is at the extreme end of the morphologic continuum of acinar atrophy that most closely mimics adenocarcinoma (Table 8.16). This continuum varies from mild acinar irregularity with a flattened layer of attenuated cells containing scant cytoplasm to that of PAH in which the lining cells are low cuboidal with moderate cytoplasm. No sharp division in this continuum exists between atrophy and PAH, thus challenging the utility of PAH as a distinct entity. However, the morphologic similarity of PAH and carcinoma creates the potential for misdiagnosis, sometimes resulting in unnecessary prostatectomy.[431,432] To avoid this potentially tragic misinterpretation, the pathologist should have an understanding of this extreme morphologic variant of atrophy. We believe that PAH is a recognizable diagnostic category for atrophic acini that most closely mimics adenocarcinoma.

PAH consists of a microscopic lobular cluster of 5 to 15 small acini with distorted contours reminiscent of atrophy. One or more larger dilated acini are usually present within round to oval clusters. The small acini appear to bud off from the dilated acinus and impart a lobular appearance to the lesion. The small acini are lined by a layer of cuboidal secretory cells with mildly enlarged nuclei with an increased nuclear-to-cytoplasmic ratio compared with adjacent benign epithelial cells. Nuclei contain evenly distributed and finely granular chromatin, and nucleoli are usually small, although mildly enlarged basophilic nucleoli are focally present in 39% of cases. The cytoplasm is often basophilic or finely granular to clear, and luminal cytoplasmic apocrine-like blebs are present in 33% of cases. Luminal mucin is occasionally present. Corpora amylacea are present in 75% of cases, but crystalloids are rare.

The basal cell layer is usually present in PAH, but it is often inconspicuous by routine light microscopy. Basal cell hyperplasia is rarely seen in foci of PAH. Immunohistochemical stains for high-molecular-weight keratin 34βE12 reveal a focally fragmented basal cell layer in some cases, but it is usually completely intact and occasionally prominent. Adjacent prostatic acini always show at least focal atrophy. MIB1 staining reveals a greater proliferative rate than in simple atrophy.[433]

Stromal changes are always present in PAH, varying from smooth muscle atrophy to dense sclerosis with compression of acini. In cases with sclerosis the acinar lumina are compressed and show marked distortion. Subtyping into lobular and postsclerotic subtypes is useful only to allow recognition of PAH and distinguish it from mimics such as low-grade adenocarcinoma, and we prefer not to use subtypes for this entity. Also, it is often associated with patchy chronic inflammation; infrequently, dilated acini contain luminal neutrophils. Elastosis is another distinctive microscopic feature of some cases.[434]

PAH is distinguished from carcinoma by its characteristic lobular architecture, intact or fragmented basal cell layer, inconspicuous or mildly enlarged nucleoli, and adjacent acinar atrophy with stromal fibrosis or smooth muscle atrophy (Table 8.16).[357] Periacinar retraction clefting represents a reliable criterion in differential diagnosis between PAH and carcinoma; it is rare in PAH and nearly constant, at least focally, in carcinoma.[379]

Low-grade adenocarcinoma is the most important differential diagnostic consideration. PAH usually has a lobular pattern on low power, like Gleason pattern 2 and 3 adenocarcinomas. However, the lobular pattern in PAH is less distinct in cases with abundant stromal sclerosis, and there may be a pseudoinfiltrative growth pattern with fibrous entrapment of acini. Nucleolar changes are also useful in separating PAH and carcinoma, although some cases of low-grade carcinoma have only scattered large nucleoli or even micronucleoli. Mildly enlarged nucleoli may be present in PAH, but only focally, and most of the cells have micronucleoli. The separation from carcinoma is most difficult in needle biopsy specimens in which only a portion of the lesion is sampled, and awareness of this entity assists in this distinction. There may occasionally be genetic changes in chromosome 8 in atrophic epithelium.[435] These

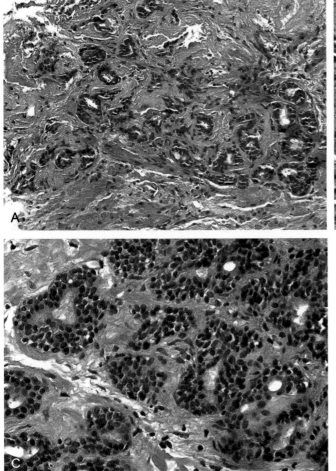

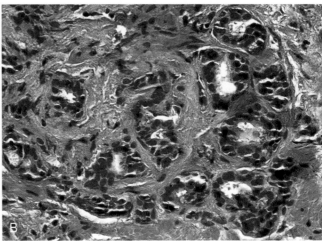

Fig. 8.51 Postatrophic hyperplasia. (A) The acini are variable in size and shape, set in a fibrous stroma. Part of the epithelium is flattened, indicating atrophy, but other areas show low cuboidal epithelium and luminal secretory blebs. (B) The epithelial lining is irregular, with hyperchromatic nuclei. (C) These elongate acini have enlarged nuclei with hyperchromasia. Nucleoli are inconspicuous.

changes were reported to be present at a similar or higher frequency in high-grade PIN and carcinoma.[436]

Is PAH associated with cancer? Anton et al. assessed a large series of radical prostatectomy and cystoprostatectomy specimens and found PAH in 32% and 27% of cases, respectively.[437] It was located in the peripheral zone (91% of cases), transition zone (8%), and central zone (1%), and had no apparent spatial association with cancer.

Prostatic Stromal Hyperplasia With Atypia

Prostatic stromal hyperplasia with atypia consists of one or more ill-defined, uncircumscribed, hyperplastic stromal proliferations, sometimes nodular, with variable numbers of atypical, bizarre giant cells, with vacuolated nuclei, smudged chromatin, and frequent multinucleation infiltrating around benign acini.[438] Despite exhibiting cytologic features that are worrisome for malignancy, this lesion is devoid of mitotic figures or necrosis. It has a hypocellular, loose, myxoid matrix. Cellularity is uniform, and the arrangement of atypical cells is haphazard. Most cells contain a moderate amount of eosinophilic cytoplasm with indistinct cellular borders. Nuclei vary in shape, but may be round. There are invariably large ectatic vessels with hyalinized thick walls within the proliferation, accompanied by lymphocytes, plasma cells, and mast cells (Figs. 8.52 and 8.53).[421] These hyperplastic growths are histologically and clinically reminiscent of benign counterparts in the myometrium, breast, vulva, vagina, and elsewhere, with degenerate smudged nuclei that may be mistaken for malignancy.

Prostatic stromal hyperplasia with atypia is a rare lesion that has been referred to by a variety of terms, including atypical stromal hyperplasia, stromal hyperplasia with bizarre nuclei, pseudosarcomatous lesion, and pseudoneoplastic lesion of the prostate gland. Some authors have suggested the acronym PSPUMP (prostatic stromal proliferation of uncertain malignant potential), later modified to STUMP (stromal tumor of uncertain malignant potential), that lumps prostatic stromal hyperplasia with atypia (benign entity), leiomyoma with atypia (benign), phyllodes tumor (malignant), and stromal sarcoma (malignant).[421,439-443] We discourage use of this terminology based on differences between these entities according to differences in light microscopic appearances, immunophenotypes, and clinical outcomes. Essentially all cases of STUMP unassociated with phyllodes tumor or sarcoma and with adequate follow-up show benign clinical behavior.

The atypical cells in prostatic stromal hyperplasia with atypia display consistent and intense nuclear immunoreactivity for androgen receptors and vimentin, moderate reactivity for desmin and actin, variable reactivity for progesterone receptors, and no reactivity for ERs and Ki-67. These findings suggest that this lesion results from local hypersensitivity to androgen, with upregulation of androgen receptors in these cells. The pattern of expression in stromal hyperplasia with atypia is like that in nodular hyperplasia except for the lack of expression of ERs.

Stromal hyperplasia with atypia has no malignant potential, and the atypical cells are degenerative myofibroblasts. Local recurrence was seen in 25% of cases in one study, with a mean follow-up of 6 years, similar to that seen with typical nodular

TABLE 8.16	Postatrophic Hyperplasia Versus Low-Grade Carcinoma	
	Postatrophic Hyperplasia	Low-Grade Adenocarcinoma
Architecture, low power	Lobular small acinar proliferation, usually with central large dilated acini or acinus	May be lobular and circumscribed
Acinar contours	Irregular, "atrophic"	May be rounded or smooth
Basal cell layer		
Light microscopy	Usually intact; may be inconspicuous	Absent
High-molecular-weight keratin (34βE12) immunoreactivity	Intact or fragmented	Absent
Stromal changes	Smooth muscle atrophy, often with dense periacinar sclerosis	With or without stromal changes
Cytology		
Nuclei	Mild enlargement	Enlarged
Nucleoli	Usually inconspicuous	Usually prominent
Cytoplasm	Basophilic	Usually pale because of greater amount of cytoplasm
Basophilic mucin	Rare	May be present
Crystalloids	Rare	May be present
Adjacent acini	Often atrophic	Variable

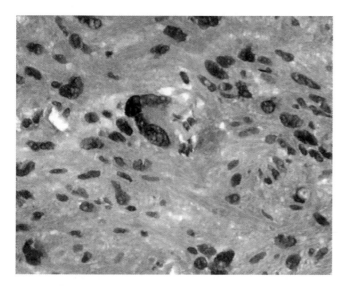

Fig. 8.52 Prostatic stromal hyperplasia with atypia. Multinucleated giant cells punctuate the stroma, with moderate cytologic atypia without mitotic figures.

hyperplasia.[421] Sarcomatous (malignant) transformation has not been described.

The differential diagnosis of stromal hyperplasia with atypia includes typical nodular hyperplasia, leiomyoma with atypia,

solitary fibrous tumor, phyllodes tumor, low-grade stromal sarcoma, leiomyosarcoma, neurofibroma, and gastrointestinal stromal tumor involving the prostate.

Basal Cell Hyperplasia and Basal Cell Proliferations

There are three patterns of basal cell hyperplasia: typical basal cell hyperplasia, atypical basal cell hyperplasia, and basal cell adenoma (Table 8.17).[283,357,444–447] These findings may be particularly challenging in biopsy specimens because of limited sampling.[448] Low-grade urothelial carcinoma involving the prostate may be mistaken for basal cell hyperplasia on biopsy.[449] Neoplastic basal cell proliferations, referred to as adenoid basal cell tumor, adenoid cystic carcinoma, and basal cell carcinoma, are described in Chapter 9.

Typical Basal Cell Hyperplasia

Basal cell hyperplasia consists of a proliferation of basal cells two or more cells in thickness at the periphery of prostatic acini (Fig. 8.54).[444] It sometimes appears as small nests of cells surrounded by compressed stroma, often associated with chronic inflammation. The nests may be solid or cystically dilated, and occasionally are punctuated by irregular round luminal spaces, creating a cribriform pattern.[448] Basal cell hyperplasia frequently involves only part of an acinus and sometimes protrudes into the lumen, retaining the overlying secretory cell layer; less commonly, symmetric duplication of the basal cell layer occurs at the periphery of the acinus. The proliferation may protrude into the acinar lumen and retain the overlying secretory luminal epithelium. Symmetric circumferential thickening of the basal cell layer is less frequent than eccentric thickening, and these changes do not result from tangential sectioning.

Basal cell hyperplasia resembles prostatic acini in the fetus, and this feature accounts for the synonyms *fetalization* and *embryonal hyperplasia*. Basal cell hyperplasia may be composed of basal cell nests with areas of luminal differentiation resembling similar lesions of the salivary gland (so-called adenoid basal form of basal cell hyperplasia).

The basal cells in basal cell hyperplasia are enlarged, ovoid or round, and plump (epithelioid), with large, pale, ovoid nuclei, finely reticular chromatin, and a moderate amount of cytoplasm. Nucleoli are usually inconspicuous (<1 μm in diameter) except in atypical basal cell hyperplasia (discussed later).

Sclerosing basal cell hyperplasia is identical to typical basal cell hyperplasia except for the presence of delicate lacy fibrosis or dense irregular sclerotic fibrosis and hyperplastic smooth muscle surrounding and distorting hyperplastic cellular aggregates. It is not associated with carcinoma, but occasionally may be confused with malignancy.

Clear cell change is common in basal cell hyperplasia, often with a cribriform pattern; a cribriform pattern without clear cell change is rare. Squamous metaplasia is infrequent, usually associated with infarction. Chronic inflammation is common, but it is nonspecific. Occasional nuclear grooves and "bubble" artifacts are observed. Focal calcification is evident in some cases and may be present within the basal cell nests (Table 8.17).

Florid basal cell hyperplasia consists of compact glandular proliferation with solid nests (Fig. 8.55).[450] The cytologic features in some areas look disturbing because the basaloid cells have moderately enlarged nuclei, often with prominent nucleoli; a few mitotic figures are present; the intervening stroma is scant and cellular; the lesion is not well circumscribed; and basaloid structures are intermingled with the surrounding glands, thus giving the impression of

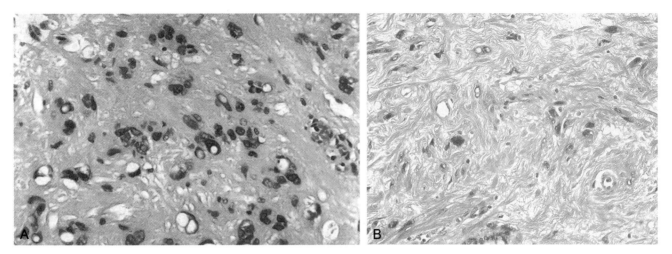

Fig. 8.53 Prostatic stromal hyperplasia with atypia. (A) Symplastic changes of many of the myocytes, including nuclear and cytoplasmic vacuolization. (B) In another case there is focal crowding of myocytes with variation in nuclear size. No mitotic figures were observed in either of these cases despite exhaustive sectioning.

TABLE 8.17	Basal Cell Proliferations of the Prostate: Diagnostic Criteria and Immunohistochemical Profile				
	Normal Basal Cell Layer	Basal Cell Hyperplasia	Atypical Basal Cell Hyperplasia	Basal Cell Adenoma	Adenoid Basal Cell Carcinoma
Architecture	Nearly continuous single-cell layer	Small cell nests (solid or cystic), usually in nodular hyperplasia, two cell layer minimum	Same as basal cell hyperplasia	Round, circumscribed nodule of basal cell hyperplasia	Infiltrating "adenoid pattern" or basaloid pattern; myxoid stroma
Cytology	Small elongate cells, ovoid nuclei, scant cytoplasm	Large ovoid nuclei, indistinct nucleoli, scant cytoplasm; may have clear cytoplasm	Same as basal cell hyperplasia, but with nucleolomegaly	Same as basal cell hyperplasia; may have nucleolomegaly	Basaloid cells with large nuclei
Immunohistochemical findings					
Basal cell–specific keratin 34βE12	+	+	+	+	+ (patchy)
Prostate-specific antigen	−	+ (patchy)	+ (patchy)	+ (focal)	+
Prostate acid phosphatase	−	+ (patchy)	+ (patchy)	+ (focal)	+
Chromogranin	−	+	+	+	−
S100 protein	−	+	+	+	−
Neuron-specific enolase	−	+	+	−	−

+, <5% of cells were positive.
Modified from Devaraj LT, Bostwick DG. Atypical basal cell hyperplasia of the prostate. Immunophenotypic profile and proposed classification of basal cell proliferations. Am J Surg Pathol 1993;17:645-659.

infiltration (this is also called *diffuse type*). The proliferation of basal cells involves more than 100 small crowded acini (per section) forming a nodule.[446]

Atypical Basal Cell Hyperplasia

Atypical basal cell hyperplasia is identical to basal cell hyperplasia except for the presence of large, prominent nucleoli (Fig. 8.56). The nucleoli are round to oval and lightly eosinophilic, like those seen in acinar adenocarcinoma of the prostate (mean diameter is 2 μm). Chronic inflammation occurs in most cases, a finding suggesting that nucleolomegaly reflects reactive changes. A morphologic spectrum of nucleolar size is observed in basal cell proliferations, and only those with more than 10% of cells exhibiting prominent nucleoli are considered atypical.[444] This lesion is significant because of the potential for misdiagnosis as high-grade PIN and adenocarcinoma.[451]

Basal Cell Adenoma

Basal cell adenoma is identical to typical basal cell hyperplasia, although the proliferating basal cell masses are usually large and circumscribed with a nodular or adenoma-like pattern. Basal cell adenoma consists of one or more large, round, usually solitary circumscribed nodules of acini with basal cell hyperplasia in the setting of nodular hyperplasia.[452] The nodules contain uniformly spaced aggregates of hyperplastic basal cells that form small solid nests or cystically dilated acini. Condensed stroma is seen at the periphery, often traverses the adenomatous nodules, and creates incomplete lobulation in some cases. Stroma is normal or slightly increased in density and may be basophilic without myxoid change adjacent to cell nests.

The basal cells in adenoma are plump, with large nuclei, scant cytoplasm, and inconspicuous nucleoli, although large prominent nucleoli are rarely observed. Many cells are cuboidal or

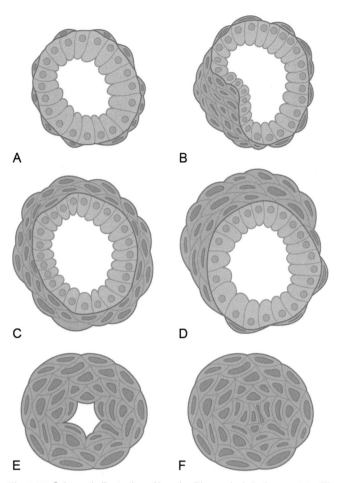

Fig. 8.54 Schematic illustration of basal cell hyperplasia in the prostate. (A) Normal prostatic gland with thin peripheral layer of basal cells and overlying columnar secretory luminal cell layer. (B) Focal basal cell proliferation with mild distortion of the glandular luminal contour. (C) Symmetric circumferential proliferation of basal cells, at least two cells in thickness. (D) Eccentric focus of atypical basal cell hyperplasia with prominent nucleoli, eccentric pattern. (E) Basal cell hyperplasia with loss of secretory cell layer (note retention of glandular lumen). Compare with (F) "solid" pattern of basal cell hyperplasia, with absence of lumen. (From Deveraj LJ, Bostwick DG. Atypical basal cell hyperplasia of the prostate: immunophenotypic profile and proposed classification of basal cell proliferations. *Am J Surg Pathol* 1993;17:645-659.)

"epithelioid," particularly near the center of the cell nests, and some contain clear cytoplasm. Prominent calcific debris is often present within acinar lumina.

Multiple basal cell adenomas are referred to as basal cell adenomatosis. Basal cell adenoma invariably arises in association with nodular hyperplasia and appears to be a variant with no malignant potential. In contrast with basal cell carcinoma, adenoma is well circumscribed, lacks necrosis, and the stroma between the basal cell nests is like that of the surrounding benign stroma.

Immunohistochemical Findings

Basal cell hyperplasia (typical and atypical forms) displays intense cytoplasmic immunoreactivity in virtually all cells with keratin 34βE12 and p63 (Table 8.17). The combination of 34βE12 and p63 improves the sensitivity for basal cell detection compared with either marker alone (Fig. 8.56).[453] Immunoreactivity for PSA, PAP, chromogranin, S-100 protein, α-smooth muscle actin, and neuron-specific enolase is present in rare basal cells in the majority of cases.

Differential Diagnosis

The differential diagnosis of basal cell proliferations includes a wide variety of benign and malignant lesions (Table 8.18).[436,454] AAH may be confused with basal cell hyperplasia, but it does not usually have a prominent basal cell layer and displays a fragmented keratin 34βE12–immunoreactive basal cell layer.[455] Sclerosing adenosis may be difficult to separate from sclerosing basal cell hyperplasia, and these lesions may coexist; however, sclerosing adenosis has no smooth muscle in the sclerotic stroma and displays myoepithelial differentiation (intense cytoplasmic immunoreactivity with keratin 34βE12, S-100 protein, and muscle-specific actin, as well as ultrastructural evidence of cytoplasmic myofilaments).

Seminal vesicle and ejaculatory duct epithelium may also be confused with basal cell hyperplasia and adenoma, particularly in small specimens such as biopsies and rarely in TURP specimens. The proliferation and stratification of lining cells with cytologic atypia may resemble small foci of solid basal cell hyperplasia. Seminal vesicle epithelium is distinguished by the presence of secretory luminal cells, significant cytologic atypia (particularly in the senile seminal vesicle), and distinctive abundant yellow to golden-brown lipochrome pigment.

The normal urothelium of the urethra and periurethral ducts resembles basal cell hyperplasia histologically and immunohistochemically. Also, urothelial metaplasia may occur in the medium and small ducts in the prostate, sometimes in association with inflammation and reactive atypia with mild nucleolomegaly.

Urethral polyp, although uncommon, may be confused with basal cell hyperplasia and adenoma, particularly in small cystoscopic specimens and needle biopsies. Urethral polyp includes proliferative papillary urethritis, ectopic prostatic tissue, nephrogenic adenoma, and inverted papilloma.

PIN may be mistaken for atypical basal cell hyperplasia and is distinguished by the presence of cytologic abnormalities in secretory luminal cells of medium to large acini, intense cytoplasmic PSA, PAP, α-methylacyl–coenzyme A racemase (P504S) immunoreactivity in the abnormal cells, and an intact or fragmented keratin 34βE12–immunoreactive basal cell layer.[359,378] The nuclei of basal cells in basal cell hyperplasia tend to be round, and, at times, the basal cells form small solid basaloid nests. In contrast, the cells in PIN tend to be pseudostratified or stratified and columnar, and do not occlude the acinar lumen.[456,457] Within areas of basal cell hyperplasia, atypical basal cells can be seen beneath the overlying benign secretory cells. PIN has full-thickness cytologic atypia, with the nuclei usually oriented perpendicular to the basement membrane.[457]

Low-grade adenocarcinoma is distinguished from basal cell hyperplasia by the presence of PSA- and PAP-immunoreactive luminal secretory cells with nucleolomegaly, frequent luminal crystalloids, and absence of a keratin 34βE12–immunoreactive basal cell layer. Similar criteria allow separation of the cribriform variant of adenocarcinoma, adenoid basal cell tumor, basal cell hyperplasia with or without clear cell change, and clear cell cribriform hyperplasia.

In contrast with basaloid carcinoma, basal cell adenoma is well circumscribed and lacks necrosis, and the stroma between the basaloid nests is like that of the surrounding normal stroma (see Chapter 9).

Cribriform Hyperplasia

Cribriform hyperplasia, including clear cell cribriform hyperplasia, is an uncommon variant of nodular hyperplasia that arises in the transition zone, so it is rarely observed in biopsy specimens (Table 8.19). It consists of an aggregate of intermediate- and large-size acini with a distinctive pattern of collapsible fenestrations

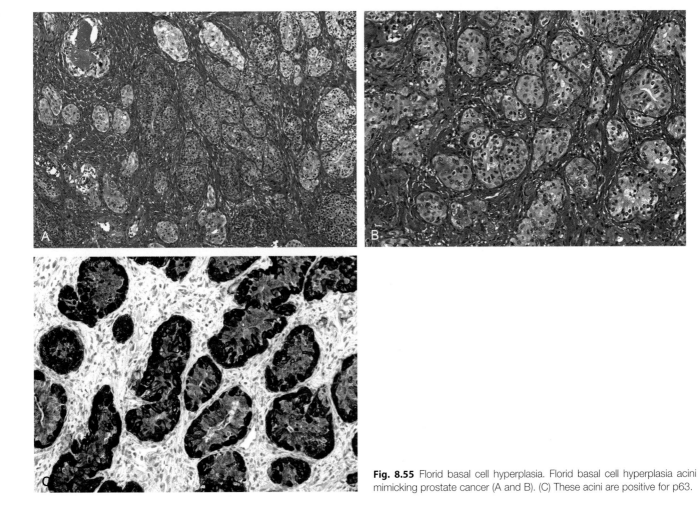

Fig. 8.55 Florid basal cell hyperplasia. Florid basal cell hyperplasia acini mimicking prostate cancer (A and B). (C) These acini are positive for p63.

(Fig. 8.57).[458-460] The secretory cells usually have pale to clear cytoplasm and small, uniform nuclei with inconspicuous nucleoli, whereas the basal cell layer is often at least focally prominent with enlarged nuclei.[458,459] This lesion is often mistaken for high-grade PIN but lacks prominent nucleoli.[436,460] Phyllodes tumor of the prostate contains foci of cribriform hyperplasia in 4% of cases.[404]

Atypical Adenomatous Hyperplasia

AAH (atypical hyperplasia) is a localized proliferation of small acini within the prostate that may be mistaken for carcinoma (Fig. 8.58 through Fig. 8.63).[187,461-464] It varies in incidence rate from 20% (TURP specimens) to 24% (autopsy series in 20- to 40-year-old men).[465] It can be found throughout the prostate but is usually present near the apex and in the transition zone and periurethral area.[463] The mean size of AAH is 0.03 cm³, although mass-forming AAH measuring 21 cm³ has been documented.[464] Some have referred to a subset of AAH adenosis, but we do not recommend use of that ill-defined term.

AAH is distinguished from well-differentiated carcinoma by (1) inconspicuous nucleoli, (2) fragmented basal cell layer, and (3) infrequent crystalloids (Table 8.20). All measures of nucleolar size allow separation of AAH from adenocarcinoma, including mean nucleolar diameter, largest nucleolar diameter, and percentage of nucleoli greater than 1 μm in diameter.[466] Despite the utility of these features, the absolute distinction between AAH and

carcinoma remains difficult in some cases. Other morphologic features are not useful in distinguishing AAH from adenocarcinoma, including lesion shape, circumscription, multifocality, mean acinar size, variation in acinar size and shape, chromatin pattern, and the amount and tinctorial quality of the cytoplasm. AAH and cancer contain acidic mucin in the majority of cases.[147]

Immunohistochemistry is often useful in the diagnosis of AAH. The basal cell layer is characteristically discontinuous and fragmented in AAH but absent in cancer, a feature that can be demonstrated in routine sections with basal cell–specific markers such as keratin 34βE12 and p63 (Figs. 8.64 and 8.65). AAH is often positive for racemase, similar to cancer, so this marker may not be useful for separation from malignancy.[211,467]

Histologic mimics of AAH include nodular hyperplasia without atypia, simple lobular atrophy (Fig. 8.66), PAH, sclerosing atrophy, basal cell hyperplasia, atypical basal cell hyperplasia, and metaplastic changes associated with radiation, infarction, mesonephric remnant hyperplasia, and prostatitis. Many mimics display architectural and cytologic atypia, including nucleolomegaly, and caution is warranted in interpretation of scant specimens, cauterized or distorted specimens, and those submitted with an incomplete patient history. AAH is uncommonly associated with sclerosis, but further study is needed to determine the relationship with sclerosing adenosis. Sclerosing adenosis differs from AAH by displaying myoepithelial features of the basal cells and an exuberant stroma of fibroblasts and loose ground substance. AAH should also be distinguished from lobular atrophy and PAH. Simple

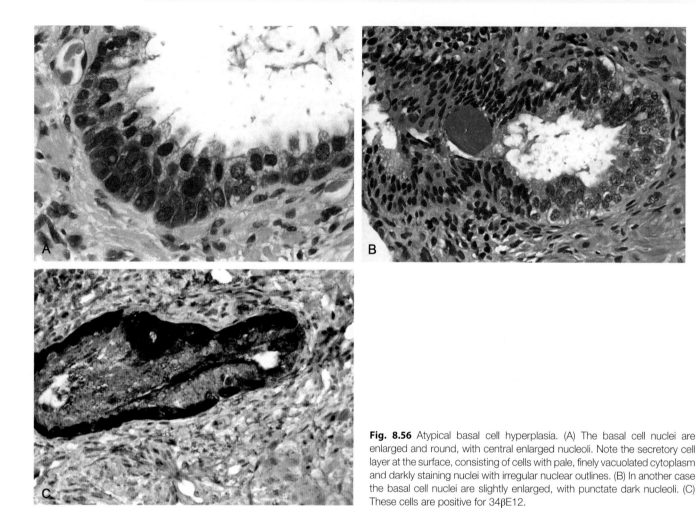

Fig. 8.56 Atypical basal cell hyperplasia. (A) The basal cell nuclei are enlarged and round, with central enlarged nucleoli. Note the secretory cell layer at the surface, consisting of cells with pale, finely vacuolated cytoplasm and darkly staining nuclei with irregular nuclear outlines. (B) In another case the basal cell nuclei are slightly enlarged, with punctate dark nucleoli. (C) These cells are positive for 34βE12.

atrophy consists of shrunken acini that demonstrate strong basal cell–specific antikeratin immunoreactivity. PAH may be difficult to separate from AAH, because proliferating luminal cells with small amounts of clear cytoplasm may occur in an atrophic background. These cells may demonstrate cytologic atypia, sometimes with luminal mucin. Both may have a fragmented basal cell layer.

Two clinical questions regarding AAH are unanswered. First, does Gleason primary grade 1 adenocarcinoma represent overdiagnosed adenocarcinoma? These lesions are uncommon; most agree that Gleason primary grade 2 adenocarcinoma (infiltrating acini) is malignant, but what is the true biologic potential of the uniform circumscribed proliferation of Gleason primary grade 1 adenocarcinoma? Most, but not all, Gleason pattern 1 cancers are now thought to represent foci of AAH, a conclusion agreed to by Gleason himself (D. G. Bostwick, personal communication). Second, is AAH a precursor of adenocarcinoma? AAH may be linked to a subset of prostate cancers that arise in the transition zone, but the evidence is circumstantial: increased incidence in association with carcinoma (15% in 100 prostates without carcinoma at autopsy, and 31% in 100 prostates with cancer at autopsy), topographic relationship with small acinar carcinoma, age peak incidence that precedes that of carcinoma, increasing silver-staining nucleolar organized region count, increased nuclear area and diameter, and a proliferative cell index similar to that of small acinar carcinoma but significantly higher than that of normal and hyperplastic prostatic epithelium.[393] Expression

of racemase in some cases of AAH has suggested possible premalignant status to some authors.[187,211]

A small but significant number of cases of AAH have genetic instability. A total of 9% of cases of AAH were abnormal using fluorescence in situ hybridization with centromere-specific probes for chromosome 7, 8, 10, 12, and Y.[467] Up to 60% of cases of AAH had highly variable allelic imbalance at chromosome 8p arm, compared with up to 90% of prostate cancers.[468] PTOV1 expression in AAH was almost three times higher than benign epithelial cells, similar to that of high-grade PIN, but lower than that of carcinoma.[469] Conversely, other studies reported that AAH does not seem to be linked closely to prostate cancer and should not be considered an obligate premalignant lesion.[470,471] AAH appears to be invariably diploid and does not display TMPRSS2-ERG rearrangements.[455,472,473]

When AAH is encountered in prostatic specimens, we believe that all tissue should be embedded and made available for examination; serial sections of suspicious foci may be useful. Biopsy specimens rarely contain AAH, and we require that most or all the focus be present for diagnosis, thus recognizing the potential for sampling AAH-like areas in adenocarcinoma. The quadruple stain (keratin 34βE12, p63, racemase, and c-myc) is useful in difficult cases. The identification of AAH should not influence or dictate therapeutic decisions; however, the clinical importance of this lesion is not fully understood, and close surveillance and follow-up may be indicated.

TABLE 8.18	Basal Cell Hyperplasia (Ordinary, Florid, and with Prominent Nucleoli): Differential Diagnosis, Morphologic Criteria, and Major Immunohistochemical Findings						
	Architecture	Cytology	34βE12	p63	Prostate-Specific Antigen	S100 Protein	α-Smooth Muscle Actin
Basal cell hyperplasia (typical, florid, and atypical)	Cell nests, two cell layers minimum, solid or cystic	Small- to medium-size nuclei, nucleoli may be prominent in some forms	+	+	±	− to ±	− to ±
High-grade prostatic intraepithelial neoplasia	Ducts and acini with various architectural patterns, ranging from flat to cribriform	Cells with enlarged nuclei, with a prominent nucleolus, similar to those in adenocarcinoma	± (basal cells)	± (basal cells)	+	−	−
Adenocarcinoma	Acini of various sizes, either separated or fused, with different architectural patterns, such as flat or monolayered or cribriform	Cells with enlarged nuclei, with prominent nucleoli	−	−	+	−	−
Sclerosing adenosis	Acinar structures, predominantly small, lined by bilayered epithelium	Small- to medium-size nuclei, inconspicuous nucleoli	+ (basal cells)	+ (basal cells)	+	+	+
Benign seminal vesicle/ejaculatory duct epithelium	Ducts lined by a bilayered epithelium	Prominent nuclear atypia and pleomorphism	+	+	−	−	−
Squamous metaplasia	Ducts and acini lined by multilayered epithelium similar to epidermis	Cells with small- to medium-size nuclei; inconspicuous nucleoli; keratinization often prominent	+	+	−	−	−
Urothelial metaplasia	Ducts and acini lined by multilayered epithelium similar to urothelium	Small- to medium-size nuclei, inconspicuous nucleoli; luminal cells larger than those in the intermediate and basal layers	+	+	− to ± (scattered luminal cells)	−	−

Sclerosing Adenosis

Sclerosing adenosis of the prostate, originally described as adenomatoid or pseudoadenomatoid tumor, consists of a benign circumscribed proliferation of small acini set in a dense spindle cell stroma.[474-478] It is an incidental finding in TURP specimens for BPH, present in approximately 2% of specimens; rare cases are associated with elevated serum PSA concentration. Sclerosing adenosis is usually solitary and microscopic, but it may be multifocal and extensive.

The acini in sclerosing adenosis are predominantly well formed and small to medium sized, but may exist as minute cellular nests or clusters with abortive lumina (Figs. 8.67 and 8.68). The cells lining the acini display a moderate amount of clear to eosinophilic cytoplasm, often with distinct cell margins. The basal cell layer may be focally prominent and hyperplastic, particularly in acini thickly rimmed by cellular stroma; hybrid cases of sclerosing adenosis and basal cell hyperplasia have been described.[479] In some areas the

acini merge with the exuberant stroma of fibroblasts and loose ground substance. The finding of a cellular stroma with myxoid features may play a role in distinguishing sclerosing adenosis from carcinoma.[480]

Sclerosing adenosis usually has no significant cytologic atypia of the epithelial cells or stromal cells, but some cases may show moderate atypia. We described five cases with significant cytologic atypia, referred to as atypical sclerosing adenosis, that were initially considered suspicious or diagnostic of adenocarcinoma.[481] Three of four cases had aneuploid DNA content by digital image analysis, whereas all cases of typical sclerosing adenosis were diploid. During a mean follow-up of 33 months (range, 5 to 73 months), none of the patients with atypical sclerosing adenosis experienced recurrence or prostatic cancer.

The unique immunophenotype of sclerosing adenosis is a valuable diagnostic clue that distinguishes it from adenocarcinoma (Table 8.21). The basal cells show immunoreactivity for S-100

TABLE 8.19	Cribriform Hyperplasia of the Prostate: Differential Diagnosis, Morphologic Criteria, and Major Immunohistochemical Findings		
	Architecture	Cytology	Basal Cell Layer
Clear cell cribriform hyperplasia	Collapsible fenestrations usually forming a nodule within the transition zone	Bland cytology with small nucleoli	Invariably present; occasionally prominent
Central zone epithelium	Complex epithelium with papillae, epithelial bridges, and cribriform growth	Benign cytology with tall stratified secretory cells with granular eosinophilic cytoplasm, round to oval nuclei	Intact
Prostatitis with reactive epithelial changes	Inflamed epithelium with reactive changes that may include cribriform growth	Reactive nuclear changes, sometimes severe, with nuclear enlargement and prominent nucleoli mimicking malignancy	Basal cell hyperplasia that may be prominent
Basal cell hyperplasia	Proliferation of small- to medium-size cribriform glands separated by loose stroma in the setting of basal cell hyperplasia; True cribriform basal cell hyperplasia consists of a nest of basal cells punctuated by multiple slits and fenestrations, whereas pseudocribriform basal cell hyperplasia has complex cribriform growth resulting from coalescence of basal cell hyperplasia nests	Benign basal cell cytology, including scant cytoplasm, round, oval or spindle hyperchromatic nuclei, finely granular uniform chromatin, inconspicuous nucleoli; sometimes with eosinophilic hyaline globules or luminal calcifications	Entire process consists of basal cells
Basal cell carcinoma	Usually seen in the adenoid cystic carcinoma variant, with irregular cribriform growth containing mucin or basement membrane–like material within the lumina; stroma is usually desmoplastic	Usually has large hyperchromatic nuclei with scant cytoplasm; nucleoli may or may not be prominent	Entire process consists of basal cells
High-grade PIN	Usually focal intraductal or intraductular proliferation without expansion; may be tufted, micropapillary, flat, or cribriform	Nuclear abnormalities, including enlargement, hyperchromasia, and prominent nucleoli in ≥10% of cells; no necrosis	At least partially intact
Intraductal carcinoma	Solid, micropapillary, or dense or loose cribriform growth, with expansile growth of acini beyond that of high-grade PIN; no definite stromal invasion	Frank anaplasia; comedo necrosis occasionally; multiple definitions (see text)	At least partially intact
Cribriform pattern of carcinoma	Same as intraductal carcinoma with invasion; associated with typical acinar carcinoma	Same as intraductal carcinoma	Loss of basal cell layer
Cribriform ductal carcinoma	Same as intraductal carcinoma with invasion; associated with typical ductal carcinoma	Same as intraductal carcinoma	Loss of basal cell layer
Secondary carcinoma (contiguous spread)	Variable; usually from contiguous spread from bladder or colon, with focal cribriform growth as well as other typical patterns	Invariably cytologically high grade	Loss of basal cell layer

PIN, Prostatic intraepithelial neoplasia.

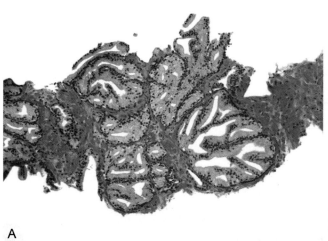 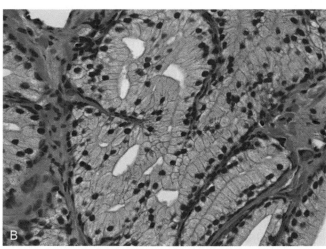

Fig. 8.57 Clear cell cribriform hyperplasia. (A) At low magnification, the fenestrations are irregular in size and shape, and are contained within expanded acini. (B) At high magnification, epithelial cells show pale finely vacuolated cytoplasm, uniform nuclei with open chromatin pattern, and small inconspicuous nucleoli.

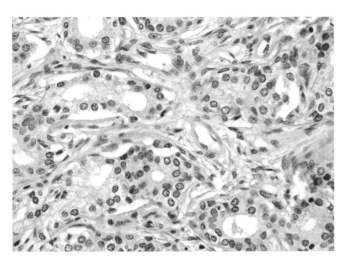

Fig. 8.58 Atypical adenomatous hyperplasia. The small acinar proliferation shows variation in size, shape, and spacing in a moderately cellular stroma.

protein and muscle-specific actin, unlike normal epithelium or carcinoma; consequently, sclerosing adenosis is considered a form of metaplasia (Fig. 8.69).[482] The basal cell layer is intact or fragmented and discontinuous in sclerosing adenosis, as demonstrated with immunohistochemical stains for keratin 34βE12 (Fig. 8.70), compared with absence of staining in carcinoma. PSA and PAP are present within secretory luminal cells. Ultrastructural studies demonstrate myoepithelial differentiation in sclerosing adenosis, with collections of thin filaments and dense bodies.[478]

Sclerosing adenosis should be distinguished from lobular atrophy and PAH. Both lesions tend to be lobulated. Simple atrophy consists of shrunken acini, whereas PAH contains proliferating luminal cells with small amounts of clear cytoplasm. The cells may demonstrate some degree of cytologic atypia, and luminal mucin may be identified. Other histologic mimics of sclerosing adenosis include sclerosing atrophy, basal cell hyperplasia, atypical basal cell hyperplasia, and metaplastic changes associated with radiation, infarction, and prostatitis.

AAH is occasionally associated with sclerosis, but it lacks the dense periacinar hyalinized fibrosis sometimes seen in sclerosing adenosis. Immunohistochemical studies reveal a fragmented and discontinuous basal cell layer in AAH, whereas sclerosing adenosis

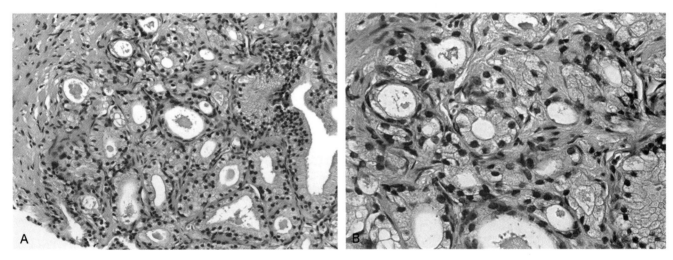

Fig. 8.59 Atypical adenomatous hyperplasia (A and B). One edge of this nodule of nodular hyperplasia consists of a proliferation of small pale acini set in a cellular stroma.

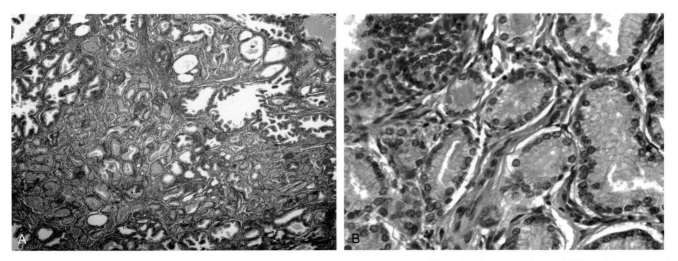

Fig. 8.60 Atypical adenomatous hyperplasia. (A) A group of small acini architecturally mimics well-differentiated adenocarcinoma. (B) The acini lack cytologic features of malignancy, without significant nuclear or nucleolar enlargement.

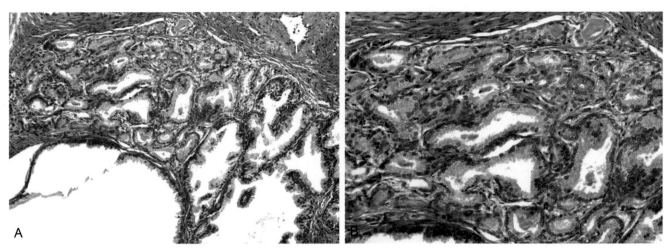

Fig. 8.61 Atypical adenomatous hyperplasia. (A) At the edge of a hyperplastic nodule is a minute nest of small acini with pale cytoplasm. (B) At high magnification the small acini contain uniform small nuclei and punctate nucleoli without significant enlargement.

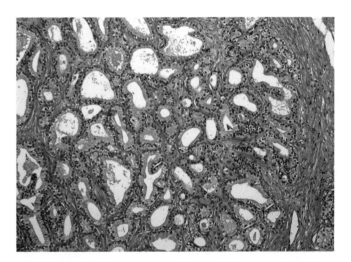

Fig. 8.62 Atypical adenomatous hyperplasia. The closely packed cluster of acini contains small nuclei and minute punctate nucleoli.

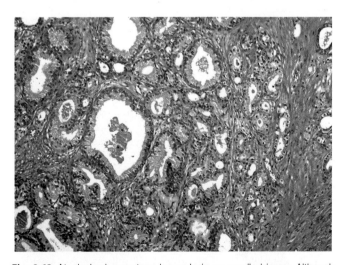

Fig. 8.63 Atypical adenomatous hyperplasia on needle biopsy. Although rare on needle biopsy, atypical adenomatous hyperplasia is occasionally observed, consisting of a small acinar proliferation in intimate association with larger acini of nodular hyperplasia. We require that most or all of the focus is present on the biopsy to diagnose atypical adenomatous hyperplasia, to avoid underdiagnosis of adenocarcinoma.

TABLE 8.20	Atypical Adenomatous Hyperplasia Versus Well-Differentiated Adenocarcinoma	
	Atypical Adenomatous Hyperplasia	Carcinoma (Gleason Grades 1 and 2)
Architectural and associated features		
Low power	Circumscribed or limited infiltration	Circumscribed or limited infiltration
Lesion size	Variable	Variable
Gland size	Variable	Less variable
Gland shape	Variable	Less variable
Crystalloids	Infrequent (16%)	Frequent (75%)
Corpora amylacea	Frequent (32%)	Infrequent (13%)
Basophilic mucin	Infrequent	Frequent
Nuclear features		
Nuclear size variation	Less variable	Variable
Chromatin	Uniform/granular	Uniform or variable
Parachromatin clearing	Infrequent	Frequent
Nucleoli	Inconspicuous	Prominent
Nucleoli (largest)	2.5 μm (rare)	3.0 μm
Nucleoli (mean)	<1.0 μm	1.8 μm
Nucleoli >1 μm	18%	77%
Basal cell layer		
Hematoxylin and eosin stain	Inconspicuous	Absent
Antikeratin stain (high molecular weight)	Fragmented	Virtually absent

usually retains an intact basal cell layer. The myoepithelial differentiation of sclerosing adenosis is distinctive. Both lesions arise chiefly in the transition zone and are usually incidental findings in TURP specimens with nodular hyperplasia.

Sclerosing adenosis can be distinguished from adenocarcinoma by: (1) a distinctive fibroblastic stroma that is rarely seen in carcinoma; (2) benign cytology, with epithelial cells and stromal cells that lack prominent nucleomegaly and nucleolomegaly usually seen in carcinoma; (3) hyalinized periacinar stroma, occasionally

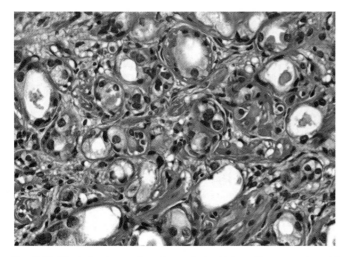

Fig. 8.64 Atypical adenomatous hyperplasia. Note uniform round nuclei without prominent nucleoli.

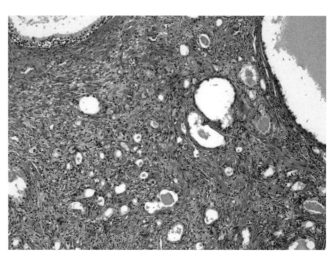

Fig. 8.67 Sclerosing adenosis with benign acini set in a cellular stroma.

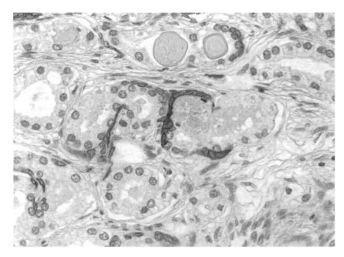

Fig. 8.65 Keratin 34βE12 immunoreactivity in the fragmented basal cell layer of atypical adenomatous hyperplasia.

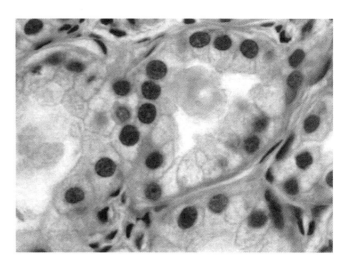

Fig. 8.68 Sclerosing adenosis. Note prominent periacinar basement membrane thickening.

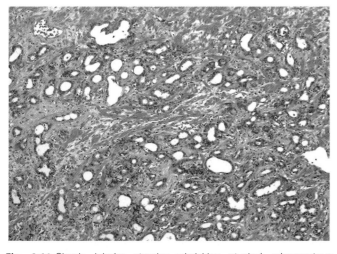

Fig. 8.66 Simple lobular atrophy mimicking atypical adenomatous hyperplasia.

seen in sclerosing adenosis; (4) intact basal cell layer; (5) frequent association with nodular hyperplasia; and (6) immunophenotype of S-100 protein and actin immunoreactivity.

Verumontanum Mucosal Gland Hyperplasia

The epithelial lining of the verumontanum may become abundant and proliferative, but criteria for separating normal and hyperplastic mucosa are not well defined.[483] This uncommon form of small acinar hyperplasia mimics low-grade carcinoma (Table 8.22).[483] It is invariably small, less than 1 mm, often multifocal, and limited anatomically to the verumontanum, utricle, ejaculatory ducts, and adjacent urethra and ducts.

The acini are small and closely packed, with an intact basal cell layer, small uniform nuclei, and inconspicuous nucleoli. The basal cells display immunoreactivity for keratin 34βE12 and are S-100 protein⁻. Although verumontanum mucosal gland hyperplasia and AAH appear histologically distinct and arise in different areas of the prostate, each is more likely to be found if the other is present.[484] This lesion is rare in biopsies and is usually not sampled by TURP because of the sparing of the verumontanum by this procedure.[484]

TABLE 8.21 | Typical and Atypical Sclerosing Adenosis Versus Adenocarcinoma

	Typical Sclerosing Adenosis	Atypical Sclerosing Adenosis	Adenocarcinoma
Architecture	Lobular small acinar proliferation; may form cell nests or clusters; prominent cellular stroma	Lobular small acinar proliferation; may occasionally have focally infiltrative margins	Small acinar proliferation infiltrating the stroma; may be lobular and circumscribed
Acini	Round and smooth; appear to merge with stroma because of pale staining	Round and smooth; may have compressed or abortive lumina	May be rounded and smooth
Basement membrane	Prominent thickening	Prominent thickening	Inconspicuous
Basal cell layer			
Light microscopy	Usually intact	Usually intact	Absent
Keratin 34βE12 reactivity	Intact or discontinuous	Intact or discontinuous	Absent
Stromal changes	Prominent myxoid cellular stroma	Prominent myxoid cellular stroma	With or without stromal sclerosis
Nuclei	May show mild enlargement	Prominent enlargement	Prominent enlargement
Nucleoli	Usually inconspicuous	Usually prominent	Usually prominent
Immunoreactivity			
S100 protein	Present (basal cells)	Present (basal cells)	Absent
Actin	Present (basal cells)	Present (basal cells)	Absent
DNA ploidy	Usually diploid	Usually aneuploid	Diploid or aneuploid

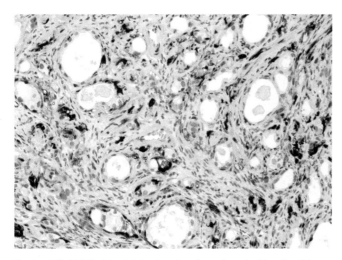

Fig. 8.69 S-100 Protein staining in sclerosing adenosis. Prominent immunoreactivity is evident in most basal cells.

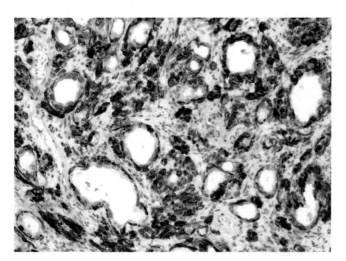

Fig. 8.70 Keratin 34βE12 stain in sclerosing adenosis. Intense cytoplasmic immunoreactivity is noted in most basal cells.

TABLE 8.22 | Verumontanum Mucosal Gland Hyperplasia Versus Adenocarcinoma

	Verumontanum Mucosal Gland Hyperplasia	Adenocarcinoma
Location	Verumontanum	Anywhere in prostate
Size	Small (<1 mm)	Any size
Architecture	Lobular small acinar proliferations; may be multifocal	May be lobular and circumscribed; usually multifocal
Basal cell layer		
Light microscopy	Usually intact; may be inconspicuous	Absent
High-molecular-weight keratin 34βE12 immunoreactivity	Usually intact	Absent
Stromal changes	With or without stromal sclerosis	With or without stromal sclerosis
Cytology		
Nuclei	Mild enlargement	Enlarged
Nucleoli	Usually inconspicuous	Usually prominent
Cytoplasm	Basophilic or clear on low power	Usually pale because of greater amount of cytoplasm
Basophilic mucin	Rare	May be present
Crystalloids	Rare	May be present

Hyperplasia of Mesonephric Remnants

Hyperplasia of mesonephric remnants in the prostate and periprostatic tissues is a rare and benign mimic of carcinoma that is usually identified in TURP specimens (Table 8.23).[18-21,485] It shares many features with mesonephric hyperplasia of the female genital tract, including apparent infiltration of the stroma and neural spaces, lobular arrangement of small acini or solid nests lined by a single cell layer, prominent nucleoli, and eosinophilic

TABLE 8.23 **Hyperplasia of Mesonephric Remnants Versus Adenocarcinoma**

	Hyperplasia of Mesonephric Remnants	Adenocarcinoma
Architecture	Lobular small acinar proliferation Two patterns: (1) small acini with colloid-like material; (2) small acini with empty lumina or solid nests	May be lobular and circumscribed
Acinar contours	May be rounded or smooth; may be atrophic or contain intraluminal micropapillary projections lined by cuboidal cells	May be rounded or smooth
Basal cell layer		
Light microscopy	Usually intact; may be inconspicuous	Absent
High-molecular-weight keratin 34βE12 immunoreactivity	Intact	Absent
Stromal changes	With or without stromal sclerosis	With or without stromal sclerosis
Cytology		
Nuclei	Mild enlargement	Enlarged
Nucleoli	Usually inconspicuous	Usually prominent
Cytoplasm	Basophilic or clear on low power	Usually pale because of greater amount of cytoplasm
Luminal contents	Often with colloid-like material	May have basophilic mucin
Immunoreactivity		
Prostate-specific antigen	No	Yes
Prostatic acid phosphatase	No	Yes

intratubular material. In one reported case, the lobular pattern was lost, and the acini were infiltrative. This process may account for the rare finding of ectopic prostatic tissue in the cervix and vagina.[486]

Two histopathologic patterns of mesonephric remnant hyperplasia are recognized, both with a lobular pattern and cuboidal cell lining. One pattern consists of small acini that contain colloid-like material reminiscent of thyroid follicles (Fig. 8.71), similar to thyroidization. The lining consists of a single layer of cuboidal cells without significant cytologic atypia. The second pattern consists of small acini or solid nests of cells with empty lumina, reminiscent of nephrogenic adenoma (Fig. 8.71). Acini may be atrophic or exhibit micropapillary projections lined by cuboidal cells. Prominent nucleoli are usually absent, but are present in rare cases, compounding the diagnostic confusion.

The diagnosis may be confirmed by immunoreactivity for keratin 34βE12 (Fig. 8.72) and lack of reactivity for PSA and PAP. One of the original cases was misdiagnosed as adenocarcinoma, resulting in unnecessary prostatectomy. In addition to cancer, mesonephric remnants should be distinguished from other benign small acinar proliferations. Differential diagnostic considerations include AAH, atrophy, PAH, basal cell hyperplasia, sclerosing adenosis, verumontanum mucosal gland hyperplasia, and atypical small acinar proliferation suspicious for but not diagnostic of malignancy.

Pseudoangiomatous Stromal Hyperplasia

We encountered a case of pseudoangiomatous hyperplasia in the biopsy of a 53-year-old man with serum PSA of 5.6 ng/mL, lower urinary tract obstructive symptoms, and a history of HIV infection treated with antiviral medications. The findings were identical to those observed in other organs, including the presence of open, slit-like, often anastomosing channels devoid of erythrocytes lined by discontinuous, often attenuated cells without atypia or mitotic activity set in a hyalinized collagenous stroma (Fig. 8.73).[487] The cells lining the sinusoidal spaces were positive for pancytokeratin, CD34, progesterone receptors, smooth muscle actin,

desmin, and vimentin but negative for PSA, factor VIII, CD31, HHV8, D2-40, synaptophysin, and chromogranin. The differential diagnosis includes angioma, angiosarcoma, Kaposi sarcoma, and leiomyoma variant. To our knowledge, pseudoangiomatous stromal hyperplasia has not been previously reported in the prostate.

Benign Nonneoplastic Conditions

Amyloidosis

Localized amyloidosis is present in 2% to 10% of prostates removed for hyperplasia or cancer, but is common in the seminal vesicles (senile seminal vesicle amyloidosis), observed at autopsy in 5% to 8% of men between 46 and 60 years old, 13% to 23% of men between 61 and 75 years old, and 21% to 34% of men older than 75 years.[488-493] It often extends bilaterally along the ejaculatory ducts to form linear or massive nodular subepithelial deposits of amorphous eosinophilic fibrillar material (Fig. 8.74). Basement membrane thickening is observed, and deposits may be seen within the vesicular lumina that occasionally cause significant narrowing. Investigation for systemic amyloidosis is not indicated.[494]

Special stains that confirm the diagnosis of amyloid include Congo red, which appears red by light microscopy with apple-green polarization birefringence; methylene blue, which reveals green polarization birefringence; crystal violet and toluidine blue, which impart a metachromatic appearance to the deposits; and PAS and sulfated Alcian blue stains, which are weakly to moderately positive. The composition of localized seminal vesicle and ejaculatory duct amyloid is histochemically unique (permanganate-sensitive, non-AA, non–β_2-microglobulin, nonprealbumin type), apparently derived from secretory protein of the epithelium; amyloid at other sites is derived from light chains or serum amyloid protein.[495]

Seminal vesicle amyloidosis may create false-positive Ga-PSMA uptake on computed tomography ERG scan.[496]

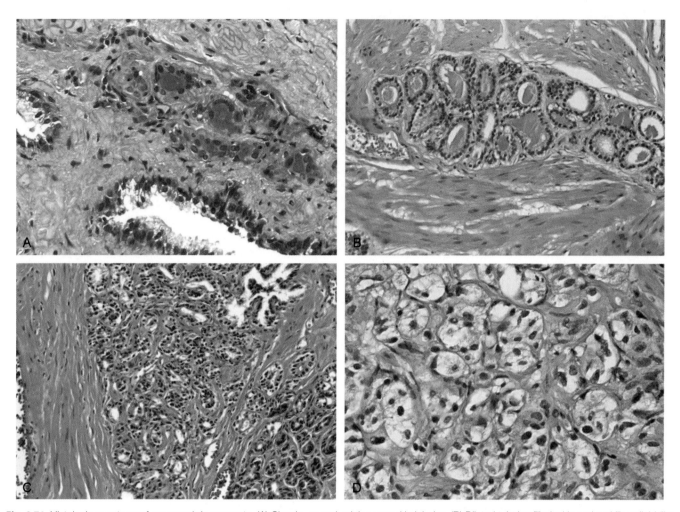

Fig. 8.71 Histologic spectrum of mesonephric remnants. (A) Closely spaced acini arranged in lobules. (B) Dilated tubules filled with eosinophilic colloid-like material. (C) Infiltrating growth pattern. (D) Small, closely spaced acini with clear cytoplasm.

Melanosis

The prostate contains two distinct types of pigment: the common melanin-like, lipofuscin-like pigment, present in benign prostate epithelium, high-grade PIN, and carcinoma; and melanin, which is rare and found only in melanocytic lesions such as melanosis, blue nevus, and malignant melanoma (see Chapter 9).[170,497-502]

Melanin-like, lipofuscin-like pigment is common in the prostatic epithelium in 89% of cases and in the stroma in 78% (Fig. 8.75).[90] It is widely distributed, including the transition zone (67%), central zone (56% to 100%), peripheral zone (89%), and periurethral glands (56%).[503] This pigment is most commonly seen in the basal portion of the secretory luminal cells, but is variable in location and amount. The reported incidence of melanin-like, lipofuscin-like prostatic pigment in the normal prostate varies from 4% to 70%.[504,505]

Pigment in the prostate has some resemblance to pigment in the seminal vesicular and ejaculatory ductal epithelium, particularly when it is present in abundance, and may cause diagnostic confusion in scant specimens such as TURP or biopsy, which may contain foci with cytologic atypia.[506] However, the pigment granules tend to be less coarse and refractile, and have a unique histochemical profile that allows them to be distinguished from seminal vesicular tissue: melanin-like (Fontana-Masson stain positive and potassium permanganate bleaching sensitive) and lipofuscin-like (prolonged Ziehl-Neelsen stain positive and S-100 protein negative), unlike pigment in seminal vesicle epithelium, which is not melanin-like (Fontana-Masson stain negative).

These findings suggest that this pigment is different from typical cutaneous melanin; the lipofuscin-like material ("wear and tear" or "old age" pigment) is probably an endogenous cellular by-product of prostate epithelium, rather than of melanocytic origin. Its only significance is to be aware of its distribution such that epithelium or stroma with pigment is not necessarily of seminal vesicle origin. Melanosis is rarely found in association with carcinoma, but when present is probably coincidental.[507]

Endometriosis

Endometriosis is a rare finding in the prostate, with fewer than a dozen cases reported, invariably after years of estrogen therapy for prostate cancer.[508,509] Patients present with hematuria and obstructive symptoms.

Treatment Changes

Treatment changes in the benign and cancerous prostate create diagnostic challenges in pathologic interpretation,

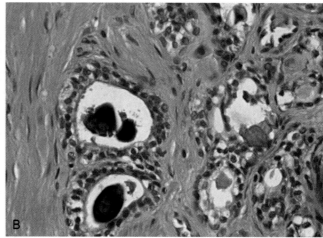

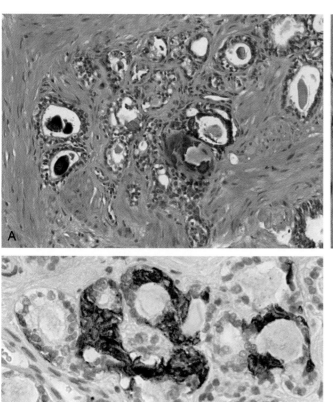

Fig. 8.72 Mesonephric remnants in transurethral resection. (A) Mesonephric remnants consist of a proliferation of closely spaced acini arranged in lobules or infiltrating between muscle bundles without stromal response. Some acini show dilated tubules filled with eosinophilic colloid-like material. (B) High-power field shows acini lined by a single layer of small- to medium-size cuboidal cells with scant amounts of eosinophilic or amphophilic cytoplasm. (C) Immunohistochemistry reveals strong positive staining for high-molecular-weight keratin (34βE12).

particularly in needle biopsy specimens. It is critical that the clinician provide the pertinent history of androgen deprivation or radiation therapy to assist the pathologist in rendering the correct diagnosis. This discussion summarizes therapy-related pathologic findings in the prostate, including those from several ablation methods.

Androgen Deprivation Therapy

One of the most popular forms of treatment for prostate cancer—androgen deprivation therapy—has been in use since the 1960s. Contemporary therapies have varying mechanisms of action, including combined androgen blockage (gonadotropin-releasing hormone agonists [e.g., goserelin and leuprolide] combined with androgen receptor antagonists [e.g., flutamide, bicalutamide, and nilutamide]), gonadotropin-releasing hormone antagonists (e.g., abarelix), and 5α-reductase inhibitors (e.g., finasteride and dutasteride). These agents are used for preoperative tumor shrinkage, symptomatic relief of metastases, cancer prophylaxis, and treatment of hyperplasia.[510-514] Current androgen deprivation therapy appears to induce an undesired expansion of the prostate cancer stem/progenitor cell population, an effect that may explain why this therapy eventually fails in patients.[515,516] Androgen deprivation also induces the transition from epithelium to mesenchyme in both normal prostate and cancer.[517] Microvessel density and expression of vascular endothelial growth factor are both significantly lower after 2 weeks of therapy.[518]

To achieve total androgen deprivation, therapy should be effective in eliminating both testicular and adrenal hormones. Typical side effects include hot flashes, loss of libido, and impotence. There are multiple methods to achieve androgen deprivation, and this form of therapy is commonly combined with radiation therapy for enhanced effect.[519,520]

The histopathologic effects of most agents are similar (Tables 8.24 and 8.25).[521-523] All modes of hormonal treatment alter the benign and cancerous prostatic epithelium and induce apoptosis characterized by fragmentation of tumor DNA, appearance of apoptotic bodies, and inhibition of cell growth. The altered epithelium displays involution and acinar atrophy, cytoplasmic clearing, nuclear and nucleolar shrinkage, and chromatin condensation, although changes with 5α-reductase inhibitors appear to be much less pronounced and variable than with other agents (discussed later).

After androgen deprivation therapy, benign and hyperplastic prostatic acini are atrophic and collapsed, typically with prominent basal cell hyperplasia and epithelial vacuolization. In some areas the lining epithelium has scant to moderate cytoplasm that is darkly eosinophilic and coarsely granular or clear. Most nuclei are small, with condensed chromatin and inconspicuous nucleoli (Fig. 8.76). Luminal secretions are inspissated, resembling corpora amylacea, but usually lack discrete laminations or angulations; multinucleated cells are infrequently present at the periphery. Squamous metaplasia is not significantly increased, but was prominent with estrogen treatment and orchiectomy. Lipofuscin pigment may

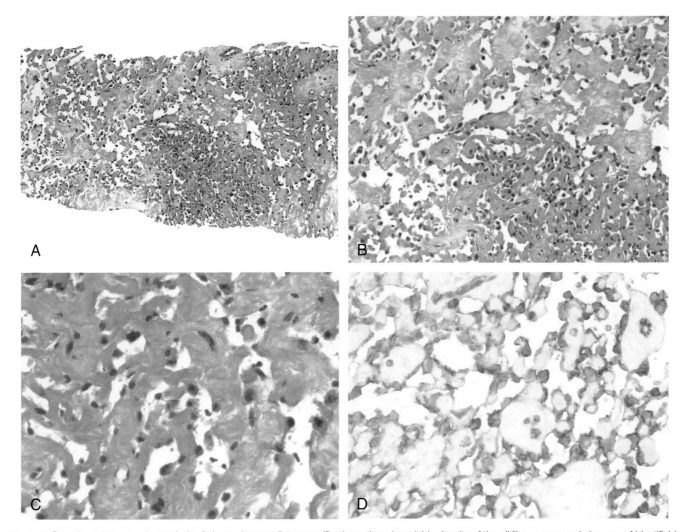

Fig. 8.73 Pseudoangiomatous hyperplasia. At low to intermediate magnifications, there is variable density of the slitlike spaces and absence of identifiable prostatic epithelium (A and B). (C) At high magnification, there is mild atypia of the cells lining the pointed elongate spaces. (D) CD34 immunoreactivity in virtually every neoplastic cell lining the slitlike spaces.

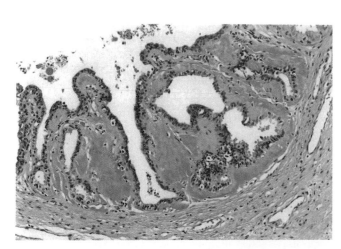

Fig. 8.74 Amyloidosis of the ejaculatory ducts.

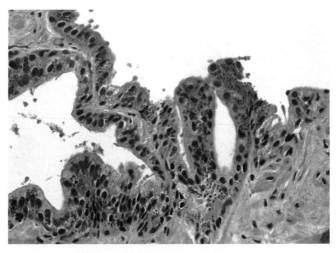

Fig. 8.75 Prostatic epithelial pigmentation. Note the granular pigment within the epithelium, reminiscent of that seen in the seminal vesicles.

TABLE 8.24 Androgen Deprivation: Comparison of Different Therapies

Therapy	Examples	Description
Orchiectomy		Eliminates androgen production by the testes but not by the adrenals
Estrogen	Diethylstilbestrol	Lowers luteinizing hormone concentration, with resulting depression of serum testosterone
Luteinizing hormone–releasing hormone agonist	Leuprolide; goserelin	Inhibits luteinizing hormone and follicle-stimulating hormone release, with resulting suppression of testosterone to castrate levels
Antiandrogen	Flutamide; bicalutamide; nilutamide; cyproterone acetate	Competitively binds to androgen receptors at the target cell level; blocks testicular and adrenal androgens
Combination	Leuprolide; flutamide	Orchiectomy or luteinizing hormone–releasing hormone agonist, plus antiandrogen
5α-Reductase inhibitor	Finasteride; dutasteride	Competitively and specifically inhibits 5α-reductase, with resulting suppression of serum and intraprostatic dihydrotestosterone concentration to castrate levels

TABLE 8.25 Androgen Deprivation Therapy: Histologic Features in the Prostate

Benign epithelium

Secretory cell layer
   Prominent acinar atrophy
   Decreased ratio of acini to stroma
   Enlargement and clearing of cytoplasm
   Prominent clear cell change
Basal cell layer
   Hyperplasia
   Prominent component of benign acini
   Squamous metaplasia
Stroma
   Edema in early stages; fibrosis in late stages
   Patchy condensation, resulting in focal hypercellularity
   Focal chronic inflammation (lymphohistiocytic)

High-grade prostatic intraepithelial neoplasia

Decrease in prevalence and extent
Nuclear shrinkage
Nuclear hyperchromasia
Nucleolar shrinkage
Other cytologic changes similar to benign secretory cell layer

Prostatic adenocarcinoma

Loss of glandular architecture
Nuclear shrinkage
Nuclear hyperchromasia and pyknosis
Nucleolar shrinkage
Mucinous degeneration
Other cytologic changes similar to benign secretory cell layer

There is some variability in these changes depending on the method of therapy.

be observed in scattered benign epithelial and stromal cells and, rarely, in tumor cells.

Histopathologic Findings After 5α-Reductase Inhibitors

The most potent nuclear androgen responsible for the maintenance of epithelial function is dihydrotestosterone (DHT).[524] By inhibiting DHT synthesis, 5α-reductase inhibitors decrease the androgen drive to hyperplastic and malignant cells while maintaining testosterone levels. Finasteride inhibits only the type 2 isoenzyme of 5α-reductase, thereby partly blocking conversion of testosterone. Unlike finasteride, dutasteride is a dual inhibitor of both 5α-reductase isoenzymes, resulting in the suppression of serum DHT by greater than 90%, compared with 70% seen

with finasteride.[525] Finasteride is somewhat less effective than other forms of androgen deprivation therapy in altering the histologic features of the benign and neoplastic prostate (Fig. 8.76), although changes have been described in all but one report.

Shrinkage of the benign prostate by 5α-reductase inhibitors has been documented in multiple preclinical and clinical studies.[523,526-528] Similarly, in the benign and hyperplastic prostate, finasteride reduces volume by 20% to 30%, with an increase in the stroma/epithelium ratio compared with untreated matched controls.[528] Ducts and acini are variable in size, and some ducts and acini retain a bistratified epithelium (Fig. 8.76). There is a 55% decline in epithelial content after 6 months of treatment that correlates with volume decrease.[529] By 24 months the epithelium involutes further, contracting from 19% to 6% of mean tissue composition (6 versus 2 cc overall mean epithelial volume; stroma/epithelium ratio from 3 to 17).[529] In another study, after 24 months of treatment the epithelial involution was similar in different zones.[528] The treated secretory cells display shrunken nuclei, condensed chromatin, inconspicuous nucleoli, and cytoplasmic clearing, and basal cells became prominent. Apoptotic bodies are occasionally present in the epithelial cells and lumina, but there are no mitotic figures. Conversely, one prospective study of needle biopsy specimens from patients who were treated for up to 4 years and matched untreated controls found no significant differences in benign epithelium.[530] These conflicting trends were noted in cancer and high-grade PIN.[514] Andriole et al. noted a reduction in epithelial cell size in the peripheral and transition zones after dutasteride treatment.[531] Epithelial androgen receptor, but not stromal androgen receptor, expression was significantly lower in patients treated with finasteride than in nontreated patients.[532] Epithelial androgen receptor expression was highly correlated with the level of atrophy.

The greater sensitivity of the peripheral zone to dutasteride may be attributed to its higher density of androgen receptors compared with the transition zone, as shown by saturation binding assays with a competitive inhibitor.[533] Nuclear androgen receptors were estimated to be present at twice the density and in 71% versus 39% of peripheral versus transition zone specimens, respectively.[453,534] These results are concordant with other studies of androgen deprivation, thus underscoring the limited repertoire of responses to androgen deprivation. Finasteride treatment in rats and dogs induces atrophy and involution, similar to humans, although the atrophy is often patchy and incomplete, a finding suggesting differential sensitivity within the gland.[526,527,535]

Prahalada et al. reported that long-term administration of finasteride resulted in a decrease in the weight of the rat prostate

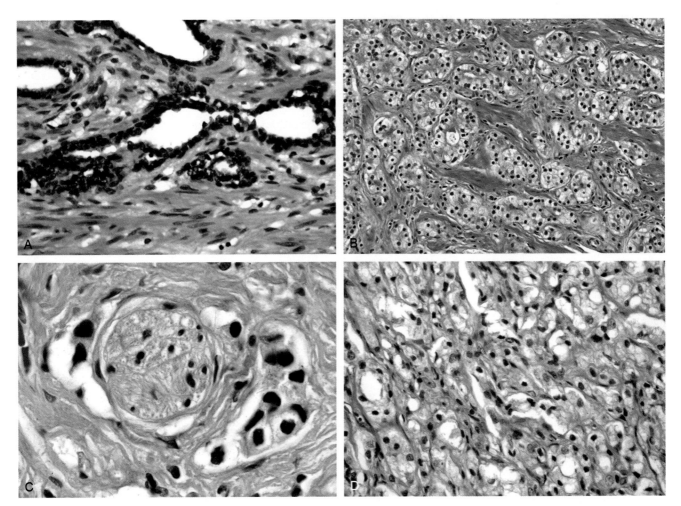

Fig. 8.76 Androgen deprivation therapy effect. (A) Benign prostatic epithelium retains the distinctive double cell layer, although the nuclei are shrunken and hyperchromatic (3 months of combined luteinizing hormone–releasing hormone agonist and antiandrogen). Finasteride-induced effects (B and C). Benign prostatic acini show mild atrophic changes (B). Compare with (D), in which the acinar basal cells are prominent and surmounted by a cuboidal to low columnar secretory cell layer.

compared with controls, and this finding correlated with a decrease in the total number of epithelial and stromal cells per acinus throughout the treated rat prostate, although these investigators found no qualitative differences in prostatic morphology between the control and finasteride-treated groups.[527] Microvessel density at the bladder neck (but not apex) was lower after 7 weeks of dutasteride treatment compared with untreated controls.[536]

Immunohistochemical Findings After Androgen Deprivation Therapy

PSA, PAP, and racemase are retained in benign and neoplastic cells after 3 months of therapy but decline with longer duration of therapy.[537] Keratin 34βE12 and p63 expression remain negative in cancer, regardless of duration, thereby indicating an absent basal cell layer. No differences are found in expression of neuroendocrine differentiation markers such as chromogranin, neuron-specific enolase, β-human chorionic gonadotropin, and serotonin.

Proliferating cell nuclear antigen immunoreactivity declines, suggesting that androgens regulate cyclically expressed proteins involved in cell proliferation.[538] Newer agents that target the androgen-signaling pathway, including abiraterone, increase survival in castration-resistant cancer after failure of taxane treatment.[539]

Radiation Therapy

The difficulty of biopsy interpretation after radiation is multifactorial and includes overlap of diagnostic findings in carcinoma and its many mimics, identification of small foci of carcinoma, and separation of treatment effects in normal tissue from recurrent or persistent carcinoma.

The degree of histologic change caused by radiation in benign, hyperplastic, and neoplastic tissues varies with the dose and duration of irradiation and the interval from therapy onset (Tables 8.26 and 8.27). Changes include acinar atrophy, distortion with loss of cytoplasm, and decreased ratio of acini to stroma (Fig. 8.77). Nuclear changes include nuclear enlargement (86% of cases) and prominent nucleoli (50%).[540] Acinar secretory cells are more sensitive to irradiation necrosis than are basal cells. Consequently,

TABLE 8.26	Histopathologic Findings in Benign Prostatic Tissue in Postirradiation Needle Biopsies at the Time of Prostate-Specific Antigen (Biochemical) Failure

Histopathologic Findings	% of Cases
Inflammation	39
Atrophy	79
Postatrophic hyperplasia	18
Acinar distortion	54
Decreased acinar-to-stromal ratio	86
Basal cell hyperplasia	68
Atypical basal cell hyperplasia	57
Hyperplastic (proliferative change)	11
Squamous metaplasia	0
Eosinophilic metaplasia	21
Stromal changes	
Stromal fibrosis	93
Stromal edema	21
Stromal calcification	21
Hemosiderin deposition	0
Atypical fibroblasts	25
Necrosis	0
Granulation tissue formation	0
Myointimal proliferation	11
Cytologic changes	
Nuclear pyknosis	75
Nuclear enlargement	86
Prominent nucleoli	50
Bizarre nuclei	54
Cytoplasmic vacuolization	29
Intraluminal contents	
Crystalloids	0
Mucin	4
Eosinophilic granular secretions	39
Corpora amylacea	32

atypical basal cell hyperplasia, often with an absent secretory cell layer, is seen in 57% of cases.[540] The stroma may be fibrotic, with paucicellular scarring, and vascular changes include intimal thickening and medial fibrosis (Tables 8.26 and 8.27). Pathologists must be aware of these changes that diminish the usual reliance on nuclear and nucleolar size to identify cancer.[541]

Changes after three-dimensional conformal therapy and other forms of radiation therapy are similar to those after conventional external beam therapy.[542,543] The addition of androgen deprivation therapy has no apparent histopathologic effect on the radiation-altered prostate, although the positive impact on survival with prostate cancer has been repeatedly confirmed.[519,542,543]

Epithelial regeneration combined with suboptimal DNA damage checkpoint responses to ionizing radiation may contribute to the high frequency of genetic lesions in the prostatic epithelium compared with the seminal vesicular epithelium.[544] Secretory luminal cells lack the prominent γH2AX DNA repair response after irradiation compared with basal cells.[545]

Immunohistochemical Findings After Radiation Therapy
PSA, P501S, and NKX3.1 are positive, respectively, in 93%, 97%, and 83% of cases of benign prostate after radiation

therapy; uroplakin 2 is invariably negative. An important diagnostic pitfall is the presence of GATA3 immunoreactivity in 100% of irradiated benign prostatic epithelium that, in combination with altered morphologic features, may be mistaken for urothelial carcinoma.[215,546]

Cryotherapy (Cryoablation)

Cryosurgical ablation refers to freezing of the prostate. Multiple cryoprobe needles filled with circulating liquid nitrogen transform the prostate into an ice ball, resulting in substantial tissue destruction and death of benign and malignant cells. The flow of liquid nitrogen through the probes is adjusted to create the desired freezing pattern and extent of tissue destruction in the prostate; no liquid nitrogen comes in contact with the tissue.

After cryosurgery the prostate shows typical features of repair, including marked stromal fibrosis and hyalinization, basal cell hyperplasia with ductal and acinar regeneration, squamous metaplasia, urothelial metaplasia, stromal hemorrhage, and hemosiderin deposition (Fig. 8.78).[541,547] Coagulative necrosis is present between 6 and 30 weeks of therapy, but patchy chronic inflammation is more common after that (Fig. 8.78). Focal granulomatous inflammation is associated with epithelial disruption resulting from corpora amylacea. Dystrophic calcification is infrequent and usually appears in areas with the greatest reparative response.

In some cases the benign prostate appears unchanged, with no definite evidence of tissue or immune response, a finding indicating lack of inclusion of that area in the ablation killing zone. As the postoperative interval increases, biopsy is more likely to contain unaltered benign prostatic tissue.

Cryotherapy is one of multiple ablation methods that vary by mechanism of tissue destruction (chemical, thermal, electrical), rapidity of cell death (apoptosis: slow, 1 to 3 days; necrosis: immediate), effect on native proteins (intact or denatured), differential sparing of adjacent structures such as blood vessels and nerves (intact or ablated), and likely impact on the immune system and abscopal effect (nonstimulatory or stimulatory) (Table 8.28).

Hyperthermia

All forms of hyperthermia (e.g., high-intensity focused ultrasound, microwave thermotherapy, laser therapy, and hot water balloon thermotherapy) result in sharply circumscribed hemorrhagic coagulative necrosis that soon organizes with granulation tissue (Table 8.28). The pattern and extent of injury are determined by the method of thermocoagulation used, the duration of treatment, tissue perfusion factors, and the ratio of epithelium to stroma in the tissue being treated.[541,548-553] Transurethral methods may be safer and more effective than transrectal methods because they appear to avoid injury to the rectal mucosa. When delivered transurethrally, laser thermocoagulation and microwave hyperthermia treatments do not usually involve the peripheral zone or neighboring structures, presumably because of differences in tissue perfusion.[554] Coagulative necrosis is greater in areas of predominantly epithelial nodular hyperplasia than of predominantly stromal hyperplasia and the dense fibromuscular tissue of the bladder neck. Confluent coagulative necrosis occurs when multiple laser lesions are created in a single transverse plane. Correlation with histopathologic

	Androgen Deprivation Therapy	Radiation	Cryoablation	Hyperthermia
Light microscopic findings				
Benign prostatic tissue				
Acini and stroma	Atrophic, collapsed, inspissated luminal secretions	Atrophic, decreased acini-to-stroma ratio	Features of repair: acinar regeneration, stromal hemorrhage and fibrosis, hyalinization; coagulative necrosis for as long as 30 wk, followed by chronic inflammation, untreated areas unaffected	Sharply circumscribed hemorrhagic, followed by granulation tissue
Secretory cells	Small nuclei, condensed chromatin, inconspicuous nucleoli, scant to moderate vacuolated, granular, or clear eosinophilic cytoplasm	Loss of cytoplasm, cell death	Absent in areas of complete effect, normal away from areas of treatment	Absent in areas of complete effect, normal away from areas of treatment
Basal cells	Hyperplastic, cytoplasmic vacuolation	Proliferation, nuclear and nucleolar enlargement	Hyperplasia at edges of damage, normal away from areas of treatment	Hyperplasia at edges of damage, normal away from areas of treatment
PIN	Regression with decreased acini-to-stroma ratio	Features preserved, sometimes with cytoplasmic vacuolation or sloughing of epithelium into the lumen	Absent in areas of complete effect	Absent in areas of complete effect
Adenocarcinoma	Conversion to higher Gleason score, neoplastic cells with abundant clear vacuolated cytoplasm, shrunken hyperchromatic nuclei, "nucleolus poor"	Features diagnostic of persistent carcinoma are architectural: infiltrative growth, perineural invasion, intraluminal crystalloids, blue mucin secretions, absence of corpora amylacea, presence of concomitant PIN	Absent in areas of complete effect	Absent in areas of complete effect
Immunohistochemical findings				
Prostate-specific antigen	+ in tumor cells after 3 months but declines later	+ in tumor cells, regardless of duration	Unaffected	Unaffected
Prostatic acid phosphatase	+ in tumor cells after 3 months but declines later	+ in tumor cells, regardless of duration	Unaffected	Unaffected
Cytokeratin 34βE12	− in tumor cells, regardless of duration	− in tumor cells, regardless of duration	Unaffected	Unaffected
p63	− in tumor cells, regardless of duration	− in tumor cells, regardless of duration	Unaffected	Unaffected
Racemase	+ in tumor cells after 3 months but declines later	+ in tumor cells, regardless of duration	Unaffected	Unaffected
c-Myc	+ in tumor cell nuclei, regardless of duration	+ in tumor cell nuclei, regardless of duration	Unaffected	Unaffected

PIN, Prostatic intraepithelial neoplasia.

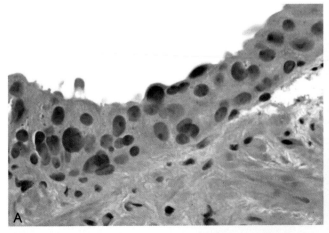
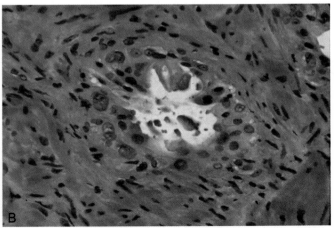

Fig. 8.77 Radiation changes. (A) Prostatic epithelium mimicking high-grade prostatic intraepithelial neoplasia. Marked nuclear abnormalities include variation in size and shape and hyperchromasia. (B) Prostatic epithelium shows nuclear abnormalities involving the basal cell and secretory cell layers.

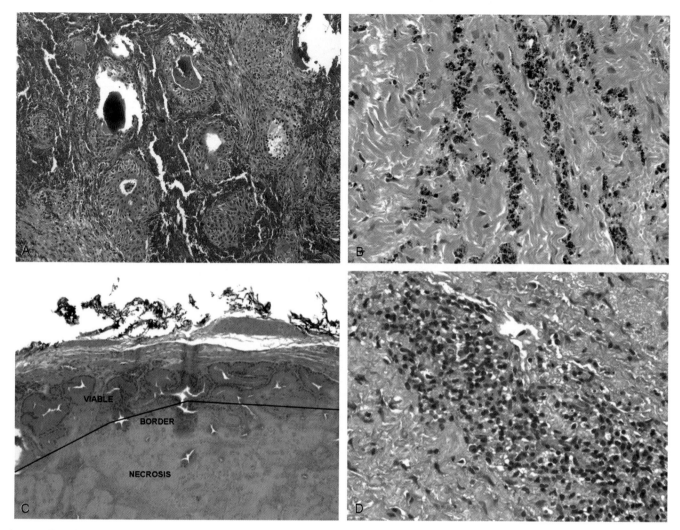

Fig. 8.78 Cryoablation effects. (A) Stromal hemorrhage with residual viable epithelium after prostatic cryoablation (human). (B) Hemosiderin deposition (ochre pigment) within the stoma after cryosurgery (human). (C) Coagulative necrosis (bottom of image) with devitalization and a thin rim of subcapsular viable tissue (*top*) after cryosurgery (dog prostate). (D) Patchy chronic inflammation within prostatic stroma is a common finding after cryoablation (human).

findings showed gadolinium-enhanced MRI to be useful for determining the location, pattern, and extent of necrosis caused within the prostate by minimally invasive techniques.[551]

Laser Therapy

Vascular-targeted photodynamic therapy is focal therapy for low-risk prostate cancer as an alternative to active surveillance that uses a low-energy laser treatment combined with soluble photosensitizer (Table 8.28).[555] After 6 months, benign tissue exposed to vascular-targeted photodynamic consists of sharply demarcated hyaline fibrotic scars punctuated by rare atrophic glands or isolated corpora amylacea rimmed by multinucleated macrophages. Mild chronic inflammation, hemosiderin, and coagulative necrosis are also observed. When present, residual cancer is never mixed with scar and has no therapy-related changes.

Irreversible Electroporation

Irreversible electroporation is a novel minimally invasive nonthermal therapy for prostate cancer using short electric pulses to ablate prostate tissue by apoptosis (Table 8.28). After 4 weeks, treated benign tissue is sharply demarcated, completely ablated, and consists only of necrotic and fibrotic tissue without viable cells.[556]

Electrical Membrane Breakdown

Electrical membrane breakdown is a novel form of nonthermal tissue ablation that induces immediate electrical pulse dose–related coagulative necrosis and nuclear pyknosis (Table 8.28).[557] Unlike cryosurgery and most other forms of tissue ablation (exception, irreversible electroporation), radiofrequency electrical membrane breakdown preserves blood vessels and nerves.

References are available at expertconsult.com

TABLE 8.28	Comparison of Common Prostatic Tissue Ablation Methods[557]		
Method	**Mechanism**	**Description**	**Expected Abscopal Effect**
Thermal			
Microwave	Heat and mechanical	Creates coagulation necrosis with friction and heat	Little or no effect because of denaturation of proteins
High-intensity focused ultrasound	Heat	Creates necrosis by focusing energy into a small area creating heat	Little or no effect because of denaturation of proteins
Laser, including vascular-targeted photodynamic	Heat	Creates necrosis with light energy	Little or no effect because of denaturation of proteins
RF thermal	Heat and mechanical	Creates cellular desiccation and protein coagulation	Little or no effect because of denaturation of proteins; marked effect in animal model when combined with immunotherapy
Steam	Heat	Creates coagulation necrosis with heat	Little or no effect because of denaturation of proteins
Cryosurgery	Cold	Creates necrosis by dehydration and ice formation	Mild to moderate effect, diminished by low temperatures or lengthy freeze; not reproducible
Nonthermal			
Alcohol, hypertonic saline, acetic acid injections	Chemical	Creates coagulative necrosis via dehydration and protein coagulation	Little or no effect because of denaturation of proteins
Photodynamic	Chemical	Creates cell damage by producing reactive oxygen species and destroying vasculature	Little or no effect in isolation; marked effect in animal model when combined with immunotherapy
Irreversible electroporation and nonthermal irreversible electroporation	Electrical	Creates apoptosis with preservation of vessels; delayed necrosis	Little or no effect because of lack of antigen release by apoptosis
Electrical membrane breakdown	Electrical	Creates necrosis with preservation of vessels	Theoretical effect because of enhanced antigen presentation and lack of denaturation of proteins

All ablation mechanisms locally and systemically stimulate components of the immune system. Expected effects are classified as mild, moderate, or marked according to comparative literature review and theoretical variables, focusing on the potential ability to vigorously and reproducibly stimulate the immune system to potentially induce an abscopal effect.

Modified from Onik GM, Bostwick DG, Miessau JA, Webb Z, Friedman MB. Electrical membrane breakdown (EMB): preliminary findings of a new method of non-thermal tissue ablation. *J Clin Exp Pathol* 2017;7:1-7.

9

Neoplasms of the Prostate

DAVID G. BOSTWICK AND LIANG CHENG

CHAPTER OUTLINE

Benign Epithelial Tumors and Tumor-like Proliferations

Prostatic Cysts

Giant multilocular prostatic cystadenoma is a large tumor composed of acini and cysts lined by prostatic-type epithelium set in a hypocellular fibrous stroma.[1-10] This rare tumor arises in men between 28 and 80 years old as a large midline prostatic or extraprostatic mass causing urinary obstruction. The epithelial lining displays prostate-specific antigen (PSA) immunoreactivity. One case was associated with high-grade prostatic intraepithelial neoplasia (PIN).[11] Surgical excision is usually curative, although it may recur if incompletely excised. The differential diagnosis includes phyllodes tumor, multilocular peritoneal inclusion cyst, multicystic mesothelioma, müllerian duct cyst, seminal vesicle cyst, lymphangioma, and hemangiopericytoma. The light microscopic appearance of the cyst lining is useful in separating these lesions (Table 9.1). One reported case was successfully treated laparoscopically.[12]

Other benign unilocular cysts that may be sampled by biopsy include seminal vesicle cyst, ejaculatory duct cyst, and müllerian duct cyst.[13-16] Location is often useful, recognizing that seminal

TABLE 9.1	Prostatic Cysts: Differential Diagnosis		
Type of Cyst	Location	Size	Contain Sperm
Prostatic cyst	Lateral	Variable	No
Seminal vesicle cyst	Lateral	Large	Yes
Diverticulum of ejaculatory duct or ampulla	Lateral	Variable	Yes
Müllerian duct cyst	Midline	Large	No

TABLE 9.2	Diagnostic Criteria for Prostatic Intraepithelial Neoplasia	
	Low-Grade PIN (Formerly PIN 1)	High-Grade PIN (Formerly PIN 2 and 3)
Acinar size	Normal; not enlarged	Normal; not enlarged
Architecture	Epithelial cells crowding and stratification, with irregular spacing	Similar to low-grade PIN; more crowding and stratification; four main patterns: tufting, micropapillary, cribriform, and flat
Cytology		
Nuclei	Enlarged, with marked size variation	Enlarged; some size and shape variation
Chromatin	Normal	Increased density and clumping
Nucleoli	Rarely prominent[a]	Prominent
Basal cell layer	Intact	May show some disruption
Basement membrane	Intact	Intact

PIN, Prostatic intraepithelial neoplasia.
[a]Fewer than 10% of cells have prominent nucleoli.

vesicle cyst is typically lateral, whereas müllerian duct cyst is midline. Seminal vesicle cyst may contain ectopic prostatic acini and urothelium.[17,18] Echinococcal cyst is usually associated with prominent inflammation, and organisms are often demonstrable.[19]

Ejaculatory Duct Adenofibroma

A case of benign adenofibroma of the ejaculatory duct has been reported.[20] This incidental autopsy finding consisted of a small polypoid mass of epithelium and stroma that projected into a cystically dilated duct. Adenomatoid tumor of the ejaculatory duct has also been described.[21]

Prostatic Intraepithelial Neoplasia

PIN refers to the preinvasive end of the continuum of cellular proliferations within the lining of prostatic ducts, ductules, and acini.[22] High-grade PIN is the earliest identifiable stage in carcinogenesis, possessing most of the phenotypic, biochemical, and genetic changes of cancer without invasion into the fibromuscular stroma.[23-25] The World Health Organization (WHO) contends that PIN is the only preinvasive lesion for prostate cancer. Other potential but unproven candidates for premalignancy in the prostate include atypical adenomatous hyperplasia (see Chapter 8), malignancy-associated changes arising in normal-appearing epithelium, and atrophy (see Chapter 8).[26-28]

Initial references to the lesion we now know as PIN were apparently made by early authors such as Kastendieck and Helpap, but they did not provide reproducible criteria and distinguish their findings from mimics of PIN.[29] McNeal emphasized the possible premalignant nature of proliferative changes in the prostatic epithelium, but his description included a variety of findings.[38] More than 21 years later, McNeal and Bostwick described reproducible diagnostic criteria for "intraductal dysplasia" and introduced a three-grade classification system.[30] The following year, Bostwick and Brawer proposed using PIN as a replacement for intraductal dysplasia, and this new term was promulgated in 1989 at a consensus workshop on prostate preneoplastic lesions sponsored by the American Cancer Society and National Cancer Institute.[31,32]

The diagnostic term *prostatic intraepithelial neoplasia* was subsequently endorsed at numerous multidisciplinary and pathology-only consensus meetings.[25,33-38] Terms such as *intraductal dysplasia*, *severe dysplasia*, *large acinar atypical hyperplasia*, and *duct-acinar dysplasia* were discouraged and have ceased to be used in routine practice.[39,40] The term *intraductal carcinoma* (IDC) was discouraged many years ago but has seen a resurgence recently as a separate entity that may be mistaken for PIN (see later).

The 1989 conference also recommended compression of the PIN classification into two grades: low-grade (formerly PIN grade 1) or high-grade PIN (formerly PIN grades 2 and 3) (Table 9.2).[32] The clinical significance of high-grade PIN was considered substantial at that time, whereas low-grade PIN was considered largely inconsequential, a belief that has been reinforced in subsequent decades and persists today.

Interobserver agreement between pathologists for high-grade PIN is "good to excellent," with 67% overall agreement between pairs of reviewers.[40-43] However, this is not true for low-grade PIN; also, it has a much lower predictive value for cancer that limits its clinical utility, and most do not routinely report this finding today except in research studies.[38,44-50] Thus, the term *prostatic intraepithelial neoplasia* is now used interchangeably with high-grade PIN by most investigators. High-grade PIN is considered a standard diagnosis that must be included as part of the reported pathologic evaluation of biopsies, transurethral resections (TURPs), and prostatectomy specimens.[38] The diagnostic utility when cancer is already present is uncertain, but 69% of urologic pathologists report PIN in this setting.[38]

Epidemiology of Prostatic Intraepithelial Neoplasia

The mean incidence rate of isolated high-grade PIN is 9% (range, 4% to 25%) of prostate biopsies. Given that there are an estimated 1,300,000 prostate biopsies performed annually, a reasonable estimate is that there are about 115,000 new cases annually of high-grade PIN without cancer and a prevalence of more than 16 million (Table 9.3).[51,52] The prevalence of PIN varies according to the population of men under study, with the lowest likelihood in those participating in PSA screening and early detection studies, with an incidence rate of PIN ranging from 0.7% to 20%.[53,54]

The relationship between the number of cores sampled and the incidence of PIN on needle biopsy is controversial, although most agree that greater sampling increases the yield of both PIN and

TABLE 9.3	Estimated Prevalence of High-Grade Prostatic Intraepithelial Neoplasia and Atypical Small Acinar Proliferation in the United States			
Age (y)	High-Grade % PIN	U.S. Population (Thousands)	PIN	ASAP[a,b]
40-49	15.2	20,550	3,123,600	822,000
50-59	24.0	14,187	3,404,880	567,480
60-69	47.3	9,312	4,404,576	372,480
70-79	58.4	6,926	4,044,784	177,040
80-89	70.0	2,664	1,864,800	106,560
	Total	**53,639,000**	**16,842,640**	**2,145,560**

ASAP, Atypical small acinar proliferation; *PIN*, prostatic intraepithelial neoplasia.

[a]The estimated value of 4% is used throughout as the prevalence of ASAP has not been determined as a function of age.

[b]It should be noted that ASAP is not a diagnostic entity but rather a diagnostic category; thus the "prevalence" shown in this table represents the theoretical detection level for this histologic finding given current methods of detection if the entire population underwent biopsy.

cancer. The incidence rate of PIN on 24-core saturation biopsy was 22% to 45%.[55,56]

Those undergoing TURP have the highest likelihood of PIN, varying from 2.8% to 33%.[44,57-59] In such cases, all tissue should be examined, but serial sections of suspicious foci are usually not necessary. Unfortunately, needle biopsies fail to show the suspicious focus on deeper levels in about one-half of cases, often precluding assessment by immunohistochemistry and compounding the diagnostic dilemma.

The prevalence and extent of PIN increase with patient age (Table 9.3).[60] An autopsy study of whole-mount prostates from older men showed that the prevalence of PIN in prostates with cancer increased with age, predating the onset of carcinoma by more than 5 years.[34,61,62] A similar study revealed that PIN is first seen in men in their twenties and thirties (9% and 22% frequency, respectively), and preceded the onset of carcinoma by more than 10 years.[61] Most foci of PIN in young men were low grade, with increasing frequency and volume of high-grade PIN with advancing age.[63]

Race and geographic location also appear to influence the incidence of PIN after controlling for patient age.[25,63] African American men have a greater prevalence of PIN than Caucasians in the 50- to 60-year-old age group, the decade preceding detection of most prostate cancers.[34,64] African American men also had the highest incidence of cancer (about 50% more than Caucasians).[34,65-67] In contrast, Japanese men living in Japan had a lower incidence of PIN than those residing in the United States, and Asians had the lowest clinically detected rate of prostate cancer.[68,69] Interestingly, Japanese men diagnosed with PIN also had an increased likelihood of development of prostate cancer, indicating that PIN is a precursor of clinical prostate cancer in Asian men.[70] Differences in the frequency of PIN in the 50- to 60-year-old age group across races essentially mirror the rates of clinical prostate cancer observed in the 60- to 70-year-old age group.[68,71]

The likely causal association of PIN with adenocarcinoma is supported by the observation that the prevalence of both increase with patient age, and that PIN precedes the onset of prostate cancer by less than one decade (Table 9.4).[61,65,71,72] The severity and frequency of PIN in prostates with cancer are greatly increased when compared with prostates without cancer (73% versus 32% frequency, respectively).[60,73,74] High-grade PIN in sextant biopsy carries a 50% risk for carcinoma on subsequent biopsy within 3 years, although this risk was lower when more than six cores are obtained; this decline in predictive value is expected given the increased sampling for cancer with a greater number of core biopsies (see later).[75]

Diagnosis of Prostatic Intraepithelial Neoplasia

PIN is characterized by cellular proliferation within preexisting ducts and acini, with cytologic changes mimicking cancer, including nuclear and nucleolar enlargement (Figs. 9.1 to 9.3).[23,76] There is inversion of the normal orientation of epithelial proliferation from the basal cell compartment to the luminal surface, similar to adenoma in the colon.[77,78] The requisite nucleolar enlargement must be present in at least 10% of cells within the focus to be considered diagnostic; however, overstaining, hyperchromasia, and nuclear overlap may obscure the nucleolar features. Overexpression of the *MYC* oncogene is responsible for increased nucleolar number and size in PIN and cancer.[79]

There are four main patterns of high-grade PIN: tufting, micropapillary, cribriform, and flat (Figs. 9.1 to 9.3).[80] The tufting pattern is the most common, present in 97% of cases, although most cases have multiple patterns. There are no known clinically important differences between the architectural patterns, and their recognition appears to be only of diagnostic utility. Sporadic retrospective reports have suggested that the cribriform or micropapillary patterns may indicate higher risk for coexistent cancer, but this has been refuted. Other unusual patterns of PIN include the signet ring cell pattern, small cell pattern, mucinous pattern, microvacuolated (foamy-gland) pattern, inverted (hobnail) pattern, and PIN with squamous differentiation (Fig. 9.4; Table 9.5).[81-83] The small cell pattern is usually negative for neuroendocrine markers and does not appear to be a precursor of small cell carcinoma.[84] The hobnail pattern usually coexists with Gleason score 7 cancer.[85]

The presence of extensive PIN appears to be more predictive of cancer than the more common isolated single acinus with PIN (see later).[86-88] The presence of intraluminal crystalloids in combination with PIN is a more compelling indication for repeat biopsy than PIN alone.[89]

PIN spreads through prostatic ducts in multiple different patterns, similar to carcinoma. In the first pattern, neoplastic cells replace the normal luminal secretory epithelium, with preservation of the basal cell layer and basement membrane. This pattern often has a cribriform or near-solid appearance. Foci of high-grade PIN may be difficult to distinguish from intraductal/intraacinar spread of carcinoma by routine light microscopy (see later).[90] In the second pattern, there is direct invasion through the ductal or acinar wall, with disruption of the basal cell layer. In the third pattern, neoplastic cells invaginate between the basal cell layer and columnar secretory cell layer ("pagetoid spread"), a rare finding. Proliferative activity according to Ki67 labeling is lower in PIN (mean, 6%; range, 2% to 15%) than in ductal adenocarcinoma; the combination of histologic features and measurements of cellular proliferation help to distinguish these findings in limited tissue samples.[91,92]

Ultrastructurally, high-grade PIN displays features between those of benign epithelium and adenocarcinoma.[93] These include the presence of cells with a variable number of cytoplasmic

TABLE 9.4	**Evidence for the Association of Prostatic Intraepithelial Neoplasia and Cancer**

Histology

They have similar architectural and cytologic features.

Location

Both are located chiefly in the peripheral zone and are multicentric. There is a close spatial association of PIN and cancer.

Correlation with cell proliferation and death (apoptosis)

Growth fraction of PIN is similar to cancer.
Apoptosis-suppressing oncoprotein Bcl-2 expression is increased in PIN and cancer.

Loss of basal cell layer

The highest grade of PIN has loss of basal cell layer, similar to cancer.

Increased frequency of PIN in the presence of cancer

Increased extent of PIN in the presence of cancer

Increased severity of PIN in the presence of cancer

Immunophenotype

PIN is more closely related to cancer than benign epithelium.
For some biomarkers there is progressive loss of expression with increasing grades of PIN and cancer, including prostate-specific antigen, neuroendocrine cells, cytoskeletal proteins, and secretory proteins.
For some biomarkers there is progressive increase in expression with increasing grades of PIN and cancer including type IV collagenase,

transforming growth factor-α, epidermal growth factor, epidermal growth factor receptor, Lewis Y antigen, and *c-erB-2* oncogene.

Morphometry

High-grade PIN and cancer have similar nuclear area, chromatin content and distribution, nuclear perimeter, nuclear diameter, and nuclear roundness.
High-grade PIN and cancer have similar nucleolar number, size, and location.

DNA content

High-grade PIN and cancer have similar frequency of aneuploidy.

Genetic instability

High-grade PIN and cancer have similar frequency of allelic loss.
High-grade PIN and cancer have similar foci of allelic loss.

Microvessel density

There is progressive increase in microvessel density from PIN to cancer.

Origin

Cancer is found to arise in the foci of PIN.

Age

Age incidence peak of PIN precedes cancer.

Predictive value of high-grade PIN

PIN on biopsy has high predictive value for cancer on subsequent biopsy.

PIN, Prostatic intraepithelial neoplasia.

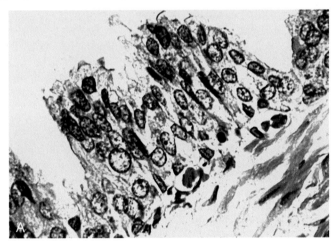 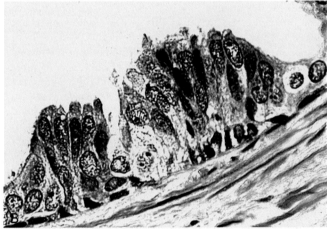

Fig. 9.1 Prostatic intraepithelial neoplasia. (A) Low grade. (B) High grade.

secretory vacuoles, luminal apocrine blebs, large nuclei with coarsely clumped chromatin, enlarged nucleoli, prominent apical microvilli, intact or discontinuous basal cell layer, and intact basement membrane. Occasional acini have luminal cells abutting the basement membrane without interposition of basal cells, and other acini with extremely attenuated basal cell cytoplasmic processes contain bundles of intermediate filaments.

Early stromal invasion, the earliest evidence of carcinoma, occurs at sites of acinar outpouching and basal cell disruption in acini with high-grade PIN (Figs. 9.5 and 9.6). Such microinvasion is present in about 2% of high-power microscopic fields of PIN and is seen with equal frequency in all architectural patterns.[36,80] At the transition from histologically normal epithelium to PIN, there is a

surge in phosphorylated Akt (prosurvival protein) and concomitant suppression of downstream apoptosis pathways (antisurvival proteins) that precedes the transition to invasive cancer.[94]

The mean volume of PIN in prostates with cancer is 1.2 to 1.3 mL, and the volume increases with increasing pathologic stage, Gleason grade, positive surgical margins, and perineural invasion (PNI).[60,95] These findings underscore the close spatial and biologic relationship of PIN and cancer, and may result from an increase in PIN with increasing cancer volume.

PIN and cancer are usually multicentric.[24,60,80,87] PIN is multicentric in 72% of radical prostatectomies with cancer, including 63% of those involving the nontransition zone and 7% of those involving the transition zone; 2% of cases have concomitant single

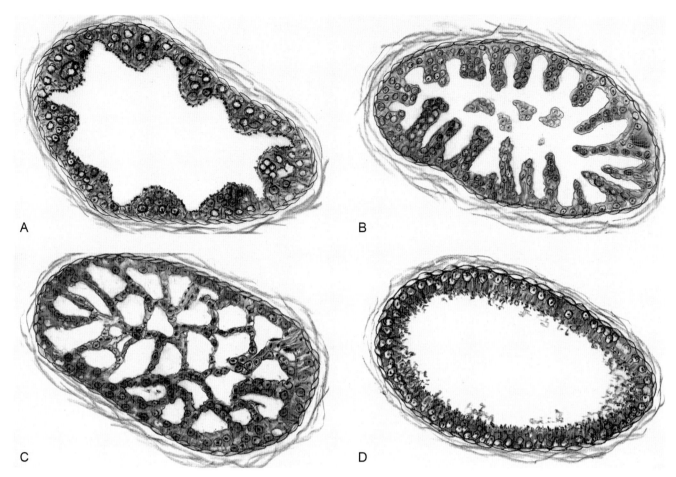

Fig. 9.2 Architectural patterns of high-grade prostatic intraepithelial neoplasia. (A) Tufting pattern. (B) Micropapillary pattern. (C) Cribriform pattern. (D) Flat pattern. (From Bostwick DG, Amin MB, Dundore P, et al. Architectural patterns of high grade prostatic intraepithelial neoplasia, Hum Pathol 1993;24:298–310, with permission.)

foci in all zones.[60] The peripheral zone of the prostate, the area in which the majority of cases of prostate cancer occur (≥70%), is also the most common location for PIN.[60,61,71,80,96] Cancer and PIN are frequently multicentric in the peripheral zone, indicating a "field" effect similar to urothelial carcinoma of the bladder. Central zone cancer is more likely to be associated with PIN in the central zone than the peripheral zone.[97] Despite common multifocality, PIN may be a monoclonal process according to similar high-resolution genomewide signatures.

High-grade PIN and prostate cancer are morphometrically and phenotypically similar (Fig. 9.7). PIN occurs primarily in the peripheral zone and is seen in areas that are in continuity with prostate cancer.[25,35,60,96,98-100] PIN and prostate cancer are multifocal and heterogeneous.[60,101,102] Increasing rates of aneuploidy and angiogenesis as the grade of PIN progresses are further evidence that high-grade PIN is precancerous.[99,103-105] Prostate cancer and high-grade PIN have similar proliferative and apoptotic indices.[68,106-109]

Swedish investigators claim that PIN cannot be diagnosed by fine needle aspiration (FNA) alone, although this has been refuted.[110,111] PIN in combination with atypical small acinar proliferation (ASAP) suspicious for but not diagnostic of malignancy is discussed later.

Biopsy remains the definitive method for detecting PIN and early invasive cancer. Serum PSA is not significantly elevated, if at all, and PIN cannot be detected by imaging methods such as ultrasound, magnetic resonance imaging (MRI), or positron emission tomography/computerized tomography (PET/CT) scans.[112-119] There is a poor correlation of PIN and PSA density.[114] Mean PSA increased from 8 to 12 ng/mL in patients with PIN who experienced development of cancer within 2 years; those with PIN who did not have cancer during this interval had an increase in PSA from 5 to 6 ng/mL. Median PSA velocity is greater in men with PIN who were subsequently diagnosed with cancer.[120] A velocity threshold of 0.75 ng/mL/year predicts which men with PIN experience development of cancer, and velocity was the only significant predictor of subsequent cancer detection on multivariate analysis.[120] The ratio of free to total PSA is the same for patients with high-grade PIN and cancer.[112,115,121,122]

Immunohistochemical Markers for Prostatic Intraepithelial Carcinoma

We routinely use a series of four immunostains that, in combination, are invaluable in separating benign and malignant conditions of the prostate (Table 9.6). Select antibodies, such as antikeratin 34βE12 (high-molecular-weight keratin) and p63 (see later), are used to stain tissue sections for the presence of basal cells, recognizing that PIN retains an intact or fragmented basal cell layer, whereas cancer does not (Fig. 9.8).[123,124] In addition, racemase

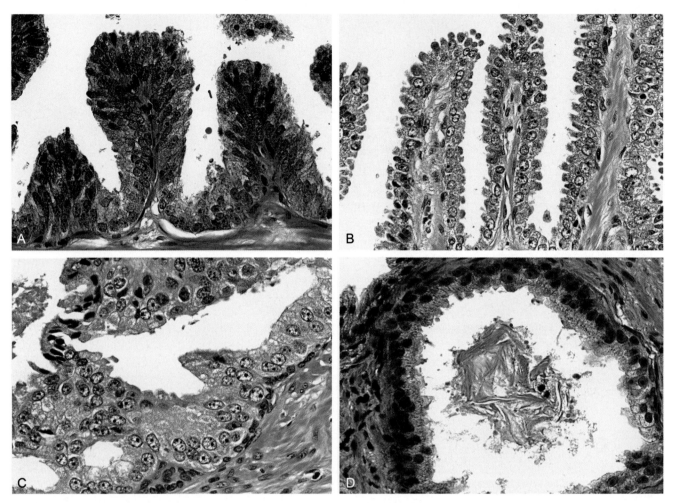

Fig. 9.3 Architectural patterns of high-grade prostatic intraepithelial neoplasia. Compare with artist's renditions in Fig. 9.2. (A) Tufting and early micropapillary patterns. (B) Micropapillary pattern. (C) Cribriform pattern. (D) Flat pattern.

and c-Myc are useful for staining of the dysplastic secretory cells of PIN (see later).

We routinely generate unstained intervening sections of all prostate biopsies for possible future immunohistochemical staining, recognizing that small foci of concern are often lost when the tissue block is recut. One study reported loss of the suspicious focus in 31 of 52 cases.[125]

Keratin 34βE12 and Other Keratins

Monoclonal basal cell–specific antikeratin 34βE12 stains the cytoplasm of most normal basal cells of the prostate, with continuous intact circumferential staining in many instances. There is no staining in secretory and stromal cells. This marker is the most commonly used immunostain for prostatic basal cells, and methods of use with paraffin-embedded sections have been optimized.[126-128] Antikeratin 34βE12 is formalin sensitive and requires pretreatment by enzymes or heat if formalin-based fixatives are used. After pepsin predigestion or microwaving, there is progressive loss of immunoreactivity from 1 week or longer of formalin fixation. Heat-induced epitope retrieval with a hot plate yielded consistent strong positive results with up to 1 month of formalin fixation.[128] Staining intensity was consistently stronger for all intervals of formalin fixation when the hot plate method was used, compared with pepsin predigestion or microwaving. Weak immunoreactivity was rarely observed in cancer cells after

hot plate treatment, but not with pepsin predigestion or microwave antigen retrieval. Steam-EDTA in combination with protease enhanced basal cell immunoreactivity compared favorably with protease treatment alone in benign prostatic epithelium.[129] Nonreactive benign acini were always the most peripheral acini in a lobule, a small cluster of outpouched acini farthest from a large duct, or the terminal end of a large duct.[130] More proximal acini had a discontinuous pattern of immunoreactivity.

Increasing grades of PIN are associated with progressive disruption of the basal cell layer, according to studies using antikeratin 34βE12. Basal cell layer disruption is present in 56% of cases of high-grade PIN and is more frequent in acini adjacent to invasive carcinoma than in distant acini. Early invasive carcinoma occurs at sites of glandular outpouching and basal cell discontinuity in association with PIN.[31] The cribriform pattern of PIN may be mistaken for the cribriform pattern of intraductal or ductal carcinoma, and the use of antikeratin staining is often useful in making this distinction, although exceptions occur (see later).[131] Cancer cells consistently fail to react with this antibody, although admixed benign acini may be misinterpreted as cancerous staining. Thus, immunohistochemical stains for antikeratin 34βE12 may show the presence or absence of basal cells in a small focus of atypical glands, helping establish a benign or malignant diagnosis, respectively. We believe that this antibody can be used successfully

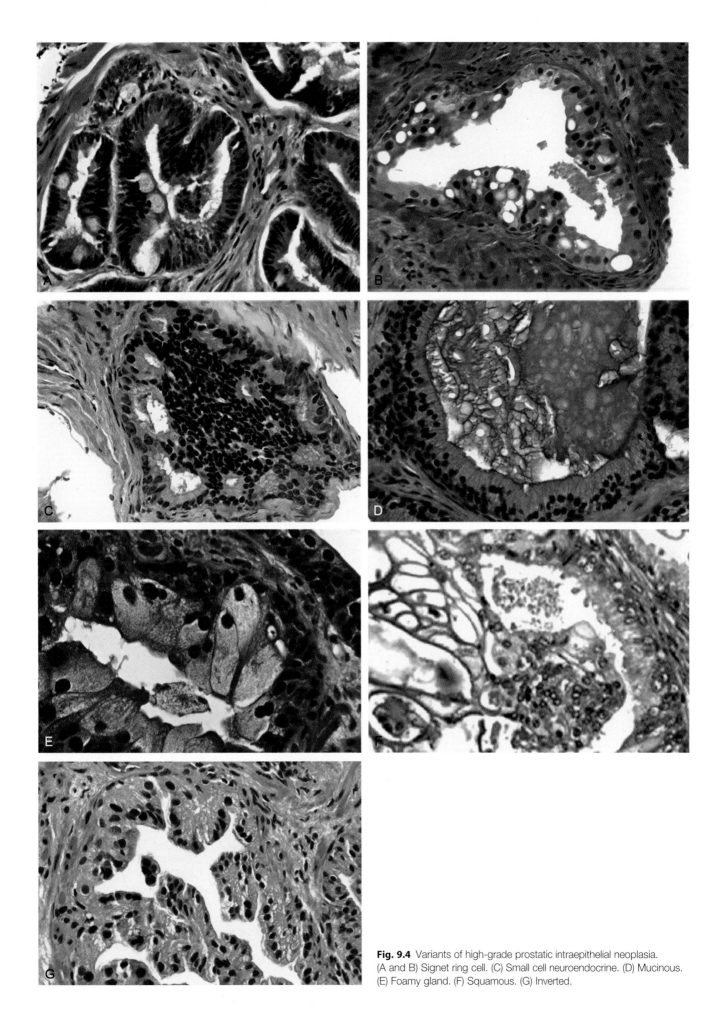

Fig. 9.4 Variants of high-grade prostatic intraepithelial neoplasia.
(A and B) Signet ring cell. (C) Small cell neuroendocrine. (D) Mucinous.
(E) Foamy gland. (F) Squamous. (G) Inverted.

TABLE 9.5	Histologic Patterns of High-Grade Prostatic Intraepithelial Neoplasia

Usual patterns[80]
  Tufting
  Micropapillary
  Cribriform
  Flat
Unusual patterns and variants
  Signet ring cell
  Small cell (neuroendocrine)[82]
  Foamy gland
    (microvacuolated)[1641]
  Hobnail (inverted)[81]
  Squamoid[83]

if one judiciously interprets the results in combination with the light microscopic findings. Relying solely on the absence of immunoreactivity (absence of basal cell staining) to render the diagnosis of cancer is discouraged.[132] Nonetheless, studies have noted that the rate of equivocal cases can be reduced considerably, by 68% or from 5.1% to 1.0%, with the addition of this immunohistochemical marker.[126,133,134] Evaluation of prostate biopsies after therapy, such as radiation therapy, may be one of the most useful roles for antikeratin 34βE12 (see later).[78]

In addition to PIN and cancer, basal cell layer disruption or loss also occurs in inflamed acini, atypical adenomatous hyperplasia, and atrophy with postatrophic hyperplasia. There may be misinterpreted as cancer if one relies exclusively on the immunohistochemical profile of a suspicious focus. Furthermore, basal cells of Cowper glands may not express keratin 34βE12, although this

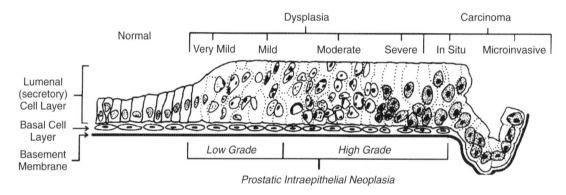

Fig. 9.5 Morphologic continuum from normal prostatic epithelium through increasing grades of prostatic intraepithelial neoplasia to early invasive carcinoma, according to the disease continuum concept. Low-grade prostatic intraepithelial neoplasia (grade 1) corresponds to very mild to mild dysplasia. High-grade prostatic intraepithelial neoplasia (grades 2 and 3) corresponds to moderate to severe dysplasia and carcinoma in situ. The precursor state ends when malignant cells invade the stroma; this invasion occurs where the basal cell layer is disrupted. Dysplastic changes occur in the superficial (luminal) secretory cell layer, perhaps in response to luminal carcinogens. Disruption of the basal cell layer accompanies the architectural and cytologic features of high-grade prostatic intraepithelial neoplasia and appears to be a necessary prerequisite for stromal invasion. Basement membrane is retained with high-grade prostatic intraepithelial neoplasia and early invasive carcinoma. (Modified from Bostwick DG, Brawer MK. Prostatic intraepithelial neoplasia and early invasion in prostate cancer, Cancer 1987;59:788–794, with permission.)

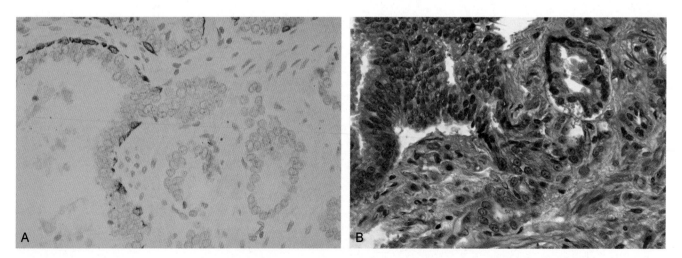

Fig. 9.6 Prostatic intraepithelial neoplasia (PIN) and microinvasion. (A) Basal cell layer disruption in high-grade PIN (*left*) and absent basal cell layer in cancer (*right*). The tongue of cells (*center*) protruding from the large acinar structure with PIN is thought to represent early invasion (basal cell–specific antikeratin 34βE12 immunostain). (B) Another case of PIN with invagination suspicious for early invasion.

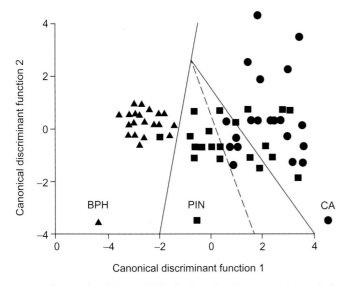

Fig. 9.7 Scatterplot of the spatial distribution of benign prostatic hyperplasia (BPH), prostatic intraepithelial neoplasia (PIN), and cancer (CA). The cases appear as continuous categories, with overlap mainly between PIN and cancer. The two lines divide the scatterplot into three parts, corresponding to three categories. The part corresponding to PIN is subdivided into two parts (*interrupted line*), separating low-grade PIN (close to BPH) and high-grade PIN (close to cancer). (Modified from Montironi R, Scarpelli M, Sisti S, et al. Quantitative analysis of prostatic intraepithelial neoplasia on tissue sections. Anal Quant Cytol Histol 1990;12:366–372, with permission.)

TABLE 9.6 Routine Immunohistochemical Stains in Atypical Small Acinar Proliferation, Prostatic Intraepithelial Neoplasia, and Cancer Diagnosis

Basal cells (benign: brown with diaminobenzidine stain)
    Cytoplasm: keratin 34 B-E12
    Nuclei: p63
Prostatic intraepithelial neoplasia and cancer cells (malignant: red with Texas red stain)
    Cytoplasm: racemase (p504S)
    Nuclei: c-Myc

has been disputed.[135,136] Rare (0.2%) cases of adenocarcinoma have been reported that focally or weakly express keratin 34βE12, including foci of metastatic high-grade adenocarcinoma.[137] Basal cell hyperplasia is a histologic mimic of cancer, and use of antikeratin 34βE12 is recommended in any equivocal cases that include this lesion in the differential considerations because it is invariably strongly immunoreactive.[138,139]

Cytokeratin (CK) 5 and CK14 messenger RNA (mRNA) and protein are expressed in the basal cells of benign acini and PIN, and CK14 mRNA is present in low levels in the luminal cells of some foci of PIN. Thus, if PIN is derived from basal cells, as is currently believed, CK14 translation is depressed and a low level of

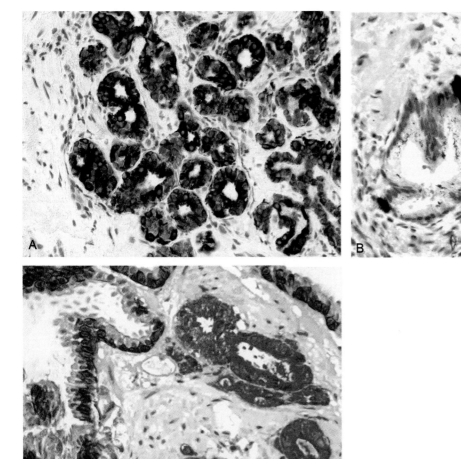

Fig. 9.8 Immunostain with antikeratin 34βE12 and racemase. (A) Intact basal cell layer in atrophic acini. (B) Basal cell layer is disrupted in high-grade prostatic intraepithelial neoplasia; note positive racemase staining (red). (C) Absent basal cell layer in cancer; note positive racemase staining (red).

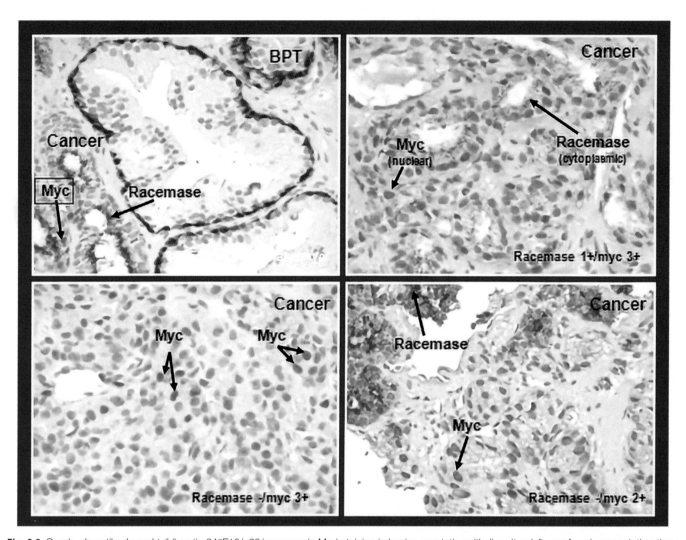

Fig. 9.9 Quadruple-antibody cocktail (keratin 34βE12/p63/racemase/c-Myc) staining in benign prostatic epithelium (*top left panel*) and cancer (*other three panels*). BPT, benign prostatic tissue.

CK14 mRNA may persist.[140] CK8 mRNA and protein were constitutively expressed in all epithelia of the normal and neoplastic prostate. CK19 mRNA and protein were expressed in both basal and luminal cells of benign acini. CK16 mRNA was expressed in a similar pattern as CK19, but CK16 protein was not detected.[140] Basal cells display immunoreactivity at least focally for keratins 10, 11, 13, 16, and 19; of these, only keratin 19 is also found in secretory cells.[44,141] Other keratins found exclusively in the secretory cells include 7, 8, and 18.

Prostatic basal cells do not usually display myoepithelial differentiation, in contrast with basal cells in the breast, salivary glands, pancreas, and other sites.[142,143]

p63

p63 is a nuclear protein that is at least as sensitive and specific for the identification of basal cells in diagnostic prostate specimens as high-molecular-weight CK staining.[123,144-153] p63 may be more sensitive than keratin 34βE12 in staining benign basal cells, particularly in TURP specimens, offering slight advantage in diagnostically challenging cases.[154] Basal cell cocktail (the combination of 34βE12 and p63) increases the sensitivity of basal cell detection and reduces staining variability.[123] Triple staining with racemase, high-molecular-weight CK, and p63 is commonly used for the diagnosis of prostate cancer (Figs. 9.8 through 9.10), although

we believe that the addition of c-Myc (quadruple stain) optimizes diagnostic yield (discussed later in this chapter).[145,147,150,151,155]

Aberrant (positive) p63 staining is occasionally observed in primary and metastatic prostate cancer, so diagnosis should not rely exclusively on this marker.[156] Normal stem cells (reserve cells) are maintained by p63, and alteration of p63 expression has an oncogenic role in prostate cancer. In contrast with usual prostatic adenocarcinomas, prostate tumors with p63 expression show a mixed luminal/basal immunophenotype, uniformly lack *ERG* gene rearrangement, and frequently express GSTP1.[157] Expression of cytoplasmic aberrance of p63 is associated with high ALDH1A1 expression.[158]

Racemase

Racemase (α-methylacyl-coenzyme A [CoA] racemase [AMACR] or P504S) is invaluable for separating benign and neoplastic acini, including evaluation of PIN, ASAP, and separation of cancer from hormonally treated benign acini. This well-characterized enzyme catalyzes the conversion of several (2R)-methyl-branched-chain fatty acyl-CoAs to (S)-stereoisomers. mRNA levels of racemase are upregulated ninefold in prostate cancer. The gene for AMACR is greatly overexpressed in prostate cancer cells.[159] Its advantage over antikeratin 34βE12 is its positive granular cytoplasmic staining in cancer cells, with little or no staining in benign acini. In PIN,

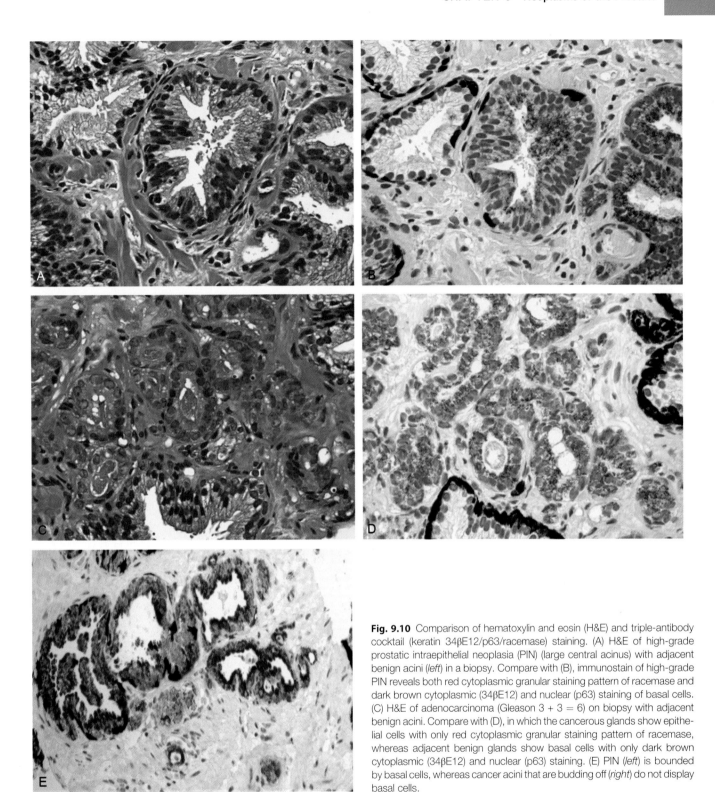

Fig. 9.10 Comparison of hematoxylin and eosin (H&E) and triple-antibody cocktail (keratin 34βE12/p63/racemase) staining. (A) H&E of high-grade prostatic intraepithelial neoplasia (PIN) (large central acinus) with adjacent benign acini (*left*) in a biopsy. Compare with (B), immunostain of high-grade PIN reveals both red cytoplasmic granular staining pattern of racemase and dark brown cytoplasmic (34βE12) and nuclear (p63) staining of basal cells. (C) H&E of adenocarcinoma (Gleason 3 + 3 = 6) on biopsy with adjacent benign acini. Compare with (D), in which the cancerous glands show epithelial cells with only red cytoplasmic granular staining pattern of racemase, whereas adjacent benign glands show basal cells with only dark brown cytoplasmic (34βE12) and nuclear (p63) staining. (E) PIN (*left*) is bounded by basal cells, whereas cancer acini that are budding off (*right*) do not display basal cells.

monoclonal and polyclonal antibodies to racemase are positive in 77% and 91% of foci, respectively (Fig. 9.10).[159-164] Because racemase is not specific for prostate cancer and is present in high-grade PIN (>90% of cases), as well as nephrogenic adenoma, this staining must be interpreted with care. The diagnosis of PIN or prostate cancer should be rendered only in combination with convincing histologic evidence.[165] Moderate to strong racemase expression in PIN is indicative of associated adenocarcinoma.[166] Racemase is negative in up to 27% of cancer cases.

Overexpression of racemase in PIN may be predictive of increased likelihood of cancer on repeat biopsy, but this has not been confirmed.[167]

c-Myc

There is a compelling need for an immunohistochemical stain for cancer nuclei that would aid in cases in which cytoplasmic racemase staining is marginal or absent. *c-Myc*, a transcription factor that regulates cell proliferation, metabolism, protein synthesis, mitochondrial function, and stem cell renewal, is highly overexpressed in PIN and cancer cell nuclei, especially in those with negative racemase staining; positive c-Myc is complementary to racemase for prostate transformation. *c-Myc* overexpression is associated with Gleason score, unlike racemase, and may be useful for both diagnosis and prognosis of prostate cancer. There is intense nuclear staining of *c-Myc* in epithelial cells in 15%, 100%, and 97% of cases of benign tissue, PIN, and cancer, respectively. Mean percentage of *c-Myc*[+] cells is 0.2% (range, 0% to 5%), 34.4% (range, 10% to 50%), and 32.3% (range, 5% to 70%), respectively. In cancer acini with negative racemase, c-Myc is usually positive.

ERG

TMPRSS2:ERG gene rearrangements are highly specific for prostatic malignancy, present in about 50% of cancers and in 10% to 29% of foci of PIN, according to both immunohistochemical staining with anti-ERG antibody and *TMPRSS2:ERG* gene rearrangement studies.[168-174] *ERG* rearrangement is associated with loss of the tumor suppressor gene *PTEN* (phosphatase and tensin homolog), and this cooperation promotes progression of PIN to invasive cancer.[175] *ERG* staining of biopsies with PIN is predictive of cancer on repeat biopsy (60% to 95% in positive cases versus 5% to 21% in negative cases).[174,176,177] However, He et al. found a 38% risk for cancer on repeat biopsy that was independent of *ERG* staining status with PIN. Immunohistochemical expression of *ERG* in PIN is strongly predictive of *ERG* status in coexistent prostate cancer, with more than 95% concordance.[178,179]

Molecular Biology of Prostatic Intraepithelial Neoplasia

PIN is associated with progressive abnormalities of phenotype and genotype, which are between normal prostatic epithelium and cancer, indicating impairment of cell differentiation and regulatory control with advancing stages of prostatic carcinogenesis.[180] There is progressive loss of some markers of secretory differentiation, cytoskeletal proteins, and multiple gene products (Table 9.7).[26,44,159,181-200] Other markers show progressive increase in expression from benign epithelium through PIN to cancer (Table 9.7). A model of prostatic carcinogenesis has been proposed based on the morphologic continuum of PIN and the multistep theory of carcinogenesis.[23,103]

High-grade PIN and prostate cancer share similar genetic alterations.[103,201,202] For example, 8p12-21 allelic loss is commonly found in cancer and microdissected PIN.[201] Other genetic changes found in carcinoma that already exist in PIN include loss of heterozygosity (LOH) at 8p22, 12pter-p12, 10q11.2, and gain

---

TABLE 9.7 **Select Markers With Progressively Altered Expression in Prostatic Intraepithelial Neoplasia and Cancer Compared With Benign Epithelium**[a]

Increased Expression	Decreased Expression
Amphiregulin[1642]	Activated caspase-3[26]
Aneuploidy[193,1643,1644]	Androgen receptor expression[193]
Apoptotic bodies[207,1645-1647]	Annexin I[186,1696]
Aurora-A (Aurora 2 kinase, STK-15), a protein found in centrosomes[1648]	Annexin II[159]
Bcl-2 oncoprotein[1649-1651]	Blood group antigens
Calcium-activated nucleotidase 1 (CANT1)[1652]	BRCA2[1689]
Cell growth regulatory protein LIM domain only 2 (LMO2)[1653]	CD10[185,1697]
Cell proliferation-associated protein Cdc46[1654]	Fibroblast growth factor-2[182]
c-erbB-2 (HER2)[321] and c-erbB-3 oncoproteins[182,1655]	Hepatocyte growth factor activator inhibitor-1[183]
c-Fes protooncogene[1656]	Inhibin[184]
Claudin-3[1657]	Insulin-like growth factor binding protein-3[194,195]
c-met protooncogene	Interstitial collagenase (MMP-1)[190]
c-Myc[1658]	Neuroendocrine cells
Cyclooxygenase-2 (COX-2)[1659-1661]	NKX3.1 homeobox gene-encoded protein[192]
Cysteine-rich secretory protein 3 (CRISP3)[1662]	Ornithine decarboxylase[191]
Dentin sialophosphoprotein[1663]	Prostate-specific antigen
Ep-Cam transmembrane glycoprotein[1664]	Prostatic acid phosphatase
Estrogen receptor α and β[1665,1666]	p-Cadherin[181]
FAS-related apoptosis signaling pathway markers FADD-FAS associating protein with death domain, pro-caspase-8, and caspase-8[1667]	Prostate-specific transglutaminase[200]
Gelatinase B (MMP-9), matrilysin-1 (MMP-7) and the membrane-type 1-MMP (MT1-MMP)[190]	Telomerase[196]
G-protein–coupled receptor PSGR2[1668]	p27KIP1[197,199,1678]
G₁ cell-cycle arrest regulator p16(INK4a)[1669]	5α-Reductase type 2[187]
Glutathione S-transferase P1[1670]	15-Lipoxygenase 1[188] and 2[189]
Heat shock protein 90[1661,1671]	
Human glandular kallikrein 2 (hK2)[1672,1673]	
Hypoxia-inducible factor 1α (HIF-1α)[1674]	

IL-6 and IL-10[1671]
Insulin-like growth factor binding protein IGFBP-rP1
Ki67 (MIB-1) expression[26,193,1678]
Lewis Y antigen
Macrophage inhibitory cytokine-1 (MIC-1)[1675]
Matriptase, a type II transmembrane serine protease[183]
Matrix metalloproteinase-26 (MMP-26)[1676]
Metallothionein isoform II[1677]
Microvessel density[219]
Minichromosome maintenance protein-2 (Mcm-2)[26]
Mitochondrial protein MAGMAS[1679]
Mitotic figures[1645]
Mammalian target of rapamycin signaling pathway markers 4E-BP1 and p-4E-BP1[1680]
Mutator (RER$^+$) phenotype[207]
Neuropeptide Y (NPY)[1675]
NOS-1 and NOS-2[1661]
Osteopontin[1681]
Polo-like kinase-1 (PLK-1)[1659]
Prolactin receptor[1682]
Promoter methylation of *GSTP1* gene[212]
Prostate-specific membrane antigen[1130,1683]
Prothymosin α[1684]
Rac-specific guanine nucleotide exchange factor Tiam1[1685]
RNase III endonuclease Dicer[1686]
Serine/threonine kinase Pim-1[1687,1688]
Skp2 (E3 ubiquitin ligase)[1689]
Slit2[1690]
Tenascin-C[1691]
Transforming growth factor-α (TGF-α)
Tissue inhibitor of metalloproteinases (TIMP-1 and TIMP-4)[1676,1692]
TXA$_2$ synthase and TXA$_2$ receptors[1660]
Type IV collagenase
Vascular endothelial growth factor (VEGF)[1674]
p21[199]
p53[1693,1694]
p62 sequestosome 1 (SQSTM1) gene product[1695]
5α-reductase type 1[187]

[a]The preponderance of reported results supports this conclusion.

of chromosomes 7, 8, 10, and 12, and the *8p24* and *PTEN* genes.[34,74,201,203-205] LOH frequencies at 13q (one of the most common chromosomal alterations in high-stage cancer) is 0% in PIN versus 49% in clinical prostate cancer.[206] Alterations in oncogene Bcl-2 expression and RER$^+$ phenotype are similar for PIN and cancer.[207,208] Up to 64% of patients with PIN have LOH for the mannose 6-phosphate/insulin-like growth factor 2 receptor (*M6P/IGF2R*) gene, a marker for glycolytic metabolism.[205]

Short telomere length in PIN and the surrounding stroma is associated with an increased risk for cancer.[209] Telomere length is also predictive of time from the original biopsy to diagnosis of cancer.[210] Overexpression of *p4EBP1* predicted cancer with sensitivity and specificity of 63% and 100%, respectively.[211]

PIN is epigenetically similar to carcinoma according to the percentage of methylated alleles for the *APC*, *GSTP1*, and *RARbeta2* genes.[212] Methylation of the apoptosis-associated *ASC* promoter region is increased in PIN and cancer.[213] TMPRSS2 exon 1 is fused in-frame with ERG exon 4 in 50% of prostate carcinomas and in 19% to 21% of cases of PIN but not in benign controls.[214,215] PIN and cancer have higher levels of oxidative stress measured by urinary F2-isoprostane than benign prostatic tissue.[216] Another mechanism associated with early prostatic carcinogenesis is deSUMOylation (SUMO refers to small ubiquitin-like modifier proteases), probably through enhanced cell proliferation resulting in PIN.[217] Overexpression of p16INK4A in PIN is reportedly an independent predictor of relapse.[218]

Microvessel density is higher in high-grade PIN than in adjacent benign prostatic tissue, and capillaries are shorter, more widely spaced, have more open lumina and curvaceous external contours. PIN vessels are lined by greater number of endothelial cells. PIN is virtually always accompanied by proliferation of small capillaries in the stroma. It is likely that PIN initially co-opts adjacent vessels, similar to other tumors, and that these vessels soon regress, only to be followed by marked angiogenesis at the cancer's edge. Microvessel density is higher in cases with PIN associated with prostate cancer than in foci of isolated PIN or benign prostatic hyperplasia (BPH).[219]

A critical balance exists between the proangiogenic vascular endothelial growth factor (VEGF) and the angiogenic antagonist angiopoietin-2. Angiogenin is a polypeptide involved in the formation and establishment of new blood vessels necessary for growth and metastasis of cancer. The percentage of cells staining positively for angiogenin in benign epithelium, PIN, and cancer is 17%, 58%, and 60%, respectively, confirming the potential role that angiogenin plays in neoplastic progression.[220,221]

Treatment Effects in Prostatic Intraepithelial Neoplasia

Radiation Therapy

The prevalence and extent of PIN is decreased after radiation therapy, although PIN persists in 9% of biopsies after a course of three-dimensional external beam conformal radiation therapy.[222,223]

After radiation therapy, PIN retains the features characteristic of untreated PIN and is readily recognized in tissue specimens. The key pathologic features include nuclear crowding, nuclear overlapping and stratification, nuclear hyperchromasia, and prominent nucleoli. The basal cell layer is present but often fragmented; racemase shows strong apical to diffuse cytoplasmic staining.[224] The most common patterns of PIN after radiation are tufting and micropapillary, similar to those reported in untreated PIN.

The long-term efficacy of radiation treatment may depend on eradication of both cancer and precancerous lesions that could induce secondary metachronous invasive cancer. Does recurrent cancer after irradiation result from regrowth of incompletely eradicated tumor or from progression of incompletely eradicated PIN?

Androgen Deprivation Therapy and Other Therapies

There is a marked decrease in the prevalence and extent of high-grade PIN after androgen deprivation therapy.[225-228] This decrease is accompanied by epithelial hyperplasia, cytoplasmic clearing, and prominent glandular atrophy, with a lower ratio of glands to stroma.

In the normal epithelium, luminal secretory cells are more sensitive to the absence of androgen than basal cells, indicating that the cells of PIN share this androgen insensitivity with basal cells. The loss of some normal, hyperplastic, and dysplastic epithelial cells with androgen deprivation is probably due to acceleration of programmed cell death (apoptosis).

There is heterogeneity in the response of PIN to therapy that probably varies with type of therapy and duration.[229] Three months of LHRH-agonist leuprolide and antiandrogen flutamide results in a 50% reduction in the incidence and extent of PIN; 6 months induces even greater reduction.[75] Flutamide decreases the prevalence and extent of high-grade PIN and induced epithelial atrophy, and cessation of therapy results in return of PIN.[230,231] A randomized prospective trial of 60 men with PIN revealed similar rates of adenocarcinoma at 1 year for those treated with flutamide or placebo (14% and 10%, respectively).[232]

Another antiandrogen, bicalutamide, lowers mean cancer volume, mean PIN volume, and incidence of PIN after a few months.[233] At prostatectomy, Gleason score is similar to the untreated control group.[227] There is no evidence of higher-grade cancer emergence after treatment.[227]

The results of 5α-reductase (finasteride) treatment of PIN are controversial, and the cumulative number of cases studied is probably too small to draw conclusions.[234] Two reports found no apparent effect on the histologic appearance or extent of high-grade PIN, whereas a third study of three cases noted atrophy, involution, and decreased prevalence.[235-237] In the Prostate Cancer Prevention Trial (PCPT), finasteride decreased the overall risk for PIN (alone and with cancer) from 12% in the placebo group to 9% in the finasteride group.[228]

Toremifene is a selective estrogen receptor modulator that eliminates high-grade PIN and reduces the incidence of prostate cancer. After 4 months of toremifene, 72% of men treated (versus 18% of controls) had no high-grade PIN on subsequent prostate biopsies.[231] In another study, cumulative risk for prostate cancer was reduced in patients taking toremifene compared with placebo (24% versus 31%) with an annualized rate of prevention equivalent to 7 cancers per 100 men treated.[238] Among patients with no biopsy evidence of cancer at baseline and at 6 months, the 12-month incidence of prostate cancer was reduced by 48% with toremifene compared with placebo (9% versus 17%).[238] The final results, however, at 3 years failed to yield a significant difference in cancer yield between untreated and treated patients (35% versus 32%, respectively).[239]

A prospective randomized 3-year trial of selenium versus placebo in men with PIN revealed no difference in cancer yield (37% versus 36%, respectively).[240]

Differential Diagnosis of Prostatic Intraepithelial Neoplasia

The histologic differential diagnosis of PIN includes a variety of benign conditions including atrophy, postatrophic hyperplasia, atypical basal cell hyperplasia, cribriform hyperplasia, and metaplastic changes associated with radiation, infarction, and prostatitis (Tables 9.8 and 9.9; see Chapter 8). Many of these display mild architectural and cytologic atypia, including enlarged nucleoli. The diagnostic difficulty is compounded when these findings appear in small, cauterized, or distorted specimens.

Neoplastic mimics of PIN include IDC (see later), cribriform adenocarcinoma, ductal carcinoma, and urothelial carcinoma. Proliferative activity is higher in ductal carcinoma than in PIN (Ki67 labeling, 33% versus 6%).[91,92] Stratified epithelium in noncribriform glands of cancer can also resemble high-grade PIN.[241]

Inflammation, Atrophy, and High-Grade Prostatic Intraepithelial Neoplasia

Inflammation may cause prostatic carcinogenesis, but the evidence to date is inconclusive or contradictory, probably because of the ubiquitous presence of inflammation in the prostate (see Chapter 8). Chronic inflammation is present in about 8% of biopsies and appears to confer a protective effect from PIN and cancer even after adjusting for age, digital rectal examination findings, serum PSA, and prostate volume.[242] Inflammation is inversely related to cancer risk, and atrophy is marginally related; whereas, PIN is a significant risk factor.[243,244]

Proliferative changes of the epithelium are linked to carcinogenesis in almost all epithelial malignancies. Proliferative regenerative change, referred to in the prostate as proliferative inflammatory atrophy, may be premalignant. The hypothesis is that cellular injury and regeneration characteristic of inflammatory atrophy is induced by inflammation and release of reactive oxygen species (oxidative stress) resulting from insult caused by chemicals (e.g., dietary carcinogens), physical factors (e.g., arteriosclerosis-induced ischemia), or bacteria. The regenerating cells are at increased risk for mutation, which predisposes them to cancerous initiation,

TABLE 9.8	Differential Diagnosis of Prostatic Intraepithelial Neoplasia
Histologic Mimic of PIN	**Differentiating Features**
Inflammatory reactive changes	• Metaplastic (eosinophilic) changes and inflammatory background
Urothelial metaplasia	• Lacks prominent nucleoli
Seminal vesicles and ejaculatory ducts	• Bizarre cells with lipofuscin pigment • Nuclear hyperchromasia, nuclear pleomorphism, and degenerative changes • Prostate-specific antigen and prostatic acid phosphatase negative
Cribriform hyperplasia	• Occurs in transition zone; sievelike pattern • Uniform cells with clear cytoplasm • Lacks nuclear and nucleolar enlargement
Postatrophic hyperplasia	• Lacks nucleolar enlargement
Atypical basal cell hyperplasia	• Small, solid nests or eccentric expansion of the basal cell layers between normal columnar secretory cells and basement membrane • The long axis of basal cells is usually parallel to the basement membrane • Enlarged nuclei with delicate stippled chromatin, occasional nuclear grooves, and nuclear "bubble" artifact • Often associated with inflammatory background • Cytokeratin 34βE12+
Low-grade PIN	• The epithelium lining ducts and acini are heaped up, crowded, and irregularly spaced • Lacks prominent nucleoli and nuclear hyperchromasia • Intact basal cell layer without disruption
Intraductal carcinoma	• Cribriform or papillary growth with significant expansion of ductal size • Frank anaplasia • Commonly adjacent to cancer
Large gland variant of Gleason pattern 3	• More extensive involvement, infiltrative growth pattern • Often associated with small acinar carcinoma • Lacks circumferential basal cell layer

PIN, Prostatic intraepithelial neoplasia.

TABLE 9.9	Mimics of High-Grade Prostatic Intraepithelial Neoplasia (Overdiagnosis of Prostatic Intraepithelial Neoplasia) in 60 Consecutive Cases[1698]
Mimic of Prostatic Intraepithelial Neoplasia	**No. of Cases (%)**
Basal cell hyperplasia	12 (20%)
Benign proliferative epithelium (noncentral zone)	10 (17%)
Low-grade prostatic intraepithelial neoplasia	10 (17%)
Reactive changes	10 (17%)
Atypical basal cell hyperplasia	7 (12%)
Central zone epithelium	5 (8%)
Urothelium	2 (3%)
Seminal vesicle	1 (2%)
Cribriform hyperplasia	1 (2%)
Postatrophic hyperplasia	1 (2%)
Atrophy	1 (2%)

promotion, and progression. The clinical implication of this hypothesis is that antiinflammatory drugs could potentially block procarcinogenic inflammatory processes.[245] Evidence to date is inconclusive as to whether atrophy is a precursor of PIN, direct precursor of cancer that bypasses PIN, or simply an epiphenomenon (see Chapter 8).

What is clear is that any association with cancer requires proliferative changes, and these changes in the setting of atrophy are most often associated with inflammation. Substantial inflammation is often linked with infectious and noninfectious prostatitis, and emerging data indicate a causative role for inflammation in prostate cancer development over time, although there are conflicting data (see Chapter 8).[246-248] The presence of CD68-immunoreactive inflammatory cells in the periprostatic white adipose tissue is associated with high-grade cancer.[249] Despite the controversy regarding the role of atrophy (or lack thereof), virtually all authors agree that inflammation-induced oxidative stress is the most plausible explanation for initiation of prostatic carcinogenesis.

Clinical Significance of Prostatic Intraepithelial Neoplasia

Predictive Value of Prostatic Intraepithelial Neoplasia

The clinical importance of recognizing PIN is based on its strong association with prostatic carcinoma. PIN in biopsies has a high predictive value for adenocarcinoma (36% in repeat biopsies within 36 months), so its identification warrants further search for concurrent or subsequent invasive carcinoma, especially when multifocal (Table 9.10).[239,250,251] This strong prediction is especially true for African American men regardless of PSA level (83% versus 7% incidence rate of cancer on rebiopsy in men with and without PIN, respectively).[252] PIN is a stronger predictor of cancer than patient age and PSA (risk ratios: 15, 4, and 4, respectively).[253]

High-grade PIN in TURP specimens is also an important predictive factor for prostate cancer.[58,254] Among 14 patients with PIN and BPH followed for up to 7 years (mean, 5.9 years), 3 (21.4%) experienced development of prostatic cancer.[58] Mean serum PSA concentration was higher than in those who did not experience cancer (8.1 versus 4.6 ng/mL, respectively). All subsequent cancers apparently arose in the peripheral zone and were detected by needle biopsy. Thus, all tissue should be submitted by the pathologist for examination when PIN is found in TURP specimens. The high predictive value of PIN for the development of subsequent cancer warrants reporting the presence of PIN in TURP specimens, according to the Cancer Committee of the College of American Pathologists. On the other hand, PIN in the transition zone and central zone from Norwegian men was not predictive of subsequent cancer development.[255]

PIN is not always predictive of adverse pathologic findings including higher Gleason grade, seminal vesicle invasion, PNI, and lymphovascular invasion (LVI).[256,257] However, Auskalnis et al. reported that PIN before prostatectomy predicted higher Gleason score and TNM stage. PIN on biopsy predicted contralateral lobe involvement.[258,259] PIN was not predictive of biochemical failure at 32 months in patients undergoing prostatectomy and androgen deprivation therapy.[225] Conversely, in a multivariate

TABLE 9.10

Suggested Clinical Responses to the Diagnosis of Prostatic Intraepithelial Neoplasia, Atypical Small Acinar Proliferation, and Intraductal Carcinoma in Biopsies[a]

Biopsy Findings	Suggested Response[b]
Isolated PIN (three or fewer sites)	Repeat biopsy after 1 year if PSA rises
Extensive or multifocal PIN (>3 foci)	Repeat biopsy
ASAP	Repeat biopsy
ASAP + PIN	Repeat biopsy
Intraductal carcinoma	Immediate repeat biopsy or definitive therapy[c]

ASAP, Atypical small acinar proliferation; *PIN*, prostatic intraepithelial neoplasia; *PSA*, prostate-specific antigen.

[a]This assumes contemporary biopsies with ≥10 cores. Other clinical and laboratory factors such as serum PSA must always be considered.

[b]Monitoring serum PSA is recommended in all cases.

[c]Intraductal carcinoma almost always coexists with Gleason pattern 4 and 5 cancer.

case-control study of 615 Swedes followed for more than 10 years, those with PIN were 89% more likely to die of prostate cancer.[260]

The extent of PIN in needle biopsies is another strong predictor of cancer.[55,86,88] The positive predictive value of PIN for existing cancer is 64%, with a sensitivity of 28% and a specificity of 81%. For those with minute foci of PIN (isolated PIN that involves only one core) identified on an extended core biopsy, repeat biopsy may not be necessary within the first year in the absence of other clinical indicators of cancer such as elevated PSA.[261] Cancer detection is greater in patients with multifocal high-grade PIN than in those with unifocal PIN (70% versus 10%, respectively).[55,87] When four or more cores contain PIN, the predictive value for cancer on subsequent biopsy is 39%.[262,263] Kronz et al. found that the number of core samples with PIN was the only independent histologic predictor of a cancer diagnosis; risk for cancer was 30.2% with one or two cores with PIN, 40% with three cores, and 75% with more than three cores.[264] Recutting of blocks with PIN reveals that 12% of patients have prostatic adenocarcinoma that was not previously detected.[265]

PIN coexists with cancer in more than 85% of prostatectomies, and the likelihood of finding cancer increases with time between procedures: 32% incidence rate of cancer on repeat biopsy performed within 1 year, compared with a 38% incidence rate after 1 year.[253]

The predictive value of PIN declines when a greater number of cores are obtained, probably contributing to the decline in predictive accuracy for cancer in recent years.[46,146,253,266] The main factor is use of extended biopsy techniques that result in more thorough prostate sampling and in higher cancer detection rates; thus, there is a smaller pool of patients with an isolated diagnosis of PIN.[267] Another factor is the lower detection rate and difficulty in the detection of the remaining small cancers; larger significant tumors may also escape detection. These factors lead to a higher frequency of negative repeat biopsies and may reflect a new steady state and a new low plateau in the predictive accuracy of this marker. In one report, the investigators demonstrated that with six core biopsies for both the initial and rebiopsy, the risk for cancer after PIN was 14.1% compared with 31.9% in the group that had

eight cores or more on follow-up with an initial six-core biopsy. The risk for cancer on biopsy within 1 year after a diagnosis of PIN (13.3%) was relatively low if good sampling (eight or more cores) was initially performed.[268]

Clinical Response to Prostatic Intraepithelial Neoplasia

Widespread PIN requires repeat biopsy, probably within 3 to 6 months. Isolated PIN probably does not require immediate repeat biopsy unless the serum PSA climbs. However, a recent survey of German urologists found that the majority undertake repeat biopsy regardless of extent of PIN.

Follow-up biopsy is suggested for patients with PIN within 1 year if the serum PSA increases or there is clinical suspicion for cancer (Table 9.10).[253,269] Some urologists perform saturation biopsies consisting of more than 16 biopsies in one session in an effort to definitively exclude cancer.[270] Most authors agree that identification of PIN in the prostate should not influence or dictate therapeutic decisions.[269] We are aware of 21 radical prostatectomies that were purposely (3 cases) or inadvertently performed (18 cases) in patients whose biopsies contained only high-grade PIN; all but two of the cases contained adenocarcinoma in the surgical specimen (D.G. Bostwick, personal communication, 2007).

Multiple chemoprevention trials using PIN as a risk factor for prostate cancer have met with variable success (Table 9.11).

Atypical Small Acinar Proliferation

Up to 6% of contemporary needle biopsies and 1% of TURP contain collections of small acini that are suspicious for cancer but fall below the diagnostic threshold.[127,271-285] These are reported as ASAP suspicious for but not diagnostic of malignancy (Figs. 9.11 to 9.13).[286] Cancer has been identified in subsequent biopsies in a significant number of cases, indicating that this finding is a useful predictor (see later). Identification of ASAP warrants repeat biopsy for concurrent or subsequent invasive carcinoma.

The prevalence of ASAP in men in the United States is estimated to be 2,145,560 (Table 9.3). It should be noted that ASAP is a diagnostic category, but not a true histopathologic entity (most cases probably represent undersampled adenocarcinoma), so the prevalence data are simply a gauge of the magnitude of the diagnostic problem of ASAP that would be encountered if all men underwent biopsy (biopsy is the only method for detection of ASAP).

Diagnosis of Atypical Small Acinar Proliferation

ASAP represents our inability to render an incontrovertible diagnosis of cancer in a needle biopsy. The focus of concern is invariably no larger than two dozen acini, less than the size of the head of a pin, so the major concern is overdiagnosis of cancer based on insufficient evidence. The diagnostic difficulty with ASAP usually results from one or a combination of the reasons listed in Table 9.12.[287] All of these may hinder the diagnosis of carcinoma, but in such cases the possibility cannot be definitively excluded. The need for this category is based on our "absolute uncertainty." That this need exists is manifested by the variety of terms or synonyms currently in use that include the word *atypical* to describe this diagnosis, although *atypical small acinar proliferation* is now the preferred term and is most widely used clinically around the world.[288] The diagnosis of ASAP indicates to the clinician that

TABLE 9.11 | Chemoprevention Clinical Trials of Men With Prostatic Intraepithelial Neoplasia

Chemopreventive Agent	Trial Phase[a]	Trial Features	Results	Reference
Green tea catechins	1	12 months of treatment; 60 men with PIN randomized to treatment or placebo	Lower incidence of cancer (3% versus 30%)	Bettuzzi et al.[1699]
Flutamide (antiandrogen)	1	12 months of treatment; 60 men with isolated PIN randomized to treatment or placebo	No reduction in cancer (14% versus 10%)	Alberts et al.[232]
Selenium, vitamin E, and soy isoflavonoids	1	6 months of treatment; 71 men with PIN; no randomization or controls	Decline in prostate-specific antigen predicted lower risk for subsequent cancer	Joniau et al.[1700]
Bicalutamide (antiandrogen)	1	6 months of treatment; 20 men with isolated PIN; control group of 22 untreated men with PIN	Lower incidence of cancer (10% versus 27%) and lower extent	Bono et al.[233]
Herbal extract Zyflamend[b]	1	18 months of treatment; 15 men; no randomization or controls	No side effects	Capodice et al.[1701]
Lycopene	1	12 months of treatment; 40 men randomized to treatment or placebo	Lower incidence of cancer	Mohanty et al.[1702]
Toremifene (antiestrogen)	2	12 months of treatment; 176 men randomized to treatment or placebo	Lower incidence of cancer (9.1% versus 17.4%)	Price et al.[238]
Flutamide (antiandrogen)	2	12 months of treatment; 172 men randomized to treatment or placebo	Lower incidence of cancer (11.2% versus 30.2%)	Zhigang et al.[1703]
Toremifene (antiestrogen)	3	36 months of treatment; 1467 men randomized to treatment or placebo	Slightly lower cancer incidence (32% versus 35%)	Taneja et al.[239]
Finasteride (5α-reductase inhibitor)	3	84 months of treatment; 9454 men randomized to treatment or placebo (secondary end point)	Lower incidence of cancer (6.0% versus 7.1%)	Thompson et al.[228]
Dutasteride (5α-reductase inhibitor)	3	48 months of treatment; 8122 men randomized to treatment or placebo (secondary end point)	Lower incidence of cancer (3.7% versus 6.0%)	Andriole et al.[1704]
Selenium, vitamin E, and soy isoflavonoids	3	36 months of treatment; 303 men with PIN randomized to treatment or placebo	No difference in risk for cancer (26%)	Fleshner et al.[1705]

PIN, Prostatic intraepithelial neoplasia.
[a]Trial phase is estimated because most of these trials were not U.S. Food and Drug Administration registration trials.
[b]Extract consists of holy basil, green tea, ginger, Baikal skullcap, rosemary, Chinese goldthread and barberry, oregano, hu zhang, and turmeric.

the biopsy in question exhibits histologic features that are neither clearly malignant nor benign, and that follow-up of the patient is warranted.

For pathologists, three questions need to be answered before the diagnosis of ASAP or cancer in a small lesion: (1) Would you be absolutely confident of this biopsy diagnosis if it were followed by a negative prostatectomy? (2) Would another pathologist agree with the diagnosis of cancer? and (3) Can you confidently support the diagnosis of adenocarcinoma based solely on this biopsy? If the answer to any of these questions is no, then we recommend use of the more conservative ASAP diagnosis. In this setting, we believe that "atypical small acinar proliferation" is a valid diagnostic category if it is used judiciously, and that maximum information has been obtained from the available tissue. Other evidence useful in supporting a cancer diagnosis, including patient age, serum PSA concentration, and results of high-molecular-weight CK, p63, racemase, and c-Myc studies, cannot substitute for convincing hematoxylin and eosin (H&E) microscopic findings. To avoid bias, the above information should be considered only in combination with microscopic examination.

The histologic features that most often preclude a definitive diagnosis of malignancy are the small size of the focus (70% of cases), disappearance on step levels (61%), lack of significant cytologic atypia such as nucleolomegaly (55%), and associated inflammation (9%), raising the possibility of one of many mimics of adenocarcinoma (Fig. 9.14).[273] Other causes include negative staining for high-molecular-weight CK or p63, atrophic changes or inflammation accompanying glands lacking a basal cell layer, and the presence of associated PIN.

Immunohistochemical stain for racemase facilitates the diagnostic support provided by antikeratin 34βE12, p63, and c-Myc, particularly in equivocal biopsies such as ASAP (Fig. 9.15).[148,160,224,289,290] These immunostains resolve 76% of ASAP diagnoses.[291] We routinely use these important techniques in the diagnostic workup of atypical prostate lesions on needle biopsies, thereby decreasing the incidence of ASAP while reducing the risk for false-negative results and the need for additional biopsies. Strand et al. demonstrated that preparing new recut sections and performing immunostains allowed definitive diagnosis of carcinoma in 22% of cases that would otherwise have been signed out as ASAP.[292]

Diagnostic criteria differ between ASAP and minimal cancer (Table 9.13).[287,293] First, the mean number of acini and length of the focus of concern in ASAP (11 acini) are about one-half of those of minimal cancer (17 acini). The small size of a focus of concern is the commonest source of difficulty in ASAP, accounting for 70% of ASAP diagnoses.[273] Infiltrative growth is a constant feature of prostate cancer, but also occurs in 68% to 75% of ASAP cases.[272] All cancers have at least mild nuclear enlargement; whereas, ASAP may have little or no significant enlargement. Prominent nucleoli may be obscured by nuclear hyperchromasia, and this occurs more commonly in ASAP than in minimal cancer. The greater frequency of mitotic figures in cancer (up to 10% of cases) stands in contrast with that of benign acini or ASAP. However, mitotic figures are too rare to be a reliable diagnostic finding in small foci of cancer. Blue-gray acidic luminal mucin may be a useful discriminator, occurring in 61% of cancers compared with 42% of ASAP cases.[272,294]

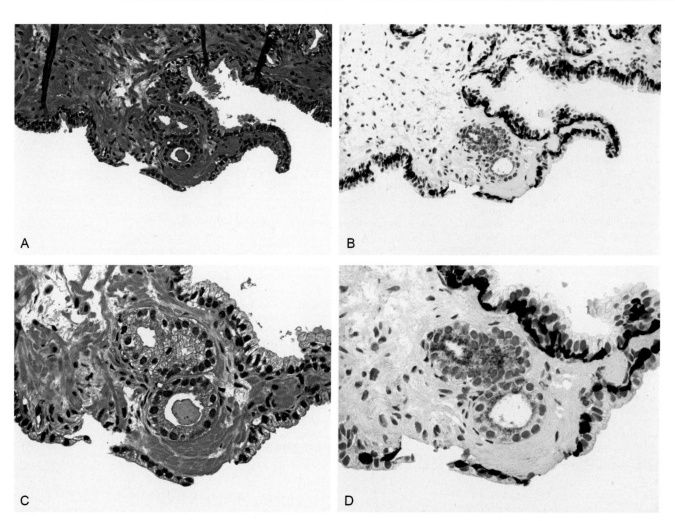

Fig. 9.11 Atypical small acinar proliferation (ASAP) highly suspicious for but not diagnostic of malignancy. This small focus consists of two to three small round to oval acini that stand in contrast with the adjacent benign epithelium; however, there is only slight nucleomegaly and minimal nucleolomegaly. Hematoxylin and eosin (H&E) sections (A and C). Matched triple stains with strong racemase staining and absence of p63 and keratin 34βE12 immunoreactivity, compounding the suspicion of malignancy (B and D). Despite the high level of suspicion, the small size of the focus and the absence of compelling cytologic features warranted diagnosis of ASAP rather than cancer.

Eosinophilic proteinaceous secretions are nonspecific, occurring with similar frequency in cancer and ASAP (73% versus 66% to 74% of cases, respectively).[272] Crystalloids are uncommon and nonspecific, occurring in 19% of cancers and 16% of cases of ASAP.[295] Prior studies reported incidence rates of crystalloids in 6%, 13%, and 22% of ASAP foci in 5% of benign biopsies.[272,273,296,297] These data confirm that crystalloids do not pose an increased risk for cancer in subsequent biopsies.[297,298] Moderate to severe atrophy accompanies more cases of ASAP than cancer. Small foci of postatrophic hyperplasia (which is invariably associated with typical atrophy and has "moderately enlarged" nuclei in 39% of cases) and typical atrophy are sometimes interpreted as ASAP.[272] Obscuring inflammation is responsible for ASAP diagnoses in 30% of cases; however, 20% of minimal cancers also have associated acute or chronic inflammation.[273]

Interobserver agreement for ASAP among urologic pathologists was higher than that of other pathologists (κ, 0.39 versus 0.21, respectively), but complete (100%) agreement was reached by the experts in only 7 of 20 biopsies. The experts diagnosed adenocarcinoma (49%) more often than the nonexperts (32%), and agreement was particularly poor for foci comprising fewer than six acini. The authors concluded that consultation would be of value with a specialized pathologist for ASAP before rendering the diagnosis of carcinoma.[299]

Subsets of Atypical Small Acinar Proliferation

Stratification of ASAP does not increase the predictive accuracy for cancer on repeat biopsy despite multiple attempts.[300,301] We stratified suspicion in each ASAP case into three levels: ASAPB (ASAP suspicious for but not diagnostic of malignancy, favor benign), ASAPS (ASAP suspicious for but not diagnostic of malignancy), and ASAPH (ASAP highly suspicious for but not diagnostic of malignancy).[301] ASAPB was used for cases in which we deemed the focus of concern unlikely to be cancer but could not with absolute certainty exclude the possibility. Conversely, ASAPH was used for cases in which the focus was almost certainly carcinoma, but a confident diagnosis of cancer could not be rendered. ASAPS was used for cases with intermediate suspicion.

In stratifying ASAP into these levels of suspicion, three criteria emerged as significant. Infiltrative growth was present in just over one-half of ASAPB cases but almost all ASAPH cases. ASAPS and ASAPH had greater degrees of nuclear enlargement than in ASAPB but were confounded more frequently by nuclear hyperchromasia.

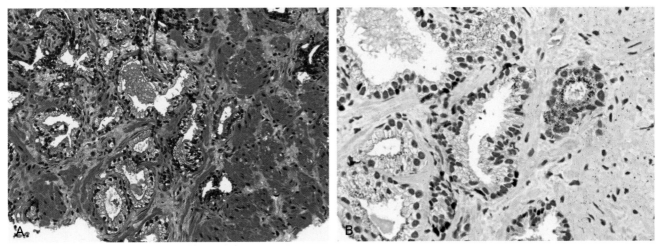

Fig. 9.12 Atypical small acinar proliferation (ASAP) highly suspicious for but not diagnostic of malignancy. The proliferation of intermediate-size acini shows variation in acinar shape and spacing (A and B). (B) A single acinus displays racemase staining with absence of p63 nuclear immunoreactivity is highly suspicious, but the small size of the focus and the absence of compelling nuclear and nucleolar abnormalities precludes a definite diagnosis of cancer.

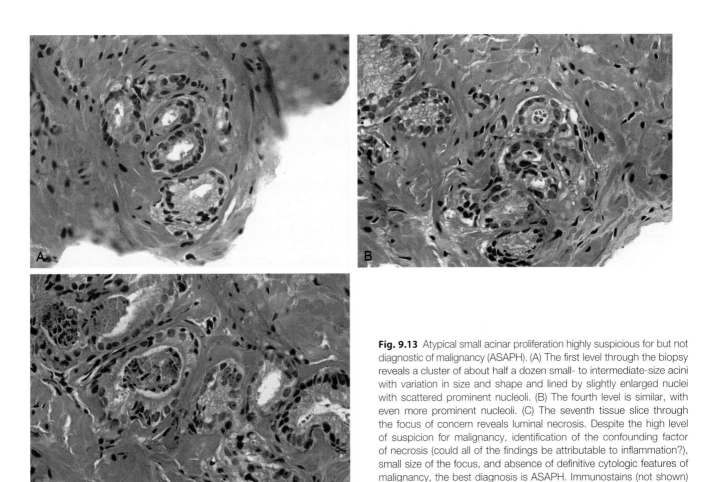

Fig. 9.13 Atypical small acinar proliferation highly suspicious for but not diagnostic of malignancy (ASAPH). (A) The first level through the biopsy reveals a cluster of about half a dozen small- to intermediate-size acini with variation in size and shape and lined by slightly enlarged nuclei with scattered prominent nucleoli. (B) The fourth level is similar, with even more prominent nucleoli. (C) The seventh tissue slice through the focus of concern reveals luminal necrosis. Despite the high level of suspicion for malignancy, identification of the confounding factor of necrosis (could all of the findings be attributable to inflammation?), small size of the focus, and absence of definitive cytologic features of malignancy, the best diagnosis is ASAPH. Immunostains (not shown) reveal scattered p63 and keratin 34βE12 immunoreactive basal cell nuclei in the focus of concern.

Hyperchromasia involved more than one-half of cases of ASAPS and ASAPH, often obscuring nuclear detail and nucleoli; nevertheless, we noted a nonsignificant trend toward prominent nucleoli in a higher percent of the cases as suspicion increased. Two other nonsignificant trends were noted with increasing suspicion for

malignancy: more frequent coexistent high-grade PIN and less frequent moderate to severe atrophy.

Multiple studies revealed nonsignificant trends for increasing risk for subsequent cancer with increasing suspicion. Stratification of ASAP also did not predict the normalized percent of involvement

TABLE 9.12	Reasons for the Diagnosis of Atypical Small Acinar Proliferation

Small Size of Focus

- Small number of acini in the focus of concern (invariably less than two dozen acini)
- Small focus size, average 0.4 mm in diameter
- Focus present at core tip or biopsy edge, indicating that the focus is incompletely sampled
- Loss of focus of concern in deeper levels

Conflicting Morphologic Findings

- Distortion of acini raising concern for atrophy
- Lack of convincing features of cancer (insufficient nucleomegaly or nucleolomegaly)
- Clustered growth pattern mimicking a benign process such as atypical adenomatous hyperplasia
- Foamy cytoplasm raising concern for foamy gland carcinoma

Conflicting Immunohistochemical Findings

- Focally positive high-molecular-weight cytokeratin
- Positive p63 staining
- Negative racemase immunostain

Confounding Findings

- Histologic artifacts such as thick sections or overstained nuclei
- Tangential cutting of adjacent high-grade prostatic intraepithelial neoplasia
- Architectural or cytologic changes (nucleomegaly and nucleolomegaly) caused by inflammation or other lesions

by cancer on positive repeat biopsy.[302] Thus at present the level of suspicion should not alter follow-up recommendations.

Clinical Significance of Atypical Small Acinar Proliferation

ASAP is predictive of prostate cancer in up 39% to 65% of repeat biopsies.[272,273,277-279,282,300-312] Saturation biopsy "substantially" increases the cancer detection rate with or without the presence of ASAP.[270,311,313-315]

ASAP represents undersampled cancer in at least 40% of cases.[277,302,316] Iczkowski et al. observed that some men with ASAP in the first set of biopsies and benign findings or high-grade PIN in the second biopsy may still contain cancer that was not detected.[277,302]

False-negative results in untreated men with documented adenocarcinoma occurred in 23% of repeat sextant biopsies.[317] These results suggest that the current practice of performing 6 to 12 biopsies per prostate does not lower the frequency of ASAP. A declining volume of cancer at prostatectomy was noted more than a decade ago and is probably reflective of increased screening and multiple sampling.[318] Thus as smaller-volume cancers are detected through increased sampling, many will be undersampled and not resolvable by immunostains, likely leading to an irreducible rate of ASAP diagnosis. Saturation biopsy increases the yield of ASAP.

What prostatic sites should be sampled at repeat biopsy? One study found that sampling only the side or site initially diagnosed as ASAP missed cancer in 39% of patients whose cancer was later detected exclusively at other sites, suggesting that the entire prostate should be rebiopsied.[302]

In a provocative report, the investigators recommended immediate prostatectomy in patients with the biopsy diagnosis of ASAP. They suggested that the risk for subsequent cancer is 100% in prostatectomy specimens.[281] We urge caution in recommending expansion of the indications for prostatectomy to include patients with ASAP. ASAP is best considered as a diagnostic risk category and not a true entity.

Atypical Small Acinar Proliferation + Prostatic Intraepithelial Neoplasia

It is often difficult with small foci in biopsies to separate cancer from suspicious foci (ASAPS) when there is coexistent high-grade PIN; the difficulty is based on the inability to separate tangential cutting of the larger preexisting acini of PIN (that may appear as small separate adjacent acini) from the smaller discrete acini of cancer (Fig. 9.16). In such cases, we prefer the term ASAP + PIN (referring to the coexistence of the two lesions, ASAP and high-grade PIN, in the same high-power microscopic field) to avoid overdiagnosis of tangential cutting of PIN and cancer.

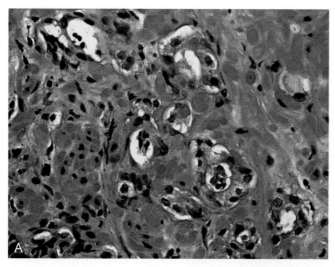
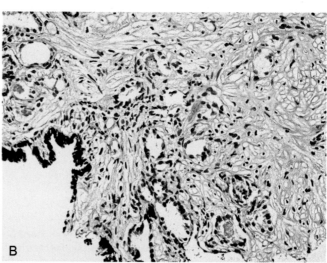

Fig. 9.14 Atypical small acinar proliferation. (A) Luminal neutrophils confound this focus that is highly suspicious for cancer by the variation in acinar size, shape, and spacing. (B) Absence of keratin 34βE12 staining (with internal positive control in adjacent benign epithelium) compounding the suspicion of malignancy.

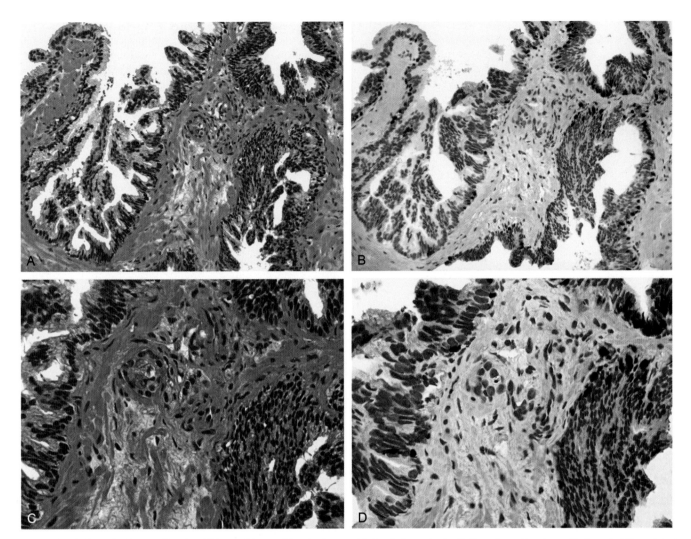

Fig. 9.15 Atypical small acinar proliferation. This small focus of two to three acini stands in contrast with the adjacent benign epithelium, but the cytologic features are obscured by the dark staining (A and C). Matched triple stains reveal absence of racemase staining, as well as p63 and keratin 34βE12 (B and D). Absence of racemase staining does little to allay the suspicion for malignancy, but the focus is simply too small and lacks cytologic support for malignancy

ASAP is placed first because of its stronger predictive value for subsequent cancer.

ASAP + PIN, found in up to 16% of all biopsies, has an intermediate predictive value of about 33% to 60% for cancer.[301,305,306,319-323] Thus it is slightly lower than isolated ASAP (37%) but higher than isolated PIN. In four studies, PIN occurred with ASAP in 17%, 23%, 31%, or 41% of cases with ASAP, but most foci were not adjacent or contiguous.[272,287,300,301] In a study of 12 patients with PIN and adjacent atypical glands (ASAP), 75% had cancer on repeat biopsy.[324] The prostate cancer risk increased in the ASAP subgroups according to the extent of PIN in the initial sample, with ASAP + multifocal PIN carrying a 71% prostate cancer risk.[325]

Differences in predictive values for cancer seen in multiple studies of PIN + ASAP arise from multiple causes. First, contiguous foci might have an intrinsically higher predictive value for cancer than those that include noncontiguous lesions. Second, selection bias present in cases referred for consultation also may have influenced some study results as compared with unselected primary cases in other cohorts. Third, the number of patients reported in some studies was so small that skewing of data in either direction might

occur. Finally, the number or method of biopsy may influence results. For example, use of transperineal template saturation biopsies at 5-mm intervals throughout the prostate revealed that ASAP for two or more cores of high-grade PIN on a previous transrectal ultrasound-guided (TRUS) biopsy strongly indicated the presence of cancer on saturation biopsy.[314] Patients who were diagnosed with high-grade PIN, or who had two or more cores with high-grade PIN or ASAP, cancer was detected in 53%, 89%, and 83%, respectively. High-grade cancer rates (Gleason score ≥7) in patients with ASAP and two or more cores of high-grade PIN were 20% and 80%, respectively.

The best available evidence today indicates that the presence of either or both lesions in needle biopsies is still a predictor for concurrent/subsequent cancer compared with patients who lack these lesions.

PIN was more than twice as frequently associated with minimal cancer (57%) than ASAP (23%). About one-half of cases of ASAP are probably undersampled cancer, and the smaller mean size of the foci in contemporary specimens decreases the likelihood of sampling accompanying high-grade PIN.

TABLE 9.13	Atypical Small Acinar Proliferation Versus Minimal Cancer	
Findings	**ASAP**	**Minimal Cancer[a]**
Architectural		
Linear extent (mm), mean ± SD	0.4 ± 0.3	0.8 ± 0.5
No. of acini, mean ± SD	11 ± 10	17 ± 14
Infiltrative growth	75%	100%
Cytologic		
Nuclear hyperchromasia	44%	9%
Nuclear enlargement (scale of 0-3), mean ± SD	1.2 ± 0.8	1.8 ± 0.7
Prominent nucleoli in at least 10% of cells	55%	100%
Mitotic figure(s)	0%	10%
Luminal		
Blue mucin	6%	33%
Stroma and adjacent acini		
High-grade prostatic intraepithelial neoplasia in same slide	23%	57%
Moderate to severe atrophy	59%	35%

ASAP, Atypical small acinar proliferation, suspicious for malignancy; *SD*, standard deviation.
[a]Adenocarcinoma involving less than 5% of total tissue.

Malignancy-Associated Changes

Although precancerous conditions are usually defined by histopathologic findings such as PIN, it is possible that nonmorphologic or subtle changes may also be predictive of either coexistent or subsequent prostate cancer. The hypothesis of malignancy-associated changes in the epithelium is based initially on subvisual architectural and nuclear chromatin features of otherwise benign epithelium adjacent to PIN or cancer according to a Bayesian belief network or image analysis.[27,28,326]

Since the original descriptions, multiple other reports have suggested field-cancerization genetic or epigenetic damage in normal-appearing epithelium adjacent to PIN and prostate cancer, analogous to the situation with the urothelium of the urinary bladder and other sites.[26,327-329] Mcm-2 expression as a measure of cell proliferation was higher in normal acini and PIN near cancer than those that were more distant.[26] Likewise expression of the apoptosis-related marker a-casp3 was also elevated in normal acini near cancer, although Bcl-2 expression was not.[26] Similar elevated field effect expression has been observed with telomerase, ERG, HOXC4, HOXC5, MME, PSMA (prostatic membrane antigen), SSTR1, BAX, Bcl-2, and the estrogen inducible protein pS2; lower expression was seen with glutathione S-transferase class π (GSTP).[330-333]

Other molecular changes in benign epithelium of biopsies may predict subsequent prostate cancer. High levels of the cell survival

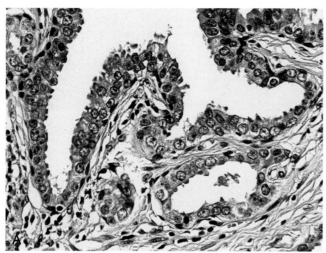

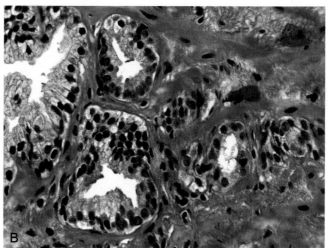

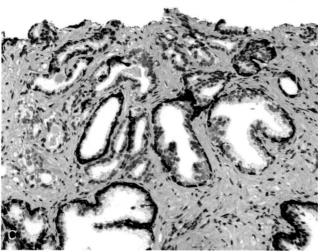

Fig. 9.16 Atypical small acinar proliferation (ASAP) + prostatic intraepithelial neoplasia (PIN). (A) Intermediate-size acini with mild architectural distortion and prominent nuclei and nucleoli in association with high-grade prostatic intraepithelial neoplasia. An unequivocal diagnosis cannot be rendered because of the small size of this focus. (B) Another example of ASAP + PIN. (C) Keratin 34βE12 revealed fragmented and absent basal cell staining in the suspicious acini.

molecule Akt-1, sometimes observed in normal epithelium, are an independent predictor of biochemical recurrence.[334,335] High expression of other markers reportedly predicted cancer in subsequent biopsies, including EPCA-1 and P2X, but our laboratory was unable to reproduce these findings (DG Bostwick, unpublished observations, 2006).[336,337] Mitochondrial DNA deletion assay was the first commercially available test of benign epithelium in biopsies that predicted prostate cancer in subsequent biopsies with a sensitivity and specificity of 84% and 54%, respectively (receiver operating characteristic [ROC] curve, 0.75).[338]

Many genes show no difference in expression of benign epithelium that was and was not associated with malignancy (lack of field effect), including racemase, hepsin, fatty acid synthase, myosin VI, SPOCK, TPD52, and EZH2.[339]

A recent study noted a fourfold increased risk for prostate cancer in men with increased number of epithelial CD4+ T regulatory cells in benign tissue.[340]

Intraductal Carcinoma

IDC remains a controversial lesion because of publication of multiple definitions (Table 9.14). The term was first introduced in 1972, but criteria were lacking and probably included numerous cases of what would be called ductal carcinoma today.[341,342] Even now the distinction between intraductal and ductal carcinoma is uncertain.

TABLE 9.14 Definitions of Intraductal Carcinoma

First Author	Definition
McNeal (1996)[343,1706]	Cancer extension within the branches of a single segment of the duct-acinar system. Three patterns of intraductal carcinoma include trabecular, cribriform, and solid/comedo, which represent progressive dedifferentiation with a reciprocal increase in proliferation. Basal cell layer is intact.
Guo (2006)[344]	Same as McNeal (1996) with addition of either marked nuclear atypia (nuclear size six times normal or larger) or comedonecrosis; also added papillary pattern without fibrovascular cores.[343,1706]
Cohen (2007)[363]	**Five major criteria:** 1. Large-caliber acini that are more than twice the diameter of normal peripheral zone glands 2. Preserved basal cells as identified with basal cell markers 3. Cytologically malignant cells 4. An expansile cell mass that spans the glandular lumen 5. Comedonecrosis (not required) **Three minor criteria:** 1. Right-angle branching; or 2. Smooth, rounded outlines; and 3. Two cell populations with an outer perimeter cell group composed of tall, pleomorphic, mitotically active cells that stain poorly for PSA, as well as a central group that is cuboidal, monomorphic, and quiescent, with abundant cytoplasm containing abundant PSA and occasional extracellular mucin.

PSA, Prostate-specific antigen.

McNeal and Yemoto defined IDC as cancer extension within the branches of a single segment of an intact duct-acinar system, usually with close proximity to cancer (Table 9.14).[343] The lumen-spanning cell masses followed normal duct contours and maintained a basal cell layer. This lesion was interpreted as being part of the evolution and spread of invasive carcinoma rather than a precursor.[343] In most cases the cribriform pattern predominated. IDC usually coexists with invasive carcinoma, and previous authors had referred to this as "noninvasive ductal carcinoma."[344]

Subsequent authors attempted to refine these criteria to include quantitative measures such as nuclear size (six times normal or larger) and duct-acinar diameter (more than twice that of normal peripheral zone acini) (Table 9.14). Similar to patterns of ductal carcinoma, IDC was noted to be either cribriform, solid, or papillary, although fibrovascular cores were absent (Fig. 9.17). Intramucosal spread to the ejaculatory ducts was described by Sanchez-Salazar et al.[345]

European urologic pathologists rely on solid intraductal growth (100% of colleagues), dense cribriform (96%), loose cribriform/micropapillary with nuclear size more than 6× normal (83%) or comedonecrosis (74%) and dilated ducts greater than 2× normal (39%). Nuclear size is interpreted as nuclear area by 74% of colleagues and nuclear diameter by 21%. Pure IDC in biopsies is reported by 100% and Gleason graded by 30% (48% assigned Gleason pattern 5 regardless of the presence or absence of basal cells). All perform immunohistochemistry in such cases to rule out invasive cancer. An intraductal component associated with invasive cancer is included in determination of tumor extent and number of cores involved by 74% and 83% of colleagues, respectively.[346]

The presence of IDC on diagnostic needle biopsy is an independent predictor of cancer-specific survival after adjusting for clinical prognostic factors and treatment modality, but is not significant after adjustment for the 2014 International Society of Urological Pathology (ISUP) grade groupings.[347]

Small cell pattern with rosettes may occur centrally within foci of IDC, similar to PIN, but has no apparent independent clinical significance.[348] Furthermore, NE markers are usually negative.[84]

Separation of Intraductal Carcinoma and Prostatic Intraepithelial Neoplasia

Unlike PIN, IDC is strongly associated with aggressive prostate cancer, including high Gleason grade and large tumor volume (Tables 9.15 and 9.16).[349] Most important are the extent of the process (PIN is usually limited in its extent to a small number of acini at most), acinar size (PIN is found within preexisting acini without significant distortion or expansion of the acinar contours, whereas IDC is usually present in greatly expanded acini and ducts), and cytologic features (PIN is rarely if ever frankly anaplastic, whereas noninvasive and invasive ductal carcinoma often exhibit high-grade nuclear abnormalities such as nucleomegaly, anisonucleosis, and marked hyperchromasia); comedonecrosis is never observed in PIN but is occasionally observed in IDC. The incidence of IDC is higher in Japanese patients than in Americans (35% versus 13%, respectively), which is independent of Gleason score and cancer stage.[350]

Unfortunately, uncertainty persists regarding precise criteria for separating IDC from PIN because of the identification of borderline cases with overlapping features or coexistent features, especially those with cribriform or near-solid growth.[351-353] IDC mixed with invasive carcinoma may occasionally share architectural

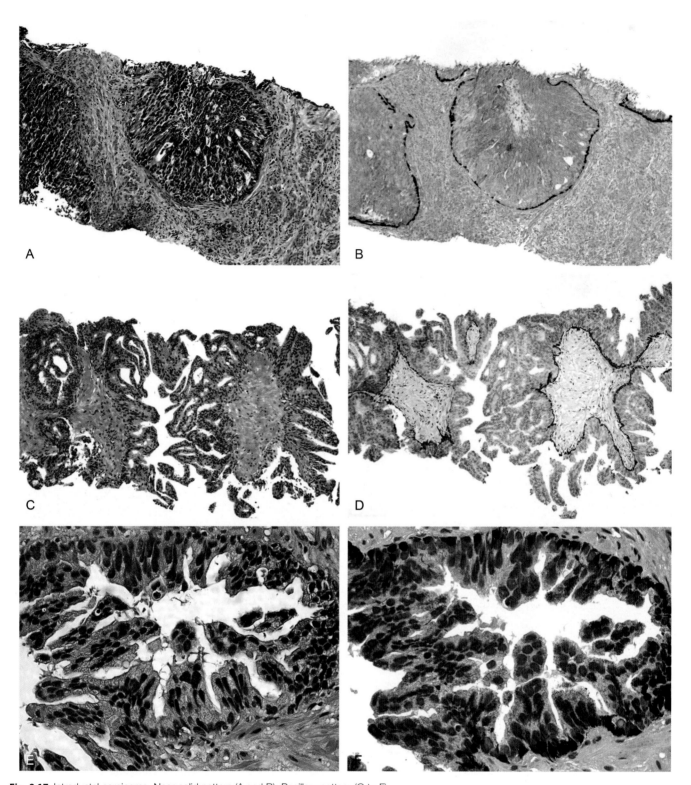

Fig. 9.17 Intraductal carcinoma. Near-solid pattern (A and B). Papillary pattern (C to F).

(Continued)

and cytologic features with cribriform PIN, and all may rarely coexist; in these cases, PIN is identified as an intraductal/intraacinar cribriform proliferation within small, smoothly rounded acini with low-grade nuclei that do not fulfill the typical criteria for IDC. Shah et al. found that the cribriform pattern of IDC was present in 18% of radical prostatectomies, was more common in cancer with Gleason score ≥7, ranged in size from 0.2 to 9.0 mm, and contained comedonecrosis in 33% of cases.[351] Pleomorphic nuclei or giant nuclei at least 6× of the adjacent nuclei were present in 28%. By comparison, isolated cribriform proliferation with malignant cells distant from cancer, referred to by some as isolated atypical cribriform proliferation (we call these IDC when the cells

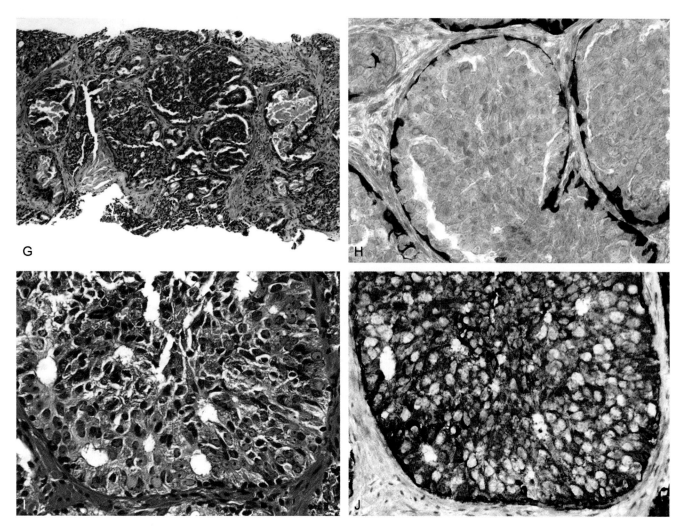

Fig. 9.17, cont'd Cribriform near-solid pattern (G to J). Hematoxylin and eosin stains (A, C, E, G, and I). Quadruple stain (brown reaction product in basal cells for keratin 34βE12 and p63; red reaction product in luminal cells for racemase and c-Myc) (B, D, H, and J).

display anaplasia), was usually associated with Gleason score 6 cancers, was smaller (range, 0.2 to 1 mm), and never displayed comedonecrosis or pleomorphic or giant nuclei. Genetic studies may be useful for borderline cases (see later). PTEN and ERG expression may be useful in separating IDC and PIN (incidence rates of 61% versus 0% and 30% versus 0%, respectively).[354]

Clinical Significance of Intraductal Carcinoma

IDC is an aggressive phenotype of prostate cancer that predicts high-grade, high-stage metastases and poor response to androgen deprivation therapy, external beam radiation therapy, and chemotherapy.[338,355-360] It should be separated from PIN and, when present, reported in prostate biopsies and prostatectomy specimens, even when there is coexistent adenocarcinoma.[356,361,362] Some authors consider IDC to be equivalent to Gleason pattern 4 or 5 adenocarcinoma, and diagnosis on needle biopsy should prompt therapeutic intervention rather than surveillance or repeat biopsy, as is the case for PIN.[363] IDC occasionally coexists with Gleason grade 3 cancer.[364]

IDC with cribriform architecture is present in 2% of autopsies and 1% of cystoprostatectomies with prostate cancer.[365]

IDC displays significant genetic abnormalities.[366] LOH is usually absent in Gleason grade 3 cancer, infrequent in PIN (9%) and

Gleason grade 4 cancer (29%), but common in IDC (60%).[367] The cribriform pattern of IDC, when present within 3 mm of invasive carcinoma, displays *TMPRSS2-ERG* gene fusion in 75% of cases, with 100% concordance with the cancerous component.[352] Cytoplasmic PTEN loss is identified in 84% of cases of IDC and 100% with the cribriform pattern; concordance with invasive carcinoma is greater than 95%.[368] IDC is associated with pathogenic germline DNA-repair gene mutations.[369]

Cribriform IDC has a higher rate of biochemical failure and cancer-specific death than acinar carcinoma with or without cribriform growth.[370,371] Gleason score 7 cancer with cribriform or IDC is independently associated with poorer biochemical recurrence-free survival after prostatectomy, but not after radiotherapy.[372] IDC using the McNeal criteria is an independent risk factor for progression after prostatectomy.[373] Androgen deprivation therapy induces regressive changes in PIN and prostate cancer but appears to have a minimal effect on IDC.

Adenocarcinoma and Other Tumors

Prostate cancer is the most common cancer of men in the United States and is third only to lung and colorectal cancer as a cause of cancer death. In 2018, an estimated 29,430 Americans died of

TABLE 9.15 Intraductal Carcinoma Versus Ductal Carcinoma Versus Cribriform Prostatic Intraepithelial Neoplasia: Microscopic Findings

Features	Intraductal Carcinoma	Ductal Carcinoma[a]	Cribriform/Papillary PIN
Acini	Large or greatly expanded (at least two to three times normal diameter); may represent true ducts and large ductules	Large or greatly expanded; may represent true ducts and large ductules	Small (normal acinar size), with smooth round contours
Lumen-spanning growth	Yes	Yes	Yes (cribriform)
Papillary growth	Papillae without fibrovascular cores	Papillae with fibrovascular cores	Papillae without fibrovascular cores
Cell shape	Pleomorphic	Variable	Relatively uniform without marked nuclear pleomorphism
Cell size	Enlarged six times normal	Enlarged, variable	Enlarged two to three times normal
Mitotic figures	Frequent	Variable	Infrequent
Comedonecrosis	Sometimes	Sometimes	Never
Solid or dense cribriform pattern	Sometimes	Sometimes	Never
Basal cell layer	Intact or fragmented	Usually absent	Intact or fragmented
Molecular genetics (Table 9.16)	Much greater abnormalities than PIN	Greater abnormalities than PIN; greater concordance with intraductal carcinoma	Some abnormalities, but not substantial

PIN, Prostatic intraepithelial neoplasia.
[a]Cribriform pattern of ductal carcinoma may be indistinguishable from cribriform pattern of acinar carcinoma.

TABLE 9.16 Comparison of Cribriform Prostatic Intraepithelial Neoplasia, Intraductal Carcinoma, and Carcinoma: Genetic Findings

	Cribriform/Papillary Prostatic Intraepithelial Neoplasia	Intraductal Carcinoma	Invasive Carcinoma
Loss of heterozygosity[367]	9%	60%	0%[a]; 29%[b]
TMPRSS2-ERG gene fusion[352]	0%	75%	75%[c]
PTEN loss[368]	0%	100%[d]	100%

[a]Grade 3.
[b]Grade 4.
[c]Carcinoma within 3 mm of intraductal carcinoma.
[d]Cribriform pattern.

prostate cancer, and 164,690 new cases will be diagnosed.[374] For all men, the overall probability is 1 in 8. Despite prevalence at autopsy of up to 80% by age 80 years, the clinical incidence is much lower, indicating that most men die *with* rather than *of* prostate carcinoma.[65] Little is known about the causes of prostate cancer despite its high incidence and prevalence. Adenocarcinoma accounts for more than 95% of prostatic malignancies.

Adenocarcinoma does not have specific presenting symptoms and is usually clinically silent, although it may cause urinary obstructive symptoms mimicking nodular hyperplasia. Consequently, cancer is occasionally manifest initially in metastatic sites such as cervical lymph nodes and bone. The diagnosis may be made in the following clinical instances: (1) routine surveillance with digital rectal examination shows a nodular or diffusely enlarged prostate (clinical stage T2, T3, or T4); serum PSA level is greater than 2.0, 2.5, or 4 ng/mL (clinical stage T1c); or imaging and biopsies are positive for malignancy (lesion-directed, random, systematic, MRI-fusion, transperineal, transrectal, or saturation needle biopsies); (2) incidental carcinoma in TURP specimens (clinical stage T1a and T1b carcinoma); (3) metastatic adenocarcinoma of unknown primary; and (4) carcinoma of the prostate presenting as a rectal mass (prostate carcinoma rarely produces an eccentric or circumferential rectal and perirectal mass with or without mucosal involvement of the rectum).

Epidemiology

Prostate cancer poses a greater risk for American men, especially African American men, than any other nonskin cancer. The veritable epidemic of prostate cancer has resulted in part from successful efforts at early detection with the use of the serum PSA test, thereby narrowing the still-enormous gap between the clinical incidence (8% lifetime risk) and autopsy-based prevalence (80% by age 80 years) (Fig. 9.18). Physicians are unable to accurately stratify patients into those who will have progressive cancer and those who will not (cannot separate the "tigers" from the "pussycats"). An equally great problem is determining which men are at greatest risk for development of clinically apparent prostate cancer.

Prostatic adenocarcinoma is rare in patients younger than 40 years.[375] Fewer than 50 cases of adenocarcinoma have been reported in each of the following groups: children younger than 12 years, adolescents, and young adults between 20 and 25 years old. In all these cases, the cancer was poorly differentiated, clinically aggressive, and unresponsive to hormonal therapy and radiation therapy.

After age 40, the incidence increases quickly. Autopsy studies of thoroughly evaluating prostates from men without clinical evidence of cancer have shown a very high level of latent (clinically

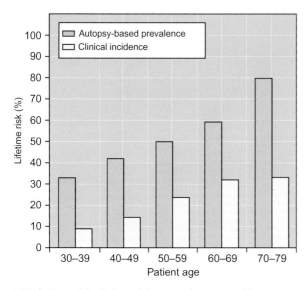

Fig. 9.18 Autopsy-detected prostate cancer increases with age.

occult) cancer. The incidence of prostatic adenocarcinoma is much higher in men of African ancestry (100 per 100,000) than in men of European ancestry (70.1 per 100,000), and men of African ancestry in the United States have the world's highest mortality rate from prostatic adenocarcinoma.[376] The prevalence of latent cancer is similar in different geographic and ethnic groups despite wide variation in the incidence of clinically apparent adenocarcinoma. The incidence is low in American Indians, Hispanics, and Asians, but high in American men of African and European ancestry.

Prostate cancer mortality varies considerably from country to country. High rates have been reported in the United States, particularly among African Americans, whereas low rates have been found in China and Japan. There are advantages and disadvantages in using mortality data to examine the underlying risk for prostate cancer. Incidence data are often unavailable, so mortality is a commonly used surrogate. However, mortality is a function of incidence, survival, and ascertainment and selection biases. International differences in mortality may reflect differences not only in the underlying risk for development of prostate cancer but also of differences in survival or ascertainment/reporting (death certificate) bias. Remarkably, the incidence of new cases surged in Japan in 2002 after the announcement that the Japanese Emperor, Akihito, had prostate cancer. Comparative autopsy study revealed a similar proportion of cancer in Russian Caucasian and Japanese men.[377] More than 50% of cancers are Gleason score ≥7 in Japanese men and nearly 25% in Russian Caucasian men, raising questions about: (1) previous assumptions related to Asian prostate cancer, and (2) the notion of significant versus insignificant cancers.

Latent Carcinoma

The prevalence of carcinoma is most strongly related to age, with the prevalence doubling about every 14 years, and the age-specific prevalence of latent cancer at autopsy is remarkably constant across countries and ethnic groups.[378] Data from the Connecticut Tumor Registry estimated the age-standardized prevalence rate to be 841.6 per 100,000 in 1994, an increase of 126% over the 1982 rate.[379] In contrast, the prevalence in Japan remained largely unchanged from 2005 to 2014 (14% and 12% and Gleason score >6 of 6% and 7%, respectively).[380] However, another report from that country

noted a great increase from 21% to 43% between 1983 to 1987 and 2008 to 2013, respectively.[381] The dramatic differences in prevalence between these autopsy studies from Japan cannot be explained. Systematic literature review concluded that "the prevalence of incidental tumors was relatively low in earlier studies of Japanese men, although more recent study estimates are similar to the rest of the world."[378]

Incidental prostate cancer is less aggressive than clinically apparent prostate cancer according to stage, surgical margin status, and Gleason score. Totally sampled cystoprostatectomy specimens with bladder cancer also contain clinically undetected incidental prostate cancer in about 42% of cases (range, 15% to 68%) with the highest incidence in older men.[382-385] Cystoprostatectomies with prostate cancer have lower stage and lower Gleason score than prostatectomy cases. Incidental prostate cancer in cystoprostatectomy cases is usually stage pT2a or pT2b (59% and 29%, respectively).[382] Incidental prostate cancer is usually low grade (Gleason scores 5 and 6 in 25% and 46% of cases, respectively), much lower than for clinical prostate cancer (5% and 21%, respectively). Only 9% of incidental cancers are Gleason scores 8 to 10. The frequency of positive margins is lower than in clinical cancer (7% versus 52%, respectively).

The relationship between incidental, latent, and clinical prostate cancer may be explained by two hypotheses.[382] One contends that incidental and latent carcinomas are identical histologically to lethal cancer, but have never acquired biologically aggressive features. The other hypothesis contends that clinically innocuous cancers are simply the smallest tumors, and cancer acquires the capacity to metastasize as a function of the passage of time, increasing volume, and "biological tumor progression," a function of the mutational instability of all cancers, which becomes manifest in proportion to the number of mitotic events. We agree with Selman that the term *latent carcinoma* is a medical misnomer and should not be used.[386]

Risk factors can be classified as endogenous or exogenous, although some factors are not exclusively one or the other (e.g., race, aging, and oxidative stress).[376] There are numerous endogenous risk factors for prostate cancer, including family history, hormones, race, and aging and oxidative stress (Table 9.17). Exogenous risk factors include diet, endocrine disrupting chemicals, and occupation.[376]

Prostate Cancer and Benign Prostatic Hyperplasia

Prostatic hyperplasia is frequently seen in association with prostatic adenocarcinoma (Fig. 9.19). There are several compelling similarities, including increasing incidence and prevalence with age, concordant natural history, hormonal requirements for growth and development, and response to androgen deprivation therapy. However, no causal relationship has been established or seriously suggested.[387,388]

Tissue Methods of Detection

Needle Core Biopsy

Introduction of the thin needle for transrectal biopsy of the prostate in the 1980s, together with the use of serum PSA, revolutionized early detection efforts for prostate cancer. These two advances were mutually beneficial, feeding off each other to effectively replace the large-bore transperineal needles and exclusive reliance on digital rectal examination for cancer detection. The rate of

TABLE 9.17	Risk Factors for Prostate Cancer

Family history
Diet
Fat
Cadmium
Zinc
Obesity
Alcohol
Hormones
Smoking
Sexual activity
Early sexual activity
Multiple sexual partners
Occupational exposure
Agricultural fertilizers and pesticides
Rubber
Ionizing radiation
Venereal diseases
Herpesvirus type 2
Cytomegalovirus
Vasectomy
Benign prostatic hyperplasia
Prostatic intraepithelial neoplasia
Atypical small acinar proliferation

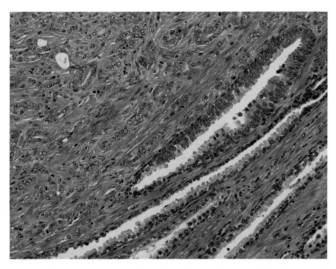

Fig. 9.19 Peripheral sinus at the edge of a nodule of nodular hyperplasia (*bottom right*) with "cancerization" of the nodule.

postbiopsy infection with the thin needle declined from 7% to 39% to 1%, and hemorrhage with urinary clot retention decreased from 3% to less than 1%. The false-negative rate declined from 25% to 11%, and there was an improvement in the quality of the tissue sample obtained, usually with little or no compression artifact at the lateral edges of the specimens. Also, the 18-gauge (18G) needle allows multiple biopsies of the prostate with minimal discomfort, particularly with the use of topical anesthetics such as lidocaine. Today it is hard to imagine practicing urology and urologic pathology without PSA and multiple biopsies.

A greater number of prostate biopsies are obtained currently, and more biopsy cores are submitted than ever before, creating a huge interpretive burden for the pathologist. It is estimated that more than one million biopsies are performed annually in the United States, with each biopsy consisting of on average about 10 to 12 cores, creating an estimated ≥10 million prostate tissue samples for the pathologist to interpret.

This burden is compounded by several factors that have increased the difficulty in prostate interpretation. First, many patients now undergo biopsy for elevated serum PSA with no other clinical evidence of cancer, resulting in an enormous number of biopsies that often contain only a small or microscopic suspicious focus. Second, numerous diagnostic pitfalls and mimics of prostate cancer have been described or refined, including postatrophic hyperplasia and IDC (see earlier in this chapter and Chapter 8). The great number of prostate biopsies being generated magnifies the risk for encountering rare or unusual lesions and the potential for misinterpretation of small foci. The concept of ASAPS was introduced in the late 1990s, accounting for about 2% of biopsy diagnoses.[302] Finally, ≥10 biopsies (≥5 from each side) have largely replaced the single bilateral cores of 20 years ago and the sextant biopsies from 10 years ago, providing multiple specimens from each patient.

Detecting Cancer: Factors That Influence Diagnostic Yield in Biopsies

How can we improve the yield of cancer from prostate needle biopsies? Table 9.18 describes the known variables that influence the diagnostic yield of prostate biopsies. Fixed, uncontrolled factors included patient-related factors and prostate-related factors; however, biopsy method-related factors are controllable by the urologist and pathologist to increase the diagnostic yield of cancer and are thus deserving of additional consideration.

TABLE 9.18	Factors That Influence the Detection Rate of Cancer in Contemporary Prostate Needle Biopsies

Uncontrolled Factors

Patient risk factors
    Patient population (e.g., screening population versus urologic practice)
    Patient symptoms
    Serum prostate-specific antigen
    Clinical stage
    Patient age
    Patient race
    Prior biopsy findings (e.g., prostatic intraepithelial neoplasia, atypical small acinar proliferation)
Prostate-related factors
    Prostate volume
    Transrectal ultrasound and other imaging findings

Controlled Factors

Urologist-controlled factors
    Number of needle cores obtained
    Method of biopsy (e.g., random, ultrasound-guided, magnetic resonance imaging–targeted, etc.)
    Location of biopsy (e.g., laterally directed biopsies versus midline, etc.)
    Amount of tissue obtained (e.g., biopsy "gun" used; operator skill)
Pathologist-controlled factors
    Histotechnologist's skill in processing and cutting prostate biopsies
    Number of needle cores embedded per cassette
    Number of tissue cuts obtained per specimen
    Pathologist's skill in prostate biopsy interpretation

Number, Length, and Location of Needle Cores Obtained

The increase from 6 to 12 cores improved prostate cancer detection by 29%, and all were greater than 0.5 cm^3 in volume.[389] By obtaining 10, 12, and 13 core biopsies, cancer detection rates increased by 26%, 22%, and 35%, respectively.[390,391] The number of biopsy cores correlates with probability of prostate cancer detection (Fig. 9.20).[392,393] Saturation biopsy (often defined as >12 or 16 cores) may be of greatest value in men with persistent suspicion of cancer after negative initial biopsy and in those with ASAP or multifocal PIN.

Cancer detection rate with the routine 18G biopsy needle (40%) is similar to that with the narrower 20G needle (35%), but pain is significantly less with 20G.[394] The diagnostic yield of biopsy is improved by ultrasound-targeted or MRI-fusion–targeted biopsies, but the magnitude of the increase in accuracy remains controversial. Use of a 29-mm cutting length increases cancer yield 18% above that of a 19-mm cutting length, although the correlation of length and cancer yield has been contested.[395,396] The combination of six transperineal and six transrectal biopsies resulted in cancer detection of 49%, and the detection rate increased 7% and 9% compared with the transperineal and transrectal groups alone, respectively.[397] Increased core length per container improves cancer detection rate and Gleason score accuracy, and 12-mm cores have optimal sensitivity (42%) and specificity (62%) for cancer detection.[398-402] Transperineal mapping biopsies are more accurate in determining clinical risk than transrectal biopsies and are less likely to induce sepsis, but transrectal biopsies are more popular in Europe than the United States.[403,404] Template-guided transperineal saturation biopsy detects 64% of clinically significant cancers.[405] Most of the undetected lesions are those with small volume. Approximately 20% to 30% of patients have clinically significant undetected lesions in a different lobe or different quadrant from the detected lesions in the biopsy.

Quantitation of cancer length in biopsies is discussed in the following paragraphs.

The detection rate of cancer in biopsies is higher with longer cores, particularly at the apex.[406] For example, a 20-mm core from the right apex has 27% probability of cancer detection versus 18% for 10 mm. Only 1% of single-core biopsies are longer than 20 mm. The amount of tissue obtained by biopsy varies widely, and cumulative core sample (likely to be an inadequate sample) is less than 50 mm in 4% of biopsies.[406] The dependence of diagnosis on tissue length is strongest at the apex. Nonglandular sampling is directly associated with shorter core lengths, with a 6-mm minimum threshold.[407] Most urologists now routinely obtain at least 10 to 12 specimen vials per biopsy for prostate biopsies.[393]

Lateral mid-gland and lateral base biopsy cores have the highest cancer detection rates for all prostate volumes, perhaps because of extensive sampling of the peripheral zone by lateral biopsies. Mid-gland and base biopsy cores have a relatively low yield, especially in small prostates, because of sampling of the central zone, where prostate cancer incidence is known to be low.[390]

Overall cancer detection rate with saturation biopsy is 44%, increasing to 52% with additional biopsies of the anterior apical region.[408] Cancer detection rate increases 23% with a modified sextant protocol by directing the needles only into the more lateral aspect.[392] Conversely, ultrasound-directed biopsies may be omitted when using 10-core biopsy protocols because the yield of these biopsies was less than 2%.[390] Rebiopsy detection rate is higher with 20 rather than 12 cores.[409]

Magnetic Resonance Imaging–Transrectal Ultrasound-Guided Fusion–Targeted Biopsies

Multiparametric magnetic resonance–transrectal ultrasound fusion–targeted biopsy may improve accuracy of: (1) detection rate of clinically significant cancer previously missed by TRUS biopsy; (2) identification of extraprostatic extension (EPE); and (3) categorization of aggressiveness based on diffusion-weighted imaging.[410-416] Accuracy is influenced by interobserver variability in imaging interpretation.[417,418] As a triage test, there may be a substantial number of false-negative cases with clinically significant cancer, suggesting that transperineal systematic biopsy may be superior for triage.[419] Combining multiparametric magnetic resonance–transrectal ultrasound fusion–targeted biopsy with systematic biopsy improves the diagnostic accuracy of either single modality without increasing the rate of insignificant prostate cancer.[420-423]

Histotechnologist's Skill in Processing Biopsies

Prostate biopsies are particularly difficult to embed and cut because of their small size and tendency to fragment and curve. Flat embedding of the biopsy cores enhances the amount of tissue that is examined by the pathologist. Laboratories that process prostate biopsies with other tissues of differing density and consistency (e.g., breast biopsies with abundant fatty tissue) usually handle all specimens the same way, optimizing results for some tissues but often resulting in prostate biopsies that are too thick to interpret or are overstained. Excessively thick tissue specimens are two or three cells in thickness rather than the optimal one to two cells in thickness, precluding adequate assessment of nuclear and cytoplasmic details in foci of concern. Similarly, overstained sections (the most common problem in our consultation practice) contain obscured nuclear chromatin without recognizable nucleoli. These problems are compounded in biopsies with small foci that are suspicious for malignancy and in younger patients (those in their 40's and 50's) who have abundant proliferative epithelium that may mimic malignancy. The problems noted here apply doubly to interpretation of high-grade PIN and ASAP, accounting for both overdiagnosis (the most common mistake in current practice, in our experience) and underdiagnosis. Separate processing of the delicate prostate needle cores is recommended by the European Society of Uropathology.[424]

Number of Needle Cores Embedded per Cassette

Multiple needle biopsies submitted in one or two containers tend to entangle and fragment and are difficult to embed in a single

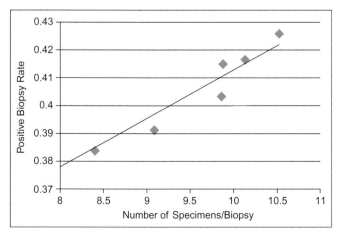

Fig. 9.20 Correlation between positive biopsy rate and number of specimen vials/biopsy.[393]

plane during processing. The resulting loss of tissue surface area makes a definitive diagnosis difficult in many cases, resulting in equivocal pathology reports.[280] If multiple cores are embedded in one cassette, it is necessary to take care that all are separated. We carefully embed up to six cores in parallel arrays per cassette after differential inking and find the cancer yield equivalent to one core per cassette with significant reduction in labor cost and effort.[425] In a study from Finland, there was no significant difference in cancer detection rate when up to nine cores were embedded per cassette.[426]

Number of Tissue Cuts Obtained per Specimen

There is variation between laboratories in the number of serial tissue cuts obtained from each needle core for routine examination. To avoid the serious problem of undersampling, we routinely obtain six separate cuts (two adjacent sections from three separate levels) from the paraffin block for H&E staining; additional intervening sections are placed on another slide and saved for immunohistochemical stains or special studies (Fig. 9.21). We consider the recommendation of the European Randomized Study of Screening for Prostate Cancer to be inadequate (they recommend only two cuts in total), probably missing up to 3% of cancers with such limited sampling.[427,428] In our experience, recutting the block for additional levels with small suspicious foci is useful in about one-half of cases, with usually no more than four additional slides before the tissue specimen is exhausted. Rogatsch et al. compared

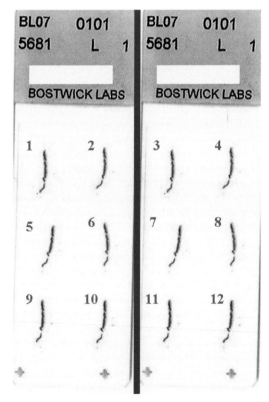

Fig. 9.21 Bostwick Laboratories' prostate biopsy slide protocol. A total of two slides are obtained, each with six tissue slices. One is stained with hematoxylin and eosin (H&E), and the second is held unstained for subsequent immunostain or, as in this case, a second H&E-stained section. The red numbers indicate the order in which the sections are placed on the slides to ensure optimal comparison of each of the two slides and standardization in every case.

biopsy cores submitted floating free in formalin with those that were stretched and oriented at biopsy and before formalin fixation, and found that the diagnostic rate of cancer increased from 24% to 31%.[429]

Future Trends in Biopsies

Select future trends in biopsy handling and clinical significance are presented in Table 9.19. Precise localization of cancer by site-specific labeling and three-dimensional mapping of extended saturation biopsies enables the use of targeted focal therapy such as cryosurgery.[430-432] Quality-assurance measures should focus on the quantity and quality of biopsy samples. The ultimate goal of cancer detection—prediction of outcome for the individual patient—can be augmented by advanced methods of database analysis, such as artificial intelligence.[376,433,434] Furthermore, there is continuing improvement in the definition and treatment of clinically insignificant cancer. Finally, molecular biology is beginning to revolutionize the field of diagnostic pathology.

Fine Needle Aspiration

Interest in FNA in the United States is minimal because of the ease of acquisition and interpretation of the 18G needle core biopsy. Both techniques have similar sensitivity in the diagnosis of prostatic adenocarcinoma, and both are limited by small sample size; they are best considered as complementary techniques. Complications of FNA occur in less than 2% of cases and are like those with needle core biopsy including epididymitis, transient hematuria, hemospermia, fever, and sepsis.

FNA produces clusters and small sheets of epithelial cells without stroma.[435] This enrichment for epithelium allows evaluation of single-cell morphology and the relationship between cells. Benign and hyperplastic prostatic epithelium consists of orderly sheets of cells with distinct margins creating a honeycomb-like pattern. Benign nuclei are uniform with finely granular chromatin and indistinct nucleoli; basal cells are often present at the edge. Prostatic carcinoma is distinguished from benign epithelium by increased cellularity, loss of cell adhesion, variation in nuclear size and shape, and nucleolar enlargement (Fig. 9.22). A recent case of prostatic synovial sarcoma was diagnosed by FNA and confirmed by fluorescent in situ hybridization (FISH) analysis for *SYT* rearrangement on the cell block.[436]

TABLE 9.19	Trends in Biopsy Reporting and Clinical Application

Location of Prostate Cancer

Site-specific labeling
3D mapping
Focal therapy

Quality Assurance in Urology

Quality of biopsies
Number of biopsies
Quality assurance in urologic pathology

Personal Outcome Predictions

Use of neural networks and advanced measures of outcome
Improved understanding of "clinically insignificant" cancer

Molecular Diagnostics From Needle Biopsies

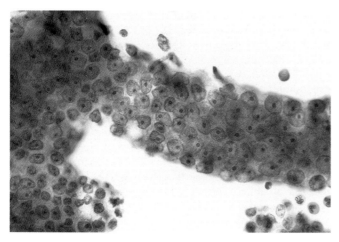

Fig. 9.22 Moderately differentiated prostatic adenocarcinoma on fine needle aspiration.

Transurethral Resection

The regions of the prostate sampled by TURP and transrectal needle biopsy tend to be different. TURP specimens usually consist of tissue from the transition zone, urethra, periurethral area, bladder neck, and anterior fibromuscular stroma. Occasionally, TURP specimens may also contain small portions of seminal vesicle tissue. Radical prostatectomies performed after TURP show that the resection does not usually include tissue from the central or peripheral zones, and not all of the transition zone is removed. Most needle biopsies consist only of tissue from the peripheral zone, seldom including central or transition zones.

The role of TURP in dealing with urinary obstructive symptoms has declined in the past decade because of the introduction of ablative techniques such as the yttrium-aluminum-garnet (YAG) laser, as well as prostate-reducing medications such as 5α reductase inhibitors (e.g., finasteride, dutasteride).

The incidence rate of cancer in TURP specimens for nodular hyperplasia is about 5%.[437] Well-differentiated adenocarcinoma found incidentally in TURP chips usually has arisen in the transition zone (Fig. 9.23). These tumors are frequently small and may be completely resected by TURP. Transition zone cancer location is associated with better biochemical recurrence-free survival.[438]

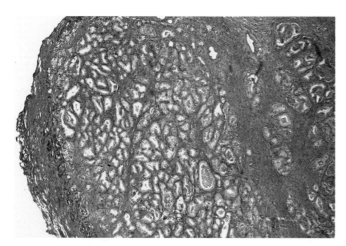

Fig. 9.23 Gleason grade 1 adenocarcinoma (pseudohyperplastic pattern) in transurethral resection.

Poorly differentiated adenocarcinoma in TURP chips usually represents part of a larger tumor that has invaded the transition zone after arising in the peripheral zone.

TMPRSS2:ERG and *ETV1* are upregulated in acini in the peripheral zone compared with the transition zone, and these fusions account for 50% to 80% and 20% of prostate cancers, respectively. These results indicate that the benign and neoplastic glands of the two zones display distinct molecular differences and zonal-specific expression, and that *ERG* and *ETV1* may play a role in the development and progression of cancer.[439]

The optimal number of chips to submit for histologic evaluation is a minimum of six cassettes for the first 30 g of tissue and one cassette for every 10 g thereafter.[440]

Prostatic Enucleation (Suprapubic Prostatectomy; Adenectomy)

In patients with massive benign hyperplasia, open surgical enucleation may be preferred to TURP. The specimen usually consists exclusively of transition zone tissue and periurethral tissue with grossly visible nodules.

Radical Prostatectomy

There are two main surgical approaches to prostatectomy. The first, retropubic prostatectomy, is the most popular approach in the United States, allowing staging of lymph node biopsies with frozen section evaluation before removal of the prostate when desired. The second surgical approach, perineal prostatectomy, does not allow lymph node biopsy during the same operation because of the anatomic approach used. Refinements in technique include nerve-sparing prostatectomy, robotic prostatectomy, and laparoscopic prostatectomy, all of which are gaining greatly in popularity.

The completeness of pathologic examination of prostatectomy specimens affects the determination of pathologic stage (Tables 9.20 and 9.21).[441-445] Partial sampling results in missing 29% of cases with positive margins and 20% of those with EPE.[446,447] There is an increase in positive surgical margin rate (12% versus 59%, respectively) and pathologic stage with complete sectioning compared with limited sampling (sections of palpable tumor and two random sections of apex and base).[448] Complete sectioning shows a higher detection rate of EPE (34% versus 55%, respectively) and seminal vesicle invasion (8% versus 15%, respectively) than lesser methods of sampling, even in prostates removed as part of a cystoprostatectomy.[449,450] Complete sectioning also correlates with greater cancer-free survival in organ-confined and specimen-confined cases. Sehdev et al. compared 10 different methods of prostatectomy sampling using complete sectioning as the gold standard and favored two partial sampling methods (Fig. 9.24) that balanced the extra time and expense of additional sections versus the risk of missing important predictive information.[441] The first method was submission of every posterior section plus one midanterior section from right and left sides; if either of these anterior sections shows sizable tumor, all ipsilateral anterior slides are examined. This method detects 98% of tumors with Gleason score ≥7, 100% of positive margins, and 96% of cases with EPE (mean, 27 slides). The second method is the same as the first but with submission only of sections ipsilateral to the previous positive needle biopsy. This method detects 92% of tumors with Gleason score ≥7, 93% of positive margins, and 85% of cases with EPE (mean, 17 slides).

The presence and extent of EPE in clinical stage T2 adenocarcinoma (and hence clinical staging error) is also related to the number of blocks processed. Current guidelines for the evaluation of

TABLE 9.20 Sample Surgical Pathology Report

Tissue Description

Prostate (5.5 × 3.8 × 3.5 cm) and seminal vesicles (4 × 3.2 × 1 cm) are submitted and weigh 40 and 15 g, respectively. Tumor is identified grossly involving both sides of the prostate extensively, chiefly on the right.

Pelvic lymphadenectomy tissue (right, 5.5 × 3 × 1 cm and 3 × 1 × 1 cm; left, 4.5 × 2 × 1 cm and 3 × 0.5 × 0.5 cm) submitted separately.

Diagnosis

Radical retropubic prostatoseminovesiculectomy:

ADENOCARCINOMA (GLEASON GRADE 4 + 3 = 7). ISUP 2014 GRADE GROUPING 3. GLEASON PATTERN 4 COMPRISES 60% OF THE CANCER. TERTIARY PATTERN 5 COMPRISES 5% OF THE CANCER.

Size: about 27.72 cm3

Location: bilateral peripheral zone and transition zone

Resection margins: negative

Perineural invasion: extensive

Capsule: bilateral invasion and extensive multifocal right-sided extraprostatic extension (cumulative 1.1-cm linear length)

Premalignant change: patchy high-grade prostatic intraepithelial neoplasia

Pelvic lymph nodes: metastases to 2 of 9 right and 1 of 6 left pelvic lymph nodes

Apex: involvement of the right anterior and posterior and left posterior quadrants without extension to the margin

Bladder base: negative

Seminal vesicles: positive on the right side

Vascular/lymphatic invasion: extensive

Other: nodular hyperplasia

DNA content (flow cytometry): tetraploid (block C8; 60% cancer)

TNM (2017 revision) stage: T3bN1M: not applicable

ISUP, International Society of Urological Pathology.

---

radical prostatectomy specimens emphasize information that should be included in the pathology report but leave the decision regarding partial or complete sampling to the pathologist.[376,451] The 2009 ISUP consensus conference recommended standardization of pathology reporting of prostatectomy specimens. In response to the question relating to how much of the prostate should be blocked, participants considered both partial and complete embedding of prostates to be acceptable if the method of partial embedding is stated. Pathologists have to balance the extra costs and time involved in processing entire specimens against the risk of missing important prognostic information.[452]

All methods begin with weighing the specimen and measuring in three dimensions: apical to basal (vertical), left to right (transverse), and anterior to posterior (sagittal), with the maximum length of each dimension recorded.[452] Prostate weight with and without the seminal vesicles should be recorded.[452,453] For ultrasonographic measurements, radiologists often describe the shape of the prostate as a prolate ellipsoid (length × height × width × 0.532), but this is only a rough estimate that shows considerable variability. Separate measurements are made of the seminal vesicles.

The gland should be fully fixed before sectioning. Several inking systems are available. It is recommended that a minimum of two different colors be used to secure correct left-side and right-side identification.[452] The number of colors may be increased to three or four to facilitate identification of anterior and posterior. The adhesion of the ink is subsequently improved by immersing the specimen in acetone or Bouin fixative.

The apical and bladder neck margins are a common location for positive margins and EPE. The cone method is preferred for blocking the apex and the base.[452] A thick section is amputated from the apex and the base, then cut and embedded sagittally. Sagittal slicing offers the advantage over radial slicing of producing uniform thickness tissue blocks. The shave method of the apical margin is no longer recommended because it causes either underdiagnosis or overdiagnosis of positive margins. Assessment of EPE is also more difficult with shave margin blocks. However, thin shave margins at the base are not as undesirable as apical shave margins. The bladder neck margin consists of thick muscle bundles outside of the prostate, so a positive thin shave margin at this site indicates EPE.

The remaining specimen is serially sectioned at 4 to 5 mm thickness by knife to create transverse sections perpendicular to the long axis of the prostate from the apex to the tip of the seminal vesicles. Partial and complete sampling differ by the amount of prostate tissue submitted.

The Bostwick Laboratories protocol using whole mount sections for preparing and reporting prostatectomy specimens is illustrated with multiple examples in Fig. 9.25. Complete and careful submission of tissue for histologic evaluation allows the following: unequivocal orientation of specimen and tumor (left, right; transition zone, peripheral zone; anterior, mid, posterior; apex, base, etc.); evaluation of the extent and location of positive surgical margins; assessment and quantitation of the extent and location of EPE and seminal vesicle(s) invasion; quality-control data for the surgeon, particularly in regard to surgical margins in nerve-sparing or robotic prostatectomy. This method also facilitates postoperative measurement of tumor volume for correlation with imaging studies, as desired; evaluation of tumor grade (percentage of poorly differentiated adenocarcinoma); fulfillment of all recommendations by the Cancer Committee of the College of American Pathologists; and comparison of results with published studies.[444,454-456]

Standard template protocols are useful because of the frequent multifocality of prostatic adenocarcinoma, the inability to fully identify the location and extent of tumor by examining randomly chosen tissue slices, and the inability to grossly identify positive surgical margins and EPE. Despite our personal preference for complete submission, most pathologists undertake partial submission, and this is practical for most cases, does not require special processing or large cassettes, and provides all necessary clinical information.

Pathologic Interpretation

Gross Pathology

Gross identification of prostatic adenocarcinoma is often difficult or impossible, and definitive diagnosis requires microscopic examination. In TURP specimens, adenocarcinoma is often difficult to identify grossly because of the confounding macroscopic features of nodular hyperplasia. In prostatectomies, adenocarcinoma tends to be multifocal, with a predilection for the peripheral zone. Grossly, apparent tumor foci are at least 5 mm in greatest dimension and may appear yellow-white with a firm consistency because of stromal desmoplasia (Fig. 9.26) that stands in sharp contrast with the normal spongy parenchyma.

Gross assessment of cancer diameter usually underestimates the microscopic extent. Of cancers that are identified grossly, 30% are tan, 30% white, 16% yellow, and 24% orange.[457] Transition zone cancer is most often orange (61%), whereas peripheral zone cancer is usually tan or white (35% and 33%). All macroscopically identifiable cancers are poorly circumscribed. Among substantial (large)

TABLE 9.21 Protocol for Processing Radical Prostatectomies

Frozen Sections of Lymph Nodes During Surgery

This is optional and at the discretion of the treating surgeon. If frozen sections are requested, then all lymph nodes and perinodal adipose tissue are submitted for evaluation. Permanent sections of all frozen tissue should be obtained.

Radical Prostatoseminovesiculectomy

Each prostate is weighed, measured in three dimensions, and inked. Inking is performed by coating with India ink (or another preferred color) and rapid (1-2 seconds) immersion in acetone to create ink adherence to the tissue. Some use more than one ink to mark different anatomic sites (e.g., left and right sides).

Apex and Base

Conization or shave margins are acceptable at the discretion of the pathologist; however, each pathologist is encouraged to use only one of these methods for all of their cases. Cancer involving the apex or base is not considered EPE even if the margins are positive (exception: when adipose tissue is present and cancer is in contact).

Conization Margins

* After fixation, the apex and base are amputated at a thickness of about 4 mm. The apical slice is divided into four quadrants, and each is serially sectioned at 3-mm intervals in the vertical parasagittal plane, similar to a cervical conization specimen, and submitted separately. The section from the bladder base is sectioned in a similar manner, although the amount of tissue was usually less, with divisions as hemispheres rather than quadrants. Cancer touching ink is considered a positive margin. For conization the apex usually requires quadrant sectioning, and we routinely use abbreviations for the right anterior apex (RAX), left anterior apex (LAX), right posterior apex (RPX), and left posterior apex (LPX). Similarly, the base is sampled, usually into left and right halves as left bladder base (LBB) and right bladder base (RBB), respectively. Advantages include greater localization of the cancer and determination of proximity to the margin when the margin is negative.

Shave Margins

* A thin, translucent shaving of the entire face of the apex and face of the bladder should be taken. Any evidence of cancer in these specimens indicates a positive margin. Advantages include encompassing the entire surface of the apex and base for analysis.

Seminal Vesicles

The seminal vesicles are amputated from the prostate at the junction of the two organs without incising the prostate itself; a slice encompassing each seminal vesicle at this junction should be submitted for routine histologic examination. If cancer is identified in the seminal vesicles or adjacent soft tissues, then the seminal vesicles should be serially sectioned in a manner similar to the prostate and submitted entirely for histologic review.

Prostate

The prostate is serially sectioned as thinly as possible (about 4- to 5-mm-thick sections) by knife in a coronal plane perpendicular to the long axis of the gland from the apex of the prostate to the site of the amputated seminal vesicles. Orientation and ordering of the slices are maintained throughout to allow spatial reconstruction later of the prostate. The transverse sections are submitted in total for routine processing through neutral-buffered formalin (or equivalent alternative fixative) and sectioning as whole-mount sections (preferred) or after subdivision into two parts, four parts, or more, depending on the size of each slice. A record should be maintained so that the prostate can be reconstructed at histologic review. Routine sections should be stained with hematoxylin and eosin.

Protocol for Results Reporting of Radical Prostatectomies

Volume of Prostate

The volume of the prostate is calculated using the formula for a prolate ellipsoid, defined as length × height × width × 0.532 (correction factor for a prolate ellipsoid); no shrinkage correction factor is necessary because these measurements are made in fresh specimens.

Cancer and Ablated Tissue Volume, Location, and Extent

On each slide the exact outlines of carcinoma and ablated tissue are dotted in different color inks. The area of EPE is measured by an ink line drawn along the prostatic surface, and sites of positive surgical margins are indicated with a plus (+) sign.

Cancer volume is calculated by the grid method. In brief, a transparent grid of premeasured squares is placed over the slides, and the number of squares overlying carcinoma is counted; the total number of squares per case is multiplied by the area of each square, and the sum is multiplied by the thickness of each slice of the prostatectomy. Slice thickness is calculated by dividing the fresh tissue measurement of the long axis of the prostate minus 4 mm for conization (accounts for apical section amputation) (2 mm for shave margins) by the total number of slices of the prostate. To include the volume of cancer in the apical and basal sections, the number of grids overlying cancer from these sections is multiplied by 0.09 cm² and then by 0.5 cm (section thickness). Final cancer volume is multiplied by 1.25, to account for tissue shrinkage caused by fixation.

The area of EPE for each case is calculated as the sum of measured line lengths on traced slides multiplied by the section thickness. The volume of tumor in the seminal vesicles is calculated by multiplying the number of grids overlying tumor in the muscular wall of the seminal vesicles by the section thickness. Positive surgical margins are defined as ink touching tumor cells (or foci of ablation); the number of separate foci with positive surgical margins is evaluated. Determinants of pathologic staging include evaluation of seminal vesicle involvement (unilateral or bilateral, as well as volume of tumor), EPE (unilateral or bilateral, as well as sites of perforation and area of EPE), and lymph node involvement (unilateral or bilateral, as well as number of nodes involved). Do not use focal versus established terminology.

The orientation of the long axis of the tumor is determined, as well as the greatest diameter of the predominant tumor nodule. Tumor location and ablated tissue location are recorded as transition zone and/or nontransition zone, with no attempt to determine precise site of tumor origin because of significant overlap of tumor and multifocality. The number of tumor foci and ablated tissue foci are counted; tumor >2 mm from a tumor nodule is considered a separate focus by convention. Perineural invasion and vascular/lymphatic invasion are considered focal (present in less than three separate foci when evaluated by ×400 microscopic fields) or extensive (three or more foci involved).

Cancer Grade

The following variables are evaluated: Gleason primary pattern, Gleason secondary pattern, Gleason score (sum of the primary and secondary patterns), and ISUP grade grouping. The percentages of Gleason primary patterns 4 and 5, and the sum of primary patterns 4 and 5 are estimated in 10% increments. The Gleason grading scheme is noted (e.g., classic Gleason grading, ISUP 2005 modification, ISUP 2014 modification).

EPE, Extraprostatic extension; *ISUP,* International Society of Urological Pathology.

---

cancers, transition zone cancer is less frequent than cancer in the peripheral zone (33% and 13%, respectively).

Mucinous (colloid) carcinomas may have a variegated appearance and are often softer than the adjacent prostate. Similar gross findings may be caused by tuberculosis, granulomatous prostatitis, and acute and chronic prostatitis.

Microscopic Pathology

Microscopically, most prostatic adenocarcinomas are composed of small acini arranged in one or more patterns. Diagnosis relies on a combination of architectural and cytologic findings, and may be aided by ancillary studies such as immunohistochemistry. The single most important consideration is whether there are

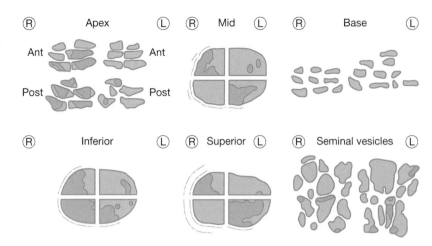

Fig. 9.24 Partial sampling protocol for preparing and reporting prostatectomy specimens.

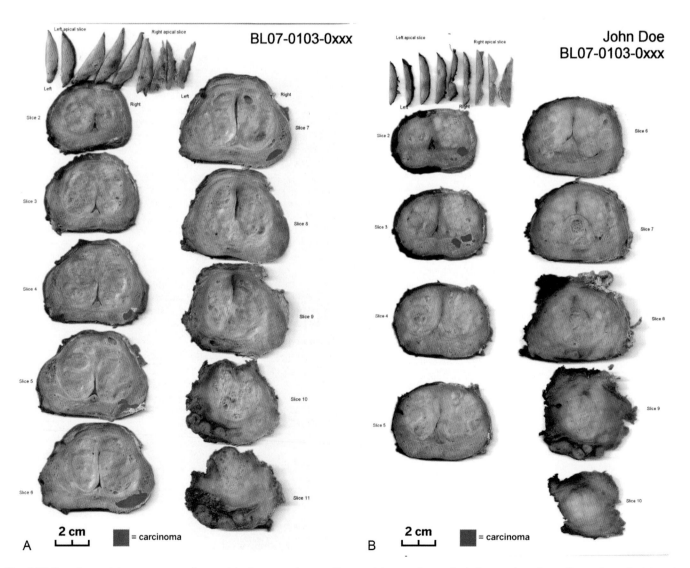

Fig. 9.25 Sample prostate cancer maps for prostatectomy specimens with complete sampling and whole-mount sections. Cancer is marked in red. (A) Unilateral, unifocal, organ-confined cancer. (B) Unilateral, multifocal (apparently), organ-confined cancer (pathologic stage T2aN0M0).

(Continued)

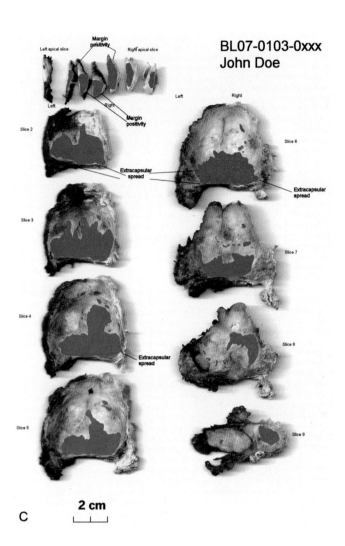

Fig. 9-25, cont'd (C) Bilateral, multifocal cancer with multifocal bilateral extraprostatic extension, seminal vesicle invasion, and multiple positive apical surgical margins.

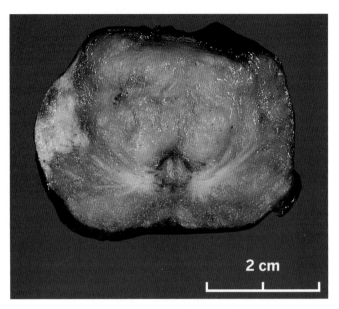

Fig. 9.26 Gross appearance of prostatic adenocarcinoma. Large firm yellow tumor mass is grossly visible on one side, but microscopic foci were present throughout the peripheral zone bilaterally. The yellow color is due to abundant cytoplasmic lipid in tumor cells, which was confirmed histochemically.

discrete single acini or fused masses, thereby distinguishing Gleason patterns 3 and 4, respectively (see later).

Architectural features are assessed at low- to medium-power magnification, with variation in size, shape, and spacing of acini (Fig. 9.27). The acini in suspicious foci are usually small or medium, with irregular or elongate contours that stand in contrast with the smooth contours of normal prostatic acini. Variable acinar size is of value, particularly when there are small, irregular, abortive acini with primitive lumens. Comparison with adjacent benign acini is always of value. The arrangement of the acini is diagnostically useful; malignant acini often have an irregular haphazard arrangement, sometimes splitting or distorting muscle fibers in the stroma, with variable spacing between acini. The stroma frequently contains young collagen that appears lightly eosinophilic, and desmoplasia may be prominent, although this is an uncommon and unreliable feature when assessed in isolation. An understanding of the Gleason grading system is of value for interpretation of small foci because of its reliance on architectural patterns (see later). Gleason taught that cancer could usually be identified by its pattern at low magnification ($10\times$), and that high-power magnification was best used to confirm the diagnosis

and avoid misdiagnosis of mimics by identification of tell-tale cytologic and luminal features (DG Bostwick, personal communication, 1984).

Cytologic features of adenocarcinoma include nuclear and nucleolar enlargement, and these features are important for the diagnosis of malignancy (Fig. 9.28). Enlarged nuclei are typically present in most malignant cells, and enlarged nucleoli are present in many. Every cell has a nucleolus, so one searches for "prominent" nucleoli, which are at least 1.25 to 1.50 μm in diameter; of greatest importance is the ratio of nucleolus to nucleus and comparison with adjacent benign acini. The identification of two or more nucleoli is virtually diagnostic of malignancy (or PIN), particularly when the nucleoli are eccentrically located and abutting the chromatinic rim. A study of three-dimensional nuclear chromatin texture revealed significant difference between PIN and its mimics.[458] Overstaining of nuclei and other artifacts may obscure nucleoli, creating diagnostic difficulty. Size of nucleoli in ASAP is a positive predictor of subsequent detection of adenocarcinoma.[459]

The basal cell layer is absent in adenocarcinoma, an important feature that may be difficult to evaluate in routine sections stained with H&E. Compressed stromal fibroblasts may mimic basal cells but are usually only seen focally at the periphery of acini. An intact basal cell layer is present surrounding benign acini, whereas carcinoma entirely lacks a basal cell layer. Sometimes, small foci of adenocarcinoma cluster around larger acini that have intact basal cell layers, compounding the difficulty. In difficult cases it may be useful to employ monoclonal antibodies directed against high-molecular-weight CK (e.g., clone 34βE12) and p63 to evaluate the basal cell layer.

Cancer-Associated Pathologic Findings

Luminal Mucin
Acidic sulfated and nonsulfated mucin is often seen in acini of adenocarcinoma, appearing as amorphous or delicate threadlike basophilic secretion (Fig. 9.29).[460-463] This mucin stains with Alcian

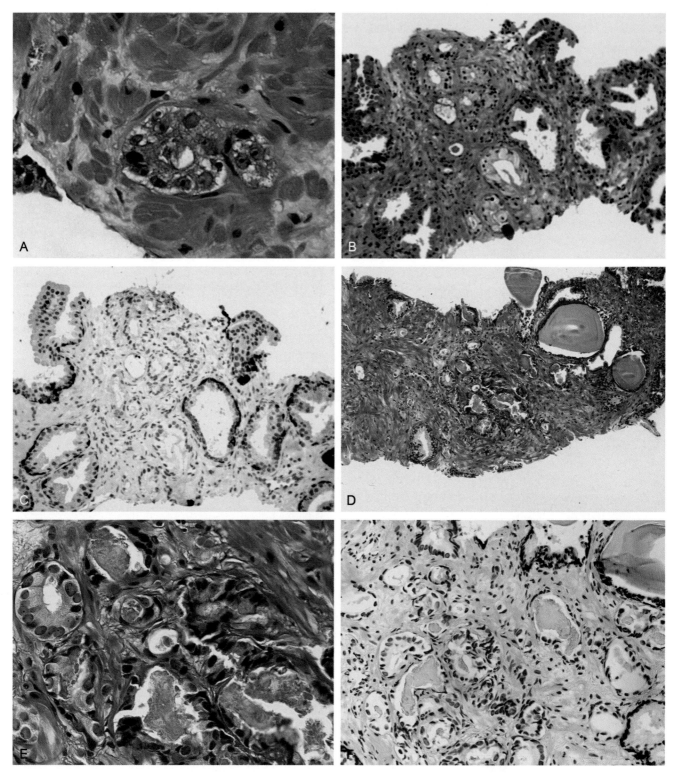

Fig. 9.27 Minimum criteria for the diagnosis of cancer on biopsy. (A) Microscopic focus contains acini with variation in size, shape, and spacing. Triple immunostain (not shown) revealed racemase staining, as well as absence of p63 and keratin 34βE12 staining. Irregular loose cluster of small to intermediate acini, including a few with foamy cytoplasm (*bottom*) that stand in contrast with the adjacent benign acini (B and C). This was diagnosed as "foamy gland prostatic intraepithelial neoplasia" at another medical center without obtaining immunostains. Compare with (C) (triple immunostain), in which there is absence of racemase staining, as well as p63 and keratin 34βE12, with intense immunoreactivity for adjacent benign acini (internal positive control). This immunoprofile effectively excludes prostatic intraepithelial neoplasia from consideration and, in combination with the architectural abnormalities, is diagnostic of adenocarcinoma (Gleason 3 + 3 = 6) with focal foamy gland pattern. (D to F) Another minimal cancer, confirmed by absence of keratin 34βE12 staining in (F).

(Continued)

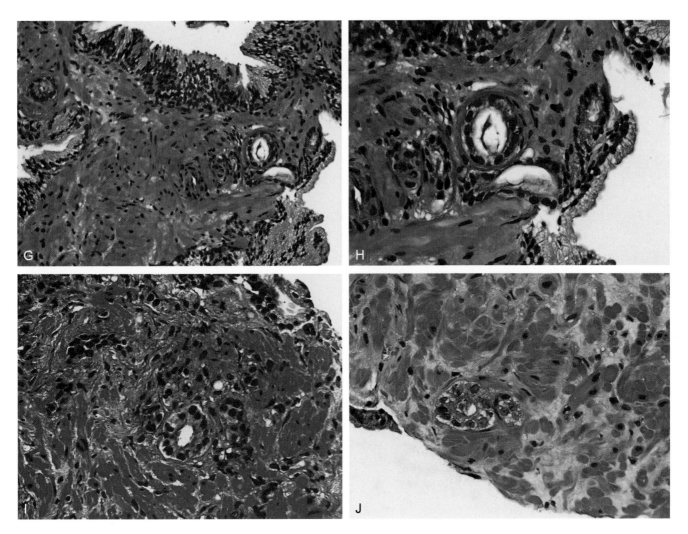

Fig. 9-27, cont'd Other cases of minimal cancer (G to J).

blue and is best demonstrated at pH 2.5, whereas normal prostatic epithelium contains periodic acid–Schiff (PAS)–reactive neutral mucin. Acidic mucin is not specific for carcinoma and may be found in PIN and rarely in BPH.[464] The predominant acidic mucin is sialomucin, and O-acetylation expression is inversely correlated with cancer grade.[465] Expression of episialin, also known as MUC1, may correlate with Gleason grade and microvessel density.[466,467]

Luminal Proteinaceous Secretions

Ill-formed secretions are more often found in the lumens of suspicious and cancerous acini than benign acini, varying from pale pink and scant to brightly eosinophilic and extensive (Fig. 9.29).[302] Although a nonspecific finding, the abundance of luminal secretions in prostate cancer is often distinctive and should spur the search for other cytologic features of malignancy. Proteinaceous secretions are often found in association with crystalloids and corpora amylacea.

Crystalloids

Crystalloids are sharp rhomboid or needle-like eosinophilic structures that are often present in the lumens of well-differentiated and moderately differentiated carcinoma (Fig. 9.29).[151,273,295,468]

They are not specific for carcinoma, and can be found in other conditions such as atypical adenomatoid hyperplasia.[469] The presence of crystalloids in metastatic adenocarcinoma of unknown site of origin is strong presumptive evidence of prostatic origin, although it is an uncommon finding.[470,471]

The pathogenesis of crystalloids is uncertain, but they probably result from abnormal protein and mineral metabolism within benign and malignant acini, including loss of acidity.[472] Ultrastructurally, they are composed of electron-dense material that lacks the periodicity of crystals, and x-ray microanalysis reveals abundant sulfur, calcium, phosphorus, and a small amount of sodium.[295] Seminal vesicles also contain inspissated secretions in many cases, including 24% of cases with predominantly crystalloid morphology.[472]

Collagenous Micronodules

Collagenous micronodules are a specific but infrequent and incidental finding in adenocarcinoma, consisting of microscopic nodular masses of paucicellular eosinophilic fibrillar stroma that impinge on acinar lumens (Fig. 9.29).[473] They are usually present in mucin-producing adenocarcinoma and result from extravasation of acidic mucin into the stroma. Collagenous micronodules are present in 2% to 13% of cases of adenocarcinoma and are not

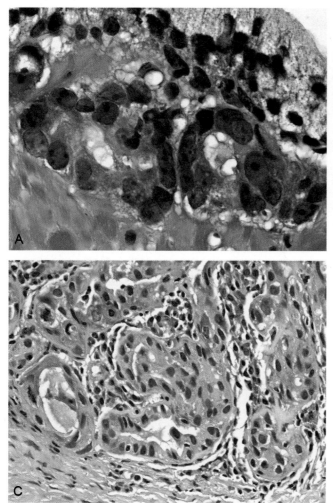

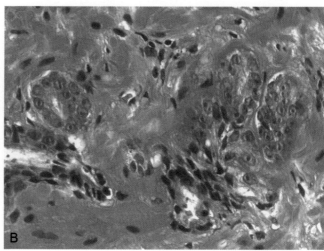

Fig. 9.28 Nuclear and nucleolar enlargement in prostate cancer (A and B). The focus of adenocarcinoma (*left*) displays marked nuclear and nucleolar enlargement when compared with adjacent benign epithelium (*right*). (C) Another case of prostate cancer with variability in size and hyperchromasia of nuclei.

observed in benign epithelium, nodular hyperplasia, or PIN.[474] They are an infrequent finding, present in 1% of needle biopsies and 13% of prostatectomies.[474,475]

They are composed predominantly of collagen fragments admixed with basement membrane material.[476] Ultrastructurally, they consist of fragmented banded collagen fibrils. Collagenous micronodules are formed by subepithelial accumulations of fragmented collagen fibers, possibly related to the digestion by collagenase produced by prostatic adenocarcinoma cells. The term *mucinous fibroplasia* has been erroneously applied by some to collagenous micronodules, but these micronodules are often not associated with mucin, so this term should be abandoned.

Perineural Invasion

PNI is the major mechanism of cancer spread outside the prostate and is present in 17% to 38% of biopsies; in some cases it is the only evidence of malignancy (Figs. 9.29 and 9.30).[474,477,478] This finding is strong presumptive evidence of cancer, but is not pathognomonic because it can occur rarely with benign acini. Complete circumferential growth, intraneural invasion, and ganglionic invasion are almost always limited to cancer. However, benign acini can rarely mimic cancer with perineural indentation, tracking, wrapping, or even intraneural spread, so caution is warranted in relying on this feature to the exclusion of all others.[479] PNI usually indicates tumor spread along the path of least resistance and does not represent lymphatic invasion. Perineural cancer cells acquire a

survival and growth advantage using the nuclear factor-κB survival pathway, so targeting PNI might retard local cancer spread and possibly influence survival.[334] Neural cell adhesion molecule is upregulated in nerves with PNI.[480]

Routine light microscopy is usually sufficient to identify prostatic nerves.[481] However, in difficult or equivocal cases, immunohistochemistry for epithelial membrane antigen (EMA) and S-100 protein may be of value in separating PNI from perineural indentation.[482] Normal peripheral nerves are continuously encircled by perineurium, which is immunoreactive for EMA. Three patterns of EMA immunoreactivity with PNI were observed in a large series of radical prostatectomies: discontinuity or complete loss of the perineurium (55% of cancers), acini in the perineural space or peripheral nerves (25%), and no changes in the perineurium (20%). In one study, no acini were observed in the perineural space with benign acini.[482]

One-half of patients with PNI on biopsy have EPE at prostatectomy, but it has no independent predictive value for stage after consideration of Gleason grade, serum PSA, amount of cancer on biopsy, or positive surgical margins.[478,483-485] About 24% of experienced academic urologists use PNI status to guide nerve-sparing surgery.[486]

The predictive value of PNI in biopsies appears to vary with different treatments. It is an independent adverse predictive factor for patients treated by external beam radiation therapy, but only in patients with pretreatment serum PSA less than 20 ng/mL,

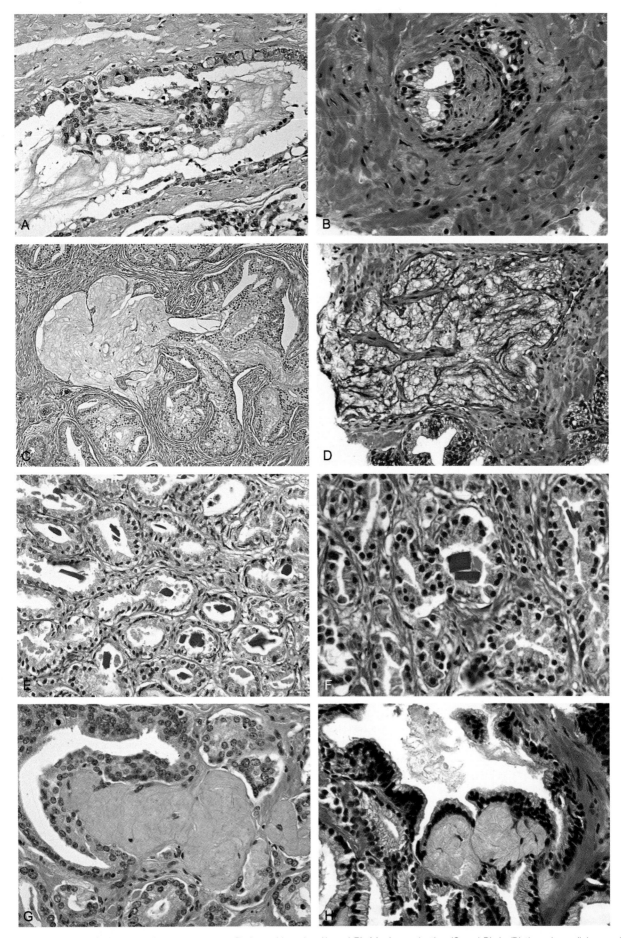

Fig. 9.29 Ancillary histologic features of prostate cancer. Perineural invasion (A and B). Mucin production (C and D). In (D) there is acellular mucin that, on levels, was shown to contain cells of mucinous carcinoma (not shown). Crystalloids (E and F). Collagenous micronodules (G and H).

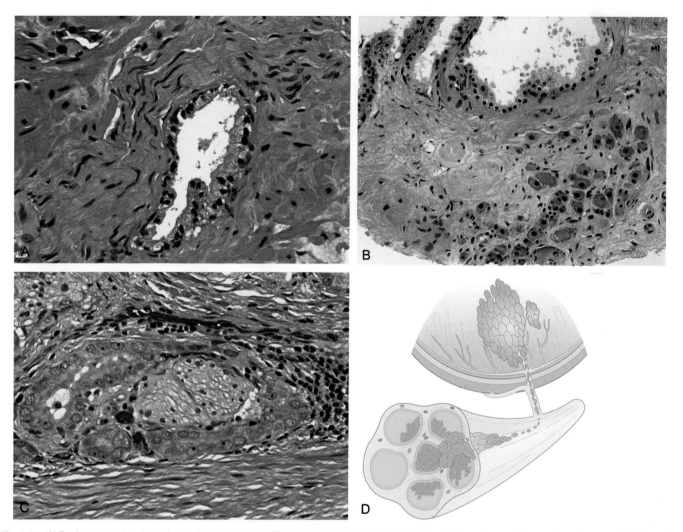

Fig. 9.30 (A) Benign prostatic acinus abuts a large nerve twig. (B) Intraprostatic ganglion cells initially misinterpreted as high-grade carcinoma. (C) Perineural invasion by adenocarcinoma. (D) Prostatic cancer invading neurovascular bundles (artist's rendering).

suggesting that the poor prognosis associated with elevated PSA overrides any additional information that PNI may provide.[487,488] PNI is not a significant predictor of biochemical recurrence in patients undergoing brachytherapy for prostate cancer.[477,489] PNI is predictive of recurrence-free survival after prostatectomy in univariate analysis, but usually not in multivariate analysis.[490-497] PNI was identified in 28% of patients after magnetic resonance–ultrasound fusion–targeted 12-core biopsy and predicted biochemical recurrence after surgery.[498-500] The predictive value of PNI has been recently reviewed.[501]

PNI was found in 46% of prostatectomy specimens, of which 74% had unifocal and 26% had multifocal PIN; an increased risk for biochemical recurrence was observed in those with multifocal PNI.[502] The diameter of PNI may be an independent predictor of cancer volume and cancer recurrence, but was not predictive of outcome after brachytherapy.[489,503,504]

Lymphatic and Vascular Invasion

LVI is defined as the unequivocal presence of tumor cells within endothelial-lined spaces with no underlying muscular walls or the presence of tumor emboli in small intraprostatic vessels. Only a few studies have attempted to distinguish between lymphatic and vascular channels because of the difficulties in differentiation by

light microscopic examination.[505,506] Stains directed against endothelial cells such as factor VIII–related antigen, CD31, CD34, D2-40, or *Ulex europaeus* may increase the detection rate.[505]

LVI is considered negative when findings are equivocal, or cancer cells merely encroach on a vascular space. Mimics include retraction artifact and PNI, cancer impinging on vascular space without actual transendothelial invasion, tangential sections of blood vessels, displacement of benign and collapsed malignant acini, retraction with erythrocytes, intravascular degenerating tumor cells, malignant glands in atrophic ducts, and rarely, myofibroblastic proliferation in thrombosed vessels.[507] Use of antibodies specific for lymphatic endothelial cells (D2-40, directed against podoplanin) revealed that intratumoral lymphatic vessel density was lower than that of the peritumoral and normal prostate compartments; peritumoral lymphatic vessel invasion had a better correlation with the presence of lymph node metastases than intratumoral lymphatic vessel invasion.[508,509]

LVI is associated with pathogenic germline DNA-repair gene mutations.[369]

Tumor present only within endothelial-lines spaces in the muscular wall of the seminal vesicles was considered as pT3b by 50% of the participants at the 2009 ISUP Conference. However, 59% report the presence of tumor in a lymphatic space adjacent to a

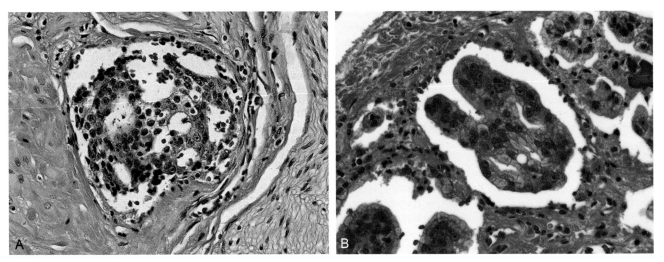

Fig. 9.31 Microvascular invasion. Note the red blood cells at the periphery of the lumen (A and B).

lymph node as a negative lymph node with a specific comment that others may report this finding as positive.[510]

LVI in biopsies usually indicates malignancy, and its presence correlates with grade and stage, although it is sometimes difficult to distinguish from fixation-associated retraction artifact of acini.[505,506] Definite LVI is present in 6% of cases and equivocal LVI in 3%; both are associated with other adverse pathologic features, including advanced stage, higher Gleason grade, and positive surgical margins.[511] LVI, present in 10% to 38% of prostatectomy specimens, is commonly associated with EPE and lymph node metastases (62% and 67% of cases, respectively) (Fig. 9.31).[505,506,512,513] There was no evidence of lymphangiogenesis. The lack of coexpression of podoplanin and receptor-3 in some lymphatic vessels suggests that there is a heterogeneous population of lymphatic endothelial cells in the prostate.[514]

LVI appears to be an important predictor of outcome after prostatectomy and carries a twofold to fourfold greater risk for tumor biochemical recurrence, progression, and death, especially when accompanied by reactive stroma.[506,511,515-522] Five-year biochemical-free survival is 38% to 76% and 84% to 87% for patients with and without LVI after surgery, respectively.[512,513] However, LVI may or may not be an independent predictor of progression when stage and grade are included in the analysis after surgical or radiation therapy.[506,523-525] LVI of the seminal vesicles is also predictive of tumor progression and lymph node metastases.[526]

Microvessel Density (Angiogenesis)

There is a significant increase in microvessel density in PIN and carcinoma when compared with benign tissue or atypical adenomatous hyperplasia (Fig. 9.32), although this assertion has been contested.[219,527-534] This increase correlates with the expression of angiogenic factors VEGF and basic fibroblast growth factor (bFGF), and the receptors FLK/KDR and Flt-1.[535] Increased microvessel density is probably related to the production of proangiogenic growth factors.[536-538] Recent studies found that CD105, Tie-2/Tek, and VEGF receptor (VEGFR) were the best markers of neoangiogenesis.[539] Microvessel density can be accurately measured in core biopsies when compared with matched prostatectomies.[540]

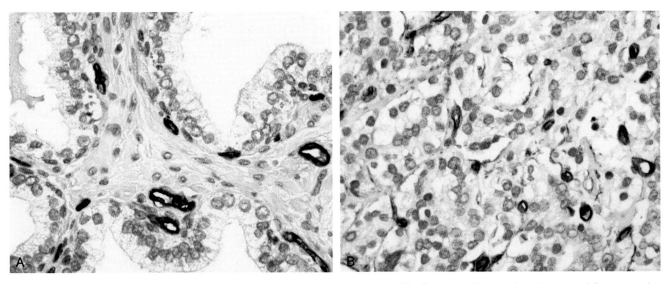

Fig. 9.32 Microvessel density in benign prostate (A) and high-grade adenocarcinoma (B). Brown reaction product decorates delicate vasculature (CD34 immunostain).

Microvessel density is lower in transition zone cancer than peripheral zone cancer and declines in those treated with androgen deprivation therapy.[541,542] The 5α-reductase inhibitor finasteride induces prostate apoptosis and reduces tissue vascularity by inhibiting epithelial cell adhesion, and these effects occur within 2 weeks of onset of therapy.[543,544]

Most studies found a positive correlation of microvessel density with Gleason grade and pathologic stage.[527,535,545-547] Microvessel density in cancer on biopsy showed a positive correlation with matched prostatectomies and was an independent predictor of EPE.[106,547] The bulk of evidence favors the relationship of microvessel density and cancer stage, although variance exists between methods and patient cohorts. Mean blood vessel count is higher in tumors with metastases than in those without metastases, and most, but not all, studies demonstrate a correlation with pathologic stage.[528-530,548-550] Increased microvessel density contributes to extraprostatic spread of adenocarcinoma, perhaps by facilitating microvascular invasion, and also promotes survival of distant metastases because tumor cells can shift angiogenic balance within the distant target. Microvessel density appears to be an independent predictor of cancer progression.[548,551-554] In patients treated by surgery or external beam radiation therapy, microvessel density and microvascular invasion predicted biochemical failure, but this has not always been confirmed by other studies.[506,517,528,548,550,552,554-560]

Glomeruloid microvascular proliferation in prostate cancer correlates with microvessel density, aggressive tumor behavior, and reduced survival in multivariate analysis.[561]

Significant Problems in Interpretation

Atypical Small Acinar Proliferation

In some needle biopsies, a proliferation of small acini is found that is highly suggestive of carcinoma but falls below the diagnostic threshold for adenocarcinoma (see Chapter 8). This is often caused by the small size of the focus, distorted acini with architectural features of malignancy that lack convincing cytologic features, and acinar atrophy or prominent inflammation in which the adjacent benign acini show distortion and reactive atypia with nuclear and nucleolar enlargement. In such cases, it may be appropriate to describe the case as "small acinar proliferation suspicious for but not diagnostic of malignancy" and to suggest rebiopsy. Such lesions are found in up to 3% of needle biopsies. In view of the serious consequences of the diagnosis of adenocarcinoma, it is prudent to diagnose adenocarcinoma only when one has absolute confidence in the histologic findings. A wide variety of lesions may mimic adenocarcinoma, particularly in small specimens (Table 9.22).

TABLE 9.22	Differential Diagnosis of Prostatic Adenocarcinoma
Atrophy	
Postatrophic hyperplasia	
Basal cell hyperplasia	
Atypical adenomatous hyperplasia	
Sclerosing adenosis	
Nephrogenic metaplasia	
Verumontanum mucosal gland hyperplasia	
Hyperplasia of mesonephric remnants	
High-grade prostatic intraepithelial neoplasia	
Intraductal carcinoma	

Prostatic Intraepithelial Neoplasia Versus Large Acinar Variant of Gleason Grade 3 and Intraductal Carcinoma

PIN encompasses the spectrum of dysplastic cytologic abnormalities within preexisting structures in the prostate that are invested with an intact basal cell layer (see earlier). In contrast, the large acinar variant of Gleason grade 3 carcinoma, including the cribriform pattern of IDC, does not have a circumferential basal cell layer and is almost always associated with areas of small acinar adenocarcinoma. In equivocal cases, diagnosis may be aided by staining with basal cell–specific antibodies to high-molecular-weight keratin 34βE12.

Clear Cell Pattern of Carcinoma Versus Benign Acini

Numerous forms of adenocarcinoma contain clear cytoplasm (Fig. 9.33). Adenocarcinoma arising in the transition zone characteristically contains clear cells and is well or moderately differentiated. In contrast, Gleason grade 3 and 4 carcinomas often contain cells with clear cytoplasm, previously referred to as the hypernephroid pattern. In addition, therapy such as androgen deprivation induces abundant clear cell change in benign and carcinomatous acini, and the diagnosis of adenocarcinoma in such cases may be difficult (see discussion later in this chapter). The clear cell pattern of carcinoma may be confused with histiocytes, vacuolated stromal smooth muscle cells, and metaplastic cells.

"Vanishing" Prostate Cancer in Radical Prostatectomies

Radical prostatectomies have no residual cancer (stage pT0) in less than 1% of cases, but this incidence may be increasing because of an upswing in the number of patients receiving preoperative androgen deprivation therapy (5% incidence), which causes apparent cancer volume reduction or even complete ablation.[562-564] Also, with increased vigilance, prostate cancer is now being detected at smaller volume and lower stage than ever before.[318,565-570] It is highly unlikely that biopsy alone can completely ablate a focus of prostate cancer, although this possibility has been considered.[570] Variance in the handling of prostatectomy specimens, including partial submission, may increase the risk of the "vanishing" cancer phenomenon. When this issue arises, it is recommended that all remaining tissue be submitted for histologic analysis to minimize the concern for incomplete sampling.

Genotypic analysis to verify patient identity in cases of "vanishing" cancer appears prudent to reassure patients.[318,569] The inability to identify residual cancer in prostatectomy specimens raises the question of accuracy of the original diagnosis. In one report, biopsies were overdiagnosed as cancer in two of four cases with no residual cancer after prostatectomy.[318]

In a series of 38 patients with pT0 cancer from totally embedded prostatectomies, we found that none experienced clinical evidence of cancer recurrence with a mean follow-up of almost 10 years.[565] Furthermore, those who died of other causes had no evidence of prostate cancer at the time of death. Another report found that 11% of patients experienced recurrence and one had systemic progression, but that retrospective report consisted chiefly of partially and incompletely sampled prostate.[562]

Grading

Histologic grade is a strong prognostic factor in prostatic adenocarcinoma. Since the 1920s, numerous grading systems have been proposed since the pioneering work of Brodersmore, and all successfully identify well-differentiated adenocarcinoma, which progresses slowly, and poorly differentiated adenocarcinoma, which

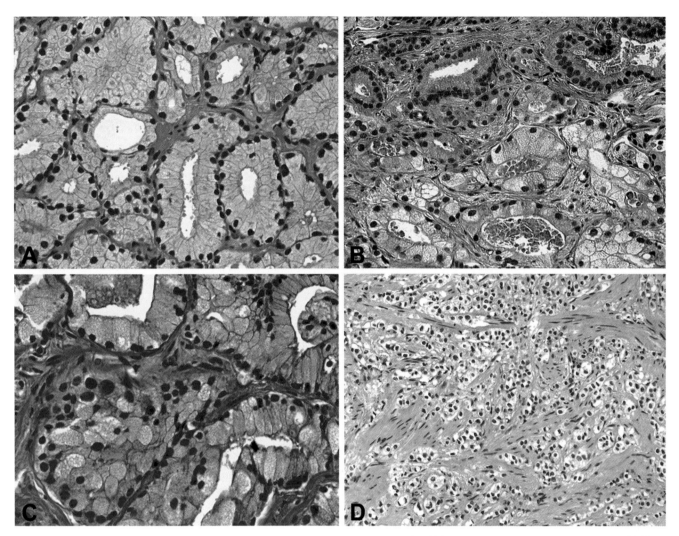

Fig. 9.33 Clear cell patterns of adenocarcinoma. (A) Gleason 2 + 2 = 4 cancer with clear cells. (B) Gleason 3 + 3 = 6 cancer with clear cells. (C) Gleason 3 + 3 = 6 with foamy gland pattern. (D) "Hypernephroid" (clear cell) pattern of Gleason 4 + 4 = 8 cancer.

progresses rapidly. However, grading systems are less successful in subdividing most moderately differentiated adenocarcinomas that have intermediate clinical and biologic potential. Since 1999, Gleason grading is the recognized international standard for prostate cancer grading and, in our experience, is now routinely used by most pathologists around the world.[25,451,571]

Problems with grading include interobserver and intraobserver variability, and imprecise predictive value. In biopsies, these problems are compounded by small sample size, tumor heterogeneity, and undergrading of biopsy samples.[572,573] Also, significant histologic changes in adenocarcinoma occur as a result of radiation and androgen deprivation therapy. The sections that follow describe the current role of grading in prostatic adenocarcinoma, including reproducibility, possible improvements in grading such as the ISUP 2005 and 2014 modified Gleason grading systems, correlation of biopsy grade with prostatectomy grade, the influence of treatment on grade, and correlation of grade with anatomic and biochemical markers of progression.

Gleason Grading System

The Gleason grading system resulted from the Veterans Administration Cooperative Urological Research Group study of more than 4000 patients between 1960 and 1975.[574,575] It is based on the

degree of architectural differentiation (Table 9.23; Fig. 9.34). Tumor heterogeneity is accounted for by assigning a primary pattern for the dominant grade and a secondary pattern for the nondominant grade; the histologic score is derived by adding these two patterns together. Early studies described the addition of the clinical stage (1 to 4 scale) to create the Gleason "sum," but this did not achieve widespread use and was abandoned decades ago. Nuclear grade was also originally considered for inclusion by Gleason but added only minimal incremental predictive accuracy for patient outcome beyond the architectural patterns and was discarded to avoid complexity (DG Bostwick, personal communication with DF Gleason, 1996).

The success of the Gleason grading system is due to four factors: (1) histologic patterns are identified by the degree of acinar differentiation without relying on morphogenetic or histogenetic models; (2) a simplified and standardized drawing is available; (3) the Veterans Administration study provided abundant prospective information that allowed objective computer-generated development of this self-defining grading system; and (4) unlike any other grading system in the body, the Gleason system provided for tumor heterogeneity by identifying primary and secondary patterns.

The Gleason score is a scalar measurement that combines discrete primary and secondary groups into a total of nine discrete

					Architecture
Pattern	**Peripheral Borders**	**Stromal Invasion**	**Appearance of Glands**	**Size of Glands**	**of Glands**
1	Circumscribed pushing, expansible	Minimal	Simple, round, monotonously replicated	Medium, regular	Closely packed rounded masses
2	Less circumscribed; early infiltration	Mild, with definite separation of glands by stroma	Simple, round, some variability in shape	Medium, less regular	Loosely packed rounded masses
3A	Infiltration	Marked	Angular, with variation in shape	Medium to large	Variable packed irregular masses
3B	Infiltration	Marked	Angular, with variation in shape	Small	Variable packed irregular masses
3C	Smooth, rounded	Marked	Papillary and cribriform	Irregular	Round to elongate masses
4A	Ragged infiltration	Marked	Microacinar, papillary, and cribriform	Irregular	Fused, with chains and cords
4B	Ragged infiltration	Marked	Microacinar, papillary, and cribriform	Irregular	Fused, with chains and cords
5A	Smooth, rounded	Marked	Comedocarcinoma	Irregular	Round to elongate masses
5B	Ragged infiltration	Marked	Difficulty to identify gland lumens	Irregular	Fused sheets

TABLE 9.23 Gleason Grading System for Prostatic Adenocarcinoma: Histologic Patterns

groups (scores 2 to 10). Optimal grading creates a continuum that incorporates the findings of a variety of diagnostic clues, including acinar formation, lumen area, acinar fusion, type of acinar fusion, acinar packing, acinar size, acinar uniformity, thickness of acinar epithelial layer, nuclear size, nuclear variability, nuclear shape, chromatin pattern, and nucleolar size.[576,577] Common misinterpretations in Gleason grading are presented in Table 9.24.

Gleason grade correlates with patient age.[578] The percentage of Gleason score 8 to 10 disease among men aged 50 to 54, 70 to 74, and 80 to 84 years is 9%, 16%, and 29%, respectively, and the percentage of high-risk cancer is 14%, 22%, and 39%.[579]

Intraobserver and interobserver variability reflects the subjective nature of grading, precluding absolute precision, no matter how carefully the system is defined. Nonetheless, significant correlation with virtually every outcome measure attests to the predictive strength and utility of grading in the hands of most investigators, including the classic Gleason grading system.

Intraobserver agreement is exact in up to 78% of cases and ±1 score unit in up to 87%.[575,580] A team of British urologic pathologists found a rate of intraobserver agreement of 77%.[581] Gleason himself noted an exact reproducibility of score in 50% of needle biopsies and ±1 score in 85%.[575]

Interobserver agreement is exact in 60% to 81% of cases and ±1 score unit in up to 86%.[582-587] One study reported a high level of disagreement among three pathologists evaluating well-differentiated and moderately differentiated adenocarcinoma.[588] Another report compared the level of interobserver agreement in a consecutive series of 100 prostatic adenocarcinomas and found complete agreement of Gleason score in only 66% of cases.[589] To perform the analysis, the authors compressed the Gleason scores into three grade groups: 2 to 5, 6 to 7, and 8 to 10. Coard and Freeman demonstrated 60% overall concordance in consensus Gleason scores.[590] The greatest discordance seemed to be in distinguishing Gleason score 6 from 7 and was more frequent among biopsies with low cancer volume, particularly among those with less than 30% involvement of the lobe.

"Substantial agreement" exists among urologic pathologists in Gleason grading of biopsies (κ, 0.56 to 0.70).[583] "Nonconsensus" cases include low-grade cancer, cancer with small cribriform proliferation, and cancer whose histology is on the border between Gleason patterns. "Moderate agreement" is found with nonurologic general pathologists examining the same cases (κ, 0.44), with consistent undergrading of Gleason scores 5 to 6 (47%), 7

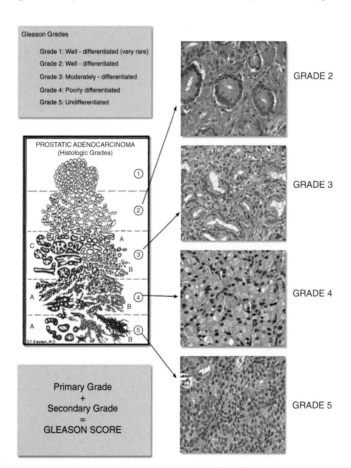

Gleason Grades

Grade 1: Well - differentiated (very rare)
Grade 2: Well - differentiated
Grade 3: Moderately - differentiated
Grade 4: Poorly differentiated
Grade 5: Undifferentiated

PROSTATIC ADENOCARCINOMA
(Histologic Grades)

GRADE 2

GRADE 3

GRADE 4

GRADE 5

Primary Grade
+
Secondary Grade
=
GLEASON SCORE

Fig. 9.34 Gleason grading of prostatic adenocarcinoma.

TABLE 9.24	Four Common Misinterpretations in Prostate Cancer Grading
Misinterpretation	**Comment**
1. If a biopsied focus of cancer is small, it is Gleason grade 1 or 2, or "well-differentiated."	Unlikely! Most cancers (>80% in Gleason's original series) are primary grade 3. When the size is too small to call cancer, *suspicious* is the prudent default. Size of the focus of cancer has no bearing on Gleason grade at prostatectomy.
2. If a biopsied focus is suspicious for cancer, it is best called Gleason grade 1 or 2, or "well-differentiated."	The prudent diagnosis in the absence of sufficient features for cancer is atypical small acinar proliferation. Optimism seems naturally to lead one to consider low Gleason grade; but if there is cancer, it is usually moderately differentiated, because most peripheral zone cancers are moderately differentiated.
3. Confusing the large gland variant of Gleason grade 3 cancer with benign acini.	Cancer acini occasionally are rounded, and medium to large, like benign acini. Look for microvacuolated cytoplasm, nuclear enlargement, and macronucleoli to diagnose cancer.
4. All cribriform acinar formations are Gleason grade 3.	Some cribriform acinar formations are grade 4. These sievelike spaces lose their round, rigid, punched-out contours and elongate; the acini collapse into solid areas.

(47%), and to a lesser extent, 8 to 10 (25%).[584] Agreement among 17 urologic pathologists for "poorly formed glands" is fair (κ, 0.34).[591,592] Poorly formed glands immediately adjacent to other well-formed glands regardless of number and small foci with less than six acini composed of poorly formed glands regardless of location were not graded as Gleason pattern 4. Predictive factors for discordance between local and central pathologist-dependent risk classification included local pathologist-dependent Gleason score 7, lower PSA (≤10 ng/mL), and lower T stage (T1 or T2a).[587]

Recent Trends in Grading

Since the introduction of PSA testing, the incidence of low-grade prostate cancer has declined.[593] Interpretive and chronological biases caused expansion of the moderately differentiated category at the expense of well-differentiated cancer and significant deviation in cancer-specific survival curves.[594,595] One report found that Gleason score rereadings in 2000 to 2002 were higher than the original readings from 1990 to 1992 (mean score increased from 5.9 to 6.8).[596] Consequently, the Gleason score-standardized contemporary mortality rate (1.5 deaths per 100 person-years) appeared to be 28% lower than standardized historical rates (2.1 deaths per 100 person-years), even though the overall outcome was unchanged. This decline in the reported incidence of low-grade prostate cancer appeared to be the result of Gleason score reclassification since the late 1990s, reflecting a statistical artifact known as the "Will Rogers phenomenon."[596] Ghani et al. noted

that all Gleason score 2 to 4 reports were upgraded to Gleason score 5 to 7 cancer.[597]

Since introduction of the ISUP 2005 modified Gleason grading system (see later), the proportion of biopsies with Gleason scores 2 to 4 declined from 21% (1990 to 1994) to 0.2% (2010 to 2013) in national cancer databases (United States).[598] Possible causes include evolving criteria for low-grade cancer and diminution of TURP surgery with lowered sampling of the transition zone.

Interobserver agreement for Gleason grade 4 is high (>80% among 23 urologic pathologists), based chiefly on cribriform and glomeruloid patterns, but rarely on ill-formed and fused glands; complex fused glands seem to constitute a borderline pattern of unknown prognostic significance on which a consensus cannot easily be reached.[599] A recent study using digital images noted highest level of agreement for Gleason score 3 + 3 = 6 (ISUP grade 1), whereas higher grades and particularly Gleason 4 + 3 = 7 (ISUP grade 3) showed considerable disagreement.[600] The presence of cribriform morphology on biopsy is strongly associated with upgrading and upstaging at prostatectomy and shows near-perfect interobserver agreement.[601] Grading is most difficult when cancer was present in multiple biopsies or contained fused patterns.

Interobserver reproducibility of percent grades 4 and 5 is at least as good as that of Gleason score.[602,603]

International Society of Urological Pathology Modifications to the Gleason Grading System

International Society of Urological Pathology 2005 Modified Gleason Grading System

The ISUP 2005 modified Gleason grading system was introduced in an effort to decrease the tendency toward undergrading observed in biopsies by resulting in higher scores for some cases than the classical system.[604] The changes were proposed as a work in progress because of the lack of validation, and meant to apply only to the grading of biopsies, not prostatectomy specimens.

Changes from classic Gleason grading included: (1) the ISUP 2005 modified score consists of the sum of the grade of the predominant pattern of the cancer and the highest grade pattern of the cancer (by comparison, the classic score combines the two most prevalent Gleason patterns); (2) there is no threshold for the amount of the highest pattern of cancer with ISUP 2005 modified Gleason score (the classic Gleason system requires ≥5% of the cancer present to warrant a secondary score); and (3) cribriform pattern is always grade 4 rather than grade 3 or grade 4, resulting in a decline in number and aggressiveness of grade 3 cancer. In addition, the clinical significance of grades 1 and 2 is greatly downplayed and should be used "rarely, if ever," although this suggestion coincided with overall decline in use of TURP because of the rise of medical therapy for nodular hyperplasia.

Reproducibility of the 2005 modified Gleason score (primary grade + highest grade) (see later) was as high as that of Gleason score, but there was clustering in odd scores (scores 5 and 7), and disagreement was more commonly observed than with classic Gleason score.[605] The authors concluded that tertiary Gleason pattern should be better defined. Nonspecialized pathologists were more likely to assign a greater ISUP 2005 modified Gleason score than a urologic pathologist, with a trend to overall Gleason pattern 4.[606]

As expected, the 2005 modified system resulted in upgrading of biopsies from 7.0 to 7.5 (mean, 7.5; κ, 0.44), especially from pattern 3 to pattern 4, diminishing the risk for progression for grade 3 (Gleason 3 + 3 = 6) cancer.[607] The proportion of cancers with score 6 declined from 48%-68% to 22%-39%, score 7 increased from 26% to 39%-68%, and scores ≥7 increased from 32% to 46%.[608-610]

Interobserver agreement among a large group of European urologic pathologists was 58% to 89% (mean, 71%) in ISUP 2005 modified Gleason score 6 cases and 46% to 64% (mean, 56%) in ISUP 2005 modified Gleason score 7 cases.[611] The largest head-to-head comparison of the classic and ISUP 2005 modified Gleason Scoring System was based on 1482 cancer-positive biopsies of the Reduction by Dutasteride of prostate Cancer Events (REDUCE) clinical trial.[612] Scores were independently assigned by two pathologists using the two different systems, with agreement in 83% of cases and 99% of cancers within ±1 of their previous score. Of discordant cases, similar numbers of biopsies were upgraded and downgraded with the two systems, with minor differences in the score distributions. Interobserver agreement was good, ranging from κ 0.62 to 0.70. The overall number of high-grade tumors ($n = 48$) remained constant between reviews, with three fewer score 8 to 10 cancers in the placebo group ($n = 16$) and three more in the dutasteride group ($n = 32$) using the ISUP 2005 modified Gleason scoring system. There was also similar concordance for cancers that received a score of 7 (either 3 + 4 or 4 + 3). Given the similar score distributions, the authors concluded that the modest differences likely reflected variance between pathologists in the interpretation of individual biopsies rather than differences resulting from the scoring system chosen.

ISUP 2005 modified Gleason was associated with reduced risk for cancer progression after surgery compared with classic Gleason grading. Five-year biochemical recurrence-free survival was 34% and 14% in the pre-ISUP 2005 and post-ISUP 2005 groups, respectively, and these differences applied to patients with Gleason scores 6 and 7 (3 + 4).[613] The C-index of the ISUP 2005 system was higher than classic Gleason grading (0.77 versus 0.64) for cancer-specific survival at 10 years postprostatectomy, but that report failed to provide the number of deaths (probably very low), rendering statistical power weak, and the authors misinterpreted classic Gleason score 4 as Gleason 3; also, one wonders why this publication appeared 2 years after the ISUP 2014 Conference in which one of the authors participated.[614]

International Society of Urological Pathology 2014 Modified Gleason Scoring System (Grade Groupings)

The ISUP 2014 Conference on modified Gleason grading introduced multiple changes to the ISUP 2005 modified Gleason grading system (Table 9.25), the most significant of which was grade groupings (Table 9.26), first introduced in 2013 by Pierorazio.[615,616] This new grade grouping system was subsequently adopted in the 2016 WHO tumor classification.[617] The new system used data from multiple large-scale databases to compress the ISUP 2005 modified Gleason grading system into five grade groupings according to the correlation with biochemical/clinical recurrence, disease-specific survival, and overall survival in patients treated by prostatectomy. Despite claims that the grade groupings represent a new grading system, it should instead be considered as a compressed derivative of the underlying modified ISUP 2014 Gleason grading system (e.g., grade group 1 is simply another name for ISUP 2014 modified Gleason grade 3 + 3 = 6, etc.). Although referred to as a consensus conference, the meeting in 2014 was dominated by a single person and not based on systematic review of the literature (DG Bostwick, personal communication, 2014). Subsequent communiqués from the original authors of the grade group system introduced changes that have created complexity and confusion (Table 9.27).

TABLE 9.25	Comparison of International Society of Urological Pathology 2005 and International Society of Urological Pathology 2014 Modified Gleason Grading Systems	
Changes	2005	2014
Name	ISUP 2005 modified Gleason grading system	ISUP 2014 modified Gleason grading system
Grade groups	No	Yes
Tertiary grade	Reported as secondary grade when higher	Revert to original Gleason scoring (tertiary grade reported when present, but not as a replacement of secondary grade[a])
Cribriform pattern[b]	Grade 3 or 4	Exclusively grade 4
Glomeruloid pattern[b]	Grade 3 or 4	Exclusively grade 4
Mucinous adenocarcinoma	Grade 4	Grade 3, 4, or 5 based on architecture

ISUP, International Society of Urological Pathology.
[a]Reverted to classic Gleason grading system. This was the agreement at the ISUP 2014 Conference (DG Bostwick, personal communication; 2014), but it has been refuted in subsequent publications.[1707]
[b]Four main architectural types comprise ISUP 2014 modified Gleason grade 4 cancer: cribriform, glomeruloid, poorly formed, and fused glands.

TABLE 9.26	International Society of Urological Pathology 2014 Grade Groups	
Grade Group	ISUP 2014 Modified Gleason Score	Non-ISUP 2017 Modification of the ISUP 2014 Modified Gleason Score
1	≤6	≤6
2	3 + 4 = 7	3 + 4 = 7
3	4 + 3 = 7	4 + 3 = 7, 4 + 4 = 8
4	4 + 4 = 8, 3 + 5 = 8, 5 + 3 = 8	3 + 5 = 8, 5 + 3 = 8, 4 + 5 = 9
5	4 + 5 = 9, 5 + 4 = 9, 5 + 5 = 10	5 + 4 = 9, 5 + 5 = 10

ISUP, International Society of Urological Pathology.
Confusion has arisen regarding which scores are placed in which groups. This table presents the original ISUP 2014 grade grouping scheme, but others now place some of the scores into different groups (4 + 4 [grade group 3] and 4 + 5 [grade group 4]), creating the non-ISUP 2017 modification of the ISUP 2014 modification (the 2017 modification is not endorsed by the ISUP).[1708,1709]

Remarkably, modified Gleason scores remain unchanged with the ISUP 2014 criteria when compared with the 2005 ISUP criteria. Biopsies in a series of 568 men were graded as score 6, 7, and 8 to 10 in 5%, 35%, and 60% of cases, respectively.[618] Grade groupings were 1, 2, 3, 4, and 5 in 5%, 13%, 22%, 22%, and 38% of cases, respectively.

Interobserver agreement with ISUP 2014 grade grouping among Japanese pathologists is good (κ, 0.64).Overall reproducibility of groups is 71%, with the highest in grade group 5 (85%), grade groups 2 and 3 (77%), and grade group 1 (64%),

TABLE 9.27	International Society of Urological Pathology 2014 Grade Groupings: Advantages and Disadvantages

Advantages

- Lower adverse psychological impact on patients with low-grade cancer (e.g., "You have grade group 1" rather than "You have Gleason 3 + 3 = 6"); labeling the lowest grade category as grade group 1 provides a greater sense of lower risk for disease progression than Gleason score 6 and can strengthen recommendation for active surveillance rather than interventional treatment
- Simplifies presentation of grade with a single number rather than multiple numbers
- Subdivides Gleason score 7 into two prognostically important groups
- Removed confusion regarding tertiary pattern replacing secondary pattern ("best and worst" now replaced by Gleason original reporting of "best and second best," with tertiary included as additional information in reports)

Disadvantages

- "Grade groups" were never endorsed by the ISUP despite claims by some authors to the contrary[1710]
- Dichotomizes continuous variables unnecessarily
- Alters grading criteria to render comparison with previous grading systems difficult or impossible, similar to ISUP 2005 (thus data are not comparable—raises the "comparing apples and oranges" problem)
- Interobserver variability persists from previous grading systems[1711]
- Will require years to be fully "embraced"[629]
- Introduces additional numbers for grade groupings, reported together with Gleason grading, creating confusion (e.g., "You have Gleason 3 + 4 = 7 [grade group 2]" and "You have grade 3 cancer" [Does this mean grade group 3 (4 + 3 = 7) or Gleason 3 + 3 = 6?])
- Original report was not validated and was based on ISUP 2005 modified Gleason grading system criteria[629,1711,a]
- Considerable overlap in grade groupings for outcome[629,d]
- Different rules for needle biopsies and prostatectomies ("Best and worst grades" rule applies only to needle biopsies, similar to ISUP 2005)[629]
- Significant differences in application of ISUP 2014 rules for grading among the original authors[629,c]
- In biopsies, no discussion whether group based on a single core or multiple cores[1711] (example: Gleason 3 + 3 = 6 on one core, Gleason 3 + 4 + 7 on another core; is this case overall group 1 or group 2?)
- In biopsies, no discussion whether group based on an overall global score or worst score[b]
- No agreement on terminology for grouping and grading[629]
- Lack of minimum required amount of pattern 4 cancer to cross threshold from 3 + 3 = 6 to 3 + 4 = 7 (original Gleason grading had 5% threshold) other than "any amount of pattern 4"[628,629,1711]

ISUP, International Society of Urological Pathology.

[a]*Groups 1 and 2 overlap because of small volume of pattern 4 in group 2 cancer tumors with outcome similar to those in group 1. Group 3 and 4 tumors overlap because of combining grade 3 + 5, 5 + 3, and 4 + 4 tumors into group 4. Some of the original authors suggest compressing the 5-bin ISUP 2014 grade groupings into 4 or even 3 bins.[629,1711]*

[b]*In subsequent reports the claim was made that this threshold is 5%, similar to the threshold used by Gleason originally in assigning a secondary grade, but such consensus was never reached at the original ISUP 2014 meeting (DG Bostwick, personal communication, 2014).[629,691]*

[c]*One author contributing to the original report included only 4 + 4 = 8 into group 4, whereas others additionally included 3 + 5 = 8 and 5 + 3 = 8.[629]*

[d]*A subsequent report found no clinical difference in cancer-specific outcome between these two scores after prostatectomy.[1712]*

and the lowest in grade group 4 (61%), indicating to the authors that further improvements are needed.[619]

Prediction of biochemical recurrence is improved with the 2014 system compared with the 2005 system. The 5-year biochemical recurrence-free survival rates are 71% to 96%, 67% to 88%, 26% to 63%, 17% to 48%, and 8% to 26% for grade groups 1 to 5 after prostatectomy.[616,620,621] Causes for the substantial range in these rates are uncertain. For radiotherapy, there is overlap between 4 + 3 and 4 + 4 (grade group 3 and grade group 4, respectively), perhaps because of confounding influence of androgen deprivation therapy.

Grade group 5 includes single cells in 100% of cases, cribriform glands 99%, cords 86%, IDC 78%, comedonecrosis 53%, sheets 49%, small solid cylinders 49%, ductal carcinoma 45%, glomerulations 35%, and solid medium to large nests with rosette-like spaces 14%.[622]

Among men with PSA ≤10 ng/mL and clinical stage T1c/T2a, those with grade group 2 with ≤2 total positive cores have similar rates of adverse pathology and recurrence as men with grade group 1 (Table 9.28).[623] Multivariate analysis confirmed that higher grade grouping was associated with risk for recurrence after prostatectomy, although ISUP grade grouping did not improve predictive value of grading and was less sensitive in separating 3 + 4 and 4 + 3 patterns in prostatectomy specimens.[624-626] Conversely, a study from Australia reported no difference in biochemical recurrence-free survival between biopsy 3 + 3 and 3 + 4 groups.[627] This is especially true when the amount of Gleason pattern 4 is less than 6%.[628] Many of the original authors are now questioning inclusion of Gleason 5 + 3 = 8 as grade group 4 when recent studies indicate that they behave more like grade group 5 cancers.[629,630]

Prediction of cancer-specific survival has shown variable improvement with the ISUP 2014 grade groupings (Table 9.28).[631] A study from the Veterans Administration showed that higher grouping was associated with cancer-specific survival.[632] Using data from the literature, Vollmer estimated the probability of survival was closely related to the new grade groupings.[633] The ISUP 2014 system was a better predictor of cancer-specific death than the 2005 system.[634] Conversely, another report found that grade groups ≥4 in cT3a patients failed to predict cancer-specific survival, although they were independent predictors for biochemical recurrence.[635] Similarly, in a series of more than 500 men initially diagnosed with hormone-sensitive bone metastatic prostate cancer, the ISUP 2014 grade groupings failed to distinguish outcomes (progression and overall survival) in those with grade group 2 (Gleason 3 + 4) and grade group 3 (Gleason 4 + 3) or accurately subdivide Gleason score 7 and Gleason score 8 to 10 patients.[618] A study of men undergoing prostatectomy at the University of Southern California revealed that those with grade group 5 (Gleason 9 to 10) had worse biochemical (hazard ratio [HR], 1.6) and clinical recurrence-free survival (HR, 1.9), but overall survival was the same.[636]

We agree with the recent conclusions of many of the original authors that "ISUP grading categories will require revision in the immediate future."[630] All pathologists using this system should explicitly state whether they are using the ISUP 2005 or ISUP 2014 modified Gleason score to avoid confusion with the classic Gleason scoring system that has remained essentially intact and unaltered since the late 1970s, and has been used successfully in more than 4000 published articles. Remarkably, this repeated recommendation by the ISUP is largely ignored, even by organizers of the ISUP 2005 and 2014 meetings (DG Bostwick, personal communication, 2017). Consequently, "Gleason scores" reported on patient reports or published articles since 2005 may not be comparable because they often use different criteria, a chaotic situation for patients and clinicians compounded by the 2014 changes.

	Patients (n)	Follow-Up, Median (months)	Outcome End Point	Results
Preprostatectomy biopsy				
Berney[1712]	988	Not given	PCSS	HRs: 1, 2.8, 8.1, 7.1, and 12.7 for grade groups 1-5, respectively
Choy[710]	585	60	BRFS	Significant correlation for grade groups 1-3
Dell'Oglio[1713]	9,728[b]	68	CR	HR: 1, 3.6, 5.9, 11.4, and 18.1 for grade groups 1-5, respectively; no additive benefit for grade group over Gleason score
Epstein[616]	16,176	36	BRFS	5-year BFRS: approximately 95%, 81%, 63%, 48%, and 27% for grade groups 1-5, respectively[c]
Ham[1714]	721	36	ACM, PCSS	10-year ACM/PCSS: 17%/88% and 36%/68% for grade groups 4 and 5, respectively
He[1715,d]	119,431	38	PCSS	7-year PCSS: 99.5%, 99.5%, 99%, 98%, and 95% for grade groups 1-5, respectively HRs: 1, 1.1, 1.9, 5, and 10.9 for grade groups 1-5, respectively
Loeb[1716]	4,325	54	BRFS	4-year BRFS: 89%, 82%, 74%, 77%, and 49% for grade groups 1-5, respectively
Mathieu[1717]	27,122[b]	29	BRFS	4-year BRFS: 91%, 82%, 70%, 60%, and 44% for grade groups 1-5, respectively
Pierorazio[615]	7,850	24	BRFS	2-year BRFS: 97%, 91%, 80%, 71%, and 52% for grade groups 1-5, respectively
Samaratunga[1718]	2,079	44	BRFS	Significant correlation of BRFS with grade groups 1-5
Spratt[621]	3,715	53	BRFS	5-year BRFS: 94%, 89%, 73%, 63%, and 55% for grade groups 1-5, respectively HRs: 1, 2, 4.2, 5.6, and 9.3, respectively
Yeong[624]	680		BRFS	Grade group system a stronger predictor than Gleason score
Preradiation therapy biopsy				
Delahunt[7,e]	496	77 (minimum)	BRFS, DMFS, PCSS	ISUP 2014 superior to ISUP 2005 for all end points
Epstein[616]	5,501	36	BRFS	5-year BFRS: approximately 95%, 90%, 80%, 80%, and 63% for grade groups 1-5, respectively[c]
He[1715]	107,148	38	PCSS	HRs: 1, 1.8, 2.9, 5, and 9.9 for grade groups 1-5, respectively
Loeb[1716]	1,555	54	BFRS	4-year BRFS: 95%, 91%, 85%, 78%, and 70% for grade groups 1-5, respectively
Huynh[743]	462	7.6	CSS	Higher PCSS for men with GS 3 + 5/5 + 3 PC than for men with GS 4 + 4 PC, indicating need for subclassification of score 8 with and without Gleason pattern 5
Prostatectomy				
Dell'Oglio[1713]	9,728[b]	68	CR	HR: 1, 5, 10, 15.3, and 25.1 for grade groups 1-5, respectively; no added benefit of grade group over Gleason score
Epstein[616]	20,845	36	BRFS	5-year BRFS: 96%, 88%, 63%, 48%, and 26% for grade groups 1-5, respectively
Erickson (2018)[1709]	831	133	PCSS	Grade group[g] superior to Gleason score for predicting survival
Grogan[634]	635	180	BRFS, CR, and PCSS	Grade group superior to Gleason score in predicting BRFS, CR, and PCSS, but impact as an independent predictor on PCSS in multivariable analysis is not reported
Ham[1714]	1,047	48	ACM, PCSS	10-yr ACM/PCSS: 17%/91% and 37%/71% for grade groups 4 and 5, respectively
Leapman[631]	5,058	81	PCSS	HRs: 1, 1.9, 2.7, 6.1, and 12.6 for grade groups 1-5, respectively
Loeb[1716,f]	4,325	54	BRFS	4-year BRFS: 92%, 85%, 73%, 63%, and 51% for grade groups 1-5, respectively
Mathieu[1717]	27,122	29	BRFS	4-year BRFS: 96%, 87%, 67%, 63%, and 41% for grade groups 1-5, respectively
Pierorazio[615]	7,869	24	BRFS	2-year BRFS: 99%, 94%, 86%, 74%, and 59% for grade groups 1-5, respectively
Spratt[621]	3,715	53	BRFS	BRFS: 96%, 93%, 74%, 64%, and 50% for grade groups 1-5, respectively HRs: 1, 2, 7, 10, and 19, respectively
Yeong[624]	680		BRFS	Grade group system had higher prognostic discrimination than Gleason score

ACM, All-cause mortality; *BRFS*, biochemical recurrence-free survival; *CR*, clinical recurrence; *CSS*, cancer-specific survival; *DMFS*, distant metastasis-free survival; *GS*, Gleason score; *HR*, hazard ratio; *ISUP*, International Society of Urological Pathology; *PCSS*, prostate cancer–specific survival.

[a]Excludes biopsy data from Leapman (2017) because the treatments are combined (preprostatectomy, preradiation, and others). For the combined biopsy cohort the HR for PCSS is 1, 1.8, 2.0, 4.4, and 5.1 for grade groups 1-5, respectively.[631]

[b]For combination of biopsies and prostatectomies.

[c]Data are approximate because they are imputed from figures 2 and 3; raw data were not provided.[616]

[d]Included patients treated surgically and others by radiation therapy.

[e]Included posttreatment androgen deprivation therapy.

[f]Postprostatectomy radiation therapy.

[g]Used 2017 modification of the ISUP 2014 modified Gleason grading system grade groupings.[1709]

Biopsy Versus Prostatectomy Grade

There is significant discordance between needle biopsy and prostatectomy grades. Biopsy underestimates grade in 22% to 45% of patients and overestimates grade in 4% to 32%.[637-642] Study of the Swedish National Prostate Cancer Registry revealed that discordance declined from 45% to 32% between 2000 and 2012, with most of the decrease occurring before publication of the ISUP 2005 modified Gleason grading system.[643] Discordance rate is independent of the number of biopsy cores in systematic biopsy.[644]

Comparison of the ISUP 2014 modified Gleason grade group criteria with the ISUP 2005 criteria revealed a lower risk for upgrading from biopsy to prostatectomy specimens (45% versus 35%, respectively), indicating less potential to miss aggressive tumors.[626,645] ISUP 2014 grade groups of biopsies and prostatectomies are discordant in 45% of cases, with 31% upgrading and 14% downgrading, with high level of variance between different hospitals.[645] Conversely, study of Swedish cases revealed greater discordance with ISUP 2014 grade group when cases from 2000 and 2012 were evaluated (32% versus 43%, respectively).[643]

Interobserver agreement with ISUP 2014 is no better than that with ISUP 2005 (63% versus 64%, respectively).[646]

Grading errors are common in biopsies with small amounts of tumor and low-grade tumor, probably because of tissue sampling error, tumor heterogeneity, and undergrading of needle biopsies when compared with matched prostatectomies.[647,648] One study showed good correlation between biopsy and resection specimens.[638]

For those with low-risk cancer defined by the D'Amico criteria (PSA level <10.0 ng/mL, cT1c-cT2a, and Gleason score ≤6) or the Prostate Cancer Research International Active Surveillance criteria (PSA level ≤10 ng/mL, T1c-T2, Gleason score ≤6, PSA density <0.2 ng/mL^2, ≤2 positive cores), upgrading to Gleason score 4 and 5 cancers occurs in 5% and 4% of cases, respectively.[649] In men followed for 6 years for active surveillance (80% were low risk), rebiopsy revealed upgrading in 31%.[650]

Gleason 3 + 3 = 6 is upgraded in up to 44% to 65% of cases, including 42% to Gleason 3 + 4 = 7, 16% to Gleason 4 + 3, and 7% to Gleason 4 + 4 = 8.[651,652] Another report found upgrading of Gleason score 6 cancer in 33%; variables predictive of upgrading included prebiopsy PSA, highest percentage of cancer at any single biopsy site, PSA density, and prostate volume.[653,654]

Among men with intermediate risk (Gleason 3 + 4 = 7) on biopsy, 13% are upgraded and 17% are downgraded; 17% harbor nonorgan-confined disease, and 25% have unfavorable disease.[655]

Men with high-risk cancer (higher PSA concentration or more positive cores) are more likely to have cancer upgraded at prostatectomy, and obtaining more biopsy cores reduces the likelihood of upgrading.[656-660] Biopsy grading error does not correlate with amount of cancer on the biopsy or with clinical staging error.[661] In one study the accuracy of biopsy was highest for the primary Gleason pattern, but the secondary pattern on biopsy appeared to be sufficiently accurate in predicting prostatectomy grade to provide useful predictive information, particularly when combined with primary pattern to create the Gleason score (Figs. 9.34 to 9.36).[662] Based on these results, Gleason grading is recommended for all needle biopsies, even those with small amounts of tumor, similar to the original recommendation of Gleason.[573] Comparison of Gleason score in biopsies with matched lymph node metastases revealed exact correlation in 40% of cases, ±1 in 76%, and ±2 in 95%.[663] The lack of an anaplastic pattern in metastatic deposits implies that factors other than loss of differentiation were responsible for the ability of the cells to metastasize.

Among patients with Gleason score 8 carcinoma, 45% have downgrading at prostatectomy specimen and a correspondingly more favorable long-term outcome.[664] Predictors of downgrading are lower clinical stage (T1c) and Gleason score 8 in the biopsy specimen. In another report, clinical stage, serum PSA, and biopsy Gleason score had a predictive accuracy of 0.80 for Gleason upgrading between biopsy and prostatectomy.[665,666]

The distribution of cancer grades is not associated with prostate volume.[667] The concordance rate between needle biopsy and prostatectomy of the Gleason scores of the greatest tumor percentage in the core, Gleason score of core with maximal tumor length, and the highest Gleason score were 64%, 62%, and 57%, respectively.[668]

Biopsy-prostatectomy upgrading rate varies between systematic biopsy only, MRI-fusion only, and combined fusion and systematic (41%, 24%, and 14%, respectively).[669] Upgrade from combined fusion and systematic biopsy results was lower in the saturated than in the nonsaturated lesion group (7% versus 18%, respectively).

Ross et al. showed that DNA ploidy analysis of biopsies predicted grade shifting, that it was a more sensitive and specific indicator of final grade at prostatectomy than the original needle biopsy grade, and ploidy status independently predicted postoperative cancer recurrence.[670]

Dedifferentiation

Histologic dedifferentiation has been reported by numerous investigators, but these studies included only cases with more than one resection, probably selecting for adenocarcinoma that is more aggressive and thus more likely to require repeat operation. Brawn reported dedifferentiation in 65% of repeat TURP.[671] Cumming et al. described 74 patients with repeated TURP after a mean interval of 2.4 years; Gleason score remained constant in 12, increased in 49, and decreased in 7, and dedifferentiation occurred in untreated adenocarcinoma and in those subjected to expectant management.[672] Dedifferentiation to high-grade adenocarcinoma is unusual in low-grade (Gleason patterns 1 to 3) small-volume (1 cm^3) adenocarcinoma, occurring in only 2% of patients in 7 years, thereby accounting for the large discrepancy in incidence of clinical cancer among populations with similar prevalence of occult cancer.[673] A study of 67 men with median time to follow-up biopsy of 22 months (range, 7 to 60) found that Gleason score was unchanged in 20 patients (30%), upgraded in 19 (28%), and downgraded in 27 (40%); 21 (31%) had no malignancy on follow-up biopsy.[674] The authors concluded that there is no consistent histologic upgrading on follow-up biopsy at 22 months in untreated, low- to intermediate-grade clinically localized prostate cancer.[675] Conversely, men with Gleason score 3 + 4 on biopsy were almost five times more likely to have upgrading on subsequent biopsy than men with an initial Gleason score of 3 + 3 at 3 years.[676] By the third surveillance year, 63% of men with Gleason score 3 + 4 had been upgraded compared with 18% who started with Gleason score 3 + 3.

Interestingly, in men older than 80 years with PSA concentration greater than 30 ng/mL, at least 97% have cancer and more than 90% have high-grade cancer.[677] Therefore, there may be ascertainment bias if one does not correct for patient age.

Epidemiologic evidence revealed that dedifferentiation is a major mechanism of progression in prostate cancer. Tumors may dedifferentiate during the screen-detectable phase; consequently, screening with PSA and early treatment may prevent dedifferentiation.[678]

There is a trend toward histologic dedifferentiation when prostate carcinoma metastasizes to regional lymph nodes.[679] Gleason score in lymph node metastases is higher than in the primary tumor in 45% of cases, lower in 12%, and matched exactly in 43%. The 5-year progression-free survival is lower in patients with histologic dedifferentiation (88% ±3) and those without dedifferentiation (94% ±2) (P = 0.04); however, dedifferentiation is not associated with progression when adjusted for lymph node cancer volume.

Gleason 3 + 3 = 6 cancer carries a minimal long-term risk for progression or mortality, whereas cancer-specific mortality increases with increasing proportions of the Gleason 4 component in the prostatectomy specimen, from 3 + 3 = 6 with tertiary 4 (i.e., <5% of a Gleason 4 component) to 3 + 4 = 7, 4 + 3 = 7, and 4 + 4 = 8.[680] This means that a smaller proportion of Gleason 4 suggests that the cancer was identified at an earlier phase in the natural history of the disease, and that this component of cancer probably increases in volume more quickly than lower-grade components. Two hypotheses were proposed to account for increasing amounts of Gleason 4 cancer in a prostate specimen: (1) preferential growth of a single clone of

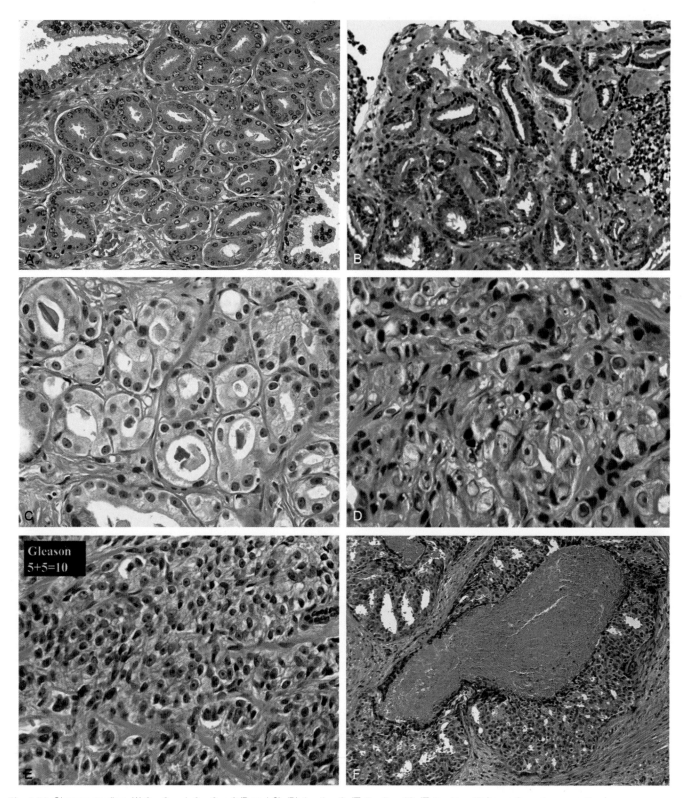

Fig. 9.35 Gleason grading. (A) 2 + 2 = 4. 3 + 3 = 6 (B and C). (D) 4 + 4 = 8. (E) 5 + 5 = 10. (F) 5 + 5 = 10 (comedocarcinoma pattern).

Gleason 4 cells, possibly with intraprostatic spread; and (2) evolution of Gleason 3 cancer cells to become Gleason 4.

Other Proposed Grading Changes
Numerous modifications have been proposed for Gleason grading to improve its discriminative capabilities (Table 9.29).[617,681,682]

Tertiary Grade
In up to 5% of biopsies and 10% of prostatectomies, three separate Gleason grades are encountered rather than the typical one or two.[683] Gleason noted that more than 50% of adenocarcinomas in his series contained two or more patterns.[574,575] Similarly, Aihara et al. found a mean of 2.7 different Gleason grades per case

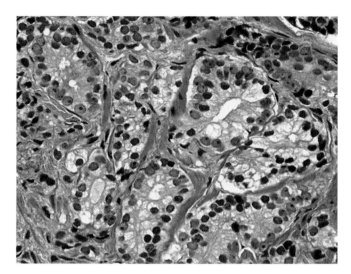

Fig. 9.36 Gleason pattern 3 adenocarcinoma, large acinar type, consisting of an irregular aggregate of rigid angulated acini with variability of size, shape, and spacing.

TABLE 9.29	Contemporary Modifications of Gleason Grading

ISUP 2014 Modified Gleason Score

Grade groupings
Primary and secondary grades are common and second most common
    (revert to original Gleason grading system), respectively
No threshold for amount of highest pattern (no 5% requirement)
All cribriform patterns are grade 4
All glomeruloid patterns are grade 4
Mucinous carcinoma grade according to architecture

WHO 2016

Percent of high-grade adenocarcinoma (Gleason patterns 4 and 5) in 10%
    increments
ISUP 2014 grade groupings

Other Proposed Modifications or Additions

Nuclear grading and morphometric grading
Grade compression
Weighted average of all Gleason scores
Reactive stromal grading
Digital whole-slide scanning and deep learning algorithms

ISUP, International Society of Urological Pathology.

(range, 1 to 5) in prostatectomies, and more than 50% contained at least three different grades.[684] The number of grades increased with greater cancer volume, and the most common finding was high-grade adenocarcinoma within a larger well-differentiated or moderately differentiated adenocarcinoma (53% of cases). Tertiary Gleason pattern 5 was the strongest predictor of an unfavorable outcome in one study of surgically treated patients with Gleason grade 7 carcinoma.[685]

Most urologists want the highest Gleason grade reported by the pathologist, even if it is the tertiary grade (as it almost always is) and accounts for only a small percentage of the cancer volume present in the specimen.[686] Our group has reported tertiary grade for two decades by providing the classic Gleason score as noted earlier and simply adding a statement such as, "In addition, there is a small (5%) tertiary component of Gleason grade 5 present."

The ISUP 2005 modified Gleason grading system includes the sum of the most common grade and the worst grade present to account for cases with three separate Gleason scores.[687] For example, if a prostatectomy has 60% Gleason grade 3 cancer, 35% grade 4, and 5% grade 5, the ISUP grade would be 3 (most common) + 5 (worst grade) = score 8; the classic Gleason score would be 3 (most common) + 4 (second most common) = score 7. However, this was abandoned in the ISUP 2014 system.

Patients with a tertiary pattern on biopsy have a 5-year risk for PSA progression of 37% versus 13% in cases in which no tertiary Gleason pattern was present.[688] Tertiary pattern 5 is an independent predictor of clinical failure after adjusting for pathologic stage, surgical margin status, EPE, and seminal vesicle invasion (HR, 4.0).[683,689] In prostatectomies, there is intermediate risk for biochemical recurrence for men with 3+4 (grade group 2) and 4+3 (grade group 3) with or without tertiary pattern 5 cancer; however, the presence of less than 5% Gleason pattern 5 in those with Gleason score 4 + 4 = 8 (grade group 4) imparts a poor prognosis equivalent to grade group 5.[690,691]

Nuclear Grading and Morphometric Grading

Nuclear and nucleolar enlargements are important diagnostic clues for the diagnosis of malignancy. The West German Pathological-Urological Working Group of Prostate Cancer validated a combined architectural and cytologic grading system that incorporates nuclear and nucleolar features to predict patient outcome and identify best candidates for active surveillance (Table 9.30).[692,693]

TABLE 9.30	Helpap Modification of the Combined Histologic and Cytologic Grading System of West German Pathological–Urological Working Group of Prostate Cancer	
	Score	**Comments**
Architecture		
Well differentiated	0	Includes classic Gleason grades 1, 2, and 3
Moderately to poorly differentiated	1	Includes classic Gleason grades
Cribriform	2	Identical to ISUP 2014 modified Gleason pattern 4
Solid/trabecular	3	Identical to ISUP 2014 modified Gleason pattern 5
Cytology		
Minimal alterations	0	Nuclei: small, round, solitary, homogeneous chromatin Nucleoli: small, solitary and centrally located
Moderate	1	Nuclei: size slightly increased, round, solitary, slightly heterogeneous chromatin Nucleoli: slightly enlarged, still solitary, mostly centrally located
Severe	2	Nuclei: large, polymorph, heterogeneous chromatin Nucleoli: enlarged, mostly multiple, eccentrically located

ISUP, International Society of Urological Pathology.

Morphometric methods allow objective evaluation of nuclear size, roundness, shape, chromatin texture, and other features. Numerous investigators have used morphometry to improve the predictive value of Gleason grading, but these methods are not routinely used.[100,571,694-697] Useful diagnostic features include nuclear enlargement (moderate to marked in 94%), nucleolar enlargement (62%), and nonuniform chromatin distribution (100%), but these do not vary with grade; conversely, pleomorphism (moderate in 59%), nuclear overlapping (63%), nuclear membrane infoldings (66.2%), and irregular contours (frequent in 94%) are significant diagnostic features that increase in frequency and extent with increasing grade.[698] Three-dimensional reconstruction is emerging as a potentially useful tool for determining cancer volume and surface area.[699]

Nuclear roundness has been the subject of considerable interest for more than 20 years, but is not routinely used.[571,694,695] Mean nuclear roundness accurately predicts prognosis in patients with untreated stage T1b prostatic adenocarcinoma. However, many of these reports are limited by small sample size (<30 patients), use of the same patient cohort in multiple publications, failure to describe the morphologic variations and nuclear roundness extremes, and bias in patient selection. Furthermore, significant problems of reproducibility have been encountered, and the results with different digitizing instruments are not comparable. Nuclear roundness predicts recurrence after radiation therapy for well-differentiated adenocarcinoma.[700] The good correlation of morphologic nuclear grade in biopsies and prostatectomies is probably due to the large number of cases that fall into the nuclear grade 2 (of 3) category.

There is similar nucleolar surface area in biopsies and matched prostatectomies in 70% of cases.[701,702] Nucleolar grading has been proposed but has not been adopted (grade 1: large and prominent nucleoli in virtually every cell; grade 2: intermediate; grade 3: tiny nucleoli that are difficult to find).[703]

Machine learning with quantitative phase imaging separated Gleason patterns 3 and 4 cancer with 82% accuracy in prostatectomy specimens.[704,705]

Grade Compression (Dichotomization) and Weighted Average Score

Many authors have simplified the Gleason grading system by compressing (lumping) the scores into groups, usually creating three groups: 2-3-4, 5-6-7, and 8-9-10.[706] Although the ISUP 2014 grade group uses five groups after ignoring primary grades 2, 3, 4, and 5, it suffers from the same loss of data because of compression. For example, grade group 3 + 4 = 7 may harbor 5% to 45% Gleason secondary pattern 4 cancer.[707] Compression of data simplifies presentation for clinical use and publication, but such conversion of data from continuous to interval variables, referred to as dichotomizing, creates significant problems: (1) reduction of statistical power available to test hypotheses; (2) inappropriate dichotomization of continuous data may create spurious significant results if the variables are correlated; and (3) the choice of grouping is often problematic; the most important "cutpoint" is between Gleason scores 6 and 7 due to the emergence of poorly differentiated adenocarcinoma (pattern 4) in score 7, yet many studies combine these scores. Fitzsimons declared "death to dichotomizing" in protesting this practice.[708] Gleason argued against grade compression except in studies with a small number of patients in which grouping is unavoidable; in such cases, a cutpoint between scores 6 and 7 is preferred.[575] The probability of lymph node metastases is greater in patients with score 7 adenocarcinoma than in those with score 6.

Percent Gleason 4 and 5

The 2016 WHO Classification of Tumours of the Urinary System and Male Genital Organs recommends that the percent of Gleason pattern 4 be reported to better reflect the extent in Gleason score 7 tumors.[617] This reaffirms the same conclusion by the 1999 WHO Consensus Conference. Our laboratory has routinely reported this for two decades.

Quantitative Gleason score, a weighted average of all Gleason patterns present in the pathology specimens, improves the correlation between biopsy and prostatectomy, as well as increasing the accuracy of prediction of biochemical recurrence in Gleason 7 cancer or greater.[709] Assessment of percent Gleason pattern 4 in 10% increments is reproducible. Percent of each Gleason pattern rather than groupings predicts continuous increase of risk for biochemical failure with increasing increments of Gleason 4, with remarkably small differences in outcome at clinically important thresholds (0% versus 5%; 40% versus 60% Gleason 4), challenging the notion of thresholds and dichotomization of continuous data in the ISUP 2014 grade grouping scheme.[707] Dividing percent Gleason 4 into quartiles showed a 5-year biochemical recurrence-free survival of 84% (1% to 20% Gleason 4), 74% (21% to 50% Gleason 4), 66% (51% to 70%), and 32% (for >70%).[710] Quantitative Gleason scoring of biopsies identified intermediate-risk groups with respect to Gleason findings in corresponding prostatectomies.[707]

The volume of high-grade adenocarcinoma is an important prognostic factor: As cancer volume increases, the frequency and volume of high-grade tumor increases. According to McNeal, Gleason grade stratifies cancer into three subgroups with different levels of aggressiveness.[711] The first subgroup, Gleason primary patterns 1 and 2, comprises adenocarcinomas that are almost always small, usually less than 1 cm^3, and are indolent, localized, and frequently limited to the transition zone. The second subgroup, grade 3 adenocarcinoma, is variable in size and very common. The final subgroup, grades 4 and 5 adenocarcinomas, is usually larger and more aggressive than lower grades, and is likely to extend beyond the prostate or metastasize. This classification is a precursor of the ISUP 2014 grade group scheme, with the latter simply subdividing the second and the third subgroups to create five groups; no credit was given to McNeal in the ISUP 2014 publication despite his original seminal contribution.

The incremental percent Gleason grade 4 cancer in biopsies is an important predictor of adverse pathology and biochemical recurrence-free survival across the entire range of percentages.[712] On multivariate analysis, percent Gleason 4 was a significant predictor of adverse pathology and time to biochemical failure. Multivariate analysis of biopsies showed that each percent increase of Gleason primary pattern 4 elevated the odds of stage T3 cancer or higher by 2%.[713] Tertiary Gleason 5 areas also have strong prognostic impact in Gleason 7 carcinoma.[714]

Gleason score and percent of patterns 4 and 5 adenocarcinoma showed a positive correlation with cancer volume.[715] The European Randomized Study of Screening for Prostate Cancer reported that the amount of high-grade cancer (Gleason patterns 4 and 5) was the strongest predictor of biochemical failure after prostatectomy, similar to the results of others.[716-719] The cumulative data suggest that the volume of high-grade adenocarcinoma is of paramount prognostic significance, refuting Gleason's contention that it behaves according to the average of histologic grades.[575,720] The extent of solid undifferentiated carcinoma (Gleason grade 5) correlates with cancer progression.[721]

Should Gleason 3 + 3 = 6 Be Called Cancer?

In contemporary biopsies, the lowest end of the Gleason grading continuum (e.g., Gleason 1 and 2 patterns) is almost never used, probably because these patterns are usually seen in transition zone and anterior cancers sampled by TURP, a method that is now used infrequently. So, what about the next step up in the Gleason scoring system, Gleason pattern 3 (grade group 1, Gleason 3 + 3 = 6)? When observed in isolation, Gleason 3 + 3 = 6 has low malignant potential, so the question has been posed whether this should be renamed as neoplasm of low malignant potential, like the argument posed with grade 1 urothelial carcinoma. Given the emergence of active surveillance as a common management for these patients, the initiative to abandon the word *cancer* in this setting is dissipating.[722,723]

Concordance between global grade grouping in biopsies and that in prostatectomies is identical in 59% of cases, with the highest concordance for global grade group 2 and global grade group 5 and lowest for global grade group 4: global grade group 1, 48%; global grade group 2, 74%; global grade group 3, 53%; global grade group 4, 21%; and global grade group 5, 68%.[724] Final grade group is upgraded or downgraded in 32% and 8% of cases, respectively; global grade group 1, 52% and 7%; global grade group 2, 19% and 31%; global grade group 3, 16% and 46%; and global grade group 4, 33% and 32%.[724] Grade group 1 (Gleason 3 + 3 = 6) in biopsies predicted the following in prostatectomies: 4% were upgraded to Gleason 7 or higher, 1% had seminal vesicle invasion, and 0.4% had lymph node metastases. PSA and age were the only predictors of adverse pathology; there was no association with number of positive cores or length of cancer in any core.[725] There was no evidence of a threshold effect between grade groups 1 and 2.

In men with Gleason 3 + 3 = 6 at prostatectomy, positive lymph node metastases were found surgically in 0.2% of Surveillance, Epidemiology, and End Results (SEER) cases (2004 to 2011) and 0.2% of National Cancer Database cases (2004 to 2013).[726] Another study found that median age of patients was 60 years (range, 44 to 76 years), 82% were cT1c, median PSA was 5 ng/dL, 28% had positive margins, and 11% had biochemical failure at a median follow-up of 93 months (range, 17 to 161, with 45% followed ≥8 years).[727] Among 451 patients with 3 + 3 = 6 cancer treated by prostatectomy, none had synchronous lymph node metastases; 10% suffered biochemical failure, but virtually all of these had at least focal Gleason pattern 4 on blinded pathology rereview.[728]

Gleason 7 Subdivision (3 + 4 Versus 4 + 3)

Gleason score 7 cancer is common and heterogeneous, perhaps because of the range of Gleason grade 4 patterns (fused, 75% prevalence of G4; ill-defined, 64%; cribriform, 48%; and glomeruloid, 25%).[729,730] Among patients with Gleason score 7, primary grade 4 indicates a likelihood of higher tumor stage and higher probability of PSA recurrence after surgery than primary pattern 3.[685,731-733] However, it does not independently predict worse outcome after controlling for other known prognostic parameters associated with disease progression, and it appears to be of less value in patients treated by brachytherapy.[685,734-737] Conversely, Rasiah et al. found that patients with primary Gleason grade 4 cancer were more likely to have seminal vesicle involvement and EPE and, along with patients with tertiary Gleason grade 5, had shorter time to cancer recurrence.[738]

Helpap and Oehler evaluated interobserver agreement for Gleason 4 with fused glands.[739] The definition of glandular fusion was complete lack of stroma between a minimum of two glands and only one line of nuclei within the area of fusion. As expected, interobserver reproducibility of fused glands by specialized observers was higher than that of nonspecialized pathologists.

Of patients with Gleason pattern 3 + 4 tumors on biopsy, 24% were upgraded to primary pattern 4 or more on final pathologic analysis.[740] Of the patients with Gleason pattern 4 + 3 tumors on biopsy, 47% were downgraded to primary pattern 3 or less on final pathologic analysis.

Grade Group 4 Heterogeneity

The 3-year progression-free survival rate for Gleason 3 + 5 = 8 is higher than that for Gleason 4 + 4 = 8 cancer, reflecting heterogeneity in ISUP 2014 grade group 4.[741] The 5-year cancer-specific mortality rate after surgery for patients with Gleason score 4 + 4 = 8, 3 + 5 = 8, 5 + 3 = 8, and 9 cancer is 6%, 7%, 14%, and 14%, respectively, suggesting that Gleason 5 + 3 should be combined with score 5 (4 + 5 and 5 + 4) rather than score 3 (4 + 4 and 3 + 5).[742] Likewise, after brachytherapy, cancer-specific survival with a median of almost 8-year follow-up is higher for men with Gleason score 3 + 5 and 5 + 3 than for men with score 4 + 4.[743] Subcategorizing Gleason 8 into prostate cancer with or without grade 5 should be considered as a stratification factor in randomized trials.

Gleason Pattern 5

The highest grade of prostate cancer, Gleason pattern 5, may be heterogeneous, appearing variably as sheets, single cells, cords, small solid cylinders, solid medium to large nests with rosette-like spaces, comedonecrosis, and near-solid cribriform glands, and is sometimes associated with ductal carcinoma and IDC. The presence of a greater number of these morphologies predicts higher risk for recurrence after surgery.[622]

Reactive Stromal Grading

A grading system for cancer-associated reactive stroma is independently predictive of biochemical recurrence and cancer-specific survival after prostatectomy on multivariate analysis, with 10-year survival rates for reactive stromal grades 0, 1, 2, and 3 of 96%, 81%, 69%, and 63%, respectively.[744]

Morphologic patterns of cancer with extravasated stromal mucin are likely overgraded in a subset of cases with more complex epithelial bridges, whereas stromogenic cancers have a worse outcome than conveyed by Gleason grade alone.[745]

Digital Pathology and Deep Learning

The first digital pathology system was cleared by the U.S. Food and Drug Administration in early 2017, heralding the start of a major disruption in workflow in anatomic pathology. The advent of deep learning algorithms is maturing rapidly and in parallel to allow accurate diagnosis by machine vision. It is likely that machine-based prostate biopsy interpretation will be among the first applications of this new technology.[746] The utility of digital image analysis has been shown for surgical margin determination and Gleason grading.[747,748]

Grading After Therapy

Grading After Radiation Therapy

Grading after radiation therapy yields conflicting results, with some observers noting no difference from pretherapy grade and others finding a substantial increase in grade. Bostwick et al. found no apparent difference in grade before and after external beam therapy in 40 patients.[749] Conversely, Wheeler et al. found an increase in grade after treatment that they attributed to time-dependent tumor progression.[750] Similarly, Siders and Lee evaluated matched tissue specimens from 58 men before therapy and more than 18 months after therapy, and found a significant increase in Gleason score.[751] There was a 24% increase in poorly differentiated adenocarcinoma (scores 8 to 10) and a shift toward aneuploid DNA content in 31% of pretreatment diploid tumors, indicating increasing aggressiveness; no outcome data were provided to support this assertion. In grade 4 cancer, radiotherapy may cause disappearance of glandular lumina, resulting in grade 5 morphology. Despite conflicting results, some investigators recommend grading of specimens after therapy, recognizing that the biologic significance of grade may be different from that in untreated cancer. We believe that Gleason grading after radiation therapy is potentially misleading because of the high risk for overgrading, and we do not report it unless requested to do so and always with the appropriate disclaimer ("Grading of adenocarcinoma after radiation therapy is not validated and may create spurious and misleading higher Gleason grade, so these results may not be predictive of patient outcome and should be interpreted with caution").

Grading systems have been proposed for therapy-induced adenocarcinoma regression, but they have not been widely adopted.[752,753] These systems are useful after androgen deprivation therapy and radiation therapy. Böcking and Sinagowitz suggested that reversible cell damage in prostate cancer is characterized by cytoplasmic vacuolization, nuclear shrinkage, and reduction in the number and size of nucleoli, whereas irreversible cell damage is characterized by rupture of the cytoplasm, nuclear pyknosis, and loss of nucleoli.[752]

Grading After Androgen Deprivation Therapy

After androgen deprivation therapy (e.g., leuprolide, flutamide), there may be an increase in Gleason grade that is accompanied by a marked reduction in nuclear and nucleolar size and prominent cytoplasmic clearing.[754] Ellison et al. found a significant increase in Gleason grade, decrease in nuclear grade, and decrease in the extent of PIN in cases treated with androgen deprivation therapy; the "uncoupling" of the architectural and cytologic pattern was considered vexing because of identification of small shrunken nuclei within malignant acini.[755] Conversely, there was no significant alteration in Gleason grade after monotherapy with the antiandrogen bicalutamide or 5α-reductase inhibitors finasteride and dutasteride.[227,234,756-759]

Despite a potential increase in grade with some agents, adenocarcinoma after androgen deprivation therapy is probably not more clinically aggressive than when untreated; however, outcome data are not available to confirm this assertion. Thus we and most investigators conclude that Gleason grading after androgen deprivation therapy is potentially misleading and is not recommended.[760]

Clinical Significance of Grading

Grade is one of the strongest predictors of biologic behavior, including invasiveness and metastatic potential, but is not reliable when used alone in predicting pathologic stage or patient outcome for individual patients. Grade is included among other prognostic factors in therapeutic decision making, including patient age and health, clinical stage, and serum PSA level. Men with smaller prostates have more high-grade cancer and more advanced disease and are at greater risk for progression after prostatectomy.[761]

Grade and Outcome

Virtually every measure of recurrence and survival is strongly correlated with grade, including overall survival, tumor-free survival

after treatment, metastasis-free survival, and cause-specific survival.[762-769] Humphrey et al. found that the Gleason score was the strongest predictor of time to recurrence after prostatectomy.[770-772] Biopsy Gleason grade is an integral component of nomograms that predict 10-year probability of recurrence after prostatectomy (in combination with PSA, clinical stage, and number of involved cores).[773]

Schroeder et al. measured the impact on cancer-specific survival of 12 histopathologic characteristics used in grading prostatic adenocarcinoma.[774] In their analysis of 346 patients treated by perineal prostatectomy, they found that four characteristics provided independent predictive value: acinar arrangement (architecture), nuclear size, nuclear shape, and the presence of mitotic figures.

Grade and Cancer Volume

The strong correlation between Gleason grade and cancer volume has been shown in biopsies, TURPs, and radical prostatectomies.[775] Low-grade adenocarcinoma (Gleason patterns 1 and 2) is rarely larger than 1 cm^3, whereas high-grade adenocarcinoma (patterns 4 and 5) is almost always larger than 1 cm^3.[711] The probability of tumor progression is best indicated by grade and volume; when cancer volume is held constant, grade has residual prognostic value, indicating that it provides additional independent information, although these two prognostic factors are closely linked.

Grade and Prostate-Specific Antigen

Adenocarcinoma associated with elevated serum PSA is more likely to be of higher grade, larger volume, and more advanced pathologic stage than adenocarcinoma associated with normal PSA. There is a positive correlation between PSA and primary Gleason grade, the percentage of Gleason patterns 4 and 5, nuclear grade, and DNA content in totally embedded prostatectomies.[776] Adenocarcinoma with Gleason score ≥7 has a higher median serum PSA and cancer volume than that with lower (<7) Gleason score. Also, patients with more than 30% Gleason patterns 4 and 5 have a higher median serum PSA and cancer volume than patients with ≤30% Gleason patterns 4 and 5. Furthermore, median PSA is greater in tumors with Gleason pattern >3 than in those with Gleason pattern <3 after controlling for tumor volume in 5-cm^3 increments. However, patients with Gleason 8 to 10 cancer and PSA less than 4.0 ng/mL have more aggressive cancer (lower overall survival at 6 years) than those with PSA levels of 4 to 9.9 ng/mL; these low PSA cancers behave more like those with PSA levels of 10 to 19.9 ng/mL.[777] It is likely that low PSA levels among men with Gleason 8 to 10 prostate cancer may result from cellular dedifferentiation rather than low cancer burden.

Serum PSA may be of limited utility for staging localized cancer because of the influence of tumor grade. After controlling for cancer volume but not gland volume (PSA/cancer volume), there is a negative correlation with the Gleason score, suggesting that PSA is determined by multiple confounding factors.[778] Conversely, Blackwell et al. found that combining PSA with gland volume and cancer volume (PSA cancer density) increases the reliability and predictive value for pathologic stage and tumor grade.[776] Although individual cells in poorly differentiated adenocarcinoma produce less PSA per cell than cells in well-differentiated and moderately differentiated adenocarcinoma, poorly differentiated cells are usually present in such large numbers (greater cancer volume) and replace so much more of the prostate than well- or moderately differentiated that serum PSA level is higher with high-grade tumors. Serial measurements of PSA suggest that cancer has a constant log-linear growth rate, with mean PSA doubling time of 2.4 years for localized adenocarcinoma and 1.8 years for metastatic adenocarcinoma.[779] Higher Gleason grade is associated with faster doubling time.

Grade and Pathologic Stage

Grade is one of the strongest and most useful predictors of pathologic stage (pT), according to numerous univariate and multivariate studies.[780-782] This predictive ability applies to virtually every measure of stage, including EPE, seminal vesicle invasion, lymph node metastases, and bone metastases. Some investigators claim that a Gleason score ≥8 on biopsy is strongly predictive of lymph node metastases and recommend dispensing with staging lymph node dissection in these cases. However, others have justified lymph node dissection even for high-grade tumors.[783,784] Despite the optimism for grading to predict clinical stage, the predictive value is not high enough to permit its application for individual patients, particularly in those with moderately differentiated adenocarcinoma.

Grade and Cancer Location

Grade may be related to the site of origin of cancer within the prostate. The majority of cancers involve the apex and are within 5 mm of the urethra.[785] Adenocarcinoma arising in the transition zone appears to be lower grade and less aggressive clinically than that arising in the peripheral zone.[541] The majority of transition zone adenocarcinomas arise in foci adjacent to nodular hyperplasia, with one-third actually originating within nodules.[96,443] These adenocarcinomas are better differentiated than those in the peripheral zone, accounting for the majority of Gleason patterns 1 and 2 tumors. However, comparison of high-grade cancer arising in the transition zone with peripheral/central zone cancer reveals higher PSA, cancer volume, and incidence of positive surgical margins, but lower incidence of IDC, extraprostatic spread, seminal vesicle invasion, lymph node involvement, and biochemical failure after prostatectomy.[786,787]

About 15% of prostatectomies have the largest cancer focus anteriorly, referred to as "anterior-predominant" cancer.[788] Of these cases, 49% were assigned to the anterior peripheral zone, 36% to the transition zone, 8% were of indeterminate zone, and 7% were of both zones. In Japanese men, anterior cancers were more likely to be pT2 positive and less likely to be high grade than posterior cancers (23% versus 4% and 16% versus 29%, respectively); no seminal vesicle invasion was found in anterior cases.[789] Comparison of anterior peripheral zone and transition zone cancers revealed no significant differences in Gleason scores, incidence of EPE, overall surgical margin positivity rate, or laterality.

Variants and Other Carcinomas, Including Neuroendocrine Tumors

Variants of adenocarcinoma arising in the prostate raise questions of tumor origin, particularly whether the tumor represents metastasis or contiguous spread from another site. Also, the clinical behavior of morphologic variants may differ from usual acinar adenocarcinoma, carrying a better or worse prognosis. These tumors are usually associated with typical acinar carcinoma, rarely occurring in pure form. The Gleason grade, pathologic criteria, and clinical significance of variants of prostatic adenocarcinoma and other carcinomas are listed in Tables 9.31 and 9.32. (Table 9.32.)

TABLE 9.31 Histologic Spectrum of Prostatic Carcinoma

Epithelial Carcinoma	Gleason Primary Pattern
Variants of acinar adenocarcinoma	
Atrophic	Underlying glandular pattern
Pseudohyperplastic	3
Microcystic[a]	3
Foamy gland (microvacuolated)	Underlying glandular pattern
Mucinous (colloid)	4
Signet ring cell	5
Pleomorphic giant cell[a]	5
Sarcomatoid (carcinosarcoma)	5
Ductal adenocarcinoma	3 or 4 (5 with necrosis)
Cribriform carcinoma	3 or 4
Papillary	3 or 4
Solid	5
Comedocarcinoma	5
Intraductal carcinoma	No grade applies
Carcinoma with NE differentiation	Underlying glandular pattern
Adenocarcinoma with NE cells with large eosinophilic granules (Paneth cell–like change)	Underlying glandular pattern
Low-grade NE (carcinoid)	Underlying glandular pattern
High-grade NE (small cell and large cell[a])	5
Adenocarcinoma with glomeruloid features	4
Carcinoma with oncocytic feature	Usually 3
Lymphoepithelioma-like carcinoma	No grade applies
Clear cell carcinoma	Underlying glandular pattern
Adenoid cystic/basal cell carcinoma	No grade applies
Squamous and adenosquamous carcinoma	Usually high grade
Urothelial carcinoma	See Chapter 6

NE, Neuroendocrine.
[a]New variants of prostatic carcinoma included in World Health Organization 2016 classification.

TABLE 9.32 World Health Organization 2016 Classification: Changes from 2004[1719]

- Inclusion of ISUP 2014 grade groupings
- Intraductal carcinoma is a newly recognized entity
- New acinar adenocarcinoma variants: microcystic adenocarcinoma and pleomorphic giant cell adenocarcinoma
- Include percent Gleason pattern 4 for score 7 cancer (same as WHO 1999 recommendation)

ISUP, International Society of Urological Pathology; *WHO*, World Health Organization.

Variants of carcinoma included in the WHO 2016 classification include atrophic, pseudohyperplastic, microcystic, foamy gland, mucinous, signet ring cell, pleomorphic giant cell, and sarcomatoid carcinoma (Tables 9.31 and 9.32).[617,790,791]

Nonacinar carcinoma variants account for about 5% of carcinomas that are primary in the prostate.[792] These types include ductal (cribriform, papillary, solid, and PIN-like), IDC, NE tumors (including adenocarcinoma with Paneth cell–like NE differentiation, well-differentiated NE tumor, small cell carcinoma, and large cell NE carcinoma), urothelial carcinoma, squamous and adenosquamous carcinoma, and basal cell carcinoma (Tables 9.31 and 9.32).[617,790]

Atrophic Adenocarcinoma

Acinar atrophy and postatrophic hyperplasia are commonly confused with adenocarcinoma.[793,794] Cancer acini with round dilated and distorted lumens and flattened lining cells with scant cytoplasm are referred to as "atrophic" cancer (Fig. 9.37).[795,796] This is an unusual pattern that is easily mistaken for atrophy. All cases have cytologic evidence of malignancy, including nuclear enlargement and prominent nucleoli, and these findings cannot be attributable to potential confounders such as inflammation or treatment effect.[795] Atrophic cancer is identified in 3% of radical prostatectomies and 2% of biopsies, comprising mean cancer proportions of 27% (range, 10% to 60%) and 24% (range, 10% to 90%), respectively.[795]

Caution is warranted in rendering this difficult diagnosis on biopsies with only a small amount of cancer.[795,796] Racemase is expressed in 70% of atrophic prostate cancers compared with weak staining in up to 13% cases of atrophy, and thus such immunostaining alone is not sufficiently discriminatory by itself; a panel of immunostains that also includes keratin 34βE12 and p63 is recommended.[797]

Pseudohyperplastic Adenocarcinoma

At low magnification, the low-grade carcinoma pseudohyperplastic adenocarcinoma (Gleason primary pattern 2 or 3 cancer) may be mistaken for an exuberant hyperplastic nodule.[798-801] It consists of large atypical glands with branching, papillary infoldings, and corpora amylacea in 20% of cases (Fig. 9.38). The incidence rate is about 2% in biopsies and 1% in TURP.[802] Features most helpful in establishing a malignant diagnosis with this variant are nuclear enlargement (95% of cases), pink amorphous secretions (70%), occasional to frequent nucleoli (45%), crystalloids (45%), and transition with typical small acinar pattern.[799,802] Immunostains for keratin 34βE12, racemase, and p63 are often required to confirm this lesion as malignant.[241] In our experience, the entire focus is often negative for basal cell stains, in striking contrast with adjacent benign glands. About 77% of cases are positive for racemase.[803] The cancer is histologically distinctive but does not warrant separation as a clinicopathologic entity.

Pseudohyperplastic carcinoma may coexist with foamy gland cancer or as a component of carcinosarcoma, exhibiting the

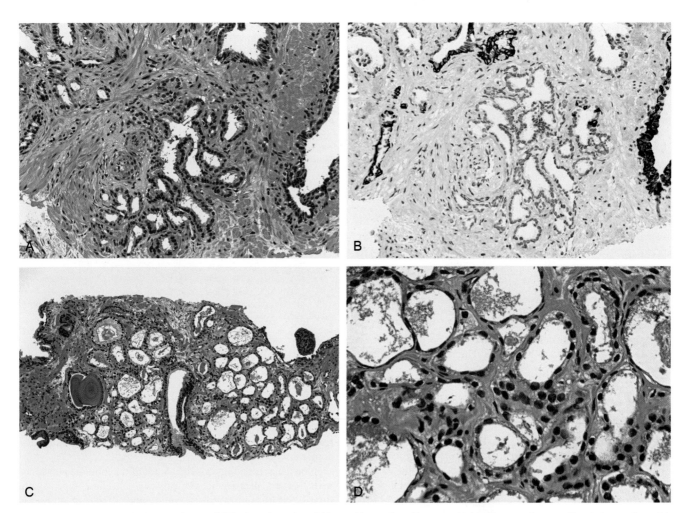

Fig. 9.37 Atrophic pattern of adenocarcinoma. (A) The large irregular acini (*center*) have dilated lumens with modest cytoplasm and hyperchromatic nuclei; at this magnification, it is difficult to distinguish between atrophy and atrophic pattern of cancer. (B) The focus of concern lacks basal cells, confirming the suspicion of cancer, with positive internal control indicating benign acini at the periphery (immunohistochemical stain for keratin 34βE12). (C) Cancer acini with round dilated and distorted lumina, showing mixed features of atrophic pattern and early microcystic pattern. (D) Higher magnification shows acini lined by flattened cells with scant cytoplasm and enlarged nuclei with prominent nucleoli.

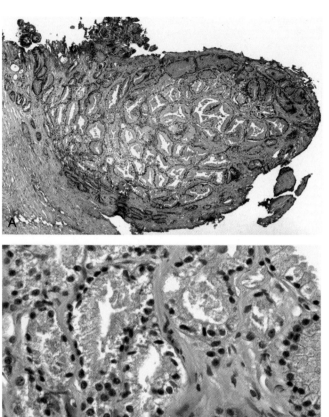

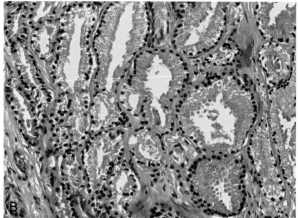

Fig. 9.38 Pseudohyperplastic carcinoma (A to C). Well-differentiated adenocarcinoma (Gleason pattern 1 or 2) in transurethral resection consists of uniformly spaced acini mimicking hyperplastic epithelium.

pseudohyperplastic nodular pattern but sharing the feature of inconspicuous cytologic atypia (discussed later in this chapter).[804,805]

Microcystic Adenocarcinoma

Microcystic adenocarcinoma represents a form of atrophic or pseudohyperplastic variant characterized by cystic dilatation and rounded expansion of glands of usual acinar adenocarcinoma with flat luminal lining layer.[806] Intraluminal crystalloids and blue mucin are present in all cases, and mean acinar/ductal size is 10-fold greater than that of usual adenocarcinoma. There is complete basal cell loss.

Foamy Gland Carcinoma (Microvacuolated)

The adenocarcinoma foamy gland carcinoma (microvacuolated) consists of cells with abundant microvacuoles in the cytoplasm that displace the nuclei basally (Fig. 9.39).[803,807-811] Patient age is similar to typical acinar adenocarcinoma, and preoperative serum PSA level in one study ranged from 3 to 38 ng/mL (mean, 15 ng/mL).[807] Incidence in radical prostatectomies varies from 15% to 23%.[812]

Diagnostic difficulty is encountered when this pattern predominates because of the small nuclear size and lack of nuclear hyperchromasia that may be interpreted as benign.[800] Nuclear enlargement and prominent nucleoli were absent or rare in 61% and 71% of foamy gland carcinomas, respectively.[809]

Foamy gland cancer is negative for mucin and lipid stains, but positive for colloidal iron and Alcian blue stain. About 68% of cases stain with racemase.[803] Ultrastructurally foamy cells displayed numerous intracytoplasmic vesicles and numerous polyribosomes.[807]

Early reports indicated that patients with foamy gland carcinoma tended to have high-volume bilateral cancer and an aggressive course, although the number of cases with long-term follow-up was limited.[807-813] Subsequent studies found the same prognosis as usual acinar adenocarcinoma.[811,813] Nonetheless, recognition of foamy gland carcinoma is important because there is a Gleason grade 4 element in the majority of cases.[812]

Mucinous (Colloid) Carcinoma

Fewer than 300 cases of mucinous carcinoma of the prostate have been reported, but the incidence is probably higher.[294,813-817] The signs and symptoms of mucinous carcinoma are similar to typical acinar carcinoma. There are no apparent differences in patient age, stage at presentation, cancer volume, or serum PSA level. Typical acinar adenocarcinoma may produce mucin after high-dose estrogen therapy.

Focal mucinous differentiation is observed in at least one-third of carcinoma cases, but the diagnosis of mucinous carcinoma requires that at least 25% of the tumor consist of pools of extracellular mucin (Fig. 9.40).[814,817,818] Those less than the 25% threshold may be referred to as "adenocarcinoma with mucinous features."[819]

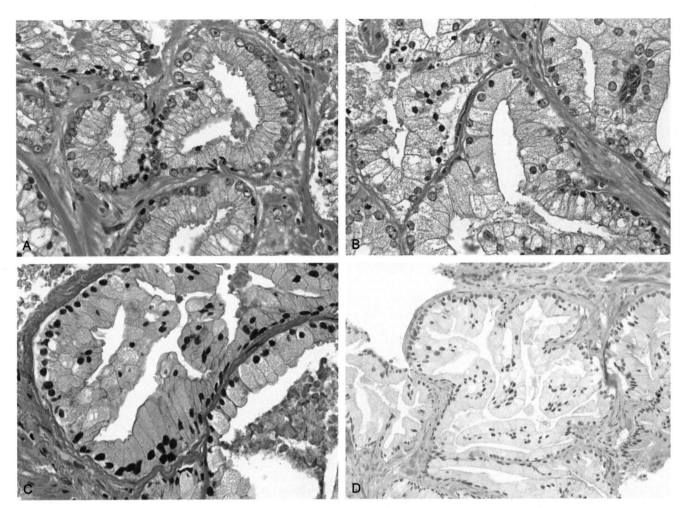

Fig. 9.39 Foamy gland carcinoma. (A) Note the pale eosinophilic with finely vacuolated cytoplasm, distinct cell membranes, basal nuclei, and small punctate nucleoli. (B) Another case with clear cytoplasm and finely vacuolated cytoplasm. (C) A third case with clear, finely vacuolated cytoplasm and hyperchromatic nuclei with indistinct nucleoli; compare with (D), showing absence of immunoreactivity for basal cell–specific keratin 34βE12, immunohistochemical confirmation of the diagnosis of carcinoma.

Mucinous carcinoma consists of tumor cell nests and clusters floating in mucin, similar to mucinous carcinoma of the breast. In small specimens such as needle biopsies, rare cases consist only of mucin pools, without identifiable tumor cells, although serial sectioning usually reveals malignant cells on deeper levels. The three patterns of mucinous carcinoma include acinar carcinoma with luminal distension, cribriform carcinoma with luminal distension, and "colloid carcinoma" with cell nests embedded in mucinous lakes.[814]

Other patterns of cancer are often present in association with mucinous carcinoma, including cribriform and comedo patterns. The cells of mucinous carcinoma usually have enlarged nuclei and display the entire spectrum of cytologic abnormalities observed in typical carcinoma. In some cases, nuclei have low-grade cytologic findings, with uniform finely granular chromatin and inconspicuous nucleoli, but their presence within mucin pools is diagnostic of malignancy. Signet ring cells are usually not present in mucinous carcinoma, although there are some cases which have such cells in abundance.[820] Mucinous carcinoma may arise in the transition zone in association with large numbers of NE cells with large eosinophilic granules. Collagenous micronodules are often an incidental finding that probably results from extracellular acid

mucin.[475] The number of collagenous micronodules is correlated with the amount of mucin production, including luminal mucin and extraacinar mucin; there is a weak negative correlation of collagenous micronodules with the percent of tumor composed of signet ring cells.

Prostatic mucin can be stained with PAS, Alcian blue, and mucicarmine. Most studies have found neutral mucin in benign acini and acidic mucin in malignant acini, although benign acini rarely produce small quantities of acidic mucin. Based on these findings, some have suggested that acidic mucin is a useful supportive feature in the diagnosis of adenocarcinoma, present in about 60% of cases.[294,813-815] In adenocarcinoma, sialomucins predominate over sulfomucins. Well-differentiated and moderately differentiated noncolloid tumors have non-O-acylated sialomucins. Poorly differentiated tumors contain mono-O-acylated (C9) sialomucins and colloid-type tumors secrete mono-, di-, and tri-O-acylated sialoglycoproteins. Acidic mucins, mainly sialomucins, constitute the major secretory component in prostatic adenocarcinoma, and O-acylation of these sialoglycoproteins inversely correlates with differentiation.[465] Well-differentiated and moderately differentiated tumor is not O-acylated, whereas poorly differentiated cancer characteristically has O-acylated sialomucins in C9. Mucinous adenocarcinoma is the

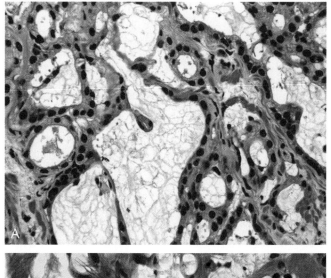
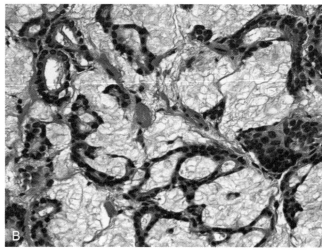
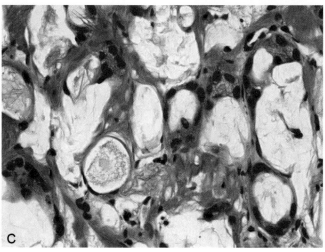

Fig. 9.40 Mucinous (colloid) carcinoma. Abundant luminal mucin expands the malignant acinar lumens (A to C).

most heavily O-acylated of the variants.[465] Acidic mucin also has been described in atypical adenomatous hyperplasia, mucinous metaplasia, PIN, sclerosing adenosis, and basal cell hyperplasia.

The cells of mucinous carcinoma express PSA and prostatic acid phosphatase (PAP), but usually do not produce carcinoembryonic antigen (CEA) unless there is prominent signet ring cell differentiation.[821] In one case, nonspecific esterase (NSE) immunoreactivity was observed, confirming histochemical results with the Grimelius stain.

Ultrastructurally, tumor cells are joined by zonula adherens junctions and set in an amorphous background. Microvilli and cytoplasmic projections are prominent. Nuclei are compressed to one side of the cells, with cytoplasmic organelles and mucinogen granules filling the remainder of the cells.

The pattern of metastases of mucinous carcinoma of the prostate is similar to typical prostatic adenocarcinoma. Early reports suggested that these tumors are less aggressive and of lower stage than other forms of adenocarcinoma, with no tendency for bone metastasis, but studies with long-term survival have effectively refuted this claim.[822-824] Patients may be treated with radiation therapy, hormonal therapy, or both. Fifty percent of patients die within 3 years, and up to 75% within 7 years, although one study reported median survival of 6.4 years, similar to acinar carcinoma.[814,817,825] There is a significant difference in survival between Caucasian and African American patients (median survival, 144 versus 99 months, respectively).[826]

Mucinous carcinoma of the rectum and urinary bladder may invade the prostate, mimicking prostatic origin. Similarly, Cowper gland carcinoma displays prominent mucinous differentiation, although this cancer is vanishingly rare. IDC and ductal carcinoma may rarely exhibit prominent mucin production, as can urethral adenocarcinoma.[827-829] These distinctions are important because of significant differences in treatment and prognosis.

Pseudomyxoma ovarii-like change is a rare mimic of mucinous carcinoma that consists of extravasated acid mucin, lacks basal cells, rarely occurs in intimate association with residual prostatic carcinoma in posttreatment prostatectomy specimens, and probably represents tumor regression secondary to androgen ablation.[830] Small or large pools of extravasated mucin dissect through the prostatic stroma with an infiltrative appearance. Secretions are basophilic in routine sections and contain occasional degenerate cells. Rare pan-CK–immunoreactive cells are present at the secretion/stroma interface, with negative staining for keratin 34βE12. Secretions are positive for mucicarmine, Alcian blue at pH 2.5, and PAS after diastase digestion. There is no correlation between the presence of pseudomyxoma-like change and dose or duration of neoadjuvant therapy, postprostatectomy clinical follow-up, Gleason score, or pathologic stage.

Signet Ring Cell Carcinoma

Signet ring cell carcinoma of the prostate is rare, with fewer than 300 reported cases.[820,831-839] The characteristic cytoplasmic

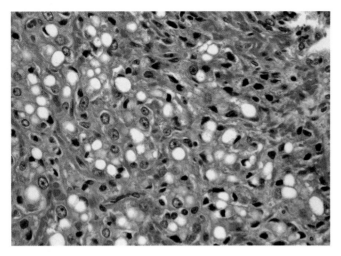

Fig. 9.41 Signet ring cell carcinoma.

clearing is rarely mucicarminophilic, in contrast with signet ring cell carcinoma of the bladder, urachus, stomach, and other sites. Presenting signs and symptoms are similar to typical acinar adenocarcinoma. Rectal examination may reveal stony-hard induration.

Signet ring cells are present in 3% of cases of acinar adenocarcinoma, but the diagnosis of signet ring cell carcinoma requires that 25% or more of the tumor be composed of signet ring cells; some authors require 50% (Fig. 9.41). Tumor cells show distinctive nuclear displacement by clear cytoplasm. Almost all cases are associated with other forms of poorly differentiated prostatic adenocarcinoma, including cribriform carcinoma, comedocarcinoma, and solid (Gleason grade 5) carcinoma. Tumor cells diffusely infiltrate

through the stroma, invading perineural and vascular spaces, and often perforate the capsule.

Histochemical and immunohistochemical results for mucin, lipid, PSA, PAP, and CEA are inconsistent, suggesting variants of signet ring cell carcinoma (Table 9.33). Giltman reported a case of pure signet ring cell carcinoma that was PAS-positive and diastase-resistant, but negative for acid mucin and fat (mucicarmine, Alcian blue, and oil red O).[840] In another case, tumor cells were shown to stain with Sudan black, indicating the presence of intracellular lipid. Mucin stains are variably positive. Ro and colleagues reported eight cases in which the tumor cells did not stain for Alcian blue, mucicarmine, or PAS with or without diastase. PSA, PAP, and keratin immunoreactivity are usually observed within signet ring cells and the non–signet ring cell component of cancer, but CEA is usually negative.[841-843] The signet ring cell appearance results from different factors in different cases, including cytoplasmic lumens, mucin granules, and fat vacuoles, thus accounting for the contradictory histochemical and immunohistochemical results.

Ultrastructurally, signet ring cells contain cytoplasmic vacuoles and intracytoplasmic lumens, sometimes lined by microvilli and without mucin or lipid vacuoles. Occasional rod-shaped intraluminal crystalloids are observed in metastatic sites, similar to crystalloids observed in typical acinar adenocarcinoma.

Most patients have clinical stage T3 or N[+] adenocarcinoma. Treatment is variable, including hormonal therapy, radiation therapy, or both. Patients with primary signet ring cell carcinoma have as little as a 27% 3-year survival rate, and none survive beyond 5 years.[825,841]

Signet ring cell carcinoma should be distinguished from similar tumors arising in other sites, particularly the gastrointestinal tract and stomach. Prostatic origin should be considered in metastatic

TABLE 9.33	**Signet Ring Cell Carcinoma of the Prostate: Laboratory Findings**										
	Number of Cases	Preoperative Serum PAP	Preoperative Serum PSA	PAS	Lipid Stain	Alcian Blue	Mucicarmine	PSA	PAP	CEA	Other Findings
Lipid-rich											
Kums and van Helsdingen[1720]	2			—	1/2	—	—	—	—	—	
Glycogen or mucin-rich											
Giltman[840] and Remmele et al.[843]	1			1/1	0/1	0/1	0/1	—	—	—	
Uchijima et al.[1721]	1			1/1	—	1/1	1/1	0/1	0/1	1/1	
Alline and Cohen[1722]	1	Normal	5.2	0/1	—	1/1	1/1	0/1	0/1	1/1	
Catton et al.[842]	1	33.6	—	—	—	0/1	0/1	1/1	1/1	0/1	
Segawa and Kakehi[1723]	1	Normal	<4.0	1/1	—	—	1/1	0/1	0/1	1/1	
Skodras et al.[1724]	1			1/1	—	1/1	1/1	1/1	1/1	1/1	
Guerin et al.[832]	5	2.4/1.5/21.9	4.6	5/5	0/1	5/5	—	5/5	5/5	1/1	
Smith et al.[1725]	1			1/1	—	—	1/1	1/1	1/1	1/2	CA19.9+
Torbenson et al.[836]	12	1.7		9/10	—	6/10	5/10	—	—	1/1	Diploid primary; aneuploid metastases
Kuroda et al.[835]	1			1/1	—	1/1	1/1	1/1	1/1		
Lipid, glycogen, or mucin-poor											
Ro et al.[841]	8			0/8	—	0/8	0/8	4/4	4/4		
Fujita et al.[1726]	1		9.3	0/1	—	0/1	—	1/1	1/1	0/4	
Jiang et al.[1727]	10			0/10	—	0/10	0/10			0/1	

PAP, prostatic acid phosphatase; *PSA*, prostate-specific antigen.

signet ring cell carcinoma of supraclavicular lymph nodes that exhibits negative mucin staining; PSA and PAP immunostaining may be useful. There are no reported cases of signet ring cell lymphoma involving the prostate.

Artifactual changes mimicking signet ring cell carcinoma have been described in TURP specimens, with lymphocytes and vacuolated smooth muscle cells causing diagnostic difficulty.[844,845] In these cases, PSA and PAP staining of the suspicious cells is negative, although LCA immunoreactivity is observed within the inflammatory cells.

Pleomorphic Giant Cell Adenocarcinoma

Giant cell carcinoma in the prostate is histologically similar to its counterpart in other organs, composed of pleomorphic giant tumor cells mixed with typical high-grade adenocarcinoma (Fig. 9.42).[791,846] Although rare, this variant of prostatic cancer should be considered in the differential diagnosis of metastatic giant cell carcinoma. Patients present with widespread metastases and die soon thereafter; this clinical presentation and aggressive behavior are characteristic of giant cell carcinoma arising in other organs. Giant cell carcinoma is unresponsive to conventional androgen deprivation therapy and is androgen receptor (AR) negative by immunohistochemistry. Giant cell carcinoma of the prostate is classified as Gleason pattern 5.

Controversy exists regarding the histogenesis of giant cell carcinoma. Lopez-Beltran et al. emphasized the importance of radiation therapy and chemotherapy as causative factors for spindle cell and giant cell carcinoma in urothelial cancer, and these factors probably apply to this cancer in the prostate.[846]

The most important differential diagnostic consideration of giant cell carcinoma is sarcomatoid carcinoma of the prostate with or without heterologous elements, which occasionally exhibits neoplastic giant cells. Sarcomatoid carcinoma is composed of spindle cells with large, pleomorphic, hyperchromatic nuclei. Other tumors that exhibit giant cells, such as giant cell carcinoma of the bladder, urothelial carcinoma with osteoclast-type giant cells or trophoblastic differentiation, and leiomyosarcoma with frank nuclear anaplasia, should also be considered. Osteoclast-type giant cells have some features of giant cell tumor of bone and are immunoreactive for vimentin and CD68, but not CK, whereas trophoblastic cells are immunoreactive for βHCG. Exceptionally, neoplastic giant cells and osteoclast-type cells may be present in the same neoplasm, although this has not been described in the prostate. Immunohistochemical stains for keratin, PSA, and PAP are useful in verifying the epithelial nature of giant cell carcinoma.

Sarcomatoid Carcinoma (Carcinosarcoma)

Sarcomatoid carcinoma is considered by most to be synonymous with carcinosarcoma.[847-853] Authors who separate these tumors define sarcomatoid carcinoma as an epithelial tumor showing spindle cell (mesenchymal) differentiation; carcinosarcoma is defined as adenocarcinoma intimately admixed with identifiable malignant soft tissue elements (Fig. 9.43). Tumors that contain areas of bone, cartilage, or striated muscle differentiation are sometimes referred to as sarcomatoid carcinoma with heterologous elements. Regardless of terminology, these tumors are rare and have a poor prognosis.

Patients tend to be older men who have symptoms of urinary outlet obstruction, similar to typical adenocarcinoma. Serum PSA may be normal at the time of diagnosis. About one-half of the patients have a prior history of typical acinar adenocarcinoma treated by radiation therapy or androgen deprivation therapy.[854]

Sixty percent of cases display an intimate mixture of sarcomatoid carcinoma and typical acinar adenocarcinoma, with transition forms.[852] Coexistent adenocarcinoma is almost always high grade (Gleason score 9 or 10). The most common heterologous elements are osteosarcoma and leiomyosarcoma.[847]

The epithelial component displays cytoplasmic immunoreactivity for keratin, PSA, and PAP, similar to typical adenocarcinoma. The soft tissue component usually displays immunoreactivity for vimentin, with variable staining for desmin, actin, and S-100 protein. ERG expression confirms epithelial derivation.[855]

Ultrastructurally, tumor cells occasionally display desmosomes and filaments, which apparently are CK. In two cases there was no ultrastructural evidence of epithelial differentiation.[852]

Treatment is variable and has no apparent influence on the poor prognosis. Dundore et al. found a 41% 5-year cancer-specific survival rate and 12% 7-year cancer-specific survival rate, similar to survival for Gleason score 9 and 10 adenocarcinoma without sarcomatoid features.[847] Of five patients reported by Shannon et al., three died of tumor within 46 months of diagnosis, one was alive with tumor at 48 months, and one was lost to follow-up after 1 month.[852] Hansel and Epstein reported that that six of seven patients died within 1 year of diagnosis.[856]

Separation of sarcomatoid carcinoma from sarcoma may be difficult and clinically unimportant, although immunohistochemical stains and electron microscopy are helpful. Weak diffuse keratin immunoreactivity has been identified in some cases of leiomyosarcoma, so this finding alone may not be sufficient to determine epithelial differentiation.

Ductal Adenocarcinoma

Ductal carcinoma classically arises as a polypoid, papillary, cribriform, or cystic mass within the prostatic urethra and large periurethral prostatic ducts, and often resembles endometrial carcinoma of the uterus.[90,370,857-863] Cytologic smears typically show cells with abundant cytoplasm and oval nuclei arranged in papillary groups or flat and folded sheets, some of which have peripheral nuclear palisading.[864] The morphologic appearance and common location of this tumor near the verumontanum suggests origin from the müllerian (female) remnant of the utriculus masculinus, implying that these tumors are estrogen dependent.[865] The therapeutic importance of estrogen-dependent prostatic carcinoma would be considerable because hormonal (estrogen) therapy would be contraindicated. However, the hypothesis of true uterine ("endometrial") carcinoma arising in the male is now abandoned, and virtually all studies have shown that endometrioid carcinoma is merely a histopathologic variant of prostatic adenocarcinoma; thus the preferred term is endometrioid carcinoma or simply ductal carcinoma. The term *endometrial* should not be used in the prostate.

Ductal carcinoma accounts for about 0.5% of cases of adenocarcinoma, although a recent report found an incidence rate of 4%.[90,866] It occurs exclusively in older men who may have symptoms of hematuria, urinary urgency, frequency, and rarely, acute retention. The clinical symptoms of pure ductal carcinoma and mixed ductal-acinar carcinoma overlap with those of typical acinar carcinoma. In some cases, adenocarcinoma is detected by digital rectal examination or PSA elevation in asymptomatic patients, usually in association with peripherally located acinar adenocarcinoma. Cystoscopically, ductal carcinoma may appear as multiple friable, polypoid, wormlike white masses protruding from ducts at or near the mouth of the prostatic utricle of the verumontanum; more often, however, there are no distinguishing cystoscopic findings. The prostate may be enlarged.

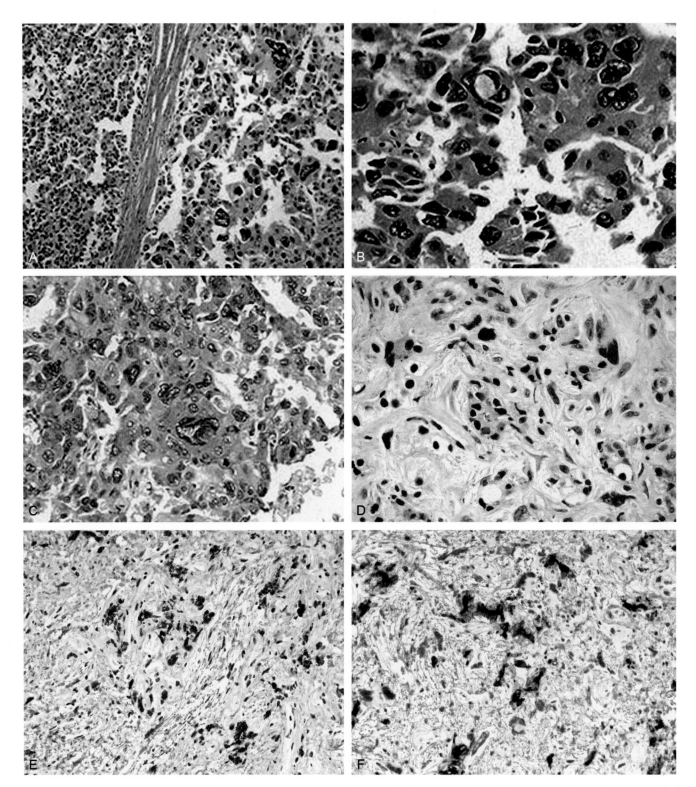

Fig. 9.42 Pleomorphic giant cell carcinoma. This unusual cancer is composed of large cells with single or multiple bizarre enlarged hyperchromatic nuclei with adjacent (*left*) typical high-grade adenocarcinoma (A and B). (C) Prostate-specific antigen immunoreactivity within most cells confirms prostatic origin. (D to F) Another case of giant cell carcinoma, demonstrating staining for racemase (E) and prostatic membrane antigen (F).

At the time of symptom presentation, most patients have tumors confined to the prostate or urethra, with concurrent invasive acinar prostatic adenocarcinoma in at least 77% of cases. Serum concentration of PSA may be normal or elevated at the time of diagnosis.

The tumor is often indistinguishable from uterine carcinoma, consisting of masses of complex papillae or anastomosing glands lined by variably stratified columnar epithelium (Fig. 9.44). The mitotic rate tends to be higher than in typical acinar adenocarcinoma. Noninvasive ductal carcinoma is a common finding, but

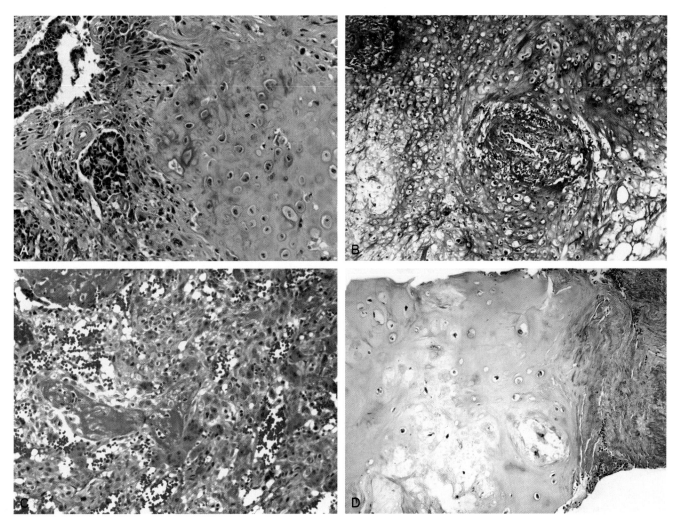

Fig. 9.43 Three cases of sarcomatoid carcinoma (carcinosarcoma) of the prostate, consisting of an intimate admixture of adenocarcinoma and chondroblastic osteosarcoma (A to C). Compare with benign chondroma (D) in a biopsy.

precise histopathologic criteria for separation from high-grade PIN and IDC have not yet been defined; nonetheless, all agree that massive expansion of large periurethral prostatic ducts by papillary and cribriform masses is best diagnosed as IDC (or what used to be called "noninvasive ductal carcinoma"), regardless of the presence or absence of scattered circumferential basal cells.[867] The papillary and cribriform patterns of ductal carcinoma coexist in about one-half of cases, and both usually display nuclear anaplasia, nucleolomegaly, and frequent mitotic figures, although there is a spectrum of cytologic abnormalities. Comedocarcinoma has the highest level of mitotic activity. Cystic growth is a less common pattern and usually occurs in the peripheral zone, often with exophytic papillary and cribriform growth within large accommodating spaces in a manner similar to endometrial tumors expanding within the uterine cavity or ovarian tumors growing within cystic spaces or the peritoneal cavity.[858,859] The expansion of potential spaces by adenocarcinoma probably accounts for the distinctive cribriform or papillary growth in large periurethral ducts and the urethra, and thus may merely represent a distinctive growth pattern of acinar adenocarcinoma. Identification of papillary or cribriform growth of cancer in biopsies usually represents peripheral zone adenocarcinoma (90% of cases with

these patterns) and not periurethral ductal involvement (10%).[90] Consequently, we refer to papillary or cribriform growth of cancer in needle biopsies as the "ductal subtype" of adenocarcinoma with a note stating that it is virtually always seen in association with typical acinar adenocarcinoma.

Subtypes include cribriform, papillary, solid, comedocarcinoma, urothelial-like cancer, mucinous cancer, and intestinal-type mucinous cancer.[829,860,868,869] The least common pattern of ductal carcinoma, urothelial-type adenocarcinoma, is a rare and newly described entity that arises from either the prostatic urethra or proximal ducts, and is most difficult to distinguish histologically from secondary colorectal carcinoma invading the prostate.[827,828,869] Urothelial-type adenocarcinoma is diffusely positive for CK7 and focally positive for keratin 34βE12, thrombomodulin, and CK20, consistent with origin from the urothelium of the prostatic urethra or proximal prostatic ducts; interestingly, weak or negative staining for PSA and PAP is also observed. The differential diagnosis includes conventional prostatic adenocarcinoma with mucin production, urothelial carcinoma with glandular differentiation, and secondary adenocarcinoma, usually of colorectal origin.[870] However, typical mucinous carcinoma is positive for PSA and PAP, and usually negative for CK7, CK20, and 34βE12. Adenocarcinoma of colonic origin is

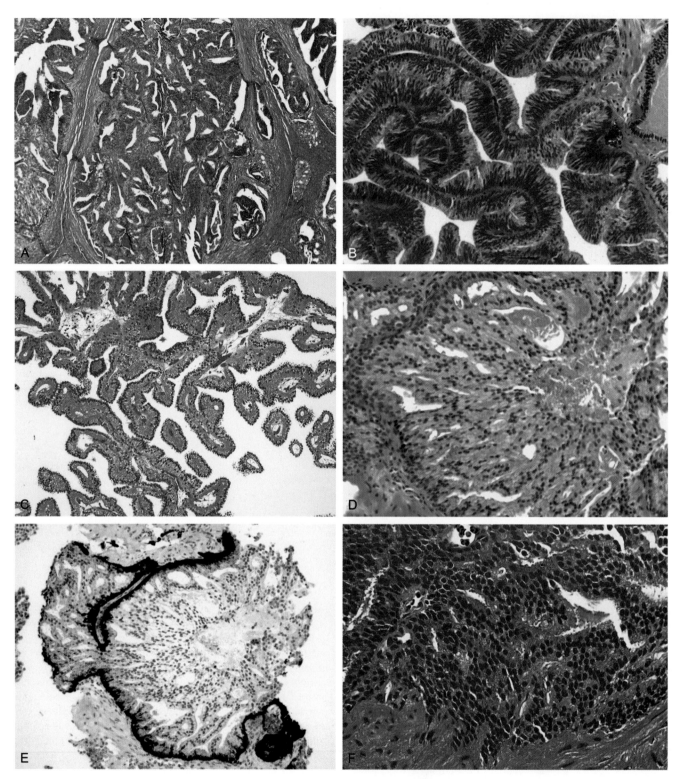

Fig. 9.44 Ductal adenocarcinoma. (A) Intraductal (noninvasive) pattern. (B) Papillary. (C) Papillary with unusual inverted pattern (nuclei are abluminal rather than typical basal location). (D) Cribriform. Compare with (E), showing scattered basal cells at the periphery, indicating noninvasive (intraductal) nature of the growth at this site. This papillary proliferation filled the large periurethral prostatic ducts and protruded into the urethra, with prostatic stromal invasion elsewhere. (F and G) Near-solid ductal carcinoma; quadruple stain on

(Continued)

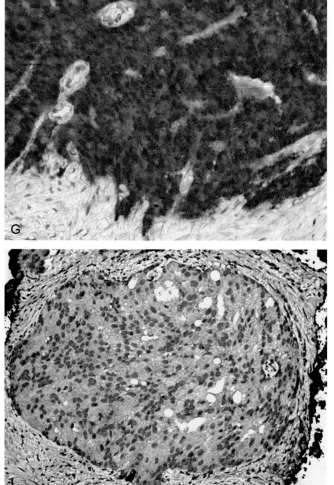

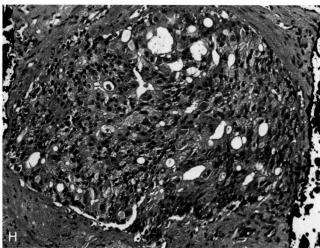

Fig. 9.44, cont'd (G) reveals intense cytoplasmic and nuclear staining (red reaction product) for racemase and c-Myc, respectively, but absence of basal cells (brown reaction product is absent) for keratin and p63. (H and I) Near-solid ductal carcinoma. Quadruple stain on (I) reveals absence of basal cells around this large mass, indicating that it is invasive.

diffusely CK20⁺ and either negative or focally positive for CK7 and negative for 34βE12.

PIN-like (ductal) adenocarcinoma resembles PIN in gland architecture, including the flat, tufted or micropapillary patterns of PIN.[790,871] However, unlike in PIN, stains for basal cells are negative in ductal carcinoma. As in PIN, racemase may be positive. The term *PIN-like ductal adenocarcinoma* has also been used because some of these cases have high columnar cells; however, not all cases appear to be of the ductal type. We do not recognize this as an entity and do not use this diagnosis, considering it is merely another name for ductal carcinoma.

Macrocystic growth of ductal carcinoma is present in 0.3% of cancers at prostatectomy and may exhibit multiple patterns: exuberant papillary proliferation with fibrovascular cores within macroscopic multilocular cysts, multilocular cysts lined by flat epithelium with foci of low papillae, and large cysts with comedonecrosis.[872] Most cystadenocarcinomas, whether the clinically apparent giant multilocular form or the incidentally identified microscopic type, are variants of ductal carcinoma.[873]

Ductal carcinoma invariably displays intense cytoplasmic immunoreactivity for PSA and PAP.[862,874] Nuclear AR staining is usually strong, whereas estrogen receptor staining is negative.[874] All ductal carcinomas express Ki67.[875] Focal CEA immunoreactivity is observed in a minority of cases. Focal patchy immunoreactivity for estrogen-regulated protein and estrogen receptor–related protein indicates prostatic origin.[876] PTEN and ERG expression

are low when compared with typical acinar cancer (18% versus 50% and 11% versus 50%, respectively).[877]

Ultrastructural findings include well-developed acini with distinct basal lamina, luminal microvilli, large nuclei with prominent nucleoli, desmosomes, secretory droplets, lysosomes, and abundant rough endoplasmic reticulum. Two types of tumor cells are distinguished on the basis of cytoplasmic differentiation: light cells are most common, containing secretory droplets, lipid-filled vacuoles, and pinocytotic vesicles; and dark cells contain electron-dense cytoplasm with abundant endoplasmic reticulum and free ribosomes. Transitional forms are also present.

Ductal carcinoma must be distinguished from urothelial carcinoma of the prostate, ectopic prostatic tissue, benign polyp, nephrogenic metaplasia, proliferative papillary urethritis, inverted papilloma, and accentuated mucosal folds. There is usually evidence of glandular differentiation in ductal carcinoma, allowing separation from urothelial carcinoma. In difficult cases, immunohistochemical stains for PSA and PAP are useful (positive in ductal carcinoma and negative in urothelial carcinoma). Benign mimics are distinguished from ductal carcinoma by the absence of nuclear abnormalities.

Subclassification of ductal carcinoma based on location is not performed in routine practice. Primary duct (large duct) and secondary duct prostatic adenocarcinomas are indistinguishable from each other, and most authors consider these as a single entity, abandoning this artificial separation. There are no clinical or pathologic criteria for separation of ductal carcinoma into utricular and nonutricular types.

Ductal carcinoma appears to have a less favorable prognosis than typical acinar adenocarcinoma, although conflicting results have been found.[863,878,879] A large, contemporary, population-based study showed that, compared with patients with Gleason 8 to 10 acinar carcinoma, those with ductal carcinoma present with lower mean PSA (10 versus 16 ng/mL), have a similar rate (12%) of clinical EPE, are more likely to undergo prostatectomy (54% versus 36%), and have more favorable pathology: stage $\geq$T3 (39% versus 52%), fewer positive lymph nodes (4% versus 11%), and fewer positive margins (25% versus 33%), but have similar 5-year survival rate (75% versus 77%, respectively).[880] Up to 36% of cases have metastases at the time of diagnosis, similar to acinar carcinoma. The 5-year survival rates range from 15% to 43%, with 46% survival rate at 6 years and 16% at 8 years.[881,882] According to the SEER cancer registry, the incidence of ductal carcinoma has increased over the past two decades, and men with ductal cancer are more likely to present with advanced cancer (30% T3 with ductal cancer, compared with 7% with acinar cancer).[883] When ductal cases were stratified by the proportion of the ductal component, the high ductal component group ($\geq$30%) had a lower biochemical recurrence rate compared with that in the low ductal component group (<30%) (60% versus 20% biochemical progression-free survival after 5 years).[866]

The pattern of metastases is identical to that of the typical acinar carcinoma. Metastases usually reveal a tumor histologically similar to ductal carcinoma, even when coexistent acinar carcinoma is present in the prostate, suggesting that the endometrioid pattern is more aggressive.

Androgen deprivation therapy provides palliative relief in many cases but does not appear to influence survival. Patients may respond to orchiectomy or estrogen therapy, albeit transiently, with marked symptomatic improvement.[882] Radiation therapy has been used to palliate voiding difficulty and hematuria, as well as to control bone pain, and these tumors appear to be sensitive to treatment with radiation. Nonetheless, the prognosis is poor.[861]

Cribriform, Papillary, and Solid Carcinomas

These histologic patterns are present in both IDC and ductal carcinoma, and often coexist. The cribriform pattern of carcinoma is characterized by masses of tumor punctuated by sievelike spaces.[884,885] Unlike cribriform PIN, cribriform carcinoma does not have a basal cell layer at the periphery of glands.[344,370,861] Some studies suggest that cribriform carcinoma and IDC/ductal carcinoma are the same entity.[886]

Up to 70% of cribriform masses of malignant cells are intraductal, and these are now classified as IDC rather than noninvasive ductal carcinoma.[30] Based on the cumulative data, we suggest that the term *cribriform carcinoma* be used only as a descriptive term, if it is used at all, and should not refer to a specific entity.

Systematic plus targeted biopsy is superior to systematic biopsy alone or targeted biopsy alone to detect cribriform morphology.[884] On final histopathology, cribriform tumor foci are associated with an increased percent of pattern 4 involvement and EPE. Only 17% of cribriform tumors in pure form were visible on multiparametric MRI. Based on final histopathology, the sensitivity of systematic biopsy, targeted biopsy, and systematic plus targeted biopsy for cribriform morphology was 21%, 29%, and 37%, respectively.

The amount of cribriform or IDC collectively in patients with Gleason 3 + 4 cancer correlates with amount of pattern 4 (6%, 22%, and 44% of cribriform/IDC in those with less than 10%,

10% to 25%, and 25% to 50% pattern 4 cancer, respectively) and biochemical recurrence-free survival after surgery and radiation therapy.[886]

PTEN loss is frequent in fused small acini, cribriform-central cells, small cribriform acini, and Gleason grade 5 cells; p27 loss is common in cribriform-peripheral cells and fused small acini in comparison with benign acini; and CD44v7/8 loss is often present in cribriform-peripheral cells.[887]

Comedocarcinoma

Comedocarcinoma is characterized by luminal necrosis within round masses of malignant cells, similar to comedocarcinoma of the breast. This variant of adenocarcinoma is considered Gleason pattern 5 carcinoma based on the degree of acinar differentiation. It is frequently aneuploid, suggesting aggressiveness.[888,889] PAP and PSA are present in the majority of tumor cells. Comedocarcinoma is invariably found in association with other patterns of adenocarcinoma and does not warrant separation as a clinicopathologic entity.

Adenocarcinoma With Neuroendocrine Differentiation

NE differentiation is present at least focally in virtually all cases of adenocarcinoma, although the number of NE cells varies according to the tissue fixative used, antibody and method of staining used, and number of tissue sections examined.[890-913] Abrahamsson and colleagues[908,911] identified NE cells in 92% of cancers fixed in formalin. Aprikian et al. found NE cells in 77% of untreated cancers, 60% of hormone-refractory cancers, and 52% of metastases, with a small number of dispersed positive cells in each.[914] About 10% of adenocarcinomas contain unique NE cells with distinctive large eosinophilic granules (adenocarcinoma with Paneth cell–like change) (see later).

NE differentiation typically consists of scattered cells that are inapparent by light microscopy but revealed by immunoreactivity for one or more markers, including the prototypical signature of positive NE markers, intense and abundant Ki67 expression, and negative nuclear AR staining caused by androgen resistance. Chromogranin and serotonin are the best markers of NE cells in formalin-fixed sections (Fig. 9.45), although these may be negative in 12% of cases and are not required for diagnosis.[915] PSA immunoreactivity is present in up to 20% of small cell carcinomas of the prostate. NE cells are apparently increased after irradiation or androgen deprivation, and they are relatively resistant to cytotoxic drugs and other therapies.[916,917]

NE cells have no apparent clinical or prognostic significance in benign epithelium, cancer, and lymph node metastases, according to most, but not all, reports.[918] Aprikian et al. found no correlation of NE differentiation with pathologic stage or metastases.[914,919] We found no apparent relationship between the number of immunoreactive NE cells in PIN and cancer and a variety of clinical and pathologic factors, including stage.[901] Allen et al. studied 120 patients and found no significant association between NE differentiation and patient prognosis.[920] Krijnen et al. reported that NE differentiation was associated with early hormone therapy failure, indicating that these cells are androgen independent.[921,922] Their findings suggested that the presence of large numbers of NE cells in cancer may indicate a poor prognosis, perhaps because of insensitivity to hormonal growth regulation, but this claim has been refuted by most studies. We determined the expression of chromogranin A and serotonin in patients with node-positive prostate cancer and found that immunoreactivity was greatest in benign epithelium, with less expression in localized cancer and

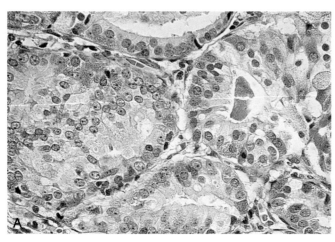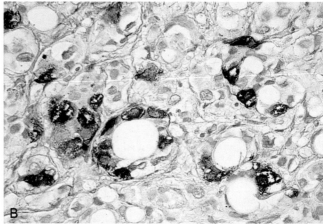

Fig. 9.45 Prostatic cancer with neuroendocrine differentiation. (A) Adenocarcinoma with large eosinophilic granules. (B) Another case, with serotonin-immunoreactive cells corresponding to the cells with granules.

metastases.[901] There was no consistent association between the expression of chromogranin A or serotonin and survival. The cumulative findings reveal no consistent association of NE differentiation in typical adenocarcinoma and any clinical outcome variable.[923,924] The number of NE cells is greatest in castrate-resistant cancer.[925]

Significant overexpression and gene amplification of AURKA and n-Myc was observed in 40% of NE cancers and 5% of non-NE cancers, and these biomarkers may cooperate to induce a NE phenotype in prostatic cells.[926]

Adenocarcinoma With Neuroendocrine Cells With Large Eosinophilic Granules (Paneth Cell–like Change)

Cells with large eosinophilic granules (Paneth cell–like change) represent an uncommon but distinct form of NE differentiation (Fig. 9.45). This finding is more common (10% prevalence rate) than previously believed, but usually consists of only rare foci of scattered cells and small clusters that may be overlooked.[905,927-934] Although cells with large eosinophilic granules in benign epithelium and adenocarcinoma resemble Paneth cells of the intestine, they are distinguished by the identification of NE differentiation and absence of lysozyme immunoreactivity. They display intense cytoplasmic immunoreactivity for chromogranin, NSE, and serotonin, and are analogous to "eosinophilic argentaffin cells" of the appendix, cervical glandular mucosa, colonic adenoma, and Sertoli cells of the testis.

A greater number of cells than those with large eosinophilic granules stain with NE markers, suggesting that there are NE cells with smaller granules that are not apparent on H&E-stained sections.[927,929] Most reports on NE differentiation in benign and malignant prostate samples have described only scattered cells that are inapparent on routine stain but are immunoreactive for NE markers.[905,927-933,935] Thus large eosinophilic granules represent a distinctive form of NE differentiation.

PSA and PAP immunoreactivity are also observed in cells with large eosinophilic granules, similar to other benign and neoplastic NE cells in the prostate.[929] Azumi et al. and others identified concomitant PSA and NE marker immunoreactivity in prostatic carcinoid and other prostatic tumors.[936,937] Abrahamsson et al. showed AR immunoreactivity in cells with NE differentiation.[938] It appears that select cells in the prostate coexpress glandular and NE differentiation. This differs from pure NE carcinoma of the

prostate in which clonal proliferation and lack of PSA expression are common (see later).

The presence of cells with large eosinophilic granules is not associated with aggressive behavior, including higher stage, serum PSA, and cancer grade, suggesting that this pattern of NE differentiation is not indicative of a poor prognosis.[927,929] We disagree with the unsubstantiated suggestion that cancer that contains such cells should not be included in Gleason grading, recognizing that grade is reflective of architectural pattern and cytologic findings.[927] The significance with cribriform pattern is uncertain. Although the functional role of prostatic cells with NE differentiation is unknown, they appear to be important in regulation of cell growth, differentiation, and secretion.[938-941]

Low-Grade Neuroendocrine Carcinoma (Carcinoid)

A spectrum of NE differentiation can be seen in prostatic adenocarcinoma, varying from the rare carcinoid-like pattern (low-grade NE carcinoma) to the unusual but more common small cell undifferentiated (oat cell) carcinoma (high-grade NE carcinoma) (see later).[942-949] Carcinoid tumor of the prostate shares similar morphologic and immunophenotypic features with its counterpart in other organs. The differential diagnosis includes metastatic carcinoid tumor from the colon or another site, paraganglioma, and nested variants of urothelial carcinoma.[950] Correlation of the clinical presentation and histopathologic features (including the immunohistochemical profile) ensures accurate diagnosis.

High-Grade Neuroendocrine Carcinoma (Small Cell and Large Cell Carcinoma)

Most cases of NE carcinoma have typical signs and symptoms of prostatic adenocarcinoma, and serum PSA usually varies according to cancer volume and stage. However, some cases of pure small cell carcinoma may progress without detectable serum PSA increase.[853,951,952] Rare cases are gigantic, enlarging the prostate to more than 500 g.[953] In addition, paraneoplastic syndromes are frequent in patients with small cell carcinoma and carcinoid of the prostate.[954] Cushing syndrome is most frequent, invariably in association with adrenocorticotropic hormone immunoreactivity in tumor cells. Other clinical conditions include malignant hypercalcemia, the syndrome of inappropriate antidiuretic hormone secretion, and myasthenic (Eaton-Lambert) syndrome.[955]

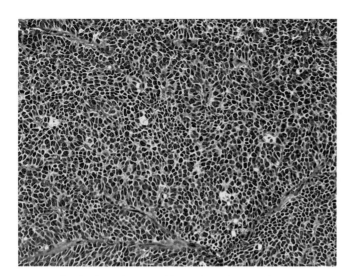

Fig. 9.46 Small cell undifferentiated (oat cell) carcinoma of the prostate.

These tumors are morphologically identical to small cell carcinoma of the lung and other sites (Fig. 9.46). Typical acinar adenocarcinoma is present, at least focally, in about 25% of cases, and transition patterns may be seen. In cases of adenocarcinoma with a solid Gleason 5 pattern suggestive of NE carcinoma, immunohistochemical stains are recommended to confirm differentiation; it should be noted that some cases will be nonreactive for NE markers, and they are not required for diagnosis. In one case, the cancer was immunoreactive for pan-CK, KIT, platelet-derived growth factor-α, p53, Ki67, PSA, and racemase, but negative for NE markers.[956] Importantly, many cases of Gleason 5 + 5 = 10 contain at least focal small cell carcinoma.[957]

Immunohistochemically, a wide variety of secretory products may be detected within small cell carcinoma cells, including serotonin, calcitonin, adrenocorticotropic hormone, HCG, TSH, bombesin, calcitonin gene-related peptide, and inhibin.[915,958] The same cells may express peptide hormones, PSA, and PAP.[955] About 45% of small cell carcinomas contain *ERG* gene rearrangements, compared with 0% in counterparts originating in the lung and bladder.[687] Interestingly, small cell carcinoma is more basal and stemlike than the adenocarcinoma phenotypes.[959]

Ultrastructurally, small cell carcinoma and carcinoid tumor display typical NE features.[893] The characteristic finding is variable numbers of round, regular 100- to 400-nm diameter membrane-bound neurosecretory granules. Well-defined cytoplasmic processes are usually present, with approximately 8 to 15 granules per process. The cells are small, with dispersed chromatin and small inconspicuous nucleoli. Acinar formation is lacking in the NE component, and no tonofilaments are present.

Small cell carcinoma is aggressive and rapidly fatal.[960] It was originally classified by Gleason as a variant of pattern 5 carcinoma. Today, many describe the histogenesis of this cancer without applying a Gleason grade, reserving grading for only adenocarcinoma and its variants; we, however, maintain Gleason grading and simply add a comment. AR expression in small cell carcinoma was predictive of a poorer outcome (median survival, 10 months) than in cases without expression (median survival, >30 months), regardless of treatment.[961] Deorah et al. found that 61% presented with metastases.[962] The 12, 24, 36, 48, and 60 months observed survival rates were 48%, 28%, 19%, 17%, and 14%, respectively.[962] In multivariate regression, age, pathology, and stage were strong predictors of survival.

Treatment is like that of small cell lung carcinoma, with the same disappointing results. One study found that addition of doxorubicin to the etoposide/cisplatin regimen improved survival, whereas another found higher toxicity and failure to improve outcome.[963,964]

Although unusual, metastases to the prostate from other sites may mimic carcinoid and small cell carcinoma of the prostate. High-grade carcinoma from the bladder that invades the prostate may be mistaken for NE carcinoma. Other rare tumors, such as peripheral neuroectodermal tumor, desmoplastic small round cell tumor, and malignant lymphoma, may be mistaken for prostatic NE carcinoma, particularly in extraprostatic sites.

Large cell NE carcinoma is an unusual variant of high-grade NE carcinoma that shares with small cell carcinoma a frequent antecedent history of adenocarcinoma treated with hormone therapy, common coexistence with adenocarcinoma, and rapid metastasis and death.[456] It consists of solid sheets and ribbons of cells with abundant pale to amphophilic cytoplasm, large nuclei with coarse chromatin, prominent nucleoli, brisk mitotic activity, and foci of necrosis. Intense immunoreactivity is seen for CD56, CD57, chromogranin A, synaptophysin, racemase, Bcl-2, MIB1 (Ki67), and p53, with focal positive staining for PSA and PAP, and negative AR staining.[965]

Adenocarcinoma With Glomeruloid Features

Prostatic cancer with glomeruloid features is characterized by the presence of acinar adenocarcinoma with round to oval epithelial buds (glomerulations) projecting into acinar lumens, architecturally mimicking renal glomeruli (Fig. 9.47).[966] There is an external layer of "parietal" cells and a conspicuous central tuft of "visceral" cells. The central tuft sometimes has a cribriform architecture; in other cases a prominent central fibrovascular core is present. Less commonly, there is a characteristic concentric infolding of epithelial cells arranged in semicircular rows with delimiting cleft-shaped spaces.

Three percent of needle biopsies and 5% of prostatectomies with prostate cancer contain glomeruloid features.[966] When present, a minority of each cancer, up to 20%, consists of glomeruloid features, and the remaining typical acinar adenocarcinoma was usually Gleason score 6 or 7.[966] The cases were equally divided between the apex and the peripheral zone.

Glomeruloid structures appear to be a specific but uncommon finding in prostate cancer.[38,474,966,967] They are not observed in any benign or hyperplastic processes in radical prostatectomies or needle biopsies. This feature appears to be a useful diagnostic clue for malignancy and may be valuable in some challenging needle biopsies.

Adenocarcinoma with glomeruloid features may be mistaken for the invasive cribriform pattern of carcinoma. In cribriform carcinoma the cellular bridges around the periphery of the nests are usually relatively evenly spaced and similar in size. In contrast, glomeruloid structures show a distinctive polarity of growth, with a dominant cellular bridge connecting the central cell mass to the periphery. Other cellular bridges may be seen focally but are thin and few. Fibrovascular cores are less common in cribriform carcinoma, and semicircular delimiting concentric cleftlik spaces are lacking. In some cases, the glomeruloid and cribriform patterns coexist. It is possible that these two patterns represent a spectrum of differentiation.

Primary Wilms tumor of the prostate also contains glomeruloid structures.[968] This tumor apparently arises from nephrogenic rests in relation to the wolffian duct system and shows the classical

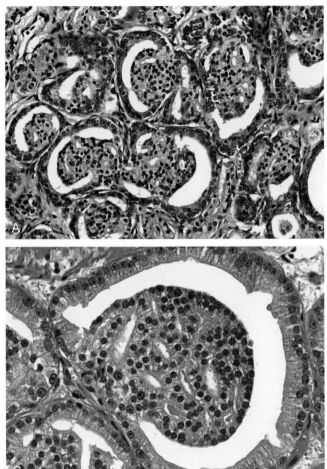

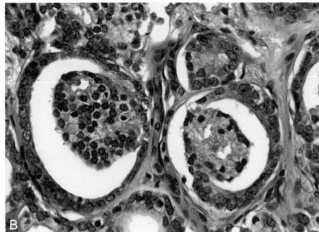

Fig. 9.47 Adenocarcinoma with glomeruloid features. (A) Multiple epithelial buds protrude into acinar spaces, reminiscent of renal glomeruli. (B) Each glomerulation shows cribriform growth with a dominant cellular bridge connecting it to the rest of the acinus; in this case, the nuclei in the glomerulation have indistinct nucleoli. Compare with (C), another case in which the nuclei in the glomerulation have prominent nucleoli.

triphasic histologic pattern typical of Wilms tumor. Glomeruloid microvascular proliferations in the prostate are related to increased microvessel density and decreased survival.[561] To our knowledge, no other processes that occur in the prostate possess glomeruloid features.

Adenocarcinoma with glomeruloid features is currently regarded as Gleason grade 3, although some consider this to be grade 4 because of the cribriform pattern and occasional coexistence with Gleason pattern 4 cancer. Further studies are needed to determine the independent prognostic value of the glomeruloid growth pattern and its correlation with Gleason grading, but this task will be difficult because the glomeruloid pattern is virtually never observed in isolation without another pattern.

Carcinoma With Oncocytic Features

Rare cases of adenocarcinoma with diffuse oncocytic change have been reported, characterized by tumor cells with abundant eosinophilic granular cytoplasm reflecting the presence of abundant mitochondria.[969,970] Tumor cells display PSA immunoreactivity. The clinical behavior appears to be the same as typical acinar adenocarcinoma. Differential diagnosis includes prostatic nodular hyperplasia with oncocytic change (oncocytoma), NE carcinoma, and rhabdoid tumor.

Lymphoepithelioma-like Carcinoma

Carcinoma accompanied by a dense lymphocytic infiltrate is termed *lymphoepithelioma*, *lymphoepithelioma-like carcinoma*, and

medullary carcinoma (Fig. 9.48). This histologically distinctive tumor is most common in the head and neck but has rarely arisen in the breast, bladder, and other sites. Rare cases have been reported in the prostate.[850,971] Although prostatic adenocarcinoma may be associated with granulomatous prostatitis or may be patchy acute and chronic, it rarely appears as solid islands of epithelial cells punctuating a sheetlike infiltrate of lymphocytes characteristic of

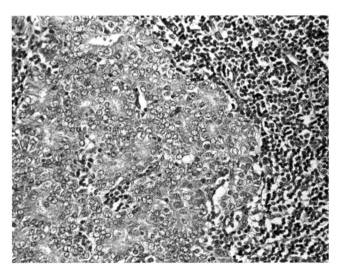

Fig. 9.48 Lymphoepithelioma-like carcinoma of the prostate.

lymphoepithelioma-like carcinoma at other sites. The tumor has large areas of typical adenocarcinoma, but the different patterns are not intermingled.

Immunohistochemistry reveals that the lymphocytic infiltrate is composed chiefly of T cells, similar to the lymphocytic response in lymphoepithelioma-like carcinoma at other sites. No atypical lymphocytes are observed, and these are not the features of malignant lymphoma or leukemia involving the prostate. Flow cytometry reveals that the tumor is aneuploid. In situ hybridization is negative for Epstein-Barr virus.

Clear Cell Carcinoma

There are single case reports of renal-type clear cell carcinoma, tubulocystic clear cell adenocarcinoma of the prostate, and clear cell adenocarcinoma resembling müllerian/urethral adenocarcinoma arising in the prostatic utricle.[972-975]

Basal Cell Carcinoma (Adenoid Cystic/Basal Cell Carcinoma)

Grossly, basal cell carcinoma (adenoid cystic/basal cell carcinoma) is white and fleshy, sometimes with microcysts, unlike acinar carcinoma, which is usually yellow. It invariably involves the transition zone with or without the peripheral zone.[976,977]

Microscopically, it consists of tumor nests or nodules of various size embedded in a desmoplastic or myxoid stroma (Fig. 9.49). The adenoid pattern is characterized by nests and clusters with keratinization that may be reminiscent of eccrine spiradenoma, with trabeculae of cells with cribriform growth and microcystic spaces with abundant basement membrane material. The basaloid pattern consists of nests of hematoxyphilic cells with microvacuolated nuclei, scant cytoplasm, and peripheral palisading, virtually identical to basal cell carcinoma of skin. There is occasional squamous metaplasia. Tumor necrosis is uncommon (Table 9.34).

PNI is often prominent, and rarely intraneural invasion is present. Metastases usually have a predominant adenoid pattern and are limited to lymph nodes, liver, lung, and bowel (bone metastases have not been reported).[976]

Immunohistochemical findings indicate that adenoid cystic/basal cell carcinoma is a biphasic ductal/myoepithelial tumor, similar to its counterpart in the salivary gland.[139,978-982] All cases are at least focally immunoreactive for CK AE1/AE3, basal cell keratin 34βE12, and p63 in up to 90% of cells (Table 9.35).[976] Staining with keratin 34βE12 is present in peripheral but not luminal cells of the adenoid nests; conversely, staining for CK7 was observed only in luminal cells, and no tumors react with CK20. Remarkably cytoplasmic reactivity is noted for S-100 protein in a small but significant number of cells (up to 20%) in 63% of cases; α-smooth muscle actin immunoreactivity is present in up to 70% of cells in a minority of cases.[976] There is also strong immunoreactivity in all cases for CD44 and HER2, and in 67% for EGFR.[983,984] Loss of PTEN expression is observed in 56%.[984] *TMPRSS2-ERG* rearrangements are not detected by molecular techniques or immunohistochemistry, and ERBB2, KIT, p53, and AR expressions are either absent or show only weak, limited reactivity.[984]

The rarity of immunoreactivity for PSA and PAP (patchy staining limited to luminal cells of adenoid nests with cribriform pattern) is consistent with the normal preoperative serum PSA usually observed with this variant. By in situ hybridization, no mRNA for PSA was detected.[980]

Adenoid cystic/basal cell carcinoma behaves aggressively, with about one-half of the cases displaying high-risk pathologic features

or local recurrence (44%) within 4 years; there is also a small but significant potential for late recurrence and metastasis.[976,984] It often coexists with typical acinar adenocarcinoma, but the absence of transition forms strongly suggests coincidental coexistence or rare collision tumor. Perineural growth is typical, similar to its counterpart in other organs. Prostatic basal cells are not androgen dependent, unlike typical acinar adenocarcinoma, so adenoid cystic/basal cell carcinoma is considered unresponsive to androgen deprivation therapy.

Squamous Cell and Adenosquamous Cell Carcinoma

Squamous cell carcinoma is rare in the prostate, with fewer than 100 published cases.[985-1005] Adenosquamous carcinoma refers to the combination of squamous cell carcinoma and typical acinar carcinoma, and appears to be even rarer than pure squamous cell carcinoma.[1005,1006]

Presenting signs and symptoms are similar to those of typical adenocarcinoma, although there is often a history of hormonal therapy or radiation therapy. Patients are older than 50 years, with a mean peak in the seventh decade of life. PSA and PAP levels are usually normal, even with metastases, and bone metastases are typically osteolytic rather than osteoblastic. Squamous cell carcinoma of the prostate may arise in patients infected with *Schistosoma haematobium*.

Squamous cell carcinoma is histologically similar to its counterpart in other organs, consisting of irregular nests and cords of malignant cells with variable keratinization and squamous differentiation, rarely with squamous pearls (Fig. 9.50). Keratinizing squamous cell carcinoma usually arises in the periurethral ducts and is rare; otherwise the site of origin of squamous cell carcinoma is unknown. Mott required an absence of acinar differentiation for the diagnosis of squamous cell carcinoma, as well as a lack of bladder involvement.[1007] Mixed tumors are best classified simply as adenosquamous carcinoma. Mott also required no prior estrogen therapy, but we consider this exclusion unnecessary.[1007] Metastases sometimes consist of adenosquamous carcinoma in cases without a squamous component in the primary tumor, perhaps because of sampling error of the initial prostate biopsy.

Saito et al. identified PAP immunoreactivity in the acinar and squamous components.[1008] Conversely, Gattuso et al. found staining only in the acinar component.[1006] Interestingly, they noted immunoreactivity in the squamous component for high-molecular-weight keratin AE3, but not in the acinar component. The adenosquamous carcinoma reported by Devaney et al. showed PSA and PAP immunoreactivity in the acinar component, but not in the squamous component; both components were diploid.[1005]

The histogenesis of squamous and adenosquamous carcinoma is unknown, but proposed origins include multipotential stem cells, basal cells or reserve cells, columnar secretory cells, prostatic urethral or periurethral urothelial cells, cells of adenocarcinoma, and metaplastic squamous cells. Most contemporary authors believe that the cancer arises from the urothelium of the urethra or large periurethral prostatic ducts.

Squamous cell carcinoma is aggressive, with a mean survival of about 14 months regardless of therapy. These tumors appear to be unresponsive to androgen deprivation therapy.

Squamous cell carcinoma may be confused with squamous metaplasia because of infarction, radiation therapy, and hormonal therapy. Rarely, adenocarcinoma may exhibit benign squamous metaplasia. Squamous cell carcinoma of the bladder may invade the prostate and must be excluded.

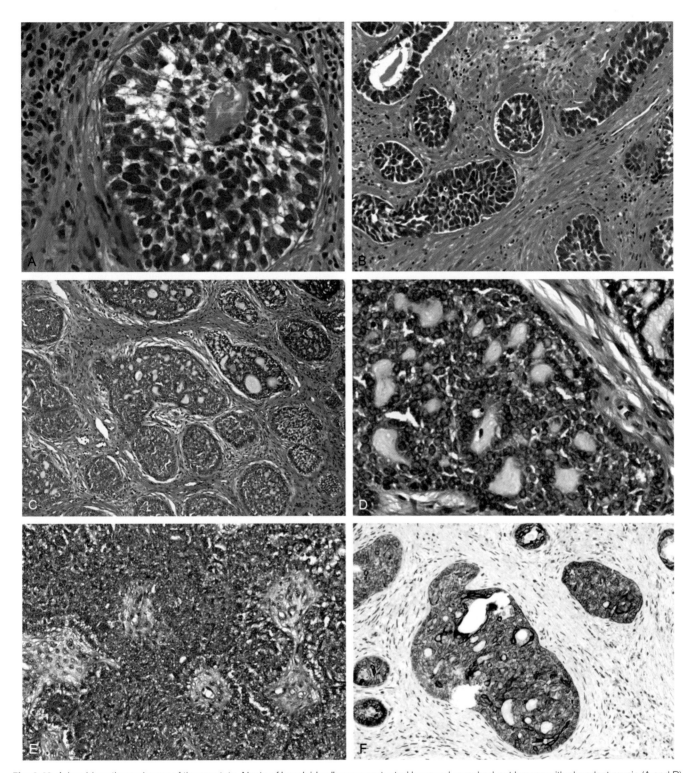

Fig. 9.49 Adenoid cystic carcinoma of the prostate. Nests of basaloid cells are punctuated by round, punched-out lumens with abundant mucin (A and B). Adenoid cystic pattern (C and D). (E) Basal cell pattern. (F) Strong immunoreactivity for basal cell–specific keratin 34βE12.

Urothelial Carcinoma

Urothelial carcinoma is rarely primary in the prostate, accounting for less than 4% of prostatic cancers, and usually represents synchronous or metachronous spread from carcinoma in the bladder and urethra (Fig. 9.51).[1009-1013] It involves the prostate in about 40% of cysto-prostatectomy specimens for bladder carcinoma. Up to 41% of patients have unsuspected coexistent prostatic adenocarcinoma.[1014]

Patients usually have symptoms of hematuria, urinary obstruction, or prostatitis. Serum PSA and PAP levels are not elevated. Clinically, urothelial carcinoma may be mistaken for prostatitis or nodular hyperplasia. Most clinical findings are due to tumor arising elsewhere in the urothelium.

Urothelial carcinoma usually involves the periurethral prostatic ducts and acini. About 62% of cases diagnosed by biopsy consist of

TABLE 9.34 Comparative Histology of Adenoid Cystic/Basal Cell Carcinoma With Benign Basal Cell Proliferations

	Benign Basal Cell Proliferations[a]	Adenoid Cystic/Basal Cell Carcinoma
Layers of cells	Multilayered	Multilayered
Contour	Rounded, circumscribed nodule	Infiltrative nests or trabeculae
Lumen formation	If present, bounded by secretory cells	Present, bounded by basal cells; prominent in adenoid pattern
Basement membrane deposits	Absent	Present in lumina
Cribriform formations	Absent	Present in adenoid pattern
Stroma	Unaltered	Myxoid or desmoplastic
Extraprostatic extension	Absent	May be present
Perineural invasion	Absent	May be present
Macronucleoli	May be present	Present

[a]Includes basal cell hyperplasia, atypical basal cell hyperplasia, and basal cell adenoma.

TABLE 9.35 Immunohistochemical Reactivity of Adenoid Cystic/Basal Cell Carcinoma

Markers	Cases Tested	Positive Cases	Range of % Cells Positive
Prostate cancer markers			
Cytokeratin 34βE12	15	15 (100%)	40%-90%
p63	7	6 (86%)	40%-100%
P540S/AMACR	3	0	
Prostate-specific antigen	10	2 (20%)[a]	<5%
Prostatic acid phosphatase	8	1 (14%)[a]	1%
Other markers			
CD44	10	9 (90%)	100%
c-kit	1	1	5%
Cytokeratin 7	12	12 (100%)[a]	30%-90%
Cytokeratin 20	7	0	
S-100 protein	8	5 (63%)	2%-20%
α-Smooth muscle actin	8	2 (25%)	30%-70%

[a]In adluminal cells.

urothelial carcinoma in situ of prostatic ducts and acini; 29% consist of both carcinoma in situ and invasive carcinoma; and 9% have widespread stromal invasion without carcinoma in situ.[1015] Diagnostic criteria are identical to those for urothelial cancer of the bladder. Most cancers are moderately or poorly differentiated and usually associated with prominent chronic inflammation. Squamous metaplasia is infrequent.

TURP containing prostatic tissue at the 5 or 7 o'clock position of the verumontanum substantially improves detection of ductal and acinar involvement.[1016] Moreover, if superficial glands are involved at the 5 or 7 o'clock position of the verumontanum, involvement of deeper glands should also be suspected.

Radical cystoprostatectomy is the treatment of choice.[1017,1018] Bladder cancer extending into the prostate can be easily missed. The 5-year cancer-specific survival rates for the locoregional categories were as follows: carcinoma in situ of the prostatic urethra and prostatic ducts and acini, 100%; stromal invasion, 45%; EPE and seminal vesicle involvement, 0%; and lymph node metastases, 30%.[1012]

Distinguishing urothelial carcinoma from adenocarcinoma is clinically important because of the estrogen unresponsiveness of the former; these tumors often coincidentally coexist. By light microscopy, adenocarcinoma usually displays some evidence of acinar differentiation, although this may be difficult to identify in high-grade cancer or cases of urothelial carcinoma with pseudoglandular pattern. Immunohistochemical stains for PSA and PAP distinguish these tumors, with immunoreactivity exclusively in adenocarcinoma. Also, keratin 34βE12 is highly specific and sensitive for urothelial carcinoma regardless of grade, as is GATA3.[1019] Other differential diagnostic considerations include urothelial-type adenocarcinoma and urothelial differentiation in carcinosarcoma.[849] In cystoprostatectomy specimens that contain carcinoma in situ in prostatic ducts, CK5/6 and CK5 immunoreactivity separated prostatic basal cells from carcinoma in situ.[1020] Low-grade urothelial carcinoma involving the prostate is particularly difficult because of the similarity to urothelial metaplasia and basal cell hyperplasia.[1021]

Urothelial carcinoma often arises in patients with previous radiation therapy for prostate cancer and is usually high grade, with a high incidence of sarcomatoid features.[1022-1024] After radiation, 40% of patients have residual prostate cancer with or without coexistent prostatic urothelial carcinoma (15% and 25%, respectively).[1025]

Immunohistochemistry of Prostate Cancer

Identifying Prostatic Origin in Metastases

The detection rate of prostate origin of metastasis for single immunohistochemical markers is 100% for NKX3.1, 98% for AR, 84% for PSMA, 81% for PSA, 66% for PAP, 60% for HOXB13, 60% for prostein and 50% for ERG.[1026] The sensitivity of HOXB13 as a marker for prostate origin in lymph node metastases is 93% and in bone metastases is 33%.[1027,1028] A panel of markers is recommended to account for occasional cases with false-positive and false-negative staining.

TMPRSS2:ERG and the ETS Family Gene Fusions

Gene fusion between the androgen-responsive gene *TMPRSS2* and members of the *ETS* family of DNA-binding transcription factor genes are found in up to 70% of prostate cancers and in a lower percentage of cases of high-grade PIN, and are specific for prostatic malignancy.[1029] Recurrent fusions are identified between the 5′-noncoding region of *TMPRSS2* and *ERG*. These fusions are the driving mechanism for overexpression of the three members of the ETS transcription factor family: *ERG* (21q22.3), *ETV1* (7p21.2), and *ETV4* (17q21). Considering the high incidence of prostate cancer and the high frequency of this fusion, the *TMPRSS2:ETS* gene fusion is the most common genetic aberration described to date in human malignancies.

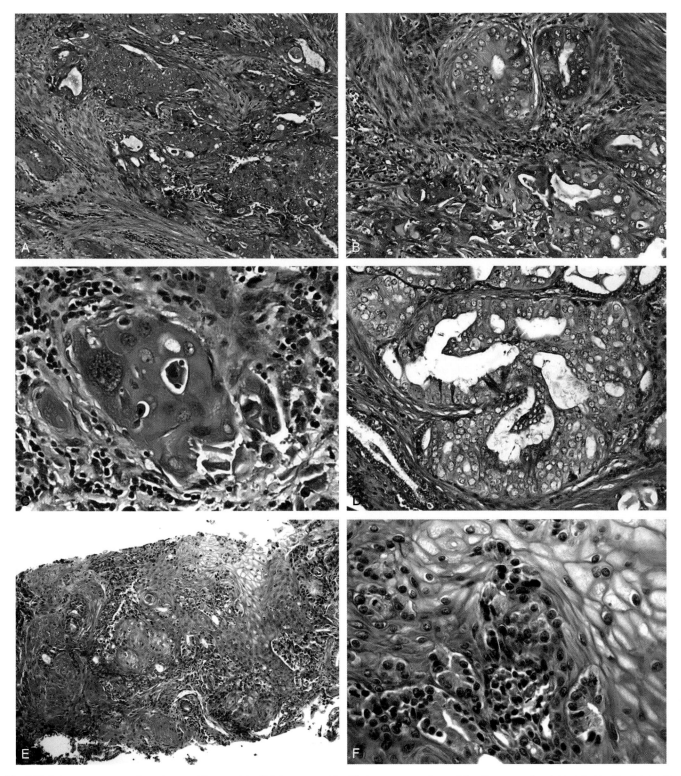

Fig. 9.50 Adenosquamous cell carcinoma of the prostate. This tumor was identified many years after radiation therapy and androgen deprivation therapy for typical acinar adenocarcinoma (A to D). Mixed glandular and squamous elements (A and B). (C) High-grade squamous cell carcinoma with keratinization. (D) Glandular differentiation. Compare with (E) and (F), an unusual case of adenocarcinoma with florid squamous metaplasia after androgen deprivation therapy.

Fusion-positive tumors are often associated with higher grade, higher stage, larger cancer volume, and poorer survival than fusion-negative tumors, although conflicting results have been obtained.[1030-1036] ERG immunoreactivity in prostatectomies is associated with younger age at diagnosis.[1037] Adjacent Gleason pattern 3 and 4 cancers in prostatectomy specimens are concordant for the *TMPRSS2:ERG* gene fusion.[1038]

Five morphologic features are associated with *TMPRSS2-ERG* fusion prostate cancer including blue-tinged mucin, cribriform growth pattern, macronucleoli, cancer spread with preexisting ducts

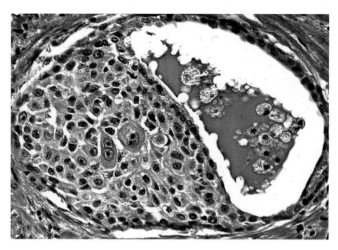

Fig. 9.51 Urothelial carcinoma showing pagetoid spread through this periurethral prostatic duct.

and ductules, and signet ring cell features.[1039] Distinct hybrid transcript patterns are found in samples taken from multifocal cancer, suggesting that *TMPRSS2-ERG* gene fusions arise independently in different foci.[1040] *TMPRSS2:ERG* gene fusions are also detected clinically in the urine of patients with prostate cancer.[1031]

Results of ERG measurement by immunohistochemistry and FISH are beset by variance in intrafocal heterogeneity, with 20% of cancer foci having intrafocal heterogeneity for protein expression by immunohistochemistry and 33% for FISH-based gene fusion status and fusion pattern.[1041] Interestingly, SPINK1 expression is mutually exclusive of ERG expression, although this has been refuted.[1036,1042,1043]

Phosphatase and Tensin Homolog

PTEN loss is present in 27% of Gleason 3 + 4 = 7 cancers and correlates with higher grade and stage.[1044,1045] PTEN inactivation and ERG overexpression are observed by immunohistochemistry in 24% and 2% of transition zone T1a cancers, respectively.[1046] There is high concordance between PTEN determination by immunohistochemistry and FISH; 93% of cancers with expression of PTEN by immunohistochemistry show absence of *PTEN* gene deletions by FISH, and 66% of those with PTEN protein loss showed *PTEN* gene deletion.[1047,1048]

Expression in biopsies correlates with rebiopsy and prostatectomy upgrading, treatment change, and adverse histopathology at prostatectomy.[1049-1052] FISH and immunohistochemistry for detection of PTEN loss are each predictive of biochemical recurrence-free survival after surgery.[1042,1048,1053] The "triple-hit" combination of PTEN loss, *TMPRSS2:ERG* expression, and *SLC45A3:ERG* expression by immunohistochemistry is strongly predictive of biochemical failure.[1054] PTEN loss is also predictive of cancer-specific survival, especially in those with negative ERG and strong AR expression.[1050,1055]

In multifocal cancer on biopsies, there is a high rate of variability in PTEN results, with intratumoral and intertumoral heterogeneity of 68% for both for loss of PTEN expression, with greatest loss in high-grade and high-volume cancer.[1056]

Subsets of PTEN based on deletion size comprise five distinct subtypes with different aneuploid signatures: (1) "small interstitial" (70 bp to 789 Kb); (2) "large interstitial" (1 to 7 Mb); (3) "large proximal" (3 to 65 Mb); (4) "large terminal" (8 to 64 Mb), and (5) "extensive" (71 to 132 Mb).[1057]

Prostate Cancer Antigen 3

The prostate cancer antigen 3 (*PCA3*) gene, located on chromosome 9q2 1-22, is overexpressed more than 60-fold in more than 90% of prostate cancers, but is not transcribed in the benign prostate. Moreover, no PCA3 transcripts are detectable in a wide range of extraprostatic tissues, indicating that PCA3 is the most specific prostate cancer gene identified to date. The PCA3 mRNA includes a high density of stop codons; thus it does not have an open reading frame, resulting in a noncoding RNA.

This test is a promising adjunct tool for the early diagnosis of prostate cancer from urine samples. The PCA3 urine test can be used after negative biopsy to determine which patients may be candidates to undergo active surveillance and, possibly, a second biopsy.

Matched prostatectomy studies indicate that PCA3 is a significant and independent biomarker of cancer that shows no correlation with serum PSA or prostate volume. However, it is predictive of cancer volume, stage, Gleason score, and positive surgical margins, and is not influenced by inflammation.[1058-1060] *PCA3* gene testing holds valuable potential in men with: (1) elevated PSA level but no cancer on initial biopsy, (2) cancer despite normal levels of PSA, (3) PSA elevation associated with prostatitis, and (4) presumed microfocal cancer undergoing active surveillance.[1061] In a large, prospective, multicenter study of biopsies, PCA3 had a specificity of 78% and sensitivity of 49% for prostate cancer detection (Fig. 9.52).[1062] PCA3 score is associated with Gleason score and cancer volume. A higher PCA3 score also correlates with increased probability of detecting prostate cancer.

c-Myc

Nuclear c-Myc (MYC) expression is observed in 73% of prostate cancers, but rarely in benign epithelium.[1063] Most studies suggest that c-Myc plays a role in the regulation of prostate growth and carcinogenesis.[101,1064-1066] c-Myc is a well-known oncogene that is activated in many human cancers, and expression is amplified with increasing grade of prostate cancer, particularly in metastases.[1067-1073] c-Myc expression correlates with growth of androgen-responsive prostate epithelium.[1074] Activation of c-Myc leads to formation of enlarged nucleoli and increased nucleolar number in luminal epithelial cells in vivo.[79] Elevated c-Myc protein expression by immunohistochemistry correlates with c-Myc amplification.[1072]

c-Myc expression, together with PTEN and Ki67 expression in primary cancer samples, is more accurate in predicting biochemical recurrence-free survival than clinical factors alone in men with high-risk prostate cancer receiving adjuvant docetaxel after prostatectomy.[1075] Conversely, a recent report found no significant association between c-Myc protein expression and stage, grade, or PSA level at diagnosis after surgery or prediction of metastases and cancer-specific survival.[1076]

Telomerase

There is consistent overexpression of telomerase occurring in PIN and persisting throughout all stages of cancer progression.[1077] Interestingly, telomerase expression correlates with c-Myc.

Apoptosis-Suppressing Oncoprotein Bcl-2

Bcl-2 is an apoptosis suppressor gene. Overexpression of the protein in cancer cells may block or delay onset of apoptosis, selecting and maintaining long-living cells, and arresting cells in the G_0 phase of the cell cycle. Expression of Bcl-2 is usually restricted to the basal cell layer of the normal and hyperplastic epithelium.[1078]

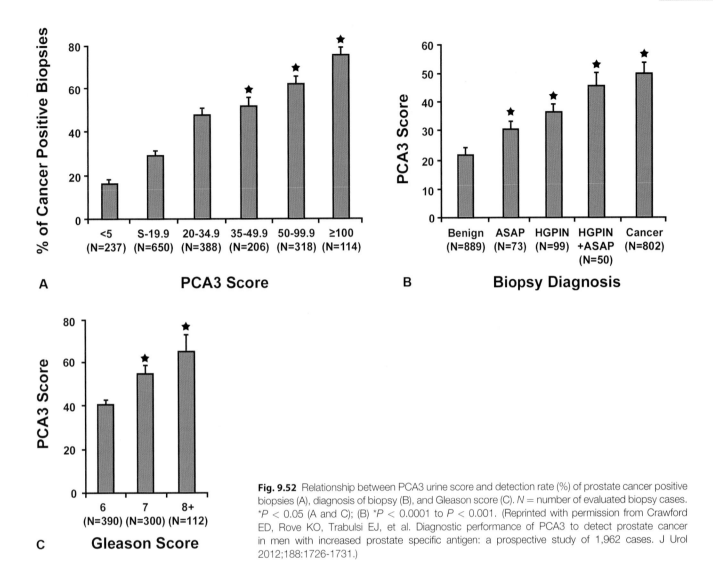

Fig. 9.52 Relationship between PCA3 urine score and detection rate (%) of prostate cancer positive biopsies (A), diagnosis of biopsy (B), and Gleason score (C). N = number of evaluated biopsy cases. *P < 0.05 (A and C); (B) *P < 0.0001 to P < 0.001. (Reprinted with permission from Crawford ED, Rove KO, Trabulsi EJ, et al. Diagnostic performance of PCA3 to detect prostate cancer in men with increased prostate specific antigen: a prospective study of 1,962 cases. J Urol 2012;188:1726-1731.)

Overexpression of Bcl-2 is present in PIN. In cancer the prevalence and expression pattern of Bcl-2 is controversial. More than 70% of prostate carcinomas are Bcl-2⁻, 18% have weak expression, and 11% exhibit strong expression.[1079] One study found moderate heterogeneous Bcl-2 overexpression in localized cancer that was inversely correlated with Gleason grade.[1080]

Expression of Bcl-2 correlates with high stage, high grade, metastases, response to therapy, biochemical recurrence-free survival, and cancer-specific survival.[1081,1082] Bcl-2 was positive in 46% of cases, and Bax expression was altered in 54% of cases after radiation therapy; abnormal Bcl-2 was not related to any of the failure end points tested.[1083] Altered Bax expression was associated with failure. The combination of negative Bcl-2/normal Bax expression seemed more robust after radiation and androgen deprivation therapy, being related to reduced biochemical failure and any failure.[1083] Androgen deprivation therapy decreased Bcl-2 expression in cancer, suggesting that these cells develop resistance to apoptotic signals.[1080] Targeted suppression of Bcl-2 antiapoptotic family members using multitarget inhibition strategies through induction of apoptosis is being investigated as a treatment option.[1084]

p53

Mutant p53 expression is a late event in localized prostate cancer, usually present in high-grade cancer and elevated in untreated metastatic cancer, hormone-refractory cancer, and recurrent cancer. p53 is an independent predictor of metastatic risk.[1085] Inactivation of p53 is associated with cancer progression and may be a marker of survival in stage T2-3N1-3M0.[1086,1087] When combined with stem cell gene expression patterns and loss of PTEN, loss of p53 expression predicts very poor survival.[1088] Docetaxel induces p53 phosphorylation, a crucial determinant of docetaxel sensitivity in prostate cancer cells.[1089] In multivariable analyses, p53 status is independently associated with survival in castrate-resistant metastatic cancer.[1090]

p16

p16 nuclear and cytoplasmic expression is observed in 0% to 16% of benign specimens and 37% to 86% of cancer specimens, with high specificity (84%) and positive predictive value (74%).[1091,1092] p16 expression was found in 58% of ERG⁺ but in only 22% of ERG⁻ cancers, and prediction of biochemical failure was strictly limited to the subset of ERG⁻ cancers.[1091]

p21

The *WAF1/CIP1* gene encodes a p21 cyclin-dependent kinase inhibitor that plays a role in regulation of the cell cycle. Upon induction by p53, *p21WAF1/CIP1* binds to cyclin-dependent kinase 2, resulting in downregulation of CDK2 activity and G_1 growth arrest. Mutations in the *WAF1/CIP1* gene abrogate this apparent tumor suppressor gene activity, thereby facilitating escape of G_1/S checkpoint control with propagation into S phase and maintenance of malignant potential.[1093] There is an increase in *WAF1/CIP1* polymorphisms in prostate cancer, but no correlation exists between *WAF1/CIP1* expression and grade, stage, or cancer progression.[1094,1095] p21 protein expression showed a significant association with cancer-specific survival and overall survival.[1096] AR primes androgen-independent prostate cancer cells to DNA damage-induced apoptosis through the PIRH2-p53-p21 axis.[1097]

p27Kip1

The cyclin-dependent kinase inhibitor p27Kip1 negatively regulates cell proliferation by mediating cell-cycle arrest in G_1 and may have an important causative role in development of aggressive prostate cancer.[1098] p27Kip1 expression decreases with higher Gleason score and seminal vesicle invasion.[1099] Furthermore, p27Kip1 expression is an independent predictor of treatment failure of node-negative cancer after prostatectomy.[1099,1100] Combined immunohistochemical analysis of c-Myc, EZH2, and p27 accurately predicted outcome for intermediate-risk prostate cancer patients after surgery.[1101]

Androgen Receptors

Androgen action in target cells is mediated by androgen receptors (AR). Mutations of AR are rare in untreated cancer and are present in up to 25% of cancers from patients treated with antiandrogens.[1102,1103] No amplifications are found in untreated cancer. AR gene amplification leads to overexpression, and almost all hormone-refractory prostate carcinomas express high levels of AR.[1104]

Molecular events in AR influence the natural history of prostate cancer, including deregulated expression, somatic mutation, and posttranslational modification.[1105-1107] The androgen-signaling pathway is co-opted in prostate cancer by genetic and epigenetic changes that alter initiation and transcriptional outcome of signaling by silencing key targets and fusing androgen-responsive promoters to new genes to create new targets for androgen signaling.[1108] ERBB appears to activate ARs, especially when androgen levels are low, promoting survival of prostate cancer cells.[1109] This might be similar to targeting HER2 in hormone-refractory prostate cancer.[1109] PSA localizes to nuclei of androgen-stimulated cancer cells and controls AR mRNA and protein levels.[1110]

Immunostaining for AR is positive in 95% of prostatic adenocarcinomas, compared with 19% of vesicular urothelial carcinomas, 16% of renal pelvic urothelial carcinomas, and 19% of primary renal cell carcinomas.[1111]

Methylation

A validated panel of 25 DNA methylation probes successfully separated aggressive and nonaggressive subclones of cancer.[1112] Another report validated a four-gene methylation signature (*AOX1*, *GSTP1*, *HAPLN3*, and *SLC18A2*) that accurately separated biopsies from patients with and without cancer (area under the ROC curve, 0.65; sensitivity, 30.8%; specificity, 100%).[1113]

An epigenetic signature of 52 differentially methylated *CpG* sites predicts recurrence-free survival after prostatectomy.[1114]

Glutathione S-transferases (GSTs) comprise a family of detoxifying enzymes that are critical for inactivation of toxins and carcinogens. *GSTP1* is the most commonly altered gene in prostate cancer. Silencing of the *GSTP1* expression by hypermethylation of the promoter region is present in 90% of prostate cancers and 70% of PIN cases. Detection of hypermethylated *GSTP1* may be useful for diagnosis and prognosis.[1115,1116] High levels of *GSTP1* promoter methylation are associated with the transition from PIN to carcinoma.[212] However, GST polymorphisms are not consistently associated with cancer risk.[1117] There was reduction or loss of immunoreactivity of all subclasses of GST with progression from benign epithelium to high-grade PIN and carcinoma.[1118] We hypothesized that carcinogenesis in the prostate results from impaired cellular handling of mutagenic agents caused by reduction or loss of expression of GST and of other detoxifying and antimutagenesis agents.

Mitochondrial DNA Testing

Mitochondrial DNA deletion by quantitative polymerase chain reaction (qPCR) predicts missed cancer and men who do not require repeat biopsy with a high degree of accuracy (sensitivity and specificity of 84% and 54%, respectively).[338]

Integrins

Integrins participate in multiple cellular processes including cell adhesion, migration, proliferation, survival, and activation of growth factor receptors.[1119] Expression of the E-cadherin/catenin complex correlates with risk for high-grade prostate cancer, and β_1 integrin activation predicts metastases.[1120] Immunohistochemical expressions of α_3 and $\alpha_3\beta_1$ correlate with recurrence after prostatectomy.[1121] Only 19% and 28% of patients were recurrence free at a mean 10-year follow-up when their tumors showed strong α_3 or positive $\alpha_3\beta_1$ immunoreactivity, respectively.

Metaanalysis of gene expression data was used from 18 gene array datasets targeting the transition from normal to localized prostate cancer and from localized to metastatic prostate cancer to functionally annotate the top 500 differentially expressed genes, and these were clustered in pathways involving integrin-based cell adhesion[1122]: integrin signaling, the actin cytoskeleton, cell death, and cell motility pathways. Integrins were downregulated in the transition from benign tissue to primary localized cancer. Based on the results, the authors developed the collagen hypothesis of prostate carcinogenesis in which the initiating event is age-related decrease in expression of collagen genes and other genes encoding integrin ligands. Concomitant depletion of integrin ligands leads to the accumulation of ligandless integrin and activation of integrin-associated cell death. To escape integrin-associated death, cells suppress the expression of integrins, which in turn alters the actin cytoskeleton, elevates cell motility and proliferation, and disorganizes prostate histology, contributing to the histologic progression and metastases of cancer.

Heat Shock Protein 90

Cell surface heat shock protein 90 (Hsp90) is involved in prostate cancer cell invasion through the integrin β_1/FAK/c-Src signaling pathway, and molecular targeting of cell surface Hsp90 may be a novel target for the effective treatment of metastases. The Hsp90 chaperone, tumor necrosis factor receptor–associated protein-1 (TRAP1), is abundantly expressed in PIN and cancer but not in the benign prostate.[1123]

Initial reports of robust preclinical antitumor activity of first-generation Hsp90 inhibitors in cancer were followed by disappointing clinical responses; however, advances in compound design and development, use of novel preclinical models, and further biologic insights into Hsp90 structure and function have now stimulated a resurgence in enthusiasm for these drugs as a therapeutic option.[1124]

Pro-PSA

Pro-PSA, the precursor of PSA, is an inactive 244-amino acid protein secreted by prostatic cells. It is a distinct molecular form of free PSA in serum, including native and truncated forms. Truncated (-2) pro-PSA accounts for up to 19% of free PSA in the serum of patients without prostate cancer, but represents up to 95% of free PSA.

Percent pro-PSA is superior to percent-free and calculated complexed PSA for early detection in the PSA range of 2 to 10 ng/mL, and it detects more aggressive cancer.[1125] However, this claim has been challenged.[1126] In multivariable logistic regression models, PSA, pro-PSA, and the combination of PSA and pro-PSA increased the accuracy of the base multivariable model by 6%, 6%, and 6%, respectively (all $P < 0.001$).[1127]

In tissue samples, we found that 100% and 99% of cases of PIN and cancer were immunoreactive for (−5/−7) pro-PSA and (−2) pro-PSA, respectively.[1128] A total of 31% of high-grade PIN and 11% of cancer cases with negative racemase staining showed strong staining for (−5/−7) pro-PSA. Both forms were sensitive markers for prostatic epithelium, making them possible candidates for investigating carcinoma with an unknown primary, particularly in cases in which PSA staining is negative and the level of suspicion is high.

Prostatic Membrane Antigen

PSMA is expressed in the prostatic epithelium and is a potential marker of progression. PSMA overexpression is detected in high-grade PIN and is associated with a higher Gleason score of prostate cancer (Fig. 9.53).[1129,1130] In Gleason patterns 4 and 5 verseus Gleason pattern 3, PSMA sensitivity is 84% and specificity is 95%.[1131] PSMA immunoreactivity is predictive of progression after surgery.[335,1132] Maximum standardized uptake value on 68Ga-PSMA PET/CT (gallium 68 PSMA PET/CT) correlates with PSMA immunohistochemical expression in cancer, enabling detection with high sensitivity and specificity.[1133]

Proliferating Cell Nuclear Antigen

Proliferating cell nuclear antigen (PCNA) is a nuclear nonhistone protein that serves as an auxiliary protein for DNA polymerase that reaches maximal expression during the S phase of the cell cycle.[1134,1135] Hence, PCNA has been widely used as an index of the proliferative activity. The PCNA labeling index is lowest in benign prostatic epithelium and organ-confined cancer, and

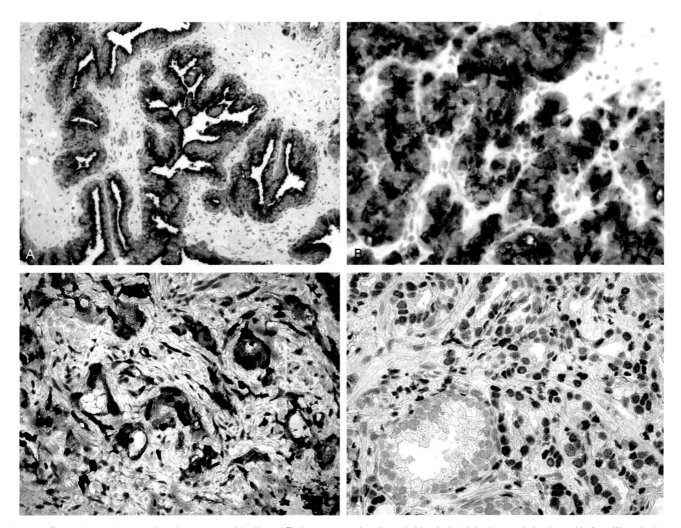

Fig. 9.53 Prostatic membrane antigen immunoreactivity (A and B). Intense cytoplasmic and abluminal staining is seen in benign epithelium (A) and adenocarcinoma (B). ERG staining in high-grade cancer (C and D).

increases from well-differentiated to poorly differentiated invasive cancer, although there is wide variance.[1136] The correlation of the PCNA index with cancer stage is strong.[1134,1136,1137] Hence, high PCNA labeling indices indicates progression and may be an independent prognostic indicator.[1135,1138-1141]

Ki67/MIB1

The Ki67 antigen, detected by the MIB1 antibody, is preferentially expressed during the late G_1, S, G_2, and M phases of the cell cycle. Expression increases with Gleason grade and predicts biochemical recurrence-free survival, overall survival, and cancer-specific survival after prostatectomy.[545,1142-1149] There is a trend for prediction after radiation therapy.[1150]

BRCA1 and BRCA2

BRCA1 and BRCA2 immunostaining is present in 93% and 42% of cancers, respectively. Multivariate analysis showed that BRCA1, BRCA2, pT3 stage, resection margin positivity, prostate size, and Gleason score are independent predictors of biochemical recurrence.[1151] BRCA2 inactivation is present by immunohistochemistry in 15% of patients with metastatic castrate-resistance cancer.[1152] Although this finding does not preclude a response to docetaxel, it predicts a poor response (25% versus 71% in men with wild-type BRCA2).

Engrailed Nuclear Protein-2

Engrailed nuclear protein-2 (EN2) gene is a homeobox-containing transcription factor overexpressed in cancer cells when compared with benign epithelial cells. Downregulation of EN2 expression by siRNA resulted in decreased PAX2 expression and cancer cell proliferation. EN2 in urine is predictive of prostate cancer, with a sensitivity of 66% and a specificity of 88%, with no relation to PSA concentration.[1153]

Sarcosine and Other Metabolites

Sreekumar et al. profiled more than 1126 metabolites across 262 clinical samples related to prostate cancer in urine samples and identified sarcosine, an N-methyl derivative of the amino acid glycine, as a differential metabolite that was highly increased during progression to metastasis.[1154] Sarcosine level was also increased in cancer cell lines relative to benign epithelium. Knockdown of glycine-N-methyl transferase, the enzyme that generates sarcosine from glycine, attenuated cancer invasion. Addition of exogenous sarcosine or knockdown of the enzyme that leads to sarcosine degradation, sarcosine dehydrogenase, induced an invasive phenotype in benign epithelial cells. AR and the ERG gene fusion product coordinately regulate components of the sarcosine pathway. However, Jentzmik and colleagues noted that sarcosine had no clinical value as a marker for prostate cancer detection or identification of aggressive cancer.[1155]

Other Immunohistochemical Markers of Prognosis in Prostate Cancer

A wide variety of other diagnostic and prognostic factors have been evaluated in prostate cancer, but none is recommended at this time for routine use.[25,454,1156]

CXCR4 protein expression is upregulated in cancer and correlates with increased stage and cancer-specific survival.[1157]

Membrane-associated guanylate kinase, WW and PDZ domain-containing protein 2 (MAGI2) may be a useful adjunct when racemase fails because it has a higher accuracy for distinguishing benign from malignant glands on the same core (95% versus 88%, respectively).[1158,1159] MAGI2 expression is reduced during cancer progression and its loss predicts biochemical recurrence.[1160]

Kinesin family member 14 (KIF14) is a novel candidate oncogene that is strongly expressed in 57% of cancer cases, with little or no expression in hyperplasia.[1161] Expression was positively correlated with Gleason score and clinical stage.

Expression of zinc-α 2-glycoprotein (AZGP1) is strong in benign acini and 62% of cancers, and correlates with higher Gleason score, higher pT, positive nodal status, and biochemical recurrence-free survival on multivariate analysis.[1162] Absence of AZGP1 expression is an independent predictor of biochemical failure, overall survival, and cancer-specific survival.[1163,1164] Expression in a phase 3 trial of prostatectomies independently predicted biochemical recurrence-free survival and metastasis-free survival.[1165]

Immune checkpoint inhibitor programmed death ligand 1 (PD-L1) expression is commonly seen in prostate cancer cells (92% of cases).[1166] Another inhibitor, programmed cell death protein 1 (PD-1), expressed in lymphocytes, is a significant negative independent prognostic factor for biochemical recurrence-free survival (HR, 2.5) in multivariate analysis. PD-L1 is not expressed in benign hyperplasia and localized cancer, and is found in up to 32% of castrate-resistant cancers and 43% of small cell carcinomas.[1167,1168] In node-positive patients at high risk for progression, those with at least 1% PD-L1–immunoreactive cancer cells have shorter metastasis-free survival than those with PD-L1⁻ cancer, and PD-L1 expression is associated with CD8⁺ T-cell density, but not with CD20⁺ B-cell density.[1169]

Transforming acidic coiled-coil (TACC3), a member of the TACC family, is upregulated in metastatic cancer, and high expression predicted stage, Gleason score, and shorter cancer-free survival than patients with low expression.[1170]

Apurinic/apyrimidinic endonuclease 1 (APE1/Ref-1) overexpression is an independent predictor of biochemical recurrence in cancer lacking TMPRSS2:ERG fusion.[1171]

DNA repair protein ERCC1 (excision repair cross-complementation group 1) expression predicts biochemical recurrence.[1172]

Oncogene epithelial cell transforming sequence 2 (Ect2) predicts higher overall survival and biochemical recurrence-free survival when expressed at low levels.[1173]

STAT3 and IL6R are expressed at varying levels in 95% of metastases of castrate-resistant cancer.[1174]

Epithelial-mesenchymal transition–related molecule Twist-1 and stem cell marker EZH2, when highly expressed, are strongly associated with higher pretreatment PSA level, Gleason score ≥7, advanced tumor stage, lymph node involvement, distant metastasis, and biochemical progression.[335,1146,1175]

Cysteine-rich secretory protein 3 (CRISP3) expression in prostatectomies is predictive of longer biochemical recurrence-free survival.[1042]

OCT4 expression in prostatectomy specimens predicted a 5-year biochemical recurrence-free survival rate of 57% when high and 91% in patients when low.[1176]

Prostate stem cell antigen expression predicts biochemical recurrence after surgery and androgen deprivation therapy.[1177]

High expression of caveolin-1 in tumor stroma was associated with longer cancer-specific survival.[1178]

ERα, ERβ, and aromatase in the epithelium and stroma each independently predicted biochemical recurrence-free survival after prostatectomy.[1179]

MUC1 is membrane-bound glycoprotein involved in cell adhesion and intracellular signaling. Expression in epithelial cells is different in benign acini, primary cancer, and lymph node metastases. High MUC1 expression in primary cancer correlates with cancer volume and T stage. In lymph node metastases, high expression corresponds with size of metastases and predicts biochemical recurrence-free survival and cancer-specific survival.[1180]

Transient receptor potential cation channel, subfamily M, member 4 (TRPM4) expression is widely expressed in prostatic epithelium, with strongest staining intensity in cancer.[1181] Overexpression is associated with increased risk for biochemical failure after surgery.

HOXB13 is expressed in 52% of prostate cancers and correlates with advanced pT stage, high Gleason grade, positive lymph node status, high preoperative PSA level, *TMPRSS2:ERG* fusion status, PTEN deletions, AR expression, cell proliferation, reduced PSA expression, and early biochemical recurrence.[1182]

Paxillin is involved in cell adhesion and is upregulated in cancer compared with normal and hyperplastic tissues.[1183] Expression predicts shorter biochemical recurrence-free survival after surgery.

Molecular Biology of Prostate Cancer

Prostate carcinogenesis involves multiple genetic changes, including loss of specific genomic sequences associated with inactivation of tumor suppressor genes and gain of other genes associated with activation of oncogenes.[1184,1185] Multiple panels of genes are commercially available for a variety of applications in diagnosis and prognosis of prostate cancer (Table 9.36).

The most common chromosomal aberrations in PIN and carcinoma are TMPRSS2:ETS translocations, gain of chromosome 7 (in particular 7q31), loss of 8p and gain of 8q, and loss of 10q, 16q, and 18q.[105] Microsatellite instability is being used to guide immunotherapy treatment for men with advanced cancer.[1186] Mitochondrial DNA content is lower in prostate cancer compared with normal adjacent prostate tissue, but tumors with high content have an unfavorable stage.[1187]

Despite decades of gene expression and sequencing studies, there is no unified molecular classification of prostate cancer.[1188] Efforts are hampered by the enormous complexity of this cancer; even when the earliest or smallest cancer is detected, it already contains hundreds of deregulated, aberrantly expressed, or mutated genes. This creates great difficulty in identifying gene-signaling pathways that are potential drivers of pathogenesis suitable for therapeutic intervention. Further, there is marked heterogeneity of prostate cancer at both the cellular level and the level of multifocality (e.g., "men don't get prostate cancer, they get prostate cancers").[1189] Despite this intratumor variation, DNA sequencing of single-cell nuclei from core biopsies is a rich source of quantitative parameters for evaluating neoplastic growth and aggressiveness, including the presence of clonal populations, phylogenetic structure of those populations, the degree of the complexity of copy number changes, and measures of the proportion of cells with clonal copy number signatures, all of which show good correlation with Gleason score.[1190]

Is it possible that there is a myriad of pathways that culminate in what we recognize as prostate cancer?

Genetics of Familial Prostate Cancer

Genomewide association studies to date have revealed about 35 single-nucleotide polymorphisms (SNPs) that are consistently associated with familial prostate cancer, although none has been linked to cancer stage or outcome.[1191,1192] Cancer risk is minimal (<1.3) for individual SNPs, accounting in total for only about 25% of inherited risk.[1193] Conversely, linkage analysis of families with hereditary prostate cancer has usually yielded inconsistent findings. A recent report found by linkage analysis in combination with targeted massively parallel sequencing a recurrent mutation in the HOXB13 G84E variant on chromosome 17 that was associated with early-onset and hereditary prostate cancer, but accounted for only a small fraction of all prostate cancer cases (3%).[1194]

The best model to predict genetic susceptibility to prostate cancer may be a mixed model of inheritance that included both a recessive major gene component and polygenic component composed of all SNPs known to be associated with cancer and a residual polygenic component due to postulated unknown genetic variants.[1195] Such a model may be able to predict the probability of cancer development based on the combination of SNP profiles and family history. Sun et al. found that the area under the ROC curve of genetic score for predicting positive biopsy was higher (0.58 to 0.62) than family history (0.51 to 0.55) in five published study populations.[1196] Likewise, Seibert et al. reported that polygenic hazard scores based on 59 SNPs accurately predict age at onset of aggressive cancer with no contribution from family history.[1197]

DNA Ploidy

DNA ploidy analysis of prostate cancer provides important predictive information that supplements histopathologic examination.[1198] Patients with diploid tumors have a more favorable outcome than those with aneuploid tumors. Among patients with lymph node metastases treated with prostatectomy and androgen deprivation therapy, those with diploid tumors survive 20 years or longer, whereas those with aneuploid tumors die within 5 years.[1199] However, the ploidy pattern of prostate cancer is often heterogeneous, creating potential problems with sampling error.[1200]

Analysis of multiple biopsies is important for correct preoperative ploidy estimation.[1200] A good correlation exists between DNA ploidy and histologic grade, and DNA ploidy adds clinically useful predictive information for some patients.[1201,1202] The incidence of aneuploidy in high-grade PIN varies from 32% to 68% and is somewhat lower than in carcinoma (55% to 62%). There is a high level of concordance of DNA ploidy of PIN and coexisting cancer. About 70% of aneuploid cases of PIN are associated with aneuploid carcinoma; conversely, only 29% of cases of aneuploid cancer are associated with aneuploid PIN. DNA ploidy pattern by flow cytometry correlates with cancer grade, volume, and stage. Most low-stage tumors are diploid and high-stage tumors are nondiploid, but numerous exceptions occur.

Biopsy ploidy status independently predicts cancer recurrence in patients treated by prostatectomy.[1087] However, 40% of patients with Gleason score ≥4 + 4 and 55% of patients with biochemical recurrence have diploid cancer.[1202] Patients with diploid lymph node metastases treated by androgen deprivation therapy alone have longer progression-free survival and overall survival than those with aneuploid metastases.[1203] Five-year cancer-specific survival is about 95% for diploid tumors, 70% for tetraploid tumors, and 25% for aneuploid tumors.[1204] Digital image analysis appears to have a high level of concordance (about 85%) with prostatectomy specimens evaluated by flow cytometry.[1205]

For T1a prostate cancer, DNA ploidy is not predictive of progression or survival, but such patients have a very favorable prognosis.[1206]

MicroRNA

MicroRNA (miRNA) are small endogenous noncoding RNA (18 to 25 nucleotides) that can block protein expression and promote or suppress cancer development and progression caused by specific tissue expression signatures. For example, miRNA-1 and miRNA-143 expression correlated with longer relapse-free survival. This topic has been recently reviewed.[1207-1210]

TABLE 9.36   Commercially Available Molecular Tests for Prostate Cancer (United States)

Test	No. of Genes or Proteins	Description	Selection Criteria	Predicted Outcome
Before diagnosis				
ConfirmMDx	3	Tissue expression of methylation biomarkers GSTP1, APC, and RASSF1	Initial negative biopsy; all risk levels	Risk for cancer and adverse pathology
ExoDx	3	Urine RNA levels of SPDEF, ERG, and PCA3 extracted from exosomes	All risk levels	Risk for cancer and adverse pathology
Mi-Score	3	Urine levels of ERG and PCA3 combined with serum PSA	All risk levels	Risk for cancer and adverse pathology
Progensa PCA3	1	Urinary RNA level of DD3 (PCA3)	All risk levels	Risk for cancer
SelectMDx	2	Urinary RNA levels of DLX1 and HOXC6	All risk levels	Risk for cancer and adverse pathology
4Kscore	4	Plasma levels of pro-PSA, active PSA, ACT-bound PSA and cleavage-inactivated PSA	All risk levels	Risk for cancer and adverse pathology
Prostate Health Index	3	Plasma levels of fPSA, tPSA, and -2 pro-PSA (p2PSA)	All risk levels	Risk for cancer and adverse pathology
Apifiny	8	Plasma autoantibodies to CSNK2A2, centrosomal protein 164 kDa, NK3 homeobox 1, aurora kinase interacting protein 1, 5′-UTR BMI1, ARF6, chromosome 3′-UTR region Ropporin/RhoEGF, and desmocollin 3	All risk levels	Risk for cancer and adverse pathology
After positive biopsy				
DeCipher	22	Tissue RNA biomarkers involved in cell differentiation, proliferation, structure, adhesion and motility, immune modulation, cell-cycle progression, and androgen signaling (LASP1, IQGAP3, NFIB, S1PR4, THBS2, ANO7, PCDH7, MYBPC1, EPPK1, TSBP, PBX1, NUSAP1, ZWILCH, UBE2C, CAMK2N1, RABGAP1, PCAT-32, GLYATL1P4, PCAT-80, and TNFRSF19)	Adverse pathology (pT3 and/or positive margins or recurrence)	Recurrence and metastases at 5 years
Oncotype Dx	12	Tissue RNA biomarkers involved in androgen pathway (AZGP1, KLK2, SRD5A2, and FAM13C), cellular organization (FLNC, GSN, TPM2, and GSTM2), proliferation (TPX2), and stromal response (BGN, COL1A1, and SFRP4)	All risk levels after diagnosis	Adverse pathology, recurrence, and metastases at 10 years
Prolaris	31	Tissue RNA biomarkers of cell-cycle progression	All risk levels after diagnosis	Recurrence, metastases, and cancer-specific survival at 10 years
Promark	8	Tissue protein expression of DERL1, CUL2, SMAD4, PDSS2, HSPA9, FUS, pS6, and YBOX1	Gleason 3 + 3 and 3 + 4 after diagnosis	Adverse pathology: Gleason ≥4 + 3 and/or non–organ-confined disease (T3a, T3b, N1, or M1)
ProstaVysion	2	Tissue PTEN and *TMPRSS2:ERG* by fluorescence in situ hybridization and immunohistochemistry	Low or intermediate risk after diagnosis	Adverse pathology
Postprostatectomy tests				
DeCipher	22	Tissue RNA biomarkers involved in cell differentiation, proliferation, structure, adhesion and motility, immune modulation, cell-cycle progression, and androgen signaling (LASP1, IQGAP3, NFIB, S1PR4, THBS2, ANO7, PCDH7, MYBPC1, EPPK1, TSBP, PBX1, NUSAP1, ZWILCH, UBE2C, CAMK2N1, RABGAP1, PCAT-32, GLYATL1P4, PCAT-80, and TNFRSF19)	Adverse pathology (pT3 and/or positive margins or recurrence)	Recurrence and metastases at 5 years
Metastatic cancer				
Oncotype Dx	1	AR-V7 protein level in blood	Metastatic castrate resistant	Resistance to androgen receptor-signaling inhibitor therapies

PSA, Prostate-specific antigen; *UTR*, untranslated region.
See reviews for comparative analysis of these tests and supportive evidence.[1728-1738]

Chromosome 7

FISH studies showed that aneusomy of chromosome 7 is frequent in prostate cancer and is associated with higher grade, higher pathologic stage, and early patient death.[1211,1212] PCR analysis of microsatellite markers identified frequent imbalance of alleles mapped to 7q31 in prostate cancer.[1212,1213] Allelic imbalance of 7q31 was strongly correlated with cancer aggressiveness, progression, and cancer-specific death.[1214] Genetic alterations of the 7q-arm may play an important role in the development of cancer.

Chromosome 8

Chromosome 8p is one of the most frequently deleted regions in prostate cancer. The rate of 8p22 loss ranged from 29% to 50% in PIN, 32% to 69% in primary cancer, and 65% to 100% in metastatic cancer.[1215] Other frequently deleted 8p regions include 8p21 and 8p12.[201,1215] Loss of 8p12 to 8p21 is observed in 63% of PIN foci and 91% of cancer foci using microdissected frozen tissue, whereas loss of 8p21 to 8p12 is present in 37% of PIN foci and 46% of cancer foci.[24,201] These findings suggest that more than one tumor suppressor gene may be located on 8p, and inactivation of these tumor suppressor genes may be important for the initiation of prostate cancer. In addition to loss of the 8 p-arm, there may be gain of the 8 q-arm.[1066,1215] Gain of 8q is found in 11% of primary cancers and 40% of lymph node metastases.[1216] There is amplification of 8q DNA sequences in 75% of cancers metastatic to lymph nodes.[1217] Also, gain of 8q is more frequent in recurrent cancer than in primary cancer and in metastatic and androgen-independent prostate cancer.[1218,1219] Target genes for 8q gain are overexpressed and amplified in 20% to 30% of the hormone-refractory carcinomas.[1220,1221] Gain of chromosome 8 centromere or 8 q-arm occurs simultaneously with loss of portions of the 8 p-arm in PIN and carcinoma.[1066,1219]

Chromosome 10

There is a high frequency of allelic imbalance at 10p and 10q in prostate cancer.[1222] The 10q23 to 10q24 region is most commonly deleted on the 10 q-arm, and this loss may inactivate the *MXI1* gene. Loss of *PTEN*, a tumor suppressor gene on chromosome 10q23, is found in 25% to 33% of advanced cancers (Fig. 9.54) and correlates with higher Gleason score and risk for clinical recurrence.[1223]

Chromosome 16

Allelic imbalance at 16q is present in about 30% of cases of clinically localized prostate cancer, and there is a high frequency at 16q23 to 16q24.[1224,1225] The most commonly deleted region is located at 16q24.1 to 16q24.2, and this deletion is associated with high stage, high grade, accelerated cell proliferation, the presence of lymph node metastases, positive surgical margin, and progression.[1225,1226] Chromosome 16p13.3 gain predicts biochemical recurrence and is frequently observed in metastases.[1227]

Other Chromosomes

The frequency of loss of 18q22.1 varies from 20% to 40%.[1228] Other regions demonstrating frequent allelic imbalance include 3p25 to 3p26, 5q12 to 5q23, 6q, 13q, 17p31.1, and 21q22.2 to 21q22.3.[1229] Loss of 10q, 16q, and 18q has also been reported in PIN.[24] There is a risk variant on chromosome 17q21 (odds ratio per allele, 1.5) that has a frequency of the risk allele of 5% in men of African descent, whereas it is rare in other populations (<1%).[1230] A recent metaanalysis of four studies identified a prostate cancer susceptibility locus, rs11672691 on chromosome 19, that is also associated with aggressiveness.[1231]

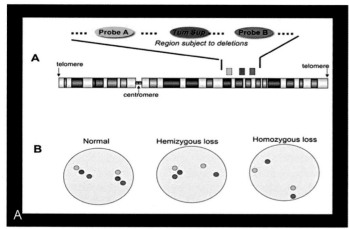

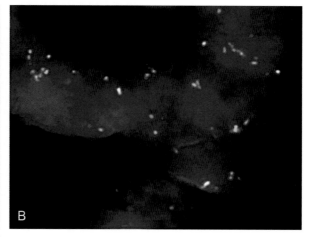

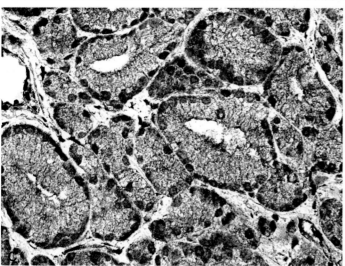

Fig. 9.54 Changes to PTEN proteins are caused by deletion of the gene (A) in cells. This deletion can be reliably detected by fluorescence in situ hybridization (B), which shows homozygous deletion detected by red FISH probe. (C) PTEN immunoreactivity is diffuse and weak in well-differentiated carcinoma.

DNA Mismatch Repair Genes

Genomic defects in DNA repair occur in up to 30% of cases of advanced castration-resistant cancer, many of which are germline aberrations and heritable.[1232] MSH6, MLH1, and PMS2 expression are immunohistochemically detectable in 90%, 85%, and 85% of cancers and are particularly strong in cancer with advanced stage, high grade, nodal metastasis, and early biochemical recurrence.[1233] High levels of *MMR* gene expression correlates with features of genetic instability such as the number of genomic deletions per cancer. The prognostic value of *MMR* genes is largely driven by the subset of cancers that lack *ERG* fusion.

Treatment Changes in Prostate Cancer

Treatment changes in the cancerous prostate tissue create diagnostic challenges for interpretation, particularly in prostate biopsies and extraprostatic metastases. It is critical that the clinician provide the pertinent history of androgen deprivation or radiation therapy to assist the pathologist in rendering the correct diagnosis.

Androgen Deprivation Therapy

One of the most popular forms of treatment for prostate cancer, androgen-deprivation therapy, has been in use for more than six decades. Contemporary therapies have varying mechanisms of action, including combined androgen blockage (gonadotrophin-releasing hormone [GnRH] agonists [e.g., goserelin and leuprolide] combined with an AR antagonist [e.g., flutamide, bicalutamide, and nilutamide]), GnRH antagonists (e.g., abarelix), and 5α-reductase inhibitors (e.g., finasteride and dutasteride). These agents are used for preoperative tumor shrinkage, symptomatic relief of metastases, cancer prophylaxis, and treatment of hyperplasia.[1234-1237]

To achieve total androgen deprivation, therapy should be effective in eliminating both testicular and adrenal hormones. Typical side effects of androgen deprivation therapy include hot flashes, loss of libido, and impotence.

Pathologic Findings After Androgen Deprivation

The histopathologic effects of most agents are similar (Table 9.37; Figs. 9.55 and 9.56).[226,235,760,1238-1242] All modes of hormonal treatment alter the cancerous epithelium, inducing apoptosis characterized by fragmentation of tumor DNA, appearance of apoptotic bodies, and inhibition of cell growth. The altered epithelium displays involution and acinar atrophy, cytoplasmic clearing, nuclear and nucleolar shrinkage, and chromatin condensation, although changes with 5α-reductase

TABLE 9.37	Androgen Deprivation Therapy: Histologic Features in Prostatic Adenocarcinoma[a]

Loss of glandular architecture
Nuclear shrinkage
Nuclear hyperchromasia and pyknosis
Nucleolar shrinkage
Mucinous degeneration
Other cytologic changes similar to benign secretory cell layer

[a]There is some variability in these changes depending on the method of therapy.

inhibitors appear to be much less pronounced and variable than with other agents (see later).

Adenocarcinoma displays distinctive histologic changes after androgen deprivation therapy. Architecturally most treated cancers have the appearance of Gleason primary grades 4 and 5, with a variety of patterns, including compressed fused glands, sheets of tumor cells, small cell clusters, and single-file ribbons of cells.

Treated tumor cells contain abundant clear vacuolated cytoplasm and central shrunken hyperchromatic nuclei obscuring the nucleoli and creating a "nucleolus-poor" appearance in many areas.[1238] Anisonucleosis is lower in treated cases than in untreated cases. Longer duration of androgen deprivation further decreases nuclear size. Necrosis and luminal crystalloids are usually absent. The combination of irregular cell clusters and single-file ribbons of tumor cells, cytoplasmic clearing, and shrunken hyperchromatic nuclei is strikingly reminiscent of lobular carcinoma of the breast. This pattern presents similar difficulties in differentiating small tumor foci from treatment-altered benign glands and lymphocytes, particularly in metastases. The uncoupling of the architectural and cytologic pattern is vexing due to the identification of small shrunken nuclei within malignant acini, particularly in lymph nodes submitted for frozen section evaluation.[757] An uncommon finding is the presence of atypical microacini with a single cell layer displaying large nucleoli, cytoplasmic vacuolation, and a "hemangiopericytoma-like" arrangement, but this was uncommon.[1243] Immunohistochemical studies with basal cell–specific markers and racemase are useful in difficult cases.

Pathologic Findings After 5α-Reductase Inhibitors

The primary nuclear androgen responsible for the maintenance of epithelial function and the most potent one is dihydrotestosterone (DHT).[1244] By inhibiting DHT synthesis, 5α-reductase inhibitors decrease the androgen drive to hyperplastic and malignant prostate cells while maintaining testosterone level. Finasteride inhibits only the type 2 isoenzyme of 5α-reductase, thereby partially blocking conversion of testosterone. Unlike finasteride, dutasteride is a dual inhibitor of both 5α-reductase isoenzymes, resulting in the suppression of serum DHT by greater than 90% compared with 70% seen with finasteride.[1245-1247] Finasteride and dutasteride are less effective than other forms of androgen deprivation therapy in altering the histology of the benign and neoplastic prostate (Fig. 9.57), although some changes have been described (details below).

Only a few reports have evaluated the histopathology of prostate cancer after 5α-reductase inhibitor treatment.[1248-1250] Civantos et al. analyzed prostatectomy specimens from patients treated for up to 24 months, and found that the effects of finasteride were more prominent in Gleason primary grade 2 and 3 cancer, making it difficult to recognize at low power and mimicking high Gleason grade cancer.[1248] Also, they noted that finasteride did not alter the cribriform pattern of primary grade 3 and 4 cancer, and noted that such foci should not be overgraded as grades 4 and 5.[1248] Conversely, Yang et al. prospectively studied 53 biopsies and found no differences between finasteride-treated and untreated cancer for a variety of histopathologic features, including Gleason score, number of cores involved, extent of cancer in the biopsies, atrophic changes in cancer cells, number of mitotic figures, amount of luminal mucin, and presence of prominent nucleoli.[1249] Their results were limited by sampling variation, but cancer was readily identifiable after finasteride treatment.

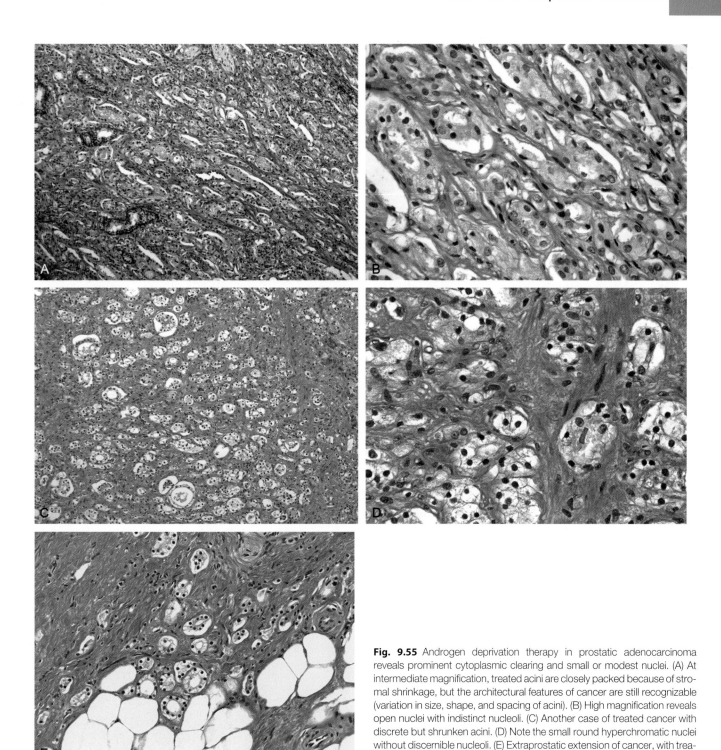

Fig. 9.55 Androgen deprivation therapy in prostatic adenocarcinoma reveals prominent cytoplasmic clearing and small or modest nuclei. (A) At intermediate magnification, treated acini are closely packed because of stromal shrinkage, but the architectural features of cancer are still recognizable (variation in size, shape, and spacing of acini). (B) High magnification reveals open nuclei with indistinct nucleoli. (C) Another case of treated cancer with discrete but shrunken acini. (D) Note the small round hyperchromatic nuclei without discernible nucleoli. (E) Extraprostatic extension of cancer, with treated acini infiltrating adipocytes.

The PCPT was the first large-scale study to provide significant evidence for the role of 5α-reductase inhibitors in the chemoprevention of prostate cancer.[1251] PCPT demonstrated that treatment with finasteride in a 7-year period was associated with a 25% decrease in the prevalence of prostate cancer versus placebo.[1252] However, tumors of higher Gleason scores (7 to 10) were detected more frequently in the treated versus placebo group (37% versus 22%), raising concerns that alteration in the androgen milieu by 5α-reductase inhibition may promote the growth of more aggressive tumors.[1252] One proven effect of finasteride is shrinkage of the prostate, and it is likely that there is increased detection of cancer (particularly large cancers), probably accounting for the appearance of higher Gleason score (an example of sampling bias).[1253] A recent retrospective study found no evidence of grade reclassification on rebiopsy when comparing treated and untreated cases.[759]

Iczkowski and colleagues reported the histopathologic effect in cancer after dutasteride therapy, comparing the pathologic findings

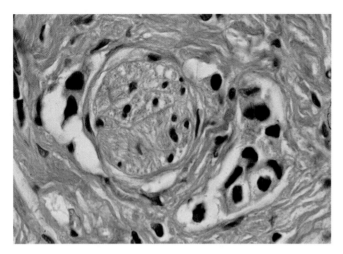

Fig. 9.56 Perineural invasion by prostatic adenocarcinoma after androgen deprivation therapy.

in radical prostatectomies from men receiving placebo and those preoperatively treated with a course of dual 5α-reductase inhibitor dutasteride.[1250,1254] They found that cancer volume was lower in dutasteride-treated men than in the placebo-treated group (15% versus 24%). Also, the percentage of atrophic epithelium was increased, and the stroma/gland ratio was doubled. The treatment alteration effect score was doubled and did not correlate with Gleason score changes.[1250] According to digital image analysis, key features associated with dutasteride treatment included greater shape and color uniformity in stroma, irregular clustering of epithelial nuclei, and greater variation in lumen shape.[1255] These findings indicate that dutasteride likely has a chemopreventive or chemoactive role.

The effect of dutasteride on the development of prostate cancer was studied prospectively in 4325 men with benign hyperplasia randomized to receive dutasteride or placebo.[234] The investigators reported that the incidence of cancer was lower in the dutasteride than in the placebo group (1% versus 3%) at 27 months.[234] Likewise, the REDUCE study found reduced relative risk for cancer with dutasteride of 23% (95% confidence interval, 15 to 30) over a 4-year study period in 8000 men randomized to receive dutasteride or placebo for 4 years.[234]

Differential Diagnosis

The main differential diagnostic considerations after androgen deprivation therapy are a variety of atrophic and hyperplastic changes in benign glands, including clear cell cribriform hyperplasia, sclerosing adenosis, acinar atrophy, postatrophic hyperplasia, atypical adenomatous hyperplasia, and atypical basal cell hyperplasia. Difficulty may be encountered in separating minute clusters and single-file ribbons of tumor cells after androgen deprivation from lymphocytes, myocytes, and fibroblasts, particularly on a cell-by-cell basis in some foci. Casual low-power scanning of some areas may fail to identify tumor because of the deceptively benign-appearing cytoplasm and nuclei after therapy. Untreated carcinoma may have a clear cell pattern, particularly when arising in the transition zone in association with nodular hyperplasia, but it is usually well differentiated (Gleason primary patterns 1 and 2) at that site, exhibits prominent nucleoli, and is not usually seen with atrophic glands with abundant clear cell change.

Stage and Surgical Margins After Androgen Deprivation Therapy

The volume of prostate cancer is reduced by more than 40% after treatment, and there is a 25% decline in positive margins at prostatectomy.[226,1242,1256] Pathologic stage is similar in untreated and treated carcinoma, although there is a trend toward lower stage in treated cases.[235,1242,1257] Occasional cases after therapy display the "vanishing cancer phenomenon" in which no residual cancer was found in the prostatectomy specimen.[566]

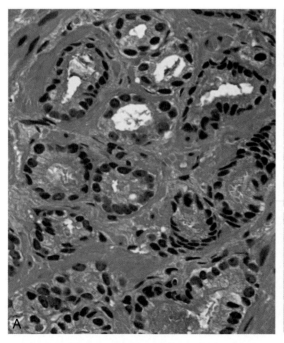
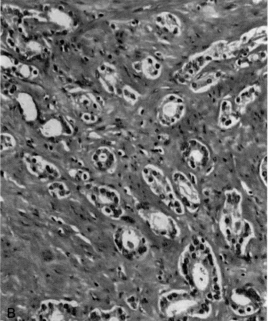

Fig. 9.57 Dutasteride changes in adenocarcinoma. (A) Untreated. (B) Three months after treatment.

Immunohistochemical Findings After Androgen Deprivation Therapy

PSA, PAP, and racemase expression are retained in tumor cells after 3 months of therapy but decline with longer duration of therapy.[1258] Keratin 34βE12 and p63 remain negative, regardless of duration, indicating an absent basal cell layer (Table 9.38).[1258] No differences were found in expression of NE markers such as chromogranin, NSE, βHCG, and serotonin after androgen deprivation therapy, although some claim a significant increase.[899,904,1259,1260] PCNA immunoreactivity declines after androgen deprivation therapy, indicating that androgens regulate cyclically expressed proteins involved in cell proliferation.[1261-1263] Some investigators reported that, after androgen deprivation therapy, residual tumoral proliferative activity in lymph nodes, assessed by PCNA staining, is greater than that in primary tumors (5% and 1%, respectively).[1262] This could be due to a metastatic phenotype that is less responsive to hormonal therapy than the primary tumor. In another study, PCNA was the same for tumors with lower and higher Gleason scores, suggesting that cellular dedifferentiation after neoadjuvant androgen deprivation represents a mere morphologic phenomenon and not a real increase in tumor aggressiveness.[1263] Untreated and treated cancer have similar levels of genetic alterations, suggesting that untreated cancer contains most of the chromosomal changes necessary for recurrence.[1264] The value of immunohistochemistry in predicting outcome after androgen deprivation is uncertain (Table 9.39).

Radiation Therapy

Irradiation creates difficulty in interpretation that includes separation of carcinoma from its many mimics, identification of small foci of carcinoma, and separation of treatment effects in normal tissue from recurrent or persistent carcinoma. As more patients choose radiotherapy and as these patients are observed for longer intervals, pathologists bear an increasing burden to discriminate irradiated benign acini from adenocarcinoma.

TABLE 9.38   Immunohistochemical Changes After Androgen Deprivation Therapy

Biomarker	Effect of Androgen Deprivation on Cancer[a]
Prostate-specific antigen	Unchanged
Prostatic acid phosphatase	Unchanged
Prostate-specific membrane antigen	Unchanged
Basal cell–specific keratin 34βE12	Unchanged
Neuroendocrine markers	Unchanged
Integrins IL-3, IL-6, M-CSF, TNF-α	Unchanged
Estrogen receptors	Increased
NM23-H2	Increased
A-80 mucin glycoprotein	Increased
Tissue transglutaminase	Increased
Oncoprotein Bcl-2	Increased
p53	Increased
p21/WAF1/CIP1	Increased
Cytokeratin 5	Increased
TGFB1 and TGF receptors I and II	Increased
Fibroblast growth factor 8	Increased
Insulin-like growth factor binding protein 2	Increased[b]
27-kDa heat shock protein	Increased[b]
Microvessel density	Unchanged or decreased
Proliferating cell nuclear antigen	Decreased
Ki67 (MIB1)	Decreased
Integrins Il-1α, Il-1β	Decreased
NM23-H1	Decreased or absent

[a]Compared with untreated prostate cancer.
[b]Studied with complementary DNA and tissue microarrays.

TABLE 9.39   Prognostic Value of Immunohistochemical Findings in Prostate Cancer Treated by Androgen Deprivation Therapy

Biomarker	Prognostic Value	Reference
Androgen receptors	Not related to cancer-specific death	Noordzij et al. (1997)[1739]
	Predictive of survival in advanced stage	Prins et al. (1998)[1740]
		Schafer et al. (2006)[1741]
		Chen et al. (2018)[1742]
	Decreased staining is predictive of failure of hormonal therapy	Tilley et al. (1996)[1743]
		Nabi et al. (2004)[1744]
Prostate-specific antigen	Increased expression predicted earlier relapse	Ryan et al. (2006)[1745]
Neuroendocrine cells	Not predictive of clinical outcome	Pruneri et al. (1998)[1746]
HER2	Predicts cancer-specific survival	Hernes et al. (2004)[1747]
	Predicts time to biochemical failure	Osman et al. (2001)[1748]
	Not predictive of cancer-specific survival	Di Lorenzo et al. (2002)[1749]
Bcl-2	Not predictive of cancer-specific survival	Noordzij et al. (1997)[1739]
Ki67	Higher values predictive of cancer recurrence	Koivisto et al. (1997)[1750]
Fibroblast growth factor 8	Predicts worse survival in patients with androgen-independent cancer	Dorkin et al. (1999)[1751]
Protein kinase C	Predicts decreased survival after relapse	Edwards et al. (2004)[1752]
BAG1	Predicts earlier relapse	Krajewska et al. (2006)[1753]
p53 immunoreactivity	Predicts androgen receptor gene amplification and cancer progression in patients with androgen independent cancer	Koivisto et al. (1999)[1754]
P21/WAF1/CIP1	Predictive of worse clinical outcome	Baretton et al. (1999)[1755]
Epidermal growth factor receptor	Increased expression predictive of earlier relapse and decreased overall survival	Schafer et al. (2006)[1741]

Most cancers grow slowly and regress slowly, so histologic changes evolve for up to 12 months after completion of radiation therapy. Thus, biopsy is of limited value before about 12 months because of ongoing cell death. Slow tumor death is attributed to the fact that radiotherapy causes necrosis only after a prostate cell has gone through cell division. After this period biopsy is a good method for assessing local tumor control, but complete histologic resolution of cancer may take 2 to 3 years.[1265] Sampling variation is minimized by obtaining multiple specimens.[223,463,750,751,1265,1266]

Evaluation of local tumor control is assisted by digital rectal examination and transrectal ultrasound. Posttherapy serum PSA correlates with posttherapy biopsy results, including degree of radiation effect.[223,1267] Crook et al. diagnosed postradiotherapy biopsies as indeterminate in 33% of first biopsies (median, 13 months), 24% of second biopsies (28 months), 18% of third biopsies (36 months), and 7% of fourth biopsies (44 months).[1265] These figures are higher than the 2% to 9% of biopsies with indeterminate findings in unselected nonirradiated series, highlighting the increased diagnostic challenge after radiotherapy.[274,302] Identification of cancer in biopsies after radiotherapy has a significant impact on patient management: positive needle biopsies portend a worse prognosis.[463,1268-1271] Study of salvage prostatectomies revealed residual cancer in sites often not biopsied, including the apex (90% of cases), within 5 mm of the urethra (69%), and seminal vesicles (42%).[785]

The histologic diagnosis of cancer without radiation effect relies on both architectural and cytoplasmic atypia (Figs. 9.58 and 9.59; Table 9.40). Radiotherapy causes cytologic atypia of benign glands, forcing the pathologist to identify cancer almost totally on architectural findings. Changes vary widely among patients.[223] Radiotherapy causes shrinkage of cancer glands and loss of cytoplasm, although some cases have voluminous foamy cytoplasm. Features most helpful for the diagnosis of cancer after radiotherapy are chiefly architectural: infiltrative growth, PNI, intraluminal crystalloids, blue mucin secretions, the absence of corpora amylacea, and the presence of concomitant high-grade PIN. Paneth cell–like change can be seen in 32% of biopsies.[223] Occasionally, cytologic findings, such as double nucleoli in a secretory cell, may be helpful. Deep rectal ulcer complicating brachytherapy may lead to distortion of the normal rectoprostatic anatomical landmarks, resulting in detection of pseudomalignant prostatic glands at the ulcer base that may be mistaken for a primary rectal malignancy in limited biopsy material.[1272]

Differential Diagnosis of Prostate Cancer After Radiotherapy

In our experience, atypical basal cell hyperplasia most frequently mimics treated cancer after irradiation. Atypical basal cell hyperplasia is defined as basal cell proliferation with more than 10% of cells exhibiting prominent nucleoli.[139] These cells were present in 57%

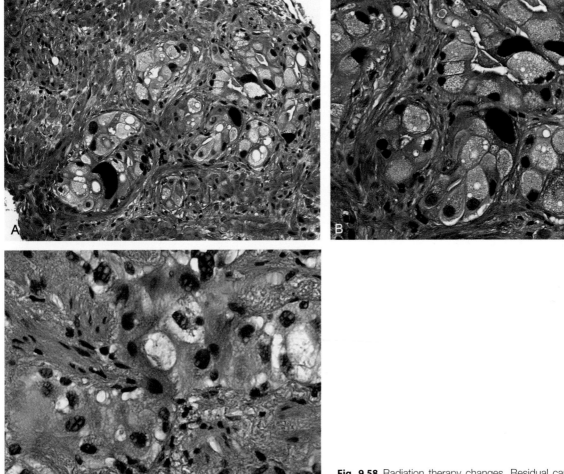

Fig. 9.58 Radiation therapy changes. Residual carcinoma after radiation therapy displays typical nuclear pleomorphism (A to C).

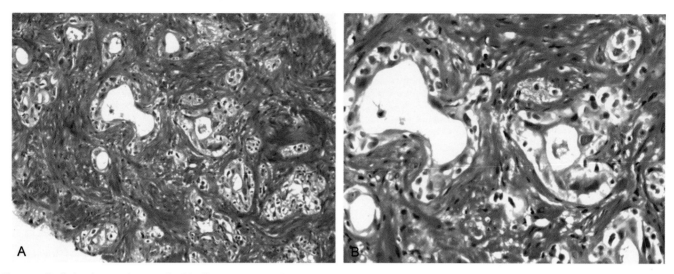

Fig. 9.59 Radiation therapy changes. Residual/recurrent prostatic adenocarcinoma 16 months after brachytherapy, with prominent acinar atrophy and cytologic atypia (A and B).

of cases in a study of salvage prostatectomies and represented a nonspecific host response to radiation injury.[1273]

Immunohistochemical Findings After Radiotherapy

PSA, PAP, keratin 34βE12, racemase, and c-Myc expressions in the prostatic epithelium are not altered by radiation therapy and are often of value in separating treated adenocarcinoma and its mimics. Prostate cancer after radiation therapy has increased p53 nuclear accumulation and Ki67 labeling index associated with a greater risk for distant metastasis and lower cancer-specific survival.[1274]

Cryotherapy

Cryosurgical ablation refers to lethal freezing of the prostate (see Chapter 8). Clinical results for cancer are encouraging, but the method is used only with select patients.[432,1275] Biopsy after cryosurgery may reveal no evidence of recurrent or residual carcinoma in the areas with treatment effect, even in patients with elevated PSA. Some investigators reported residual malignant cells in 7% to 23% of men, with areas of viable benign glands in 45% to 70% of patients.[1276] Positive biopsy findings were reported in 13% and 18% of patients after cryosurgery with or without androgen deprivation therapy, respectively.[430,1277] Some authors reported persistence of cancer cells in the 6- and 12-month biopsies in 11% and 6% of cases, respectively; all 24-month biopsies were negative, suggesting continued destruction over time, similar to radiation therapy.[1278] High-risk patients (defined as either a PSA level >10 ng/mL or a Gleason sum score >8, or both) who were unwilling to undergo radical surgery or radiation therapy had positive postcryosurgical biopsies in 13%.[1279] No patient progressed, and the overall survival rate was 100%.[1279] One series reported that, after cryosurgery, serum PSA reached a nadir of less than 0.5 ng/mL and did not increase by more than 0.2 ng/mL on at least two occasions. However, biopsies were positive after 38% of procedures.[1280]

Cryotherapy induces coagulative necrosis regardless of tissue, with mummification and complete cell death, marked vascular congestion, and occasional scattered intermediate size and large cellular vacuoles. There is no thrombosis, but vessels are devitalized, with pyknotic endothelial nuclei as well as loss of staining, creating pale "ghost" nuclei. At the margins, there is a thin 1- to 2-mm line of demarcation between altered and unaltered tissue (Fig. 9.60). In some cases the cancer appears unaltered, with no change in grade and no evidence of tissue or immune response, probably indicating lack of inclusion of that area in the ablation killing zone. Outcome is independent of DNA ploidy status.[1281] There is no consensus regarding grading after cryoablation therapy, and most pathologists, including us, routinely report Gleason grade.

Several studies have reported positive salvage cryotherapy results with biopsy-proven local failure after external beam radiotherapy.[1282-1287] The most worrisome clinical finding is positive postcryotherapy biopsy; the presence of residual or recurrent cancer is considered evidence of inadequate cryotherapy and inadequate radiotherapy. In one study of patients with biopsy-proven local failure after external beam radiotherapy, the combination of neoadjuvant androgen deprivation therapy with salvage cryotherapy resulted in residual cancer, viable benign acini, and viable stroma in 14%, 42%, and 27% of cases, respectively.[1283] These biopsy results were obtained with four-core sampling and therefore likely underestimate the true incidence of residual cancer.[1283] A cohort of 59 patients treated with radiation therapy and rising PSA underwent salvage cryoablation for localized, histologically proven, recurrent cancer.[1287] Remarkably, no biopsies (0%) showed evidence of residual or recurrent disease.[1287]

No definitive method exists for assessment of tumor viability after cryoablation. PSA and PAP expression persist in benign and malignant epithelium, suggesting that tumor cells capable of protein production probably retain the potential for cell division and consequent metastatic spread. Keratin 34βE12, p63, racemase, and c-Myc expression also persist after cryoablation and are of diagnostic value in separating treated adenocarcinoma and its mimics.

There is a strong correlation between MRI with gadolinium defects and amount of coagulation necrosis caused within the prostate by minimally invasive techniques.[1288] However, gadolinium defects were not seen in areas of viable tissue as determined by histopathologic evaluation.[1288] Some investigators reported that findings of postoperative gadolinium-enhanced MRI were not predictive of 6-month biopsy results or follow-up PSA level.[1289]

TABLE 9.40	Histopathologic Findings in Prostatic Adenocarcinoma in Postirradiation Needle Biopsies at the Time of Prostate-Specific Antigen (Biochemical) Failure

Histopathologic Findings	% Cases
Gleason score	
<7	17
7	48
>7	35
% of cancer involvement	
≤10%	31
11%-40%	28
41%-80%	35
81%-100%	7
No. of cancer foci	
1	36
2-4	50
≥5	14
Combined score of radiation effect[a]	
0-2 (minimal)	52
3-4 (moderate)	38
5-6 (severe)	10
Infiltrative growth	100
Perineural invasion	31
Atrophic change	10
Nuclear pyknosis	72
Nuclear enlargement	93
Prominent nucleoli	79
Cytoplasmic vacuolization	
<10%	45
10%-50%	45
>50%	10
Inflammation	0
Stromal desmoplasia	76
Necrosis	0
Intraluminal contents	
Crystalloids	3
Mucin	21
Eosinophilic	24
Corpora amylacea	0
Concomitant high-grade prostatic intraepithelial neoplasia	7

[a]Radiation effect was quantified using the scoring system described by Crook et al.[1265]

Ultrasound Hyperthermia, Microwave Hyperthermia, Laser Therapy, and Hot Water Balloon Therapy

All forms of hyperthermia result in sharply circumscribed hemorrhagic coagulative necrosis that soon organized with granulation tissue. The pattern and extent of injury is determined by the method of thermocoagulation used, the duration of treatment, tissue perfusion factors, and the ratio of epithelium to stroma in the tissue being treated.[1290,1291]

High-Intensity Focused Ultrasound

Necrosis is observed in 13% to 72% of cases after high-intensity focused ultrasound, usually in association with varying amounts of acute and chronic inflammation.[1292] Mild or moderate fibrosis is present in all biopsies. In benign glands, there is heterogeneous cellular damage and cellular response including cytologic atypia

and basal cell hyperplasia. There are no apparent alterations in prostate cancer cells. Treatment effects do not preclude assignment of Gleason score or use of immunohistochemistry.[1293]

Salvage after high-intensity focused ultrasound after failed radiation therapy results in extensive coagulative stromal necrosis in 100% of cases, smudgy chromatin of cancer nuclei in 82%, and markedly enlarged bizarre nuclei in 55% of cases of residual cancer.[1294]

Irreversible Electroporation

Irreversible electroporation (IRE) is a novel nonthermal electrical ablation method that induces apoptosis without immediate necrosis. After 4 weeks, IRE ablation is characterized by sharply delineated zones of fibrosis and all-inclusive devitalized tissue without skip lesions, mild to moderate inflammation, fibrinoid necrosis of the neurovascular bundles, and denuded acini.[1295,1296] Hemorrhage was present outside this zone at the site of the electrode placement, and the prostatic urethra urothelium was denuded. A variant of IRE, high-frequency IRE, creates apoptosis combined with necrosis.

Predictive Factors in Prostate Cancer

Multifactorial analysis improves prediction of all outcome variables, including pathologic stage, cancer recurrence, and survival.[451,1297]

Prostate-Specific Antigen

PSA is a 34-kDa, single-chain glycoprotein of 237 amino acids produced almost exclusively by prostatic epithelial cells. PSA is a serine protease, a member of the kallikrein gene family, and has high sequence homology with human glandular kallikrein 2. It has chymotrypsin-like, trypsin-like, and esterase-like activity. In the serum, PSA is present mainly as a complex with α_1-antichymotrypsin. It is secreted in the seminal plasma and is responsible for gel dissolution in freshly ejaculated semen by proteolysis of the major gel forming proteins, semenogelin I and II, and fibronectin. A small amount of PSA in semen is complexed. The free, noncomplexed form of PSA constitutes a minor fraction of the serum PSA. Production of PSA appears to be under the control of circulating androgens acting through the ARs. PSA is routinely used for early detection of prostate cancer.

Serum PSA may be elevated by conditions other than cancer, including prostatitis, PIN, acute urinary retention, and renal failure. The value of PSA as a screening tool has been questioned by some investigators because of the overlap of PSA concentration between BPH and prostate cancer.[1298-1301] PSA is particularly sensitive and accurate in the detection of prostate volume, residual cancer, recurrence, and cancer progression after treatment, irrespective of the treatment modality.[1302-1304] PSA accurately predicts cancer status and can detect recurrence several months before detection by any other method.[1305]

Multiple derivatives of PSA have been proposed as adjuncts or replacements for total PSA, including free PSA, complex PSA, age-specific reference ranges, PSA density, pro-PSA, BPSA, and PSA velocity.[120,1306-1310] Androgen deprivation therapy predictably decreases serum PSA and hampers its predictive value for cancer.[1311]

PSA is a sensitive and specific immunohistochemical marker for tumors of prostatic origin (Fig. 9.61). Staining for PSA is useful in identifying poorly differentiated cancer near the bladder and the rectum; it can also verify prostatic origin of metastatic carcinoma.

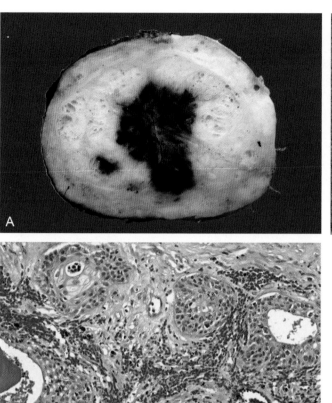

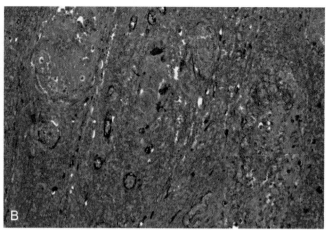

Fig. 9.60 Cryotherapy. (A) The prostate displays sharp demarcation of devitalized tissue (brown-black) around urethra from surrounding viable tissue (tan). (B) Hemorrhagic necrosis with diffuse devitalized prostatic tissue. (C) At border of treated and untreated tissue, there is basal cell hyperplasia with stromal hemorrhage.

The intensity of PSA immunoreactivity often varies from field to field within a tumor, and the correlation of staining intensity with tumor differentiation is inconsistent.[241,1312,1313] PSA expression is generally greater in low-grade tumors than in high-grade tumors, but there is significant heterogeneity from cell to cell. Up to 5% of poorly differentiated cancers are negative for both PSA and PAP.[1314,1315] The presence of PSA-immunoreactive tumor cells in poorly differentiated carcinoma suggests that these tumors retain subpopulations of cells with properties of normal secretory prostatic epithelial cells. Extraprostatic expression of PSA has been reported in several tissues and tumors, including breast tissue, periurethral gland adenocarcinoma in women, rectal carcinoid, and extramammary Paget disease (Table 9.41).

Stage

Staging separates patients with early carcinoma into two main groups: those with palpable tumors and those with nonpalpable tumors.[1316-1318] This reliance on palpability as determined by digital rectal examination is unique among organ-staging systems and is hampered by low sensitivity, low specificity, and low positive predictive value.[75,1318-1320] Clinical staging categorizes men with tumors detected by biopsies secondary to elevated PSA as cT1c and men with palpable but localized cancer as cT2.[1318] The current TNM staging system implies that patients with prostate cancer detected by PSA screening have a better prognosis than those with palpable prostatic tumors. The data, however, suggest that prostate cancer detected by PSA screening (cT1c) and tumor detected on digital rectal examination (cT2) may have the same prognosis after treatment.[1321]

The TNM classification, endorsed by the American Joint Committee on Cancer, is considered the international standard for staging and was updated for January 1, 2018, implementation (Fig. 9.62; Tables 9.42 and 9.43).[1322] Changes in pathology factors include: (1) deletion of subclassification of organ-confined cancer (pT2) for radical prostatectomies based on bilaterality and extent of involvement, although it is important to note that clinical pT2 is still subclassified as cT2a, cT2b, and cT2c; (2) addition of histologic grade groupings and update to ISUP 2014 modified Gleason score; (3) inclusion of nonanatomic factors PSA and grade grouping into AJCC stage III group; and (4) incorporation of select statistical prediction models.[1322]

Cancer-specific mortality rate at 10 years for all patients is 5% for clinically localized lesions, 7% for T3aN0M0, 14% for T3bN0M0, 26% for T4N0M0, 27% for TanyN1M0, and 66% for TanyNanyM1.[1323] For pathologically staged patients, mortality rate at 10 years is 1% for localized lesions, 4% for T3aN0M0, 9% for T3bN0M0, 9% for T4N0M0, and 19% for TanyN1M0.

The previous TNM staging scheme divided pT2 disease into T2a, T2b, and T2c subcategories, but these subdivisions are deleted for 2018; however, the subdivisions are retained for clinical staging (cT2a, cT2b, cT2c).[1319] Many investigators questioned the existence or utility of T2b cancer, and study of prostatectomy specimens concluded that the three-tiered T2 classification system was not necessary, taking into consideration the biology and anatomy

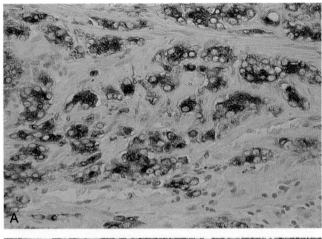

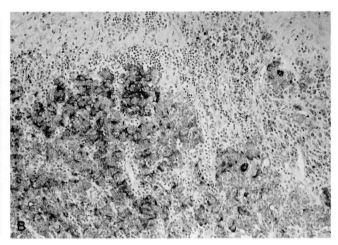

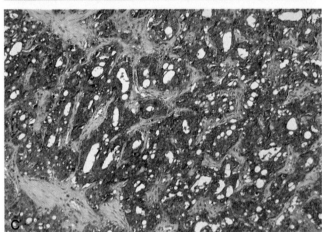

Fig. 9.61 Prostate-specific antigen immunoreactivity. (A) Prostate-specific antigen expression in the cytoplasm of poorly differentiated adenocarcinoma. (B) Metastatic prostatic adenocarcinoma in cervical lymph nodes. (C) Skene gland adenocarcinoma of the female urethra.

of prostate cancer.[495,1324-1328] Chun et al. studied more than 1700 patients with stage T2 cancer, and found that T2 substages were equally predictive of pretreatment PSA, margin status, and Gleason score.[1329] pT2 substaging has no prognostic significance for biochemical recurrence-free survival after prostatectomy.[1330,1331] As currently classified, cT2b cancer probably represents pathologically bilateral disease, either through contiguous involvement by the primary tumor, de novo lesions of independent origin, or satellite lesions derived from intraglandular dissemination. Concordance of cT and pT category at prostatectomy for localized cancer is 15% for cT2a, 11% for cT2b, and 55% for cT2c, with EPE missed in cT1 and cT2 in 24% and 36%, respectively.[1332] Such low agreement between clinical and pathologic T category often results in understaging.

Other 2018 changes enhance the prognostic ability of TNM staging and consist chiefly of additions of contemporary nonanatomic findings, including serum PSA, ISUP 2014 grade groupings, and statistical models. These alterations are a substantial departure from the original goal of staging based chiefly on anatomic factors, and they greatly increase complexity.

National Comprehensive Cancer Network/American Urological Association Risk Classification

The National Comprehensive Cancer Network/American Urological Association guidelines identify three risk groups defined by the combination of histologic grade group, clinical stage, PSA level, and PSA density (Table 9.44).[1333,1334] In Japanese men,

National Comprehensive Cancer Network classification groups predict tumor stage ≥pT3, Gleason score ≥8, and biochemical recurrence.[1335]

Pathology of Prostate-Specific Antigen–Detected Adenocarcinoma (Clinical Stage T1c)

Before widespread clinical use of PSA, most organ-confined adenocarcinoma was discovered by digital rectal examination or at the time of TURP.[1336] Routine use of PSA increased the detection rate of cancer and uncovered some cases that would not have been detected by digital rectal examination. There is no pathologic stage equivalent for clinical stage T1c, and such tumors are invariably upstaged at surgery, usually to pathologic stage T2 or T3. Clinical stage T1c, T2a, and T2b adenocarcinomas had similar diameters, frequencies of multifocality, tumor grades, DNA content results, pathologic stages, and tumor locations; interestingly, they had different serum PSA values, tumor volumes, positive surgical margins, and prostate gland sizes, with the T1c tumors having higher values for each feature.[1337-1339] These findings indicate that PSA detects adenocarcinoma that is clinically important, potentially curable, and heterogeneous.[1340] Also, PSA-detected tumors that are visible on TRUS have similar pathologic features as those that are not visible.[1341]

Patients with clinical stage T2 tumor have higher Gleason score and advanced pathologic stage than those whose cancer is detected because of high serum PSA (T1c). These results suggest that cT1c tumors should be separated from cT2 disease, but the

TABLE 9.41	Immunoreactivity of Prostate-Specific Antigen in Extraprostatic Tissues and Tumors

Extraprostatic Tissues

Urethra, periurethral glands (male and female)
Bladder, cystitis, cystica, and glandularis
Urachal remnants
Neutrophils
Anus, anal glands (male only)

Extraprostatic Tumors

Mature teratoma
Urethra, periurethral gland adenocarcinoma (female)
Bladder, villous adenoma, and adenocarcinoma
Penis, extramammary Paget disease
Salivary gland, pleomorphic adenoma (male only)
Salivary gland, carcinoma (male only)

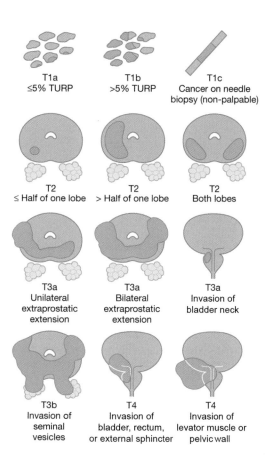

Fig. 9.62 Prostate cancer staging using the TNM system, 2018 revision. Red indicates extent of cancer.

TABLE 9.42	2017 TNM Staging System for Pathologists[1322,d]

Primary Tumor (T)

TX: Primary tumor cannot be assessed
T0: No evidence of primary tumor
T1: Clinically inapparent tumor not palpable
   T1a: Tumor incidental histologic finding in ≤5% of tissue resected
   T1b: Tumor incidental histologic finding in >5% of tissue resected
   T1c: Tumor identified by needle biopsy found in one or both sides, but not palpable[a]
T2: Tumor confined within prostate[b]
T3: Extraprostatic tumor that is not fixed or does not invade adjacent structures
   T3a: Extraprostatic extension (unilateral or bilateral) or microscopic invasion of bladder neck
   T3b: Tumor invades seminal vesicle(s)
T4: Tumor is fixed or invades adjacent structures other than seminal vesicles such as external sphincter, rectum, bladder, levator muscles, and/or pelvic wall[c]

Regional Lymph Nodes (N)

NX: Regional lymph nodes were not assessed
N0: No regional lymph node metastasis
N1: Metastasis in regional lymph node(s)

Distant Metastasis (M)

MX: Distant metastasis cannot be assessed
M0: No distant metastasis
M1: Distant metastasis[e]
   M1a: Nonregional lymph node(s)
   M1b: Bone(s)
   M1c: Other site(s) with or without bone disease

[a]Tumor that is found in one or both lobes by biopsy, but is not palpable or reliably visible by imaging, is classified as pT1c.
[b]In the new 2017 TNM staging system (also Fig. 9.62), pathologically organ-confined tumor is considered pT2 and no longer subclassified by extent of involvement or laterality. Invasion into the prostatic apex or into (but not beyond) the prostatic capsule is not classified as T3, but as T2.
[c]Microscopic invasion into the bladder neck is not classified as T4, but as T3a.
[d]Took effect on January 1, 2018.
[e]When more than one site of metastasis is present, the most advanced category (pM1c) is used.

TABLE 9.43	Changes to TNM 2018 Staging for Pathologists[1322]

- Deletion of subclassification of organ-confined cancer (pT2) for radical prostatectomies (clinical subclassification [cT2a, cT2b, cT2c] retained)
- Addition of ISUP 2014 grade groupings and update to ISUP 2014 modified Gleason score
- Prognostic stage group 3 incorporates nonanatomic factors (serum prostate-specific antigen level and ISUP 2014 grade groupings)
- Statistical prediction models included

ISUP, International Society of Urological Pathology.

PSA recurrence rate for both stages is similar, indicating a need for further evaluation and refinement of the current clinical staging system.[1338]

Extraprostatic Extension

The term *extraprostatic extension* (EPE) was accepted at an international conference to replace other terms, including capsular invasion, capsular penetration, and capsular perforation.[1342]

Extension of cancer beyond the edge or capsule of the prostate is diagnostic of EPE. There are four criteria for EPE, depending on the site and composition of the extraprostatic tissue: (1) cancer in adipose tissue, (2) cancer in perineural spaces of the neurovascular bundles, (3) cancer in anterior muscle, and (4) cancer invading periseminal vesical soft tissue (Fig. 9.63). Seminal vesicle invasion is usually discussed separately from EPE (see later), despite frequent cooccurrence. Because cancer in large neurovascular

TABLE 9.44

National Comprehensive Cancer Network/American Urological Association/American Society for Radiation Oncology/Society of Urologic Oncology 2018 Guidelines for Risk Stratification of Localized Prostate Cancer[1333,1334]

Risk Status	Criteria
Very low risk	PSA <10 ng/mL AND grade group 1 (Gleason score ≤6) AND clinical stage T1-T2a AND <34% of biopsy cores positive AND no core with >50% involved, AND PSA density <0.15 ng/mL/cc
Low risk	PSA <10 ng/mL AND grade group 1 AND clinical stage T1-T2a
Intermediate risk	PSA 10 to <20 ng/mL OR grade groups 2-3 (Gleason score 7) OR clinical stage T2b-T2c • **Favorable:** grade group 1 with PSA 10 to <20 ng/mL OR grade group 2 (Gleason score 3 + 4) with PSA <10 ng/mL • **Unfavorable:** grade group 2 (Gleason score 3 + 4) with either PSA 10 to <20 ng/mL or clinical stage T2b-T2c) OR grade group 3 (Gleason score 4 + 3) with PSA <20 ng/mL
High risk	PSA ≥20 ng/mL OR grade groups 4-5 (Gleason scores 8-10) OR clinical stage >T3

PSA, Prostate-specific antigen.

bundles or in anterior muscle is less common, recognition of EPE usually depends on finding carcinoma cells in periprostatic adipose tissue. Although pathologists tend to report the location(s) of EPE, there is no evidence that the location has prognostic significance with respect to therapy.

EPE is rare in biopsies (<1% of cases) and is typically found at the base in association with palpable, high-grade/high-volume cancer.[1343] In patients treated by prostatectomy for localized cancer, the frequency of EPE (stage pT3 cancer) is reported between 23% and 52%.[571,1344-1349] There is a strong association of tumor volume with EPE and seminal vesicle invasion.[1350,1351] An autopsy study showed EPE in 2% of cancers less than 0.5 cm³ in volume, compared with 52% of larger cancers.[442] There is "good" concordance between central and local pathology review for EPE (pT3a/b, 94%; κ, 0.8), as well as seminal vesicle invasion (pT3b, 91%; κ, 0.9) and positive surgical margin status (87%; κ, 0.7).[1352] However, urologic pathologists display only "moderate" consensus, with concordance in 68% of cases (κ, 0.6).[1353]

Patients with EPE have a worse prognosis than those with organ-confined cancer.[1345] Cancer-specific survival rate 10 years after surgery in patients with pT3 cancer is between 54% and 80%; at 15 years, survival rate was 69%.[763,1354-1356] By comparison, cancer-specific survival 10 years after radiation therapy in patients with clinical stage T3 is 44% or 59%, and at 15 years, survival rate varies from 33% to 39%.[1357-1359]

Many patients with EPE also have positive surgical margins, with a frequency rate of 41% to 81%.[1345,1349,1360] The combination of EPE and positive margins predicts a worse prognosis than EPE alone.[1360,1361] Positive surgical margin should be indicated in staging by an R1 descriptor (residual microscopic disease).[1362] Close proximity of EPE to the margin without touching is not associated with recurrence.[1363]

Some investigators report that a prostate biopsy core with a tumor length of at least 7 mm plus a positive basal biopsy core of any length and tumor grade is predictive of ipsilateral EPE; these criteria may be of value for predicting EPE and selecting patients for nerve-sparing prostatectomy.[1364]

Detection of cancer cells within the adipose tissue of needle biopsies is rare but, when present, indicates EPE. Sung et al. reviewed 313 consecutive prostatectomy specimens, and none revealed adipose tissue within the most peripheral boundary of normal prostatic acini in the prostate.[1365] The authors concluded that the occurrence of fat within the prostate is rarely, if ever, found. Accordingly, the finding of carcinoma invading adipose tissue in biopsies should continue to be considered EPE and stage pT3a assigned.[1365]

Because there is little periprostatic adipose tissue at the apex and anterior prostate, it is difficult to identify EPE in these areas. For practical purposes the diagnosis of EPE should not be made at the apex. The anterior fibromuscular stroma of the prostate interdigitates with external smooth muscle and skeletal muscle adjacent to the pubic bone. EPE can be diagnosed in these areas only when there is unequivocal evidence of tumor extension beyond the normal confines of the prostate and beyond the rounded interface between the fibromuscular stroma and skeletal muscle.[510,1366]

Seminal Vesicle Invasion (Stage pT3b Prostate Cancer)

Cancer arising in the base is more likely to exhibit seminal vesicle invasion than that in the apex or anteromedial region.[1367] Five-year biochemical recurrence-free survival rate in patients with pT3b tumors with or without bilateral seminal vesicle invasion is 4% or 20%, respectively, and bilateral seminal vesicle invasion is an independent prognostic factor in multivariate analysis together with PSA level and lymph node status.[1368] Seminal vesicle invasion indicates a higher likelihood of cancer-specific death after prostatectomy than EPE alone.[1369]

Microscopic Bladder Neck Invasion (Stage pT3a Prostate Cancer)

In the 2002 TNM staging system, bladder neck invasion was designated as pT4 disease, whereas in the 2010 and 2017 TNM scheme, microscopic bladder neck invasion is assigned as pT3a cancer.[1318,1322] In the past, prostate cancer with bladder neck invasion was considered as advanced disease, similar to external sphincter or rectal involvement, based on the concept that tumor invading surrounding structures is more aggressive and warrants higher staging. Microscopic bladder neck invasion is defined as the presence of neoplastic cells within the smooth muscle bundles of the coned bladder neck or as the presence of microscopic invasion of the muscular wall of the bladder neck by cancer cells in the absence of benign prostatic glandular tissue in the section. The prognosis of this subset of patients seems to be different from that of men with rectal or striated sphincter muscle invasion (Fig. 9.64), and most studies have shown that bladder neck invasion carries a risk for progression similar to EPE and lower than that of seminal vesicle invasion.[1370-1375] However, in multivariate models, bladder neck invasion was found not to be an independent predictor of PSA recurrence after prostatectomy.

Surgical Margins

Positive surgical margins are defined as cancer cells touching the inked surface of the prostate (Fig. 9.65). This definition was reiterated by pathologists at the 2009 ISUP Conference, and locations of positive margins should be indicated as either posterior, posterolateral, lateral, anterior at the prostatic apex, mid-prostate, or base.[1376] Other items of consensus included specifying the extent of any positive margin as millimeters of involvement. The concept of considering a surgical margin as negative if the carcinoma does not reach the surface of the prostatectomy specimen despite proximity of less than 0.1 mm has been supported by studies that have documented an absence of residual tumor with a lack of any postoperative progression.[1377] Even a very close margin is likely to be truly negative, because surgery results in considerable tissue destruction from cautery, vascular disruption, and subsequent inflammation.[1378,1379]

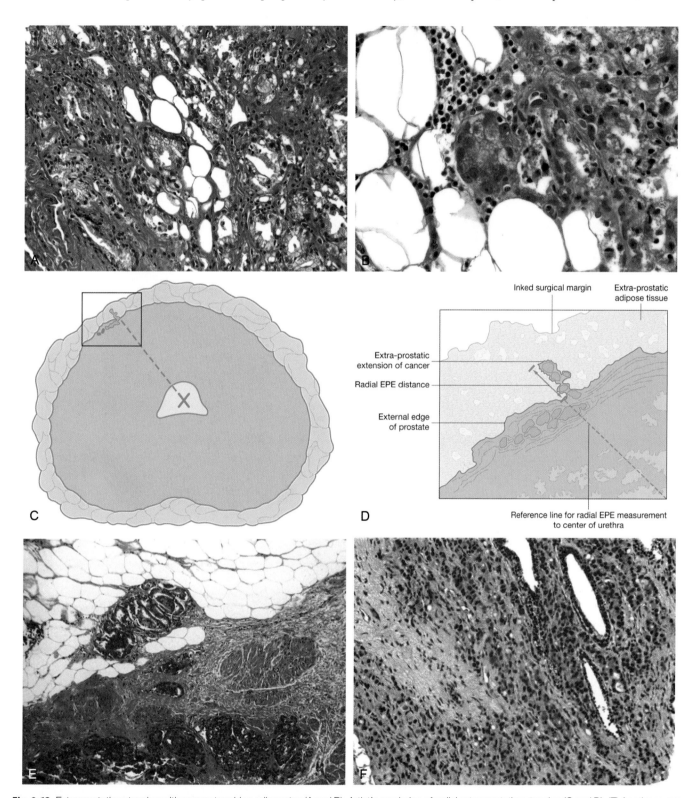

Fig. 9.63 Extraprostatic extension with cancer touching adipocytes (A and B). Artist's rendering of radial extraprostatic extension (C and D). (E) Another example of focal extraprostatic extension. (F) Seminal vesicle invasion by high-grade adenocarcinoma; note the pigmented epithelium.

(Continued)

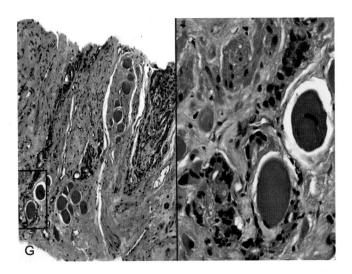

Fig. 9.63, cont'd (G) Cancer in anterior muscle on biopsy (*left*; *inset* is on *right*)-assigned stage pT3a.

Conversely, one report found that close but negative margin less than 1 mm is tantamount to positive margin.[1380] Surgical margin status is not included in pathologic staging.[1345] However, many studies have erroneously equated positive margins and EPE, particularly in cases in which the surgeon has cut into the prostate and intraprostatic cancer.[1342] Frozen sections have a final margin predictive accuracy rate of 81% when compared with results of permanent sections, with the conclusion that frozen sections should not be used to predict final margin status.[1379]

The frequency of positive surgical margins has steadily declined in the past decade, probably because of refinements in surgical technique and earlier detection of cancer at smaller volume and lower stage.[1381] Ohori et al. found positive surgical margins in 24% of whole-mount radical prostatectomies obtained at their hospital before 1987, usually in the posterolateral region near the neurovascular bundles; by surgically approaching the neurovascular bundles laterally and widely dissecting the apex, they lowered the positive surgical margin rate to 8% within 6 years despite similar volume grade and pathologic stage of cancer.[1347] The frequency of positive surgical margins is reported between 8% and

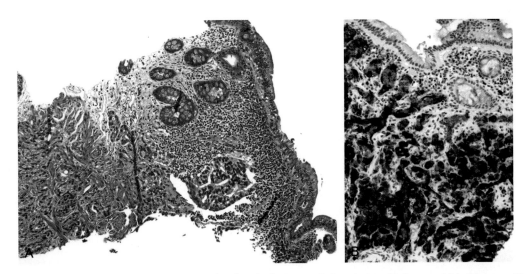

Fig. 9.64 (A) Contiguous spread of prostate cancer into the rectal wall and submucosa. Note colonic epithelium on right of image, with abundant cancer beneath. (B) Immunostain for prostatic acid phosphatase.

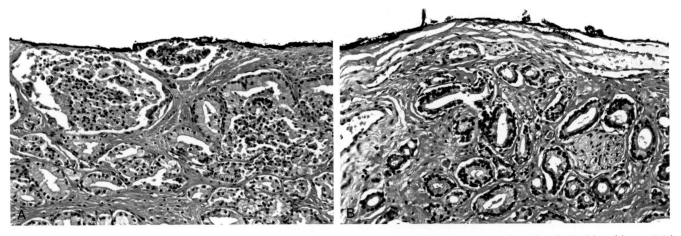

Fig. 9.65 Surgical margins. (A) Positive surgical margin, with cancer touching the inked surface without extraprostatic tissue (surgical incision of the prostate). (B) Negative surgical margin. Cancer is close to the surface but does not make contact. Note perineural invasion on right side.

57%, with no difference in specimens from nerve-sparing and non–nerve-sparing operations.[1345,1381-1386]

Positive surgical margins strongly correlate with cancer volume and number of cores containing cancer.[717,1347,1350,1361,1383,1387-1389] Most positive margins with cancer smaller than 4 cm^3 are caused by surgical incision.[1345,1389] Predictors of positive margins include abnormal digital rectal examination, preoperative PSA greater than 10 ng/mL, biopsy Gleason score greater than 7, more than one positive biopsy core, clinical suspicion of EPE, and presence of cancer in skeletal muscle in biopsies.[1390,1391] Positive margins are located at the apex (48%), rectal and lateral surfaces (24%), bladder neck (16%), and superior pedicles (10%).[1383]

Adjuvant radiation therapy in patients with positive surgical margins with or without EPE appears to be beneficial.[1392,1393] Patients have biochemical failure rate at 5 years of 12% compared with 41% of patients matched by age, the site of positive surgical margins, DNA ploidy status, Gleason score, and PSA who were not given adjuvant radiotherapy.[1394]

Surgical margin status is an important predictor of patient outcome after prostatectomy and is the only predictor of cancer progression other than Gleason score or DNA ploidy in patients without seminal vesicle invasion or lymph node metastases.[764,1345,1360,1395-1398] Positive margin at the base has the highest risk for biochemical recurrence.[1399,1400] In a multivariable model that adjusted for pathologic variables and year of prostatectomy, positive surgical margin was a modest independent predictor of prostate cancer–specific mortality (HR, 1.4), when compared to Gleason score (HR, 6) and pathologic stage (HR, 11).[1401] The actuarial 5-year and 10-year biochemical disease-free survival rates were 71% and 60% for patients with negative and positive surgical margins, respectively.[1402] The extent of margin positivity correlates with biochemical recurrence-free survival in univariate analysis, although it has no predictive value independent of Gleason score.[1378,1382] Grading of tumor at positive margins is left to the discretion of the reporting pathologist, although a recent report noted that, on multivariate analysis, Gleason grade 4 or 5 at the margin remained an independent predictor of recurrence (HR, 2.1).[1376,1403] In men with positive surgical margins, Gleason score is the only factor predictive of biochemical recurrence.[1404,1405]

The presence, extent, and location of each margin should be specifically reported.[571] However, there is no current agreement or recommendation as to the specific method of quantifying the amount of cancer in these locations.

Perineural Invasion

PNI is common in adenocarcinoma, present in 11% to 38% of biopsies, and may be the only evidence of malignancy in a needle core.[477,478,484] Among low-risk patients (stage T1c-T2a, Gleason 6 or less, three or fewer positive cores, 50% or less of any core involved, and PSA ≤11 ng/mL), the incidence rate is 4%.[1406] Only one-half of patients with intraprostatic PNI on biopsy have EPE. In univariate analysis, PNI is predictive of EPE, seminal vesicle invasion, positive surgical margins, and pathologic stage in patients treated by prostatectomy.[478,1407-1409] However, in multivariate analysis, PNI has no predictive value after consideration of Gleason grade, serum PSA, and amount of cancer on biopsy.[478,484,1409,1410] PNI is not a significant predictor of biochemical recurrence in patients undergoing brachytherapy or low-risk patients treated by external beam therapy, although this has been debated.[477,488,1411,1412] These findings indicate that there is no value in routinely reporting PNI in biopsies, although this has also been contradicted.[501,1413] We still report PNI because it is quick and reproducible.

PNI in prostatectomy specimens appears to provide no significant prognostic information, although a recent quantitative approach subdividing PNI into four groups based on circumference of nerve involvement (0%, 1% to 49%, 50% to 99%, and 100%) was predictive of survival.[496,497,1414-1416] Immediate treatment rather than watchful waiting may be more appropriate for patients with localized prostatic cancer and PNI.[501]

Biopsy Cancer Volume

Biopsy cancer volume depends on multiple factors, including prostate volume, cancer volume, cancer distribution, number of biopsy cores obtained, the cohort of patients being evaluated, method of quantitating cancer length, and the technical competence of the investigator. Biopsy extent of tumor provides predictive value for extent in prostatectomy specimens and probably should be reported, although its predictive value for an individual patient is limited.[1377,1398,1417-1428] Reliance on this measure alone is often be misleading. There is a fair to good correlation between amount of cancer reported in matched biopsies and prostatectomies, especially for large cancers.[1419,1422] High cancer burden on biopsy is strongly suggestive of large-volume, high-stage cancer.[1398,1417-1420]

Quantitation of total cancer length in biopsies may be continuous, in which intervening stroma is included in measurement of multiple foci, or discontinuous, in which the length of each focus is measured individually, then measurements of that core are summed, excluding the length of any normal intervening stroma; we have always used the latter. About 25% of biopsy cores containing multiple foci show discordant ERG/SPINK1 status, consistent with multiclonal cancer (likely to be separate and distinct).[1429]

Reporting may include positive core number, percent of positive cores, greatest percentage of cancer in a single core, greatest length of cancer in cores, and total length of cancer in all cores. We provide total percentage and length for each core, allowing the other measures to be easily determined by anyone examining the biopsy report. On multivariate analysis, total length of cancer in cores is an independent predictor of index cancer volume and total volume.[1430] Percent positive biopsy cores independently predicts biochemical recurrence-free survival after radiation treatment beyond traditional pretreatment risk factors.[1431]

Low tumor burden on needle biopsy does not necessarily indicate low-volume, low-stage cancer at surgery. Patients with fewer than 30% of cores involved by cancer had a mean volume in the prostatectomy of 6.1 cm^3 (range, 0.2 to 16.8 cm^3), indicating that the amount of tumor on biopsy was not a good predictor of total tumor volume.[1422] In another report, patients with less than 10% cancer in the biopsy had a 30% risk for positive surgical margins, 27% risk for EPE, and 22% risk for PSA biochemical progression; these risks were higher in patients with more than 10% cancer.[1428] Patients with less than 3 mm cancer and Gleason score 6 or less on biopsy had a 59% risk for cancer volume exceeding 0.5 cm^3.[1418] Those with less than 2 mm of cancer had 26% risk for extraprostatic cancer, and those with less than 3 mm had 52% risk.[1425,1426] The College of American Pathologists recommends that the volume of cancer in biopsy should be reported as the percentage of tissue involved by cancer. A recent report found that percentage of total carcinoma length in millimeters in all cores of a biopsy had the strongest positive predictive value for stage greater than pT2 and risk for biochemical recurrence after prostatectomy.

Cancer volume should also be recorded in prostatectomy specimens, although there is no accepted universal approach.[440] The

2009 ISUP Conference concluded that there should be reporting of some quantitative measure of tumor volume without prescribing a specific methodology.[299] Methods of cancer volume measurement include computer-assisted morphometric determination, simple measurement of length × height × section thickness of the cancer (some measure the largest "index" focus, whereas others report the aggregate volume), greatest cancer dimension, grid method, and visual estimate of the percentage of cancer.[428,557,1419,1432-1439] Measurements performed on fixed tissue sections may include formalin shrinkage correction factor, which varies from 1.15 to 1.5, representing tissue shrinkage of 18% to 33%; conversely, Schned et al. demonstrated that shrinkage correction is unnecessary.[1440,1441]

Cancer volume is a critical element in the distinction between clinically significant and insignificant prostate cancer.[1432,1438] Up to 84% of men undergoing prostatectomy are found to have multifocal cancer, a finding that is a major theoretical objection to focal ablation (Table 9.45).[1442] However, about 80% of incidental tumors are less than 0.5 cm^3, indicating that a significant percentage of multifocal tumors, other than the largest or index cancer identified preoperatively, may not be of clinical significance. Until now, however, little attention has been paid in trying to differentiate patients with unifocal and multifocal disease because it had little clinical significance; all treatments are aimed at total gland ablation. Small-volume prostate cancers are often multifocal and bilateral, with predilection for the peripheral zone. Of these small-volume prostate cases, 16% had Gleason pattern 4 and might therefore be clinically significant.[1443] Importantly, Noguchi et al. found that smaller cancers in multifocal prostate tumors did not adversely influence prognosis, and they concluded that only the largest (index) cancer was significant.[720,1444]

At the 2009 ISUP Conference, incorporation of the zonal or anterior location of the dominant/index tumor in the pathology report was accepted by most participants, but a formal definition of the identifying features of the dominant/index tumor remained undecided.[299] Tumor size and Gleason grading were considered the two most important parameters when defining the dominant or index tumor. This means that if two tumor nodules each have a similar Gleason score, then the larger tumor should be the dominant/index tumor. In the case of two tumor nodules with differing Gleason scores, the nodule with the higher score should be the dominant/index tumor, regardless of size. It was also suggested that the tumor with the highest grade or stage might be more appropriately considered to be the dominant/index tumor. Billis et al.

showed that total and index cancer extent predicted time to biochemical recurrence on univariate analysis, but only index tumor extent was an independent predictor on multivariate analysis.[1445]

Cancer volume was usually but not always predictive of cancer recurrence after prostatectomy.[496,717,1398,1439,1446] In a screening population, median cancer volume in men with biochemical progression after prostatectomy was 2.6 cm^3 versus 0.9 cm^3 in men who were free of disease 5 years after surgery.[1447] Cancer volume and percentage of high-grade cancer volume are independent predictors of recurrence-free survival.[1448,1449] In most multifocal tumors, the largest nodule contains the highest Gleason score (91% of cases).[1450] Total tumor and index tumor volumes are significant predictors of biochemical recurrence.[1450]

In patients with nodal metastases, very small tumor size predicts higher cancer-specific death compared with larger tumors in multivariate analysis. There was a significant association of cancer volume and nodal involvement. In the absence of nodal involvement the 10-year mortality risk increased monotonically with increasing tumor size, whereas among those with nodal involvement, patients with the smallest tumors (<2 mm diameter) had increased 10-year mortality rate compared with patients with tumors 2 to 15 mm or 16 to 30 mm, and similar 10-year mortality rate as those with tumors larger than 30 mm.[1451]

Location of Cancer

Cancer is predominant in the transition zone in 10% to 35% of prostatectomies and anteriorly in 1% to 51%.[1452] The site of origin of cancer appears to be a significant prognostic factor (Table 9.46). Transition zone and anterior cancer tends to be less aggressive than typical peripheral zone carcinoma, although this has been contested (Fig. 9.66).[1453-1455] It is usually lower grade than cancer in the peripheral zone, including Gleason primary grade 1 and 2 tumors, and has lower rate of EPE; conversely, it has higher positive surgical margins rate.[1456] Interestingly the volume of low-grade transition zone cancer tends to be larger than that arising in the peripheral zone, although conflicting findings have been reported.[1456-1459] The confinement of transition zone carcinoma to its anatomic site of origin may account in part for the favorable prognosis of clinical stage T1 tumors. Therefore outcome is more dependent on the features of cancer in the peripheral zone than in the transition zone.[1460] The transition zone boundary probably acts as a relative barrier to tumor extension, because malignant acini appear to frequently fan out along this boundary before invasion into the peripheral and central zones.

TABLE 9.45	Incidence of Multifocal Prostate Cancer in Radical Prostatectomies		
Prostatectomy Handling	**Reference**	**No. of Subjects**	**Multifocality (%)**
Stanford protocol[a]	Villers et al.[1756]	234	50
Whole-mounted	Miller et al.[1757]	151	56
4-mm specimen sections	Djavan et al.[1758]	308	67
Stanford protocol[a]	Noguchi et al.[1444]	222	76
Whole-mounted	Song et al.[1759]	132	33
Whole-mounted	Ng et al.[497]	364	85
Whole-mounted	Eichelberger et al.[1327]	312	85
4-mm specimen sections	Horninger et al.[1760]	80	65
Whole-mounted	Cheng et al.[1458]	62	69
Stanford protocol[a]	Torlakovic et al.[1761]	46	65
Totally embedded	Hollman et al.[1442]	61	84

[a]Stanford protocol is using serial transverse sections at 3-mm intervals.[1756]

TABLE 9.46 Prostatic Carcinoma: Comparison Based on Anatomic Site of Origin[a]

	Transition Zone	Peripheral Zone Cancer
Incidence		
Stage T1a	75%	—
Stage T1b	79%	—
All stage T1	78%	—
All stages	24%	70%
Origin		
In or near BPH	Yes	No
Near apex	Yes	Yes
Detection rate by TURP	78%	—
Pathologic features		
Tumor pattern	Alveolar-medullary	Tubular
Tumor grade (primary Gleason grade)	Usually 1 or 2	Usually 2, 3, or 4
Clear cell pattern	Common	Uncommon
Stromal fibrosis	Uncommon	Uncommon
Associated putative premalignant changes	AAH or PIN	PIN
Aneuploidy	6%	31%
Clinical behavior		
Extraprostatic extension	11%	44%
Site of extraprostatic extension	Anterolateral and apical	Lateral
Average tumor volume with extraprostatic extension	4.98 cm^3	3.86 cm^3
Risk for seminal vesicle invasion	0%	19%
Risk for lymph node metastases	Low	High

AAH, Atypical adenomatous hyperplasia; *BPH*, benign prostatic hyperplasia; *PIN*, prostatic intraepithelial neoplasia; *TURP*, transurethral resection of the prostate.
[a]Central zone cancer (5%-10% of total) excluded.

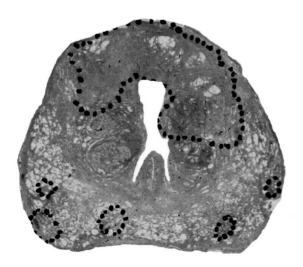

Fig. 9.66 Transition zone cancer. Whole-mount section showing large transition zone cancer (*top*) and smaller foci in the peripheral zone (*bottom*).

Transition zone cancer has a lower rate of positive biopsies in the middle (63% versus 80%) and base (50% versus 80%) of the prostate than peripheral zone cancer.[1461] Positive biopsies are exclusively obtained from the apex in 20% of transition zone and 5% of peripheral zone cancers. There is exact agreement between Gleason scores of needle biopsies and those of prostatectomy specimens in 15% of transition zone and 55% of peripheral zone cancers, respectively. The concordance rate for detection of cancer by location in matched biopsy and resected specimens is 59%.[1462]

It is important to clinically determine whether there is involvement of the anterior part of the prostate, because cancers of peripheral or transition zone origin may also be predominantly located anteriorly.[788] All transition zone cancers are located in the anterior half of the prostate: 3% at the base, 69% in the mid-gland, and 28% at the apex.[1463] These tumors are less likely to be detected by routine biopsy and may be associated with a higher incidence of margin positivity and increased risk for biochemical failure.[496]

Peripheral zone cancer tends to spread along the prostate capsule and is most extensive transversely.[711,1464] Above 4 cm^3 in volume, there is a progressive increase in incidence of bilateral spread, transition zone invasion, and nodularity. Dominant growth is toward the base along nerves to the superior pedicle, the most likely site of EPE. Transition zone cancer arises mainly in the anterior mid-transition zone, invading the anterior fibromuscular stroma, and when larger than 4 cm^3, the anterolateral peripheral zone.

The WHO recommends that prostate biopsies be submitted separately, the anatomic site of each prostate biopsy be labeled, and each specimen be reported separately.[451] Thus, the anatomic site and the amount of high-grade carcinoma within each prostate biopsy are included in the pathology report.

Lymph Node Metastases

Thirty years ago the incidence of lymph node metastases (Fig. 9.67) in patients with prostate cancer evaluated for surgical treatment was as high as 40%. In the modern era of screening and improved patient selection the incidence is now less than 10%. The risk for nodal metastases is influenced by stage, PSA concentration, Gleason grade, and the aggressiveness of lymph node dissection.[1465,1466] Staging pelvic lymph node biopsy may be performed before prostatectomy, and many urologists discontinue surgery if metastases are identified. Lymph node dissection is performed by an open, laparoscopic, or robotic procedure. Perineal prostatectomy and lymph node dissection are performed as separate procedures because the surgical approaches are different, whereas retropubic prostatectomy and lymphadenectomy may be performed as a single procedure. Extended dissection reveals a higher rate of metastases than limited dissection.[1467]

Sentinel-guided pelvic lymph node dissection allows detection of small lymph node metastases.[1468-1470] The accuracy of sentinel pelvic lymph node dissection is comparable with that of extended pelvic lymph node dissection; sentinel nodes are identified outside of the extended dissection field in 4% to 25% of cases.[1471,1472] False-negative rate is 0% to 24%.[1472] A nomogram based on pretreatment PSA, clinical stage, and biopsy Gleason score accurately predicts nodal metastases.[1473] The number of removed sentinel nodes and the PSA level are independent predictors of biochemical recurrence-free survival and metastases-free survival.[1474]

At the 2009 ISUP Conference, there was no consensus on sampling of a pelvic lymph node dissection specimen, although there was agreement that all lymph nodes should be completely blocked.[1475] It may not be necessary to submit obvious adipose

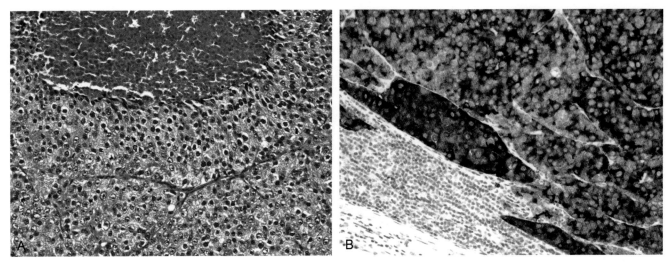

Fig. 9.67 (A) Pelvic lymph node with complete effacement by high-grade cancer with necrosis. (B) Immunostain for prostatic acid phosphatase confirms prostatic primary origin.

tissue, although it is our policy to do so. Sampling error by frozen section accounts for a false-negative rate of lymph node metastases of 2% to 3% in our experience (DG Bostwick, unpublished observations; 1999). The surgical pathology report should include the number and sites of all submitted lymph nodes, as well as the sites of involvement and size of cancer foci. Remarkably it has been shown that nodal metastases are more often detected in smaller lymph nodes (excluding massive involvement of nodes).[1476]

The diameter of the largest nodal metastasis appears to be more predictive of cancer-specific survival than the number of positive nodes alone, whereas the presence of extranodal extension is not predictive on multivariate analysis.[1477-1479] Patients with up to two positive lymph nodes have a clinical recurrence-free survival rate of 73% at 10 years compared with 49% in those with five or more involved lymph nodes.[1478] Patients undergoing excision of at least 4 lymph nodes (node-positive and node-negative patients) or more than 10 nodes (only node-negative patients) had a lower risk for cancer-specific death at 10 years than did those who did not undergo lymphadenectomy.[1480] As expected, the removal of a greater number of nodes is associated with a greater likelihood of the presence of positive nodes.[1480] There is a 3% to 13% incidence rate of occult prostatic carcinoma in pelvic lymph nodes that cannot be detected by routine H&E staining.[1481-1483] In patients treated surgically and with adjuvant androgen deprivation therapy, micrometastasis is an independent factor predicting biochemical recurrence.[1484]

Thirty percent to 40% of lymph node metastases occur contralateral to the dominant (index) cancer.[1485] Nodal metastases are usually associated with high-grade, high-stage, and large-volume cancer, and only rarely with anterior dominant cancer.

Lymph node metastases are heterogeneous and have a close relation to the corresponding primary tumor. Independent predictors of PSA recurrence among patients with positive lymph nodes include LVI in the lymph nodes and the nuclear grade of the primary tumor.[1443,1486]

Extranodal extension of nodal metastasis, defined as growth of neoplastic cells through the lymph node capsule into the perinodal adipose tissue, is predictive of biochemical recurrence.[1487]

Benign müllerian-type glandular inclusions in lymph nodes are a benign mimic of metastases that are histologically identical to endosalpingiosis in women. Identification of PAX8 and

WT1 immunoreactivity in these glands in men supports the theory that this entity results from müllerian metaplasia of the peritoneal mesothelium rather than displacement of tubal-type epithelium.[1488]

Distant Metastases

The usual sites of metastases are pelvic lymph nodes, bone (chiefly osteoblastic), and lungs (Fig. 9.68).[1489-1491] However, many unusual sites of metastases have been described including kidney, breast, and brain. No important differences in the pattern of metastases at autopsy have been reported in Japan and the United States. The number of metastatic sites is similar in those who do and do not receive estrogen therapy, although treated patients are more likely to experience brain metastases. Cluster analysis of metastases revealed a subset of men of African ancestry who experienced distant metastases with minimal local spread of cancer.[1489]

Morphometric Markers

Morphometric markers provide useful predictive information in prostate cancer but are infrequent in routine practice and are considered investigational.[451] The most popular morphometric

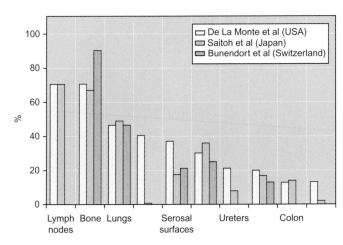

Fig. 9.68 Most common sites of prostate cancer metastases at autopsy in the United States, Japan, and Switzerland.

markers are nuclear size, nuclear shape and roundness, chromatin texture, size and number of nucleoli, and number of apoptotic bodies.[697,1492-1513] Volume-weighted mean nuclear volume is independently predictive of cancer-specific survival in combination with Gleason score and clinical stage.[1514] Morphometric alterations demonstrated by quantitative nuclear grade combined with pro-PSA immunohistologic localization independently predict significant differences between native Japanese and Japanese American men with prostate cancer, indicating a basis for biologic and molecular alterations in the adjacent benign and malignant epithelia between these two groups.[1515]

The recent rapid expansion in use of digital pathology is likely to spark a resurgence of interest in morphometric markers in coming years.

Benign Mesenchymal Tumors and Tumor-like Conditions

Table 9.47 summarizes the current classification of soft tissue tumors of the prostate. The dominant soft tissue in the prostate, smooth muscle, accounts for the wide diversity of benign and neoplastic tumors, most of which have a counterpart in other muscle-rich organs such as the uterus and gastrointestinal system.[1516]

Nodular hyperplasia of the prostate (BPH) accounts for most tumor-like conditions in the prostate (see Chapter 8). A brief discussion of two variants of hyperplasia, stromal hyperplasia and leiomyoma, is presented later because of the potential for misdiagnosis as malignancy. Both are described in detail in Chapter 8.

Stromal Hyperplasia (Stromal Subtype of Nodular Hyperplasia)

The most common tumor of the prostate, nodular hyperplasia, usually consists of a mixture of epithelial and stromal elements (see Chapter 8). The presence of atypical stromal cells warrants consideration of stromal hyperplasia with atypia (Table 9.48).

In our experience, the stromal subtype of nodular hyperplasia creates the greatest diagnostic difficulty for pathologists in separation from low-grade leiomyosarcoma and is the most frequent soft tissue tumor referred for second opinion. Size alone is usually of great value, because stromal hyperplasia rarely is larger than 1 cm in greatest dimension, whereas leiomyosarcoma is virtually always much larger and is usually high grade. A rare round cell pattern of stromal hyperplasia was recently reported, although the clinical impact of this finding is uncertain.[1517]

TABLE 9.47	Soft Tissue Tumors of the Prostate: Classification
Benign	**Malignant**
Stromal hyperplasia (stromal subtype of benign nodular hyperplasia)	Rhabdomyosarcoma
Stromal hyperplasia with atypia	Leiomyosarcoma
Leiomyoma	Phyllodes tumor
Leiomyoma with atypia	Stromal sarcoma
Postoperative spindle cell nodule	
Inflammatory myofibroblastic tumor	
Solitary fibrous tumor	

Leiomyoma

The distinction between nodular hyperplasia and leiomyoma is often difficult in biopsies and TURP, but this separation appears to have no practical clinical importance. Leiomyoma is defined as a well-circumscribed, encapsulated, solitary smooth muscle nodule greater than 1 cm in diameter (Figs. 9.69 and 9.70).[1518-1522] It is histologically identical to leiomyoma occurring in the uterus and other sites, and is composed of spindled or epithelioid smooth muscle cells separated by variable amounts of collagen. The tumor cells are often arranged in an orderly pattern of intersecting fascicles. Individual cells have blunt-ended nuclei with evenly distributed nuclear chromatin. Variants of leiomyoma include epithelioid leiomyoma, cellular leiomyoma, atypical leiomyoma, and leiomyoblastoma.[1523,1524]

Distinguishing leiomyoma from low-grade leiomyosarcoma is a difficult but uncommon problem in the prostate because most sarcomas are high grade and easily identified. Infiltrative growth, cellularity, nuclear atypia, tumor necrosis, and increased mitotic activity are the most important distinguishing features, and the diagnosis of sarcoma should be made if at least two or more of these features are present.[1518,1525] Treatment has shifted from surgery to embolization and other minimally invasive approaches.[1526]

Pseudosarcomatous Myofibroblastic Proliferation

Pseudosarcomatous myofibroblastic proliferation, a rare benign pathologic entity of unknown etiology (probably reactive), occurs in the bladder, prostate, urethra, and other sites without a history of prior surgery.[1527] It has a multitude of names including inflammatory myofibroblastic tumor, inflammatory pseudotumor, myofibroblastoma, low-grade inflammatory fibrosarcoma, spindle cell proliferation with no prior operation, pseudosarcoma, nodular fasciitis, and pseudosarcomatous fibromyxoid tumor. Patients range in age from 16 to 73 years (mean, 41 years). Mean tumor size is 4 cm but can measure up to 8 cm in diameter. The stroma is loose, edematous, and myxoid, with abundant small, slitlike blood vessels resembling granulation tissue (Figs. 9.71 and 9.72). Mitotic figures are infrequent, with less than 3 per 10 high-power fields; none is atypical. Ulceration and focal necrosis are present in most cases but are not prominent.

There is intense vimentin immunoreactivity and variable staining for smooth muscle actin, desmin, and keratin. S-100 protein and myoglobin are negative. Positivity for anaplastic lymphoma kinase-1 protein (ALK1) has been reported in some cases of inflammatory myofibroblastic tumor, suggesting a neoplastic rather than a reactive process.[1528,1529] Ultrastructural studies reveal myofibroblastic differentiation including cytoplasmic microfilaments and dense bodies. Tumors are usually diploid, with low S-phase fraction.

Recurrence may occur, particularly if incompletely excised, but no reported case in the prostate has metastasized. It should be noted that the clinicopathologic features of lesions associated with and without instrumentation are similar and inseparable, so many now believe that these are essentially the same entity.[1529,1530] Accordingly, Harik et al. proposed the term *pseudosarcomatous myofibroblastic proliferation*.[1529] Even in the face of atypical histologic features, the prognosis is excellent. Differential diagnostic considerations are identical to those of postoperative spindle cell nodule (Table 9.49).

TABLE 9.48	Prostatic Stromal Hyperplasia With Atypia: Differential Diagnosis[a]			
Characteristic Features	Stromal Hyperplasia With Atypia (Infiltrative Pattern)	Leiomyoma With Atypia (Symplastic Leiomyoma)	Phyllodes Tumor	Leiomyosarcoma
Clinical features				
Mean patient age, years (range)	69 (59-80)	68 (57-80)	55 (25-86)	61 (41-78)
Presenting symptoms	Urinary obstructive symptoms or incidental finding	Urinary obstructive symptoms or incidental finding	Urinary obstructive symptoms, hematuria, or incidental finding	Urinary obstructive symptoms; perineal pain
Cystoscopic/ macroscopic	Stromal nodule	Stromal nodule		Mass measuring 3-21 cm in diameter (mean, 9 cm)
Serum PSA	Normal range	Normal range	Normal range	Normal range
Architecture	Ill-defined hyperplastic stromal nodule with atypical cells diffusely and uniformly infiltrating around typical hyperplasia acini; hypocellular loose myxoid matrix with large ectatic vessels	Solid circumscribed expansile stromal nodule with abundant smooth muscle and atypical stromal cells	Biphasic pattern, including distorted cystically dilated or slitlike epithelial glands, often with leaflike projections, together with condensed stroma	Large, bulky nodular tumor composed of spindle cells
Cytology	Bizarre giant stromal cells with vacuolated nuclei and frequent multinucleation; no mitotic figures or necrosis	Bizarre giant stromal cells with vacuolated nuclei and frequent multinucleation; no mitotic figures or necrosis	Benign epithelium; variable number of bizarre stromal cells with vacuolated nuclei and multinucleation; mitotic figures and necrosis indicate higher grade	Spindle or epithelioid tumor cells with variable pleomorphism, mitotic figures, and frequent necrosis
Immunohistochemistry				
Vimentin	+++	+	Usually +++	++
Desmin	Usually +	+++	Usually -; rare +++	Usually -; rare +
Actin	+	+++	+	Usually -; rare +
Estrogen receptors	-	-	-	NT
Progesterone receptors	Usually +++	Usually ++	Usually -; rare +	NT
Androgen receptors	+++	+++	Usually -; rare ++	NT
Keratin AE1/AE3	-	-	++ (epithelium)	Usually - (+ in 27% of cases)
Keratin 34βE12	-	-	++ (epithelium)	NT
PSA	-	-	+++	-
Prostate acid phosphatase	-	-	+++	-
S-100 protein	-	-	-	-
Follow-up	Benign; rare solitary recurrences	Benign; rare solitary recurrences	Frequent recurrences with late onset of stromal overgrowth	Malignant; mean of 22 months to death (3-72 months)

NT, Not tested; *PSA,* prostate-specific antigen.
[a]Radiation therapy is also in the differential diagnosis but can easily be distinguished by clinical history and the diffuse nature of the changes, unlike the focal findings in these neoplasms.

Postoperative Spindle Cell Nodule (Postsurgical Inflammatory Myofibroblastic Tumor)

Postoperative spindle cell nodule, a rare benign reparative process, is considered clinically and histopathologically identical to pseudosarcomatous fibromyxoid tumor except for the antecedent history of surgery or trauma. It occurs 4 to 12 weeks after surgery and typically consists of small nodules measuring less than 1 cm in diameter with spindle cells arranged in fascicles with occasional or numerous mitotic figures (up to 25 mitotic figures/10 high-power fields).[1531] However, atypical or bizarre mitotic forms have not been reported. The cells have central elongate to ovoid nuclei, small prominent nucleoli, and abundant cytoplasm. There is mild to moderate acute and chronic inflammation. Necrosis may be present but is usually not a prominent feature.

The cells are strongly positive for vimentin and smooth muscle actin. This immunohistochemical profile cannot differentiate postoperative spindle cell nodule from leiomyoma or low-grade leiomyosarcoma. The key feature in recognizing postoperative spindle cell nodule is the clinical history of surgery or instrumentation within the previous few months. Most prostatic sarcomas is sufficiently cytologically pleomorphic that differentiation from postoperative spindle cell nodule is usually not a problem. Sarcomatoid carcinoma is also pleomorphic and may display immunoreactivity for CK and rarely PSA and PAP.[848,852]

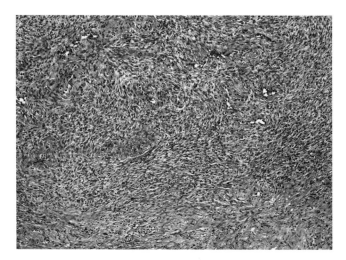

Fig. 9.69 Stromal nodule. This circumscribed cellular lesion is characterized by vascular and spindle cell proliferation without atypia.

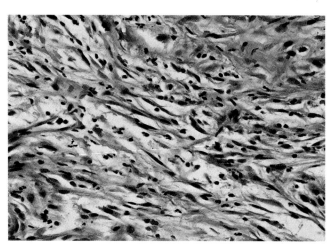

Fig. 9.71 Pseudosarcomatous fibromyxoid tumor. The loose myxoid stroma contains spindle cells, small slitlike blood vessels, and inflammatory cells, mainly lymphocytes and plasma cells.

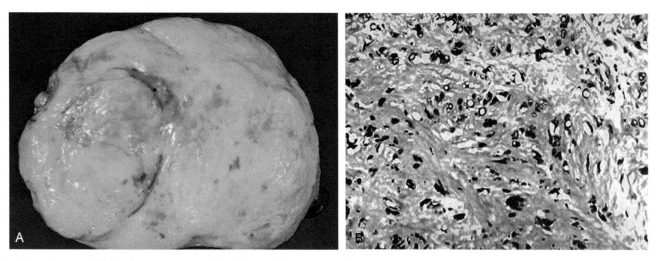

Fig. 9.70 Leiomyoma. (A) Simple prostatectomy with rubbery bulging nodules reminiscent of uterine leiomyoma. (B) Stromal hyperplasia with atypical giant cells. Note the prominent nuclear vacuolization.

Solitary Fibrous Tumor

Solitary fibrous tumor is a rare neoplasm, with fewer than 100 reported cases in the prostate, and is usually benign but can rarely exhibit malignant behavior.[1532] It more commonly arises on serosal surfaces (solitary fibrous mesothelioma) such as the visceral pleura.[1533,1534]

Solitary fibrous tumor is grossly well circumscribed. It is variable in cellularity, consisting of a mixture of haphazard, storiform, or short fascicular patterns of benign-appearing spindle cells with paucicellular dense collagenous bands (Fig. 9.73). A hemangiopericytoma-like growth pattern is typically seen. Positive immunostains for CD34, Bcl-2, and CD99 are invaluable in confirming the diagnosis, whereas S-100 protein, CD31, and CK are negative. STAT6 is sensitive and specific for diagnosis of solitary fibrous tumor (91% and 75%, respectively), and coexpression with ALDH1 yielded the same sensitivity but improved specificity to 100%.[1535]

Blue Nevus

Blue nevus of the prostate is characterized by the presence of melanin pigment within dendritic bipolar cells in the stroma, whereas in prostatic melanosis, it is chiefly in the epithelium (Fig. 9.74).[1536-1550] Premelanosomes and melanosomes are present ultrastructurally in the cells of prostatic blue nevus, indicating that they are melanocytic. Conversely, only stage IV melanosomes occur in the epithelial cells. S-100 protein immunoreactivity was demonstrated in the stromal cells, confirming the ultrastructural findings.[1545]

Other Rare Benign Soft Tissue Tumors

Other benign tumors that reflect the vast spectrum of mesenchymal tissues may rarely arise in the prostate including hemangioma, lymphangioma, neurofibroma, neurilemoma, chondroma, gastrointestinal stromal tumor, hemangiopericytoma, paraganglioma (pheochromocytoma) (Fig. 9.75), and myxoma.[1551-1561]

Sarcoma of the Prostate

Sarcoma accounts for less than 0.1% of prostatic neoplasms.[1516] One-third occur in children, and most of these are

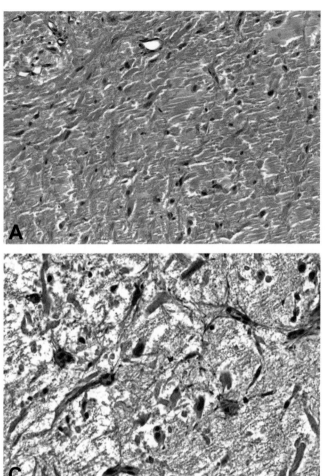

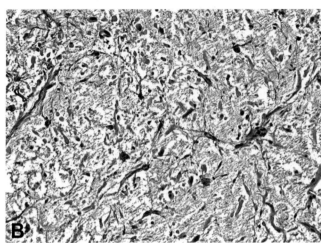

Fig. 9.72 Pseudosarcomatous fibromyxoid tumor. This tumor was from a 65-year-old man with a history of prostatitis who underwent transurethral resection of a mass in the prostate protruding into the urethral lumen (A to C). The tumor consisted of a loose spindle cell proliferation with abundant granular myxoid background stroma.

rhabdomyosarcoma; leiomyosarcoma is most common in adults. Symptoms include prostatism and pelvic pain. Tumors may be ≥15 cm in diameter and are usually soft with focal necrosis.

Patients with prostatic stromal sarcoma or rhabdomyosarcoma have worse 5-year local control (47% versus 55%, respectively) and overall survival (49% versus 58%, respectively) than those with other types of sarcoma.[1562]

Rhabdomyosarcoma

Rhabdomyosarcoma has a peak incidence between birth and 6 years of age, but sporadic cases have been reported in men as old as 80 years. Median age is 34 months (range, 2 to 176 months).[1563] Origin in the prostate, bladder, and vagina accounts for 21% of cases in children, second only to head and neck. Serum PSA and PAP are normal. Three affected adults had hypercalcemia caused by bone metastases.[1564]

The tumor is usually large and bulky, with a mean diameter up to 9 cm. It often involves the prostate, bladder, and periurethral, perirectal, and perivesicular soft tissues. Urethral involvement may not be apparent cystoscopically. Symptoms include acute or chronic urethral obstruction, bladder displacement, and rectal compression. The prostate may be palpably normal, although large tumors often fill the pelvis and can be palpated suprapubically.

Most are embryonal rhabdomyosarcoma, and the remainder are alveolar, botryoid, and spindle cell subtypes.[1565] Tumor cells are arranged in sheets of immature round to spindle cells set in a myxoid stroma (Figs. 9.76 and 9.77). Polypoid tumor fragments ("botryoid pattern") may fill the urethral lumen, covered by intact urothelium with condensed underlying tumor cells creating a distinctive cambium layer. Nuclei are usually pleomorphic and darkly staining. Scattered rhabdomyoblasts may be present, with eosinophilic cytoplasmic processes containing cross striations.

Rhabdomyosarcoma is immunoreactive for markers of muscle differentiation, and myogenin and myo-D1 are the most sensitive and specific.[1566] Tumor cells also display immunoreactivity for myoglobin, desmin, and vimentin but are negative for PSA and PAP. Alveolar subtype contains translocations t(2;13) and t (1;13) in 80% of cases, indicative of more aggressive behavior.[1567]

Ultrastructural study reveals two cell types, similar to rhabdomyosarcoma at other sites. Large oval or elongate tumor cells contain segments of sarcomere with abundant glycogen, and smaller round cells contain abundant cytoplasmic organelles but lack myofibrils. All tumors are aneuploid.[1568]

Combination chemotherapy, together with surgery and radiotherapy, results in a 3-year survival rate greater than 70%, according to the Intergroup Rhabdomyosarcoma Study.[1569] Long-term survival has been reported.

Leiomyosarcoma

Leiomyosarcoma is the most common prostatic sarcoma in adults. Patients range in age from 40 to 71 years (mean, 59 years), with sporadic reports in younger patients.[1570] The sarcoma presents

TABLE 9.49   Differential Diagnosis of Myxoid Lesions of the Prostate

	Pseudosarcomatous Fibromyxoid Tumor	Postoperative Spindle Cell Nodule	Sarcomatoid Carcinoma	Myxoid Leiomyosarcoma	Myxoid Rhabdomyosarcoma	Myxoid Malignant Fibrous Histiocytoma
Light microscopic findings						
Cellularity	Variable, often low	Variable, often low	High	Variable	Variable	Variable
Growth pattern	Tissue culture-like	Tissue culture-like	Biphasic	Intersecting fascicles	Subepithelial condensation	Storiform
Pleomorphism	+	-	+++	+/-	++	+++
Vessels	Slitlike	Unremarkable	Unremarkable	Unremarkable	Unremarkable	Unremarkable
Necrosis	+/-	+/-	++	++	+	++
Mitotic figures	+	++	++	+ (variable)	++	+++
Atypical mitotic figures	+	-	+	+	+	+
Immunohistochemical findings						
Cytokeratin	- (rarely +)	- (rarely +)	+	- (rarely +)	- (rarely +)	- (rarely +)
Vimentin	+	+	+	+	+	+
Desmin	+/-	+/-	+/-	+	+	- (rarely +)
Smooth muscle actin	+	+	+/-	+	-	-
S-100	-	-	+/-	-	-	-
Myogenin	-	-	-	-	+	-
Myoglobin	-	-	-	-	+/-	-

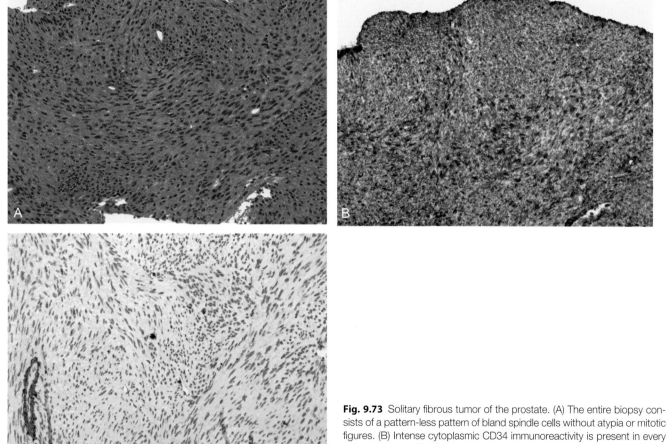

Fig. 9.73 Solitary fibrous tumor of the prostate. (A) The entire biopsy consists of a pattern-less pattern of bland spindle cells without atypia or mitotic figures. (B) Intense cytoplasmic CD34 immunoreactivity is present in every cell. Compare with (C), showing absence of smooth muscle actin staining (note the focal positive blood vessel serving as internal control).

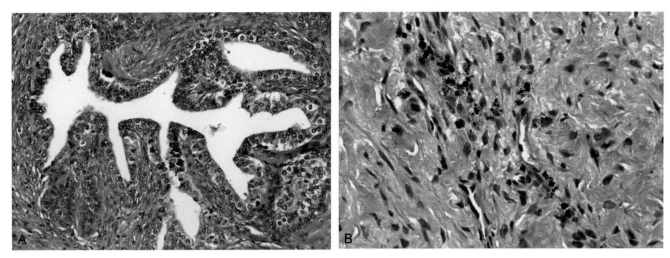

Fig. 9.74 Prostatic pigment. (A) Melanosis, with melanin pigment limited to the benign epithelium. (B) Blue nevus, with dusty and granular melanin pigment within myofibroblasts in the stroma.

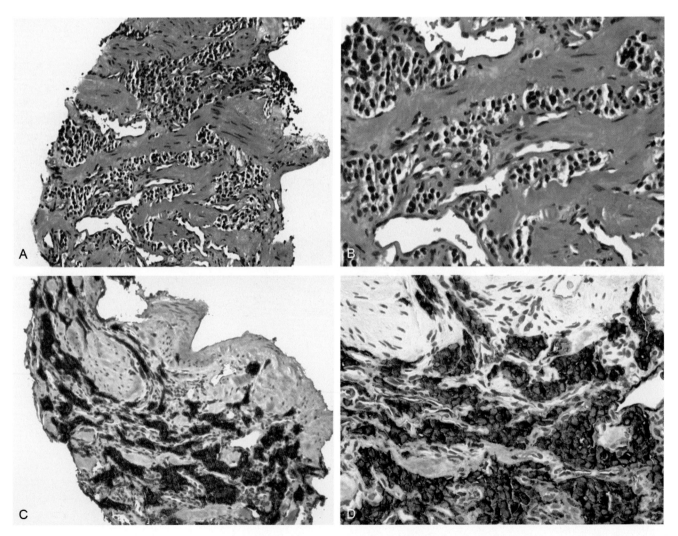

Fig. 9.75 Paraganglioma on biopsy. Irregular anastomosing cellular proliferation (A and B). (C) Synaptophysin immunoreactivity. (D) Chromogranin immunoreactivity.

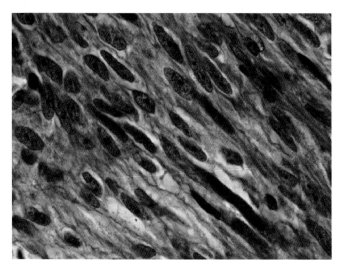

Fig. 9.76 Rhabdomyosarcoma of the prostate arising in a child.

as a large mass that replaces the prostate and periprostatic tissues, ranging in size from 3 to 21 cm in diameter. In a series of 23 cases, no tumors were grade 1, 7 were grade 2, 10 were grade 3, and 6 were grade 4, all histologically similar to leiomyosarcoma at other sites (Fig. 9.78).[1570] Prominent sclerotic stroma was noted in two cases. Five tumors had epithelioid features, and one had a focal area

reminiscent of neurilemoma. Necrosis may be extensive. Although the criteria for separating leiomyoma from low-grade leiomyosarcoma have not been precisely defined in the prostate, they are probably like those in other organs, including degree of cellularity, cytologic anaplasia, number of mitotic figures, amount of necrosis, vascular invasion, and size.

Tumor cells usually display intense cytoplasmic immunoreactivity for smooth muscle–specific actin and vimentin, and weak desmin immunoreactivity. Most are negative for keratins and S-100 protein, but exceptions have been described, particularly in those with epithelioid features in which keratin immunoreactivity may be seen.[1570] Local recurrence and distant metastasis are frequent, and the prognosis is poor. Mean survival after diagnosis is less than 3 years (range, 0.2 to 7 years), and most patients die of sarcoma.[1570]

Phyllodes Tumor

Phyllodes tumor (cystic epithelial-stromal tumor; phyllodes type of atypical hyperplasia; cyst adenoleiomyofibroma; cystosarcoma phyllodes; stromal tumor of uncertain malignant potential) of the prostate is a rare lesion that should be considered a neoplasm rather than atypical hyperplasia because of frequent early recurrences, infiltrative growth, and potential for extraprostatic and metastatic spread in some cases.[1571] Dedifferentiation (stromal overgrowth) with multiple recurrences in some cases is further

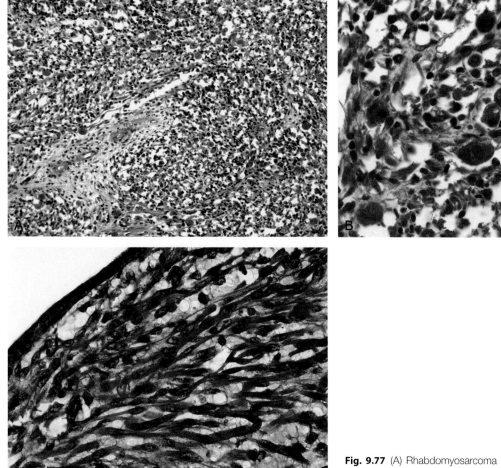

Fig. 9.77 (A) Rhabdomyosarcoma of the prostate. (B) Rhabdomyoblasts display intensely eosinophilic cytoplasm. (C) Another case, in which striated muscle differentiation is not evident.

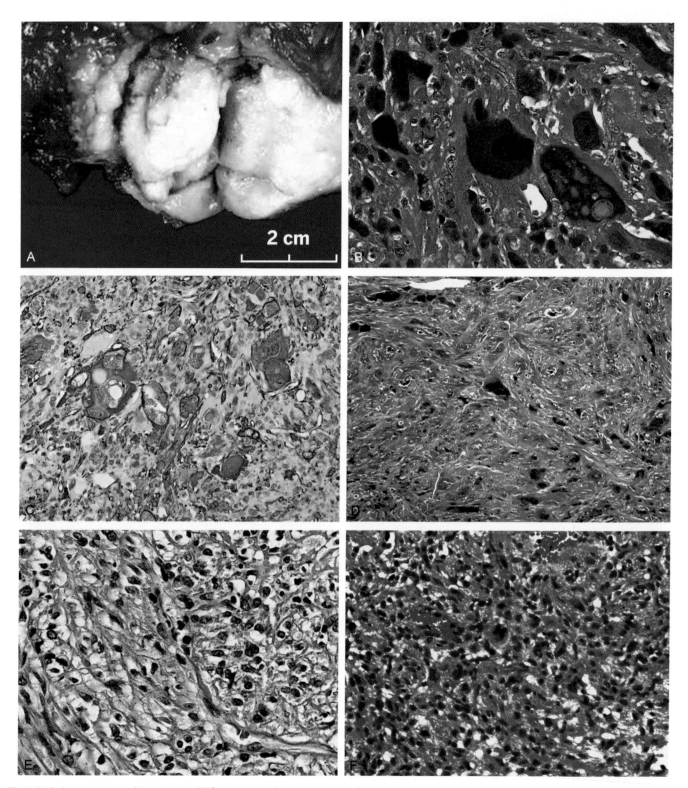

Fig. 9.78 Leiomyosarcoma of the prostate. (A) Gross examination reveals a large, fleshy tan mass replacing most of the prostate. (B) Bizarre giant cells punctuate this spindle cell proliferation. (C) Intense cytoplasmic immunoreactivity for actin in most tumor cells. Other examples of leiomyosarcoma, revealing typical high-grade cytologic findings (D to F).

evidence of the potentially aggressive nature of this tumor.[1571] A benign clinical course has been suggested by some, but a significant number of patients experience local recurrences and metastases.[1571]

Patients with prostatic phyllodes tumor typically present with urinary obstruction, hematuria, and dysuria. Most tumors range in size from 4 to 25 cm. At the time of TURP, there may be an unusual spongy or cystic texture of the involved prostate.

The diagnosis of phyllodes tumor is usually made on resected tissue, and it may be overlooked on biopsy in which it is difficult to appreciate the pattern of the tumor. Important diagnostic clues include diffuse infiltration, variably cellular stroma surrounding cysts, and compressed elongate channels that often have a leaflike configuration (Fig. 9.79). Prostatic phyllodes tumor exhibits a spectrum of histologic features, similar to its counterpart in the breast.[1571] High-grade phyllodes tumor has a high stromal/epithelial ratio, prominent stromal cellularity and overgrowth, marked cytologic atypia, and increased mitotic activity. A sarcomatous component may arise within a low-grade tumor over time, invariably after multiple recurrences over many years.[1571] The lining epithelium is benign but may show various metaplastic and proliferative changes such as basal cell hyperplasia or squamous metaplasia.[1572,1573]

Immunohistochemical studies reveal intense cytoplasmic immunoreactivity in stromal cells for vimentin and actin; in luminal epithelial cells for PSA, PAP, and keratin AE1/AE3; and in basal epithelial cells for high-molecular-weight keratin 34βE12; no staining was observed for desmin and S-100 protein.

Phyllodes tumors are clonal, and the epithelial and stromal components have different clonal origins and appear to be true neoplasms.[1574] EGFR and AR are frequently and strongly expressed in both epithelial and stromal components.[1575] *EGFR* gene amplification may account for one of the mechanisms leading to protein overexpression in some but not all cases. Anti-EGFR or antiandrogen agents may be potentially useful for management of patients with tumors expressing EGFR or AR.

Stromal Sarcoma

Undifferentiated sarcoma of the prostatic stroma is rare.[1576-1580] Most sarcomas arising in the prostate are classified along the known lines of differentiation for soft tissue sarcomas; those that do not fit within the known lines of differentiation are simply called *stromal sarcoma* or *sarcoma, NOS (not otherwise specified).*[1572,1581] Stromal sarcoma may arise in patients of all ages but is usually seen in adults and the elderly. Prognosis depends on grade and stage, but all are malignant and potentially very aggressive.

Microscopically, stromal sarcoma varies from a diffuse proliferation of round and plump cells (low-grade stromal sarcoma) to spindle cells with a considerable degree of nuclear atypia and hyperchromasia (high-grade stromal sarcoma) (Fig. 9.80). There are invariably more than 2 mitotic figures/10 high-power fields, even in needle biopsies. Areas of necrosis are frequently seen. The cells are arranged in miscellaneous architectural patterns ranging from diffuse sheets to short fascicles that often show a storiform pattern.

The neoplastic stromal cells are immunoreactive for vimentin and CD34, but are usually negative for smooth muscle actin, desmin, and S-100 protein. Progesterone receptors are occasionally positive, whereas estrogen receptors are invariable negative. Some cases showed a similar immunohistochemical profile: positivity for vimentin and desmin, but negativity for smooth muscle actin.[1582-1585] In contrast, Yum et al. reported a case that was positive for vimentin, smooth muscle actin, and desmin, and classified the tumor as leiomyosarcoma arising in phyllodes tumor.[1586]

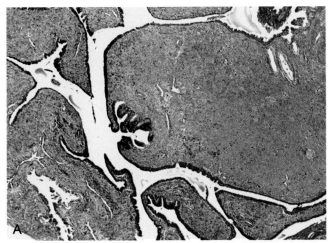

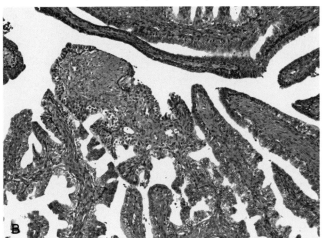

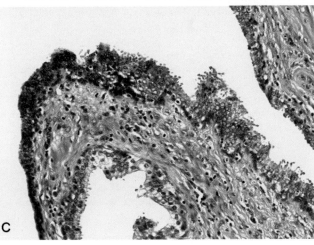

Fig. 9.79 Phyllodes tumor. Low-grade prostatic phyllodes tumor with leaf-like intraluminal epithelial-lined stromal projections (A and B). (C) Low-grade prostatic phyllodes tumor with a low cellularity, a low stroma-to-epithelium ratio, moderate cytologic atypia, and no mitotic figures.

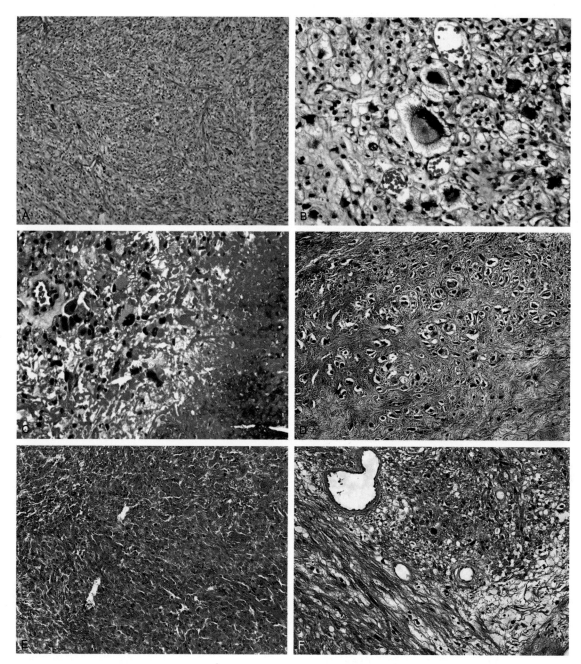

Fig. 9.80 Multiple examples of stromal sarcoma (A to F).

Other Sarcomas

Other sarcomas reported in the prostate include fibrosarcoma, osteosarcoma, undifferentiated pleomorphic sarcoma (malignant fibrous histiocytoma) (Fig. 9.81), angiosarcoma, chondrosarcoma, primitive neuroectodermal tumor (Fig 9.82), neurofibrosarcoma, liposarcoma, and synovial sarcoma.[436,1587-1595] Regardless of classification, the prognosis is poor. There appears to be no association of radiation therapy and prostatic angiosarcoma.[1596]

Other Malignancies of the Prostate

Hematologic Malignancies

Hematologic malignancies are rare in the prostate, with primary involvement or secondary spread from systemic lymphoma, leukemia, or myeloma.

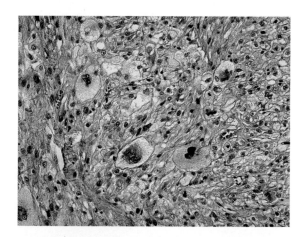

Fig. 9.81 Undifferentiated pleomorphic sarcoma (malignant fibrous histiocytoma) replacing most of the prostate.

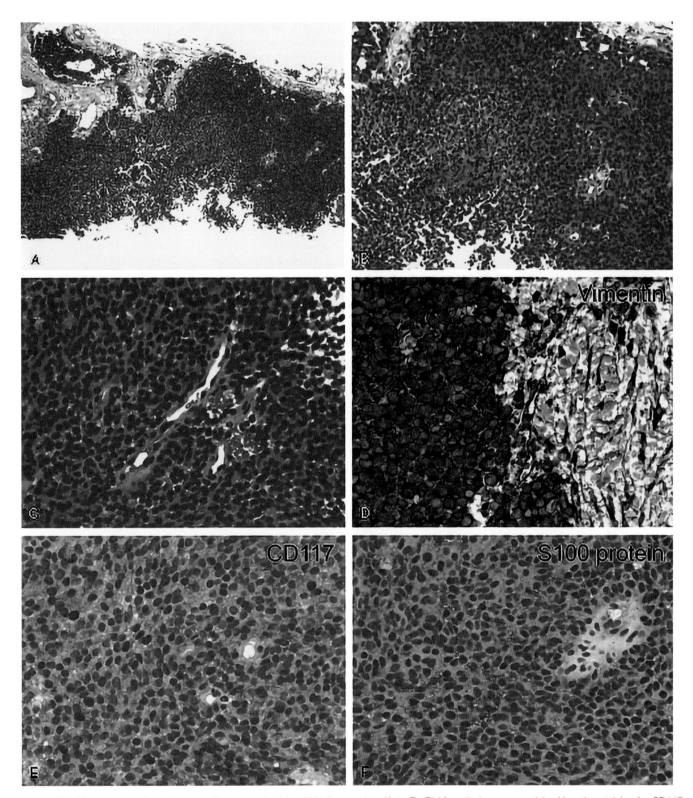

Fig. 9.82 Primitive neuroectodermal tumor with apparent origin within the prostate (A to F). (D) Vimentin immunoreactivity. Negative staining for CD117 and S-100 protein, respectively (E and F).

Leukemia

Chronic lymphocytic leukemia is the most common leukemia involving the prostate, with more than 300 reported cases. Many are incidentally discovered during investigation of prostatic enlargement or adenocarcinoma.[1597-1599] The autopsy prevalence rate is about 20% of cases of leukemia.[1600] The clinical symptoms and histologic pattern in the prostate are similar to malignant lymphoma, and leukemia is distinguished chiefly from lymphoma by the presence of blood involvement. An unusual case was described of late relapse of granulocytic sarcoma (chloroma) detected by urinary obstructive symptoms and TURP caused by prostatic enlargement after 9 years of remission.[1601] Bladder neck obstruction in patients with leukemia may respond to surgery if chemotherapy is ineffective, although others have successfully used radiation therapy.[1602,1603]

Malignant Lymphoma

Patients with malignant lymphoma involving the prostate are usually older men (mean, 62 years) who have urinary obstructive symptoms including urinary urgency, frequency, acute retention, infections, and hematuria.[1604] Systemic symptoms, including fever, chills, night sweats, and weight loss, are infrequent and are found only in patients with widespread lymphoma. Occasional cases are discovered incidentally at biopsy or prostatectomy for adenocarcinoma.[1597,1599] Grossly, the prostate is diffusely enlarged, nontender, and firm or rubbery. PSA is usually not elevated.

Primary lymphoma is much less frequent than secondary involvement.[1597,1604,1605] Ewing and others challenged the existence of primary extranodal lymphoma because of the paucity of lymphoid tissue in the prostate.[1606] However, identification of rudimentary lymphoid nodules in the prostate by Fukase, the recognition of malignant lymphoma arising in extranodal sites, and histologic documentation of cases with involvement limited to the prostate confirmed the existence of lymphoma apparently arising in the prostate.[1607] The prevalence rate of primary lymphoma at autopsy is 0.2% of extranodal lymphomas.[1605] Diagnostic criteria for primary lymphoma include symptoms attributable to prostatic enlargement; lymphoma chiefly involving the prostate with or without involvement of adjacent tissues, and lack of liver, spleen, lymph nodes; and peripheral blood involvement within 1 month of diagnosis (sufficient time to allow for staging studies).[1608]

Microscopically, the lymphomatous infiltrate may be diffuse or patchy within the stroma, with characteristic preservation of prostatic acini (Fig. 9.83); by contrast, granulomatous prostatitis causes acinar destruction.[1604] The infiltrate is usually extensive but may be irregular and patchy, often extending into the extraprostatic soft tissues; involvement of the acinar epithelium is uncommon and rarely includes aggregates in the lumens. The most frequent lymphoma involving the prostate is diffuse non-Hodgkin

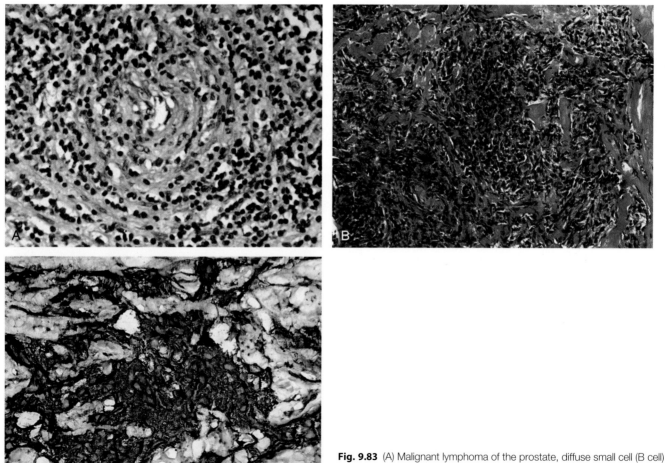

Fig. 9.83 (A) Malignant lymphoma of the prostate, diffuse small cell (B cell) type, with prominent angiotropism. (B) Another case, displaying dense monomorphic cellular infiltrate. Compare with (C), showing intense immunoreactivity for CD20.

lymphoma, including small cleaved cell, large cell, and mixed-cell types. Hodgkin disease is rare, with fewer than 10 documented cases.[1597,1604] Angiotropic lymphoma, mantle zone lymphoma, Burkitt lymphoma, and mucosa-associated lymphoid tissue lymphoma have also been described. Occasional cases have coincidental adenocarcinoma.[1609-1615]

The prognosis is usually poor regardless of patient age, stage, or histologic classification. Lymphoma-specific survival rate is 64% at 1 year, 33% at 5 years, 33% at 10 years, and 16% at 15 years.[1604] There is no difference in median survival after diagnosis of prostatic involvement between primary and secondary lymphoma (23 versus 28 months, respectively). Long-term survival is possible with combination chemotherapy, whereas surgery is used chiefly for symptomatic relief of urinary obstruction.

The differential diagnosis of lymphoma includes leukemia, granulomatous prostatitis, chronic prostatitis with follicular hyperplasia, and NE carcinoma. A 68-year-old man with prostatic pseudolymphoma was described by Peison et al. The patient had no prior history of lymphoma and showed symptoms of acute urinary obstruction and normal blood count.[1616] Histologically, there was prominent lymphoid hyperplasia in the TURP specimen without evidence of malignancy. Long-term follow-up was not available. Extramedullary hematopoiesis of the prostate was reported in a 75-year-old man with a history of myelofibrosis and progressive outlet obstruction.[1617] The TURP revealed a diffuse stromal infiltrate of atypical megakaryocytes, immature myeloid elements, and normoblasts; the epithelium was preserved. Chloroacetate esterase stain was useful in confirming the myeloid nature of the infiltrate.

Multiple Myeloma

Multiple myeloma involving the prostate is rare, with less than 10 cases reported.[1618] Most are diagnosed at autopsy, usually after systemic diagnosis. Immunoglobulin D and A myelomas have been described and rarely may cause urinary obstructive symptoms. The incidence of prostatic involvement by myeloma is uncertain.

Germ Cell Tumors

Rare cases of germ cell tumor apparently arising in the prostate have been reported, invariably with metastases and massive prostatic involvement.[1619-1625] These tumors probably arise from sequestration of germ cells during migration, usually occurring in the midline. This theory also accounts for germ cell tumors in the vagina, mediastinum, liver, retroperitoneum, and liver. Alternatively, some cases probably represent regressed or burned out testicular germ cell tumor with retrovesicular metastasis.

A patient with retroperitoneal seminoma and simultaneous occurrence in the prostate was described, as well as a 40-year-old with mixed germ cell tumor (embryonal carcinoma and teratoma) who was alive 2 years after treatment.[1626,1627] Choriocarcinoma involving the prostate is exceedingly rare.[1628]

The main differential diagnostic considerations include sarcomatoid carcinoma (carcinosarcoma), mucinous carcinoma, typical acinar adenocarcinoma, ductal carcinoma, and metastases from testicular or retroperitoneal primary. The diagnosis of primary germ cell tumor of the prostate should be considered only after all other possibilities are excluded. The usual histologic features of germ cell tumor at other sites are present. For yolk sac tumor these include Schiller-Duval bodies, hyaline PAS+ globules, and elevated AFP. PSA and PAP are normal. Fewer than 10 cases of prostatic yolk sac tumor have been reported.[1629,1630]

Other Rare Malignancies

Rhabdoid tumor is a poorly differentiated malignant neoplasm with light microscopic features of rhabdomyosarcoma that displays epithelial differentiation including intense cytoplasmic immunoreactivity for keratin proteins and EMA, rare cell junctions, occasional intracytoplasmic lumens, and distinctive paranuclear aggregates of intermediate filaments. Most cases occur in the kidney, but extrarenal tumors have been identified, including rare cases in the prostate.[1631] Peripheral neuroectodermal tumor has also been described in the prostate.[1632,1633]

Malignant melanoma of the prostate is histologically identical to its counterpart arising at other sites.[1634,1635] Bladder and urethral mucosal origin is much more common.

A single case of primary Wilms tumor of the prostate was reported, arising in a 32-year-old man with hemospermia and obstructive symptoms.[968] The characteristic triphasic pattern was observed, including blastema, epithelial tubules, and spindled stroma. The patient had pulmonary metastases 1 year after presentation. Extrarenal Wilms tumor is thought to arise from embryonic rests of metanephric blastema, explaining the occurrence of this tumor in other urogenital areas such as the scrotum, spermatic cord, and in an ovotestis. The differential diagnosis includes sarcoma such as rhabdomyosarcoma, sarcomatoid carcinoma, and teratoma.

Metastases to the Prostate

Tumors arising in other organs occasionally involve the prostate, usually because of contiguous spread, but metastases may occur, with involvement at autopsy in 0.5% to 2% of men dying of malignancies.[834,1636,1637] The most common tumor metastasizing to the prostate is pulmonary squamous cell carcinoma, accounting for almost one-half of all metastases. Malignant melanoma accounts for approximately 27% of prostatic metastases, with an incidence rate of prostatic involvement of 1% of patients with malignant melanoma at autopsy.[1638] An unusual case was reported of tumor-to-tumor metastasis of malignant melanoma to prostatic adenocarcinoma.[1638] A 63-year-old man experienced development of metastatic breast cancer to the prostate that was positive for GATA3 and ER and negative for PSA, P501S, p63, and high-molecular-weight keratin.[1639] The remaining 25% of metastases to prostate arise from a variety of sites including skin, pancreas, and stomach.[1640]

References are available at expertconsult.com

10
Seminal Vesicles

DAVID G. BOSTWICK

Introduction

The seminal vesicles were described by the Italian anatomist Berengario a Carpi in 1521. These paired androgen-dependent accessory sex glands were first regarded simply as storage sites for semen, but their milky alkaline secretions are now known to constitute the majority of the ejaculate, promoting sperm function and providing a variety of potent antibacterial factors to the male genital tract.[1-3] Cross-sectional area increases with duration of abstinence from ejaculation.[4] Infections, cysts, and neoplasms of the seminal vesicles are rare, in sharp contrast with their anatomic neighbor, the prostate.

Embryology and Anatomy

Under the influence of testosterone, the seminal vesicles appear during the thirteenth week of development as outpouchings of the lower mesonephric ducts. They are bounded by the prostate distally, the base of the bladder anteriorly, and Denonvilliers fascia and the rectum posteriorly. Their anatomic position in this region is variable, and they are sometimes found within or adherent to the posterior capsule of the prostate gland.[2,3,5] The seminal vesicles may be palpable on digital rectal examination and, when adherent to the prostate, may be mistaken for prostatic nodularity or induration. Approximately 5% of prostate biopsies for nodularity contain fragments of seminal vesicle epithelium, a potential source of diagnostic confusion (Fig. 10.1).[6,7] In adults the seminal vesicles average 6 cm long and 2 cm wide, with a capacity of up to 4.5 mL, although there is wide variation in size, shape, and volume.[5] Interestingly, α blockers, such as silodosin, tamsulosin, and alfuzosin used for treating prostatic nodular hyperplasia, create loss of seminal emission and seminal vesicular enlargement.[8]

The muscular wall of the seminal vesicles consists of a thick circumferential coat of smooth muscle, which contracts during ejaculation. Contraction is regulated by excitatory adrenergic and modulatory neuropeptide Y-encephalin-peptidergic nerve fibers.[5] Tangential cuts through this wall frequently reveal irregular clusters of epithelial tubules, which may be mistaken for adenocarcinoma.

The ducts of the seminal vesicles merge with the ampullae of the vasa deferentia on each side to form the ejaculatory ducts, and these structures compose a functional unit that develops slowly until the onset of puberty.[5] These ducts immediately enter the central zone of the prostate and converge as they approach their outlets at either side of the verumontanum in the prostatic sinus of the prostatic urethra. Unlike the seminal vesicles, the ejaculatory ducts lack a thick muscular wall, surrounded by a collagenous stroma. Luminal and wall dimensions are remarkably uniform among adult men, with diameter greater than 2.3 mm the cutpoint for dilatation.[9]

Histologically the seminal vesicular mucosa consists of complex papillary folds and irregular convoluted lumens lined with nonciliated, pseudostratified tall columnar epithelium. The cells are predominantly secretory, containing microvesicular lipid droplets and characteristic lipofuscin pigment granules.[10] The pigment is golden-brown and refractile, increasing in amount with age; similar pigment may be seen in prostatic epithelium, but is usually less conspicuous and abundant.[11] These cells also contain androgen receptors, similar to the prostatic epithelium. Secretory products include glycoproteins, protein kinase inhibitor, protein C inhibitor, fructose, prostaglandins, ascorbic acid, sperm motility factor, transferrin, lactoferrin, lysozyme, and metallothionein. Secretion is regulated by nerves from the pelvic plexus, which are cholinergic postganglionic, sympathetic, and possibly parasympathetic.[5,12,13] Nerves are arranged in a vertical plate lateral to the seminal vesicles. Mean ± SD distance of nerves to the seminal vesicles was 1.68 ± 0.84, 1.50 ± 0.12, and 1.76 ± 0.37 mm at the tip, middle, and

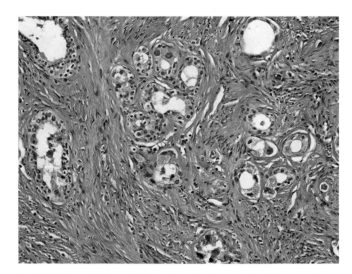

Fig. 10.1 Tangential needle biopsy through the seminal vesicles, which may be mistaken for adenocarcinoma.

base, respectively.[14] Up to 85% of the seminal fluid originates in the seminal vesicles, and the semen volume varies from 2 to 5 mL. It takes 3 days for the epithelium to refill the seminal vesicles after ejaculation.

MUC6 is selectively expressed in benign seminal vesicle epithelium, in contrast with benign prostate and adenocarcinoma.[15] Likewise, intense immunohistochemical expression of GATA binding protein 3 (GATA3) in seminal vesicle epithelium may help distinguish from mimics, although this marker is also positive in prostatic basal cells and, with less intensity, in secretory cells, and rarely in prostatic adenocarcinoma.[16]

Age-Associated Changes

The seminal vesicles begin to shrink in the seventh decade.[17] The tall columnar cells lining the mucosa in young men are replaced over time by flattened cuboidal cells, comprising only 50% of the epithelium in men in the fifth decade of life and 2% in octogenarians. With advancing age, the stroma of the seminal vesicles becomes hyalinized and fibrotic. In sexually active middle-aged

men, the volume of the seminal vesicles was significantly larger in those who had a sexual frequency once every 3 months than in those who had a sexual frequency once every 6 months or less.[18]

The flattening of the epithelium is accompanied by striking nuclear abnormalities, and highly atypical cells are present in about 75% of older men (Fig. 10.2).[19-26] These cells have large irregular hyperchromatic nuclei with coarse chromatin and prominent nucleoli. Multinucleated cells are also present, as well as giant ring-shaped nuclei with large intranuclear cytoplasmic inclusions. Mitotic figures are absent. These nuclear abnormalities, not observed before age 20 years, are probably degenerative changes reflecting hormonal influences. When encountered in needle biopsies, such "pseudomalignant" cytologic atypia may lead to a mistaken diagnosis of prostate cancer.[27] Difficulty may also be encountered in cytologic evaluation of fluids obtained by prostatic massage because seminal vesicular cells are frequently shed intact into the lumens. The distinctive lipochrome pigment aids in their recognition.[21-23,25] Cells in prostatic aspirates derived from the seminal vesicles and ejaculatory ducts may be cytologically indistinguishable. DNA ploidy analysis reveals aneuploidy in up to 48% of seminal vesicles.[19,28] Consequently DNA analysis of prostate cancer specimens may yield false-positive results if contaminated by seminal vesicle tissue. It is uncertain why there is such a low level of aneuploidy in an organ with frequent and substantial cytologic atypia.

Seminal vesicular cells are found as contaminants of cervical smears in 10% of specimens with spermatozoa, and they may be diagnostically confusing.[29] These cells contain foamy cytoplasm, scant pigment, vesicular hyperchromatic nuclei, sievelike chromatin pattern, and mild anisokaryosis.

Congenital and Acquired Malformations

Malformations of the seminal vesicles are frequently associated with abnormal development of other mesonephric derivatives, although isolated hypoplasia, agenesis, and cysts have been reported.[30,31] Unilateral absence of one seminal vesicle may be associated with ipsilateral prostatic central zone agenesis, renal agenesis, or vas deferens anomalies or agenesis.[32,33] Unilateral agenesis is often associated with decreased semen volume, hypospermia or azoospermia, impaired sperm motility, acidic

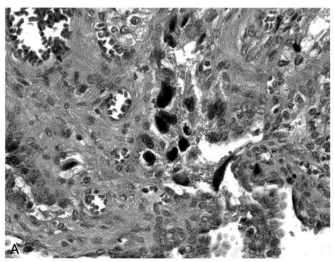

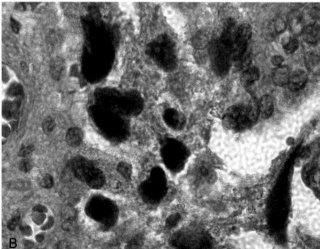

Fig. 10.2 Seminal vesicle from an 80-year-old man that shows distinctive highly atypical epithelial cells. (A) low power. (B) oil immersion.

ejaculate, and absence of fructose and coagulation activity. Up to 37.5% of these men are infertile, implying that the single vas is abnormal. Bilateral dilation or absence of the seminal vesicles is sometimes observed in patients with cystic fibrosis, reportedly caused by an unexplained failure of development.[34] Unilateral duplication of the seminal vesicles is an unusual anomaly. Seminal vesicle surgery is usually undertaken for evaluation of congenital malformations.

Maldevelopment of the ureteric bud results in ureteral ectopy, with the ureters terminating in the seminal vesicles, prostatic urethra, vas deferens, epididymis, or ejaculatory ducts.[35-49] Ureteral ectopy is frequently seen in association with ipsilateral renal dysgenesis or contralateral renal hypertrophy, and the seminal vesicles become enlarged and dilated with accompanying ureterocele.

Cysts

Seminal vesicle cysts are rare and may be congenital or acquired.[50-53] Symptoms are vague, including perineal pain during ejaculation or defecation, dysuria, urinary retention, and recurrent epididymitis. Congenital cysts are associated with ipsilateral renal agenesis in 80% of cases and commonly with ureteral ectopia or agenesis (Zinner syndrome), with more than 100 reported cases.[35,52,54-65] These paired anomalies are caused by the close association of the ureteric bud and mesonephric duct during embryogenesis; the ureteric bud is more cephalad, and the elongated ureter may fail to connect with and stimulate the differentiation of the nephrogenic blastema. Hajji et al. described a unique variant of inverted Y ureteral duplication with concurrent ectopic ureteral insertion into a seminal vesicle cyst, ureterocele, and renal dysgenesis in a 29-year-old man with lower urinary tract symptoms, hematospermia, and postcoital discomfort.[66] Other cases of congenital cysts are associated with ipsilateral absence of the testis or hemivertebra.[39,67] Congenital cysts of the seminal vesicle are usually detected in patients between 18 and 41 years of age, the period of maximal sexual and reproductive activity; most have arisen in Caucasian patients.[68] Cysts may be asymptomatic or cause ill-defined lower urinary tract symptoms.[69] Magnetic resonance imaging (MRI) is useful for detecting cysts and associated urogenital tract anomalies.[70] Interestingly, 23% of men with adult polycystic kidney disease have seminal vesicle ectasia (cystic changes).[71]

The cyst is usually unilateral and unilocular, lateral to the midline, up to three times larger than the normal seminal vesicle, and considerably smaller than müllerian duct cyst (Table 10.1), although rarely the cyst is gigantic and may cause rectal obstruction.[72-74] Enlargement is caused by insufficient drainage with accumulation of seminal fluid. The unilocular cyst contains viscous pale-white fluid, similar to the usual secretions of the seminal

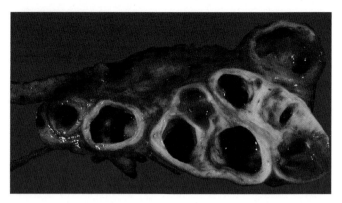

Fig. 10.3 Incidental acquired cyst of the seminal vesicles found at autopsy in a 70-year-old man.

vesicles, and is lined by cuboidal or flattened epithelium with a fibrous wall of variable thickness. Rarely there may be intracystic papillary adenoma.[75] Massive enlargement has been called hydrocele or hydrops.[76] Bilateral congenital cysts are rare and may be associated with absent vasa deferentia.[77]

Acquired cyst is usually associated with inflammation and obstruction of the ejaculatory ducts and seminal vesicles (Fig. 10.3). This fluctuant cyst may be palpable on digital rectal examination and often contains red cells, white cells, and spermatozoa. The epithelial lining is inflamed or sloughed, depending on the duration and severity of inflammation. In one case, endoscopic removal of a small calculus lodged at the orifice of the ipsilateral ejaculatory duct caused complete resolution of a 14-cm seminal vesicle cyst, evidence for an obstructive etiology and demonstration of the utility of preoperative imaging techniques to detect stones.[78] One unique case presented as an inguinal hernia, with the cyst extending through the inguinal canal.[79]

Echinococcal (hydatid) cyst can occur in the retrovesicular region, invariably in association with infection in another organ; cyst excision is curative.[80-85] Megavesicles are characterized by marked dilation of the seminal vesicles. The cause of megavesicles is unknown, but this condition is sometimes seen in individuals with diabetes.[86] Cystadenoma is a benign neoplasm mimicking acquired cyst (see later).

The differential diagnosis of seminal vesicle cyst includes prostatic cyst, ejaculatory duct diverticulum, and cystic dilation of wolffian and müllerian duct remnants (Table 10.1).[86-89] The cyst may produce hydronephrosis caused by displacement of the lower ureter toward the midline with obstruction. Radiographic evaluation of seminal vesicle cyst includes vasoseminovesiculography, ultrasonography, computerized tomography (CT), and MRI.[60,90] Aspiration of congenital or acquired cysts relieves symptoms, but surgical removal or marsupialization is preferred.

Ectopic Prostatic Tissue

Benign ectopic prostatic tissue rarely arises in seminal vesicle tissue and may be mistaken for extraprostatic adenocarcinoma.[91] Ectopia may involve prostatic or urothelial tissue, and most frequently is identified in the wall of seminal vesicle cyst, sometimes forming a nodular mass.[92,93] In one case, prostate cancer arose within the prostatic ectopia in the seminal vesicles.[94] The intimate spatial coexistence of endoderm-derived prostatic tissue and mesonephric duct-derived seminal vesicle tissue is rare.[95]

TABLE 10.1	Differential Diagnosis of Seminal Vesicle Cyst		
Type of Cyst	Location	Size	Contains Spermatozoa
Seminal vesicle cyst	Lateral	Large	Yes
Diverticulum of ejaculatory duct	Lateral	Variable	Yes
Prostatic cyst	Lateral	Variable	No
Müllerian duct cyst	Midline	Large	No

Nonneoplastic Abnormalities

Amyloidosis

Localized amyloidosis of the seminal vesicles, which may also include the ejaculatory and deferent ducts (referred to as senile seminal vesicle amyloidosis or senile seminal tract amyloidosis), is observed at autopsy in 5% to 8% of men between 46 and 60 years of age, 13% to 23% between 61 and 75 years, and 21% to 34% over 75 years.[96-99] The clinical incidence in men with hematospermia is 33%; at radical prostatectomy, the incidence rate is 1.1%.[100,101] There may be an association with prior androgen deprivation therapy for prostate cancer, but this has been refuted.[101,102]

Amyloidosis often extends bilaterally along the ejaculatory ducts, forming linear or massive nodular subepithelial deposits of amorphous eosinophilic fibrillar material (Fig. 10.4). Basement membrane thickening is observed, and deposits may be seen within the vesicular lumens, occasionally causing significant luminal narrowing. Rare cases are associated with calcification or a florid foreign body giant cell reaction.[103] By contrast, systemic amyloidosis rarely affects the seminal vesicles, involving vascular walls, smooth muscle, and stroma.[104] Vesicular amyloidosis is usually asymptomatic but may cause hematospermia, chronic perineal pain, or mimic seminal vesiculitis.[105,106] It is best visualized by MRI, and it may mimic tumor invasion from bladder or prostate cancer, including after Ga-prostate-specific membrane antigen uptake on positron emission tomography/CT scans.[100,107-110] Localized and systemic amyloidosis may coexist.[111]

Special stains that confirm the diagnosis of amyloid include Congo red, which appears red by light microscopy with apple-green polarization birefringence; methylene blue, which reveals green polarization birefringence; crystal violet and toluidine blue, which impart a metachromatic appearance to the deposits; and periodic acid–Schiff and Alcian blue stains, which are weakly to moderately positive. The composition of localized seminal vesicle amyloid is histochemically unique (permanganate-sensitive, lactoferrin- and amyloid P component–positive, and non-AA, non-B2M, non-κ or -λ, non–prealbumin type), apparently derived from secretory protein of the seminal vesicles; amyloid at other sites is derived from light chains or serum amyloid protein.[99,100,103,111-113]

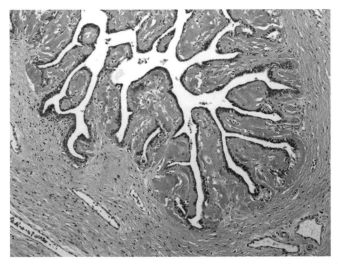

Fig. 10.4 Amyloidosis of seminal vesicles.

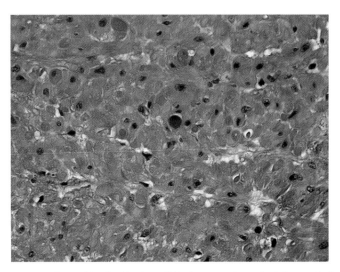

Fig. 10.5 Stromal hyaline bodies within the muscular wall of the seminal vesicles.

Stromal Hyaline Bodies

Small 15- to 20-μm eosinophilic hyaline bodies are sometimes observed within the muscular wall of the seminal vesicles, vas deferens, and prostate, and are designated stromal hyaline bodies (Fig. 10.5).[24,114,115] These round-to-oval structures probably result from degeneration of smooth muscle fibers, and transition forms can be seen arising from smooth muscle cells. They stain red with Masson trichrome and pink with periodic acid–Schiff, but fail to stain with phosphotungstic acid–hematoxylin, methyl green pyronine, Feulgen, Alcian blue at pH 2.5, or Congo red.

Fibrosis

Rarely, seminal vesicle fibrosis may be associated with retroperitoneal and mediastinal fibrosis.[116]

Inflammation

Seminal vesiculitis is associated with infection and inflammation of adjacent organs, including the prostate, bladder, ejaculatory ducts, vas deferens, and epididymis.[117] Acute vesiculitis is usually caused by retrograde infection with or without indwelling catheter, ureteral or ejaculatory duct stenosis or anatomic anomaly, calculi, or surgical trauma. The seminal vesicles are highly resistant to infection unless their secretory capability is decreased, as occurs with androgen deprivation.[118] Decreased expression of clusterin is closely related to seminal vesiculitis, perhaps as a result of concomitant downregulation of semenogelin I that may weaken the antibacterial activity of the seminal vesicles, thereby inducing disease.[119] Antibiotic therapy is usually effective, using the same agents used for acute prostatitis; biopsies are rarely obtained in such cases and may be contraindicated because of complications of abscess formation and stricture. Protracted acute and chronic seminal vesiculitis results in atrophy and ejaculatory duct stricture. Abscess presents with irritative voiding symptoms, fever, and pain in the scrotum, testis, perineum, or rectum; purulent ejaculation may also occur.[120] Ultrasonography, CT, and MRI are useful in verifying the diagnosis and directing transurethral incision and drainage.[121,122]

Chronic vesiculitis is associated with chronic prostatitis, and both respond poorly to antibiotic therapy. Before the antibiotic era, the most common cause of vesiculitis was tuberculosis, which resulted in perineal fistula, fibrous adhesions, ejaculatory duct stricture, and massive circumferential calcification of the walls of the seminal vesicles at the site of previous necrotizing granulomas. Malakoplakia should be excluded.[123,124] Seminal vesicle dilation and congestion may occur after prostatectomy, resulting in persistent dysuria.[125]

Seminal hyperviscosity is associated with increased oxidative stress in infertile men and increased proinflammatory interleukins in patients with male accessory gland infection, more when the infection was extended to the seminal vesicles.[126]

Schistosomiasis, usually secondary to *S. haematobium* infection of the bladder, involves the seminal vesicles more commonly than the prostate. Viruses (e.g., cytomegalovirus), fungi, and parasites are rare causes of seminal vesiculitis.[127,128] Echinococcal cyst of the seminal vesicles and prostate has been reported.[80] Rare cases have been described of localized necrotizing vasculitis.[129]

Surgery for seminal vesiculitis is unnecessary unless complicated by abscess, fistula, or stricture. In the early 1900s the seminal vesicles were thought to be the cause of inflammatory rheumatoid disease, and perineal seminal vesiculotomy was popular at that time. This was also the treatment of choice for vesicular tuberculosis until the advent of antibiotic therapy.

Calcification and Calculi

Calcification often follows seminal vesiculitis, particularly with tuberculosis. Patients with a history of diabetes mellitus or uremia also experience dystrophic calcification of the seminal vesicles and other mesonephric derivatives. Most foci of calcification are idiopathic and asymptomatic, and imaging studies of the pelvis may detect them incidentally (Fig. 10.6).[130] Calcification may be unilateral or bilateral and usually coexists with calcification of the vas deferens.[131-139] Calcification is present within the muscular wall, often forming concentric rings; the mucosa is rarely involved. Osseous metaplasia is also rarely observed in the wall.

Calculi are more frequent in the seminal vesicles than in the vas deferens, appearing as brown stones of variable number, and measuring up to 1 cm in diameter (Fig. 10.7). They usually consist of phosphate and carbonate salts. The mechanism of formation is

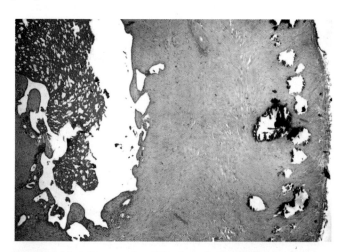

Fig. 10.6 Idiopathic mural calcification of the seminal vesicle in a patient undergoing radical prostatoseminalvesiculectomy for prostatic adenocarcinoma.

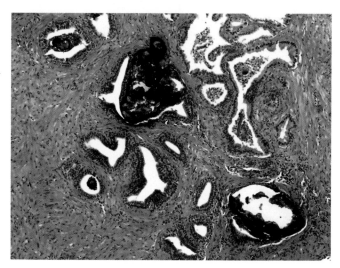

Fig. 10.7 Calculi within the seminal vesicular lumen.

uncertain, but it may be caused by reflux of urine up the ejaculatory ducts.[140,141] Cutaneous fistula is a rare complication that can be treated by fulguration and lithotripsy.[142] Calculi may cause spermolithiasis.[143]

Radiation Changes

Radiation therapy for prostatic carcinoma causes atrophy and fibrosis of the seminal vesicles and perivesicular fat in 89% of patients.[144] The golden-brown lipochrome pigment characteristic of the seminal vesicle epithelium is retained. MRI shows decreased luminal fluid and stromal fibrosis in about 37% of cases.[145]

Neoplasms

The seminal vesicles are frequently involved secondarily by tumors originating elsewhere, particularly prostatic carcinoma. However, fewer than 1000 primary neoplasms of the seminal vesicles have been reported. Clinical documentation of many is poor, and the pathologic diagnosis is often questionable.

Adenocarcinoma

Adenocarcinoma is the most common primary malignancy of the seminal vesicles, but it is rare, with fewer than 100 acceptable cases reported.[132,146-156] Mean patient age is 62 years (range, 17 to 90 years), and presenting symptoms include urinary obstruction and hematospermia.[150,151,154] Seminovesiculography and CT are useful in identifying these tumors.

The diagnosis of seminal vesicle adenocarcinoma requires: (1) tumor located primarily in the seminal vesicle; (2) no evidence of carcinoma in the prostate, bladder, or colon; (3) architectural features of adenocarcinoma, usually with papillary or sheetlike growth and mucinous differentiation; (4) in situ adenocarcinoma in the adjacent seminal vesicle epithelium; (5) cytoplasmic immunoreactivity for carcinoembryonic antigen; and (6) absence of staining for prostate-specific antigen (PSA), prostatic-specific acid phosphatase (PSAP), and other prostate-specific markers.[157] Tumor cells may be hobnail, columnar, or polygonal, with clear cytoplasm, and they rarely contain lipofuscin. Immunoreactivity for CA-125 and PAX8 may distinguish seminal vesicle adenocarcinoma from prostatic primary.[158-160] CA-125 also serologically fluctuates with growth and recurrence.[161] Some antibodies may display weak or focal immunoreactivity for PSA and PSAP, so appropriate controls should always be run in parallel.[157] MUC6 is an immunohistochemical marker of seminal vesicle epithelium (negative in benign prostatic epithelium and adenocarcinoma), but it has not been studied in seminal vesicle malignancy.[15] With high-stage, poorly differentiated adenocarcinoma, the precise site of origin may be impossible to determine.

Radical surgery and external beam radiation therapy have been used in many cases, but the prognosis is poor. Androgen deprivation therapy may also be of value.[162,163] Combination chemotherapy that included platinum-based agent was somewhat effective.[164] Recent results with immunotherapy found that chimeric antigen receptor–modified T (CAR-T) cells were injected intratumorally into two independent metastatic lesions of the same patient with MUC1$^+$ seminal vesicle cancer as part of an interventional treatment strategy; the initial results indicated no side effects of the MUC1-targeting CAR-T cell approach, and patient serum cytokine responses were positive.[165]

Two cases of noninvasive well-differentiated adenocarcinoma were reported within seminal vesicle cysts, including one in a 19-year-old with an acquired cyst and another in a 17-year-old with congenital cyst and ipsilateral renal agenesis.[150,166] A case of combined seminal vesicle adenocarcinoma, prostatic adenocarcinoma, and carcinosarcoma was reported with autopsy documentation.[167] A single case of apparent primary squamous cell carcinoma of the seminal vesicles was reported in a 54-year-old with painless hematuria.[168]

Adenocarcinoma of the seminal vesicles and prostate can be induced experimentally in Lobund-Wistar rats using a combination of testosterone propionate and nitrosamine compounds. A system for grading these tumors stratifies them into three groups: in situ, invasive without desmoplasia, and invasive with desmoplasia.[169] Montironi et al.[170] described the first case of seminal vesicle intraepithelial neoplasia or basal cell hyperplasia in 1 of 3000 radical prostatoseminalvesiculectomy specimens (incidence rate of 0.003%). This finding was easily distinguished from intraepithelial spread by prostatic adenocarcinoma. The epithelial lining was thicker than the surrounding normal ducts with obliteration of the acinar lumen, with varying degrees of cell stratification. Immunostains were negative for PSA, PSAP, prostate-specific membrane antigen, prostein (P501S), α-methylacyl-coenzyme A racemase, and GATA binding protein 3, but positive for p63, keratin 34βE12, cytokeratin 5/6, and p53 in cells in basal and suprabasal positions, whereas CA-125 was expressed in the luminal cells. The case shows morphologic and immunohistochemical features like those of basal cell hyperplasia of the prostate and was different from the early neoplastic epithelial changes of the seminal vesicle in the transgenic adenocarcinoma mouse prostate model (i.e., seminal vesicle intraepithelial neoplasia).

Metastasis and Contiguous Spread

Seminal vesicle involvement by prostatic adenocarcinoma is common, observed in about 12% of contemporary radical prostatectomy specimens from patients with cancer clinically confined to the prostate (Fig. 10.8). There are three patterns of seminal vesicle invasion: (1) direct spread along the ejaculatory duct complex into the seminal vesicles; (2) prostatic capsular perforation followed by extension into the periprostatic soft tissues and spread into the seminal vesicles; and (3) isolated deposits of cancer in the seminal vesicles (see Chapter 9).[171-175] Intraepithelial spread most likely results from direct invasion of carcinoma from the muscular wall of seminal vesicles rather than extension from the ejaculatory duct system in the invaginated extraprostatic space.[176] Endorectal coil MRI is accurate in detecting seminal vesicle invasion according to radical prostatectomy correlation studies, with loss of architectural contour as a dominant feature.[177] Bilateral invasion portends a worse prognosis (biochemical recurrence-free survival) than does unilateral invasion.[178]

Urothelial carcinoma of the bladder may also invade the seminal vesicles by direct extension or mucosal spread, occurring in up to 28% of patients undergoing radical cystectomy.[179,180] Direct extension is usually observed in cancer of the trigone and inferoposterior wall and indicates pathologic stage T4 cancer. Mucosal involvement by in situ urothelial carcinoma is rare, present in only 1% of cases.[181] It spreads along the mucosa of the prostatic urethra, the prostatic and ejaculatory ducts, and seminal vesicles by intraepithelial replacement and pagetoid spread along the basement membrane.[182] Five-year recurrence-free survival rate for seminal vesicle involvement was significantly worse than prostatic involvement (14% versus 68%, respectively).[180] In those with prostatic

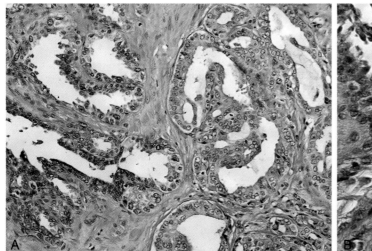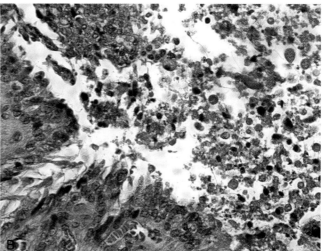

Fig. 10.8 Prostatic adenocarcinoma invading the seminal vesicles. (A) low power. (B) cancer within lumen.

stromal invasion, concomitant seminal vesicle invasion adversely affected cancer-specific survival.[183]

Rectal adenocarcinoma occasionally invades the seminal vesicles and prostate, and may cause diagnostic difficulty.[184] Metastases to the seminal vesicles and retrovesicular space from other organs are rare, including renal cell carcinoma, seminoma, malignant thymoma, and melanoma.[185-189]

Soft Tissue Tumors and Other Tumors

A variety of benign soft tissue tumors have been described in the seminal vesicles, including leiomyoma, fibroma, schwannoma, fibrous pseudotumor, gastrointestinal stromal tumor, paraganglioma, and solitary fibrous tumor (one case of solitary fibrous tumor was reported as malignant).[190-206] There is a spectrum of mixed epithelial and stromal neoplasms arising in the seminal vesicle, analogous to fibroadenoma and phyllodes tumor in the breast and prostate, and these have been referred to as cystadenoma, cystomyoma, low-grade phyllodes tumor, benign mesenchymoma, adenomyosis, and mesonephric hamartoma.[207-217] Reikie et al. suggested categorizing this group of mixed epithelial and stromal

tumors (MEST) as low-grade MEST, intermediate-grade MEST (uncertain malignant potential), and high-grade MEST, similar to suggestions made for prostatic mixed tumors; however, critics claim that the value of lumping disparate tumor histologies into such "bins" may compress and distort existing data without any clinical benefit.[218] Cystadenoma is a rare benign tumor composed of cysts lined with a simple columnar epithelium with chronically inflamed loose fibrous stroma or fibromuscular stroma (Fig. 10.9). The cysts are grossly multiloculated, ranging in size from 5 to 15 cm in diameter. Ultrasound and CT scan reveal a characteristic "honeycombing" pattern.[219] The patients' average age is 60 years, and most cases are incidental findings at autopsy.[207-210] One case of cystadenoma did not recur in the 25 years after the initial resection (D. G. Bostwick, unpublished observations).[210] Phyllodes tumor consists of a mixture of variably cellular stroma and glandular elements (Fig. 10.10). The density and cytologic features of the stroma determine whether the tumor is a fibroadenoma, low-grade phyllodes tumor, or high-grade phyllodes tumor (cystosarcoma phyllodes).[220,221] Features considered predictive of malignancy for phyllodes tumor in the breast may apply in the seminal vesicles, including infiltrating margins, stromal atypia, increased numbers of mitotic features, and overgrowth of glands by stroma; however, too few cases have been reported in the seminal vesicles to determine prognosis based on histologic features alone. One case of low-grade phyllodes tumor displayed stromal pleomorphism without mitotic activity; 2 years after excision, the tumor recurred in the pelvis, but it did not recur with 18-month follow-up after second excision.[222] Another report described a benign tumor consisting of glands with epithelium arranged in leaflike clefts and slits with subepithelial stromal condensation.[210] Less than a dozen cases of cystosarcoma phyllodes have been reported, including one that metastasized to the lungs after 5 years despite radical surgery.[214,223,224] This tumor was considered malignant because of its expansive and destructive growth pattern, densely cellular stroma, moderate stromal atypia, focal hemorrhage and necrosis, and numerous mitotic figures. Heterologous differentiation was not apparent histologically or ultrastructurally, although desmin reactivity was observed in 30% of the stromal cells, particularly in the looser myxoid regions, suggesting muscular differentiation.[214] The transgenic adenocarcinoma mouse prostate model (TRAMP) consistently developed low-grade phyllodes tumor of the seminal vesicles.[225]

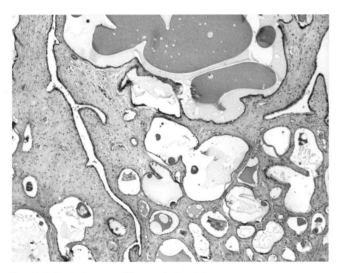

Fig. 10.9 Cystadenoma of the seminal vesicles.

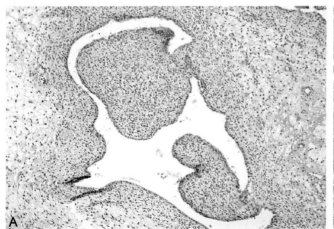
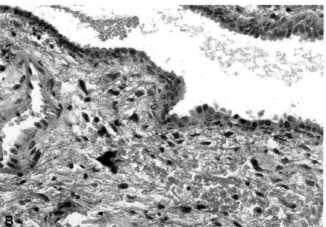

Fig. 10.10 Cystosarcoma phyllodes of the seminal vesicle. At low magnification (A), there is a proliferation of slitlike epithelial spaces with a cellular stroma. At high magnification (B), the stromal cells display varying degrees of cytologic atypia.

Other sarcomas of the seminal vesicle are also rare, including leiomyosarcoma, and usually present with symptoms of pelvic pain, urinary obstruction, rectal obstruction, and symptoms from distant metastases.[226,227] Unlike prostatic sarcoma, seminal vesicle sarcoma rarely presents with hematuria unless the tumor is large and advanced. These tumors grow locally and compress adjacent pelvic organs such as the prostate, bladder, and rectum.[228] Primary sarcomas of the seminal vesicle include leiomyosarcoma, fibrosarcoma, liposarcoma colliding with prostatic carcinoma, "primary sarcoma," "large cell alveolar sarcoma," "pleomorphic cell sarcoma," "malignant myoblastoma," leiomyoma of vascular origin with "some suggestion of malignant potential," "round cell sarcoma," and "fibrosarcoma with evidence of smooth muscle differentiation by electron microscopy."[229] Amirkhan et al. reported a high-grade leiomyosarcoma of the right seminal vesicle arising in a 68-year-old man with urinary obstructive symptoms, low-back pain, and impending rectal obstruction.[230] The tumor appeared to arise from the muscular wall of the seminal vesicle and displayed immunoreactivity for muscle-specific actin, smooth muscle actin, and focally for keratin AE1/AE3. The patient was reported well 13 months after radical surgery. Other malignant soft tissue tumors of the seminal vesicle include angiosarcoma, fibrosarcoma, and rhabdomyosarcoma.[190,231-234] Malignant lymphoma rarely involves the seminal vesicles.[235]

Rare primary germ cell tumors have been reported in the seminal vesicles, presumably caused by midline entrapment of primitive germ cells in the fetus. Primary choriocarcinoma was reported in a 28-year-old, forming a hemorrhagic 12-cm diameter mass; at autopsy the testes were normal on serial sectioning, and no other primary site was found.[236] Primary seminoma was found in a 48-year-old, which required cystoprostatectomy; the testes were clinically normal.[237] Primary carcinoid tumor has also been reported in the seminal vesicles.[26] Recurrent adnexal tumor of probable wolffian origin arose in a 20-year-old man.[238] Primary squamous cell carcinoma presented in a 69-year-old man with seminal vesicle cyst.[239]

References are available at expertconsult.com

11
Urethra

VICTOR E. REUTER AND HIKMAT A. AL-AHMADIE

CHAPTER OUTLINE

Embryologic Development and Normal Anatomy

The urethra serves as a conduit for urine from the urinary bladder to the exterior through the external urethral meatus. In males it also serves as a conduit for semen. The epithelium of the urethra is derived from the urogenital sinus, which is formed when the endodermal cloaca divides into the rectum dorsally and the urogenital sinus ventrally, separated by the urorectal septum.[1] In females the epithelium of the urethra is derived from the endoderm of the urogenital sinus, whereas the surrounding connective tissue and smooth muscle arise from splanchnic mesenchyme. In males the epithelium also is derived from the urogenital sinus, except in the fossa navicularis, where it is derived from ectodermal cells migrating from the glans penis. As in females, the connective tissue and smooth muscle surrounding the male urethra are derived from the splanchnic mesenchyme.

In men the urethra is 15 to 20 cm long and is divided into three anatomic segments (Fig. 11.1). The prostatic urethra is approximately 3 to 4 cm long and begins at the internal orifice at the bladder neck and extends through the prostate to the prostatic apex.[2] Most prostatic ducts open along the posterior and lateral walls of the prostatic urethra adjacent to the urethral crest, the longitudinal ridge along the dorsal wall of the prostatic urethra. In the central part of the urethral crest is an eminence called the verumontanum or colliculus seminalis. The verumontanum contains a slitlike opening that leads to an epithelial-lined sac called the prostatic utricle, a Müllerian vestige. The ejaculatory ducts empty into the urethra on either side of the prostatic utricle. The membranous urethra is the shortest segment, only 1 cm long. It extends from the prostatic apex to the bulb of the penis, traversing the musculature of the urethral sphincter and inferior fascia of the urogenital diaphragm. Cowper glands, small paired bulbomembranous urethral glands, are located on the left and right sides of the membranous urethra and secrete into it.[2-6] The penile urethra is the longest segment (10 to 15 cm) and extends from the lower surface of the urogenital diaphragm to the urethral meatus in the glans penis. The orifices of the bulbomembranous urethral glands are located on the lateral surfaces of the proximal (bulbous) portion of the penile urethra. The penile urethra is surrounded by the corpus spongiosum along its length. Scattered mucus-secreting periurethral glands (Littré glands) are present at the periphery of the penile urethra except anteriorly.

The female urethra is approximately 4 cm long (Fig. 11.2). At its periphery are paraurethral glands (Skene glands), which empty into the urethra through two ducts near the external urethral orifice.

The type of epithelium lining the urethra varies along its length.[2-4] In general, urothelium lines the prostatic urethra, pseudostratified columnar epithelium lines the membranous segment and most of the penile urethra, and nonkeratinized stratified squamous epithelium lines the fossa navicularis and external urethral orifice. In females the proximal third of the urethra is lined by urothelium and the distal two-thirds by nonkeratinized stratified squamous epithelium. However, it should be noted that most urethral tissues submitted for surgical pathologic examination are diseased or altered by instrumentation, both of which may cause metaplastic changes.

The lymphatic drainage of the male urethra arises from a rich mucosal network that extends the entire length of the urethra.[5] This network is continuous proximally with that of the prostate and urinary bladder, and distally with that of the penis. The lymphatics of the prostatic and bulbomembranous segments drain to the obturator and medial external iliac lymph nodes, whereas those of the distal penile urethra drain to the superficial inguinal nodes. In females the proximal urethra drains to the external iliac, hypo-

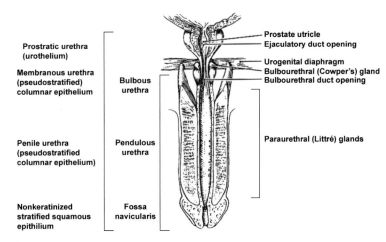

Prostratic urethra
(urothelium)

Membranous urethra
(pseudostratified)
columnar epithelium

Bulbous
urethra

Penile urethra
(pseudostratified
columnar epithelium)

Pendulous
urethra

Nonkeratinized
stratified squamous
epithilium

Fossa
navicularis

Prostate utricle
Ejaculatory duct opening
Urogenital diaphragm
Bulbourethral (Cowper's) gland
Bulbourethral duct opening

Paraurethral (Littré) glands

Fig. 11.1 Anatomy of the male urethra.

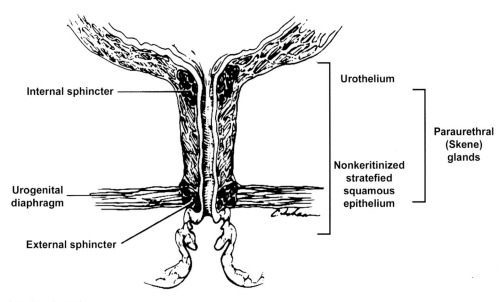

Internal sphincter

Urogenital
diaphragm

External sphincter

Urothelium

Nonkeritinized
stratefied
squamous
epithelium

Paraurethral
(Skene)
glands

Fig. 11.2 Anatomy of the female urethra.

gastric, and obturator lymph nodes. The distal urethral lymphatics communicate freely with vulvar lymphatics and drain to the superficial inguinal nodes.

Congenital Anomalies

Urethral Valves

Several congenital anomalies may affect the urethra but are rarely encountered by surgical pathologists. Urethral valves are mucosal folds that project into the urethral lumen and may cause obstruction, hematuria, or inflammatory symptoms, although they are usually asymptomatic.[7,8] Urethral valves are usually covered by normal urothelium but may be inflamed. The submucosa may also be inflamed and edematous. The so-called posterior urethral valves, usually seen in adult males, are associated with bladder neck hypertrophy.[7] One study reported prenatal diagnosis in monochorionic twins.[9]

Urethral Diverticula

Urethral diverticula are uncommon and often overlooked or misinterpreted. The overwhelming majority occur in women.[10-13]

They may be asymptomatic but can present with irritative symptoms or urinary incontinence, sometimes with localized pain.[14] On physical examination diverticula present as a paraurethral mass that can sometimes be palpated through the vagina. It is thought that urethral diverticula may be either acquired or congenital, but there are no clear morphologic criteria to make this distinction. Most urethral diverticula in adults are acquired as sequelae of infection, trauma, calculi, obstruction, dilation, or inflammation of paraurethral glands.[12,13,15,16]

Diverticula are usually lined by urothelium, although they often undergo squamous or glandular metaplasia. Nephrogenic adenoma may also arise in diverticula.[17,18] The submucosa often is edematous and inflamed. Most patients with clinically apparent urethral diverticula have a major complication such as infection, stricture, lithiasis with subsequent obstruction, or carcinoma (Fig. 11.3).[12,19,20] The percentage of urethral diverticula that develop cancer is unclear, with reported incidence rates ranging from 2% to 15% of symptomatic diverticula.[21,22] Carcinoma that develops in this setting is usually squamous cell carcinoma or adenocarcinoma, but may also be urothelial.[23,24] Adenocarcinoma may be of the conventional type or of the clear cell type (see the section on clear cell carcinoma later in this chapter).[25,26]

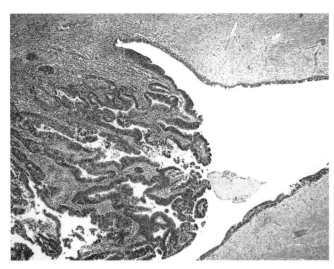

Fig. 11.3 Adenocarcinoma arising in a urethral diverticulum. Note transition from normal urothelium to adenocarcinoma in situ.

The main differential consideration for diverticulum is urethral cyst.[27,28] An unusual case of endometriosis presented in a woman as a diverticulum.[29]

Duplication of the Urethra

Duplication of the urethra is rare and usually comes to the attention of the surgical pathologist at autopsy.[30-32] The first description of a case of duplication of the urethra is attributed to Aristotle. Duplication of the urethra may be complete, extending from the bladder to the dorsum of the penis, or partial, extending from the dorsal surface or, less commonly, the ventral surface of the penis and ending blindly.[31,33] Only 15% of cases of duplicated urethra, whether complete or partial, connect with the functional urethra. Most cases are asymptomatic, but the most common complication is infection.[34,35] Patients may have urinary obstruction caused by compression of the functional urethra by a mass of desquamated material in the blind accessory urethra. In other cases, patients may complain of incontinence or double urinary stream.

Congenital Urethral Polyp

Also known as fibroepithelial polyp, congenital urethral polyp, a rare lesion, occurs almost exclusively in males.[36-44] Patients usually come to clinical attention between the ages of 3 and 9 years, but rarely they may present during infancy or adulthood.[7] For this reason it has been suggested that congenital urethral polyp is secondary to poorly understood congenital defect in the urethral wall. Congenital urethral polyp usually arises in the prostatic urethra adjacent to the verumontanum (posterior urethral polyp). Signs and symptoms include hematuria, difficulty voiding, urinary retention, and infection. Symptoms are similar to other obstructing urethral lesions, including the urethral valve, stricture, and lithiasis.

Morphologically, congenital urethral polyp is covered by urothelium that may be inflamed, ulcerated, or exhibit squamous metaplasia. This differs from the more common prostatic urethral polyp occurring in adults, which is covered by prostatic epithelium (see the later Ectopic Prostatic Tissue and Prostatic Urethral Polyp section).

Anterior urethral polyp is rare and arises in the membranous or penile urethra.[42] It produces the same symptoms and has the same morphology as posterior polyp. The subepithelial stroma consists of loose fibrous tissue that may be highly vascular and may contain a few fascicles of smooth muscle. If it has a long stalk, it may "telescope" into the bladder and produce bladder outlet obstruction.

Polyps in prepubertal girls and women probably arise from prolapsing urothelium that has evolved into a polyp.[45]

Nonneoplastic Diseases

Urethritis

Urethritis is defined morphologically as an inflammatory response within the urethra. In men they are usually asymptomatic, and the diagnosis is made by the presence of a urethral discharge and the finding of neutrophils in the urethral smear. Women are often symptomatic; the symptoms are like those of cystitis and include dysuria, urinary urgency, and urinary frequency.[46-48] A urethral smear will also aid in the diagnosis in women. Urethritis may be caused by sexually transmissible agents such as *Neisseria gonorrhoeae, Chlamydia trachomatis, Gardnerella vaginalis, Ureaplasma urealyticum, Mycoplasma hominis, Trichomonas vaginalis,* and *Candida* species. In women, urethritis secondary to *Neisseria, Trichomonas,* or *Candida* rarely occurs without concomitant cervical infection.[47]

Reiter syndrome is characterized by the triad of urethritis, conjunctivitis, and arthritis.[49] The cause is uncertain, but it is usually preceded by an enteric or venereal infection. The syndrome occurs predominantly in men between the ages of 18 and 40 years, but women occasionally are affected. Urethritis is the most common initial symptom. Other urologic manifestations of Reiter syndrome include prostatitis and hemorrhagic cystitis. In the acute phase the mucosa appears congested and may contain shallow ulcers. Symptoms commonly subside within 2 to 4 weeks but recur at irregular intervals in 50% to 75% of cases. It is important to recognize that not all involved organ systems may be symptomatic at the same time, so this syndrome should always be included in the differential diagnosis of urethritis in young adults.

Caruncle

Urethral caruncle is a pedunculated or sessile polypoid lesion in women located in the distal urethra near the meatus. Grossly, it has a fleshy, pink-red appearance and bleeds readily (Fig. 11.4). Patients may be asymptomatic, although commonly they experience dysuria, urinary frequency, or obstructive symptoms.[50-53] Three histologic subgroups are described: papillomatous, angiomatous, and granulomatous. This separation is based on the most prominent component (surface epithelial, vascular, and inflammatory, respectively), but this distinction has no apparent clinical relevance. The surface epithelium may be urothelial or squamous and is invariably inflamed (Fig. 11.5); caruncle covered by metaplastic columnar epithelium has been reported. The epithelium may be hyperplastic and constitute the bulk of the lesion. The underlying stroma is richly vascular and inflamed, occasionally containing glandular elements thought to be derived from Skene glands.

Rarely the stroma of urethral caruncle may contain atypical mesenchymal cells, actually reactive myofibroblasts, mimicking sarcoma (pseudosarcomatous fibromyxoid tumor) (Fig. 11.6).[54]

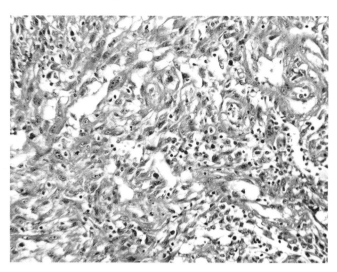

Fig. 11.6 Pseudosarcomatous fibromyxoid lesion (Postoperative spindle cell nodule). The patient experienced development of a hemorrhagic polypoid mass several months after an endoscopic procedure. Note myofibroblasts with epithelioid nuclei and abundant eosinophilic cytoplasm, scattered inflammatory cells, and prominent vascularity.

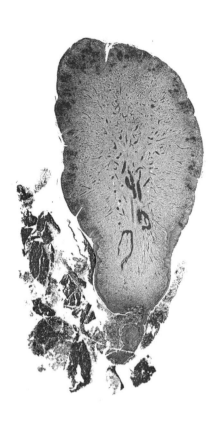

Fig. 11.4 Whole-mount appearance of caruncle. This reactive erythematous polypoid mass may be confused with a true neoplasm at the time of urethroscopy.

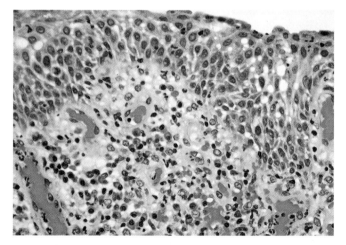

Fig. 11.5 Caruncle. Inflamed mucosa and lamina propria with extravasated red blood cells and prominent vascularity.

The mixed inflammatory infiltrate and rich vascularity, in combination with the clinical setting, should establish the correct diagnosis. Pseudosarcomatous fibromyxoid tumor may appear spontaneously or follow a pelvic surgical procedure by weeks or

months (postoperative spindle cell nodule) and present not only as a polypoid lesion but also as a paraurethral mass.[55] Like other pseudosarcomatous lesions involving the urothelial tract, these atypical but reactive myofibroblasts may display cytokeratin, actin, and IgG-4.[56,57] Epithelial membrane antigen is invariably negative.

Polypoid Urethritis

Polypoid urethritis is the urethral counterpart of polypoid cystitis, although an association with indwelling catheter has not been noted with urethral lesions.[58,59] Polypoid urethritis is a nonneoplastic inflammatory lesion that usually resolves spontaneously after removal of the inflammatory stimulus. It is commonly found in the prostatic urethra near the verumontanum, appearing as single or multiple polypoid or papillary growths. Morphologically it is characterized by abundant edematous stroma containing distended blood vessels and a chronic inflammatory infiltrate (Fig. 11.7). The overlying urothelium may be ulcerated or exhibit metaplastic and proliferative changes such as squamous metaplasia, Brunn nests, or urethritis cystica.[58,59]

Polypoid urethritis does not usually recur after resection unless the cause of the irritation persists. At the time of urethroscopy, it may be confused with papillary urothelial tumor, although experienced urologists will recognize it as a benign, reactive, or low-grade lesion and rarely confuse it with high-grade, aggressive neoplasm.

Nephrogenic Adenoma (Metaplasia)

Similar to Brunn nests and urethritis cystica, in most cases, nephrogenic adenoma is a reactive, proliferative lesion that may occur anywhere along the urothelial tract as a consequence of local irritation.[60-63] It is most common in the urinary bladder, but occasionally arises in the urethra. Nephrogenic adenoma is thought to arise through metaplasia of the urothelium in response to an inflammatory stimulus or local injury, and some investigators prefer the term *nephrogenic metaplasia*. However, Mazal et al.

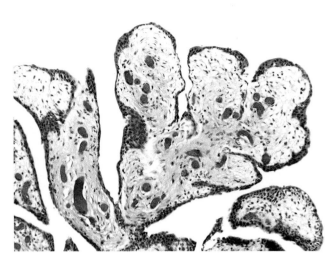

Fig. 11.7 Polypoid urethritis. This reactive fibroepithelial lesion results from chronic local insult.

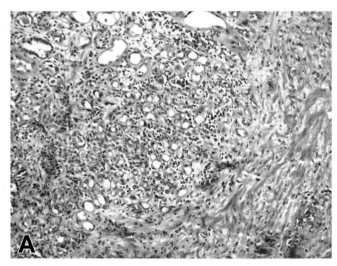

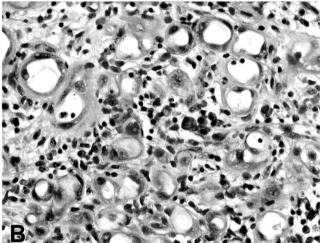

Fig. 11.8 Nephrogenic adenoma. (A) Low-power magnification. (B) High-power magnification. Note the small tubules, which may be confused with adenocarcinoma.

described cases of nephrogenic adenoma in patients who had undergone renal transplant from donors of the opposite sex and demonstrated that the lesions were of donor origin.[64] Thus it is likely that some lesions represent implantations from shed renal tubules. Often this lesion is an incidental finding at surgery for other reasons. The most common symptom is hematuria. It appears grossly as flattened, erythematous areas or as discrete papillae. Microscopically the latter architecture consists of complex papillary structures covered by cuboidal epithelium with basophilic or eosinophilic cytoplasm that may be vacuolated. The nuclei are round to oval, hyperchromatic, centrally located, and may contain small nucleoli. Mitotic figures are uncommon. The same epithelium may form discrete tubules in the underlying stroma. These have distinct lumina that are usually empty but may contain deeply eosinophilic secretions or pale basophilic material (Fig. 11.8A and B). These tubules are thought to arise through a process of invagination from the surface epithelium, much like Brunn nests. Each is surrounded by a distinct basement membrane.[60] Infrequently, cuboidal cells are present in the stroma singly or in small groups lacking a visible lumen, or they may have a signet ring cell appearance. The luminal secretions may be periodic acid–Schiff positive, diastase resistant, or mucicarminophilic, but intracytoplasmic mucin is less frequent. In a study of 26 cases of nephrogenic adenoma involving the prostatic urethra, Allan and Epstein found that 77% of cases extended into smooth muscle, which is not surprising given the anatomy of this site.[65] The lesion often appears infiltrative and may be confused with adenocarcinoma, especially in cases lacking a papillary component and composed primarily of tubules in the stroma. The surrounding stroma may be edematous and inflamed, but there is no desmoplastic reaction to the epithelial cells. Allan and Epstein reported focal immunoreactivity for prostate-specific antigen and prostatic acid phosphatase in 36% and 55% of cases, respectively, although others have not confirmed this finding.[65] However, strong PAX2/PAX8 and cytokeratin 7 positivity, combined with attention to the cytomorphologic features, should be sufficient to arrive at the correct diagnosis.

No convincing evidence has been reported that nephrogenic adenoma is a preneoplastic condition, although rare cases coincidentally coexist with or precede the development of carcinoma.[62] Nevertheless, it is possible to have common predisposing conditions and consequently experience development of nephrogenic adenoma independently. For example, nephrogenic adenoma and adenocarcinoma have been reported in association with urethral diverticulum.[18] Like other proliferative lesions of the urothelium, nephrogenic adenoma may recur after resection if the inflammatory stimulus is not removed.

Malakoplakia

Malakoplakia is a rare condition that mainly affects the urothelial tract but has also been described in other sites such as the testes, gastrointestinal tract, and retroperitoneum.[66-68] Although it may occur anywhere along the urothelial mucosa, most cases occur in the urinary bladder, and urethral involvement is rare.[69-72] Women are affected more often than men in a 4:1 ratio. Patients usually present with irritative symptoms or urinary obstruction, and endoscopy may reveal an erythematous plaquelike lesion or polypoid or nodular mass that is clinically suggestive of neoplasm. Microscopically malakoplakia is characterized by a mixed inflammatory infiltrate dominated by histiocytes with abundant granular, eosinophilic cytoplasm (von Hansemann cells).

The cytoplasm contains Michaelis-Gutmann bodies, laminated calcospherites that are basophilic and targetoid in appearance, measuring 5 to 10 μm in diameter. These stain for iron, as well as calcium, and may occasionally be found within the stroma. The overlying urothelium may be ulcerated, hyperplastic, or metaplastic. In chronic lesions the characteristic infiltrate may be replaced by fibrosis and scar.

The cause of malakoplakia is unknown, although current knowledge suggests that it is an unusual response to infection, perhaps the result of a disturbed immune response or abnormal macrophage or lysosomal function in the host.[66-68]

Amyloidosis

The urothelial tract can be involved in cases of systemic amyloidosis but rarely is the primary site of disease.[73-78] In descending order of frequency, amyloid deposits have been described in the urinary bladder, ureter, renal pelvis, and urethra. The usual clinical presentation is hematuria, although dysuria, partial obstruction, or a deviated urinary stream has also been reported. At cystoscopy the lesion may appear anywhere along the urethra as an elevated plaque or mass that is commonly confused with neoplasm. The overlying mucosa may be ulcerated or hyperemic. The amyloid deposits appear as eosinophilic, homogenous material within the lamina propria, often extending into the underlying muscle and connective tissue. Perivascular amyloid deposits are uncommon in tumoral amyloidosis but common in systemic amyloidosis. Inflammation is usually absent except adjacent to ulcerated mucosa. Special stains, such as Congo red, crystal violet, or van Gieson solution of trinitrophenol and acid fuchsin, are useful in establishing the diagnosis. Localized lesions may be managed by transurethral resection, but cases with diffuse involvement and intractable symptoms may require radical surgery.[79]

Condyloma Acuminatum

Condyloma acuminatum is a common sexually transmitted infectious squamoproliferative growth caused by human papillomavirus that is not related to squamous papilloma.[80] It usually occurs on the mucocutaneous surfaces of the external genitalia, perineum, or anus, but extension into the urethra occurs in up to 20% of cases.[81-84] It is often multifocal or diffuse. Macroscopically, condyloma is smooth, pink-tan, and often papillary. Flat condylomata may be difficult to visualize cystoscopically. Microscopically, it consists of papillary fronds or flat mucosa containing hyperplastic squamous epithelium that may be hyperkeratotic. The squamous epithelial cells typically have clear perinuclear halos and the nuclei are eccentrically placed, hyperchromatic, and pleomorphic (koilocytic atypia) (Fig. 11.9). Many cases can be diagnosed by these morphologic features alone, although in subtle cases the diagnosis can be confirmed by immunohistochemistry, viral culture, in situ hybridization, or polymerase chain reaction.[85-88] The antibodies currently available to identify human papillomavirus are rather insensitive; in situ hybridization and polymerase chain reaction are more sensitive and specific than morphology, even from paraffin-embedded sections.[89] More recently, RNA chromogenic in situ hybridization assays have been shown to be highly sensitive and specific.[90] The human papillomavirus serotypes most commonly found in urothelial condylomata are 6, 11, 16, and 18, although high-risk genotypes usually predominate.[84] These often coincide with the type in the patient's sexual partner.[84-87,91]

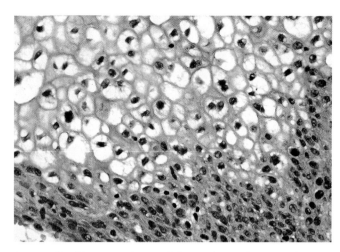

Fig. 11.9 Condyloma acuminatum. Cells contain vacuolated cytoplasm and irregular nuclei with perinuclear halos.

Condyloma of the urinary tract may cause hematuria and irritative symptoms. Surgical management may include transurethral resection, laser, or cryotherapy or a more radical procedure, depending on the extent of disease. It is important to remember that condylomata may undergo transformation to verrucous or infiltrating squamous cell carcinoma.[83,86,87]

Metaplasia of the Urothelium

Urothelium frequently undergoes squamous or glandular metaplasia as a response to chronic inflammatory stimuli like urinary tract infection, diverticula, calculi, or repeated instrumentation. This is very common and is not preneoplastic per se. Nevertheless, under certain conditions, carcinoma may arise in metaplastic epithelium, as in adenocarcinoma or squamous carcinomas arising in diverticula. Glandular metaplasia is more common in the urinary bladder but may occur along the urethra. The morphology of the metaplastic urothelium is usually tall columnar with goblet cells, strikingly similar to enteric epithelium.

Ectopic Prostatic Tissue and Prostatic Urethral Polyp

Prostatic acinar epithelium may line the urothelial tract focally. This is seen mostly in adult males but occasionally occurs at younger ages.[92-97] This process is most common in the prostatic urethra (prostatic urethral polyp) but has also been described at the bladder neck and bulbous and penile urethra.[98-101] This ectopic tissue is usually asymptomatic and discovered at urethroscopy for other causes. Hematuria is the most common symptom. Cystoscopically the lesions appear as discrete small papillary growths that may be solitary or extensive, producing a velvety coating of the mucosa (Fig. 11.10). The papillary fronds contain a thin, fibrovascular core and are covered by prostatic acinar epithelium with abundant clear or faintly eosinophilic apical cytoplasm and small, basally located round or oval nuclei without visible nucleoli (Fig. 11.11). Occasionally foci of residual urothelium are intermingled with the prostatic epithelium. Immunohistochemical stains for prostate-specific antigen are positive.[94,96,98]

The cause of this phenomenon is controversial. Prostatic urethral polyp probably results from hyperplasia and overgrowth of the overlying urothelium by prostatic acinar epithelium. It is important to carefully examine the underlying prostatic urethral

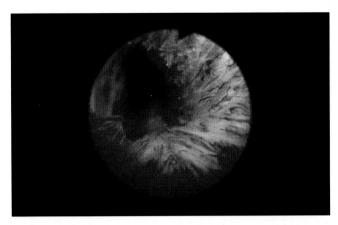

Fig. 11.10 Prostatic urethral polyp. Endoscopically the small papillae are clearly identifiable.

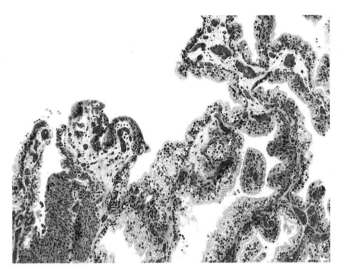

Fig. 11.11 Prostatic urethral polyp. The urothelium of the prostatic urethra is replaced by papillary fronds lined by benign prostatic acinar cells.

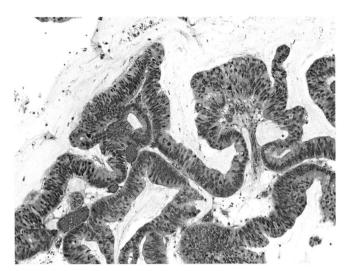

Fig. 11.12 Urethral implant from urachal adenocarcinoma. After partial cystectomy the patient experienced urethral mucosal implants, which were treated by transurethral resection. Given the low-grade appearance of this lesion, it was confused with a prostatic urethral polyp until the pathologist compared it with the original lesion and performed immunohistochemical stains for prostate-specific antigen, the results of which were negative.

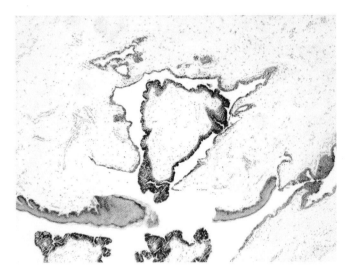

Fig. 11.13 Benign polyp arising at the fossa navicularis (immunohistochemical stain for prostate-specific antigen).

tissue because there may be an associated acinar-type prostatic adenocarcinoma. Also, the cytologic features of epithelial cells must be evaluated because prostatic adenocarcinoma may extend to the mucosal surface and take on a papillary growth pattern. Rarely, low-grade papillary adenocarcinoma of the bladder or urachus may seed the prostatic urethra, mimicking prostatic urethral polyp (Fig. 11.12). The origin of ectopic prostatic tissue in the penile urethra is less clear and may represent implantation, metaplasia, or an embryologic abnormality (Fig. 11.13). These lesions are benign and, if symptomatic, should be managed conservatively by urethroscopic resection or electrocauterization. Urologists commonly see these lesions during endoscopic evaluation for other causes and seldom perform biopsies on them unless they believe that they are the source of the patient's symptoms.

Neoplastic Diseases

Benign Neoplasms

Papilloma

Papilloma, like other papillary urothelial tumors, rarely arises de novo within the urethra.[102] The definition of papilloma has evolved over the years.[103-106] This benign tumor is characterized by discrete exophytic papillary projections with thin fibrovascular cores covered by urothelium indistinguishable from normal urothelium. The urothelial cells maintain their polarity perpendicular to the basement membrane and exhibit abundant eosinophilic cytoplasm, which commonly contains perinuclear vacuoles. Nuclei are elongate or round, depending on the plane of sectioning; they may be slightly enlarged compared with normal urothelium but show little or no pleomorphism. The chromatin pattern is homogeneous, and nucleoli are absent or small and sparse. Mitotic figures are usually absent, although a few normal mitotic figures may be observed in the basal layer. The thickness of the epithelium (the number of cell layers) is variable due to the plane of sectioning. Umbrella cells may be prominent and hyperchromatic.[103,104,106]

The main feature of papilloma is its discrete nature and lack of cytologic features of malignancy. Papilloma may rarely recur, very infrequently, as carcinoma. Nevertheless, it is incapable of invasion (progression) without showing definitive cytologic and architectural evidence of malignancy. Urothelial papilloma should be managed with transurethral resection alone. Although clinical surveillance is warranted, the time interval between visits and the length of surveillance is not established.

Inverted Papilloma

Inverted papilloma rarely occurs along the urethra, but when it does, it shares all the morphologic features of the more common vesicular inverted papilloma.[107,108] Patients usually have hematuria, and on urethroscopy the lesion appears as a polypoid or nodular growth with a smooth, glistening surface. It measures up to 2.5 cm in diameter and is easily confused with carcinoma, even by experienced endoscopists.[109,110] Microscopically it is covered by compressed benign invaginated interconnected cords and nests of urothelium that proliferate and expand the lamina propria, giving the lesion its characteristic bulging or polypoid gross appearance.[109] The urothelial cells are cytologically benign but more closely packed than normal because of the endophytic growth pattern. Some cells may be spindle-shaped, especially near the center of the cords (Fig. 11.14). Occasionally the centers of the cords become dilated, forming microcysts lined by flattened or cuboidal cells. Rarely, there is focal squamous metaplasia. The anastomosing cords of urothelium that make up this lesion result from invagination rather than invasion. There is no reactive fibrosis in the surrounding stroma. Mitotic figures are rare and, if present, are normal and in the basal layer. Inverted papilloma is well circumscribed.

The cause of this lesion is controversial. Most investigators conclude that they are neoplasms, but others suggest that they are an unusual reactive, proliferative response to inflammation. A few cases have been coincidentally associated with carcinoma.[110] In support that at least some of these lesions are neoplastic in nature, Cheng et al. reported TERT mutations in 15% of inverted

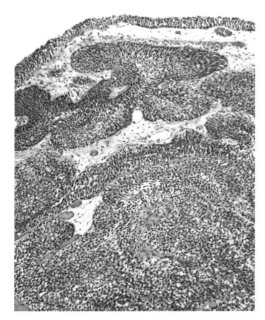

Fig. 11.14 Inverted papilloma. Anastomosing nests and cords of urothelial cells extend into the periurethral tissue but lack cytologic or architectural evidence of malignancy.

papilloma. Management of inverted papilloma should be limited to transurethral resection.[111]

Malignant Neoplasms

Urothelial Carcinoma in Association With Carcinoma of the Urinary Bladder

Secondary involvement of the urethra by urothelial carcinoma of the bladder is much more common than primary urethral carcinoma. As with vesicular neoplasms, it occurs more often in men. The reported incidence of urethral involvement varies according to the study design and patient population. For example, an autopsy study by Gowing[112] reported an incidence rate of 20% in patients who had been treated with cystectomy for bladder cancer. Clinical series have reported the incidence rate of urethral involvement in patients with bladder cancer to be between 8% and 22%.[113-122] Liedberg et al. concluded that the incidence of urothelial carcinoma in the prostatic urethra and prostate is probably underestimated.[123] Recurrent urethral involvement by carcinoma is not an issue in female patients because total urethrectomy is part of the cystectomy procedure. In males total urethrectomy is not routinely performed because of the increased morbidity caused by this procedure. It is standard to leave the membranous, bulbous, and penile urethra intact. Recurrence is possible in the immediate postoperative period or as late as 9 years after cystectomy. For this reason it is important for the clinician to routinely evaluate the urethra by urethroscopy, cytology, flow cytometry, or a combination of these.[124,125] Most patients with invasive urethral recurrences die within 5 years. Urologists routinely assess the status of the prostatic urethra before cystectomy because most of them believe that patients with prostatic urethral involvement are not candidates for a "urethra-sparing" procedure.[121]

Multifocal papillary carcinoma and multifocal carcinoma in situ in the bladder predispose the patient to urethral involvement or subsequent recurrence. In a study of male patients, De Paepe et al. reported that 9 of 20 (45%) patients had prostatic duct involvement by urothelial carcinoma at the time of cystoprostatectomy.[126] Carcinoma in situ of the bladder was observed in each of the nine patients. Pettus et al. reported prostatic urethral or periurethral duct involvement by urothelial carcinoma in 33% of patients in which the prostate gland was submitted in toto as whole-mount sections.[127] In a study dealing with female patients, 4 of 22 patients (18%) had carcinoma in situ in the urethra. These four patients represented 24% of the patients with multifocal carcinoma in situ in the bladder.[128] Interestingly three of these patients had carcinoma in situ extending into periurethral glands, and 17% of patients with invasive disease in the bladder also had stromal invasion in the urethra. This fact confirms that urethrectomy should be performed along with cystectomy in female patients. Pathologic staging of urothelial carcinoma that involves the prostatic urethra and prostate differs from staging for primary urethral neoplasms (Table 11.1).[129] Microscopically, secondary urethral involvement by urothelial carcinoma may take the form of papillary carcinoma or carcinoma in situ (Fig. 11.15). The tumors may be single or multiple and may occur at the surgical stump or anywhere along the urethra, including the meatus.[126,128,130]

Papillary urothelial carcinoma is characterized by papillary fronds lined by epithelial cells that show little or no orientation in relation to their basement membrane. The cells are crowded and have variable amounts of eosinophilic cytoplasm with an increased nuclear/cytoplasmic ratio. Nuclei are irregular and

TABLE 11.1 — TNM Pathologic Staging of Primary Urethral Tumors

Primary tumor (T) (male and female)

TX Primary tumor cannot be assessed
T0 No evidence of primary tumor
Ta Noninvasive papillary carcinoma
Tis Carcinoma in situ
T1 Tumor invades subepithelial connective tissue
T2 Tumor invades any of the following: corpus spongiosum, periurethral muscle
T3 Tumor invades any of the following: corpus cavernosum, anterior vagina
T4 Tumor invades other adjacent organs (e.g., invasion of the bladder wall)

Urothelial carcinoma of the prostate

Tis Carcinoma in situ, involvement in the prostatic urethra or periurethral or prostatic ducts without stromal invasion
T1 Tumor invades urethral subepithelial connective tissue
T2 Tumor invades the prostatic stroma surrounding ducts
T3 Tumor invades the periprostatic fat
T4 Tumor invades other adjacent organs (e.g., invasion of the bladder wall, rectal wall)

Regional lymph nodes (N)

NX Regional lymph nodes cannot be assessed
N0 No regional lymph node metastasis
N1 Single regional lymph node metastasis in the inguinal region or true pelvis (perivesical, obturator, internal/external iliac, or presacral lymph node)
N2 Multiple regional lymph node metastasis in the inguinal region or true pelvis

Distant metastasis (M)

M0 No distant metastasis
M1 Distant metastasis

Used with permission of the American College of Surgeons, Chicago, Illinois. The original source for this information is the AJCC Cancer Staging Manual, Eighth Edition (2017) published by Springer International Publishing

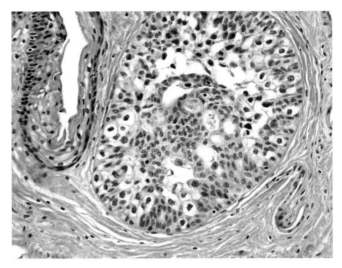

Fig. 11.16 Urothelial carcinoma extending into periurethral ducts. Duct involvement must be distinguished from stromal invasion.

contain nucleoli. Mitotic figures may be present, are sometimes atypical, and may be located well above the basal layer. Carcinoma in situ is characterized by flat mucosa that contain similarly atypical cells occupying virtually the entire thickness of the mucosa (for a more complete description of papillary and flat urothelial carcinoma, see Chapter 6). Carcinoma in situ may extend into periurethral ducts and glands along the entire length of the urethra, as well as into prostatic ducts (Fig. 11.16).[131] It is important for the pathologist to distinguish between ductal involvement and stromal invasion, because extension into periurethral glands does not affect prognosis, whereas periurethral or prostatic stromal invasion confers a worse prognosis.[115] Although controversial, some investigators advocate transurethral resection with or without instillations with bacillus Calmette–Guérin as sufficient treatment for patients with intramucosal or periurethral prostatic duct involvement.[132] It is generally agreed that total urethrectomy is the treatment of choice in cases with periurethral involvement.

A subtle but important morphologic pattern of urothelial carcinoma in the urethra is intramucosal pagetoid spread (Fig. 11.17). This pattern occurs most frequently in association with multifocal carcinoma in situ of the bladder and is characterized by individual or small groups of carcinoma cells percolating through an otherwise benign urothelium.[128,133,134] The carcinoma cells may have minimal or abundant cytoplasm but have large round or irregular hyperchromatic nuclei with prominent nucleoli that closely resemble the cells of Paget disease of the breast. The surrounding urothelium often undergoes squamous metaplasia. The tumor cells are unreactive for S100 protein and prostate-specific antigen. Occasionally they may be weakly mucicarmine positive. This variant of carcinoma in situ may be seen in the surface urothelium, metaplastic squamous epithelium, or periurethral or prostatic ducts. It is rare in primary urethral carcinoma. For this reason, when encountered in a urethral biopsy, the differential diagnoses for this pattern should include urothelial carcinoma arising in the urinary bladder, malignant melanoma, and periurethral or prostatic adenocarcinoma.[135] Radiation-induced changes may mimic urothelial carcinoma.[111,136] In these cases, the patient usually presents with hematuria and, on cystoscopy, is seen to have an area of ulceration and hemorrhage, suspicious for carcinoma. On microscopy the remaining urothelium is atypical and may exhibit squamous metaplasia with nests of cells extending into the subepithelial connective tissue, mimicking invasive disease. Stromal inflammation and

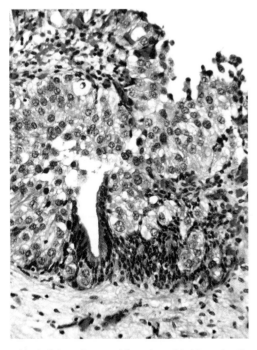

Fig. 11.15 Urothelial carcinoma of the urinary bladder extending into the urethra. The tumor partially replaces the benign urothelium.

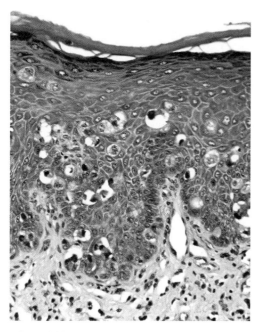

Fig. 11.17 Pagetoid intramucosal spread of urothelial carcinoma in the membranous urethra. This pattern of spread is most commonly seen in association with multifocal urothelial carcinoma in situ in the urinary bladder.

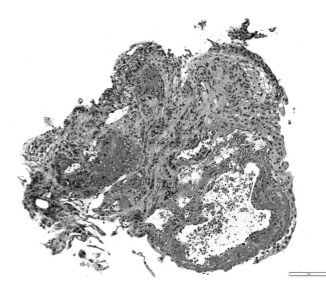

Fig. 11.18 Radiation-induced urethritis. The surface urothelium is partially denuded but atypical. Dilated blood vessels with fibrin thrombi are present in the subepithelial connective tissue.

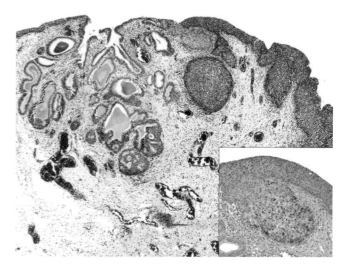

Fig. 11.19 Human papillomavirus–associated carcinoma of the female urethra. Notice basaloid features of the in situ carcinoma and the presence of integrated viral particles visible by RNA in situ hybridization directed toward high-risk human papillomavirus (inset).

fibrin thrombi are common (Fig. 11.18). Practically speaking, these changes could be seen under any situation that causes chronic local injury.

Primary Urethral Carcinoma

Primary carcinoma of the urethra is rare. The incidence is higher in women than in men, and the age distribution is similar to that of other urothelial carcinomas (mean incidence in the seventh decade of life).[106,119,137-142] In general, tumors arising in the proximal (prostatic urethra in males, proximal one-third in females) have the morphology of typical urothelial cancer, whereas distal carcinomas (membranous, bulbous or penile in men, distal two-thirds in women) are likely to be squamous cell carcinoma. These findings coincide with the epithelial lining in those sites, although it must be noted that the morphology and anatomic distribution of "normal" mucosa may be quite variable. This is especially true in patients with irritative symptoms in whom squamous and glandular metaplasia is quite common. Moreover, it may be morphologically impossible to differentiate moderate- to high-grade urothelial carcinoma from nonkeratinizing squamous carcinoma.

Tumors related to human papillomavirus infection may be encountered in the urethra in females as well as in males. They may arise de novo at this site or as an extension from a genital primary.[142-144] It is common for these tumors to have basaloid or basaloid-squamous features, at least in the noninvasive component of the tumor (Fig. 11.19). Risk factors include prior history of genital human papillomavirus, recurrent catheterization, and chronic indwelling catheters.

Adenocarcinoma may arise anywhere along the urethra but is most commonly associated with diverticula, prostatic adenocarcinoma, or, in women, may arise in periurethral glands and extend to the urethral mucosa secondarily. The latter is rarely seen in men. Because the incidences of histologic types are different, primary carcinoma in males and females will be discussed separately.

Primary urethral carcinoma is rare in males, a finding underscored by the article from Memorial Sloan-Kettering Cancer Center, an institution that treats hundreds of new bladder cancer patients each year but reported only 23 urethral tumors in a series spanning 30 years.[118] Two were adenocarcinomas, and the rest were either urothelial or squamous cell carcinomas. The symptoms are usually dysuria, hematuria, decrease in urinary stream, urinary obstruction, or fistula.[118,119,130] A history of infection, diverticulum, fistula, or stricture is common. Ray et al. found that prognosis correlated with the anatomic location and pathologic stage of the primary, but not with grade or histologic subtype (Table 11.1).[118] Stage for stage, cancer arising in the distal (bulbous and pendulous) urethra had a better prognosis than cancer arising in the membranous or prostatic urethra.[145,146] In one study, in the former group, 6 of 9 patients (67%) survived 5 years, whereas only 3 of 14 (21%)

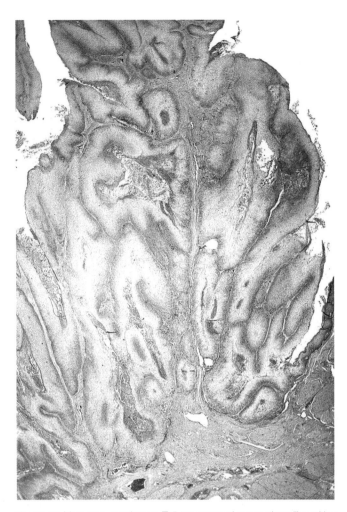

Fig. 11.20 Verrucous carcinoma. Tall compressed mucosal papillae with a broad infiltrative base. These lesions tend to arise in the distal urethra.

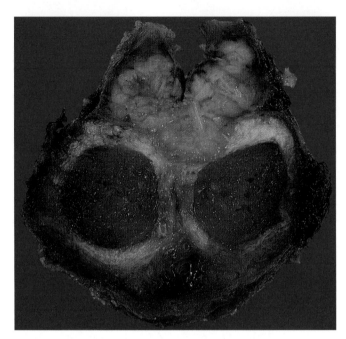

Fig. 11.21 Squamous carcinoma of the penile urethra. The tumor invades through the corpus spongiosum into the septum but spares the corpora cavernosa (pT2). (From Reuter VE, Melamed M. The lower urinary tract. In: Sternberg S, ed. *Diagnostic surgical pathology*, 2nd ed. New York: Raven Press, 1994.)

of the latter group survived 5 years. Tumors arising in the distal urethra are commonly diagnosed at an earlier stage. Well-differentiated squamous cell or verrucous carcinoma is common in the distal urethra (Fig. 11.20). Invasion into vascular spaces of the corpus spongiosum (Fig. 11.21) or corpora cavernosa is common, and metastasis, if present, involves inguinal lymph nodes. Wide dissemination at the time of presentation is rare. Partial penectomy and inguinal lymph node dissection is usually the treatment of choice.

Tumors arising in the proximal urethra in males commonly present at a higher stage and can infiltrate into the prostatic stroma or pelvic soft tissues to the point that establishing adequate surgical margins of resection may be difficult (Fig. 11.22).[119] In these tumors the histologic distinction is difficult to ascertain between high-grade urothelial carcinoma and nonkeratinizing squamous cell carcinoma (Fig. 11.23). Metastases may be to inguinal or pelvic lymph nodes, and if operable, treatment usually requires a cysto-prostatectomy and urethrectomy. If the scrotal skin, soft tissues, or deep pelvic tissues are involved, total emasculation may be required, although heroic surgical procedures rarely ensure long-term survival.

Urethral Carcinoma in Women

Primary urethral carcinoma in women is rare, although more common than in men.[147-150] The clinical histories and symptoms of

these patients are similar to those seen in male patients. In women, urethral carcinoma is frequently initially misdiagnosed as caruncle. For this reason biopsy should be performed on any presumed caruncle that does not respond successfully to therapy or is associated with persistent bleeding. Approximately 75% of urethral carcinoma cases in women are nonkeratinizing or keratinizing squamous carcinoma; the remaining 25% to 30% are split between urothelial carcinoma and adenocarcinoma, some of which have the morphology of clear cell carcinoma. In the cases of adenocarcinoma and clear cell carcinoma, it may be very difficult to establish whether they arise within the urethral surface epithelium, periureteral glands, or female genital tract because of overlapping morphology and immunophenotype. Tumors arising in the distal one-third of the female urethra are commonly low-grade squamous cell or verrucous carcinomas (Fig. 11.20). If invasive, metastasis is usually to inguinal lymph nodes. Treatment usually consists of distal urethrectomy and inguinal lymph node dissection. Cancer arising in the proximal urethra is usually urothelial and typically metastasizes to pelvic lymph nodes. Treatment includes total urethrectomy as well as inguinal and pelvic lymph node dissection. Wide dissemination at presentation is quite rare, although metastases to regional lymph nodes are common. In two large series approximately 28% of patients who underwent inguinal lymphadenectomy and approximately 50% of patients who underwent pelvic lymphadenectomy had metastases.[148,151] Histologic type and grade were not significant predictive factors when corrected for stage.

Adenocarcinoma

Urethral adenocarcinoma is more common in women than in men.[119,152-160] Stage for stage, it has the same prognosis as squamous cell and urothelial carcinomas of the urethra. Adenocarcinoma may arise from the surface mucosa through metaplasia or

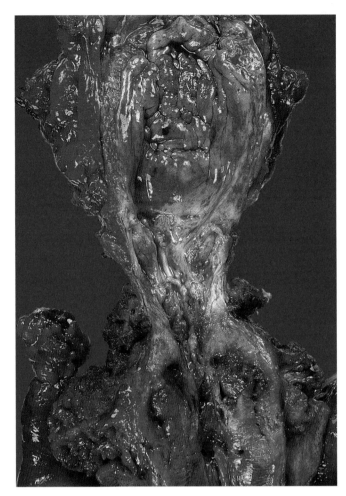

Fig. 11.22 Squamous cell carcinoma arising in the bulbomembranous urethra. Tumors that arise at this site tend to be at an advanced stage at diagnosis. This lesion infiltrated the cavernous urethra, periurethral, and periprostatic soft tissues; it required cystoprostatourethrectomy and total emasculation.

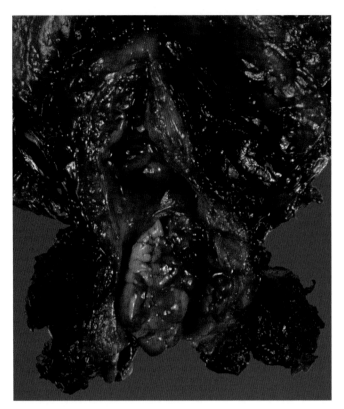

Fig. 11.24 Adenocarcinoma of the female urethra presenting as an exophytic mass. It is easy to understand how a lesion such as this can lead to dysuria, hematuria, and urinary obstruction.

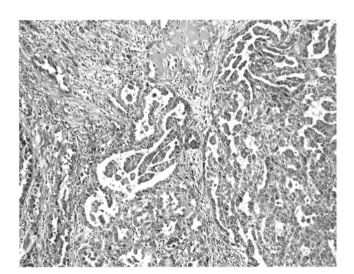

Fig. 11.25 Adenocarcinoma arising in periurethral (skene) glands. The tumor is predominantly papillary and exhibits high nuclear grade.

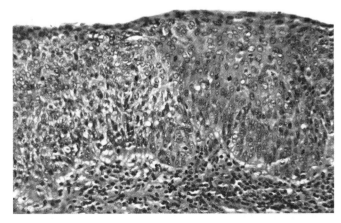

Fig. 11.23 Squamous carcinoma in situ of the penile urethra. The full thickness of the mucosa is replaced by neoplastic cells with significant cytologic and architectural disorder.

from periurethral glands (Figs. 11.24 and 11.25).[161-165] Those arising from the surface urothelium are usually associated with a chronic inflammatory insult such as stricture, diverticulum, infection, or fistula (Fig. 11.3), and present with irritative symptoms, hematuria, or urinary obstruction. On urethroscopy, adenocarcinoma appears as papillary or polypoid masses. Microscopically it is composed of simple or pseudostratified columnar epithelium with apical cytoplasm and basally located hyperchromatic nuclei. Occasionally the cytoplasm is vacuolated and contains mucin,

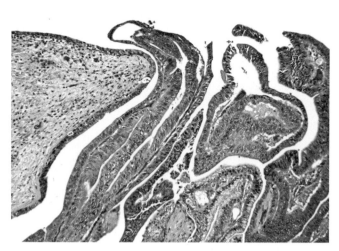

Fig. 11.26 Prostatic adenocarcinoma, ductal type, extending through periurethral ducts and into the urethra. This phenomenon may be confused with a primary urethral neoplasm.

giving the tumor a colonic appearance (Fig. 11.26). Rarely, urethral adenocarcinoma is frankly mucinous.[166] High-grade lesions exhibit greater pleomorphism and numerous mitotic figures. Glandular metaplasia, urethritis cystica, and urethritis glandularis are often present in the adjacent mucosa. This tumor does not react with antibodies to prostate-specific antigen. It must be distinguished from intraurethral papillary prostatic (ductal) adenocarcinoma, which usually arises adjacent to the verumontanum.[94,167] Papillary prostatic adenocarcinoma tends to have prominent eosinophilic nucleoli and is associated with typical prostatic adenocarcinoma in the underlying periurethral tissue. Extension of other adenocarcinomas into the urethra, such as rectal adenocarcinoma in males or rectal, endometrial, endocervical, vaginal, or Bartholin glands adenocarcinoma in females, must be considered in the differential diagnosis.

Adenocarcinoma of Accessory Glands

In males there are a few reports of adenocarcinoma arising in Cowper glands and Littré glands.[161-164,168,169] These diagnoses are very difficult because the tumor has usually destroyed the local anatomic landmarks and extended to or ulcerated the overlying mucosa. Adenocarcinoma arising in Cowper glands is located in the bulbomembranous region, whereas that arising from Littré glands tends to originate in the distal portion of the penile urethra but may arise at any point along its length. Both present with hematuria, dysuria, and progressive urinary obstruction. It is common for these patients to be treated for urethritis before the proper diagnosis is established. Microscopically these neoplasms share features with adenocarcinoma arising from the urethral mucosa. The tumor may have a tubular or micropapillary growth pattern, and tumor cells are either cuboidal or columnar with clear or eosinophilic cytoplasm and large hyperchromatic nuclei. Intracytoplasmic mucin vacuoles or a frank mucinous component are uncommon. Cytoplasmic clearing, if present, is usually due to glycogen production (see later Clear Cell Carcinoma section).

In women, adenocarcinoma arising from periurethral or Skene glands displays the same symptoms as the accessory gland in adenocarcinoma in men (Fig. 11.24).[119,156,165] It may arise at any point in the urethra but is more common distally. In that location, patients often have a perineal mass that may be confused with an infected cyst or uterine prolapse. Microscopically, tumors may have a glandular, papillary, or micropapillary architecture, and the tumor cells are either columnar or cuboidal with eosinophilic or clear cytoplasm (Fig. 11.25). Cytoplasmic clearing is usually caused by glycogen deposition or, less frequently, intracytoplasmic mucin. Intraluminal mucin is common. The nuclei are large and hyperchromatic, and often exhibit prominent nucleoli. It should be noted that the diagnosis of adenocarcinoma arising in periurethral glands is usually very difficult because of extension or ulceration of the overlying urethral mucosa and obliteration of anatomic landmarks.[119,156] The best indication of periurethral gland origin is partial involvement of recognizable periurethral glands. Even then, this may represent downward extension from the surface. The prognosis in all cases of urethral adenocarcinoma, whether of surface or periurethral gland origin, is determined by pathologic stage at the time of presentation rather than the site of origin.

Clear Cell Carcinoma

Clear cell carcinoma is an unusual variant of urethral adenocarcinoma that may arise from the mucosa or from periurethral glands.[156,159,160,170-175] It is also called *mesonephric adenocarcinoma* and *glycogen-rich carcinoma*.[172,175] Its morphologic features are identical to those of clear cell carcinoma of the genital tract. Nevertheless, several authors have concluded that urethral clear cell carcinoma arises through metaplasia of the surface mucosa or from periurethral glands rather than from Müllerian or mesonephric remnants.[170,176]

Microscopically, clear cell carcinoma may have a tubular, papillary, micropapillary, acinar, or diffuse growth pattern (Fig. 11.27). Commonly, it exhibits a combination of growth patterns. The cells often have abundant clear or eosinophilic cytoplasm that contains glycogen and little or no mucin. Mucicarmine positivity is usually evident only in the luminal secretions. In a few cases prostate-specific antigen and prostatic acid phosphatase immunoreactivity have been demonstrated in clear cell carcinoma in women.[177-181] The nuclei are large, pleomorphic and hyperchromatic, and, if luminally located, give the tubules a distinct hobnail appearance. Several cases have presented with paraneoplastic hypercalcemia similar to that seen with other clear cell tumors

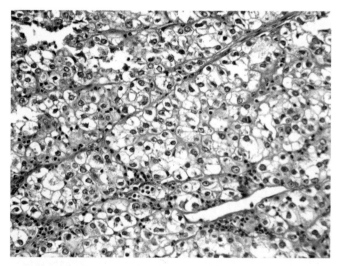

Fig. 11.27 Clear cell carcinoma. This tumor may arise from the surface mucosa or periurethral glands. Morphologically it may be difficult to differentiate from clear cell carcinomas arising in the female genital tract or metastatic from the kidney.

such as renal cell carcinoma.[170] Clear cell carcinoma of the urethra is distinguished from gynecologic clear cell carcinoma and metastatic renal cell carcinoma by clinical history and diagnostic workup. Gynecologic clear cell carcinoma tends to occur in younger patients exposed to nonsteroidal estrogens before birth. Cantrell et al. reported a case of papillary prostatic adenocarcinoma occupying the prostatic urethra and exhibiting clear cell features.[182] The diffuse pattern may be confused with amelanotic melanoma. Also, clear cell carcinoma must be distinguished from nephrogenic adenoma.[176,183,184] Nephrogenic adenoma lacks the nuclear pleomorphism and hyperchromasia and infiltrative and destructive growth pattern seen in adenocarcinoma. Mitotic figures are rare in nephrogenic adenoma but usually are readily apparent in clear cell carcinoma. This distinction may be difficult to establish on small biopsy.

The prognosis of clear cell carcinoma of the urethra is uncertain because of the rarity of this tumor and limited follow-up in reported series. A series from MD Anderson Hospital suggests that these patients may have a somewhat better prognosis than those with adenocarcinoma of other types, although the numbers did not reach statistical significance.[156] In general, prognosis correlates with pathologic stage at presentation. Clinical management has varied, including transurethral resection, radical excision, and radiation therapy, or a combination of these.[185]

Other Histologic Types of Carcinoma

Other epithelial neoplasms arising within the urethra include adenosquamous carcinoma, adenoid cystic carcinoma, carcinoid, small cell carcinoma, and so-called cloacogenic carcinoma.[186-192] All cases have been single-case reports with limited follow-up. Their morphologic features are similar to their counterparts arising at other sites.

Malignant Melanoma

Although rare, the urethra is the most common site of origin of malignant melanoma in the urinary tract.[193-206] In 1988, Manivel and Fraley reviewed the literature and found only 26 cases.[194] The urethra is more commonly involved by spread from melanoma arising in the glans penis and vulva. Urethral melanoma occurs in

males and females, and has been described in black patients.[196,198] The tumor may be associated with melanosis, although precursor lesions are rarely identified. Most cases occur in older patients. Begun et al. reported a 13-year-old boy who had melanoma of the penis.[193]

Patients usually present with hematuria, dysuria, deviated urinary stream, or urinary obstruction. Melanuria is an uncommon finding. Endoscopic examination reveals a nodular mucosal mass or masses that are usually pigmented and frequently ulcerated. As with other mucosal melanomas, the growth pattern is commonly lentiginous, although all other patterns may be represented (Fig. 11.28). Mucosal melanoma is more likely to be amelanotic than cutaneous melanoma. Extensive radial growth is common, accounting for the frequency of local recurrence. Metastasis is usually to inguinal and pelvic lymph nodes and common in advanced lesions. Hematogenous spread to liver, lungs, and brain is common.

Treatment is surgical and includes urethrectomy or penectomy with regional lymph node dissection. The role of immunotherapy, radiation therapy, and chemotherapy remains uncertain.[199,201] Staging for urethral melanoma has not been standardized because most reports deal with isolated cases. Prognosis depends on the thickness of the lesion, similar to melanoma at other mucosal sites. Pathologists should carefully evaluate the status of the mucosal margin of resection because local recurrence at the surgical bed is common. Skip lesions involving the urinary bladder and ureter may occur and should be investigated before extirpative surgery.

Soft Tissue Tumors

Leiomyoma is the most common soft tissue tumor of the urethra, although fewer than 30 cases have been reported.[207-215] Leiomyoma may also involve the paraurethral soft tissue, but the exact site of origin is uncertain. Urethral leiomyoma ranges in size from 1 to 40 cm and may present as an asymptomatic mass or with dysuria and urinary obstruction.

Other nonepithelial neoplasms are rare in the urethra and periurethral soft tissues. These include hemangioma, papillary endothelial hyperplasia, paraganglioma, plasmacytoma, and

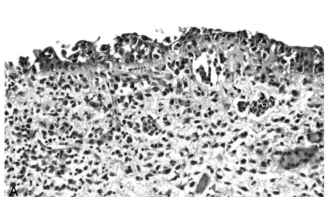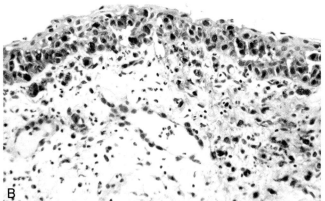

Fig. 11.28 Urethral malignant melanoma. (A) Neoplastic melanocytes occupy the surface mucosa and extend into the submucosa. (B) Tumor cells are immunoreactive with S100 protein.

neurofibroma.[216-227] Lymphoma may involve the urethra but usually is a manifestation of systemic disease, with only a few cases asserted to be primary in the urethra.[228,229]

Even though sarcoma has been described in the pelvic and paraurethral tissues, it is difficult to establish whether it is truly of urethral origin. Steeper and Rosai described a soft tissue tumor arising in the pelvis and perineal soft tissues of women, *aggressive angiomyxoma*, consisting of vascular fibromyxoid tissue that is locally infiltrative with a tendency to multiple recurrences.[230] These patients present with urinary obstruction or dysuria.

References are available at expertconsult.com

12

Nonneoplastic Diseases of the Testis

MANUEL NISTAL, RICARDO PANIAGUA AND PILAR GONZÁLEZ-PERAMATO

CHAPTER OUTLINE

Embryology and Anatomy of the Testis

Embryology

Development of the Testis

Genetic Mechanisms Involved in Sex Determination and Testicular Differentiation

Sexual differentiation is the result of complex genetic and endocrine mechanisms that are closely associated with the development of both the genitourinary system and the adrenal glands. Formation of the bipotential gonad—and subsequently the testis or the ovary—depends on gene expression in both sex and autosomal chromosomes. Testes secrete steroid and peptide hormones, both of which are necessary for the development of internal and external genitalia. These hormonal actions are mediated by specific receptors that function as transcription regulators. Alteration of genetic events results in sexual dimorphisms involving the internal and external genitalia and may hinder development of other organs.[1]

Determination of chromosomal gender takes place at the time of fertilization, with formation of an embryo of either 46,XY (male) or 46,XX (female) karyotype. The subsequent cascade of genetic events leads to development of either female (ovaries) or male (testes) gonads, referred to as gonadal gender. Hormonal secretions from the ovaries or testes are essential for development of external genitalia, thereby determining phenotypic gender. The relationship between the individual and the environment determines social gender.

Gonadal development comprises two phases. The first phase is characterized by the appearance of the bipotential gonad, or genital ridge, which is an indifferent gonad that is identical in males and females. Cells in the bipotential gonad may develop into either female or male gonads. The second phase is the development of a testis or an ovary.

Development of the Bipotential Gonad

Formation of the Gonadal Ridge

In the fourth week of gestation the urogenital ridges appear as two parallel prominences along the posterior abdominal wall. This process is apparently driven by the expression of transcription factors Lim1 and Odd1. Each urogenital ridge gives rise to two important pairs of structures: the genital ridges arising from the medial prominences and the mesonephric ridges deriving from the lateral prominences. The genital ridges are the first primordium of the gonad, appearing as a pair of prominences about the midline. In 30- to 32-day embryos, each genital ridge is lateral to the aorta and medial to the mesonephric duct. The coelomic epithelium lining the genital ridges undergoes proliferation and thickening, protrudes into the coelomic cavity, and grows into cordlike structures giving rise to the gonadal ridges, the primary sex cords. Expression of steroidogenic factor 1 (SF1), triggered by the *WT1* gene (Wilms tumor 1) (+KTS isoform), the transcription factor Pbx1, and the homeobox proteins Emx2 and Lhx9, is essential for cell survival and proliferation during this period.

The coelomic epithelium also proliferates to invade the subjacent mesenchymal tissue. Cell proliferation in this phase also depends on Lhx9 expression. The basement membrane underlying the coelomic epithelium appears discontinuous and is rich in laminin content. As the coelomic cells proliferate, laminin production in the gonadal ridge increases, an apparently essential element for germ cell colonization. Immediately beneath the coelomic epithelium are several mesonephric tubules and glomeruli (Figs. 12.1 and 12.2).

Primordial Germ Cells: Origin, Migration, and Formation of the Gonadal Blastema

Initially the genital ridges are devoid of primordial germ cells, but they are detected in the third week of gestation in the extraembryonal mesoderm that lines the yolk sac posterior wall near the allantoic evagination. The germ cells are ovoid, 12 to 14 μm in diameter, and immunohistochemically express alkaline phosphatase, OCT3/4, NANOG, and LIN28.[2,3] Nuclei are spherical and possess one or two large and prominent central nucleoli.[4] The cytoplasm contains mitochondria with tubular cristae,

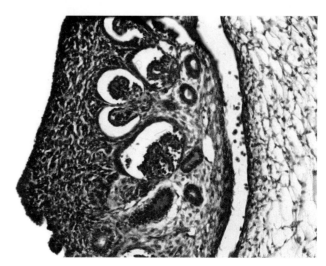

Fig. 12.2 Longitudinal section of the gonad showing the close relationship between gonadal blastema and mesonephric glomeruli.

lysosomes, microfilaments, lipid inclusions, numerous ribosomes, and abundant glycogen granules. Attracted by chemotactic factors, the primordial germ cells migrate along the mesenchyma of the mesentery and reach the genital ridge by 32 to 35 days.[5,6] The appearance of these cells coincides with the expression of several proteins in the extraembryonal mesoderm, including Bmp4, Bmp8, and Blimp1.

Primordial germ cells begin to express two membrane proteins, fragilis and brachyurus, and the cells migrate through the primitive streak to settle into the developing endoderm (hindgut).[7] The hindgut then invaginates into the future abdominal cavity and approaches the gonadal ridges. Primordial germ cells migrate by ameboid movements along the hindgut mesentery to reach the gonadal ridges. This emigration process occurs along autonomic nerve fibers that support them and requires the interaction of several factors: the integrin CXCR4-β1 (expressed by primordial germ cells), stromal cell–derived factor 1 (expressed by the body wall mesenchyma and gonadal ridges), and several extracellular matrix proteins.[8–12] An essential mechanism for adequate primordial germ cell migration, survival, and chemoattraction is the interaction between CD117, expressed in the germ cell surface, and the stem cell factor present in the surrounding tissues.[13–15] After entering the gonadal ridges, primordial germ cells colonize them; this process involves the expression of E-cadherin and germ cell interaction with a rich laminin network produced by organizing coelomic cells in the gonadal ridges.[16] The association of coelomic-derived somatic cells, primordial germ cells, and a laminin-rich stroma in the gonadal ridge characterizes the gonadal blastema. Once inside the genital ridge, germ cells lose their motility and begin to aggregate.

Male–Female Determination

Normal male determination depends on the expression of the *SRY* (*sex-determining region Y*) gene, located on the Y chromosome. In the absence of *SRY*, an ovary is formed. In the testicular blastema, *SRY* is exclusively expressed by the coelomic-derived somatic cells induced to differentiate into pre–Sertoli cells, which form the sex cords.[17–19] These cells are believed to act as the organizing center of the male gonad, orchestrating differentiation of all other cell types.

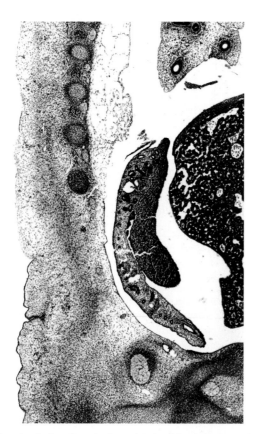

Fig. 12.1 Longitudinal section of a fetus showing the primitive gonad as an elongate structure along mesonephros. In the upper corner of the image the lung can be recognized, and the liver is in front of the gonad.

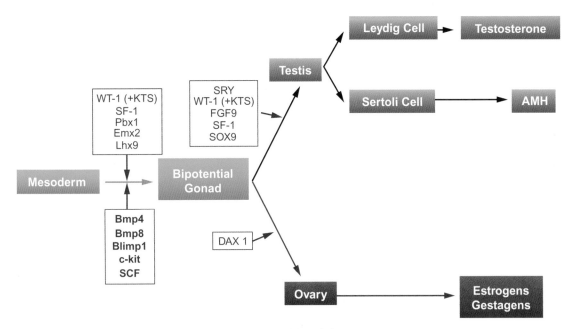

Fig. 12.3 Genetic mechanisms involved in sex determination and testicular differentiation.

SRY expression is transient, ceases when sex cords form, and is activated by *WT1* (+KTS isoform), which is consistently expressed in the coelomic epithelium and the proliferating coelomic-derived somatic cells.[20,21] Gonads lacking *WT1* (+KTS) show lower *SRY* levels per cell and also fewer *SRY*-positive cells. This observation led investigators to hypothesize that *WT1* (+KTS) contributes to SRY activation by increasing the number of pre–Sertoli cells.[22] SRY expression is observed first in the anterior and central portions of the gonad and then in the poles.[18] Expression of *SRY* requires proliferating gonadal somatic cells, and both SF1 and fibroblast growth factor 9 (FGF9) play a role in this proliferation.[23,24] Immediately after *SRY* expression begins, FGF9 contributes to maintenance of cell proliferation necessary for sex cord formation.[25,26] FGF9 regulates male-specific proliferation that produces pre–Sertoli cells.[27]

The origin of sex cord formation, and thus the first morphologic distinction between a testis and an ovary, also depends on the expression of *SRY-box containing gene 9* (*SOX9*). This expression occurs in the cytoplasm of somatic elements in the bipotential gonadal ridge. *SOX9* is expressed in the pre–Sertoli cells in the same dynamic wave as *SRY*; it originates in the center of the gonad and then continues to the rostral and caudal poles. Its transcription is activated by the synergistic action of *SRY* and *SF1*. *SOX9* also stimulates other factors that induce differentiation of Sertoli cells such as FGF9 and prostaglandin D$_2$.[28] *SOX9* is also expressed in the female gonad, but there are important differences from the male gonad.[19,20,29,30] Only males have an increase in *SOX9* gene transcription and translocation of its protein product into the nucleus. This event occurs simultaneously with the initiation of sex cord formation. Therefore, like *SRY*, *SOX9* is necessary and sufficient for both Sertoli cell differentiation and testis development.[31] *SOX9* expression in pre–Sertoli cells remains after sex cord formation, a finding indicating that *SOX9* may have additional roles during proliferation and maturation of the testis, although it is dispensable for the development of embryonic and early postnatal testis.[32] Contacts among pre–Sertoli cells during sex cord formation are regulated by neurotropic tyrosine receptor kinases (Fig. 12.3).[33]

Testis Differentiation: Development of Seminiferous Cords and Interstitium

Early Organization of the Gonadal Blastema. Somatic coelomic epithelium-derived cells expressing nuclear *SOX9* organize into clusters of pre–Sertoli cells as migrating primordial cells aggregate. These clusters are fused and transformed into tubular structures that form the primitive testis cords.[17,20,29] The interaction of pre–Sertoli cells with peritubular myoid cells, which appear early, results in acquisition by pre–Sertoli cells of epithelial characteristics, polarization of organelles, and synthesis and deposition of collagen IV and small amounts of laminin.[34–37] Myoid peritubular cells secrete fibronectin and collagens I and IV to form the basement membrane of the primitive testis cords. These pre–Sertoli cells express antimüllerian hormone under the synergistic action of *SOX9* and *SF1*.[20,38] The primitive testis cords have a toroid structure, parallel to each other and aligned along the testicle.[39] All have a point of contact in the dorsomedial part of the testicle, anastomosing to form a plexus that will be the future rete testis. The plexus has perforations through which vessels of the mesonephros penetrate.

For such development to occur, specific interactions are necessary between germ cells, Sertoli cells, endothelial cells, macrophages, and interstitial cells. Shortly after formation of the gonadal blastema in male gonads, cells of the adjacent mesonephros begin to migrate to the gonadal blastema. This migration depends on *SRY* expression by coelomic-derived cells and is controlled by the expression of FGF9.

The main emigration involves endothelial cells; they originate from the gonad-mesonephros border and migrate radially into the gonadal blastema parallel to the involution of the vascular mesonephric plexus from which they originate.[40] When the endothelial cells reach the antimesonephric region, the celomic vessel forms under the coelomic epithelium, the male-specific main testicular artery. Branches of this vessel penetrate the gonad, delimiting about 10 avascular domains that form the cords and subsequently the seminiferous tubules.[41] The process is mediated by platelet-derived growth factor receptor A (PDGFA) and vascular endothelial growth factor (VEGF).[42,43] The action of VEGF and endothelial cells is a requirement for pre–Sertoli cells to organize into testis cords.[44,45]

Macrophages play an important role at this stage of testicular differentiation. They arise from primitive yolk sac–derived progenitors and initially are in direct contact with pre–Sertoli cells and germ cells. Once the primitive cords form, macrophages remain extratubular with active involvement in regulation of vascularization, morphogenesis of cords, and phagocytosis of pre–Sertoli and germinal cells that remain to be incorporated into the cords (Fig. 12.4).[46]

It is uncertain whether other cells are incorporated into the testicle from the mesonephros. Undifferentiated cells may penetrate the gonad following the endothelial cells and differentiate into a population of Leydig cells.[47] The vessels not only contribute to Leydig cell progenitor migration but also affect their proliferation.[48] Most stem Leydig cells arise directly from coelomic epithelium directly.[25,36]

Leydig cell progenitors express LIM homeobox gene 9, but not gonadal somatic markers such as transcription factors *GATA4* and *SF1*. Fetal Leydig cell differentiation is regulated, at least in part, by three signaling molecules and pathways: desert hedgehog, PDGFA, and Notch signaling.[49]

The same may apply to peritubular myoid cells that may differentiate either from the coelomic epithelium or from undifferentiated perivascular cells that migrate into the gonad from the mesonephric border, following the endothelial cells.

Differentiation of Primordial Germ Cells. Primordial germ cells (that have proliferated in the seminiferous cords) that have undergone mitotic arrest in the G_1 and G_0 stages of the cell cycle are called *gonocytes*. Mitotic arrest depends on adequate cord formation and is probably mediated by inhibitory signals provided through gonocyte interactions with Sertoli cells.[50] These cells remain in mitotic arrest until a few days after birth, when they resume proliferation.

Initially, gonocytes are in the central ("luminal") portion of seminiferous cords. Later, during fetal and neonatal periods, gonocytes migrate toward the cord basement membrane because of gonocyte–Sertoli cell adhesion that is mediated by neural cell adhesion molecule.[51,52] Gonocyte mitoses resume as soon as migration begins and may be identified at the basement membrane. These divisions result in the first generation of spermatogonia. Gonocytes that fail to migrate to the basement membrane undergo apoptosis. It has been suggested that Antimüllerian hormone (AMH) plays a role in gonocyte migration and the start of mitotic activity.[53]

Sertoli Cell Differentiation. Near the end of the seventh week, pre–Sertoli cells differentiate from somatic cells in the sex cords, creating seminiferous cords. It was previously believed that interaction of peritubular myoid cells and pre–Sertoli cells was essential for seminiferous cord formation to promote basal lamina deposition and tubular organization.[35,37] However, recent evidence indicates that peritubular myoid cells are not involved in the initial partitioning of the XY gonad into cord regions, which consist of clusters of both pre–Sertoli cells and germ cells.

As soon as seminiferous cords are formed by the interaction of peritubular myoid cells and pre–Sertoli cells, primordial germ cells become "entrapped" in tubules. This entrapment is mediated by interactions between primordial germ cells and pre–Sertoli cells through expression of E-cadherin and P-cadherin on the cell surfaces.[16]

The differentiation of pre–Sertoli cells into Sertoli cells appears as polarization in which they form aggregates that assemble into seminiferous cords. Early events include the following:

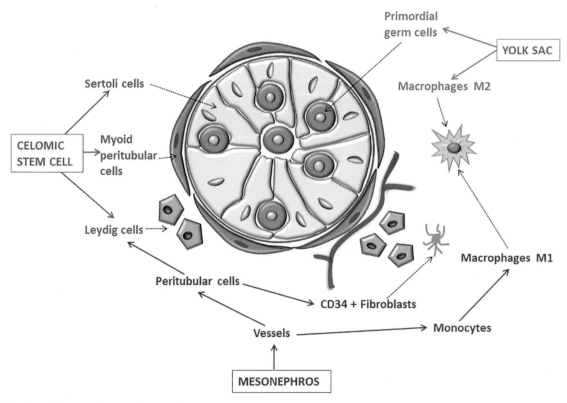

Fig. 12.4 Origin of the different cell types of the testicle.

development of intercellular junctions between adjacent Sertoli cells; formation of a basal lamina that surrounds the external surface of seminiferous cords; and expression of AMH, sulfated glycoprotein-2, and clusterin by the Sertoli cells.[54] Activin A, the major transforming growth factor-β protein, produced by fetal Leydig cells, acts directly on Sertoli cells to promote proliferation during late embryogenesis and plays an essential role in seminiferous cord morphogenesis in the murine testis (Figs. 12.5 to 12.7).[55]

Peritubular Myoid Cell Differentiation. Peritubular myoid cells share expression of many genes with interstitial cells from early fetal development, so it has been hypothesized that they have an interstitial origin either from the mesenchymal cells that populate the initial genital ridge or from the somatic cells that proliferate from the coelomic epithelium.[44]

Peritubular myoid cells form a single layer of flattened cells that surround the Sertoli cells and rim the seminiferous cords. Basal lamina formation by peritubular myoid cells is regulated through *DHH* homologue gene expression by the myoid cells themselves.[56] Survival of peritubular myoid cells, and therefore seminiferous cord formation, depends on *DAX1* (dosage-sensitive sex reversal,

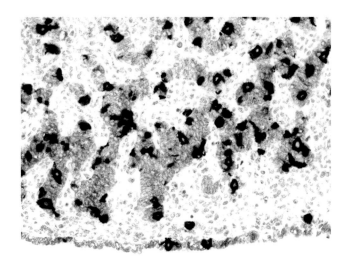

Fig. 12.7 Testis from an 8-week-old fetus. Primordial germ cells, located in sex cords, show intense expression of D2–40. Note that some are situated in the celomic epithelium itself.

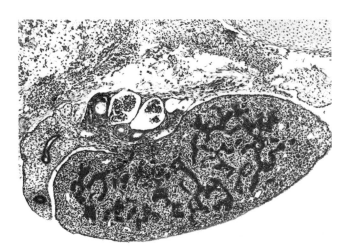

Fig. 12.5 Longitudinal section of an 8-week-old fetal testis showing sex cord configuration. In the hilum, there are several glomeruli and nephric tubules.

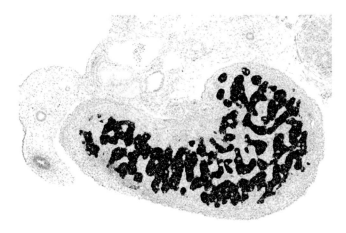

Fig. 12.6 An 8-week-old fetal testis showing intense expression of inhibin in pre–Sertoli cells that form sex cords.

adrenal hypoplasia critical region, on chromosome X, gene 1) nuclear receptor expression, induced in turn by *SF1* expression.[57–59] *DAX1* expression ceases in seminiferous cords after formation, whereas it is maintained in ovaries, a finding suggesting that dosage and stage-specific expression of this protein may be responsible for ovarian differentiation. Seminiferous cords lose their connection with the coelomic epithelium, whose height decreases to one or two cell layers.

Leydig Cell Development. Leydig stem cells proliferate actively and begin differentiation in the eighth week of gestation. Most originate from the same pool of *NR5A1*[+] precursor cells from which Sertoli cells derive; others are perivascular *NR5A1*[−] cells from the mesonephros.[39,60] Differentiation is independent of hormonal stimulation, caused by two Sertoli cell–derived signaling molecules: *DHH* and *PDGFA*.[61] Other factors involved in control of the development and functions of fetal human Leydig cells are *GATA4* (transcription factor that recognizes the GATA consensus DNA sequence), insulin-like growth factor-1 (IGF1) (both are stimulatory factors), and the basic helix–loop–helix transcription factor *POD1* (suppressive factor).[61,62] Histochemical detection of 3β-hydroxysteroid dehydrogenase (3β-HSD) is the apparent first signal of differentiation and is completed with acquisition of ultrastructural characteristics of steroidogenesis.

As fetal development progresses, new cells differentiate from precursor Leydig cells located in the outer of the two peritubular layers (Fig. 12.8). At 12 weeks of gestation, they begin to express LHCGR. Between weeks 14 and 18, Leydig cell number and testosterone level peak.[63] After week 22, tubular walls are reduced to the internal layer. Differentiating Leydig cells are identified by characteristic expression of the androgen receptor (AR) at this stage. Fetal Leydig cells produce androstenedione, which in turn is converted into testosterone by HSD17B3 in Sertoli cells in a gonadotropin-independent process.[64] Pituitary gonadotropins control Leydig cell function throughout the second and third trimesters, especially luteinizing hormone (LH).

Rete Testis Formation. Rete testis develops from residual cords that persist from the mesonephros in continuity with seminiferous cords. The mesonephros and its testicular connection become progressively thinner and appear circular in cross sections. The testis remains between two ligaments: the cranial suspensory ligament

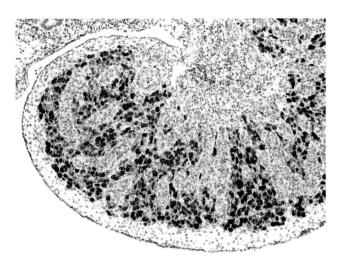

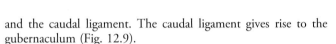

Fig. 12.8 Fetal Leydig cells form large accumulations under the albuginea and among the testicular cords in a 10-week-old fetus. Calretinin immunostaining was used.

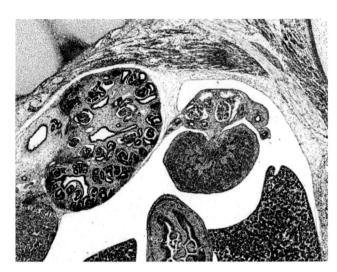

Fig. 12.9 Transverse section of a fetus showing the relationship of the testis to abdominal organs such as liver, kidney, and digestive tract.

and the caudal ligament. The caudal ligament gives rise to the gubernaculum (Fig. 12.9).

Development of the Urogenital Tract. The development of the urogenital tract begins at the stage of the undifferentiated gonad, with the appearance of two different pairs of ducts: the wolffian ducts and the müllerian ducts (Fig. 12.10).

Wolffian ducts arise inside the mesonephros, accounting for the close relationship between the reproductive and urinary systems. This pair of ducts originates in the third week of gestation, when the cranial region of the segmented intermediate mesoderm gives rise to 10 pairs of tubules, the nephric tubules, arranged with a segmental distribution. One end of each nephric tubule opens to the coelomic cavity, and the other end empties into an excretory duct.

There are thus two excretory ducts, longitudinally placed at both sides of the embryonal axis, named pronephros. In the fourth week, the pronephros disappears and is replaced by another tubular excretory system, the mesonephros, derived from nonsegmented intermediate mesoderm. The medial ends of the mesonephric tubules are connected to glomeruli at one end and the wolffian ducts at the other end. The caudal ends of the wolffian ducts drain into the urogenital sinus.[65] At the end of the second month, the mesonephros is replaced by the metanephros, the definitive kidney. In the male the most caudally located mesonephric tubules persist and give rise to the efferent ducts, whereas the wolffian ducts are the source of the epididymides, vas deferens, seminal vesicles, and ejaculatory ducts.

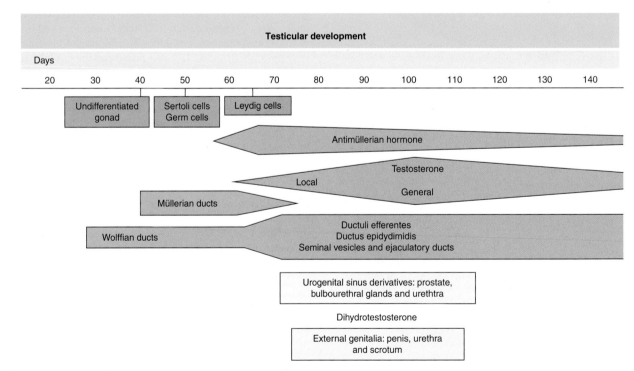

Fig. 12.10 Development of the genital system during the first months of intrauterine life.

Both *müllerian ducts* originate from two longitudinal invaginations of the coelomic epithelium in the anterolateral aspects of the genital ridges. The cranial end of each duct is a funnel that opens into the coelomic cavity. The initial segments of both ducts run parallel and lateral to their respective wolffian ducts, and as they pass caudally, they cross over to lie medial to the wolffian ducts. Finally, in the distal portions, both müllerian ducts fuse into a single duct that serves as origin for the uterovaginalis duct. This duct elongates caudally to reach the posterior aspect of the urogenital sinus, forming a dilation named the Müller tubercle. Each wolffian duct drains at one side of this tubercle.[66]

The remaining structures of the male genital system are derived from the urogenital sinus. Epithelium of this sinus with endodermal origin forms the prostate, the bulbourethral glands, the urethra, and the periurethral glands.

The primitive urogenital sinus derives from the cloaca, a structure that appears at the end of the first month and consists of a dilation of the final portion of the primitive posterior intestine. The cloaca is closed by the cloacal membrane.

During the third week, a crown of mesenchymal cells develops on the outer aspect of the cloacal membrane and gives rise to the cloacal folds. A knob in the middle of the cloacal fold is known as the cloacal eminence. In the sixth week the cloacal folds enlarge to form the genital folds, also known as the urethral folds. The cloacal eminence gives rise to the genital tubercle. External to the genital folds, two mesenchymal outgrowths develop to form the genital prominence or genital swellings.

In the fifth week the cloaca is divided by a septum into two cavities. The anterior cavity is the primitive urogenital sinus, which is covered by the urogenital membrane. The posterior cavity is the anorectal channel, which is covered by the anal membrane.

The primitive urogenital sinus divides further into two new compartments; the anterior compartment, the vesicourethral channel, becomes the urinary bladder and the urethra, whereas the posterior compartment, the definitive urogenital sinus, later differentiates according to gender.

Hormonal Control of Male Genital Tract Differentiation

Subsequent development of the male genital system is under hormonal control. The mammalian fetal testis is initially independent of hormonal control, but then becomes LH (and possibly follicle-stimulating hormone [FSH]) dependent in the second half of gestation.[67] At this point the most important hormones are AMH, testosterone, dihydrotestosterone (DHT), FSH, and LH.

AMH, also called müllerian-inhibiting substance, is secreted by Sertoli cells. It consists of a glycoprotein polymer with two identical subunits linked by a disulfide bridge.[68–71] AMH is a member of the TGFB superfamily and is synthesized as a precursor peptide with proteolytic cleavage, which is required for hormone activation. AMH is encoded by a 2.75-kb gene, which comprises five exons and is located in the p13.3 region of chromosome 19.[72–74]

AMH is secreted only by somatic gonadal cells that include male Sertoli cells and female granulosa cells. It is detected from the sixth week of development (eighth to ninth week of gestation), probably as soon as primordial germ cells come in contact with Sertoli cell precursors exactly 1 week before the müllerian ducts lose their responsiveness.[75,76] AMH is at high concentration during the second trimester and drops markedly in the third trimester.[77] Levels increase again during the first year of postnatal life and decrease during infancy and childhood. At the onset of puberty, AMH drops dramatically to low or undetectable levels, and

this persists through adult life. The amount of hormone secreted by Sertoli cells is inversely proportional to their degree of maturation.[68,78,79]

The regulation of AMH production is incompletely understood. Its expression is regulated by *SOX9*; *SF1* (also called Ad4BP) also seems to be involved.[80] *SF1* is an orphan nuclear receptor that functions as a transcriptional regulator of all the steroidogenic genes within the P450 complex. It also has a regulatory effect on the *SRY* factor because *SRY* expression in Sertoli cells is detected shortly before AMH expression is detected.[81] During puberty, AMH is negatively regulated by androgen levels.[82]

AMH regulates the testis, genital tract, and extragenital structures, causing involution of the ipsilateral müllerian ducts that begins at the caudal end of the testis and progresses rapidly. In adulthood, remnants of this duct may be observed near the cranial (testicular hydatid) and caudal (prostatic utricle or verumontanum) ends of the testis. AMH is also responsible for formation of tunica albuginea, with accumulation of mesenchyma between the coelomic epithelium and the sex cords. The mesenchyma gives rise to collagenized connective tissue that contains several layers of fibers arranged parallel to the testicular surface.[83] AMH also hinders spermatogonial proliferation into meiotic spermatocytes and has a paracrine role regulating fetal androgen production.[84,85] The most important extragenital function of AMH involves maturation of the fetal lungs.[86]

Testosterone synthesis by Leydig cells is regulated by human chorionic gonadotropin (hCG) and LH. hCG secretion reaches a peak between 11 and 14 weeks, whereas testosterone peaks between 11 and 17 weeks. From the 18th week forward, hCG declines markedly. hCG-dependent testosterone production plays an important role in genital differentiation. Wolffian duct differentiation occurs only in response to testosterone secretion by the ipsilateral testis, and this differentiation gives rise to the ipsilateral epididymis, vas deferens, and seminal vesicle.[87,88] Anomalies of androgen synthesis during embryogenesis lead to incomplete masculinization and cryptorchidism.

DHT is formed from testosterone by the action of the enzyme 5α-reductase and causes differentiation of the prostate and development of the external genitalia, including the male urethra, penis, and scrotum. The scrotum is formed by the fusion of the labioscrotal folds in the midline, the so-called scrotal raphe. The penile urethra, initially a urethral groove, is formed by the fusion of urethral folds. The genital tubercle enlarges to form the glans penis. The terminal segment of the penile urethra is derived from an ectodermic invagination of the glans end. The urogenital sinus gives rise to the urinary bladder, the prostatic urethra, and the prostate.[66] The first effects of DHT are observed on day 70; by about day 74, the urethral groove is closed; and between the 18th and 20th weeks, development of the external genitalia is complete.[89]

The actions of testosterone and DHT on the male genital system must occur at precisely programmed times. Failure or delay of secretions or lack of responsiveness to these hormones are the main causes of genital malformations in disorders of sexual differentiation.

The fetal hypophyseal hormones FSH and LH play important roles in the last months of gestation. LH is first detected in the blood in the 10th week, peaking in the 18th week. Thereafter, levels decrease slowly until birth. LH controls androgen production in the second half of fetal life; fetal Leydig cells are devoid of luteinizing hormone receptors (LHRs) in the first half of gestation. LH does not exert negative control over LHRs and androgen production by fetal Leydig cells, whereas the converse occurs in the adult; also, the steroidogenic ability of fetal Leydig cells is higher than that in the adult.[64] Fetal Leydig cells are insensitive to the inhibitory effects of estrogen.

FSH is an essential mitogen for Sertoli cells, which undergo maximal mitotic activity at the end of fetal life.[90,91] This hormone appears to activate transcription factors such as *GATA4*, which shows intense Sertoli cell expression from the nineteenth to the 22nd week following an increase in serum FSH. GATA transcription factors are structurally related zinc finger proteins that recognize a consensus DNA sequence (A/T)GATA(A/G), known as GATA motif, which is an essential *cis*-acting element in promoters and enhancers of multiple genes.[92]

Fetal Testis Structure

The structure of the fetal testis evolves under the influence of placental hormones and the hypophysis. Changes include modifications in external morphology (from elongate to ovoid) and development and differentiation of the cell types. The degree of development is uniform in both testes, and growth varies with gestational age.[93]

Supporting Structures. The testicular covering, the tunica albuginea, increases in thickness 10-fold from the 10th to the 41st week of gestation. From the 29th week onward, two layers may be distinguished: an outer fibrous layer and an inner loose layer. Interlobular septa begin to appear between the 17th and 21st weeks and are completely formed between the 25th and 28th weeks. These septa support blood vessels. Nerve fibers are seen for the first time in the 16th week within the loose connective tissue of the albuginea (tunica vasculosa) and in the 20th week in the septa.[94]

Seminiferous Cords. These irregular compact structures gradually acquire a cylindrical shape as they elongate and become convoluted. The diameter increases slowly up to the 16th week and stabilizes until birth. During fetal life the seminiferous cords consist of Sertoli cells and germ cells, surrounded by a tunica propria. The seminiferous cords are solid structures devoid of lumina. Between the cords the connective tissue forms the testicular interstitium, which contains numerous Leydig cells (Fig. 12.11).[95]

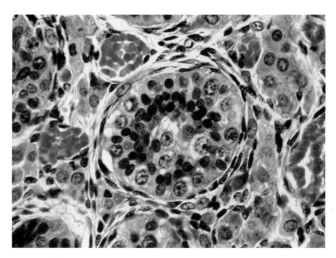

Fig. 12.11 Testis From a 24-week-old fetus. The seminiferous tubules contain Sertoli cells (small dark nuclei) and gonocytes (spherical cells with larger nuclei and central nucleoli). At this age the interstitium contains numerous Leydig cells.

Germ Cells. In contrast with other species, germ cells in the human fetal testis are not homogeneous, with several cell types that form the basis of different classifications.[95a,96–98] Three cell types are identified by immunohistochemistry: gonocytes, intermediate cells, and fetal spermatogonia (prespermatogonia) (Table 12.1).[99]

Gonocytes refers to the primordial germ cells once they reside in the gonadal ridge. They are prominent for the large size (twice that of the surrounding cells) and location in the center of the seminiferous cords during most of fetal life. Nuclei are spherical and possess prominent central nucleoli.[100,101] The cytoplasm contains well-developed Golgi complex, lipid droplets, short rough endoplasmic reticulum cisternae, and microfilaments. Gonocytes connect with Sertoli cells by gap junctions and desmosome-like junctions. Adhesion molecules are present, including neural cell adhesion molecule (NCAM), PB-cadherin, and connexin 43. Immunoreactivity includes octamer-binding transcription factor 4

TABLE 12.1	Evolution Through Fetal Life and First Year of Life of the Immunoexpression of Different Markers in Germ Cells				
Marker	Germ Cell Type	First Trimester	Second Trimester	Third Trimester	First Year of Life
PLAP	Gonocyte	+++	++	+	+
	Prespermatogonia	++	+	−	−
Kit	Gonocyte	+++	+++	++	+
	Prespermatogonia	+++	+++	++	+
OCT3/4	Gonocyte	+++	+++	+	+
	Prespermatogonia	−	−	−	−
TSPY	Gonocyte	−	−	−	−
	Prespermatogonia	++	++	++	++
Ki67	Gonocyte	+++	+++	+	+
	Prespermatogonia	++	++	+	−

PLAP, Placental alkaline phosphatase.
Data are taken from Honecker et al. (2004).[99]
+, Less than one positive cell per tubule (isolate); ++, one to three positive cells per tubule; +++, four to six positive cells per tubule.

(OCT4), KIT, placental alkaline phosphatase (PLAP), serine/threonine-protein kinase 2 (CHK2), and proliferating cell nuclear antigen (PCNA), with absence of melanoma-associated antigen 4 (MAGE-A4).[102–104]

Intermediate cells are morphologically similar to gonocytes, although the cytoplasm-to-nucleus ratio is lower, the number of cytoplasmic processes is higher, and rough endoplasmic reticulum cisternae are more numerous. Intermediate cells are connected by cytoplasmic bridges. They express PCNA, weakly express OCT4, but are negative for KIT and MAGE-A4.

Fetal spermatogonia are also joined by intercellular bridges, are grouped at the periphery of seminiferous cords, and differ from gonocytes by exhibiting more condensed nuclear chromatin and a higher cytoplasm-to-nucleus ratio. The cytoplasm is pale, and mitochondria are adjacent to one side of the nucleus and joined by electron-dense bars. Rough endoplasmic reticulum and lipid droplets are scant. Immunohistochemically, these cells are MAGE-A4+ and are negative for KIT and PCNA, indicating a quiescent phenotype.

The three germ cell types are rich in glycogen granules, polysomes, and chromatoid bodies. Chromatoid bodies consist of finely granular material intermingled with other larger granules, which are similar in size to ribosomes; their mission is to accumulate regulatory RNAs to be used during transcription.

The germ cell number per cross-sectional cord reaches a peak between the 12th and 22nd weeks.[105] In the 10th week, most germ cells are gonocytes; at approximately the 15th week, many intermediate cells are present together with gonocytes, and fetal spermatogonia may be observed for the first time. From the 16th to the 20th week, germ cell degeneration occurs with Sertoli cell phagocytosis.[106] From the 22nd week onward, most germ cells are fetal spermatogonia. Mitotic activity is high in the last trimester of gestation.[107] Approximately 22% of testes between 14 and 33 weeks contain ectopic germ cells located beneath the coelomic epithelium, in the connective tissue that separates the testis from the epididymis, or in the rete testis.[108] Some gonocytes persist after birth. The majority will be transformed into Ad spermatogonia during the 30th to 90th postnatal days (minipuberty).

Sertoli Cells. Fetal Sertoli cells are the most numerous cells in the seminiferous cords, where they form pseudostratified epithelium that rests on the basal lamina. At approximately the 13th week of gestation, Sertoli cells exhibit an indented outline and long cytoplasmic processes, and are connected by desmosomes. Nuclei are spherical and contain small nucleoli. The cytoplasm is electron dense and contains numerous lysosomes, actin microfilaments, and intermediate filaments. Other organelles include microtubules, mitochondria, and well-developed Golgi complexes. In the apical region are numerous, parallel rough endoplasmic reticulum cisternae. The Sertoli cells progressively elongate, their cytoplasm becomes less electron-dense, and filaments predominate in the basal region.[5] They express vimentin filaments throughout life, whereas low-molecular-weight cytokeratins (8, 18, and 19) are present until the 20th week.[109,110] Desmin filaments may be observed from the 11th to the 14th week.[111] Fetal Sertoli cells express inhibin and Stem cell factor (SCF) to secure a niche for gonocytes.[112,113]

During gestation, the number of Sertoli cells increases even though mitoses are only occasionally observed. The number of Sertoli cells per cross-sectioned cord does not increase during this period, but their proliferation contributes to increased length and tortuosity of the cords. Sertoli cell proliferation and testicular cord expansion take place in response to activin A, which is secreted by Sertoli cells. At the end of gestation, there are approximately 260 million Sertoli cells per pair of testes. In the fetal and early postnatal period, the absence of AR expression in Sertoli cells characterizes androgen insensitivity within the male gonad during this period.[114] Fetal Sertoli cell functions include AMH secretion, fetal Leydig cell differentiation induction, and prevention of entry of germ cells into meiosis.[115,116]

Peritubular Myoid Cells. From the 14th week, two types of peritubular cells may be observed: inner myoid cells and fibroblast-like cells. Fibroblast-like cells occupy the outermost layers. In total, there are four to five layers of peritubular cells. At this time the number of myoid cells is low, but are predominate by the 34th week. The probable precursors of myoid cells are the fibroblast-like cells because both coexpress Ki67.[111] In the final weeks of gestation the number of peritubular cell layers decreases to only two, perhaps because of intense lengthening of seminiferous cords and Leydig cell differentiation from peritubular cell precursors. The presence of the AR in peritubular myoid cells suggests an important role in Sertoli cells control.[117]

Leydig Cells. Leydig cells first appear among the seminiferous cords in the eighth week of gestation, and increase in number to 48 million per pair of testes (~50% of testicular volume at this moment) between the 13th and 16th weeks, coinciding with the testosterone peak (Fig. 12.12).[118,119] Leydig cell number is maintained up to the 24th week, although the testicular volume occupied by Leydig cells is lower at this time because the seminiferous cords have grown markedly during this period. From the 24th week to birth, the number of Leydig cells progressively decreases to 18 million.[67,106,120]

Leydig cells are polyhedral and measure between 30 and 37 μm in diameter. They have eccentric and pale nuclei, with voluminous nucleoli, and eosinophilic cytoplasm. There is an abundance of smooth endoplasmic reticulum, numerous mitochondria with tubular cristae, and a variable number of lysosomes and lipid droplets. The rough endoplasmic reticulum consists of some groups with a few short, parallel cisternae.[121] These cells differ from adult Leydig cells by the absence of Reinke crystals and paracrystalline structures, and by the lesser amount of lipid droplets.[122] Histochemical expression included acid phosphatase, glucose-6-phosphatase, and 3β-HSD. In addition to testosterone, these cells secrete several peptides that play important roles in endocrine and

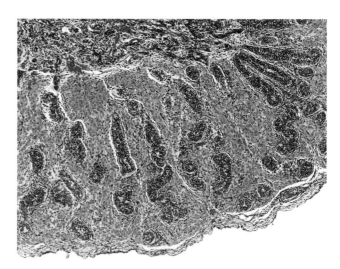

Fig. 12.12 A 16-week-old fetal testis showing numerous Leydig cells in the interstitium and slightly convoluted seminiferous tubules.

paracrine control of testicular function.[119] One of these peptides, insulin-like factor 3 (INSL3), is important in testicular descent.[123]

Other Testicular Cell Types. Macrophages and hematopoietic cells are usually observed in the testicular interstitium of the fetal testis. They derive from yolk sac hematopoietic progenitors and migrate to colonize the testis and other organs.

Macrophages are more numerous at the end of the fetal period, probably because of involution of Leydig cells. These cells are likely involved in Leydig cell paracrine regulation.

Hematopoietic cells appear in isolated clusters at 17 to 20 weeks in the testis, chiefly located beneath the tunica albuginea or near the testicular mediastinum. In the final weeks of gestation, more than two-thirds of testes show hematopoietic foci.

Vascularization of the Fetal Testis. Most fetal testes (72%) receive blood through three arteries: the testicular (inner spermatic) artery, which originates from the abdominal aorta; the deferential (vassal) artery, which originates from the inferior vesical artery; and the cremasteric (outer spermatic) artery, which is a branch of the inferior spermatic artery. In 23% of fetal testes, only two arteries (testicular and deferential) are present, whereas 5% of testes have four arteries.[124]

Fetal Epididymis. The testis and epididymis form an anatomic and functional complex, but the anatomic relationships vary widely. The most frequent finding (almost 90%) is connection of the testis limited to the caput and cauda of the epididymis. In other cases (about 8%) the testis is intimately attached to all parts of the epididymis (caput, corpus, and cauda), and uncommon cases (3%) have deficiencies in the testis-epididymis junction in the caput or the cauda.[125] These variations are not related to the position of the testis or to the side of the body (right or left). During fetal life, androgenic receptors are observed in epithelial cells of both efferent ducts, the epididymal duct, and the peritubular stroma.[117]

Testicular Descent

Testicular descent results from hormonal and mechanical influences that mediate migration through the abdominal wall and the inguinal canal to the scrotum.[126] The process of descent begins between weeks 8 to 15 of gestation, accelerating from weeks 24 to 26.[127] At week 23, most testes (90%) are still in the abdomen, and from weeks 26 to 28 they pass through the deep inguinal ring. Testicular displacement through the inguinal canal lasts a few days. At approximately week 28, they pass through the superficial inguinal ring and reach the scrotum, a process completed within 4 weeks. After week 35, descent is normally complete.[128]

Anatomic Structures Involved in Testicular Descent. Three phases are classically recognized in testicular descent: nephric, transabdominal, and inguinal. In the nephric phase the gonad detaches from the metanephros (primitive kidney) by week 7. Transabdominal descent consists of the displacement from the posterior abdominal wall to the future inguinal region (inner inguinal ring, also called the deep ring) by week 15. This displacement is associated with regression of the cranial suspensory ligament and enlargement of the caudal suspensory ligament (gubernaculum). At the same time, marked growth of the lumbar backbone takes place, and as a result the testis moves away from kidneys.[129] Inguinal descent refers to the entry into the inguinal canal and complete descent into the scrotal pouch, occurring between week 28 of gestation and birth.

Testicular descent is directed by the gubernaculum testis, a structure that appears at approximately week 6 of gestation as an elongate condensation of mesenchymal cells (the caudal ligament) extending from the genital ridge to the presumptive inguinal

region. This dynamic formation undergoes multiple morphologic changes. At this level of the abdominal wall, the gubernacular cells persist as simple mesenchyma, whereas the remaining abdominal wall cells differentiate into muscle. The mesenchymal cells give rise to the inguinal canal. Thus the testis lies on a continuous column of mesenchyma (plica gubernaculum) limited by the cranial testicular ligament in the upper pole and the plica gubernaculum joining the testis to the future scrotal region in the inferior pole. The periphery of this mesenchyma is invaded by the vaginal process, which develops from a blind peritoneal pouch that opens cranially into the abdominal cavity. The pouch partially encircles the gubernaculum except for its dorsal aspect, and divides the gubernaculum into two portions: central (plica gubernaculum) and peripheral (pars vaginalis gubernaculum).

Once the inguinal canal and the plica gubernaculum are formed, development slows. In the seventh month the processus vaginalis undergoes active growth, the cremasteric muscle develops from the mesenchyma outside the processus vaginalis, and the distal end of the gubernaculum enlarges markedly.

Gubernacular thickening occurs from weeks 16 to 24 of gestation, produced by an increase in number of cells and quantity of glycosaminoglycans and hyaluronic acid.[130] This tissue later absorbs water to create the final volume of the gubernaculum. The tissue is reminiscent of Wharton jelly of the umbilical cord. By this time the testis-epididymis complex is pear shaped, and its largest component is the gubernaculum. The inguinal descent of the testis behind the gubernaculum begins in week 25. The testis and epididymis slide through the inguinal canal behind the gubernaculum. Simultaneously, development of the processus vaginalis concludes, and the gubernaculum begins to shorten and fibrose, located caudal to the testis and epididymis (gubernacular regression); the epididymis develops further, with lengthening of testicular blood vessels and vas deferens (Figs. 12.13 and 12.14).[126]

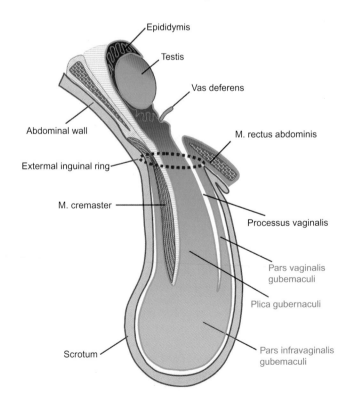

Fig. 12.13 Development of the gubernaculum and related anatomical structures.

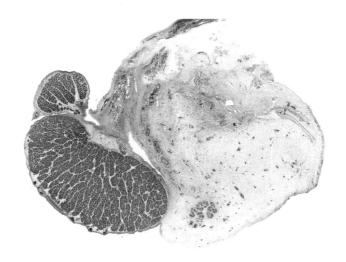

Fig. 12.14 Panoramic view of testis, epididymis, and gubernaculum of a 34-week gestation newborn. The size of the gubernaculum exceeds that of the testis and epididymis combined.

Prerequisites for Testicular Descent. Testicular descent is a complex process integrating several essential factors that probably act sequentially and synergistically. The main prerequisites are normal hormonal stimulation, intraabdominal pressure, development of epididymis and spermatic vessels, development of the gubernaculum, and harmonic development of the processus vaginalis.

Normal Hormonal Stimulation. The critical role of hormonal function in testicular descent is exerted through placental gonadotropins, the hypothalamic–pituitary-testicular axis function, and successful synthesis and action of testosterone produced by the testis.[131] In animal models, destruction of the pituitary blocks testicular descent. Anencephalic fetuses and patients with familial hypogonadotropic hypogonadism usually have undescended testes. Many cryptorchid patients have transient neonatal hypogonadotropic hypogonadism. Some cryptorchid testes descend after treatment with hCG or gonadotropin-releasing hormone (GnRH). Defective Leydig cell function caused by absence of LH, defective testosterone synthesis, or defective ARs interferes with testicular maldescent.

Adequate Intraabdominal Pressure. Another important prerequisite for the testicular descent is adequate abdominal pressure.[132–134] In prune belly syndrome, bilateral abdominal cryptorchidism is associated with urologic malformations and lack of abdominal wall musculature. In a variant termed pseudo–prune belly syndrome, a positive correlation is seen between the development of abdominal wall musculature and testicular descent. The more developed the abdominal wall musculature is, the further the testes descend.[135]

Adequate Development of the Processus Vaginalis. Development of the processus vaginalis also plays a critical role in testicular descent. Growth of the processus vaginalis into the gubernaculum takes place harmoniously. If this structure is invaded, even partially, by fibrous tissue, the testis will descend in an abnormal direction, thus giving rise to ectopia. If fibrous tissue completely replaces the gubernaculum, the processus vaginalis and cremasteric muscle fail to develop fully, and as a result the testis is mechanically blocked in its route of descent.[136]

There is a close relationship between the development of the processus vaginalis and descent. If the processus does not extend far from the abdominal wall, then the testis remains intraabdominal. The processus protrudes throughout the outer inguinal ring only when testicular descent is initiated, and descends into the scrotum only after the testis has entered the inguinal canal.

Factors That Regulate Testicular Descent. Given that nephric displacement consists only of detachment of the testis from the mesonephros, descent may also be classified as occurring in two phases, each regulated by different factors. The most important factor for transabdominal displacement is androgen-independent peptide INSL3 (also called INSF3 or IGF3), a member of the relaxin-insulin family that is produced by fetal Leydig cells.[136–139] This peptide reaches high levels in the first half of gestation, stimulating gubernacular swelling by the production of hyaluronic acid and glycosaminoglycan that trap large amounts of water.[140–145] In animal models, mutations in the genes that encode INSL3 or its receptor LGR8 (leucine-rich repeat-containing G protein–coupled receptor 8) or another receptor called RXFP2 (relaxin/insulin-like family receptor 2) cause cryptorchidism by disrupting transabdominal descent.[146,147]

In humans, however, mutations in the genes that encode INSL3 or its receptors have been found in only 1% of cryptorchid patients, even in studies of familial cryptorchidism.[148–150] The low frequency of such mutations in human cryptorchid patients may account for the infrequent disruption of the first phase of descent in humans, but the inguinoscrotal phase is usually impaired.[149] Analyses of other potential candidate genes for human cryptorchidism, such as homeobox genes *HOXA10* and *HOXA11*, and the estrogen receptor ESR1, also fail to elucidate mechanisms underlying cryptorchidism.[150] Androgens facilitate regression of the cranial suspensory ligament, which also seems to contribute to positioning of the gonad.

In contrast, the inguinoscrotal phase of testicular descent depends on androgenic action, as explained by the genitofemoral nerve (GFN) hypothesis.[151,152] The nucleus of the GFN is located in the spinal cord. The nerve courses along the anteromedial surface of the psoas muscle, and the genital branch crosses the inguinal canal to innervate the cremaster muscle, whose rhythmic contractions are likely transmitted to the gubernaculum, orienting it in a scrotal direction. Based on this hypothesis, androgens act on the GFN nuclei rather than directly on the gubernaculum. Under androgenic action, GFN neurons then undergo masculinization.[151] Male mice have a greater number of neurons than females, and the neurons secrete calcitonin gene–related peptide (CGRP), which is a GFN neurotransmitter. The gubernaculum tip may contain an area of primitive mesenchymal cells. Growth of the gubernaculum apparently results from CGRP-induced cell proliferation and prevention of apoptosis.[153] The range of GFN-mediated androgenic effects is broad and may include obliteration of the processus vaginalis, inguinal canal differentiation, cremaster muscle myocyte differentiation, and initiation of transabdominal descent through involution of the testicular cranial suspensory ligament.[126]

Other factors that influence testicular descent include epidermal growth factor (EGF) and estrogens.[154,155] EGF has a positive effect on descent through stimulation of the placental-gonadal axis. Maternal EGF levels increase just before fetal masculinization.[154] The placenta has an elevated concentration of EGF receptors, and placental stimulation by EGF may stimulate hCG production, which in turn may stimulate Leydig cells to produce androgens that, alone or combined with other factors, may stimulate descent. In contrast, estrogens play a competing role in descent by preventing regression of the cranial gonadal ligament, gubernaculum growth, and Leydig cell proliferation, resulting in a decrease in androgen and INSL3 secretion.[156–160] Exposure to environmental

Transabdominal phase   Inguinoscrotal phase

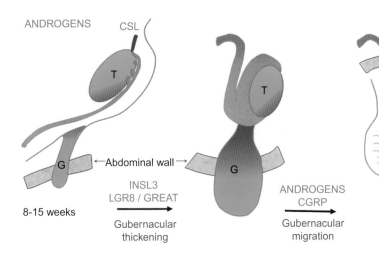

Fig. 12.15 The main factors involved in testicular descent. *CGRP*, calcitonin gene–related peptide; *CSL*, cranial suspensory ligament; *INSL3*, insulin-like factor 3; *LGR8*, leucine-rich repeat-containing G protein–coupled receptor 8.

endocrine disrupters such as estrogen in utero has a negative effect on male genital tract development. During the first trimester of gestation, mothers of cryptorchid infants have free estradiol serum concentrations that are significantly higher than those of controls.[156] Experimental studies have shown that estradiol diminishes gubernaculum swelling and stabilizes müllerian ducts; therefore estradiol may inhibit the cell proliferation that causes swelling through a reduction of INSL3 secretion by Leydig cell damage (Fig. 12.15).[158,159,161]

After birth the gubernaculum and processus vaginalis involute. The gubernaculum is replaced by fibrous tissue that forms the scrotal ligament. Once the testis has descended, the processus vaginalis undergoes atrophy and reabsorption, mainly in its cephalic portion. Failure of the processus vaginalis to regress may be a common cause of acquired cryptorchidism.[162] In some patients a noticeable and wide processus vaginalis is associated with inguinal hernia and cryptorchidism, whereas a narrow processus vaginalis appears associated with hydrocele; if there is partial obliteration of the lumen with persistence of the processus vaginalis, the testis could be retractile.[163]

Prepubertal Testis

From birth to puberty the testis is a dynamic structure, an important consideration when interpreting biopsy results in children. All testicular components undergo waves of proliferation and differentiation before puberty.[164,165] Morphometric analyses and endocrinologic studies in infants and children revealed that the number of Sertoli cells and germ cells increases during this period, accompanied by significant production of AMH and inhibin.[166,167]

During the prepubertal period, three waves of germ cell proliferation occur: during the neonatal period, in infancy, and at puberty. Germ cell proliferation at puberty gives rise to the adult testis with complete spermatogenesis. Leydig cell proliferation also has three waves (fetal, neonatal, and pubertal), the last of which corresponds to the pubertal wave of germ cell proliferation.

Development of the Testis From Birth to Puberty
The Testis at Birth
The newborn testis has a volume of approximately 0.6 mL, and it is covered by a thin tunica albuginea from which the intratesticular

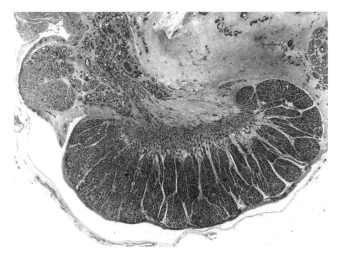

Fig. 12.16 Longitudinal section of the testis and the caput and tail of epididymis from a newborn. Intratesticular septa split the testis into lobules that converge in the mediastinum.

septa arise.[168] These septa divide the testis into approximately 250 lobules containing the seminiferous tubules and testicular interstitium (Fig. 12.16). The seminiferous tubules measure 60 to 65 μm in diameter, form solid cords with no apparent lumina filled with Sertoli cells and germ cells, and are surrounded by a thin basement membrane and isolated myoid cells and fibroblasts.

Sertoli cells are the most abundant cells, with 26 to 28 per tubular cross section (Fig. 12.17). They form a pseudostratified cellular layer and have elongated to oval nuclei with darker chromatin than that of mature Sertoli cells, as well as one or two small peripheral nucleoli. The apical cytoplasm contains abundant rough endoplasmic reticulum, several Golgi complexes, and numerous vimentin filaments, with inhibin B expression (Fig. 12.18). Interdigitations and small junctions of the occludens and adherens types join adjacent Sertoli cells, and desmosome-like junctions are present between Sertoli cells and germ cells. Mitotic figures are occasionally seen. These cells express AMH and vimentin, as well as weak staining for M2A oncofetal antigen.[169] Also, in the apical pole, spherical

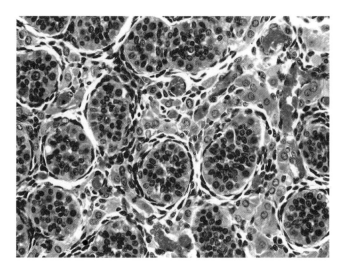

Fig. 12.17 The seminiferous tubules contain Sertoli cells, the most numerous ones and two germ cell types: gonocytes and spermatogonia. The gonocytes have large nuclei with large central nucleoli. The spermatogonia have smaller nuclei and pale cytoplasm. Several Leydig cells are seen in the interstitium.

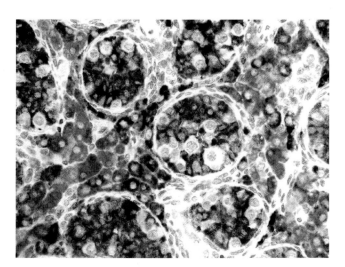

Fig. 12.18 Newborn testis. Both Sertoli cells and Leydig cells are intensely immunoreactive for inhibin.

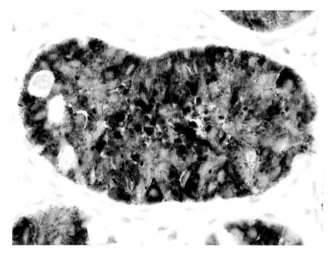

Fig. 12.19 Newborn testis. Inhibin inclusion in the apical pole of Sertoli cells. The clear unstained spaces correspond to germ cells.

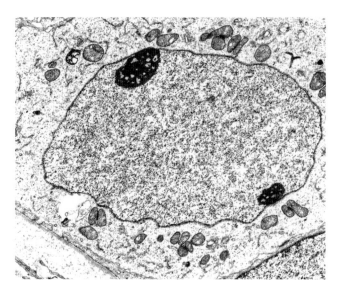

Fig. 12.20 Spermatogonia show wide cytoplasm and regularly outlined nuclei with eccentric nucleoli. The cytoplasm contains mitochondria joined by electron-dense bars.

or ovoid bodies show intense immunostaining with inhibin (Fig. 12.19).[170]

Germ cells comprise fetal spermatogonia, spermatogonia A dark (Ad), and gonocytes. Spermatogonia are present chiefly on the basal lamina in a discontinuous pattern, possessing smaller nuclei and less cytoplasm than gonocytes; nucleoli are peripheral and small. At birth, most spermatogonia correspond to the adult type A (Germ cell-Spermatogonia) (Fig. 12.20). Spermatogonia Ad have smaller nuclei, and barely visible nucleoli are peripherally distributed. Gonocytes are usually located near the center of the tubules, with spherical and voluminous nuclei and large central nucleoli.[171] Most gonocytes are immunoreactive with PLAP and KIT.

Seminiferous tubules are surrounded by the *tunica propria*, which comprises a basal lamina, myoid cells, fibroblasts, collagen fibers, and extracellular matrix. The peritubular myoid cells express intense nuclear immunostaining for AR, with expression similar to

interstitial cells, easily distinguished from the negative staining in Sertoli cell nuclei.[167]

The *testicular interstitium* is a loose connective tissue that contains fetal Leydig cells that resemble adult Leydig cells but lack Reinke crystalloids (Fig. 12.21).[172,173] These cells have well-developed smooth and rough endoplasmic reticulum, filament bundles, and lipid droplets. In addition, mast cells, macrophages, and hematopoietic cells are present.[170]

Neonatal Development of the Testis

Minipuberty is first important postnatal development. It involves changes in germ cells, Sertoli cells, and Leydig cells caused by a transient increase in secretion of FSH and LH during the third postnatal month.[174–180]

Testicular weight and volume increase twofold from birth to 5 months of age.[181–183] FSH induces Sertoli cell proliferation, increasing fivefold to sixfold during the first year of life.[184–186] Under the influence of LH, resident Leydig stem cells undergo

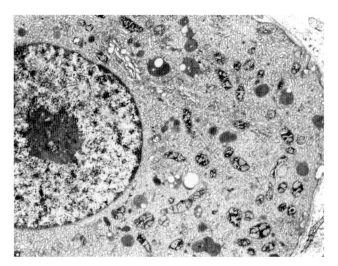

Fig. 12.21 Leydig cells have eccentric, round nuclei, abundant smooth endoplasmic reticulum and mitochondria, lysosomes, and stacks of rough endoplasmic reticulum cisternae.

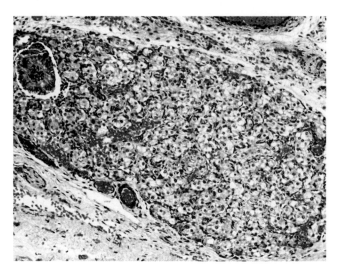

Fig. 12.23 Newborn epididymis showing a paraganglion around the epididymal duct.

stimulation, with new ones differentiating from peritubular myoid cells, and the number increases, peaking between 2 and 4 months after birth.[173,187] In the following months, this cellular population declines rapidly so that by the end of the first year, Leydig cells are rare. As a consequence of the changes in Sertoli and Leydig cells, serum levels of inhibin B, testosterone, and INSL3 increase.[136] Inhibin B, a Sertoli cell marker, remains elevated even when FSH and LH levels have decreased.[180]

The total number of germ cells per testis increases up to three-fold in the first months of life to the end of the neonatal period, and drops later.[171,188] Gonocytes move from the center of the seminiferous tubule toward the basal lamina. This migration is probably facilitated by cell adhesion molecules on the immature Sertoli cell surface, including P-cadherin.[189] Transformation of gonocytes into spermatogonia Ad is enhanced by testosterone and probably also by AMH, which is found at high levels between the 4th and 12th months of life (Fig. 12.22).[53] This transformation is complete by age 6 months and coincides with total loss of fetal germ cell markers PLAP and KIT by the end of the year one.

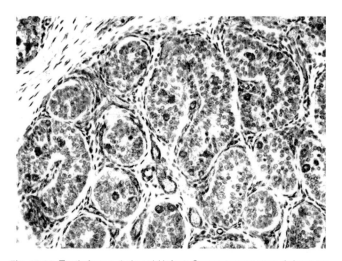

Fig. 12.22 Testis from a 4-day-old infant. Gonocytes are strongly immunoreactive for KIT.

Paraganglia are often observed in epididymides and spermatic cords in newborns. This finding is not surprising because paraganglia are the main source of catecholamine before birth (Fig. 12.23).[190]

Testis in Infancy

From the sixth month to approximately the second half of the third year of life, the testis is in a *resting period*. Tubular diameters decrease (from 80 to 60 μm), and spermatogonial proliferation is rarely observed. Leydig cells involute so that by the end of this period, only a few of these cells persist and are not easily detected in routine specimens. The thickness of the albuginea diminishes to 250 μm. Despite these findings, which permit investigators to define a resting period of the testis, Sertoli cells maintain active hormone synthesis. During these years Sertoli cells produce high levels of AMH and inhibin.[180,191,192] AMH modulates the number and function of Leydig cells by hindering the differentiation of these cells from their mesenchymal precursors and diminishing synthesis of steroidogenic enzymes.[193] Inhibin B plays a role in the inhibition of FSH during infancy. Immunohistochemically, its expression is observed throughout the cytoplasm and in a granular pattern in the apical pole.

This quiescence is broken at the end of the third year by the second wave of germ cell proliferation, the so-called growth period.[168] The number of Ap spermatogonia increases, and B spermatogonia (derived from Ap spermatogonia) appear. In some normal testes from children who are older than 4 years, meiotic primary spermatocytes and round spermatids (Sa + Sb types) are observed (Fig. 12.24).[194] This second spermatogenic attempt fails, and many degenerate germ cells may be present but are phagocytosed by Sertoli cells.[195,196] The testis continues to produce AMH (by Sertoli cells) and inhibin B.[180,191] AMH modulates the number and function of Leydig cells by regulating differentiation of the mesenchymal precursors and expression of steroidogenic enzymes.[193] Inhibin B plays a role in FSH inactivation during infancy.

The cause of this second wave of germ cell proliferation is unknown; no elevation of FSH or LH serum concentrations occurs between 6 months and 10 years of life. After the sixth year, there is a slight increase in adrenal androgens, but testicular testosterone levels increase only after the tenth year.[197,198] By the third year, most Leydig cells have degenerated: from a peak of approximately

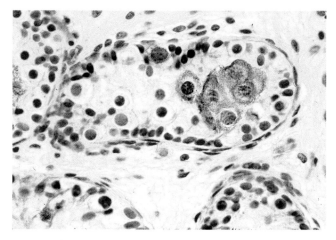

Fig. 12.24 Testis from a 4-year-old infant. The seminiferous tubules have spermatogonial proliferation and contain a central group of primary spermatocytes.

18 million at birth, only 60,000 remain by the age of 6 years. At this age, testosterone levels are similar to those of girls, and most androgens are of adrenal origin.[197] Testosterone levels during infancy are much higher in the tunica vaginalis than in plasma.[199] It also could be important that Sertoli cells begin to express the AR in their nuclei at this age (Fig. 12.25).[167] Expression is probably related to development of this wave of proliferation and differentiation of germ cells.

The Testis in Childhood

From the fourth to the ninth year of life, the seminiferous tubules and testicular interstitium undergo active growth and development. The seminiferous tubules increase in length, width, and diameter, and the epithelium changes from pseudostratified to columnar. Sertoli cell nuclei remain ovoid, but the outlines become increasingly irregular. The number of cells decreases gradually while the seminiferous tubules lengthen, and the result is that the total number of Sertoli cells per testis increases. At the same time, all spermatogonia types (Ad, Ap, and B) increase in number. The lamina propria now contains one to four fibroblasts embedded in collagen fibers.

Cholinergic and adrenergic nerves are observed, with cholinergic nerves ending in the tubular basal lamina.[200,201]

The testicular interstitium apparently lacks classic morphologic Leydig cells. Isolated Leydig cells persist that are fetal in origin or else developed during minipuberty, with pronounced signs of dedifferentiation, alongside a large number of fibroblast-like cells corresponding to adult Leydig stem cells.[202] The tunica albuginea becomes progressively thicker and more collagenized.

At the end of the growth period, between the fourth and ninth years of life, moderate degeneration of spermatogonia occurs. During this period the control of gonadotropic secretion is likely mediated by inhibiting neuroendocrine secretions, whereas testicular hormone levels are low.[203]

There is autonomic innervation of Leydig cells, with three different types of nerve endings. Type I contains many small agranular vesicles (30 to 60 nm) and occasionally large granular vesicles (100 nm); they are probably cholinergic fibers. Type II nerve endings, with many small granular vesicles (30 to 60 nm) and occasionally large granular vesicles (100 nm), are probably adrenergic fibers. Type III contains large granular vesicles of the mixed type. Most of these nerve fibers are "boutons en passant," characterized by fibers are separated from Leydig cells by at least 150 nm, but true contact (20 nm) has also been reported.[204]

At approximately 9 years of age, the *maturation period* begins. The third and definitive wave of spermatogenesis occurs, coinciding with a significant elevation of LH.[205] This is followed by additional increases in the level of this hormone between 13 and 15 years of age. LH induces fibroblast-like Leydig cell precursors to differentiate into mature Leydig cells in the seminiferous tubule walls and in the interstitium.[206] By the end of puberty, the number of Leydig cells per testis is estimated to be 786 million. Leydig cells secrete androgens that, together with the rise in FSH between 11 and 14 years of age, cause Sertoli cell maturation, germ cell development, and appearance of tubular lumina (Fig. 12.26), thus increasing the size of the testes between the ages of 11.5 and 12.5 years.[207,208] At 10 years of age, the testicular volume is 1.5 mL (three times that of the first year of life).[209] This enlargement is assumed to be the first clinical manifestation of puberty. The spermarche, defined as the first spermaturia, occurs early, and may precede other androgen effects such

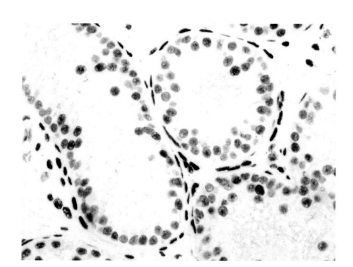

Fig. 12.25 Testis from an infant at the end of the third year of age showing androgen receptor–positive immunostaining in myoid peritubular cells and some nuclei of Sertoli cells.

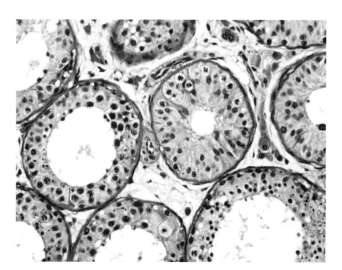

Fig. 12.26 Testis from an 11-year-old boy. Germ cell development varies from one tubule to another. The number of spermatogonia is lower than that of the adult testes. Residual immature Sertoli cells show elongate nuclei with small nucleoli. Leydig cells are scant.

as the development of secondary sex characteristics and the pubertal growth spurt.[210–214] Spermaturia is a constant finding when testicular volume is greater than 4 mL (or even lower).[215]

Morphologic changes occurring at puberty involve all testicular structures. Sertoli cells undergo active proliferation in the prepubertal period, a prerequisite to ensure normal spermatogenesis, beginning at about 11 years of age, but is not completed until 13 years of age.[172,216,217] Sertoli cell nuclei become enlarged and irregular with indentations; the chromatin becomes looser, and nucleoli acquire a tripartite structure.[218] Prominent cytoplasmic changes include development of endoplasmic reticulum (smooth and rough), elongation of mitochondria with longitudinal cristae, increase in the amount of lysosomes and lipid droplets, appearance of annulate lamellae and Charcot-Böttcher crystals, and development of inter-Sertoli junctional specializations that form the blood-testis barrier.[219] The degree of Sertoli cell maturation may be deduced from AMH levels: high levels when Sertoli cells are immature, with marked decrease after puberty with the advent of meiotic spermatocytes and rise of testosterone.[220,221]

Proliferation of Sertoli cells is accompanied by an increase in the number of peritubular myoid cells induced by PDGF ligands. The myoid cells in turn contribute to elongation of the seminiferous tubes.[222]

Germ cell proliferation finally achieves efficient spermatogenesis, although morphologic anomalies of spermatozoa are frequent up to the end of puberty. The mean age for appearance of spermatozoa is 13.4 years.

Leydig cell differentiation is rapid, and many interstitial Leydig cell clusters are seen before seminiferous epithelium development is complete.[202]

Collagenization of the tunica albuginea progresses up to the end of puberty, when thickness reaches 400 to 450 μm. Final testicular volume is approximately 20 mL.[223]

Relationship of Testis and Epididymis During Infancy, Childhood, and Puberty

From the first month of postnatal life to the 18th year of age, the most common testis-epididymis configuration is connection by the caput and cauda epididymidis (84% of cases), resulting in a digital fossa present between testis and epididymis.[224] A less frequent configuration (12%) is complete testis-epididymis union. Other configurations are pathologic.

Interpretation of Testicular Biopsy From Prepubertal Testes

Testicular biopsy in children is necessary to determine the nature of the gonads in those with ambiguous genitalia, a history of leukemia or lymphoma whose testes underwent rapid enlargement, or precocious testicular maturation of unknown cause. Testicular biopsy has been replaced by fine needle aspiration in the study of enlargement in patients with leukemia or lymphoma. In other situations the value of biopsy is less clearly established. For example, biopsy of cryptorchid testes during orchidopexy is controversial, although routine performance of such biopsies provided information on precocious development of lesions in cryptorchidism, including explanations of the causes of cryptorchid lesions such as testicular dysgenesis or transient hypogonadotropic hypogonadism, and to abandon the disproven hypothesis of temperature-induced lesions.

Evaluation of biopsy samples of the prepubertal testis should involve assessment of tunica albuginea thickness, mean tubular diameter (MTD), and the number of germ cells, Sertoli cells, and Leydig cells.

Tunica Albuginea

The most frequent anomaly of the tunica albuginea is the presence of thin, poorly collagenized, altered tissue layers arranged parallel to the surface resembling ovarian stroma. There may be irregular seminiferous tubules protruding from the testicular surface, a configuration classically known as *testicular dysgenesis*, including mixed gonadal dysgenesis, dysgenetic male pseudohermaphroditism, and persistent müllerian duct syndrome (PDMS).[83] This alteration results from insufficiency or defective action of AMH.[225] This anomaly may affect all or part of the tunica albuginea.

This lesion should not be misinterpreted as simple seminiferous tubule ectopy, such as that seen in an otherwise normal, well-collagenized tunica albuginea and an orderly arrangement of layers. Focal ectopy of seminiferous tubules is a frequent finding in both normal and cryptorchid testes.[226,227] In these testes, ectopic seminiferous tubules after puberty may undergo normal germ cell development or become hyalinized. Occasionally, ectopic tubules have cystic dilation that forms a bulbous zone that may be macroscopically visible (Table 12.2).

In patients with disorders of sex differentiation, groups of ovocytes may replace the tunica albuginea, the characteristic structure of ovotestis.

Seminiferous Tubules

Evaluation of seminiferous tubules includes qualitative study of the morphology of the epithelial cells and quantitative estimates of MTD and number of germ cells and Sertoli cells.

Mean Tubular Diameter. The MTD is an excellent indicator of development of the seminiferous epithelium. In the prepubertal testis, tubular diameter depends principally on the number and trophism of Sertoli cells, thus indicating whether there is adequate stimulation by FSH. Tubular diameter varies throughout, being smallest at the end of the third year of life, slowly enlarging up to 9 years of age, and rapidly enlarging thereafter up to 15 years, when the tubule reaches its definitive diameter (160 to 190 μm) (Fig. 12.27).

The most frequent abnormality in the prepubertal testis is a low MTD. This is seen in undescended testes and hypogonadotropic or hypergonadotropic hypogonadism (Table 12.3). In the latter condition the lesion results from anomalous Sertoli cell responsiveness to FSH.[211]

The three levels of severity of low tubular diameter are slight tubular hypoplasia (≤10% reduction in relation to the diameter normal for the age), marked tubular hypoplasia (from 10% to 30% reduction), and severe tubular hypoplasia (>30% reduction).

High MTD is observed in precocious puberty.[228] There is a focal increase in diameter (precocious tubular maturation) of tubules at the periphery of Leydig cell tumors. This enlargement seems to be produced by elevated androgen concentration, which would also be responsible for precocious tubular maturation.[229] The same occurs with some Sertoli cell tumors.

Diffuse increase in MTD may be unilateral or bilateral (Table 12.3). Unilateral increase is found in monorchidism (compensatory testicular hypertrophy), as well as in some testes that are

TABLE 12.2	**Frequent Anomalies of the Tunica Albuginea**

- Thin, poorly collagenized albuginea, ovarian-like stroma
- Focal ectopy of testicular parenchyma
- Presence of ovocytes in an ovarian-like stroma

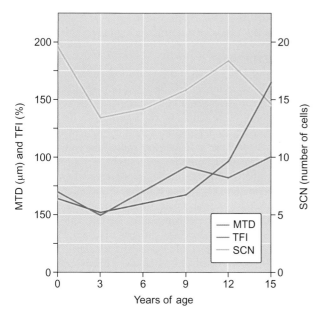

Fig. 12.27 Changes in mean tubular diameter (MTD), tubular fertility index (TFI), and Sertoli cell number per cross-sectioned tubule (SCN) from birth to puberty.

TABLE 12.3 Anomalies in Tubular Diameter

Decrease in tubular diameter

Hypogonadotropic hypogonadism
Hypergonadotropic hypogonadism
Undescended testis

Increase in tubular diameter

Diffuse
Compensatory hypertrophy
Precocious puberty
Benign idiopathic macroorchidism
Macroorchidism associated with fragile X chromosome
Familial testotoxicosis
Macroorchidism associated with hypothyroidism

Focal
Megatubules, ring-shaped tubules, tubules with eosinophilic bodies with microliths
Sertoli cell intratubular neoplasia

contralateral to cryptorchid testes.[230,231] Most frequently, diffuse enlargement occurs in benign idiopathic macroorchidism, macroorchidism associated with fragile X chromosome, familial testotoxicosis, hypothyroidism, and other forms of precocious puberty.[232–235] Focal increase in MTD is usually associated with precocious maturation of the seminiferous epithelium in tubules at the periphery of Sertoli cell tumors and Leydig cell tumors.

Frequently, infantile testicular biopsies of undescended testes contain several types of malformations such as nearly straight tubules or ramified tubules. Other findings are large tubules (megatubules or ring-shaped tubules), which are malformed tubules displaying a tight spiral course, or bell-shaped deformities (bell-shaped tubules). Megatubules may surround and isolate connective tissue that often develop eosinophilic bodies or microliths.[236] These tubules are likely an indicator of poor prognosis in those with infertility.

The presence of one or more groups of enlarged tubules with marked thickening of the basal lamina in infant testes suggests

intratubular Sertoli cell neoplasia. This pattern is frequently seen in infants with Peutz-Jeghers syndrome.

Some infantile testicular biopsies show enlarged tubules with prominent lumina or cystically dilated tubules. Testicular fluid is not produced before puberty, so normal prepubertal tubules do not contain lumina. Therefore the observation of such findings suggests *cystic dysplasia of the rete testis*. This disorder may include absence or dysplasia of the ipsilateral kidney and urinary excretory ducts.

Germ Cell Number. Germ cells may be counted in two ways: calculation of the number of cells per tubular cross section or determination of the tubular fertility index (TFI). The first method counts the number of germ cells in a light microscopic field and divides this by the number of cross-sectioned tubules. In the first 6 months of postnatal life, the normal testis has two germ cells per cross-sectioned tubule, dropping to 1.5 at the end of the first year and to 0.5 at the end of the third year. The number then increases to 1.8 cells at the age of 3 to 4 years, which coincides with the appearance of spermatocytes in some tubules.[237] This number then increases slowly up to 8 years of age, decreases again up to 9 to 10 years, and increases once more, rising markedly from 12 years of age to the end of puberty.[195,238] Separation of spermatogonia and gonocyte counts reveals time of last transformation of gonocytes into Ad spermatogonia.

TFI reflects the percentage of tubular sections containing germ cells. In newborns, 68% of tubular sections contain at least one germ cell. From birth to 3 years, this decreases to 50%, followed by a progressive increase to 100% at puberty.[168] The most accurate measure is calculation of total germ cell number per testis. This is more difficult because it requires morphometric assessment of intratubular volume and careful clinical measurement of the three axes of the testis.

Three levels of severity of germinal hypoplasia are recognized: slight (TFI > 50), marked (TFI between 50 and 30), and severe (TFI < 30). Marked and severe germinal hypoplasia is usually associated with marked or severe tubular hypoplasia, in most cases resulting from tubular dysgenesis. It may also be useful to determine whether the seminiferous tubules devoid of germ cells are randomly distributed. If grouped, they probably belong to the same lobule or group of lobules that will never develop normally.

Congenital decrease of germ cells occurs in numerous conditions, including trisomies 13, 18, and 21; some forms of primary hypogonadism such as Klinefelter syndrome; anencephaly; cryptorchid testes and posterior urethral valves; and severe obstruction of urinary ducts (Table 12.4).[239,239a,240] Congenital germ cell

TABLE 12.4 Variation in Tubular Fertility Index

Decrease in tubular fertility index

Congenital
13, 18, 21 trisomies.
Klinefelter syndrome.
Anencephalia.
Cryptorchidism.
Patients with posterior urethral valves.

Acquired
Treatments with antitumoral chemotherapy.
Treatments with immunosuppression.
Therapies in transplantation.

Increase in tubular fertility index

Parenchyma close to either germ cell tumors or gonadal-stroma tumors.

decrease may result from deficient colonization of genital ridges by primordial germ cells, reduced germ cell proliferation, or increased germ cell loss. In Klinefelter syndrome, defective germ cell colonization has been suggested as the cause because of the high incidence of extragonadal germ cell tumors in such patients.[240]

During infancy and childhood a significant reduction in the number of spermatogonia occurs in children undergoing chemotherapy or immunosuppression. An increased number of germ cells may be seen at the periphery of germ cell tumors, gonadal-stromal tumors, and paratesticular sarcomas.[241,242]

Other altered germ cells include multinucleate or hypertrophied spermatogonia and gonocyte-like cells. Multinucleate spermatogonia have two to four nuclei, and Ap and Ad nuclei may coexist within the same cell, representing a failure of cytokinesis. Hypertrophic spermatogonia are located over the basal lamina and exhibit large, usually hyperchromatic nuclei and abundant cytoplasm, findings indicating polyploid cells that are unable to complete cellular division. Most of the hypertrophic spermatogonia degenerate rapidly. Gonocyte-like cells are located among Sertoli cells in the center of tubules, appearing as large cells with ovoid nuclei, large central nucleoli, and small heterochromatin granules. These cells should not be misinterpreted as cells from germ cell neoplasia in situ (GCNIS). Tumoral cells of GCNIS, which share with gonocytes immunoreactivity for PLAP, KIT, and OCT3/4, also show immunoreactivity for SCF.[243] The presence of gonocytes is common in gonads of patients with disorders of sexual differentiation, and this finding often indicates delay in germ cell maturation.

Complete maturation of the seminiferous epithelium at early ages may occur in patients with precocious puberty, as well as in the testicular parenchyma at the periphery of Leydig cell tumors.

Sertoli Cell Number. The number of Sertoli cells per tubular cross section varies during childhood as a result of slow proliferation from 4 to 12 years and redistribution as seminiferous tubules become longer and broader.[185] An apparent decrease in Sertoli cell number results from cellular displacement as a consequence of slow growth in length and tortuosity of tubules and not from degeneration. The pseudostratified cellular pattern characteristic of Sertoli cells at birth and the first months of life changes slowly to a columnar pattern during later infancy. During puberty, three phenomena occur: proliferation of Sertoli cells with emergence of pseudostratified seminiferous epithelium that ensures growth of tubules; Sertoli cell maturation; and subsequent transformation of pseudostratified epithelium into the columnar epithelium that is characteristic of the adult testicle.[244] Proliferation is under the control of FSH and testosterone, ensuring optimum sperm production.[245]

Testicular biopsies may reveal hypoplasia or hyperplasia of Sertoli cells. Hypoplasia may indicate congenital hypogonadotropic hypogonadism, Kallmann syndrome, Prader Willi syndrome, DAX1 mutation, or multiple pituitary hormone deficiency. Hyperplasia may be observed in several pathologic states and manifests itself at different moments of development. In childhood, hyperplasia is observed in most cases of macroorchidism, because most of the volume of the testis at this time depends on the number of Sertoli cells. This also applies for patients with the syndrome of fragility of the X chromosome and in those with peripheral precocious pseudopuberty, a component of McCune-Albright syndrome (MAS). Sertoli cell hyperplasia seen at the beginning of puberty is characteristic of cryptorchid testicles and reflects the inability of the growth in length and tortuosity of the seminiferous tubules, and, to a lesser extent, an absolute increase in number of Sertoli cells. This is considered a sign of tubular dysgenesis.[246] Biopsies may reveal one or several tubular sections containing Sertoli cells with eosinophilic and granular cytoplasm that is positive for CD68 and

α_1-antitrypsin, oncocytic changes that result from lysosomal accumulation; this is considered a primary anomaly.[247]

Leydig Cell Number

Calculation of Leydig cell number during childhood is difficult because of the low numbers.[206] Use of semithin sections or immunohistochemistry to detect cells containing testosterone or calretinin may be helpful.[207] Selection of the appropriate denominator to express the Leydig cell population is another problem. The most frequent measures are Leydig cell number per tubular section or per unit area, or total Leydig cell number per testis.[208]

Low numbers of Leydig cells are observed in undescended testes, hypogonadotropic hypogonadism, disorders of sexual differentiation caused by an anomaly in LHRs, and anencephaly.[248] High numbers occur in congenital Leydig cell hyperplasia, triploidy, variants of precocious puberty, and several syndromes such as leprechaunism and Beckwith-Wiedemann syndrome (Table 12.5).[249–251] Focal accumulation of Leydig cells with broad and microvacuolated cytoplasm caused by the presence of lipids is characteristic of patients with sexual developmental disorders secondary to mutations of the *NR5A1* (*SF1*) gene.[252] They may also be seen in patients with defects in androgen synthesis.

Intertubular Connective Tissue

The seminiferous tubules are normally closely packed, separated only by a small amount of loose connective tissue that maintains cohesion among the tubules and contains scant Leydig cells, macrophages, mast cells, blood vessels, and nerves. This intertubular connective tissue may be altered, including increased amount, increased cellularity, abnormal development of lymphatic vessels, and the presence of cell types that are unusual in this location.[253]

An apparent increase in loose connective tissue is found in patients with marked tubular hypoplasia. The cellular basis for increased connective tissue is uncertain. Some testes have thick fusiform cell bundles that separate groups of closely packed seminiferous tubules. These cells are reminiscent of the cells that form ovarian stroma and are the most characteristic histologic finding in Botella-Nogales-Morris syndrome (a sex differentiation disorder secondary to androgen insensitivity).[254]

Other alterations include the presence of overly developed lymphatic vessels (congenital testicular lymphangiectasis), focal hematopoiesis, leukemic infiltrate, and the presence of cells reminiscent of the adrenal cortex (tumors of the adrenogenital syndrome).

Adult Testis

Anatomy

The adult testis is an egg-shaped organ suspended in the scrotum from the spermatic cord, the retroepididymal surface, and the

TABLE 12.5	Variation in Leydig Cell Number

Decrease in Leydig cell number

Hypogonadotropic hypogonadism.
Undescended testes.
Defects in luteinizing hormone receptors.
Anencephalic fetuses.

Increase in Leydig cell number

Congenital hyperplasia of Leydig cells (maternal diabetes mellitus).
Malformative syndromes (Beckwith-Wiedemann syndrome, leprechaunism).
Precocious puberty.

scrotal ligament. Mean weight in white men is 21.6 ± 0.4 g for the right testis and 20 ± 0.4 g for the left. Mean testicular diameter is 4.6 cm (range, 3.6 to 5.5 cm) for the longest axis and 2.6 cm (range, 2.1 to 3.2 cm) for the shortest.[255–258] Testicular volume varies from 15 to 25 mL. Testicular volume correlates with height, weight, body mass index, and body surface area, and it decreases in adulthood.[259]

Supporting Structures

The tunica albuginea and interlobular septa make up the connective tissue framework of the testis. The *tunica albuginea* consists of three connective tissue layers: an outer layer of mesothelium apposed to the basal lamina (*tunica vaginalis*), a middle layer of dense fibrous tissue, and an inner layer of loose connective tissue (*tunica vascularis*) with nerve fibers and abundant blood and lymphatic vessels. From the outer to the inner layers, the amount of collagen fibers decreases, whereas the number of cells increases. The fibers and cells in the two outermost layers form planes parallel to the testicular surface; cell types include fibroblasts, myofibroblasts, mast cells, and nervous fibers. Myofibroblasts are more numerous in the posterior portion of the testis (Fig. 12.28). The thickness of the tunica albuginea increases with age from 400 to 445 μm in young men to more than 900 μm in older men.[260] The tunica albuginea acts as a semipermeable membrane that produces the fluid of the vaginalis cavity. The presence of many contractile cells showing high concentrations of guanosine monophosphate suggests that the tunica albuginea undergoes cycles of contraction and relaxation. The cells may regulate testicular size and favor the transport of spermatozoa into the epididymis.[261,262] The *interlobular septa* consist of fibrous connective tissue with blood vessels supplying the testicular parenchyma. The interlobular septa divide the testis into approximately 250 pyramidal lobules, with the bases at the tunica albuginea and vertices at the mediastinum testis. Each lobule contains two to four seminiferous tubules and numerous Leydig cells.[263]

Seminiferous Tubules

Adult seminiferous tubules are 180 to 200 μm in diameter and 30 to 80 cm long. The total combined length of the seminiferous tubules is approximately 540 m (range, 299 to 981 m).[264] These tubules are highly convoluted and tightly packed within the lobules. The seminiferous tubules comprise approximately 80% of testicular volume.[265] The tubular lining of germ cells and Sertoli cells is surrounded by a lamina propria (tunica propria) (Fig. 12.29).

Sertoli Cells

Sertoli cells are columnar cells that extend from the basal lamina to the tubular lumina, with 10 to 12 cells per cross-sectioned tubule. They are easily identified by their nuclear characteristics. Nuclei are located near the basal lamina and appear triangular with an indented outline. They are euchromatic, as expected of cells that express a great proportion of the genome to synthesize a large variety of substances required for its multiple functions. Nucleoli are central and voluminous (Fig. 12.30). The cytoplasm has lateral

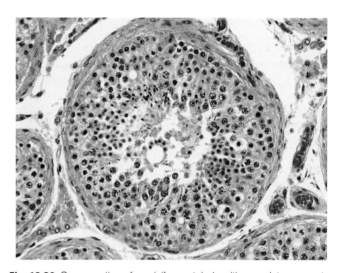

Fig. 12.29 Cross section of seminiferous tubule with complete spermatogenesis surrounded by tunica propria. Both interstitium and tunica propria blood vessels may be observed. Among seminiferous tubules, small groups of Leydig cells may be observed.

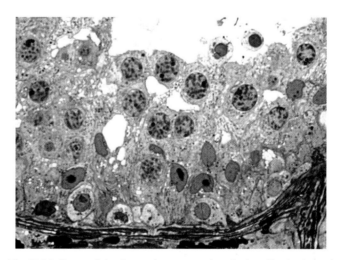

Fig. 12.30 Germ cell development progresses from the basal lamina toward the lumen of the tubule. Each germ cell type forms a different layer in the seminiferous tubules and may be identified by its nuclei. Spermatogonia are basal cells with pale cytoplasm, round nuclei, and eccentric nucleoli. Above these cells, the Sertoli cell nuclei may be recognized by their large central nucleoli. The inner layers consist of primary spermatocytes showing the chromatin pattern characteristic of meiosis (semithin section).

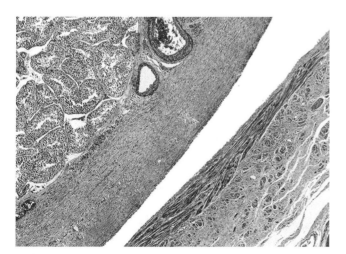

Fig. 12.28 Testis located in vaginal cavity. It is externally covered by tunica albuginea, which is a thick layer formed by collagenized fibrous tissue. The parietal layer has abundant smooth muscle fibers, whereas the innermost layer of albuginea contains large vessels (tunica vasculosa).

processes that spread out and surround adjacent germ cells and touch other Sertoli cells, facilitating direct contact with 40 to 50 germ cells and 6 to 7 adjacent Sertoli cells. Charcot-Böttcher crystals and lipid droplets often are visible in the cytoplasm.[266–269]

The number of Sertoli cells per testis decreases from approximately 250 million in young men to 125 million in men who are older than 50 years of age.[270,271] A positive correlation exists between the number of Sertoli cells and daily sperm production.[272] Sertoli cells are the target of FSH and androgen action.[273–275] In adulthood these cells produce testicular fluid through an active transport mechanism, creating and maintaining the lumen of the seminiferous tubule. Testicular fluid is isosmotic, with a high content of potassium that exposes various membrane and water transporters.[276] The fluid provides an optimal milieu for developing spermatozoa and a vehicle to transport them from the testis.

Ultrastructurally, Sertoli cells have characteristic nucleoli, plasma membranes, and cytoplasmic components. Nucleoli have a tripartite structure with round fibrillar centers, compact granular portions, and three-dimensional nets composed of intermingled fibrillar and granular portions.[218,277,278] The plasma membrane has two types of intercellular junctions that develop at puberty: junctions between adjacent Sertoli cells and junctions between Sertoli cells and germ cells.[279] The ectoplasmic junction is a unique and specific junction that consists of Sertoli-Sertoli cell junctions (basal ectoplasmic specializations) and Sertoli-germ cell junctions (apical specializations). Sertoli-Sertoli junction specializations consist of adherens, tight junctions, and gap junctions that are dynamically remodeled to allow the movement of germ cells across the seminiferous epithelium and the timely release of spermatids into the tubular lumens.[219] This dynamic remodeling of cell junctions is mediated by several mechanisms at transcription and posttranslation.[280] In addition, ectoplasmic specializations also confer cell orientation and polarity in the seminiferous epithelium.[281] Within the plasma membrane are adhesion molecules such as connexin 43 that may regulate other proteins of intercellular junctional complexes that occur between adjacent cells.[282] The presence of connexin depends on the seminiferous epithelium stage, absent at stages II and III when primary spermatocytes cross from the basal to the adluminal compartment.[283]

Three different types of membrane protein have been identified in the testis: occludin, claudins, and adherens junction molecules.[280,284,285] In addition, beneath the Sertoli cell plasma membrane and cisterns of the endoplasmic reticulum, several molecules are recognized: actin filaments, anchorage molecules, vinculin, zonula occludens 1 (ZO-1) and ZO-2, plakoglobin, radixin, and nectins.[286,287]

The inter-Sertoli cell junctions are the morphologic basis for the blood-testis barrier and divide the seminiferous epithelium into two compartments; the basal compartment contains spermatogonia and newly formed primary spermatocytes, whereas the adluminal compartment contains meiotic primary spermatocytes, secondary spermatocytes, and spermatids.[288] These junctions permit each compartment to have its own microenvironment for spermatogenic development.[219,289,290] The Sertoli cells, the only cell types present in both compartments, together with primary spermatocytes, become the key to control the passage of information from one compartment to another.[291] There is a transient compartment between the basal and adluminal compartments, where preleptotene and leptotene spermatocytes linger before entering the adluminal compartment. The blood-testis barrier is always secured by the existence of tight junctions both apically and basally to the cells.[292] Definitive establishment of the blood-testis barrier is

complete when Sertoli cell proliferation and maturation ceases, features coinciding with the initiation of meiosis. Terminal differentiation of Sertoli cells is regulated to a great extent by retinoblastoma protein.[293]

Sertoli cell-germ cell junctions (desmosomes and tight junctions) persist from the primary spermatocyte stage through spermatozoon release. Adhesion of Sertoli cells and germ cells is mediated by N-cadherin.[294] These glycoproteins are involved in maintaining the seminiferous epithelium architecture and germ cell migration from the basal to the adluminal compartment. These junctions may also be present between spermatogonia.[292,295]

Sertoli cell basal cytoplasm contains abundant smooth endoplasmic reticulum (involved in steroid synthesis), scant rough endoplasmic reticulum (involved in protein synthesis), annulate lamellae, Golgi complex, lysosomes, residual bodies, glycogen granules, lipid droplets in amounts that vary with the seminiferous tubule cycle, Charcot-Böttcher crystals (structures several micrometers long, formed of multiple parallel laminae of protein), and ribosomes.[296–298] The apical cytoplasm contains elongate mitochondria, numerous microtubules, and large numbers of vesicles with degraded cytoplasmic fragments derived from phagocytosis of residual bodies of spermatids.[299]

Sertoli cells are immunoreactive for inhibin, WT1 (Fig. 12.31), GATA4, SOX9, follicle-stimulating hormone receptor (FSHR), vimentin, nuclear AR (Fig. 12.32), F-actin filaments, and α-tubulin in the cytoplasm. Actin filaments appear in both inter-Sertoli cell junctions and ectoplasmic specializations that surround germ cells.[300] F-actin bundles contribute to formation of Sertoli-Sertoli cell junctions arranged at regular intervals beneath the plasma membrane and cistern of the endoplasmic reticulum connected to microtubules.[301] Actin distribution varies during the cycle of the seminiferous epithelium. It is more abundant next to the heads of elongate spermatids (ectoplasmic specializations) and in the Sertoli cell cytoplasm that surrounds spermatids.[302,303] Actin filaments, intermediate filaments (vimentin), and microtubules make up the cellular cytoskeleton, one of the more developed somatic cell cytoskeletons (Fig. 12.33).[304]

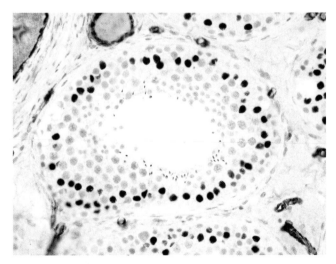

Fig. 12.31 Cross section of a seminiferous tubule. Immunostaining in the nuclei of Sertoli cells and in endothelial cells with the WT1 antibody is observed.

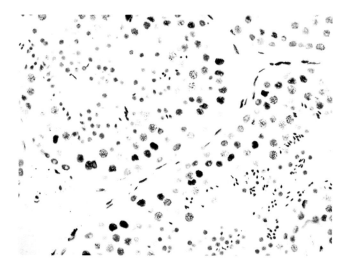

Fig. 12.32 Sertoli cells and peritubular myoid cells show immunoexpression of androgen receptor in the nuclei.

TABLE 12.6	Sertoli Cell–Leydig Cell Regulatory Interactions		
Paracrine Factor	**Origin**	**Receptor**	**Action**
Androgens	Leydig cell	Sertoli cell	Regulate/maintain function and differentiation
Proopiomelanocortin peptides	Leydig cell	Sertoli cell	Decrease FSH actions
β-Endorphin	Leydig cell	Sertoli cell	Decrease steroidogenesis
GnRH-like factor	Sertoli cell	Leydig cell	Decrease steroidogenesis
Estrogens	Sertoli cell	Leydig cell	Decrease steroidogenesis
TGFA	Sertoli cell	Leydig cell	Decrease steroidogenesis
Interleukin-1	Sertoli cell	Leydig cell	Decrease steroidogenesis
IGF1	Sertoli cell	Leydig cell	Increase steroidogenesis
Inhibin	Sertoli cell	Leydig cell	Increase steroidogenesis

FSH, Follicle-stimulating hormone; *GnRH*, gonadotropin-releasing hormone; *IGF1*, insulin-like growth factor; *TGF*, transforming growth factor A.

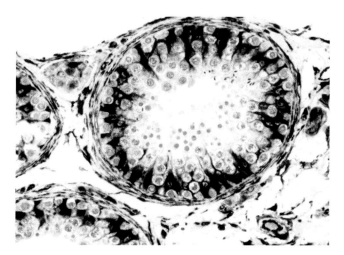

Fig. 12.33 Cross section of seminiferous tubule showing Sertoli cells that are intensely immunoreactive for vimentin. Positive staining is also observed in peritubular and endothelial cells.

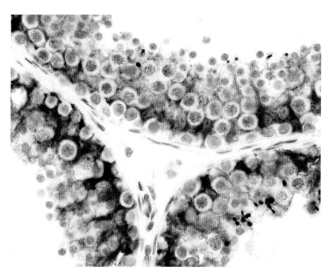

Fig. 12.34 Cross section of part of three seminiferous tubules showing intense immunoreactivity for inhibin in the cytoplasm of Sertoli cells.

Sertoli cells synthesize multiple products to ensure the nutrition, proliferation, and maturation of germ cells; they also stimulate other cells such as Leydig cells and peritubular cells, and contribute to hormonal regulation (inhibin secretion) (Table 12.6).[305,306] Transport of small molecules (<600 to 700 Da) such as pyruvate, lactate, and probably choline from the Sertoli cell to germ cells occurs through gap junctions. Large or small soluble molecules are transported by proteins that are synthesized by Sertoli cell and include androgen-binding protein (ABP), transferrin, ceruloplasmin, sulfated glycoproteins, α2-macroglobulin, and γ-glutamyl transpeptidase.[307,308] Activin and inhibin are Sertoli cell–secreted proteins that induce proliferation and differentiation of germ cells. Activin stimulates FSH production and resultant spermatogonial proliferation, and controls the seminiferous epithelium cycle, whereas inhibin B inhibits FSH secretion and is an important marker of spermatogenesis (Fig. 12.34).[309,310] Other Sertoli cell secretions include interleukins, mainly IL1, and growth factors such as TGFB, IGF1 and IGF2, and seminiferous growth factor.[311] Some of these growth factors, such as TGFA, TGFB, and IGF1,

are involved in regulation of Leydig cell function. Other secreted substances include clusterin, the steroid 3-α-4-pregnen-20-one, and prostaglandin D synthase (PGDS) (Table 12.7). Sertoli cells are also involved in migration of differentiating germ cells toward the tubular lumens. This movement leads to continuous remodeling of the plasma membrane and requires synthesis of several proteases, including urokinase, tissue-type plasminogen activator, cyclic protein 2, collagenase IV, other metalloproteins, and several antiproteases, such as cystatin C, tissue inhibitor of metalloproteinase type 2, and α2-macroglobulin.[312] Differentiation of germ cells

TABLE 12.7 Major Sertoli Cell Secretory Products

Products	Functions/Characteristics
Transport-Binding Proteins	
Androgen-binding protein (ABP)	Androgen transport
Transferrin	Iron transport
Ceruloplasmin	Copper transport
Sulfated glycoprotein-1	Sphingolipid binding
Regulatory Proteins	
Inhibin	Endocrine-paracrine agent
Müllerian duct inhibitory agent	Development
Sulfated glycoprotein-2	Sperm coating, immunosuppressant
Growth Factors	
GDNF	Glial cell–derived neurotrophic factor
FGF2	Fibroblast growth factor 2
TGFA	Growth stimulation
TGFB	Growth inhibition
IGF1	Maintain growth/differentiation
Interleukin-1	Growth regulation
Metabolites	
Lactate-pyruvate	Energy metabolites
Estrogens	Steroid hormone, endocrine-paracrine agents
Proteases/Inhibitors	
Plasminogen activator	Plasminogen activation
Cyclic protein-2	Cathepsin activity
α_2-Macroglobulin	Protease inhibitor
Extracellular Matrix Components	
Laminin	
Collagens I and IV	
Proteoglycans	

IGF1, Insulin-like growth factor; *TGFA*, transforming growth factor A; *TGFB*, transforming growth factor B.

of adjacent Sertoli cells. Nuclei are spherical, contain several peripheral nucleoli, and have four different patterns according to their shape, size, and nuclear staining features: Ad (dark), Ap (pale), Al (long), and Ac (cloudy).[314,315] The cytoplasm of Type A spermatogonia contains a moderate number of ribosomes, small ovoid mitochondria joined to each other by electron-dense bars, and Lubarsch crystals. These are several micrometers long and are composed of numerous 8- to 15-nm parallel filaments intermingled with ribosome-like granules. Ad spermatogonia are thought to be stem cells in spermatogenesis, and under normal conditions do not divide.[316] Some Ad spermatogonia replicate their DNA and acquire an elongate shape (Al spermatogonia). They later divide to make another Ad (maintaining the stem cell reservoir) and an Ap spermatogonia. During replication, Ap spermatogonia become Ac and then divide by mitosis to form two type B spermatogonia.[317–319]

Type B spermatogonia are the most numerous, and their contact with the basal lamina is less extensive than that of type A. Nuclei usually are more distant from the basal lamina than are those of type A spermatogonia and contain one or two large central nucleoli. The cytoplasm contains more ribosomes than type A spermatogonia, and intermitochondrial bars are usually not observed. Type B spermatogonia divide to form primary spermatocytes.

Although all type A spermatogonia are located on the basal membrane, their distribution varies in the seminiferous tubules from one area to another. Spermatogonial stem cells (SSCs) are in specific areas of the basal membrane known as the SSC niche.[320] The niche may be defined as a space limited by somatic cells (Sertoli cells) and basal membrane. The number of SSCs and niches is determined by the Sertoli cells.[321] The niches are preferably located in those segments of seminiferous tubules that line the small intertubular spaces between three or four seminiferous tubules that frequently contain small blood vessels and Leydig cells. In contrast, the spermatogonia in differentiation reside along the basal membrane, where seminiferous tubules are in contact with each other (Fig. 12.35).

Sertoli cells, Leydig cells, myoid cells, macrophages, and endothelial cells with several growth and transcription factors participate, either directly or indirectly, in regulation of self-renewal or

requires different molecules such as SCF, bone morphogenetic protein 4, and retinoic acid. Sertoli cells also regulate germ cell apoptosis. Approximately one-half of spermatogonia in differentiation undergo apoptosis. Dead cells are degraded by Sertoli cells and then recycled.[313] Regulation of apoptosis occurs by production of Fas-ligand, which binds to its receptor (APO-1, CD95) in germ cell plasma membranes. In addition, Sertoli cells possess receptors for several factors such as the nerve growth factor produced by spermatocytes and young spermatids, underscoring the complexity of the Sertoli cell–germ cell relationship. Sertoli cells also produce steroid hormones (estradiol and testosterone) and several components of the seminiferous tubule wall, including laminin, type IV collagen, and heparin sulfate–rich proteoglycans.

Germ Cells

Germ cells of the adult testis include spermatogonia, primary and secondary spermatocytes, and spermatids (Fig. 12.29).

Spermatogonia. There are two types of spermatogonia: A and B. Type A spermatogonia are approximately 12 μm in diameter, rest on the basal lamina, and are surrounded by the cytoplasm

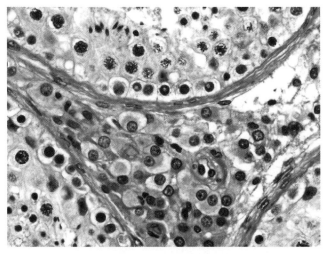

Fig. 12.35 Leydig cells may be observed in the space among three seminiferous tubules. Seminiferous tubules show numerous type A spermatogonia in the center and type B spermatogonia in the peripheral areas.

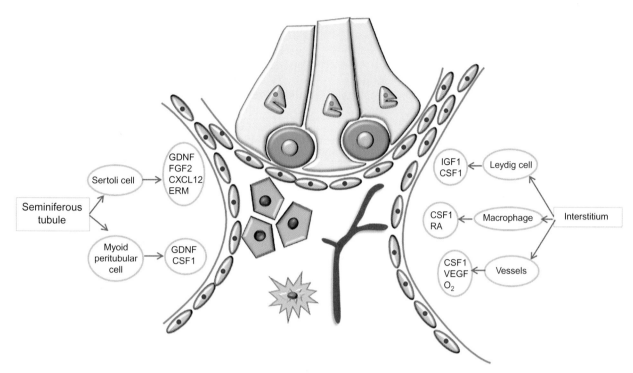

Fig. 12.36 Regulation of proliferation, self-renewal, and expansion of spermatogonial stem cells. *GDNF,* glial cell line–derived neurotropic; *FGF2,* fibroblast growth factor 2; *CXCL12,* C-X-C motif chemokine ligand 12; *ERM,* ezrin-radixin-moesin protein family; *CSF1,* colony-stimulating factor 1; *IGF1,* Insulin like growth factor 1; *VEGF,* Vascular Endothelial Growth Factor.

differentiation of spermatogonia. The best-known growth factors are glial cell line–derived neurotropic factor (GDNF), FGF2, SCF, activin A, bone morphogenic protein 4 (BMP4), and colony-stimulating factor 1 (CSF1). GDNF and FGF2 are secreted by Sertoli cells, and CSF1 is secreted by Leydig cells, myoid cells, macrophages, and endothelial cells. Different factors regulate proliferation, self-renewal, and expansion of SSCs.[322] Among transcription factors, the following have similar actions: Bcl6c, Etv5, and Lhx1 dependent on GDNF, Taf4b (TATA box-binding protein-associated factor 4b), and Plzf. Activin A, SCF, and BMP4, produced by Sertoli cells, seem to be involved in stem cell differentiation (Fig. 12.36).[323] Each step in differentiation of spermatogonia, including formation of spermatocytes and spermatids, is regulated by the microenvironment.

Spermatocytes. *Primary spermatocytes* at interphase of the cell cycle lose contact with the basal lamina and inhabit cavities formed by the Sertoli cell cytoplasm. Their cytoplasm contains more rough endoplasmic reticulum than that of spermatogonia, and the Golgi complexes are more developed.[324] Meiotic primary spermatocytes are tetraploid and are readily identified by their chromatin pattern. The leptotene spermatocyte, with filamentous chromatin, leaves the basal compartment and migrates first to an intermediate compartment and then to the adluminal compartment.[325] In the zygotene spermatocyte, chromosomes are shorter, and pairing of homologous chromosomes begins. Ultrastructural studies show coarse chromatin masses in which synaptonemal complexes and sex pairs may be present. Nucleoli acquire a peculiar pattern of segregation of the fibrillar and granular portions. Associated with nucleoli are the round bodies that contain proteins but no nucleic acids.[314] In pachytene spermatocytes, homologous chromosomes are completely paired, and ultrastructurally show chromatin masses that are larger and less numerous than in zygotene spermatocytes. In diplotene spermatocytes, the larger spermatocytes, paired

homologous chromosomes begin to separate and remain joined by the points of interchange (chiasmata); neither synaptonemal complexes nor sex pairs are observed. Diakinesis spermatocytes show maximal chromosome shortening, and the chiasmata begin to resolve by displacement toward the chromosomal ends. Nuclear envelopes and nucleoli disintegrate. The spermatocytes complete the other phases of the first meiotic division (metaphase, anaphase, and telophase), thus forming two secondary spermatocytes; the first meiotic division lasts 24 days.[326] Prophase of the first division usually lasts from 1 to 3 weeks, whereas the remaining phases of the first meiotic division occur in less than 2 days.

Secondary spermatocytes are haploid cells, smaller than primary spermatocytes, and contain coarse chromatin granules and abundant rough endoplasmic reticulum cisternae.[327] These cells rapidly undergo second meiotic division and within 8 hours give rise to two spermatids. The newly formed spermatids have smaller nuclei with homogeneously distributed chromatin, unlike secondary spermatocytes.

Spermiogenesis. Transformation of spermatids into spermatozoa is called spermiogenesis. During this process pronounced changes occur in the nuclei and the cytoplasm.[328] Nuclei become progressively darker and elongate, and chromatin is rearranged before it becomes completely condensed.[329,330] The cytoplasm develops the acrosome and flagellum, mitochondria cluster around the first portion of the spermatozoon tail, and the remaining cytoplasm is phagocytized by Sertoli cells.[299,331,332] By electron microscopy, four transient stages of spermatid development are seen: Golgi, cap, acrosome, and maturation. These stages correspond to those defined by light microscopy of nuclear morphology: Sa, Sb, Sb$_1$, Sb$_2$, Sc, Sd$_1$, and Sd$_2$.[333,334] These phases may be grouped as early (or round) spermatids that comprise the stages with round nuclei (Sa + Sb) and as late (or elongate) spermatids that comprise the stages with elongate nuclei (Sc + Sd). Mature spermatids (Sd$_2$) are the spermatozoa released into the tubular lumens (spermiation). The presence of spermatids and phagocytosis of their residual bodies stimulates the Sertoli cells to initiate a new cycle of the seminiferous epithelium and to produce tubular fluid, inhibin, ABP, IL1, and IL6.[335,336] All germ cells derived from the same stem cell remain interconnected by cytoplasmic bridges to ensure synchronous maturation during the spermatogenic process.[337]

Cycle of the Seminiferous Epithelium. At first glance the germ cells in the seminiferous tubules appears disordered. However, closer study reveals that these cells are grouped into six successive steps, designated I to VI. In contrast with other mammals, in humans the volume occupied by each step is small, so several steps may be observed in the same tubular cross section. Stereologic studies have shown that the successive steps are organized helically along the length of the seminiferous tubule.[269,337–339] Each association persists for a specific number of days (I, 4.8 days; II, 3.1 days; III, 1 day; IV, 1.2 days; V, 5 days; and VI, 0.8 days), and each successively transforms into the following association. Finally, at the end of step VI, the cycle is repeated; the spermatogenic process requires several cycles.[340] The time from initiation of spermatogenesis to the appearance of sperm in the ejaculate is only 64 days, instead of 74 days, as was formerly believed (Fig. 12.37).[325,326,341,342]

The succession of different steps probably depends on cyclic Sertoli cell activity. Cyclic changes in the mitochondria, rough endoplasmic reticulum, Golgi complexes, lysosomes, and lipid droplets have been reported.[297,343,344] This cyclic activity is probably regulated by numerous factors, both intrinsic (Sertoli and germ cells) and extrinsic (androgens and retinoic acids).[345,346]

The efficiency of spermatogenesis (daily sperm production per gram of parenchyma) in humans is only 25% to 35% of that found in most species, including other primates, and is no more than 3 to 7 million per gram of testis per 24 hours. Germ cell degeneration at the end of meiosis is important.[347,348] The ratio of spermatids to primary spermatocytes is 2.45:1 instead of the expected 4:1 because of a high degree of spontaneous apoptosis, which mainly

affects primary spermatocytes but also involves spermatogonia and spermatids.[349] When spermatogenesis is defective, the number of stages that may be observed in the same cross-sectioned tubule decreases.

Tunica Propria

The seminiferous tubules are surrounded by a 6-μm-thick lamina propria (tunica propria) consisting of a basement membrane, myofibroblasts (peritubular myoid cells), fibroblasts, collagen and elastic fibers, and extracellular matrix.[218,350] The basement membrane measures 100 to 200 nm in thickness and has three layers: the lamina lucida (beneath the Sertoli cells), lamina densa (basal lamina), and lamina reticularis (a discontinuous layer containing fibers). The basal lamina contains laminin, type IV collagen, entactin (nidogen), and heparan sulfate.[351] External to the basal lamina are five to seven discontinuous layers of flat elongate peritubular cells.[352] The two outer layers are formed by fibroblasts and the remainder by peritubular myoid cells.[353]

Peritubular myoid cells, also known as myofibroblasts, form three or five innermost layers of the tubular walls. Ultrastructurally these cells have numerous actin and myosin-immunoreactive filaments, dense plaques, an abundance of free ribosomes, small mitochondria, and poorly developed rough endoplasmic reticulum and Golgi complexes. Peripheral borders of myofibroblasts are divided into laminar prolongations arranged in two planes. Myofibroblasts express ARs, smooth muscle cell antigens (smooth muscle actin, α-actin, desmin, GB-42, and myosin) (Fig. 12.38), and fibroblast antigens (vimentin, fibroblast surface protein).[302,354] The cells are contractile and secretory, facilitating rhythmic tubular contractions that propel spermatozoa toward the rete testis.[355–357] They also synthesize numerous products, including those involved in paracrine regulation of Sertoli cells such as PModS (peritubular modifies Sertoli) that modulates the secretion of ABP, transferrin, inhibin, IGF1, bFGF, and many interleukins. Others such as GDNF and CSF1 are involved in regulation of SSC renewal. Finally, myoid cells contribute to formation of tubular walls, secreting fibronectin, collagens, proteoglycans and entactin, and

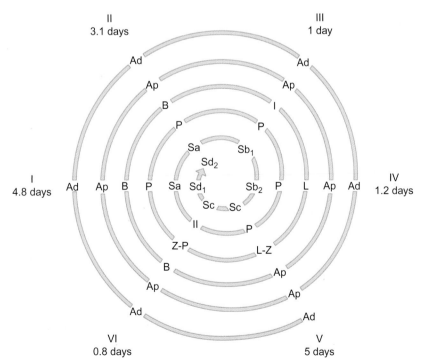

Fig. 12.37 The six different germ cell associations of the seminiferous tubules and the sequence of spermatogenesis. Completion of spermatogenesis requires more than four cycles and lasts for approximately 64 days. Each association is indicated by Roman numerals with its corresponding duration. *Ad,* Dark type of A spermatogonia; *Ap,* pale type of a spermatogonia; *B,* B spermatogonia; *I,* interphase primary spermatocyte; *II,* secondary spermatocyte (only in stage VI); *L,* leptotene primary spermatocyte; *P,* pachytene primary spermatocyte; *Z,* zygotene primary spermatocyte. Sa, Sb1, Sb2, Sc, Sd1, and Sd2 represent the progressive stages of spermatid differentiation into spermatozoa.

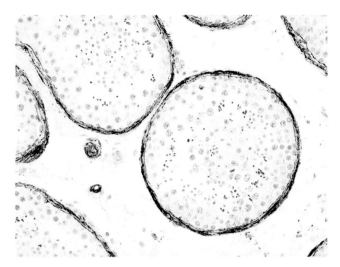

Fig. 12.38 The three to five layers of myofibroblasts surrounding seminiferous tubules show intense immunostaining for muscle-specific actin.

TABLE 12.8	Major Peritubular Myoid Cell Secretory Products and Target Structures	
Products	**Functions/Characteristics**	
Paracrine Regulation of Sertoli Cells		
P-mod-S	Modulate ABP, transferrin, and inhibin secretion	
IGF1, βFGF, several interleukins	Regulate multiple functions	
Plasminogen activator inhibitor	Inhibition of plasminogen activator activity	
Niche		
CDNF and CDF1	Self-renewal of spermatogonia stem cells	
Tubular Wall Formation		
Fibronectin, collagen I, proteoglycans, and entactin	Extracellular matrix component	
Angiogenic (VEGF-C) and antiangiogenic (PEDF) factors	Prevent seminiferous tubule vascularization	

ABP, Androgen-binding protein; *EGF*, epidermal growth factor; *IGF1*, insulin-like growth factor; *P-mod-S*, protein modulating Sertoli cell; *TGF*, transforming growth factor; *βFGF*, Fibroblast growth factor; *CDNF*, Cerebral dopamine neurotrophic factor; *CDF1*, Cycling DOF factor 1; *VEGF-C*, Vascular endothelial growth factor; *PEDF*, Pigment epithelium-derived factor.

angiogenic factors such as vascular endothelial growth factor-C and antiangiogenic pigment epithelium-derived factor involved in the avascularity of the seminiferous tubules (Table 12.8).[358,359]

Most functions of peritubular cells are under androgenic control. Contractile function is regulated by angiotensin II activin via type angiotensin receptor, oxytocin, PDGF, neurotransmitters, and prostaglandins.[360–363] Tumor necrosis factor-α strongly upregulates production of proinflammatory interleukins.[364]

Fibroblasts in the two outermost layers lack desmin filaments and have less actin and myosin than the myofibroblasts.[354] Two types of fiber may be found: collagen and elastic fibers. Collagen fibers are present among the peritubular cells and are abundant between the basal lamina and the peritubular cells. Elastic fibers are located mainly at the periphery of peritubular cells. Elastic fibers appear at puberty, so their absence in adults is a sign of tubular immaturity or dysgenesis.[365] In addition, the tubular walls may

contain capillaries and Leydig cells. These cells are similar to interstitial Leydig cells and are referred to as peritubular Leydig cells.

Testicular Interstitium

The interstitium between the seminiferous tubules contains Leydig cells, macrophages, neuron-like cells, mast cells, blood vessels, lymphatic vessels, and nerves, accounting for 12% to 20% of testicular volume.[366]

Connective Tissue Cells

The most numerous connective tissue cells are fibroblasts and myofibroblasts. Fibroblasts are also known as interstitial dendritic cells or CD34+ stromal cells. They display a network around the seminiferous tubules and Leydig cells, and form the outermost layers of the tubular wall (Fig. 12.39).[367] This distribution begins in fetal life. Some of these cells are in contact with typical macrophages, so it has been suggested that they may be involved in immune surveillance. Myofibroblasts, in addition to their presence in the inner layer of the tubular wall, are numerous in the tunica albuginea.

Leydig Cells

Leydig cells are distributed singly or in clusters, comprising approximately 3.8% of testicular volume.[368,369] Most are in the interstitium, although they may also be found in ectopic locations such as inside the tubular tunica propria, mediastinum testis, tunica albuginea, epididymis, and spermatic cord. Extratesticular Leydig cells are usually seen within or near nerve trunks.[368,370–372]

Leydig cells have spherical eccentric nuclei with one or two eccentric nucleoli and prominent nuclear lamina. The cytoplasm is abundant and eosinophilic, containing lipid droplets and lipofuscin granules (residual bodies) (Fig. 12.40). Reinke crystalloids are found only in adults. Although it was formerly believed that these crystals were present exclusively in humans, they have also been observed in the wild bush rat. Reinke crystalloids dissolve completely in formalin and partially in alcohol. They stain with anti–3β-HSD antibodies.[373] Reinke crystalloids are rodlike, up to 20 μm long and 2 to 3 μm wide, consisting of a complicated meshwork of 5-nm filaments with a trigonal lattice arrangement. Depending on the plane of section, three basic aspects of this lattice may be discerned. Frequently the crystalloids display pale lines,

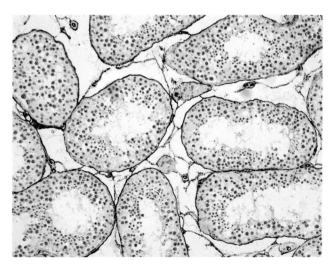

Fig. 12.39 A network of CD34+ stromal cells forms the frame of testicular interstitium surrounding seminiferous tubules, Leydig cell groups, and blood vessels.

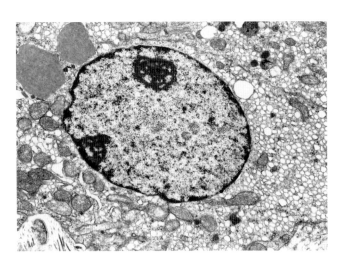

Fig. 12.40 Leydig cells with round nuclei, abundant smooth endoplasmic reticulum, mitochondria with tubular cristae, and Reinke crystalloids.

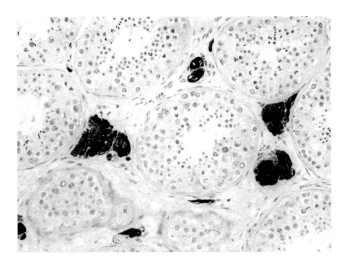

Fig. 12.41 Leydig cells form small intertubular clusters that are immunostained for calretinin.

considered to be potential planes of cleavage. The filaments are grouped into 19-nm-wide hexagons visible on cross section. Some areas have aggregates of electron-dense, rod-shaped structures. Leydig cells may harbor other types of paracrystalline inclusions, the most common of which are multiple parallel-folded laminae.[374]

Leydig cells contain abundant, well-developed smooth endoplasmic reticulum, pleomorphic mitochondria with tubular cristae, numerous lysosomes, and peroxisomes. Marked morphologic changes in Leydig cells occur during the six stages of the seminiferous epithelium cycle.[375]

Leydig cells in the adult originate at puberty from fibroblast-like precursor cells under LH stimulation.[82,376] Studies in adult rats reveal that Leydig cells originate from peritubular cells, vascular smooth muscle cells, and blood capillary pericytes.[377,378] Leydig cell precursors resemble nervous system stem cells because of their expression of nestin and some neuron and glial cells features.[379] Adult Leydig cells infrequently undergo mitosis.[380] The human testis contains approximately 200 million Leydig cells. This number decreases with age; the testes of 60-year-old men contain approximately one-half as many Leydig cells as do those of 20-year-old men.[381,382] Leydig cells in aging men often show cytoplasmic hypertrophy to balance the loss in number, and some of these cells are giant and multinucleate.[382] Lipids and lipofuscin increase progressively. Testosterone production is maintained at normal levels up to the end of the fifth decade because of the high number of persistent Leydig cells.[383] Most elderly men have increased LH levels, but only 22% have low testosterone levels.[384]

Leydig cells comprise a specialized population of cells with endocrine, neuroendocrine, and paracrine functions.[385] They are immunoreactive for LHRs, 3β-HSD, relaxin-like factor, inhibin, and ghrelin.[93,386,386a] Relaxin-like factor, more commonly known as INSL3, is a peptide involved in testicular descent that may be found in serum.[387] Its concentration is a marker of Leydig cell functional status.[388] As occurs with testosterone, INSL3 production is associated with LH.[389a] Leydig cells are immunoreactive for calretinin, a 29-kDa calcium-binding protein that has a buffering effect to avoid abnormal increase in intracellular calcium.[389] Calretinin is a more sensitive, albeit less specific, marker than inhibin (Fig. 12.41).[390] Leydig cells also contain VEGF and its two receptors (Flt-1 and KDR) and endothelin and its two receptors (α and β). VEGF and endothelin are involved in paracrine and autocrine control of Leydig cells. These cells also contain certain

substances that suggest neuroendocrine function, including oxytocin, proopiomelanocortin, substance P, endorphin, NCAM, and microtubule-associated protein-2 (MAP2). Immunohistochemical studies have demonstrated synaptophysin, chromogranins A and B, neurofilament proteins, neuron-specific enolase, S100 protein, and gliofibrillary acidic protein expression in Leydig cells adjacent to nerves, justifying inclusion in the diffuse endocrine system or paraneuron family.[391–394] Leydig cells are the targets of LH and several paracrine and growth factors produced by Sertoli cells and other cells, including IGF1 (secreted by Sertoli cells and by the Leydig cell itself) that improves Leydig cell response to hCG administration; inhibin and activin, which enhance Leydig cell function; and IL1 (synthetized by Sertoli cells, germ cells, Leydig cells, and macrophages), a stimulant of DNA synthesis in immature Leydig cells. TGFB (produced by Leydig cells and Sertoli cells) is a potent Leydig cell inhibitor. In response to LH stimulation, Leydig cells produce testosterone and other androgens necessary for maintenance of spermatogenesis and many structures of the male genital tract and other tissues of the body (bone, muscle, and skin).[369,383,395,396] Mean daily testosterone production by Leydig cells is 6 to 7 mg, representing more than 95% of the circulating testosterone, reaching levels of intratesticular concentration more than 100 times serum levels.[397] These cells are also the main source of estrogen in adult males.[398] Testosterone influences Sertoli cells either directly or indirectly through the P-mod-S (protein modulating Sertoli cell) factor secreted by peritubular myofibroblasts in the tunica propria.[358,375,399–401a] Nuclear testosterone receptors are found in Sertoli cells, Leydig cells, and peritubular myofibroblasts.[402]

Leydig cells also secrete numerous nonsteroidal factors, including oxytocin, which acts on myofibroblasts and stimulates seminiferous tubule contraction; β endorphin, which inhibits Sertoli cell proliferation and function; and other factors with less certain actions such as angiotensin, proopiomelanocortin-derived peptide, which inhibits Sertoli cell proliferation and function, some other proopiomelanocortin peptides, and α-melanotropic–stimulating hormone (Table 12.9). EGF is secreted in the testes mainly by Leydig cells, modulating spermatogenesis by stimulating germ cell differentiation and reducing spermatogonial proliferation. EGF is also an autocrine regulator of Leydig cells.[385] Together with Sertoli cells, peritubular cells, and endothelial cells, Leydig cells produce Nitrous oxide (NO), which has a relaxing effect on smooth muscle

TABLE 12.9   Major Leydig Cell Secretory Products

Products	Functions/Characteristics
Androgens	Steroid hormone/endocrine-paracrine agent
Estrogens	Steroid hormone/endocrine-paracrine agent
Insulin-like growth factor 3 (INSL3)	Maintenance growth/differentiation Self-renewal of spermatogonia stem cells
Colony-stimulating factor 1 (CSF1)	Self-renewal of spermatogonia stem cells
Proopiomelanocortin peptides	Opiates/proopiomelanocortin regulatory agents

of seminiferous tubules and blood vessels, thus regulating spermatozoon transport and testicular blood flow, respectively.[403]

Leydig cells are spatially related to adrenergic and cholinergic nerve fibers.[201] Varicosities containing synaptic vesicles have been found near Leydig cells, and nerves that end on Leydig cells have been identified. The functional meaning of this innervation is unknown.[404]

Macrophages, Neuron-like Cells, and Mast Cells

Macrophages are a normal component of the testis.[405,406] Young adult men have one macrophage per 10 to 50 Leydig cells, and this number increases with age.[407] They are classified by phenotype into two groups: resident (M2 macrophages), which are the most numerous, and activated (M1 macrophages). Both express CD68, but only resident macrophages express CD163.[408] Resident macrophages appear in the testis early in development, present in the urogenital ridges, and are believed to be derived from fetal yolk sac progenitors.[46] Activated macrophages are likely derived from circulating monocytes.

Macrophages help maintain normal testicular function and homeostasis, including interaction with Leydig cells. Slender Leydig cell cytoplasmic expansions penetrate deep into the cytoplasm of the macrophages.[405] One of the factors that favorably influence steroidogenesis in Leydig cells is 25-hydroxycholesterol.[409,410] Macrophages regulate spermatogenesis through CSF1 and enzymes involved in the synthesis of retinoic acid, and participate in proliferation and differentiation of Leydig cell fibroblastic precursors and in the proliferative activity of newly formed cells.[411] Activated macrophages secrete abundant antiinflammatory cytokine IL10, and produce IL1 and IL6, tumor necrosis factor-α, and TGFA, which is important in the control of bacterial infections.[412,413]

Immunohistochemistry has revealed the presence of fusiform or star-shaped cells known as *neuron-like cells* in the interstitium. Their number is low in adult testes.[414] These cells express neuron-specific intermediate filament NF-200, voltage-activated sodium (Na) channel, and intratesticular catecholamines, which appear to be increased in some disorders such as Sertoli cell–only syndrome and hypospermatogenesis.

Mast cells are a normal finding in the interstitium, in peritubular and perivascular locations, among Leydig cells, and inside interlobular septa and the tunica vasculosa.[415,415a] The number decreases with age, and this change seems not to be influenced by Sertoli Growth Factor (SGF) produced by Sertoli cells. The main product of mast cells is tryptase. Among mast cell functions, participation in intercellular matrix formation may be fundamental.[414] The number of mast cells increases in several diseases, and it is greatly increased in patients with nonobstructive azoospermia.[416–418]

Blood and Lymphatic Vessels

The testis is supplied by the testicular artery, which arises from the abdominal aorta. In the spermatic cord the testicular artery gives rise to two or three branches that obliquely penetrate the tunica albuginea, spawning multiple branches that run along the intralobular septa of the testis.[419,420] These centripetal arteries lead to the mediastinum testis. Along their course the centripetal arteries give off branches that abruptly reverse direction, the so-called centrifugal arteries. At puberty, both the centripetal and centrifugal arteries develop pronounced spiral architecture.[421,422] The centrifugal arteries develop additional branches in the interstitium that give rise to arterioles and capillaries that form intertubular plexuses, some of which are apposed to the tunica propria.[423,424] Capillaries are of the continuous type, except for the seminiferous tubule capillaries, which are partially fenestrated, and their endothelial cells are similar to those of brain capillaries, with scant pinocytosis, intercellular junctions of the fascia adherens type, and low permeability.[425] The mediastinum testis is poorly vascularized.

The inner two-thirds of the testicular parenchyma is drained by veins that follow the interlobular septa to the mediastinum testis (centripetal veins). The outer one-third is drained by veins that lead to the tunica albuginea (centrifugal veins). Both centripetal and centrifugal veins join and anastomose, exiting the testis by the veins of the pampiniform plexus, which drains the testis via the spermatic cord.

Lymphatic vessels are poorly developed in the testis and are limited to the tunica vasculosa, interlobular septa, and mediastinum, where they accompany arterioles and venules.[426] Prelymphatic vessels have been reported in the interstitium and probably drain interstitial fluid into the true interlobular lymphatic vessels.

Nerves

Efferent innervation of the testis is mainly supplied by neurons of the pelvic ganglia, where contralateral and bilateral neural connections occur. Postganglionic nerve fibers enter the testis via the pelvic nerves, extend throughout the tunica vasculosa, and follow the interlobular septa to reach the interstitium. These nerve fibers end in the walls of arterioles, the walls of seminiferous tubules, and the Leydig cells.[190] Adrenergic nerve fibers innervate the tunica albuginea and blood vessels of the tunica vasculosa, but do not enter the testicular parenchyma.[427,428] Most nerve fibers are peptidergic.[429] Afferent nerve endings form corpuscles like those of Meissner and Pacini in the tunica albuginea.

In summary, testicular histology may be understood only by considering the different autocrine, endocrine, and paracrine relationships that occur among the different cells of the testicular parenchyma. Only in that way may we understand the complex processes of cellular interrelation that take place in spermatogenesis and that culminate in spermatozoon production with adequate morphology, vitality, and fertilizing capacity.

Rete Testis

The rete testis is a network of channels and cavities that connects the seminiferous tubules with the ductuli efferentes. Differences in the configuration and size of channels and cavities distinguish three

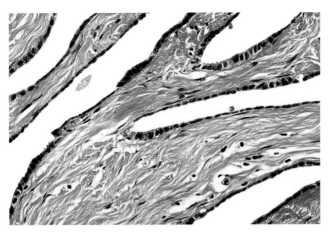

Fig. 12.42 Rete testis showing cavities lined by flat squamous epithelium interspersed with small groups of columnar cells, which are usually located in angles. Connective tissue among cavities is dense.

portions of the rete testis: septal (intralobular), composed of the tubuli recti; mediastinal, composed of a network of interconnected channels; and extratesticular, composed of dilated cavities (≤3 mm in diameter) termed the *bullae retis*.

The tubuli recti are short tubules (0.5 to 1 mm long) that connect the seminiferous tubules to the mediastinal rete, although some seminiferous tubules, principally those in the central region of the testis, may connect directly to the mediastinal rete. The tubuli recti are lined by cuboidal epithelium. There are approximately 1500 tubuli recti (or their analogous seminiferous tubule segments). The tubuli recti in the cranial, central, and anterior testis are perpendicular to the mediastinal rete testis channel into which they drain, and those in the caudal testicular region are parallel to their respective channels. The transitional segments between the seminiferous tubules and the tubuli recti are formed by modified Sertoli cells.[430]

The epithelium of the mediastinal rete testis consists of flattened cells interspersed with small areas of columnar cells (Fig. 12.42). Both cell types have a single centrally located cilium and numerous microvilli on their free surfaces and contain keratin and vimentin filaments.[431] Interdigitations are present between adjacent cells. The epithelium rests on a basal lamina surrounded by a layer of myofibroblasts and a rim of fibroblasts and collagen and elastic fibers.

The rete channels and cavities are traversed by the chordae rete, columns 15 to 100 μm long and 5 to 40 μm wide, arranged obliquely to the long axis of the cavity. The chordae rete consists of fibrous connective tissue and fibroblasts covered by flattened epithelium. The rete testis probably has the following functions: damping of differences in pressure between the seminiferous tubules and the ductuli efferentes; reabsorption of protein and potassium from tubular fluid; and, occasionally, phagocytosis of spermatozoa.

Congenital Anomalies of the Testis

Alterations in Number, Size, and Location

Anorchidism

Anorchidism refers to absence of one (monorchidism) or both testes (testicular regression syndrome). Unilateral anorchidism may present as true congenital testicular absence or vanishing testis. Monorchidism is estimated to occur in approximately 4.5% of cryptorchid testes, in 40% of the testes that are impalpable on physical examination, and in 1 in 5000 males. Bilateral anorchidism occurs in approximately 1 in 20,000 males.[432–435] Evaluation of a child with a solitary palpable testis begins with scrotal palpation. Laparoscopy is required for patients in whom no apparent testicular nubbin tissue is found in the scrotum or for those with a patent vaginal processus.[436]

Monorchidism

The hormonal pattern in prepubertal patients with monorchidism is similar to that of normal children, whereas children lacking both testes have undetectable levels of AMH and elevated levels of gonadotropins that fail to respond to stimulation with hCG even in the first months of postnatal life.[78,435,437–442] Although hCG stimulation challenge is often positive in children with bilateral cryptorchidism, it is negative in some children with bilateral intraabdominal cryptorchidism, further complicating the differential diagnostic separation of anorchidism and cryptorchidism.[443] Exceptionally, anorchidism may be associated with hypogonadotropic hypogonadism.

For unknown reasons the left testis is more frequently absent (69%) than the right. In such cases the contralateral scrotal testis undergoes compensatory hypertrophy, and its volume increases to more than 2 mL.[444] Compensatory hypertrophy has also been reported in association with abdominal cryptorchid testis.[231]

The absence of testicular parenchyma should be confirmed before diagnosing monorchidism. Laparoscopy has been proposed as the usual procedure to localize a nonpalpable or absent testis.[445] At exploration the finding of a vas deferens ending near or in a hypoplastic epididymis is not sufficient for the diagnosis of monorchidism. The only acceptable finding is blind-ending spermatic vessels. If inguinoscrotal exploration fails to identify these vessels, intraabdominal exploration is required to exclude undescended testis and avoid development of a testicular tumor.[446] All remnants found at exploration should be removed.[447]

Testicular Regression Syndrome

Testicular regression syndrome refers to a variety of conditions, including agonadism, anorchidism, testicular agenesis, rudimentary testes, hypoplastic testes, and embryonal testicular dysgenesis.[448–450] Each syndrome shares complete absence or involution of both testes, but they differ in the time of testicular disappearance during development.[451] The most frequently observed are Swyer syndrome (see discussion of Disorders of sex development (Gonadal dysgenesis)), true agonadism, rudimentary testes, bilateral anorchidism, vanishing testes syndrome, and Leydig cell–only syndrome (Table 12.10).

True Agonadism (46,XY Gonadal Agenesis Syndrome). Patients are phenotypically girls, and the male gender may be discovered only at the time of referral for other symptoms such as primary amenorrhea.[452,453] External genitalia are female with or without clitoromegaly, labioscrotal fusion, and short vagina. Examination of the internal genitalia demonstrates the absence of müllerian and wolffian derivatives, although the presence of uterine and uterine fallopian hypoplasia may occur. No gonads (not even in an ectopic location) are found. Early testicular regression occurs between the seventh and eighth weeks of embryonal development, just after the onset of AMH secretion.

Sporadic and familial cases are both with associated extragenital anomalies. In some cases the cause is heterozygous mutation

TABLE 12.10 Testicular Regression Syndromes

| | EMBRYONAL PERIOD | | FETAL PERIOD | | |
	Early	Late	Early	Middle	Late
Müllerian structures	Vestigial	Differentiated	Differentiated/vestigial	Vestigial	Vestigial
Wolffian structures	Vestigial	Vestigial	Vestigial/differentiated	Differentiated	Differentiated
External genitalia	Female	Female	Ambiguous	Ambiguous-male	Male

of *WT1*.[454] In most familial cases, inheritance is either recessive autonomic or X-linked, and the cause seems to be either unknown anomalies in the *WT1* gene or known anomalies in other genes involved in development.[455] SRY molecular defect has never been observed.[456] Agonadism may be associated with several syndromes, including PAGOD (hypoplasia of lungs and pulmonary artery, agonadism, omphalocele/diaphragmatic defect, dextrocardia), Seckel, and CHARGE (ocular coloboma [C], heart disease [H], choanal atresia [A], retarded growth or development [R], genitourinary defects or hypogonadism [G], and ear anomalies or deafness [E]).[457–460]

Rudimentary Testes Syndrome. Patients with rudimentary testes have a normal male phenotype. Müllerian remnants are absent, and wolffian derivatives are usually present.[461] The testes are cryptorchid and small, less than 0.5 cm long. Seminiferous tubules are few in number (Fig. 12.43). Testicular regression occurs between the weeks 14 and 20 of gestation. This syndrome has been reported in several members of the same family, a finding suggesting genetic transmission, but this is not a constant feature.[462–464]

Congenital Bilateral Anorchidism. Congenital bilateral anorchidism is defined as complete absence of testicular tissue in a patient with a normal male karyotype and phenotype.[441] Congenital bilateral anorchidism occurs in 1 in 20,000 newborns.[465–468a] Patients have male external genitalia, but the internal genitalia consists only of normal wolffian derivatives without müllerian derivatives, a finding suggesting that the testes were present and functionally active up to approximately the 20th week of gestation, thus producing sufficient amounts of AMH and

androgens. Patients have male external genitalia with hypoplasia of both the scrotum and penis.[469] The disorder may be associated with other malformations, such as anal atresia, rectourethral and rectovaginal fistula, and urinary exstrophy. Patients diagnosed in adulthood have male phenotype, androgen insufficiency symptoms, and elevated levels of both FSH and LH.[442,470] The cause of congenital bilateral anorchia is uncertain, with numerous hypotheses, including intrauterine torsion of both testes, endocrinologic or immunologic disfunction, or genetic abnormality. The possibility of genetic anomaly was suggested by the occurrence of several familial cases.[471] However, isolated mutations in the *SF1* gene have been identified in only one case to date, and no mutations have been found in the *SRY* gene, the *INSL3* gene (necessary for correct testicular descent), or in the gene of its receptor.[472–475]

The basal plasma concentration of AMH, inhibin B, and testosterone is undetectable in anorchic patients.[476] The increase in testosterone levels after GnRH or hCG administration is low or undetectable.[442,443,477,478] FSH and LH levels are abnormally high during the first months of life and then progressively decrease. LH decreases more rapidly to normal levels than does FSH in 70% of anorchic patients until pubertal age, when gonadotropins increase to high levels.[479] A case of bilateral anorchidism was reported in association with hypogonadotropic hypogonadism in a pubertal patient with Kallmann syndrome.[480]

Vanishing Testes Syndrome. Vanishing testes syndrome applies to disappearance of one or both testes between the last months of intrauterine life and the beginning of puberty.[481–484] Two criteria are required for diagnosis: (1) absence of a palpable testis on examination with the patient under anesthesia; and (2) blind-ending spermatic vessels visualized within the retroperitoneum, or spermatic vessels and vas deferens seen exiting a closed internal inguinal ring. Testicular regression occurs after the seventh month of embryonal life, so exploration finds the vas deferens in the inguinal canal or high in the scrotum; it may be accompanied by the epididymis and less frequently by testicular remnants consisting of small groups of seminiferous tubules (Figs. 12.44 and 12.45). Patients who lack both testes experience hypergonadotropic hypogonadism after puberty, with gynecomastia, infantile phallus, hypoplastic scrotum, and impalpable prostate. The condition is usually secondary to perinatal scrotal torsion, although rarely it has a genetic cause.[436,475,485]

Leydig Cell–Only Syndrome. Patients with Leydig cell–only syndrome have agonadism without eunuchoidism and normal male phenotype, although meticulous surgical exploration fails to find testicular remnants. Study of serial sections from the spermatic cord reveals clusters of Leydig cells.[486] Detection of testosterone in spermatic vein blood indicates that these ectopic Leydig cells are functionally active and synthesize testosterone in amounts sufficient to induce a rudimentary male phenotype but are insufficient to support complete development of secondary sex characteristics.[467]

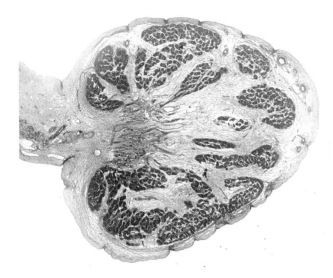

Fig. 12.43 Cross-sectioned rudimentary testis from a 2-year-old infant. Testicular lobules are separated by wide septa and contain scant seminiferous tubules.

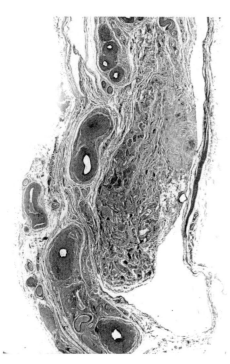

Fig. 12.44 Spermatic cord in anorchidism. Fibrous connective tissue with dystrophic calcification that probably would correspond to the testis adjacent to the distal end of the vas deferens.

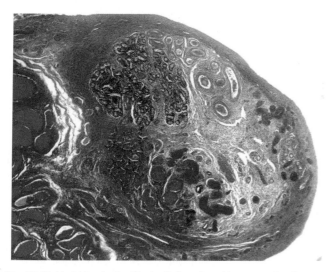

Fig. 12.45 Vanishing testis. The testis is reduced to connective tissue, a small group of seminiferous tubules, the rete testis, numerous blood vessels, and a thickened albuginea.

Macroscopic and histologic findings in patients with testicular absence differ according to the cause of anorchidism (true congenital absence or disappearance of a former testis). In true congenital absence the lack of testis is associated with absence of both the ductus epididymis and ductus deferens. In acquired testicular absence, the morphology of spermatic cord remnants is similar to monorchidism and testicular regression syndrome occurring after the 20th week of gestation.[487–490] The ductus deferens, testicular artery, and a venous plexus may usually be identified in spermatic cord sections.[491] Grossly, a small, firm mass is found at the end of the spermatic cord (Fig. 12.44). Histologic examination reveals vas deferens, epididymis, or small groups of seminiferous tubules in 69% to 83% of cases.[492] Vas deferens is the most constant finding (79%), followed by epididymis (36%) and seminiferous tubules (0% to 20%).[447,493–496] These tubules may or may not contain germ cells.[497–499] Small vessel groups are present in 83% of patients, but in only 24% is the number of vessels sufficient to identify them as spermatic vessels. Blind-ending cord structures have been found in the abdomen (21% of cases), the inguinal canal (59%), the superficial inguinal ring (18%), and the scrotum (2%).[500]

Areas of dystrophic calcification, hemosiderin deposition (Fig. 12.46), and giant cell reaction may be found within the mass in place of the testis. Other reported findings include arterial and venous vessels (88%), fat (44%), and nerves that may resemble traumatic neuroma (56%).[501]

The minimum requirement for diagnosis is identification of either a vascularized fibrous nodule with calcification or hemosiderin, or a fibrous nodule with cord elements.[502]

There are few histologic studies of evanescent testes removed in adulthood that refer to residual testicular parenchyma. In three cases from our files, we have not observed areas of calcification or macrophages with hemosiderin. All contained tubules with complete spermatogenesis mixed with Sertoli cell–only tubules with dysgenetic characteristics (mixed atrophy [MAT]); the interstitium had significant Leydig cell hyperplasia (Figs. 12.47 and 12.48). No GCNIS cells were observed.

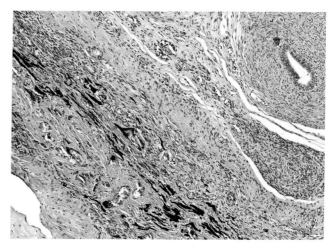

Fig. 12.46 Next to the vas deferens, fibrous tissue with numerous macrophages with hemosiderin may be observed where the testis should have been.

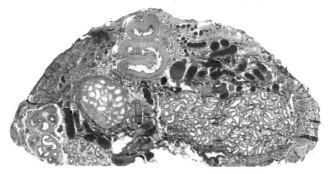

Fig. 12.47 Vanishing testis in an adult. The central nodular formation corresponds to the testis. It is surrounded by the body and tail of the epididymis. In the upper part the onset of the vas deferens may be observed.

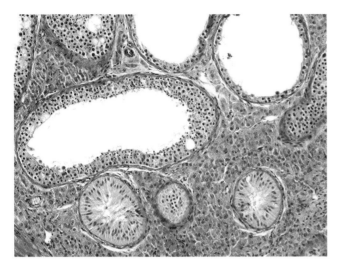

Fig. 12.48 Vanishing testis (same case as Fig. 12.47). Testicular parenchyma shows mixed atrophy. Tubules with spermatogenesis have marked ectasia, and the remaining only Sertoli cells. Note also a diffuse hyperplasia of Leydig cells.

Optimal management of the testicular remnant associated with the vanishing testis syndrome is controversial.[503] Some urologists advocate surgical exploration, either laparoscopic or through an inguinal scrotal approach, whereas others believe these procedures are unnecessary based on the low percentage (21%) of seminiferous tubules found in the removed testicular nubbins; only 14% contain seminiferous tubules with germ cells, and thus the probability of a tumor is minimal.[493,496,498] Only one case of GCNIS has been reported.[497] Thus some authors defend conservative management, whereas others believe that these remnants should be removed, given the potential for malignant degeneration.[493,496,498,504]

Most cases of unilateral and bilateral testicular loss apparently occur during the fetal period after the testis has inhibited the müllerian ducts and induced differentiation of wolffian duct derivatives, or else postnatally. Two hypotheses account for the disappearance of the testes. The first involves atrophy secondary to a vascular lesion such as thrombosis or intrauterine torsion, trauma, or neonatal scrotal hematoma.[505–508] The presence of macrophages with hemosiderin and dystrophic calcification suggests a vascular event.[469] In addition, the morphology of the contralateral testis is normal. If the disappearance resulted from hormonal influences, the contralateral testis would show abnormalities, as is typical in the contralateral testis in cryptorchidism.[471] The second hypothesis of disappearance invokes a primary anomaly of the gonad such as a true congenital testicular absence, which would be responsible for only 27% of nonpalpable testes. This theory is supported by multiple factors: histologic presence of dysgenetic lesions in the residual testicular parenchyma; absence of evidence of old hemorrhage or ischemia; evidence of disturbance in endothelial development leading to a reduction in vascular formation; and the occasional presence of malformations of the urogenital system, such as absence of the kidney, cystic seminal vesicles, or ipsilateral renal dysgenesis.[509–511]

Microorchidism

The clinical term *microorchidism* refers to diverse conditions characterized by small testicular size, including Klinefelter syndrome, hypogonadotropic hypogonadism, and bilateral cryptorchidism.[512,513] In adulthood, microorchidism refers to testes with a volume ≤ 12 mL. Patients with microorchidism are candidates for genetic or hormonal studies to identify the underlying disease or syndrome. For example, some patients with Kenny-Caffey syndrome exhibit short stature, cortical thickening and medullary stenosis of long bones, delayed closure of anterior fontanelles, hypoparathyroidism, and ocular abnormalities. FSH serum level is elevated in some cases, whereas LH and testosterone levels are normal. Adult testes are small, with seminiferous tubules showing complete but diminished spermatogenesis. Leydig cells are hyperplastic. Unlike patients with the rudimentary testes syndrome, a patient with microorchidism has a normal-sized penis and no epididymal or prostatic atrophy.[514]

The most frequent causes of adult microorchidism are Klinefelter syndrome, testicular maldescent, varicocele, secondary atrophy, and other idiopathic clinical disorders. Most patients have azoospermia or oligoasthenoteratozoospermia.[515]

Polyorchidism

Polyorchidism refers to congenital presence of more than two testes. It is a rare condition, with slightly more than 200 reported cases.[516,517] The first histologic description appeared in 1880, and the first case treated surgically and confirmed histologically was reported in 1895.[518,519] Although the existence of three testes is the most common presentation, four testes have been reported in 10 patients, and five testes in one case report that lacked histologic confirmation.[520–532] The age at diagnosis varies from newborn to 74 years, with a mean of 17 years. Most patients are phenotypically similar to persons of their age. With the exception of isolated cases with 46,XX karyotype with XY mosaicism and deletion of the long arm of chromosome 21, patients typically do not have chromosomal abnormalities. Testicular duplication is usually an incidental finding during surgery for inguinal hernia, cryptorchidism, or testicular torsion, but has also been detected in patients with infertility or unexplained fertility after bilateral vasectomy.[533–535] The extra testis is often intrascrotal (75%) and less frequently inguinal (20%), abdominal, or retroperitoneal (5%).[536–540] Duplication is three times more frequent on the left side than on the right.[541] Testicular maldescent (40%), inguinal hernia (30%), hydrocele (9%), varicocele, and contralateral cryptorchidism are the most frequently associated anomalies.[542–547] Testicular torsion (13%) and testicular cancer (6.4%) are occasional complications.[534,543,548] In isolated cases, imperforate anus, idiopathic infertility, and contralateral anorchidism have been observed.[549–553] High-resolution sonography is indicated, followed by magnetic resonance imaging (MRI) when sonographic findings are inconclusive.[521,554,555]

The extra testis may be histologically normal, but usually is not, containing Sertoli cell–only tubules, hypospermatogenesis, maturation arrest, or microlithiasis.[311,542,556–558] Lack of spermatogenesis has been attributed to the anomalous location of the testis and the absence of communication between the testis and excretory ducts, although in some cases the lesions are probably primary.[557,559]

Embryologic origin of polyorchidism remains uncertain, and the following mechanisms have been proposed to account for the variety of findings in different cases (Fig. 12.49):

- *Duplication of the genital ridge.* All structures of the genital ridge and mesonephric ducts are duplicated. Each of the two testes resulting from duplication has an excretory duct and develops active spermatogenesis.[519,535,560–562]
- *Longitudinal division of the genital ridge.* Of the two resulting testes, the medial loses its connection with the mesonephric ducts and undergoes atrophy.
- *High transverse division of the genital ridge.* The two resulting portions are in continuity with the mesonephric ducts that give

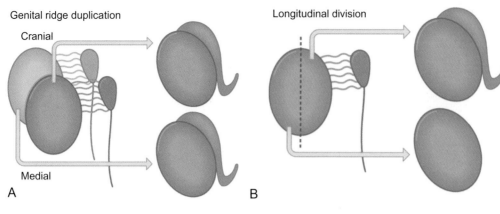

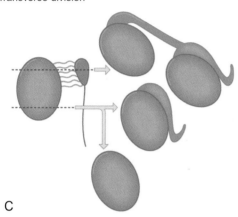

Fig. 12.49 Possible mechanisms of polyorchidism. (A) Genital ridge duplication gives rise to two testes with their respective epididymides. (B) Longitudinal division of the genital ridge. The testis derived from the medial region has no epididymis. (C) Transverse division of the genital ridge. The resulting testes either share a single epididymis or one testis is devoid of epididymis.

rise to the ductuli efferentes. Each testis may have its own ductus epididymidis or shares a common one, but there is a separate vas deferens for each.[557,563]

• *Low transverse division of the genital ridge.* The more caudal testis has no excretory ducts.[544]

Several classifications of polyorchidism have been proposed, including one based on embryology and another on reproductive potential.[564–566] In embryologic classification, type II is the most frequent variation (Table 12.11), and types II and III together comprise more than 90% of cases.[564] This classification does not consider certain isolated cases such as the occurrence of double testes on one side, each connected to their own epididymis and vas

deferens. This finding may be explained embryologically by complete splitting of the genital ridge and entire mesonephros with wolffian duct elements along the dorsoventral line of cleavage. Embryologic classification also fails to consider double testes on one side that are not connected with an epididymis or vas deferens; this anomaly is explained by horizontal splitting of the genital ridge to form the gonad.

In the reproductive potential classification (Table 12.12), type I includes types II, III, and IV of the embryologic classification, but excludes type II and all ectopic testes (types IB and IIB).[565] Supernumerary testis type IA may be excluded if the patient has at least one intrascrotal testis with normal drainage, if the testicular biopsy of the supernumerary testis shows a Sertoli cell–only pattern or malignancy, or if difficulties in patient follow-up are expected.[567]

TABLE 12.11	**Embryologic Classification of Polyorchidism**

Type I: A supernumerary testis lacks an epididymis or vas deferens and has no attachment to the usual testes (division of the genital ridge only).

Type II: The supernumerary testis drains into the epididymis of the usual testis, and they share a common vas deferens (division of genital ridge occurs in the region where the primordial gonads are attached to the metanephric ducts, although the mesonephros and metanephric ducts are not divided; i.e., incomplete division).

Type III: The supernumerary testis has its own epididymis, and both epididymides (that of the supernumerary testis and that of the ipsilateral testis) drain into one vas deferens (complete transverse division of mesonephros, as well as the genital ridge).

Type IV: Complete duplication of the testes, epididymis, and vas deferens (vertical division of the genital ridge and mesonephros).

Data are from Leung AK. Polyorchidism. Am Fam Physician 1988;38:153–156.

TABLE 12.12	**Reproductive Potential Classification of Polyorchidism**

Type I: The accessory testis (supernumerary testis) is attached to the draining epididymis and vas deferens with reproductive potential (30% of polyorchidism).

   Type IA: The accessory testis is intrascrotal.

   Type IB: The accessory testis is in an ectopic location.

Type II: The testis lacks such an attachment and has no reproductive potential.

   Type IIA: The accessory testis is intrascrotal.

   Type IIB: The accessory testis is in an ectopic location.

Data are from Singer BR, Donaldson JG, Jackson DS. Polyorchidism: functional classification and management strategy. Urology 1992;39:384–388.

TABLE 12.13 Modified Reproductive Potential Classification of Polyorchidism

Type A1: The drained supernumerary testis has its own epididymis and vas.
Type A2: The drained supernumerary testis may have its own epididymis but shares a common deferens duct with its neighbor.
Type A3: The drained supernumerary testis may share a common epididymis (and duct) with its neighbor.
Type B1: The undrained supernumerary testis does have its own epididymis.
Type B2: The undrained supernumerary testis does not have its own epididymis and thus consists of testicular tissue only.

Data are from Bergholz R, Koch B, Spieker T, Lohse K. Polyorchidism: a case report and classification. *J Pediatr Surg* 2007;42:1933–1935.

Proposed modification of the reproductive potential classification is shown in Table 12.13.[566]

The clinical differential diagnosis of polyorchidism includes other conditions that enlarge the scrotum and spermatic cords, including spermatocele, hydrocele, cyst and tumor of the spermatic cord, crossed testicular ectopia, adrenal cortical ectopia, and splenogonadal fusion. Orchidectomy has been replaced as treatment of choice for atrophic and nonscrotal testes by fixation of the testis to the scrotal pouch and re-creation of a "simple testis" when permitted by the anatomic condition and after exclusion of malignancy.[568] This treatment may allow spermatogenesis, as well as psychological and cosmetic benefits.[569] Intrascrotal rhabdomyosarcoma, testicular teratoma, and seminoma have been reported in patients with polyorchidism.[570–572]

Testicular Hypertrophy (Macroorchidism)

Macroorchidism may be unilateral or bilateral, and is caused by excessive development of seminiferous tubules, Leydig cells, or both. It may be associated with chromosomal anomalies, tumors, or endocrine alterations. An increase in the testicular parenchyma occurs in several conditions, including congenital Leydig cell hyperplasia, compensatory hypertrophy, benign idiopathic macroorchidism, bilateral megalotestes with low gonadotropins, fragile X chromosome, and testicular hypertrophy observed in juvenile hypothyroidism.[573]

Congenital Leydig Cell Hyperplasia

Congenital Leydig cell hyperplasia is uncommon and may be diffuse or nodular.[544] Diagnosis of diffuse Leydig cell hyperplasia requires quantification of Leydig cells by morphometry using normal newborn testes as controls (Fig. 12.50). Nodular Leydig cell hyperplasia is characterized by the presence of nonencapsulated cellular aggregates in the mediastinum testis, adjacent testicular parenchyma, and connective tissue among the ductuli efferentes (Figs. 12.51 and 12.52).

The differential diagnosis of nodular Leydig cell hyperplasia includes intratesticular adrenal rests and bilateral Leydig cell tumor. Excluding adrenogenital syndrome, intratesticular adrenal rests are rare. Rests are encapsulated, except with adrenogenital tumors, and consist of radially arranged cells with vesicular nuclei and small nucleoli displacing the rete testis or seminiferous tubules. Leydig cell tumors may be bilateral, poorly circumscribed, and surrounded by testicular parenchyma, features making it difficult to distinguish from Leydig cell hyperplasia. However, Leydig cell tumors are rarely congenital, whereas those occurring during infancy often induce precocious maturation of the adjacent seminiferous tubules and early macrogenitosomia.

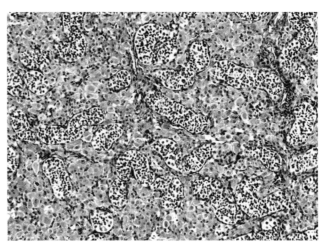

Fig. 12.50 Congenital Leydig cell hyperplasia. Fetal Leydig cells form large clusters surrounding groups of seminiferous tubules.

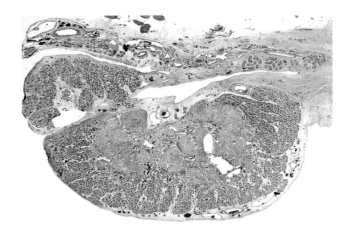

Fig. 12.51 Congenital Leydig cell hyperplasia. Multiple nodules of Leydig cells are present in the mediastinum testis, as well as deep in the parenchyma.

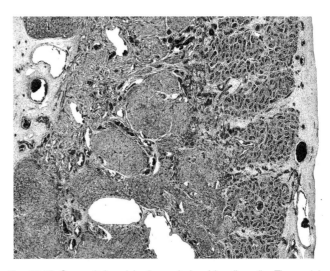

Fig. 12.52 Congenital nodular hyperplasia of Leydig cells. The nodules occupy much of the section. They are located between the rete testis and the scarce peripheral testicular parenchyma.

Congenital Leydig cell hyperplasia is caused by large quantities of hCG entering the fetal circulation.[574] Mothers with diabetes, particularly those with hypertension, may experience development of hyperplacentosis; the resulting edema in the placental villi alters vascular permeability and allows passage of hCG to the fetus. Congenital Leydig cell hyperplasia decreases rapidly during the first months of postnatal life after maternal hCG is gone. Combined diffuse and nodular Leydig cell hyperplasia occurs in several malformative syndromes, including Beckwith-Wiedemann syndrome, leprechaunism, triploid fetuses, and fetuses with Rh isoimmunization, as well as in several complications of pregnancy.[544,545,575,576]

Compensatory Hypertrophy of the Testis

Compensatory hypertrophy may occur in monorchidism, cryptorchidism (Fig. 12.53), and varicocele, as well as after testicular injury.[544,577,578] The disorder is characterized by increased volume of the descended testis, defined as more than two standard deviations of the corresponding size in normal children. A volume greater than 2 mL or even lower is considered to be predictive of monorchidism.[579,580] Compensatory hypertrophy develops between birth and 3 years of age, and the testis may reach a volume twice normal when the other testis is absent.[231] Hypertrophy persists and may increase during childhood and puberty, but ceases thereafter; the hypertrophied testis then becomes normal or remains slightly enlarged.[230,581] The degree of compensatory hypertrophy is determined by three factors: (1) volume of the remaining testicular parenchyma, (2) age at which the underlying pathologic event occurred, and (3) functional ability of the descended testis.[208] Compensatory hypertrophy results from alteration of hypophyseal hormonal feedback, followed by an increase in secretion of FSH, evidence that the hypertrophied testis is normal. In monorchidism, it is likely that the absent testis was initially of normal size during fetal development, but later underwent progressive shrinkage.[433]

When 50% reduction of testicular mass occurs (probably before birth), endocrine feedback changes, and the resulting secretion of FSH (before or immediately after birth) causes accelerated growth of the contralateral testis. The hypertrophied testis contains an increased number of germ cells, explaining why patients with solitary testis may not necessarily be at additional risk for infertility.[582] In cryptorchidism the reduction in overall testicular mass is less pronounced than in monorchidism, and the scrotal testis may also be abnormal, resulting in less marked compensatory hypertrophy.

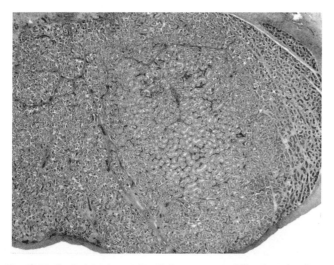

Fig. 12.53 Contralateral scrotal testis from a cryptorchid patient showing a group of large seminiferous tubules that stands out from the surrounding small tubules.

Idiopathic Benign Macroorchidism

Some prepubertal and pubertal patients have pronounced unilateral or bilateral testicular hypertrophy in the absence of other pathologic findings.[583-586] This condition probably results from hormonal receptivity in the testicular parenchyma. Clinical manifestations are usually related to the onset of the puberty.

Several disorders, such as bilateral testicular tumor (germ cell, stromal tumor, leukemia, or lymphoma), adrenal rest tumor, X-linked mental retardation, hypothyroidism, and idiopathic or cerebral precocious puberty, should be excluded before testicular enlargement is diagnosed as idiopathic benign macroorchidism.

Morphometric studies indicate that testicular enlargement results from an increase in length of the seminiferous tubules, although increases in tubular diameter and Sertoli cell number have also been observed. Elevated FSH serum level, reported in some cases, or hyperactive FSH receptors (FSHR) could cause excessive Sertoli cell proliferation and lengthening and thickening of seminiferous tubules.[232,587,588] In addition, Leydig cell hyperplasia and deficient spermatogenesis are frequent findings in adult life. In some cases the underlying mechanism is unclear because the sequential analysis of 10 exons of the FSHR was normal.[589]

The development of the two testes may be asynchronous during puberty, so some cases of unilateral macroorchidism may reveal differences that are unusually exaggerated. This situation is also known as transitory unilateral testis enlargement of puberty. The enlarged testis, usually on the right (75% of cases), may reach 20 mL in volume at the onset of puberty. The contralateral testis grows during puberty until it reaches the same volume as the hypertrophic testis, whereas growth of the hypertrophic testis slows. After puberty neither testis is larger than 25 mL in volume.[590]

Bilateral Megalotestes With Low Gonadotropins

Approximately 2% of adults with fertility problems have enlarged testes, with volumes greater than 25 mL, and low levels of FSH, LH, testosterone, prolactin, and estradiol.[591] Despite these important hormonal changes, sperm concentration and total number of spermatozoa are higher than normal. Low FSH levels may be attributable to increased inhibin secretion because the number of Sertoli cells is elevated, but reduction in other hormone levels is of unknown cause.

Fragile X Chromosome; Martin-Bell Syndrome

Fragile X chromosome is the best-known form of inherited mental retardation, with an incidence of 1 in 4000 males and 1 in 6000 females.[592] Inheritance is dominant and X-chromosome linked, with a low penetrance in females and variable expression in males.[593] In addition to facial dysmorphia (large ears, prognathism, high forehead, and arched palate), macroorchidism (Martin-Bell syndrome) is often an associated finding first described in 1943.[594-604]

The impaired gene, the *fragility mental retardation 1* gene (*FMR1* gene), is mapped to Xq27.3, which is genetically fragile in these patients. The gene alteration is caused by lengthening of trinucleotide CGG repeat that results in FMR1 gene silencing. The repeat is present in the 5'-untranslated region of the *FMR1* gene and shows 5 to 50 CGC units in the normal population.[605-607] If the CGG sequence is repeated fewer than 200 times, the disorder is considered a premutation, and males show no symptoms; if the number of repetitions exceeds 200, mutation is complete, and all affected persons show the disorder.[599,601,602] Full mutations involve hypermethylation of the gene promoter and lead to transcriptional silencing of the gene, with resulting total or partial loss of the FMR1 protein. This protein is present in many cells and regulates the translation of numerous proteins with a central role for cerebral maturation and function.[608] Genotype and phenotype are associated in patients with fragile X chromosome. Great CGC unit repeats correlate with the most severe forms of the phenotype. Conversely, nonmethylated CGC repeats show little or no semiologic repercussion.[609] Some syndromes result from intragenic FMR1 variants.[610]

In affected men, mean testicular volume is more than 70 mL (four times greater than normal). The penis is larger than normal, and both anomalies are apparent in infancy. Testicular enlargement probably begins during fetal life.[611] The scrotum is also enlarged and prematurely pigmented. This precocious genital development is difficult to explain because the hypothalamopituitary-gonadal axis is normal, but the condition may be caused by increased sensitivity to stimulation by FSH.[612] Testicular biopsies from adults may be normal or show interstitial edema and hypospermatogenesis (Fig. 12.54). Usually, one sees normal testicular parenchyma with focally reduced spermatogenesis and Sertoli cell hyperplasia (Fig. 12.55) or tubules containing only immature Sertoli cells. In other cases, severe pathologic changes have been reported, including

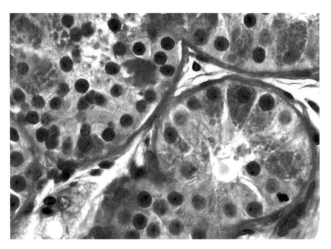

Fig. 12.56 Martin-bell syndrome (fragile X chromosome). Seminiferous tubules with immature Sertoli cells with granular changes.

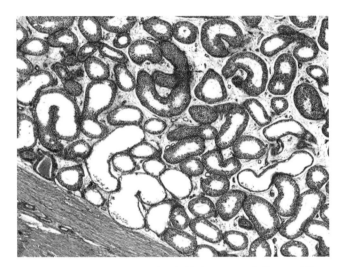

Fig. 12.54 Martin-bell syndrome (fragile X chromosome). The seminiferous tubules show variable degrees of dilatation and marked hypospermatogenesis.

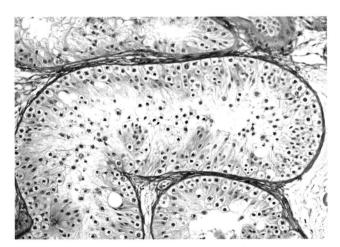

Fig. 12.55 Martin-bell syndrome (fragile X chromosome). The seminiferous tubules show marked hypospermatogenesis. Several groups of dysgenetic Sertoli cells are seen near the lumen.

marked tubular ectasia and atrophy of the seminiferous epithelium, granular changes in Sertoli cells (Fig. 12.56), MAT with or without Sertoli cell hyperplasia, and Sertoli cell nodules. Testicular enlargement is chiefly the result of lengthening and coiling of seminiferous tubules as a consequence of Sertoli cell proliferation.[232] The low number of spermatids is attributed to atrophy caused by compression of the seminiferous epithelium by marked increase in intratubular fluid.[613] Meiotic anomalies have been excluded. The fragile X syndrome is second in frequency only to Down syndrome as a cause of mental retardation.[593,604,614] However, this chromosomal anomaly is not always associated with mental retardation or macroorchidism, and some men with fragile X syndrome are otherwise normal.[611]

The terms *fragile X–negative Martin-Bell syndrome* and *mental retardation–macroorchidism* refer to patients with X-linked mental retardation–macroorchidism or X-linked mental retardation and macroorchidism who have the Martin-Bell syndrome phenotype, but not the fragile X site. The gene responsible for this disorder is mapped to Xq12-q21.[615] Isolated patients with fragile X chromosome have experienced testicular torsion or neoplasms (testicular or extratesticular).[616,617]

Other Causes of Testicular Hypertrophy

Testicular hypertrophy is associated with several glandular disorders such as FSH-secreting pituitary adenoma, hyperprolactinemia, hypoprolactinemia, and hypothyroidism.[468,618,619] The most frequent association of testicular hypertrophy is with hypothyroidism.

Children with *hypothyroidism* often show testicular enlargement without virilization.[619] Approximately 80% of these patients have macroorchidism, most have elevated FSH levels, and one-half have increased LH levels.[235,620,621] Testosterone levels are normal during infancy. The response of FSH and LH to GnRH is altered, and no pulsatile LH release occurs (Fig. 12.57).[622] Testicular biopsies before puberty show accelerated development with pubertal maturation of seminiferous tubules, but not Leydig cells. Testicular biopsies in untreated adults show tubular and interstitial hyalinization with few Leydig cells.[623–625] Testicular size in this type of macroorchidism diminishes as soon as substitution therapy starts.[620,626,627]

The etiopathogenesis of macroorchidism associated with primary hypothyroidism may be explained by several hypotheses:

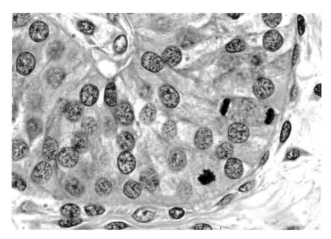

Fig. 12.57 Macroorchidism in a 3-year-old infant with hypothyroidism. The Sertoli cells have spherical nuclei that contain small heterochromatin granules. Two mitotic figures are seen. The testicular interstitium has no Leydig cells.

increase in gonadotropin secretion caused by thyrotropin-releasing hormone (TRH) stimulation of gonadotropic cells[628,629]; direct thyroid-stimulating hormone (TSH) effect on the testis resulting from structural similarity between TSH receptors and FSHRs in the testis[630,631]; and lack of steroid hormones that are required for testicular maturation (in their absence, Sertoli cell proliferation is excessive, giving rise to testicular enlargement).[632–635] Macroorchidism associated with secondary hypothyroidism is related to loss-of-function mutations in IGSF1, hyperprolactinemia, and alterations in steroid metabolism of testicular cells.[636–638]

Testicular Hypertrophy Secondary to Follicle-Stimulating Hormone–Secreting Pituitary Adenoma

Most adenomas that are considered nonfunctioning secrete variable amounts of FSH, although only exceptionally do they have any clinical manifestations.[639,640] Functioning pituitary adenoma, with FSH secretion during infancy and puberty, gives rise to variable clinical symptoms in relation to size and accelerated development of pubic hair and genitalia. In adults, macroorchidism secondary to length growth of the seminiferous tubules is accompanied by normal spermatogenesis.[641] Once the most frequent causes of macroorchidism have been ruled out, diagnosis is suggested by a discrepancy between normal or elevated FSH and decreased LH, as well as by the detection of elevated inhibin B. Atypical cases of FSH-secreting pituitary adenoma are accompanied by hypogonadism with erectile dysfunction, loss of libido, and absence of macroorchidism.[642]

Precocious Puberty

Precocious puberty is defined by the onset of secondary sex characteristics at a chronologic age that is younger than the mean middle age for the population, 2.5 standard deviations lower than the mean of a defined population. For practical purposes, this is before 8 years of age in girls and 9 years in boys. The incidence is estimated at between 1 in 5000 and 1 in 10,000, with a female-to-male ratio higher than 20:1. In boys the first symptom is rapid testicular enlargement followed by growth of pubic and axillary hair, enlargement of the penis, and acceleration of skeletal growth.[643] According to hypothalamopituitary-gonadal axis function, precocious puberty may be classified into three groups: central or gonadotropin dependent, which results from activation of this axis; peripheral

or gonadotropin independent, mediated by sex steroid hormones secreted by the testis or adrenal glands; and a mixed group that first appears as peripheral precocious puberty and, thereafter, because of the secondary response of the hypothalamus, becomes gonadotropin dependent.

Central Precocious Puberty

Central precocious puberty (CPP), also known as *true precocious puberty*, is isosexual. CPP is caused by premature activation of the hypothalamic-hypophyseal-gonadal axis. The first manifestation in boys is an increase in volume (>4 mL) or length (>2.5 cm) of the testes. It is the most common form of precocious puberty in girls and accounts for more than 50% of cases in boys. Age of presentation is between 4 and 10 years.[644]

The cause is known in only 60% of cases; most are related to lesions in the central nervous system, whereas others are usually idiopathic.[645] Increasingly, cases previously considered idiopathic are found to have an underlying genetic basis.[646]

Lesions in the central nervous system that cause CPP share alterations of specific areas, including the posterior hypothalamus (median eminence and tuber cinereum), mammillary bodies, the bottom of the third ventricle, or the pineal gland.[647,648] The most frequent causes are as follows:

- Tumor of the hypothalamus (astrocytoma, ganglioneuroma, ganglioglioma, craniopharyngioma, cyst of the third ventricle, and suprasellar cyst of the arachnoid space), pineal cyst, hamartoma (gangliocytoma) of the tuber cinereum and mammillary body, tumor of the pineal gland (teratoma and pinealoma), tumor of the optic nerve (glioma), cerebral and cerebellar astrocytoma, and granular cell tumor of the neurohypophysis[649–653]
- Cerebral trauma (including postpartum and accidental trauma) that stimulates extrahypothalamic areas responsible for hypothalamic activation[654–656]
- Infections such as meningitis, encephalitis, toxoplasmosis, and syphilis
- Cerebral malformations, including hydrocephaly, microcephaly, and craniosynostosis, pituitary duplication, and midline defects[657,658]
- Hereditary diseases such as neurofibromatosis and tuberous sclerosis; children with type I neurofibromatosis often also have optic pathway tumors[659]
- Cerebral irradiation, as occurs in hypothalamopituitary selective irradiation, prophylactic irradiation in children with acute lymphoblastic leukemia, and irradiation of cerebral tumor that is far from the hypothalamopituitary region[660–663]

Knowledge of the etiology in male patients has expanded with the use of computed tomography (CT) and MRI.[664,665] One of the most important contributions of these techniques is the finding of high numbers of hamartomas in children with precocious puberty.[666–668] These lesions, also known as gangliocytomas, consist of abnormally located neurons and glial cells. Lesions are usually multiple, small, and located on the hypothalamus between the anterior part of the mammillary body and the posterior part of the tuber cinereum. These neurons contain LH-releasing hormone–positive neurosecretory granules, a finding suggesting that this hormone may be released into the blood draining the hypophyseal portal system and reach the gonadotropic cells.[669] Other hamartomas associated with CPP do not show immunohistochemical reactivity to GnRH, but they do show reactivity to TGFA protein and its messenger RNA (mRNA), as well as to the receptors for TGFA and EGF, which could also be involved in precocious pubertal development.[670]

Precocious puberty resulting from cerebral tumors usually occurs at an advanced stage of the tumor, preceded by symptoms such as hydrocephaly, papillary edema, or psychic alterations. The same occurs when precocious puberty results from cerebral inflammation or malformation.

Although pineal gland tumor is rare in children, 30% of these produce precocious puberty, principally in boys. This tumor is usually a teratoma or nonparenchymatous tumor that destroys the pineal gland, thus hindering its antigonadotropic action and initiating puberty.[671] In contrast, pinealocyte-derived tumor secretes great amounts of melatonin, which delays the onset of puberty.

Idiopathic precocious puberty. The cause of CPP cannot be determined in approximately 80% of girls and 40% of boys. This difference between the sexes may be attributed to the higher sensitivity of female gonadotropic cells to GnRH stimulation. The presentation of idiopathic precocious puberty is familial in nearly 50% of cases, and puberty starts after 7 years in most of these boys. Inheritance may be autosomal recessive or sex linked with variable penetrance.[672] Genetic causes may play an important role in the development of some cases.[673] Activating mutation (P745) in the *KISS1* gene, encoding GPR54s ligand (Kisspeptin), may occur in boys with CPP.[674,675] Mutations resulting in MKRN3 gene deficiency induce pulsatile secretion of GnRH, and that triggers precocious puberty.[676,677]

The diagnosis of CPP is easy when there are elevated gonadotropins (both basal values and in response to GnRH) associated with high testosterone levels and an increase in either the LH/FSH ratio or in LH and FSH values after stimulation with GnRH agonists. However, in some cases it is necessary to measure nocturnal LH secretion to identify secretion pulses before a dynamic test may reveal the pubertal pattern. The treatment of choice is GnRH agonists.[678]

Associated disorders that have been reported are intrauterine growth retardation, Silver-Russell syndrome, bilateral retinal degeneration, epilepsy, cryptorchidism, and inguinal hernia.[679]

Peripheral Precocious Puberty

Peripheral precocious puberty is also known as precocious pseudopuberty. It may be caused by a primary testicular disorder, lesion in other endocrine glands, or hormonal treatment. Primary testicular disorders causing precocious pseudopuberty include familial testotoxicosis, functioning testicular tumor, excessive aromatase activity, and Leydig cell hyperplasia with focal spermatogenesis. The principal secondary anomalies include adrenal cortical anomaly (congenital adrenal hyperplasia, virilizing tumor of the adrenal, and Nelson syndrome) and hCG-secreting tumor, which accounts for one-half of cases of precocious pseudopuberty; testicular germ cell tumor and tumors of the retroperitoneum, mediastinum, and pineal gland are responsible for the other one-half (Table 12.14).[680–685] The best-known treatment that may cause precocious puberty is long-term administration of hCG.[684]

Familial Testotoxicosis: Gonadotropin-Independent Precocious Puberty or Familial Male-Limited Precocious Puberty. Familial testotoxicosis is a form of male sexual precocity characterized by early differentiation of Leydig cells and initiation of spermatogenesis in the absence of stimulation by pituitary gonadotropin. This condition is assumed to be a primary testicular abnormality with autosomal dominant inheritance that is limited to male patients.[251,686,687] Some cases occur sporadically. The patients, usually 1 to 4 years of age, have signs of pubertal development, including rapid virilization, acceleration of growth with eventual closure of epiphyses, and short adult stature. Although the testes are enlarged, testicular size does not correlate with the degree of

TABLE 12.14	Causes of Peripheral Precocious Puberty

Familial testotoxicosis

Gonadotropin-independent precocious puberty
Familial male-limited precocious puberty

Precocious pseudopuberty secondary to functioning tumors

Leydig cell tumor
Intratubular hyalinizing large cell Sertoli cell tumor
Large cell calcifying Sertoli cell tumor
Adrenal cortex virilizing tumors
Hepatoblastoma
Extratesticular human chorionic gonadotropin–secreting germ cell tumors
  Teratoma
  Choriocarcinoma
  Seminoma.

Precocious pseudopuberty secondary to disorders of aromatase activity.

Precocious pseudopuberty secondary to Leydig cell hyperplasia with focal spermatogenesis.

virilization. Histologic and ultrastructural studies confirm adult Leydig cell pattern and complete spermatogenesis, although many spermatids are abnormal (Fig. 12.58).[688,689]

The cause of familial testotoxicosis is a constitutive activating mutation of the *LH/CGR* gene.[234,690–693] This gene comprises 11 exons and has been mapped to 2p21, and approximately two dozen *LH/CGR* gene mutations have been reported.[694,695]

Hormonal measurements show elevated serum levels of testosterone and low levels of dehydroepiandrosterone sulfate, androstenedione, 17-hydroxyprogesterone, GnRH, and LH, as well as absence of a pulsatile pattern. In addition, serum level of inhibin B appears elevated before the normal age of onset of puberty.[696] In some patients a mutation in the LHR may induce Leydig cell hyperplasia.[689,697]

Patients do not respond to treatment with GnRH analogues, which are used for treatment of CPP. Therapy with the antifungal drug ketoconazole is effective, but patients may experience significant hepatotoxicity and, in some cases, suffer escape phenomenon (secondary CPP), which requires additional therapy with

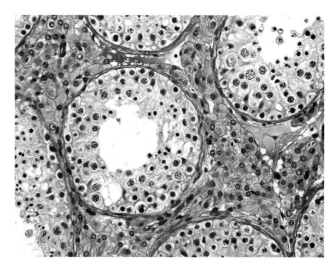

Fig. 12.58 Testotoxicosis. Leydig cell hyperplasia and seminiferous tubules with deficient spermatogenesis.

GnRH agonists.[698] A proposed alternative to GnRH analogue therapy is administration of cyproterone acetate or the aromatase inhibitor anastrozole, as well as bicalutamide, a nonsteroidal antiandrogen.[699–701] Inactivating mutations of GnRH cause male undermasculinization as a result of the absence or hypoplasia of Leydig cells.

Precocious Pseudopuberty Secondary to Functioning Tumors. Precocious pseudopuberty may be caused by Leydig cell tumor, Sertoli tumor, adrenal cortex virilizing carcinoma, and extratesticular hCG-secreting germ cell tumor.

With *Leydig cell tumor*, the involved testis is enlarged in response to tumor growth and maturation of the seminiferous tubules adjacent to the tumor; such maturation results from androgen secretion by tumor cells (Figs. 12.59 and 12.60).[702] An activating mutation of the LHR gene, Asp578His has been detected in some patients with Leydig cell tumors.[703] In most cases the contralateral testis is not enlarged.[704,705] Occasionally, tumors cause only precocious tubular maturation, and symptoms of precocious pseudopuberty are absent, probably because of early diagnosis.[705]

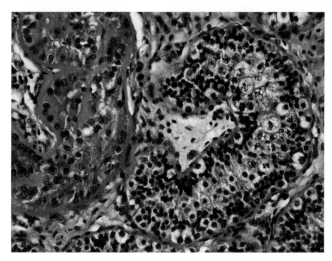

Fig. 12.61 Seminiferous tubule with abundant spermatogonia and first-order spermatocytes in a 3-year-old child at the periphery of a hyalinizing intratubular Sertoli cell neoplasia.

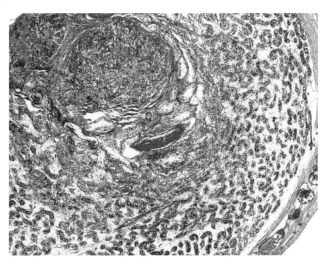

Fig. 12.59 Precocious pseudopuberty secondary to a Leydig cell tumor.

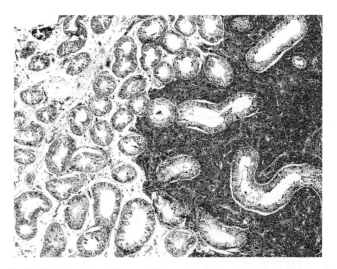

Fig. 12.60 Maturation of the seminiferous tubules located at the periphery of a Leydig cell tumor.

Intratubular large cell hyalinizing Sertoli cell neoplasia and large cell calcifying Sertoli cell tumor may give rise to precocious pseudopuberty that is isosexual (development of musculature and axillary and pubic hair) and heterosexual (gynecomastia). This precocious testicular maturation and the development of the tumor itself cause testicular enlargement (Fig. 12.61). Tumor cells may stimulate Leydig cells to produce androgens that are aromatized to estrogens by the Sertoli tumor cells themselves, thus accounting for the clinical symptoms.[706,707] These tumors are frequently observed in Peutz-Jeghers syndrome and Carney complex.[708–711]

Most infants with *adrenal cortex virilizing tumor* have small testes, but hypertrophy has also been observed.[712] Testicular development in these cases is attributed to adrenal androgenic action on seminiferous tubules.[713] In untreated (or maltreated) congenital adrenal hyperplasia, both testes may be enlarged because of growing masses of cells resembling adrenal cortex.[714] Patients with Nelson syndrome may have a similar condition. Surgical removal of virilizing adrenocortical carcinoma may induce CPP that requires treatment.[715]

Testicular enlargement is modest in paraneoplastic precocious pseudopuberty secondary to *hepatoblastoma* or *extratesticular hCG-secreting germ cell tumor*, although nodular or diffuse precocious maturation has been occasionally reported.[716–720] These nodules consist of hyperplastic Leydig cells and seminiferous tubules that may show complete spermatogenesis. Outside the nodule the seminiferous tubules maintain their prepubertal pattern. In some cases, only diffuse Leydig cell hyperplasia is observed.[721]

Precocious Pseudopuberty Secondary to Disorders in Aromatase Activity. Biosynthesis of C18 estrogens from C19 androgens occurs by three consecutive oxidative reactions that are catalyzed by an enzymatic complex known as estrogen synthetase or aromatase.[722] This complex has two components: P450 arom (a product from the *CYP19* gene located on 15p21.1), which joins C19 substrate and catalyzes the insertion of oxygen in C19 to form C18 estrogens; and reduced nicotinamide-adenine dinucleotide phosphate–cytochrome P450 reductase, a ubiquitous flavoprotein that conveys reducing equivalents to any form of cytochrome P450 it meets.[723,723a] Aromatase is in the endoplasmic reticulum of estrogen-synthesizing cells and is expressed in placenta, ovarian granulosa, Sertoli cells, Leydig cells, adipose tissue, and several central nervous system regions, including the hypothalamus, amygdala, and hippocampus.

Aromatase Excess Syndrome. Excessive aromatase causes massive conversion of androgens to estrogen.[723] It is a genetic disorder with autosomal dominant inheritance caused by gain-of-function mutation in the aromatase (CYP19A1) gene that results in heterosexual precocious pseudopuberty with gynecomastia in boys and isosexual precocity and macromastia in girls. Ultimately, patient stature is short because of the potent ability of androgens to accelerate epiphyseal closure. FSH, LH, and serum testosterone are decreased.[724] Although many patients have mild hypogonadotropic hypogonadism, testicular size in adults is normal, and most are fertile and have normal libido.[725] Generally the inhibitory estrogenic effect on testicular function is less than that observed with estrogen-producing tumors or in patients treated with exogenous estrogens.[726] Patients with aromatase excess syndrome are effectively treated with aromatase inhibitors.[727]

Aromatase Deficiency Syndrome. Aromatase deficiency syndrome, a rare recessive autosomal disorder, was first reported in 1991.[727] It is the result of several mutations in the coding region of the CYP19A1 gene that lead to decrease or loss of enzymatic function with subsequent estrogenic deficit. Most patients are homozygous for inactivating mutations because they are sons of consanguineous parents. Other patients are compound heterozygous from nonrelated patients.

In both sexes the first symptom appears in the mothers during pregnancy; these women become progressively virilized because of the placental incapacity to aromatize androgens. In a female fetus, excessive exposure to androgens in utero leads to ambiguous external genitalia. In puberty, normal adrenarche is present; however, these patients have primary amenorrhea, absence of mammary development, and progressive hypergonadotropic hypogonadism with hyperandrogenism.

In children, FSH and LH levels and the gonadotropin response to GnRH are normal findings suggesting that the role of estrogens in pituitary regulation is weak during infancy.[728] Most cases are diagnosed at puberty.[729] The most significant symptom is continuous linear growth in adulthood. In both genders, epiphyseal closure is delayed because the absence of estrogen results in failure of growth plate fusion despite high levels of androgens, and patients develop a eunuchoid habitus.[730] Men have small testes, severe oligozoospermia, and complete asthenozoospermia; FSH and LH levels are high, testosterone levels are normal, and serum estrogen levels are low. All patients with aromatase deficit have tall stature, with continuing linear growth into adulthood, unfused epiphyses, osteoporosis, bilateral genu valgum, and eunuchoid proportions.[731] Many male patients are obese with dyslipidemia, hyperinsulinemia, acanthosis nigricans, and diabetes mellitus. Estrogens play an important role in pituitary regulation in male adults, so men with aromatase deficit have low libido and infertility.[732] Hormonal analysis reveals undetectable estradiol and estrone levels and elevated gonadotropins, findings suggesting a lack of negative regulation of both FSH and LH by estrogens.[733] Androstenedione and testosterone may be normal or increased.[734] There is macroorchidism with normal consistency in some cases, and the testes are small with severe oligozoospermia and 100% immotile spermatozoa in other cases.[735,736]

A syndrome like that in men with aromatase deficit is found in patients with estrogen resistance caused by *disruptive mutations of the ER gene*. These patients have macroorchidism, increased testosterone level, and increased levels of FSH, LH, estradiol, and estrone.[737] The spermiogram reveals a low number of spermatozoa (25 million/mL) with decreased viability (18%).[738]

Estrogen therapy in patients with aromatase deficit is effective in achieving epiphysial closure, but this treatment does not improve spermatogenesis.[735-737,738a] The role of estrogens in male infertility has yet to be discussed.[739,740]

Precocious Pseudopuberty Secondary to Leydig Cell Hyperplasia With Focal Spermatogenesis. This entity may manifest with clinical symptoms like those of functioning Leydig cell tumor; this is a form of precocious pseudopuberty with ipsilateral testicular enlargement.[741,742] The testis contains hypertrophic Leydig cell nests associated with normal spermatogenesis. No tumor mass is present. Leydig cells do not contain Reinke crystalloids and do not compress seminiferous tubules. Tubules with spermatogenesis and infantile immature tubules are clear delimited. The differential diagnosis between this entity and Leydig cell tumor with precocious pseudopuberty is based on histologic pattern. Open excisional testicular biopsy is recommended; if the patient has a Leydig cell tumor, or if the diagnosis by frozen section is not conclusive, testicular removal is advisable.[743,744] There is no evidence to suggest that this hyperplasia may develop into Leydig cell tumor.

Mixed Precocious Puberty

The best-known form of mixed precocious puberty is the MAS, characterized by the association of "coffee and milk" pigmentary lesions in the skin, bone lesions (polyostotic fibrous dysplasia), enlarged testes, prepubertal size of the penis, and the absence of pubic and axillary hair.[745,746] Although testicular enlargement is usually bilateral, unilateral macroorchidism may be the first symptom.[747] The diagnosis may be delayed until adulthood.[748] This syndrome is caused by mutations that activate the guanine nucleotide–binding protein α-subunit gene (GNAS1), which encodes the α subunit of the trimeric G protein (20q13.32).[749] Because these mutations are lethal in utero, male patients with MAS bear mosaicism chromosomal constitution for this deficiency.[750,751] The anomaly is followed by inactivation of both LHR and FSHR.[752]

An interesting finding is that the onset of testicular maturation is induced by the testis itself, which produces steroid secretion secondary to autonomous hyperfunction of Sertoli cells without evidence of Leydig cell involvement.[753] This secretion causes early maturation of the hypothalamopituitary-testicular axis and subsequently true precocious puberty.[754] The testicular parenchyma shows maturation of both seminiferous tubules and Leydig cells. Testicular microlithiasis is a frequent finding (62%).[755,756]

The previously described developmental pattern is the rule. However, some cases with a different hormonal or clinical pattern have been reported. Some patients have isolated Sertoli cell hyperfunction, whereas others have only Leydig cell hyperfunction. The macroorchidism resulting from autonomous Sertoli cell hyperfunction shows abnormally elevated serum levels of inhibin B and AMH in correlation with decreased FSH and testosterone. Therefore pubertal inhibin B serum level suggests Sertoli cell hyperfunction that would exert negative feedback on FSH secretion. These testes show Sertoli cell hyperplasia and absence of maturation of both germ cells and Leydig cells, with subsequent lack of steroidogenesis (Figs. 12.62 and 12.63).[753] This peculiar condition has been related to the presence of a somatic mutation in the GNAS1 gene in Sertoli cells, but not in Leydig cells.[757] The different early embryologic origin of precursor cells that contribute to Sertoli cell and Leydig cell lineages may underlie the differential occurrence of the mutated GNAS1 gene. In other cases, and preferentially in late childhood and adult patients, clinical, biochemical, and histologic data suggest isolated Leydig cell hyperfunction with Leydig cell hyperplasia but without precocious activation of Sertoli cells;

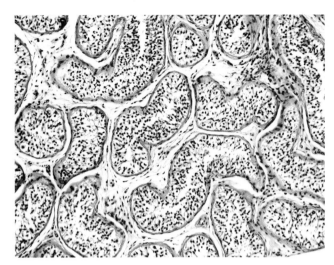

Fig. 12.62 Precocious puberty in a 5-year-old child. The seminiferous tubules are cellular. The interstitium lacks Leydig cells.

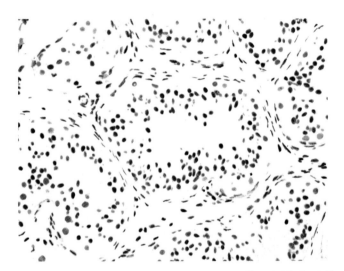

Fig. 12.63 Sertoli cell hyperplasia (same patient as in Fig. 12.62). Seminiferous tubules contain more than twice as many Sertoli cells as controls. Immunostaining for androgen receptor was performed.

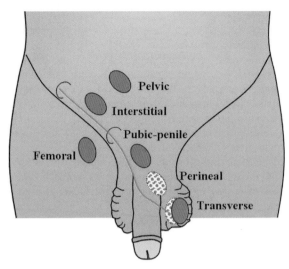

Fig. 12.64 Different locations of ectopic testis.

this condition leads to complete spermatogenesis in some tubules.[758,759] In these cases, autonomous testicular function and the gonadotropin suppression may persist for a long time.

Therapy in MAS is symptomatic. Precocious puberty is treated with aromatase inhibitors, which block the conversion of testosterone into estradiol; hypophyseal surgery in some cases of fibrous dysplasia; and bromocriptine, cabergoline, and long-acting somatostatin analogues to stop growth hormone (GH) secretion.[760]

Testicular Ectopia

A testis is ectopic when it is located outside the normal path of descent. Unlike cryptorchidism, ectopic testes are nearly normal in size and accompanied by spermatic cord that is normal or even longer than normal, as well as by a normal scrotum.[761] Testicular ectopia is estimated to account for about 5% of all undescended testes. Testicular ectopia is classified according to location (Fig. 12.64).[762–766] In decreasing order of frequency, major sites are:

- *Interstitial or inguinal superficial ectopia.* This is the most frequent form and may be confused with inguinal cryptorchidism. After passing through the external inguinal ring, the testis ascends to the anterosuperior iliac spine and remains on the aponeurosis of the major oblique muscle. These testes are more likely to be normal histologically than cryptorchid testes.

- *Femoral or crural ectopia.* After passing through the inguinal canal, the testis lodges in the high crural cone in the Scarpa triangle.

- *Perineal ectopia.* The testis is located between the raphe and the genitocrural fold in a subcutaneous location.[762,764,765] Bilateral cases have been reported.[767]

- *Transverse or crossed ectopia.* This condition is also referred to as pseudoduplication, unilateral double testis, and transverse aberrant maldescent, first reported in 1886.[768] Both testes descend through the same inguinal canal and lodge in the same scrotal pouch. The ectopic testis may be located in the internal inguinal ring, the inguinal canal, or the contralateral hemiscrotum. Each testis possesses its own vascular supply, epididymis, and vas deferens. In addition, ipsilateral hernia is present.[769–778] More than 150 cases have been reported, mostly in adults. External genitalia ranges from normal to severe undermasculinization.[77,779–782] Most cases are diagnosed during herniotomy surgery; others are identified by sonography, CT, or MRI.[783] Isolated cases have been identified through treatment of incarcerated inguinal hernia or testicular torsion.[784–787] Transverse ectopia must be suspected in cases of inguinal hernia associated with the absent contralateral testis. Treatment consists of transseptal orchiopexy or extraperitoneal transposition of the testis. Between 20% and 40% of patients have PMDS.[77,780,788] Müllerian remnants must be removed with caution, if at all. It is better to leave them in place than to perform extensive dissection that may harm spermatic cord structures.[789] High incidence of germ cell tumor (18%) has been reported.[790–792]

- *Pubopenile ectopia.* The ectopic testis is on the back of the penis near the symphysis pubis.[793–796] Penile ectopy associated with groin testicular ectopy and scrotal absence was reported in a patient with popliteal pterygium syndrome.[797] Approximately 60% of patients show genital anomalies.[798]

- *Pelvic ectopia.* The testis is in the pelvis, usually deep in the Douglas cul-de-sac.

- *Other unusual testicular ectopias* include retroumbilical, craniolateral to the inner inguinal opening between the outer and inner oblique muscles, subumbilical, and anterior abdominal wall.[799–805]

Ectopic testes in locations other than the superficial inguinal region typically exhibit histologic changes similar to cryptorchid testes. Findings include low germ cell number, low testicular volume, persistence of the vaginal process, and epididymal anomalies. Microlithiasis may occur in a patient with transverse testicular ectopy.[806] Approximately 8% of patients with ectopic testes have contralateral cryptorchid testis.[807]

There are multiple hypotheses explaining the different types of ectopia.[808–810] Accepting that testicular descent occurs in two phases, some ectopias may be explained by failure in the first phase and others by a failure in the second phase. The first phase requires the gubernaculum to be attached to the abdominal wall at the site of the future inguinal canal. Attachment to the wrong side or disruption of that attachment would result in the following ectopias: attachment to femoral canal would result in femoral ectopia; attachment to the Spigelian triangle would result in Spigelian ectopia; absence or loss of attachment to the inguinal canal would result in transverse ectopia or pelvic ectopy. In the second phase of descent the gubernaculum must emigrate from the inguinal canal to the scrotum. This event is under the control of CGRP from the GFN. The GFN has two main branches, the genital branch supplying the scrotum and the femoral branch supplying the inner side of the thigh. Erroneous distribution of GFN sensory fibers or altered secretion of CGRP occurring in the wrong branch would disrupt the usual path of emigration of the gubernaculum. If the femoral branch of the GFN directs migration, femoral ectopia occurs; if the genital branch reaches the perineum instead of the scrotum, perineal ectopia occurs; and if the genital branch supplies the penis instead of the scrotum, pubopenile ectopia occurs.

Finally, there are ectopias that occur despite normal attachment of an abnormally developed gubernaculum. This occurs in patients with defects in AMH in whom an excessively long gubernaculum allows ample displacement that may lead the testicle even to the contralateral vaginal process.

Testicular Exstrophy (Scrotoschisis)

In testicular exstrophy the testis and the spermatic cord are prolapsed externally through a defect in the scrotal wall.[811–815] The lesion may be unilateral or bilateral. The gubernaculum is normal, and testicular descent is not impaired. Testicular exstrophy may result from mesodermal failure, similar to what causes the defect of the anterior abdominal wall in newborns with gastroschisis, scrotal wall necrosis secondary to meconium peritonitis, and iatrogenic trauma during cesarean section.[813,816,817]

Testicular Fusion

Testicular fusion is a rare anomaly characterized by fusion of the testes to form a single structure, usually in the midline. Each testis has its own epididymis and vas deferens. This anomaly is often associated with other malformations such as fusion of the adrenal glands or horseshoe kidney. Testicular fusion was also observed in a patient with transverse testicular ectopia and PMDS. The fused testes had a single vas deferens.[818]

Bilobed Testis

Bilobed testicle is a rare malformation, with only four cases reported.[819–822] Patients have enlarged hemiscrotum related to testicular enlargement and hydrocele formation. The contralateral testis is normal. Sonography may exclude a tumor and thus avoid surgical exploration and testicular biopsy. This condition is considered an incomplete expression of polyorchidism. As in polyorchidism, follow-up with ultrasound imaging is recommended because of the higher risk for testicular tumor development.

Hamartomatous Testicular Lesions

Hamartoma is a term used to refer to abnormal and excessive development of structures that usually form part of the testis, epididymis, or spermatic cord. Hamartomatous lesions of the testis and sperm excretory ducts include cystic dysplasia of the rete testis, hamartoma of the rete testis, fetal gonadoblastoid testicular dysplasia (FGTD), Sertoli cell nodule, tubular hamartoma, congenital testicular and epididymal lymphangiectasis, and muscular hyperplasia of paratesticular structures. The main concern with hamartoma is not the biologic behavior, which is always benign, but their significance, because most are associated with specific disorders or are markers of complex syndromes.

Cystic Dysplasia of the Testis

Cystic Dysplasia of the Rete Testis

Cystic dysplasia of the rete testis is a congenital lesion characterized by cystic transformation of an excessively developed rete testis that may extend to the tunica albuginea of the opposite pole. It was first reported in 1973 as "cystic dysplasia of the testis," arising in a 4-year-old with right renal agenesis.[823] To date, approximately 50 cases have been reported, mostly in children, with median age at presentation of 6 years (range, 0 to 23 years).[824–826] The most remarkable clinical symptom is scrotal swelling, followed by scrotal pain suggesting testicular tumor in some cases. Approximately 35% have abdominal cryptorchidism. Ultrasound images are characteristic: small cystic formations of variable size, located in the testicular mediastinum, extend to the proximal testicular parenchyma and cause its compression. In addition, small hyperechoic foci, originating in the interphase between the walls of distal cystic and adjacent parenchyma, are observed. The observation of ipsilateral renal anomalies in ultrasound exploration may be of great importance for diagnosis.[827]

Macroscopically the testis in adult patients has a cut surface reminiscent of the thyroid, with cysts of varying size filled with colloid-like material (Fig. 12.65). The extent of the cystic transformation is widely variable. Small groups of cysts may be limited to

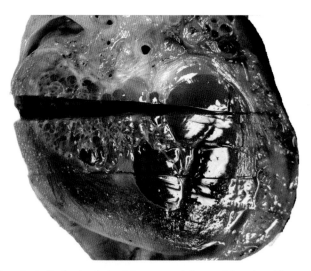

Fig. 12.65 Cystic dysplasia of the rete testis in an adult patient. The testis consists of numerous variable-sized cysts filled with a colloid-like material except for a peripheral crescent.

the region of the mediastinum testis, or cysts may extend throughout the entire testis. In extensive cases, residual seminiferous tubules occupy only a small crescent beneath the tunica albuginea, and the testis is grossly spongy.[828]

Cysts, which may be of variable size (from microscopic to several millimeters), arise in the septal and mediastinal rete testis (Fig. 12.66). They are interconnected and contain acellular, eosinophilic, periodic acid–Schiff[+] (PAS[+]) material. The cavities are lined by cuboidal cells that resemble those of normal rete testis both immunohistochemically (expressing both cytokeratin and vimentin) and ultrastructurally.[829–832] Immunoreactivity to epithelial membrane antigen, which is usually not expressed in the normal rete testis, has been reported in some cases.[833] Connective tissue between the cysts is scant and histologically similar to interstitial connective tissue. In some cases this tissue is so abundant that it partially collapses the cavities, and psammoma bodies and small inflammatory infiltrates may be present beneath the epithelium.

In cystic dysplasia, during infancy and childhood the residual testicular parenchyma may mature normally, and cryptorchid testes with cystic dysplasia have a marked decrease in spermatogonial number (Fig. 12.67). However, in all cases the proximal end (the opening to the rete testis) of the seminiferous tubules shows a small dilatation. The seminiferous tubules may be dilated and atrophic; this is more evident after puberty.[834–838]

Cystic dysplasia occurs in normally descended and cryptorchid testes, both in children and adults, and may affect one or both testes.[839] In adults, residual parenchyma often shows morphologic characteristics of obstructive lesions: complete tubular sclerosis or hypospermatogenesis with intratubular accumulation of spermatozoa and Leydig cell pseudohyperplasia. In most cases the epididymis is altered.[840] The head of the epididymis is small and contains few ductuli efferentes with irregular, usually dilated lumina, and abundant loose stroma. The ductus epididymidis is dilated, with atrophic epithelium consisting of cuboidal cells lacking stereocilia. Thick connective tissue replaces the muscular layer (Fig. 12.68). Marked epididymal hypoplasia has been described. The ductus deferens may also be dilated. Ipsilateral absence of the ductus deferens occurs infrequently.

Cystic dysplasia is frequently associated with severe anomalies of the kidney or the urinary system. These problems greatly

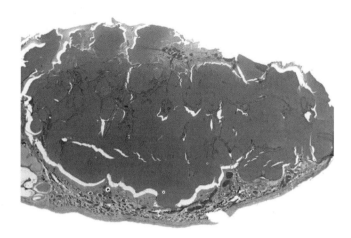

Fig. 12.67 Cystic dysplasia of the rete testis in a newborn. There is cystic transformation of the rete testis and adjacent seminiferous tubules.

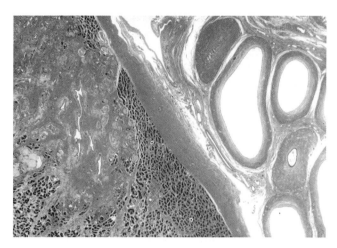

Fig. 12.68 Marked luminal dilation of the ductus epididymidis in an infant with cystic dysplasia of the rete testis.

overshadow the significance of the testicular changes. Renal agenesis (51%), renal dysplasia (21%), hydronephrosis (8%), hydroureter, dilated or cystic epididymis (8%), absence of ipsilateral ureteric orifice (6%), ureteral duplication (4%), urethral stenosis, ectopic ureter draining to the seminal vesicle, ipsilateral renal agenesis and contralateral crossed ectopia, and genitourinary manifestations of VATER (vertebra/anus/cardiac/trachea/esophagus/radius/renal anomalies) syndrome have been reported ipsilateral to testicular cystic dysplasia.[823,832,839,841–847]

The clinical differential diagnosis consists of all cystic lesions involving the prepubertal testes, including epidermoid cyst, cystic teratoma, juvenile granulosa cell tumor, testicular lymphangiectasis, simple cyst of the testis, and posttorsion cystic degeneration of the testis.[848,849] Previously, total or partial orchiectomy was the treatment of choice.[850] Currently, conservative therapy is recommended if the ultrasound diagnosis is highly suggestive, and results of α-fetoprotein and hCGβ subunit assays are negative.[851,852] Spontaneous regression may occur.[826,853–855] However, it is uncertain whether attempts to save the testis preserve spermatogenesis.

The etiology and pathogenesis of cystic dysplasia are uncertain. Given that the rete testis is a mesonephric derivative and most of

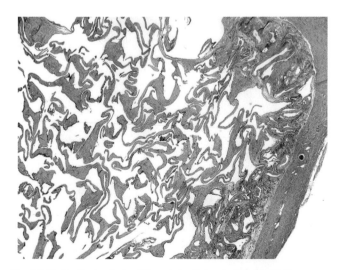

Fig. 12.66 Cystic dysplasia of the rete testis in an adult patient. Transverse section of the testis showing numerous anastomosed cavities that reach the albuginea.

the associated renal malformations are apparently caused by failure of induction of renal blastema by the mesonephros, cystic dysplasia is the result of abnormal mesonephros. During childhood the normal rete testis has no lumina because these form during puberty. The adult rete testis is a conduit for the passage of tubular fluid and spermatozoa, and actively reabsorbs part of this fluid while adding ions, proteins, and steroids.[856] Primary lesion of mesonephric cells that form the rete testis could result in abnormal function of the rete testis epithelium, which could produce fluid with abnormal composition at an inappropriate time.

Lesions similar to cystic dysplasia of the rete testis have been experimentally induced by sodium intoxication after administration of salt-retaining hormones or deoxycorticosterone acetate in fowls, as well as by estradiol administration in newborn rats.[857,858]

Cystic Dysplasia of the Epididymis

Cystic dysplasia of the epididymis (CDE) is a recently described anomaly characterized by the presence of irregular, segmental cystic dilatation of the epididymal ducts with aberrant forms and immature appearance (Fig. 12.69).[859] There is a significant decrease in the number of sections of efferent ductules without lesions in the lining epithelium. The irregular cystic dilatations cause loss of epididymal head architecture (loss of typical hemispherical shape). It may affect one segment of the epididymal duct in association with lesions in the head of the epididymis or as an isolated lesion.

CDE was observed in 19 fetal and neonatal autopsies of males from 27 weeks of gestation to 10 days of life, and in one surgical specimen from a 4-year-old. The lesion was bilateral in all evaluable cases. Eighteen of 20 cases had renal or urinary tract anomalies, including renal dysplasia (8 cases), renal agenesis (4 cases), autosomal recessive polycystic renal disease (1 case), and renal hypoplasia (1 case). In eight cases, testes were cryptorchid. One patient had associated ipsilateral testicular cystic dysplasia.

CDE is a novel congenital anomaly of mesonephric differentiation that should be added to the spectrum of male excretory system disorders associated with renal and urinary malformations.

Hamartoma of the Rete Testis

Only one case of rete testis hamartoma has been reported. It was in a 3-year-old who presented with a testicular mass. The lesion

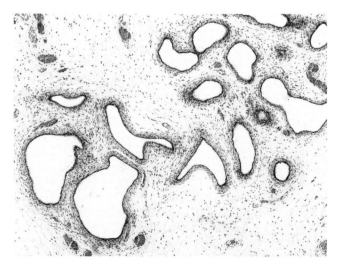

Fig. 12.69 Cystic dysplasia of the epididymis. The caput of the epididymis is formed by a few efferent ducts showing irregular dilations.

consisted of a disordered tubular proliferation lined by epithelium like that of the rete testis within a loose connective tissue stroma.[860] A peculiar hamartoma that consisted of three separate components (cystic dilatation of the rete testis, diffuse interstitial smooth muscle proliferation, and extensive stroma with myxoid areas) was reported in a 26-year-old.[861]

Fetal Gonadoblastoid Testicular Dysplasia

FGTD refers to abnormally differentiated testicular parenchyma. This disorder was first described in 1986 in a 28-week premature newborn who died 1 hour after delivery.[862] The only remarkable antecedent during pregnancy was polyhydramnios. The karyotype was 46,XY. The most relevant data from autopsy were hypertelorism, low-set ears, fenestrated secundum-type atrial septal defect, idiopathic bilateral hydronephrosis without apparent urinary duct obstruction, unilateral double renal collecting system, and pleural effusion. Genitalia were characteristic of a normal male infant.[863] Three other cases (18-week-old fetus, 22-week-old fetus, and a 3-year-old) were later reported, all in association with Walker-Warburg syndrome (WWS; https://www.omim.org/entry/236670), including left ureter malformations and ipsilateral renal cystic dysplasia. Two additional cases of FTGD were observed. The most interesting autopsy findings were hydrops, muscular lesions suggesting mitochondrial myopathy that did not fit the diagnostic criteria of WWS, and undescended testes lodged near the inferior pole of both kidneys.[864] Weinberg reported a 10-month-old with WWS whose gonads were located in the inguinal canal and consisted of epididymis, vas deferens, and a rete testis that ended blindly in fibrous streaks; "follicle-like structures" were noted microscopically.[865] This observation lends support to the notion of an association between WWS and FGTD. Incidentally, Weinberg's case appears to describe the oldest patient in whom FGTD has been identified. In contrast, Whitley and colleagues reported a patient with WWS in whom testicular abnormalities included small size attributed to shortening of seminiferous tubules and low numbers of Leydig cells.[866] No features resembling FGTD were present. WWS represents the most severe of the dystroglycanopathies, in which defective interaction between membrane receptors and extracellular matrix components results in muscle, brain, and nerve derangements.[867] Two new cases of GTD have been reported in association with Noonan syndrome.[868]

In all cases of FGTD, the testes were grossly unremarkable, with normal tunica albuginea, and the histologic testicular pattern was similar. Seminiferous tubules were well developed (number of germ cells and Sertoli cells per cross section within normal limits) only in the central zone of the testicular parenchyma, although with reduced numbers of seminiferous cords. Beneath the tunica albuginea, the peripheral testicular parenchyma showed a crescent-like zone with large malformed tubules, cords, and solid nodules of spherical or irregular shape embedded in fibrous connective tissue reminiscent of ovarian stroma organized into several concentric layers. Each of these solid nodules was surrounded by a delimiting basement membrane (Fig. 12.70). Each structure was composed of three cell types: cells with vesicular nuclei and vacuolated cytoplasm, cells with hyperchromatic nuclei, and germ cell–like cells. The former two cell types were arranged at the periphery, forming a pseudostratified epithelium with the long axes perpendicular to the nodule periphery. The third cell type resembled fetal spermatogonia and was fewer in number, although number varied from one tubular formation to another. These structures contained eosinophilic, PAS⁺ material, similar to Call-Exner bodies

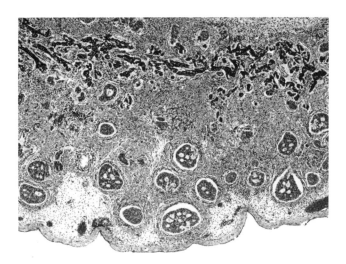

Fig. 12.70 Fetal gonadoblastoid testicular dysplasia. Several nodules are present at the periphery of the testicular parenchyma.

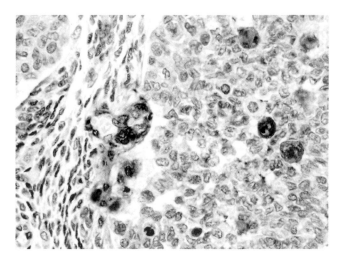

Fig. 12.72 Fetal gonadoblastoid testicular dysplasia. There is positive expression for collagen IV both in the bodies and the wall of the vessels that penetrate the nodules.

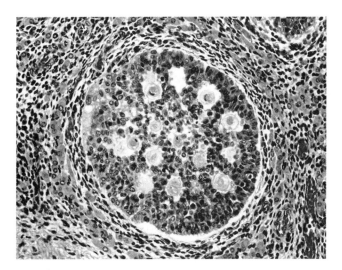

Fig. 12.71 Fetal gonadoblastoid testicular dysplasia. A nodule contains numerous Sertoli-like cells, Call-Exner bodies, and isolated germ cells. The nodule is surrounded by two cell layers: fusiform cells (inner layer) and Leydig cells (outer layer).

(Fig. 12.71). There may be continuity between these structures and normal seminiferous tubules.

Immunohistochemically, cells within the nodular lesions revealed a gradient in the expression of inhibin, most strongly at the periphery and negative in the center. The surrounding spindle stromal cells expressed vimentin and muscle-specific actin. Laminin and collagen type IV were expressed in the basement membrane and revealed deep invaginations of basement membrane material toward the center of the nodules, resembling Call-Exner bodies (Fig. 12.72). Only isolated cells morphologically resembling germ cells expressed PLAP, but most were negative for all markers. Cytokeratin (AE1/AE3) expression was only focally positive. The remaining parenchyma showed normal development according to age and revealed expression of vimentin in Sertoli cells. Inhibin was intensely and diffusely expressed in Sertoli and Leydig cells.[864]

The differential diagnosis includes conditions with anomalous seminiferous tubules at the gonadal periphery, including dysgenetic testis and gonadoblastoma. Dysgenetic testis also exhibits

tubular or cordlike structures, but these are differentiated (some form true seminiferous tubules) and may also be present within a poorly collagenized tunica albuginea. Both contain intertubular stroma consisting of fibrous connective tissue similar to the ovarian-like stroma characteristic of dysgenetic gonads. However, patients with dysgenetic testis are 46,XY disorder of sex development (DSD) with müllerian remnants, a condition that is absent in FGTD.

Distinguishing FGTD from gonadoblastoma is more difficult. Gonadoblastoma is usually found in an ovarian streak gonad or dysgenetic gonad and contains granulosa–Sertoli cells and germ cells that are like those of dysgerminoma or seminoma; these cells are absent in FGTD.

FGTD has been reported in patients with WWS, so one could hypothesize that the genetic deficiency causing this syndrome may also be responsible for normal testicular development.[863] Other hypotheses suggest a defect in segmentation of primitive cords secondary to poor fetal development of the vascular system or mutations in the *PTPN11* gene because two patients were carriers of Noonan syndrome.[869]

One may also speculate about the potential progression pathway of FGTD. Given that no patient has survived beyond a few months of life, it is not possible to ascertain how the lesion would have progressed. Incidentally, it is puzzling to recognize the vague resemblance between FGTD and granulosa cell tumor of the juvenile type, another congenital testicular tumor. The determination whether FGTD is a precursor lesion of full-blown gonadoblastoma, juvenile granulosa cell tumor, or another neoplasm, or would rather undergo atrophy, as may be surmised by the observations of Weinberg, awaits identification of FGTD in patients with longer survival.[865]

Sertoli Cell Nodule (Hypoplastic Zones or Dysgenetic Tubules)

Sertoli cell nodule consists of the presence in the adult testis of one or several foci of infantile (immature) seminiferous tubules. The term "Sertoli cell nodule" was first reported in 1973, although Pick described a lesion in 1905 known as Pick adenoma that has similar characteristics.[870,871] This lesion has also been reported as Sertoli cell hyperplasia, tubular dysgenesis, or hypoplastic zones.[872–874]

Each group of tubules appears well delimited but unencapsulated. Nodule size usually varies from microscopic to 5 mm; however, in at least 10 reported cases, size has reached up to 10 mm, termed *macroscopic Sertoli cell nodule*.[875–877] These patients may have palpable nodules at presentation. The nodules may be single or multiple. On section, each nodule is distinguished by its whitish color. Ultrasonography may suggest testicular tumor.

Sertoli cell nodule is found in about 60% of adult cryptorchid testes, regardless of when the testes descended.[878] It is also present in 22% of normal scrotal testes in some series and is an occasional finding in men with idiopathic infertility and in the parenchyma surrounding germ cell tumor.[874] The seminiferous tubules have a prepubertal diameter and may be anastomotic. The epithelium is columnar or pseudostratified, devoid of lumina, and usually consists only of Sertoli cells (Fig. 12.73). The cells have elongate hyperchromatic nuclei with one or several peripherally placed small nucleoli.[874]

The interstitium varies from scant to well collagenized. Leydig cells are usually absent in these areas, and, if present, their numbers are low; exceptionally, they are abundant (Fig. 12.74). In some nodules, isolated germ cells may be observed (Fig. 12.75). Study of serial sections sometimes reveals continuity between some tubules and normal tubules. Sertoli cell nodules change with advancing age. These changes are not related to a significant enlargement of the size because that remains unaltered, but rather reflect development of structures inside the lesions. The Sertoli cells produce large amounts of basal lamina that become intensely PAS+ and protrude inside the hypoplastic tubules. In transverse and oblique sections, these protrusions may be misinterpreted as intratubular accumulations of basal lamina material (Fig. 12.76). This material may undergo calcification to form microliths. Immunohistochemical study reveals two components of the basal lamina (collagen IV and laminin), thus confirming extracellular origin; the protrusions consist mainly of laminin, whereas collagen IV delimits the outer profile of the seminiferous tubules. So, although the amount of collagen IV is uniform around the tubules, the depth of laminin varies within the same tubule and from one to another tubule. Sertoli cells in this lesion also show immunohistochemical markers of immature cells, including expression of D2–40,

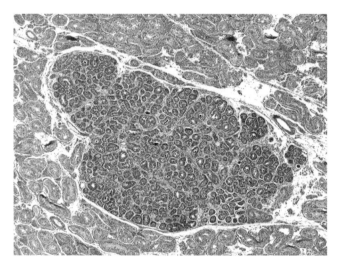

Fig. 12.73 Sertoli cell nodule. This adult cryptorchid testis contains compact groups of small seminiferous tubules with pseudostratified cell layers without lumina.

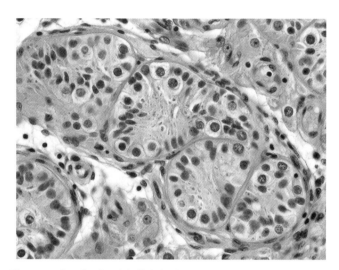

Fig. 12.75 Sertoli cell nodule. Tubular formations with immature Sertoli cells and spermatogonia.

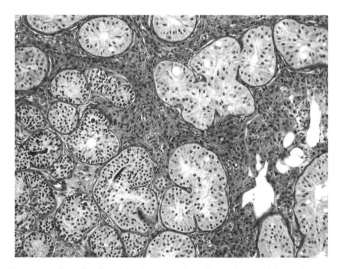

Fig. 12.74 Sertoli cell nodule. Among tubular formations with irregular contours and prepubertal maturation, abundant Leydig cells are observed.

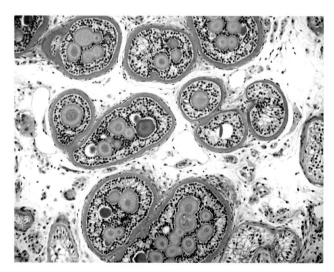

Fig. 12.76 Sertoli cell nodule. Sertoli cell–produced material, similar to the basal lamina material, forms finger-like protrusions inside the hypoplastic tubules. The Sertoli cells are arranged in a ring around this material.

AMH, calretinin, and inhibin bodies.[170] The diameter of hypoplastic tubules is usually smaller than that of the adjacent tubules, but in some cases the inverse occurs because of hypertrophy of Sertoli cells, which show some evidence of pubertal maturation without reaching full maturation of adult cells.

Sertoli cell nodules are assumed to be primary testicular lesions and are included in the spectrum of testicular dysgenesis syndrome.[879] They represent seminiferous tubules that are unable to undergo pubertal development despite the same hormonal stimuli as adjacent normal tubules. This dysgenesis includes immature Sertoli cell pattern showing D2–40 immunoexpression, low inhibin secretion, absence of ARs, and lack of maturation of peritubular myoid cells that fail to synthesize elastic fibers (Fig. 12.77).[880] The presence of hypoplastic zones (Sertoli cells nodules) in a testicular biopsy is an adverse prognostic sign for fertility, as is the presence of isolated dysgenetic tubules or hypoplastic tubules in testicular parenchyma. Attempts have been made to identify the precursor zones of these hypoplastic zones in prepubertal biopsies to obtain an additional predictor of fertility in cryptorchidism. Infantile precursor hypoplastic zones are not as well delimited as definitive hypoplastic zones of adults. Differences in diameter between hypoplastic tubules and the other tubules of the testicular parenchyma are not as clearly marked in infants as in adults. Although small tubules predominate in the hypoplastic zone precursors of the infantile testis, the degree of maturation of these tubules may be similar to or more advanced than the outer tubules of the parenchyma (Fig. 12.78). The most reliable histologic findings for identifying the precursor zones in infant testes are the cordlike arrangement of these tubules, occurrence of anastomoses among the cords, scant cellularity (Sertoli number is lower than in the remaining testicular parenchyma), and wide Sertoli cell cytoplasm, which often shows granular changes.

The differential diagnosis includes Sertoli cell adenoma, tubular hamartoma in androgen insensitivity syndrome (AIS), testis with focal Sertoli cell–only tubules (MAT of the testis), Sertoli cell neoplasm, and gonadoblastoma.

Sertoli cell adenoma and tubular hamartoma are characteristic findings in AIS. Like Sertoli cell nodule, adenoma and tubular hamartoma contain nodules composed of solid tubules of immature Sertoli cells without a capsule. The three lesions differ macroscopically in size; adenoma and tubular hamartoma are usually larger than Sertoli cell nodule. Histologically, both Sertoli cell

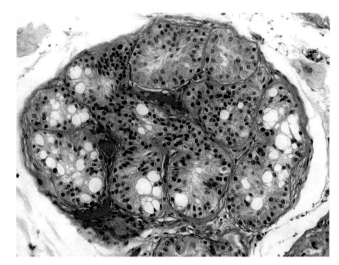

Fig. 12.78 Sertoli cell nodule. Group of anastomosed tubules lined by Sertoli cells with prepubertal maturation showing spherical nuclei, central nucleoli, and vacuoles in the cytoplasm.

adenoma and tubular hamartoma are formed by Sertoli cells with spherical, rather than elongate, nuclei that do not display pseudostratification. Although the tubular wall may be widened, it does not have nodular intratubular projections. In Sertoli cell adenoma, tubules are back to back, and the sparse interstitium does not usually contain Leydig cells. The interstitium may be densely cellular in tubular hamartoma, with fusiform cells. Tubular hamartoma always has many Leydig cells, whereas these cells are lacking or scant in Sertoli cell nodule.[254] The parenchyma surrounding tubular hamartoma has the same grade of development as the lesion. In contrast, the testes in patients with Sertoli cell nodule are always delayed in development.

Testes with focal Sertoli only–cell tubules show two seminiferous tubule types: Sertoli cell–only tubules and tubules with germ cells, although the spermatogenetic degree may vary widely in the tubules with germ cells. Sertoli cell–only tubules do not form clusters such as those seen in the hypoplastic tubules of Sertoli cell nodules. In addition, the tubular size and the degree of Sertoli cell maturation are higher in Sertoli cell–only tubules to such an extent that even lumina may be observed in some tubules. Finally, the usual cell components of the testicular interstitium (Leydig cells, macrophages, and some mast cells) are found in these Sertoli cell–only tubules.

Sertoli cell tumor not otherwise specified consists of larger cells with vesicular nuclei and prominent nucleoli with isolated atypical nuclei and mitotic figures arranged in cords and tubules without significant widening of basal membrane that is characteristic of Sertoli cell nodule.

Intratubular large cell hyalinizing Sertoli cell neoplasia may resemble Sertoli cell nodule at low magnification because both may produce multiple nodules and show widened basal membranes and intratubular projections of basal membrane–derived material. However, the tubules in intratubular large cell hyalinizing Sertoli cell neoplasia are not anastomotic and are larger in diameter than those seen in Sertoli cell nodule. Sertoli cells have an apparent higher grade of maturation (vesicular nuclei with central nucleoli and large eosinophilic cytoplasm). Immunohistochemically the cells express cytokeratin that is usually absent in Sertoli cell nodule. Also, intratubular hyalinizing Sertoli cell neoplasia does not contain germ cells, usually develops in scrotal testis, and is associated with Peutz-Jeghers syndrome.[710,881,882]

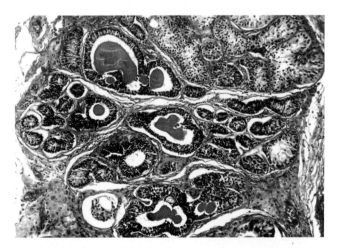

Fig. 12.77 Sertoli cell nodule. Tubular organization is complex and may show different patterns. Note the ring-shaped tubules in some areas and anastomosed tubules in others, both with immature Sertoli cells.

Sex cord tumor with annular tubules is exceptionally rare in the testis. The resemblance to Sertoli cell nodule is high, but features favoring this diagnosis include large size of the lesion and greater complexity of the tubular organization, with solid areas and hyalinized stroma.

When Sertoli cell nodule contains germ cells, the differential diagnosis of gonadoblastoma should be considered. Most germ cells in Sertoli cell nodules are spermatogonia; these cells are scant, do not show signs of proliferation, and are TSPY+ (testis-specific protein Y-encoded+). In rare cases, Sertoli cell nodule contains gonocyte-like cells in both the basal membrane and the center of the tubules; these cells express OCT3/4. These gonocyte-like cells thus represent GCNIS (Fig. 12.79). In these cases the lesion itself is like gonadoblastoma. Criteria for ruling out gonadoblastoma are as follows: Sertoli cell nodule with GCNIS is surrounded by or near germ cell tumor, and gonadoblastoma characteristically arises in malformed gonads (gonadal dysgenesis, dysgenetic testis in DSDs), whereas Sertoli cell nodule is found in well-configured testes. The disposition of tumor cells is also important. In Sertoli cell nodule, tumor cells are preferentially disposed at the center of the lesion, whereas in gonadoblastoma, the distribution is more diffuse.[883]

Another entity that should be included in the differential diagnosis is sex cord–stromal tumor of the testis with entrapped germ cells. These tumors measure several centimeters in diameter. The cells are arranged in cords and tubules and may show germ cells without atypia, mainly at the periphery.[884]

Tubular Hamartoma (Androgen Insensitivity Syndrome)

Tubular hamartoma consists of unencapsulated whitish nodules that are well delimited from the parenchyma containing small seminiferous tubules and numerous Leydig cells. It is also known as Sertoli–Leydig cell hamartoma (see later discussion of Androgen Insensitivity Syndromes).

Lymphangiectasis

Congenital Testicular Lymphangiectasis

Congenital testicular lymphangiectasis is characterized by abnormal and excessive development of lymphatic vessels in the tunica albuginea, mediastinum testis, interlobular septa, and testicular interstitium.[253,885,886] Ultrastructurally these dilated vessels are similar to normal lymphatic capillaries, although some are markedly dilated, and the testicular interstitium is slightly edematous

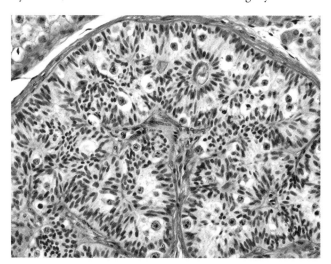

Fig. 12.79 Sertoli cell nodule showing atypical gonocytes among prepubertal Sertoli cells in an adult patient with germ cell tumor.

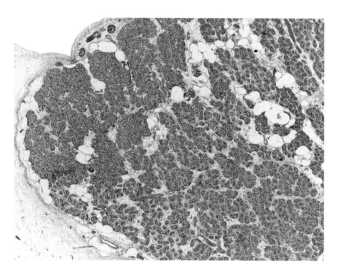

Fig. 12.80 Congenital testicular lymphangiectasis. Ectatic lymphatic vessels are seen in the tunica vasculosa and interlobular septa, as well as among the seminiferous tubules, causing compression.

(Fig. 12.80). Testicular lymphangiectasis occurs in both cryptorchid and scrotal testes. One patient had Noonan syndrome.

It does not seem to affect the seminiferous tubules, and low numbers of spermatogonia and reduced tubular diameters are observed only in cryptorchid testes. The epididymis and spermatic cord are not affected, and congenital testicular lymphangiectasis is not associated with pulmonary, intestinal, or systemic lymphangiectasis. During fetal life, lymphatic vessels are visible only immediately beneath the tunica albuginea and in the interlobular septa.[887] During childhood the number and size of the septal lymphatic vessels decrease.[426] By adulthood the vessels are inconspicuous, although ultrastructural and immunohistochemical evidence of their presence is visible in the interstitium, and they are easily identified by staining with monoclonal antibody D2–40.[888]

In lymphangiectasis, septal lymphatic vessels are large and often massively dilated. It occurs only in childhood, a finding suggesting that these dilated vessels undergo involution at puberty or that pubertal development of the seminiferous tubules masks the lymphangiectasis.

Testicular lymphangiectasis may result from alterations in lymphatic drainage caused by surgical treatment of the inguinal region, radiation therapy of retroperitoneal lymph nodes, or chronic inflammation of the spermatic cord. Lymphatic dilatation involves vessels that were previously normal, resulting in development of small cysts chiefly in the tunica vasculosa and epididymis. Similar dilatations have been observed in cryptorchid testes and in patients with Morris syndrome.

Epididymal Lymphangiectasis

Epididymal lymphangiectasis has been described in adults as "lymphangiectasis" and "lymphangioma," terms referring to pseudotumoral lesions consisting of abnormal development of lymphatic vessels in the caput epididymis. Dilated vessels compress the ductuli efferentes and cause irregular dilation by compression, thereby distorting the normal architecture (Fig. 12.81). In some cases, these malformative or hamartomatous lesions are likely primary, and the diagnosis is made by examination of orchiepididymectomy for suspected tumor or lesion.[889–891] In other cases, it is considered secondary to previous herniorrhaphy, and only epididymectomy is performed.[891]

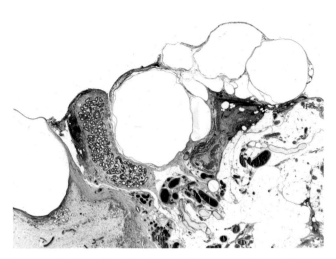

Fig. 12.81 Epididymal lymphangiectasis. There are multiple cystic formations of different size, apparently without content surrounding the epididymis.

Other Hamartomatous Testicular Lesions

Smooth muscle is a normal component of sperm excretory ducts, as well as of two other specific structures: the tunica albuginea of the inferior pole and the interstitial tissues of the cauda epididymis among the numerous folds of the ductus epididymis. Muscular hyperplasia involving any of these structures has been reported in patients from puberty to 81 years of age. The minimum size required for diagnosis is not well defined, but previously reported cases indicate that the width of muscular proliferation was 0.6 to 7 cm.

In young men, smooth muscle hyperplasia is especially frequent in those with AIS. The lesion has been reported as leiomyoma, and it may be associated with multiple tubular hamartomas.[892,893] This smooth muscle proliferation is located in the inferior pole, involves the tunica albuginea and the adjacent soft tissue (i.e., in the zone that should be occupied by the cauda epididymis), and may form nodules measuring more than 1 cm in diameter (Fig. 12.82).

In other adult patients the reported distribution of smooth muscle hyperplasia has been related to the ductus deferens (periductal), the surrounding vessels (perivascular), the different structures of the cauda epididymis (interstitial), the seminiferous tubules (peritubular hamartoma) (Fig. 12.83), or the tunica albuginea (Fig. 12.84). In periductal hamartoma, ductus deferens thickness (normally 3 mm) can reach 10 mm. The cauda epididymis (normally 0.5 to 0.7 mm) may enlarge up to 2 mm. Smooth muscle cells create a concentric pattern around sperm excretory ducts and blood vessels. In other hamartomas such as those in the tunica albuginea and the interstitial tissue of the cauda epididymis, muscle bundles are irregularly arranged and intermingled with variable amounts of connective tissue (Fig. 12.85).[894]

Most muscular hyperplasias are assumed to be hamartomas, similar to smooth muscle proliferations in other organs, including the gingiva, palate, esophagus, gastric pylorus, small intestine, large intestine, trachea, and breast.[895–902] Differential diagnosis includes leiomyoma, but hyperplasia lacks characteristic features of leiomyoma such as the cohesive pattern of smooth muscle bundles, nodularity, and well-defined delimitation from the adjacent tissues.

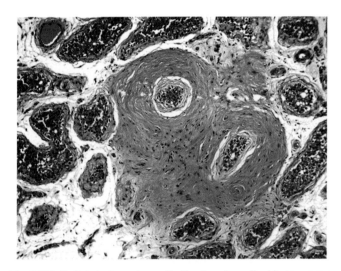

Fig. 12.83 Peritubular hamartoma. Proliferation of myofibroblasts concentrically arranged around two seminiferous tubules.

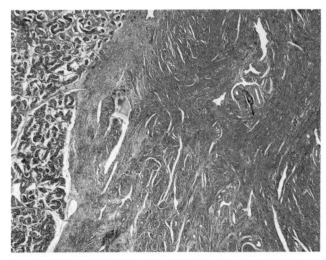

Fig. 12.82 Smooth muscle hamartoma in the lower pole of the testicle. The lesion is in continuity with the albuginea.

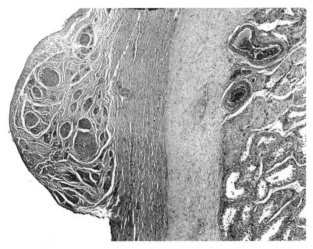

Fig. 12.84 Smooth muscle hamartoma within enlarged tunica albuginea.

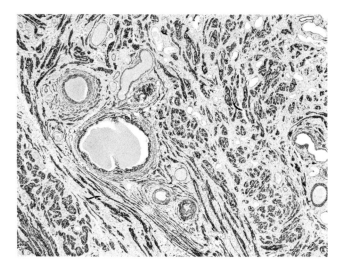

Fig. 12.85 Smooth muscle hamartoma in the lower pole of the testicle. There are bundles of loose compact muscle cells and abundant vessels (immunostaining for smooth muscle actin).

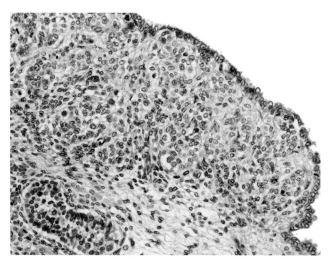

Fig. 12.86 The blastema is located between the lining epithelium of the testis and the seminiferous tubules occupying an expansion of the albuginea. The major population consists of small nucleus cells (pre-Sertoli), among which there are larger ones (gonocytes).

Ectopias

Persistence of Gonadal Blastema

The term *persistence of testicular blastema* refers to the presence of gonadal blastema in an otherwise normal testis for age. Testicular blastema includes immature sex cords, germ cells, and mesenchymal components. The primitive tissue gives rise to testicular parenchyma and is not expected to be present in completely developed testes.

This infrequent ectopia occurs in newborns as a rare autopsy finding. It was present in both testes of three fetuses from a total of more than 3000 consecutive autopsies: one fetus was spontaneously aborted as a result of chorioamnionitis; one was electively aborted because of a neural tube defect, omphalocele, and asymmetric arthrogryposis; and a third had trisomy 18 and classic phenotypic features of Edwards syndrome.[227]

The blastema is near the upper testicular pole at the implantation site of the caput of the epididymis. It has a crescent shape and extends throughout the depth of the tunica albuginea and the adjacent parenchyma.

Blastema consists of epithelial cords of cells or solid masses in continuity with mesothelium (Fig. 12.86). These cells are intermingled with others that are larger, with pale cytoplasm, vesicular nuclei, and prominent nucleoli. This second population, resembling germ cells, is less frequently seen, sparsely distributed among the cords. The remaining parenchyma, tunica albuginea, and epididymis are normal for age. Blastomatous epithelial cells display immunoreactivity for vimentin, laminin, type IV collagen, and cytokeratin; the expression of cytokeratin in the most superficial cells is like that of mesothelial cells and decreases in intensity in the deeper cells. This characteristic suggests that these may be pre–Sertoli cells. The cordlike structures are delimited by laminin and type IV collagen. The larger cell type is immunoreactive for PLAP on the surface, and lacks vimentin and cytokeratin expression, suggesting that it is related to the gonocyte. Leydig cells have not been observed among the cords of gonadal blastema.[227]

The differential diagnosis of gonadal blastema ectopia includes ovotestes. The small size of the gonocytes distinguishes these cells from ovocytes, which are several times larger. In addition, no intersex condition is observed.

The most likely evolution of blastema is differentiation toward testicular parenchyma. This possibility is supported by two features: the disorder may occur only in newborns, and in the zone where blastema cells are found (superior testicular pole), ectopic seminiferous tubules or ectopic Leydig cells have also been observed.

Seminiferous Tubule Ectopia

The presence of seminiferous tubules within the tunica albuginea is a rare and usually incidental histologic finding.[226] Ectopic tubules are present in approximately 0.8% of pediatric autopsies and 0.3% of adult autopsies. The lower incidence in adults may be explained by proportionally less sampling. The lesion ranges from microscopic to a few millimeters in diameter, and it may be visible in children as rounded macules on the surface of the testis as minute bulges in which multiple small vesicles protrude through a thin tunica albuginea.[903,904] Histologically, there are groups of seminiferous tubules in the tunica albuginea, sometimes accompanied by Leydig cells. In children, ectopic tubules appear normal (Fig. 12.87), whereas in adults they are usually slightly dilated (Fig. 12.88), although some tubules may be hyalinized. Serial sections reveal continuity with the intraparenchymatous seminiferous tubules.

Ectopia of the seminiferous tubules is probably congenital, although it has been found in older men.[905] It does not appear to be the result of trauma. The malformation probably arises in the sixth week of gestation, when the primordial sex cords have formed and are branching toward the gonadal surface, and the developing testes are covered by only one to three layers of coelomic epithelium. Later, the tunica albuginea forms around the sex cords and under the coelomic epithelium. Failure of insertion of the tunica albuginea between the sex cords and coelomic epithelium may entrap seminiferous tubules.

Ectopia differs from testicular dysgenesis, a distinctive form of 46, XY DSD with müllerian remnants. Numerous features characteristic of ectopic seminiferous tubules distinguish ectopia from other conditions, including normal thickness and collagenization of the tunica albuginea, absence of interstitial tissue resembling ovarian stroma (characteristic of testicular dysgenesis), and clear delimitation of

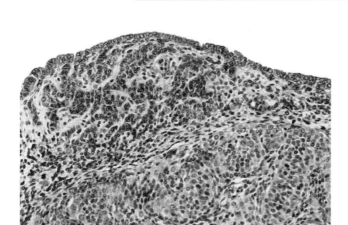

Fig. 12.87 Testis from 2-month-old infant showing ectopic seminiferous tubules within the tunica albuginea in the upper testicular pole.

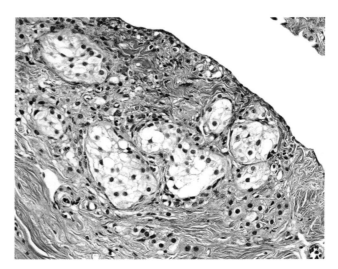

Fig. 12.89 Cluster of ectopic seminiferous tubules and Leydig cells in the wall of a hernia sac in an adult as an incidental finding.

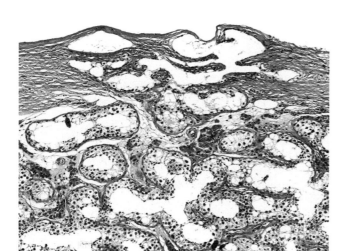

Fig. 12.88 Ectopic seminiferous tubules in albuginea in an adult. Seminiferous tubules show ectasia, and ectopic tubules have markedly atrophic seminiferous epithelium.

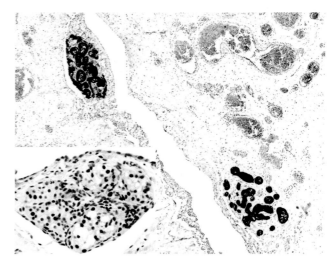

Fig. 12.90 Ectopic seminiferous tubules in the wall of a hernia sac. Two clusters of seminiferous tubules with intense immunoexpression of inhibin. (*Inset*) androgen receptor immunoreactivity in Sertoli and Leydig cells of the ectopic cluster.

the tunica albuginea and testicular parenchyma (see discussion of Disorders of Sex Development (Dysgenetic testis), below).

In a unique case, multiple clusters of seminiferous tubules and Leydig cells were present in the wall of a hernia sac that accompanied an undescended testis removed from an adult. The ectopic tubules were not surrounded by tunica albuginea and were like those in cryptorchid testicular parenchyma with only dysgenetic Sertoli cells (Fig. 12.89).[906] Sertoli cells in the tubules expressed inhibin and ARs (Fig. 12.90). In another case, ectopic seminiferous tubules immunoreactive for inhibin were in the epididymis next to extratesticular rete testis (Fig. 12.91). These extratesticular seminiferous tubules were surrounded by loose stroma and seemed to be connected to the extratesticular rete testis.

Leydig Cell Ectopia

Leydig cells occur normally in the testicular interstitium (interstitial Leydig cells) and in the wall of the seminiferous tubules (peritubular Leydig cells).[375] However, clusters of cells are often observed in other locations in the testis, in the epididymis, or in the spermatic cord.[907,908] In men the incidence rate is 40% to 90%.[909]

Inside the testis, ectopic Leydig cells may be found in the interlobular septa, rete testis, or tunica albuginea (Figs. 12.92 to 12.94), as well as within hyalinized seminiferous tubules.[370,910–916a] Intratubular Leydig cells are found only in tubules with advanced atrophy and marked thickening of the tunica propria, including the tubules in adult cryptorchid testes, those of men with Klinefelter syndrome, and in some other primary hypogonadisms (Fig. 12.95). Immunohistochemical studies suggest that the endocrine function of these Leydig cells is low.[917] Several theories have been offered to account for these ectopic cells, including in situ differentiation, migration from the testicular interstitium, and trapping of peritubular Leydig cells in the tunica propria during its thickening and seminiferous tubule shortening in atrophy progression.[917] The presence of small capillary vessels within the intratubular Leydig cell clusters would favor the last hypothesis.

Leydig cells are commonly found in the epididymis, as well as in the spermatic cord, both in newborns and adults.[910,918,919] Extratesticular Leydig cells usually form small groups within or adjacent to nerves (Fig. 12.96), present in 41% of autopsies.[368,920,920a]

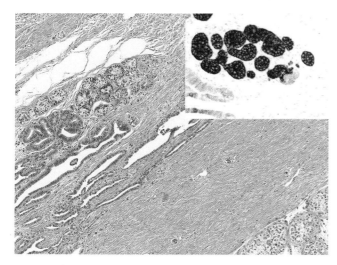

Fig. 12.91 Ectopic seminiferous tubules in epididymis. (*Inset*) Seminiferous tubules with prepubertal development showing immunoexpression for inhibin.

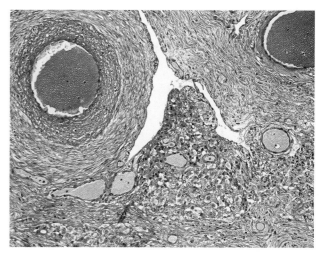

Fig. 12.94 Ectopic Leydig cells in the tunica vasculosa protruding inside a lymphatic vessel.

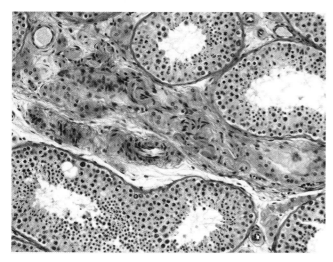

Fig. 12.92 Ectopic Leydig cells in an interlobular septum associated with nerve fibers.

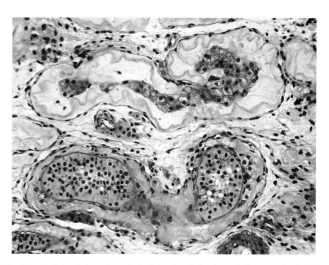

Fig. 12.95 Ectopic Leydig cells inside a hyalinized seminiferous tubule. This picture contrasts with that of the dysgenetic Sertoli cell–only tubule, which shows a patent basal membrane located between the dysgenetic Sertoli cells and the tubular wall.

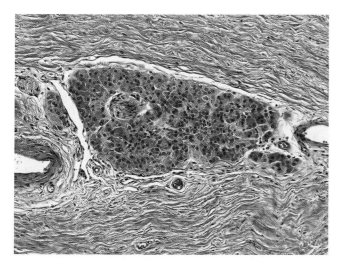

Fig. 12.93 Ectopic Leydig cells around a nerve in albuginea.

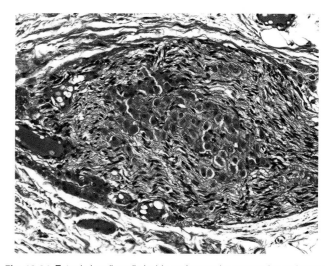

Fig. 12.96 Ectopic Leydig cells inside and around a spermatic cord nerve. Ectopic Leydig cells are distinguished from neuronal ganglion cells by their smaller size.

Extraparenchymal Leydig cells arise in more than 90% of orchiectomy specimens, and study of tissue microarrays found an incidence rate of 35%.[847] Extratesticular location of Leydig cells is apparently common, and thus finding them depends only on the number of sections obtained. In most cases, these cells are in proximity to small nerves or even inside the nerves and vegetative nervous system ganglia.[370] These cells, probably originating from in situ differentiation of Leydig cell precursors, express testosterone.[908] Inhibin and calretinin are other useful immunohistochemical markers to enhance detection of ectopic Leydig cells. Calretinin is more sensitive but less specific than inhibin.

Ectopic Leydig cells, both intratesticular and extratesticular, suffer the same atrophic and hyperplasic alterations as their eutopic counterparts, including disappearance during childhood. In older men and in those with chronic alcoholism, ectopic Leydig cells may show atrophic features, whereas in patients with hCG-secreting germ cell tumors, they show hyperplasia.

The occurrence of ectopic Leydig cells in the tunica albuginea, epididymis, or spermatic cord may account for rare cases of Leydig cell tumor in these paratesticular structures.[907] Ectopic Leydig cells should not be misinterpreted as tumor cells (infiltration or metastasis) when malignancy of a testicular Leydig cell tumor is suspected.

Adrenal Cortical Ectopia

Adrenal cortical ectopia is a frequent finding outside of the testis, although it has also been observed inside. Ectopic adrenal cortex is the most frequent incidental finding in male urologic surgery.[921] In a series of boys who underwent inguinoscrotal surgery the incidence rate of this finding varied from 3% to 3.8%.[922,923] The frequency was higher (5.1%) in a series of children with cryptorchid testis who underwent more complete exploration of the spermatic cord.[924] Most adrenal cortical ectopias are found in extratesticular locations such as the epididymis (Figs. 12.97 and 12.98), tunica albuginea, and hernia sacs (Fig.12.99).[925,926] Macroscopically, ectopic adrenal tissue forms firm yellowish nodules, measuring 1 to 4 mm in diameter, spherical or ovoid, and sometimes umbilicated. The nodules are covered by a capsule, have three well-defined layers of adrenal cortex, and lack medulla. Adrenal ectopia represents aberrant adrenal tissue that has accompanied the testis in its descent.[927]

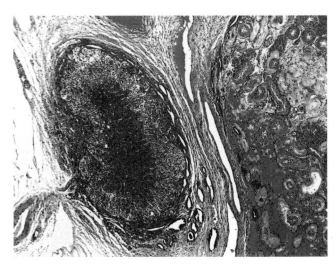

Fig. 12.98 Cortical adrenal ectopia surrounded by extratesticular rete testis cavities in a cryptorchid testis with immature and hyalinized tubules.

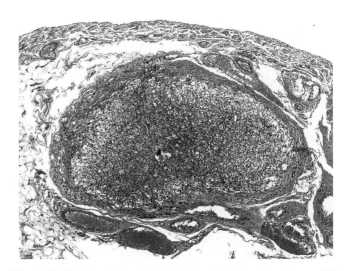

Fig. 12.99 Ectopia of adrenal cortex in the wall of a hernia sac in an adult. The ectopic adrenal tissue is surrounded by a thick capsule and still retains a radial structure.

Ectopia of cells similar to adrenal cortex may also be found inside the testis. Adrenal ectopia has been observed between the rete testis and adjacent seminiferous tubules, as well as in the parenchyma near the tunica albuginea.[928–930] Adrenal ectopic nodule may be solitary or multiple. Cytomegalic cells have been observed in newborns with adrenal cytomegaly, both in patients with Beckwith-Wiedemann syndrome and in isolated cases of adrenal cytomegaly (Fig. 12.100). The origin of these intratesticular nodules may be pluripotential testicular hilus steroid cells.[931,932]

Intratesticular nodules may undergo hyperplasia, thus causing testicular enlargement that suggests a tumor in two disorders: adrenogenital syndrome and Nelson syndrome (see later).

Other Ectopias

Other rare forms of ectopia are found within and outside the testis. Osseous and adipose tissue and ectopic ductus epididymis may be formed within the testis. Extratesticular ectopia includes splenic ectopia (splenogonadal fusion), hepatic ectopia (hepatotesticular fusion), and renal blastema ectopia.

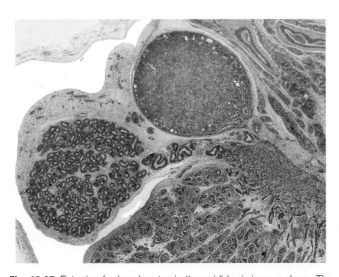

Fig. 12.97 Ectopia of adrenal cortex in the epididymis in a newborn. The adrenal cortex nodule is the same size as the caput of the epididymis.

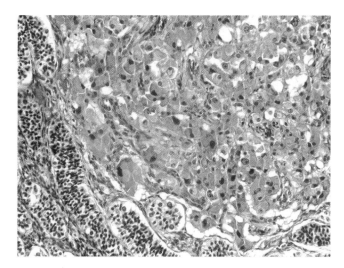

Fig. 12.100 Intratesticular adrenal cortical ectopia next to the rete testis in a boy. Adrenal-like cells show cytomegalic changes.

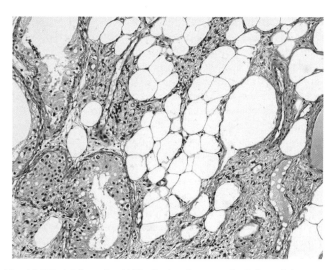

Fig. 12.102 Adult cryptorchid testis showing metaplastic fat cells between the seminiferous tubules and the rete testis.

Cartilaginous heterotopia, which may appear as small immature cartilage nodules in the caput of the epididymis, has been attributed to metaplasia of metanephric rests.

Osseous heterotopia (testicular osteoma, stone in the testicle, testicular calculus) is a rare type of metaplasia that occurs in areas of the parenchyma with fibrosis. It is possible that some cases are secondary to prior tuberculosis, hematoma resorption, or traumatic injury. In some cases, such lesions cannot be distinguished from a tumor, prompting orchiectomy (Fig. 12.101).[933-936] Reported cases and our own observations reveal that osseous metaplasia manifests as hard intraparenchymatous nodules that vary from a few millimeters to several centimeters. These nodules consist of compact osseous tissue surrounded in all cases by cholesterol clefts and a fibrous pseudocapsule. They probably represent a metaplastic process in response to testicular trauma or damage.

Adipose metaplasia is frequent in undescended testes and older men. Adipose cells are preferably located in the proximity of the rete testis (Fig. 12.102). Adipocytes are frequently found at the periphery of intratesticular adrenal cortical tumors and in some Leydig cell tumors.[937] Testicular lipomatosis is associated with

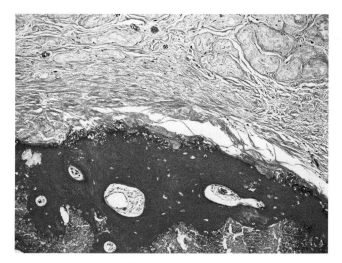

Fig. 12.101 Osseous metaplasia in an ischemic testis. Compact osseous tissue is surrounded by hyalinized seminiferous tubules and absence of Leydig cells.

Cowden syndrome (usually bilateral), Proteus syndrome, and Bannayan-Riley-Ruvalcaba syndrome.[938] These syndromes, together with adult Lhermitte-Duclos disease and autism spectrum disorders associated with macrocephaly, collectively form the PTEN hamartoma tumor syndrome (PHTS), which is related to *PTEN* gene mutations.[939] Intratesticular lipomatosis associated with these syndromes is visualized by ultrasound as multiple bilateral hyperechoic lesions.[940,941] Given the rarity of intratesticular lipoma, the presence of lipomatosis may be an indicator of underlying PTEN mutation.[942]

Intratesticular and paratesticular mesonephric remnants. Most of the structures derived from embryonic remnants (testis and epididymis hydatids, aberrant upper and lower ducts, the Giraldes organ) have a specific location and are well-known wolffian or müllerian derivatives. However, in systematic study of surgical specimens of testis, epididymis, spermatic cord, and hernial sacs, glandular or tubular formations may frequently be found that are reminiscent of the epididymis but may be misinterpreted as either normal structures of the spermatic pathways or, more significantly, as primary or secondary neoplasm. These mesonephric remnants may be found in other parts of the urogenital tract, including the kidney, renal pelvis, prostate, prostatic urethra, and paratesticular and intratesticular regions.[943]

Histologically, mesonephric remnants have variable patterns, ranging from small acini or tubules lined by low columnar epithelium with or without colloid type material inside. They resemble both histologically and immunohistochemically the efferent ducts, the main duct of the epididymis or the vas deferens, but differ by smaller size and absence of a well-structured muscular cell layer.[944]

Mesonephric remnants in the spermatic cord are the most frequent and are observed in 28% of cords at autopsy. Most are incidental, but some present clinically as cystic structures with or without papillary formations.[945] Most glandular inclusions in the wall of hernial sacs represent mesonephric remnants, with an incidence rate of 1.5% to 6%. Less frequent is the presence of mesonephric remnants in the testicular tunic, where these remnants, whose epithelium usually resembles that of efferent ducts, may produce cysts in the tunica albuginea.[946] Even rarer is the appearance of remnants inside vestigial structures of müllerian origin, as is the case of aberrant epididymal tissue reported in a testicular hydatid.[947,948]

Intratesticular mesonephric remnants are of special interest with respect to histogenesis and because they may be confused with neoplasm. Intratesticular structures reminiscent of efferent ducts or the main epididymal duct were found bilaterally in 5 of 1442 autopsies, and in 1 patient from a series of 271 orchiectomies.[949] Patient age ranged from 69 to 75 years. In autopsy cases, both testes were shrunken. The lesion was found in an orchiectomy specimen from a 67-year-old with suspected testicular tumor. The testicles showed multiple whitish areas located in the central part, as well as near the rete testis and under the tunica albuginea. Most of the mesonephric remnants corresponded to epididymis-like or efferent ductile-like structures. The luminal size varied from that of seminiferous tubules to cystic formations. Interiorly, there was granular or fibrillar PAS⁺ eosinophilic material with microcalcifications and Liesegang rings. A muscular layer surrounded most of the formations. Frequently the intratubular material was extravasated, triggering a minimal inflammatory reaction. The number and extent of these formations was so great in the reported orchiectomy specimen that in comparison with remnants observed in other organs, one could speak of florid hyperplasia of intratesticular mesonephric remnants. In most testes the adjacent parenchyma had large areas of tubular hyalinization, likely of ischemic origin (Figs. 12.103 through 12.105).

The differential diagnosis includes teratoma and burned-out germ cell tumor, but the distinction is not difficult. The location of these epididymal-like tubular formations within the parenchyma is difficult to explain from an embryologic point of view. Such displacement would have to occur at an early stage, before differentiation of the albuginea by AMH secreted by the Sertoli cells. Mesonephric cords would be trapped between nests consisting of pre–Sertoli and germ cells. An alternative hypothesis is metaplastic change in Sertoli cells.

Undescended Testes

Testicular descent is not always complete at birth, and approximately 3% of full-term newborns have incompletely descended testes. Most of these testes descend within 3 months, and only 1% of infants have incompletely descended testes 12 months after birth.

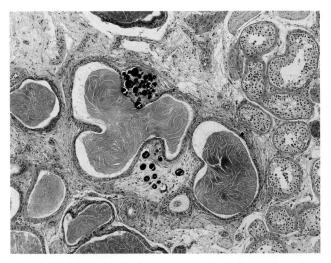

Fig. 12.103 Intratesticular mesonephric remnants. Much of the testicular parenchyma is replaced by tubular formations showing cystic transformation, eosinophilic material, and intratubular and extratubular calcifications.

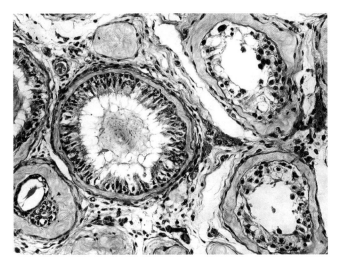

Fig. 12.104 Transverse section of an adult testis showing two tubular formations with characteristics of epididymal duct (pseudostratified epithelium with stereocilia) surrounded by seminiferous tubules with decreased spermatogenesis.

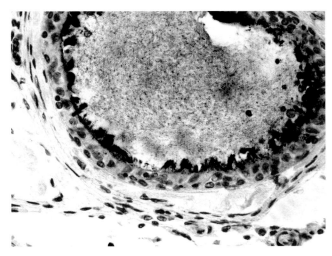

Fig. 12.105 Ectopic epididymal-like formation showing positive CD10 expression in adluminal border and stereocilia.

Spontaneous testicular descent is exceptional after the first year. In recent decades there has been a significant increase in the incidence of cryptorchidism.[950]

Only 5% of patients with impalpable testes are devoid of testes. Other causes include true cryptorchidism, testicular ectopia, and retractile testes.[951] True cryptorchidism includes abdominal, inguinal, and high scrotal testes that cannot be moved to the scrotum on physical exploration.[482] Ectopic testes are those located out of the normal path of testicular descent, most frequently in the superficial inguinal pouch. Other rare locations of ectopia include the abdominal wall, upper thigh, perineum, and base of the penis. Retractile testes may be moved to the scrotum at exploration and account for approximately one-third of clinically diagnosed undescended testes.

True Cryptorchidism

Patients with true cryptorchidism account for approximately 25% of cases of empty scrotum. These testes most frequently are found in the inguinal canal or upper scrotum; arrest within the abdomen is less frequent and accounts for only 5% to 10% of cases. Cryptorchidism is slightly more frequent on the right side than on the left (46% versus 31%, respectively), and in approximately 23% of cases is bilateral.[952] Family history of cryptorchidism is present in 14%.[953,954] Cryptorchid testis is usually smaller than the contralateral one, and this difference is often discernible at 6 months of age.[955] One-third of cryptorchid testes are soft.

Etiology

The causes of testicular maldescent are probably multiple and have not been fully elucidated. Several conditions are predictive of high risk for cryptorchidism, including increased maternal age, maternal obesity, pregnancy toxemia, bleeding during late pregnancy, exposure to phthalates, alcohol consumption and smoking, tall stature, paternal subfertility antecedents, cesarean birth, low birth weight, preterm birth, twin birth, hypospadias, other congenital malformations, and birth from September to November, as well as May to June.[956–958] Of these associations, low birth weight seems to be the most important.[959] Cryptorchidism may be congenital or acquired.

Congenital Cryptorchidism. This type of cryptorchidism is mainly caused by anomalies of development or hormonal mechanisms involved in testicular descent (see earlier). Impalpable undescended testes are infrequent because the transabdominal phase follows the simple mechanism of relative movement of the testis. Conversely, palpable undescended testes are more frequent because the second phase of testicular descent is more complex. Unilateral cryptorchidism may be caused by androgen failure, which leads to either an ipsilateral lesion in the development of GFN neurons or defect in CGRP release that hinders normal migration of the gubernaculum.[960]

Acquired Cryptorchidism. Normally descended testis may become cryptorchid and may even settle in the abdominal cavity.[961] Acquired cryptorchidism has a prevalence rate of 1% to 7% and peaks at approximately 8 years of age.[962] Two categories of acquired undescended testis have been described: postoperative trapped testis and spontaneous ascent from unknown causes.

Postoperative trapped testis is a normally descended testis that leaves the scrotal pouch after surgery for inguinal hernia or hydrocele.[963–965] This iatrogenic cryptorchidism occurs in 1% of children after herniotomy. Adherence of the testis or the cremasteric muscle to the surgical incision causes testicular ascent when the incision heals and undergoes retraction.

Various mechanisms have been proposed for *spontaneous ascent from unknown causes*, including inability of spermatic blood vessels to grow adequately, anomalous insertion of the gubernaculum and reabsorption of the vaginal process, failure in postnatal elongation of the spermatic cord, and prenatal and postnatal androgen disruption because boys with severe hypospadias are at increased risk for acquired and retractile testes.[966–973] The spermatic cord measures 4 to 5 cm at birth and reaches 8 to 10 cm by 10 years of age. This growth does not occur if the peritoneal-vaginal duct becomes a fibrous remnant. The cause may be a defect in postnatal CGRP release by the GFN.[960,974,975] Acquired undescended testis spontaneously descends at puberty in 78% of cases.[976]

Pathogenesis

Testicular maldescent has multiple causes, including anatomic anomalies of the gubernaculum testis, hormonal dysfunction (hypogonadotropic hypogonadism), mechanical impairment (insufficient intraabdominal pressure, short spermatic cord, underdeveloped processus vaginalis), dysgenesis (primary anomaly of the testis), neuromuscular conditions (CGRP and cremaster nucleus), genetic factors (mutations in INLS3 or its receptor), and other hereditary or acquired conditions.[977–979]

Most cases of cryptorchidism likely appear to be caused by a deficit of fetal androgens or an excess of maternal estrogens. Androgen insufficiency seems to be slight and transient because anomalies other than hypoplasia of the epididymis are not seen.[142] It may result from deficient gonadotropic pituitary stimulation or low production of placental gonadotropins. Elevated maternal estrogens could cause diminution of FSH secretion by the fetal pituitary, thus leading to low Sertoli cell proliferation, and could create decreased testosterone production because of the inhibitory effect of estrogens on Leydig cells.[980,981] Three mechanisms seem to be involved in this process:

- *Primary testicular anomaly.* Cryptorchid testes may bear an anomalous germ cell population.[982] More than 40% of cryptorchid patients have a marked decrease in the TFI, even with nearly normal numbers of spermatogonia; these cells also have abnormal DNA content.[239,983]
- *Lesions secondary to transient perinatal hypogonadotropic hypogonadism.* Cryptorchid patients do not have gonadotropin elevation, which normally occurs between 60 and 90 days after birth, and this deficiency of LH could cause Leydig cell involution. Subsequent androgen deficiency could account for failure of gonocytes to differentiate into spermatogonia.[984–986]
- *Injury caused by increased temperature.* This was suggested in the past based on animal studies. In follow-up biopsies from testes that were descended surgically or with hormonal treatment, the sole factor that improved during childhood was tubular diameter. Diameter depends on Sertoli cells, so temperature may be more important for Sertoli cells than for spermatogonia.[239]

The most frequent findings in congenital and acquired cryptorchidism in infancy are decreased germ cell numbers and diminished tubular diameter.[987,988] In the normal testis, transient formation of spermatocytes occurs at 4 to 5 years of age. This meiotic attempt is probably an androgenic event that does not occur in cryptorchid testes and corresponds to the characteristic low numbers of spermatogonia in the prepubertal age.[989]

Histology

Prepubertal Testes: Morphologic Classification. Undescended testis is usually smaller than contralateral, descended testis, a difference that is already significant at 6 months of age.[955,990] However, no functional studies have revealed the existence and severity of congenital lesions in cryptorchid testes. Numerous biopsy studies of cryptorchid testes in the first years of life have been conducted, but no agreement exists about the severity of damage or time of onset.[989,991,992] The presence of lesions in the first year of life in most suggests that they are primary rather than acquired as a consequence of long-standing cryptorchidism. One should not forget that the testis is a dynamic structure, with waves of proliferation and differentiation from birth to puberty. Moreover, the parameters usually applied to studies of the adult parenchyma should not be used for the prepubertal testis.[709]

The pathologist should evaluate both semiquantitative and qualitative parameters to obtain as much information as possible from histologic study of biopsies from undescended testes. Semiquantitative morphometric parameters include MTD, TFI, number of germ cells per cross-sectioned tubule, Sertoli cell index (SCI), and number of Leydig cells in the interstitium. Qualitative findings include the pattern of germ cell distribution in the parenchyma (regular or irregular), abnormal spermatogonia

TABLE 12.15	Classification of Histologic Lesions in Prepubertal Cryptorchid Testis According to Morphometric Parameters				
Type of Lesion (Incidence Rate)	MTD	TFI	SCN	Spermatogonia Distribution	
Type I (31%)	Slightly decreased (90% normal values)	>50%	Normal	Regular	
Type II (29%)	Markedly decreased (60%–90% normal values)	30%–50%	Decreased	Irregular	
Type III (40%)	Severely decreased (<60% normal values)	0%–30%	Low	Irregular	

MTD, Mean tubular diameter; *SCN*, Sertoli cell number (average Sertoli cell number per cross-sectioned tubule); *TFI*, tubular fertility index (percentage of tubules containing germ cells).

(multinucleated, hypertrophic, or atypical), focal granular changes in Sertoli cells, abnormal tubules (megatubules, ring-shaped tubules), microliths, and ARs in children who are older than 4 years. Based on the evaluation of four parameters (TFI, MTD, SCI, and the spermatogonial distribution pattern), most testicular biopsies from cryptorchid testes of children may be classified into one of three groups (Table 12.15).[239]

- *Type I (testes with slight alterations)* (about 31% of cases). TFI is higher than 50, and MTD is normal or slightly (<10%) decreased (Fig. 12.106).
- *Type II (testes with marked germinal hypoplasia)* (about 29% of cases). TFI is between 30 and 50, and MTD is 10% to 30% lower than normal. The spermatogonia are distributed irregularly, and most are in tubular sections that are grouped in the same testicular lobule (Fig. 12.107).[993]
- *Type III (testes with severe germinal hypoplasia)* (about 40% of cases). TFI is less than 30, and MTD is less than 30% of normal. Many spermatogonia are giant with dark nuclei (Fig. 12.108). The testicular interstitium is wide and edematous.

The seminiferous tubules of testes with type II or III lesions have a thickened lamina propria during childhood and, at puberty, Sertoli cell hyperplasia, and more than 30% of these testes have microliths (Fig. 12.109), ring-shaped tubules, and granular changes in Sertoli cells (Fig. 12.110).[991] Intense immunoexpression for inhibin is observed in Sertoli cells in all types of cryptorchid testes (Fig. 12.111). Patients with bilateral cryptorchidism have a higher incidence of type II and III lesions than those with unilateral cryptorchidism. Approximately 8% of testes with type I lesions contain many multinucleated spermatogonia (with three or more nuclei; Fig. 12.112), and both KIT expression and PLAP expression persist in approximately 5% of immature germ cells.[994]

Type I lesions are comparable with those seen in experimental cryptorchidism: normal testes in which lesions are induced by increased temperature.[992] Testes with type II or III lesions bear

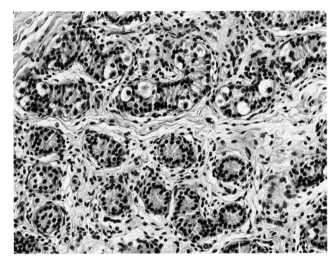

Fig. 12.107 Cryptorchidism. Seminiferous tubules with type II lesions show markedly decreased diameters and an irregular distribution of germ cells.

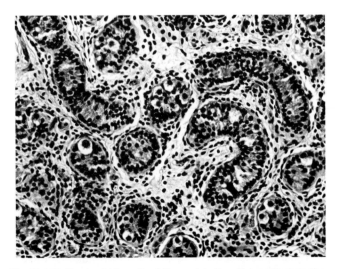

Fig. 12.106 Cryptorchidism. Seminiferous tubules with type I lesions show slightly decreased diameters and a normal tubular fertility index.

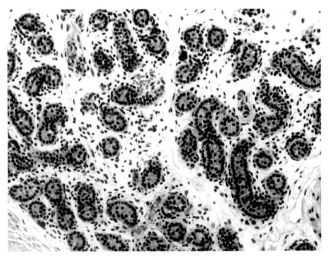

Fig. 12.108 Cryptorchidism. Seminiferous tubules with type III lesions show severe reduction in both tubular diameter and tubular fertility index.

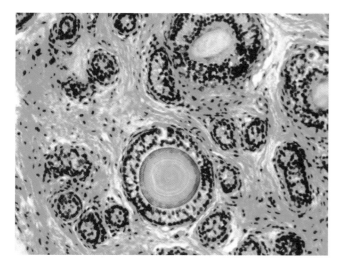

Fig. 12.109 Microlithiasis in an infant cryptorchid testis. The seminiferous tubules show type III lesions and contain numerous microliths.

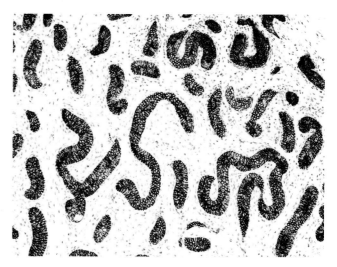

Fig. 12.111 Cryptorchidism. Slightly tortuous seminiferous tubules with decreased diameter showing intense immunoexpression of inhibin. Only one germ cell may be seen at the left lower corner.

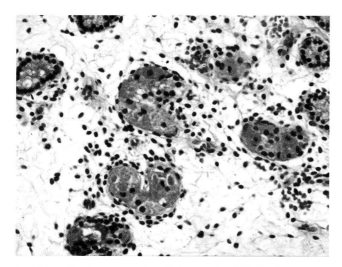

Fig. 12.110 Cryptorchidism. Type III lesions, in which the interstitium is expanded by edema. The cytoplasm of the Sertoli cells contains numerous eosinophilic granules of variable size.

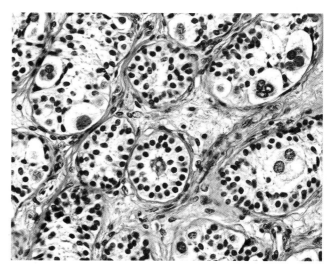

Fig. 12.112 Prepubertal cryptorchid testis. The seminiferous tubules have Sertoli cells with elongate nuclei, pseudostratified growth pattern, and isolated spermatogonia, some of which are multinucleate or contain hypertrophic nuclei.

variable degrees of dysgenesis that, in addition to germ cells, involves Sertoli cells, peritubular myofibroblasts, and Leydig cells. The dysgenesis of these other cell types is evident only after puberty and is more severe in intraabdominal testes.[995,996] In approximately 25% of cases the contralateral scrotal testis also has histologic lesions of variable severity. This finding supports the hypothesis of bilateral defect in many cases of unilateral cryptorchidism. Microdeletions in the long arm of Y-chromosome genes (DAZ, RBM, [azoospermic factor] AZFa, b, and c) are not increased in cryptorchidism.[997]

Unilateral cryptorchidism with normal contralateral testis may result from end-organ failure.[998] In cryptorchidism secondary to spontaneous ascent, lesions are like those of congenital cryptorchidism, whereas in cryptorchidism secondary to herniotomy, germ cell depletion is slight and becomes important only after 5 years of age.[999–1001]

Pubertal and Adult Testes. Most pubertal and adult cryptorchid testes have anomalies in all testicular structures. During puberty, undescended testes show severe maturation delay in both tubular and interstitial components (Fig. 12.113).[246] Seminiferous tubules display apparent Sertoli cell hyperplasia as a result of failure in lengthening and coiling of the seminiferous tubule during pubertal development, and tubules also have decreased diameter and delayed germ cell proliferation when these cells are present. Frequently, as puberty progresses, testicular development is irregular, varying from one lobule to another. Seminiferous tubules that have initiated spermatogenesis are adjacent to other tubules showing prepubertal maturative pattern. Careful study reveals a delay in Sertoli cell maturation, estimated by nuclear morphology. Irregular expression of ARs is found in these Sertoli cells (Fig. 12.114).[880] Tubules with a prepubertal pattern also show delayed maturation in mural myofibroblasts, which are unable to express muscle-specific actin.

Surgically removed cryptorchid testes from adults reveal that most have histologic lesions in all structural components and the rete testis and epididymis. Seminiferous tubules have decreased

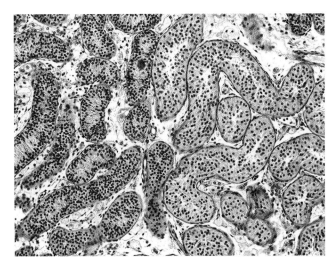

Fig. 12.113 Pubertal cryptorchidism. Testis from 12-year-old boy showing irregular maturation of the parenchyma. Tubular diameter and Sertoli cell maturation varies from one to another area. interstitium shows scarce Leydig cells.

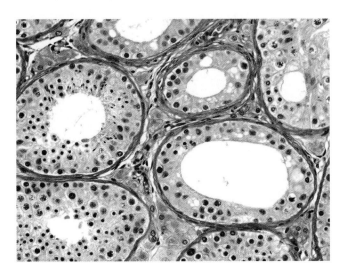

Fig. 12.115 Adult ex-cryptorchid testis that was surgically descended at the age of 2 years. Tubular sections show a pattern varying from spermatogonial maturation arrest to complete, although decreased, spermatogenesis.

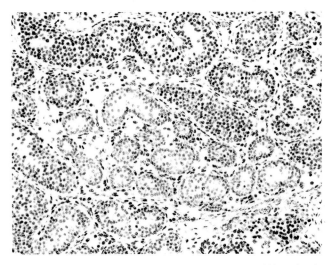

Fig. 12.114 Pubertal cryptorchidism. Testis from 12-year-old boy showing a correlation between Sertoli cell delayed maturation and androgen receptor immunoexpression. Central area shows lower androgen receptor immunoexpression than surrounding areas.

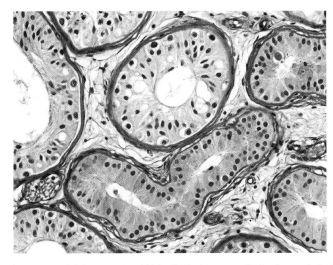

Fig. 12.116 Adult ex-cryptorchid testis that was surgically descended at infancy. Seminiferous tubules with spermatogonial maturation arrest and dysgenetic Sertoli cells adjacent to hypoplastic seminiferous tubules lined by tall Sertoli cells with granular changes in their cytoplasm.

diameters and deficient spermatogenesis. In decreasing order of frequency, the most common germ cell lesions are tubules with a Sertoli cell–only and spermatogonia-only pattern, tubules with Sertoli cells (dysgenetic) only, tubular hyalinization, and MAT. The lamina propria has scant elastic fibers, as well as irregular deposits of collagen IV and laminin in the basal lamina.[995,1002] Peritubular myoid cells in experimental cryptorchidism show disorganization of actin filaments.[1003] Sertoli cells are present in greater number and do not mature normally except in tubules with germ cells (Fig. 12.115).[246,993] In tubules with advanced spermatogenesis, the morphology of Sertoli cell nuclei is normal.[1004] In addition to being immunoreactive for vimentin, similar to normal adult Sertoli cells, the dysgenetic Sertoli cells in Sertoli cell–only tubules immunoexpress cytokeratins and desmin in the basal cytoplasm. These immunoreactions are also positive in intraluminal accumulations of sloughed Sertoli cells.[1005] Often, groups of tubules containing only Sertoli cells with a prepubertal pattern (small

diameter and total absence of maturation) may be found and are considered hypoplastic (showing a small lumen and a thick wall lined by a tall columnar epithelium, formed only by Sertoli cells of eosinophilic cytoplasm) (Fig. 12.116), dysgenetic, or hamartomatous; seminiferous tubules with granular changes in Sertoli cells may also be present.[1006] Areas of apparent Leydig cell hyperplasia are frequent (Fig. 12.117), and many of these cells contain vacuolated lipid-laden cytoplasm (Fig. 12.118).

The rete testis is hypoplastic in most cases, lined by columnar epithelium with rare areas of flattened cells. Cystic dilation is common, and adenomatous hyperplasia may be present.[1007] Most cryptorchid testes, and especially those with Sertoli cell–only tubules, contain underdeveloped rete testis whose epithelium has not differentiated between squamous and columnar cells (conversely to what normally occurs during puberty), retaining an infantile pattern referred to as "dysgenetic" (Fig. 12.119). Near the rete testis, the parenchyma frequently contains metaplastic

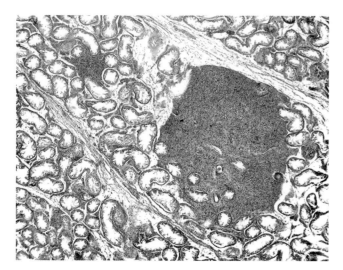

Fig. 12.117 Nodular Leydig cell hyperplasia in an adult ex-cryptorchid testis.

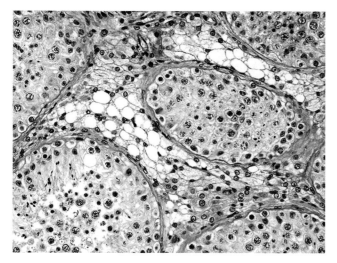

Fig. 12.118 Contralateral testis of an adult ex-cryptorchid patient with infertility. Spermatogenesis is complete. Leydig cells are increased in number and show intense cytoplasm vacuolization with a signet ring morphology.

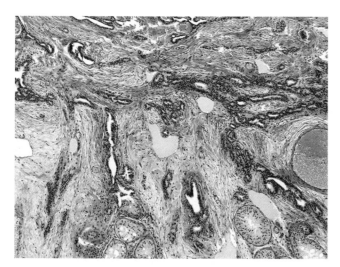

Fig. 12.119 Undescended testes of an adult. In the panoramic view a hypoplastic rete testis and enlarged interlobular walls may be observed.

fat. In some cryptorchid testes, several tubular segments are destroyed by inflammation that probably has an autoimmune cause (focal orchitis).[1008] Epididymal tubules are poorly developed, and peritubular tissue is immature.

Needle aspiration biopsy of the normally descended contralateral testis shows a variety of histologic patterns, varying from normal to with alterations like those of cryptorchid testes.[1009] This variability is probably related to the cause of cryptorchidism. Bilateral lesions suggest congenital or genetic cause, whereas normal contralateral testis suggests local anatomic anomalies.[1010]

Validation of the Morphologic Classification of the Prepubertal Undescended Testes Lesions

Study of serial sections of bilateral testicular biopsies allow comparison of histologic findings in boys with cryptorchidism at the time of orchidopexy and in adulthood (performed for evaluation of infertility).[1011] One report described diffuse and complete spermatogenesis in such testes with higher TFI (normal testes and those with type I lesions) in more than two-thirds of cases, accompanied by a quantitatively abnormal number of germ cells; MAT developed in the other one-third of cases.[993] MAT is defined as synchronous occurrence of tubules containing germ cells (with variable degrees of spermatogenesis) and Sertoli cell–only tubules (Fig. 12.120).[1012] All testes with type II lesions and 85% of those with type III lesions experience development of MAT, indicating that MAT is the most frequent lesion (68%) in adult ex-cryptorchid patients presenting with infertility (Table 12.16). In most patients with unilateral cryptorchidism, MAT is observed in both the undescended testis and contralateral descended testis, even if the surgical correction occurred at an early age. There is an inverse correlation between severity of the lesions in childhood and amount of spermatogenesis in adulthood. Approximately 85% of adult testes with type III lesions in infancy experience MAT, with spermatogenesis in less than 50% of tubules; another 5% develop hypospermatogenesis and spermatocyte I sloughing; and the remaining 10% have Sertoli cell–only tubules. Patients whose prepubertal testes had clustering of germ cell–containing tubules usually had incomplete spermatogenesis in adulthood, and when

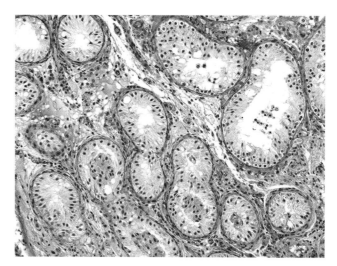

Fig. 12.120 Adult ex-cryptorchid testis that was surgically descended at infancy showing mixed atrophy. Most seminiferous tubules contain only Sertoli cells. The remaining show complete spermatogenesis, although quantitatively decreased.

TABLE 12.16 Postpuberal Evolution of the Lesions in Testes Descended in Infancy

Type of Lesion	Postpubertal Testicular Pathology
Type I	Adluminal compartment lesions (57%)
	Mixed testicular atrophy (29%)
	Basal and adluminal compartment lesions (14%)
Type II	Mixed testicular atrophy (100%)
Type III	Mixed testicular atrophy with <50% tubules with spermatogenesis (85%)
	Sertoli cell–only tubules (10%)
	Hypospermatogenesis + spermatocyte I sloughing (5%)

spermatogenesis was complete, it occurred in less than 50% of tubules.[1011]

Sperm excretory duct anomalies occur in 9% to 36% of cryptorchid patients.[1013–1015] These anomalies may cause obstruction of the excretory ducts, so biopsies may also reveal an obstructive pattern superimposed on the seminiferous tubule lesions.

In summary, the classification of testicular lesions in childhood into three types (I, II, and III) correlates with the amount of spermatogenesis found in postpubertal biopsies. The most important parameter is TFI. Spermatogenesis may also be impaired by an obstructive process that is complete or incomplete, and functional or organic. Biopsy allows adequate evaluation of congenital or obstructive lesions, and detects testes with focal spermatogenesis to establish the possibility of treatment with assisted reproductive techniques.

Effectiveness of Treatment in Undescended Testes

Optimal treatment of undescended testis is controversial. The European Association of Urology recommends mandatory surgical treatment in infancy; patients with palpable inguinal cryptorchid testes should undergo orchidopexy within 1 year and no later than 2 years of age.[1016–1020] The Nordic Consensus statements recommend anticipating orchidopexy as early as the first 6 to 12 months of life.[1021] Surgical treatment benefits all patients with primary cryptorchidism and retractile testis, even those whose testes are surgically descended at an older age.[1022]

The efficacy of hormonal treatment after orchidopexy remains controversial. Results are contradictory because great variations in the effects of hormonal treatment have been reported. Whereas use of hCG and GnRH in the treatment of cryptorchidism was found effective in some cases, it was useless in others.[1021,1023–1025] Meta-analysis showed that approximately 15% to 20% of retained testes descend during hormonal treatment, although one-fifth subsequently reascend. Moreover, treatment with hCG increases germ cell apoptosis, with subsequent damage to future spermatogenesis.[1026] Testicular biopsy is the only sure method for identification of cryptorchid boys who need hormonal treatment with luteinizing hormone-releasing hormone (LHRH) after successful surgery; consequently, some advocate mandatory biopsy during orchidopexy.[1027] Neonatal gonocytes transform into type A spermatogonia at 3 to 12 months, and this process is disrupted in undescended testes, although there is a chance of reversal by orchidopexy at an early age. The presence of Ad spermatogonia at surgery is an excellent prognostic parameter for future fertility. Cryptorchid boys who lack these cells experience infertility despite successful orchidopexy at an early age.[1024] In those whose testes contain a low number of Ad spermatogonia and suboptimal response to hCG stimulation, hormonal treatment is advised to increase the number of germ cells. It is uncertain whether different modalities and periods of hormonal therapy in patients with impaired Leydig cell response can improve histologic features prognosis for future fertility.[1028,1029]

In childhood the chance of detecting occult cancer or precancer by biopsy is low because intratubular germ cell neoplasia is not diffusely distributed throughout the testis. Nonetheless, testicular biopsy should be performed in all patients with intraabdominal testes, abnormal external genitalia, or abnormal karyotype.[1030]

Autotransplantation has been used in some patients with high intraabdominal testes as an alternative to the Fowler-Stephens technique.[1031–1033] These testes represent approximately 5% of all undescended testes.[1034] Histologic studies performed after autotransplantation reveal evidence of Leydig cell development, tubular diameter increase, and spermatogenetic development, although paternity has not been reported.[1035,1036]

Congenital Anomalies Associated With Undescended Testes

Most cryptorchid patients have a patent processus vaginalis, and 65% to 75% have a hernia sac, although most hernias are not clinically visible.[445] Urologic anomalies are present in 11%, the most frequent being hypospadias, complete duplication of the urinary tract, nonobstructive ureteral dilatation, kidney malrotation, and posterior urethral valves.[1037] Cryptorchidism is more frequent in those with microcephaly, myelomeningocele, bifid spine, omphalocele, gastroschisis, micropenis, imperforate anus, and cloacal exstrophy.[1038–1041]

The incidence of sperm excretory duct anomalies is high in patients with undescended testes, and these anomalies involve both the intratesticular and extratesticular ducts. Dysgenesis of the rete testis is observed in more than 80% of adult undescended testes.[1042] The incidence of extratesticular spermatic duct anomalies varies from 9% to 79%.[482,1013,1043–1048] Sperm excretory duct anomalies are classified into three types[1014]:

- *Ductal fusion anomalies* (25% of cases). These consist of anomalous fusion of the caput of the epididymis to the testis or segmental atresia of the epididymis and vas deferens. This category is chiefly associated with intraabdominal or high scrotal cryptorchid testes.
- *Ductal suspension anomalies* (59% of cases). The caput of the epididymis is attached to the testis, whereas the corpus and the cauda of the epididymis are separated from the testis by a mesentery. A variant consists of excessively long cauda of the epididymis that descends along the inguinal duct to the scrotum (Fig. 12.121).
- *Anomalies associated with absent or vanishing testes* (16% of cases).

The ductuli efferentes and the ductus epididymidis of cryptorchid patients show evidence of abnormal development from infancy. Remarkably, epithelial cell height of both types of ducts is low, and the muscular wall is poorly developed. In adults, ductuli efferentes show an inner circular outline instead of the wavy outline that is characteristic of normal caput of epididymidis, reflecting different epithelial cell heights.[1049] Incomplete development of the muscular wall suggests that propulsion of testicular fluid is compromised, resulting in stasis of ductuli efferentes, rete testis, and even seminiferous tubules.

Patent vaginal process is associated with epididymal anomalies, regardless of the location of the cryptorchid testis, with an incidence rate as high as 80%, compared with only 5% in those with descended testes with a closed vaginal process.[1050]

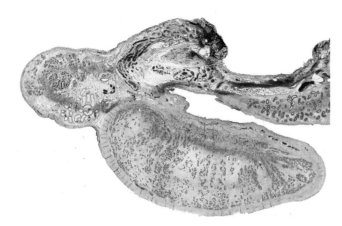

Fig. 12.121 Undescended testicle of a 3-year-old boy with marked enlargement of the interstitium showing small tortuous seminiferous tubules. Epididymis is elongate with hypoplasia of the caput and separation of the body and tail of the epididymis from the testis.

Anomalies of the gubernaculum are also frequent in cryptorchidism. Comparative studies between normal fetuses and cryptorchid infants reveal differences in the union of the gubernaculum to the testis and epididymis (72% vs 99% incidence rate, respectively). The gubernaculum is joined exclusively to the testis (the cauda epididymis is free) in 22% of cryptorchid testes and in 1% of normal fetal testes. The gubernaculum is joined exclusively to the cauda epididymis in 6% of cryptorchid testes, whereas this condition is not observed in normal fetuses.[1051]

Another anomaly is the occurrence of short spermatic vessels that hinder testicular descent. This is a frequent finding in cryptorchid testes with type III lesions and, to a lesser extent, in those with type II lesions. This observation further supports the dysgenetic nature of these testes.[1052]

Many unfavorable results obtained after surgical descent of these testes may be explained by ultrasonographic images that reveal anomalies associated with undescended testes.[1053]

Cryptorchidism may be isolated, or is often be associated with congenital, endocrine, or chromosomal disorders, as well as with disorders in sexual differentiation.[1054,1055] Cryptorchidism may occur in patients with GnRH deficit; Kallmann, Prader-Willi (PWS), Klinefelter, Noonan, Smith-Lemli-Opitz (SLOS), Aarskog-Scott, Rubinstein-Taybi, prune belly (Fig. 12.122), Cornelia de Lange, and caudal regression syndromes; testicular feminization syndromes caused by AR anomalies such as 5α-reductase deficiency (an enzyme required for conversion of testosterone to DHT); several types of undermasculinization caused by AMH absence; DiGeorge syndrome; Beckwith-Wiedemann syndrome; CHARGE association; and trisomies 13, 18, and 21. The association of impalpable testes with hypospadias suggests a disorder of sexual differentiation (this suggestion was confirmed in 27% to 30% of cases).[1056-1058]

Cryptorchidism is part of the *testicular dysgenesis syndrome*, first described in 2001.[1059-1063] This syndrome consists of a spectrum of male reproductive disorders with a range of clinical presentations, including abnormal testicular development that predisposes to cryptorchidism, hypospadias, spermatogenetic alterations, and testicular cancer. The association of these disorders with cryptorchidism has been corroborated by numerous clinical, epidemiologic, and genetic studies. The least severe form of this syndrome is defect in spermatogenesis; the most severe is testicular cancer.

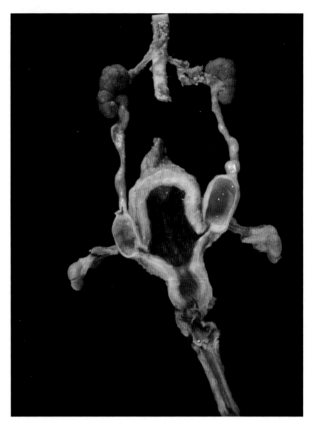

Fig. 12.122 Prune belly syndrome in a boy with the triad: renal dysplasia, megaureter-megabladder, and bilateral cryptorchidism.

A constellation of histologic lesions is common in the testes of men with testicular dysgenesis, including Sertoli cell–only pattern, MAT, hypoplastic tubules (Sertoli cell nodules), testicular microlithiasis, malformed tubules, granular changes in Sertoli cells, nodular Leydig cell hyperplasia, and GCNIS. It is assumed that the lesions develop prenatally as a result of several genetic, environmental, or endocrine disruptor factors that would interfere with the estrogen-to-androgen ratio and possibly lead to disruption of Sertoli or Leydig cell function.[1063-1066] The initial disorder is probably an imbalance between estrogens and androgens during fetal life related to increased estrogen exposure in utero.[1067] Exposure to environmental toxins, acting as endocrine disruptors, could disrupt fetal sexual differentiation by an estrogenic or antiandrogenic effect.[1068] Various environmental chemicals may alter endogenous levels of androgens (certain phthalates) and estrogens (polychlorinated biphenyls, polyhalogenated hydrocarbons).[980,1069,1070] Estrogens may induce cryptorchidism and hypospadias by suppressing androgen production or action, or by suppressing INLS3.[1064-1066,1071,1072] Although testicular dysgenesis syndrome still raises many questions of epidemiology and pathogenesis, it is accepted as a single unifying hypothesis, particularly when so little is known of etiology.[1073-1075]

Complications of Cryptorchidism

The main complications of cryptorchidism are testicular cancer, infertility, testicular torsion, and psychological problems derived from an empty scrotum.[1076]

Testicular Cancer. Approximately 1% of 1-year-olds have cryptorchidism, and approximately 10% of patients with testicular cancer had cryptorchidism. Cancer risk of undescended testis is 6.3

versus 1.7 of the contralateral testis by metaanalysis.[1077] The risk for testicular cancer in cryptorchid boys and men is 4 to 10 times higher than that of the general population.[1078,1079] Cancer risk in abdominal testes is six times higher than that of other cryptorchid testes in an inferior location.[1080,1081] Testes with an elevated number of multinucleated spermatogonia have a higher risk for cancer during adulthood.[994] The risk increases when cryptorchidism is bilateral and associated with external genitalia anomalies or chromosomal anomalies such as 45,X/46,XY.[1082] Approximately 5% of biopsies in children contain cells similar to those seen in GCNIS, although possible evolution to invasive malignancy remains a subject of controversy (Fig. 12.123).[1083,1084] The presence of GCNIS may be missed in infancy because in the prepubertal testis atypical gonocytes may not be located directly on the basal lamina; instead, these gonocytes may be present in the center of the tubules, and their number may be low.[1085] Approximately 2% to 3% of adult cryptorchid testes have evidence of GCNIS, and the most frequent tumor in these patients is seminoma.[1086–1089] Regardless of timing, orchidopexy does not reduce the risk for cancer, although it facilitates early detection because the intrascrotal testis is palpable.[1090] Twenty percent of testicular tumors arise in properly descended testes contralateral to cryptorchid testes; this finding suggests a primary bilateral testicular anomaly in cryptorchidism. Intraabdominal testes also have a higher incidence of tumors, with a similar prognosis.[1080–1087,1089–1091]

Infertility. Infertility is the most frequent problem caused by cryptorchidism. In a series of patients with infertility, almost 9% had cryptorchidism (Fig. 12.124).[1092] Hormonal serum levels in ex-cryptorchid patients show high levels of FSH, normal LH, and low testosterone.[1093]

Infertility is influenced by several factors, including bilaterality, number of germ cells, location and size of the testis, germ cell distribution, anomalous DNA content in germ cells, Leydig cell dysfunction, congenital anomalies of sperm excretory ducts, and possible iatrogenic injury to the testes, epididymis, ductus deferens, or spermatic cord during orchidopexy.[1094]

The most important risk factors are bilaterality and germ cell number; 16% to 25% of men with bilateral cryptorchidism have

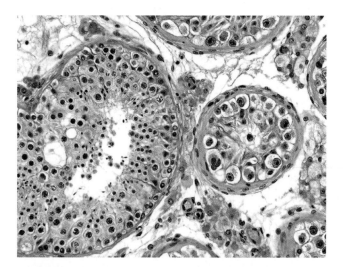

Fig. 12.123 Adult ex-cryptorchid testis that was surgically descended at infancy. The patient was infertile. The smallest seminiferous tubule shows intratubular germ cell neoplasia, undifferentiated type. The relative tumor cell homogeneity contrasts with the variety in shape and size of the cells in the adjacent seminiferous tubule with complete spermatogenesis.

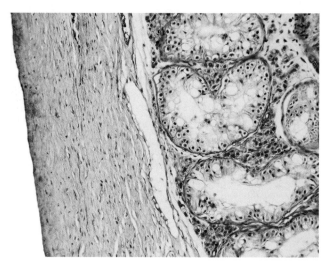

Fig. 12.124 Ex-cryptorchid testicle of an adult patient. The albuginea is thin. The seminiferous tubules contain only Sertoli cells and spermatogonia. The interstice shows a normal number of Leydig cells.

normal sperm counts (≥20 million/mL).[1095,1096] Highest sperm counts occur with testes in the superficial inguinal pouch. Patients with bilaterally impalpable testes are usually azoospermic.[1097] Fertility rates in unilateral cryptorchidism vary from 25% to 81%.[1098] Many patients with repaired bilateral cryptorchidism require assisted reproductive techniques such as intracytoplasmic sperm injection to obtain successful fertilization.[1099]

The number of germ cells per cross-sectioned tubule is the most important prognostic factor. Patients with no increase in inhibin B during the postoperative period usually have a low number of spermatogonia and low TFI.[1100] Usually a cryptorchid boy with less than 0.2 spermatogonia per cross-sectioned tubule will have a deficient spermiogram in adulthood, and fertility will be decreased. In unilateral cryptorchidism, fertility depends on the number of spermatogonia in the contralateral testis. However, if the number of germ cells per cross-sectioned tubule in the cryptorchid testis is less than 1% of normal, the risk for infertility is 33%, increasing to 75% to 100% in bilateral cryptorchidism.[1095,1101–1105] Spermatogonial number correlates with sperm number in the spermiogram, volume of surgically repaired testis, inhibin B serum level, and volume of this testis in adulthood. In a series of 142 azoospermic men with history of cryptorchidism, testicular sperm extraction (TESE) was successful in 62% of cases overall and 63% of those with bilateral cryptorchidism, favorably altering the prospect of fertility. Those patients whose FSH level is normal or testicular volume is higher than 10 cm³ have an even better prognosis because the rate of TESE with positive sperm retrieval is 75%.[1106]

Preoperative location of the unilaterally cryptorchid testis and the small size of the testis at the time of orchidopexy cannot predict likelihood of fertility.[1107–1109] Patients with high scrotal testes or superficial inguinal pouch testes have the best spermiograms, whereas those with intraabdominal or canalicular testes are oligozoospermic or azoospermic. Testicular damage may result either from the presence of more severe histologic lesions or injury produced during orchidopexy because these testes require more mobilization those in lower locations.[1097–1110] Patients whose testes are nearly normal in size also have better spermiograms.[1096] An important fertility factor is the permeability of sperm excretory ducts. Between birth and 4 years of age, patient age at orchidopexy may also influence fertility, although this has not been proven. Beyond 4 years, orchidopexy does not enhance fertility.[1102,1111]

Testicular Torsion. Undescended testes have a 10-fold higher risk for spermatic cord torsion than do normally located testes. This increased risk results from the abnormal suspension system.[1112–1115] Fixation of the contralateral testis should be performed using orchidopexy if anomalies in testicular suspension are observed.[1116] The percentage of testes that may be preserved is low because of the delay in seeking consultation and making the diagnosis.[1117]

Tunica albuginea calcifications, coinciding with site of fixation, are found in adult testes that were fixed at orchidopexy. These calcifications appear mainly when chromic suture material was used, and tare not related to pathologic features present in the cryptorchid testis at the time of orchidopexy or will develop later. Intraabdominal testes may also undergo torsion.[1118,1119]

Iatrogenic Atrophy. The high number of children subjected to orchidopexy has led to knowledge of postsurgical atrophy. The frequency of this complication is estimated to be 1% to 5% for inguinal canal testes and 25% for intraabdominal testes (Fig. 12.125).[1105,1120]

Psychological Problems. The importance of having two testes should be considered before orchidopexy because of potential damage to the male identity.[1121] Studies carried out in adults whose testes were surgically descended before puberty revealed normal male development and behavior, although these men seemed to be sexually less active than controls. This observation does not appear to be related to treatment method or age when treated.[1122] Patients should be offered testicular prosthesis and information on the risks involved (infection, migration).[1123]

Benefit of Testicular Biopsy in Patients With Cryptorchidism

Testicular biopsies of infantile testes at orchidopexy are useful for determining baseline germ cell status and whether surgery should be supplemented by hormonal treatment.[1124,1125] However, even if biopsy supplies significant data, it is not considered a routine procedure.

When the number of spermatogonia is nearly normal, spermatogenesis may not occur because of deficient spermatogonium development during childhood or failure of spermatogenesis at puberty, even in the best of cases. If complete spermatogenesis occurs, this may be associated with obstruction of sperm excretory ducts.

In childhood, risk for occult cancer or precancer at biopsy is low because GCNIS is not diffusely distributed throughout the testis. Testicular biopsy is recommended in patients with intraabdominal testes, abnormal external genitalia, or abnormal karyotype.[1126]

The situation is different in adults because GCNIS is present in 2% to 3% of cases and is diffuse.[1086,1087] When GCNIS is detected in a child, further examination of the testis and repeat biopsy after puberty are recommended.[1088] In adults, if GCNIS is unilateral, orchiectomy should be performed, but if bilateral, radiation therapy may be used to eradicate neoplasm while maintaining Leydig cell function.[1088]

Obstructed Testes

Obstructed testes are in the superficial inguinal pouch (Denis-Browne pouch) and are considered ectopic by some authors and cryptorchid by others.[501,1127] Histologic studies reveal that most obstructed testes bear the same lesions as true cryptorchid testes. Type I lesions are observed in one-half, type II lesions are seen in more than one-third, and the remaining lesions are type III. The higher proportion of type I lesions suggests a better prognosis than in true cryptorchidism.

Retractile Testes

Some authors assume that retractile testes are normal and exclude them from studies of cryptorchidism.[974,1128] However, these testes may have significant lesions, and many consider them to be a form of cryptorchidism.[1126,1129,1130] Retractile testes may not always be movable to the lower scrotum (70 to 75 mm from the pubic tubercle), and in 50% of cases are smaller than scrotal testes.[1131] Approximately 50% of retractile testes remain high after age 6 years, when cremasteric activity declines.[1132] Retractile testes have a 32% risk for becoming ascending or acquired undescended testes. The risk is higher in boys younger than 7 years or when the spermatic cord is tight or inelastic.[1133] During childhood, MTD and TFI decrease.[1126] Adults with retractile testes that descended spontaneously but late may be fertile or infertile.[1134,1135,1135a] Usually there is germ cell atrophy that varies in severity from lobule to lobule (Fig. 12.126).[1126] Regular examination of retractile testes is

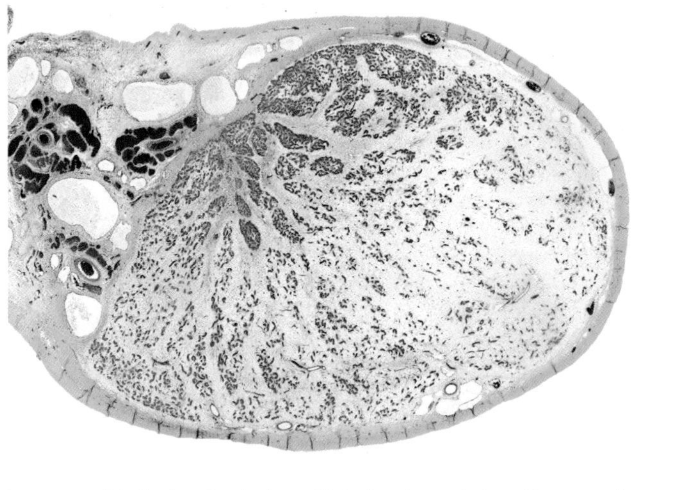

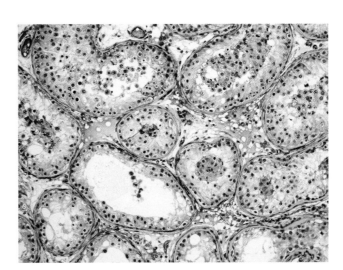

Fig. 12.125 Testicular atrophy in a child after descent done 3 years earlier. The most affected parenchyma is the peripherally situated parenchyma in which the seminiferous tubules are barely distinguished in the testicular stroma.

Fig. 12.126 Infertile patient with oligozoospermia and retractile testicles. Seminiferous tubules with slight thickening of the basal membrane, marked variation in size, and variable spermatogenesis from one tubule to another.

advisable during childhood, and if complete testicular descent does not occur, orchidopexy is indicated. In 14% of patients with retractile testicles treated by orchiopexy, abnormalities of the epididymis are similar to those observed in cryptorchid testes.[1136]

Testicular Microlithiasis

Calcifications may arise in the testis, but the high frequency of this finding has emerged with routine use of ultrasonography. Histologic studies combined with ultrasonography have elucidated the nature and significance of microliths, macroliths, clumps or calcified scars, phleboliths, stones, or calculus.

Testicular microlithiasis is characterized by the presence of numerous calcifications diffusely distributed throughout the parenchyma. Classically the term *testicular microlithiasis* was used to describe cases containing a large number of microliths.[1137] Microlithiasis may occur in infancy or adulthood, associated with tumoral and nontumoral pathologic features. In infancy, it may be seen in undescended testes, Klinefelter syndrome, Down syndrome, developmental delay and testicular asymmetry, undermasculinization XY testicular hydatid torsion, polyorchidism, congenital adrenal hyperplasia, and secondary hypogonadism, as well as in otherwise normal patients studied for other conditions.[239,755,1138–1147] In adults, microliths are frequently observed in cryptorchid and ex-cryptorchid testes, in seminiferous tubules located at the periphery of germ cell tumors, in patients with GCNIS, in testicular dysgenesis, in testes with ischemic injury, in infertile men, and in some with orchialgia.[1148–1158] Isolated cases associated with pulmonary microlithiasis and calcifications in the vegetative and central nervous system have been reported.[239,1159]

Ultrasonography is used to quantify calcifications, usually revealing multiple < 2-mm diameter hyperechoic foci without posterior acoustic shadow and diffusely distributed throughout the parenchyma ("snowstorm" pattern), or radiography is used, usually revealing multiple uniformly distributed microcalcifications.[1143,1160–1164] Ultrasonography identifies two types of testicular microlithiasis: classic type, in which the number of microliths is five or more; and limited type, with fewer than five microliths (Fig. 12.127).

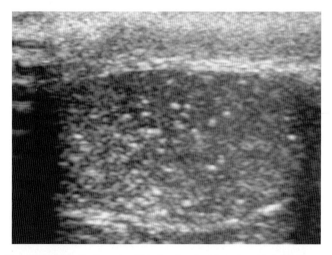

Fig. 12.127 Testicular microlithiasis showing the characteristic "snowstorm" pattern.

Incidence

The incidence of testicular microlithiasis varies according to the diagnostic method used (light microscopy, radiography, or ultrasonography), whether the population is symptomatic or asymptomatic, and the nature of the disease process being studied (cryptorchidism, infertility, or testicular tumor).

In histologic studies, testicular microlithiasis is found in approximately less than 1% of testicular pediatric biopsies, in 1% of biopsies of infertile men, and in 4% of adult male autopsies.[239,1153,1165] The incidence rate in two radiologic series varied from 1% to 74%.[1149,1166]

The real incidence of testicular microlithiasis has been established by the routine use of ultrasonography in evaluating intrascrotal abnormalities. The prevalence rate of testicular microlithiasis in infants is less than 3%. Classic testicular microlithiasis is found in 2% and limited testicular microlithiasis in 2% of asymptomatic boys.[1142] The prevalence rate of classic testicular microlithiasis in children with disorders such as cryptorchidism, hydrocele, scrotal swelling, chromosomal anomalies, orchialgia, and testicular torsion who were evaluated ultrasonographically varied from 1% to 3%.[1077,1167–1169] Several cases of testicular microlithiasis have also been observed in infant testes with neoplasm.[1168,1170] The prevalence seems to increase from birth to adolescence.

The prevalence of classic testicular microlithiasis in asymptomatic young men varies from 2% to 6% in the general population between 18 and 35 years of age, and is bilateral in 66% of affected patients.[1171,1172] The incidence shows ethnic differences; it is low in whites (4%), high in blacks (14%), and intermediate in Hispanics (9%) or Asian or Pacific Island men (6%). Ultrasonographic studies performed in adults with several disorders showed a prevalence rate varying from 1% to 4%.[1169,1173–1176] In adults, testicular microlithiasis is most often identified during investigations for infertility, pain, or testicular asymmetry.[1154] In series of infertile patients, the incidence varied from 2% to 18%.[1177,1178] The incidence ranged from 5% to 20% in subfertile patients, and it was 10% in ex-cryptorchid testes.[1156,1179,1180]

Testicular microlithiasis is observed in 30% to 50% of adult testes with germ cell tumor.[1176,1181–1184] It has also been observed in the contralateral, apparently normal testis, sometimes in association with GCNIS.[1185–1187]

Pain is the most common clinical symptom in patients without a palpable testicular mass, attributed to dilation of seminiferous tubules secondary to obstruction by microliths.

Pathology and Histogenesis

In the prepubertal testis, microliths are surrounded by a double layer of Sertoli cells and measure up to 300 μm in diameter. When microliths are large, the seminiferous epithelium may be destroyed, and the microlith is surrounded by peritubular cells. Testes with microliths have subnormal MTD and TFI.[239,1137]

Adult testes with microliths have incomplete spermatogenesis (Fig. 12.128). Microliths may appear in the tubular wall, in the seminiferous epithelium, or free in the tubular lumen. Some seminiferous tubules with microliths are cystically dilated and lined by markedly thin atrophic epithelium (Fig. 12.129). The cause of this cystic transformation may be the obstruction caused by microliths that pass through the thin tubuli recti. Microliths are also numerous in the conglomerates of hypoplastic tubules of the so-called Sertoli cell nodule or hypoplastic zone (Fig. 12.130), which are mainly observed in cryptorchid testes. However, microliths may also be observed in seminiferous tubules away from these areas.

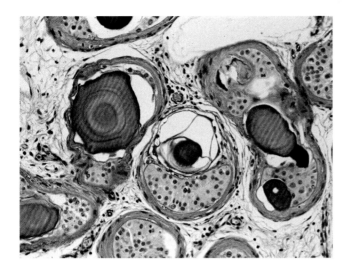

Fig. 12.128 Extratubular and intratubular microliths in an adult testis with isolated spermatogonia and Sertoli cells.

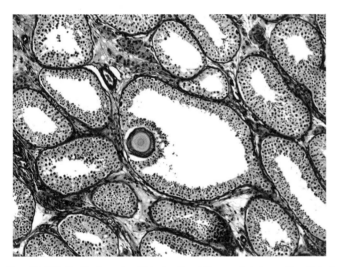

Fig. 12.129 Testicular microlithiasis. Seminiferous tubules with dilated lumina in a patient who underwent biopsy for infertility. The central tubule contains a microlith that developed in the tubular wall and protrudes into the lumen.

The origin of microliths is hypothesized to represent sloughed germ cells or glycoprotein secretions concentrated inside seminiferous tubules.[1140,1147,1188,1189] Some have hypothesized that they arise from disordered tunica propria, forming extratubular eosinophilic bodies that mineralize and pass into tubular lumina.[236] The material surrounding microliths expresses laminin and type IV collagen, both important components of basal lamina, which suggests an extratubular origin.[236,1190] This observation has led to the hypothesis that microliths originate from eosinophilic basal lamina material, giving rise initially to a spherical body, which advances toward the center of the tubule, displacing the basal lamina components and Sertoli cells that are in the path. Microliths thus become surrounded by these two elements. After internalization the nodular eosinophilic material becomes mineralized. In infantile testes, nonmineralized round eosinophilic bodies may be observed in normal and malformed seminiferous tubules. Many of the largest malformed tubules are known as ring-shaped tubules. Study of serial sections of these tubules reveals that they have a bell shape and contain eosinophilic bodies showing different degrees of mineralization, embedded in connective tissue. X-ray diffraction and Raman spectroscopy studies suggest that the mineralized material corresponds to hydroxyapatite crystals.[1191,1192]

Microlithiasis and Testicular Cancer

The possible association between microlithiasis and testicular cancer is controversial.[1151,1187,1193,1194] Testicular microlithiasis is associated with both GCNIS and germ cell tumors (Figs. 12.131 through 12.133). In infancy, it is associated with GCNIS and gonadal stromal tumors, but only in isolated cases.[1168,1170,1195–1197] Several findings favor this association: (1) nearly one-half of testes with germ cell tumors also show testicular microlithiasis; (2) patients with testicular microlithiasis may later experience development of testicular tumor; (3) patients with testicular microlithiasis and extratesticular germ cell tumor, either retroperitoneal or mediastinal, have been reported; and (4) increased prevalence of testicular microlithiasis is noted in men with familial testicular cancer and in their relatives.[1196,1198–1205] The most important finding that mitigates against an association between testicular microlithiasis and cancer is the unquestionably

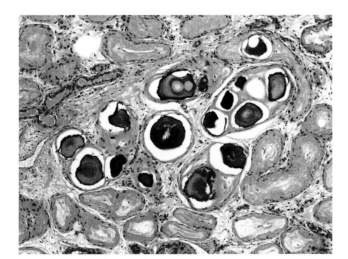

Fig. 12.130 Testicular parenchyma with hyalinized tubules. In the center of the image a hypoplastic zone with microliths may be recognized.

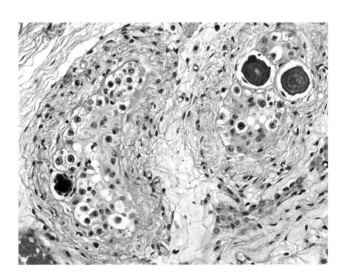

Fig. 12.131 Seminiferous tubules containing both GCNIS and microliths in the periphery of a seminoma.

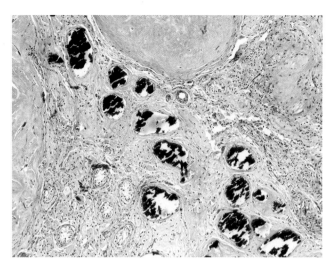

Fig. 12.132 Testicular parenchyma with fibrosis of a burned-out tumor next to intratubular calcifications of an intratubular germ cell neoplasia.

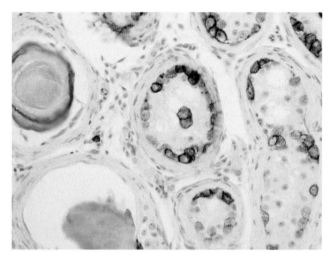

Fig. 12.133 Microlithiasis associated with germ cell neoplasia in situ. Immunostaining for placental alkaline phosphatase.

high incidence of testicular microlithiasis compared with the low incidence of testicular germ cell tumors in adults.

Isolated microlithiasis that is not associated with another disorder does not require follow-up.[1152,1198-1200,1202,1206] Three methods have been proposed for surveillance of patients with testicular microlithiasis when needed: abdominal and pelvic CT, ultrasound and testicular tumor marker study, or simple ultrasonography and physical examination every 6 months.[1181,1183,1186,1202,1207,1208] The risk for malignancy is higher in classic than in limited testicular microlithiasis.[1209] The surveillance policy may be modified depending on the associated disorders.[1206] Patients found in infancy to have isolated testicular microlithiasis without other associated disorders warrant yearly physical examination, whereas follow-up sonography should be limited to the subgroup of patients with other associated risk factors.[1210,1211] Yearly ultrasound examination is recommended in patients with testicular microlithiasis associated with cryptorchidism, infertility, atrophic testes, or contralateral testis with germ cell tumor.[1185,1212] Testicular biopsy should be performed when clinically indicated.

When testicular microlithiasis is associated with infertility, the incidence of cancer varies according to the unilateralism or bilateralism of testicular microlithiasis.[1179] Subfertile patients with unilateral and bilateral microlithiasis have GCNIS in 0% and 20%, respectively. Therefore only patients with bilateral testicular microlithiasis should undergo rigorous follow-up.

The nexus between testicular microlithiasis and cancer does not seem to be the predisposition of one disorder toward the other, but rather the predisposition of both to develop in abnormal testes, accounting for frequent coincidence. This may also explain the association between testicular microlithiasis and infertility or subfertility, and these entities may be expressions of testicular dysgenesis syndrome.[1213]

In patients with germ cell tumor, other forms of calcification may be observed. The most frequent are conglomerates of microcalcifications around the tumor or amorphous intratubular calcifications in necrotic intratubular tumors such as embryonal carcinoma, calcifications in the scar of burned-out tumors, and calcifications associated with intratubular hyalinizing Sertoli cell tumor or calcifying large cell Sertoli cell tumor. Dystrophic calcifications and ossification may be observed in the testis and paratesticular structures in patients with a history of orchitis, epididymitis, trauma, or testicular infarction.

Rete Testis, Epididymis, and Vaginal Microlithiasis and Calcifications

Microlithiasis also occurs in the rete testis or sperm excretory ducts. The disorder is asymptomatic and in most cases is not associated with testicular cancer (Figs. 12.134 and 12.135). Calcifications in the epididymis or in diverticula of the cauda of the epididymis have long been observed.[1214–1216] More than 70% of young adults undergoing kidney transplant experience development of calcifications (Fig. 12.136).[1217]

Idiopathic microlithiasis of the epididymis and rete testis is much less frequent than testicular microlithiasis in adults. Incidence is 1 case per 1000 autopsies, and it is found in 3% of orchidoepididymectomy specimens. Epididymal microlithiasis is characterized by the presence of multiple and small calcifications with lamellated structures like those of psammoma bodies. This asymptomatic process is not related to testicular cancer.[1214,1218]

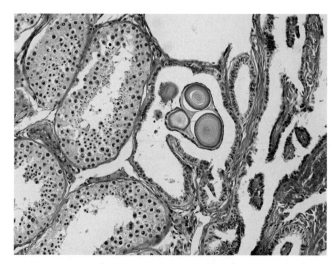

Fig. 12.134 Microlithiasis of rete testis. The three microliths are probably located in the thickness of a tendinous cord of the rete testis. The seminiferous tubules show abundant spermatogenesis.

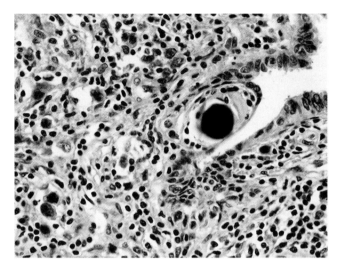

Fig. 12.135 Microlithiasis of the rete testis associated with infiltration of the testicular mediastinum by seminoma. Microliths were also observed in the conserved testicular parenchyma. The rete testis does not present pagetoid infiltration by germ cell neoplasia in situ cells.

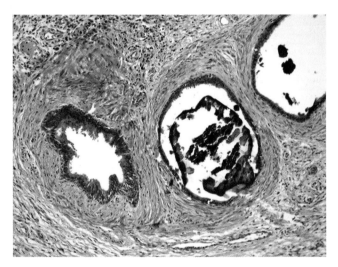

Fig. 12.136 Calculus at the tail of the epididymis. There are two diverticula. The central one contains a partial calcification of the intratubular material.

occurring with testicular microliths. They may also be formed by Liesegang ring calcifications. These eosinophilic bodies range from 10 to 800 μm in diameter and have characteristic concentric laminated cores with radial striations that are observed in obstructive processes of the spermatic pathway (Fig. 12.137).[1220]

Interstitial microlithiasis is mainly located in the body and tail of the epididymis. Epididymal rupture and extravasation into the interductal tissue may cause a histiocytic reaction around microliths that resembles malakoplakia (Fig. 12.138). The larger size and the radial structure of microliths enable correct diagnosis. As in malakoplakia, the inflammatory infiltrate is eventually replaced by fibrosis. Interstitial microlithiasis may arise after perforation of diverticula that are frequently present in the tail of the epididymis.[1221] After perforation, microliths derived from total or partial mineralization of Liesegang rings make contact with the immune system in the interstitium and may induce an immune response. The histologic differential diagnosis of Liesegang rings and microliths includes Michaelis-Gutmann bodies seen in

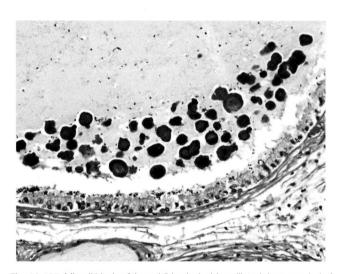

Fig. 12.137 Microlithiasis of the epididymis. Inside a dilated duct a myriad of microliths are observed (many with laminated structure) surrounded by an amorphous material with abundant spermatozoa.

Sonographic appearance is characteristic, with multiple comet-shaped foci of microcalcification throughout the epididymis.[1219] In infancy, rete testis microlithiasis is associated with paratesticular embryonal remnants, cystic dysplasia of the rete testis, and undescended testes. In adulthood, rete testis microlithiasis is infrequently associated with testicular microlithiasis and malignancy. It is also found in older men, possibly related to ischemic injury. Characteristic rete testis calcium deposits, known as intracystic polypoid nodular proliferation, have been reported only in adults with poor peripheral circulation.

Epididymal microlithiasis may occur both in association with testicular microlithiasis in prepubertal boys and as an isolated finding. Histologic studies have been reported only for the isolated form. Microliths may be found in three different locations: subepithelial, intraluminal, and interstitial. Although some microliths may originate from the testis or rete testis, most form under the epithelium and are cleared into the lumen by a mechanism like that

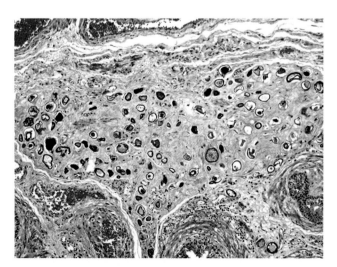

Fig. 12.138 Epididymal microlithiasis. Numerous microliths displaying a psammoma body–like appearance are set in hyalinized stroma.

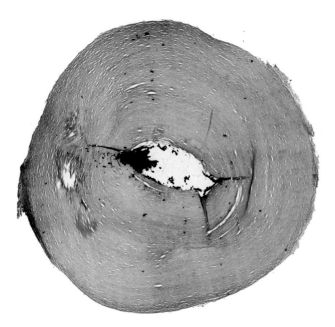

Fig. 12.139 Scrotal pearl. Concentric lamina formation with central calcification in a patient operated on for hydrocele.

malakoplakia, calcium deposits, and parasites such as the giant kidney worm *Dioctophyma renale.*[1222]

In infancy and adulthood, "pearls" or scrotal calculi may appear that are freely mobile, spheroid, <7-mm calcified bodies lying between the layers of the tunica vaginalis (Fig. 12.139). They are observed in 2% to 3% of cases during routine ultrasound examinations.[1223] The incidence rate is as high as 5% in hydrocele patients, 7% in equestrians, and 81% in extreme mountain bikers.[1224,1225] Scrotal calculi consist of calcium deposits, oxalate or phosphorous, covering nondescript material that may originate from torsion of hydatid, small hemorrhage, or desquamated mesothelial cells. Fewer than one-half of the cases are associated with scrotal pain.[1223] The effect of scrotal calculi on testicular function is unknown.[1226]

Disorders of Sex Development

Gonadal Dysgenesis

Classically, *gonadal dysgenesis* refers to disorders characterized by amenorrhea and streak gonads in phenotypically female patients with hypoplastic uterus and fallopian tubes. Streak gonad, when understood as a pathologic concept, allows syndromes with different clinical phenotypes (Turner, Swyer, and Sohval) to be included within the spectrum of disordered gonadal dysgenesis. Clinical manifestations, which are grouped under the term *male pseudohermaphroditism with müllerian rests*, should also be considered syndromes of gonadal dysgenesis, including Sohval syndrome, male with uterus, and dysgenetic male pseudohermaphroditism with preferential testicular differentiation of one or both gonads.

Consensus classification of intersex disorders was reported by the International Consensus Conference on Intersex in 2005 (Table 12.17).[1227] Conferees considered use of some terms (e.g., pseudohermaphroditism, hermaphroditism, sex reversal, and intersex situation) obsolete and introduced the term DSDs to designate all intersex disorders. This classification has given rise to numerous critical comments because it is based on chromosomal constitution (peripheral karyotype of leukocytes) and phenotype.[1228]

Specifically, in cases of gonadal dysgenesis, entities with completely different histopathologic features, such as 45,X0 Turner syndrome and its variants and mixed gonadal dysgenesis (45,X0/45,XY), are included together with Klinefelter syndrome and variants under the same term DSDs. The same may be said of the unfortunate inclusion of congenital adrenal hyperplasia in females as DSD.[1229] Several inconsistencies contribute to the unresolved problem of classification. The same karyotype may give rise to different phenotypes. Furthermore, it is increasingly understood that instead of having one cellular line, gonadal dysgenesis has mosaicisms or more complex chromosomal constitutions. This problem is complicated further with the results of chromosomal studies of the gonads. Finally, the same clinical entity may be produced by different karyotypes as occurs in patients with ovotesticular DSD (46,XX, 46,XY, mosaicisms, or genetic abnormalities).[1230] Therefore classification of these disorders that encompasses different points of view (e.g., genetic, endocrinologic, clinical, and histopathologic) remains elusive.

Pathologists rely on critical assessment of the nature of the gonad they are examining. This vantage point places them at the center of the controversy. On one side, pathologists understand which genetic mutations contribute to the condition of the gonad, and on the other side, they can explain the variability of clinical symptoms in terms of the anatomy of the gonad.

Gonadal dysgenesis may be defined as incomplete or defective gonadal differentiation because of disturbance in germ cell migration or its correct organization in the gonadal ridge. This anomaly is morphologically expressed as levels of differentiation toward ovary, testis, or both. The term *gonadal dysgenesis* comprises a broad spectrum of lesions ranging from absence of the gonad or persistence of undifferentiated gonadal tissue (UGT) to classic streak gonad or the presence of a testis surrounded by stroma similar to the ovarian cortex. In other words, the term includes the spectrum of gonads observed before the architecture of the ovary or the testis is fully defined. It is possible that all forms of gonadal dysgenesis are part of a spectrum of the same disorder.[1231]

Patients with DSDs can be classified into two groups: (1) those with gonadal dysgenesis including 45,X0 gonadal dysgenesis, 46,XX gonadal dysgenesis, 46,XY gonadal dysgenesis, mixed gonadal dysgenesis, dysgenetic male pseudohermaphroditism, PMDS, and ovotesticular dysgenesis (Fig. 12.140); and (2) patients with architecturally normal testes and different degrees of undermasculinization, which includes androgen synthesis deficiencies and impaired androgen metabolism in peripheral tissues (Table 12.18).

Types of Gonads in Patients With Gonadal Dysgenesis and Correlation With Clinical Syndromes

To gain a better understanding of gonadal dysgenesis, the pathologist should realize the utility of considering that several histologic patterns may arise from an undifferentiated gonad. When differentiation is toward ovary, two different stages may be seen: streak gonad with or without ovarian follicles and hypoplastic ovary. When differentiation is toward testis, streak gonad with epithelial cords and dysgenetic testis may be observed. If the gonad has incomplete differentiation toward either testis or ovary, but without forming ovotestis, streak testis is formed, or the undifferentiated gonad may even disappear (Fig. 12.140).

At the beginning of differentiation, the gonad may manifest as UGT arrested at the fetal stage. In the literature, these gonads have been considered either as streak gonad or as ovary. In fact, UGT may appear as a streak gonad with epithelial cord–like structures

TABLE 12.17	New Nomenclature of Disorders of Sex Development after Chicago Consensus Meeting 2005				
	46,XY DSD		**46,XX DSD**		
Sex Chromosome DSDs	Disorders of Testicular Development	Disorders of Androgen Synthesis/Action	Disorders of Ovarian Development	Fetal Androgen Excess	
45,X Turner and variants	Complete gonadal dysgenesis	Androgen synthesis defect	Ovotesticular DSD	*CAH*	*Non-CAH*
47,XXY Klinefelter and variants	Partial gonadal dysgenesis	Luteinizing hormone receptor defect	Testicular DSD	21-OH-deficiency	Aromatase deficiency
45,X/46,XY MGD	Gonadal regression	Androgen insensitivity	Gonadal dysgenesis	11-OH deficiency	P450 oxidoreductase gene defect
Chromosomal ovotesticular DSD	Ovotesticular DSD	5α-Reductase deficiency			Maternal luteoma
		Disorders AMH			Iatrogenic
		Timing defect			
		Endocrine disrupters			
		Cloacal exstrophy			

DSD, Disorder of sex development; *MGD*, Mixed gonadal dysgenesis; *CAH*, Congenital adrenal hypertrophia; *AMH*, Antimüllerian hormone.

TYPES OF GONADS IN DISORDERS OF SEXUAL DIFFERENTIATION

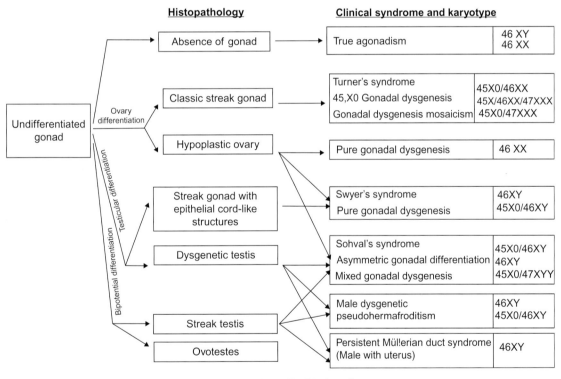

Fig. 12.140 Gonadal dysgenesis. Different types of gonads and correlation with clinical syndromes.

or focally in several types of gonads such as dysgenetic testis, streak testis, or ovotestis. UGT recognition is of great interest because of the high incidence of transformation into gonadoblastoma.[1232] The most significant characteristics of this peculiar gonad are discussed later with streak gonad with epithelial cord–like structures. Numerous germ cells are arranged neither in follicles nor in seminiferous cords, but are rather enclosed in an ovarian-like stroma or in cords of immature Sertoli cell–like/granulosa cells (Fig. 12.141).

Grossly, regardless of differentiation, the streak gonad is an elongate, fibrous, pearly formation located at the site of the normal ovary. The streak gonad measures 2 to 3 cm in length and 0.5 cm in width in the adult and may contain hilar cells or rete ovarii.

Classic Streak Gonad

Microscopically, streak gonad may consist of bundles of fibrous connective tissue or as whorled, ovarian-like stroma. This is the classic gonad seen in 45,X0 gonadal dysgenesis or Turner

			Wolffian Derivatives	Müllerian Derivatives	Leydig Cells		
	Cause	Phenotype				Spermatogenesis	Entity
Defect in Sertoli cells	Androgen receptor absence	Female	Absent or hypoplastic	Absent or rudimentary	Diffuse hyperplasia	Absent	Morris syndrome
Defect in Leydig cells	Defect in androgen synthesis	Female	Normal	Absent	Xanthomized	Absent	Congenital adrenal hyperplasia
	Lutein hormone receptor inactivating mutation	Female	Hypoplastic	Absent	Absent	Absent	Absence of response to gonadotropins
Defect in Sertoli cells, Leydig cells, and germ cells	Chromosomopathy	Male	Normal	Absent	Nodular hyperplasia	Absent or focal	XXY Klinefelter syndrome
	Androgen insufficiency	Male	Normal	Absent	Focal hyperplasia	Absent Maturation arrest Mixed atrophy	Cryptorchidism
Defects in target organs	5-α reductase deficiency	Female	Hypoplastic	Absent	Hyperplasia	Absent Hypospermatogenesis	5-α Reductase deficiency

TABLE 12.18 Disorders of Sex Development With Architectural Normal Testis and Undermasculinization in Adult Patients

Data are referred to complete forms.

syndrome. Some classic streak gonads may contain germ cells enclosed in primordial and eventually primary follicles (Fig. 12.142). These germ cells express VASA and KIT, and are negative for OCT3/4, PLAP, and TSPY. In some patients, regardless of age, atretic follicles, multiple cortical cysts (Figs. 12.143 and 12.144), abundant hilar cells, or glandular-like groups of clear cells in the hilus may be observed. This gonad is observed in patients with Turner syndrome with chromosomal mosaicism, as well as in 46,XX pure gonadal dysgenesis.

Hypoplastic Ovary (Dysgenetic Ovary)
The development of the ovary is an active process that is based, at least in part, on the absence of *SRY*, the testis-determining gene on the Y chromosome. Dysgenetic ovaries or hypoplastic ovaries do

not have the form of a streak gonad, but are ovoid, small, with a smooth surface. Primary follicles, and occasionally follicles in development, may be observed in the cortex with a regular pattern of distribution. This gonad is characteristic of 46,XX pure gonadal dysgenesis and some cases of ovotesticular dysgenesis (ovotesticular disorder).

Streak Gonad With Epithelial Cord–like Structures
The gonad consists of ovarian cortex-like stroma traversed in all directions by epithelial cord–like structures (sex cords) that form an anastomosing network. The cords may be thin or thick with coarse outlines (Fig. 12.145). These cordlike structures contain two types of cells (Fig. 12.146). Most numerous are small cells with hyperchromatic nuclei that are likely pre–Sertoli cells or immature

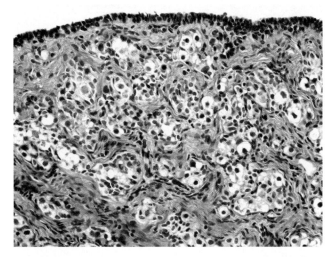

Fig. 12.141 Gonadal dysgenesis. Undifferentiated gonadal tissue. Streak gonad showing nests and cords with two types of cells: the most numerous, small-sized cells and large cells with voluminous nuclei and pale cytoplasm (germ cells).

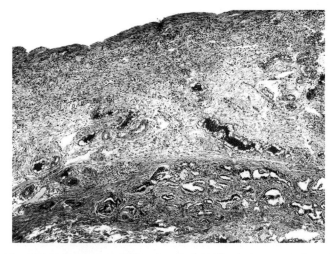

Fig. 12.142 Streak gonad. The elongate formation lacks germ cells and consists of an ovarian cortex-like stroma and tubular structures resembling rete ovarii in the deeper part.

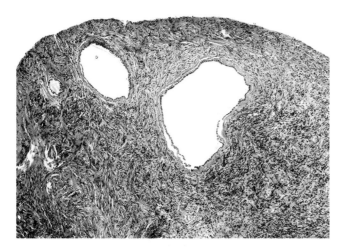

Fig. 12.143 Streak gonad with inclusion cysts lined by cuboidal epithelium.

Sertoli/granulosa cells. These cells are intensely positive for AE1/AE3 and calretinin (Fig. 12.147) and moderately positive for inhibin (Fig. 12.148); D2–40 and AMH are weakly expressed. The epithelial cord–like structures abut a basal membrane of variable thickness. In the thickest areas, spiculated or nodular projections inside the cords may be observed. The second type of cells are germ cells, which may be isolated within the stroma, forming cords, or in between Sertoli/granulosa cells. The number is variable, and some cords may even form small nests. These germ cells are immunoreactive for OCT3/4, KIT, PLAP, TSPY, and VASA. The histologic pattern of the gonad is that of UGT. Some streak gonads with epithelial cord–like structures are devoid of germ cells, although it is probable that the gonad contained germ cells at some point in development, but the cells were eliminated by apoptosis.

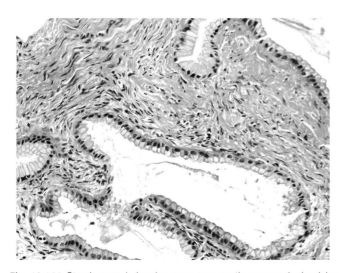

Fig. 12.144 Streak gonad showing numerous cystic or pseudoglandular formations lined by mucous epithelium.

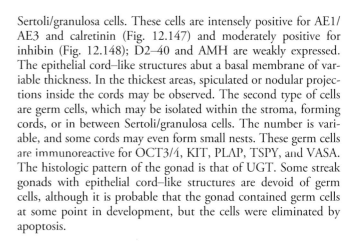

Fig. 12.146 46XY gonadal dysgenesis. Solid cords anastomosed with cells of hyperchromatic nucleus (Sertoli/granulosa) and larger cells of pale cytoplasm (gonocytes).

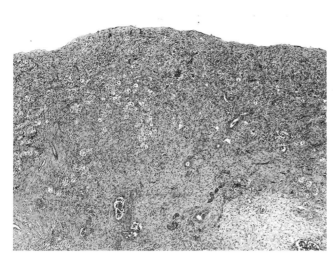

Fig. 12.145 46XY gonadal dysgenesis. Streak gonad with epithelial cordlike structures containing Sertoli/granulosa and germ cells.

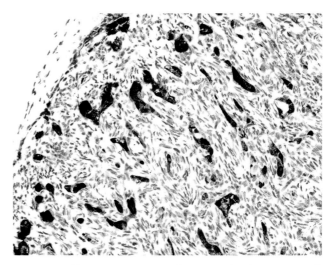

Fig. 12.147 46XY gonadal dysgenesis. Streak gonad with epithelial cordlike structures showing intense immunoexpression of calretinin in Sertoli/granulosa cells of the cords.

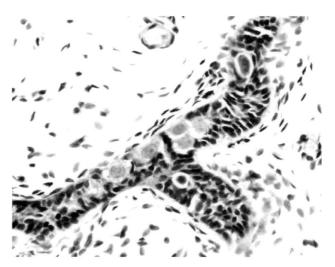

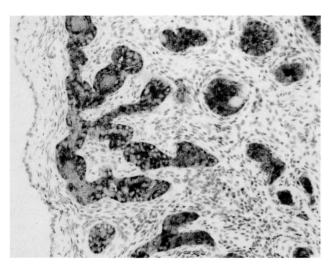

Fig. 12.148 46XY gonadal dysgenesis. Sertoli/granulosa cells from the epithelial cords show intense immunostaining for inhibin.

Dysgenetic Testis

This gonad is usually cryptorchid and small, with a compact central core containing seminiferous tubules with or without germ cells. The peripheral zone, instead of showing a well-collagenized tunica albuginea as occurs in normal testes, has an ovarian stroma with or without malformed seminiferous cords (Fig. 12.149). The seminiferous cords have strange anastomoses, and diameter varies from superficial to deep areas without exact topographic features. Seminiferous tubules or cords are separated by a wide and loose stroma. Sertoli cells express inhibin, D2–40, AMH, and, like Leydig cells, calretinin, preferentially in superficial seminiferous cords. However, in the central areas of the testis, calretinin is expressed only in small tubules usually devoid of germ cells and in Leydig cells. Germ cells are found in seminiferous tubules and adjacent to the basal membrane. The germ cell phenotype is positive for VASA, TSPY, and D2–40, and a subpopulation is positive for OCT3/4, KIT, and PLAP.

There are a modest number of studies of dysgenetic testes in pubertal and adult patients. The whorled stroma in the tunica albuginea and irregular contour with distorted seminiferous tubules are conserved. Maturation of Sertoli cells is incomplete, as expressed by absence of tubular lumina and nuclei characteristic of dysgenetic cells (round or ovoid nuclei instead of triangular nuclei with deep grooves of adult Sertoli cells). Most tubules are devoid of germ cells. The interstitium shows apparent Leydig cell hyperplasia that is diffuse and peritubular. Immunohistochemical techniques allow a better understanding of the peculiar relationships among Leydig cells, peritubular cells, and Sertoli cells. Anti-calretinin and antiinhibin antibodies may show the number of Leydig cells that form concentric circles in the tubular wall. Leydig cells are located among peritubular cells or between peritubular cells and the basal membrane. Although most tubules are devoid of germ cells, as previously mentioned, some groups of tubules with GCNIS may be observed.

This gonad corresponds to that described as "dysgenesis," and is observed in the three syndromes that are classically included in male pseudohermaphroditism with müllerian rests: (1) mixed gonadal dysgenesis (Sohval syndrome or asymmetric gonadal differentiation), whose usual karyotypes are 45,X0/46,XY, 46,XY, and 45,X0/47,XYY; (2) male dysgenetic pseudohermaphroditism, which usually shows the karyotype 46,XY or 45,X0/46,XY; and (3) müllerian duct persistence syndrome (male with uterus), which has 46,XY karyotype. Both the degree of müllerian duct regression and the AMH levels may be correlated with number of seminiferous tubules present in the dysgenetic testis.[1233,1234]

Streak Testis

This gonad has two intimately joined zones. The largest zone consists of dysgenetic testis with ovarian cortex–like stroma close to the tunica albuginea. The stroma is in continuity with streak gonad, which may or may not contain epithelial cords or ovarian follicles (Fig. 12.150). This gonad is observed in some of the three previously mentioned syndromes: mixed gonadal dysgenesis, dysgenetic male pseudohermaphroditism, and müllerian duct persistence syndrome.

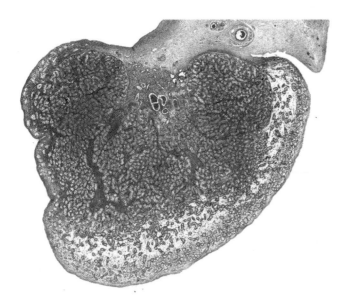

Fig. 12.149 Dysgenetic testis. The gonad consists of a central part with compact packing of seminiferous tubules and an outer part with irregular seminiferous tubules reaching the surface of the gonad.

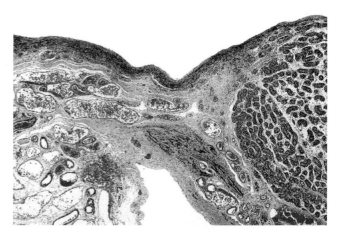

Fig. 12.150 Streak testis consisting of a streak gonad connected to a testis that shows the characteristic lesions of testicular dysgenesis.

True Agonadism

True agonadism is characterized by the absence of both gonads in patients who show female external genitalia. These patients usually present with 46,XY karyotype (46,XY gonadal dysgenesis syndrome), although a few patients with 46,XX karyotype have been reported. Internal genitalia usually include a uterus and uterine tubes, although both müllerian and wolffian remnants may be absent. Gonads are not present anywhere, even in ectopic locations. These patients are raised as girls. The diagnosis may be delayed until puberty or adulthood, when patients seek medical care for other symptoms such as absence of mammary development, small stature, or hypergonadotropic hypogonadism.[452,1235] No androgenic response is observed after hCG stimulation test, and AMH is undetectable. Cases may be sporadic or familial, and associated extragenital anomalies have also been observed. In some cases the cause is heterozygous *WT1* mutation.[452] In most familial cases, inheritance is autosomal recessive or X-chromosome linked, and the cause seems to be either other *WT1* anomalies or anomalies in other genes involved in development.[455] No molecular defect in the *SRY* gene may occur in this syndrome.[456] Agonadism may be associated with other syndromes, including PAGOD, Kennerknecht, Seckel, CHARGE and congenital adrenal hyperplasia.[457–460,1236–1239]

45,X0 Gonadal Dysgenesis

45,X0 gonadal dysgenesis is one of the most common chromosomal anomalies (from 1 in 2500 to 1 in 5000 in female newborns), although 99% of zygotes with this karyotype abort in the first stages of embryonal development.[1255,1256] The incidence among patients with delayed growth rises to 5% in some series.[1257] Patients with 45,X0 gonadal dysgenesis have characteristic stigmata of Turner syndrome, including short stature, pterygium coli, lymphedema, and cardiac malformations. External genitalia are female and infantile, with typical streak gonads (Figs. 12.151 and 12.152). Turner syndrome is defined by the combination of physical features and complete or partial absence of one or both X chromosomes, frequently associated with mosaicism.[1258] Most patients have a characteristic neurocognitive profile.[1259] Other anomalies, known as turnerian stigmata, may also be present and are classified into four groups: skeletal anomalies such as cubitus valgus, shortening of the fourth metacarpal, and Madelung

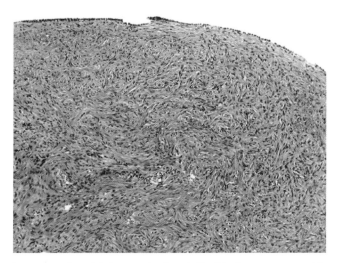

Fig. 12.151 Gonadal dysgenesis. Streak fibroblastic stroma resembling ovarian cortex.

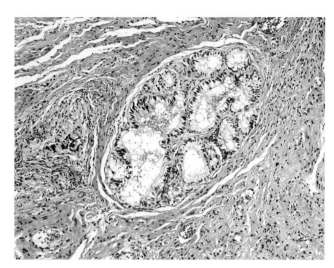

Fig. 12.152 Streak gonad in Turner syndrome (45,X0 gonadal dysgenesis) showing a glandiform proliferation lined by Sertoli-like cells.

deformity characteristic of Leri-Weill dyschondrosteosis; soft tissue anomalies such as webbed neck, low posterior hair line, and puffy hands and feet; visceral anomalies such as aortic coarctation, horseshoe kidney, polycystic kidney, urethral stenosis, and vesicourethral reflux; and miscellaneous anomalies such as nevus pigmentosus.[1251,1260–1263] SHOX (short stature homeobox-containing gene) haploinsufficiency is likely responsible, at least in part, for short stature and turnerian stigmata.[1264]

Most patients have 45,X0 chromosomal constitution that results from loss of the paternal sex chromosome.[1265,1266] Molecular techniques, such as fluorescence in situ hybridization and polymerase chain reaction (PCR), show that 50% to 75% of patients have chromosomal mosaicisms or structurally abnormal X or Y chromosomes. The most frequent mosaicisms are 45,X0/46,XX (10% to 15%), 45,X0/46,XY (2% to 6%), 45,X0/46,Xi (Xq), 45,X0/46,X,del(Xp), and 45,X0/46,XX/47,XXX. Alterations of sex chromosomes may include aberration of X structure, total or partial deletion of the short arm of the X chromosome (46,X0,del[Xp]), isochromosome of the long arm of the X chromosome (46,X,i[Xq]), ring chromosome (46,Xr[X]), and marker chromosome (46,X + m).[1267–1269] Some authors consider mosaicism in Turner syndrome to be a prerequisite for survival in early pregnancy.[1270] More than 85% of patients have Y chromosome, or at least material derived from this chromosome.[1242,1271] Internal genitalia with 45,X0 karyotype are female but infantile. Streak gonads consist of ovarian-like stroma, which may contain hilar cells and rete ovarii (Fig. 12.142).[1272] During embryonic life, gonads show normal germ cell number up to the third month, when germ cell proliferation ceases.[1233,1273] Ovogenesis stops in meiosis I, usually before the pachytene stage. The cause seems to be generalized meiotic pairing errors with the start of apoptosis to avoid formation of abnormal gametes.[1274] Massive apoptosis of ovocytes occurs between the 15th and 20th weeks.[1275] Surviving germ cells disappear throughout fetal life, and the number at birth is usually low.[1276] About 3% of patients retain scattered germ cells after puberty. This feature explains the occurrence of menstruation for a few years.[1277,1278] The rare reported cases of pregnancy result in a high rate of miscarriages, stillbirths, and malformed babies.[1279] These statistics are changing with the practice of ovocyte donation and good uterine preparation before implantation.[1280] During adulthood, the usual condition is

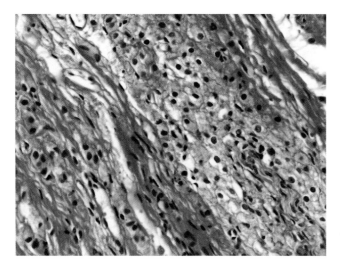

Fig. 12.153 Streak gonad in Turner syndrome. Group of hilar cells in the vicinity of nerve fibers.

hypergonadotropic hypogonadism, but isolated cases of hypogonadotropic hypogonadism have been reported.[1281,1281a] Streak gonads may contain inclusion cysts, rete ovarii cysts, and clusters of Leydig cells (Fig. 12.153).

Molecular testing detects different Y-specific sequences (SRY, Ycen, and Yq12) in different tissues (oral epithelial cells, lymphocytes, and ovarian tissue) from 10% to 20% of 45,X0 patients.[1282] The *SRY* gene is a marker of testicular tissue and of gonadoblastoma, so gonad removal has been recommended in such patients, as well those with 45,X0/46,XY karyotype.[1283,1284] Gonadoblastoma, dysgerminoma, and mixed germ cell tumor have also been reported.[1285,1286]

Patients With Chromosomal Mosaicisms

The most frequent chromosomal mosaicisms associated with this gonadal dysgenesis are 45,X0/46,XX, 45,X0/47,XXX, 45,X0/46,XX/47,XXX, and 45,X0/46,XY. The first is most common, whereas the last two are rare.[1240] The second cell line of each mosaicism may be present in a few cells only. Phenotype depends on the ratio between the Y portion and 45,X0 cells lines in the body.[1241] No two patients with mosaic Turner syndrome have the same genotype–phenotype.[1242] In general, anomalies associated with mosaicisms are less severe and fewer in number than are those of 45,X0 patients.[1243] Approximately 12% of patients with mosaicism menstruate, but only 3% of 45,X0 patients menstruate. This finding suggests the possibility of a short period of fertility.[1244] Approximately 18% of patients show breast development; this percentage is also lower (5%) in 45,X0 patients. Stature is also higher than in 45,X0 patients.

Patients with 45,X0/46,XY comprise 1.5 in 10,000 consecutive newborns, and their phenotype varies widely.[1245] There is no relationship between the degree of mosaicism and somatic features, genital development, or gonadal structure These patients may present with Turner syndrome, varied forms of undermasculinization DSD, ovotesticular disorder, hypospadias, dysgenetic streak ovaries, or mixed gonadal dysgenesis. Among patients diagnosed by prenatal amniocentesis, 95% have normal male genitalia, although only 27% presented with normal gonadal histology.[1246–1248] Overall, the estimated incidence rate of germinal tumors for patients with 45,X0/46,XY is 15%; however, if only patients with

Turner syndrome without signs of virilization are taken into account, the risk for tumor is lower.[1249,1250]

Patients with 46,Xi(Xq) have streak gonads and somatic anomalies similar to those of 45,X0 patients. Half of 46X,del(Xq)(p11) patients have amenorrhea and gonadal dysgenesis.[1251,1252]

Patients with Turner syndrome have a high frequency of autoimmune diseases such as hypothyroidism, celiac disease, and diabetes mellitus.[1253]

Long-term estrogen administration for patients with this or other forms of gonadal dysgenesis is a risk factor for endometrial carcinoma.[1254]

46,XX Gonadal Dysgenesis

Patients with 46,XX gonadal dysgenesis have normal stature, female phenotype, well-developed external genitalia, and absence of turnerian stigmata.

The anomaly is usually detected when patients present with primary amenorrhea, delayed puberty, infertility, and hypergonadotropic hypogonadism. This syndrome is sporadic and familial, and may be linked to recessive autosomal inheritance.[1287–1289] Gonadal development varies, even among members of the same family, from streak gonads to severe ovarian hypoplasia (only a few ovocytes are present) (Fig. 12.154).[1290] Patients have no predisposition to gonadal neoplasia because the incidence of tumors in these patients is low, and the most common tumor is dysgerminoma.[1291–1293]

Approximately two-thirds of cases have a genetic cause, and the remainder are secondary to infection, infarct, or infiltrative or autoimmune disease.[1294–1296] The syndrome may result from absence of a hypothetical substance that induces gonadal development, failure in germ cell formation, defective germ cell migration, or excessive germ cell loss in ovaries during fetal life. Genes responsible for ovarian development seem to be located in proximal regions of Xp and distal regions of Xq.[1297] Some patients with familial cases have balanced translocation in the X chromosome (from the long arm to the short arm).[1298,1299] Gonadal dysgenesis or early ovarian failure may occur in patients with Xq26-qter deletion, Xp28 mutations (QM gene), or balanced translocations occurring either in X;autosome or 1;11 chromosomes.[592,1300–1302] Given that FSH is necessary for ovarian follicle development, investigation has also been focused on mutations of the FSHR gene located on chromosome 2. These mutations have been observed in familial cases, as well as in unrelated cases, but they are absent in other patients.[1302a,1303–1305]

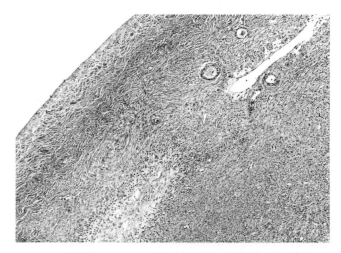

Fig. 12.154 46,XX gonadal dysgenesis in an 18-year-old patient. Streak gonad showing isolated primordial follicles and one atresic follicle.

Because FSH is necessary for ovarian follicle development, investigation has also focused on mutations of the FSHR gene located in chromosome 2. Several autosomal recessive mutations of the *WNT4*, *R-spondin*, *PSMC3IP/HOP2*, *MCM9*, *MCM8*, and *STAG3* genes have been described for FSHR genes and SYCE1, X-linked recessive mutations in BMP15, or recessive missense mutation in nucleoporin-107 (NUP107).[1306] Association with somatic anomalies is rare. The most frequent anomaly is neurosensory hearing loss (phenotype known as Perrault syndrome).[1307,1308] Other anomalies observed in isolated cases are achondroplasia and fatal lung fibrosis with immunodeficiency.[1309,1310]

46,XY Gonadal Dysgenesis

46,XY gonadal dysgenesis (Swyer syndrome) is characterized by female phenotype and external genitalia, absence of turnerian stigmata, occasionally fused labia majora, and hypertrophic clitoris.[1311] The incidence of Swyer syndrome is 1 in 100,000.[1312] Breasts develop at puberty when most cases are diagnosed. Sexual infantilism persists in adulthood, and eunuchoidism and amenorrhea appear. These patients have elevated serum gonadotropins, low estradiol, and normal female levels of androgens. Some have mosaic karyotype with one of the lines containing Y chromosome.

46,XY gonadal dysgenesis may be complete and incomplete. Patients with the *complete type* have female external genitalia and classic streak gonads with epithelial cord–like structures, although cases with ovarian tissue have been reported.[1313] Internal genitalia reflect well-developed müllerian structures. The cause is unknown in approximately 70% to 80% of cases.[1314] In 80% of patients with 46,XY gonadal dysgenesis, *SRY* is apparently normal. In the remainder, multiple genetic abnormalities are observed, including mutations in the *DHH*, *WT1*, *SOX9*, *ARX*, *AXX*, *CBX2*, *DMRT1*, *GATA4*, *MAMLD1*, *MAP3K1*, *NR0B1*, *WNT4*, *WWOX*, and *WNT4* genes.[1315] *SRY* gene is deleted in up to 10% to 15% and mutated in an additional 10% to 15%.[1316–1323]

SRY genotype is related to gonadal histology. SRY mutation is associated with *complete type* of dysgenetic gonad, whereas immature seminiferous tubules may be observed when SRY is normal. The degree of masculinization and the development of internal genitalia mirror the degree of testicular differentiation. In most cases, there is failure in early gonadal development (sixth to eighth week of gestation) that results in absence of müllerian duct inhibiting factor, testosterone, and DHT, culminating in development of female phenotype.

Patients with *incomplete* 46,XY gonadal dysgenesis have ambiguous external genitalia and variable degrees of development of the müllerian and wolffian structures. Gonads vary from a classic streak gonad, streak gonads with epithelial cord–like structures, and dysgenetic testes. Patients do not have mutations in the two major genes required for gonadal development: *SRY* and *WT1*, although some have altered *NR5A1* gene.[1324–1328] Epithelial cords of the most streak gonad express cytokeratins (AE1/AE3), inhibin, and D2–40, whereas germ cells are positive for PLAP and OCT3/4. Clitoromegaly may be caused by androgens secreted by hyperplastic Leydig cells in the streak gonad.[1329]

Cases of 46,XY gonadal dysgenesis may occur with coexistence of normal testes and ambiguous external genitalia, well-developed müllerian structures, and poorly differentiated wolffian structures. This genital pattern likely results from late testicular determination rather than testicular differentiation defect. Although the testis produces testosterone and AMH, both hormones are inefficient because the critical period of hormonal receptiveness has passed.[1330]

Some patients with 46,XY gonadal dysgenesis present with extragonadal anomalies and multiple syndromes, including camptomelic dysplasia and renal disorder; myotonic dystrophy and terminal renal disease; progressive renal insufficiency and gonadoblastoma (Frasier syndrome) (Figs. 12.155 through 12.158); mental retardation with or without facial anomalies or short stature; renal insufficiency and Wilms tumor (Denys–Drash syndrome); combination of cleft palate, micrognathia, kyphosis, scoliosis, and clubfoot (Gardner-Silengo-Wachtel syndrome or genitopalatocardiac syndrome); multiple pterygium syndrome; Graves disease; and congenital universalis alopecia, microcephaly, cutis marmorata, short stature, and peripheral neuropathy.[1330–1347]

Most cases are sporadic, although the syndrome has been reported in several members of the same family, and multiple forms of inheritance (X-linked, autosomal recessive, and male-limited autosomal dominant) have been proposed.[1238,1321,1348–1357] In addition to infertility, patients with 46,XY gonadal dysgenesis have

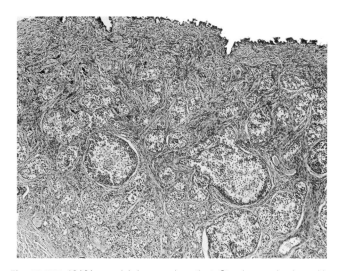

Fig. 12.155 46,XX gonadal dysgenesis patient. Streak gonad enlarged by several nodules of variable size corresponding to a gonadoblastoma.

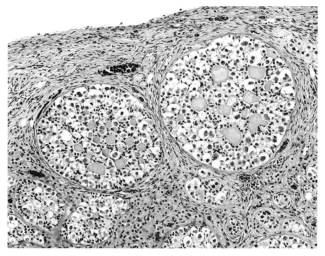

Fig. 12.156 Frasier syndrome in a 16-year-old patient. The two streak gonads contain gonadoblastoma. The nodules consist of Sertoli/granulosa cells and gonocytes. In the interstitium there are numerous Leydig cells.

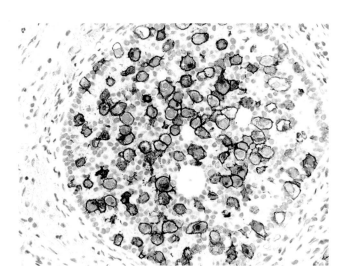

Fig. 12.157 Frasier syndrome. The cell surface and golgi zone of the atypical gonadoblastoma germ cells are immunoreactive for KIT.

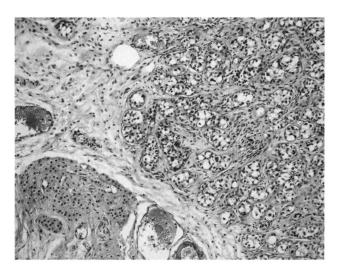

Fig. 12.158 Streak gonad with a dissecting gonadoblastoma. The lesion is characterized by the presence of solid epithelial cords and small nests in which, two cell types, Sertoli/granulosa cells and gonocytes, are identified. There is a nodule of Leydig cells.

a high risk for germ cell tumor, including gonadoblastoma, dysgerminoma, teratoma, and choriocarcinoma.[1358–1364] The presence of calcifications, regardless of whether associated with gonadoblastoma, is a frequent finding. No relationship between *SRY* status and gonadoblastoma has been found. This risk is approximately 5% in the first decade of life and 25% to 30% overall, and thus prophylactic gonadectomy is recommended.[1287,1365–1367] A few patients have had successful pregnancy and delivery of a healthy infant after in vitro fertilization using donor oocytes and embryo transfer.[1368]

Mixed Gonadal Dysgenesis

Mixed gonadal dysgenesis, also known as asymmetric gonadal differentiation or Sohval syndrome, is characterized by streak gonad with or without UGT, streak testis on one side and contralateral testis (often cryptorchid), or streak testis on both sides.[1369,1370] Classically, it is included in the categories of gonadal dysgenesis and male pseudohermaphroditism with müllerian remnants, attributed to AMH gene mutations or target organ insensitivity.[77]

AMH, also known as müllerian duct inhibiting factor or MIS, is a dimeric protein that belongs to the TGFB family and consists of two identical subunits of 72 kDa each, joined by disulfide bridges. The hormone is synthesized by the Sertoli cell. Its type II receptor is a serine/threonine kinase homologous to the receptors of other members of the same superfamily.[1371] The AMH gene is located on the short arm of chromosome 19.[72] The best-known AMH functions occur in fetal life and include müllerian duct inhibition and tunica albuginea collagenization. Both actions are ipsilateral to the testis that produces the hormone. Patients with this type of undermasculinization, in addition to the AMH defect, may also present with androgenic deficiency.

This syndrome accounts for approximately 15% of DSDs. A few patients are raised as boys, although their external genitalia are usually ambiguous as a result of fetal virilization. The penis is clitoriform, and the urethra opens in the perineum (Fig. 12.159). Most have cryptorchid testes and are raised as girls, becoming virilized at puberty. The diagnosis is not always made in infancy, and diagnosis as late as 66 years of age has been reported.[1372] In adult patients, spermatogenesis is absent or deficient, and infertility is a common symptom.[1373] Leydig cells show variable development and produce sufficient androgens to ensure pubertal virilization and lengthening of the phallus.[1374]

The etiology is heterogeneous: one-third of patients have turnerian features, in accordance with the presence of the 45,X0/46,XY karyotype in more than 50% of patients.[1375–1377] Other observed karyotypes are 46,XY (13.6%) and 45,X0/47,XYY, 45,X0/46,XX/46,XY, 45,X0/46,XYq-, 45,X0/46,XYp-, 45,X0/46,X add (Y) (p11.3), 45X/46,Xr(Y), and 45,X0/46,X dic (Yp), and "inverted" Y chromosome.[1378–1381] Approximately 81% of patients have one Y chromosome.[1382,1383] Mutation in the SRY gene has not been found.[1384]

If the gonads are intraabdominal, the labioscrotal folds may appear as either normal labia or empty scrotal sacs (Fig. 12.159). In the former, the syndrome cannot be recognized in the newborn unless a peniform clitoris is present. If the gonad is descended, it is usually testis accompanied by hernia. Müllerian derivatives such as fallopian tubes are usually associated with streak gonad (95% of cases), but may also be associated with testicular tissue (74%). Ipsilateral to the testis are one epididymis and vas deferens. On the

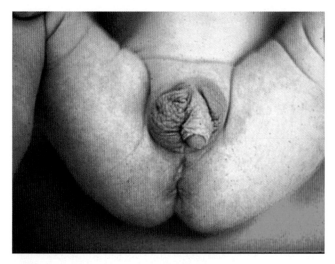

Fig. 12.159 Mixed gonadal dysgenesis in a 3-year-old child with ambiguous external genitalia, hypoplastic uterus, dysgenetic testis on the right side, and streak gonad on the left side.

contralateral side, no gonad or a streak gonad and a fallopian tube are present. Hypoplastic uterus and poorly developed vagina are frequent findings.

The gonads have three different patterns: testicular dysgenesis (Fig. 12.160), streak gonads, and streak testis. The testes in mixed gonadal dysgenesis are incapable of müllerian duct inhibition and allow complete differentiation of wolffian derivatives, virilization of external genitalia, and in most cases, testicular descent. Patients with mixed testicular dysgenesis do not produce AMH or produce it in scant amounts. Nevertheless, some cases of dysgenetic testis with normal AMH levels and normal regression of müllerian ducts have been reported.[1385] Differentiation of isolated ovocyte contained in streak testis and ovotestis remains controversial.[1386,1387]

Tumors arise in these gonads in 15% to 25% of cases, with increase in relation to age with a marked increase after puberty.[1388–1392] The most frequent tumor is gonadoblastoma, although all germ cell tumor types (except for spermatocyte seminoma) have been reported, including juvenile granulosa cell tumor.[1393,1394] Removal of all streak gonads is recommended, as well as intraabdominal testes, except for testes that may be moved into the scrotum and are not associated with ipsilateral müllerian derivatives. Scrotal testes should be retained.

Dysgenetic Male Pseudohermaphroditism

Dysgenetic male pseudohermaphroditism is a DSD characterized by bilateral dysgenetic testes or streak testis, persistent müllerian structures, cryptorchidism, and incomplete virilization. This syndrome is considered a variant of mixed gonadal dysgenesis (Fig. 12.161).[1395,1396] The karyotype may be 46,XY or 45,X0/46,XY, and turnerian stigmata may be present. The uterus and fallopian tubes are present, and both are usually hypoplastic.[1397] The testes show lesions characteristic of dysgenetic testis, decreased tubular diameter, TFI, and increased number of Sertoli cells during infancy (Figs. 12.162 through 12.164).[1397] In adults, spermatogenesis is reduced in some tubules and is incomplete, usually reaching maturation up to spermatocyte I. The remaining seminiferous tubules contain only Sertoli cells that are frequently immature. Sertoli cell number varies from one tubule to another, from markedly decreased to hyperplastic. Tubules with low number of Sertoli cells show higher maturation (Fig. 12.165). Tubules with immature Sertoli cells show an absence of immunoexpression of AR. Diffuse

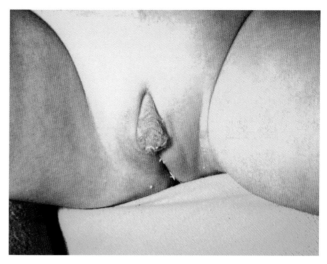
Fig. 12.161 Dysgenetic male pseudohermaphrodite with bilateral dysgenetic testis.

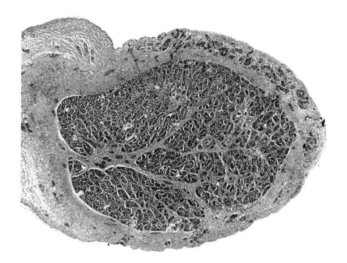
Fig. 12.162 Dysgenetic testis. The gonad has a central portion showing a testicular pattern and a peripheral band consisting of poorly collagenized connective tissue that contains seminiferous tubules that reach the gonadal surface.

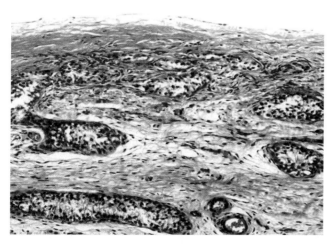
Fig. 12.160 Dysgenetic testis. Several irregularly shaped seminiferous tubules are observed within a thin, poorly collagenized tunica albuginea.

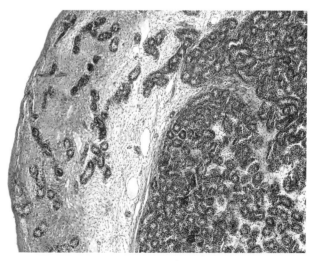
Fig. 12.163 Dysgenetic testis. The albuginea is scored by seminiferous tubules and epithelial cords in all directions.

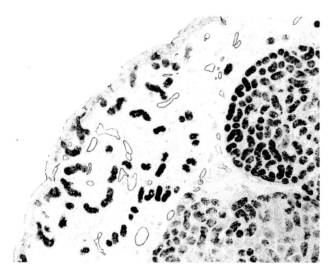

Fig. 12.164 Dysgenetic male pseudohermaphroditism. Strong positive immunostaining for D2–40 in seminiferous tubules, located both in the peripheral loose stroma and in the central part, as an expression of tubular immaturity.

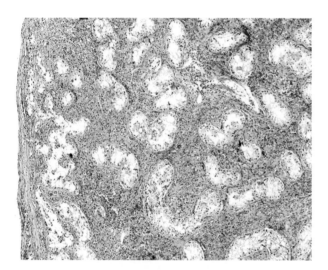

Fig. 12.165 Dysgenetic male pseudohermaphroditism in an adult patient showing pubertal maturation in Sertoli-only seminiferous tubules with irregular contours and diffuse Leydig cell hyperplasia.

or nodular Leydig cell hyperplasia is present. Leydig cells show nuclear pyknosis, grooves in the nuclear membrane, and empty nuclei. The incidence rate of germ cell tumors is high: 46% of 40-year-old patients.[1398] Approximately 25% of patients experience development of gonadoblastoma and 10% experience GCNIS.[1399]

Persistent Müllerian Duct Syndrome

PMDS has many names, including male with uterus, tubular hermaphroditism, inner male pseudohermaphroditism, persistent oviduct syndrome, and hernia uteri inguinalis.[1400] It is a rare form of gonadal dysgenesis characterized by the presence of müllerian derivative structures (fallopian tube, uterus, and upper part of the vagina) in an otherwise genetically and phenotypically normal male. The vagina opens into the posterior urethra in the verumontanum. It is the most characteristic form of isolated AMH deficiency, and more than 200 cases have been reported. Androgen-

dependent structures (penis, scrotum, vas deferens, epididymis, prostate, and seminal vesicles) are well developed. Hormonal assays reveal that testosterone and response to hCG stimulation are normal. Plasma AMH levels vary according to the molecular basis of the syndrome. Measurement of this hormone in prepubertal patients is useful for diagnosis.[1401] Exceptional cases of hernia uteri inguinalis occur in patients whose phenotype is that of normal female, and the gonads are normal ovaries.[1402] PMDS is sporadic or familial, with autosomal recessive or X-linked inheritance.[1403,1404] The incidence is estimated at 0 to 1 per 100,000 live births.[1405]

Although the external genitalia are male, one (25% of cases) or both testes (75% of cases) are cryptorchid. The syndrome usually also includes inguinal hernia contralateral to the undescended testis, with uterus and fallopian tubes within the hernia sac.[1406] Presenting complaints are inguinal hernia, cryptorchidism, infertility, or testicular tumor.[1396,1407–1410] The anatomy of the syndrome is varied and complex.[163]

Based on the location of the testicles and müllerian duct derivatives, PMDSs have been classified into three types. Type 1, the "male form," is most frequent (60% to 80%) and includes those patients with at least one testis present in the hernia sac. The contralateral testis is lodged in a hernia sac or scrotum, which also contains both a uterus and a fallopian tube (hernia uteri inguinalis (Figs. 12.166 through 12.168).[1400,1411–1413]

Type 2, "male with transverse testicular ectopy," accounts for 20% to 30% of cases of PMDSs, presenting with both testes in the same scrotal pouch, within a hernia sac that also contains a fallopian tube and uterus.[147,782,1414–1419]

Type 3, the "female form," is characterized by the presence of intraabdominal testes located in the anatomical site of the ovaries. Each is attached to its vas deferens and is associated with a uterine tube connecting with a uterus in the normal female pelvic position. Patients other than these with bilateral cryptorchidism do not usually present with inguinal hernias. They represent between 10% and 20% of cases.[1406]

The molecular basis of PMDSs is heterogeneous and recognized in almost 85% of cases. Most "males forms" (45% of cases) are due to defect in AMH synthesis caused by mutation in the AMH gene.[1420] The "female form" is due to resistance of target organs

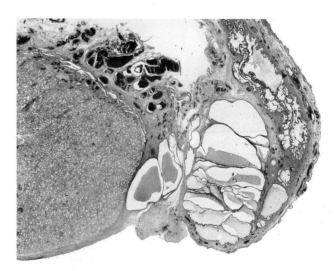

Fig. 12.166 Persistent müllerian duct syndrome. Fimbria portion of the uterine tube with follicular hydrosalpinx image fused to the lower pole of the testis.

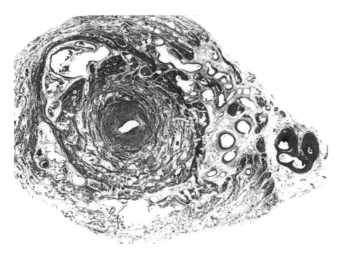

Fig. 12.167 Persistent müllerian duct syndrome. Cross-sectioned hypoplastic uterus. In its tunica adventitia and parallel to it, a folded vas deferens is seen.

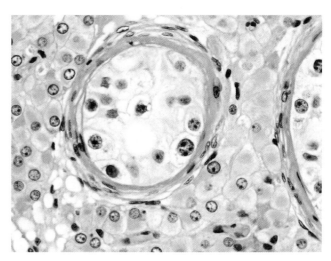

Fig. 12.169 Persistent müllerian duct syndrome. Seminiferous tubules containing germ cell neoplasia in situ (GCNIS) cells that stand out by large nuclei with several large nucleoli. Leydig cell hyperplasia is shown in the interstitium.

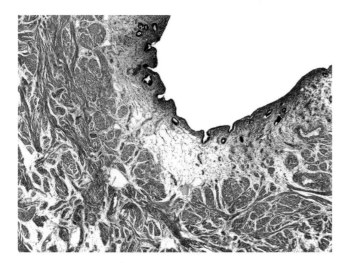

Fig. 12.168 Persistent müllerian duct syndrome. Uterus with atrophic endometrium and hypoplastic myometrium within a hernia sac.

to this hormone caused by mutations in the receptor II for this hormone (40% of cases).[1371,1420,1421] Other cases arise from failure in the action of AMH immediately before the eighth week of gestation (16% of cases).

Variation in the site of the testes results from absence of AMH, in which patients undergo normal regression of the cranial suspensory ligament (which is under androgen control) and feminization of the gubernaculum (elongate and thin gubernaculum). These two features permit great mobility of the testis.[163,1421a,1421b] Some patients present with strong connections between the müllerian structures and both the testis and the spermatic cord, thus hindering normal testicular descent and even causing ectopy.

In childhood the testes have low TFI and decreased tubular diameter. In adults the tunica albuginea is variably thickened, contains connective tissue resembling ovarian stroma, and may contain tubular structures, alterations typical of dysgenetic testes. The seminiferous tubules are usually atrophic and hyalinized. Tubules with reduced spermatogenesis or patterns suggesting MAT (seminiferous tubules with spermatogenesis intermingled with Sertoli cell–only tubules) have also been reported.[1422] The Leydig cells appear hyperplastic. Azoospermia or oligozoospermia are common, and

paternity is exceptional.[1423] These patients have a higher risk for testicular tumor (18%) than that associated with simple cryptorchidism (Fig. 12.169). All types of germ cell tumors have been observed.[1419,1424–1427] These tumors usually develop in the undescended testis, and in some cases tumors are bilateral.[225,1428–1430] Other tumors observed in the syndrome are colonic adenocarcinoma and medullary carcinoma of the thyroid gland.[1371]

Orchidectomy should not be performed during infancy because these patients have male phenotype and the virilizing ability of testes should be preserved, but it is important that the testes occupy a scrotal location. The fallopian tube and rudimentary uterus should be maintained because these structures rarely produce symptoms, and their removal may injure the vas deferens.[72,1431] Despite orchiopexy, as is the case in simple cryptorchidism, germ cell tumors may occur in later life.[1428,1432,1433] Orchidectomy is performed only in testes that cannot be mobilized to a palpable location. Another potential complication is testicular torsion secondary to testicular hypermotility.[1412]

Other Forms of Gonadal Dysgenesis

Of the dysmorphic syndromes associated with incomplete virilization of external genitalia, the best-known are Denys–Drash, WAGR (Wilms tumor, aniridia, genital anomalies, and mental retardation), and camptomelic dysplasia.

In *Denys–Drash syndrome*, undermasculinization is associated with nephroblastoma and renal insufficiency.[1434,1435,1436] The DSD is usually mixed gonadal dysgenesis, dysgenetic male pseudohermaphroditism, 46,XY pure gonadal dysgenesis, or ovotesticular DSD.[1437–1441] The most common nephropathy is diffuse mesangial sclerosis.[1442,1443] Although the most common gonadal types are streak gonads and dysgenetic testes, at least three cases with normal testes have been reported, two in patients with müllerian structures.[1444–1447] Most have mutations in the *WT1* gene, which is expressed in the genital ridge in the sixth week of gestation.[1448] Mutations in this gene may give rise to streak gonads or dysgenetic testes; if there is a delay in testicular determination, normal testes form.[1449] Testes in Denys–Drash syndrome produce testosterone and AMH, but this production is delayed, and hormonal actions are not ineffective.

The prevalence rate for *WAGR syndrome* is estimated at between 1% and 2% of patients with Wilms tumor. The syndrome is related to the syndromes of Denys–Drash and Frasier (a variety of 46,XY gonadal dysgenesis).[1335,1450,1451] All share mutations in the *WT1* gene located on chromosome 11 (11p13).[1452,1453]

WT1 product is a transcription factor expressed in different tissues which participates in embryogenesis and cell differentiation such as glomeruli precursor cells in fetal kidney, stromal cells of spleen and gonads, and mesothelial cell precursors of pleura, pericardium, and peritoneum. Mutations lead to the production of an anomalous protein that causes alterations in renal function, gonadal anomalies, and loss of tumor suppressor function. Six variants of alleles have been described: isolated Wilms tumor, mesothelioma, isolated diffuse mesangial sclerosis, Denys–Drash syndrome, Frasier syndrome, and WAGR syndrome. Frasier syndrome is caused by mutations in the donor zone of the intron 9 link, with subsequent loss of the +KTS isoform (imbalance in KTS isoforms), whereas large deletions or loss of genetic material that comprises the *WT1* gene and other contiguous genes (PAX6 or AN) will lead to the WAGR syndrome.[1454–1456] The most frequent genitourinary anomalies are cryptorchidism (60%) and ambiguous external genitalia.

Camptomelic dysplasia is an autosomal dominant syndrome with multiple osseous malformations, including bowing of long bones, especially the femora and tibiae; winging of the scapulae; the presence of fewer ribs than normal; narrow iliac wings; and clubbed feet.[1457,1458] Patients have the 46,XY karyotype and external genitalia that are ambiguous or female.[1459] Gonadal histology varies from testes to dysgenetic ovaries with primary follicles, streak testes, and even ovotestes.[1460–1464] Gonadal pathology may be present even in the absence of skeletal dysplasia.[1465] The incidence of gonadoblastoma is low.[1465a,1466] Dysgerminoma may occur in the gonad contralateral to the streak gonad.[1466] The syndrome is caused in 75% of cases by mutations in SOX9, located in 17q24.3–25.1; this gene has pleiotropic effects on the skeletal and genital systems.[1467–1470] Death usually occurs in the neonatal period from respiratory insufficiency. Only 5% to 10% survive.

Ovotesticular Disorder (True Hermaphroditism)

Ovotesticular disorder of sexual development is an abnormality of gonadal differentiation characterized by the presence in the same individual of both testicular and ovarian tissue. This disorder affects less than 10% of the population with DSDs, with an incidence of 1 in 100,000 live births.[1471–1474] This rare condition is usually difficult to diagnose because these patients do not show characteristic phenotype. As a result, only 25% of male hermaphrodites are identified before age 20 years.[1475] The age spectrum at the time of diagnosis varies from newborns to 60-year-old patients.[1476] Failure to recognize this disorder may lead to repeated surgical intervention for hernia or hypospadias repair or orchidopexy.[1477]

The most frequent karyotype is 46,XX (60%), followed by several mosaicisms (33%) that, in decreasing order of frequency, are 46,XX/46,XY, 46,XY/47,XXY, 45,X0/46,XY, 46,XX/47,XXY. The 46,XY karyotype is the least common (7%). Isolated cases with the following karyotypes have been reported: 47,XYY/46,XY/45,X0 and 46, XderY/45,X0 with rearranged Y chromosome.[1478,1479] The incidence of some karyotypes varies around the world. Mosaicism is found in 41% of European cases, but in only 21% of North American cases. Conversely, most African true hermaphrodites (97%) have 46,XX karyotype. The karyotype

46,XY is rare and its frequency is similar in Europe, Asia, and North America.[1480,1481]

Most cases are sporadic, and families with several affected members also have 46,XX males without ovotesticular disorder. This finding suggests that both genetic anomalies are alternative forms of a single genetic defect, which probably consists of an autosomal dominant mutation with incomplete penetrance or an X-chromosome–linked mutation.[1482–1486]

Pathogenetic theories proposed to explain true hermaphroditism begin with the understanding that, if patients have testes, TDF (produced by the *SRY* gene) is present. The following mechanisms are easy to explain when the karyotype is 46,XY, mosaicism 46,XX/45,XY, or chimera 46,XY. However, the presence of testicular parenchyma in the karyotype 46,XX (the most common) may result from: (1) hidden mosaicism including a line with the Y chromosome; (2) translocation of paternal Y chromosomal material that includes the *SRY* gene to the X chromosome; (3) autosomal mutation with variable penetrance; and (4) X-chromosome–linked mutations that either are coupled with a rare X-chromosome inactivation or permit testicular differentiation in the absence of *SRY*, or mutations in genes such as *SOX9* and *FGF9* that regulate the action of *SRY*, NR5A1, a transcriptional regulator of genes involved in adrenal and gonadal development, RSPO1, partial deletion of DMRT1, and SOX3 duplication.[1487–1494] Molecular studies have shown that only a few 46,XX true hermaphrodites have Y-DNA chromosome sequences, in contrast with the so-called XX males, who have Y-chromosome material including TDF in 80% of cases.[1483,1495,1496] Some 46,XX true hermaphrodites who are *SRY⁻* in lymphocyte studies show positive reactions to *SRY* in DNA obtained from the testicular parenchyma of the ovotestis.[1497–1499]

The phenotype of true hermaphrodites varies from normal male to female. Hermaphrodites with male phenotype do not exceed 10% of the total.[1482,1500] The phenotype is related to the presence of the *SRY* gene. In XX patients the phenotype could depend on two features: the length of Y translocated material (the higher the length of Yp fragment, the more complete is the masculinization) or the X chromosome where the SRY gene is translocated. If the translocation involves the active X chromosome, phenotype will be XX male (with masculinized external genitalia), whereas if the translocation involves the inactive X chromosome, the phenotype will be ambiguous genitalia. Most patients raised as boys display symptoms for the first time at puberty because of breast development (95% of hermaphrodites have some degree of gynecomastia), periodic hematuria (if they have a uterus ending in the urinary tract), or cryptorchidism.[1501–1503] 46,XX male without SRY and complete male phenotype with absence of female internal genitalia and presence of a prostate has been reported.[1504] Hermaphrodites raised as girls initially present with irregular menstruation or clitoromegaly and, rarely, cyclic pain in a descended or undescended gonad.[1505] True hermaphroditism should be suspected in all children with ambiguous sex characteristics (Fig. 12.170).[1506]

The gonads of these patients are ovotestes (44%), ovaries (33%), or testes (22%), with all possible combinations.[1507] True hermaphroditism may be: (1) unilateral, if there are both testicular and ovarian tissues (forming one ovotestis or two separate gonads) on one side and a testis or an ovary on the other side (50%)[1475,1508]; if there is no gonadal tissue on the latter side, unilateral hermaphroditism is incomplete; (2) bilateral, if testicular and ovarian tissues are present on both sides (20%); or (3) alternate, if there is a testis on one side and an ovary on the other side. Other rare presentations include patients with ovotestis and

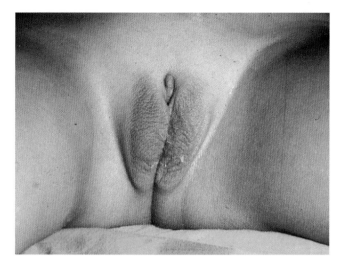

Fig. 12.170 Patient with ovotesticular disorder showing external genitalia that display transverse folds and a slightly hypertrophic clitoris.

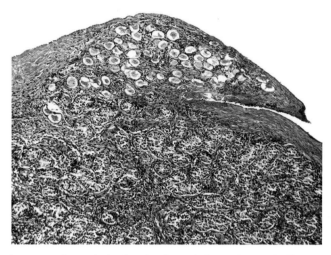

Fig. 12.172 Ovotesticular disorder. Ovotestis from a 2-year-old. The ovarian and testicular tissues are sharply demarcated.

contralateral streak gonad and those with crossed ectopy consisting of a left-sided ovotestis that is displaced to the right scrotum.[1509,1510] The degree of gonadal descent mirrors the amount of testicular tissue present. The gonadal nature may be suspected during physical examination. High testosterone levels suggest the presence of Leydig cells, and therefore the presence of a testis. High levels of estradiol after human menopausal gonadotropin stimulation suggest the presence of an ovary.[1511]

Ovotestis is the most frequent gonadal type in true hermaphroditism. It is more common on the right side and is in the abdomen (50% of cases), labioscrotal folds, inguinal canal, or external inguinal ring. Only 5% of patients with bilateral ovotestis show complete gonadal descent.[1512,1513] The ovotestis has a bilobate or ovoid shape (Fig. 12.171). In the bilobate ovotestis the testis and ovary are connected by a pedicle, whereas in the ovoid ovotestis the ovarian tissue forms a crescent capping the testicular parenchyma. The proportion of ovary to testis varies widely (Figs. 12.172 and 12.173). Clear-cut separation between ovarian and testicular tissue is evident in some cases, or ovocytes may be diffusely distributed between seminiferous tubules or even inside the tubules. The testicular zone next to the ovarian component

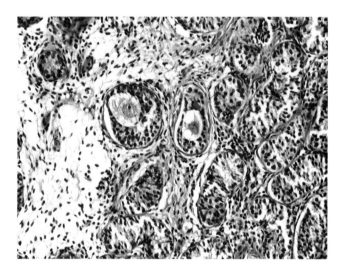

Fig. 12.173 Ovotestis. Oocyte inside a seminiferous tubule.

shows important changes in interstitium and tunica albuginea. Interstitial tissue has a stroma similar to ovarian stroma, instead of the characteristic loose connective tissue of normal testes. The tunica albuginea that covers the testicular zone shows poor differentiation, with persistence of tubular structures within it, or tubules that cross the tunica albuginea to reach the mesothelial surface. The mesothelial lining of this zone may be columnar, instead of flattened. These findings are like those observed in male pseudohermaphrodites with persistence of müllerian structures.[1479] In a large series of South African true hermaphrodites, three different types of ovotestes were observed. The ovotestes were separated by gross appearance into mixed type and bipolar (89% and 11%, respectively). The mixed-type ovotestes had an outer mantle consisting of ovarian tissue, which encapsulated an inner core of two distinct types of gonad. The first was an admixed ovotestis (constituting 44% of the mixed ovotestes); the central core consisted of gonadal stroma, with scattered foci of separate ovarian and testicular tissue. The second type was the compartmentalized ovotestis (constituting 56% of the mixed ovotestes); here, the outer mantle was thickened in the upper pole and encapsulated a large core of testicular tissue in the lower pole of the gonad. Histologically the bipolar ovotestis had a strictly polar distribution of ovarian

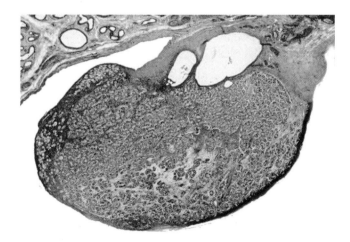

Fig. 12.171 Ovotesticular disorder. The ovotestis contains ovarian follicles arranged in a crescent. There is cystic transformation of the rete testis. The epididymis is hypoplastic.

and testicular tissue, which had an irregularly interdigitating junction between the two types of tissue. There is no correlation between the type of gonadal tissue and any clinical or genital features.[1514]

During adulthood, ovarian follicles mature and corpora lutea or corpora albicantia may be seen. The seminiferous tubules rarely develop complete spermatogenesis, often contain a higher number of dysgenetic Sertoli cells only, and frequently undergo hyalinization (Figs. 12.174 and 12.175). The interstitium usually contains Leydig cells (Fig. 12.176). Ovotestis is associated with the fallopian tube in 65% of cases (Fig. 12.177) and with the vas deferens in the

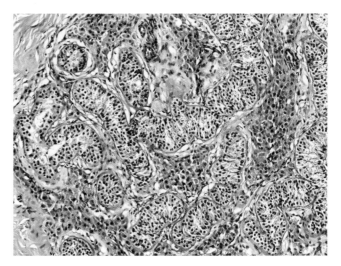

Fig. 12.176 Ovotestis. Irregularly anastomosed seminiferous tubules showing prepubertal features characterized by Sertoli cell pseudostratification and eosinophilic bodies in the apical cytoplasm of Sertoli cells. The interstitium shows Leydig cell pseudohyperplasia.

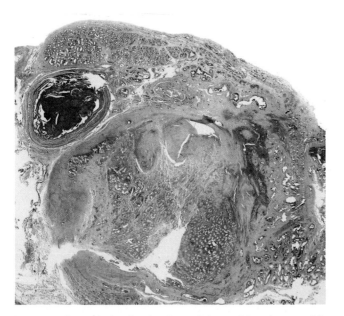

Fig. 12.174 Ovotesticular disorder. Ovotestis in an adult patient containing several corpora albicans in the periphery and seminiferous tubules in the center of the gonad. In the outer portion of the gonad, there is a cystic formation that corresponds to the uterine tube; in its periphery, epididymal ducts are observed.

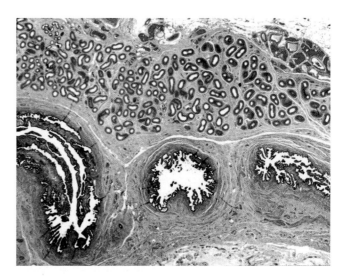

Fig. 12.177 Ovotesticular disorder. Epididymis and fallopian tube in an adult hermaphrodite raised as a female.

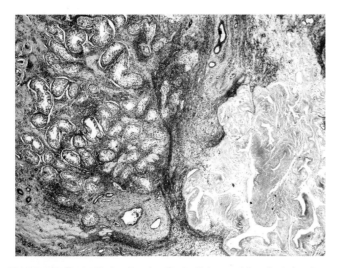

Fig. 12.175 Ovotesticular disorder. Ovotestis in an adult patient showing a clear delimitation between ovarian and testicular areas of the gonad that consist of one corpus albicans and seminiferous tubules with deficient spermatogenesis and hyalinization, respectively.

remainder. If the patient has ovotestis/ovary, a completely developed uterus is present. If the patient has bilateral ovotestis (13%), uterine agenesis is frequent.[1480]

The testis of patients with ovotesticular disorder is most often on the right side (60%) and is located anywhere from the abdomen to the scrotum. These testes have low TFI during childhood (Fig. 12.178). After puberty the seminiferous tubules remain small, often containing only dysgenetic Sertoli cells, similar to the tubules of cryptorchid testes. Isolated groups of microvacuolated Leydig cells are also observed. Incomplete spermatogenesis has been reported, but complete spermatogenesis is exceptional.

The ovary of hermaphrodites is most frequently on the left side (63%) and usually is hypoplastic with few primordial follicles (Fig. 12.179). However, in occasional patients the ovary is histologically and functionally normal.

More than two dozen pregnancies in patients with ovotesticular disorder have been reported.[1515–1523] This contrasts with the

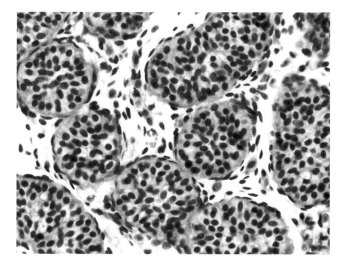

Fig. 12.178 Infantile testis contralateral to ovotestis showing apparent Sertoli cells hyperplasia, immature Sertoli cells, and isolated spermatogonia.

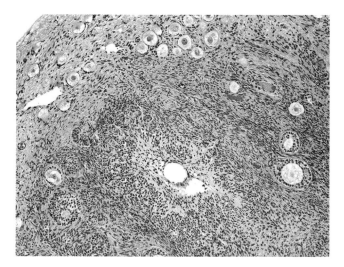

Fig. 12.179 Infantile ovary contralateral to ovotestis showing numerous primordial and primary follicles and one atretic follicle.

exceptional cases of paternity. The origin of oocytes could be an ovotestis or an ovary.[1524,1525] Most patients develop hypergonadotropic hypogonadism.

The treatment of ovotesticular DSD is complex because it involves the patient's relatives and several medical specialties, given that genetic sex, gonadal sex, social gender, and psychological gender must be considered.[1526] Management of patients with ovotesticular disorder depends on the patient's age at the time of diagnosis, the nature and location of the gonads, and the developmental stage of the external genitalia.[1527] Genetic sex determined by karyotype and Y-chromosome sequence detection are not considered useful criteria.[1528] Although bilateral castration may be justified to avoid the risk for neoplasia, gonadal preservation may be desirable until adulthood. In this case, if the patient is raised as a girl, puberty will occur spontaneously, and there is a small chance of fertility.[1527] However, the high risk for malignancy (estimated at 4.6% for those with 46,XX karyotype and 10% when the karyotype is 46,XY or mosaicism 46,XX/XY) should be taken

into account.[1283,1481] Many of these patients experience development of a gonadal tumor after long-term follow-up. The most frequent tumors are gonadoblastoma, dysgerminoma/seminoma, choriocarcinoma, and yolk sac tumor. Other reported tumors are mature teratoma, carcinoid, and granulosa cell tumor.[1507,1529–1534] Tumors that develop in these gonads, like tumors in cryptorchid testes, may reach a great size before their diagnosis. The risk for cancer may be reduced if some precautions are taken, including removal of the testis if it has not descended and surveillance of the residual gonad with periodic ultrasound studies, especially in patients with chromosomal mosaicisms.

Undermasculinization (Male Pseudohermaphroditism)

Normal male development requires adequate differentiation of the testes in the fetal period, synthesis and secretion of testicular hormones, and proper response of target organs. AMH produced by Sertoli cells inhibits development of müllerian derivatives that would otherwise form the uterus and fallopian tubes. Testosterone produced by Leydig cells stimulates differentiation of wolffian ducts into male genital ducts. Conversion of testosterone into DHT by the enzyme 5α-reductase ensures development of male external genitalia. Alterations in these processes may cause varying degrees of undermasculinization.

Impaired Leydig Cell Activity

Impaired Leydig cell activity may be present in two different conditions: insufficient androgen synthesis caused by enzymatic defects and absence or hypoplasia of Leydig cells.

Androgen Synthesis Deficiencies

These autosomal recessive syndromes are characterized by an error in testosterone synthesis that results in incomplete or absent virilization.[1535,1536] Five enzymes are responsible for testosterone synthesis. The absence of or deficit in one of these enzymes decreases androgen production. Three (20,22-desmolase, 3β-HSD, and 17α-hydroxylase) are also involved in synthesis of adrenal androgens, and deficit results in congenital adrenal hyperplasia. Deficit or absence of either of the other two (17,20-desmolase and 17β-HSD) mainly impairs gonadal synthesis of testosterone and estrogens. Cholesterol is the source of synthesis of androgens, estrogens, and other steroid hormones through multiple steps. First, the steroidogenic acute regulatory (*STAR*) protein transfers cholesterol into mitochondria; STAR gene mutations cause congenital lipoid adrenal hyperplasia. Second, within mitochondria, the cholesterol side-chain cleavage enzyme P450scc transforms cholesterol into pregnenolone; a disorder of this enzyme is rare because it is highly lethal in embryonic life. Third, pregnenolone undergoes 17α-hydroxylation by microsomal P450c17; deficiency in 17α-hydroxylase causes female sexual infantilism and hypertension. Fourth, 17-OH-pregnenolone is converted into Dehydroepiandrosterone (DHEA) by 17,20-lyase activity of P450c17. The ratio of 17,20-lyase to 17α-hydroxylase activity of P450c17 determines the ratio of C21 to C19 steroids produced. The ratio is regulated by at least three factors, including the electron-donating protein P450 oxidoreductase (POR), cytochrome b5, and serine phosphorylation of P450c17. Mutations in POR are present in Antley-Bixler skeletal dysplasia syndrome, as well as in a variant of polycystic ovarian syndrome. Fig. 12.180 shows the enzymes involved in the previously mentioned steps. The enzyme 3β-HSD transforms

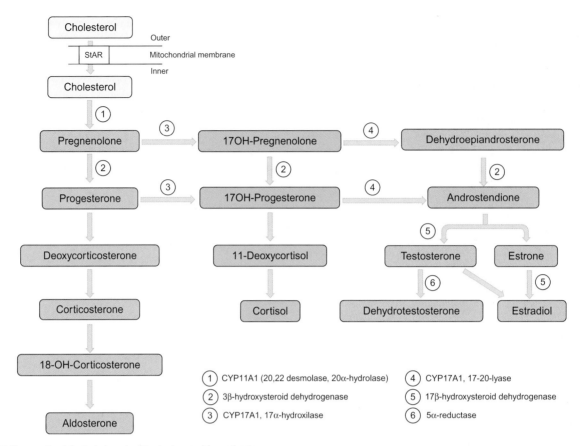

Fig. 12.180 Enzymatic defects in impaired testosterone biosynthesis.

DHEA to androstenedione, and the enzymatic complex called aromatase transforms androstenedione into estrone and testosterone into estradiol.

In some patients, cholesterol synthesis is also impaired, and congenital adrenal hyperplasia is superimposed on androgen deficiency. Deficient testosterone synthesis may result from abnormalities in the enzymes involved in pregnenolone formation (congenital lipoid adrenal hyperplasia), including 3β-HSD, 17α-hydroxylase, 17,20-desmolase, and 17β-HSD (Fig. 12.180).

Congenital Lipoid Adrenal Hyperplasia. Congenital lipoid adrenal hyperplasia is the most severe form of congenital adrenal hyperplasia.[1537,1538] The disorder is characterized by a deficit in steroid hormone synthesis in the adrenal cortex and gonads that produces 46,XY genetic males with female phenotype and severe salt-loss syndrome. Conversion of cholesterol to pregnenolone requires the enzymes 20α-hydroxylase, 20,22-desmolase, and 22α-hydroxylase. Failure of any of these leads to deficits in cortisol, aldosterone, and testosterone.[1539]

The enzymatic defect is usually caused by a deficit in the StAR protein; in other cases the deficit is in P450ssc.[1540] The mitochondrial StAR protein promotes cholesterol transfer from the outer to the inner mitochondrial membrane, where cholesterol serves as a substrate for P450scc and initiates steroidogenesis.[1541–1543] Any of 48 possible mutations in the STAR gene result in congenital lipoid adrenal hyperplasia.[1544–1547] As a result, cholesterol is not converted to pregnenolone, which is required for the synthesis of mineralocorticoids, glucocorticoids, and sex hormones.

The disorder is rare in most countries, but it is common in Japan and Korea.[1548,1549] The mutation p.Q258X accounts for 70% of affected alleles in Japan and 95% of the alleles reported to date in Korea. The disorder is also observed in Palestinian Arabs in bearers of different mutations, in Arabs from the Eastern Province of Saudi Arabia and nearby Qatar, all of whom carry the mutation p.R182H, and in the Swiss by the mutation p.L260P. Patients usually present with salt-losing crisis in the first 2 months of life.[1550,1551] In most cases, males have female external genitalia, reflecting absence of testosterone synthesis between weeks 6 and 12 of gestation. A few patients have ambiguous external genitalia and a blind-sac vagina, hypoplastic wolffian derivatives, absence of müllerian structures, and cryptorchidism.[1552] The adrenals usually appear enlarged and contain lipid accumulations that eventually diminish with age, and the adrenals shrink.[1553,1554]

Histologic studies of the testes of these patients are limited in number and lack consistency. In childhood, seminiferous tubules usually show Sertoli and germ cells or only Sertoli cells.[1539,1555] In the testes, lipid accumulations may be absent or present in Leydig cells (Fig. 12.181).[1537,1553,1556–1561] The testes of pubertal patients are usually normal for age, or lipid accumulation in Sertoli cells is noted.[1559,1560,1562] The epididymis and vas deferens are normally developed. GCNIS was reported in one case.[1563] Given that these patients are infertile, early gonadectomy may avoid development of testicular tumor.[1564]

Most patients die of adrenal insufficiency. Survivors have female phenotype and require administration of glucocorticoids, mineralocorticoids, and gonadal steroids.[1539,1562] Prenatal diagnosis may be made by several methods.[1565]

Nonclassic congenital lipoid adrenal hyperplasia is a new term to designate a disorder of the StAR protein that is caused by

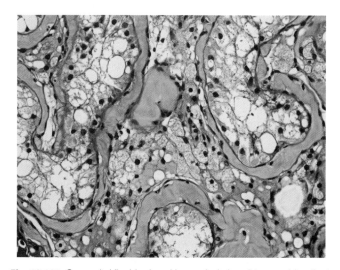

Fig. 12.181 Congenital lipoid adrenal hyperplasia in a 21-year-old patient. Seminiferous tubules show thickening of the basement membrane and contain only Sertoli cells with some cytoplasmic vacuoles. Leydig cells show large and microvacuolated cytoplasm.

mutations that retain 10% to 25% of function.[1566] This disorder is characterized by the onset of glucocorticoid deficiency after 2 years of age, as well as mild defects in mineralocorticoids and sex steroid synthesis. Rare mutations in P450scc result in both classic and nonclassic hormonal syndromes that are indistinguishable from congenital lipoid adrenal hyperplasia, but with small adrenals.[1567]

3β-Hydroxysteroid Dehydrogenase Deficiency. 3β-Hydroxysteroid dehydrogenase deficiency, first reported in 1961, is also known as type VI adrenal hyperplasia.[1568] Patients have two main problems: salt-loss syndrome produced by reduced aldosterone secretion and incomplete virilization.[1568] At puberty, virilization increases and gynecomastia develops.[1569,1570]

The enzyme 3β-HSD catalyzes the conversion of 5-3β-hydroxysteroids such as pregnenolone, 17-hydroxypregnenolone, and DHEA into 4-3β-ketosteroids progesterone, 17-hydroxyprogesterone, and androstenedione, respectively.[1571] There are two 3β-HSD genes located on the p11-p13 region of chromosome 1. The type I gene is expressed in the placenta, kidney, and skin, whereas the type II gene is expressed only in the gonads and adrenal glands. Complete absence of the 3β-HSD gene is lethal; therefore most reported cases have only partial 3β-HSD deficits.[1536,1572-1575] These deficits account for approximately 10% of cases of congenital adrenal hyperplasia.

The classic form of salt-losing 3β-HSD deficit is diagnosed in the first months of life because of insufficient aldosterone synthesis and subsequent loss of salt. The other form of 3β-HSD deficit does not involve salt loss, and its diagnosis may be delayed until puberty. Both forms are caused by mutations in the type II 3β-HSD gene (*HSD3B2*).[1570]

Severe forms of 3β-HSD deficiency are associated with deficits in aldosterone, cortisol, and estradiol. Symptoms may vary widely because enzymatic activity in the adrenal gland is not the same as in the testis. Most patients show salt loss and adrenal insufficiency; they have incomplete masculinization and may develop premature puberty and gynecomastia.[1569,1576,1577] Patients with mild forms have normal genitalia and normal mineralocorticoid levels. Some patients have only hypospadias or micropenis.[1578,1579] The testes are smaller and softer than normal. The diagnosis is made by serum and urine determinations of elevated levels of 17α-hydroxy-5-pregnenolone, DHEA, DHEAS, and other 3β-hydroxy-5 steroids.[1580]

17α-Hydroxylase/17,20-Lyase Deficiency. This deficit, also known as type V congenital adrenal hyperplasia, was first described in a woman in 1966.[1581] The first reported male patient was a 24-year-old man with male pseudohermaphroditism, ambiguous external genitalia, absence of male secondary characteristics, and prominent breast development at puberty.[1582] Testicular biopsy performed at 16 years of age showed a delay in seminiferous tubule development with the presence of early spermatogenesis and Leydig cell hyperplasia.

Deficits in the enzymes 17α-hydroxylase and 17,20-lyase are caused by mutations of the *CYP17* gene that encodes cytochrome P450c17.[1583] The *CYP17* gene is located on chromosome 10q24-q25, and 50 different mutations have been described.[1584-1586] P450c17 catalyzes the 17α-hydroxylation of pregnenolone to 17-OH-pregnenolone and of progesterone to 17α-OH-progesterone. This enzyme also catalyzes 17,20-lyase activity, thus transforming 17-OH-pregnenolone to DHEA. The P450c17 microsomal enzyme is expressed in the reticularis and fasciculate zones of the adrenal glands, Leydig cells, and theca cells of the ovary. It has two distinct activities: (1) 17α-hydroxylase, which catalyzes the 17α-hydroxylation of C21 steroids necessary for the synthesis of cortisol; and (2) 17,20-lyase, which catalyzes cleavage of the C17–21 bond and converts C21 compounds to C19 steroids in the androgen-estrogen synthesis pathway.[1587]

The classic form of 17α-hydroxylase deficit is caused by severe deficiencies in CYP17; less severe defects give rise to the isolated 17,20-lyase deficit. 17α-Hydroxylase deficit impairs the synthesis of both cortisol and testosterone.[1588] Low cortisol levels stimulate ACTH secretion, thereby causing hypersecretion of aldosterone precursors and the development of hypokalemic hypertension.[1589] The deficit in testosterone secretion by fetal testes leads to male undervirilization. Patients are raised as girls. At puberty, patients may have amenorrhea, scant axillary and pubic hair, eunuchoid appearance, and gynecomastia.[1590,1591] Elevated levels of progesterone, pregnenolone, and corticosteroids are detected in plasma.

17,20-Desmolase Deficiency. 17,20-Desmolase deficiency was first described in three male siblings.[1592] The enzyme 17,20-desmolase cleaves the side chain of 17-hydroxypregnenolone and 17-hydroxyprogesterone to form DHEA and androstenedione, respectively. This enzyme is encoded by a gene that has been mapped on chromosome 10. Varying degrees of 17,20-desmolase deficiency are seen, resulting in varied development of external genitalia that ranges from female phenotype to virilization with microphallus, bifid scrotum, perineal hypospadias, and cryptorchidism, secondary to insufficient testosterone production during fetal life.[1593] In childhood the testes contain reduced numbers of spermatogonia (Figs. 12.182 and 12.183).[1592,1594] At puberty, complete masculinization without gynecomastia occurs. Patients have low levels of testosterone, androstenedione, DHEA, and estradiol, and high levels of pregnanetriolone (a metabolite of 17α-hydroxyprogesterone).[1594] In adulthood, some patients with 17,20-desmolase deficit may develop an additional deficiency of 17α-hydroxylase with hypertension.[1595,1596] The cause may be mutations in one of the genetic loci encoding P450c17, flavoprotein POR, or cytochrome b5.[1597]

17β-Hydroxysteroid Dehydrogenase Deficiency. This syndrome was first reported in 1970.[1598,1599] The highest incidence (1 in 100 to 1 in 150 males) may occur in the Arabian population

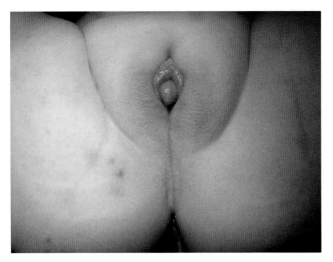

Fig. 12.182 Undermasculinization with androgen synthesis deficiency. The external genitalia are ambiguous.

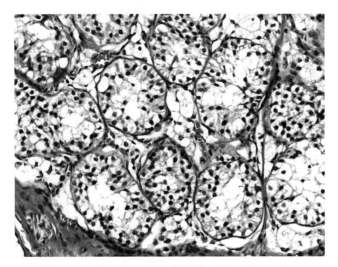

Fig. 12.183 Intense Leydig cell vacuolation in an infant with androgen synthesis deficiency.

of Israel (Gaza).[1600] The enzyme transforms androstenedione into testosterone and converts estrone into estradiol, with deficit caused by mutations in the *HSD17B3* gene located on 9q22.[1601–1604] The enzymatic defects are sex linked and have a familial occurrence. Most patients have female phenotype at birth and are raised as girls, but at puberty undergo virilization.[1605–1608] Androstenedione serum levels are increased, in contrast with low testosterone levels that do not rise after hCG stimulation. One or both testes may be cryptorchid or located in the labia majora. Normal spermatogenesis has never been observed. The most common testicular patterns are hypospermatogenesis, MAT, or Sertoli cell–only tubules, and Leydig cell hyperplasia is constant.[1609–1612] Germ cell injury was initially attributed to cryptorchidism, but is now thought to be due to a primary testicular disorder because even young patients lack germ cells.[1613]

Leydig Cell Hypoplasia

Leydig cell hypoplasia is also known as inherited defect in Leydig cell gonadotropin receptors, Leydig cell agenesis, Leydig cell

hypoplasia, absence of response to gonadotropins, abnormal Leydig cell differentiation, Leydig cell hypofunction, and Leydig cell hypogenesis.[1614–1621] This variant of undermasculinization DSD is defined by insufficient testosterone secretion; predominance of female external genitalia; absence of secondary sex characteristics (male or female) at puberty; absence of a uterus and fallopian tubes; and presence of an epididymis and vas deferens; 46,XY karyotype; low serum testosterone in spite of the increased gonadotropin levels; lack of response to hCG stimulation; absence of an enzymatic defect in testosterone synthesis; and small undescended testes that are gray and mucoid on sectioning.[1616,1617,1619,1621–1623] Age at diagnosis varies from 4 months to 35 years, although most cases are diagnosed at puberty. The syndrome is sporadic and familial.[1618,1624]

The best-known cause of Leydig cell hypoplasia is inactivating mutation of LHR in these cells.[1625–1627] Both LH and hCG have essential roles in male sexual differentiation. The action of both hormones is mediated by the LH/CG receptor (LHCGR), a member of the G protein–coupled receptor family that is expressed in Leydig cells, granulosa-lutein cells, and theca cells. The *LHCGR* gene is located on chromosome 2p21 and consists of 11 exons and 10 introns resulting in overall protein length of 674 amino acids.[1628,1629] In 50% of cases, the cause seems to be an inactivating mutation in *LHCGR,* although there are isolated cases of mutations only in certain exons such as 4, 6A, 7, and 8 or coexistence of two mutations in the same *LHCGR* gene locus.[1630–1632] In the remaining cases with clinical symptoms of Leydig cell hypoplasia, no mutations have been found, suggesting the possibility of defects in other genes or other unexplored regions of *LHCGR.*[1633,1634]

During fetal life, there is inadequate response to placental hCG initially and subsequently to pituitary LH.[1626,1627,1635] Patients with 46,XY with inactivating mutations of LHR show abnormal Leydig cell differentiation, resulting in reduced production of testosterone and, subsequently, DHT.[1625] Phenotypes vary widely according to the presence of complete or partial loss of receptor function, ranging from male undermasculinization with female external genitalia in type I Leydig cell hypoplasia (LCHT1) to male phenotype with micropenis, hypospadias, pubertal delay, and primary hypogonadism in type II Leydig cell hypoplasia (LCHT2). The different mutations detected may give rise to partial or complete loss of LHR function and explain the variability in phenotypes.[1636,1637]

In LCHT1 the testes contain small seminiferous tubules with Sertoli cells, spermatogonia, and thickened basement membranes. Leydig cells are rare, absent, or immature, in contrast with Leydig cell hyperplasia seen in other types of undermasculinization, such as those arising from defects in androgen synthesis or androgen action on peripheral tissues (e.g., 5α-reductase deficit).[1638–1641] Some patients with Leydig cell hypoplasia possess androgen-dependent structures, including epididymis and ductus deferens, although these structures are usually hypoplastic or atrophic. This finding suggests a certain amount of androgenesis during embryonal development or involvement of other factors in addition to androgens in wolffian duct differentiation.

Leydig cell hypoplasia results in low serum testosterone, lack of virilization, and lack of spermatogenesis. The absence of müllerian derivatives suggests normal function of Sertoli cells, which synthesize AMH. In LCTH2, adult testes show maturation arrest of spermatogenesis in young spermatids, as well as a few incompletely differentiated Leydig cells.[1623,1638,1642]

Impaired Androgen Metabolism in Peripheral Tissues

Androgens exert their function on differentiation and development of the normal male phenotype via a single receptor protein, the AR. AR is expressed in fetal tissues as early as 8 weeks of gestation, before the onset of androgenic action, and is activated in a ligand-dependent manner to coordinate expression of suitable responsive genes. In the human embryo, testes begin to secrete androgens by the ninth week of gestation. Testosterone reaches a peak between 11 and 18 weeks of gestation and is responsible for wolffian duct differentiation into the epididymis, ductus deferens, and seminal vesicles. Testosterone conversion into a more powerful androgen, DHT, by the 5α-reductase enzyme initiates prostate development from the urogenital sinus and masculinization of the primordial external genitalia into the penis and scrotum. Deficiencies in the peripheral actions of androgens result in complete and incomplete testicular feminization syndromes, as well as 5α-reductase deficiency syndrome.

Androgen Insensitivity Syndromes

Testosterone penetrates target tissues by passive diffusion. A small amount of this hormone is converted to DHT by the enzyme 5α-reductase. Both hormones have high binding affinity for AR located in the cytoplasm (cytosol receptors). AR complexes enter the nucleus and stimulate transcription of mRNAs involved in the synthesis of proteins responsible for peripheral androgen effects.

Resistance to androgen stimulation is the cause of several syndromes with phenotypes varying from female (complete testicular feminization) to normal male, with intermediate degrees of undermasculinization.[1643–1645] The karyotype is usually 46,XY, but 47, XXY and several mosaicisms have been observed.[1646]

These syndromes are caused by partial or complete lack of response by the target organs to androgen effects, because of the absence, diminution, or impairment of AR, abnormality of intracellular AR, or postreceptor anomaly.[254,1646a,1647–1649] The gene for AR is located on the X chromosome (Xq11-q12). It contains eight exons, and X-linked transmission occurs in two-thirds of cases. Molecular analysis of the gene for AR reveals that varied clinical presentations result from different mutations in this gene. More than 800 AR mutations have been reported in AIS.[1650–1656] The four main mutations are interruptions of AR open reading frame, mutations in the DNA-binding domain of AR, amino acid substitutions in the hormone-binding domain of AR, and amino acid substitutions causing absent ligand binding.[1657–1659] These syndromes affect 1 in 20,000 to 1 in 40,000 newborns, and transmission is recessive X-linked in two-thirds of cases.

The diverse phenotypes associated with androgen insensitivity may be classified as complete AIS (CAIS) or testicular feminization syndrome; partial AIS (PAIS) or partial testicular feminization syndrome, which includes the syndromes of Lubs, Gilbert-Dreyfus, Reifenstein, and Rosewater, as well as Kennedy disease; and mild AIS (MAIS), which includes infertile men with minimal androgen insensitivity. Classification of AIS similar to that of congenital adrenal hyperplasias has been proposed in which patients with a normal male phenotype comprise type 1 and those with female phenotype comprise types 6 and 7 according to the presence (type 6) or absence (type 7) of axillary and pubic hair (Table 12.19).[1650]

Complete Androgen Insensitivity Syndrome (Complete Testicular Feminization Syndrome). CAIS, formerly known as testicular feminization syndrome, first described in 1952, is characterized by female phenotype with testes.[1660] It accounts for 15% to 20% of all DSDs. Karyotype is usually 46,XY, although mosaicisms

and 47,XXY patients have been reported.[1646,1661–1664] Mutations in AR are present in 95% of patients. CAIS is rarely diagnosed during childhood. Exceptions include children with hernia (1% to 2% of female patients with inguinal hernia have CAIS), repair of which reveals testes, inguinal tumor, or family history of male undermasculinization.[1665–1670] Puberty is usually delayed, and stature is above the median. Primary amenorrhea is the principal presentation in adults.

The testes may be in the abdomen, inguinal canal, or labia majora. Seminiferous tubules with scant germ cells and hypertrophy and hyperplasia of Leydig cells may be seen on histologic examination of the testicular parenchyma.[1671] The incidence of abdominal testes is higher in patients with complete female phenotype and absence of pubic hair.[1672] During the first year of life, the testis may be normal histologically except for reduced tubular diameter and low TFI. Thereafter, decreased germ cell numbers become evident, and the few remaining spermatogonia are concentrated in clusters of seminiferous tubules.[1673] The interstitium contains numerous spindle cells arranged in bundles that recall ovarian stroma, and during the first year of life, there are Leydig cells with abundant eosinophilic or vacuolated cytoplasm (Figs. 12.184 and 12.185). At puberty, patients have female external genitalia, a short and blind-ended vagina, feminine breast development, and sparse pubic and axillary hair.[1643,1674] The testes show delay in seminiferous tubule maturation in relation to the interstitium. Seminiferous tubules retain an infantile morphology, whereas the interstitium has adult Leydig cells (Fig. 12.186). There is intense cytoplasmic immunoreactivity for AMH and diffuse nuclear staining of SOX9 in Sertoli cells, as well as focal weak cytoplasmic PGDS expression. Spermatogonia show focal weak nuclear PGDS

TABLE 12.19	Spectrum of Phenotypes in Androgen Insensitivity Syndromes

Androgen insensitivity syndromes and phenotype grade

Complete

Type 7: Complete androgen insensitivity syndrome without axillary or pubic hair.

Type 6: Complete androgen insensitivity syndrome with axillary or pubic hair.

Incomplete

Type 5: Lubs syndrome.
    Female phenotype, clitoromegaly, or minimal posterior labial fusion.

Type 4: Gilbert-Dreyfus syndrome.
    Ambiguous phenotype, small phallus, intermediate between penis and clitoris, urogenital sinus without perineal opening, labioscrotal folds with or without wrinkles and posterior fusion.

Type 3: Reifenstein syndrome.
    Predominant male phenotype, micropenis, perineal hypospadias, cryptorchidism, or bifid scrotum.

Type 2: Male with hypospadias.
    Male phenotype, mild defect in fetal virilization, isolated hypospadias.

Type 1: Rosewater syndrome.
    Normal male phenotype, gynecomastia, infertility.

Kennedy disease.
    Normal male phenotype, spinal and bulbar muscular atrophy, X-chromosome linked.

Infertile male syndrome.
    Normal male phenotype, infertility.

Modified from Quigley CA, De Bellis A, Marschke KB, et al. Androgen receptor defects: historical, clinical and molecular perspectives. Endocr Rev 1995;16: 271–321.

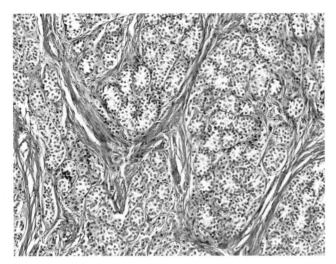

Fig. 12.184 Complete androgen insensitivity syndrome. Seminiferous tubules with prepubertal maturation separated by thick septa of hyalinized stroma.

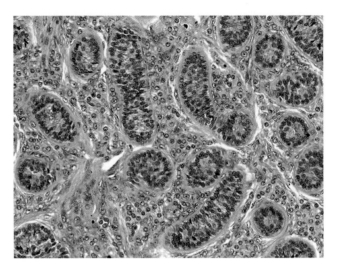

Fig. 12.186 Complete androgen insensitivity syndrome in an adult. Small seminiferous tubules with immature Sertoli cells surrounded by thick basement membranes and numerous Leydig cells.

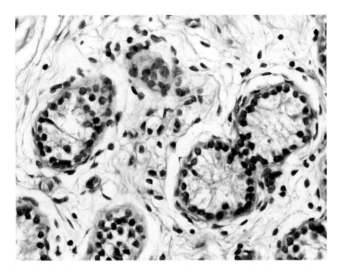

Fig. 12.185 Complete androgen insensitivity syndrome in a 5-year-old boy. Seminiferous tubules lack germ cells. The interstitium shows a group of Leydig cells with highly vacuolated cytoplasm.

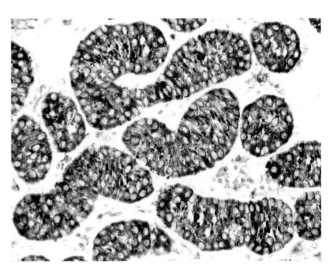

Fig. 12.187 Complete androgen insensitivity syndrome. Inhibin immunostaining showing intense expression in seminiferous tubules with prepubertal features. Note the inhibin-positive bodies in the apical pole of Sertoli cells.

expression. No AR immunoreactivity is observed.[1675] Hormonal studies show increased levels of testosterone, Sex Hormone Binding Globulin (SHBG), LH, β-estradiol (a by-product of peripheral conversion of testosterone), and AMH (which remains increased in spite of the presence of testosterone because normal AR signaling in Sertoli cells is a prerequisite for the repressive effect on AMH).[1676] FSH levels are normal or decreased.[1677] The SHBG androgen sensitivity test is a simple diagnostic tool for detection of AR malfunction.[1678]

In adults, both in complete and partial forms of androgen insensitivity, the testes vary from small to large, are tan brown, and have small seminiferous tubules without lumina and usually contain only Sertoli cells.[1679,1680] Most tubules contain Sertoli cells that show immunoexpression for inhibin, have inhibin positive bodies (Fig. 12.187), variable positivity for D2–40 and calretinin, and are negative for AR immunostaining. Leydig cells are sometimes arranged diffusely, and others surround groups of seminiferous tubules (Fig. 12.188). Focally, seminiferous tubules appear as epithelial cords two to three cells wide in cross section. In one-third of

patients, both Sertoli cells and spermatogonia are present.[1681] Ultrastructurally, Sertoli cells lack Charcot-Böttcher crystals and annulated lamellae; inter–Sertoli cell specialized junctions are not well developed, and in cryofracture studies the arrangement of membrane particles has an immature pattern.[1682,1683] Leydig cells are abundant and contain lipid inclusions, but few contain Reinke crystalloids. Frequently, spherical or ovoid eosinophilic inclusions larger than nuclei may be observed in the cytoplasm. Focally, Leydig cells show intense immunostaining for cytokeratin AE1/AE3. Ectopic Leydig cells are frequent. Often, areas in the testicular interstitium resemble ovarian stroma. Some patients, probably with a form of androgen sensitivity, have more complete tubular development and a certain degree of spermatogenesis.

In approximately two-thirds of patients with CAIS, the testes contain grossly visible prominent white nodules, referred to as Sertoli-Leydig hamartomas (Figs. 12.189 and 12.190). Histologically the nodules are well delimited from the parenchyma and consist of clusters of small seminiferous tubules with immature Sertoli cells, hyalinized lamina propria, numerous Leydig cells, and an

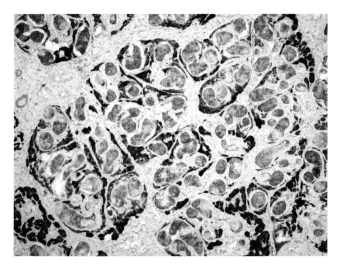

Fig. 12.188 Complete androgen insensitivity syndrome. Leydig cells, demonstrated with calretinin, are preferably distributed around groups of seminiferous tubules in contact with the ovarian-like stroma.

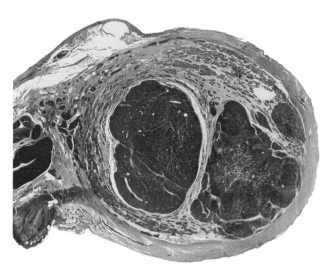

Fig. 12.190 Complete androgen insensitivity syndrome. Cross-sectioned testis with multiple well-demarcated nodules.

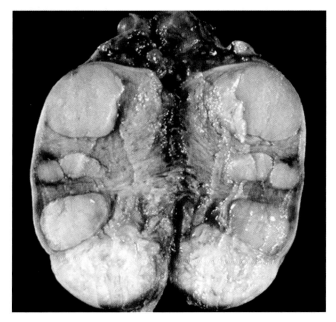

Fig. 12.189 Complete androgen insensitivity syndrome. Both testes are enlarged and contain several gray-white nodules. The poorly delimited nodule in the lower pole corresponds to a muscular hamartoma.

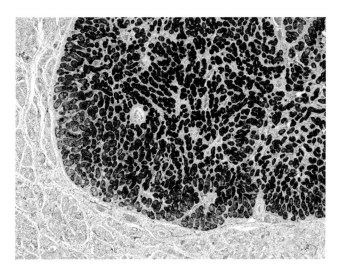

Fig. 12.191 Sertoli-Leydig hamartoma. Immunostaining for D2–40 shows that Sertoli cells of the hamartoma are even more immature than Sertoli cells in the rest of the parenchyma.

absence of elastic fibers. α-Inhibin is expressed in the Sertoli cells and Leydig cells of nodules and the parenchyma, and there is stronger immunoreactivity for D2–40 in Sertoli cells of the nodules than in those of the surrounding tubes (Fig. 12.191).[1684] Approximately 25% of testes contain Sertoli cell adenoma, which may measure up to 14 cm in diameter and up to 1 kg in weight (Fig. 12.192).[1685–1687] These tumors consist of tubules resembling infantile testis but lack germ cells and peritubular myofibroblasts. No Leydig cells are present between the tubules (Fig. 12.193).[1686] Other benign tumors include Sertoli cell tumor (large cell calcifying Sertoli cell tumor and sex cord tumor with annular tubules), Leydig cell tumor, leiomyoma, and fibroma.[1680]

Approximately 60% of patients with CAIS have small cystic structures closely apposed to the testes that may be several

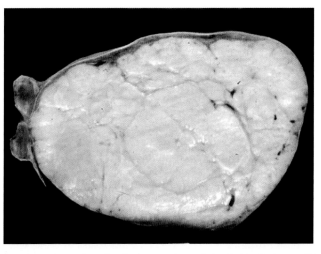

Fig. 12.192 Large Sertoli cell adenoma in an abdominal testis from a 65-year-old patient with complete androgen insensitivity syndrome.

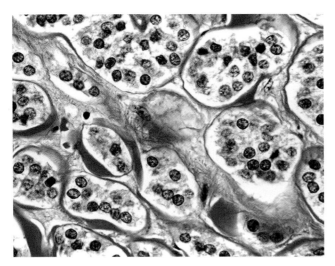

Fig. 12.193 Sertoli cell adenoma showing tubular clusters with a hyalinized wall in a stroma devoid of Leydig cells.

centimeters in diameter, and approximately 80% of patients have thick bundles of smooth muscle fibers resembling myometrium near the testis.[1688,1689] These structures may fuse in the midline of the body and suggest bicornuate uterus, which in rare instances may exhibit a uterine cavity.[1690] True myometrium has been demonstrated in a patient who underwent estrogen treatment for several years.[1691,1692] Hypoplastic fallopian tubes are present in approximately one-third of cases. In approximately 70% of patients, the epididymis and vas deferens are rudimentary; the only explanation for this is residual activity of the mutated AR.[1693] Exceptionally, some testes show spermatogenesis within apparently normal seminiferous tubules admixed with hyalinized tubules with Sertoli cells only.

Approximately 10% of testes from patients with testicular feminization syndrome develop malignancy. The frequency increases with age, but tumors rarely appear before puberty. The risk for tumor is estimated at 4% in 25-year-old patients and 33% in 33-year-old patients.[1388] These tumors include GCNIS (Fig. 12.194), several types of germ cell tumor, which is bilateral

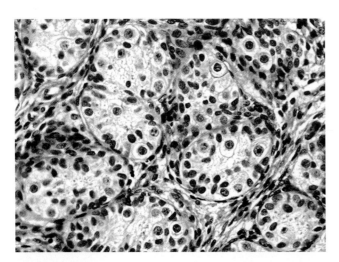

Fig. 12.194 Germ cell neoplasia in situ, undifferentiated type, in a phenotypically female patient with inguinal testes. The tumor cells stand out by virtue of their large size, pale cytoplasm, and prominent nucleoli.

in some cases, and sex cord tumor.[1598,1689,1694–1700] Thus the gonads should be removed immediately after puberty.[1701]

Partial Androgen Insensitivity Syndrome (Partial Testicular Feminization Syndrome). The phenotype of patients with PAIS varies from normal female to normal male, with several intermediate forms giving rise to the following well-defined syndromes[1640]:

- Lubs syndrome, characterized by partial fusion of labioscrotal folds, a definitive introitus, clitoromegaly, pubic and axillary hair, male skeletal development, and poor breast development[1702–1706]
- Gilbert-Dreyfus syndrome, characterized by progressively greater male phenotypic features with general male habitus that include small phallus, hypospadias, incomplete development of wolffian derivatives, and gynecomastia[1707]
- Reifenstein syndrome, or male with micropenis, characterized by hypospadias, weak or absent virilization, cryptorchidism, testicular atrophy, gynecomastia, azoospermia, and infertility[1640,1708–1714]
- Rosewater-Gwinup-Hamwi syndrome, characterized by infertile men whose only abnormal feature is gynecomastia[1715]

The correlation between genotype and phenotype has been studied in patients with AIS. There is no phenotype variation in CAIS-affected families, whereas the phenotype in PAIS is extremely variable and is rarely predicted by the AR genotype.[1716] Patients with completely defective AR function have some pubic hair, Tanner stage P2, and vestigial wolffian duct derivatives despite the absence of AR expression.[1674] PAIS must be differentiated from other entities in patients with karyotype 46,XY such as testosterone biosynthesis defects, 5α-reductase deficiency, and partial gonadal dysgenesis. Serum determinations of testosterone, DHT, and AMH are useful. Normal or high levels of testosterone and DHT suggest PAIS and rule out defects in testosterone biosynthesis. Low testosterone levels suggest partial or complete gonadal dysgenesis. AMH is elevated in PAIS, and its values are low in gonadal dysgenesis.[1717] In adult patients the presence of streak gonads and functioning müllerian structures in the absence of spontaneous breast development suggest gonadal dysgenesis.[1718] Only 25% of patients have mutations in the AR gene.[1719]

Mild Androgen Insensitivity Syndrome. Spermatogenesis requires high levels of intratesticular testosterone. A minor form of androgen insensitivity may be observed in some patients with male phenotype who present with infertility.[1720] The frequency of androgen resistance among azoospermic and oligozoospermic men is estimated at approximately 19% or lower.[1721–1723] MAIS is also observed in phenotypically male patients whose external genitalia are underdeveloped or who have subtle alterations such as simple coronal hypospadias or prominent midline raphe of the scrotum.[1724]

At puberty, MAIS has two phenotypic forms, although both present with variable degrees of gynecomastia, high-pitched voice, sparse pubic and axillary hair, and impotence. In some patients, spermatogenesis is normal or at least sufficient for fertility, whereas others are infertile, with impaired spermatogenesis.[1654,1725]

Some patients have loss of AR gene exon 4, which encodes a protein subunit that enhances the transport of the AR-androgen complex from the cytoplasm to the nucleus in target cells. In the absence of this exon, transport also occurs, but with markedly lower efficiency.[1726] Mutations in exons 6 and 7 and larger trinucleotide repeat size have also been reported.[1723,1727,1728] The ranges vary for ejaculate volume, testosterone level, estradiol level, and androgen sensitivity index significantly between men with and without AR gene mutations.[1715,1729] Patients with mild forms of androgen insensitivity may show improvements in spermiogram after treatment with tamoxifen, clomiphene citrate, or mesterolone.[1710,1730,1731]

Kennedy Disease. Kennedy disease (spinal and bulbar muscular atrophy) is an X-linked recessive disorder of adult men.[1732,1733] It is characterized by loss of motor neurons in the spinal cord and brainstem, and is associated with less significant loss of sensory neurons and atrophy caused by skeletal muscle denervation.[1732,1734] Onset occurs at approximately 20 years of age with muscular weakness, cramps, and fasciculations.[1735] Disease progression is usually slow. Atrophy and muscular weakness begin in the proximal leg muscles and then involve the muscles of the superior extremities and face; if laryngeal or pharyngeal muscles are damaged, dysarthria or dysphagia may occur.[1736,1737] The most frequent cause of death is pneumonia secondary to respiratory difficulties. In most cases the male reproductive system is impaired.[1735,1738,1739] The testes may be normal in initial stages, and many patients are fertile; however, as the disease progresses, secondary testicular atrophy and gynecomastia develop. Testosterone levels are decreased in some cases.

The disease results from mutations in the first exon of the AR gene.[1740] The SMBA gene, located on Xq11–12, has expansion of a repetitive CAG sequence in exon A coding for a polyglutamine (PolyQ) tract in the N-terminal transactivation domain of the AR protein. The number of CAG repeats is 21 (range, 17 to 26) in control men and more than 40 in men with Kennedy disease.[1733,1741–1744] Neuronal alterations are thought to result from the action of PolyQ AR, whereas muscular anomalies are secondary to denervation.[1745] Severity of the disease increases in successive generations (genetic anticipation).[1746,1747] Patients with CAG repetitive sequence between 26 and 35 have male infertility, hirsutism, and cryptorchidism.

Intranuclear inclusions corresponding to mutant AR protein have been identified in motor neurons of the spinal cord and brainstem, as well as in nonnerve cells of other tissues such as skin, scrotum, dermis, kidney, heart, and testis.[1748,1749] These inclusions show epitope features, detectable by antibodies that recognize a small portion of the N terminus of the AR protein. Immunoultrastructural studies reveal clusters of granular, AR-positive, membrane-unbound material.[1750]

5α-Reductase Deficiency

5α-Reductase deficiency is a rare variant of male undermasculinization DSD caused by a lack of the enzyme 5α-reductase, with failure of conversion of testosterone to DHT in peripheral tissues such as external genitalia and prostate.[1751,1752] It was first noted and described in 24 affected individuals in 13 families living in an isolated rural community in the Dominican Republic.[1751] The same syndrome was diagnosed in two sibling black men and was described as *incomplete male pseudohermaphroditism type 2.*[1752]

Patients with the 46,XY karyotype have two isoenzymes: isoenzyme 1 is encoded by the gene *SRD5A*, located on 5p15, and isoenzyme 2 is encoded by the gene *SRD5A2* on 2p23.[1753–1754] Deficit in 5α-reductase has been demonstrated in more than 50 families, and more than 90 mutations have been reported in all of the five exons of gene *SRD5A2*, including missense, non-sense, regulatory, gross deletions, small deletions, small insertions, small indels, or splicing mutations.[1755] A correlation between genotype and phenotype has not been established yet.[1754,1756–1761] Transmission is autosomal recessive.

During childhood, patients have a clitoriform penis, bifid scrotum, and a vagina that opens into the urethra or urogenital sinus, as well as testes in the inguinal canal or labioscrotal folds. These malformations led investigators to designate this syndrome *pseudovaginal perineoscrotal hypospadias.*[1751,1752] Wolffian duct derivatives are present, but müllerian derivatives are absent. Many patients grow up as girls. In some cases the phenotype is male, or the only malformation is hypospadias.[1762,1763] The main differential diagnostic consideration is incomplete androgen insensitivity because both diseases may show a similar phenotype and elevated basal testosterone levels. The presence of well-developed androgen-dependent structures (epididymis, ductus deferens) supports the diagnosis of 5α-reductase deficit, confirmed by analysis of steroid 5a-reductase type 2 gene (*SRD5A2*).

At puberty, these patients acquire the male phenotype, with development of male habitus, enlargement of the penis and scrotum, and change of the voice.[1764] Adults have normal libido and are capable of penile erection and ejaculation. They have scant body hair, thin beard, small prostate, and lack of temporal hairline recession (male pattern baldness). Male sexual behavior acquired after puberty may be maintained with adequate treatment.[1611,1763a,1765] Serum levels of FSH, LH, and testosterone are increased, but DHT is decreased.[1766,1767] The ratios of 5α-steroids to 5β-steroids and etiocholanolone to androsterone are reduced, and there is excessive response to gonadotropin stimulation with LHRH. Some patients also have hyperprolactinemia.

In the first years of life, testes may show normal histologic features.[1768] Later, primary spermatocytes, which are usually observed at 4 to 6 years of age, are absent.[1769] As in normal boys, Sertoli cells manifest gradual loss of cytokeratin 18, D2–40, and AMH near puberty, and residual Leydig cells have vacuolated cytoplasm (Fig. 12.195).[1770] After onset of puberty, important changes occur. The seminiferous tubules show reduced diameter, and most of them lack lumina; the only cell components of the seminiferous epithelium are numerous Sertoli cells showing incomplete maturation.[1767] Spermatogenesis is rarely evident. The testicular interstitium contains an increased number of Leydig cells, which have apparently normal morphology or vacuolated

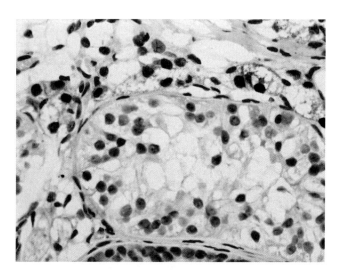

Fig. 12.195 Testis from an infant with 5α-reductase deficiency showing hyperplastic Leydig cells that have marked cytoplasmic vacuolation and surround a seminiferous tubule lacking germ cells (immunostain for calretinin).

cytoplasm. In contrast with AISs, the epididymis is well developed, and its epithelial cells show AR immunoexpression similar to normal epididymis.

The defect in 5α-reductase is genetically heterogeneous. This feature explains why cultured fibroblasts obtained from nongenital skin show either normal or defective 5α-reductase activity, and root hair cells show variable activity of this enzyme.[1751,1766,1771,1772]

Other Forms of Male Undermasculinization

Many dysmorphic syndromes are associated with incomplete masculinization of external genitalia including RSH syndrome, Opitz syndrome (GBBB syndrome), ATR-X syndrome, Gardner-Silengo-Wachtel syndrome, Meckel syndrome, brachioskeletogenital syndrome, Down syndrome, and other trisomies. These syndromes are directly associated with mutations in genes that regulate different steps of sexual differentiation.

Smith-Lemli-Opitz Syndrome

SLOS, or RHS syndrome, is a disorder with multiple malformations, dysmorphic facial features, and mental retardation.[1773] It is caused by mutation in the gene encoding for 7-dehydrocholesterol reductase (*DHCR7*). The gene *DHCR7* maps to chromosome 11, q12–13 band, and its product is a microsomal, membrane-bound protein. Many different missense, non-sense, and splice-site mutations, as well as duplications and deletions, have been reported.[1774–1779]

Defective *DHCR7* impairs cholesterol synthesis, resulting in accumulation of the steroid precursor, 7-dehydrocholesterol, with a subsequent lack of cholesterol.[1780–1783] SLOS is an autosomal recessive disorder frequent in the white population, with an estimated incidence of 1 in 20,000 to 40,000 births. SLOS is rare in African and Asian populations.[1784–1786] There is little correlation between genotype and phenotype.[1787]

The most severe forms are lethal before birth, and fetuses show postnatal oligodactyly (instead of polydactyly) and, sometimes, severe hydrops.[1788] Postnatal lethal forms are characterized by severe growth failure, semiobtunded state, lack of psychomotor development, microcephaly, congenital cataracts, characteristic facies, broad anteriorly rugose alveolar ridges with cleft palate, unilobulate lungs, male undervirilization or female external genital phenotype in 46,XY patients, postaxial polydactyly of the hands and feet, congenital heart defects, and renal anomalies.[1789] Hepatic and renal insufficiency are also frequent.[1790]

Boys with the least severe forms may have normal genitalia, but 70% exhibit genital anomalies. These anomalies include hypospadias (sometimes severe) with or without cryptorchidism and numerous small anomalies that, together, are characteristic of the syndrome. Most patients suffer from mental retardation and severe behavioral problems.[1349]

Prenatal diagnosis is possible by a combination of ultrasonographic, cytogenetic, and biochemical analyses in the second trimester in pregnant woman with abnormal maternal serum screening results, specifically low levels of unconjugated estriol.[1791]

Opitz Syndrome

Patients with Opitz syndrome (GBBB syndrome) are typically males with ventral midline anomalies: hypertelorism and severe unilateral or bilateral labial cleft, laryngeal cleft, severe dysphagia with major or minor life-threatening aspiration, hypospadias, and, occasionally, imperforate anus. Internal anomalies of the tracheobronchial tree, cardiovascular system (defects in heart septation), and gallbladder are prominent, suggesting subjacent defect of the developing ventral midline. The syndrome is genetically heterogeneous, combining two entities formerly described separately. The syndrome is caused by at least two mutant genes: the *ADOS* gene (autosomal dominant Opitz syndrome or G syndrome characterized by gastrointestinal anomalies), which maps to 22q11.2; and the *XLOS* gene (X-kinked Opitz syndrome or BBB syndrome characterized by labial or palatal cleft and mental retardation), which is located in Xp22.3 and is caused by mutations in the RING finger protein MID1.[1349,1792–1796]

ATRX Syndrome

ATRX syndrome is characterized by the presence of mild α-thalassemia (not from deletion of the α genes), severe mental retardation, facial dysmorphism, and X-linkage.[1797] The association between α-thalassemia and mental retardation was first observed in 1981.[1798] The disease is rare, with an estimated incidence lower than 1 in 100,000 liveborn boys.[1799] Facial anomalies are associated with genital abnormalities, including undescended testes, small or dysgenetic testes, shawl-like or hypoplastic scrotum, penile hypoplasia, and hypospadias. The most severely affected boys grow up as girls; puberty may be delayed, and gonads vary from dysgenetic testes to streak gonad. Patients usually present with gastrointestinal problems, especially feeding difficulties, regurgitation and vomiting, abdominal pain or distention, and chronic constipation. Death in early childhood from aspiration of vomitus or pneumonia presumed to be secondary to aspiration has been recorded.[1800] Hemoglobin H inclusions in red blood cells are characteristic.[1801] The syndrome is caused by mutations in the *ATRX* gene (synonyms XNP, XH2), locus Xq13.3, that belongs to the helicase superfamily whose protein products have a number of regulatory functions ranging from DNA recombination and repair to control of transcription.[1802–1806]

Infertility

Infertility affects not only the healthcare system but also the social environment.[1807] It is defined as inability of a couple to conceive naturally after 12 months of regular unprotected sexual intercourse. Infertility affects 13% to 15% of couples worldwide. In more than one-half, the cause lies in the male partner with or without a concomitant female partner problem. Causes include varicocele, spermatic pathway obstruction, primary testicular failure, cryptorchidism, gonad toxin exposure, genetic anomalies, infections, hormonal dysfunction, immunologic conditions, ejaculatory or sexual dysfunction, cancer, and systemic disease.[1808] In 28% of cases of male infertility, the cause is idiopathic.[1809] Approximately one-half of infertile males have conditions that are potentially correctable by surgical or medical treatment.

Testicular Biopsy

Testicular biopsy as a tool to diagnose infertility began in the 1940s, and most of the diagnostic terms used today were created at that time.[1810–1812] These terms are usually descriptive and reflect subjective analysis except for a few (e.g., normal testes, Sertoli cell–only tubules, tubular hyalinization). The terms *maturation arrest* and *hypospermatogenesis* apply to biopsies in more than 50% of cases of infertility, but the criteria for these conditions vary widely among pathologists.[1813–1815]

There are two forms of maturation arrest: spermatogenic arrest and spermatocytic arrest, or its equivalent, meiotic arrest. True spermatogenic arrest is rare because germ cell maturation usually does not arrest at the level of a defined germ cell type.[1816] To avoid confusion, the term *irregular hypospermatogenesis* has been proposed for testicular biopsies with decreased numbers of germ cells, subclassified as slight, moderate, or severe.[1817] However, this diagnosis is of little help to clinicians. The reported frequency of spermatocytic (meiotic) arrest in infertile men varies from 12% to 32%, and this disorder is present in one or both testes in approximately 18% of oligozoospermic or azoospermic patients.[1814,1818–1819] If observed in only one testis, the contralateral testis contains histologic changes ranging from normal spermatogenesis to hyalinized tubules.

Disorganization of the seminiferous tubular cell layers is another frequent diagnosis in biopsies, but this term is rejected by many pathologists.[1812,1820,1821] Actual disorganization of the seminiferous tubular cells is unlikely and has not been demonstrated in ultrastructural studies. In most cases the apparent disorganization is an artifact induced by handling or fixation.[1822,1823]

Tubular blockage was used to describe biopsies with at least 50% of seminiferous tubules devoid of central lumina and showing spatial disorganization of germ cells.[1821] This morphology was found in 28% of testicular biopsies from infertile men, mainly men with obstructive azoospermia.[1824] Although this appearance may result from improper fixation, accumulation of Sertoli cells and immature germ cells in the centers of the tubules suggests a specific lesion, a variant of germ cell sloughing.[1825]

Diagnostic confusion decreased the interest and trust of urologists and andrologists in the study of testicular biopsies. Subsequent studies attempted to correlate semen spermatozoa concentration with testicular size and biochemical findings such as serum levels of FSH, and biopsies were undertaken only in a limited number of oligozoospermic and azoospermic patients.[1822,1825,1826] However, these studies were also disappointing because FSH was found to correlate poorly with number of spermatozoa in the semen but better with numbers of spermatogonia in the seminiferous tubules.[1827] Normal numbers of spermatozoa may be produced by relatively small testes, whereas some large testes have no spermatogenesis. Flow cytometry studies to evaluate the presence of germ cells in seminal fluid have not yielded satisfactory results.[1828] Inhibin B serum levels correlate positively with both spermatozoon number and serum FSH levels.[1829,1830] Evaluation of semen for the presence of cell-free mRNA and specifically DEAD (Asp-Glu-Ala-Asp) box polypeptide 4 (DDX4 or VASA) is considered an excellent marker for the presence of germ cells in the testis.[1831,1832] Although such studies may have relevance, they do not always allow correlation with histology in nonobstructive azoospermia or oligozoospermia, and therefore serve only a complementary function in evaluating infertility.[1833,1834]

The development of morphometry caused a resurgence of interest in biopsies, and many semiquantitative and quantitative studies were conducted.[1817,1835–1842] The greatest achievements were enhanced reproducibility and better evaluation of the reversibility of lesions. Morphometry has emerged as the best method for objectively evaluating seminiferous tubular cells.[1843] The scoring method of Johnsen, estimation of the germ cell/Sertoli cell ratio for each germ cell type, and the calculation of germ cell number per unit length of seminiferous tubules are reliable and useful.[1836,1851–1855]

Several methods are available to evaluate the Leydig cell population, including mean number of Leydig cells per seminiferous tubule and per Leydig cell cluster, mean number of Leydig cell clusters per seminiferous tubule, the ratio of Leydig cell area to seminiferous tubule area, and the ratio of Leydig cells to Sertoli cells.[1844,1845] These methods have shown that the appearance of Leydig cell hyperplasia described in many conditions is false, and that true Leydig cell hyperplasia is rare.

In summary, histologic study of the parenchyma is the only method to determine conditions inside the testis. The more information biopsy may give us, the higher its value will be. Histologic study may provide information not only on the real condition of the parenchyma but also on the reversibility or progression of lesions and their causes. Nonetheless, the practice of biopsy has been criticized as lacking cost-effectiveness, and is subject to complications related to its invasive nature.[1135]

Indications

Indications for testicular biopsy may be diagnostic, prognostic, or therapeutic.

Diagnostic biopsy is recommended in all cases of obstructive azoospermia to confirm the presence of normal spermatozoa if surgical correction is considered. Patients who have previously undergone vasectomy or those with congenital absence of the vas deferens are not included unless they also have testicular atrophy or high FSH levels. Diagnostic biopsy is also indicated if there is clinical concern for the possibility of GCNIS in patients with small testis associated with microlithiasis, history of cryptorchidism or contralateral germ cell tumor, or inhomogeneous testicular echogenicity. GCNIS occurs in 1% to 5% of infertile men.[1846]

Prognostic biopsy is recommended in all patients with cryptorchidism, regardless of the time at which the testis becomes located in the scrotum (prepubertal or pubertal). In both unilateral and bilateral cryptorchidism, when Ad spermatogonia are not detected, the patient will be infertile despite surgical treatment. Hormonal treatment increases the number of germ cells.[1847]

Therapeutic biopsy is used to extract spermatozoa from men with nonobstructive azoospermia.[1848] Histologic study enables identification of the testicular lesion and exclusion of GCNIS.[1849]

Optimal interpretation of biopsies depends on the surgical technique by which the sample is taken, the care and delicacy with which it is handled, and proper fixation and processing. The size of the sample should not be larger than a grain of rice (i.e., no diameter should be >3 mm). This amounts to approximately 0.1% of testicular volume (normal volume is approximately 20 mL). The biopsy should be bilateral because in more than 28% of patients the findings differ between the testes. At the time of the biopsy the testicular axes should be measured as the basis of quantitative studies. The tissue should be taken opposite the rete testis through a 4- to 5-mm incision in the tunica albuginea. Parenchyma herniates through the incision and may be carefully snipped off. If only light microscopy is to be performed, the specimen should be fixed in either Bouin fluid for 24 hours or Stieve solution, as the European Germ Cell Cancer Consensus Group recommends.[1084] Both fixatives allow excellent conservation of spermatogenesis, although they have the disadvantage of false-negative results in some cases when immunohistochemistry is used to detect GCNIS. One alternative is neutral-buffered formaldehyde, which diminishes the shrinkage artifacts of formalin.[1850] If electron microscopy is indicated, a small biopsy fragment should be fixed in glutaraldehyde-osmium tetroxide or similar fixative. To perform meiotic studies, biopsy should be processed according to air-drying or surface-spreading methods. Examination includes qualitative and quantitative evaluation, and correlation between the biopsy and spermiogram.

Qualitative and Quantitative Evaluation

Various methods of analysis of biopsies have been proposed, but most are of limited clinical utility.[1836,1851–1855] A method developed by our group provides information on the number of each type of germ cell and the proportions among these cells, thus achieving functional exploration of spermatogenesis and associated disorders of the Sertoli cells or interstitium.[709]

Examination of biopsies involves several steps: first, quantitative evaluation of seminiferous tubular cells, which permits the identification of the affected germ cell or cells, when the numbers are compared with normal values; second, qualitative evaluation, which may provide additional data on a particular type of cell; and finally, establishment of a correlation between elongate spermatids (Sc + Sd) and the number of spermatozoa per milliliter in the ejaculate, to evaluate the permeability of the spermatic pathway.

Light microscopy at low magnification immediately reveals whether the lesion is focal or diffuse. If focal, the percentage of tubules showing each lesion (e.g., Sertoli cell–only, hyalinization, tubular hypoplasia) should be calculated. It is useful to evaluate elastic fibers with a special stain because this highlights groups of small tubules that may be missed with hematoxylin and eosin. A minimum of 30 cross-sectioned tubules should be studied (this is usually possible when 5 or 6 histologic sections are available). The diameter of each seminiferous tubule should be measured, and the numbers of spermatogonia, primary spermatocytes, young spermatids (also called *round spermatids or Sa + Sb spermatids*), mature spermatids (also called *elongate or Sc + Sd spermatids*), Sertoli cells, and, in some cases, peritubular cells counted. The presence of tubular diverticula, maturation of Sertoli cells, and morphologic anomalies in germ cells should also be noted.[1856,1857] Evaluation of the testicular interstitium should include the number of Leydig cells per tubule (or the number of Leydig cell clusters per tubule), the presence of angiectasis (phlebectasis), and the occurrence of peritubular or perivascular inflammation. Normal values are tabulated in Table 12.20. For a clear and rapid understanding of the results, data may be presented using cartesian axes.

Common Lesions

The most frequently observed lesions are Sertoli cell–only tubules, tubular hyalinization, alterations in spermatogenesis in either the adluminal or basal compartments of seminiferous tubules, and mixed tubular atrophy.

Sertoli Cell–Only Syndrome

Sertoli cell–only syndrome includes any azoospermia in which the seminiferous epithelium consists only of Sertoli cells. To understand this syndrome, it is necessary to consider morphologic and functional changes induced in the Sertoli cell by hypophyseal gonadotropin secretion during puberty. During childhood, Sertoli cells are pseudostratified, and nuclei are dark, small, and round or elongate, with regular outlines and one or two small peripherally placed nucleoli. The cytoplasm lacks specialized organelles.[216] The apical cytoplasm contains one or several inhibin bodies.[170] Adult Sertoli cells have characteristically pale, triangular nuclei with irregular, indented outlines. Nucleoli are large and have tripartite structures. The cytoplasm contains abundant smooth endoplasmic reticulum and specialized structures, including annulated

TABLE 12.20	Testicular Parameters in Normal Adult Testes (Per Cross-Sectioned Tubule)
Parameter	Mean ± SD
Seminiferous Tubules	
Mean tubular diameter (μm)	193 ± 8
No. of spermatogonia	21 ± 4
No. of primary spermatocytes	31 ± 6
No. of young (Sa + Sb) spermatids	37 ± 7
No. of mature (Sc + Sd) spermatids	25 ± 4
No. of Sertoli cells	10.4 ± 2
No. of Sertoli cell vacuoles	0.8 ± 0.3
Lamina propria thickness (μm)	5.3 ± 1
No. of peritubular cells	21 ± 4
Testicular Interstitium	
No. of Leydig cell clusters per tubule	1.2 ± 0.3
No. of Leydig cells per tubule	5 ± 0.2

Sa+Sb, Round spermatids; *Sc+Sd*, elongate spermatids.

lamellae, Charcot-Böttcher crystals, and specialized junctional complexes with other Sertoli cells. The pubertal increase in both length and width of the seminiferous tubules replaces the infantile pseudostratified pattern with a simple columnar distribution.

Five variants of the Sertoli cell–only syndrome are identified by morphology, the degree of development of seminiferous tubules, and the presence or absence of interstitial lesions.[1858] These variants are designated by the appearance of the predominant Sertoli cell population: immature Sertoli cells, dysgenetic Sertoli cells, adult Sertoli cells, involuting Sertoli cells, and dedifferentiated Sertoli cells (Fig. 12.196). Each type is associated with other tubular and interstitial alterations (Table 12.21).

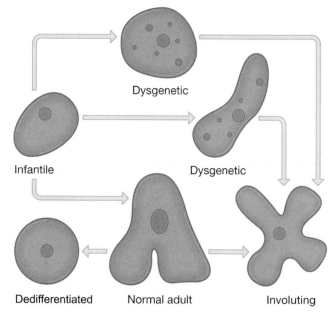

Fig. 12.196 Sertoli cell types.

TABLE 12.21 Differential Diagnosis of the Sertoli Cell–Only Syndrome

Testis Pattern	VARIANTS OF THE SERTOLI CELL–ONLY SYNDROME				
	Immature Sertoli Cells	Dysgenetic Sertoli Cells	Adult Sertoli Cells	Involuting Sertoli Cells	Dedifferentiated Sertoli Cells
Tubular diameter	Markedly decreased	Decreased	Decreased	Decreased	Decreased
Tubular lumen	Small or absent	Small or absent	Normal	Normal	Normal
Lamina propria thickness	Thin	Enlarged	Normal or enlarged	Normal or enlarged	Enlarged
Elastic fibers in lamina propria	Absent	Decreased	Normal	Normal	Normal
Sertoli cells					
Number	Markedly increased	Increased	Normal or increased	Normal or increased	Increased
Distribution	Pseudostratified	Pseudostratified	Columnar	Columnar	Columnar or pseudostratified
Nuclear shape	Ovoid	Round or ovoid	Triangular	Lobated	Round
Nuclear outline	Regular	Regular	Few indented	Markedly indented	Regular
Chromatin	Dark	Pale with granules	Pale	Pale	Pale
Nucleolus	Small, peripheral	Developed, central	Developed, central	Developed, central	Small, central or peripheral
Vacuoles	Absent	Present	Present	Abundant	Abundant
Lipids	Absent	Absent	Decreased	Abundant	Abundant
Vimentin filaments	Basal	Basal	Basal and perinuclear	Basal and perinuclear	Basal
Inhibin bodies	Present	Absent	Absent	Absent	Present
Antimüllerian hormone	Present	Present	Absent	Absent	Absent
Interstitium	Scant	Increased	Normal	Normal/fibrosis	Fibrosis
Leydig cells	Absent	Pleomorphic, vacuolated, increased or decreased	Normal	Decreased, many lipofuscin granules	Decreased, many lipofuscin granules
Clinical symptoms	Hypogonadotropic hypogonadism	Infertility	Infertility, orchitis	Infertility, hypergonadotropic hypogonadism, chemotherapy or radiation therapy	Treatment with estrogens, antiandrogens, or cisplatinum; chronic hepatopathy

The most frequent types of Sertoli cell–only syndrome in patients with infertility are dysgenetic Sertoli cells, adult Sertoli cells, and involuting Sertoli cells. The clinical manifestations are similar, including normal external genitalia, well-developed secondary male characteristics, azoospermia, elevated serum FSH levels, normal or elevated serum LH levels, and normal or slightly low testosterone levels. These clinical and histologic features were long thought to constitute a single syndrome, Del Castillo syndrome, but more recent ultrastructural, histochemical, immunohistochemical, and cytogenetic studies showed that this condition results from a variety of syndromes that may be primary or secondary (Table 12.22).[334,1859–1862]

Some patients with adult Sertoli cell or dysgenetic Sertoli cell variant have a few spermatozoa in the spermiogram. This discrepancy between oligozoospermia and histologic findings is caused by the presence of some seminiferous tubules with complete spermatogenesis elsewhere in the parenchyma.[1863] In these patients the assessment of DDX4 cell-free seminal mRNA is of great value.[1864]

Sertoli Cell–Only Syndrome With Immature Sertoli Cells. Sertoli cells in adult testes with this variant of Sertoli cell–only syndrome have an immature prepubertal appearance with pseudostratification. The number of cells per cross-sectioned tubule is greater than normal. Other tubular and interstitial features suggest immaturity, including small tubular diameters (<80 μm), tubules lacking central lumina, thin lamina propria lacking elastic fibers, and interstitium lacking mature Leydig cells.[404,1865,1866] Immunohistochemistry shows that these Sertoli cells have prepubertal characteristics with expression of cytokeratin 18, AMH, and inhibin bodies.[170]

This syndrome is caused by a deficiency of both FSH and LH. This deficit begins in childhood and is responsible for lack of maturation of Sertoli cells, tubular walls, and interstitium. Subsequently, no renewal or differentiation of germ cells occurs, and these cells eventually disappear. When patients have been treated with hormones, the biopsy may show some degree of spermatogenesis or thickening and hyalinization of the tubular basement membrane.

Biopsies from patients with CAIS also show seminiferous tubules with only immature Sertoli cells, but differ from the condition described earlier in several important respects. Sertoli cells in CAIS lack AR, the interstitium contains abundant spindle cells that simulate the ovarian stroma, and there are a large number of Leydig cells.[1867]

Sertoli Cell–Only Syndrome With Dysgenetic Sertoli Cells. Dysgenetic Sertoli cells begin pubertal differentiation but variably deviate from normal maturation, so that the morphology of dysgenetic Sertoli cells differs among tubules and even among Sertoli

TABLE 12.22   Differential Diagnosis in Tubular Hyalinization

	Dysgenetic	Hormonal Deficit	Ischemia	Excretory Duct Obstruction	Postinflammatory Hyalinization	Physical or Chemical Agents
Hyalinized tubule size	Minimum	Minimum	Minimum	Markedly decreased	Minimum	Markedly decreased
Tubular lumen	Absent	Absent	Absent	Present	Absent	Absent
Peritubular cells	Decreased	Decreased	Decreased	Increased	Decreased or increased	Decreased
Elastic fibers	Decreased	Normal	Normal	Normal	Normal	Normal
Leydig cells	Increased or decreased, pleomorphic	Absent	Absent	Normal	Pseudohyperplasia	Decreased
Follicle-stimulating hormone	Increased	Decreased	Increased	Increased	Increased	Increased
Luteinizing hormone	Increased	Decreased	Increased	Increased	Increased	Increased
Testosterone	Normal or decreased	Decreased	Normal or decreased	Normal	Normal	Normal or decreased

cells within the same tubule. Nuclei usually have both mature features (pale chromatin and a centrally located, tripartite nucleolus) and features of immaturity (in some cases, they are small, ovoid, or round with regular outlines; in others, elongate, with major axis perpendicular to the basal lamina). Both types of nuclei may contain dense chromatin granules (Figs. 12.197 through 12.200).[246] These Sertoli cells show immunoexpression of vimentin, AMH, and cytokeratin 18.[1868,1869] Immunoreactivity for AMH and cytokeratin 18 is assumed to be a sign of immaturity because, under normal conditions, it is not detected after puberty. Other signs of immaturity are poor development of the hematotesticular barrier and absence of tubular lumina.[1870]

Tubular lumina are small or even absent in most dysgenetic Sertoli cell–containing tubules because the ability to produce testicular fluid is greatly reduced. Sertoli cell number per cross-sectioned tubule is high, and MTD is lower than 120 μm. Tubular walls have few elastic fibers, and most show a variable degree of tunica propria hyalinization.[1002]

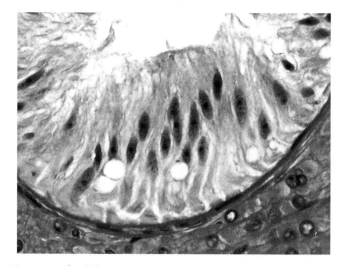

Fig. 12.198 Seminiferous tubule with dysgenetic Sertoli cells only. Elongate nuclei, pseudostratified arrangement.

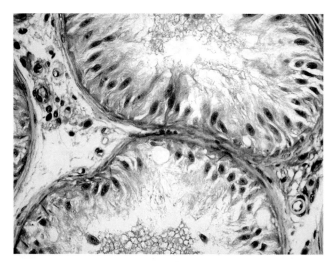

Fig. 12.197 Sertoli cell–only syndrome with dysgenetic Sertoli cells. Seminiferous tubules show slightly thickened tunica propria. The Sertoli cells are increased and have elongate nuclei and abundant apical cytoplasm.

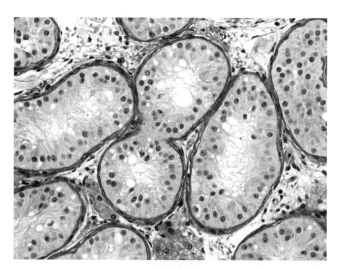

Fig. 12.199 Sertoli cell–only syndrome with dysgenetic Sertoli cells. The seminiferous tubules are small and lack lumens. The interstice contains isolated groups of Leydig cells.

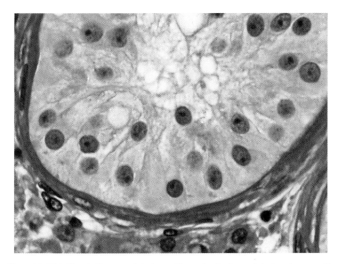

Fig. 12.200 Seminiferous tubule with spherical nuclei in dysgenetic Sertoli cells. Thickening of tubular wall and isolated Leydig cells.

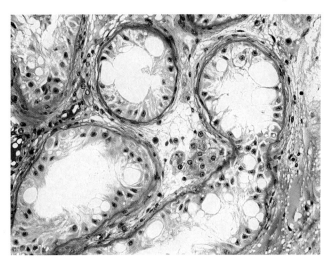

Fig. 12.201 Sertoli cell–only syndrome with mature Sertoli cells. The seminiferous tubules are lined by normal adult Sertoli cells, many with cytoplasmic vacuoles.

Completely hyalinized tubules are common. The testicular interstitium contains a variable number of Leydig cells (normal, decreased, or apparently increased), many of which are pleomorphic with abundant paracrystalline inclusions.[1770,1871]

The morphologic findings may be observed in biopsies from men with cryptorchid testes, at the periphery of germ cell tumors in biopsies from men with chromosomal anomalies such as 46,XX 48,XYYY, Y-chromosome anomalies, and in biopsies from men with idiopathic infertility.[1872,1873]

Sertoli Cell–Only Syndrome With Mature Sertoli Cells. In this variant, most Sertoli cells appear mature, with nuclei like those of normal mature Sertoli cells, but are present in increased numbers (14 ± 0.8 Sertoli cells per cross-sectioned tubule).[1874] The seminiferous tubules have small diameters, but larger than in the two variants described above, and central lumina are visible. The lamina propria is normal or slightly thickened. Leydig cells are normal. Ultrastructurally the cytoplasm of the Sertoli cells contains abundant vacuoles that communicate with the tubular lumina (Figs. 12.201 and 12.202). The lateral cell surfaces have many unfolding and extensive specialized junctions with other Sertoli cells (from the basement membrane to the apical cytoplasmic portion). Lipid droplets, usually derived from phagocytosis of spermatid tubulobulbar complexes and dead germ cells, are scant.[1859] Vimentin filaments are abundant in the basal and perinuclear cytoplasm.[110]

Serum testosterone is normal or nearly normal, and FSH and LH levels are elevated.[1875–1877] This syndrome is probably caused by failure of migration of primordial germ cells from the primitive yolk sac to the gonadal ridge.[1878] This failure may result from deletion in the AZFa region in Yq11, a mutation in the genes that encode KIT or its ligand (SCF), responsible for the migration, proliferation, and survival of germ cells or PLK4 mutations.[1879,1880]

Sertoli Cell–Only Syndrome With Involuting Sertoli Cells. Testes with this variant of Sertoli cell–only syndrome have numerous changes. Sertoli cell nuclei may have lobulated shapes with irregular outlines, coarse chromatin granules, and inconspicuous nucleoli. Seminiferous tubules have central lumina, decreased diameters, and variable thickening of the basement membrane (Figs. 12.203 and 12.204). Elastic fibers are present in normal or diminished amounts. Leydig cells are variably involuted.

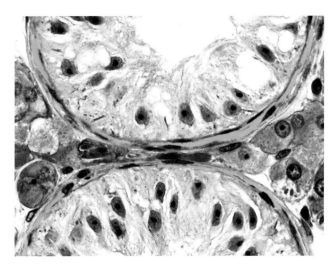

Fig. 12.202 Sertoli cell–only syndrome with adult Sertoli cells. Note the presence of triangular nuclei of Sertoli cells with large nucleoli and Charcott Böttcher subnuclear crystals.

This syndrome may be a primary disorder or secondary to irradiation or cytotoxic therapy, such as cancer chemotherapy or treatment for nephrotic syndrome.[1881] It is not usually possible to determine the etiology from the biopsy findings alone. Changes in the tubular walls are more pronounced in patients with a history of cyclophosphamide treatment, combination chemotherapy, or radiation therapy. The interstitium may be fibrotic in patients treated with *cis*-platinum or cyclophosphamide.[1882] Syndromes with involuting Sertoli cells associated with decreased amounts of elastic fibers are an expression of primary testicular anomaly with involuting and dysgenetic Sertoli cells within the same tubule.

Sertoli Cell–Only Syndrome With Dedifferentiated Sertoli Cells. The presence of immature-appearing Sertoli cells in otherwise mature tubules is the most striking feature of this variant of Sertoli cell–only syndrome. Sertoli cells appear abnormally numerous because of shortening of the tubule, and nuclei are either

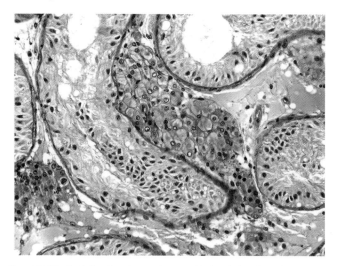

Fig. 12.203 Sertoli cell–only syndrome with involuting Sertoli cells. The Sertoli cell nuclei are hyperchromatic and have irregular outlines.

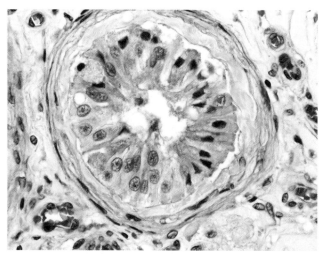

Fig. 12.204 Sertoli cell–only syndrome with involuting Sertoli cells. More than one-half of the cells have retracted hyperchromatic nuclei with irregular surface. Marked thickening of the tubular wall. Leydig cell atrophy is shown.

round or elongate. Round nuclei have single, small, central, or peripheral nucleoli, whereas elongate nuclei have dense, clumped chromatin and small peripheral nucleoli.

The tubular wall is thickened and contains elastic fibers, increased amounts of collagen fibers, and elevated numbers of peritubular cells as a result of shortening. MTD is markedly decreased to <90 µm. The interstitium contains few Leydig cells, and these appear dedifferentiated or contain increased amounts of lipofuscin. This variant may occur after androgen deprivation therapy for prostatic cancer, estrogen treatment for transsexuality, and cancer chemotherapy with *cis*-platinum.

In summary, most patients seeking consultation for infertility who have Sertoli cell–only pattern have one of the following variants: dysgenetic, adult, or involutive Sertoli cells. Clinical features of all are similar: azoospermia, normal external genitalia, well-developed male sexual characteristics, elevated levels of FSH, normal or increased levels of LH, and normal or low-normal

levels of testosterone.[1883,1884] The use of ultrastructural, histochemical, immunohistochemical, cytogenetic, and molecular biology studies has increased our knowledge of these syndromes.[1859–1862,1872,1885,1886]

Tubular Hyalinization

A few azoospermic patients have diffuse hyalinization of seminiferous tubules. The incidence is difficult to estimate, given that these patients usually do not undergo biopsy because their testes are small, and the diagnosis is obtained from clinical, hormonal, or cytogenetic data. Hyalinization of seminiferous tubules is the end point of tubular atrophy and includes the absence of both germ cells and Sertoli cells with alterations in the lamina propria and Leydig cells. The etiology may be determined from several histologic features and clinical data, including the following:

- *General histologic appearance:* the extent and topography of the hyalinized tubules and the presence of isolated tubules containing germ cells or Sertoli cells only (dysgenetic, adults, involuting, or dedifferentiated)
- *Appearance of atrophic tubules, all showing the same pattern or variable degrees of atrophy:* tubular diameter; trophism of peritubular cells; the presence of elastic fibers; the degree of collagenization of the lamina propria; and the presence of cell remnants or unusual cells in the tubules.
- *Appearance of the interstitium:* the number and morphology of Leydig cells; vascular lesions; and lymphoid infiltrates
- *Chronology of testicular shrinkage*

The most common causes of tubular hyalinization include dysgenetic hyalinization, hormonal deficit, ischemia, obstruction, inflammation, and physical or chemical agents. The differential diagnosis is given in Table 12.22.

Dysgenetic Hyalinization. Dysgenetic hyalinization is a diffuse lesion in which most tubules are uniformly hyalinized (Fig. 12.205). There is a lack seminiferous tubular cells and a reduced number of peritubular cells. The few preserved tubules usually contain only Sertoli cells, although rarely a few tubules with spermatogenesis are present. Dysgenetic hyalinization is seen in Klinefelter syndrome, in testes that remain cryptorchid through puberty, and in some, hypergonadotropic hypogonadisms associated with myopathy. Focal lesions are seen in MAT of the testis.

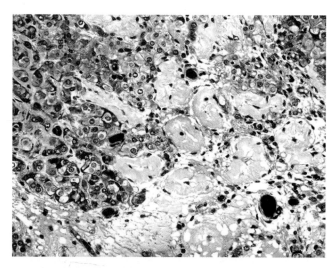

Fig. 12.205 Dysgenetic hyalinization. Fully hyalinized seminiferous tubules and a few peritubular cells among Leydig cell clusters.

Tubular hyalinization is pronounced in Klinefelter syndrome, and from infancy the seminiferous tubules are small, containing reduced numbers of Sertoli cells and few or no spermatogonia. At puberty the dysgenetic Sertoli cells fail to mature and soon disappear. The tubules collapse, thus giving the appearance of phantom tubules.[1887] Peritubular cells fail to differentiate, and their number is low.[1888] They form a discontinuous ring around the hyalinized tubules and are incapable of synthesizing elastic fibers and other components of the lamina propria. Dysgenesis also involves the interstitium; Leydig cells exhibit a characteristic adenomatous pattern, although the total number is decreased. The morphology of the Leydig cell is not uniform, with shrunken, normal, and large forms. Most Leydig cells contain reduced amounts of lipofuscin granules and lipid droplets. Reinke crystalloids are uncommon, and paracrystalline inclusions are abundant.[1871] Despite the hyperplastic adenomatous appearance of the Leydig cells, testosterone secretion is markedly decreased, and the resulting hypogonadism is the most important clinical feature of Klinefelter syndrome.

Tubular hyalinization in the cryptorchid testis is also dysgenetic. However, in contrast with the atrophic collapse seen in Klinefelter syndrome, cross sections of the hyalinized tubules in cryptorchidism are targetoid. This morphology, which results from the arrangement of the peritubular cells into two layers, suggests an atrophic process that has evolved over a longer period than in Klinefelter syndrome or has a lesser degree of dysgenesis.[995] Elastic fibers are diminished.[1002] Leydig cells appear hyperplastic, forming large aggregates, although their absolute number is decreased. Leydig cell pleomorphism is less intense than in Klinefelter syndrome. Many Leydig cells have abundant vacuolated cytoplasm. Whereas tubular hyalinization in Klinefelter syndrome is secondary to the effect of pubertal gonadotropin secretion on dysgenetic tubules, tubular hyalinization in cryptorchidism probably results from the effect of increased temperature on the dysgenetic tubules. However, other mechanisms are also involved in cryptorchid tubular hyalinization, including obstruction of sperm excretory ducts (anomalies in these ducts are frequent in cryptorchidism) and ischemia (principally in testes that could be only incompletely descended at surgery).

Hyalinization Caused by Hormonal Deficit. Hormonal deficit causes diffuse tubular hyalinization, although the tubules may be recognized as cellular cords surrounded by hyaline material. Sertoli cells, a few spermatogonia, and rare primary spermatocytes may be identified in these cords. When hyalinization is complete, only the elastic fibers in the lamina propria indicate the structure of the previously normal adult testis. Peritubular myofibroblasts decrease in number and form a ring at the periphery of the lamina propria. Leydig cells disappear as hyalinization progresses, and the few remaining cells have pyknotic nuclei and shrunken cytoplasm with abundant lipofuscin granules.

This process manifests clinically as postpubertal hypogonadotropic hypogonadism and is usually caused by lesions in or near the pituitary, such as adenoma, craniopharyngioma, and trauma to the cranial base or sella turcica (see later discussion of Hypogonadism Secundary to Sndocrine Gland Dysfuction and Other Disorders (Hypothalamus-hypophysis-Hypopituitarism)).

Ischemic Hyalinization. Ischemic atrophy is usually caused by torsion of the spermatic cord, vascular injury during inguinal surgery, polyarteritis nodosa (PAN), and severe arteriosclerosis.[1889,1890] Except for cases caused by torsion of the spermatic cord, these patients usually are not seen in infertility clinics.

Torsion of the spermatic cord is often not listed among the causes of infertility. However, follow-up of those with torsion reveals marked alteration in the spermiogram. Several hypotheses have been offered to explain the low number of sperm produced by the contralateral normal testis; the most promising hypotheses include response to release of antigens by the ischemic testis and primary lesions of the contralateral testis (see earlier Testicular Torsion section).[1891]

Testicular anoxia caused by torsion rapidly produces severe lesions that are irreversible without adequate treatment. After 8 hours, intense hemorrhagic infarction of the seminiferous tubular cells occurs. Chronic anoxia leads to tubular hyalinization and loss of Leydig cells (Fig. 12.206).

Testicular atrophy secondary to inguinal hernia surgery may occur in <1% of patients in the first repair, and in 1% to 5% of patients who undergo surgical repair of recurrent hernia. Atrophy is most frequent in cases that require extensive dissection of the spermatic cord.

Postobstructive Hyalinization. Obstruction of the sperm excretory ducts may cause atrophy of seminiferous tubules. To produce tubular hyalinization, the obstruction must be close to the testis because the ductuli efferentes in the caput of the epididymis absorb approximately 90% of tubular fluid and protect the testis from excessive intratubular pressure. Obstructive tubular hyalinization is usually focal and secondary to varicocele and other disorders involving dilation of the channels of the rete testis. These disorders may be congenital, as in epididymis-testis dissociation, or acquired, as rete testis dilation secondary to epididymal atrophy caused by arteritis, arteriosclerosis, or androgen insufficiency. Obstructive tubular hyalinization also occurs in the seminiferous tubules at the periphery of the testis in patients who have had orchitis.[1892]

Obstructive hyalinization has a mosaic distribution: lobules of completely hyalinized tubules are intermingled with lobules of normal tubules (Fig. 12.207). The diameter of the hyalinized tubules is not as small as in hyalinization of other causes, and the tubules occasionally contain Sertoli cells. In the center of many is a small lumen, or a vacuole may be present in the cytoplasm of a residual Sertoli cell.[1893] The lamina propria is thick and contains hypertrophic peritubular cells and abundant extracellular material. Finally,

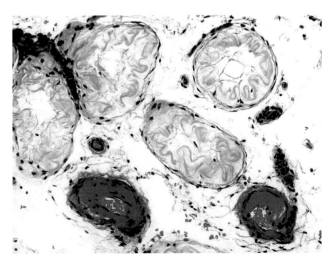

Fig. 12.206 Ischemic tubular hyalinization. Fully hyalinized seminiferous tubules are surrounded by peritubular cells. The testicular interstitium lacks Leydig cells and shows arteriolar hyalinization.

the peritubular cells dedifferentiate, and only fibroblasts remain.[1888,1893a] The interstitium contains a normal number of Leydig cells, forming small clusters, some of which are among hyalinized tubules. This feature is not seen in other patterns such as ischemic hyalinization. In addition, dilated veins with eccentrically hyalinized walls may be seen in testes associated with varicocele. This lobular pattern of tubular atrophy causes a peculiar ultrasound image that has been described as striated pattern.[1894,1895] This pattern is nonspecific and has also been described in patients with neoplasia, fibrosis, and orchitis.[1896]

Postinflammatory Hyalinization. Many infections of the testis cause irreversible lesions in the seminiferous tubules. In bacterial infections the epididymis is usually involved, resulting in obstructive azoospermia. In viral infections the testis is often affected, even without symptoms. Two types of viral orchitis often cause infertility: mumps orchitis and coxsackie B orchitis.

Tubular atrophy caused by viral infection has a mosaic topography in which hyalinized and normal tubules are intermingled. In fully hyalinized tubules the only recognizable cells are peritubular cells that form an incomplete peripheral ring around the hyalinized material. The presence of elastic fibers in these tubules distinguishes this condition from dysgenetic hyalinization. Leydig cells form clusters of variable size, but total number is normal. In bacterial infections the pattern of tubular hyalinization is variable.

Tubular atrophy of unknown etiology may be caused by an autoimmune response. This occurs in hypogonadism associated with disorders in other endocrine glands, including Addison disease associated with gonadal insufficiency, adrenal-thyroid-gonadal insufficiency, diabetes, hypogonadism, adrenal insufficiency, and hypothyroidism. The testicular lesions are morphologically like those seen in seminiferous tubules at the periphery of germ cell tumors and with burned-out germinal cancer. In the initial stages of hyalinization associated with germ cell neoplasm, tubules are small and contain GCNIS and dysgenetic Sertoli cells, and the lamina propria is infiltrated by macrophages, lymphocytes, and plasma cells. In the final stages the intratubular cells have degenerated, inflammation has disappeared, and seminiferous tubules are replaced by areas of hypocellular or acellular fibrosis (Fig. 12.208). Obstructive, ischemic, and dysgenetic types of

hyalinization are more than autoimmune hyalinization in association with testicular tumors.

Hyalinization Caused by Physical or Chemical Agents. Radiation and a wide variety of chemicals cause tubular hyalinization. Prolonged chemotherapy combined with radiation therapy invariably causes hyalinization. Children's testes are most sensitive to radiation. Radiation therapy for testicular leukemia frequently causes tubular hyalinization. In addition, radiation induces dense interstitial fibrosis and loss of peritubular cells, thus obscuring the borders between the interstitium and tubules. This makes the tubules difficult to see in hematoxylin and eosin–stained sections. Leydig cells are atrophic and decreased in number. Ischemia secondary to radiation-induced vascular injury also contributes to hyalinization.

In tubular hyalinization associated with chemotherapy, in addition to direct toxicity of drugs in seminiferous tubular cells (see earlier Sertoli Cell–Only Syndrome With Involuting Sertoli Cells section), nutrition deficiencies cause hypogonadotropic hypogonadism.[1897,1898]

Diffuse Lesions in Spermatogenesis

Histophysiologic studies identify two compartments in seminiferous tubules: basal and adluminal. The blood-testis barrier separates these compartments, and each contains different cell types with diverse hormonal and nutrition requirements. On this basis, lesions may be classified as involving only the adluminal compartment or both the basal and adluminal compartments. The following discussion of spermatogenic lesions uses this newer concept of tubular pathophysiology while conserving the classic terminology as much as possible.

Lesions in the Adluminal Compartment of Seminiferous Tubules. This category includes all infertile testes with normal number of spermatogonia, normal or decreased number of spermatocytes and young spermatids, and variable number of adult spermatids. A descriptive term for this disorder is *immature germ cell sloughing.*

A few immature germ cells are normally seen in the lumina of seminiferous tubules, a finding that correlates with the presence of these cells in the ejaculates of fertile men.[1898,1899] When such cells make up more than 4% of cells in the ejaculate, this finding is

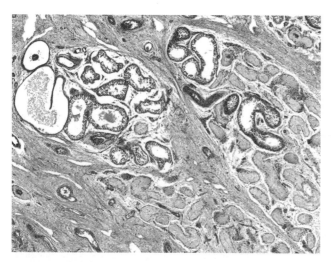

Fig. 12.207 Postobstructive hyalinization. Seminiferous tubules with marked ectasis with hyalinized tubules. Leydig cell clusters are seen among the hyalinized tubules.

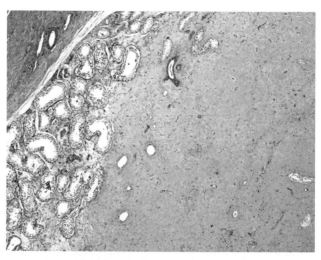

Fig. 12.208 Postinflammatory hyalinization. Most of the testis consists of cicatricial tissue with no recognizable seminiferous tubules.

abnormal and results from premature sloughing of spermatids and, in some cases, of spermatocytes.[1900,1901] Some authors have attempted to establish a correlation between the number of sloughed immature germ cells and severity of lesions of seminiferous epithelium by using light and electron microscopy.[1902,1903]

Lesions in the adluminal compartment are classified according to the most abundant type of germ cell whose maturation is arrested and that then sloughs young spermatids, late primary spermatocytes, or early primary spermatocytes (Fig. 12.209).

Young Spermatid Sloughing. Young spermatid sloughing is present when the ratio of elongate (Sc + Sd) spermatids to round (Sa + Sb) spermatids is lower than normal. The implication of this pattern is that many round spermatids are incapable of further differentiation and slough (Fig. 12.210).

Late Primary Spermatocyte Sloughing. In this condition, spermatogenesis develops normally to the level of interphase primary spermatocytes, which are present in normal numbers. These spermatocytes later degenerate without achieving meiosis and slough into the tubular lumen. All types of spermatids are greatly reduced in number. When biopsies are not properly fixed, seminiferous tubules acquire target-like appearance, with numerous cells in the lumen, an appearance that sometimes has been referred to as *tubular blockage* or *spermatogenic arrest.* The latter term is often inadequate because some spermatids are present, and the number of primary spermatocytes is usually not increased as would occur if the transformation of spermatocyte into spermatid were blocked (Fig. 12.211). *Late spermatocyte sloughing* more accurately names this condition and is preferred. Primary spermatocyte sloughing occurs at the pachytene or diplotene stage of meiosis.

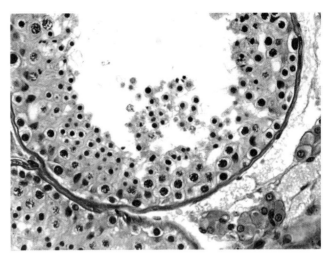

Fig. 12.210 Seminiferous tubule showing a dilated lumen and moderate young spermatid sloughing.

Early Primary Spermatocyte Sloughing. This lesion is characterized by the presence of a normal number of spermatogonia and decreased number of primary spermatocytes (Fig. 12.212). Seminiferous tubules may contain a few spermatids. The term *early primary spermatocyte sloughing* does not necessarily imply an early meiotic lesion, which is quite rare.[1819,1901] Rather, it refers to sloughing of newly formed spermatocytes. Sertoli cells may show vacuolation of the apical cytoplasm as an expression of germ cell loss. This lesion is more severe than that in testes with late primary spermatocyte sloughing and likely results from failure of the Sertoli cells to maintain the adluminal compartment.

Etiology Overview. The mechanisms causing adluminal compartment lesions may be classified as obstructive or nonobstructive. Obstruction is present in more than 70% of cases and is characterized by the variability of involvement among lobules and the presence of at least two of the following abnormalities: enlargement of tubular diameter and lumen with remarkable differences among lobules; Sertoli cells with adherens germ cells protruding into the lumen, thus giving an indented outline; intense apical

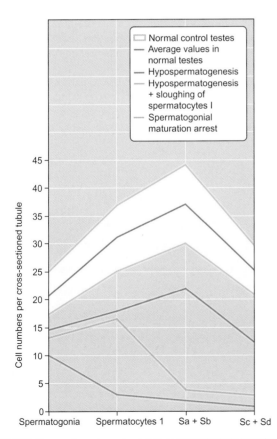

Fig. 12.209 Germ cell numbers per cross-sectioned tubule in patients with lesions in the adluminal compartment of seminiferous tubules.

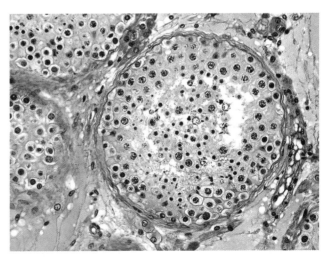

Fig. 12.211 Seminiferous tubule showing sloughing of both primary spermatocytes and young spermatids.

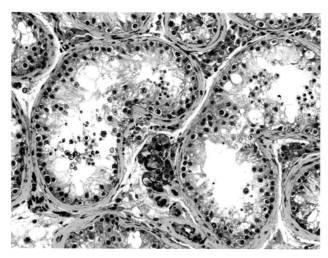

Fig. 12.212 Seminiferous tubules showing dilated lumens, apical vacuolation of Sertoli cells, normal number of spermatogonia, and decreased number of other germ cell types.

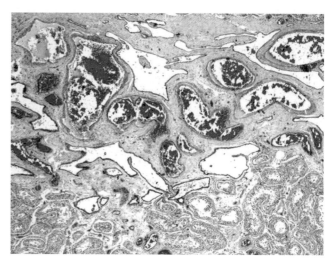

Fig. 12.213 Mediastinum testis from a young man with varicocele. Marked venous dilation (intratesticular varicocele) disrupts and compresses rete testis cavities, causing partial obstruction of the tubuli recti.

vacuolation of Sertoli cell cytoplasm; accumulation of spermatozoa in lumina of some tubules; or number of spermatids Sc + Sd higher than that of Sa + Sb (see the later discussion of Correlation Between Testicular Biopsy and Spermiogram (Obstructive Azoospermia and Oligozoospermia)).[1903a]

The three levels of severity of adluminal compartment lesions emphasized by the terms *young spermatid sloughing*, *later primary spermatocytes sloughing*, and *early primary spermatocyte sloughing* depend on the degree (total or partial) of obstruction and the level of the sperm excretory duct obstruction; the closer the obstruction is to the testis, the greater the severity. Obstruction may be extratesticular (epididymis, vas deferens, and ejaculatory ducts) or intratesticular (rete testis or any level of the seminiferous tubule length). The most frequent causes of extratesticular excretory duct obstruction are vasectomy, inflammation (epididymitis, prostatitis), mucoviscidosis (congenital bilateral absence of vas deferens), and testis-epididymis dissociation.

Rete Testis Obstruction. Varicocele is the most frequent cause of obstruction of the rete testis. More than 50% of testes with varicocele have a mosaic pattern of tubular lesions, together with marked dilation and eccentric mural fibrosis of intratesticular veins. In normal testes, walls of veins are extremely thin, and lumina are nearly collapsed. Patients with varicocele also often have spermatozoa with characteristically elongate heads with thin bases.[1904] Initially, abnormalities are confined to the testis ipsilateral to the varicocele, but eventually both testes are affected, although abnormalities are more severe in the ipsilateral testis. Elevated pressure in the pampiniform plexus is transmitted to the veins within the testes, principally to the centripetal veins that cross the testicular mediastinum and drain most of the parenchyma (Fig. 12.213).[1905] Dilated centripetal veins compress the intratesticular sperm excretory ducts, a finding that explains the mosaic distribution of the tubular lesions.[1905a]

Seminiferous Tubule Obstruction. Obstruction at the level of seminiferous tubules may be dysgenetic or postorchitic. Dysgenesis may be suspected in specimens with mosaic distribution of lesions and seminiferous tubules with small diameters, thickened lamina propria, and an unusual tubular cell layer consisting of cuboidal Sertoli cells and spermatozoa that clog the lumina (Fig. 12.214). Diagnosis is confirmed by study of serial sections demonstrating

continuity between the altered tubules and those with conserved spermatogenesis.[1821,1906] This tubular stenosis appears to result from primary anomaly of Sertoli cells and peritubular cells.

Postorchitic obstruction should be suspected in cases of tubular atrophy with a mosaic pattern without dysgenetic tubules or varicocele. Some patients have histories of orchitis associated with parotiditis, whereas in others the only findings are oligozoospermia and small testes.[1907] Biopsy with sampling of the periphery reveals the consequences of obstruction, similar to lesions observed with varicocele. However, some postinflammatory changes are also present, including hyalinized tubules, dilated tubules lined by cuboidal Sertoli cells, or complete spermatogenesis. Occasionally, modest perivascular or peritubular inflammation and angiectasis are noted.[1908,1909]

Approximately 30% of testes with lesions in the adluminal compartment have no obstruction, and most have primary anomalies of germ cells. This claim is supported by the pronounced decrease of germ cell type when the preceding type is greatly increased in

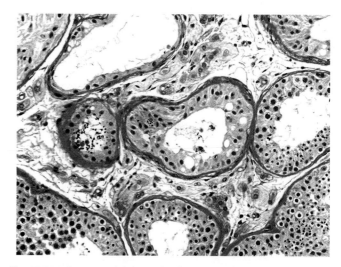

Fig. 12.214 Segmented dysgenesis of seminiferous tubules. The two central tubules, which display only dysgenetic Sertoli cells, contain numerous spermatozoa that come from adjacent seminiferous tubules with normal spermatogenesis.

number, the normal correlation between number of mature spermatids in the biopsy and number of spermatozoa in the spermiogram, and the presence of numerous malformed germ cells in the adluminal compartment.

Decrease in the number of germ cell types may be so significant that spermatogenesis is arrested, with subsequent azoospermia. In some cases, maturation arrest is only partial and results in severe oligozoospermia. This maturation arrest is observed mainly in primary spermatocytes and young spermatids.

Primary spermatocyte sloughing may also result from meiotic anomalies (Fig. 12.215). The observation of increased number of spermatocytes arrested in preleptotene-leptotene or, more frequently, pachytene, suggests the diagnosis.[1819,1901] The lesion is always bilateral. Spermatocytes arrested in pachytene are usually increased in size and later degenerate. In addition, some spermatids have large, diploid, spherical, hyperchromatic nuclei. The anomaly does not always affect all spermatocytes, and a higher number of spermatids is produced.[1819] Primary meiotic arrest may result from lack of expression of several genes such as the absence of BOULE protein expression, altered expression of heat shock transcription factor, Y chromosome (HSFY), HSPA2, downregulation of microRNA-383, lack of expression of survivin, or lack of expression of *BET* genes.[1910–1915] Meiotic arrest is also associated with copy number variations and TEX11 deletions and mutations.[1916,1917] Young spermatid sloughing not associated with obstruction may result from meiotic anomalies or defective spermiogenesis. Meiotic anomalies give rise to the appearance of many multinucleate, polyploid, hyperchromatic young spermatids. In defective spermiogenesis, young spermatids are incapable of transforming into mature spermatids, and only round spermatids appear in the ejaculate.

Lesions in the Basal and Adluminal Compartments of Seminiferous Tubules. Lesions in the basal and adluminal compartments of seminiferous tubules are the most frequent finding in biopsies from infertile men and are classified as hypospermatogenesis or spermatogonial maturation arrest (Fig. 12.216).

Hypospermatogenesis: Types and Etiology. Hypospermatogenesis is defined as reduced number of spermatogonia and primary spermatocytes, with primary spermatocytes outnumbering spermatogonia. Most seminiferous tubules contain few spermatids. Approximately 8% of patients with hypospermatogenesis have focal tubular hyalinization.[1918] Two variants of hypospermatogenesis have been quantitatively distinguished: pure hypospermatogenesis and hypospermatogenesis associated with sloughing of primary spermatocytes.

Pure hypospermatogenesis is defined as a proportionate decrease in the number of all types of germ cells. The number of spermatogonia per cross-sectioned tubule is lower than 17 and usually higher than 10. The number of primary spermatocytes is equal to or higher than that of spermatogonia. The number of round spermatids is higher than that of primary spermatocytes, and the number of elongate spermatids is equivalent to that of spermatogonia (Fig. 12.217).

Hypospermatogenesis associated with primary spermatocyte sloughing is characterized by two features: low numbers of spermatogonia and primary spermatocytes (with spermatocytes more numerous than spermatogonia), and degeneration and sloughing of many primary spermatocytes. The remaining spermatocytes give rise to the few spermatids observed in the tubules (Fig. 12.218).

Etiology of Hypospermatogenesis: Overview. Hypospermatogenesis may result from hormonal dysfunction, congenital germ cell deficiency, Sertoli cell dysfunction, Leydig cell dysfunction, androgen insensitivity, exposure to chemical or physical agents, and vascular malfunction.

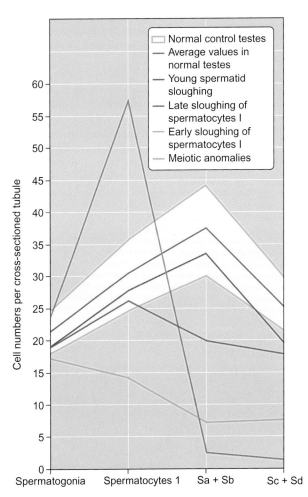

Fig. 12.216 Germ cell numbers per cross-sectioned tubule in patients with lesions in the basal and adluminal compartments of seminiferous tubules.

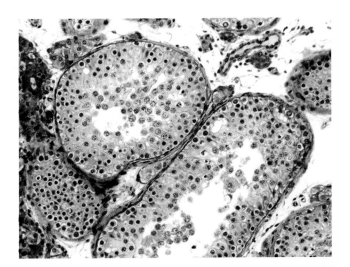

Fig. 12.215 Meiotic abnormalities. The seminiferous tubules contain a normal number of spermatogonia and a disproportionately high number of primary spermatocytes, which do not complete meiosis. No spermatids are seen.

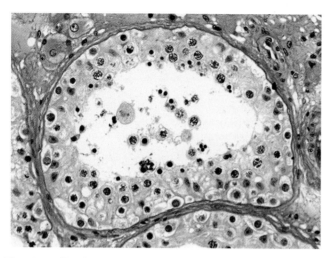

Fig. 12.217 Pure hypospermatogenesis in a patient with severe oligozoospermia. The seminiferous tubule shows slight ectasis and a proportionate decrease of all germ cell types.

Hormonal Dysregulation. Although complete spermatogenesis may be observed in men with low levels of FSH and LH, production of normal numbers of spermatozoa requires normal gonadotropin levels. Hypospermatogenesis may occur in patients with abnormal pulsatile secretion of FSH and LH, low gonadotropin secretion, biologically inactive gonadotropins, mutation in the gonadotropin β subunit, inactivating mutations of the FSHR gene, hyperprolactinemia, and adrenal and thyroid dysfunction (see later Hypogonadism Secondary to Endocrine Gland Dysfunction and Other Disorders section).[1753,1919–1922]

Congenital Germ Cell Deficiency. Testicular biopsy of cryptorchid patients after orchidopexy reveals that spermatogonial proliferation is decreased and germ cell development is insufficient in adulthood even if the number of spermatogonia was normal in infancy. This poorly understood primary anomaly of germ cells is likely present in some cases of hypospermatogenesis.

Sertoli Cell Dysfunction. For many years, primary germ cell deficiency was considered the most common cause of hypospermatogenesis; today, Sertoli cell failure is recognized as the cause of

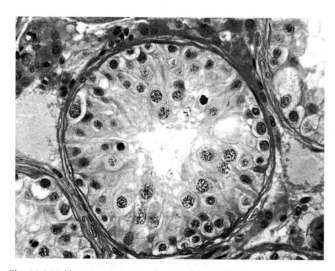

Fig. 12.218 Hypospermatogenesis associated with primary spermatocyte sloughing in an azoospermic patient. Spermatogonia and primary spermatocytes are the sole germ cell types.

many cases of germ cell deficiency. This conclusion is based on several findings. Sertoli cells of infertile patients are often markedly abnormal, with increase in number of glycogen granules and acid phosphatase activity, decrease in number of lipid droplets, and alterations in the cytoskeleton, nucleus, and cytoplasmic organelles.[1753,1859,1923–1925] Sertoli cells may have abnormal maturation, with elongate nuclei containing coarse chromatin masses instead of triangular nuclei with pale chromatin. Anomalies in Sertoli cell FSHRs may be present in idiopathic oligozoospermia associated with elevated levels of FSH.[1926] Serum inhibin B concentration may be used as a marker to estimate Sertoli cell function.[1927]

Leydig Cell Dysfunction. Testosterone synthesis by Leydig cells is necessary for normal spermatogenesis, and abnormal Leydig cell function is detected in 10% to 20% of patients with azoospermia or oligozoospermia and idiopathic infertility.[1928–1931] Leydig cell dysfunction should be suspected when the cells appear diffusely hyperplastic. Patients have elevated serum LH with depletion of rapid-release testosterone, revealing lack of early response of Leydig cells to GnRH stimulation. The ratio of testosterone to LH in plasma indicates the severity of Leydig cell dysfunction. Decreased ratio with normal testosterone suggests compensated dysfunction. Patients with a ratio less than 1:5 and otherwise normal parameters may complete spermatogenesis.[1931] In development of this dysfunction of Leydig cells, overexpression of CYP19A1 aromatase by chronic stimulation of LH may play an important role. This situation would lead to higher production of estradiol, which would negatively affect androgen biosynthesis by Leydig cells.[1932]

Androgen Insensitivity. Some patients with severe oligozoospermia or azoospermia have a defect in AR responsiveness, similar to that noted in Reifenstein syndrome.[1700,1933,1934] The abnormality may arise from a genetic defect in the eight exons that code for this receptor, mapped to Xq11–12, or from posttranslational errors.[1726,1730,1935] This defect is also referred to as *infertile male syndrome* and *MAIS*, and patients have male phenotype with somatic features of slight androgen deficit.[1936] Histologically the testis is similar to that observed in Leydig cell dysfunction or MAT, although the mechanism causing Leydig cell hyperplasia is quite different (Fig. 12.219). Peripheral resistance to testosterone action alters regulation of the hypothalamohypophyseal-testicular axis, and LH and testosterone levels are elevated. The frequency of RA mutations in patients with azoospermia or oligozoospermia who consult for infertility is estimated at 2% to 3%.[1937] In such cases, spermatogenesis improves with administration of tamoxifen citrate, clomiphene citrate, or androgen therapy.[1710,1731,1938] Calculation of the index of androgen insensitivity may be helpful: plasma LH (mIU/mL) × plasma testosterone levels (ng/mL). In patients with androgen insensitivity the index is greater than 200 (normal is ~102).

Physical and Chemical Agents. The number of chemicals implicated in infertility increases daily. Detailed history is invaluable in evaluating these patients. The same is true of physical agents such as prolonged exposure to heat, ionizing radiations, or microwave radiation.[1939]

Etiology of Hypospermatogenesis Associated With Primary Spermatocyte Sloughing. Most testes with primary spermatocyte sloughing have varicocele, and this is commonly associated with infertility.[573,1940–1942] Varicocele is found in 15% of the general population and is present in 30% to 40% of infertile men. The mechanism by which varicocele affects fertility is unknown. Clinical varicocele may occur without a testicular lesion (or only phlebectasis), and subclinical varicocele may be associated with severe spermatogenic lesions. Increased testicular temperature and

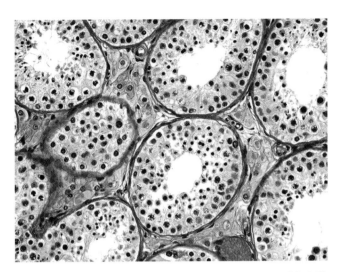

Fig. 12.219 Hypospermatogenesis due to androgen receptor defect. The seminiferous tubules show hypospermatogenesis associated with diffuse Leydig cell hyperplasia.

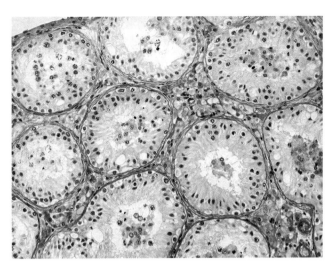

Fig. 12.220 Spermatogonial maturation arrest. The seminiferous tubules have increased numbers of Sertoli cells and nearly normal number of spermatogonia, whereas the remaining germ cell types are scant. The testicular interstitium shows diffuse Leydig cell hyperplasia.

compression of intratesticular sperm excretory ducts by dilated veins are the most plausible mechanisms.[1905a,1943,1944] In other cases, primary spermatocyte sloughing results from anomalies of primary spermatocytes and spermatids, a finding suggesting meiotic anomaly. Finally, in some patients the cause may be the presence of involuting Sertoli cells.

Spermatogonial Maturation Arrest. Spermatogonial maturation arrest is defined by the presence of fewer than 17 spermatogonia per cross-sectioned tubule and even fewer primary spermatocytes. Spermatids are usually absent. Attempts have been made to correlate the etiology of spermatogonial maturation arrest with the Sertoli cell type.[1945] Immature Sertoli cells are characteristic of hypogonadotropic hypogonadism and some AISs (Fig. 12.220). Mature Sertoli cells, if their presence is unilateral, are observed in varicocele, epididymitis, and ipsilateral testicular traumatism, but if they appear in both testes, the etiology is unknown. Involuting Sertoli cells are usually present bilaterally; some cases are idiopathic, whereas others are associated with a history of alcoholism or chemotherapy. Dedifferentiated Sertoli cells are found in spermatogonial maturation arrest caused by gonadotropin inhibition in treatment with estrogen, GnRH agonists, or antiandrogen.[1946,1947]

Focal Lesions in Spermatogenesis (Mixed Atrophy). *Mixed atrophy (MAT)* is a descriptive term for the coexistence, in the same testis, of Sertoli cell–only tubules and tubules with complete or incomplete spermatogenesis (Fig. 12.221).[1948] This disorder includes patchy failure of spermatogenesis and partial Del Castillo syndrome.

The extent of Sertoli cell–only tubules varies widely. Tubules with spermatogenesis may be normal or partially atrophic. Tubular hyalinization is occasionally seen. The interstitium shows an increase in mast cell number.[1949] MAT is more common than suggested by the literature, and many cases are included under other diagnoses, such as "hypospermatogenesis with severe germ cell depletion in such a way that some Sertoli cell–only tubules are seen" and "Sertoli cell–only syndromes with focal spermatogenesis."[1950]

Serial sections from testes with MAT reveal that the two different types of tubules are grouped according to their histologic pattern, a finding suggesting that their distribution is by testicular

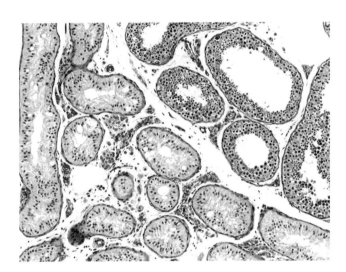

Fig. 12.221 Mixed atrophy. Seminiferous tubules showing slight ectasis and complete spermatogenesis adjacent to Sertoli cell–only pattern. The tubular lesions probably belong to a different lobule.

lobules. In cases of MAT the percentage of tubules with spermatogenesis, the degree of spermatogenic development in these tubules, and the type of Sertoli cells present should be reported. Correlation of the first two with the spermiogram gives an indication of prognosis, whereas the Sertoli cell type identifies the nature (primary or secondary) of the lesion (Fig. 12.222).[245]

MAT (probably primary) is observed in idiopathic infertility, cryptorchidism (even if orchidopexy was done in infancy, in both the cryptorchid and contralateral descended testes), retractile testes, macroorchidism, intravaginal torsion of the spermatic cord (in both twisted and contralateral testis), and chromosomal anomalies such as Down syndrome, 47,XYY karyotype, 46,XX karyotype, giant Y chromosome, Klinefelter syndrome with chromosomal mosaicism, Y-chromosome microdeletions, PAIS, some undermasculinization male (DSD), and in parenchyma peripheral to germ cell tumor.[1951,1952] Secondary MAT is sometimes seen in patients undergoing chemotherapy, receiving glucocorticoid

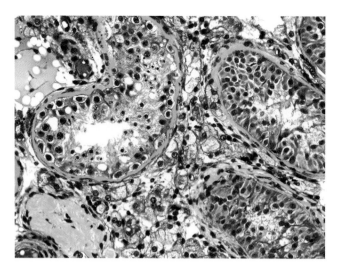

Fig. 12.222 Mixed atrophy. Tubules on the left have complete although quantitatively abnormal spermatogenesis, and Sertoli cell–only tubules on the right have Sertoli cells with nuclei of dysgenetic characteristics and intensely eosinophilic cytoplasm suggesting a primary lesion. Leydig cells show microvacuolated cytoplasm.

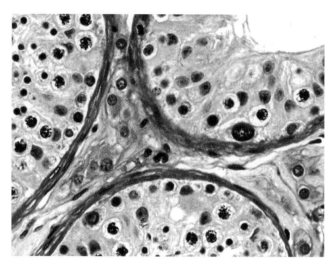

Fig. 12.223 Hypertrophic spermatogonia in a seminiferous tubule showing marked decrease in the number of spermatogenetic cells.

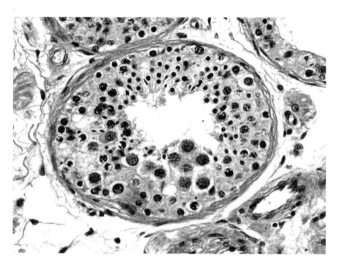

Fig. 12.224 Megalospermatocytes. The seminiferous tubule contains a group of large primary spermatocytes displaying fine chromatin and eosinophilic cytoplasm.

therapy, with a history of viral orchitis, and in the parenchyma peripheral to a germ cell tumor.[1882]

Germ Cell Anomalies in Infertile Patients

In addition to identifying anomalies in seminiferous tubules, examination of the biopsy should include morphology of the germ cells.

Giant Spermatogonia

Isolated giant spermatogonia are normal components of the seminiferous epithelium. These cells may be altered spermatogonia in the S or G_2 phase of the cell cycle. They rest on the basal lamina, and have pale cytoplasm and ovoid nuclei measuring at least 13 μm in diameter. The frequency of these cells in normal and infertile men is approximately 0.65 cells per 50 cross-sectioned tubules, although the number is usually higher in MAT. These cells should not be mistaken for GCNIS; they are also present in normal numbers in tubules at the periphery of germ cell tumor (Fig. 12.223).[1953]

Multinucleate Spermatogonia

Multinucleate spermatogonia are common in cryptorchid testes that were surgically corrected, in infertile patients, and in old men. Nuclei of both Ad and Ap spermatogonial types may be seen within the same cell.

Dislocated Spermatogonia

Normally, spermatogonia are present in the transition zone between the seminiferous tubule basal layer and tubuli recti. Dislocated spermatogonia may be found throughout the testis in old age, in infertile patients with a variety of lesions, after long-term estrogen therapy, and in seminiferous tubules with intratubular germ cell neoplasia.[1954–1956]

Megalospermatocytes

Megalospermatocytes are large primary spermatocytes arrested in the leptotene stage (Fig. 12.224), which exhibit asynapsis of chromosomes.[1957,1958] Joined by cytoplasmic bridges, they form small groups. These cells may be clones of synchronously degenerating spermatocytes.[1959] They are frequently found in older men and are a nonspecific finding in infertile patients.

Multinucleate Spermatids

The presence of spermatids with multiple nuclei (from 2 to 86) is frequent in old age.[1960] Similar cells with fewer nuclei have also been reported in infertility secondary to cryptorchidism or hyperprolactinemia, as well as in idiopathic infertility (Fig. 12.225).[1961]

Malformed Spermatids

At least four teratozoospermic syndromes may be easily identified by biopsy, although the diagnosis of most previously relied on morphologic study of the spermiogram: (1) round-headed spermatids (characteristic of spermatozoa lacking acrosomes) (Fig. 12.226); (2) Sc + Sd spermatids with elongate head (characteristic of varicocele) (Fig. 12.227); (3) macrocephalic Sc + Sd spermatids whose DNA content suggests an anomaly in the first meiotic division; and (4) Sc + Sd spermatids with voluminous eosinophilic cytoplasmic droplets (syndrome of spermatozoa with short, thick flagella or fibrous sheath dysplasia[1962]).

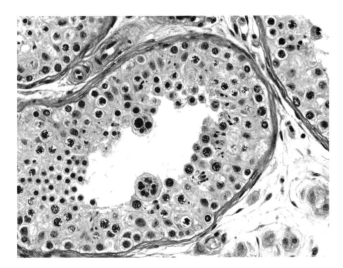

Fig. 12.225 Multinucleation of both spermatids and spermatocytes.

In some patients, Sa + Sb spermatids are present in the initial phases of spermiogenesis and eventually become sloughed.[1963] Other testes have macrocephalic Sc + Sd spermatids with anomalous DNA content, findings suggesting an anomaly in the first meiotic division.

Morphologically Abnormal Spermatozoa

Ultrastructural study of spermatozoa is sometimes necessary to determine the cause of male infertility. Some morphologically abnormal spermatozoa are seen in all semen samples, including those from fertile men, but abnormal spermatozoa are most numerous in infertile patients. Ultrastructural study of spermatozoa is valuable for identifying spermatozoal disorders, but it is also useful for assisted reproductive technology and genetic risk assessment; it is advised in all cases of asthenozoospermia, in teratozoospermia when the number of spermatozoa showing the same morphologic anomaly is high, and in cases with apparently normal spermatozoa that fail to fertilize in vitro.[1964–1966] Classification is based on light microscopic findings of lesions in the head and tail.[1967]

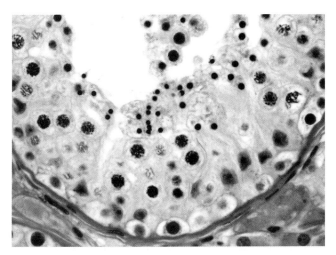

Fig. 12.226 Testicular biopsy showing spermatids with small spherical nuclei, a finding characteristic of round spermatozoa lacking acrosomes. The remaining germ cells are morphologically normal.

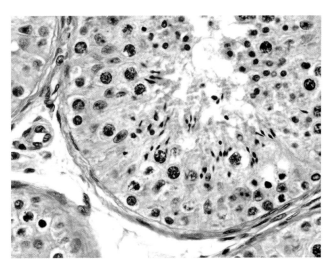

Fig. 12.227 Elongate spermatids showing a bell-clapper nucleus in a varicocele patient.

Anomalies of the Spermatozoal Head

Anomalies of the spermatozoal head are defined by changes in the shape of the spermatozoal head and usually involve both the nucleus and acrosome. Some anomalies, such as pear-shaped, candle-shaped, or egg-shaped heads, are regarded as minor variants of normal.[426,1968] Significant abnormalities are the elongate, microcephalic, macrocephalic, and crater defect forms. The most frequent abnormal head shape is elongate with a narrow base (tapered head spermatozoa), commonly associated with varicocele.[1969]

Microcephalic spermatozoa have spherical (globozoospermia) or irregularly shaped heads. Microcephalic spermatozoa with spherical heads contain round nuclei with poorly condensed chromatin and lack acrosomes, postacrosomal sheaths, and a nuclear ring (Figs. 12.228 and 12.229). Most cases are sporadic, but this lesion was also reported in two pairs of infertile brothers.[1970–1972] Microcephalic spermatozoa with irregularly shaped heads have small and irregular acrosomes that usually are not in contact with the nucleus. This anomaly may be congenital, as in Aarskog-Scott syndrome, or secondary to heat exposure or hashish smoking.[1973] In both types of microcephaly, loss of connection between the acrosomal vesicle and spermatozoal head is attributed to a deficiency in basic proteins of the sperm perinuclear theca that promotes nuclear envelope organization and adhesion of the acrosomal vesicle.[1974] Acrosin is reduced or absent in spermatozoa lacking acrosomes and in those with small acrosomes.[1975] Motility may be normal. The occurrence of aneuploidy and disomy of sex chromosomes in some cases should be evaluated before performing Intracytoplasmatic sperm injection (ICSI).[1976–1978]

The responsible genetic defect of most cases is 200-kb homozygous deletion of DPY19L2.[1979] This transmembrane protein, located in the inner nuclear membrane, ensures attachment of the acrosome to the nucleus. Because of defect, the acrosome is not formed and manchette does not produce elongation of the nucleus. Other genes responsible of globozoospermia are *SPATA16*, *PICK1*, and *DPY19L2*.[1980–1982]

Macrocephalic spermatozoa (macronuclear spermatozoa) have enlarged, irregular heads and deficient chromatin condensation. Both types (multiple tails and aflagellate) have abnormal DNA content (many are tetraploid), a finding suggesting meiotic anomaly, and are associated with increased frequency of

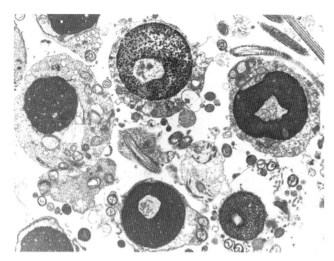

Fig. 12.228 Microcephalic spermatozoa with spherical nuclei lacking acrosome and poorly condensed chromatin. Ultrastructural anomalies are observed.

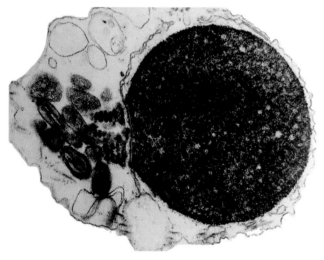

Fig. 12.229 Microcephalic spermatozoa without acrosome (globozoospermia).

aneuploidy.[1983–1987] Most patients harbor homozygous truncating mutations in the aurora kinase gene (*AURKC*), which acts preferentially in meiotic chromosomal segregation and cytokinesis.[1988,1989]

Irregular spermatozoa are characterized by altered shape of the nucleus or acrosome.[1990] In crater defect syndrome the acrosome penetrates an invagination of the nuclear envelope. The tail is morphologically normal, and motility is only slightly reduced. In spermatozoa with spoon-shaped nuclei the defect is probably genetic. Other anomalies include double-headed spermatozoa with two nuclei sharing a single acrosome.[1991]

Anomalies of the Spermatozoal Tail

Spermatozoal tail anomalies are classified as generalized anomalies or anomalies of defined tail components such as the connecting piece, the axoneme, or periaxonemal structures.[1992]

Cytoplasmic Remnants. The presence of cytoplasmic droplets is normal during spermiogenesis. Increased number of spermatozoa with cytoplasmic droplets in semen is associated with premature sloughing, as occurs in varicocele, and should not be misinterpreted as spermatozoa with excess residual cytoplasm.[1993] These spermatozoa are often abnormal, and the residual cytoplasm may be located around the intermediate piece or surrounding the head. These spermatozoa also have other flagellar anomalies.

Bent Tail. A bend in the tail may occur at the level of the connecting piece or the intermediate piece. In bends of the connecting piece the tail is laterally implanted and forms an angle with a nucleus that displays a thin base. Bends of the intermediate piece are associated with cytoplasmic droplets, malposition of mitochondria, and loss of parallel arrangement of the dense outer fibers. Spermatozoa with bent tail may show anomalies secondary to a mutation in *Septine12*, a testis-specific gene critical for terminal differentiation of male germ cells.[1994]

Coiled Tail. Spermatozoa with coiled tail are a frequent finding in centrifuged semen, but may also be a true abnormality. These spermatozoa have a perinuclear cytoplasmic remnant containing a flagellum that is coiled around the nucleus and along the middle or principal pieces (Fig. 12.230). This finding is frequently associated with abnormalities of the periaxonemal structures.

Tail Stump (Short-Tail Spermatozoa). The presence of many spermatozoa with short, thick tails in semen represents a well-defined teratozoospermic syndrome (Fig. 12.231).[1995] Ultrastructural examination reveals hypertrophy and hyperplasia of the fibrous sheath (Figs. 12.232 and 12.233), hence this syndrome has also been termed *fibrous sheath dysplasia*.[1996,1997] Additional axonemal malformations may be identified, including absence of the central pair of microtubules, lack of dynein arms, and anomalies in head–neck junction.[1998,1999] Anomalies in the fibrous sheath may be demonstrated using antibodies against antiacetylated tubulin and anti-FSC1 (the major protein components of the fibrous sheath).[2000] Approximately 24% of patients have respiratory disease from an early age, including rhinosinusitis, bronchitis, and bronchiectasis. Similar findings have been reported in the cilia of the upper respiratory tract, and thus a relationship between fibrous sheath dysplasia and immotile cilia syndrome has been assumed. The clinical presentation may be sporadic or familial. The cause of the fibrous sheath dysplasia and subsequent lack of motility in spermatozoa is probably related to deletions in *AKAP3*

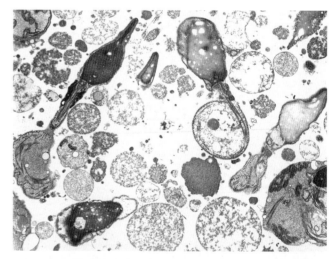

Fig. 12.230 Spermatozoa with coiled tails. The anomaly occurs in the principal pieces. The intermediate pieces show variable lengths, absence of parallelism in the outer dense fibers, and large cytoplasmic droplets. This teratozoospermia was found in two infertile brothers.

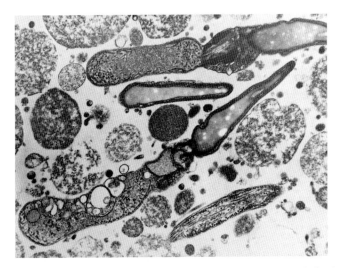

Fig. 12.231 Dysplasia of the fibrous sheath associated with hypoplasia of the intermediate piece in a patient with short and thick spermatozoa under light microscopy.

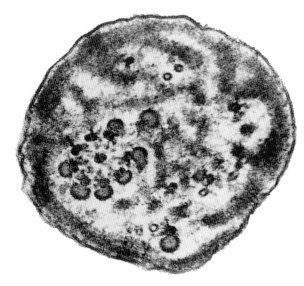

Fig. 12.233 Dysplasia of the fibrous sheath associated with disorganization of dense fibers and microtubules.

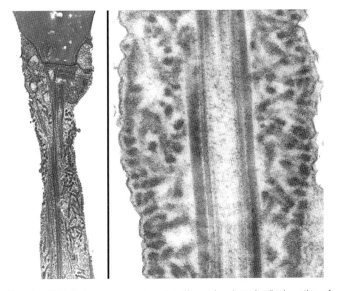

Fig. 12.232 Tail-stump spermatozoal malformation. Longitudinal section of two spermatozoa showing a marked thickening of the principal piece with both hypertrophy and hyperplasia of the fibrous sheath. The one on the left also shows a short intermediate piece.

and *AKAP4* genes and absence of AKP4 protein in the fibrous sheath.[2001]

Multiple Tails. The presence of more than two tails is associated with macrocephalic spermatozoa.[1135]

Sperm Tail Agenesis. Teratozoospermia with 100% sperm tail agenesis has been reported in patients with a high degree of consanguinity. These spermatozoa also have defects in chromatin condensation and residual cytoplasmic droplets.[2002]

Sperm With Abnormal Elongation of the Tail. Abnormally elongate tails are associated with frequent ruptures at different levels, coiled tails, and a strongly rolled axoneme, among other malformations. These abnormalities are considered to have a genetic origin.[2003]

Anomalies of the Connecting Piece

Anomalies of the connecting piece are classified as acephalic spermatozoa, deficient organization of the connecting piece, or separation between the head and the tail.

Acephalic spermatozoa are known as "pin-headed," although they lack a true head; the small, cephalic, knoblike thickening is actually a cytoplasmic droplet with variable degree of mitochondrial organization giving rise to variable degree of motility.[2004] This anomaly is secondary to early failure in spermiogenesis. It may be familial in some cases.[2005,2006] Spermatozoa with deficient organization of the connecting piece have narrowing at this level, with loss of alignment of the head and flagellum axes. This may occur through one of the following mechanisms: (1) failure in the postnuclear region to form the basal plaque and the implantation fossa, (2) chemical anomaly of the filamentous material present between the capitellum and the basal plaque, or (3) abnormal position of the tail over the caudal pole of the nuclei during flagellum development.[2007,2008] Spermatozoa with a separated head and flagellum, known as decapitated and decaudated spermatozoa, also result from an anomaly in spermiogenesis, but separation between head and tail may occur during spermiation or at any level of the sperm excretory ducts. Failure of the head-tail coupling apparatus is caused by centriole dysfunction and deficient assembly of the manchette.[2009,2010]

Anomalies of the Axoneme

Abnormalities of the axoneme are classified as numeric anomalies, microtubule ectopia, or the immotile cilia syndrome. The most common numeric anomalies are the absence of one or both microtubules of the central pair and the complete lack of the axoneme. Spermatozoa lacking the central microtubule pair also lack the central sheath and are immotile, although they appear normal by light microscopy (Fig. 12.234). Familial cases have been reported.[2011] This anomaly may be associated with ciliary dyskinesia.[2012]

The immotile cilia syndrome (primary ciliary dyskinesia) refers to patients having low mucociliary clearance associated with otitis, sinusitis, bronchitis, bronchiectasis, and immotile spermatozoa.[2013] Most patients have the same defect in the axoneme and cilia of the respiratory mucosa. The frequency of this syndrome

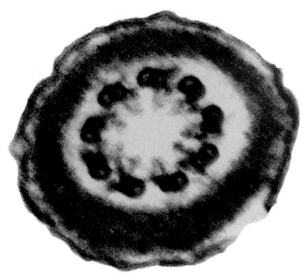

Fig. 12.234 Cross section of the main piece of a spermatozoid showing absence of the pair of central microtubules and the central sheath.

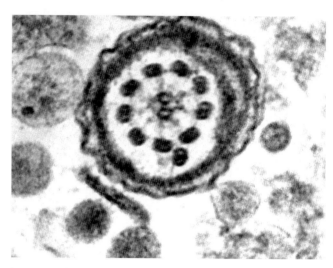

Fig. 12.236 Cross section of the principal piece from spermatozoa lacking in dynein arms and showing a supernumerary microtubule doublet.

is estimated at between 1 in 20,000 and 1 in 60,000 men. Clinical symptoms consist of reduced clearance of ciliary mucus in the airway, with onset in infancy. To prevent subsequent development of bronchiectasis, ultrastructural study of the respiratory mucosa is advisable if other disorders have been excluded, including cystic fibrosis (CF), allergy and other immune disorders, α_1-antitrypsin deficiency, and cardiovascular and metabolic diseases.[2014] The most frequent anomalies are absence of the following: microtubule doublets and peripheral junctions, central microtubule pair, outer dynein arms, central junctions, the two dynein arms, and the inner dynein arm plus the peripheral junctions (Figs. 12.235 and 12.236). Spermatozoa lacking the two dynein arms or peripheral junctions are immotile. Reduced motility is seen in spermatozoa with only one dynein arm.

Kartagener syndrome is a variant of the immotile cilia syndrome characterized by the classic triad of situs inversus, bronchiectasis, and chronic sinusitis. It is autosomal recessive, and found in 20% to 25% of patients with situs inversus.[2015,2016] Although spermatozoa are immotile, pregnancy has been achieved with assisted reproductive techniques such as subzonal insemination; ICSI, either isolated or associated with hypoosmotic swelling test; and in vitro fertilization.[2017–2020]

The cause of primary ciliary dyskinesia has been identified in 50% of cases, particularly in mutations of several genes and chromosomal loci. The most common causes are mutations in DNAH5 (28%).[2021–2022] Other genes responsible for isolated cases are DNAI2, DNAH11, TXNDC3, DNAAF3, mutations in RSPH9 and RSPH4A encoding two radial spoke head proteins that produce defects in the central pair, and mutations in CCDC39 and CCDC40 causing misplacement of the central pair of microtubules.[2023,2024] Mutations in genes encoding cytoplasmic proteins such as KTU and LRRCSO may also be implicated in assembly of dynein arms.[2025]

Anomalies of Periaxonemal Structures

Periaxonemal abnormalities include mitochondrial sheath defects; malposition or the annulus; alteration in number, shape, or length of the outer dense fibers; and absence, thickening, or disruption of the fibrous sheath.[1997,2026,2027]

Many of the asthenozoospermias, present in 30% of infertile men, may be attributable to deficient mitochondrial function that is measured by respiratory control ratio.[2028] The 7436-bp deletions of mitochondrial DNA are one of the most common causes of nonmotile sperm.[2028,2029] Abnormalities of dense fibers are associated with deficient motility. Abnormalities of the fibrous sheath include previously mentioned dysplasia, absence, and redundant fibrous sheath material associated with deficit or lack of mitochondria.[2030,2031] The three defects are probably inherited. Spermatozoa with fewer mitochondrial gyres have a shorter midpiece, whereas spermatozoa with a great number of gyres have a larger midpiece.[2032]

Presence of Tumoral Cells

The incidence rate of GCNIS in infertile patients is 0.4% in England, 0.7% in Spain, 0.73% in Germany, and 1.1% in Denmark.[2033–2036] A higher risk occurs in patients with severe oligozoospermia (<10 million spermatozoa/mL), azoospermia associated with unilaterally or bilaterally diminished

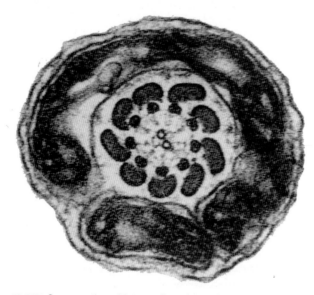

Fig. 12.235 Cross section of intermediate piece of a spermatozoid with absence of both dynein arms.

testicular volume, history of maldescent, or unilateral testicular cancer.[1078,2037–2039]

The cells of GCNIS are in seminiferous tubules with decreased tubular diameter that lack spermatogenesis. The cells are large, have pale cytoplasm, and display large and irregular nuclei with one or several prominent nucleoli. They stain intensely with PAS and express PLAP, KIT, OCT3/4, and the cell adhesion molecule CD44.[2040]

Anomalies of Leydig Cells

Absence or paucity of Leydig cells is infrequent in infertility. It occurs in hypogonadotropic hypogonadisms secondary to LH deficit and in patients with biologically inactive LH.

Leydig cell hyperplasia is common.[1656] It may occur in Klinefelter syndrome, cryptorchidism, undermasculinization, minor androgen insensitivity, infertility secondary to Leydig cell dysfunction, varicocele, after treatment with 5α-reductase inhibitors or nonsteroidal antiandrogens, and in older men. Hyperplasia may give rise to hypoechoic or hyperechoic images that may be misdiagnosed as tumor.[2041]

Mast Cells

A close relationship exists between testicular dysfunction and elevated mast cell number in the testis, epididymis, and seminal fluid. An increase in interstitial and peritubular mast cells occurs in many patients with azoospermia or oligozoospermia.[417,2042–2044] A significant increase in mast cells has also been observed in semen from patients with varicocele and idiopathic asthenozoospermia.[2045,2046] Surgical treatment of varicocele and daily administration of ketotifen, an antihistamine-like drug with mast cell–stabilizing effect, significantly improves spermiogram parameters in some patients.[2047,2048]

Macrophages

Macrophages are a common component of the interstitium, maintaining a paracrine relationship with Leydig cells. The CD68+ macrophage count is increased in patients with obstructive azoospermia when compared with patients with nonobstructive azoospermia.[2049]

Correlation Between Testicular Biopsy and Spermiogram

For effective therapy, it is important to know whether azoospermia or oligozoospermia is the result of obstruction.[1826,2050]

Obstructive Azoospermia and Oligozoospermia

Azoospermia caused by obstruction is usually easily diagnosed, but identification is more difficult with oligozoospermia. Obstruction of the ductal system should be suspected when there are more than 20 mature spermatids (Sc + Sd) per cross-sectioned tubule and fewer than 10 million spermatozoa in the spermiogram (Fig. 12.237).[2051,2052] Obstructive azoospermia is implicated in 7% to 14% of cases of male infertility.

Classification of Obstructive Azoospermia by Location

Obstruction is classified as proximal, distal, or mixed according to the distance from the testis to the point of obstruction in the ductal system.

Proximal Obstruction. Obstruction is considered proximal when the lesion lies between the seminiferous tubules and the distal end of the ampulla of the vas deferens. Epididymal obstruction,

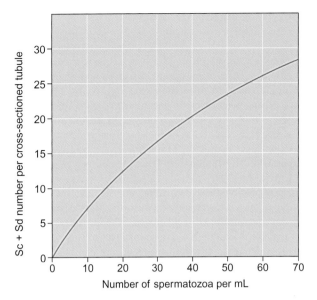

Fig. 12.237 Power curve showing the correlation between the number of spermatozoa in the spermiogram and the number of mature spermatids (Sc +Sd) per cross-sectioned tubule. If the number of mature spermatids is correlated to that of spermatozoa in spermiogram, the oligozoospermia is of the pure secretory type. If the number of mature spermatids is higher than that of spermatozoa in spermiogram, the disorder is either an obstructive azoospermia with "normal" testicular biopsy or a mixed obstructive secretory oligozoospermia.

principally of the caput-corpus transition zone, accounts for 66% of cases. Rarely, defective connection is present between the rete testis and epididymal ductuli efferentes. The seminal vesicles are normal, so men with proximal obstruction have normal volume of semen (the testicular contribution to semen is only 5% of the total volume). When obstruction is in the cauda of the epididymis, levels of epididymal markers, including carnitine, glycerophosphorylcholine, and α-glycosidase, are low.[2053] The nearer the obstruction is to the caput of the epididymis, the higher the levels.

Distal Obstruction. Distal obstruction is located between the ampulla of the vas deferens and the junction of the ejaculatory ducts and urethra. These patients present with sacral, perineal, or scrotal pain on ejaculation. Rectal examination often reveals enlarged seminal vesicles. The volume of semen is low and consists of watery fluid that fails to coagulate. Seminal vesicle secretions are lacking. The concentration of prostatic secretions, such as acid phosphatase and citric acid, is increased because of the lack of semen dilution. Vasography may help in the diagnosis because higher segments fail to fill.[2054] Transrectal ultrasonography is the most accurate imaging modality for the diagnosis of ejaculatory duct obstruction. Needle aspiration of seminal vesicle fluid may show spermatozoa that have entered the seminal vesicles by reflux.

Mixed Obstruction. Mixed obstruction refers to lack of patency of the vas deferens or the epididymis and alterations in ejaculatory ducts or seminal vesicles (low ejaculate volume and absence of fructose). The most frequent cause is mucoviscidosis. One-third of patients with congenital bilateral absence of vas deferens have agenesis or hypoplasia of seminal vesicles. The cause of epididymal obstruction in patients with anomalies of the prostate-vesiculodeferential junction is difficult to determine.

Etiology of Obstructive Azoospermia

Obstructive azoospermia may be caused by congenital or acquired lesions.

Congenital Azoospermia. The most frequent anomalies associated with congenital azoospermia are testis-epididymis dissociation, epididymal malformation in cryptorchidism, bilateral absence of the vas deferens, congenital unilateral absence of the vas deferens associated with a pathologic process of the contralateral testis or its sperm excretory ducts, seminal vesicle agenesis, and ejaculatory duct obstruction (Table 12.23).

Agenesis of All Mesonephric Duct Derivatives. Agenesis of all mesonephric duct derivatives is a rare disorder that gives rise to varied anatomic anomalies, depending on the stage of embryonic development at which the mesonephric duct derivatives disappear. If failure occurs before the fourth week, the ipsilateral kidney and ureter are absent, although the testis may be present, or other renal anomalies may occur. If failure occurs during the fourth week and the ureteral bud is already formed, the ureter and kidney may develop normally. If failure occurs between the 4th and 13th weeks, there is a variable constellation of anomalies that most frequently include normal development of the testis and globus major, and hypoplasia of the other excretory duct segments or agenesis of an excretory duct segment (epididymis, vas deferens, or seminal vesicle).

Epididymal Anomalies. The most frequent epididymal anomalies are absence of the epididymis, testis-epididymis dissociation, defective connection of the vas deferens and the epididymis, epididymal cysts, and anatomic abnormalities of the epididymis.

Complete absence of the epididymis is frequent in monorchidism and anorchidism. The epididymis is replaced by a small mass of cellular connective tissue with abundant blood vessels at the blind end of the vas deferens.

Partial absence of the epididymis is more frequent than complete absence. Absence of the corpus of the epididymis gives rise to a characteristic malformation called *bilobed epididymis*. This varies from simple strangulation to complete separation of the caput and cauda. These anomalies are often associated with absence of the vas deferens.

Testis-epididymis dissociation is found in 1% of cases of obstructive azoospermia and is usually associated with cryptorchidism. Defects in connection of the ductuli efferentes and ductus epididymidis are rarely complete. In the incomplete form, some of the 5 to 30 ductuli efferentes in the epididymis are short and end blindly.

Epididymal cyst usually arises from blind-ending ductuli efferentes and contains spermatozoa. Spermatocele retains its epithelial lining, although it becomes atrophic (Figs. 12.238 through 12.240). Spermatozoa may be obtained from such a cyst. Some epididymal cysts arise from embryonic remnants, do not contain spermatozoa, and are lined by columnar or pseudostratified epithelium. Wolffian cysts, unlike müllerian cysts, are immunoreactive in the apical border of epithelial cells for CD10, with linear immunostaining.[2054] Cysts lined by clear cells with or without papillae raise concern for von Hippel–Lindau disease.[2055] Large epididymal cysts require removal and must be excised with great care to avoid damaging the ductuli efferentes and creating obstruction. Epididymal cysts are present in approximately 5% of male patients, and

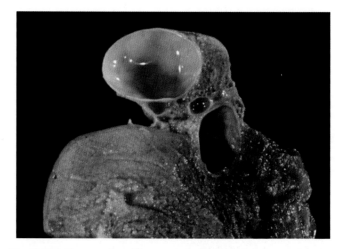

Fig. 12.238 Gross section of the caput of epididymis showing several cysts.

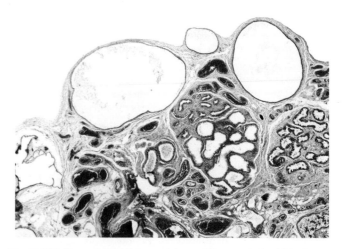

Fig. 12.239 Several cysts in the periphery of the caput of epididymis.

TABLE 12.23	Congenital Anomalies of the Male Mesonephric Ducts

I. Agenesis of All Mesonephric Duct Derivatives

II. Epididymis

Agenesis of the epididymis.
Testis-epididymis dissociation.
Failure in the connection between ductuli efferentes and ductus
    epididymidis.
Cysts of the epididymis.
Anomalies in epididymal configuration.
    Elongate epididymis.
    Angulated epididymis.
    Free epididymis.

III. Vas Deferens

Agenesis of the vas deferens.
Persistent mesonephric duct.

IV. Seminal Vesicle

Agenesis of the seminal vesicle.
Cysts of the seminal vesicle.
Opening of the ureter into the seminal vesicle.

V. Ejaculatory Duct

Agenesis of the ejaculatory duct.

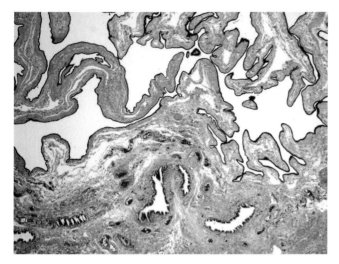

Fig. 12.240 Infertile patient with bilateral epididymal cysts. The cystic wall appears collapsed and folded on the epididymis.

the incidence rate is high (21%) in those exposed to diethylstilbestrol during gestation.[2056]

Anomalies in epididymal configuration that alter its shape and location are frequent in men with cryptorchidism and uncommon in those with descended testes. The most common malformations are elongate epididymis, angulated epididymis, and free epididymis. Elongate epididymis is found in approximately 68% of undescended testes. The length of the epididymis may be several times that of the testis, and in abdominal or inguinal cryptorchidism the epididymis extends several centimeters below the testis. Angulated epididymis is characterized by long epididymis that has a sharp bend in the corpus, with or without stenosis. With free epididymis, all or part of the epididymis is unattached to the testis. The most common variant is epididymis with free cauda.

Vas Deferens Anomalies. The most frequent anomalies of the vas deferens are congenital absence, segmental aplasia, ectopia, duplication, diverticula, and crossed dystopia.[2057]

Congenital absence is defined as unilateral or bilateral absence of the whole vas deferens or only a segment. Obviously, azoospermia occurs with bilateral absence. The frequency of this malformation varies among populations. At autopsy the prevalence rate is 0.5%, but the clinical incidence rate is 1% in infertile men and 10% to 25% in patients with obstructive azoospermia.[2058] Unilateral complete absence is three times more frequent than bilateral, and absence of only a segment is even more frequent. The affected segment may be absent or reduced to a fibrous cord. Absence of the vas deferens may be associated with other malformations of the sperm excretory ducts or the urinary system. The most frequent malformations of the excretory ducts are absence of the ejaculatory ducts (33% of cases) and, less frequently, absence of the seminal vesicles. Approximately 71% of patients with bilateral absence of the vas deferens have partial aplasia of the epididymis. The most frequent malformations of the urinary system are absence of the ipsilateral kidney and other renal anomalies. Complete or partial absence of the vas deferens occurs frequently in patients with CF.

Persistent mesonephric duct consists of the ureter joined to the vas deferens, forming a single duct that opens into an ectopic orifice between the trigone and verumontanum. This malformation may be associated with cystic transformation or absence of the seminal vesicle. The kidney may be normal or dysplastic.

Anomalies of Seminal Vesicle and Ejaculatory Duct. The most frequent anomalies are agenesis of the seminal vesicles or ejaculatory ducts, cyst of the seminal vesicle, and ectopic opening of the ureter into the seminal vesicle. The last anomaly is the most common and often is associated with ipsilateral renal dysplasia.[2059]

Acquired Azoospermia. Inflammation and trauma are the main causes of acquired azoospermia. Epididymitis is a frequent cause; *Chlamydia trachomatis* and *Escherichia coli* are currently the most common infectious causes.[2060–2062] Infections with *Neisseria gonorrhoeae* and mycobacteria also are implicated, and nonspecific epididymitis is significant.[2063] Apart from elective vasectomy the most frequent traumatic causes of azoospermia are surgical accidents during herniorrhaphy in children, orchidopexy, varicocelectomy, hydrocelectomy, deferentography, and removal of epididymal cyst.[2064–2066] Obstructive azoospermia may also result from blockage of the ejaculatory ducts after transurethral resection or as a result of long-term urethral catheterization.

Testicular and Epididymal Lesions Resulting From Obstruction of Sperm Excretory Ducts. Lesions of the testis and epididymis may result from obstructed sperm excretory ducts, depending on the location, origin (congenital or acquired), and duration of the obstruction (Fig. 12.241).

Location of Obstruction. Obstruction at the level of the ampulla of the vas deferens, seminal vesicles, or ejaculatory ducts does not usually cause significant lesions in the testis or epididymis. More proximal obstruction at the level of the vas deferens, epididymis, or testis-epididymis junction usually causes severe lesions in both the sperm excretory ducts and the testicular parenchyma. Obstruction of the vas deferens causes increased pressure within the ductus epididymis. As a result the epididymal lumina dilate, the epithelium atrophies, and fluid containing few spermatozoa and some spermiophages accumulates in the lumina (Fig. 12.242). The most dilated epididymal segment is the caput. The ductuli efferentes often become cystically dilated and filled with spermatozoa and macrophages. Reabsorption and lysosomal degradation of this protein-rich fluid occurs, causing the epithelium to accumulate lipofuscin granules or acquire apical eosinophilic granules (Paneth-like change) (Fig. 12.243).[2067] Rupture of the wall gives rise to spermatic granulomas (Fig. 12.244) or granulomas rich in histiocytes with eosinophilic and granular cytoplasm that mimics malacoplakia (Fig. 12.245). Rupture of the vas deferens gives rise to microgranulomas and ceroid granulomas

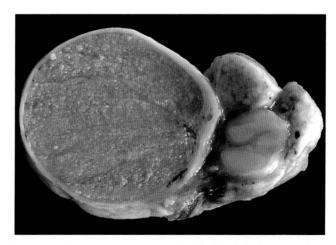

Fig. 12.241 Gross section of testis and epididymis. A marked cystic dilatation may be observed in the tail of epididymis.

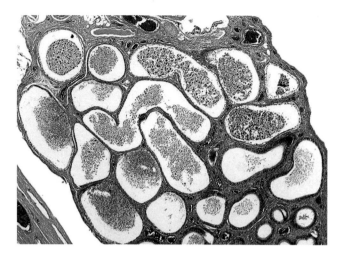

Fig. 12.242 Obstructive azoospermia in a patient with history of epididymitis. The caput epididymidis shows a marked dilation of the ductuli efferentes that contain numerous spermatozoa.

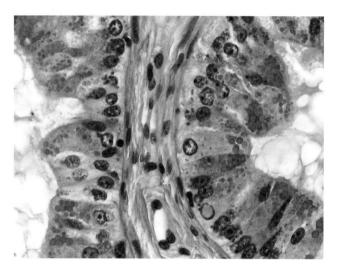

Fig. 12.243 Paneth-like changes in the epithelial cells of the efferent ducts. Abundant eosinophilic granulations at the apical pole of the cells.

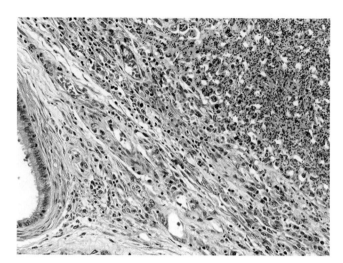

Fig. 12.244 Spermatic granuloma. Abundant spermatozoa in the intertubular interstitium of the epididymis both free and inside the cytoplasm of macrophages.

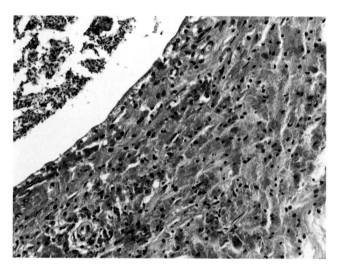

Fig. 12.245 Granuloma in the epididymis with abundant histiocytes of eosinophilic and granular cytoplasm suggesting malacoplakia. The lesion is located in the wall of a dilated efferent duct with abundant spermatozoa.

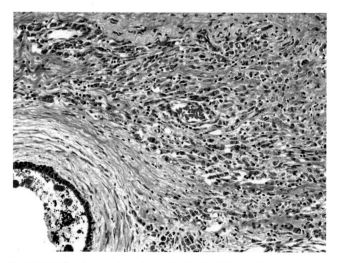

Fig. 12.246 Ceroid granuloma in a patient with a history of sperm excretory duct obstruction.

(Fig. 12.246). Macrophages and lymphocytes often are present in the intertubular connective tissue.[2068]

The most frequent testicular lesions in proximal obstructions involve the adluminal compartment. These lesions result from the negative effect of hydrostatic pressure on the seminiferous epithelium and, in particular, on the Sertoli cell (Figs. 12.247 through 12.249).

Etiology of Obstruction. Congenital ejaculatory duct obstruction and congenital absence of the vas deferens usually causes minimal testicular injury, mainly dilation of the seminiferous tubules, and an increase in number of mature (Sc + Sd) spermatids.[2069] Lesions resulting from vasectomy are more important. Increased intraluminal pressure in the epididymis may give rise to pain (late postvasectomy syndrome).[2070,2071] Testicular lesions depend on the surgical technique used: they are slight if the proximal end of the vas deferens is not ligated or a sperm granuloma forms at the site of vasectomy. Spermatogenic rhythm in the testis is slower than before vasectomy, and lesions characteristic of obstruction develop, including thickening of the lamina propria and fibrosis

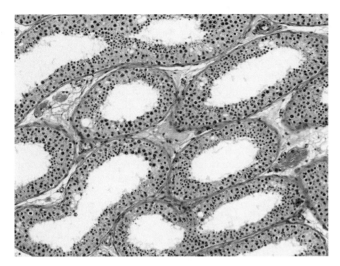

Fig. 12.247 Seminiferous tubules with marked luminal dilation, moderate decrease in cellularity, and occasional vacuolation of the Sertoli cell cytoplasm.

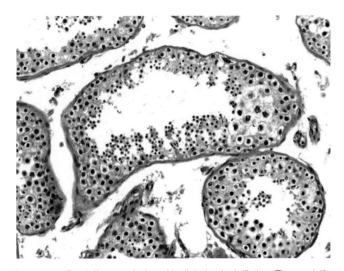

Fig. 12.248 Seminiferous tubules with slight luminal dilation. The seminiferous tubular cell layers have a "toothed" pattern. Degenerating megalospermatocytes may be seen in the seminiferous epithelium.

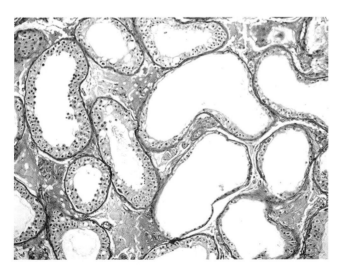

Fig. 12.249 Seminiferous tubules with marked ectasis and atrophy of the seminiferous epithelium in a patient with epididymal obstruction.

of the interstitium.[397] In testicular obstruction secondary to herniorrhaphy in infancy, lesions are mild. Lesions may be significant if the epididymis is damaged by hydrocelectomy, consisting mainly of primary spermatocyte sloughing. Hyalinized tubules may also be present when obstruction is caused by inflammation.

Duration of Obstruction. In acquired obstruction, testicular lesions worsen with time. Obstruction in the caput of the epididymis causes disappearance of all germ cells in the adluminal compartment of seminiferous tubules. The tubules become dilated, and Sertoli cells become vacuolated. Testicular alterations after vasectomy may not be related to the duration of the obstruction, but rather to the initial injury, and may disappear with time as the intraluminal pressure decreases.[2072,2073] However, if a significant amount of time elapses after vasectomy, the possibility of attaining a normal spermiogram with vasovasostomy is low. Vasal patency is restored in most cases of reanastomosis, but paternity rates are markedly lower (25% to 51%) than normal (85%).[2074] Results improve with the use of robotic microsurgery, novel instrumentation, and adhesive sealants.[2075] The best results are obtained in patients with high inhibin B levels. At first, spermatozoa obtained from the testis are of better quality than those from the epididymis.[2076]

Functional Azoospermia and Oligozoospermia

Some azoospermic patients have biopsies with minimal histologic abnormalities or minor tubular dilation without detectable excretory duct obstruction. These findings are characteristic of two main conditions: Young syndrome and alterations in spermatozoal transport.

Young Syndrome

Young syndrome is defined by the following constellation of findings: azoospermia, sinusitis, bronchitis or bronchiectasis, and normal spermatozoal flagella.[2077] The incidence is probably higher than that recorded in the literature, and Young syndrome should be suspected in all patients with obstructive azoospermia without a history of epididymitis or scrotal trauma. Patients have a lesion at the junction of the caput and corpus that gives the epididymis a characteristic gross appearance of distension, with the ductuli efferentes containing yellow fluid and numerous spermatozoa, whereas the remaining epididymal segments are normal. The ductus epididymidis is blocked by thick fluid.[2078] Young syndrome should be distinguished from other causes of infertility also associated with chronic sinusitis and pulmonary infections, including ciliary dyskinesia and CF. Ciliary dyskinesia consists of morphologic, biochemical, and functional alterations in cilia and flagella, including immotile cilia syndrome, Kartagener syndrome, and miscellaneous syndromes characterized by imperfectly defined abnormalities of cilia and flagella.[2079] In Young syndrome, sinusitis and pulmonary infections develop in childhood and stabilize or improve in adolescence; in other conditions the pulmonary damage increases with age, and cilia and flagella are ultrastructurally abnormal.[2080]

Alterations in Spermatozoon Transport

Normally, spermatozoa detach from Sertoli cells and traverse the intratesticular and extratesticular excretory ducts, where they are stored, mainly in the cauda of the epididymis, and ultimately released from the corpus by ejaculation or eliminated by phagocytosis. Only approximately 50% of spermatozoa are ejaculated. Whereas the release of spermatozoa from the corpus is intermittent, transit through the sperm excretory ducts is continuous.

Transit is accomplished by peristaltic contractions of myofibroblasts in the wall of the seminiferous tubules and ductuli efferentes, and by smooth muscle cells in the wall of the ductus epididymidis and vas deferens. Spermatozoa are propelled along the length of the epididymis in a mean of 12 days (range, 1 to 21 days). The walls of the seminiferous tubules and extratesticular excretory ducts are under hormonal and neural control. The myofibroblasts in the seminiferous tubules have oxytocinic, α_1-adrenergic, β-adrenergic, and muscarinic receptors. Unmyelinated nerve fibers penetrate the tubular lamina propria, pass among the myofibroblasts, and end near the Sertoli cells.[200] Along their length the nerve fibers have varicosities containing sympathetic vesicles.

The ductus epididymidis is innervated by sympathetic adrenergic nerve fibers that end among smooth muscle cells. Several hormones, including oxytocin, endothelin-1, vasopressin, and prostaglandins, act on the musculature of the ductus epididymidis. The peristaltic contractions begin in the caput and propagate toward the cauda. The frequency and amplitude of contractions vary from region to region; they are higher in frequency near the caput and of maximal amplitude in the initial portion of the cauda. The progressive increase in amplitude parallels the progressive increase in the thickness of the muscular wall and the requirement for greater force to propel the fluid as it becomes progressively more viscous with a higher concentration of spermatozoa. The distal portion of the cauda is usually at rest because it is the main reservoir of spermatozoa between ejaculations. Several times daily, vigorous contractions of the distal cauda impel the spermatozoa from the cauda toward the vas deferens.[2081] Several drugs that favor contraction of the muscular wall (α_1-blocking agents and $F_2\alpha$ prostaglandins) have been successfully used in the treatment of alterations in the spermatozoon transport.[2082]

Summary of Diagnostic Groups Suggested by Testicular Biopsy

Testicular biopsy provides enough information to identify three types of pathologic processes: obstructive disorders of spermatic pathways (posttesticular causes), primary testicular disorders (testicular causes), and disorders secondary to alterations in hypophyseal-pituitary-testicular axis or other endocrine disorders. Clues for diagnosis are given in Table 12.24.

Biopsy provides prognostic information regarding the fertility of the patient. When findings associated with a poor prognosis are present, patients may require assisted reproductive techniques. Prognostic factors are listed in Table 12.25.

Infertility and Chromosomal Anomalies

Knowledge about the incidence of chromosomal abnormalities in male infertility has progressed in parallel with advances in technology, including karyotype studies in peripheral blood, meiotic and chromosomal studies of biopsies, analysis of chromosomes in spermatozoa, and analysis of DNA in blood and spermatozoa for detection of chromosome Y deletions.[2083] The incidence rate of chromosomal anomalies in the infertile population is 2% to 7%, whereas in the general population it is less than 0.5%. The frequency of chromosomal abnormalities increases in an inverse relationship with the number of spermatozoa in the ejaculate.[2084]

Abnormalities in Sex Chromosomes
Klinefelter Syndrome
Genetic and Clinical Aspects. Klinefelter syndrome is characterized by an abnormal number of X chromosomes and primary

TABLE 12.24 Keys to Classify Diagnostic Groups in Testicular Biopsy for infertility

Obstructive Pathology of Spermatic Pathway

Data from quantitative study

Increased MTD and remarkable differences in MTD and lumen among lobules.
Lesions in the adluminal compartment: most are obstructive (exception: absence or markedly decreased Sa + Sb with normal or increased spermatocytes I).
Lesions in the basal compartment: only those testes with better conserved MTD and hypospermatogenesis with mild spermatocyte I sloughing.
Number of Sc + Sd spermatids higher than that of Sa + Sb.

Data from qualitative study

Mosaic pattern of spermatogenesis lesions.
Tubular ectasis.
Tubules with indented outline.
Accumulation of spermatozoa in the lumen of some tubules.
Intense apical vacuolation of the Sertoli cell cytoplasm.
Tubular hyalinization of obstructive mechanism.
Primary testicular pathology.

Data from quantitative study

Decreased MTD.
All lesions in the basal compartment.
Some lesions in the adluminal compartment (sharp interruption in spermatocytes I or round spermatid maturation).

Data from qualitative study

Testis with germ cell abnormalities.
Anomalies in spermatogonia: high number of hypertrophic, multinucleate, and dislocated spermatogonia.

Anomalies in spermatids: high number of multinucleate, macrocephalic, round, without acrosome, or short- and thick-flagellum spermatids.
Testis with Sertoli cell abnormalities.
All Sertoli cell–only syndromes with dysgenetic Sertoli cells.
Most Sertoli cell–only syndromes with adult and involutive Sertoli cells.
All mixed atrophies with dysgenetic Sertoli cells.
Most of the mixed atrophies with adult and involutive Sertoli cells.
Testis with tubular hyalinization of dysgenetic mechanism.
Tubules with absent or decreased elastic fibers.
Testis with Leydig cell anomalies.
Dysgenetic Leydig cells.
Some Leydig cell hypertrophies and hyperplasias.
Testicular pathology secondary to alteration in hypothalamopituitary-testicular axis and other endocrine disorders.

Data from quantitative study

Markedly decreased MTD (<120 μm).
Lesions in the basal compartment.

Data from qualitative study

Testis with infantile or pubertal pattern.
Testis with immature Sertoli cells.
Testis with dedifferentiated Sertoli cells.
Tubular hyalinization by hormonal deprivation.
Absence or decrease of Leydig cells.

MTD, Mean tubular diameter; Sa + Sb, round spermatids; Sc + Sd, elongate spermatids.

TABLE 12.25

TABLE 12.25 Predictors of Poor Prognosis in Testicular Biopsy

More than 25% of hyalinized tubules.
More than 50% of Sertoli cell–only tubules.
Diffuse thickening of tunica propria.
Adluminal and basal compartment lesions with disproportionate sloughing of spermatocytes or round spermatids.
Most of maturation arrest in spermatogonia.
Testis with meiosis anomalies and anomalies in spermiogenesis.
Presence of interstitial and peritubular inflammatory infiltrates.

testicular insufficiency. The original description was of a man with eunuchoidism, gynecomastia, small testes, mental retardation, and elevated levels of serum gonadotropins.[2085] His case drew attention to the significant lesions observed in the testes of such patients. Lesions involve seminiferous tubules and interstitium: (1) tubular atrophy may lead, through a hyalinization process, to complete disappearance of tubules, with only ghost tubules remaining; and (2) there is an apparent increase in the number of Leydig cells, which form characteristic nodules that tend to coalesce and delete the testicular structure.

This syndrome is the most common genetic cause of male infertility.[2086] Frequency varies according to the population studied: 1 in 500 newborns and infants, 1 in 100 of patients in mental institutions, 3.4 in 100 of infertile men, 0.7 in 100 oligozoospermic patients, and 11% of azoospermic patients.[2087–2089] At least 11% of azoospermic men have Klinefelter syndrome, although the initial pathologic investigations of the lesions were focused on adult patients studied for infertility.[2090–2093] Later, when the primary dysgenetic nature of the testicular lesions was known, studies extended to infancy and childhood. Even though the estimated incidence of this disorder is 1 in 600 male newborns, and many children with Klinefelter syndrome present with language and behavior problems, as well as mental retardation, only a few patients (10%) are diagnosed before puberty.[2094–2097] With increasingly frequent use of amniocentesis and histologic studies of fetuses, testicular lesions can now be identified before birth.

Study of Klinefelter syndrome currently involves a search for X-chromosome genes involved in triggering and development of testicular lesions.[2098–2100] In about 80% of cases, the karyotype is 47,XXY. The remaining 20% have chromosomal mosaicism with at least two X chromosomes, most frequently 46,XY/47,XXY (10%). The other uncommon karyotypes include 46,XY/48,XXXY, 46,XX/47,XXY, 47,XXY/46,XX/46,XY, 46,XY/45,XO/47,XXY, 46,XX/47,XXY/48,XXXY, 48,XXXY/49,XXXXY, and 47,XXi(Xq)Y.[1571,2101–2104] The 47,XXY lesion results from nondisjunction of sex chromosome migration during the first or second meiotic division of the spermatocyte or ovule. Mosaicisms are caused by mitotic nondisjunction in the zygote after fertilization.[2105] Study of the Xg antigen in blood revealed that the extra X chromosome is maternal in 73% of cases and paternal in 27%. Advanced maternal age increases the incidence of children with the 47,XXY karyotype.

The diagnosis of Klinefelter syndrome in infants, who may have few clinical stigmata of the disorder, calls for other techniques besides microscopic analysis of G-banded chromosomes. Although this technique is the gold standard, it is time consuming, requires experience, and is expensive. Screening for transcripts of the *XIST*

(*X-inactive–specific transcript*) gene by PCR may be helpful. Somatic cells express gene products only when they have more than one X chromosome.[2106] Up to 20% of cases with Klinefelter syndrome are not detected with this technique because of RNA instability. Alternatively, copy number of the AR gene located in Xq11.2-q12 may be measured by quantitative real-time PCR technique. This method is specific and accurate.[2107]

Most 47,XXY patients with Klinefelter syndrome are diagnosed in adulthood. Only 25% are recognized in the pediatric age group, principally during adolescence.[2108] The most common clinical findings are as follows[2109]:

- *Eunuchoid phenotype with increased stature.* Increased height is caused by disproportionate lengthening of lower extremities. The ratio of span to height is less than 1.
- *Incomplete virilization.* This is variable and ranges from normal development to the absence of secondary sex characteristics.
- *Gynecomastia, usually bilateral.* This is present in 50% of patients.
- *Mental retardation.* This is seen in many patients, although 80% have an intelligence quotient (IQ) that permits them to be functional in society. These patients have been described as immature, lacking in initiative, and emotionally unstable, with poor concentration capacity.[2110]

Two classic stigmata, female escutcheon and gynecomastia, are present in 32% and 12% of patients, respectively.[2111]

Other commonly associated conditions include the following: chronic bronchitis; varicose veins; cervical rib; kyphosis; scoliosis or pectus excavatum; and a high incidence of hypothalamic, hypophyseal, thyroid, and pancreatic dysfunction.[2112]

External genitalia often appear to be normal. The testes are usually less than 2.5 cm long, although in some cases of chromosomal mosaicism they are of normal size.[2113] Consistency is firm in 50% of cases and soft in 20%. The incidence of cryptorchidism is low in 47,XXY patients, but increased in mosaicism variants with more than two X chromosomes.[2114]

Supernumerary X-chromosome material is associated with reduction of gray matter in the left temporal lobule, a finding correlated with verbal and language deficits.[2115]

Histochemical, immunohistochemical, and ultrastructural studies from testes of pubertal and adult 47,XXY patients reveal diffuse abnormalities. A better knowledge of Sertoli and Leydig cell physiology has led investigators to establish a strong correlation between hormonal changes and lesions.[2116]

In adults the testes show the classic histologic picture of tubular dysgenesis with small, hyalinized seminiferous tubules lacking elastic fibers and pseudoadenomatous clustering of Leydig cells (Figs. 12.250 and 12.251).[2085] Most biopsy samples show some tubules with a few Sertoli cells.[2092] Two types of Sertoli cell–only tubules may be distinguished: (1) type A tubules, whose Sertoli cells have dysgenetic morphology (pseudostratified distribution, elongate hyperchromatic nuclei with small, peripherally placed nucleoli, absence of annulate lamellae, and weak immunoreaction to AMH); and (2) type B tubules, which display central lumina and whose Sertoli cells show an adult, mature pattern or some signs of involution (many nuclear folds). In some testes, both types are present.[2090,2092] Dysgenetic Sertoli cells of type A tubules are sex chromatin negative, whereas adult mature Sertoli cells of type B tubules may be either positive or negative.[2117] This finding suggests either testicular mosaicism of the X chromosome or heterochromatinization of both X chromosomes. In mosaicism the Sertoli cell–only tubules may be more numerous than hyalinized tubules.

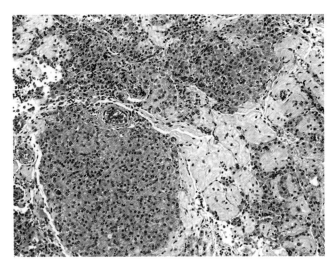

Fig. 12.250 Klinefelter syndrome. Leydig cell nodules mingle with hyalinized tubules.

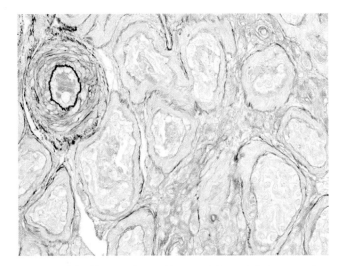

Fig. 12.251 Klinefelter syndrome. Most seminiferous tubules, even those with Sertoli cell only, have scant elastic fibers that may be demonstrated with orcein stain. The intense staining observed in the inner elastic lamina of arterioles provides a positive control.

Reduced testicular volume imparts an appearance suggestive of Leydig cell hyperplasia, but quantitative studies show that the total number of Leydig cells is lower than normal.[2091,2093] Many are pleomorphic, and some are multivacuolated. Immature fibroblast-like Leydig cells may be present, and cells with hypertrophic cytoplasm and those with signs of exhaustion may also be observed.[1871,2118] The abnormally differentiated Leydig cells have nuclei with coarsely clumped chromatin, deep unfolding of the nuclear envelope, multiple paracrystalline inclusions instead of Reinke crystalloids, multilayered concentric cisternae of smooth endoplasmic reticulum, large masses of microfilaments, and scant lipid droplets.[2119] Sex chromatin is apparent in 40% to 70% of Leydig cells. Leydig cell function is insufficient, and androgen levels are less than 50% of normal. Basal FSH and LH levels are markedly increased.[2112,2120,2121] In a few patients, testicular damage is less prominent; biopsies show isolated groups of Sertoli cell–only tubules or even some tubules show spermatogenesis.[2122] Exceptionally, complete spermatogenesis and even paternity have

been reported.[2123] Although 47,XXY patients are classically azoospermic and have been considered infertile, 8% have some spermatozoa in their ejaculates.[2124] This finding opens new expectations regarding potential fertility, and 50% of patients with Klinefelter syndrome may have offspring as a result of TESE and assisted fertilization technologies.[2125]

In these patients, prepubertal Sertoli cells do not mature into adult Sertoli cells at puberty, and the cells that focally persist have dysgenetic or involutive features.[246,2090] This finding correlates with the low synthesis of inhibin B. Peritubular cells have impaired myoid differentiation and are unable to produce elastic fibers.[1888] Despite the presence of Leydig cells, most patients do not produce normal levels of testosterone.[517]

The causes of early germ cell loss and inability of spermatogonia to proliferate and complete meiosis in 47,XXY patients are uncertain. It is likely that an abnormal proportion of some genes in the X chromosome changes germ cell division or apoptotic rate.[2126] The presence of XIST expression in blood cells of patients with Klinefelter syndrome (absent in 46,XY males) suggests that somatic cells inactivate the supernumerary X chromosome, as do somatic cells in normal females.[2106,2127] Inactivation of some X-linked genes (an essential process in meiosis regulation) could hypothetically explain the inability to complete meiosis. Focal spermatogenesis, as occurs in some patients, may originate in euploid germ cells.[2128]

Klinefelter Syndrome 46,XY/47,XXY. The 46,XY/47,XXY karyotype is the most frequent variant of Klinefelter syndrome. In this setting, clinical abnormalities may be attenuated. Gynecomastia is present in 33% of cases, compared with a frequency of 55% in men with 47,XXY karyotype. Azoospermia is found in 50% of cases (93% in XXY men). The testes are larger and spermatogenesis is more developed than in men with 47,XXY because spermatogonia with normal chromosomal constitution are present (Fig. 12.252).[2129] Patients with 47,XXY karyotype who have spermatozoa in seminiferous tubules have 46,XY spermatogonia and also 47,XXY spermatogonia, whereas those who have no spermatozoa harbor only 47,XXY spermatogonia; these 47,XXY spermatogonia may include some spermatozoa with 23,X or 23,Y chromosomal complement, elevated numbers of both 24,XY and 24,XX spermatozoa, and a high frequency of spermatozoa with 21 disomy. This 21 disomy may be an important risk factor for gonosomy, as well as for trisomy 21.[2130,2131]

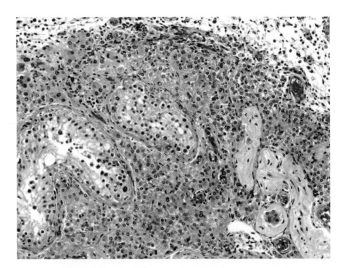

Fig. 12.252 Klinefelter syndrome mosaicism showing focal spermatogenesis in two seminiferous tubules located within a Leydig cell nodule.

Although a few decades ago patients with Klinefelter syndrome were considered sterile, currently successful sperm recovery rate with micro-TESE is 57% and pregnancy rates with TESE plus ICSI per embryo transfer are greater than 25%.[2132,2133] The risk for aneuploidy in children is low.

Klinefelter Syndrome 48,XXYY. In 1960 the first report of the chromosomal constitution 48,XXYY was published and annotated as the "double male."[2134,2135] The incidence of the 48,XXYY karyotype is estimated to be approximately 1 in 17,000 to 1 in 50,000 males, or 2% of patients with Klinefelter syndrome.[2136–2140] This karyotype may be associated with aggressive character, antisocial behavior, significant mental retardation, and a higher frequency of congenital malformations than the 47,XXY karyotype.[2141–2144] Foot ulcers are observed in some cases.[2145] Men with 48,XXYY karyotype also have characteristic dermatoglyphics with increase in arches, decrease in total finger ridge count, and ulnar triradii associated with changes in the hypothenar region.[2146] Male patients with 48,XXYY are tall, with an adult height of more than 6 feet. They have eunuchoid habitus with long legs, small penis and testicles, gynecomastia, and hypergonadotropic hypogonadism. Testicular biopsy shows hyalinized tubules, dysgenetic Sertoli cell–only tubules, and Leydig cell hyperplasia (Fig. 12.253). A peculiar finding is the presence of concentric lamellae of smooth endoplasmic reticulum cisternae in the Leydig cell cytoplasm (Fig. 12.254).[2118]

Klinefelter Syndrome 48,XXXY and 49,XXXYY. Patients with 48,XXXY karyotype were first reported in 1964.[2147] They may be of average or tall stature, with hypertelorism, epicanthus, flat nasal bridge, simplified ears, and mild prognathism. Men with 48,XXXY or 49,XXXYY karyotype often have skeletal malformation, principally fifth-finger clinodactyly, elbow malformations with radioulnar synostosis, and slow molar development.[2148] Their IQs are between 40 and 60 with severely delayed speech, and are typically passive and immature, but may be aggressive.[2149] Cryptorchidism is frequent.[2150] Hypergonadotropic hypogonadism, gynecomastia, and in 25% of cases, hypoplastic penis may also be present.[2151] Testes show tubular hyalinization and occasionally focal spermatogenesis.[2152]

Pentasomy 49,XXXXY is one of the rarest chromosomal defects and is associated with a clinical syndrome characterized by delayed

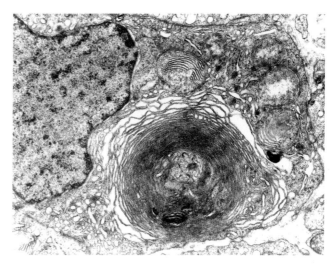

Fig. 12.254 48,XXYY Klinefelter syndrome showing a Leydig cell that contains giant mitochondria and a wheel of smooth endoplasmic reticulum.

prenatal and postnatal growth, microcephaly with short stature, and severe mental retardation.[2153] Patients are typically shy and friendly, and their IQs range between 20 and 60.[2154] They have hypoplasia of the external genitalia, cardiac malformations, radioulnar synostosis, proximal tibiofibular synostosis, and high arched palate.[2153,2155–2161] The incidence is 1 in 85,000 male births.[2162] The syndrome results from maternal nondisjunction during both meiosis. Cryptorchidism is frequent. Testes show decreased or normal germ cell numbers in the fetal period.[2163–2165] At puberty, patients experience hypergonadotropic hypogonadism with low testosterone levels, tubular hyalinization, and Leydig cell hyperplasia. Many patients require hormonal replacement therapy.[2166] One of the 176 reported patients had Leydig cell tumor.[2167]

Association With Malignancy. Patients with Klinefelter syndrome have a higher incidence of malignancy than the general population, related to higher incidence of leukemia and lymphoma, and a 20-fold increase in the incidence of breast carcinoma because of hormonal imbalances (Fig. 12.255).[2168–2174] Although testicular germ cell tumors are rare in these patients, extragonadal germ cell tumor is 30 to 40 times more frequent than in the general population.[2175–2177] Most tumors occur in the mediastinum (~71%).[2178] This means that approximately 8% of chromatin-positive men will experience development of these tumors.[2179] Less commonly, germ cell tumors have been observed in the pineal gland, the spinal cord, the retroperitoneum, gastrointestinal tract, and prostate.[2180–2184] The most frequent types are teratoma associated with yolk sac tumor, followed by choriocarcinoma.[2185] Pure embryonal carcinoma, seminoma, and yolk sac tumor are rare.[2186–2192] In patients younger than 8 years, a gain of chromosome 20 or 20p is frequent (70%), whereas in adolescents older than 8 years, gains of 12p (69%) and X (59%) are most common.[2187,2193] Extragonadal origin of germ cell tumors has been attributed to abnormal germ cell migration from the yolk sac. In the mediastinum, possible origin from primordial thymus cells has been postulated.[2193a] Development of malignancy has been attributed to either high hormonal levels or the abnormal chromosomal constitution of germ cells.[2172,2194–2196]

The incidence of other solid tumors in patients with Klinefelter syndrome (bronchogenic carcinoma, urothelial carcinoma of the bladder, adrenal carcinoma, prostatic adenocarcinoma, testicular

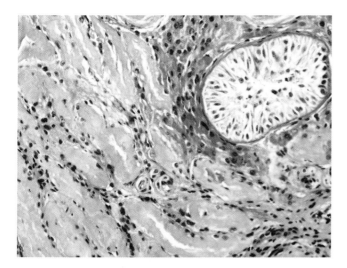

Fig. 12.253 Postpubertal patient with 48,XXXY Klinefelter syndrome showing diffuse tubular hyalinization except for on Sertoli only–cell tubule with dysgenetic Sertoli cells surrounded by abundant Leydig cells.

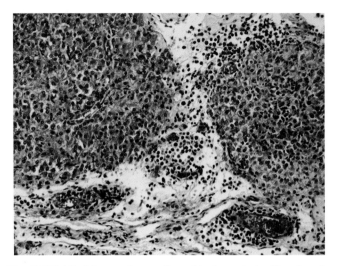

Fig. 12.255 Klinefelter syndrome with nodular hyperplasia of Leydig cells. Perivascular and interstitial leukemic infiltrates.

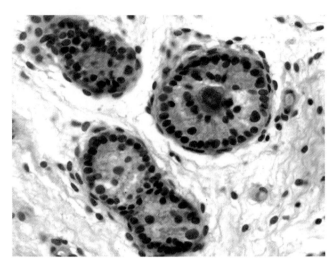

Fig. 12.256 Klinefelter syndrome at infancy. Seminiferous tubules showing decreased diameters, isolated germ cells, and a ring-shaped tubule that contains a microlith.

Leydig cell tumor, and epidermoid cyst) is comparable with that of the general population.[2185,2197–2202]

Occurrence in Childhood. Early identification of Klinefelter syndrome is possible through systematic cytogenetic study of newborns with positive sex chromatin or mental retardation.[2203] Several clinical stigmata suggest Klinefelter syndrome, including decreased muscle tone, delayed speech, poor language skills, reading difficulties, dyslexia, mental retardation, psychiatric problems, excessive stature for age, disproportionately long legs, micropenis, and small testes with advancing age.[1536,2095,2109,2204–2206] Infants often have low body weight at birth, and 6% show incomplete descent in one or both testes. Androgen deficiency is an early finding.[2207]

Prepubertal children show a slight increase in FSH, whereas LH and inhibin levels are normal.[2208,2209] In pubertal boys, LH level increases markedly, although testosterone remains low.[203]

Testicular lesions occur early in Klinefelter syndrome. Biopsy reveals few or no germ cells. Germ cell number in genital ridges does not differ from normal, but early cell loss takes place once testis differentiation begins.[2210] The number of germ cells in 47,XXY fetuses is significantly lower than in normal 46,XY fetuses. This fact has been confirmed in 47,XXY fetuses at abortion between weeks 18 and 22 of gestation. Most 47,XXY newborns have TFI of less than 30% and decreased germ cell number per tubular section. Germ cell loss is associated with irregular distribution of germ cells: tubules with germ cells alternate with vacant tubules. Neither the Leydig cells nor the remaining testicular structures show lesions. Testosterone levels in the umbilical cord vary from low to normal.[2208,2211]

Seminiferous tubules have reduced diameters, particularly those devoid of germ cells. The number of Sertoli cells is reduced. Megatubules, ring-shaped tubules, and intratubular eosinophilic bodies are common (Fig. 12.256). In some cases of Klinefelter syndrome associated with Down syndrome, tubular hyalinization is observed in childhood.[1139] The interstitium is wide and contains few Leydig cell precursors. If one testis is undescended, its histologic features do not differ from those of the contralateral testis. The testicular pattern remains constant through childhood.[2155] At puberty, before maturation of the tunica propria, the seminiferous tubules rapidly hyalinize, and Leydig cell precursors differentiate into Leydig cells.[2212]

The first two waves of germ cell proliferation (at "minipuberty" and at ~4 years of age) that occur in normal testis are not observed in 47,XXY patients. On the contrary, germ cells decrease in number (or even totally disappear) from the second year of life onward in cases with associated cryptorchidism despite the presence of testosterone.[2213] FSH, LH, AMH, and inhibin B levels are similar to those in normal boys, and even testosterone peak may occur in the first months of life coinciding with "minipuberty.[2214] During infancy, tubular diameter remains low and static, with subsequent small testicular volume (1 to 1.5 mL instead of 1.8 mL that is reached at the end of childhood).[2155,2203,2208] However, secretion of inhibin B and AMH by Sertoli cells continues normally, and FSH and LH serum levels do not differ from those of controls.[2208,2214,2215] Based on small testicular volume in Klinefelter syndrome, we may assume that, in infancy, these testes have at least two impaired cell types: Sertoli cells and germ cells. Whether the defect is in both or only in Sertoli cells remains speculative.

In early adolescence, testicular size increases to greater than 3 mL, coinciding with normal hypothalamic–pituitary-testicular axis activation and increase in FSH, LH, testosterone, and inhibin B levels. Permanent hypergonadotropic hypogonadism is rapidly established. When a new wave of germ cell proliferation would be expected, if it actually takes place, it occurs only in some tubules, where a few spermatocytes may be observed; otherwise germ cells completely disappear.[2212,2216–2218] In most cases, as puberty progresses, residual spermatogonia disappear and Sertoli cell degeneration becomes evident. Between 12 and 14 years of age, there is onset of tubular hyalinization and progressive increase in Leydig cell number; however, in occasional cases, isolated seminiferous tubules with Sertoli cell–only pattern persists (Fig. 12.257). Testicular volume stabilizes. The levels of inhibin B and AMH are normal at the onset of puberty, but decrease soon thereafter. The decline in inhibin B occurs in parallel with Sertoli cell involution, whereas the decrease and ultimate cessation of AMH production in adult men is the result of both Sertoli cell loss and testosterone increase.[2215]

Association With Precocious Puberty. Precocious puberty refers to development of secondary sex characteristics in a boy before the age of 9 years.[2219] Mean age of puberty is earlier with Klinefelter syndrome than in unaffected boys.[2209] 47,XXY

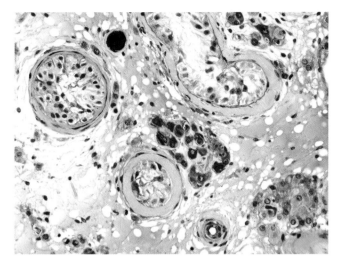

Fig. 12.257 Pubertal patient with klinefelter syndrome showing Sertoli only–cell pattern, variable thickening of tubular walls, and groups of Leydig cells.

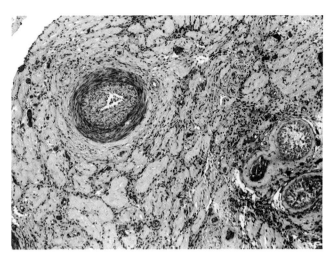

Fig. 12.258 Klinefelter syndrome with hypogonadotropic hypogonadism showing diffuse tubular hyalinization associated with absence of Leydig cells. Only tubules with dysgenetic Sertoli cells are present.

Klinefelter syndrome and its variants may begin clinically with CPP, but this is not a characteristic finding in Klinefelter syndrome. Karyotyping in older boys with mental retardation, gynecomastia, small testes, and precocious puberty is advisable. Typically the cause of precocious puberty is hCG-secreting germ cell tumor in the mediastinum.[2220–2222] Infrequently, precocious puberty is idiopathic, and it rarely results from hamartoma in the third ventricle.[2223,2224]

Association With Hypogonadotropic Hypogonadism. Klinefelter syndrome is often associated with pituitary disorders such as panhypopituitarism or incomplete hypopituitarism.[2225,2226] Deficits in FSH, LH, or both have been reported.[2227–2231] The cause of this association is unknown, and diverse causative factors such as trauma, immunologic disorders, and genetic deficiencies have been postulated. Alternatively, the syndrome may result from exhaustion of pituitary gonadotropin-secreting cells after years of GnRH stimulation.[2226]

In patients deficient in both gonadotropins, testicular biopsy shows diffuse tubular hyalinization and marked reduction or absence of Leydig cells. The histologic picture is similar to that of hypogonadotropic hypogonadism occurring after puberty except for the presence of isolated tubules containing only dysgenetic Sertoli cells and absence of elastic fibers in the hyalinized tubular wall (Figs. 12.258 and 12.259).[2230] In patients with isolated LH deficit, the histologic picture is that of Sertoli cell–only tubules with dysgenetic Sertoli cells and variable number of hyalinized tubules.[2227] In patients with isolated FSH deficit, the histologic findings are similar to classic 47,XXY Klinefelter syndrome.

46,XX Males (XX Sex Reversal, Testicular Disorder of Sex Development)

The 46,XX karyotype may be present in three phenotypes: male phenotype including normal external genitalia; male undermasculinization, with a variable degree of ambiguity in external genitalia ranging from hypospadias to micropenis; and true male hermaphroditism.

46,XX Males With Male Phenotype and Normal External Genitalia. The first case of a 46,XX male with male phenotype and normal external genitalia was reported in 1964.[2232] Some considered this a variant of Klinefelter syndrome.[1680] Men with

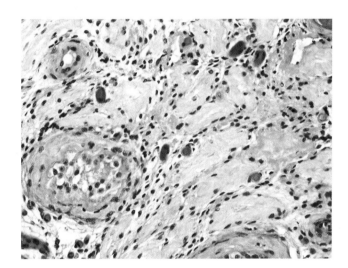

Fig. 12.259 Klinefelter syndrome with hypogonadotropic hypogonadism. Absence of Leydig cells between hyalinized tubules.

46,XX karyotype have clinical features similar to those of Klinefelter syndrome, including small testes, small or normal penis, azoospermia, gynecomastia, and minimal development of secondary sex characteristics. However, these men exhibit normal body proportions, normal or slightly short stature, and normal intelligence, in contrast with men with Klinefelter syndrome.[2233–2235] The incidence of 46,XX males is low: 1 in 10,000 to 1 in 25,000 live births, accounting for approximately 0.2% of infertile men.[1245,2234,2236–2238] Most cases are sporadic, although familial cases have been reported.[1485,2239,2240]

Male patients with 46,XX karyotype have hypergonadotropic hypogonadism with elevated serum level of FSH and, to a lesser degree, elevated LH, with normal or slightly decreased testosterone. All patients are infertile. The probable cause is absence of AZF, a locus of the Y chromosome where several genes required for primordial germ cell migration and maintenance of spermatogenesis are found.

During childhood, testicular biopsy in 46,XX males reveals decreased numbers of germ cells.[2234,2241] Biopsies from adults show one of the three patterns: histologic features similar to those of 47,XXY men, including diffuse tubular hyalinization with prominent Leydig cell populations (Fig. 12.260); Sertoli cell–only tubules with numerous dysgenetic Sertoli cells (Fig. 12.261); or both patterns intermingled with less prominent Leydig cell population.[2242–2247] The last pattern is the most frequent. Some tubules in any of the patterns may show isolated spermatogonia and even primary spermatocytes (Fig. 12.262). Ultrastructural studies reveal an increase in intermediate filaments and absence of annulate lamellae in Sertoli cells, absence of Reinke crystalloids, and an abundance of intracytoplasmic and intranuclear paracrystalline inclusions in Leydig cells.[2247,2248]

46,XX Males With Ambiguous External Genitalia. Some males with the 46,XX karyotype have ambiguous external genitalia or hypospadias and are assumed to have male undermasculinization.[2249] Such patients are found in families whose members have ovotesticular DSD, suggesting that these disorders are different manifestations of the same genetic defect.[2250] Several authors have

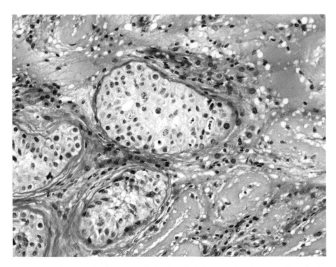

Fig. 12.262 Testicular biopsy of a XX male. The predominant pattern is that of dysgenetic Sertoli-only cell. There are isolated hyalinized tubules and a slightly increased number of Leydig cells.

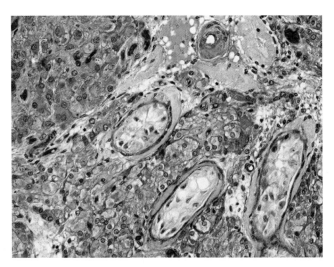

Fig. 12.260 Testis from a 46,XX male showing Sertoli cell–only tubules together with hyalinized tubules, and nodular and diffuse Leydig cell hyperplasia.

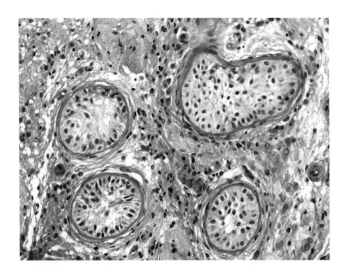

Fig. 12.261 Testicular biopsy of a XX male. Next to fully hyalinized tubules, other tubules show spermatogonia and first-order spermatocytes.

found that different phenotypes are compatible with the same 46,XX genotype.[2251–2253]

Etiology. The origin of 46,XX male status may be difficult to determine. Given that testicular differentiation requires genes located on the Y chromosome, 46,XX males have been classified by cytogenetic studies as those having the SRY gene, those lacking the SRY gene, and those with XX/XY mosaicism.

Male patients with the SRY gene comprise 80% of 46,XX males.[2254] This likely occurs by translocation of the short arm of the Y chromosome to the X chromosome.[2255] The amount of translocated Y-chromosome material is variable.[2256] According to this hypothesis, during paternal meiosis the homologous pseudoautosomal regions in the short arms of X and Y chromosomes interchange the terminal portions of their short arms, thus giving rise to X chromosome with translocated *SRY* gene.[2257,2258] Infertility would be the consequence of deletion of Yq involving the *DAZ* gene.[2259–2268] Alternatively, the SRY region may be inserted into an autosome.[2269,2270] Most 46,XX patients who are *SRY*+ have normal male phenotype.[2271,2272]

Approximately 10% of *46,XX* males are SRY⁻, and most have ambiguous genitalia.[1488,2273–2275] Some have a normal male phenotype but are infertile.[2276–2278] The underlying basis of a 46,XX SRY⁻ male phenotype is unknown. Although SRY is assumed to be the most important regulatory factor of testicular determination, possible causes include unknown X-linked or autosomal gene involved in testis differentiation or hidden Y-chromosome mosaicism limited to the gonad.[2251,2279–2281] A few cases result from duplication of SOX9, which is sufficient to initiate testis differentiation in the absence of SRY.[2282] The same occurs in partial duplication of chromosome 22q or overexpression of the *SOX10* gene at 22q13, mutations in the *RSPO1* gene, translocation 12;17, and SOX3 gain of function.[2280,2283–2285] Testes show diffuse tubular hyalinization and Leydig cell hyperplasia.[2243]

Approximately 10% of *46,XX* males have XX/XY mosaicism or another karyotype with the chromosomal complement Y.[1495,2286] In these cases, detection of the specific DNA sequences of the Y chromosome may be difficult because this chromosome may be present in only some tissues or in small numbers of cells, including testes or skin, but not lymphocytes.[2234,2270,2287]

47,XYY Syndrome

47,XYY syndrome was first described in 1961 in the father of a girl with Down syndrome.[2288] The only clinical findings were excessive height and pustular acne. Study of other cases suggests that some have a predisposition to psychopathic and antisocial behavior, and may exhibit neurodevelopmental disorders such as delayed speech, reading difficulties, and motor difficulties.[2289,2290] Aggressive behavior was found in only 1% to 2%, a finding that questions whether an extra Y chromosome by itself predisposes to aggressive behavior.[2291,2292]

The incidence rate of 47,XYY patients is estimated to be 0.01%, including 0.2% of men who smoke, 0.7% to 0.9% of men in prison, and 1.8% of sexual homicide criminals.[1571,2293-2295]

Since 2000, many cases of 47,XYY syndrome have been diagnosed prenatally. From birth, patients have weight, stature, and cephalic circumferences greater than mean values and a higher risk for delayed language or motor development. Approximately 50% of children have psychological and psychiatric problems such as autism; although intelligence is normal, many are referred to special education programs.[2296] As adults, they have normal external genitalia and secondary sex characteristics. Some patients have decreased fertility, and others are infertile, although, as in the first reported case, paternity may occur.[2297,2298]

Serum levels of LH and testosterone are normal.[2299] FSH may be elevated in patients with small testes and severe lesions of the seminiferous epithelium.[2300] Hypogonadotropic hypogonadism has exceptionally been observed.

Most patients have normal testicular size.[2301] Biopsies typically reveal mixed tubular atrophy characterized by spermatogenesis associated with Sertoli cell–only tubules (Fig. 12.263).[2302-2304] Tubules with spermatogenesis may show normal spermatogenesis or have lesions in the adluminal or basal compartments; about 64% of pachytene cells have three sex chromosomes, and many XYY spermatocytes degenerate during meiosis.[2305] The number of normal spermatozoa in the ejaculate is low. The incidence of both YY and XY spermatozoa and disomy 18 is high.[2306]

The extra Y chromosome originates from nondisjunction during paternal second meiotic division. The presence of different tubular types (normal spermatogenesis, maturation arrest of primary spermatocytes, and Sertoli cell–only tubules) in the same biopsy is explained by postulating the disappearance of spermatocytes that were unable to pair their sexual chromosomes during meiosis or, later, during the round spermatid stage.[2307-2310] Typically, there is a high rate of XYY cell degeneration during meiosis. Germ cells with X or Y chromosomes that fail to pair in the pachytene stage would be eliminated during the first or second meiotic division, or even later in the stage of round spermatids.[2310-2312] Spermatocytes that form trivalent chromosomes (instead of bivalents) would be more protected and are initially viable.[2311] The ultimate trivalent chromosome segregation yields aneuploid and euploid cells in equal numbers. Sertoli cell–only tubules are attributed to either spermatogonial damage by substances released from degenerated spermatocytes or absence of testicular colonization by primordial germ cells.[2313]

One concern is whether the spermatozoa of these patients have a high rate of aneuploidy. This has not been observed in XO/XYY, whereas men with other constitutions such as 47,XYY/46,XY have a higher risk for fathering children with a hyperdiploid chromosomal constitution.[2314] Spermatozoa should be studied genetically to evaluate this risk before an ICSI program is begun.[2315] The 47,XYY syndrome has been reported to be associated with 21 trisomy and fragile X syndrome.[2316,2317]

Men with three and four Y chromosomes have been reported.[2318] Men with the 48,XYYY karyotype are tall and have a normal male phenotype, slight mental retardation, azoospermia, and, during childhood, frequent infections of the upper respiratory tract.[2319] Mosaicisms with 48,XYYY line produce additional anomalies. Biopsy shows Sertoli cell–only tubules, severe hyalinization of the tubular basement membranes, and diffuse Leydig cell hyperplasia. The chromosomal complement of parents may be normal.[2320] This karyotype probably results from fertilization of a normal ovule by a YYY spermatozoon.[2321]

Men with 49,XYYYY have no significant phenotypic abnormalities (except for cases of chromosomal mosaicism). Slight mental retardation, infertility, and antisocial behavior are reported.[2322] Rarely patients have facial dysmorphism and various skeletal abnormalities.[2323] Because the fathers of these patients have a normal karyotype, the explanation for this anomaly is nondisjunction in spermatogonial mitosis followed by a second nondisjunction in meiosis.[2324]

Structural Anomalies of the Y Chromosome

The Y chromosome is essential for gender determination and spermatogenesis, and Y-chromosomal abnormalities often lead to infertility. Cytogenetic studies showed that deletion of the distal euchromatic region is associated with infertility.[2325] The relationship between Y-chromosomal abnormalities and infertility is best understood in azoospermic men with alterations in the distal region of the euchromatic part of the long Y arm. This region contains the gene (or genes) assumed to be responsible for spermatogenesis and named the azoospermic factor gene or AZF gene, located in the bands that extend from Yq11.21 to Yq11.23 (Fig. 12.264).[2326-2331]

DNA of the Y chromosome contains approximately 60 megabases (Mb), equivalent to 60 million base pairs (bp). The euchromatic transcriptionally active region contains 30 to 40 Mb and comprises the short arm, the centromere, and the proximal portion of the long arm. The heterochromatic (condensed) region has a variable length and no known important functions. The short arm euchromatic region starts in the telomere, with a pseudoautosomal region (2.7 Mb), which is homologous with the X chromosome

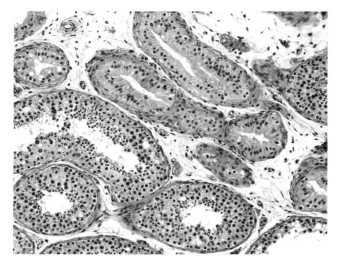

Fig. 12.263 47,XYY syndrome. The testis shows tubules with complete spermatogenesis, Sertoli cell–only tubules, and tubules with spermatogonial maturation arrest.

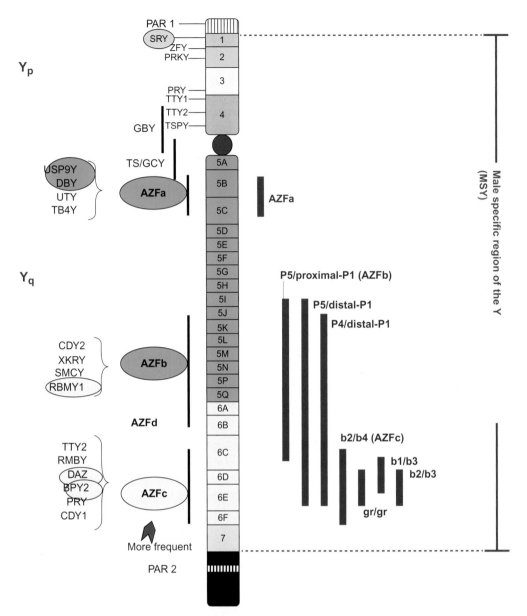

Fig. 12.264 Scheme of Y chromosome showing azoospermic factor (AZF) regions.

short arm terminal region and contains genes that encode the granulocyte-monocyte colony-stimulating factor receptor α subunit (SCFrRA) and T cell adhesion factor (MICS). This euchromatic region continues with a 280-kilobase (kb) region that contains the sex determining genes (*SRY*), a ribosomal protein gene (RPS4Y), and a zinc finger protein (ZFY). Next is a region that is homologous with Xp21, as well as a short segment that is homologous with Xp22 and contains the amelogenin gene (*AMGL*). This region is followed by the centromere, a region homologous with Xp22, and the long arm heterochromatic region. The long arm proximal portion begins with the gene responsible for Kallmann syndrome (*KAL1*), followed by the genes that encode steroid sulfatase (*STDP*), the AZF, the gonadoblastoma factor, and the growth factor.

Y-chromosome sequencing was completed in 2003; to date, 122 genes and 110 pseudogenes have been identified.[2332] The following deletions and microscopically visible rearrangements affecting Yq11 region are recognized clinically: monocentric Yq-chromosomes, dicentric Yq-chromosomes of the short arm (dic-Yp), Y chromosomes with ring structure (rin-Y), Y/Y translocation chromosomes, and translocation of Y chromosome to an autosome or the X chromosome.

Deletions and Microscopically Visible Rearrangements in Infertile Patients

Monocentric Deleted Yq Chromosome. Partial deletion of the distal portion of the Yq11 euchromatic region is associated with azoospermia secondary to loss of AZF.[2333,2334] Men have normal external genitalia except for small testes, normal testosterone and LH serum levels, and increased FSH.[2325] The most frequent finding is Sertoli cell–only pattern, although many other patterns have been reported.[2335] The number of Leydig cells is normal or increased. These findings suggest that adequate AZF function is required for early spermatogenesis.[2336] If the breakpoint of Yq11 is proximal to the centromere, patients are short because the gene that controls stature is close to that for AZF.[2337,2338]

Dicentric Yq Isochromosomes. Dicentric chromosomes are the most common structural change in the Y chromosome. Sterility is frequent.[2339] This anomaly is usually associated with the 45,X cell line. The proportion of this line varies among patients and between cell types (fibroblasts and lymphocytes). When the point of breakage and fusion of the two Y chromosomes is in the distal region, Yq11 and the second centromere are inactivated. The Y isochromosome is of normal size but does not stain with quinacrine, and thus is called nonfluorescent Y chromosome (Ynf). Because the breakpoint is in the Yq11 region, AZF function is altered.[1872,2340,2341] Development of external genitalia varies from ambiguous to normal. Some patients have sex reversal and short stature, whereas others have turnerian stigmata.[2342–2345] This variability is probably related to the extent of XO present.[2342] Biopsy findings are similar to those of men with monocentric deleted Yq chromosomes (i.e., Sertoli cell–only tubules with dysgenetic Sertoli cells and Leydig cell hyperplasia) (Fig. 12.265).[2346–2348] Patients with dicentric Y chromosome without mosaicism may show male phenotype and maturation arrest of primary spermatocytes.[2349,2350]

Ring Y Chromosome. Men with ring Y chromosomes have a normal male phenotype, azoospermia, and in some cases, short stature.[2351] Most have a mosaic karyotype with 45,X line.[2352] In some cases, biopsy resembles that of men with monocentric deleted Yq chromosome, but in other cases one sees premeiotic arrest of spermatocyte maturation.[2353,2354] This finding is attributed to difficulty in pairing the X and Y chromosomes during meiosis. Many patients have deletion of some AZF regions.[2355,2356] Vertical transmission following assisted reproductive technology and ICSI has been reported.[2357]

Y/Y Translocation Chromosome. Patients have azoospermia, small and soft testes, and primary spermatocyte maturation arrest as a result of defective pairing of the X and Y chromosomes. The karyotype may be a mosaic with 45,X line.[2358]

Translocation of Y Chromosome to X Chromosome. This anomaly comprises two groups of patients: those with nonvisible or visible X;Y translocations. Nonvisible translocations are most common and have been observed in infertile patients with 46,XX karyotype.[2359] The phenotype differs from that of patients with Klinefelter syndrome by shorter stature, absence of mental retardation, and small tooth size. Biopsy reveals Sertoli cell–only pattern.

The clinical characteristics of patients with visible translocations resemble those of patients with Klinefelter syndrome more than patients with nonvisible translocations. Biopsy reveals tubular hyalinization and nodular Leydig cell hyperplasia.

Autosomal translocation of Y Chromosome. Translocation of the distal heterochromatic portion of the Y chromosome to the short arm of an acrocentric chromosome occurs occasionally. The most frequent translocations are to chromosomes 5, 18, 13, 15, and 22.[2360–2362] Fertility of these men depends on the site of breakage.[2363] If breakage occurs in the Yq12 heterochromatic region, the patient has a male phenotype and is fertile. If the point of breakage is in the Yq11 region, the patient is infertile and has small testes.[2363,2364] Seminiferous tubules may show only Sertoli cells, spermatogenetic arrest in the early stages of meiosis followed by apoptosis and primary spermatocyte sloughing, or an infantile pattern.[2365,2366] Other Y-chromosome abnormalities associated with infertility include paracentric and pericentric inversions.[2367,2368]

Microdeletions of Y Chromosome. The Y chromosome is divided into seven deletion intervals: numbers 1 to 4 correspond to the short arm and centromeric region, and numbers 5 to 7 correspond to the long arm. Most deletions in infertile patients occur in three nonoverlapping subregions of Y chromosome (Yq11), located at intervals 5 and 6: AZFa, AZFb, and AZFc. AZFa is located in the proximal portion of the deletion interval 5, AZFb is present in the proximal end of interval 6 and the distal part of interval 5, and AZFc is in the distal portion of interval 6.[2369,2370]

Y-chromosome microdeletions are observed in up to 18% of cases of idiopathic male infertility, with ethnic and geographic differences, as well as differences related to the method of investigation. When only patients with idiopathic azoospermia are studied, the incidence rate is estimated between 14% and 15%.[2371,2372] In Asia the incidence is even higher: 21% in Hong Kong, 24% in Taiwan, 30% in northwestern Iran, and 52% in southern Iran.[2373–2376] Among patients with severe oligozoospermia, the incidence is also variable: 2% in Germany; 5% in Italy; up to 14% in Australia, Scandinavia, China, India, Japan, and Russia; and up to 18% in the United States.[2377] Some patients present with complete deletion of the AZF region, but most have deletion of only one subregion.

AZF deletions result from recombination of large palindromic sequences that have an identity greater than 99.9% and consist of long direct or indirect repeats called amplicons.[2332] The ampliconic portion of the masculine-specific region of the Y chromosome contains a high density of genes from nine gene families, with each gene existing in multiple (2 to 35), nearly identical copies. These genes are predominantly or exclusively expressed in the testis. Clinically, 90% of patients with Y-chromosome microdeletion have small testes, increased FSH level, and azoospermia or severe oligozoospermia.

Microdeletions of the AZFa subregion represent 5% of Y-chromosome microdeletions. This subregion contains single copies of the *DFFRY* (*Drosophila* fat-facets related Y) and *DBY* genes. The *DFFRY* gene has been mapped to Yq11.2.[2378–2380] This gene is a member of a gene family that encodes deubiquitinating enzymes (which remove ubiquitin from protein-ubiquitin conjugates), and it is ubiquitously expressed in embryonal and adult tissues, including the testis.[2381] Although this gene does not appear to be essential for spermatogenesis, it may play an important role in normal development.[2382] Complete deletion produces a Sertoli cell–only pattern.[2383,2384] Partial microdeletions do not alter spermatogenesis.[2385]

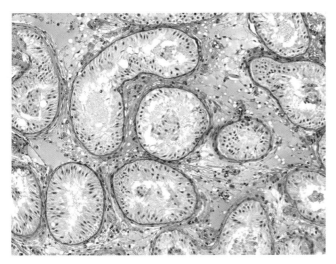

Fig. 12.265 Testis from a male with dicentric Yq isochromosome showing seminiferous tubules with Sertoli cell–only pattern and slight Leydig cell hyperplasia.

Microdeletions of the AZFb subregion represent 10% to 16% of Y-chromosome microdeletions. RBM1 and RBM2 are located in this region, and both are specifically expressed in the testis and germ cells. These genes codify RNA-binding proteins that localize to the nucleus of all germ cells and are involved in spermatogenesis.[2386,2387] Patients with complete deletion of the AZFb subregion have azoospermia, and biopsy shows either Sertoli cell–only pattern or maturation arrest (Fig. 12.266).[2388] In a study of patients with incomplete AZFb deletion, 50% had spermatozoa in the ejaculate.[2389,2390]

Microdeletions of the AZFc subregion are the most frequent of all microdeletions (80%), present in 5% to 10% of all patients with azoospermia or severe oligozoospermia.[2391–2396] The *DAZ* (deleted in azoospermia) gene family is the most important in terms of infertility in deletions of this subregion.[2397] Four functional copies (*DAZ1, DAZ2, DAZ3,* and *DAZ4*) are arranged in two clusters.[2398] *DAZ* encodes a testis-specific RNA-binding protein containing 8 to 24 amino acids sequences, known as DAZ repeat. *DAZ* gene deletions produce a variety of effects on the testis. *DAZ1/DAZ2* deletion is associated with incomplete maturation arrest of primary spermatocytes (Fig. 12.267), maturation arrest of spermatids, or MAT, whereas *DAZ3/DAZ4* deletion may be observed in fertile and infertile patients.[2369,2397,2399,2400] Partial deletion of the AZFc subregion known as gr/gr leads to subfertility because it removes at least two copies of *DAZ* and one copy of chromodomain protein Y-linked 1 (CDY1) and several other transcription units.[2401–2403]

Investigation for microdeletions of chromosome Y is recommended in all patients with severe oligozoospermia or azoospermia before intervention using ejaculated sperm and any surgical procedure to identify spermatozoa in the setting of azoospermia.[2404] Sons conceived with sperm from men with Y-chromosome microdeletions are expected to inherit the abnormal Y chromosome and infertility problems.[2394,2405,2406] They also have a potential risk for development of 45,X0 Turner syndrome or other forms of sex chromosome mosaicism, including hermaphroditism.[2407] Clinically, primary use of donor sperm rather than TESE is recommended for men with deletions that involve complete loss of the AZFa or AZFb subregion.[2377]

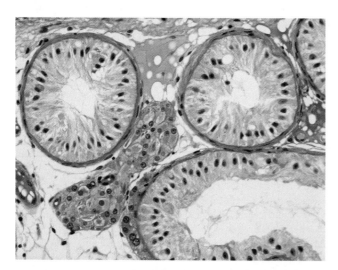

Fig. 12.266 Microdeletion of the AZFb in a patient with azoospermia. Seminiferous tubules with only Sertoli cells. In the intestinum there is a large cluster of Leydig cells and in the wall of a tubule, between the myoid cells, there are several peritubular Leydig cells.

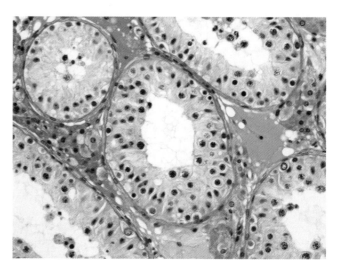

Fig. 12.267 Microdeletion of AZFc region of Y chromosome in an infertile patient with severe oligozoospermia. Seminiferous tubules show maturation and scarce spermatogenesis with isolated adult spermatids.

The correlation between genotype and phenotype is inexact, but most microdeletions in AZFa, AZFb, and AZFc are associated with Sertoli cell–only syndrome, maturation arrest, and spermatid maturation arrest or mixed testicular atrophy, respectively.[2408,2409]

Structural Anomalies of the X Chromosome

46,XY patients with duplication of distal Xp may exhibit male, female, or ambiguous genitalia, and gonadal dysgenesis is frequent. Male genitalia, when present, are hypoplastic, and these patients have hypogonadotropic hypogonadism and frequently multiple congenital anomalies and mental retardation.[2410] Clinical symptoms are related to the genetic content of the duplicated segment.[2411] Male patients with translocation of the X chromosome to an autosome may have disturbed spermatogenesis with subfertility or infertility.[2412–2414]

47,XXX patients have mental retardation, gynecomastia, normal stature, scrotal hypoplasia, well-formed small penis, small testes, and scant pubic hair. Serum testosterone level is markedly decreased. Seminiferous tubules show severe hyalinization. The 47,XXX genotype results from abnormal X-Y interchange during paternal meiosis and X-X nondisjunction during maternal meiosis.[2415] Transcriptionally inactive X chromosome is required for adequate spermatogenesis. It is possible that, in patients with translocation of the X chromosome to an autosome, this latter anomaly reactivates the X chromosome.[2416]

Anomalies in Autosomes

Autosomal anomalies are frequently linked with infertility. However, the causes are not fully understood because the same anomaly is associated with infertility in some patients, but not in others.

Chromosomal Translocations and Inversions

Robertsonian translocations are found in 0.7% of infertile men (9% higher than in the normal population) and are more frequent in oligozoospermic than in azoospermic men; 25% of patients have normal sperm parameters.[2417] The most common balanced Robertsonian translocations are 13;14 and 14;21.

The incidence rate of reciprocal translocations in infertile patients is 1% (0.1% in the general population) and increases to 0.8% in patients with azoospermia or severe oligozoospermia.[2418]

The most frequent reciprocal translocations in infertile men are 11;22 and 17;21.

Paracentric and pericentric inversions (except for the pericentric inversion of the heterochromatic region in chromosome 9) are eight times more frequent in infertile patients (0.16%) than in the general population. The highest risk for infertility is associated with pericentric inversion of chromosome 1.[2419,2420]

The presence of small supernumerary marker chromosomes in the infertile population is much more frequent than in the general population. Partial trisomy of some genes and mechanical alteration of meiosis might account for infertility.[2421]

The most common testicular lesions in men with autosomal anomalies are spermatogonial maturation arrest, primary spermatocyte sloughing sometimes associated with hypospermatogenesis, and Sertoli cell–only pattern.[1886]

Down Syndrome

The most frequent autosomal trisomy associated with prolonged survival is found in Down syndrome, with an estimated incidence of 1 in 1000 newborns. More than 80% patients reach or exceed 50 years. In addition to trisomy 21 and the characteristic appearance, patients with Down syndrome usually have cryptorchidism, small testes, hypoplasia of the penis and scrotum, and hypospadias.[2422] Patients experience development of leukemia more frequently, and testicular, brain, and hepatocellular tumors less frequently.[2423] Adults have oligozoospermia or azoospermia secondary to primary testicular deficiency. Levels of FSH and LH are elevated, but testosterone level is normal or slightly diminished.[2424] Isolated cases of paternity have been reported.[2425,2426]

In utero, there is marked delay in germ cell development.[2427] Histologic studies of prepubertal testes at autopsy reveal decreased tubular diameter and TFI. Eosinophilic bodies or microliths may be present in some tubules (Fig. 12.268). Adult testes have deficient spermatogenesis and MAT, with some tubules showing complete spermatogenesis and others containing only Sertoli cells.[2428] Isolated cases of azoospermia associated with trisomy 18 have been reported.[2429]

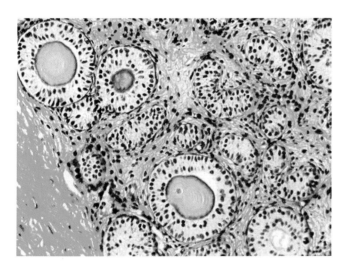

Fig. 12.268 Prepubertal testis in down syndrome. There are megatubules, ring-shaped tubules, and small seminiferous tubules. Germ cell number is low in all these tubules. Eosinophilic bodies or microliths are present in some tubules.

Other Syndromes Associated With Hypergonadotropic Hypogonadism

Hypergonadotropic hypogonadism is found in several myopathies (myotonic dystrophy and progressive muscular dystrophy) and dermopathies (Bloom, Rothmund-Thomson, Werner, Cockayne, and Tay syndromes), with histologic features resembling those of Klinefelter syndrome. Hypogonadism is also observed in Noonan syndrome, cerebellar ataxia (with milder testicular lesions), and a miscellaneous group of syndromes with variable histologic findings.[2430]

Myotonic dystrophy accounts for approximately 30% of men with muscular disorders, and approximately 80% have testicular atrophy. The estimated incidence is 1 in 8000 live births. The abnormality involves the distal muscles of the extremities. Patients may also have premature baldness, posterior subcapsular cataracts, cardiac conduction defects, impotence, gynecomastia (rarely), and dementia (at later stages).[2431] Myotonic dystrophy is autosomal dominant inherited with variable penetrance. Two loci are associated with the disease phenotype: DM1 in 19q13.3 and DM2 in chromosome 3. Mutation in DM1 results in serine/threonine protein kinase deficiency that causes expansion of the CTG repeat (from 50 to several hundred repeats) located on the 3'-untranslated region of the dystrophy myotonic–protein kinase gene. The number of repeats correlates with the severity of the disease and is negatively correlated with age of clinical onset.[2432–2434] DM2 is caused by mutation in 3q21.3 of the *ZNF9* gene and accounts for CCTG-repeat expansion (from 75 to 11,000 repeats) in intron 1 of this gene. Common clinical symptoms result from gain of function of RNA mechanism in CUG and CCUG repeats altering cellular function, including alternative splicing of various genes.[2435] The severity of the disease increases in successive generations.[2436] The number of CTG repeats is not associated with male subfertility.[2437] Hypogonadism is hypergonadotropic in most cases and not related to the number of CTG repeats.[2438,2439] Testicular lesions probably begin late because 65% of patients father children. Biopsies have variable findings, ranging from nearly normal to fully hyalinized tubules, with the number of Leydig cells varying from increased to decreased. The cause of germ cell disappearance is related to decrease in SIX5 level. The *SIX5* gene is necessary for germ cell survival and spermatozoa maturation, and is silenced by CTG expansion in DM1.[2440] In some patients, hypogonadism is hypogonadotropic, and the testes show an infantile pattern. Infertility may be the first symptom of myotonic dystrophy.[2441]

Progressive muscular dystrophy is a multisystemic X-linked recessive disease. It is usually associated with gonadal atrophy caused by a defective locus in chromosome 19. Patients rarely live more than 20 years. The incidence is approximately 1 in 4000 live births. In both Duchenne and Becker forms, the cause is a defect in the dystrophin gene located in Xp21. Dystrophin is a structural protein of skeletal and myocardial muscular cells.[2442–2446] The most common endocrine alteration is hypogonadotropic hypogonadism with delayed puberty and low serum testosterone.[2447,2448] Several cases of an association between Becker progressive muscular dystrophy and Klinefelter syndrome have been reported.[2449]

Bloom, Rothmund-Thomson, and *Werner syndromes* are caused by a homozygous defect in human RECEQ helicases in chromosome 15. The RecQ family of DNA helicases comprises essential proteins in prokaryotes and eukaryotes because these helicases catalyze unwinding of double-stranded DNA to provide simple-stranded templates for replication, repair, recombination, and transcription.[2450,2451] Of the five members of this gene family

(*RECQ1*, *BLM*, *WRN*, *RECQ4*, and *RECQ5*), three produce autosomal recessive inherited diseases. Mutations of the *BLM* gene have been identified in patients with Bloom syndrome, *WRN* has been shown to be mutated in Werner syndrome, and mutations of *RECQ4* have been associated with Rothmund-Thomson syndrome.[2452-2454] Despite similar genetic abnormalities in the three syndromes, the syndromal elements are different. *Bloom syndrome* is characterized by short stature, narrow face with prominent nose, facial patchy skin color changes that become more marked with sunlight exposure, high-pitched voice, and increased susceptibility to respiratory diseases, cancer, and leukemia.[2455] Severe oligozoospermia and azoospermia are common. Leydig cell function is conserved.[2456] *Rothmund-Thomson syndrome* is characterized by poikiloderma, juvenile cataracts, sparse hair, short stature, skeletal defects, dystrophic teeth and nails, and hypogonadism. These patients are predisposed to skin cancer and osteogenic sarcoma.[2457-2459]

Werner syndrome (progeria adultorum) manifests in young adults who appear much older than their chronologic age. The prevalence in the United States is estimated to be 1 in 200,000.[2460] The youngest confirmed patient was diagnosed at the age of 6 years.[2461] However, most patients have normal development up to the end of the first decade of life. In the second decade, symptoms develop that may include low stature, premature graying hair and baldness, cataracts, atrophy followed by fibrosis and calcification of muscular and adipose tissues, wrinkling of the skin, keratosis, osteoporosis, telangiectasis, atheroma, diabetes mellitus type 2, gynecomastia, and hypergonadotropic hypogonadism. Fertility declines soon after sexual maturity. Nonetheless, paternity at a young age has been reported.[2462] Inheritance is autosomal recessive. Experiments with cultured cells from these patients have shown that several cell types, such as fibroblasts, have a shorter life than that of control cells.[2463] The gene mutated in Werner syndrome, *WRN*, encodes both a $3' \rightarrow 5'$ DNA helicase and a $3' \rightarrow 5'$ DNA exonuclease.[2453,2464,2465] These patients have a high incidence of sarcoma.

Cockayne syndrome is a rare autosomal recessive neurodegenerative disorder.[2466] Signs and symptoms include failure to thrive in infancy; short stature; poorly developed trunk; premature aging; neurologic alterations; retinitis pigmentosa; optic atrophy; cataract; deafness; microcephaly; micrognathia; photosensitivity; delayed eruption of primary teeth; congenital absence of some permanent teeth; partial macrodontia; atrophy of the alveolar process and caries; limited articular movements in elbows, knees, and fingers; abnormally small eccrine glands; and hypergonadotropic hypogonadism.[2467,2468] Three general presentations have been reported: Cockayne syndrome type I or classic Cockayne syndrome, in which the major features of the disease become apparent by 1 or 2 years of age; Cockayne syndrome type II, the most severe form, whose symptoms are recognized at birth or in the early neonatal period; and Cockayne syndrome type III, a milder and later-onset form. This rare disease is linked to biallelic mutations in the *CSB/ERCC6* and *CSA/ERCC8* genes. Mutations of *CSB* and *CSA* genes jeopardize transcription-coupled repair of damaged nuclear and mitochondrial DNA, and the resumption of replication and transcription-encoding proteins involved in the transcription-coupled DNA repair pathway.[2469-2471]

Tay syndrome was first described in 1980, with an account of two Asian siblings whose parents were first cousins.[2472] The term *trichothiodystrophy* (TTD) was introduced in 1980 to describe the hair anomalies in these patients.[2473] Patients with TTD have brittle hair and nails (associated with reduced content of cysteine-rich matrix proteins), ichthyosis, cataracts, and physical and mental growth retardation. Hair from patients with TTD, when examined under polarized light microscopy, reveals alternating light and dark bands known as the "tiger tail" anomaly. The diagnosis may be confirmed by sulfur content analysis of hair shafts, which show decreased sulfur and cysteine content. Approximately one-half of patients with TTD have photosensitivity and are designated as TTD-photosensitive patients; the rest are nonphotosensitive patients and are designated as TTD-nonphotosensitive patients.[2474] TTD is part of a more broadly defined group of diseases identified as IBIDS (ichthyosis, brittle hair, impaired intelligence, short stature). Photosensitive cases are also identified as PIBIDS (photosensitivity with IBIDS). These syndromes are caused by mutations in genes encoding subunits of the transcription/repair factor IIH.[2475] In both forms of TTD, patients have decreased fertility. Hypergonadotropic hypogonadism has been reported in one patient.[2476]

Noonan syndrome is characterized by multiple malformations reminiscent of Turner syndrome, including short statute, pterygium coli, and cubitus valgus, although patients have normal male karyotype. Pulmonary artery stenosis has been found in 62% and hypertrophic myocardiopathy in 20%.[2477-2479] As in Turner syndrome, aortic coarctation may also be present.[2478,2480] Malformations in the peripheral vascular system may be occasionally observed.[2481,2482] The incidence is 1 in 1000 to 1 in 2500 live births and autosomal dominant inheritance, with sporadic occurrence in approximately 50% of cases. Fathers of one-half of the patients show some of the characteristic features of this syndrome.[2483,2484] A locus for dominant forms has been mapped to 12q24.1.[2485] Mutation in PTPN11 (protein-tyrosine phosphatase, nonreceptor type 11) accounts for one-half of the cases, although similar germline mutations also cause Leopard syndrome, Costello syndrome, and cardiofaciocutaneous syndrome.[2486,2487] These syndromes are genetically heterogeneous, but they share several symptoms. Noonan syndrome is caused by activating mutations in genes encoding upstream factors of the Ras–mitogen-activated protein kinase pathway, including PTPN11 that encodes *SHP2* and *SOS1*, as well as *KRAS*, *SHOC2*, and *NRAS* genes.[2488-2493] The characteristic Noonan stigmata are likely the result of a malformative sequence caused by a failure in one or more lymphogenic genes.[1251] Aberrant lymphatic endothelial differentiation produces lymphatic stasis, and subsequent distention and lymphedema exert mechanical pressure on the adjacent tissues and organs.[2494,2495]

Cryptorchidism is present in approximately 70% of patients and is usually bilateral.[2496] Testes are small and, in the first year after birth, show delayed disappearance of gonocytes.[2497] Biopsies from infants have low TFI and decreased MTD.[2498] Patients may present with testicular and epididymal lymphangiectasis. Puberty is usually delayed.[2499] Laboratory data from pubertal patients, either with or without cryptorchidism, show that LH level is normal, whereas FSH is increased, and inhibin B is low or just above the lower limit of normality. These findings suggest Sertoli cell dysfunction.[2500] Puberty is often delayed, and hypogonadotropic or hypergonadotropic hypogonadism occurs during adulthood. Ultrastructural studies reveal morphologic anomalies in germ cells.[2501] Although spermatogenesis is generally impaired, some patients are fertile (Fig. 12.269).

Noonan syndrome may be associated with Klinefelter syndrome and Becker muscular dystrophy.[2502,2503] Patients with Noonan syndrome, as well as those with Costello syndrome or cardiofaciocutaneous syndrome, have a high incidence of malignancies.[2504,2505] In rare instances, germ cell tumor has been reported.[2506]

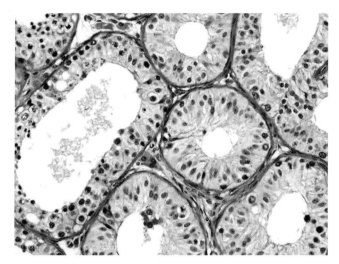

Fig. 12.269 Testis from a 15-year-old boy with Noonan syndrome. Most seminiferous tubules are small and contain Sertoli cells and isolated spermatogonia. The most dilated tubules have complete, although quantitatively decreased, spermatogenesis.

Cerebellar atrophy may be associated with hypogonadism. Patients are infertile and have moderate ataxia. Infertility results from morphologic abnormalities of spermatozoa caused by decreased expression of MAP2 (the most important microtubule-associated protein) and a defect in erythroid ankyrin.[2507,2508] Both proteins are involved in cytoskeletal protein assembly and are essential for normal germ cell morphogenesis. The most frequent malformations are nuclear deformation, acrosome separation or loss, rolling of the tail inside the cytoplasm, and loss of mitochondrial and dense fibers. Although hypogonadism observed in ataxia patients is usually hypogonadotropic, patients with cerebellar ataxia and hypergonadotropic hypogonadism have been reported.[2509,2510]

Many other syndromes also manifest with primary hypogonadism. The best known are Alström, Weinstein, Börjeson-Forssman-Lehmann, Marinesco-Sjögren, Richards-Rundle, Robinow, and Silver-Russell syndromes.

Secondary Idiopathic Hypogonadism

Age of onset of puberty depends on genetic (ethnic and familial) and environmental factors. Genetic factors determine an estimated 50% to 80% of these age differences.[2511] The onset of puberty depends on many genes; among them, the KISS1/GPR54 system stands out.[2512] Mutations in many genes impair hypothalamo-hypophyseal-testicular axis development at different levels. SF1 and DAX-orphan nuclear receptors are expressed at multiple levels throughout the reproductive axis. KAL, FGFR1, and NELF are related to anosmia or hyposmia and abnormal GnRH neuron migration from the nasal cavity to the hypothalamus. Leptin, leptin receptor, ghrelin, and PC1 are related to obesity. HESX1, LHX3, and PROP1 impair differentiation or function of pituitary gonadotropic cells, thus causing mutations in the GnRH receptor and in gonadotropic genes *LHB* and *FSHB*, with resulting structural anomalies in these hormones and in gonadotropin actions.[674,2513,2514] Hypogonadotropic hypogonadism or hypogonadism of hypothalamohypophyseal origin is classified according to whether the hypothalamohypophyseal failure occurs before or after puberty. Eunuchoidism, present only in the former, is the

basis of the distinction. The most frequent types of hypogonadism caused by hypothalamohypophyseal failure are those resulting from a deficit of GnRH, bioinactive FSH and LH, or a deficit in GH, as well as those types associated with PWS and Laurence-Moon-Rozabal-Bardet-Biedl syndrome.

Gonadotropin-Releasing Hormone Deficit

The onset and maintenance of the hypothalamohypophyseal-gonadal axis depend on pulsatile GnRH secretion by approximately 1500 neurons of the nucleus arcuatus hypothalamus, with release into the pituitary portal system and subsequent stimulation of GnRH receptors on the surface of gonadotropin-secreting cells in the anterior pituitary lobule. The GnRH gene is located on 4q13.[2515]

Patients with GnRH deficit have partial or complete absence of GnRH-induced pulsatile LH secretion and normalization of pituitary and gonadal secretions after exogenous GnRH administration. Imaging studies of the hypothalamohypophyseal region are normal, as are findings in the remaining hypothalamopituitary axes. GnRH secretion starts early in embryonal life. LH and FSH are detected in the pituitary during the 19th week. GnRH levels in fetal blood reach a peak approximately halfway through gestation and decrease later, when the mechanisms for negative feedback are developed. During the neonatal period, evidence of GnRH secretion is based on persistence of pulsatile gonadotropin secretion.[2516] In boys, 6 months after birth, GnRH secretion begins to decrease to low levels. During infancy the hypothalamohypophyseal-testicular axis remains quiescent.

At the beginning of puberty the hypothalamohypophyseal axis starts to secrete. This activity is characterized by an increase in the amplitude of pulsatile, GnRH-induced, LH secretion during sleep. With advancing puberty, gonadotropin secretion occurs night and day. In adulthood, LH pulses are produced in men approximately every 2 hours.

Clinical symptoms vary by age at presentation (congenital or acquired) and severity (complete or partial deficit). Clinical presentations include delayed puberty, idiopathic hypogonadotropic hypogonadism (IHH; isolated gonadotropin deficit), Kallmann syndrome, isolated FSH deficit, and isolated LH deficit (fertile eunuch syndrome).

Congenital GnRH deficit may be diagnosed occasionally in the neonatal period, during investigation for cryptorchid patients who have micropenis associated with low serum gonadotropin levels. During adolescence the diagnosis is prompted by failure of the onset of puberty and failure to develop secondary sex characteristics.

Acquired GnRH deficit has been reported in patients who, after going through normal puberty, experience diminished libido and fertility. In some cases the hormonal pattern resembles that of congenital GNRH deficit.[2517] In other cases, hormonal deficits are not so pronounced. This disorder may occur in athletes during training and may be reversed with clomiphene citrate.[2518]

Constitutional Delay of Growth and Puberty

Normal puberty is a period of development that results in complete growth and maturation to adulthood. It includes sexual development and acquisition of specific psychosocial behaviors. Delayed puberty is one of the most common reasons why adolescent boys are referred to an endocrinologist.

The most common cause of delayed puberty in males is constitutional delay of growth and puberty (CDGP), followed, in decreasing order of frequency, by delayed puberty secondary to underlying chronic disease (functional hypogonadotropic hypogonadism), permanent hypogonadotropic hypogonadism, and permanent hypergonadotropic hypogonadism.[2519]

CDGP is assumed to be a minor form of GnRH deficit.[2520] Many cases are likely inherited as an autosomal dominant, recessive, or X-linked trait. Single-gene defects have not yet been identified.[2521,2522] CDGP is characterized by delayed sexual maturation in otherwise healthy adolescent boys. Patients are short and usually have a family history of delayed puberty. Puberty usually begins at 13 to 14 years of age and progresses over 2 years. If a 14-year-old boy has not begun pubertal changes such as testicular enlargement (the testis has not reached 4 mL in volume or the major axis measures <2.5 cm), growth in height, and development of secondary sex characteristics, delayed puberty should be suspected.[2523-2527] Among the different causes invoked to explain delayed sexual maturity in adolescent boys with CDGP is conjunction of elevated serum ghrelin and decreased leptin concentration.[2528] Ghrelin is mainly synthesized in the stomach, and among its numerous functions is control of GH secretion, food intake, energy balance, and adiposity.[2529] Leptin is secreted by adipose tissue and directly acts on hypothalamic nuclei to suppress food intake and increase energy expenditure.[2530]

Biopsy reveals delayed development at the tubular and interstitial level and a great variety of tubular patterns. Tubules of prepubertal diameter predominate, devoid of lumina and containing only immature Sertoli cells or isolated spermatogonia (Fig. 12.270). Sertoli cells still express D2-40 and show focal immunoreactivity to AR (Fig. 12.271). Other irregularly distributed tubules contain a greater number of spermatogonia, spermatocytes I, and even some spermatids.

The main problem in patients with CDGP is that different types of hypogonadotropic hypogonadism require different treatments. Simple pubertal delay that spontaneously resolves quickly without treatment must be distinguished from hypogonadotropic hypogonadism. The latter should be suspected when any of the following symptoms are present in the patient or his family: midline defect, anosmia, or pubic hair without testicular development. In addition, low testicular volume (<3 mL) is much more frequent in hypogonadotropic hypogonadism than in CDGP. Hormonal assays may also assist in the diagnosis. Valuable tests include

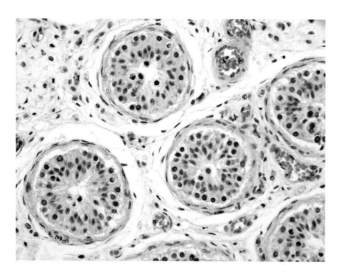

Fig. 12.270 Testis from a 15-year-old boy with delayed puberty. Seminiferous tubules have initial pubertal maturation, showing spermatogonia and isolated spermatocytes. The interstitium has scarce Leydig cells.

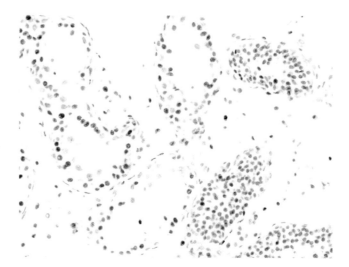

Fig. 12.271 Testis from a 15-year-old boy with delayed puberty. Seminiferous tubules with variable immunoexpression of androgen receptor. Some tubules have intense expression adjacent to other tubules showing minimal or absent expression.

nocturnal LH sampling, Prolactin (PRL) response to TRH, daily urine excretion of FSH and GnRH, and hCG stimulation, although no single test is absolute.[2531] The most useful test seems to be the combination of GnRH test with 3-day (short) hCG and 19-day (extended) hCG stimulation.[2532] This differential test may also be made on the basis of plasma inhibin B and AMH concentrations.[2533,2534] Inhibin B and AMH remain high in patients with CDGP, a fact that does not occur in patients with hypogonadotropic hypogonadism.[2535] If a patient between 16 and 18 years old has prepubertal gonadotropin levels, he probably has hypogonadotropic hypogonadism.

The incidence of delayed puberty associated with chronic illness is unknown. Delayed puberty may be associated with recurrent infections, immunodeficiency, gastrointestinal disease, renal disturbances, respiratory illnesses, chronic anemia, or endocrine disease. Malnutrition is probably the most important mechanism responsible for delayed puberty.[2536,2537] The degree of growth and pubertal development impairment in chronic illness depends on the type of disease, patient age at onset of illness, duration and severity of the disorder, and individual factors.

In milder cases of delayed puberty, treatment is often not required. However, evidence indicates the efficacy and safety of short courses of low-dose testosterone therapy in select individuals.[2538]

Isolated Gonadotropin Deficit

A variant of hypogonadotropic hypogonadism, isolated gonadotropin deficit (IHH), is characterized by absence of pubertal development, low levels of gonadotropins secondary to hypothalamus-hypophyseal axis abnormalities, and infertility. IHH results from defects in GnRH neuron fate, specification, or migration, as well as from anomalies in GnRH secretion or action causing defects in synthesis or release of FSH and LH; other hypophyseal functions are normal. The estimated incidence is 1 in 10,000 males and 1 in 50,000 females.[2539] The disorder is heterogeneous both clinically and genetically.[2540] Only 15% to 20% of patients with IHH have a demonstrable genetic basis. KAL1, GNRHR, and FGFR1 mutations are the most frequently detected abnormalities. Other genes implicated are nuclear receptor subfamily 0, group B member 1

(NR0B1), G protein–coupled receptor 54 (GPR54), leptin (LEP), leptin receptor (LEPR), proprotein convertase subtilisin/kexin type 1 (PCSK1), KISS1 metastasis suppressor (KISS1), nasal embryonic LHRH factor (NELF), prokineticin 2 (PROK2), prokineticin receptor 2 (PROKR2), chromodomain helicase DNA-binding protein (CHD7), tachykinin B (TAC3), and tachykinin B receptor (TAC3R).[2541,2542] The IHH phenotype may also be observed in combined hypophyseal deficiencies resulting from mutations in HESX homeobox 1 (HESX1), prophet of PIT1 (PROP1), and Lim homeobox gene 3 (LHX3).[2543–2545]

Patients with IHH may be normosmic, anosmic (in Kallmann syndrome), or suffer from LH deficit (fertile eunuch syndrome).

Idiopathic Normosmic Hypogonadotropic Hypogonadism

This form of IHH has classically been reported in patients who have eunuchoid phenotype, with small testes and penis, scant body and facial hair, high-pitched voice, and poorly developed muscles.[2523] It is caused by defective GnRH action on gonadotropin secretion. Genetic anomalies implicate the following genes: GnRH receptor (*GNRHR*), FGF receptor 1 (*FGFR1*), G protein–coupled receptor 54 (*GPR54*), cadherin 7 (*CDH7*), and the genes that encode tachykinin B (*TAC3*) and its receptor NK3R (*TAC3R*).[2546] Of these, the gene most frequently involved is GNRHR, of which nearly two dozen different mutations have been reported.[2547–2549] The frequency of FGR1 mutations varies from 3% to 7%.[2550,2551] Loss-of-function mutations of the *GPR54* gene have been reported in several members of the same family.[2552]

Patients have low levels of FSH, LH, testosterone, and estrogen. AMH levels are greatly elevated in this and other forms of hypogonadotropic hypogonadism. This finding is expected because Sertoli cells are immature. In normal boys, AMH concentrations decrease to undetectable levels at puberty when adequate testosterone synthesis is established. The same occurs in hypogonadotropic hypogonadism after treatment with hCG or testosterone.[2553]

Clomiphene citrate treatment fails to increase FSH and LH.[2339] Pulsatile administration of GnRH is useful to promote both androgen production and spermatogenesis. The LH–Leydig cell–testosterone axis is usually normal, but normalization of the FSH–Sertoli cell–inhibin axis is not achieved in all cases. Basal inhibin levels higher than 60 pg/mL, preceding a history of sexual maturation and absence of cryptorchidism, are favorable predictors of acquisition of normal testicular size and acceptable spermatogenesis.[2554]

Biopsy reveals an immature pattern (Fig. 12.272). Seminiferous tubules have neither lumina nor elastic fibers (Fig. 12.273). Sertoli cells are immature, and differentiated Leydig cells are lacking.[1866] Spermatogonia are found in low numbers and do not undergo proliferation. Some patients have Sertoli cell–only testes with immature Sertoli cells.[1865]

Hypogonadism Associated With Anosmia

Two syndromes are included: Kallmann syndrome and CHARGE syndrome.

Kallmann Syndrome

Kallmann syndrome is a specific type of IHH characterized by hypogonadotropic hypogonadism, anosmia, neurologic defects, facial midline defects, and renal abnormalities. A syndrome characterized by the association of hypogonadism with anosmia was first described in 1856.[2555] Eighty-eight years later the same syndrome was reported in three families, and the suggestion was made regarding genetic transmission.[2556] In 1954, testicular atrophy was

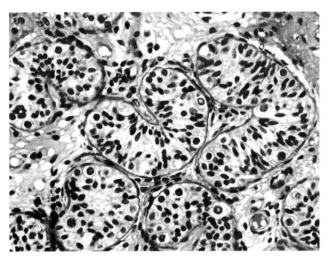

Fig. 12.272 Isolated gonadotropin deficit. The seminiferous tubules have prepubertal diameter, pseudostratified distribution of the Sertoli cells, and several spermatogonia per tubular section.

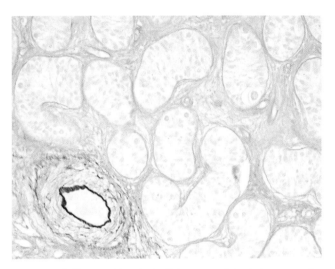

Fig. 12.273 A 17-year-old patient with hypogonadotropic hypogonadism. Absence of elastic fibers in the wall of seminiferous tubules (orcein).

identified in 14 of 31 patients with olfactory bulb agenesis, and the condition was named "olfactory-genital dysplasia."[2557] Patients may have hypogonadotropic hypogonadism and anosmia, or only one. Hypogonadism is caused defective hypothalamic GnRH secretion that causes failure in pituitary secretion of LH and FSH. Anosmia may be caused by olfactory bulb agenesis or neuronal dysfunction, because olfactory bulbs are present in 25% of patients.[2558] The anosmia may be unilateral by aplasia of the ipsilateral olfactory tract and bulb.[2559] Although many patients experience delayed puberty, the diagnosis is usually made in the third decade of life.[2560]

Autopsy studies in patients with anosmia and hypogonadism reveal agenesis of the olfactory bulbs that may be partial or complete and unilateral or bilateral, together with an apparently normal hypophysis and normal or hypoplastic hypothalamus. This syndrome is the least severe form of holoprosencephaly-hypopituitarism complex, a spectrum of developmental anomalies associated with impaired midline cleavage of the embryonic forebrain, aplasia of olfactory bulbs and tracts, and midline dysplasia of the face. Associated abnormalities include cryptorchidism, mental retardation, color blindness, facial asymmetry, nerve deafness, epilepsy, shortening of the fourth metacarpal, tarsal navicular fibrous dysplasia, diabetes mellitus, hyperlipidemia, gynecomastia, lip, maxillary or palate cleft, choanal atresia, dental agenesis, cardiovascular abnormalities, and neurologic disorders such as cerebellar ataxia, sensory-neural hearing loss, oculomotor abnormalities, and synkinesis (mirror movements of extremities).[2561–2564] Renal agenesis has also been reported.[2565] One patient experienced development of seminoma.[2566]

Kallmann syndrome may be associated with X-linked ichthyosis or punctata chondrodystrophy. Both disorders form part of a contiguous gene syndrome caused by large terminal or interstitial deletions of the Xp22.3 region.[2567–2569]

Presentation is heterogeneous and, within the same family, may include the full spectrum, anosmia only, hyposmia or anosmia limited to certain odors, and IHH only. Heterogeneity is also seen with associated somatic defects, as well as in the severity of hypogonadotropic hypogonadism. Many cases occur spontaneously, but others have a genetic cause. In the latter cases, inheritance may be X-linked recessive, autosomal dominant with variable expression, or autosomal recessive.[2570–2573] Inheritance pattern may correlate with mutations in specific genes.

Most patients with X-linked inheritance (30% to 70%) and 5% of patients without a family history have mutations in the *KAL1* gene, mapped to the Xp22.3 region.[2574] This gene encodes the protein anosmin-1, similar to other nerve cell adhesion molecules (NCAM, NCAMLI, TAGI, and contactin) involved in axonal growth and development.[2575] KALIG-1 seems to be involved in spatial orientation of growth in GnRH neurons and may have various mutations (termed *Kal-X*, *KALIG1*, and *ADMLX*), complete deletion, and point mutations.[2576] Autosomal-dominant presentation (occurring in 10% of cases) results from loss of function of *FGFR1*. Interaction between *KAL1* and *FGFR1* is required for neuronal migration. The predominant mutations are in *FGFR1*, prokineticin receptor 2 (*PROKR2*), prokineticin 2 (*PROK2*), *FGF8*, and nasal embryonic LHRH factor (*NELF*).[2577,2578] The autosomal recessive form is caused by mutations in *PROKR2* and *PROK2*. Currently, KS is classified into six subtypes: type 1 or X-linked KS associated with KAL1 mutation; subtypes 2, 3, 4, 5, and 6 linked, respectively, with mutations in *FGFR1*, *PROKR2*, *PROK2*, *CHD7*, and *FGF8*.[2579]

For a full understanding of the importance of these proteins, it is best to keep in mind a summary of embryonal development of some anatomic structures.[2580] Olfactory sensory neurons originate from the olfactory placode (embryo) or neuroepithelium (postnatal life). Projections of these neurons occur in a stereotyped manner. Olfactory sensory neurons that express receptors for specific odors cross the cribriform lamina and converge to form a few glomeruli in the olfactory bulb.[2581] These glomeruli establish synapses with dendrites of mitral cells whose axons form the olfactory tract. Mitral cells secrete a glycosylated 600-amino acid protein, referred to as KAL or anosmin, that induces odor-sensitive olfactory sensory neuron axons to grow and penetrate the olfactory bulb to establish synapses with mitral cells.[2582] The neuroepithelium also gives rise to a population of neuroblasts that migrate to reach the medial basal hypothalamus, where they originate in cells that secrete GnRH.[2583] GnRH reaches the anterior lobule of the hypophysis by the portal system. This migration occurs in two stages. First, neuroblasts exit the olfactory placode, cross the cribriform lamina, and reach the vicinity of olfactory sensory neurons. Second, the neuroblasts migrate from the olfactory bulb to the hypothalamus

following the vomeronasal nerve and produce GnRH neurons. Axons of the vomeronasal nerve secrete cell adhesion molecules of the CAM type to ensure this migration.[2584] These neurons secrete GnRH, the peptide that controls FSH and LH secretion by gonadotropic cells in the hypophyseal anterior lobule. In Kallmann syndrome, mitral cells fail to secrete KAL protein, and axons of the olfactory bulb neurons do not penetrate the brain but instead form a tangle between the cribriform lamina and forebrain. Migration of GnRH neurons also remains blocked. This anomaly is not limited to patients with Kallmann syndrome, but has also been observed in arhinencephalic disorders such as CHARGE syndrome, trisomy 13, and trisomy 18.[2585]

In human fetuses with Kallmann syndrome, GnRH neurons, as well as the axons of olfactory neurosensory neurons, vomeronasal nerves, and axon terminals, end in the meninges and form an abnormal neural tangle.[2583] GnRH neurons do not penetrate the brain and may be found in nasal cavities or the dorsal surface of the cribriform lamina. These alterations lead to aplasia or agenesis of the olfactory bulb and olfactory tract and to hypothalamic aplasia, and may be easily demonstrated by MRI.[2586] Pituitary structure and its response to pulsatile GnRH stimulation are normal.

In infancy and puberty, the most important findings suggesting the diagnosis of Kallmann syndrome are anosmia or hyposmia, hypoplasia of the penis (65%) and cryptorchidism (73%), cleft lip/palate (13% to 14%), hearing loss (28%), renal agenesis, or synkinesis.[2587] Diagnosis is confirmed by the absence of olfactory bulbs and olfactory tract on MRI.

Adult patients are classified into two groups according to the partial or complete absence of GnRH. Complete absence is diagnosed by the absence of spontaneous pulses of LH, FSH, and testosterone during a 24-hour period.[2588] These patients show an increase in FSH only after GnRH administration.[2589] Testes are histologically infantile; tubules have small diameters that may be even smaller than that of infantile seminiferous tubules, lack lumina, and contain immature Sertoli cells and isolated spermatogonia.[2590] The interstitium is wide and consists of acellular connective tissue with no recognizable Leydig cell precursors (Fig. 12.274).[2591] Partial absence of GnRH is diagnosed by the

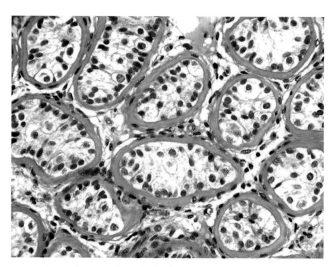

Fig. 12.274 Hypogonadism associated with anosmia in a previously treated patient. The testis shows marked hyalinization of the tubular wall. Some spermatogonia may be observed among the Sertoli cells. The testicular interstitium lacks Leydig cells.

presence of spontaneous pulses of LH, FSH, and testosterone during a 24-hour period, and biopsies show some degree of pubertal maturation.

Treatment also varies. If only virilization is desired, androgenic therapy is sufficient. If the aim is to promote fertility, hCG alone or in combination with recombinant human FSH or hMG or pulsed administration of GnRH may be used.[2592]

CHARGE Syndrome

The term *CHARGE syndrome*, proposed in 1987, incorporates letters from the most characteristic anomalies of this disorder: coloboma, congenital heart disease, choanal atresia, retarded growth, mental retardation, or central nervous system anomalies, genital hypoplasia, and ear anomalies or deafness.[2593] Most cases are sporadic; in familial cases, autosomal dominant inheritance is suggested. The syndrome is caused by mutations in the *CHD7* gene (chromodomain helicase DNA-binding protein 7) located on chromosome 8q12.1, which belongs to a protein family that participates in chromatin organization in fetal development.[2594–2596] CHARGE syndrome is present in 1 in 10,000 newborns and has no gender distinction. Micropenis and cryptorchidism are frequent findings, indicative of hypogonadotropic hypogonadism, and associated with anosmia by olfactory bulb hypoplasia or aplasia in 81% of patients.[2597–2600]

Isolated Luteinizing Hormone Deficiency

The first reports of patients with eunuchoid habitus, conserved spermatogenesis ("fertile eunuchs"), LH deficit, spermatozoa, and absence of Leydig cells appeared in the 1950s.[2601–2603] Patients have eunuchoid habitus, small testes, decreased libido, female distribution of pubic hair, and high-pitched voice. Other frequent findings include gynecomastia, anosmia, ocular lesions, and pituitary tumor.[2603] FSH level is normal, but LH and testosterone are low.[2604] The negative response to clomiphene citrate suggests hypothalamic anomaly.[2605,2606] Mutations in the LH β-subunit gene and the GnRH receptor have been reported.[2607–2611]

The clomiphene test result is usually negative, and GnRH stimulation produces a normal response, increased LH, and to a lesser degree, FSH, and suggests that pituitary gonadal function is normal.[2612] Biopsy shows seminiferous tubules with normal or slightly decreased diameters and complete spermatogenesis; however, the number of all germ cell types is lower than normal. Leydig cells are rare or absent (Fig. 12.275). Maintenance of spermatogenesis in the absence of Leydig cells and serum testosterone may be explained only by assuming occurrence of testosterone secretion sufficient for spermatogenesis, but not high enough to be detectable in the blood. LH increase, produced by pulsatile GnRH secretion, occurs during monitored sleep.[2613] Under FSH stimulation, Sertoli cells secrete large ABP amounts, which induce testosterone level elevation that is enough to maintain spermatogenesis.[2614] Treatment with testosterone or hCG improves spermatogenesis.

Isolated Follicle-Stimulating Hormone Deficiency

Isolated FSH deficiency is a rare syndrome characterized by azoospermia or oligozoospermia in normally virilized patients with normal sexual potency.[2615] It is an exceptional clinical situation caused by FSH β-subunit gene mutations.[2616–2619] Serum levels of LH and testosterone are normal, but FSH is low or undetectable.[2620] Clomiphene stimulation gives variable results, whereas the GnRH test induces only normal LH response.[2621] Biopsy in puberty shows a reduced number of Sertoli cells, absence of germ cells, Leydig cell hyperplasia, and thickened basement membrane in

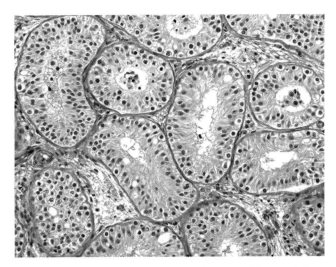

Fig. 12.275 Isolated deficiency of luteinizing hormone. Most seminiferous tubules have a central lumen, numerous spermatogonia, and increased number of Sertoli cells. Spermatocytes and spermatids are observed only in isolated tubules. The testicular interstitium lacks Leydig cells.

seminiferous tubules.[2622] Biopsy in adults shows maturation arrest at the spermatocyte level, hypospermatogenesis, or partial Sertoli cell–only pattern.[2623] Gonadotropin treatment increases spermatozoal numbers in most cases, and fertility may be induced after as little as 20 weeks of treatment.[2624]

Bioinactive Follicle-Stimulating Hormone and Luteinizing Hormone

In addition to adequate hypothalamic function, spermatogenesis requires that FSH and LH be biologically active for adequate Leydig cell stimulation.[2625,2626] LH is a heterodimer, composed of two subunits: α (common to FSH and LH) and β (specific for LH). The genes for the β subunit are on 19q13.32, close to another cluster of genes and pseudogenes that encode the hCGβ subunit. If both alleles are mutated, LH is biologically inactive, although it may be detectable in standard hormone assay. Homozygous patients have an elevated serum level of LH, normal FSH, and testosterone, failure of puberty, infantile testes, and infertility. Heterozygous patients are infertile but otherwise normal.[2627] Patients with mutation in the β subunit of the FSH gene are oligozoospermic or azoospermic.[2628] Low-bioactive FSH has been detected in patients with idiopathic oligozoospermia.[2629]

Mutations in Gonadotropin Receptor Genes

Activating and inactivating mutations of gonadotropin receptor genes may occur.[2630–2632] Activating mutation of the LH/hCG receptor gene causes familial precocious puberty (see earlier Familial Testotoxicosis section).[690,2633] Complete inactivation of this gene by mutation results in a male with completely female phenotype secondary to poor differentiation and activity of Leydig cells (see Disorders of Sex Development (Leydig Cell Hypoplasia)). Partial LH/hCG resistance results in male phenotype with micropenis and hypospadias.

Inactivating mutation of the *FSHR* gene produces only mildly impaired spermatogenesis, a finding emphasizing the limited role of FSH in spermatogenesis.[1922] Activating mutation of this gene was reported in a patient who experienced panhypopituitarism after surgical removal and irradiation of pituitary adenoma. Despite low gonadotropin levels, the patient had a normal seminal study.[2634]

Growth Hormone Deficit

GH plays an important role in the development and functional maintenance of male and female reproductive systems.[2635] Patients with GH deficit (isolated GH deficit, resistance to GH action, multiple hormonal pituitary deficiencies, or men with dwarfism such as the Laron type) may have delayed puberty and hypogonadotropic hypogonadism.[2636,2637] Some patients with spermatogenetic maturation arrest or idiopathic oligozoospermia have relative deficit of GH.[2638,2639] This hormone apparently directly stimulates Sertoli cells or Leydig cells to secrete IGFI, which likely stimulates spermatozoa maturation in a paracrine-autocrine way.[2640]

Prader-Willi Syndrome or Hypotonia-Hypomentia-Hypogonadism-Obesity Syndrome

PWS or hypotonia-hypomentia-hypogonadism-obesity syndrome is characterized by hypogonadism, obesity, muscular hypotonia, mental and physical retardation, acromicria, and hyperphagia.[2641] Other frequent findings include strabismus, non–insulin-dependent diabetes mellitus, hypothyroidism, and short stature.[2642–2644] Symptoms begin during gestation, during which negligible fetal motility is seen. Difficulties in delivery and postnatal feeding have also been observed. The incidence is estimated at between 1 in 12,000 and 15,000 newborns, and is higher in boys (60% of cases). Most cases are sporadic, but familial inheritance has been reported.[2645] In infants, there is a transient rise in postnatal testosterone levels that gives rise to "minipuberty," but hereafter, delayed and incomplete puberty is the norm. During infancy the penis and testes may be either normal or hypoplastic, and cryptorchidism is present in approximately 70% of cases (bilateral in 45% of cases) (Fig. 12.276).[2646–2648]

Hypogonadism is present in 87% of adult patients with PWS and has classically been described as hypogonadotropic. However, hormonal data and biopsy findings suggest a special form of hypogonadism consisting of a combination of central and peripheral hypogonadism. Hormonal assays show low serum levels of LH, testosterone, estradiol, and B inhibin, whereas FSH is high.[2649] Patients frequently have deficits in other hypophyseal hormones, findings in accord with the small size of the anterior pituitary.[2650]

At birth the gubernaculum shows altered concentrations of collagen and elastic fibers.[2651] During infancy and childhood the testes have reduced tubular diameters for age, and spermatogonia are scant or completely absent.[2652,2653] Adult patients have small testes with infantile tubular diameters and common absence of spermatogonia.[2654] Despite normal serum levels of FSH, Sertoli cells do not undergo pubertal maturation.

This syndrome is caused by an anomaly of chromosome 15, usually in the 15p11-q13 band, a chromosomal region that contains the imprinted genes *SNRPN*, *PAR1*, *PAR5*, *ZNF127*, and *IPW7*. Cytogenetically, deletions in this region of chromosome 15 occur in 70% of patients.[2655] These deletions always occur in the paternal chromosome.[2656–2660] Chromosome 15 deletions are demonstrable either by G-banding techniques or fluorescence in situ hybridization.[2661] Maternal uniparental disomy of chromosome 15 is observed in 25% of cases, and mutations altering the imprinting process are found in 5%.[2662,2663] These latter mutations usually alter the small nucleolar ribonucleoprotein N gene (*SNRPN* gene) or involve translocations in chromosome 15.[2664–2670]

Diagnosis by molecular testing revealed that 17% of patients do not fulfill clinical criteria established in 1993. To avoid overdiagnosis, an adequate, age-related evaluation of the patient's clinical symptoms is recommended when molecular techniques are not available.[438,2671] Association of PWS and 47,XYY syndrome has been reported.[2672]

Bardet-Biedl Syndrome

Bardet-Biedl syndrome (BBS), first described in 1920, is a pleiotropic disorder characterized by obesity (72% to 96%), mental retardation (>50%), postaxial polydactyly (69%), retinal dystrophy or retinitis pigmentosa (>90%), hypogonadism (98%), and renal structural abnormalities or functional impairment (100%).[2673–2675] Expression and severity of the various clinical BBS features show interfamilial and intrafamilial variability.[2676] The prevalence of BBS in Europe and North America varies from 1 in 125,000 to 175,000 newborns, and is markedly increased (1 in 13,500) in highly consanguineous Arab-Bedouin communities and in Newfoundland, Canada.[2677] Mean age at diagnosis is 9 years, but BBS may be suspected in patients with associated polydactyly, precocious obesity, and hyperechogenic kidneys.[2678] BBS is more frequent and severe in males. Men are infertile, and approximately 74% show hypogonadism that is usually characterized by cryptorchidism, which is found in 42% of male patients and is bilateral in 28%; hypoplastic or bifid scrotum; and small penis. Testes are prepubertal, in keeping with the hypothalamic origin of this hypogonadotropic hypogonadism.[2679] However, three exceptions have been reported: (1) patient with normal serum testosterone, increased FSH, and tubular hyalinization and germinal aplasia; (2) patient with normal testosterone and gonadotropins, as well as germinal aplasia; and (3) patient who presented with delayed puberty, followed by hypogonadotropic hypogonadism that reversed, ending with normal gonadotropins and normal spermatogenesis.[2680–2682] Patients are infertile except for isolated cases.[2683]

There is a high incidence of pituitary anomalies by MRI (63%) and hormonal derangements (45%). Prominent structural pituitary abnormalities include tumoral changes, hypoplastic hypophysis, and Rathke cleft cysts. Endocrinologic anomalies include delayed puberty, hypogonadotropic hypogonadism, GH deficiency, and hyperprolactinemia.[2684]

Mutations in 21 genes (*BBS1* to *BBS20* and *NPHP1*) have been cloned to date and are present in 70% to 80% of BBS-affected families.[2685] In whites, mutations in *BBS1* and *BBS10* genes are responsible for 45% to 50% of cases.[2686,2687] Mutated proteins in BBS are ones involved in regulation of microtubule-based

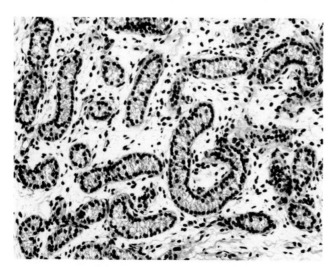

Fig. 12.276 Testis from a 7-year-old child with Prader-Willi syndrome. The seminiferous tubules have a reduced diameter and lack germ cells.

transport processes and are included in the ciliopathy family of disorders that also includes Joubert syndrome and Meckel-Gruber syndrome.[2688] Dysfunction of these proteins is responsible at least for the ocular and renal lesions.[2678,2689–2698]

Hypogonadotropic Hypogonadism Associated With Dermatologic Diseases

Associations between ichthyosis, hypogonadism, epilepsy, mental retardation, dwarfism, and macrocytic anemia have been reported since 1927.[2699] Inheritance is heterogeneous. Currently, several different ichthyosis types are recognized, each with its own characteristics.[2700]

Most cases of ichthyosis associated with hypogonadism are X linked. Approximately 15% of patients have cryptorchidism, small testes, micropenis, and a high risk for testicular cancer. The cause is a defective microsomal enzyme, steroid sulfatase, which catalyzes hydrolysis of several sulfated 3β-hydroxysteroids in fibroblasts, leukocytes, and keratinocytes. Hydrolysis causes accumulation of cholesterol sulfate that hinders sloughing of the cornified layer of the epidermis. The gene responsible for this enzyme is mapped to Xp22.3. The associated hypogonadism is usually hypogonadotropic. Some patients also have anosmia or hyposmia because involvement of adjacent genes causes a contiguous gene defect.[2701–2703]

Johnson-McMillin neuroectodermic syndrome is a rare autosomal dominant disorder characterized by alopecia, hypogonadotropic hypogonadism, anosmia or hyposmia, deafness, prominent ears, microtia, or atresia of the external auditory meatus, and pronounced tendency to dental caries. Both genders are affected.[2704–2706]

Hypogonadotropic Hypogonadism Associated With Ataxia

Hypogonadism associated with ataxia is rare.[2707–2709] Most are children from a consanguineous marriage. Inheritance is autosomal recessive.[2710,2711] Patients show eunuchoidism, absence of secondary sex characteristics and libido, firm and small testes, and infertility.[2712,2713] The most frequent syndromes are Louis-Bar syndrome (ataxia-telangiectasia) and Friedreich ataxia.

Ataxia-Telangiectasia

Ataxia-telangiectasia is the most common inherited ataxia (autosomal recessive; 1 in 50,000), with an estimated carrier frequency of 1 in 110 in the European population. It is characterized by cerebellar ataxia that begins in infancy and develops progressively to include mucocutaneous telangiectasis, anomalies of the immune system that cause pulmonary infection, hypersensitivity to ionizing radiation resulting from impairment of DNA repair, and high risk for lymphoid neoplasia.[2714] Immunologic anomalies involve both humoral and cellular immunity, and cause low T cell response to mitogens and antigens, decreased number of CD4 cells, increased numbers of γ-δ T cells, low serum levels of immunoglobulin A (IgA), IgE, and often IgG, and elevated IgM.[2715–2718] Bronchiolitis obliterans is the most characteristic disease resulting from the immunologic impairment.[2719] Cytomegalic cells with telescoped nuclear inclusions have been observed in the pituitary. This disorder starts with progressive gait and limb ataxia; symptoms begin before 25 years of age. Other symptoms are loss of vibration and position sense, areflexia, dysarthria, skeletal abnormalities, and hypertrophic cardiomyopathy that frequently leads to precocious death.[2720] Gonadal alterations are more important in females and are manifest by precocious puberty and early menopause.[2721] The gene responsible is on 11q22-q23.1.[2722] Ataxia results from inactivation of A-T mutated kinase, a critical protein kinase that regulates the response to DNA double-strand breaks by selective phosphorylation of a variety of substrates.[2723]

Friedreich Ataxia

Friedreich ataxia is a neurodegenerative disorder characterized by degeneration of dorsal root ganglia and spinocerebellar tracts.[2724] Its onset typically occurs during childhood or adolescence.[2725] The disease is characterized by gait and limb ataxia, dysarthria, usually absent tendon reflex, bilateral Babinski sign, impairment of position and vibratory senses, scoliosis, pes cavus, and a high incidence of hypertrophic cardiomyopathy. The incidence is estimated at 1 in 40,000 children.[2726] Symptoms and the rapidity of disease development vary even within members of the same family. The associated hypogonadism is usually hypogonadotropic, although cases of hypergonadotropic hypogonadism have also been reported.

This syndrome is the first trinucleotide disease with autosomal recessive inheritance. It is caused by defects in the *FXN* gene, which encodes a 210-amino acid mitochondrial protein that is a precursor of frataxin.[2727] *FXN* mRNA levels in these patients are reduced to 13% to 30% and to 40% in carriers. The residual level of frataxin protein in patients with this disorder varies between 5% and 30% of normal levels, whereas healthy heterozygous carriers express more than 50% of normal frataxin levels.[2728,2729] Frataxin deficiency causes a range of metabolic disturbances, which include oxidative stress, deficit of iron–sulfur clusters, and defects in heme synthesis, sulfur amino acid and energy metabolism, stress response, and mitochondrial function.[2730] Mitochondrial iron deposition in the heart usually accompanies hypertrophic cardiomyopathy, the main cause of death.[2731] Approximately 95% of patients are homozygous for unstable trinucleotide (GAA) expansion located in the first intron of the *FXN* gene on chromosome 9q13.[2732] The normal gene has up to 35 or 40 triplet repeats, whereas patients with ataxia carry 70 to more than 1000 GAA triplets.[2733] Extent of the expanded allele is directly proportional to severity of disease, early onset, and development of cardiac abnormalities.[2734] Other ataxias associated with hypogonadism are Kearns-Sayre (see later), Boucher-Neuhäuser, and Gordon-Holmes syndromes.

Boucher-Neuhäuser Syndrome

Characteristics of the autosomal recessive Boucher-Neuhäuser syndrome are cerebellar ataxia, hypogonadotropic hypogonadism, and chorioretinal dystrophy.[2711,2735,2736] Boucher-Neuhäuser syndrome is caused by mutations in the *PNPLA6* gene.[2737] A characteristic finding in these patients is the occurrence of hypersegmented neutrophils. Although this finding is frequent in other processes, it may be useful to support the diagnosis in the presence of other symptoms suggestive of Boucher-Neuhäuser syndrome.[2738]

Gordon-Holmes Syndrome

Gordon-Holmes syndrome is characterized by progressive cerebellar ataxia and hypogonadotropic hypogonadism. This rare autosomal recessive disorder was first recognized more than 100 years ago. The genetic causes of this syndrome are biallelic inactivating mutations in the *RNF216* gene or the combination of deleterious mutations in *RNF216* and *OTUD4* genes.[2739] GnRH pulsatile administration does not increase gonadotropins because of a hypothalamic defect.[2740] However, treatment with exogenous gonadotropins is efficacious in establishing spermatogenesis.[2741]

Carpenter Syndrome

The autosomal recessive disorder Carpenter syndrome, also known as acrocephalopolysyndactyly type II, was first reported in 1901.[2742] Carpenter syndrome is characterized by craniosynostosis, peculiar facies, prolonged retention of primary teeth or hypodontia, brachysyndactyly of fingers, preaxial polydactyly, syndactyly, congenital heart disease, obesity, mental retardation, umbilical hernia, cryptorchidism, and hypogonadism.[2743,2744] The disorder is caused by mutations in the *RAB23* gene, which encodes a member of the RAB-family of small guanosine triphosphatase involved in vesicle trafficking.[2745,2746]

Biemond Syndrome

Biemond syndrome is characterized by hypogonadotropic hypogonadism, coloboma of the iris, short stature, severe mental retardation, and postaxial polydactyly.[2746a] This is one of the syndromes included in retinal ciliopathies.[2746b]

Fraser Syndrome (Meyer-Schwickerath Syndrome or Ullrich-Feichtiger Syndrome)

Fraser syndrome is an inherited autosomal recessive multisystemic disorder first reported in 1962.[2747] Its incidence is estimated to be 0.43 in 100,000 live-born infants and 11 in 100,000 stillbirths.[2748,2749] The syndrome is characterized by unilateral or bilateral cryptophthalmus, facial anomalies (abnormal hairline, coloboma of alae nasi, midfacial cleft, cleft lip and palate, ankyloglossia, small ears), conductive hearing loss, syndactyly, umbilical hernia, cryptorchidism, and hypogonadotropic hypogonadism.[2750] It is genetically heterogeneous, and three genes are involved: *FRAS1* on 4q21.21, *FREM2* on 13q13.3, and *GRIP1* on 12q14.3. In 50% of cases, a causative mutation is detected.

Approximately one-half of the families with Fraser syndrome carry mutations in the *FRAS1* gene on chromosome 4, and the remainder have about an equal incidence of mutations in the other two genes.[2751,2752] FRAS1 and FREM proteins are expressed on the basal surface of epithelial cells in many embryonic tissues and contribute to embryonic epithelial-mesenchymal integrity. Its function is replaced once terminated in embryogenesis by type VII collagen.[2753]

Hypogonadism Secondary to Endocrine Gland Dysfunction and Other Disorders

Maintenance of spermatogenesis requires synchronous actions of several endocrine glands and proper functioning of other tissues. Although only 2% of infertile men have stigmata of endocrinopathy, more than 9% have abnormal endocrine studies.[2754] Hypogonadism may be present in disorders involving the hypothalamus-hypophysis, thyroid, adrenals, pancreas, liver, kidney, and gastrointestinal tract, and may be associated with AIDS, chronic anemia, obesity, starvation, inherited metabolic diseases, and neoplasia. Hypogonadotropic hypogonadism may also be found in some patients (especially women) who perform rigorous sports (long-distance runners, swimmers, dancers, and rhythmic gymnasts).[2518]

Hypothalamus-Hypophysis

Hypopituitarism

Hypogonadism may result from destruction of the hypothalamus or hypophysis caused by primary or secondary hypothalamic tumor; granulomatous disease (histiocytosis X or Langerhans cell histiocytosis) (Figs. 12.277 and 12.278); fracture of the cranial

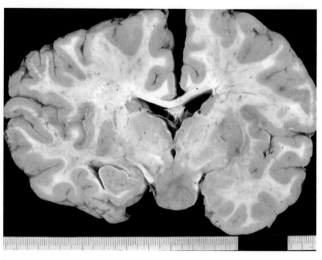

Fig. 12.277 Frontal section from an 18-year-old patient showing destruction of the hypothalamus caused by Langerhans cell histiocytosis.

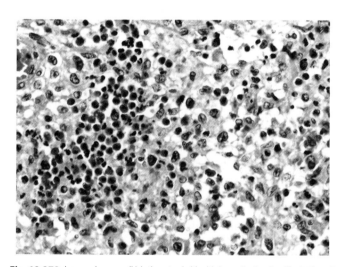

Fig. 12.278 Langerhans cell histiocytosis X with hypothalamic affectation. A severe infiltrate with large cells with grooved nuclei and abundant eosinophilic leukocytes may be observed.

base; radiation therapy for malignancy of the nasopharynx, central nervous system, or orbit; pituitary adenoma (Fig. 12.279) and cyst; aneurysm of the internal carotid artery; and chronic and nutrition disease. Many of these processes cause panhypopituitarism with varied symptoms, and sometimes lead to a selective decrease in secretion of LH and FSH.[2755–2757]

Clinical manifestations of hypogonadism in patients with pituitary lesions vary according to the time of onset (childhood or after puberty).[2758] In prepubertal hypopituitarism the testes retain an infantile appearance into adulthood. Proliferation of spermatogonia and development of primary spermatocytes are rare. Biopsy shows variable hyalinization of tubules. In postpubertal hypopituitarism, there is a decrease in ejaculate volume and testicular volume, as well as low testosterone, FSH, and LH levels. Histology ranges from complete spermatogenesis to tubular hyalinization (Fig. 12.280). The presence of elastic fibers in tubular walls indicates that pubertal maturation occurred before the development of hypopituitarism. Leydig cells have pyknotic nuclei and retracted cytoplasm with abundant lipofuscin.[2756] In some patients, recovery of spermatogenesis occurs after administration of hCG.[2759] In

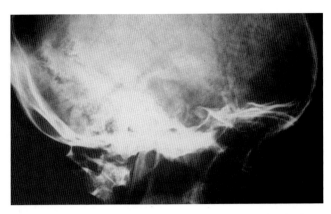

Fig. 12.279 Radiologic image of a pituitary macroadenoma showing important enlargement of sella turcica.

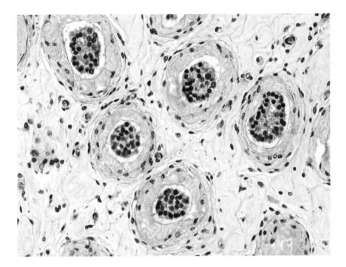

Fig. 12.280 Tubular hyalinization caused by hormonal deprivation and decreased Leydig cell number in a 28-year-old patient who underwent surgery because of pituitary adenoma. The seminiferous tubules contain dedifferentiated Sertoli cells and isolated spermatogonia.

some cases, pituitary adenoma secretes FSH and LH, thus inducing testosterone hypersecretion and elevated sperm count.[2760] A significant number of patients have macroorchidism. Testicular enlargement is due to an increase in the length of the seminiferous tubules.[618,641]

Hyperprolactinemia

PRL inhibits GnRH secretion and hence FSH and LH secretion. In addition, PRL has a direct inhibitory effect on androgens in target tissues. In men, hyperprolactinemia causes impairment of spermatogenesis, impotence, loss of libido, and depressed serum testosterone.[2761] Some patients seek treatment because of oligozoospermia and infertility. Hyperprolactinemia is also associated with dysfunction of PRL receptors.[2762] The spermiogram usually shows oligozoospermia and an elevated level of fructose, although not all male patients with hyperprolactinemia have subnormal testicular function.[2763,2764]

Biopsy reveals variable testicular atrophy. The most frequent lesion is in the tubular adluminal compartment, with degenerative changes in the apical cytoplasm of Sertoli cells, sloughing of young spermatids, and increased lipid droplets in Leydig cells.[2763,2765] In addition to prolactinoma, two other conditions associated with

abnormal PRL secretion have been reported in boys: one is characterized by hyperprolactinemia, testicular enlargement, and primary hypothyroidism; the other consists of PRL deficiency, obesity, and enlarged testes.[621,2766–2769] In adults, testicular hypertrophy may also be secondary to FSH-secreting pituitary adenoma.[2770]

Thyroid Gland

Thyroid hormone plays an important role in testicular development and function by influencing steroidogenesis and spermatogenesis, mainly in infancy. Triiodothyronine (T_3) is involved in control of Sertoli cell proliferation and functional maturation, as well as postnatal Leydig cell differentiation and steroidogenesis.[2771]

Infertility caused by thyroid gland malfunction is rare but reversible. It accounts for approximately 0.5% of cases of male infertility. Testicular function is impaired more by hypothyroidism than by hyperthyroidism. Patients with hyperthyroidism may have gynecomastia, impotence, and infertility. Levels of FSH and LH in serum are normal or increased, with elevated SHBG, increased testosterone concentration, reduced non-SHBG–bound testosterone, and little or no change in free testosterone.[2772,2773] Patients with Graves disease have pronounced inhibition of gonadal steroidogenesis.[2774] In patients with hyperthyroidism, spermatozoa may be normal or reduced in number, and progressive motility is low. Primary hypothyroidism in adults causes hypergonadotropic, hypogonadotropic, or normogonadotropic hypogonadism, but testicular function is rarely impaired, and patients are usually fertile.[2775,2776] The cause of testicular damage is decreased gonadotropins or hyperprolactinemia.[2777]

Congenital central hypothyroidism is characterized by impaired secretion of TSH, which may or may not be accompanied by impaired secretion of other pituitary hormones. Testes are small. A form of central X-linked congenital hypothyroidism known as immunoglobulin superfamily member 1 (IGSF1) deficiency syndrome characterized by loss-of-function mutations in the *IGSF1* gene apart from hypothyroidism shows variable prolactin deficiency, occasional GH deficiency and, frequently, macroorchidism.[636]

Prepubertal hypothyroidism may impair function by causing precocious or delayed puberty. In delayed puberty, hypothyroidism leads to hypogonadotropic hypogonadism, with testes showing incomplete maturation arrest and hydrocele in severe myxedematous hypothyroidism.[623] In experimental hypothyroidism, enlargement is frequently associated with increased spermatid production.[2778a] Children with hypothyroidism usually have precocious pseudopuberty, and frequently have testicular enlargement without virilization.[619,2778] Approximately 80% have macroorchidism, most have increased FSH level, and 50% have elevated LH level.[620,621,2779] Testosterone level is normal during infancy. Prepubertal biopsy shows accelerated development with pubertal maturation of seminiferous tubules, but not Leydig cells. Testicular size in this type of macroorchidism diminishes as soon as substitutive therapy starts.[620,626,627] Etiopathogenesis is based on three hypotheses: increase in gonadotropin secretion caused by TRH stimulation of gonadotropic cells, direct TSH effect resulting from structural similarity between TSH receptors and FSHRs present in the testis, and lack of steroid hormones required for testicular maturation (in their absence Sertoli cell proliferation is excessive, giving rise to testicular enlargement).[628–630,632–635]

Adrenals

Adrenal disorders most frequently associated with infertility are adrenal hypoplasia, adrenal hyperplasia, Cushing syndrome (CS), and adrenal cortical tumors.

Congenital Adrenal Hypoplasia With Hypogonadotropic Hypogonadism

Congenital adrenal hypoplasia with hypogonadotropic hypogonadism, first reported in 1975, is an X-linked recessive disorder that gives rise to adrenal insufficiency in the first months of life with symptoms such as delayed growth, poor feeding, vomiting, weight loss, muscular weakness, and lethargy: all symptoms run parallel to involution of the fetal adrenal cortex.[2780,2781] The disorder is also characterized by cryptorchidism and delayed puberty.[2782,2783]

This rare disorder is caused by mutations or complete deletion of the *NROB1* gene that encodes the DAX-1 protein. The responsible gene, *DAX1* on Xp21, is expressed in the adrenals, testes, pituitary, and hypothalamus.[2784] DAX-1 protein has 470 amino acids, and the N-terminal portion contains four incomplete repeats of a new structural motif encoding DNA-binding function. The C-terminal half of the protein has high homology with the ligand-binding domain (E domain) of the nuclear hormone receptor superfamily, especially with the E domain of the retinoid x receptor and orphan receptor subfamily.[2785] Most patients have deletions or point mutations of DAX-1.[2786-2789] Large mutations may also alter genes located next to DAX-1. This could explain the association of congenital adrenal hypoplasia with hypogonadotropic hypogonadism and Duchenne muscular dystrophy, glycerol kinase deficiency, short stature, and psychomotor delay.[2790,2791] The resulting hypogonadism may be either pure or mixed (hypophyseal and testicular). In the mixed form, hypogonadism is partial.[2789] In some patients the cause of hypogonadism seems to be pituitary failure because levels of FSH, LH, and testosterone are low, and FSH and LH increase in response to GnRH stimulation.[2792,2793] Other patients present with mixed and partial hypogonadism, both pituitary and testicular; basal levels of FSH and LH are normal or high, and do not increase after GnRH stimulation.[2794] It is conceivable that, during the first years of life, the hypothalamohypophyseal-testicular axis acts properly.[2795] Then, at the onset of puberty, transient hypergonadotropic hypogonadism occurs, and in adulthood, hypogonadotropic hypogonadism is established.[2796,2797] Cases of precocious puberty with testicular and penile enlargement likely secondary to persistent ACTH stimulation have been reported.[2798,2799]

Autopsy studies of infants who died with congenital adrenal hypoplasia suggest that adrenal lesions are like those of the so-called fetal or cytomegalic form of adrenal hypoplasia.[2800] The adrenal glands are small and have abnormal architecture. The adrenal cortex is poorly developed, and no clear distinction between the zona glomerulosa and zona fasciculata may be established. Adrenal cortical cells are abnormally large and pleomorphic.[2801]

Most adult patients have azoospermia or oligozoospermia. Biopsy from one of our adult patients (Fig. 12.281) demonstrated lesions that suggested primary testicular alteration consisting of seminiferous tubules with only dysgenetic Sertoli cells, together with tubules showing spermatogonial maturation arrest, as well as hypertrophy and hyperplasia of Leydig cells (Fig. 12.282).[2802-2804] Exogenous gonadotropin treatment is ineffective in reestablishing spermatogenesis.[2805]

Congenital Adrenal Hyperplasia

Infertility is common in patients with minor forms of congenital adrenal hyperplasia (Fig. 12.283), and these patients often seek consultation regarding infertility. Most patients present with a deficiency of 21-hydroxylase or 11β-hydroxylase.[2806] In untreated patients, the testes become enlarged by testicular adrenal rest

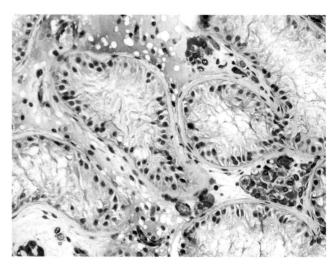

Fig. 12.281 Congenital adrenal hypoplasia with hypogonadotropic hypogonadism treated. Seminiferous tubules lacking lumen with only Sertoli cells.

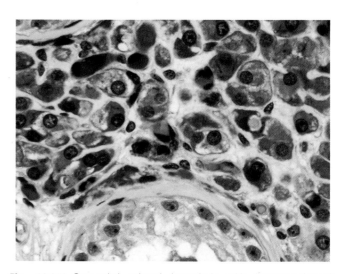

Fig. 12.282 Congenital adrenal hypoplasia with hypogonadotropic hypogonadism treated. Leydig cell hyperplasia; many cells have vacuolated cytoplasm.

tumors (TARTs), the so-called tumors of the adrenogenital syndrome first described in 1940 (Figs. 12.284 through 12.288).[2807-2811] Some TARTs are palpable, but others require ultrasonographic or MRI studies for detection. Grossly the tumors consist of well-delimited, but not encapsulated, yellow nodules, up to several centimeters in greatest dimension located in the parenchyma. They are composed of large, microvacuolated cells that are similar to cells that comprise Leydig cell tumors. Distinction of TART from Leydig cell tumor may be difficult (Table 12.26).[2812] Although CD56 immunoexpression has been reported to be diffuse and strong in tumors of adrenogenital syndrome and focally weak to moderate or negative in Leydig cell tumors, this finding is inconsistent and unreliable.[2813] Delta-like 1 homolog (DLK1) is expressed in TART, whereas INSL3 is expressed in Leydig cell tumors.[2814]

Patients seeking consultation for infertility present with oligospermia (60%) or azoospermia (40%). Parenchyma shows complete spermatogenesis with reduced numbers of all germ cells. The characteristic histologic finding is decreased number of Leydig

Fig. 12.283 Congenital adrenal hyperplasia. Adrenal gland with cerebroid surface.

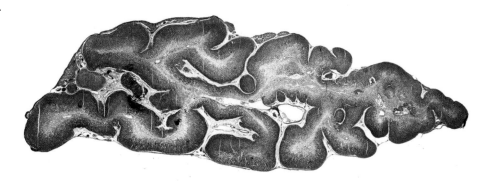

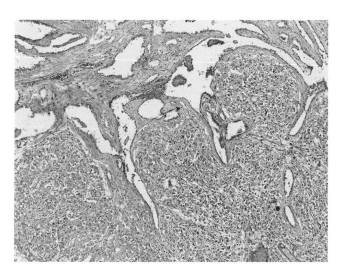

Fig. 12.284 Tumor of the adrenogenital syndrome in an adult patient. Nodules in testicular mediastinum protruding into rete testis cavities.

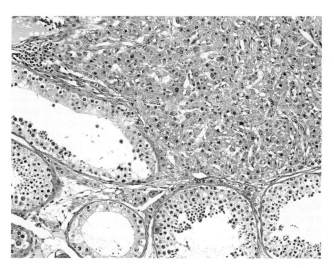

Fig. 12.286 Tumor of the adrenogenital syndrome in an adult patient. Tumoral cells with severe pleomorphism and granular eosinophilic cytoplasm. Surrounding seminiferous tubules show variable grades of spermatogenesis.

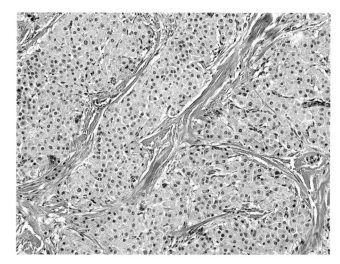

Fig. 12.285 Tumor of the adrenogenital syndrome in an adult patient. Trabeculae of tumoral cells with spheric nuclei separated by thick hyalinized conjunctive tracts.

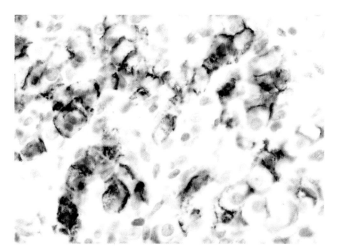

Fig. 12.287 Tumor of the adrenogenital syndrome in an adult patient. Tumoral cells show CD56 immunoexpression, typically in basal membrane and peripheral cytoplasm.

cells.[2807–2810] Infertility has been explained by: (1) hypogonadotropic hypogonadism, because the high levels of adrenal androgens would be aromatized to estrogens either peripherally or in the central nervous system, and thus suppress gonadotropin secretion; and (2) rete testis obstruction by tumor nodules.[2815,2816]

Treatment with glucocorticoid therapy corrects adrenal insufficiency and, in many cases, improves the spermiogram by decreasing nodule size. If treatment fails to diminish TART size, testis-sparing surgery may be performed, but it is not always successful in improving function.[2817]

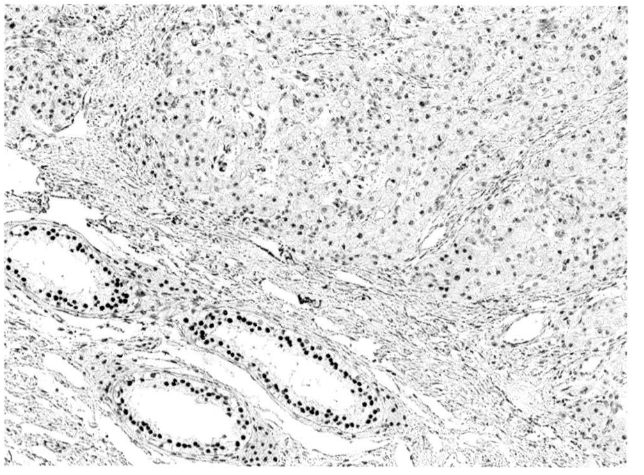

Fig. 12.288 Tumor of the adrenogenital syndrome in an adult patient. Tumoral cells do not show immunoreactivity for androgen receptors, contrasting with intense expression in Sertoli cells of adjacent seminiferous tubules.

Deficit in 17β-Hydroxylase. The enzyme 17β-hydroxylase transforms 12-hydroxyprogesterone and 11-deoxycortisone (also known as deoxycorticosterone) into cortisone. Enzyme deficiency results in increased levels of deoxycorticosterone, which leads to water and salt retention, renal activity suppression, decreased aldosterone secretion, and hypertension in one-half of affected patients. The high concentration of ACTH stimulates testosterone precursors and gives rise to virilization. In some cases, virilization is not evident before puberty. Testes show the same alterations as in patients with 21-hydroxylase deficit.[2810,2818]

Deficit in 20α-Hydroxylase. 20α-Hydroxylase deficiency, also known as Prader syndrome or lipoid congenital adrenal hyperplasia, results in defective conversion of cholesterol to 20α-cholesterol, resulting in deficiency in all three types steroid hormones that are synthesized by the adrenal gland and testes. External genitalia are female. Histologic study of the testes and adrenals reveals excessive lipid deposits. Affected patients typically have short a life span despite adequate treatment.

Deficit in 3β-Hydroxysteroid Dehydrogenase. 3β-Hydroxysteroid dehydrogenase is an enzyme that converts pregnenolone to progesterone, 17-OH-pregnenolone to 17-OH-progesterone, and DHEA to androstenedione in the adrenal glands and gonads. Deficiency of this enzyme hinders formation of cortisol, aldosterone, and testosterone.[2819,2820]

Patients have salt-loss syndrome and ambiguous external genitalia. Gynecomastia develops at puberty, probably because of lack of testosterone during fetal life, resulting in failure of inhibition of the mammary anlage.[2821]

Steroid 17α-Hydroxylase Deficiency. Deficiency of 17α-hydroxylase (CYP17A1, also known as P450c17) accounts for 1% of cases of congenital adrenal hyperplasia. CYP17A1 catalyzes two different paths in the steroidogenesis pathway: 17α-hydroxylase and 17,20-lyase.[2822] CYP17A1 deficiency results in hypermineralocorticoidism and low androgen level. The low androgen level results in ambiguous external genitalia. At puberty, adequate virilization does not occur, patients experience development of hypergonadotropic hypogonadism, and gynecomastia is frequent.[2823]

Cushing Syndrome

Physiologic levels of glucocorticosteroids are necessary for maintenance of gonadal function. Patients treated with long-term corticoid therapy, such as those with Crohn disease, Cushing disease, ulcerative colitis, rheumatoid arthritis, or asthma, may have reduced fertility (Fig. 12.289). The mechanism by which corticosteroids act is twofold. First, they induce an inhibitory effect on the hypothalamic–pituitary-gonadal axis through direct or indirect action on synthesis and release of GnRH, LH, and FSH. Second, they are powerful inhibitors of testosterone synthesis because most testicular receptors for corticoids are in Leydig cells.

CS may be endogenous or exogenous. Endogenous CS has adrenocorticotropic hormone (ACTH)-dependent and ACTH-independent causes. ACTH-dependent CS results from either ACTH-secreting adenoma or ectopic ACTH syndrome. ACTH-secreting adenoma is the most frequent cause of endogenous CS in children older than 5 years and adolescent boys, comprising 75% to 80% of pediatric cases. Ectopic ACTH syndrome is rare in children; it may occur in those with carcinoid tumor in different locations, clear cell sarcoma, malignant neuroendocrine tumor of

TABLE 12.26	Differential Diagnosis of Tumors of the Adrenogenital Syndrome and Leydig Cell Tumor							
	Gross Features	Bilaterality	Location	Trabeculae	Reinke Crystals	Immunology	Regression After Dexamethasone Treatment	Association
Tumors of the adrenogenital syndrome	Multiple extratesticular frequent	Usually	Adjacent to rete testis	Frequent	No	CD56 + Synapto +++ AR - AR + DLK1 +++ INSL3 -	Decrease	Congenital adrenal hyperplasia
Leydig cell tumor	Single	Rarely	No preference	Infrequent	40%	CD56 + Synapto + AR +++ DLK1 - INSL3 +	No regression	Precocious pseudopuberty

AR, Androgen receptor; *Synapto*, synaptophysin.
Findings without value in the differential diagnosis: adipose metaplasia, osseous metaplasia, lymphocyte infiltrate, or lipofuscins.

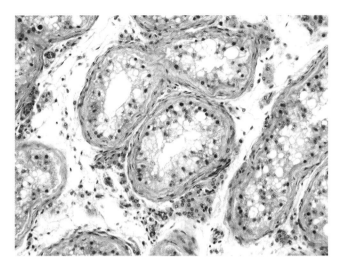

Fig. 12.289 Patient with rheumatoid arthritis treated with corticoids for several years. The seminiferous epithelium is reduced to Sertoli cells of vacuolated cytoplasm and spermatogonia. The tubular wall is thickened. Leydig cells show signs of atrophy.

the pancreas, Wilms tumor, adrenal neuroblastoma, and pheochromocytoma.[2824] Median age at presentation is 9.5 years.

ACTH-independent CS is produced by adrenocortical tumor (adenoma and carcinoma) and primary bilateral adrenal hyperplasia (micronodular and macronodular).

Exogenous CS is caused by long-term glucocorticoid therapy (e.g., treatment of asthma, eczema, and arthritis).[2825] To avoid negative effects on fertility, administration should be limited in time and restricted to the acute stage of disease.

Adrenal Cortical Tumors

Adrenal carcinoma is often associated with excessive secretion of hormones that cause hyperaldosteronism, CS, virilization, or feminization. Virilizing tumors in infancy have their own characteristics that differ from those of the same tumors in adults. The infantile form may be associated with other disorders, such as hemihypertrophy and Beckwith-Wiedemann syndrome, and may be included in the spectrum of families with cancer predisposition as a result of abnormalities in genes that encode transcription factors implicated in cell proliferation, differentiation, senescence, apoptosis, and genomic instability. Less than 10% of pediatric adrenal cortical tumors occur in Li-Fraumeni syndrome.[2826,2827] Disorders in which adrenal cortical tumors may be observed include multiple endocrine neoplasia type I (mutations in the *MEN1* gene), familial adenomatous polyposis (mutations in *APC* gene), Beckwith-Wiedemann syndrome (deregulation of imprinted genes in the 11p15.5 chromosomal region), Carney complex (mutations in *PRKAR1A*), and MAS (mutations in the *GNAS1* gene).[2828–2830]

Most adrenal tumors are clinically benign. The differential diagnosis between adenoma and carcinoma may be difficult even for an experienced pathologist.[2831] Both tumors may be hormonally active, thus giving rise to hyperaldosteronism, CS, virilization, or feminization. Tumors secreting androgens and cortisol simultaneously are frequent. Virilizing tumors produce precocious pseudopuberty in infancy.[2832] Feminizing tumors in infancy produce gynecomastia and pubic hair development.[2833,2834] Even small tumors may produce significant clinical manifestations.[2835] One-third of pediatric patients have hypertension.[2836]

In adults, adrenal carcinoma may cause marked reduction in fertility as a result of conversion into estrogen of large amounts of DHEA produced by the tumor. Feminizing tumor has striking clinical manifestations because of elevated estrogen, including progressive loss of male secondary sexual characteristics and gynecomastia. Testicular atrophy results from the inhibitory effect of estrogen on pituitary gonadotropins. Similar symptoms may be observed in patients with prostatic adenocarcinoma treated with estrogens or those receiving long-term estrogen therapy for gender change, as well as in other conditions with excessive estrogen production such as Sertoli cell or Leydig cell tumor.[2837]

Primary Pigmented Adrenocortical Disease

Primary pigmented adrenocortical disease represents 10% of cases of ACTH-independent CS. Two types are distinguished clinically and histopathologically: bilateral micronodular and macronodular adrenal hyperplasia. Primary pigmented nodular adrenocortical disease is an infrequent form of bilateral micronodular hyperplasia characterized by the presence of multiple, small (from submicroscopic to 10 mm in diameter), unencapsulated cortical nodules. These nodules, usually black and brown, are formed by large cells with abundantly pigmented eosinophilic cytoplasm. The internodular cortical tissue is usually atrophic. Half of patients with primary pigmented adrenocortical disease have familial association with Carney complex, an autosomal dominant multiple neoplasia syndrome characterized by cardiac myxoma, spotty skin pigmentation, and endocrine overactivity.[2838] The presence of testicular tumor in Carney complex, mainly large cell calcifying Sertoli cell tumor, is a well-known feature.[2839]

Adrenocorticotropic Hormone–Independent Macronodular Adrenal Hyperplasia

CS in MAS often occurs in the first year of life, is ACTH independent, and may spontaneously resolve.[2840] ACTH-independent macronodular adrenal hyperplasia, a rare condition that occurs in children, consists of massive enlargement of both adrenal glands and is frequently associated with hypogonadism and gynecomastia in boys.[2841,2842]

When adrenal hyperplasia develops in MAS (adrenocortical hyperplasia associated with MAS), it has an aggressive course and frequently requires unilateral or bilateral adrenalectomy.[2843,2844]

Pancreas

Diabetes Mellitus

Alterations in carbohydrate, lipid, and protein metabolism characteristic of diabetes mellitus adversely affect the genital system, although most patients with diabetes are fertile. Gonadal impairment depends on the type of diabetes and time of disease onset (infancy and childhood, puberty, or adulthood).[2845,2846] Even the newborn of a diabetic mother has a high mortality rate; there is typically Leydig cell hyperplasia in the fetal testis.[249]

Puberty may be delayed in patients with diabetes, although the cause is unknown. Other gonadal alterations appear at puberty, and men with diabetes who have not been adequately treated may be infertile and have sexual dysfunction. Serum levels of FSH, LH, and testosterone are decreased, and spermatozoan mitochondrial function is abnormal.[2847–2849] Spermiograms reveal low number and progressive decline in motility of spermatozoa.[2850] PRL levels are increased, and testosterone level is low or nearly normal.

Seminiferous tubules have reduced diameter, thickening of the lamina propria, and alterations in the adluminal compartment consisting of degenerative changes in the Sertoli cell apical cytoplasm and sloughing of immature germ cells. The major lesions are in the interstitial connective tissue and Leydig cells. Small interstitial blood vessels show diabetic microangiopathy characterized by enlargement and duplication of the basal lamina, pericyte degeneration, and endothelial cell alterations. There is an increase in the number of fibroblasts and amount of collagen and intercellular matrix in the interstitial connective tissue.[2851] Leydig cells are decreased in number and contain an abundance of lipid droplets and lysosomes.

Tubular lesions are attributed to low serum testosterone level, probably because of deficient Leydig cell stimulation by insulin (or a decrease in insulin-dependent FSH) and abnormal carbohydrate metabolism of Sertoli cells. Sexual dysfunction is present in more than one-half of patients, who complain of impotence, decreased libido, disorders of intercourse, and retrograde ejaculation.[2852] Hypogonadotropic hypogonadism has been associated with obesity, but not duration of diabetes, elevated glycosylated hemoglobin, or the presence of microvascular lesions.[2853] Causes of impotence are multiple, including microangiopathy and macroangiopathy, hormonal deficiencies, psychological factors, and autonomic neuropathy affecting the parasympathetic system. Neuropathy is probably chiefly responsible for erectile failure in men with diabetes.[2854] Alterations in sperm excretory ducts may be associated with diabetes. The most frequent are enlargement and calcifications of seminal vesicles and vasa deferentia. Calcifications are found in the muscular layers and display a concentric arrangement (Fig. 12.290).[2855]

Mucoviscidosis

The principal symptoms of mucoviscidosis, also called *cystic fibrosis (CF)*, are progressive chronic pulmonary disease, pancreatic insufficiency, and increased level of chlorine in sweat. Although CF was recognized before 1940, its effects on the male genital system were not recognized until the 1970s.[2856,2857] This may be explained by improvements in medical care during childhood that allowed survival of many patients to adulthood and recognition of CF in patients who had been diagnosed with chronic bronchitis and hepatic or digestive dysfunction. In the United States, CF is the most lethal congenital disease, with a prevalence of 1 in 2500 children and carrier status of 1 in 25 white men.[2858] In some countries

such as Japan, this disease is extremely rare.[2858a] Lesions in sperm excretory ducts involve (in decreasing order of frequency) the vas deferens (congenital bilateral absence, unilateral absence), ejaculatory ducts (bilateral obstruction), epididymis (diffuse or segmental hypoplasia), and seminal vesicles (incomplete development). The most proximal part of the epididymis is usually present.[2859,2860] Thus most patients with CF (99%) are infertile owing to obstructive azoospermia.[2861,2862] Most patients with CF have congenital bilateral absence of the ductus deferens, sometimes associated with agenesis or atresia of the epididymis and seminal vesicles. Those with congenital bilateral absence of the ductus deferens, even without other characteristic symptoms of CF, are usually carriers of a minor form (genital form) of CF.[2863] Before initiating treatment for infertility, the possibility that the patient is a carrier of the *CF* gene should be evaluated.[2864,2865] The second most frequent presentation of CF is unilateral absence of the ductus deferens, although this disorder may also appear without CF. The third presentation, in order of frequency, comprises a group of healthy infertile patients with abnormal seminal parameters or nonobstructive azoospermia. These patients have an increased frequency of cystic fibrosis transmembrane regulator (*CFTR*) mutations, with an incidence rate of 17% versus 1% to 4% in the general population.[2866] The possibility of this form of CF should be considered during genetic counseling in patients who desire ICSI.[2867]

Malformation of the genital system plays the most important role in infertility in CF.[2868] Lesions begin in the 10th week of gestation when the wolffian duct forms the sperm excretory ducts.[2857] Variable penetrance of the CF gene accounts for the diversity of malformations affecting different regions of the male genital system. Whether the lesions of sperm excretory ducts correspond to agenesis or atresia remains controversial. The finding that 12- to 18-week aborted fetuses with CF show ductus deferens, as well as ultrasonographic assessment of the presence of sperm excretory ducts in many infants, supports the hypothesis that initial normal development is interrupted by accumulation of inspissational secretions in the lumina of the ducts and culminates in atresia.[2869] This process of atresia may be of early onset in some patients and is found at birth in some newborn autopsies. As a result, epididymides are small, ductus deferentia are only epithelial cords, and the walls contain only some rings of loose connective tissue. Testicular development in patients with CF is often delayed at puberty.

Histologic studies in children reveal that the vas deferens and ductus epididymis are absent or reduced to small ductuli with reduced or absent lumina and thin, poorly muscularized walls (Fig. 12.291). The testes are normal during childhood, but show hypospermatogenesis and spermatid malformations by adulthood (Fig. 12.292). The spermiogram is characteristic of obstructive azoospermia, with acid pH, decreased semen volume and fructose concentration, and increased citric acid and acid phosphatase.[2870] In adulthood, slight diminution of testicular size occurs, although some degree of spermatogenesis is maintained. Most testes show tubular ectasia with minimal lesions of the adluminal compartments. These lesions are probably secondary to obstruction, which may be superimposed on those derived from chronic nutrition deficiency. Whether these secondary lesions are superimposed on primary lesions of spermatogenesis has been debated because the CFTR protein also plays a role in spermatogenesis and sperm maturation.[2866] Given that the median life expectancy of patients with CF is approximately 40 years, some patients desire assisted reproductive techniques, and it is mandatory that they receive appropriate genetic, medical, and psychological counseling.[2860,2871]

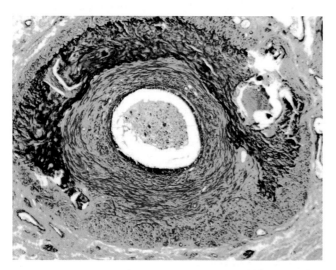

Fig. 12.290 Patient with diabetes with dystrophic calcification in the ductus deferens muscular wall.

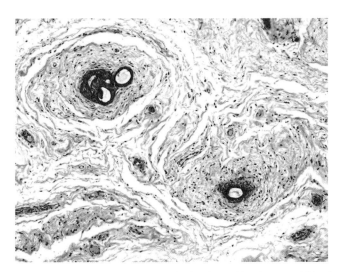

Fig. 12.291 Epididymis in cystic fibrosis. Sections of the ductus epididymidis show decreased lumen diameter with surrounding concentric rings of loose connective tissue.

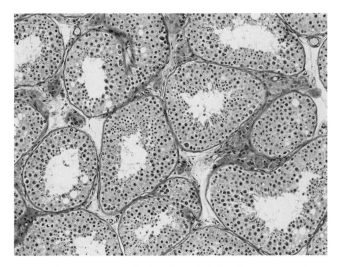

Fig. 12.292 Patient with cystic fibrosis and obstructive azoospermia. The seminiferous tubules show only slight ectasia.

The disease is a genetic disorder with autosomal recessive inheritance. The impaired gene (the *CF* gene) is on chromosome 7 (7q31), consists of 27 exons, and encodes the 1480-amino acid CFTR protein.[2872] In CF the deficiency results from mutations altering *CFTR* gene function. More than 1500 CF-causing *CFTR* mutations have been identified.[2872a] The most frequent mutation in whites is D-F508, caused by deletion of Phe-508 and responsible for 70% of cases. The protein product controls chlorine ion flux throughout the plasma membrane and plays an important role in hydration of epithelial secretions.[2873] The epithelia showing absence or dysfunction of CFTR are impermeable to chlorine ions. Secretions subsequently become thick and sticky, producing obstructions in the excretory ducts of many glands (respiratory tract, pancreas, sweat glands), as well as in the developing sperm excretory ducts, such as the ductus epididymis and ductus deferens.[2864] Patients with CF usually present with delayed puberty, which is a result of both the disease itself and malabsorption secondary to pancreatic insufficiency.

Liver

The liver has a primary role in metabolism, detoxification, and excretion of sex steroid hormones. Chronic hepatic failure damages the hypothalamohypophyseal-testicular axis and consequently all related endocrine glands. Hypogonadism is frequent in the final stages of severe chronic liver diseases, including alcoholism and nonalcoholic fatty liver diseases.

Hypogonadism, Liver Disease, and Excessive Alcohol Consumption

The association of atrophy with gynecomastia and hepatic cirrhosis is referred to as Silvestrini-Corda syndrome.[2874,2875]

Alcohol has a direct toxic effect on Leydig cells. Acute alcoholic intoxication suppresses serum testosterone level in male nonalcoholic volunteers and laboratory animals. Long-term alcohol ingestion, even in the absence of cirrhosis, causes hypogonadism, with symptoms of Leydig cell failure, including testicular atrophy, infertility, decreased libido, impotence, and reduced size of the prostate and seminal vesicles.[2876] Patients with chronic alcoholism with cirrhosis also have symptoms of hyperestrogenism, including gynecomastia, female escutcheon, and female fat distribution pattern.

Most men with chronic alcoholism, with or without cirrhosis, have significant testicular lesions. Seminiferous tubules have reduced diameters, thickened lamina propria, and decreased or absent germ cells. Leydig cells are reduced in number and contain abundant lipofuscin granules (Fig. 12.293). The epididymis becomes atrophic, mainly in the ductuli efferentes, as a result of androgen deprivation. The epithelium of the rete testis becomes cuboidal or columnar in response to estrogens. The spermiogram correlates with variability of histologic findings, and usually shows marked reduction in number and motility of spermatozoa and increase in the percentage of morphologically abnormal spermatozoa.[2877,2878] Approximately 20% of patients initially have an elevation in serum testosterone; with advanced disease, testosterone level decreases. The initial increase is caused by an elevation in SHBG concentration and reduced testosterone metabolism by the liver.[2879] Serum estrogen level also increases because of increased conversion of testosterone to estrogen in peripheral adipose and muscular tissue.[2880]

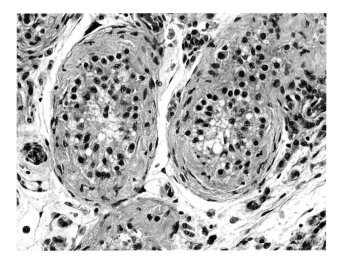

Fig. 12.293 Testis from a patient with alcoholic cirrhosis. The seminiferous tubules show decreased diameter, thickening of the tubular wall, and spermatogonia and Sertoli cells exhibiting intense vacuolation of the adluminal compartment. The testicular interstitium shows marked Leydig cell atrophy and numerous macrophages.

Nonalcoholic Liver Diseases and Infertility

Different clinical situations are grouped under the term *nonalcoholic fatty liver diseases:* steatosis, nonalcoholic steatohepatitis, liver fibrosis, and cirrhosis.[2881] Effects on gonadal function vary according to the severity of disease.[2882] Patients have decreased level of total and biologically active free testosterone. Hormonal alterations are not as severe as in alcoholics, a finding emphasizing the direct action of alcohol on Leydig cells. Hypogonadism in young patients may result from severe chronic liver disease. Patients with viral hepatic cirrhosis have increased serum estradiol, androstenedione, and SHBG levels, and reduced serum testosterone and DHEA levels. In α_1-antitrypsin deficiency, testicular function and fertility are conserved for years; only in advanced stages of the disease do minor biochemical alterations occur.[2883] In Alagille syndrome (intrahepatic biliary duct hypoplasia), hypogonadism is associated with cholestasis; frequent vertebral, cardiac, and facial malformations; and mental retardation. Hypogonadism is manifest by small testes, delayed puberty, and, in adults, lack of germ cell development.[2884]

Kidney

Autosomal Dominant Polycystic Renal Disease

Autosomal dominant polycystic kidney disease (ADPKD) is a systemic disease characterized by the presence of multiple cysts in both kidneys leading to renal failure. It is associated with cysts in liver and pancreas, cardiovascular pathology (aneurysms), and infertility. It is caused by mutation in *PKD1* or *PKD2* genes. The condition affects 1 in 1000 in the general population. Patients with this disease comprise 10% of those with end-stage renal failure.[2885] Infertility may become apparent even before renal insufficiency begins. Oligoteratozoospermia and necrospermia are frequent findings.[2886,2887] Serum levels of FSH, LH, PRL, testosterone, and estradiol remain normal for a long time before the onset of renal insufficiency. The most frequent causes of infertility in patients with ADPKD are thought to be obstruction of the spermatic pathway by epididymal cysts or seminal vesicle cysts, which have a high incidence in patients with polycystic renal disease (5.2%); abnormal spermatogenesis as a result of abnormal polycystins; uremia; and stationary cilium syndrome described in some patients.[591,2011,2888,2889]

Chronic Renal Insufficiency

Chronic renal insufficiency is associated with disturbed endocrine function in the pituitary, thyroid, parathyroids, and testes. The associated sexual dysfunction consists of erectile dysfunction, diminution of libido and semen volume, oligozoospermia or azoospermia, and infertility. In children, skeletal development and puberty are delayed.[2890]

In adults, bilateral testicular volume is decreased in patients undergoing hemodialysis. Hormonal studies reveal elevated levels of FSH, LH, and PRL, but testosterone level is low.[2891,2892] Biopsy shows seminiferous tubules with reduced diameters and reduced or absent germ cells (Fig. 12.294).[2893,2894] The interstitium contains a normal number of Leydig cells, increased number of macrophages, and fibrosis.[2895] Hypospermatogenesis, late maturation arrest, and germ cell aplasia are the most frequent histologic findings in patients undergoing hemodialysis.[2896] In addition, patients with chronic renal insufficiency secondary to glomerulonephritis have thickening of the tubular lamina propria and decreased number of Leydig cells. Patients with end-stage renal disease who undergo dialysis, especially older patients and those receiving prolonged dialysis, show calcifications in several organs and tissues, including the male genital system (epididymidis, tunica albuginea,

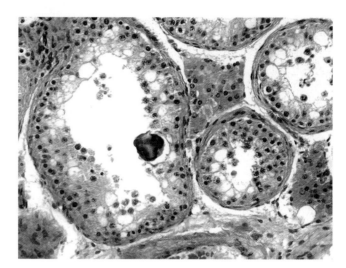

Fig. 12.294 Testis from a patient with chronic renal insufficiency. The seminiferous tubules show premature sloughing of primary spermatocytes and Sertoli cells with vacuolation of the apical cytoplasm. An intraepithelial microlith is present.

and cavernous tissue) in 87% of cases, with isolated cases of calcification of the testicular parenchyma and microlithiasis.[2897] Elevated serum level of phosphorus, increased calcium-phosphorus product, and severe hyperparathyroidism contribute to the development of calcifications. Uremic calcification is a cell-mediated process in which elevated levels of TGF, vitamin K–dependent proteins such as osteocalcin and atherocalcin, and defects in calcium-regulatory proteins such as fetuin are implicated.[2898] Uremic patients receiving dialysis exhibit decreased testicular function, low serum testosterone level, low ejaculate volume, and azoospermia. Dialysis does not restore spermatogenesis. Accumulations of urate and oxalate crystals are found in the rete testes and ductuli efferentes (Fig. 12.295). These crystals are deposited beneath the epithelium and are often sloughed into the lumen. Reactive changes in the rete testis, including cystic transformation, are frequent.[2899] Some patients with chronic renal insufficiency show enlargement of the caput of the epididymis (Fig. 12.296).

The etiology of gonadal dysfunction in this condition is unclear. Several factors are probably involved, including impaired testicular

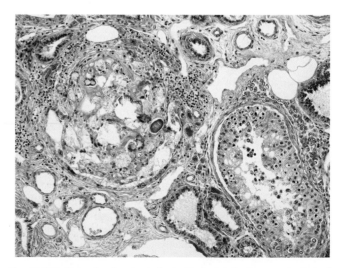

Fig. 12.295 Deposits of urates in the testicular mediastinum and rete testis walls. Minimum lymphoid infiltrate.

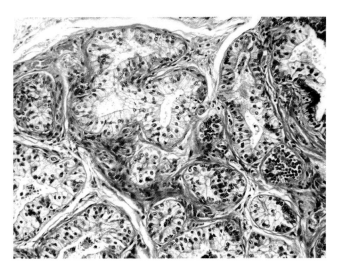

Fig. 12.296 Hyperplasia of caput of the epididymis in a chronic renal insufficiency patient. Ductules efferentes show pseudostratified epithelium of large columnar cells with clear cytoplasm.

steroidogenesis, reduced clearance of pituitary hormones, secretory defects of the pituitary and hypothalamus, and oxidative stress.[2900–2906] The response to renal transplantation is not immediate and is related to the glomerular filtration rate. Patients with rates lower than 50 mL/min experience atrophy of the seminiferous epithelium.[2901] Patients with long-term and early-onset uremia along with corticosteroid or cyclosporine combined with azathioprine treatments experience the most severe gonadal dysfunction.[2907]

Chronic Inflammatory Bowel Disease

Celiac Disease

Celiac disease is associated with numerous disorders, including type 1 diabetes mellitus, autoimmune thyroid disease, Addison disease, osteoporosis, secondary hyperparathyroidism, vitamin D or iron deficiency, fertility problems, hypogonadism in men, and autoimmune hypopituitarism.[2908,2909]

The relationship of celiac disease with subfertility has been a matter of controversy, and some affected men are infertile. Earlier studies suggested that hypogonadism is a frequent finding in men with celiac disease and results in clinical symptoms in 5% to 10% of untreated patients. Spermiograms show reduced motility and numerous morphologic anomalies in spermatozoa. Hormonal studies show elevated serum FSH level in more than 25% of men with celiac disease. LH also is increased in more than 50%. The response of FSH and LH to GnRH stimulation is excessive. Affected men have signs of tissue resistance to androgens. The cause of pituitary derangement is unknown, but one possible cause is deficiency of fat-soluble vitamins, such as A and E. Vitamin A is important for Sertoli cell function, as well as for early spermatogenetic phases. Vitamin E supports proper differentiation and function of epididymal epithelium, spermatic maturation, and secretion of proteins by the prostate.[2910] Sperm anomalies are not always corrected by a gluten-free diet.

Recent studies suggest that celiac disease is not a risk factor for infertility in men, whereas in females it is responsible for delayed puberty, infertility, and predisposition to spontaneous abortion, conditions that are rapidly corrected with a gluten-free diet.[2911–2913]

Inflammatory Bowel Disease

Patients with *quiescent Crohn, ulcerative colitis,* or *indeterminate (unclassified) colitis* are usually as fertile as the general population, although those with active Crohn disease and ulcerative colitis have problems with fertility (27% and 24% of patients, respectively).[2914,2915] Those with ulcerative colitis and regional enteritis have low sperm count, impaired motility, and ultrastructural alterations, including nuclear pleomorphism and chromatin malcondensation and decondensation. Zinc deficit may be responsible for similar alterations in Crohn disease, apparently related to the extent of intestinal involvement and severity of symptoms.[2916,2917] Younger patients who undergo pharmacologic treatment or pelvic or abdominal surgery frequently exhibit pubertal delay and impaired spermatogenesis without involvement of endocrine function.[2918] The main drugs used for inflammatory bowel disease (sulfasalazine, methotrexate, or infliximab) adversely affect semen parameters. Spermiogram parameters improve when treatment ceases.[2919] Surgical treatment does not seem to affect erectile function, sexual desire, orgasm, or sexual satisfaction, although retrograde ejaculation is common.[2920]

AIDS

More than 17% of HIV-infected men have hypogonadism, which may be present even in those whose viral replication is under control and have a normal number of CD4 lymphocytes.[2921] Patients frequently experience early andropause, marked by dysregulation of the hypothalamopituitary-testicular axis.[2922] Hypogonadism is more frequent in HIV-infected men with wasting syndrome, and may warrant physiologic androgen replacement therapy.[2923–2926]

The incidence rate of hypogonadism in men with AIDS is estimated to be 50%.[2927–2929] According to autopsy studies, this percentage increases to 100% in the 3 to 24 months before death.[2929] Histologic studies reveal that 28% of patients have complete but quantitatively abnormal spermatogenesis, and the remainder have spermatocytic arrest or Sertoli cell–only pattern.

Chronic Anemia

In patients with chronic anemia who require multiple transfusions, excess iron accumulates in tissues and forms reactive oxygen species causing irreparable damage (secondary hemochromatosis). Pituitary, thyroid, liver adrenals, and testes are the most compromised organs (Fig. 12.297). The latter show reduced spermatogenesis and iron storage in Leydig cells. The most frequent chronic anemias are β-thalassemia, sickle cell anemia, and Fanconi anemia.

β-Thalassemia

β-Thalassemia is autosomal dominant with three manifestations: thalassemia trait (heterozygous β-thalassemia), intermediate thalassemia, and major β-thalassemia. The cause is mutation in the β-globin gene, resulting in ineffective erythropoiesis, hemolysis, and anemia. The β-thalassemia trait is present in 2% to 3% of the general population, and incidence is higher in Mediterranean and African people. Nearly 20% of patients with major thalassemia have delayed puberty.[2930–2932] Loss of libido with erectile or ejaculatory dysfunction is common, and 69% of patients have hypogonadotropic hypogonadism.[2933–2941] Gonadal dysfunction persists in most patients despite improvements in intensive chelation therapy (Fig. 12.298).[2942,2943] Spermiogram studies demonstrate poor quality of most seminal parameters.[2944] Hypogonadism probably has multiple causes: extensive iron deposition in the pituitary and testis as a result of multiple transfusions, hypoxia

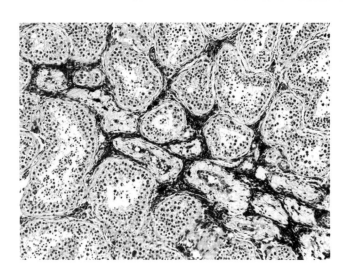

Fig. 12.297 Major thalassemia in a patient who underwent multiple blood transfusions. The testicular interstitium and atrophic tubules show Perl stain–positive iron deposits.

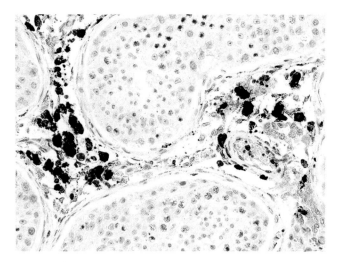

Fig. 12.298 Testis from a man with chronic anemia with chelation therapy showing complete spermatogenesis and abundant macrophages in the interstitium that are negative for Perl stain and intensely immunoreactive for CD68. Leydig cells do not show significant alterations.

subsequent to ineffective erythropoiesis in spite of marked erythroid hyperplasia, liver disorders, diabetes mellitus, and zinc deficiency.[2945] Testosterone replacement therapy is indicated.[2946]

α-Thalassemia

α-Thalassemia has two different clinical presentations: hemoglobin Bart hydrops fetalis (Hb Bart) syndrome and hemoglobin H disease. Patients with Hb Bart syndrome, the most severe form, are affected during gestation and are born with generalized edema, pleural and pericardial effusions, and severe hypochromic anemia. Hydrocephaly, hepatosplenomegaly, extramedullary erythropoiesis, urologic defects (ambiguous genitalia, undescended testis, and hypospadias), and cardiac defects are common. Most die during the neonatal period.[2947,2948] Patients with hemoglobin H disease are only mildly affected and do not have genital anomalies.[2949]

Sickle Cell Anemia

Sickle cell anemia is autosomal recessive with a constellation of findings resulting from abnormal synthesis and structure of hemoglobin. The gene responsible for the disease is located on chromosome 11, and more than 90% of synthesized hemoglobin is type A. Homozygous sickle cell anemia (SS) is found in 0.2% of the African American population, whereas heterozygous sickle cell trait (AS) is present in 8%. Patients may present with delayed puberty, hypogonadism that varies from slight to severe, eunuchoid habitus, decreased libido, erectile dysfunction, priapism, and poor semen quality. In most patients, hypogonadism is hypogonadotropic, although 25% have increased FSH level, and 50% of these patients also have increased LH and low testosterone. Testicular size may be normal but is usually diminished.[2950]

Causes of hypogonadism in these patients may be multiple and include CDGP, hypothalamic dysfunction, pituitary infarcts, primary testicular failure, and zinc deficit. Testicular function usually improves with advancing age.[2951–2957]

Fanconi Anemia Syndrome

Fanconi anemia is a rare inherited disorder characterized by chromosomal instability, bone marrow failure, developmental defects, and predisposition to cancer. Fanconi anemia, together with ataxia telangiectasia, Nijmegen breakage syndrome, Bloom syndrome, xeroderma pigmentosum, Cockayne syndrome, and TTD, belongs to a group of genetic disorders termed *chromosomal breakage syndromes* or *DNA-repair disorders*. These disorders share susceptibility to chromosomal breakages and increased frequency of breaks and interchanges, occurring either spontaneously or after exposure to various DNA-damaging agents.[2958]

Patients with Fanconi anemia show hypogenitalism with small penis and testes, as well as delayed puberty. Fertility has not been routinely studied.[2959] Autopsy study of an adolescent boy showed seminiferous tubules containing only Sertoli cells and isolated spermatogonia.[2960] During adulthood, hypergonadotropic hypogonadism may occur.[2961]

Obesity

A high percentage of people in developed countries are overweight, and the incidence of obesity has increased considerably in recent decades. Nonetheless, few studies have addressed the effect of obesity on gonadal development in childhood, recognizing that there may be an effect on hypothalamopituitary-gonadal function.[2962] The brain constantly monitors nutrition state by glucose level and circulating factors such as leptin, insulin, and ghrelin. In obese boys, testosterone level is decreased, including basal testosterone or testosterone level after hCG administration.[2962,2963] Basal PRL level is normal, but mean peak PRL response and mean increment in PRL level after TRH administration are significantly lower in prepubertal obese children. These findings suggest that neuroendocrine regulation of PRL is impaired in prepubertal children even with mild to moderate obesity. This impairment could be secondary to altered neurotransmitter status at the hypothalamic level.[2964]

Obesity is a component of certain complex syndromes with specific genetic defects that are responsible for abnormalities of spermatogenesis. Examples include Alström syndrome, which results from a loss of function of a simple gene (*ALMS1* gene); and PWS and Angelman syndrome, which are caused by chromosomal anomaly in 15q11-q13.

It is generally agreed that obesity has adverse effects on fertility. The underlying problems likely include erectile dysfunction, decreased sexual intercourse, and alterations of the hypothalamic–pituitary-testicular axis. Obesity causes alterations in most semen parameters, including sperm morphology, sperm concentration, total sperm count, total motility sperm count, and DNA fragmentation, independent of development of other disorders associated with obesity, such as hypertension, diabetes mellitus, heart disease, and stroke. Patients with morbid obesity have hypogonadotropic hypogonadism.[2965] Hormonal measurements demonstrate important alterations in the hypothalamic-hypophyseal-testicular axis. Obesity is associated with decreased levels of free and total testosterone and SHBG, increased level of serum estradiol, and decreased FSH/LH ratio and inhibin B, as well as a lower amplitude of LH pulses and increased circulating estrogen.[2966–2968] Testosterone reduction is not followed by a compensatory increase in gonadotropins, thus resulting in hypogonadotropic hypogonadism.[2969–2971] Numerous hormones are involved in regulation of food intake, including leptin, adiponectin, ghrelin, resistin, and endocannabinoids.[2972,2973]

Testicular abnormalities begin with the adluminal compartment and later involve the basal compartment. Patients also have Leydig cell atrophy, cuboidal metaplasia of the rete testis, and epididymal atrophy. Fertility rate improves after weight loss.[2974] The utility of bariatric surgery for improving male fertility in obese patients is uncertain.[2975,2976]

Starvation

Starvation inhibits GnRH secretion, resulting in hypogonadotropic hypogonadism. Inhibition appears to be mediated by leptin. Low serum FSH, LH, and testosterone levels usually normalize when normal weight is reached.[2977]

Autoimmune Polyglandular Syndrome

Autoimmune polyglandular syndromes, also known as autoimmune polyendocrine syndromes, affect endocrine glands and nonendocrine organs, characterized by coexistence of more than one organ-specific autoimmune disorder. Pluriglandular autoimmune syndromes are relatively frequent among patients who are seeking consultation in endocrinologic centers.[2978] The four types of autoimmune polyglandular insufficiency syndromes are PGA1 (Blizzard syndrome), PGA2 (Schmidt syndrome), PGA3, and PGA4; the most frequent are PGA1 and PGA2.[2979,2980]

PGA1 is autosomal recessive, also known by the acronym APECED (autoimmune polyendocrinopathy, candidiasis, ectodermal dystrophy) or MEDAC (multiple endocrine deficiency autoimmune candidiasis syndrome) or Whitaker syndrome, defined by the presence of at least two of three characteristic features, including Addison disease, hypoparathyroidism, and chronic mucocutaneous candidiasis.[2981–2984]

The spectrum of associated diseases includes other autoimmune endocrinopathies (hypergonadotropic hypogonadism, insulin-dependent diabetes mellitus, autoimmune thyroid and anterior hypophysis diseases), autoimmune or immune-mediated intestinal diseases (atrophic chronic gastritis, pernicious anemia, malabsorption), active chronic hepatitis, autoimmune skin diseases (vitiligo and alopecia), ectodermal dystrophy, keratoconjunctivitis, cellular and humoral immunologic diseases, asplenia, and cholelithiasis.[2985]

PGA1 starts early and affects males and females equally. The syndrome is more frequent in Iranian Jews (1 in 6500 to 9000) and Finnish people (1 in 25,000), whereas low frequency is observed in Norway with an incidence of 1 in 80,000.[2986–2988]

The *AIRE* gene (autoimmune regulator), responsible for PGA1, is on 21q22.3, and the disorder is autosomal recessive.[2989–2991] The syndrome is genetically homogeneous, although phenotype varies widely.[2992,2993] R257X mutation is responsible for 82% of Finnish PGA1 alleles.[2994a]

Chronic mucocutaneous candidiasis manifests in children younger than 5 years, followed by hypoparathyroidism (<10 years of age), and, finally, Addison disease (<15 years of age). Hypergonadotropic hypogonadism is frequent.[2995] Patients with PGA1 syndrome have antibodies against many autoantigens, intracellular enzymes including the P450 side-chain cleavage enzyme 17α-hydroxylase, 21-hydroxylase, glutamic acid decarboxylase 65, aromatic L-amino acid decarboxylase, tyrosine phosphatase–like protein IA-2, tryptophan hydroxylase (TPH), tyrosine hydroxylase, and cytochrome P450 1A2.[2996,2997] Testing for antibodies is recommended for diagnosis in patients whose clinical symptoms suggest a polyglandular autoimmune syndrome and to establish which organs may be affected.[2994,2995,2998,2999] Abnormal T-cell–mediated immunity is the likely underlying deficit.[3000]

PGA2 or Schmidt syndrome is mainly observed in adult patients. Prevalence is 1.4 to 4.5 per 100,000 persons. Male-to-female ratio is 3:1. PGA2 is defined by the presence of two or more disorders, including primary adrenal insufficiency; Graves disease or Hashimoto thyroiditis; insulin-dependent diabetes mellitus; primary hypogonadism; myasthenia gravis; celiac disease; and other relatively frequent conditions such as vitiligo, alopecia areata, serositis, pernicious anemia, and essential thrombocythemia.[3001,3002] PGA2 is a complex polygenetic disease that shows familial aggregation and is associated with HLA-DR3 and HLA-DR4 and environmental factors.[3003] The incidence rate of hypogonadism is 5%, and is hypergonadotropic in most cases.[3004,3005]

PGA3 is defined by the association of thyroiditis with diabetes mellitus, pernicious anemia, vitiligo, or alopecia.[3006] Adrenal cortical insufficiency is not part of this syndrome.

PGA4 includes patients who do not meet the diagnostic criteria of PGA1 to PGA3.[3007]

Features of Hypogonadism in Patients With Polyglandular Autoimmune Syndrome

Hypogonadism is present in 14% of male patients and 60% of female patients with primary adrenal insufficiency; hypogonadism in these patients is hypergonadotropic. The testes appeared atrophic, and seminiferous tubules show reduced diameter, absence of elastic fibers, and only some dysgenetic Sertoli cells in numbers that vary widely from one tubule to another. Spermatogonia are only occasionally seen. Deposits of immunoglobulin in basal membrane may be observed. In patients without adrenal insufficiency, the hypogonadism is usually hypogonadotropic. Even patients with better-conserved testicular function are infertile because they have oligozoospermia or antisperm antibodies.[1281,2983] Hypogonadism may result from autoimmune destruction of testicular cells or pituitary gonadotropin-secreting cells (Fig. 12.299).[3008,3009]

Inherited Metabolic Diseases

Hereditary metabolic diseases affecting the testis may be classified as: (1) diseases associated with accumulation of toxic substances (hemochromatosis and galactosemia); (2) diseases associated with disturbances in energy required for hormone synthesis (mitochondrial disorders); and (3) defects in degradation or synthesis of complex molecules (comprising both peroxisomal diseases [adrenoleukodystrophy (X-ALD), primary hyperoxaluria, and D-bifunctional protein (DBP) deficiency] and lysosomal diseases [Fabry disease, Wolman disease, Niemann-Picks disease, and cystinosis], as wells as disorders of intracellular trafficking and abnormal transverse protein [Alström syndrome and selenoprotein deficiency disorders]).[3010]

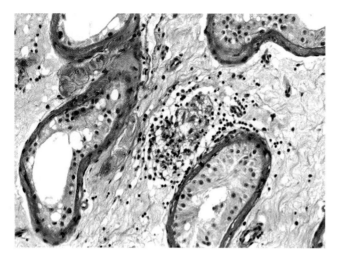

Fig. 12.299 Testis from a man with autoimmune polyglandular syndrome showing selective lymphoid infiltrates in a Leydig cell cluster. Reinke crystalloid may be recognized. The seminiferous tubules contain Sertoli cells and isolated spermatogonia.

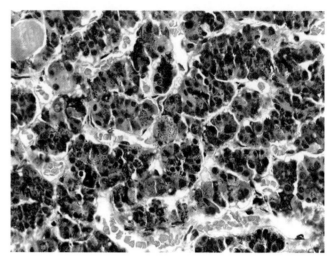

Fig. 12.300 Perl stains decorate the voluminous iron deposits in cells of the anterior pituitary in a patient with hemochromatosis.

Hemochromatosis and Infertility

Hereditary hemochromatosis is the most frequent genetic disease in the Northern Hemisphere. It results from excessive iron absorption and accumulation in multiple tissues and organs, and leads to cirrhosis, diabetes, hypogonadism, and arthralgia. It is estimated that 1.5 million Americans are affected, although most patients remain undiagnosed.[3011] This figure represents 1 in 124 to 133 U.S. residents. In northern Europe and Australia, data are similar.[3012–3015] The prevalence is lower in African Americans, southern Europeans, Ashkenazi Jews, and Australian aborigines.[3016] The male-to-female ratio is 1.5:1. In men the disease appears at a younger age than in women and usually is more severe.[3017]

Iron homeostasis depends on many genes that act in a coordinated manner, and the exact function is not well known. Iron balance depends on intestinal absorption, regulated by the hepatic peptide hormone hepcidin through its receptor, the cellular exporter ferroportin, and adequate iron recycling.[3018] It is assumed that normal individuals absorb 1 to 2 mg/day of iron, whereas homozygous patients with hereditary hemochromatosis absorb up to 3 to 4 mg/day. Excessive iron absorption is due to hepcidin deficiency or insensitivity of ferroportin to hepcidin. Iron deposits accumulate in the liver, pancreas, hypophysis, heart, adrenals, and gastric mucosa. Once intracellular ferritin saturation occurs, excess free iron participates in generating intracellular redox reactions, generating toxic reactive oxygen species, and causing cell injury or cell death. Eventual consequences include liver dysfunction (cirrhosis and cancer in 5% to 10% of patients), pancreatic dysfunction (diabetes in 80% of patients), cardiac pathology (myocardiopathy), musculoskeletal disorders (arthritis), and hypophyseal injury (hypogonadism) (Fig. 12.300).[3019]

Five types of hereditary hemochromatosis have been described based on genetic, biochemical, and clinical characteristics.[3020–3023] Type 1, the most frequent, is caused by mutation in type 1 hereditary hemochromatosis gene (HFE) (*C282Y*), which encodes the high iron HFE protein, thus leading to increased intestinal absorption of iron, supersaturation of iron deposits, and damage in multiple organs. This type mainly affects male patients, and the clinical course is slow. The HFE gene is located on the short arm of chromosome 6.[3020,3024] A cysteine-tyrosinase amino acid substitution, caused by a G8945A transition at codon 282 (C282Y), is found in

85% to 100% of patients with inherited hemochromatosis who have northern European ancestors.[3024] Other mutations observed in gene HFE are H63D and S65C.[3022] The protein encoded by HFE is expressed mainly in intestinal crypt epithelial cells, and its function is to interact with the transferrin receptor to decrease affinity of this receptor for iron-bound transferrin. Therefore HFE is a negative regulator of transferrin-iron capture.

Type 2 gene is a juvenile form of hereditary hemochromatosis that manifests before the age of 30 years in both sexes and has a rapidly progressive course; it is associated with severe cardiomyopathy and hypogonadism.[3025,3026] Two subtypes of juvenile hemochromatosis are distinguished: type A and type B. Type A juvenile hemochromatosis is related to mutations in the *HJV* gene (formerly named *HFE2*) encoding the hemojuvelin protein. Type B juvenile hemochromatosis is related to the *HAMP* gene (formerly named *HFE3*) encoding the hepcidin protein.[3027] Type 3 gene defects on chromosome 7q22 impair the transferrin 2 receptor. Consequences are like those of the type I receptor defect. Type 4 hemochromatosis is caused by mutation in the ferroportin (*SLC40A1*) gene on 2q32. It is autosomal dominant and affects the basolateral iron carrier ferroportin 1, resulting in iron deposition in macrophages. Types 1, 2, and 3 have recessive autosomal inheritance and show a similar distribution pattern of iron deposits. In all five types, there may be alteration of gonadal function.

Hypogonadism may be the first sign of disease when it starts in adult life as in type 2 hemochromatosis and may be the initial symptom.[3028] With age, hypogonadism becomes hypogonadotropic, with low serum levels of testosterone, LH, and FSH in more than 40% of patients, except when early treatment is initiated.[3029,3030] The most frequent findings are atrophy with diminished MTD, tubular wall thickening, progressive decrease in spermatogenesis, and increased lipofuscin granules in Leydig cells. The cause of these testicular disorders may be preferential deposition of iron in gonadotropic cells.[3031] Iron deposits are not observed in the testis.

Given that early diagnosis is possible in all types of hemochromatosis, clinicians in countries with a high prevalence of the disease should be vigilant, thereby allowing affected patients to begin treatment at an early age and thus avoid later complications.[3032] Deferasirox treatment and aggressive phlebotomy therapy decrease iron deposits and improve hormonal dysfunction.[3030,3033–3037] Liver transplantation in patients with cirrhosis restores hormonal balance in a high percentage of cases, with recovery of libido within 6 weeks and gradual return of spermatogenesis in one-half.[3038] ICSI enables paternity in some cases.[3039] Testosterone administration may be useful to treat impotence and failure of ejaculation.[3040,3041]

Galactosemia

Classical galactosemia is a rare autosomal recessive galactose metabolism disorder caused by mutation in the *galactose-1-phosphate uridyltransferase* (*GALT*) gene. Galactosemia may produce important abnormalities of the genital system. In infancy the incidence rate of cryptorchidism is high (25%).[3042] Pubertal development is delayed in up to 20% of patients.[3043] In adult males, there is low seminal volume, and the levels of testosterone and inhibin B are at the lower limits of normality, whereas gonadotropin levels are normal, suggesting a subtle defect in Leydig and Sertoli cell function.[3044]

Kearns-Sayre Syndrome

Kearns-Sayre syndrome primarily affects the neuromuscular and endocrine systems and manifests before the age of 20 years. The principal characteristics of this syndrome are progressive external ophthalmoplegia, pigmentary retinopathy, cardiac conduction defects, and cerebellar ataxia. Disorders of the reproductive system, including cryptorchidism, delayed puberty, testicular hypoplasia, and low gonadotropin levels, are found in 20% to 30% of cases.[3045] Other endocrine alterations are hypothyroidism, short stature with or without GH deficit, diabetes mellitus, and hypoparathyroidism.[3046] The syndrome belongs to a group of multisystemic disorders (Kearns-Sayre syndrome, Pearson marrow-pancreas syndrome, and chronic progressive external ophthalmoplegia) caused by mutations in the mitochondrial genome. In Kearns-Sayre syndrome, most mitochondrial DNA deletions are sporadic and probably occur at the germ cell level or early in embryonic development.[3047–3049] As in other mitochondrial disorders the syndrome is inherited exclusively from the mother because all mitochondria in the zygote have maternal origin, and spermatozoa do not contribute to this cell organelle.[3050] Presentation of this syndrome depends on the level of dysfunction of the conduction system, which appears in most of the patients aged between 15 and 20 years.[3051,3052]

Adrenoleukodystrophy (Adrenal Testicular Myeloneuropathy)

Adrenoleukodystrophy (X-ALD) is a rare and progressive sex-linked recessive disorder that chiefly involves the central nervous system and causes progressive demyelization, adrenal insufficiency, and testicular failure.[3053] It is caused by a defect in β-oxidation of very-long-chain fatty acids (VLCFA), principally hexacosanoic (C26:0), pentacosanoic (C25:0), and tetracosanoic (C24:0) acids.[3054,3055] These acids are easily detected in serum.[3056,3057] Their accumulation in various tissues results in disease manifestations. The incidence is estimated to be 1 in 20,000, with no differences among ethnic groups.[3058,3059] The gene responsible for X-ALD, *ABCD1*, is located on the terminal end of the X-chromosome long arm (Xq28) and occupies approximately 26 kb of genomic DNA, with 10 exons encoding 745 amino acids.[3060] The gene product, ALDP, is a peroxisomal transmembrane protein belonging to the family of adenosine triphosphate–binding cassette (ABC) transporters. It acts to transport VLCFA into peroxisomes, where VLCFA is subject to β-oxidation.[3061] X-ALD is the most common peroxisomal disorder. More than 1000 mutations in the *ABCD1* gene have been registered in the international database (http://www.x-ald.nl).

Despite being X-linked, disease effects are not limited to males; 20% to 50% of female carriers experience symptoms. The phenotype is varied, but no correlation exists between genotype and phenotype. Six phenotypes were initially recognized, based on age of onset and clinical manifestations: the childhood cerebral form (CCALD), with cerebral demyelization and childhood onset; the adolescent cerebral form; the adult cerebral form; adrenomyeloneuropathy (AMN), with axonopathy of the pyramidal and somatosensory tracts and peripheral neuropathy; the olivopontocerebellar form; and Addison disease only. Today, at least nine phenotypes are identified in male patients and two in female patients.[3062,3063] Only CCALD and AMN are discussed in this chapter.

CCALD is the most common form, with onset in school age. Cerebral demyelization is initially manifest by attention-deficit/hyperactivity disorder, ophthalmic or ear abnormalities, and psychological problems.[3064] In many patients, diagnosis is confirmed by the onset of seizures, gait disturbances, and other neurologic symptoms. Ultimately, demyelization leads to a vegetative state, and patients do not reach adulthood.[3063–3066] Testes are small. Seminiferous tubules have greatly reduced diameters, with thickened walls and an epithelium with low number of Sertoli cells and few spermatogonia. The interstitium lacks Leydig cells. In addition to atrophy of seminiferous tubules, there is marked atrophy of the efferent ductule, which presents as cellular cords (Figs. 12.301 through 12.304).

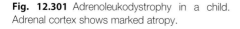

Fig. 12.301 Adrenoleukodystrophy in a child. Adrenal cortex shows marked atropy.

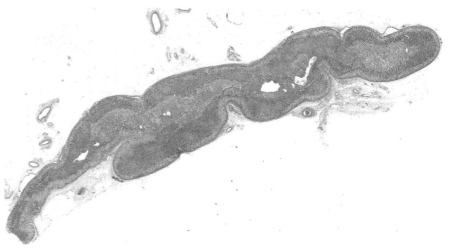

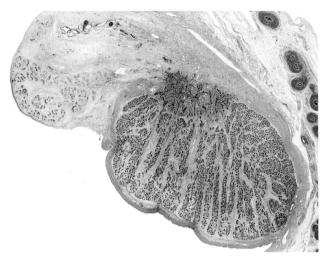

Fig. 12.302 Adrenoleukodystrophy. Testis of a child with marked atrophy. The caput of the epididymis is reduced to a loose connective tissue in which the silhouettes of the efferent ducts are hardly observed.

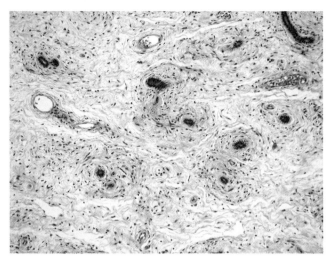

Fig. 12.304 Sections of efferent ducts of the same patient of the previous figures. Most of the ducts lack lumens and show significant peritubular fibrosis.

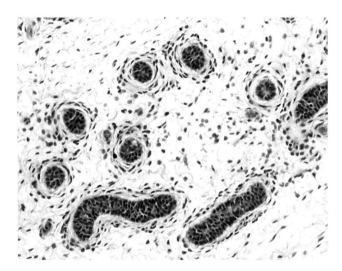

Fig. 12.303 The seminiferous tubules of this prepubertal patient with adrenoleukodystrophy are reduced to epithelial cords. The interstitium appears greatly enlarged.

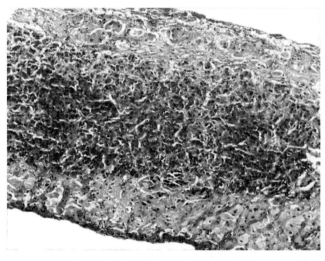

Fig. 12.305 Adrenoleukodystrophy. Adrenal gland showing severe atrophy of the cortex and globoid cells at the periphery. Medulla is preserved in the center of the figure.

AMN presents clinically at approximately 30 years of age, and one-half of patients show cerebral effects within 10 years of onset.[3067] The first symptoms include progressive paraparesis, thin scalp skin, alterations in sphincters, peripheral neuropathy, and adrenocortical failure.[3068] Most men have symptoms of gonadal dysfunction, including decreased libido (46%), erectile dysfunction (58%), and testicular descent failure (15%). Physical examination shows scant pubic hair (50%), gynecomastia (35%), and small testes (12%).[3069] Spermiogram reveals azoospermia or oligozoospermia and low ejaculate volume. Most patients experience primary testicular failure. FSH serum level is elevated in 32% to 57% of patients, and increased LH level is observed in 16% to 63% of patients. Response of LH to GnRH stimulation is abnormally high in 47% of patients, whereas response of FSH to stimulation is excessively low in 16%. Testosterone level is similar to controls, although free testosterone level is lower. Testosterone/LH ratio, a sensitive marker of Leydig cell function, is decreased in most patients (82%).[3069–3072]

Histologic changes follow the development of the disease. At the onset, spermatogenesis and sperm count may be normal, although teratozoospermia and asthenozoospermia are frequent. Later, spermatogenesis undergoes rapid deterioration, with variable degree of germ cell arrest and azoospermia.[3073] Characteristic findings in biopsies are observed in Leydig cells, which have specific lamellar cytoplasmic inclusions that are also found in adrenal cortical cells and cerebral cells (Figs. 12.305 and 12.306).[3070,3074]

Treatment of patients with X-ALD consists of steroid replacement therapy to counteract the clinical effects of adrenal cortical insufficiency, although treatment does not alter neurologic deterioration. Patients in the early phases may benefit from hematopoietic cell transplantation, whereas those with advanced disease are candidates for experimental therapies.[3075–3078]

Primary Hyperoxaluria

Primary hyperoxaluria is an autosomal recessive disease of glyoxylate metabolism that results in excessive production of oxalate. The

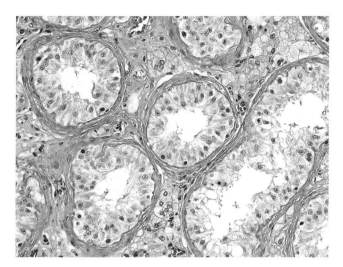

Fig. 12.306 Testis from a patient with adrenoleukodystrophy. Seminiferous tubules contain mainly Sertoli cells with only isolated spermatogonia. In the interstitium, Leydig cells with vacuolated cytoplasm may be observed.

and cerebrovascular dysfunction develop. Patients usually have cutaneous angiokeratomas, posterior capsular cataracts, and tortuous retinal veins. Death occurs between the third and fourth decades of life. All endocrine glands tend to accumulate Gb3.[3090]

Through systematic pedigree analysis, the incidence of the disease and clinical manifestations in pediatric patients are better understood. The most frequent clinical symptoms in children are acroparesthesia, hypohidrosis, and cornea verticillata. Other symptoms such as tinnitus, recurrent vertigo, headache, diminished level of activity, fatigue, and depression may also be observed. Renal disease may appear in adolescence. Age of onset is the same between sexes.[3091] Diagnosis is made by the presence of marked decrease of activity of α-galactosidase A in white blood cells or cultured skin fibroblasts.[3092]

Testes and excretory spermatic ducts are significantly damaged. Some alterations, including those in endothelial cells, smooth muscle cells, and fibroblasts, are nonspecific; other changes are specific, including those in myofibroblasts, Leydig cells, and epididymal epithelium (Figs. 12.307 and 12.308). Patients have asthenozoospermia, oligozoospermia, or both. Seminiferous tubules show

most frequent form of primary hyperoxaluria is type I, caused by deficient or absent activity of liver-specific peroxisomal alanine/glyoxylate aminotransferase enzyme. Renal effects include recurrent nephrolithiasis, nephrocalcinosis, and early renal failure. Massive deposition of calcium oxalate in tissues is known as oxalosis.[3079] Neither dialysis nor kidney transplantation permanently eliminates renal oxalate deposition. Liver transplantation is the most effective therapy. Only a single report of an effect is recorded: a man with obstructive azoospermia related to seminiferous tubule obstruction by calcium oxalate crystals achieved paternity after TESE-ISCI.[3080]

D-Bifunctional Protein Deficiency

DBP deficiency is an autosomal recessive disorder that compromises beta fatty acid oxidation in the peroxisome caused by mutations in the *HSD17B4* gene. The most frequent clinical symptoms are neonatal hypotonia, altered psychomotor development, dysmorphism, loss of hearing and vision, and abnormalities of the central nervous system Most patients die before the age of 2 years, but when DBP deficiency is incomplete, patients are able to reach adulthood. Involvement of the genital tract varies from hypergonadotropic hypogonadism with azoospermia and low serum testosterone to patients with normal testicular function and paternity.[3081,3082]

Fabry Disease

Fabry disease is an X-linked metabolic disorder first reported in 1898, characterized by intralysosomal deposits of globotriaosylceramide (Gb3) resulting from α-galactosidase deficiency due to mutation in the *GLA* gene.[3083,3084] The incidence of Fabry disease may be as high as 1 in 3100 live births.[3085,3086] Symptoms depend on the type of mutation of α-galactosidase A and residual enzymatic activity.[3087–3089] Progressive accumulation of Gb3 in endothelial cells, pericytes, smooth muscle cells, renal epithelial cells, myocardium, and nervous system cells of dorsal ganglia produces most of the symptoms.

Clinical manifestations may begin with what it is known as "Fabry crisis" (strong, burning pain in the palms and feet associated with fever and elevated erythrocyte sedimentation rate). After that, severe painful neuropathy and progressive renal, cardiovascular,

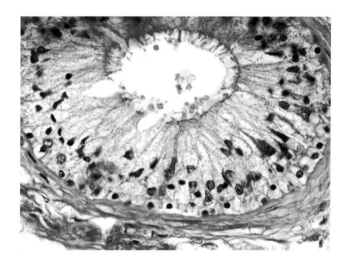

Fig. 12.307 Fabry disease. Both basal and principal cells of the epididymis show pale and vacuolated cytoplasms, due to lipid deposits.

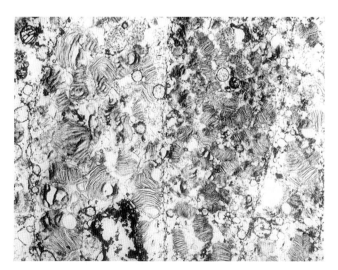

Fig. 12.308 Fabry disease. The deposits observed in the ductus epididymidis epithelium consist of multiple, parallel-arranged laminae (zebra bodies).

decreased diameter and tunica propria thickening. Sertoli cells accumulate lipids, and germ cells are limited to a few spermatogonia. Leydig cells are normal in number; nuclei are small, and cytoplasm contains numerous lipofuscin granules.[3093] All damaged cell types except germ cells contain large cytoplasmic vacuoles, consisting of deposits of complex lipids that stain with oil red O, Sudan black, or acid hematein. Ultrastructurally, the deposits appear as multiple, concentrically arranged lamellae surrounded by membrane (myelin-like bodies). Deposits are scant in Sertoli cells and Leydig cells, but myelin-like bodies are abundant in the epithelia of the ductus deferens and ductus epididymidis. Cell organelles are scant, and stereocilia are absent. Similar myelin-like bodies have been observed in endothelial cells, smooth muscle, fibroblasts, and myofibroblasts. The placenta shows significant deposits of Gb3 in the intermediate trophoblast, amniotic epithelial cells, and endothelial and muscular cells of the decidua and umbilical cord vessels.[3094]

Enzyme replacement with α-galactosidase prevents glycosphingolipid deposition and reduces glycosphingolipid levels, so this therapy is recommended as soon as possible.[3095–3099]

Wolman Disease

Wolman disease is a rare inherited lysosomal disease characterized by deficit in acid lipase/cholesteryl ester hydrolase whose genetic mutation is mapped to 10q23.2-q23.3.[3100] Complete enzymatic deficiency (Wolman disease) causes death in infancy as a result of accumulation of cholesterol esters and triglycerides in numerous organs such as the liver, adrenal cortex, and intestines.[3101,3102] Partial deficiency is known as cholesteryl ester storage disease. Patients tend to experience premature atherosclerosis.[3103] The diagnosis should be suspected when a child exhibits hepatomegaly, vomiting, diarrhea, failure to thrive, adrenal calcifications, and elevated levels of low-density lipoprotein-cholesterol or low levels of high-density lipoprotein-cholesterol with elevated transaminase activity.[3104]

Histologic examination reveals deposits in the interstitium. Leydig cells appear hypertrophic and foamy, containing autofluorescent and birefringent lipid material that consists ultrastructurally of giant lysosomes containing acicular inclusions. Cell organelles are scant. Increased numbers of interstitial macrophages are present, bearing granular cytoplasm that contains ceroid material. Cholesteryl ester accumulates in Leydig cells because these cells use large amounts of lipoprotein-bound cholesteryl ester as substrate for hormonal synthesis. Cholesteryl ester accumulation is not apparent in macrophages in tissues other than the testis. This finding suggests that testicular macrophages play an important role in normal protein turnover and emphasizes the relationship between testicular macrophages and Leydig cells.[3105]

Fertility is not usually decreased in patients with cholesteryl ester storage disease.[3106] Enzyme replacement therapy with sebelipase alfa delays the appearance of complications and increases life expectancy.[3107]

Niemann-Pick Disease

Niemann-Pick disease consists of a heterogeneous group of autosomal recessive diseases characterized by storage of different kinds of lipids in the reticuloendothelial system and other tissues. Four types (A, B, C, and D) are recognized, according to the clinical and biochemical characteristics of the disease.[3108] Type A (NP-A) is a neuropathic infantile form, and type B (NP-B) is a non-neuropathic infantile form. In NP-A and NP-B the principal storage lipid is sphingomyelin. The genetic defect is recessive mutation in the *sphingomyelin phosphodiesterase 1* (*SMPD1*) gene located in

11p15.1–4, which encodes a lysosomal hydrolase. NP-A is the most frequent of the four types, comprising 75% to 80% of all cases. NP-A is a severe neurodegenerative form that usually leads to death by 3 years of age. Patients with type B (NP-B) experience hepatosplenomegaly and respiratory disorders, but have little or no neurologic involvement and may survive into adolescence or adulthood.[3109] Type C (NP-C) is the neuropathic juvenile form, and type D (NP-D) is a geographic variant of NP-C involving several families in Nova Scotia; in both types, patients have massive accumulation of cholesterol, glycosphingolipids, and other lipids within the endosomal-lysosomal system caused by failure of intracellular trafficking of cholesterol and consequent failure of lipid homeostasis.[3110] The mutant gene responsible for more than 95% of the cases is in the 18q11–12 region and termed NPC1.[3111] The remaining cases are caused by mutations in the *NPC2* gene.[3112] NP-C is heterogeneous clinically.[3113]

NPC1 mutant mice (models of NPC disease) and *Drosophila* NPC1 mutants are infertile. Mutant mice show decreased steroidogenesis and decreased number of spermatozoa with a high frequency of morphologic anomalies. The *Drosophila* NPC1 mutants have larval death and infertility.[3114] Histologic studies show partial arrest of spermatogenesis.

Testicular findings in boys consist of lipid accumulations in interstitial macrophages. Ultrastructural studies show abundant lipid vacuoles in Sertoli cells, Leydig cells, macrophages, epididymal epithelial cells, and spermatozoa.[3115,3116]

Cystinosis

Cystinosis is an autosomal recessive metabolic disease characterized by alteration in cystine transport from lysosomes to the cytosol that results in intralysosomal accumulation of cystine. The incidence is estimated at 0.5 to 1 per 100,000. The main gene responsible for the disease (*CTNS*) is on chromosome 17p13 and encodes a lysosomal membrane protein named cystinosin, which is involved in transport.[3117] A second gene (*CARKL*), which encodes a protein with carbohydrate kinase activity, has also been identified.[3118] Neither gene is expressed in one-half of the patients with cystinosis. Cystine storage occurs in all body tissues, but predominantly in bone marrow, lymph nodes, kidney, thyroid, endocrine pancreas, muscles, central nervous system, cornea, conjunctiva, and testis. Renal parenchymal deposits result in nephropathic cystinosis, a form of renal failure that may present in infancy, adolescence, or adulthood. Severity of the disease is widely variable; it may be asymptomatic in adults and may even be incidentally diagnosed by the presence of corneal deposits.[3119]

Testicular function is severely altered in those with nephropathic cystinosis, many of whom have azoospermia. Patients experience hypergonadotropic hypogonadism with elevated serum levels of FSH and LH, and reduced response of testosterone to hCG stimulation. Paternity has not been reported.[3120] Cystine crystals stand out by their hexagonal pattern, appear doubly refractive under polarized light, and are located in the cytoplasm of interstitial macrophages. Involvement of the testicular interstitium may be massive.[3120] Associated lesions include hypospermatogenesis, interstitial fibrosis, and hydrocele.[3121]

Treatment with cysteamine probably worsens testicular function by an effect on Sertoli and Leydig cells through somatostatin and ghrelin.[3122] Testosterone replacement is possible.[3123]

CDG1 (Abnormal Glycosylated Proteins)

Congenital disorders in glycosylation comprise a group of metabolic diseases, previously identified as glycogenosis, that result from deficiency in synthesis of N-linked oligosaccharides. More than 85 congenital disorders in glycosylation are identified. Twenty-one different enzymes are involved in synthesis.[3124] The most frequent variant of this disorder (83%), CDG-Ia, is produced by deficiency in phosphomannomutase (PMM) caused by mutation in the *PMM2* gene, mapped to chromosome 16p13. Most patients (more than 700 reported to date) are diagnosed in infancy, and about 20% do not reach adulthood. Most organs are affected. The most important clinical symptoms are mental retardation, cerebellar hypoplasia, peripheral neuropathy, hepatic dysfunction, strokelike episodes, growth retardation, hemorrhagic episodes, and seizures.[3125] Men exhibit decreased testicular volume and hypogonadotropic or hypergonadotropic hypogonadism.[3126]

Alström Syndrome

Alström syndrome is a rare autosomal recessive disorder that is characterized by pigmentary retinal degeneration, sensorineural hearing loss, obesity, insulin-dependent diabetes mellitus, and chronic nephropathy.[3127,3128] Hypergonadotropic hypogonadism, acanthosis nigricans, hepatic dysfunction, hepatic steatosis, alopecia, hyperlipidemia, hypothyroidism, short stature, and dilated myocardiopathy are occasionally present.[3129,3130] Estimated prevalence rate is less than 0.001%.[3131] ALMS is caused by mutations in the *ALMS1* gene located on the short arm of chromosome 2 (2p13.1). Most mutations are located in exons 8, 10, and 16.[3130,3132] This gene encodes a protein linked with centrosomes and ciliary basal bodies implicated in formation, maintenance, and function of primary cilia (including hypothalamic neurons).[3133] ALMS is included in the list of disorders known as ciliopathies.[3134] Phenotypic expression varies widely, and not all symptoms are evident in early childhood, but eventually develop during the first and second decades of life. There is no correlation of genotype and phenotype.[3135]

In male adolescents, testes and penis are small. Onset of puberty is sometimes delayed. Secondary sexual characteristics are usually normal.[3136] The presence of normal to high FSH and LH levels and low testosterone level suggest primary hypogonadism. Gynecomastia and low sperm counts are frequent. Histologically, seminiferous tubules show atrophy and fibrosis, whereas the interstitium has scant Leydig cells.[3131] An association between ALMS and Klinefelter syndrome has been reported.[3137]

Selenoprotein Deficiency Disorder

Selenium is a component of the SBP2 selenoprotein that is essential for human health. More than 200 selenoproteins have been identified, functioning as oxidases involved in thyroid hormone metabolism.[3138] Development of effective spermatogenesis requires an optimal level of selenium in the testis. Selenium deficiency and excess are both deleterious to spermatogenesis and sperm maturation. Lack of testis-enriched selenoproteins produces delayed puberty and oligoasthenozoospermia.[3139] Serum testosterone level is normal, whereas inhibin B is markedly decreased, suggesting alteration of Sertoli cells.[3140] Selenoproteins such as mGPx4 and snGPx4 are structural components of mature spermatozoa, whereas others such as GPx1, GPx3, mGPx4, cGPx4, and GPx5 protect spermatozoa during maturation against oxidative damage.[3141]

Infertility Secondary to Physical and Chemical Agents

Physical and chemical agents may impair testicular function by direct action on the pituitary, testes, or sperm excretory ducts.

In the pituitary, damage to gonadotropic cells may be caused by estrogen. In the testes, gonadotoxic agents may selectively impair a select cell type, but global dysfunction occurs later. For example, there is direct toxicity to Sertoli cells by phthalates used as plasticizers, nitroaromatic compounds used in production of dyes and explosives, and γ-diketones used as solvents. Cadmium and bisphenol A perturb the blood-testis barrier. Direct toxicity on spermatogenesis is seen with ionizing radiation. Many drugs that impair epididymal fluid or spermatozoon transport damage sperm excretory ducts, with subsequent loss of fertility.[2965,2966]

Occupational Exposure

The relationship between infertility or subfertility and certain professions or exposures to environmental agents is well known.[1939,3142,3143] Adverse effects on spermatogenesis have been demonstrated for organic solvents such as carbon disulfide, chlorinated solvents, aromatic solvents and varnishes, degreasers, thinners, and adhesives; certain pesticides, notable DDT, linuron, and polychlorinated biphenyls; metals such as lead, cadmium, mercury, arsenic, copper, manganese, and molybdenum; industrial wastes such as dioxins and ethylene dibromide; phthalates and polyvinyl chloride; oral contraceptives; radiation or high temperature; recreational drugs and those used for athletic doping; and many other agents with potentially harmful effects on testicular function.[3142,3144–3150]

Carbon Disulfide

Carbon disulfide is used as a solvent in the production of rayon. Continuous exposure is toxic to the nervous system and causes decreased spermatogenesis and libido, and increased FSH and LH serum levels because of direct damage to Sertoli cells via an endoplasmic reticulum apoptotic pathway.[3150–3154]

Dibromochloropropane

Dibromochloropropane is used as a soil fumigant to control nematodes. Lengthy exposure causes oligozoospermia, azoospermia, increased FSH and LH levels, and Y-chromosome nondisjunction.[3155,3156] Workers exposed to 2-bromopropane (used as an alternative to ozone-depleting cleaning solvents) have reduced number of premeiotic spermatocytes because of germ cell apoptosis.[3157]

Lead

Inorganic lead is more dangerous than the organic form. Exposure of workers to inorganic lead in smelting, battery, and stained-glass plants may cause direct spermatogenic damage.[3158] Affected patients have asthenospermia, teratozoospermia, and oligozoospermia.[3159,3160] In addition to impaired spermatogenesis, lead toxicity affects steroidogenesis and the redox (reduction–oxidation reaction) system.[3161]

Oral Contraceptive Manufacture

Workers in pharmaceutical plants generating synthetic estrogens and progestins may experience hyperestrogenism with gynecomastia, decreased libido, and impotence.[3162] Neonatal exposure of boys to diethylstilbestrol (DES) may induce cryptorchidism, testicular hypoplasia, epididymal cysts, and severe anomalies in semen production.[437,3163,3164] However, the risk for infertility is only slightly increased.[3165]

Endocrine-Disrupting Compounds

Estrogen-like effects are produced by a variety of naturally occurring estrogens (so-called phytoestrogens) and numerous synthetic compounds such as phthalates, pesticides, and polychlorinated biphenyls.[3166–3170] These endocrine disruptors mimic natural hormones, inhibit the action of hormones, or alter the normal regulatory function of the endocrine system. These substances have potential hazardous effects on the male reproductive axis, including possible infertility, because they target testicular spermatogenesis, steroidogenesis, and the function of both Sertoli and Leydig cells[3171]; they also affect testicular function through induction of oxidative stress and apoptosis.[3172] Principal modes of contact with potential endocrine-disrupting compounds are environmental exposure and the dietary ingestion of milk, fish, meat, fruits and vegetables, and soy.[3173–3175] Heightened risk for cryptorchidism, hypospadias, testicular cancer, and poor semen quality may be related to the negative influence of environmental factors on the testis during fetal life.[3176] The term *testicular dysgenesis syndrome* has been proposed to designate this constellation of putative syndromes.[1059]

Estrogen exposure in utero may disrupt development of the testes and the entire male reproductive tract. Estrogen may hinder FSH secretion by the fetal pituitary and may also interfere with subsequent Sertoli cell proliferation, and hence secretion of AMH required for regression of müllerian ducts. Persistence of müllerian derivatives is associated with failure of testicular descent. Changes in AMH secretion may also account for altered germ cell proliferation during fetal life. Exposure to high concentrations of estrogen may compromise testosterone production, as well as masculinization of external genitalia (hypospadias) and inguinal descent of the testis (cryptorchidism). Abnormal development of Sertoli cells and low germ cell number may cause diminished spermatozoon production and infertility.[3177]

Recreational Drugs and Doping

Drug use may be an important cause of male infertility, and adverse effects have been reported on the hypothalamopituitary-testicular axis, sperm function, and testicular structure.[3178] Marijuana decreases sperm density, motility, and the acrosomal reaction, and increases the number of morphologically abnormal spermatozoa. Inhibitory effects are mediated by dysregulation of the hypothalamic-hypophyseal-testicular axis and direct action of cannabinoids on sperm through the activation of the cannabinoid receptor subtype CNR1 that has been shown to be expressed in mature sperm.[3179–3181] Marijuana is also a potent inhibitor of mitochondrial oxygen consumption in human sperm.[3182] Cocaine induces apoptosis in the rat testis.[3183] Approximately 20% of injectable drug users have low serum testosterone level. Consumption of more than 80 g/day alcohol adversely affects spermatogenesis in two-thirds of patients.[3184] Biopsy showed maturation arrest of germinal cells at the pachytene stage with no mature sperm cells. Rapid and dramatic improvement of semen characteristics may occur after alcohol withdrawal. Patients should be questioned about alcohol intake before assisted reproductive technology is performed.[3185] Smoking causes deterioration of all sperm parameters.[3186,3187] Abuse of anabolic steroids by athletes causes hypogonadotropic hypogonadism and transient azoospermia.[3188–3190]

Radiation

The testicular parenchyma is one of the most radiosensitive tissues of the body, and germ cells are the most radiosensitive testicular cells at all ages, including male fetuses.[3191] Ionizing radiation causes alterations in spermatogenesis and hormonal regulation. Men treated with brachytherapy for prostate cancer have abnormal sperm DNA fragmentation index, indicating likely infertility.[3192] Some patients recover fertility a few years after radiation exposure.[3193] The effects of nonionizing radiation are less severe, although increased use of newer technologies may decrease fertility potential by increasing long-term exposure to nonionizing radiation.[3194] Electromagnetic radiation from cell phones carried in the pocket of trousers near the testis impairs spermatozoon motility.[3195–3198] Reduced libido and reduced number of spermatozoa have been reported in men exposed to microwaves.[3199] Laptop computers with Wi-Fi connect through radiofrequency electromagnetic waves may damage spermatozoa through microwave radiation.[3200,3201] Whether laptop computers connected wirelessly to the Internet decrease sperm motility and increase sperm with DNA fragmentation by a nonthermal effect is debated.[3202–3205] Magnetic and electromagnetic fields induce oxidation of phospholipids, which are a major component in the sperm mitochondrial sheath.[3206] Additionally, portable computers generate high temperatures, thus increasing scrotal temperatures, which may produce deleterious effects on spermatogenesis.[3207,3208]

Heat

Normal intratesticular temperature is 31 °C to 33 °C, approximately 4 °C to 6 °C lower than core body temperature. Deterioration in the quality of semen has been verified in taxi drivers, welders, and habitual users of the sauna.[3209] Conditions causing higher testicular temperature, such as varicocele and cryptorchidism, also cause damage, with decreased numbers of spermatozoa and an elevated percentage of spermatozoa with abnormal forms and low motility.[3210,3211] Exposure to intermittent heat in healthy people produces greater damage in spermatogenesis than continuous heat exposure.[3212] Scrotal heat stress produces alterations in semen quality, DNA integrity chromatin condensation, and caspase-3.[3213] Primary spermatocytes at the end of the pachytene stage are most sensitive to heat. The mechanism by which heat produces testicular lesions is uncertain, although heat stress is closely associated with oxidative stress, and that is followed by apoptosis of germ cells.[3214] Hyperthermia affects the activity of enzymes such as ornithine decarboxylase and carnitine acetyl transferase, both necessary for metabolism and proliferation of seminiferous tubular cells.[3215–3217] Synthesis of DNA and RNA by germ cells also depends on temperature. DNA synthesis by spermatogonia and preleptotene primary spermatocytes is higher at 31 °C than at 37 °C. RNA and protein synthesis is normal at temperatures between 28 °C and 37 °C, but both decrease markedly at 40 °C.[3218]

Testicular Trauma

Injury to male external genitalia is uncommon when compared with injury in other parts of the body, accounting for <1% of all trauma-related injuries, with a peak between 10 and 30 years of age.[3219] Testicular trauma most commonly results from sports injuries, road traffic accidents, and gunshot wounds, and is especially frequent among athletes.[3220–3222] Testicular trauma to the newborn during breech birth, whether by vaginal delivery or not, adds to the statistics.[507,3223] Protection from damage is afforded by relative seclusion and mobility of the genitalia. Testes have some mechanisms for protection from injury such as mobility, the cremasteric reflex, toughness of the elastic tunica albuginea, and, in infancy, the small size. However, testes may be injured by wounds or penetrating force against the pubic symphysis, the pubic ramus, or the upper thigh. Trauma may result in a wide variety of lesions, including hematoma (Figs. 12.309 and 12.310)

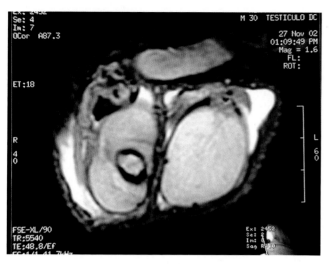

Fig. 12.309 Magnetic resonance image of a hematoma in the central region of right testis showing a target pattern.

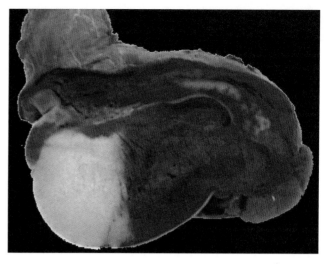

Fig. 12.311 Testicular traumatism. Extrusion of dark-colored testicular parenchyma through an albuginea break.

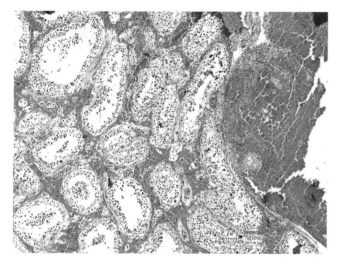

Fig. 12.310 Histologic section of a testicular hematoma showing a blood collection among seminiferous tubules.

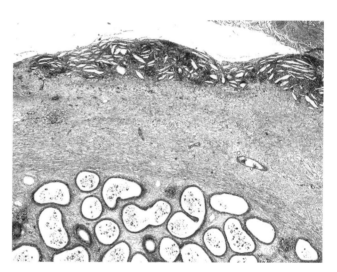

Fig. 12.312 Hematocele in reabsorption phase. Granulomatous reaction with abundant cholesterol crystal in the epididymis surface.

contusion with or without hematocele, rupture, dislocation, and spermatogenic impairment.

Traumatic Hematocele

Traumatic hematocele usually results from testicular rupture (80% of cases) or a tear in the pampiniform plexus veins.[3224,3225] It is important to distinguish between hematocele that follows blunt testicular contusion with an intact tunica albuginea that would not require surgery and hematocele secondary to testicular rupture that requires immediate repair (except for selected cases) to avoid ischemic necrosis or abscess formation.[3226] Approximately 45% of patients with blunt testicular trauma present with tunica albuginea break (Fig. 12.311). Special care should be taken to evaluate the testes of children and adults who have suffered blunt abdominal trauma to avoid delayed diagnosis of significant testicular injury.[3227,3228]

Differential diagnosis of hematocele includes testicular tumor, testicular torsion, and epididymoorchitis.[3229] In hematocele of recent occurrence the tunica sac contains coagulated fresh blood. If the hematocele is older, the tunica sac appears filled with spongy material several times larger than the testicular volume. Most of this material is fibrin and cholesterol granulomas (Fig. 12.312).[3230–3232] In chronic hematocele the blood clot is totally or partially organized and consists of connective tissue that contains numerous newly formed blood vessels and hemosiderin-laden macrophages. Connective tissue facing the tunica cavity is lined by fibrin remnants. In its final stages the lesion consists of a thickened, fibrosed, and calcified tunica sac (Fig. 12.313), which may also show osseous metaplasia (Fig. 12.314).[3233]

Hematocele should be evacuated as quickly as possible to avoid pressure atrophy of the parenchyma.[3234] Rare complications include infection, suppuration, and scrotal gangrene. Repair of rupture may be difficult, especially if it is circumferential. In such cases a large portion of parenchyma is herniated and may already be necrotic.[3235,3236] Newer surgical techniques are used to preserve as much viable testicular tissue as possible.[3237] In some patients who have suffered penetrating trauma, the testis herniate through the scrotal skin lacerations. Many patients with scrotal injuries also have epididymal and spermatic cord lesions.[3238] Diagnostic ultrasonography is generally useful but does not allow an exact diagnosis

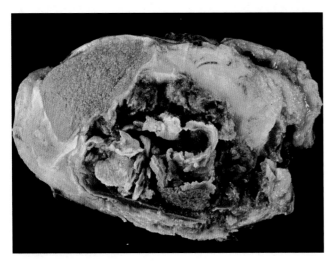

Fig. 12.313 Old hematocele. Vaginal cavity is filled up with calcified laminar formations that compress an atrophic testis.

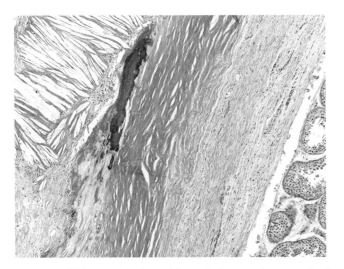

Fig. 12.314 Old hematocele. Around the testicular parenchyma an albuginea with marked fibrosis, a trabecular bone parallel to it, and fissures of cholesterol in the periphery are observed.

in all cases.[3239,3240] The same is true of CT, whereas MRI usually provides the correct diagnosis.[3241,3242] In children, peritumoral and retroperitoneal hemorrhage, splenic rupture, and adrenal cortical hemorrhage have reportedly caused hematocele by tracking of blood into a communicating hepatocele.[3243–3245]

Testicular Dislocation or Luxation

Testicular dislocation or luxation, first reported in 1818, involves displacement of one or both testes to a nonscrotal location such as the inguinal canal, abdominal cavity, or acetabular area, or distant locations such as the perineum, subcutaneous tissues, or superficial to the outer oblique fascia.[3246–3250] This injury is characteristic of motorcycle accidents and is caused by direct testicular contusion against the gas tank or the handlebars.[3251,3252] Widespread use of motorcycles in Asian countries accounts for the high frequency of reported cases in the Asian literature. Most cases are unilateral (90%).[3253] In displacement, muscular attachments of the spermatic cord are broken and the testis becomes lodged between the external oblique fascia and subcutaneous tissue in more than

50% of cases.[3254] Other reported sites of displacement include tissues adjacent to the superficial inguinal ring; suprapubic, inguinal canal, perineum, intraabdominal, and retrovesical sites; and acetabular or crural areas.[3249,3255–3257] Canalicular or intraabdominal dislocation occurs only in the setting of preexisting patent processus vaginalis.[3246–3248] Dislocation has also been reported in cases of pelvic fractures.[3258] More force is necessary to produce luxation in an adult than that which causes rupture of the tunica albuginea.[3259] Manual reduction is the treatment of choice for acute traumatic dislocation of the testis. Open reduction is advisable for delayed cases when testicular rupture or possible torsion is suspected, or if manual reduction fails.[3260] Prompt surgical intervention is crucial because the testis may be salvaged if surgical repair is performed within 72 hours of injury.[3261] In one remarkable case, bilateral orchiopexy 13 years after traumatic dislocation was successful in restoring spermatogenesis.[3262]

Testicular Trauma and Infertility

Few studies have addressed the relationship between testicular injury and infertility. Direct testicular injury is not considered a classic cause of spermatogenic impairment and testicular dysfunction. However, 17% of reported patients with unexplained infertility have a history of trauma. The spermiogram of such patients usually shows low number of spermatozoa, decreased motility, and high number of abnormal forms. In one report of patients with bilateral testicular trauma, all had more than 20 million/mL spermatozoa.[3235] Conversely, another study revealed that less than 50% of patients who underwent unilateral orchiectomy or open repair had decrease in sperm density and motility several months later, whereas those who underwent conservative treatment had minimal alterations.[3263,3264] Therefore it is compulsory to protect testes adequately while engaging in some sports.

Biopsies show decreased spermatogenesis and groups of completely hyalinized tubules. These observations suggest that testicular lesions are underestimated. The most constant hormonal finding is an increase in estradiol level.[3265] Possible causes of altered spermatogenesis include direct effect of trauma, formation of antisperm antibodies in response to disruption of the blood-testis barrier, and sperm excretory duct lesion.

Cancer Therapy

Sexual dysfunction occurs in 25% to 50% of patients treated for cancer.[3266] Testicular cancer, Hodgkin disease, and leukemia are the most frequent malignancies during the reproductive years. Other cancers in children are Wilms tumor, non-Hodgkin lymphoma, germ cell tumor, Ewing sarcoma, osteosarcoma, soft tissue sarcoma, retinoblastoma, and brain tumors.[3267] Approximately 1 in 600 children experiences development of cancer before the age of 15 years. Remarkable progress has been made in the treatment of cancer in infants and children, and up to 80% are now cured.[3268] In 2010, it was estimated that 1 in 250 young adults between the ages of 20 and 29 years was a survivor of childhood cancer.[3269,3270] Concerns have been raised about the possible mutagenic effect of chemotherapy on sperm. Therefore preservation of fertility requires selection of less gonadotoxic therapeutic regimens; if paternity is planned, cryopreservation of semen before treatment may be considered. Cancer treatments such as surgery, radiation therapy, and chemotherapy may achieve relatively high rates of remission and long-term survival. Despite continuous improvement in cancer treatment, altered testicular function and infertility frequently represent major adverse effects. Gonadal damage in boys treated for cancer may result from chemotherapy or radiation therapy involving the spinal or pelvic area. The testis is highly susceptible to the toxic effects of cancer therapy throughout life.[3271] Damage may involve the somatic cells of the testis (Sertoli and Leydig cells), as well as the germ cells. The main risk factors that adversely affect fertility in child cancer survivors are age at the time of the treatment, use of alkylating agents, and irradiation of reproductive organs or the hypothalamus/pituitary.[3272]

Many other aspects of cancer treatment also impair fertility, and the disease itself may contribute to male gonadal dysfunction. For example, up to 70% of patients with Hodgkin disease, assessed before the beginning of treatment, have impaired semen quality.[3273–3275] This impairment also seems to occur with other malignancies to a lesser extent. Patients with testicular germ cell tumor bear the highest risk for having poor semen quality before cancer treatment.[3276,3277] The association of testicular germ cell tumor and impaired spermatogenesis is well known, and both are included in the testicular dysgenesis syndrome. In patients with testicular cancer, individuals with certain genotypes may be more susceptible to treatment.[3278] Delayed maturation in spermatogenesis may be found in prepubertal patients before treatment of solid mesenchymal tumors.[3279]

The mechanisms involved in testicular dysfunction in patients with cancer are poorly understood, but are likely multifactorial. Possibilities include primary germ cell deficiency, release by tumor cells of substances that are toxic to seminiferous tubules and Leydig cells, and alteration of the hypothalamohypophyseal axis.[3280,3281] Paraneoplastic phenomena, such as fever, anorexia, and pain, may also impair semen quality.[3282,3283]

Radiation Therapy

Testicular parenchyma is one of the most radiosensitive tissues of the body, and germ cells are the most radiosensitive cells of the testis at all ages.[3191] In children, radiation-induced gonadal damage is most often encountered after direct irradiation used for management of testicular relapse of leukemia, or after total body irradiation that is given before bone marrow transplantation. The degree and persistence of damage depend on the total dose, patient age, extent and site of the treatment field, and the fractionation schedule. Fractionation may be more harmful to testicular function because it reduces the time available for repair.[3193,3284] Experimental irradiation of volunteers with a single dose revealed that late spermatogonia (Ap and B) are more radiosensitive than early (Ad) spermatogonia. Ap and B spermatogonia may be destroyed with doses as low as 0.1 to 1.2 Gy (1 Gy = 100 rad), whereas Ad spermatogonia tolerate doses higher than 4 Gy. Type A spermatogonia, spermatids, and spermatozoa are, respectively, 100, 200, and 10,000 times less radiosensitive than B spermatogonia. Doses of more than 4 Gy may produce permanent damage to spermatogenesis, and doses higher than 6 Gy produce Sertoli cell–only pattern.[3285] Testicular irradiation (16 to 18 Gy) therapy as used to treat GCNIS is associated with a high rate of permanent sterility.[3276] Leydig cells are more resistant to damage than the germinal epithelium, and function of these cells is usually preserved up to 20 Gy in prepubertal boys and at up to 30 Gy in men. This finding explains why development through puberty with normal testosterone level is the rule, and why many patients develop secondary sexual characteristics despite severe impairment of spermatogenesis.[3286] Patients treated for Wilms tumor, retroperitoneal ganglioneuroblastoma, or paratesticular rhabdomyosarcoma may have delayed puberty and, in adulthood, oligozoospermia or azoospermia with elevated level of FSH; these findings suggest that Leydig cells are also damaged (Figs. 12.315 and 12.316).

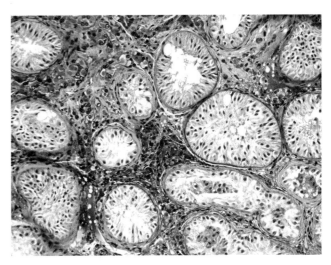

Fig. 12.315 A 27-year-old patient who consulted for infertility. He had a history of radiotherapy treatment for a retroperitoneal ganglioneuroblastoma. Seminiferous tubules of variable caliber with only Sertoli cells whose number varies from one tubule to another. Diffuse Leydig cell hyperplasia.

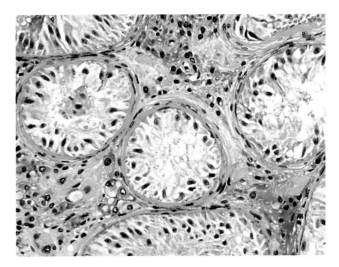

Fig. 12.316 Testis from a 26-year-old patient who, at the age of 9 years, underwent surgery followed by radiotherapy for paratesticular rhabdomyosarcoma. The testicular biopsy shows postirradiation lesions, including germ cell absence and peritubular and interstitial fibrosis.

A special case is that of children with acute lymphoblastic leukemia involving the testis. Radiation therapy with doses of 20 to 25 Gy, either alone or with chemotherapy, causes irreversible damage to Leydig cells and induces hyalinization of seminiferous tubules. Patients experience azoospermia and hypogonadotropic hypogonadism with low serum testosterone level. In addition, radiation induces dense interstitial fibrosis and loss of peritubular cells, thus obscuring the border between the interstitium and tubules. This makes the tubules difficult to identify in hematoxylin and eosin–stained sections. Leydig cells are atrophic and decreased in number. Ischemia secondary to radiation-induced vascular injury also contributes to hyalinization.

Tumors of the central nervous system are the most common solid malignancy in the pediatric population. Cranial irradiation is frequently used as a therapeutic modality in these children. Although this treatment does not harm the gonads directly, fertility may be impaired by disruption of the hypothalamopituitary-gonadal axis. Patients receiving radiation doses of 35 to 45 Gy experience deficiencies in FSH and LH secretion. The clinical sequelae of gonadotropin deficiency vary in severity from subclinical abnormalities detectable only by an abnormal GnRH test to significant reduction in circulating sex hormone levels, delayed puberty, and infertility.[3282,3287]

Sertoli cells tolerate up to 60 Gy, although they show ultrastructural alterations after low doses of radiation, as well as increased phagocytosis of germ cell remnants.[3282] Recovery of spermatogenesis takes place from surviving stem cells (type A spermatogonia) and depends on the dose of radiation. Complete recovery requires 9 to 18 months after irradiation of ≤ 1 Gy, 30 months after exposure of 2 to 3 Gy, and 5 years or more after exposure of ≥ 4 Gy.[3285]

Despite optimal protection, the contralateral testis absorbs 0.2 to 1.4 Gy during adjuvant therapy for rectal cancer or when the opposite testis is irradiated,[3288,3289] a dose sufficient to cause temporary azoospermia. Similarly, irradiation of iliac or inguinal lymph nodes for Hodgkin disease or other forms of lymphoma exposes the testes to approximately 5 Gy.[3290] Restoration of testicular function is time dependent, requiring at least 2 years.[3291,3292] Fertility in patients with thyroid cancer who received radioiodine-131 (^{131}I) therapy decreases transiently.[3293]

Chemotherapy

Use of cytotoxic chemotherapy is associated with a wide variety of adverse side effects, including gonadotoxicity. The prepubertal testis is especially vulnerable, probably because of the steady turnover of early germ cells that undergo spontaneous degeneration before the haploid stage is reached.[3294] It is postulated that this activity is essential for normal adult function, and thus reduced fertility (as a consequence of cytotoxic treatment) is anticipated when children receive chemotherapy. Chemotherapeutic agents kill rapidly proliferating cells, differentiating spermatogonia, and stem cells. In addition, stem spermatogonia that do survive fail to differentiate, resulting in permanent infertility. Leydig cells are more resistant than germ cells due to lower turnover rate. Leydig cell dysfunction after chemotherapy is usually limited to elevated LH concentration with normal or low normal testosterone level, and thus secondary sexual characteristics develop normally. Less frequently, patients show hypogonadism.[3295]

Numerous chemotherapeutic agents are gonadotoxic, and the nature and extent of gonadal injury depend on the drug administered, cumulative dose, treatment duration, combination used, age, pretreatment gonadal status, and individual sensitivity (Fig. 12.317).[3296,3297] The adverse effects of chemotherapy on spermatogenesis are caused by chromosomal aberrations (platinum antineoplastic agents and topoisomerase inhibitors), maturation arrest by inhibiting microtubule polymerization (vinca alkaloids), mutagenic effect in all stages of spermatogenesis (alkylating agents), and impairment of spermatozoa motility. Taxanes inhibit microtubule function, thereby inhibiting cell division, and cause reduction of inhibin B and reciprocal elevation of FSH, which are associated with significant gonadal damage.[3298]

Certain treatment regimens, such as that used for Hodgkin disease, are especially prone to infertility. Combination chemotherapy makes it difficult to ascertain which specific agent is responsible for azoospermia and Leydig cell dysfunction. Comparative studies of chemotherapy for acute lymphoblastic leukemia, extragonadal solid tumors, Hodgkin disease, Ewing sarcoma, and other soft tissue sarcomas in children and pubertal boys have shown that alkylating agents (chlorambucil, cyclophosphamide, and melphalan) cause the most severe testicular damage.[1080,3299–3302] Injuries are

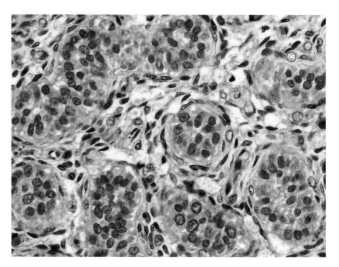

Fig. 12.317 A 12-month-old child with severe combined immunodeficiency who had received bone marrow transplantation. Small-sized seminiferous tubules with absence of germ cells. Note decreased Leydig cells.

dose dependent and occur regardless of tumor type, age, or pubertal status at diagnosis. Seminiferous epithelium is the most vulnerable cell type to the detrimental effects of this chemotherapy. Alkylating agents destroy the seminiferous tubular cells and induce tubular atrophy, thus shrinking the testis and increasing FSH serum concentration.[3303] These agents also impair Leydig cell function and lower testosterone level despite normal or elevated serum level of LH and an exaggerated response of LH to GnRH administration.[3304]

Cyclophosphamide appears to be responsible for the greatest incidence of temporary or permanent cases of azoospermia after chemotherapy. This agent acts directly on the spermatogenic stem cells, and recovery depends on the number of surviving cells.[3301] In children, cyclophosphamide reduces seminiferous tubule diameter and germ cell number; nuclei in the residual spermatogonia are enlarged. Puberty may progress, even during treatment, and the adult testis may show a Sertoli cell–only pattern.[1080] In adults, cyclophosphamide treatment may cause irreversible testicular damage (Figs. 12.318 and 12.319). Administered alone, 20 g/m^2 produces permanent azoospermia in 50% of men. If cyclophosphamide is administered with doxorubicin, vincristine, dacarbazine, or dactinomycin (drugs that alone do not cause azoospermia), doses of 7.5 g/m^2 will cause azoospermia in 50% of patients. Fludarabine, used for the treatment of chronic lymphocytic leukemia, produces testicular damage with diminution of ejaculate volume, oligozoospermia, increased serum levels of FSH and LH, and decreased testosterone level. DNA in spermatozoa is markedly abnormal, an effect that persists for several months.[3305] High dosage of ifosfamide-based therapy for osteosarcoma causes a high rate of azoospermia.[3306] Cisplatin-based regimens used in the treatment of testicular germ cell tumor cause azoospermia at high dosage (400 to 600 mg/m^2).[3307] There are few data for newer drugs such as taxanes, oxaliplatin, irinotecan, monoclonal antibodies. and tyrosine kinase inhibitors. Inhibin B was slightly reduced after treatment with oxaliplatin.[3308] Experimental studies in prepubertal mice found that Irinotecan metabolite SN38 induces marked dose-dependent sensitivity in germ cells.[3309] Imatinib mesylate (tyrosine kinase inhibitor), used in the treatment of chronic myeloid leukemia, produces severe oligozoospermia.[3310]

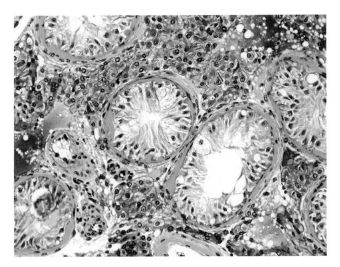

Fig. 12.318 Testis from a patient with Hodgkin disease after chemotherapy. The seminiferous tubules are small and contain only vacuolated Sertoli cells. The testicular interstitium has pseudohyperplasia of Leydig cells.

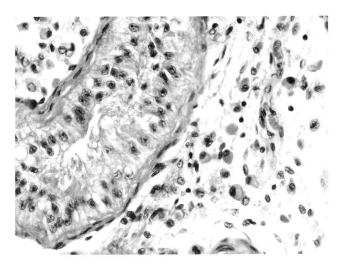

Fig. 12.319 A 36-year-old patient with Hodgkin disease who required bone marrow transplantation. He died of infectious complications. Seminiferous tubule with only Sertoli cells. The interstitium contains abundant macrophages and lymphocytes.

Combinations of chemotherapy drugs heighten the negative effects on testicular function. Procarbazine, used alone to treat Hodgkin disease, causes permanent azoospermia in 30% of patients; however, when combined with mustine, vincristine, and prednisolone, it causes 97% of male patients to became permanently sterile.[3285] LH concentration is raised, suggesting Leydig cell impairment. Patients treated with procarbazine, cyclophosphamide, vincristine, and prednisone do not recover spermatogenesis even if the cyclophosphamide dose does not exceed 4.8 g/m². Newer protocols with different drugs and doses are constantly introduced to reduce gonadotoxicity.

Studies of young adults add negative data about fertility restoration in patients with cancer. Approximately 17% those who received chemotherapy are azoospermic at the initial diagnosis.[3311] In a different way, damage may impair the number, morphology, and motility or DNA integrity of spermatozoa. The causes of this damage may be more complex than increased catabolic state,

malnutrition, or increase in stress hormones and decrease in gonadotropic levels.[3281]

Chemotherapeutic regimens that include neither alkylating agents nor procarbazine, such as the ABVD (doxorubicin, bleomycin, vinblastine, and dacarbazine) or VBM (vinblastine, bleomycin, and methotrexate) regimens produce reversible azoospermia in 36% of patients. Alternating use of MOPP (mechlorethamine, vincristine, procarbazine, and prednisone) and ABVD causes testicular dysfunction in 87% of patients, but spermatogenesis recovers in 40%.[3312]

Patients with germ cell malignancy who received chemotherapy with BEP regimens (cisplatinum, etoposide, and bleomycin) become azoospermic 7 to 8 weeks after starting treatment. When the total doses reach 600 mg/m², infertility is irreversible; at lower dosages, fertility may be recovered over a period of approximately 2 to 5 years (50% and 80% of patients, respectively), although a high percentage of spermatozoa with DNA abnormalities will persist.[3313,3314]

Therefore fertility preservation after cancer treatments requires careful selection of the least gonadotoxic therapeutic regimen, as well as male fertility preservation surgical approaches.[3315,3316] International guidelines recommend discussion with the patient or parents about infertility, fertility preservation options, and potential need for contraception before initiating therapy.[3317,3318] Cryopreservation of semen is now standard practice and should be offered to all men who are about to receive potentially sterilizing therapy. Advances in assisted reproductive techniques increase the likelihood of successful pregnancy using cryopreserved spermatozoa.[3297] Cryopreservation of immature testicular tissue or isolated germ cells from prepubescent males to achieve restoration of fertility after treatment, either by germ cell transplantation or by in vitro maturation of the germ cells harvested, remains experimental.[3279,3282,3319–3321] Research in the field of spermatogenic stem cells offers promise with options such as autotransplant of stem cells for repopulation of the testes after treatment.[3298] Research efforts are also concentrated on techniques for maturation and proliferation of immature gametes after thawing.[3322] However, effective gonadal function-preserving drugs are not yet available for use in male patients.[3323] A recent animal study reported the protective effect of humanin analog on germ cells during chemotherapy in male mice, but clinical studies have not yet begun.[3324]

Apart from causing gonadotoxicity, other treatments may also impair gonadal function by inducing endocrine disorders. Opioids used for pain management inhibit gonadal function and cause hyperprolactinemia.[3316] Hypogonadism in childhood cancer survivors may be related to local or brain irradiation.[3325]

Potential for Fertility After Cancer Treatment in Childhood

The wide spectrum of gonadal insults after chemotherapy or radiation therapy makes it difficult to accurately predict potential fertility for individual patients. Risk for subfertility may be categorized according to the type of malignancy and the associated treatment (Table 12.27).[3295,3315,3326] Low risk for development of subfertility is observed after treatment of acute lymphoblastic leukemia, Wilms tumor, stage 1 sarcoma, germ cell tumor (with opposite gonadal preservation and no radiation therapy), retinoblastoma, and brain tumor treated with surgery only or cranial irradiation lower than 24 Gy. Medium risk for subfertility is observed with acute myeloblastic leukemia, hepatoblastoma, osteosarcoma, Ewing sarcoma, high-stage sarcoma, neuroblastoma, non-Hodgkin lymphoma, Hodgkin disease treated with "alternating therapy,"

TABLE 12.27 Risk for Gonadal Subfertility due to Cytotoxic Drugs and Current Treatments for Disease

High Risk	Medium Risk	Low Risk	Limited Data
Drugs			
Alkylating drugs	Platinum analogues	Plant derivatives	Taxanes
Cyclophosphamide	Cisplatin	Vincristine	Oxaliplatin
Ifosfamide	Carboplatin	Vinblastine	Irinotecan
Busulfan	Doxorubicin	Antibiotics	Tyrosine kinase
Melphalan	BEP	Bleomycin	inhibitors
Chlorambucil	ABVD	Dactinomycin	Monoclonal
Chlormethine		Antimetabolites	antibodies
Procarbazine		Methotrexate	
		Mercaptopurine	
		5-Fluoruracil	
Disease/Treatment			
Total body irradiation	Acute myeloblastic leukemia	Acute lymphoblastic leukemia	
Localized radiotherapy: pelvic/testicular	Hepatoblastoma	Wilms tumor	
Chemotherapy conditioning for bone marrow	Osteosarcoma	Soft tissue sarcoma: stage 1	
transplant	Ewing sarcoma	TGCT (gonadal preservation and no	
Hodgkin disease: alkylating agent-based therapy	Soft tissue sarcoma	radiotherapy)	
Soft tissue sarcoma: metastatic	Neuroblastoma	Retinoblastoma	
	Non-Hodgkin lymphoma	Brain tumor (surgery only)	
	Hodgkin disease: "alternating	Cranial irradiation <24 Gy	
	therapy"		
	Brain tumor: craniospinal		
	radiotherapy		
	Cranial irradiation >24 Gy		

BEP, Cisplatinum, etoposide and bleomycin; *ABVD*, Doxorubicin, bleomycin, vinblastine and dacarbazine; *TGCT*, Testicular germ cell tumor.
Adapted from Brydoy M, Fossa SD, Dahl O, Bjoro T. Gonadal dysfunction and fertility problems in cancer survivors. Acta Oncol 2007;46:480-489; and Brougham MF, Kelnar CJ, Sharpe RM, Wallace WH. Male fertility following childhood cancer: current concepts and future therapies. Asian J Androl. 2003;5:325-337.

and brain tumor treated with craniospinal radiation therapy or cranial irradiation higher than 24 Gy. High risk for development of subfertility is associated with total body irradiation, localized radiation therapy either in the pelvic or testicular region, chemotherapy conditioning for bone marrow transplant, alkylating agent–based therapy in Hodgkin disease, and treatment of metastatic sarcoma.[3282]

A high percentage of children with cancer reach adulthood, so infertility is a serious potential long-term side effect of treatment (Fig. 12.320). Prevention of sterility in survivors of childhood cancer is a major challenge. However, early detection of gonadal damage is not currently possible because there is no sensitive or specific marker of gonadal function in the prepubertal age group. At present, there is great interest in plasma inhibin B or the inhibin B/FSH ratio as a potential marker of gonadotoxicity in this age group.[3282,3327–3329] Interdisciplinary cooperation among patients, pediatric oncologists, surgeons, immunologists, and endocrinologists is required on a routine basis to provide individualized options for fertility preservation.[3330–3333]

Estrogen and Antiandrogen Therapy

Estrogen treatment is used for adults with prostate cancer and those with gender dysphoria undergoing sex reassignment surgery to female. In the latter group, cross-sex hormone treatment is a prerequisite for sex reassignment surgery.

Patients with prostate cancer treated with estrogens have reduced spermatogenesis, Sertoli cell–only pattern, or spermatogonia-only–containing tubules, reduced Leydig cell number, and hyalinized tubules (Fig. 12.321).[3334]

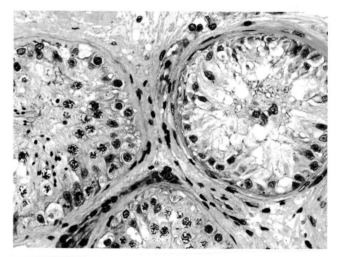

Fig. 12.320 Adult man consulting for infertility who was treated with chemotherapy for a nephroblastoma in his infancy. The testicular parenchyma shows mixed atrophy with one seminiferous tubule with Sertoli cell–only pattern and Sertoli cells of adult type and the other two tubules with spermatogenesis. *BEP*: Cisplatinum, etoposide and bleomycin; *ABVD*: Doxorubicin, bleomycin, vinblastine and dacarbazine; *TGCT*: Testicular germ cell tumor.

In *patients with gender dysphoria changing from male to female*, testicular changes have been studied in bilateral orchiectomy specimens after sex reassignment surgery. Estrogen exposure during adulthood causes atrophy and induces true dedifferentiation of adult human Sertoli cells, including induction of immature

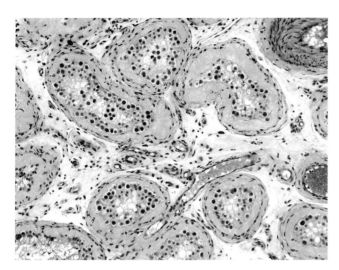

Fig. 12.321 Hypogonadism caused by estrogen therapy for prostate cancer. The seminiferous tubules contain isolated spermatogonia and dedifferentiated Sertoli cells with spherical nuclei, small nucleoli, and pseudostratified infantile distribution. The interstitium contains scattered Leydig cells.

immunophenotype such as reexpression of antimüllerian hormone, D2–40, and inhibin bodies.[1947,3335] Histologic findings in these patients may be classified into three groups: (1) complete but quantitatively decreased spermatogenesis with low number of spermatocytes and spermatids; (2) predominantly pubertal-like seminiferous tubules (the most frequent pattern); and (3) mainly infantile seminiferous tubules. In 72% of cases, spermatogenesis is pubertal-like, with seminiferous tubules containing Sertoli cells and spermatogonia only, or spermatogonia and primary spermatocytes, as the only germ cells. Spermatogonial numbers are highly variable; Sertoli cell nuclei are round instead of indented as in normal adults, and tubular walls are thickened (Fig. 12.322).

Sertoli cell–only tubules in patients treated with estrogens contain dedifferentiated Sertoli cells. A correlation exists between the degree of Sertoli cell dedifferentiation and the dose and timing of treatment with estrogens or antiandrogens. Brief treatment induces germ cell loss and inconspicuous Sertoli cell changes, and up to

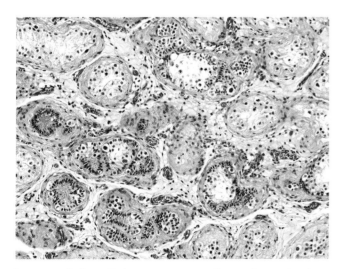

Fig. 12.322 Patient with long-term estrogen therapy for gender change showing tubular structures reminiscent of Sertoli cell nodules.

48% of patients show spermatogenesis.[3336] Long-term treatment causes pronounced Sertoli cell changes, initial nuclear rounding followed by elongation with the development of dark chromatin masses.[3337] Eventually, nuclei come to resemble those of infantile Sertoli cells, including pseudostratification. Tubules become hyalinized and peritubular cells increase, whereas Leydig cells may disappear,[3335,3338] decline or increase in number, or remain unchanged.[1947,3335,3338]

Estrogens act on the pituitary, by inhibiting LH secretion, and on Leydig cells.[3339] The action of GnRH agonist analogues is limited to the pituitary. Treatment with nonsteroid antiandrogens, which are highly selective, do not produce alterations in Leydig cells or seminiferous tubules.

Surgery

Sexual function is often adversely affected in patients who undergo bilateral retroperitoneal lymph node dissection for nonseminomatous testicular cancer. Up to 90% lose antegrade ejaculation, although libido, erection, and orgasm are normal. Loss of antegrade ejaculation results from removal of or injury to sympathetic ganglia and the hypogastric nervous plexus during surgery. Unilateral surgery, especially if limited to the right side, and modern nerve-sparing techniques reduce this complication by preserving antegrade ejaculation and fertility.[3340–3343] Hypospermatogenesis may develop after surgery for rectal cancer, perhaps as a result of vascular compromise.

Infertility in Patients With Spinal Cord Injury

Spinal cord injury is common, with more than 10,000 new cases annually in the United States, predominantly involving young adults.[3344] Fertility is impaired in 90% of male patients with spinal cord injury. Major sexual dysfunctions in these patients include lack of erection and ejaculation and poor semen quality.[3345–3351] Failure of ejaculation occurs in 95% of patients. Most of these men demonstrate defective seminal emission as well (entrance of semen into the posterior urethra).[3352] Erectile dysfunction is successfully treated with oral and injectable medications, the use of vacuum devices, and penile prosthetic implants. Semen may be obtained by means of vibratory stimulation of the penis or electro-ejaculation in more than 90% of cases, but quality is low, with increased number of dead spermatozoa, markedly low motility, and reduced fertilization rate.[3353–3355]

Low semen quality does not seem to be related to changes in scrotal thermal regulation, frequency of ejaculation, or duration of spinal cord damage, but rather to factors related to the seminal plasma.[3065] Possible explanations include genitourinary tract infection, endocrine anomaly, and impaired spermatogenesis because men with spinal cord injuries experience defects in the secretory function of Leydig cells, Sertoli cells, and male accessory genital glands.[3352] Recurrent infection occurs in 60% to 70% of patients. Compared with controls, semen in these patients has significantly increased numbers of neutrophils and macrophages, and markedly higher levels of reactive oxygen species.[3356,3357] These findings, coupled with the presence of elevated cytokine levels, are likely linked to the low quality of semen.[3358] Neutralization of target cytokines does not damage sperm DNA or sperm viability, a finding indicating that this method may hold promise for improving sperm motility in these men.[3359] Endocrine anomalies are transient, and hormone levels return to normal a few months after cord injury. More than 50% of patients have abnormalities of the adluminal compartment of the seminiferous tubules, with varying degree of immature germ cell sloughing.[3360] In 50% of patients, the number of mature spermatids per cross-sectioned tubule is less than 10 (normal is >21).

Possible etiologies include increase in testicular temperature resulting from vascular dilation or alteration in scrotal thermoregulation secondary to impaired sympathetic innervation from prolonged wheelchair restraint; alteration in sperm transport secondary to nerve injury that results in sperm stagnation in seminal vesicles, a hostile environment that normally is devoid of spermatozoa; and abnormal composition of seminal fluid with consequent deterioration of spermatozoa that, in the epididymis and ductus deferens, had good motility.[3361,3362]

More than 25% of patients with spinal cord injury have brown-tinged semen in some ejaculations.[3363] Although the cause is unknown, it could be related to seminal vesicle dysfunction.

When spermatozoa cannot be obtained by electroejaculation or vibratory stimulation, vasal aspiration or surgical sperm retrieval may be offered.[3364] Most patients have at least a few mature spermatids in some seminiferous tubules; therefore TESE followed by intravaginal insemination, intrauterine insemination, or ICSI is a reasonable consideration in azoospermic patients.[3360,3365] Successful pregnancy with sperm from male partners with spinal cord injury may occur despite abnormal semen quality.

Inflammation and Infection

Infectious agents may reach the testis and epididymis through blood vessels, lymphatics, sperm excretory ducts, or directly from a superficial wound. Infection transmitted through the blood mainly affects the testis and causes orchitis, whereas infection ascending through sperm excretory ducts usually causes epididymitis. Acute inflammation is accompanied by enlargement of the testis or epididymis. The tunica albuginea is covered by a fibrinous exudate, and the testicular parenchyma is yellow or brown. Bacterial infection may cause abscess formation. In some cases the infection heals with deposition of granulation tissue and fibrosis; in others, infection may persist as an active process, resulting in chronic orchiepididymitis.[3366]

Orchitis

Viral Orchitis

The most common viral causes of orchiepididymitis are mumps virus and coxsackie B virus; others include influenza, infectious mononucleosis, echovirus, lymphocytic choriomeningitis, adenovirus, coronavirus, Rio Bravo virus, varicella, vaccinia, rubella, dengue, and phlebotomus fever. Subclinical orchitis probably occurs during other viral infections (Fig. 12.323).

Before vaccination was widely used, mumps orchiepididymitis complicated 14% to 35% of adult mumps cases and was bilateral in 20% to 25% of cases (Fig. 12.324). Nevertheless, miniepidemics still occasionally occur.[3367,3368] Japan has one of the highest incidences among developed countries with more than 1 million annual cases.[3369] Incidence is also high in other countries where vaccination is not obligatory.[3370] In approximately 85% of cases of mumps orchitis, the epididymis is also involved, but epididymal involvement alone is rare.[3371] Clinical symptoms of orchitis usually appear 4 to 6 days after symptoms of parotitis, but orchitis may also appear without parotid involvement.[3372] Testicular involvement is diffuse and consists of acute inflammation of the interstitium and seminiferous tubules. The tubular lining is destroyed, leaving behind only hyalinized tubules and clusters of Leydig cells.[3373]

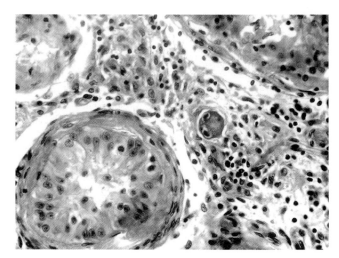

Fig. 12.323 Orchitis caused by cytomegalovirus in a patient with HIV. The inflammatory infiltrate of the testicular interstitium has two characteristic intranuclear inclusions.

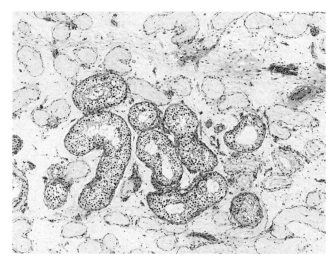

Fig. 12.324 Orchitis secondary to mump virus infection in a patient consulting for infertility. A group of tubules with complete spermatogenesis surrounded by completely hyalinized tubules may be observed.

With time the testes shrink and become soft. If infection is bilateral, the patient usually becomes infertile, with severe oligozoospermia or azoospermia, although biopsy may reveal the presence of mature spermatids in some tubules, thus allowing sperm extraction for paternity.[3374,3375] If only one testis is affected, sperm concentration may be normal or slightly decreased and fertility is maintained. Occasionally, testicular damage is so severe that testicular endocrine function is impaired, causing hypergonadotropic hypogonadism, with low testosterone level and regression of secondary sex characteristics. Mumps orchiepididymitis is infrequent in childhood.

Bacterial Orchitis

Most cases of bacterial orchitis are associated with bacterial epididymitis (Fig. 12.325). Orchitis secondary to suppurative epididymitis caused by *E. coli* is most common.[3376] Tubules are effaced by intense acute inflammation (Fig. 12.326). Chronic orchitis with microabscesses is caused by *E. coli*, streptococci,

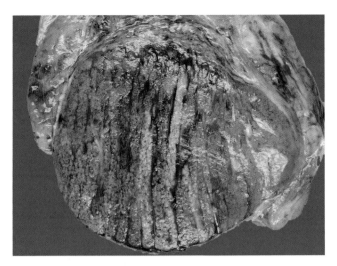

Fig. 12.325 Bacterial orchitis in an adult patient. Gross image of the testis showing congestion and separation of lobules by intense edema.

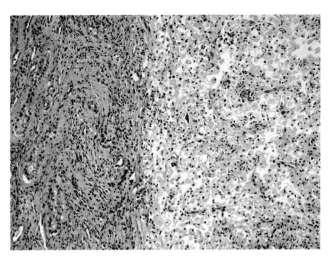

Fig. 12.327 Xanthogranulomatous orchitis showing a dense infiltrate of macrophages with vacuolated cytoplasm surrounded by atrophic seminiferous tubules.

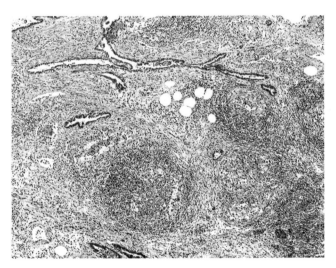

Fig. 12.326 Bacterial orchitis. Inflammatory infiltrate as microabscesses directly related to seminiferous tubules. The interstitium also shows abundant inflammatory infiltrate.

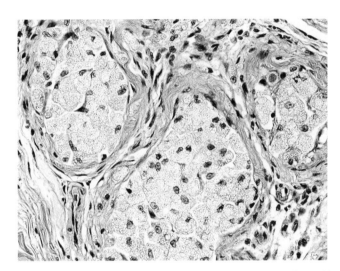

Fig. 12.328 Whipple disease. Seminiferous tubules and interstitium with histiocytes showing microvacuolated cytoplasm.

staphylococci, pneumococci, *Salmonella enteritidis*, and *Actinomyces israelii*.[3377–3379] In some cases of chronic bacterial orchitis the testis contains an inflammatory infiltrate consisting of numerous histiocytes with foamy cytoplasm (xanthogranulomatous orchitis) (Fig. 12.327), similar to that of idiopathic granulomatous orchitis but lacking intratubular giant cells.[3380–3382] Rarely, as in Whipple disease, large numbers of bacilli are present in histiocytes in the interstitium, vascular walls, and seminiferous tubules (Fig. 12.328).

The most frequent complications of pyogenic bacterial orchiepididymitis are abscesses (Fig. 12.329), involving the testis or tunica sac, and chronic draining scrotal sinus. Small fragments of testicular parenchyma may be eliminated through the scrotal skin, a condition known clinically as fungus testis. Another complication is testicular infarct (Fig. 12.330), resulting from compression or thrombosis of veins in the drainage system of the scrotal contents.[3383,3384]

Granulomatous Orchiepididymitis

Most cases of chronic orchiepididymitis are associated with granulomas in the testis. Specific causes may require special stains, cultures, or serologic tests and include tuberculosis, syphilis, leprosy, brucellosis, mycoses, and parasitic diseases. In sarcoidosis and idiopathic granulomatous orchitis the causative agent is unknown.

Tuberculosis

The incidence of tuberculous orchiepididymitis declined after the development of effective antibiotics, but it has experienced resurgence among people who have emigrated from countries with a high incidence of the disease, as well as in the increasing population of immunologically compromised patients.

Most cases of tuberculous orchiepididymitis are associated with involvement elsewhere in the genitourinary system.[3385] Tuberculous epididymitis is usually the result of ascent of mycobacteria from tuberculous prostatitis, which in turn is often secondary to renal or pulmonary tuberculosis, although tuberculous epididymoorchitis without renal involvement has also been observed.[3386] The pattern of spread is different in children: more than one-half

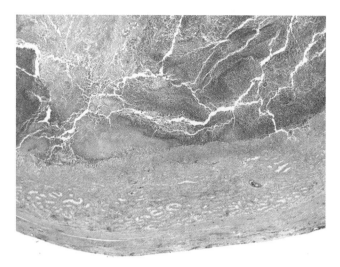

Fig. 12.329 Testicular tissue abscess secondary to orchiepididymitis. Note a peripheral subalbugineal crescent of testicular parenchyma.

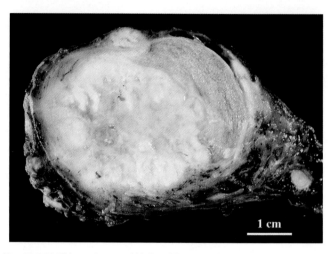

Fig. 12.331 Tuberculous orchitis in a 38-year-old patient with a white-gray nodule that has a pseudotumoral pattern and caused testicular enlargement.

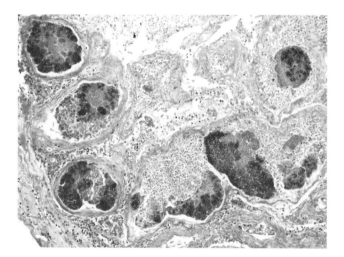

Fig. 12.330 Testicular necrosis showing silhouettes of seminiferous tubules occupied by bacterial colonies.

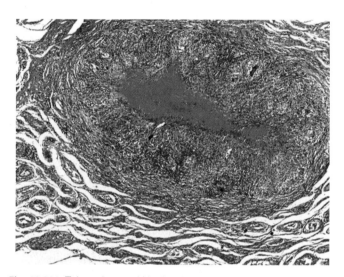

Fig. 12.332 Tuberculous orchitis showing central necrosis surrounded by numerous granulomas, some of which contain giant cells in their centers.

have advanced pulmonary tuberculosis, and the testis is infected through the blood.[3387] More than 50% of patients with renal tuberculosis experience development of tuberculous epididymitis, and orchitis occurs in approximately 3% of patients with genital tuberculosis, usually secondary to epididymal tuberculosis. Tuberculous orchiepididymitis may be sexually transmitted.[3388] It occurs mainly in adults: 72% of patients are older than 35 years, and 18% are older than 65 years. Signs and symptoms may be mild, consisting only of testicular enlargement and scrotal pain or enlargement mimicking tumor.[3389] In such cases, fever is infrequent, and constitutional symptoms may be absent.[3390]

Typical caseating and noncaseating granulomas destroy the seminiferous tubules and interstitium (Figs. 12.331 and 12.332). In immunosuppressed patients the granulomas consist of epithelioid histiocytes and a few lymphocytes with rare giant cells. Acid-fast bacilli tend to be more numerous in immunosuppressed patients. Similar lesions may be observed in orchiepididymitis caused by bacillus Calmette-Guérin, which is usually used for intravesical instillation in patients with vesicular urothelial carcinoma.[3391,3392]

Syphilis

Syphilitic orchitis may be congenital or acquired, with similar histologic findings. In congenital syphilitic orchitis, both testes are enlarged at birth. If diagnosis is delayed until puberty, the testis often shows retraction and fibrosis. In adults, acquired orchitis is a complication of the tertiary stage of syphilis and has two characteristic histologic patterns: interstitial inflammation and gumma formation.

Early in the disease, patients with interstitial orchitis have painless enlargement. Grossly the parenchyma is gray with translucent areas. Plasma cells are abundant. Inflammation begins in the mediastinum testis and septa, and later extends through the parenchyma as the tubular cellular lining sloughs and undergoes sclerosis. Initially, arteries show obliterans type of endarteritis.[3393] Small gummas may be observed. Eventually, inflammation subsides and is replaced by fibrosis. The epididymis is usually not affected.

Gummatous orchitis, a rare entity with only 11 reported cases since the 1950s, is characterized by the presence of one or several well-delineated, grossly gray-yellow zones of necrosis.[3394,3395] Histologically, ghostly silhouettes of seminiferous tubules are visible within the gumma, surrounded by inflammation consisting of lymphocytes, plasma cells, and scattered giant cells. In most cases spirochetes may be demonstrated histochemically with Warthin-Starry silver stain, immunohistochemical stains, or by using PCR in paraffin-embedded material.[3396]

Leprosy

The testis may be infected in patients with lepromatous or borderline leprosy. Frequent involvement results from the relatively low intrascrotal temperature that promotes growth of the bacilli. Orchitis is usually bilateral, although the degree of involvement may differ. Occasionally, testicular involvement may be the sole indication of the infection, and diagnosis may be made by biopsy.[3397] Histologic findings vary with the duration of the infection. Initially, there is perivascular lymphocytic inflammation and interstitial macrophages that contain numerous acid-fast bacilli. Later, seminiferous tubules undergo atrophy, Leydig cells cluster, and blood vessels show endarteritis obliterans. Final stages are characterized by fibrous tissue with scattered lymphocytes and macrophages containing acid-fast bacilli. Most patients with lepromatous leprosy show hypogonadism and are infertile, even if the orchitis was clinically mild.[3398,3399]

Brucellosis

Brucellosis is common in some parts of the world, including the Middle East.[3400,3401] Orchitis occurs in some patients and may be the first sign of disease. Brucellosis should be suspected when enlargement occurs in young patients with undulating fever, malaise, sweats, weight loss, and headache.[3402] Occasionally it may mimic testicular tumor. There is dense lymphohistiocytic inflammation with occasional noncaseating granulomas in the interstitium. Seminiferous tubules are infiltrated by inflammatory cells and undergo atrophy. The diagnosis is made by clinical and laboratory findings, including blood culture, the Bengal rose test, and high *Brucella* agglutination titers, or by reverse transcriptase PCR assay of urine.[3403–3405] Sexual transmission of *Brucella* from male to female has been reported.[3406]

Sarcoidosis

Sarcoidosis is a systemic granulomatous disease of unknown etiology that preferentially affects young black adults. Clinical involvement of the genitourinary tract occurs in only 0.5% of patients with sarcoidosis, but involvement of the genitourinary tract is evident in 5% at autopsy. Fewer than 30 cases of isolated epididymal involvement have been reported, and approximately 12 of these also involved the testis.[3407,3408]

Isolated testicular involvement is exceptional.[3407,3409,3410] Testicular sarcoidosis is usually unilateral and nodular, and is often asymptomatic and found at autopsy.[3411] The testis contains noncaseating granulomas similar to sarcoid granulomas at other locations, noncaseating epithelioid cell granulomas with multinucleate giant cells, minimal lymphocyte infiltrate, and Schaumann and asteroid bodies (Fig. 12.333). Before confirmation of diagnosis, other granulomatous lesions should be excluded, including tuberculosis, sperm granuloma, granulomatous orchitis, and seminoma. Seminoma may induce an intense, sarcoid-like reaction, and examination of multiple histologic sections may be necessary to find diagnostic foci.[3412] Mediastinal sarcoidosis and testicular cancer may be linked.[3413] Genital involvement by sarcoidosis may cause temporary or intermittent azoospermia that may improve after corticosteroid therapy.[3414]

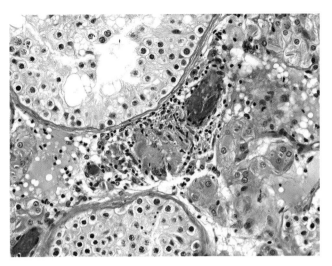

Fig. 12.333 Nonnecrotic granuloma composed of multinucleated giant cells, epithelioid cells, and minimal lymphocytic infiltrate in a patient with sarcoidosis.

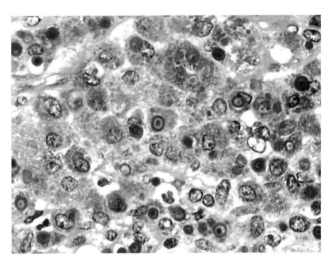

Fig. 12.334 Malakoplakia of the testis showing macrophages with granular and eosinophilic cytoplasm that contains several Michaelis-Gutmann bodies.

Malakoplakia

Malakoplakia is a chronic inflammatory disease that was initially described in the bladder, although subsequently found in most other organs.[3415] The testes (alone or together with the epididymis) are involved in 12% of cases involving the urogenital system.[3416,3417] Grossly the testes are enlarged and have brown-yellow parenchymal discoloration, often with abscesses.[3418] Malakoplakia causes tubular destruction associated with dense infiltrates of macrophages with granular eosinophilic cytoplasm, often containing Michaelis-Gutmann bodies (Fig. 12.334).[3419,3420]

The etiology is probably multifactorial. Inefficient phagocytosis by a lysosomal deficit, generally against gram-negative organisms (*E. coli* in 76% of the cases), has been proposed, similar to Whipple disease. Imbalance of cyclic adenosine monophosphate (cAMP) and guanosine monophosphate in favor of cAMP would give rise to deficient lysosomal degranulation and, consequently, impaired ability of phagocytes to digest bacteria completely. This hypothesis is supported by the high incidence of malakoplakia in immunosuppressed patients and others with chronic debilitating diseases.[3421,3422]

The differential diagnosis includes idiopathic granulomatous orchitis and Leydig cell tumor. Inflammation in idiopathic granulomatous orchitis includes intratubular multinucleated giant cells; in malakoplakia it is difficult to identify the tubular outlines, and giant cells are usually absent. Leydig cell tumor is not usually associated with inflammation, but may contain mononucleated or binucleated cells with abundant eosinophilic cytoplasm. Reinke crystalloids are identified in up to 40% of cases of Leydig cell tumor but are absent in malakoplakia. Leydig cell tumors do not contain Michaelis-Gutmann bodies.

Orchiepididymitis Caused by Fungi and Parasites

Fungal orchitis is rare; most cases are associated with blastomycosis, coccidioidomycosis, histoplasmosis, and cryptococcosis.[3423] The genital tract may be involved in widespread blastomycosis. Organs most frequently affected (in decreasing order) are the prostate, epididymis, testis, and seminal vesicles. Grossly, there are small abscesses that may have caseous centers. Fungi are present measuring 8 to 15 µm in diameter with double refringent contours in giant cells rimming granulomas, and these stain with PAS and methenamine silver.[3424]

Coccidioidomycosis is endemic in California, the southwestern United States, and Mexico, and may manifest as epididymal disease after remission of systemic symptoms.[3425] Granulomas are similar to those of tuberculosis and contain 30- to 60-µm diameter sporangia with endospores that stain with PAS.

Dissemination of histoplasmosis and cryptococcosis frequently occurs after steroid therapy and may give rise to granulomatous orchitis with extensive necrosis.[3426,3427] *Histoplasma capsulatum* measures 1 to 5 µm in diameter and may be demonstrated with silver stain. *Cryptococcus* is identified by its thick wall that stains with mucicarmine.

Most parasites that reach the genital tract, such as *Filaria* and *Schistosoma*, are in the spermatic cord, and testicular lesions are secondary to vascular injury.[3428] Testicular infection has also been reported in patients with visceral leishmaniasis, congenital and acquired toxoplasmosis (Figs. 12.335 and 12.336), *Echinococcus* infection, and orchitis caused by *Trichomonas vaginalis*.[3429,3430]

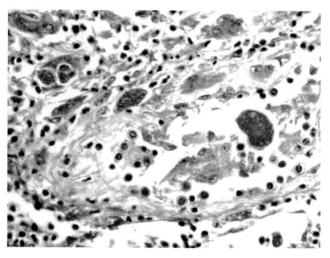

Fig. 12.336 Orchitis caused by toxoplasmosis. The giant cells in the testicular interstitium and those in the seminiferous tubules or walls contain numerous organisms.

Idiopathic Granulomatous Orchitis

Idiopathic granulomatous orchitis is a chronic inflammatory condition of older adults (mean, 59.2 years). It was first described in 1926.[3431] The most prominent clinical symptom is unilateral enlargement suggesting malignancy.[3432] Most patients have a history of scrotal trauma, surgical procedure, or epididymitis; 66% have symptoms of urinary tract infection with negative cultures, and 40% have sperm granuloma in the epididymis. An autoimmune etiology has been suggested.

The testis is enlarged, with a nodular cut surface and areas of necrosis or infarction. Two histologic forms are seen, according to whether the lesion is predominantly in the tubules (tubular orchitis) or interstitium (interstitial orchitis). In tubular orchitis, germ cells degenerate, and Sertoli cells have vacuolated cytoplasm and vesicular nuclei. Plasma cells and lymphocytes infiltrate the walls of the seminiferous tubules to form concentric rings. Multinucleated giant cells are present in tubular lumina and sometimes in the interstitium (Figs. 12.337 and 12.338). Vascular

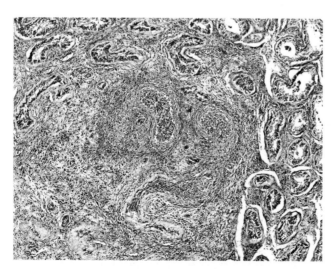

Fig. 12.335 Well-delimited necrotizing lesion affecting both the seminiferous tubules and the interstitium in an adult patient with toxoplasmosis.

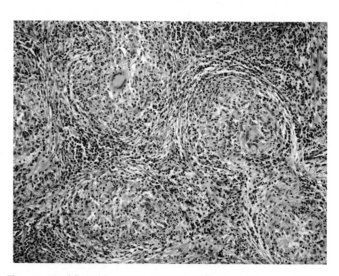

Fig. 12.337 Idiopathic granulomatous orchitis showing seminiferous tubules with peritubular fibrosis. Numerous lymphocytes and macrophages are present in the interstitium and within seminiferous tubules. Multinucleated giant cells are present in some tubules.

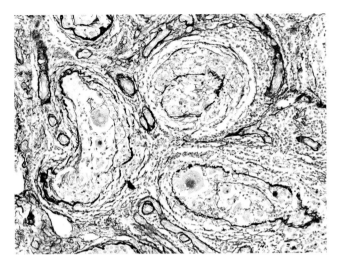

Fig. 12.338 Idiopathic granulomatous orchitis. Selective destruction of seminiferous tubules by inflammatory infiltrate with giant cells (silver methenamine).

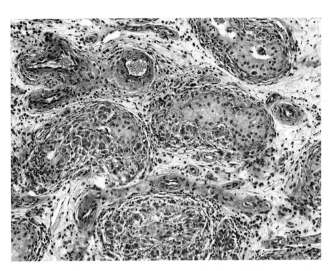

Fig. 12.339 Peritumoral granulomatous orchitis. The infiltrates are preferably located in the wall of the seminiferous tubule. In none of the tubular sections is germ cell neoplasia in situ observed (peripheral testicular parenchyma to a seminoma).

thrombosis and arteritis are common. In interstitial orchitis, inflammation is predominantly interstitial. Ultimately, tubular atrophy and interstitial fibrosis prevail in both forms, which may arise from different immune mechanisms.[3433] Tubular orchitis histologically resembles experimental orchitis caused by injection of serum from animals with orchitis, whereas interstitial orchitis resembles orchitis produced by the transfer of cells from immunized animals.

The differential diagnosis of idiopathic granulomatous orchitis is infectious orchitis caused by bacteria, spirochetes, fungi, or parasites. A useful clue in the tubular form is the presence of giant cells within seminiferous tubules without caseation.

Peritumoral Granulomatous Orchitis

This lesion resembles idiopathic granulomatous orchitis and specifically tubular orchitis. It is observed in the parenchyma adjacent to some germ cell tumors, especially seminoma, characterized by the presence of giant cell epithelioid granulomas in the walls of seminiferous tubules. It differs from idiopathic granulomatous orchitis in the topography of the lesions and the density of the inflammatory infiltrates. Inflammation occurs in tubular walls between myoid cells and the basal lamina (Fig. 12.339 and 12.340). The seminiferous epithelium, often consisting only of Sertoli cells, is displaced toward the tubular lumen. Eventually, inflammatory cells including multinucleated giant cells exfoliate into the tubule. The tubular and interstitial infiltrates are not as prominent as in idiopathic granulomatous orchitis. The topography of the lesions suggests an immune response to components of the tubular walls.

Focal Orchitis (Primary Autoimmune Orchitis)

This lesion is characterized by the presence of inflammation around one or more seminiferous tubules. Initially, neutrophils form microabscesses between the peritubular cells and the basal lamina. Later, T lymphocytes predominate, followed by B lymphocytes and macrophages (Figs. 12.341 and 12.342). Clinical manifestations are infertility, asymptomatic orchitis (rarely with testicular mass), and the presence of antisperm-specific antibodies (ASA).[3434] The occurrence of focal lymphoid cell infiltrates in the interstitium is common in infertile patients, after surgical treatment for bilateral inguinal hernia, after vasectomy complicated

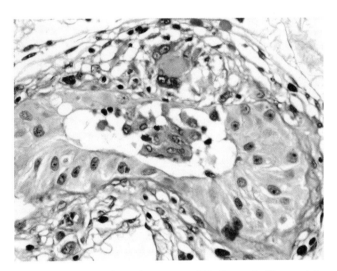

Fig. 12.340 Peritumoral granulomatous orchitis. The wall of the seminiferous tubule shows in the thickness of the peritubular cells layer a giant multinucleated cell and some lymphocytes. Inside the tubule some macrophages and lymphocytes have penetrated.

by post-infection obstruction, after testicular piercing, and in cryptorchidism.[1008,3435–3439] The topography of the inflammation suggests an immunologic response to components of the seminiferous epithelium that have gained access to the interstitium by alteration of the hematotesticular barrier (Fig. 12.343).

Testicular Pseudolymphoma

Pseudolymphoma is a benign reactive process with a lymphoid cell proliferation so intense that it may be mistaken for lymphoma; it consists of an abundance of lymphocytes and plasma cells that partially or totally destroy the parenchyma.[3440–3442]

The differential diagnosis includes lymphoma, various forms of orchitis, and seminoma. The diagnosis of lymphoma may be excluded by the lack of atypia and polyclonal nature of the inflammation. Syphilitic orchitis also produces a plasma cell–rich inflammatory infiltrate, but pseudolymphoma does not have other

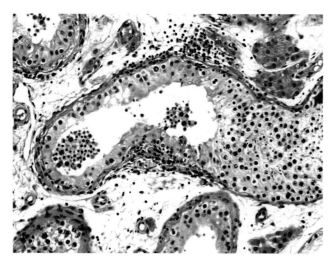

Fig. 12.341 Focal orchitis showing infiltrates of lymphoid cells and macrophages within a seminiferous tubule. There is persistence of Sertoli cells and isolated spermatogonia.

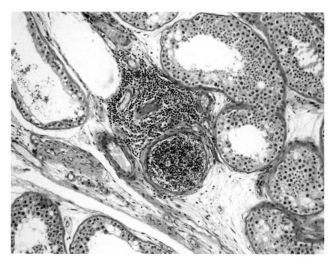

Fig. 12.343 Focal orchitis. Infertile patient with obstructive azoospermia. Marked ectasia of some seminiferous tubules. Dense lymphocytic infiltrates in relation to a tubule full of spermatozoa.

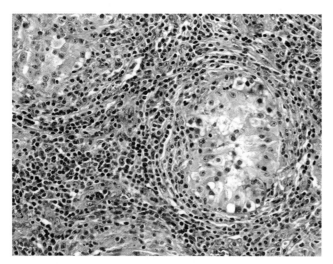

Fig. 12.342 Focal orchitis. A predominantly peritubular and interstitial lymphoid infiltrate that mimics a leukemic infiltrate or lymphoma.

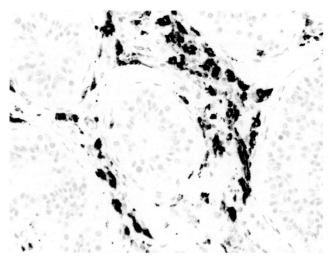

Fig. 12.344 Testis of a prepubertal patient with liver transplantation showing abundant macrophages that express CD68.

characteristic features of syphilitic orchitis such as endarteritis obliterans; spirochetes cannot be demonstrated by special stains. The absence of granulomas or significant numbers of macrophages, together with the negative results of specific histochemical stains, also helps exclude idiopathic granulomatous orchitis, tuberculosis, leprosy, sarcoidosis, and fungal infection. Finally, although the presence of a prominent inflammatory infiltrate and, in many cases, numerous lymphoid follicles may suggest the diagnosis of seminoma, the presence of seminoma cells can be easily demonstrated with Best carmine stain, PAS, PLAP, SALL4, or OCT 3/4. The term *plasma cell granuloma* refers to a reactive process characterized by the presence of polyclonal adult plasma cells that are absent in testicular plasmacytoma.[3443,3444]

Histiocytosis With Testicular Involvement

Increased number of interstitial macrophages may be observed in autopsy material from more than two-thirds of adult males. A history of previous abdominal surgical procedure or peritonitis is common in such cases (Fig. 12.344). Accumulation of macrophages has also been observed in the parenchyma at the periphery of burned-out germ cell tumor (Fig. 12.345). Three situations deserve special comment: sinus histiocytosis with massive lymphadenopathy, Erdheim-Chester disease, and histiocytosis in treatment with hydroxyethyl starch plasma expander.

Sinus histiocytosis with massive lymphadenopathy (or *Rosai-Dorfman disease*) is a benign proliferation of S-100 protein immunoreactive histiocytes that uniquely contain numerous lymphocytes in their cytoplasm. Involvement of the urogenital system is rare; the organ most frequently affected is the kidney followed by the testis. Lesions may be unilateral or bilateral.[3445,3446] Some cases are associated with systemic hematopoietic diseases.[3447]

Erdheim-Chester disease is a non-Langerhans cell histiocytosis of unknown etiology. It affects the long bones of lower extremities, central nervous system, heart, lung, liver, spleen, retroperitoneum, skin, orbit, and testicles. Patients experience development of hypogonadotropic hypogonadism with testicular atrophy. The lesion is characterized by an interstitial infiltrate of lipid-laden foamy

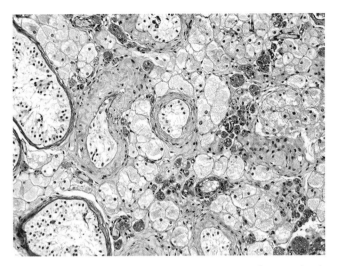

Fig. 12.345 Cryptorchid testis with burned-out germ cell tumor showing seminiferous tubules with dysgenetic Sertoli cells, hypertrophic and hyperplasic Leydig cells, and macrophage accumulations intensely stained with periodic acid–Schiff.

histiocytes. The cells have spherical nuclei without folds. Macrophages are immunoreactive for CD68, but not CD1a or S-100 protein, distinguishing this condition from other histiocytoses.[3448]

Histiocytosis in treatment with hydroxyethyl starch plasma expander. Interstitial macrophages are prominent owing to large size and multivacuolated cytoplasm, suggesting thesaurosis. There is no evidence of mucin glycoproteins, proteoglycans, starch, lipids, glycogen, or foreign body material. Most patients lack clinical symptoms other than pruritus and persistent erythema.[3449]

Other Testicular and Epididymal Lesions

Epididymitis Nodosa

Epididymitis nodosa is a proliferation of small, irregular ducts whose epithelium lacks characteristic features of the epididymal epithelium. The disorder is associated with inflammation and

fibrosis. The lesion and its pathogenesis are similar to vasitis nodosa (Fig. 12.346).[3450,3451]

Epididymitis Induced by Amiodarone

Amiodarone is widely used in the treatment of arrhythmias. In several tissues, including the testis, amiodarone is concentrated up to 300 times its plasma level, with resulting testicular atrophy and increased serum levels of FSH and LH in some patients.[3184,3452] The incidence rate of epididymitis during amiodarone therapy varies from 3% to 11% depending on dosage and duration of usage, and more than 35 cases (in several cases involvement was bilateral) have been reported.[3453–3457] The disorder may occur at any age.[3458] Epididymitis induced by amiodarone is clinically characterized by chronic epididymalgia without fever or leukocytosis. Although etiology is unknown, the disorder has been attributed to the ability of epididymal tissue to concentrate amiodarone and its metabolites.[3459] Autopsy studies show focal areas of fibrosis and nonspecific lymphoid cell infiltrates. When amiodarone dosage is cut in half to 300 mg/day, symptoms resolve within a few weeks.[3460] Recognition of this side effect of amiodarone is important to avoid unnecessary antibiotics or aggressive surgery.

Ischemic Granulomatous Epididymitis

Ischemic granulomatous epididymitis refers to a lesion preferentially located in the head of the epididymis and characterized by noninfectious necrosis with production of polypoid masses of inflamed granulation tissue. It usually arises in elderly patients or those with advanced arteriosclerosis (Fig. 12.347). Granulomas containing multinucleated giant cells with cholesterol crystals develop within the efferent ducts or walls of epididymal ducts. There may be sperm microgranulomas with ductal neoformation like that of epididymitis nodosa and ceroid granulomas (Fig. 12.348). Cause is unknown, but it may result from ischemia.[3461]

Vasculitis

The testicular arteries may be affected by systemic disorders such as Schönlein-Henoch purpura, Wegener disease, Cogan disease,

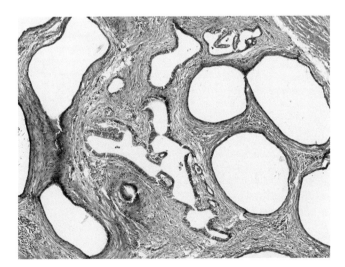

Fig. 12.346 Epididymitis nodosa. Some ducts with regenerative epithelium and variable size and shape may be observed among ecstatic epididymal ducts.

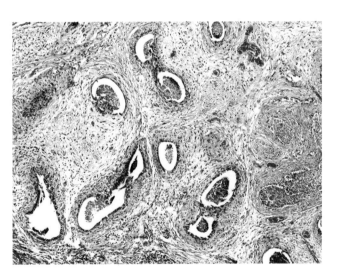

Fig. 12.347 Ischemic epididymitis. Caput of the epididymis showing ducts with necrotic epithelium that is total or partially sloughed in the lumens of efferent ducts.

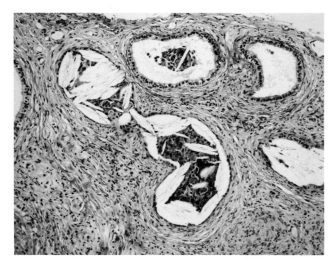

Fig. 12.348 Efferent ducts with epithelial necrosis, cholesterol crystals inside, and an infiltrate with abundant macrophages in the interstitium.

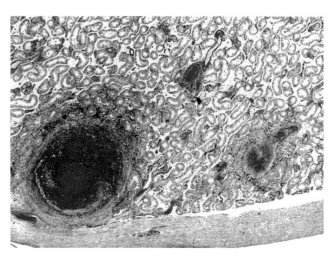

Fig. 12.350 Polyarteritis nodosa involving several intraparenchymal arteries.

Behçet disease, thromboangiitis obliterans, giant cell arteritis, relapsing polychondritis, rheumatoid arthritis, and dermatomyositis, but most frequent involvement is with PAN.[3462–3467]

Polyarteritis Nodosa

Approximately 80% of patients with PAN have testicular or epididymal involvement, but only 2% to 18% of these cases are diagnosed during life; rarely, these sites are the first manifestation of the disease. Symptoms may suggest orchitis, epididymitis, testicular torsion, or tumor.[3467–3471]

The testis usually shows arterial lesions in different stages of evolution, including fibrinoid necrosis, inflammatory reaction, thrombosis, or aneurysm. The parenchyma initially has zones of infarction (Figs. 12.349 and 12.350). Histologic findings similar to those of PAN may occasionally be observed as an isolated finding, referred to as *isolated arteritis of the testis and epididymis*, differing from classic polyarteritis by lack of vascular thrombosis, aneurysm, or infarct.[3472] The etiology of isolated arteritis is unknown, but the prognosis is excellent.[3473] The etiology and pathogenesis of both systemic and localized PAN are unknown.

Some patients with systemic PAN have autoimmune (erythematous lupus, rheumatoid arthritis) or infectious diseases (hepatitis B or C, HIV). Only three patients with PAN in the male reproductive tract have malignancy in other organs (prostatic adenocarcinoma, myeloid leukemia, and hepatocellular carcinoma). Isolated arteritis of the testis and epididymis coexisted with associated germ cell tumor.[3474] We have observed similar findings in other germ cell tumors, both seminomas and nonseminomatous tumors. It may be possible that antigens of tumor cells cross-react with those of the endothelium in an appropriate environment to trigger the inflammatory reaction. Identification of necrotizing arteritis in the testis or epididymis should be followed by clinical, hematologic, and biochemical studies to exclude systemic arteritis.[3475,3476]

Wegener Disease

Testicular involvement in this multisystemic disease associated with cytoplasmic antineutrophil antibody is rare, occurring in less than 1% of affected individuals.[3463,3464,3477,3478] The testis and epididymis may be affected separately or jointly. Vessels contain

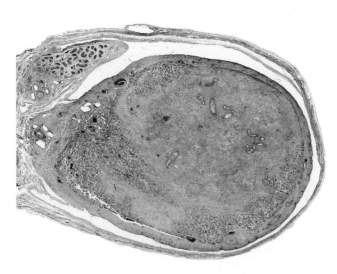

Fig. 12.349 Necrosis of most of the testicular parenchyma secondary to polyarteritis nodosa lesions in testicular vessels and epididymis.

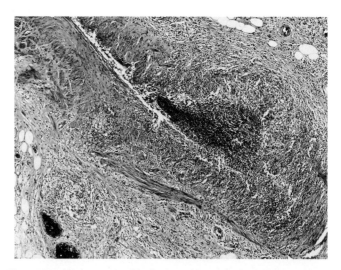

Fig. 12.351 Wegener vasculitis. Patient with spermatic cord tumor. Necrotizing lesion of the wall of a longitudinally sectioned vessel. Granulomas are seen both in the wall and in the periadventitial tissue.

fibrinoid necrosis, intense infiltration of neutrophils, and numerous giant cells both within and at the periphery of the vessel wall (Fig. 12.351).[3479] Multiple infarcts develop in the testis.

A peculiar form of nonsystemic granulomatous vasculitis affecting the testis and epididymis may occur in patients with classical seminoma in both the ipsilateral and contralateral testes. The most important features of the lesion are circumferential inflammation, preferential involvement of the media and adventitia, an abundance of epithelioid cells and multinucleated giant cells, and stenosis of the vascular lumen. It is possible that the lesions are secondary to circulating tumor antigens.

Thromboangiitis Obliterans

Thromboangiitis obliterans is a rare disease that may affect the vessels of the spermatic cord, and this may be the only site of involvement. The clinical findings may mimic tumor.[3480] Indurations are found along the spermatic cord, representing involvement of arteries and veins. In early lesions, thrombi and microabscesses with

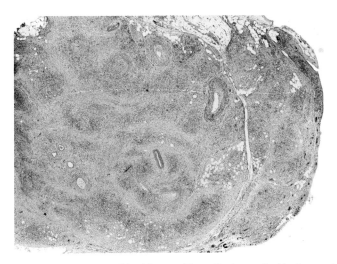

Fig. 12.352 Thromboangiitis obliterans. The patient consulted for tumor of the spermatic cord. Most vessels in the spermatic cord are not recognized. A fibrosis that includes the different structures of the cord stands out.

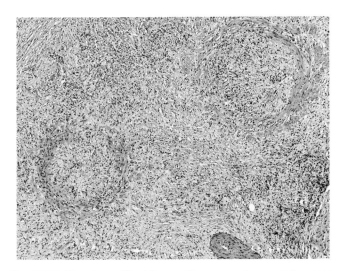

Fig. 12.353 Thromboangiitis obliterans. The vessels show partially recanalized thrombosis and an inflammatory infiltrate extending into the perivascular tissue.

multinucleated giant cells predominate. In later lesions the inflammatory infiltrate involves all layers of the cord. Eventually, thrombi recanalize and fibrosis develops, affecting the arteries, veins, and nerves (Figs. 12.352 and 12.353).

Giant Cell Arteritis

The vessels of the spermatic cord, epididymis, and testis are sometimes affected in this condition. Clinical findings may mimic neoplasm.[3481] Lesions are characterized by an inflammatory reaction with giant cells that are preferentially located in the intimae, destroying and phagocytizing the internal elastic lamina.

Henoch-Schönlein Purpura

Henoch-Schönlein purpura disease is characterized by the classic triad of purpura, arthritis, and abdominal pain, and is most frequent in 4- to 6-year-old boys. Involvement of scrotal content is reported in up to 38% of cases.[3482] Patients experience scrotal pain that invokes all the entities that constitute the clinical picture of acute scrotum.[3483–3485] It is histologically characterized by the presence of leukocytoclastic vasculitis as a consequence of the deposition of immune complexes containing IgA antibody.

Cogan Disease

Systemic vasculitis may occur in this autoimmune disease that preferably affects the eye (interstitial keratitis) and auditory system (sensorineural deafness and vestibular dysfunction).[3486] About 5% of patients have testicular involvement.[3465]

Behçet Disease

This systemic vasculitis is characterized by recurrent aphthous oral and genital ulcers, relapsing uveitis, and cutaneous lesions. The epididymis and testis are affected with an incidence rate that varies widely, from 2% in France to 44% in Russia.[3466] Clinical presentation is that of epididymoorchitis. Testicular infarction may ensue.[3487,3488]

Amyloidosis

The testis is frequently affected in amyloidosis, which may alter testicular function. Up to 77% of patients have secondary infertility, and only 6% have normal spermatogenesis.[3489] Testicular involvement is present in 85% of patients with secondary amyloidosis (type AA amyloidosis), in which it may be the first manifestation of the disease,[3490,3491] in 91% of patients with primary systemic amyloidosis (amyloidosis with AL deposits), and in most patients with hereditary apolipoprotein A-I amyloidosis, in which testicular involvement may also be the first manifestation of the disease. The testis is less frequently affected in amyloidosis with beta-2 M deposits and in amyloidosis with transthyretin deposits. In amyloidosis with AA and AL deposits, the media and adventitia of arteries and veins are preferentially affected, but amyloid deposits in walls of capillaries and seminiferous tubules may also be observed (Figs. 12.354 and 12.355).[3492] In beta-2 M amyloidosis, deposits are located under the endothelium of the veins; when massive deposition occurs, the adventitia and interstitium are also involved (Fig. 12.356). In amyloidosis with AL deposits and apolipoprotein A-I hereditary amyloidosis, deposits may be so massive that, instead of producing small atrophic testis, as is typically the case, they induce macroorchidism.[3493,3494]

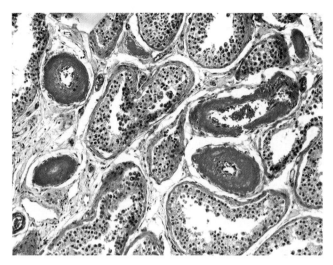

Fig. 12.354 Amyloid deposits on the wall of intraparenchymal vessels. The amyloid material is circularly arranged. Seminiferous tubules still retain spermatogenesis.

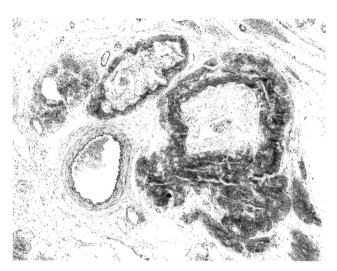

Fig. 12.356 Amyloid beta-2 M deposits in the vessels of the pampiniform plexus (Congo red).

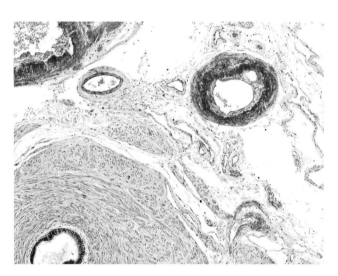

Fig. 12.355 Cross section of the spermatic cord showing several vessels with amyloid deposits on their wall (Congo red).

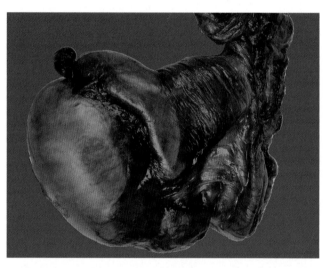

Fig. 12.357 Highly evolved intravaginal testicular and epididymal torsion in a prepubertal patient.

Testicular Infarct

Torsion of the spermatic cord is the most frequent cause of testicular infarct, followed by trauma, incarcerated inguinal hernia, epididymitis, and vasculitis.

Spermatic Cord Torsion

Spermatic cord torsion is a surgical emergency. If repair is delayed more than 8 hours, testicular viability is usually compromised. It may appear at any age; peak incidences are in the perinatal period and puberty. The annual incidence of torsion is estimated at 4 to 5 in 100,000 males up to 25 years of age.[3495]

Factors that predispose to testicular torsion are anatomic anomalies in testicular suspension and abnormal position of the testis. Many affected men have abnormally high reflection of the tunica vaginalis that gives rise to the "bell-clapper" deformity. Other anomalies include elongate mesorchium, separation between the epididymis and testis, and absent or elongate gubernaculum. The frequency of torsion is high in cryptorchid and retractile testes.

There are two classic anatomic forms of testicular torsion: high (supravaginal or extravaginal) and low (intravaginal). Each appears at a different age. Extravaginal torsion typically occurs in infancy and childhood, whereas intravaginal torsion is more frequent at puberty and in adulthood.

Neonatal torsion is bilateral in 12% to 21% of cases.[3496] Most torsion observed during the first years of life is intrauterine.[3497] Pubertal and adult torsion cause testicular pain that may radiate to the abdomen or other sites. Approximately 36% of patients have a previous history of pain or swelling in one or both testes. The differential diagnosis includes all causes of acute scrotum (Fig. 12.357).[3498,3499]

Torsion causes hemorrhagic infarction of the testis (Fig. 12.358). In old neonatal torsion the histologic findings are so advanced that only collagenized tissue containing calcium and hemosiderin deposits is seen. In adults, three degrees of histologic lesion may be distinguished.[3500] Degree I (26.5% of adult twisted

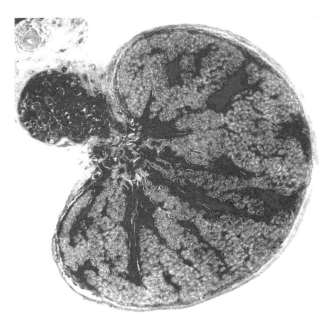

Fig. 12.358 Hemorrhagic infarct in a newborn testis. The hemorrhagic areas are near the rete testis and follow the course of the centripetal veins.

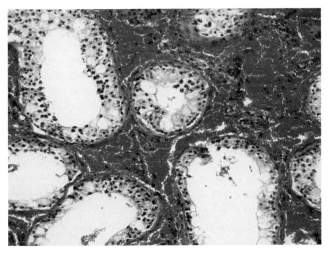

Fig. 12.359 Hemorrhagic infarct grade ii in a 13-year-old boy. There is interstitial hemorrhage, focal sloughing of the seminiferous tubular cells, and intense Sertoli cell vacuolation.

testes) is characterized by edema, vascular congestion, and focal hemorrhage. Seminiferous tubules are dilated, with sloughed immature germ cells, apical vacuolation of Sertoli cells, and dilated lymphatic vessels.[1764] Degree II (26.5% of testes) has pronounced interstitial hemorrhage and sloughing of all germ cell types in the seminiferous tubules. The lesion is more severe in the center of the testis, and thus biopsy could provide erroneous information (Fig. 12.359). Degree III lesions (45% of testes) are characterized by necrosis of the seminiferous epithelium. The duration of torsion correlates with severity of the histologic findings.[3501] Degree I occurs in torsion with a duration of less than 4 hours, degree II occurs in torsion lasting between 4 and 8 hours, and degree III occurs in torsion lasting more than 12 hours. Exceptions may relate to the number of twists in the spermatic cord (degrees of testicular rotation) and other factors. The testicular salvage rate, defined as testicular growth and development that reflect the age of the

patient and the contralateral testis, is approximately 50%.[3502] Testes that do not bleed into the albugineal incision within 10 minutes are assumed to be nonviable and should be removed.[3503]

Little attention has been paid to intermittent testicular torsion, and only a few cases are reported in adults.[3504] However, at least 50% of boys with testicular torsion have antecedent testicular pain caused by intermittent torsion.[3505] Early orchiopexy not only eliminates the pain in most cases but also eliminates testicular loss at a later date. It is hypothesized that testes that undergo intermittent torsion become progressively smaller and excessively mobile because most have the bell-clapper deformity.[3506] Intermittent testicular torsion is thought to cause vascular congestion with or without decreased arterial flow, leading to histologic damage such as decreased spermatogenesis and tubular hyalinization.

Histologic diagnosis of torsion does not usually pose a problem (Fig. 12.360). However, we have observed two histologic findings that may cause diagnostic difficulties. One set of findings resembles lymphoma (Fig. 12.361), and the other resembles sarcoma. In the

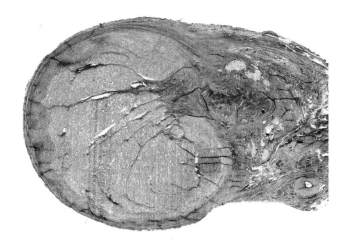

Fig. 12.360 Hemorrhagic infarct. The entire testicular parenchyma is necrotic. Peripherally, at the level of the albuginea there is a dense ring of myofibroblastic proliferation. At the epididymis level there are several whitish areas with a geographical outline of lipomembranous fat necrosis.

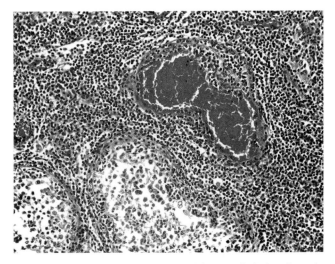

Fig. 12.361 Dense lymphoid infiltrate resembling a testicular lymphoma in a recurrent testicular torsion.

first instance, some testes of patients in the early stage of hemorrhagic infarcts have, apart from testicular enlargement, dense, interstitial, and intratubular inflammation consisting of lymphocytes, usually T lymphocytes. The lesion varies from lobule to lobule. The presence of macrophages and multinucleate giant cells may mimic idiopathic granulomatous orchitis. The second set of histologic findings consists of reactive myofibroblastic proliferation surrounding necrotic parenchyma (Figs. 12.362 and 12.363). Mitotic figures are frequent. The myofibroblastic cells express specific muscle actin. A polymorphous infiltrate of polymorphonuclear leukocytes, lymphocytes, and macrophages is typically present as well.

Some adults with untreated testicular torsion experience fat necrosis of the spermatic cord.[3507] Patients report pain in the high scrotum. At this level a small nodule corresponds to remnants of the twisted testis. The epididymis and proximal spermatic cord characteristically exhibit fat necrosis (Fig. 12.364).

Adults with prior spermatic cord torsion often seek consultation for infertility. The mechanisms underlying spermiogram alteration are not well established, and three hypotheses have been proposed:

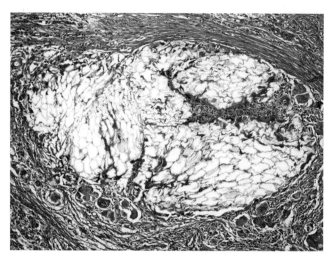

Fig. 12.364 Lipomembranous fat necrosis in a 14-year-old boy who presented with a history of several weeks of intense scrotal pain. Giant cell granulomatous reaction around the membranes had developed.

- *Autoimmune process.* Ischemic injury breaks the blood-testis barrier, and antigens released from the necrotic germ cells activate macrophages and lymphocytes in the interstitium, thus stimulating the formation of antibodies against these antigens. The antibodies enter the blood circulation and may presumably damage the contralateral testis.[3508]
- *Alterations in microcirculation.* After testicular torsion, blood flow decreases in the contralateral testis and causes an increase in the characteristic products of hypoxia, such as lactic acid and hypoxanthine.[3509] Intense apoptosis involving mainly spermatocytes I and II may occur.[3510] The long-term effects are unknown.
- *Primary testicular lesions.* Many torsed testes have lesions that are obviously preexisting, such as hypoplastic tubules, testicular microlithiasis, and focal spermatogenesis. In addition, more than one-half of biopsies from the contralateral testis show significant spermatogenetic abnormalities.[3511] These findings suggest that torsion occurs in congenitally abnormal testes.

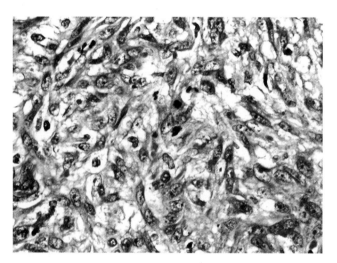

Fig. 12.362 Pseudosarcomatous reaction in testicular covers in a degree III testicular torsion.

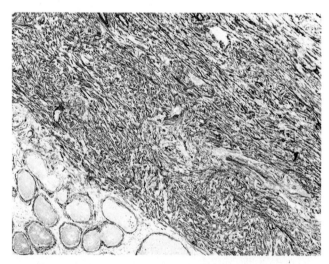

Fig. 12.363 Pseudosarcomatous myofibroblastic reaction with intense expression of actin adjacent to seminiferous tubules with necrosis of the epithelium.

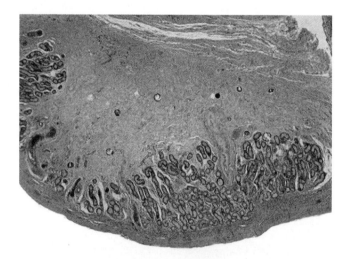

Fig. 12.365 Longitudinally sectioned testis from a 4-year-old infant who had previously undergone orchidopexy. The testis shows marked fibrosis and numerous calcifications except for the periphery of the testicular parenchyma.

Other Causes of Testicular Infarct

Trauma and disease affecting vessels of the spermatic cord may also cause infarction.[3263] Ischemic atrophy is a risk for inguinoscrotal surgical procedures, including herniorrhaphy, varicocelectomy, hydrocelectomy, and orchiopexy for undescended testis (Fig. 12.365). The incidence rate of atrophy after inguinal herniorrhaphy varies from 0.1% in primary herniorrhaphy up to 8% after surgical treatment of recurrent hernia, depending on the difficulty of the procedure and extent of the hernia (Fig. 12.366).[1889,3512] Atrophy may rarely follow thrombosis of the vena cava or spermatic artery.[3513]

Segmental infarction must be included in the differential diagnosis of acute testicular pain in males of all ages, but is most common in adulthood. It may be associated with vasculitis, epididymitis, intimal fibroplasia of spermatic artery, polycythemia, sickle cell disease, trauma, and laparoscopic inguinal hernia repair.[3514,3515] However, in most cases the cause is unknown. Clinical symptoms of infarct mimic tumor and torsion. Diagnostic strategies include tumor biomarker testing and radiologic imaging. Color Doppler ultrasound confirms diagnosis in most cases, revealing an avascular, wedge-shaped, hypoechoic lesion with well-defined borders.[3516–3518] Complementary evaluation with contrast-enhanced ultrasound and real-time tissue elastography are useful.[3519] Accurate evaluation of clinical and imaging symptoms may prevent unnecessary orchiectomy (Fig. 12.367).

Other Testicular Diseases

Cystic Malformation

Cystic malformation of the tunica albuginea and testicular parenchyma was first described in the nineteenth century and was considered rare.[3520–3522] With systematic use of ultrasonography the incidence rate of cysts is much higher than previously believed.[3523] Nonneoplastic cysts are found in 2% to 10% of testes.[3524–3527]

Cyst of the Tunica Albuginea

Cyst of the tunica albuginea is usually an incidental finding in patients in the fifth or sixth decade of life. It is located in the anterolateral aspect of the testis and may be unilocular or multilocular, ranging from 2 to 4 mm and containing clear fluid without spermatozoa.[946,3528] Some cysts may become calcified or contain small crystals of carbonate-apatite, hydroxyl apatite, or calcium carbonate (milk of calcium) associated with low-grade inflammation or psammoma bodies.[3529] The cyst may be embedded within the connective tissue of the tunica albuginea, protrude from the inner surface of the tunica albuginea into the testicular parenchyma (Fig. 12.368), or protrude from the outer surface forming a blue lump in the tunica albuginea (Fig. 12.369). The epithelium lining the cyst may be simple columnar or stratified cuboidal, supported by a thin layer of collagenized connective tissue. The columnar epithelium usually includes ciliated cells, and the cuboidal epithelium is composed of two layers of nonciliated cells (Fig. 12.370).[3530] Cysts may be numerous and enlarge sufficiently to cause atrophy of the parenchyma. Cystic change restricted to the parietal layer of the tunica vaginalis results in formation of large clusters of cysts that protrude into the tunica sac (Fig. 12.371).

Tunica albuginea cysts, previously thought to result from trauma or inflammation, are now believed to represent mesothelial inclusions, mesothelial metaplasia, or embryonic remnants.[3531–3533] Mesothelial cysts are lined by flat epithelium whose cells express

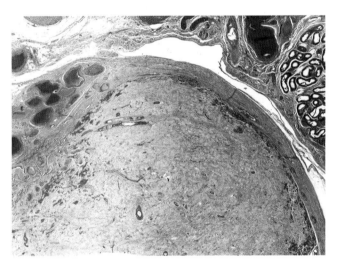

Fig. 12.366 Ischemic atrophy of the testis in an adult patient with a history of herniorrhaphy.

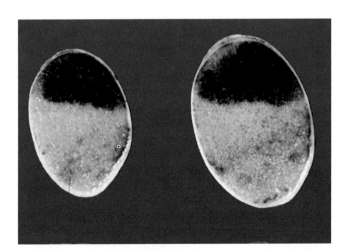

Fig. 12.367 Segmental infarct showing sharp delimitation between necrotic and conserved testicular parenchyma.

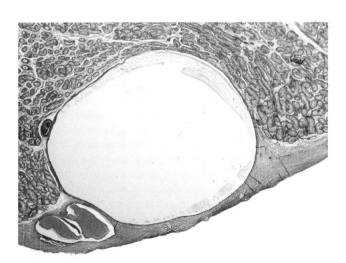

Fig. 12.368 Multilocular cyst in the tunica albuginea. The largest cavity protrudes into the testicular parenchyma.

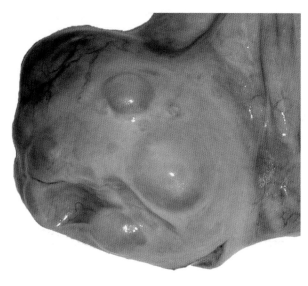

Fig. 12.369 Multiple cysts of the albuginea in a patient with hepatorenal polycystic disease.

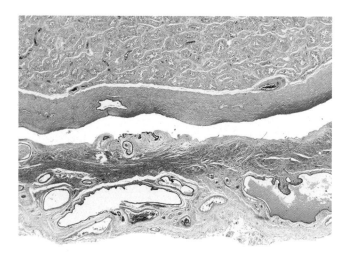

Fig. 12.371 Multiple cysts in testicular vaginal associated with a cyst of the albuginea.

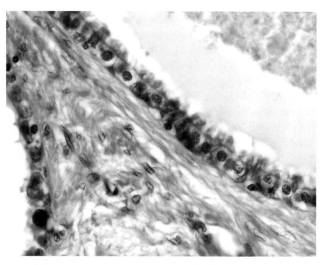

Fig. 12.370 Cyst of embryonic remnants. The epithelium with ciliated and nonciliated cells is like that of the efferent ducts (same case as in Fig. 12.368).

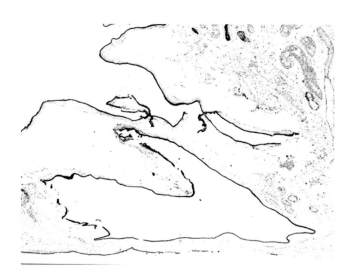

Fig. 12.372 Partially collapsed mesothelial cyst protruding into the testis (immunostaining for D2–40).

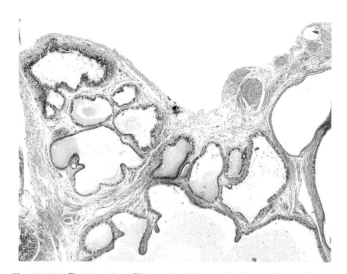

Fig. 12.373 Florid cystic müllerianosis of the vaginal tunic. The epithelium that covers the multiple cysts presents characteristics similar to that of the uterine tube.

calretinin, cytokeratins 8, 18, and 19, and D2–40 (Fig. 12.372).[946] Areas of cuboidal or tall columnar epithelium with ciliated and non-ciliated cells may be identified and may be in continuity with meso-thelium, but do not express mesothelial markers. Such cells may express androgen and progesterone receptors, but do not express estrogen receptor. The morphology and immunoprofile of these cells is like that of the fallopian tubes and areas of endosalpingiosis in women, and therefore likely represent mesothelial metaplastic changes. Extreme examples of this type of change have been described as *florid cystic müllerianosis of the testis* (Fig. 12.373).[3534] Cellular inclusions and cysts of the tunica albuginea that resemble von Brunn nests of the urothelium also likely represent metaplastic change (Fig. 12.374). Cysts lined by pseudostratified epithelium are likely in most instances to have originated from remnants of meso-nephric ducts.[3530,3535–3537]

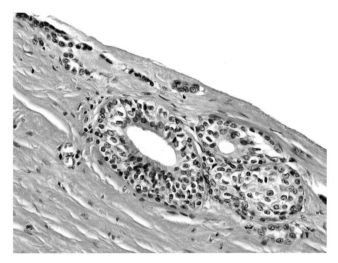

Fig. 12.374 The tunica albuginea presents small mesothelial inclusions parallel to the surface and two epithelial formations with central lumens reminiscent of von brown nests.

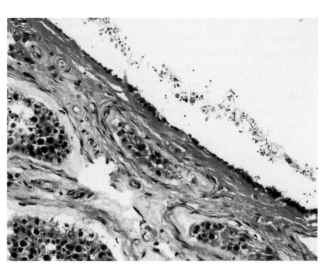

Fig. 12.376 Rete testis cyst. It is lined by flat cells alternating with islets of cylindrical cells. It contains abundant sperm.

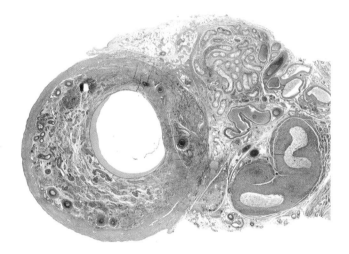

Fig. 12.375 Rete testis cyst. Cystic formation located in the lower pole of the testis near the testicular mediastinum in an elderly patient.

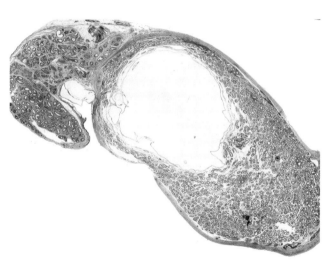

Fig. 12.377 Simple cyst of the testicle. Half of the testicular parenchyma is occupied by a cystic formation with thin walls. No content is observed.

Cyst of the Rete Testis

Cyst of the rete testis exhibits a distinctive epithelial lining composed of areas of flattened cells intermingled with tall columnar cells. Spermatozoa are frequently found within such cysts; hence cyst of the rete testis is also called *intratesticular spermatocele* (Figs. 12.375 and 12.376).[3538,3539] It may be associated with cystic transformation of the rete testis and multiple epididymal cysts. Rete testis cyst is not always attached to the rete and may be found distant from it.

Simple Cyst of the Testis

Simple cyst of the testis is usually lined by cuboidal epithelium and contains no spermatozoa (Fig. 12.377).[3540,3541] Simple cyst ranges from 2 to 18 mm in diameter.[3542,3543] It may appear from 5 months of age to 84 years, with a bimodal distribution with peaks at 8 months and 60 years.[3544] It may occur bilaterally, and two simple cysts have been reported in the same testis.[3531,3545] Simple cyst

of the testis may be of mesothelial origin or may arise from ectopic rete testis epithelium.[3546] These cysts are unrelated to epidermoid cyst and differ in their ultrasonographic and histologic features (see earlier Hamartomatous Testicular Lesions section).[3547,3548] Ultrasound studies indicate that simple testicular cyst has little potential for growth.[3547,3549] Currently, excision is recommended in children only when there is concern that the cyst may impair testicular development.[3550]

Disorders of the Rete Testis

Dysgenesis

Dysgenesis of the rete testis is characterized by inadequate maturation and persistence of infantile or pubertal characteristics in adults.[1007] This disorder is frequent in undescended adult testes. The lesion involves the rete testis segments referred to as septal, mediastinal, and extratesticular. There is poor development of the cavities and their epithelial lining, which become cuboidal or

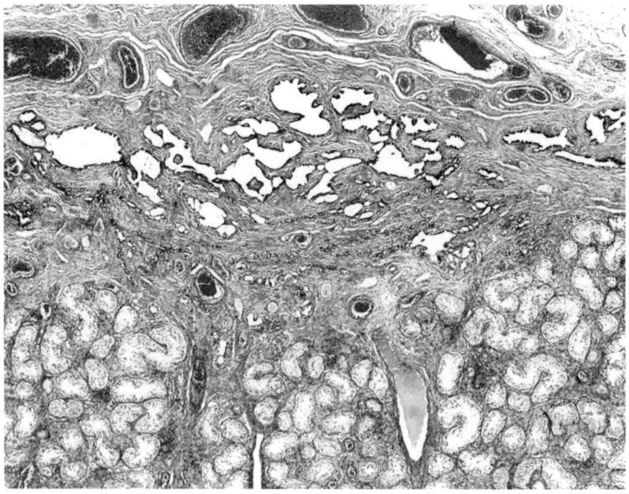

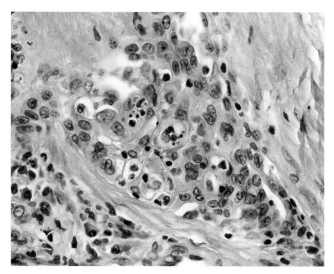

Fig. 12.378 Dysgenesis of the rete testis. Rete testis with microcystic hypoplasia. The most important characteristic is the presence in an adult of a rete testis that retains characteristics of the prepubertal rete testis with cubic or cylindrical epithelia and low and abnormal development of the mediastinal rete testis.

Fig. 12.379 Reactive hyperplasia of rete testis. The cavity of the rete testis is occupied by a proliferation of epithelial cells associated with isolated inflammatory cells in a patient with orchitis. Hyperplasia mimics carcinoma.

columnar instead of flattened with areas of columnar cells. The lumina of the rete testis cavities may be completely absent (simple hypoplasia) or, conversely, may undergo microcystic dilation (cystic hypoplasia) (Fig. 12.378). In a few cases the rete testis develops papillary, cribriform, or tubular formations (adenomatous hyperplasia).

Acquired Disorders of the Rete Testis

Metaplasia

The epithelium of the rete testis is usually flattened, with scattered areas of columnar cells. Metaplasia of the rete testis is characterized by replacement of the flattened epithelium by cuboid or columnar cells. This change occurs in mouse testis exposed to DES.[3551,3552] In estrogen-treated patients and in those with chronic hepatic insufficiency or functioning tumor that secretes estrogens or hCG, the rete testis epithelium may diffusely transform into tall columnar epithelium. Except for the last group, metaplasia of the rete testis seems to be an estrogen-dependent process, and estrogen receptors are present in the rete testis epithelium.[3553] Rete testis epithelial metaplasia may also be related to inflammatory processes in the vicinity (orchitis or epididymitis), severe hydroelectrolytic changes such as those observed in acute renal insufficiency, marked testicular atrophy, or associated with other cystic lesions of the rete testis.

Reactive Hyperplasia of the Rete Testis

Reactive hyperplasia of the rete testis is characterized by proliferation of the rete testis epithelium that completely or partially fills most of the cavities of the septal and mediastinal rete. This proliferation may take different patterns of growth: solid, trabecular, or cribriform (Figs. 12.379 through 12.381). The cells have morphologic characteristics (polyhedral cells, deep folded nuclei, eosinophilic cytoplasm) and immunophenotype (positivity for cytokeratins and vimentin) reminiscent of normal rete testis epithelium. Some cells contain eosinophilic bodies in the cytoplasm. Mitotic activity is generally limited. The proliferation is confined

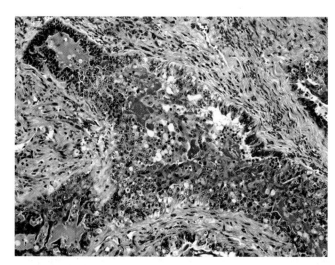

Fig. 12.380 Reactive hyperplasia of rete testis secondary to testicular torsion in an adult. Epithelial proliferation associated with accumulation of red cells both within the cavities and in the testicular mediastinum.

to luminal spaces. In many cases, reactive hyperplasia of rete testis is associated with adjacent lymphoid infiltrates or granulation tissue.

Reactive hyperplasia of the rete testis is a nonspecific finding that may be associated with various inflammatory and neoplastic testicular entities such as testicular torsion, orchitis, epidermoid cyst, sex cord/gonadal stromal tumor, germ cell tumor, testicular sarcoma, or primary testicular lymphoma.

When a solid or cribriform pattern predominates, the differential includes intratesticular adenomatoid tumor, adenocarcinoma of the rete testis, and extension of germ cell tumor. The intracavitary location of the reactive hyperplasia and its multicentric disposition excludes adenomatoid tumor. The absence of infiltrating growth or invasion of adjacent testicular parenchyma excludes adenocarcinoma. Germ cell tumors may involve the rete testis either

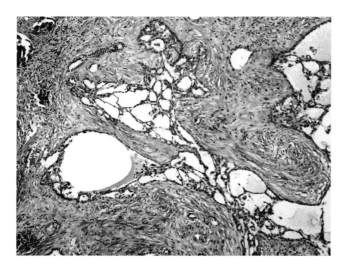

Fig. 12.381 Reactive hyperplasia of rete testis in a patient with embryonal carcinoma associated with yolk sac tumor. The nontumor nature of intracavitary reticular proliferation was confirmed by immunohistochemical study.

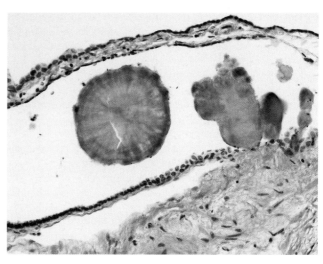

Fig. 12.383 Inside the cavities, apart from isolated spermatozoa, we may observe nodular formations of radial structure reminiscent of colonies of actinomyces (same case as in Fig. 12.382).

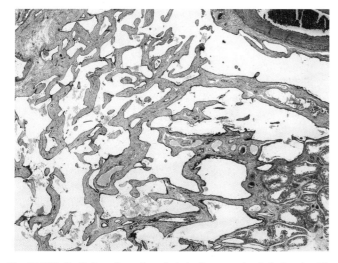

Fig. 12.382 Cystic transformation of rete testis secondary to ischemia of the caput of the epididymis. The cavities of the rete testis are lined by a highly flattened epithelium.

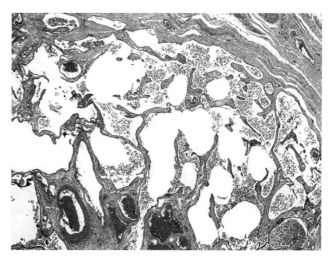

Fig. 12.384 Cystic transformation of the rete testis secondary to a lesion in the caput epididymidis in a patient with chronic epididymitis.

by pagetoid spread or direct extension from an adjacent tumor. Immunohistochemical staining may help resolve the diagnostic dilemma.

Cystic Ectasia of the Rete Testis (Acquired Cystic Transformation)

Acquired cystic transformation of the rete testis is common, and incidence increases with age and associated disorders.[3554] Ultrasound and MRI studies reveal characteristic images that suggest the diagnosis without biopsy or orchiectomy.[3555–3558] The lesion has three forms: simple, associated with epithelial metaplasia, and with crystalline deposits.

Simple Cystic Transformation

Simple cystic transformation is the most frequent form and consists of dilated cavities with normal epithelium. It is a diffuse and homogeneous lesion causing symmetrical dilatation, resulting from

obstruction that obliterates efferent ducts at the epididymal-testis union, the epididymis, or the initial portion of the vas deferens. The obstruction may be explained by three different mechanisms:

- *Ischemia.* In aging men with arteriosclerosis, the superior epididymal artery, a small collateral branch of the testicular artery, is frequently affected and causes ischemia of the majority of the head of the epididymis.[1890] Efferent duct atrophy causes loss of the absorptive capacity of their cells and obstruction of fluid that accumulates in a retrograde manner in the rete testis (Figs. 12.382 and 12.383).
- *Mechanical obstruction.* Epididymal obstruction occurs in two situations. One situation is extrinsic compression by epididymal and spermatic cord cyst or tumor, long-term hematocele, or congested veins in varicocele. Ectasia of the rete testis in varicocele may be either at the extratesticular level by varicose vein compression of the ductuli efferentes or at the intratesticular level by compression or distortion of centripetal veins.

Dilatation of the rete testis in this situation is not pronounced, and it is always asymmetric. The other situation is interruption of epididymal outflow in patients who have undergone epididymectomy.[3559]

- *Inflammation.* Ectasia is produced in patients with previous epididymitis by direct inflammatory swelling of acquired fibrotic obstructive changes in the head of the epididymis (Fig. 12.384).
- *Malformation.* The most common of such entities are testis-epididymis dissociation, partial or total agenesis of epididymis, and absence of the initial portion of the vas deferens.[3560]
- *Iatrogenic causes.* Epididymectomy or excision of epididymal cyst results in outflow obstruction.[3559,3561]

Cystic Transformation With Epithelial Metaplasia

Cystic transformation with epithelial metaplasia is a frequent finding at autopsy.[3562] It is the combination of two lesions, cuboidal or columnar metaplasia and cystic transformation of the rete testis, produced by the same etiologic mechanism or by several mechanisms. It is probably caused by the concurrence of sperm excretory duct obstruction and conditions with increased serum estrogen level, such as chronic liver insufficiency and hormonally active testicular tumor. Another possible cause is inflammation of the rete testis. Two mechanisms may be involved in this form of cystic ectasia of the rete testis:

- *Hormonal.* Estrogens cause cystic transformation of the rete testis when they are experimentally administered in the neonatal period.[858] Epithelial changes of the rete testis observed in chronic hepatic insufficiency may also result in increased estrogen levels, whereas cystic transformation may be the consequence of atrophy of the head of the epididymis or hypoandrogenism.[2879] The same hormonal mechanism causes metaplasia of the epithelium of the rete testis in testicular tumors producing estrogens or hCG. Cystic transformation in the absence of atrophy of the epididymis or spermatic pathway obstruction could be explained by hyperproduction of fluid by tumoral testis that would create imbalance in production, transport, and reabsorption.
- *Inflammatory.* In some cases of chronic orchitis involving the mediastinum testis, and in testicular tumor with abundant lymphoid infiltrates, cystic transformation of the rete testis may be observed. It is usually irregular and asymmetric. Epithelial changes are reactive. Inflammatory exudates are frequently present in cystically dilated lumens.

Cystic Transformation With Crystalline Deposits

Cystic transformation with crystalline deposits has also been called *cystic transformation of the rete testis secondary to renal insufficiency.*[3562] It is a bilateral lesion of adult testes characterized by the concurrence of three findings: cystic transformation of the rete testis, cuboidal or columnar metaplasia of the epithelium, and the presence of urate and oxalate crystalline deposits that may be recognized using polarized light. The lesion is seen exclusively in patients with chronic renal insufficiency who are receiving dialysis. Crystalline deposits are initially formed beneath the epithelia of the rete testis and efferent ducts; later they protrude into the lumina, where they are finally released. Inflammation is absent or minimal, although there may be scattered giant cells and small fibrotic areas (Figs. 12.385 and 12.386). Large quantities of deposits in secondary oxalosis may simulate testicular tumor.[3563]

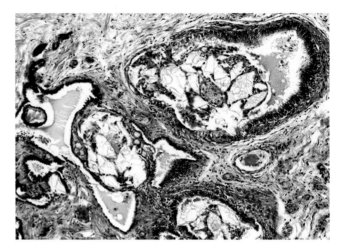

Fig. 12.385 Changes in the rete testis associated with dialysis. Dilation of the rete testis and initial portion of the efferent ducts may be observed. Crystalline structures, mainly rhomboidal in shape, accumulate inside and outside the tubules.

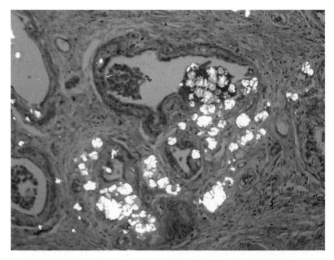

Fig. 12.386 Renal dialysis-associated cystic transformation of the rete testis with oxalate crystals demonstrated by polarized light.

Cystic transformation of the rete testis in these patients is related to efferent duct obstruction by the deposits or efferent duct atrophy caused by ischemia secondary to arteriosclerosis or hypertension that is frequently present. This lesion resembles the cystic lesion described in kidneys of these patients.[3564] This is hardly surprising because embryologic origin of mesonephric ducts and their derivatives in the testis (rete testis and ductuli efferentes) are related to embryologic origin of the kidney.

Cystic transformation with crystalline deposits develops slowly. In most cases, lesions usually arise 30 months or more after the start of dialysis.

Cystic ectasia of the rete testis should be differentiated from cystic dysplasia of the rete testis. Criteria for diagnosing cystic ectasia of the rete testis are bilaterality, occurrence in older patients, absence of genitourinary malformations, and presence of spermatozoa inside the cavities.

Adenomatous Hyperplasia

Adenomatous hyperplasia is characterized by diffuse or nodular proliferation of tubular or papillary structures derived from rete testis epithelium. It may arise in both cryptorchid or normally descended testes in newborns, children, and adults.[1042,3565]

Adenomatous hyperplasia in newborn and infantile testes consists of enlargement of the mediastinum testis by cordlike or tubular structures derived from rete testis epithelium. The lesion may occupy up to one-third of the testicular volume. Despite hyperplastic changes, normal connections with seminiferous tubules and efferent ducts remain intact. Presentation may be unilateral or bilateral. When unilateral, it is associated with cryptorchidism or vanishing testis. When bilateral, it is associated with bilateral renal dysplasia. Efferent ducts may show luminal dilation and irregular outlines. The origins of the lesion may be like those of cystic dysplasia of the testis.[1042]

Adenomatous hyperplasia in adults is usually an incidental finding at autopsy, in cryptorchid testes, or in testes with germ cell tumor.[3566,3567] The rete testis epithelium forms nonencapsulated proliferations that are either nodular or diffuse. Nodules may be large enough to raise concern for neoplasia. The epithelium consists of cuboidal cells with ovoid nuclei, deep nuclear folds, and peripheral nucleoli. Atypia and mitotic figures are absent (Fig. 12.387). The ultrastructure and immunophenotype of the epithelium are like that of normal rete testis. Spermatozoa may be present inside the lumina. In most instances the testis shows varying degrees of tubular atrophy.

When found incidentally, etiology is unknown, although it may be related to hormonal or chemical agents.[860,3568,3569] In cryptorchid testes and in cases associated with testicular tumor the most probable cause is a primary anomaly that is part of the testicular dysgenesis syndrome.[1061]

Adenomatous hyperplasia should be distinguished from three entities: rete testis pseudohyperplasia, which appears in atrophic testes; primary rete testis tumor; and metastatic adenocarcinoma. In pseudohyperplasia, lesions are focal, microscopic, and usually located in the septal rete, although the mediastinal rete shows few or no alterations. Benign rete testis tumor such as adenoma (solid and papillary variants) and cystadenoma are isolated and focal, whereas rete testis hyperplasia is diffuse.[3570] Adenocarcinoma of the rete testis is a tumor that displays abundant mitotic activity, cytologic atypia, and infiltrates adjacent structures.[3571] Metastatic prostatic adenocarcinoma alters the rete testis architecture; immunostains for prostate specific membrane antigen (PSMA) and NKX3.1 may aid in establishing that diagnosis.

Hyperplasia With Hyaline Globule Formation

This reactive lesion is characterized by the presence of intracytoplasmic accumulation of hyaline eosinophilic globules in epithelial cells of the rete testis. The epithelium may be hyperplastic, but does not contain mitotic figures or nuclear atypia. Globules are up to 15 μm in diameter (Fig. 12.388). This lesion is associated with tumors and inflammatory processes occurring near the mediastinum testis, and may be observed in association with 75% of cases of mixed testicular germ cell tumor, 47% of seminomas, and 20% of nongerm cell testicular tumors such as adenomatoid tumor of the testis.[3572] Yolk sac tumor infiltrating the rete testis may closely resemble this type of rete testis hyperplasia. Positive immunoreactions for α-fetoprotein, SALL4, and OCT4 are helpful to distinguish germ cell neoplasia from this rete testis hyperplasia.[3573]

Intracavitary Polypoid Nodular Proliferation

Intracavitary polypoid nodular proliferation, described as nodular proliferation of calcifying connective tissue in the rete testis, is characterized by the presence of multiple nodules that originate from the rete testis lining and subjacent connective tissue, protruding into channels of the rete testis. These nodules consist of cellular connective tissue covered by several layers of fibrin-like material, which in turn is covered by rete testis epithelium. The nodules may be totally or partially calcified (Fig. 12.389), or may take the form of a myriad of spherical or ovoid calcifications simulating parasite eggs (Fig. 12.390).[3574] The lesion is an incidental finding at autopsy in patients with impaired peripheral perfusion.

Selective location of the lesion in the walls of the cavities and chordae rete testis is probably related to poor vascularization of these structures. The etiopathogenetic mechanism may be anoxia, necrosis, fibrin deposition, proliferation of connective tissue, or

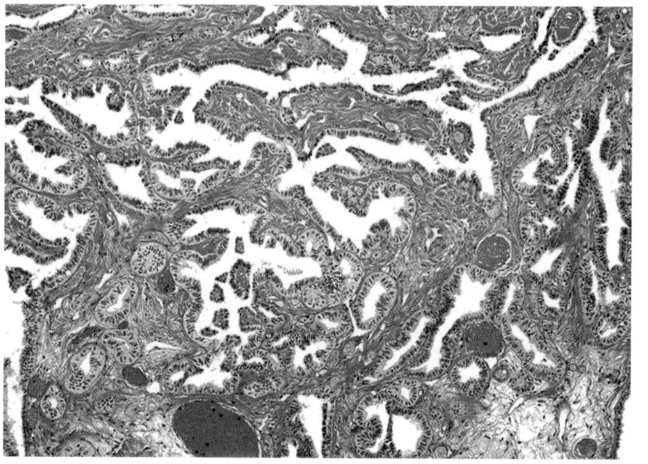

Fig. 12.387 Adenomatous hyperplasia of the rete testis. The epithelium is columnar and supported by a well-collagenized stroma.

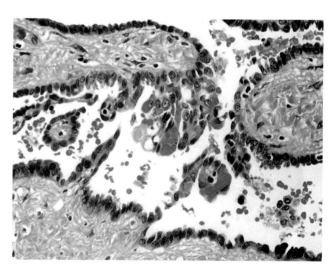

Fig. 12.388 Rete testis hyperplasia with hyaline globules. The globule-containing cells protrude into the lumina of the rete testis channels.

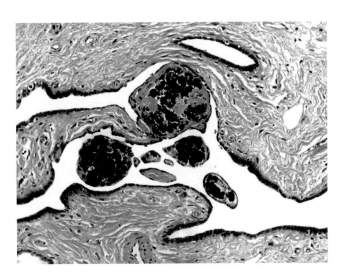

Fig. 12.389 Nodular proliferation of calcifying connective tissue in the rete testis with large calcium deposits.

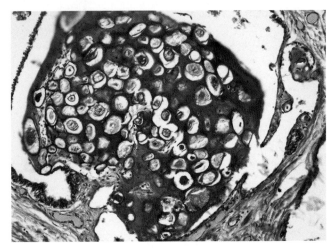

Fig. 12.390 Intracavitary polypoid nodular calcification simulating parasite eggs.

dystrophic calcification. Intracavitary growth could result from the lower intracavitary pressure and from the stiff structure of the mediastinum testis.

References are available at expertconsult.com

13

Neoplasms of the Testis

ROBERT E. EMERSON AND THOMAS M. ULBRIGHT

CHAPTER OUTLINE

Although weighing only about 19 grams, the testis is responsible for a complex array of neoplasms.[1] The rapidly proliferating spermatogenic cells give rise to the majority of testicular tumors, 95% of which are of germ cell derivation. Most are malignant and usually occur in young men, but they can be cured by current therapies; therefore accurate diagnosis is essential. The supporting cells and interstitial cells of the testis are responsible for the less common sex cord–stromal tumors that comprise a disproportionate number of diagnostic problems. Some of these are associated with clinical syndromes that may be suspected based on the testicular pathology.[2-7] A number of tumors of soft tissue origin may be identified in the paratestis, and secondary tumors are relatively frequent in both the testis and paratestis. The spectrum of lesions and the capacity of many tumors to mimic others make testicular neoplasia a continuing challenge to surgical pathologists, and this topic has been the subject of several recent reviews.[8-13]

Staging

The currently recommended staging system for testicular cancer is the eighth edition of the Cancer Staging Manual of the American Joint Committee on Cancer (AJCC), published in 2017 (Table 13.1), which replaces the seventh edition, published in 2010.[14,15] Interpretation of two difficult areas of staging using 2010 AJCC criteria (tunica vaginalis invasion and hilar fat invasion without vascular invasion) was identified as the most significant area of variation in practice with regard to handling and reporting testicular cancer specimens in a recent survey.[16] These points have been clarified in the 2017 AJCC staging manual.[14] In the eighth edition, changes include subdivision of the T1 category, for seminoma only, into T1a (tumor less than 3 cm) and T1b (tumor 3 cm or larger), assignment of stage T2 for epididymal or hilar soft tissue invasion independent of vascular invasion, and classification of discontinuous involvement of the spermatic cord by vascular-lymphatic invasion as M1 disease.[14] Serum marker studies play a key role in the evaluation of patients with testicular germ cell tumors, so the values of serum α-fetoprotein (AFP), human chorionic gonadotropin (hCG), and lactate dehydrogenase (LDH) are incorporated into the determination of the stage groupings.

Patterns of Metastasis

Testicular neoplasms usually first metastasize to retroperitoneal lymph nodes. There tends to be selective lymph node involvement with early-stage tumors, which depends on whether the right or left

TABLE 13.1 Eighth Edition AJCC Pathologic Staging System for Testicular Cancer

pT Category	Criteria
pTX	Unknown status of testis
pT0	No apparent primary (includes scars)
pTis	Germ cell neoplasia in situ
pT1a	Tumor limited to testis (including rete testis invasion) without lymphovascular invasion, tumor smaller than 3 cm[a]
pT1b	Tumor limited to testis (including rete testis invasion) without lymphovascular invasion, tumor 3 cm or larger[a]
pT2	Tumor either: limited to testis (including rete testis invasion) with lymphovascular invasion *or* involving hilar soft tissue or epididymis or penetrating visceral mesothelium of tunica albuginea with or without lymphovascular invasion
pT3	Tumor invading spermatic cord (although discontinuous involvement of the spermatic cord soft tissue via a vascular thrombus is regarded as pM1)
pT4	Tumor invading scrotum

pN Category	Criteria
pNX	Unknown nodal status
pN0	No regional node involvement
pN1	Node mass or single nodes ≤2 cm; ≤5 nodes involved; no node >2 cm
pN2	Node mass >2 but <5 cm; or >5 nodes involved; none >5 cm; or extranodal tumor
pN3	Node mass >5 cm

pM Category	Criteria
pM0	No distant metastases
pM1a	Nonregional nodal or lung metastases
pM1b	Distant metastasis other than nonregional nodal or lung

S Category	Criteria
SX	No marker studies available
S0	All marker studies normal
S1	LDH <1.5 × upper limit of normal and hCG <5000 mIU/mL and AFP <1000 ng/mL
S2	LDH 1.5-10 × upper limit of normal or hCG 5000-50,000 mIU/mL or AFP 1000-10,000 ng/mL
S3	LDH >10 × upper limit of normal or hCG >50,000 mIU/mL or AFP >10,000 ng/mL

Stage Grouping	
0	pTis, N0, M0, S0
I	pT1-4, N0, M0, SX
IA	pT1, N0, M0, S0
IB	pT2-4, N0, M0, S0
IS	Any pT, N0, M0, S1-3
II	Any pT, N1-3, M0, SX
IIA	Any pT, N1, M0, S0-1
IIB	Any pT, N2, M0, S0-1
IIC	Any pT, N3, M0, S0-1
III	Any pT, any N, M1, SX
IIIA	Any pT, any N, M1a, S0-1
IIIB	Any pT, N1-3, M0, S2 *or* Any pT, any N, M1a, S2
IIIC	Any pT, N1-3, M0, S3 *or* Any PT, any N, M1a, S3 *or* Any pT, any N, M1b, any S

[a]Subclassification based on size criterion applies only to seminomas.

Used with permission of the American College of Surgeons, Chicago, Illinois. The original source for this information is the AJCC Cancer Staging Manual, Eighth Edition (2017) published by Springer International Publishing.

testis is involved. For right-sided tumors, the interaortocaval nodes at about the level of the second lumbar vertebra are usually first involved, although right paracaval and precaval involvement may also occur.[17,18] In early stage involvement from right-sided tumors, there is absence of both suprahilar nodal involvement and involvement of the left paraaortic nodes below the inferior mesenteric artery (Fig. 13.1).[18] For left-sided tumors, the left paraaortic nodes, in an area bounded by the left ureter, left renal vein, aorta, and origin of the inferior mesenteric artery, are first involved.[17] Suprahilar nodal metastases may be seen in early-stage disease from left-sided testicular tumors, in contrast with right-sided lesions (Fig. 13.2).[18] As metastases become more widespread, right-sided lesions develop suprahilar and contralateral spread and left-sided tumors develop interaortocaval and precaval involvement, as well as a greater frequency of suprahilar involvement. As the volume of retroperitoneal disease increases, retrograde involvement of iliac and inguinal nodes may be seen.[18] Inguinal lymph node involvement may also be seen when the primary tumor has extended to the scrotal skin or a transcrotal approach was used for the primary resection. The extension of the primary tumor to the epididymis also correlates with the development of external iliac nodal spread. Eventually, supradiaphragmatic spread occurs to the mediastinum and supraclavicular and cervical lymph nodes, tending to involve the left supraclavicular nodes much more commonly than the right.[19]

Seminoma tends to metastasize in an orderly pattern through lymphatics, whereas choriocarcinoma more frequently spreads by hematogenous routes. The other germ cell tumors, such as embryonal carcinoma, tend to have a lymphatic pattern of spread, although hematogenous spread can also be seen. Hematogenous spread is most commonly reflected by lung, liver, central nervous system, and bone involvement.[20] Brain involvement is most common with choriocarcinoma and, perhaps unexpectedly, bone involvement with seminoma.[20]

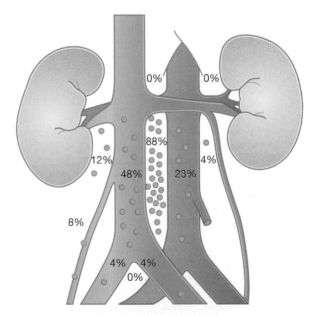

Fig. 13.1 Pattern of early retroperitoneal lymph node involvement from right-sided testicular tumors. (From Donohue JP. Metastatic pathways of nonseminomatous germ cell tumors. *Semin Urol.* 1984;2:217–229, with permission.)

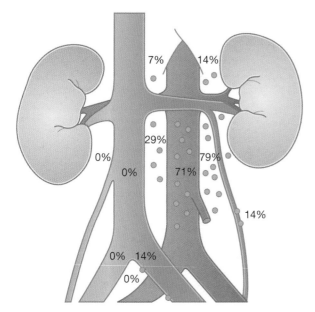

Fig. 13.2 Pattern of early retroperitoneal lymph node involvement from left-sided testicular tumors. (From Donohue JP. Metastatic pathways of nonseminomatous germ cell tumors. *Semin Urol.* 1984;2:217–229, with permission.)

Gross Examination

Gross examination and proper handling of the orchiectomy specimen are often neglected, and many diagnostic problems at the microscope can be traced to suboptimal processing of the gross specimen. Under the best circumstances, the testis and accompanying tunics and spermatic cord should be received fresh, dissected, and allowed to thoroughly fix before tissue blocks are submitted. What often happens, however, is that the urologist places the radical orchiectomy specimen intact into fixative, and only hours later is the specimen dissected. The testicular tunics are resistant to penetration of fixative, so this approach results in autolytic changes. It is preferable for the urologist to make a single, nearly through-and-through incision in the specimen before placing it into fixative if it is not feasible to send it to the laboratory immediately in the fresh state.

A radical orchiectomy specimen consists of the testis, tunica vaginalis, and a portion of spermatic cord. The specimen should be weighed, measured in three dimensions, and the length of the cord noted. We recommend examination of the spermatic cord next, before incision of the testis, to avoid the common contamination by "buttered" tumor of the cord, with submission of the cord resection margin and a cross-section adjacent to the testis, just superior to the head of the epididymis.[8,21] The tunica vaginalis should then be incised, any abnormalities described, the quantity and nature of any intratunical fluid recorded, and the tunica albuginea carefully inspected and palpated for penetration by neoplasm. The testis should then be bisected in the plane of its long axis, through the testicular hilum, by a long, sharp knife. Fresh tissue may then be harvested for special studies such as cytogenetics, flow cytometry, electron microscopy, and molecular studies, although these are not routinely needed for diagnosis. Photographs may be obtained, and then multiple, serial, parallel cuts at 3-mm intervals should be made, leaving the tunica albuginea intact posteriorly to keep the specimen together. The specimen should then be placed in a generous volume of 10% neutral buffered formalin

and allowed to thoroughly fix before further processing. After fixation, the neoplasm should be described and measured, with attention paid to the relationships to the tunica albuginea and the testicular hilum. Most examples of extratesticular spread occur by extension through the hilum.[22] Multiple blocks of neoplasm should be submitted, because many tumors are quite heterogeneous. Blocks of all the different-appearing areas should be made, including hemorrhagic and necrotic areas, with attention to the testis/parenchymal interface, where lymphovascular invasion is often most apparent. A minimum of one block of neoplasm for every centimeter of maximum tumor dimension or a total of 10 blocks, whichever is greater, is a general rule of thumb. It is prudent to submit blocks quite generously if the gross appearance suggests seminoma, because the discovery of nonseminomatous elements may change therapy. Hence, small seminomas should be totally submitted, and at least 10 blocks of larger tumors (or one block for every centimeter of maximum tumor dimension) should be submitted. The nonneoplastic testis should also be sampled, as well as a block to include the testicular hilum. The epididymis should be incised by multiple, parallel cuts perpendicular to its long axis, any abnormalities noted, and the appropriate blocks submitted.

Germ Cell Tumors

Classification

About 95% of testicular neoplasms are of germ cell origin. The 2016 World Health Organization (WHO) classification of testicular germ cell tumors (Table 13.2) incorporates recent advances in the understanding of the pathogenesis of these tumors, specifically separating the germ cell neoplasia in situ–related and germ cell neoplasia in situ–unrelated tumors.[23] This classification replaces previous classifications including the British Testicular Tumor Panel (BTTP) classification that was sometimes used in Europe.[24,25]

Histogenesis

The histogenesis of testicular germ cell tumors has been clarified over the past several decades by several clinical, morphologic, and immunohistochemical observations. Gene expression profiling and other molecular techniques have allowed a great increase in understanding of the molecular changes in the most common testicular cancers, the germ cell neoplasia in situ–associated tumors, which have also been described as type II germ cell tumors.[26-28] Perhaps foremost in importance is the recognition that all of the adult germ cell tumors, with the exceptions of spermatocytic tumor, rare benign teratomas (a category now including epidermoid and dermoid cysts), and even more rare yolk sac tumors, are derived from a common precursor that Skakkebaek originally recognized and described as "carcinoma in situ" of the testis.[23,29-32] *Intratubular germ cell neoplasia of the unclassified type* (IGCNU) had later been considered the appropriate term for this lesion, given the nonepithelial nature of the constituent cells, but the preferred term in the recent WHO classification is germ cell neoplasia in situ (GCNIS).[23,33,34] GCNIS consists of a basilar proliferation of seminoma-like cells (occupying the "spermatogonial niche") with clear cytoplasm and enlarged, hyperchromatic nuclei having one or two prominent nucleoli (Fig. 13.3). Additionally it has many features, apart from its light microscopic appearance, that it shares with seminoma, including ultrastructure, immunohistochemical reactions with various antibodies (M_2A/podoplanin/ D2-40, TRA-1-60, placental-like alkaline phosphatase [PLAP],

TABLE 13.2 Classification of Testicular Tumors

Germ Cell Tumors

Germ cell tumors
  Germ cell neoplasia in situ
  Germ cell tumors derived from germ cell neoplasia in situ
    Tumors of a single histologic type
      Seminoma (including seminoma with syncytiotrophoblast cells)
      Nonseminomatous germ cell tumors
        Embryonal carcinoma
        Yolk sac tumor, postpubertal type
        Trophoblastic tumors
          Choriocarcinoma
          Nonchoriocarcinomatous trophoblastic tumors
        Teratoma, postpubertal type
        Teratoma with somatic-type malignancy
      Nonseminomatous germ cell tumors of more than one histologic
        type
        Mixed germ cell tumors
      Germ cell tumors of unknown type
        Regressed germ cell tumors
  Germ cell tumors unrelated to germ cell neoplasia in situ
    Spermatocytic tumor
    Teratoma, prepubertal type
    Mixed teratoma and yolk sac tumor, prepubertal type
    Yolk sac tumor, prepubertal type

Sex Cord–Stromal Tumors

Pure tumors
  Leydig cell tumor
  Sertoli cell tumor, not otherwise specified
  Large cell calcifying Sertoli cell tumor
  Intratubular large cell hyalinizing Sertoli cell neoplasia
  Granulosa cell tumor
    Adult granulosa cell tumor
    Juvenile granulosa cell tumor
  Tumors in the fibroma-thecoma group
  Myoid gonadal stromal tumor
Mixed and unclassified sex cord–stromal tumors

Tumors Containing Both Germ Cell and Sex Cord–Stromal Elements

Gonadoblastoma

Miscellaneous tumors of the testis and paratesticular tissue

Ovarian-type epithelial tumors
Juvenile xanthogranuloma
Hemangioma and other stromal tumors

Hematolymphoid tumors

Modified from Moch H, Humphrey PA, Ulbright TM, Reuter V. *WHO Classification of Tumours of the Urinary System and Male Genital Organs.* 4th ed. Lyon, France: IARC; 2016.

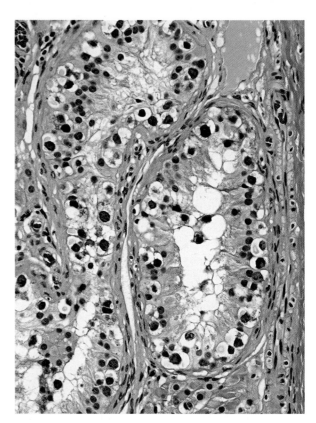

Fig. 13.3 GCNIS in seminiferous tubules. There are cells with clear cytoplasm and enlarged, hyperchromatic nuclei along the basilar aspect of tubules lacking spermatogenesis. Sertoli cells are displaced luminally.

glutathione-S-transferase [isoenzyme π], the 14–3–3 beta protein, OCT3/4, NANOG, stem cell factor, TSPY protein, SOX17+/ SOX2– immunophenotype), its DNA content, the number of nucleolar organizer regions, and lectin-binding patterns.[35-53]

The strong similarities between GCNIS and seminoma imply that seminoma is also a precursor for other germ cell tumors. This interpretation is supported by several morphologic, immunohistochemical, and molecular observations. These include autopsy studies showing nonseminomatous elements in patients who died of metastatic germ cell neoplasm after orchiectomy of pure testicular seminoma.[20,54] Additionally, seminoma may undergo subtle transition to either embryonal carcinoma or yolk sac tumor.[55,56] Also,

10% to 20% of seminomas contain syncytiotrophoblast cells, and some trophoblastic hormone–containing cells in seminoma are not easily distinguished histologically from the surrounding seminoma cells.[57-59] Ultrastructural studies of seminoma have demonstrated evidence of epithelial differentiation (*seminoma with early carcinomatous features*) in some light microscopically typical cases.[60] Furthermore, the DNA content of seminoma is consistently higher than in nonseminomatous germ cell tumors, suggesting that nonseminomatous tumors evolve from seminoma as a consequence of gene loss, perhaps caused by loss of cancer suppressor genes.[51,61,62] Karyotypic analyses have shown a striking tendency for certain chromosomes to be in parallel excess or deficiency in seminoma and the nonseminomatous germ cell tumors, and loss of heterozygosity studies also show similar patterns of allelic imbalance between coexisting seminoma and nonseminoma in the testis.[61,63] These data indicate that seminomas transform to nonseminomatous tumors.

Genetic changes precede the development of an invasive germ cell tumor from GCNIS.[26,64,65] Although overrepresentation of gene sequences from the short arm of chromosome 12, mostly in the form of an isochromosome [i(12p)], is consistent in invasive germ cell tumors of adult patients, such overrepresentation is not found in the associated GCNIS.[66-68] It is believed that additional 12p sequences are essential for invasive growth by inhibiting apoptosis and thereby permitting survival of invasive tumor cells outside of the microenvironment of the seminiferous tubules.[67] There are marked similarities between many of the genetic changes in GCNIS and the associated invasive tumor, in support of the precursor role of the former.[63,64] Immunohistochemical study has shown that loss of the cell cycle–dependent kinase inhibitors, p18 and p21, accompanies invasive growth, as does gain of the ubiquitin ligase murine double minute-2 (mdm-2) and increased production of cyclin E.[69,70]

Transformation of GCNIS to nonseminomatous tumor may apparently occur at the time of invasion, because pure embryonal carcinoma, yolk sac tumor, or choriocarcinoma are associated with GCNIS. Alternatively, these elements may overgrow a small focus of seminoma from which they arose. The common occurrence of seminoma with nonseminomatous elements also supports transformation from invasive seminoma. Allelotyping analysis supports this concept, as loss of heterozygosity is seen at progressively more loci from GCNIS to seminoma and then to embryonal carcinoma.[71] Loss of heterozygosity at various loci was frequently shared among the seminoma and embryonal carcinoma components, and heterozygosity was retained in GCNIS, further supporting that the embryonal carcinoma component arose from the seminoma.[71]

Additional data show that GCNIS adjacent to seminoma or nonseminomatous tumors shares chromosomal abnormalities with the invasive tumor that differ depending on whether the adjacent tumor is seminomatous or nonseminomatous, an observation that supports genetic transformation within the tubules before morphologic change.[72] Collectively, these observations led to a revised model of testicular germ cell tumor histogenesis based on the tetrahedron model proposed by Srigley et al. (Fig. 13.4).[60]

The histogenesis of testicular germ cell tumors in children (excluding those with disorders of sex development) is different from that of postpubertal patients. This is reflected in epidemiologic studies that documented a progressive increase in the incidence of testicular germ cell tumors throughout the twentieth century in postpubertal patients but not in the prepubertal group.[73] Unlike the postpubertal tumors, the examples in children (confined to two types of neoplasm, yolk sac tumor and teratoma) lack association with GCNIS.[74-78] Furthermore, the teratomas have a diploid DNA content and a normal karyotype, unlike those of postpubertal patients, and the yolk sac tumors lack consistent 12p abnormalities.[79-81] The pediatric germ cell tumors therefore have a fundamentally different pathogenesis. These observations and others have led one group to propose that there are five fundamentally different forms of germ cell tumor: type I represented by the pediatric types, type II consisting of the usual postpubertal germ cell tumors, type III consisting only of spermatocytic tumor, type IV represented by ovarian dermoid cyst, and type V consisting of gestational choriocarcinoma.[82] Each has its own unique pattern of gene activation and genomic imprinting.

Epidemiology

Germ cell tumors of the testis (with the notable exception of spermatocytic tumor) occur mostly in young men, with the incidence accelerating rapidly after puberty and peaking close to 30 years of age (Fig. 13.5). There is a small peak in early childhood, but many cases of "testicular cancer" in elderly men correspond to lymphoma or secondary tumors rather than to germ cell tumors (Fig. 13.5). Whites have a much higher frequency of testicular germ cell tumors than do non-whites, with the exception of the Maori of

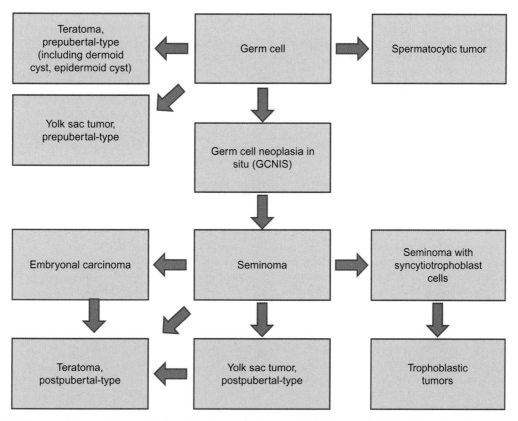

Fig. 13.4 New model of germ cell tumor histogenesis, based on the tetrahedron model of Srigley et al. (Srigley JR, Mackay B, Toth P, Ayala A. The ultrastructure and histogenesis of male germ neoplasia with emphasis on seminoma with early carcinomatous features. *Ultrastruct Pathol.* 1988;12:67–86). In this model, seminoma plays a pivotal role as a precursor for many other forms of germ cell tumor. Note the absence of GCNIS for prepubertal-type teratoma, prepubertal-type yolk sac tumor, and spermatocytic tumor.

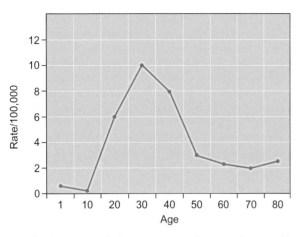

Fig. 13.5 Incidence of testicular tumors according to patient age. Note a small peak in infancy, a nadir at 10 years of age, and a rapid rise after puberty. The peak incidence occurs at 25 to 30 years. The cases in older patients often correspond to nongerminal tumors, mainly lymphoma. (Data from the Surveillance, Epidemiology and End Results [SEER] Program).

New Zealand who have an incidence comparable to white populations.[83,84] Native Hawaiians, Native Alaskans, and Native Americans are also at higher risk than other non-whites.[85] The rates of increase of testicular cancer in black men (+1.67%/year), Hispanic men (+2.94%/year), and American Indian/Alaska Native men (+2.96%/year) in the United States are, however, increasing faster than that of white men (+1.23%/year) in recent decades.[86] Denmark and Switzerland have the highest rates of testicular cancer, about 9 cases per 100,000 males per year, compared with the rate in the US white population of 5 to 6 per 100,000 males.[86] The rates in Africans and Asians are generally about 1 per 100,000 males.[87] In a study of over 1 million Israeli males, risk was strongly associated with birthplace, with odds ratios of 0.10 for those born in North Africa and 0.35 for those born in Asia compared with those born in Israel.[88]

The incidence of most testicular germ cell tumors increased steadily in the United States during the twentieth century, and recent National Cancer Institute Surveillance, Epidemiology, and End Results Program (SEER) data indicate an increase in the rate of testis cancer in 15- to 39-year-old males in the United States at a time when the incidences of most other cancers in this age group are decreasing.[89-91] Increasing testicular cancer rates have been noted in several other countries, including Denmark, Norway, England, Germany, Scotland, New Zealand, Australia, Canada, Iceland, and Japan, although, as noted, the rate remained steady in children.[73,84,92-104] Eastern Europe, which previously had a lower rate, has had the most rapid increase in testicular cancer incidence in recent years and now has a rate similar to Northern and Western Europe.[105]

Numerous studies have demonstrated a higher frequency of testicular germ cell tumors in professional workers or those of higher socioeconomic class compared with laborers or those of lower socioeconomic status.[84,85,106-112] Higher rates have also been observed in those with occupational exposures to fertilizers, phenols, heat, smoke, or fumes; farm workers; draftsmen; those involved in food manufacture and preparation; leather workers; pesticide applicators; those exposed to insect repellants; metalworkers; police exposed to handheld radar; aircraft repairmen; motor vehicle mechanics; fishermen; electrical workers, paper and printing workers, and foresters; men of tall stature; and

physicians.[84,106,107,113-123] Other studies have implicated in utero exposure to high estrogen levels, dietary iron, testicular trauma, various HLA-haplotypes, a family history of breast cancer, early puberty, early birth order, dizygotic twinship, ichthyosis, Marfan syndrome, the Li-Fraumeni syndrome, the dysplastic nevus syndrome, and HIV infection.[124-146] One study has shown a correlation between testicular cancer and a variant allele of the glutathione-S-transferase π gene.[147] Another study demonstrated increased risk in the sons of fathers who were wood processors, metalworkers, or employed in the food product industry.[148] Recently, baldness and a history of severe acne, both associated with high androgen levels at puberty, have been associated with testicular germ cell tumors.[149] Marijuana use has been associated with a 1.7 to 2.2-fold increased risk for testicular nonseminomatous germ cell tumors.[150-152] Most of these associations, however, are weak and fail to account for the general increase in testicular germ cell tumors. It is hypothesized that important causative factors in testicular cancer occur in the antenatal period, with a protective effect in European countries for men born during the World War II era.[92,153,154] This protective effect leads to the hypothesis that testicular cancer is causally related to prosperity, probably secondary to in utero effects. Environmental endocrine-disrupting chemicals have attracted interest as a possible causative factor for germ cell tumors (and the other components of the proposed testicular dysgenesis syndrome).[28,65,155,156] Phthalates, chemicals present in plastics, have attracted interest as an environmental endocrine disruptor, but a causative role remains unproven.[65,156] A potential unifying thread to several of the most compelling observations is that maternal obesity (leading to elevated estrogens) and/or maternal exposure to estrogen simulators or antiandrogens lead to testicular maldevelopment with impaired Sertoli cell function that is key to germ cell neoplasia. The use of alcohol and tobacco, prior vasectomy, radiation exposure, and maternal and paternal occupational pesticide exposure have not been associated with testicular germ cell tumors.[83,157-161]

Despite the weak correlation of most etiologic factors with testicular germ cell tumors, four contributing factors are proven: cryptorchidism, prior testicular germ cell tumor, family history of testicular germ cell tumors, and certain disorders of sex development.[83,162] An estimate of the increased risks associated with these disorders is provided in Table 13.3.

Cryptorchidism

An increased frequency of cryptorchidism, varying from 6.5% to 14.5%, has been found in patients with testicular germ cell tumors, which has led to increased risk calculations of 2.5 to 35 times higher among cryptorchid patients.[89,125,163-176] Such risk does not manifest before 20 years of age and is probably most accurately assessed as 3.5 to 5.0 times increased over a control population.[167,173] If cryptorchidism is unilateral, the noncryptorchid testis is also at increased risk for a testicular germ cell tumor, although at a lower rate than the cryptorchid testis.[85,169,171,177-179] Ectopia alone cannot explain the association of cryptorchidism and testicular germ cell tumor, a fact reinforced by the failure of orchiopexy to reduce the risk to that of the general population (although there is probably insufficient experience with orchidopexy in the very young to rule out an ameliorating effect).[85,168,169,180,181] Early surgical correction, at 6 to 18 months of age, has been recommended as treatment for cryptorchidism, as the risk reduction is related to age, with a relative risk for developing cancer of 2.2 if orchiopexy is performed before 13 years of age compared with 5.4 if performed after 13 years of age.[182-184]

	Estimated Increased Risk for Testicular Germ Cell Tumors Associated With Certain Conditions		
TABLE 13.3			
Condition	**Estimated Increased Risk**	**References**	
Cryptorchidism	3.5–5X	Pottern, 1985[167]	
		Giwercman, 1987[173]	
Prior testicular germ cell tumor	5–10X	Giwercman, 1991[1]	
		Dieckmann, 1999[195]	
		Giwercman, 1987[218]	
		Loy, 1993[219]	
Family history (first-degree male relative)	3–10X	Dieckmann, 1997[236]	
		Fuller, 1986[237]	
		Tollerud, 1985[238]	
		Forman, 1992[239]	
Gonadal dysgenesis with a Y-chromosome	50X[a]	Giwercman, 1991[1]	
		Rutgers, 1987[253]	
		Hughesdon, 1970[254]	
Androgen insensitivity syndrome	15X	Giwercman, 1991[1]	
		Manuel, 1976[260]	
		Morris, 1953[261]	
		Rutgers, 1991[262]	
		Rutgers, 1991[265]	

[a]Includes cases of gonadoblastoma.

It seems likely that cryptorchidism is a marker of patients with a general defect in testicular and genital development and that cryptorchid testes are "dysgenetic," as supported by abnormalities of the external genitalia or sex chromosomes in some cryptorchid patients with germ cell tumors.[179,185-187] This has been conceptualized as the "testicular dysgenesis syndrome," a collection of findings including cryptorchidism, infertility, disorders of sex development, GCNIS, and germ cell tumors that may share common etiologic factors.[65,188,189] A distinctive array of testicular lesions may be seen in the parenchyma adjacent to germ cell tumors, including Leydig cell hyperplasia, microlithiasis, angiopathy, Sertoli cell nodules, tubular atrophy, and multinucleated spermatogonia, supporting an underlying developmental problem.[190] Cryptorchidism may disproportionately predispose to seminoma compared with nonseminomatous tumors.[163,174,191,192] GCNIS has been estimated to be present in about 2% to 4% of patients with cryptorchidism.[193-196] At least 50% of such patients develop germ cell tumor within 5 years.[197] Thus bilateral testicular biopsy at 18 to 20 years of age has been recommended for cryptorchid patients.[198] A negative result is good evidence of no increased risk, although there are infrequent false-negative results.[193,199,200] A positive biopsy should prompt orchiectomy of the affected testis. In testes with extreme atrophy, the biopsy should be directed to sample the region near the rete testis.[201] Apart from germ cell tumors, cryptorchid testes have an increased frequency of nodules composed of small tubules lined by immature Sertoli cells, often with central deposits of basement membrane. These Sertoli cell nodules have been termed *Pick adenoma,* which is a misnomer because they are not true neoplasms.[202,203]

Prior Testicular Germ Cell Tumor

A second germ cell tumor occurs in the remaining testis of 1% to 5% of patients with a previous germ cell tumor.[204-217] The risk for

a second germ cell tumor is higher in patients with seminoma, especially in men 30 years of age or younger.[216] Similarly, there is a 3.2% to 6.6% frequency of GCNIS in the opposite testis of patients with a germ cell tumor.[210,211,217-220] There is a low risk in the absence of GCNIS on biopsy because of occasional false-negative biopsies.[220] In one study, 5 of 1859 patients (0.3%) who had negative testicular biopsies opposite a germ cell tumor developed a second tumor on follow-up.[200] Sensitivity is improved if three biopsies of the contralateral testis are performed.[221] If the residual testis is either atrophic or cryptorchid, the risk is greater, with a 23% frequency of GCNIS.[218-220,222,223] Unfortunately, almost 50% of cases of contralateral GCNIS would be missed if contralateral biopsies were restricted to patients with atrophy or cryptorchidism.[219] One study suggested that atrophy rather than maldescent is the important predictor of contralateral GCNIS.[224] Young (but postpubertal) age at onset of the first tumor and bilateral cryptorchidism are also associated with an increased risk for bilateral occurrence.[211,224] It is estimated that biopsy of an atrophic testis opposite a germ cell tumor in a patient younger than 31 years of age will detect GCNIS in one-third.[224] Prepubertal testicular germ cell tumors, in contrast, do not appear to be associated with an elevated risk for second gonadal cancers.[203]

About 50% of second primary tumors of the testis occur within 3 to 5 years after diagnosis of the initial germ cell tumor, with a mean of 5.6 to 6.5 years, but intervals of more than a decade can occur.[207,215,216,225-227] Concordant or discordant neoplastic types may occur, with some tendency for concordance of pure seminoma.[207] The risk for bilateral tumors is increased about fourfold with a positive family history.[228,229] Chemotherapy administered for the first tumor has been observed to decrease the risk for a contralateral tumor, but not in all studies.[209,212,217] Contralateral tumors may occur even in the absence of GCNIS in biopsies of the opposite testis performed at the time of the first germ cell tumor diagnosis.[230] An increased frequency of rare alleles of the *HRAS* gene is seen in patients with testicular germ cell tumors, and such alleles are associated with bilaterality and early age of onset.[231] Androgen receptor polymorphisms (with high or low numbers of CAG repeats) have been associated with testicular cancer risk.[232] In one study, 64% of bilateral germ cell tumors had *KIT* mutations compared with 6% of unilateral tumors, suggesting a causative role for *KIT* mutations occurring early in embryonal development in patients with bilateral tumors.[233] Genetic associations with germ cell tumor risk have been reviewed, and the association with *KIT* signaling has been confirmed with genome-wide association studies that have found associations with five molecular pathways: *KIT* signaling, other pathways of male germ cell development, telomerase function, microtubule assembly, and DNA damage repair.[234,235]

Family History

First-degree male relatives of patients with germ cell tumor of the testis have a 3 to 10 times greater risk for a testicular germ cell tumor than the general population.[236-239] The risk is highest for brothers (10 times), intermediate for sons (6 times), and lowest for fathers (4 times).[240] Also, a family history of testicular germ cell tumor is associated with an 8% to 14% frequency of bilaterality, compared with the 1% to 5% frequency in the general population of patients with testicular germ cell tumors.[205-208,216,228,237,240] The occurrence of an unexpected number of testicular germ cell tumors in the relatives of children with soft tissue sarcomas has raised the question of whether testicular germ cell tumors may represent part of the spectrum of the Li-Fraumeni cancer syndrome.[241,242] It appears, however, that neither germline nor somatic *TP53* mutations occur in these cases.[243,244] Immunohistochemical demonstration of p53 protein therefore indicates overexpression of nonmutated protein.[245,246] Segregation analysis of data regarding familial cases has suggested the presence of a major gene that conveys risk in a recessive model.[247] Genetic linkage analysis has implicated a susceptibility gene localized to Xq27 in one study, but this was not confirmed in a second.[248,249] Single nucleotide polymorphisms in *BAK1, DMRT1, KITLG,* and *TERT-CLPTM1L* genes have been associated with testis cancer risk odds ratios of 1.6 to 2.3.[250] In a study including 147 families with either two or more cases of testis cancer or one case of bilateral testis cancer, no rare, highly penetrant susceptibility gene was identified.[251] It is believed that, instead, familial testis cancer most likely results from multiple, common, low-penetrance alleles in a manner more similar to type 2 diabetes or familial prostate cancer than to the more well-known adult cancer susceptibility disorders with high-penetrance genes associated with breast, ovarian, and colorectal carcinoma.[251] No increase in overall risk for nontesticular cancers was seen in relatives of familial testicular tumor patients in a recent study of 1041 first-degree relatives from 66 multiple case testicular germ cell tumor families, suggesting that tumors other than testis cancer are not part of the association.[252]

Disorders of Sex Development

Patients with some disorders of sex development are at increased risk for germ cell tumors. Patients with gonadal dysgenesis in the presence of a Y-chromosome, including patients with pure 46,XY gonadal dysgenesis (Swyer syndrome) and mixed gonadal dysgenesis, commonly develop gonadal germ cell tumors.[253-257] About 25% to 30% of such patients develop gonadoblastoma, and this may serve as the precursor lesion for the development of an invasive germ cell tumor (discussed later in this chapter).[253,254,256] GCNIS is also present in about 8% of children and adolescents with gonadal dysgenesis.[258] Because an invasive tumor may develop in childhood, gonadectomy is indicated as soon as the diagnosis is established. Patients with androgen insensitivity syndrome, caused by various mutations in the androgen receptor gene, develop a malignant germ cell tumor in 5% to 10% of cases overall.[259-263] The tumor usually develops after puberty, and this may permit delayed gonadectomy until full feminization has occurred, although this remains controversial because of an occasional case of invasive germ cell tumor developing at an early age. Delay of prophylactic gonadectomy beyond the early postpubescent period in patients with androgen insensitivity syndrome (AIS) is risky, with a 22% frequency of malignant germ cell tumor in such patients beyond 30 years of age.[260,264] Not all testicular masses in patients with the AIS are germ cell tumors; these patients commonly develop hamartomatous nodules composed of Sertoli cell–lined tubules with intervening clusters of Leydig cells in the interstitium, as well as pure Sertoli cell adenomas and occasional juvenile granulosa cell tumors.[253,255,262,265] In addition to patients with mutations in the androgen receptor gene, there is a single report of GCNIS in a phenotypic female patient with an XY karyotype and a nonsense mutation in the gene for steroidogenic acute regulatory protein.[266]

Infertility

Patients with infertility have an increased but less than 1% frequency of testicular germ cell tumor.[35,195,218,267-269] The relative risk for germ cell tumor in patients with infertility is much lower than that associated with cryptorchidism or a history of contralateral germ cell tumor.[270] It is not clear, however, if infertility is a risk factor for germ cell tumor that is independent of cryptorchidism or gonadal dysgenesis.[271] Impaired semen quality, hypospadias, cryptorchidism, and germ cell tumors are the components of the testicular dysgenesis syndrome theoretical construct and are each related to the other.[155] Semen quality may be a highly sensitive marker for environmental exposures, which are also related to germ cell tumor incidence.[155]

Other Associations

Testicular microlithiasis, seen ultrasonographically as hyperechogenic foci without shadowing, is observed in about 13% of patients evaluated by this method.[272,273] Rare cases of germ cell tumor have been reported in patients, including teenage boys, being followed for testicular microlithiasis.[274] It is unusual for a patient with testicular microlithiasis but without other risk factors to have GCNIS on biopsy, so biopsy is only recommended if other risk factors, such as infertility, cryptorchidism, or contralateral tumor, exist.[272]

Inguinal hernia and genital malformations other than cryptorchidism including hypospadias have also been associated with testicular germ cell tumor risk, although not as strongly as cryptorchidism.[272,275]

Germ Cell Neoplasia in Situ and Related Germ Cell Tumors

Germ Cell Neoplasia in Situ

Grossly, the testis with GCNIS may be unremarkable or appear atrophic and fibrotic. Microscopically, intratubular germ cell neoplasia consists of a proliferation of undifferentiated germ cells resembling primitive gonocytes or, less frequently, may be composed of cells of a specific neoplastic type, such as intratubular embryonal carcinoma.[32] The primitive gonocyte-like form of intratubular germ cell neoplasia is confined to the basilar aspect of the seminiferous tubules (in the so-called "spermatogonial niche") and is associated with all types of the postpubertal germ cell tumors, except for spermatocytic tumor and the rare benign teratomas (including dermoid/epidermoid cyst) and prepubertal-type yolk sac tumors.[29,30] GCNIS cells have enlarged, hyperchromatic nuclei, often with one or two prominent nucleoli, thickened nuclear membranes, and clear cytoplasm (Fig. 13.3). The median nuclear diameter is 9.7 µm, compared with a median nuclear diameter of spermatogonia of 6.5 µm.[276] Spermatogenesis in the affected tubules is usually decreased or absent, and the tubules may have a thickened peritubular basement membrane. Sertoli cells are often displaced luminally (Fig. 13.3). The distribution of GCNIS is characteristically patchy, and adjacent profiles of seminiferous tubules may appear unremarkable with intact spermatogenesis (Fig. 13.6). The patchy distribution has implications for biopsy diagnosis, as a small volume sample may result in a false-negative diagnosis.[277] Leydig cell hyperplasia may occur in the interstitium. GCNIS often spreads into the rete testis in a "Pagetoid" fashion, intermixing with nonneoplastic epithelium, which is displaced toward the lumen (Fig. 13.7).[278] The strong similarity of the cells of seminoma and GCNIS suggests that GCNIS could be termed *intratubular seminoma;* however, this term may falsely suggest that GCNIS is the precursor lesion only for seminoma rather than for virtually all postpubertal germ cell tumors. The term *intratubular seminoma* has been applied to those proliferations of GCNIS-like cells that fill and distend seminiferous tubules (Fig. 13.8), although such lesions may simply be a more advanced stage of GCNIS.[279]

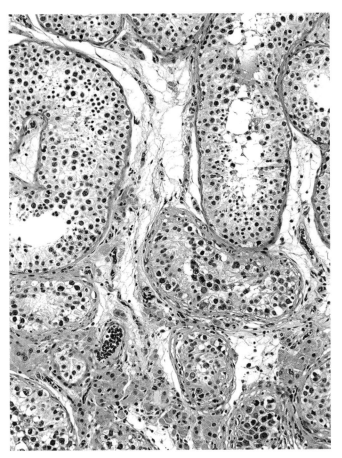

Fig. 13.6 Patchy distribution of GCNIS. Tubules without GCNIS have spermatogenesis, whereas adjacent tubules with GCNIS lack spermatogenesis.

Special Studies

Glycogen is present in the cytoplasm of 98% of cases of GCNIS (Fig. 13.9), and its demonstration is diagnostically helpful but nonspecific because nonneoplastic spermatogonia and Sertoli cells may also contain glycogen.[280,281] The current best immunohistochemical marker for GCNIS is OCT3/4, a nuclear transcription factor with a key role in maintaining pluripotency in embryonic stem cells. OCT3/4 is uniformly sensitive for GCNIS (Fig. 13.10).[45,50,282,283] It, as well as other GCNIS markers, is also seen in germ cells with delayed maturation in gonadal dysgenesis, Down syndrome, and undervirilization syndromes that have different features from GCNIS. PLAP is also a good marker for GCNIS.[284-287] It highlights the cytoplasmic membranes of most cases (reported sensitivity: 83%-100%; Fig. 13.10A).[40,281,288,289] Only rarely (less than 1%) are isolated nonneoplastic spermatocytes (which are unlikely to be confused with GCNIS) PLAP positive, with spermatogonia being PLAP negative.[288] Immunohistochemical staining for NANOG, a regulatory factor upstream to OCT3/4, similarly marks GCNIS.[46] GCNIS has also been found to react with monoclonal antibodies M₂A (D2-40/gp36/podoplanin), 43-9F, TRA-1-60, HB5, HF2, HE11, and with antibodies directed against glutathione-S-transferase, isoenzyme π, CD117 (Fig. 13.10C), angiotensin-converting enzyme, p53, growth differentiation factor 3 (GDF3), stem cell factor, and Krüppel-like factor 4.[37,42,47,233,283,289-298] It is negative for the RNA-binding motif protein, in contrast with nonneoplastic germ cells.[299] GCNIS is SOX17 positive and SOX2 negative, but SOX17 also marks nonneoplastic germ cells, a problem we have

also encountered with CD117.[49,300,301] In contrast, intratubular embryonal carcinoma is SOX17 negative and SOX2 positive.[49] The positive reactions for PLAP, OCT3/4, CD117, and TRA-1-60 support the idea that GCNIS resembles fetal gonocytes.[38,40,293] There is some heterogeneity in expression of germ cell markers in cells in GCNIS tubules, and it is the OCT3/4⁺/MAGEA4⁻ population of cells that has the higher proliferative activity (relative to OCT3/4⁺/MAGEA4⁺ cells) and is thought to progress to invasive tumor.[302] By electron microscopy, GCNIS has evenly dispersed chromatin, intricate nucleoli, and sparse cytoplasmic organelles with prominent glycogen deposits. Occasional rudimentary intercellular junctions may be identified.[35,303-306] These features are essentially the same as those of seminoma.[307] The DNA content of GCNIS is similar to that of seminoma, usually in the triploid and hypotetraploid range.[51,308] Some of the genetic features of GCNIS have been previously mentioned.

Differential Diagnosis

GCNIS should be distinguished from specific forms of intratubular germ cell neoplasia. Intratubular seminoma fills and distends the tubules, whereas GCNIS is restricted to the basilar area, although the cells are histologically identical. Atypical germ cells that do not resemble GCNIS cells may also occur in seminiferous tubules. These cells may have large nuclei or be multinucleated. They lack the cytoplasmic clarity and nucleolar prominence of GCNIS cells and do not stain for the usual GCNIS markers. Although they may indicate a perturbation in testicular development, as evidence by increased frequency in cryptorchid boys and adjacent to testicular germ cell tumors, their significance is not clear, unlike GCNIS.[190,309]

Despite some controversy, GCNIS does not occur in prepubertal patients except for those with disorders of sex development. Many purported cases represent germ cells with delayed maturation (Fig. 13.11). These cells may occur in young children who have conditions that place them at increased risk for germ cell tumors, including cryptorchidism, gonadal dysgenesis, Down syndrome, and undervirilization syndromes.[285-287,310] They, however, are distinguished from GCNIS by their nonbasilar location in the tubules (Fig. 13.11) and tendency to cluster in areas of the parenchyma. More recently, "pre-GCNIS" has been put forth as a lesion intermediate between maturation delay and GCNIS.[23] It differs from them by having the lesional cells in both basilar and nonbasilar loci (Fig. 13.12) and, unlike maturation delay, is associated with expression of stem cell factor in the affected tubules, a feature shared by GCNIS. The full clinical significance of maturation delay is not clear, meaning it is not known how frequently it progresses to an invasive germ cell tumor. It is important to distinguish such cells from GCNIS because it is known that GCNIS will progress in virtually all cases. If GCNIS or pre-GCNIS is found in a prepubertal patient, it is in the context of a disorder of sex development.[311] Pre-GCNIS in patients with a disorder of sex development has also been termed *infantile GCNIS*.[312]

Prognosis

The practical importance of GCNIS is its progression to an invasive germ cell tumor (either seminomatous or nonseminomatous) in about 50% of cases within 5 years after identification.[313] Only a small fraction of patients remain free of an invasive tumor by 7 or 8 years of follow-up (Fig. 13.13), although some patients may not develop a tumor for more than 15 years.[314,315] Furthermore, there is no documented case of spontaneous regression of typical GCNIS.[315] GCNIS is identified with increased frequency in

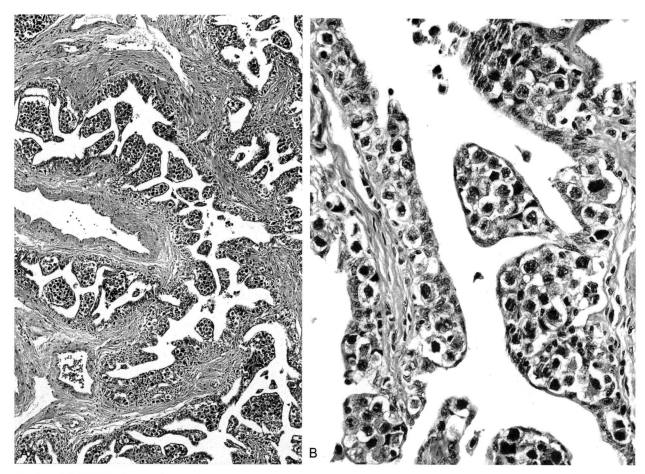

Fig. 13.7 (A and B) GCNIS cells have extended in a pagetoid fashion into the rete testis, with a layer of rete epithelium stretched over them.

patients with cryptorchidism, a previous history of a testicular germ cell tumor, gonadal dysgenesis, androgen insensitivity syndrome, and infertility.[35,193,194,197,198,220,224,316-325] GCNIS is also identified in the residual seminiferous tubules of virtually every postpubertal patient with a testicular germ cell tumor, with the exceptions of spermatocytic tumor, prepubertal-type teratoma/dermoid cyst/epidermoid cyst, and prepubertal-type yolk sac tumor.[30,280,326-329] The prepubertal-type germ cell tumors, as mentioned previously, lack association with GCNIS. In our opinion, many reported cases in children (Figs. 13.14 and 13.15) represent reactive enlargement of nonneoplastic germ cells induced by a mass lesion, as described by Hawkins and Hicks, atypical but nonneoplastic germ cells of unknown significance, or examples of delayed maturation of germ cells.[330]

Biopsy Diagnosis

Testicular biopsies are a sensitive method for detecting GCNIS. Fixatives such as Bouin, B-5, and Stieve enhance cytologic detail and may permit easier detection of GCNIS compared with formalin fixation. Formalin, Bouin, and Stieve fixatives permit immunohistochemical detection of placental alkaline phosphatase, whereas Cleland fluid yields inconsistent results.[1] Nonformalin fixation may result in weaker immunohistochemical staining, so formalin may be preferred if immunohistochemical staining is expected.[277] Berthelsen and Skakkebaek concluded that one or two 3-mm biopsies of a testis harboring GCNIS will detect virtually every case, although rare false-negative results do occur (0.3% in one study of 1859 biopsies that were initially interpreted as negative).[200,331]

Two site biopsies have a 17% improvement in sensitivity over one site and have been recommended as standard.[332] Another study supported three biopsies, each 5 mm in length, as optimal.[221] In cases of severe atrophy, with obliteration of many tubules, it may be necessary to sample the region near the hilum, where GCNIS is more frequently preserved within the epithelium of the rete testis.[201] Recently, some authors have considered OCT3/4 immunohistochemistry mandatory for the evaluation of testis biopsies, as it identifies GCNIS in approximately 20% more cases than hematoxylin and eosin staining alone.[277] It should be noted that positivity for immunohistochemical markers, including OCT3/4 and D2-40, may be seen before 2 years of age in the absence of GCNIS, so, in younger patients, positive immunohistochemical staining alone does not indicate a positive diagnosis.[333] Potential indications for screening biopsies include patients with cryptorchidism (2% to 4% positivity for GCNIS), a prior testicular germ cell tumor (4% to 5% positivity), somatosexual ambiguity (25% positivity), and, less strongly, oligospermic infertility (0% to 1% positivity).[195,268,276,315,332,334] A recent study of 4130 germ cell tumor patients found a rate of metachronous germ cell tumor of 1.9% in the cohort who had prior screening biopsies (and treatment if positive) and 3.1% in the unscreened cohort, but this did not reach statistical significance.[334] Sperm concentration, contralateral testis volume, and ultrasound echo pattern have been proposed to estimate the risk for contralateral GCNIS in germ cell tumor patients and to select patients for biopsy.[335]

GCNIS in a biopsy from a patient with retroperitoneal germ cell tumor probably indicates the regression of a prior invasive tumor

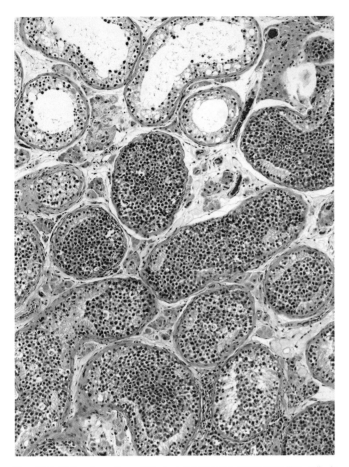

Fig. 13.8 Distension of seminiferous tubules by seminoma-like cells is referred to as "intratubular seminoma."

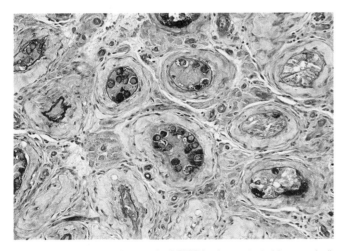

Fig. 13.9 Cytoplasmic glycogen in GCNIS is demonstrated by a periodic acid-Schiff stain.

that metastasized to the retroperitoneum.[336,337] Therefore, a patient with presumed primary germ cell tumor of the retroperitoneum may benefit from testicular biopsy.[196]

Treatment

Because of the high rate of progression of GCNIS to invasive testicular germ cell tumor, these patients should receive appropriate ablative treatment, either orchiectomy or low-dose external beam radiation.[338] Unilateral GCNIS is usually managed by orchiectomy and bilateral GCNIS with radiation. Because GCNIS is very radiosensitive, low doses are used, permitting preservation of androgen function. Chemotherapy, often given to patients with metastatic disease from a contralateral testicular tumor, may ablate GCNIS in the remaining testis but is not a consistently effective therapy.[276,339-342] In a German cooperative group study, radiation treatment was highly effective in curing GCNIS, although failures occur in about 2% of patients.[332,343] Chemotherapy reduced the incidence of subsequent germ cell neoplasia, but was much less effective than radiotherapy.[343]

Seminoma

Clinical Features

Seminoma is the most common pure testicular germ cell tumor, and pure seminoma accounts for about 50% of all cases, although its relative proportion may be declining.[344-346] In one study, the percentage of seminomas decreased from 52% to 43% over the 20-year study period.[347] It occurs in patients at an average age of 40 years, which is about 10 years older than those with nonseminomatous germ cell tumor.[39,55] African Americans may have an earlier age of onset.[348] Most patients present with a painless testicular mass, but there may be a dull, aching sensation. Up to 11% have normal-sized or atrophic testes.[349] Occasional patients (2% to 3%) present with symptoms of metastases, usually back pain caused by retroperitoneal involvement, but gastrointestinal bleeding, bone pain, central nervous system dysfunction, dyspnea and cough, and other symptoms may rarely be presenting complaints.[17] Gynecomastia may occur as a result of elevation of serum hCG caused by intermingled syncytiotrophoblast elements in seminoma and is rarely a presenting feature.[350] Very rarely, a paraendocrine form of exophthalmos can be a presenting complaint, as can paraneoplastic hypercalcemia, hemolytic anemia, and limbic encephalopathy.[351-355] About 30% of seminoma patients have metastases at the time of diagnosis, and this is probably decreasing as a result of an overall trend for earlier detection of germ cell tumors.[39,347]

Patients with seminoma usually lack serum AFP and hCG elevations that occur commonly in patients with nonseminomatous germ cell tumors. AFP levels should be normal, although concomitant liver disease (including seminomatous metastases to the liver) may cause modest AFP elevation, and "borderline" elevated AFP levels have been seen in some cases without evidence of nonseminomatous elements.[356,357] Most oncologists regard significant AFP elevation in a patient with apparently pure testicular seminoma as evidence of nonseminomatous elements and treat accordingly. About 10% to 20% of patients with clinical stage I "pure" testicular seminoma have elevated serum hCG, and 25% or more with advanced seminoma have hCG elevations.[358] At initial diagnosis, 7% to 25% of patients with seminoma have elevated hCG.[223,356,359-363] If blood is sampled from the testicular vein, 80% to 85% of patients have elevated hCG.[364,365] Such elevation reflects the presence of intermingled syncytiotrophoblast elements in these tumors, and the elevations are generally modest. Although rare, large seminomas with abundant syncytiotrophoblast cells may produce elevations of over 4000 IU/L.[366] Elevations of serum hCG exceeding 40 IU/L have been correlated with a poorer prognosis, although this is controversial.[359,367,368] Peripheral venous elevations of hCG have been correlated with larger tumors, perhaps explaining the relationship of elevated hCG with adverse prognostic features.[365] Elevation of serum levels of lactate dehydrogenase, PLAP, and neuron-specific enolase may also occur in patients with seminoma. Such elevations, however, are neither specific nor

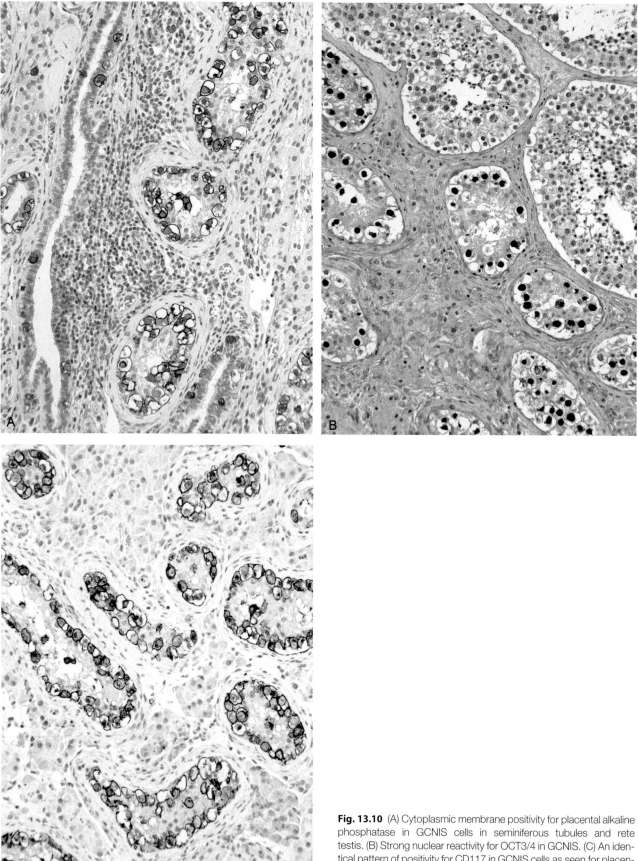

Fig. 13.10 (A) Cytoplasmic membrane positivity for placental alkaline phosphatase in GCNIS cells in seminiferous tubules and rete testis. (B) Strong nuclear reactivity for OCT3/4 in GCNIS. (C) An identical pattern of positivity for CD117 in GCNIS cells as seen for placental alkaline phosphatase.

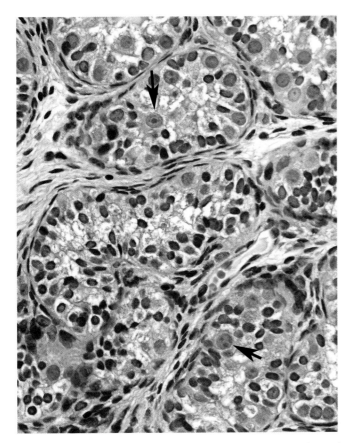

Fig. 13.11 Delayed maturation of germ cells. Gonocyte-like cells *(arrows)* are present in the center and parabasal positions.

especially sensitive, which limits their clinical utility.[358,367,369-372] MicroRNA-based evaluation for miR-371-3 and miR-367 as a potentially more sensitive marker of tumor recurrence is currently being investigated.[373,374]

Pathologic Findings

Grossly, seminoma is usually cream to tan to pale pink and often multinodular (Fig. 13.16), with occasional yellow foci of necrosis. Infrequently, necrosis is extensive. In some cases, the tumor is diffuse, fleshy, and encephaloid, similar to testicular lymphoma (Fig. 13.17). In contrast with lymphoma, however, only about 10% of seminomas extend into paratesticular structures.[375] Intraparenchymal hemorrhage may cause red discoloration.[34] The cut surface usually bulges from the surrounding parenchyma (Fig. 13.16). Punctate foci of hemorrhage often correspond to intermingled foci of syncytiotrophoblast elements.[376] A fibrous consistency is uncommon but results when prominent fibrous septa develop in the tumor or if there is extensive intratumoral sclerosis.

Microscopically, seminoma is usually arranged in a diffuse, sheetlike pattern interrupted by branching, fibrous septa containing an inflammatory infiltrate (Fig. 13.18) consisting chiefly of lymphocytes but often containing plasma cells and sometimes eosinophils. Distinct nodules may be apparent, sometimes with confluent growth imparting a lobulated pattern. In some cases, a prominent cordlike arrangement of cells is present (Fig. 13.19), often at the periphery of nodules showing a sheetlike pattern. Foci of intertubular growth may be seen, with preservation of seminiferous tubules. This pattern is usually most apparent at the

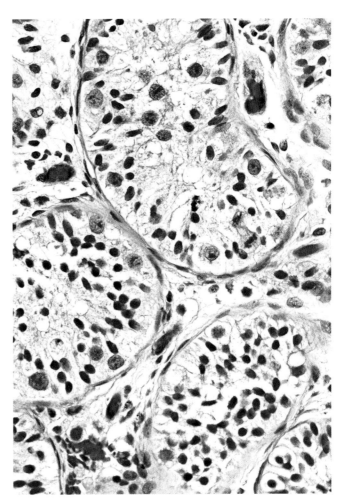

Fig. 13.12 "Pre-GCNIS" gonocyte-like cells occupy both central and basilar loci in the tubules. Simultaneous expression of stem cell factor (KIT-ligand, *not shown*) in the same tubule is also required.

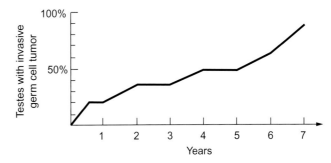

Fig. 13.13 Follow-up of patients with GCNIS on biopsy. About 90% have invasive tumor after 7 years. (Data from Skakkebaek NE, Berthelsen JG, Visfeldt J. Clinical aspects of testicular carcinoma-in-situ. *Int J Androl.* 1981;4 Suppl s4:153–160).

periphery of neoplastic nodules and may be associated with rete testis invasion and aggressive behavior.[377] In rare seminomas, an intertubular pattern may predominate (Fig. 13.20), with well-preserved seminiferous tubules even in the central portions of the neoplasm. Such cases are prone to being overlooked because they do not destroy the seminiferous tubules, and they often do not form a discrete gross mass.[378] The presence of a lymphocytic infiltrate may be a clue to intertubular seminoma (Fig. 13.20). This

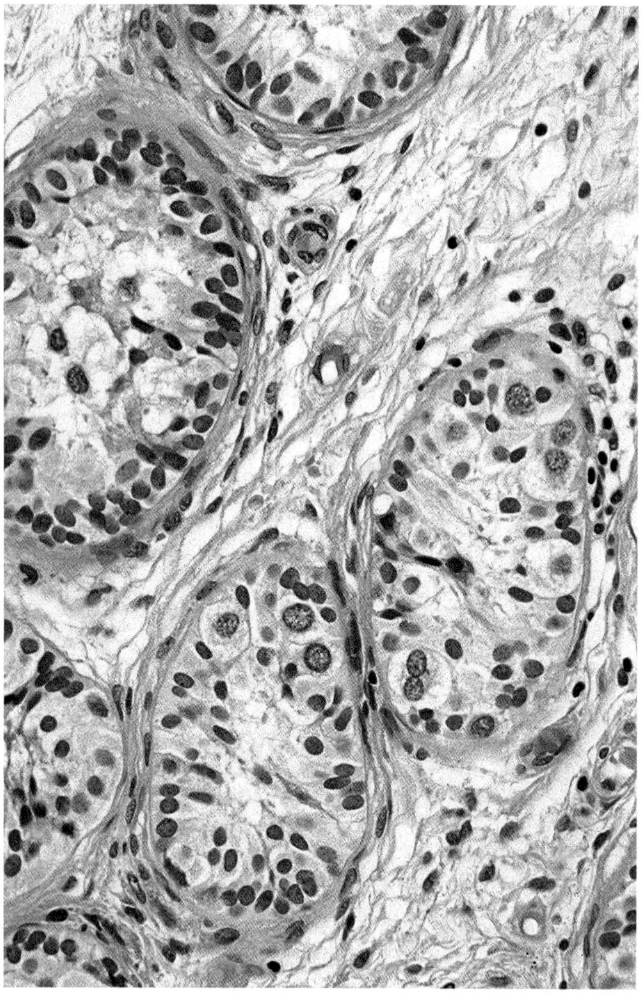

Fig. 13.14 Abnormal germ cells, some binucleated, adjacent to teratoma in a pediatric patient. These cells lack the features of GCNIS.

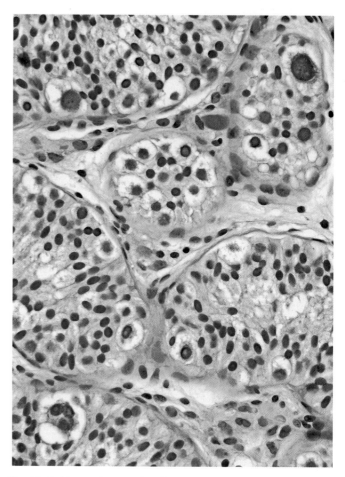

Fig. 13.15 Abnormal germ cells adjacent to teratoma in a pediatric patient. These cells lack the features of GCNIS.

pattern is much more common, however, in testicular lymphoma. With time, many seminomas develop foci of scarring. Hyalinized deposits of collagen may separate the neoplastic cells into small nests resembling solid pseudotubules (Fig. 13.21). Extensive collagen deposits may result in broad scars with only a few scattered neoplastic cells. Calcification and even ossification may rarely occur in hyalinized fibrous trabeculae of seminoma.[379] Rarely, seminoma may show a distinctly tubular pattern in which a palisade-like arrangement of neoplastic cells occurs at the periphery of tubule-like structures that may contain loosely cohesive neoplastic cells in their "lumens" (Fig. 13.22).[380-383] Seminoma may also develop intercellular edema with separation of neoplastic cells and formation of microcystic spaces (Figs. 13.23 and 13.24). These spaces are generally, but not always, irregular in outline and frequently contain visible edema fluid and intracystic exfoliated neoplastic cells that contrast with the "cleaner," more round and regular microcystic spaces commonly identified in yolk sac tumor.[384] Foci of coagulative necrosis are present in about one-half of seminomas and may be extensive in a minority of cases.[349]

A lymphoid infiltrate is a virtually constant feature of seminoma and is usually most evident in perivascular areas and around fibrous trabeculae, which also contain many capillaries (Fig. 13.25). Lymphocytes are also frequently intermingled with the seminoma cells elsewhere. A florid lymphoid reaction, with formation of germinal

centers, occurs in a minority of cases, but most of the lymphocytes in seminomas are T cells.[385-391] Ultrastructural studies have demonstrated a cytolytic effect of the lymphocytes on the seminoma cells, correlating with the observation of some investigators of a better prognosis in cases associated with a prominent lymphocytic reaction.[390,392]

A variable granulomatous reaction occurs in up to 50% of seminomas. In most cases, it consists of small clusters of epithelioid histiocytes scattered among neoplastic cells (Fig. 13.25). Langhans-type giant cells and other multinucleated giant cells may be present. Intratubular collections of epithelioid histiocytes may also be seen. Rarely, the granulomatous reaction can be extensive and virtually efface the neoplasm (Fig. 13.26); in such cases, it may be difficult to distinguish a florid granulomatous reaction in a seminoma from granulomatous orchitis, and careful search for residual seminoma and GCNIS is indicated. Intravascular granulomas have been reported in 15% of seminomas but were not a significant predictor of tumor recurrence.[393]

The cells of seminoma have generally clear to lightly eosinophilic cytoplasm, measuring 15 to 25 µm in diameter. The nuclei are relatively uniform, polygonal, usually centrally or slightly eccentrically placed, with finely granular chromatin and one or two prominent nucleoli (Fig. 13.27). Many nuclei have a relatively flat edge that has been described as "squared-off," lending the nuclei a "boxy" appearance. The nuclear membranes are irregularly thickened. The cell borders are typically well defined in adequately fixed specimens (Fig. 13.27). Abundant cytoplasm separates the

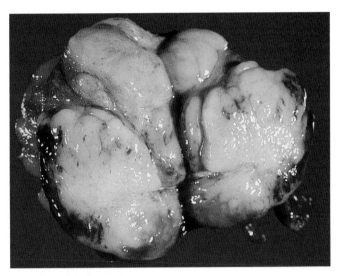

Fig. 13.16 Cut surface of a seminoma demonstrating a cream-colored, multinodular neoplasm bulging from the surrounding testicular parenchyma.

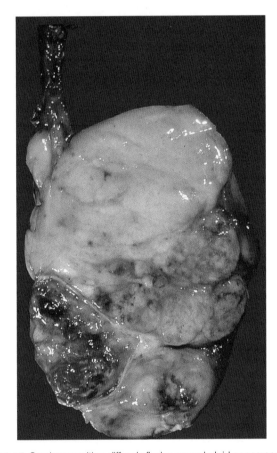

Fig. 13.17 Seminoma with a diffusely fleshy, encephaloid appearance and foci of hemorrhage. (Courtesy of RH Young, MD, Harvard Medical School, Boston, MA).

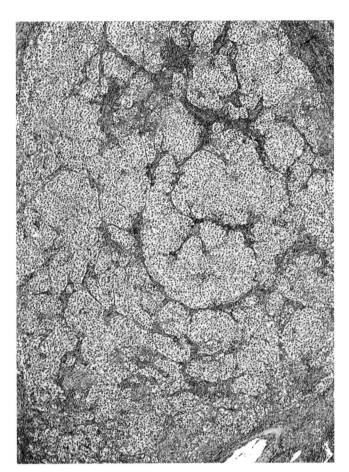

Fig. 13.18 Sheetlike pattern of a seminoma is interrupted by branching, fibrous septa containing lymphocytes.

nuclear fragments. Such isolated foci, in the absence of distinct epithelial differentiation, do not exclude a diagnosis of seminoma. Rarely seminoma cells develop intracytoplasmic vacuoles that cause a signet ring cell morphology (Fig. 13.30).[394] This may be a focal finding in an otherwise usual-appearing tumor. We have also seen prominent aggregates of glycogen create a signet ring cell appearance (Fig. 13.31).[394]

Mitotic figures in seminoma are prominent, and in the past, when present in sufficient numbers, were considered as evidence of "anaplastic seminoma."[170] Now it is clear that mitotic rate in seminoma does not correlate with prognosis.[395-397] Furthermore, there is no immunohistochemical difference between typical and "anaplastic" seminomas.[398] Use of the term *anaplastic seminoma* is therefore discouraged. Although some seminomas behave more aggressively than most, it remains unclear if such cases can be identified prospectively. Tickoo et al. described cases of "seminoma with atypia" based on nuclear pleomorphism and crowding, paucity of lymphocytes, and darker-staining cytoplasm.[399] In their experience, such tumors were more likely to present at advanced clinical stage, to express CD30, and to lose KIT expression. It remains unclear, however, if such cases should receive different treatment.

Seminoma With Syncytiotrophoblast Cells

Syncytiotrophoblast cells are present in 10% to 20% of seminomas.[58] The morphology of these cells is variable, ranging from typical syncytiotrophoblast cells with cytoplasmic lacunae and multinucleation (Fig. 13.32) to large mononucleated or binucleated cells that may not be easily distinguished from the background

nuclei so that overlapping nuclei are usually not seen. Occasionally, seminoma displays foci of increased cellular atypia with less well-defined cytoplasmic membranes, darker cytoplasm, and enlarged, crowded nuclei (Fig. 13.28). These changes may impart a plasmacytoid appearance to the tumor cells (Fig. 13.29). Such changes may be seen in association with early necrosis and contain pyknotic

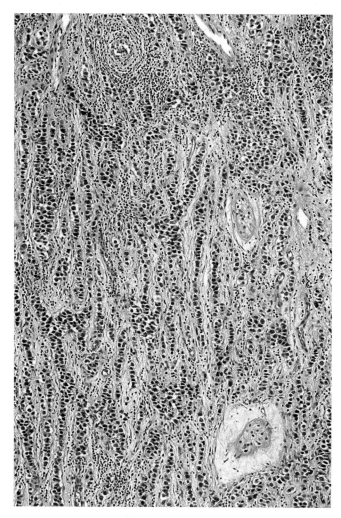

Fig. 13.19 Prominent cordlike pattern in a seminoma.

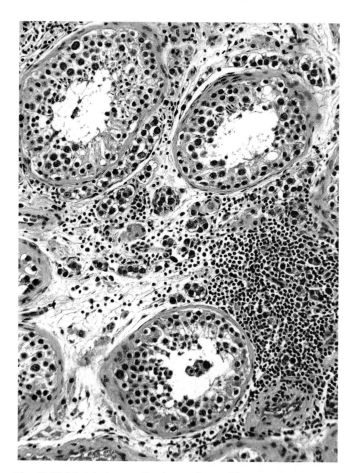

Fig. 13.20 Intertubular growth of a seminoma. There are small nests of seminoma cells between tubules. The lymphocytes are a helpful clue.

seminoma cells but that are highlighted by immunostains against hCG.[400] Intermediate between these extremes are cells containing multiple nuclei in a "mulberry" pattern. Syncytiotrophoblast cells are often located close to capillaries, and microhemorrhages may be seen in these foci. Unlike choriocarcinoma, the syncytiotrophoblast cells are not intermingled with a mononucleated trophoblast cell component but are randomly admixed as single cells or small clusters with seminoma cells. With hCG immunohistochemistry, intratubular trophoblasts can be detected in a substantial fraction of seminoma cases, indicating that differentiation toward trophoblastic elements may occur before invasion.[401]

Special Studies
Glycogen is usually prominent in seminoma (Fig. 13.33), and most cases show immunoreactivity for PLAP, generally in a peripheral, "membranous" staining pattern (Fig. 13.34A); cytoplasmic staining may also be identified.[41,281,402,403] Seminomas are uniformly reactive for OCT3/4 (Fig. 13.34C), a nuclear transcription factor identified in nonneoplastic stem cells and embryonic cells that plays an important role in the maintenance of a pluripotential capacity.[282,404,405] OCT3/4 staining is also seen in embryonal carcinoma but not in other testicular tumors.[50,282,404,405] Angiotensin-converting enzyme was demonstrated in 100% of 91 seminomas in one study.[296] Reactivity for CD117 (c-kit protein) occurs in most seminomas, with a cytoplasmic membrane

pattern similar to PLAP (Fig. 13.34B).[406,407] Podoplanin (D2-40) is positive (Fig. 13.35), as is SALL4, a general germ cell tumor marker.[408,409] The NANOG protein, a product of a gene located at 12p13, a region frequently amplified in testicular germ cell tumors, is similarly detectable by immunohistochemistry in GCNIS, seminoma, and embryonal carcinoma, but not in teratoma or yolk sac tumor.[46,410] SOX17, a nuclear transcription factor, was identified in 95% of seminomas but not in embryonal carcinomas.[49,300,301] Many seminomas also express limited degrees of cytokeratin immunoreactivity, although such staining may only be demonstrable using frozen sections, with frequent negativity in routinely processed tissue.[411] The most common cytokeratins in seminoma are cytokeratins 7, 8, and 18, although others, including cytokeratins 4, 17, and 19, can be identified occasionally.[411,412] Cytokeratin 20 is negative.[412] Epithelial membrane antigen (EMA) is only rarely expressed in seminoma, and the combination of positivity for PLAP and negativity for EMA and cytokeratin AE1/AE3 in formalin-fixed, paraffin-embedded tissue is a relatively specific pattern for seminoma.[41,170,412,413] Vimentin, LDH, and NSE may be present in seminoma but are not specific.[41,411,414] A minority of seminomas may stain for Leu-7, α-1-antitrypsin, desmin, and neurofilament protein.[41,411] Desmoplakins and desmoglein are usually present in seminoma.[411,415] The syncytiotrophoblast cells that occur in some seminomas contain hCG, and some cells containing hCG may not have an overtly "syncytiotrophoblastic" appearance in routine sections.[41,57-59,416] CD30 is usually negative in seminoma, which contrasts with its virtually uniform presence in embryonal carcinoma, except after

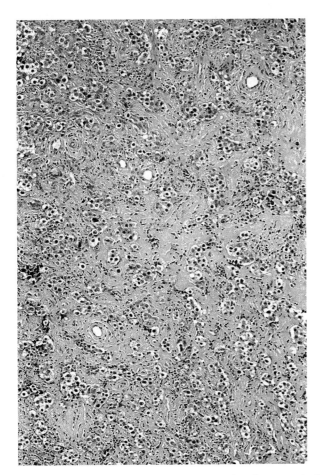

Fig. 13.21 Scarring in a seminoma creates a pattern of small nests and solid pseudotubules separated by hyalinized stroma.

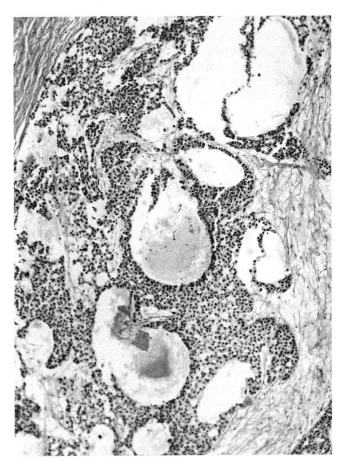

Fig. 13.23 Edema in a seminoma creating an irregular, microcystic pattern.

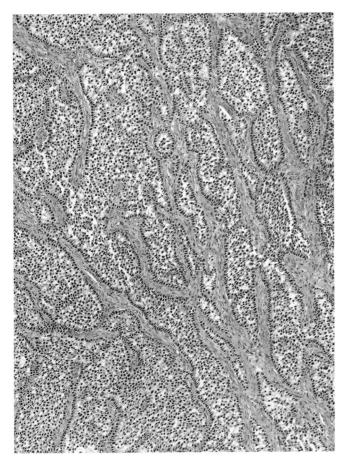

Fig. 13.22 Tubular pattern of a seminoma, with palisade-like arrangement of cells at the periphery of tubule-like structures.

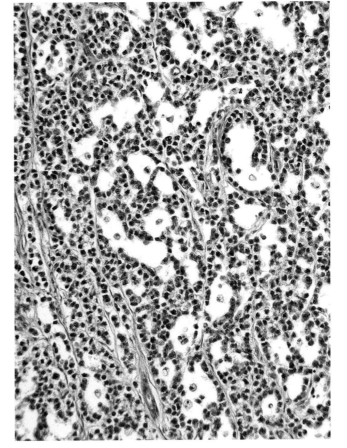

Fig. 13.24 Microcystic pattern in a seminoma.

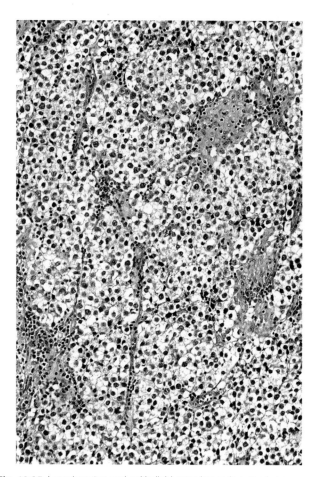

Fig. 13.25 Lymphocytes and epithelioid granulomas in a seminoma.

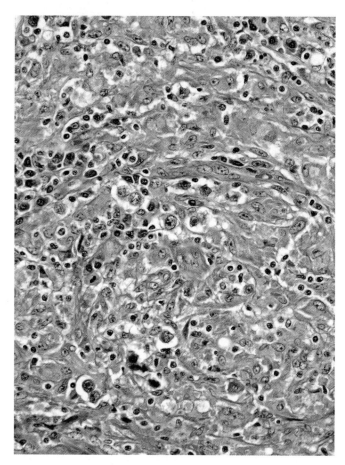

Fig. 13.26 An extensive granulomatous reaction in a seminoma, leaving only rare tumor cells.

chemotherapy, in which case loss of CD30 expression is frequently seen.[412,417]

Ultrastructurally, seminoma has closely apposed cytoplasmic membranes that usually show only sparse, primitive, intercellular junctions. The cellular organelles consist of scattered mitochondria, occasional cisternae of smooth and rough endoplasmic reticulum, ribosomes and polyribosomes, occasional membrane-bound lysosome-like structures, and occasional Golgi bodies. Glycogen may be present in large quantities but may also be sparse. It is common for the cytoplasmic organelles to be polarized eccentrically in the cytoplasm. The nuclei are round and have evenly dispersed chromatin and intricate, large nucleoli.[60,418,419] Occasional seminomas that are typical-appearing at the light microscopic level may show evidence of epithelial differentiation, with small, extracellular lumens, microvilli, and well-defined junctional complexes.[60] Such cases, despite "transitional" morphology at the ultrastructural level, appear to behave as typical seminoma.[60]

The DNA content of seminoma is generally in the triploid to hypotetraploid range and is greater than that of nonseminomatous tumors.[51,62,420] The DNA content of seminoma with syncytiotrophoblast cells does not differ from seminoma lacking them, supporting classification as seminoma.[421] Evolution of seminoma to other types of germ cell tumor may occur as a result of gene loss.[51,62,420,422] As in many testicular germ cell tumors, seminoma frequently contains an isochromosome derived from the short arms of chromosome 12, i(12p).[423,424] Numerous other cytogenetic abnormalities have also been described; certain chromosomes are commonly overrepresented (1q, 7, 8, 12, 14q, 15q, 17, 21q,

22q, and X) and others underrepresented (3, 4, 5, 10, 11, 12q, 13q, 16, 18q, and Y).[423,425-427]

A number of molecular observations are reported in seminoma, including absence of Fas, loss of p18^{INK4C}, upregulation of cyclin E, cyclin D2 expression, and activation of p16^{INK4} by hypermethylation.[70,428-430] Activating exon 17 mutations of the *KIT* gene are seen in 12% to 13% of cases and about 20% have *KIT* gene amplification.[431,432] Seminomas are reported to have loss of Notch 1, Jagged 2, and Fhit expression, show *SMAD4* and *ras* mutations, and express DAZL1 protein, hst-1, N-myc, Krüppel-like factor 4, and *MAGE* genes.[298,433-443] The *MAGE* gene products, along with NY-ESO-1, are members of a group known as "cancer testis antigens" which show variable, low-level expression in seminoma.[444-446] These antigens are consistently strongly expressed in spermatocytic tumors and are infrequently expressed by nonseminomatous germ cell tumors and GCNIS.[444-446] Gene expression studies have confirmed significant upregulation of genes previously known to be upregulated in seminoma such as *POU5F1* (*OCT4*), *KIT*, *ALPL*, and *PROM1* and have also identified upregulation of a number of other genes including *BOB1*, *CD9*, *THY1*, and *PUM2*.[447]

Differential Diagnosis

Seminoma can be misinterpreted as the solid pattern of embryonal carcinoma, especially in poorly fixed preparations. The formation of glands, true tubules, or papillae argues against the diagnosis of seminoma; the nuclei of seminoma are more uniform, less crowded, and more evenly spaced than those of embryonal carcinoma, which are pleomorphic, irregularly shaped, crowded, and appear to abut or

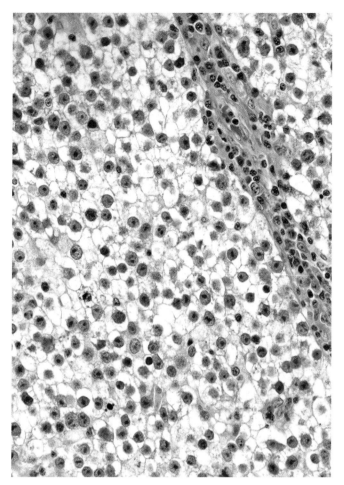

Fig. 13.27 Seminoma cells with clear cytoplasm, well-defined cell borders, and nuclei with one or two prominent nucleoli. Lymphocytes are present in a fibrous septum, and some tumor nuclei have "squared-off" edges.

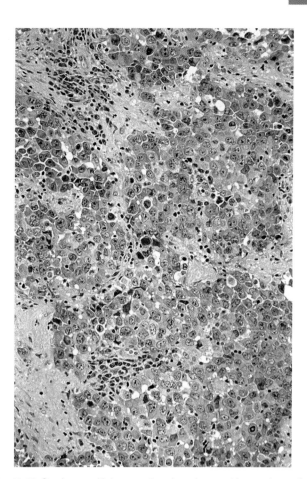

Fig. 13.28 Seminoma with increased nuclear pleomorphism and crowding and denser cytoplasm than usual.

even overlap. The cytoplasmic borders of seminoma are well defined and those of embryonal carcinoma are mostly poorly defined, with occasional exceptions in foci.[448] The cytoplasm of embryonal carcinoma is typically denser. Embryonal carcinoma lacks the regular fibrous septa of many seminomas. Cytokeratin reactivity is usually weaker and PLAP reactivity stronger in seminoma than in embryonal carcinoma. CD30 reactivity is rare in seminoma and positive in embryonal carcinoma, and CD30 immunohistochemistry may be especially useful in combination with CD117 (c-kit) to distinguish seminoma (CD30–/CD117+) from embryonal carcinoma (CD30+/CD117–).[283,412,449] Weak staining of embryonal carcinoma for c-kit has been seen in up to 32% of tumors in one study, however.[450] Podoplanin (M2A, D2-40), similar to CD117, is typically diffusely positive in seminoma and usually negative or focally reactive in embryonal carcinoma.[290,450-452] Monoclonal antibody 43-9F is reported to be strongly reactive in embryonal carcinoma and negative or only weakly positive in seminoma, but additional experience is necessary to confirm this finding.[453] An antibody to SOX2, a nuclear transcription factor, appears to be a highly sensitive nuclear marker for embryonal carcinoma and is consistently negative in seminoma.[49,283] A related protein, SOX17, in contrast, is positive in seminoma and negative in embryonal carcinoma.[49] Immunohistochemical staining for AP-2γ, another nuclear transcription factor, marks a higher percentage of nuclei in embryonal carcinoma than

seminoma, but is probably not of use in differentiating these two tumors, although it may, like OCT3/4, be a useful marker for the two as a group.[450] AFP is occasionally positive in embryonal carcinoma and is negative in seminoma.

The distinction of seminoma from spermatocytic tumor is discussed in the Spermatocytic Tumor section later in this chapter.

Yolk sac tumor with a solid pattern may mimic seminoma. Such cases are usually distinguished from seminoma by the presence of typical patterns of yolk sac tumor, the tendency for microcyst formation in the solid areas, intercellular bandlike deposits of basement membrane, intracellular hyaline globules, nuclear pleomorphism, and absence of lymphocytes and fibrous septa.[454] Edematous seminomas, however, may produce a microcystic pattern reminiscent of yolk sac tumor, but the cystic spaces are usually more irregular and contain edema fluid and exfoliated neoplastic cells, in contrast with those of yolk sac tumor, although there are exceptional seminomas with regular and uniform microcysts.[384] The typical polygonal cells of seminoma in microcystic areas, however, contrast with the flattened cellular profiles and more variable nuclear appearance of yolk sac tumor cells lining microcystic spaces. AFP is negative in seminoma and usually positive in yolk sac tumor; glypican-3 has a similar pattern of reactivity but is more sensitive for yolk sac tumor.[455-457] Cytokeratin is often negative or weak in seminoma (in routinely processed tissues), whereas it is almost always strongly positive in yolk sac tumor. OCT3/4 and podoplanin are strongly positive in seminoma but negative in yolk sac tumor. CD117 is not useful in this differential diagnosis because it is often positive in both.

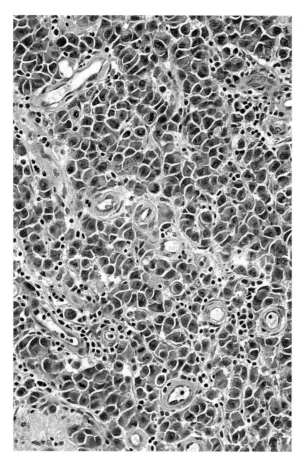

Fig. 13.29 Plasmacytoid seminoma. Many cells have dense cytoplasm and eccentric nuclei.

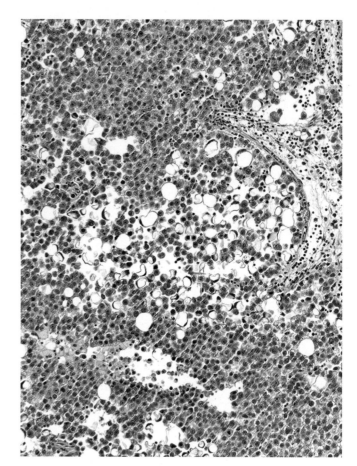

Fig. 13.30 Seminoma with signet ring cells.

Lymphoma must be distinguished from seminoma; most patients with testicular lymphoma are older than 50 years of age, whereas patients with seminoma are usually younger.[458-465] Bilateral involvement is more likely in lymphoma than in seminoma.[459,461-463,466] Lymphoma usually infiltrates the interstitium, preserving the seminiferous tubules, whereas most seminomas do not show as prominent a degree of intertubular growth, although there are exceptions.[378,461,462,467] GCNIS is seen in seminoma but not in lymphoma. Lymphoma often is more pleomorphic than seminoma and may be composed of cells with cleaved and irregularly shaped nuclei that stand in contrast with the polygonal and relatively uniform nuclei of seminoma. The cytoplasm of lymphoma is usually amphophilic and less distinct than that of seminoma. Immunostains directed against PLAP and OCT3/4 are positive in seminoma and negative in lymphoma, whereas leukocyte common antigen (LCA) and other lymphoid markers show opposite results.[41,413]

Rarely, seminoma with a tubular pattern may be confused with Sertoli cell tumor, a neoplasm that frequently has a tubular architecture.[8,380,381,383,468] The cytoplasmic clarity in seminoma is caused by glycogen, whereas lipid is mainly responsible for this appearance in Sertoli cell tumor. Most Sertoli cell tumors have low-grade cytologic atypia and infrequent mitotic figures that contrast with the high-grade atypia and conspicuous mitotic activity of seminoma. GCNIS is present in almost all seminomas but is not associated with Sertoli cell tumor. Tubular patterns in seminoma are usually focal but may be widespread in Sertoli cell tumor.[381] Immunostains for PLAP, OCT3/4, and SALL4 are positive in

seminoma but negative in Sertoli cell tumor, whereas inhibin and nuclear β-catenin are positive in a substantial proportion (but not all) of Sertoli cell tumors but negative in seminomas. This differential diagnosis may be further complicated by those Sertoli cell tumors that show a mostly diffuse growth pattern, frequently associated with a lymphocytic infiltrate.[469]

Treatment and Prognosis

Although patients with early seminoma (clinical stage I or nonbulky stage II) have traditionally been treated with orchiectomy and radiation to the paraaortic and paracaval nodes, frequently with ipsilateral pelvic nodal radiation (so-called "dogleg" field) (although the pelvic field component may not be necessary for clinical stage I patients), current American and European treatment guidelines for clinical stage I seminoma consider surveillance an appropriate option, with adjuvant treatment also being discussed.[470-476] The American National Comprehensive Cancer Network (NCCN) guidelines state that active surveillance is preferred, but they do not make recommendations between chemotherapy and radiation treatment.[475] In contrast, the European Association of Urology Guidelines state that surveillance and carboplatin chemotherapy are recommended and that radiotherapy is not recommended.[476] Stratification by risk factors has also been employed, with carboplatin recommended for patients with two risk factors (tumor size >4 cm and rete testis involvement) and surveillance for those with zero or one of these risk factors, and use of a nomogram considering these two factors has been proposed, but others have found this model for risk stratification to be inadequately predictive and have found only tumor size to be associated with recurrence.[477-479]

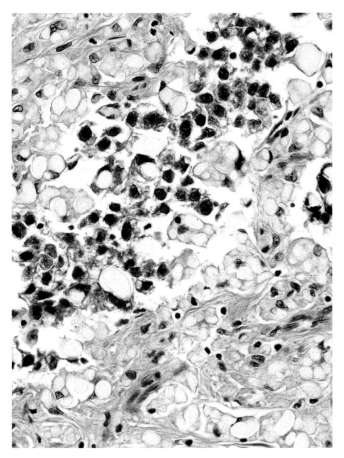

Fig. 13.31 Seminoma with prominent aggregates of glycogen creating a signet ring cell appearance. Many histiocytes with phagocytosed glycogen aggregates are also present.

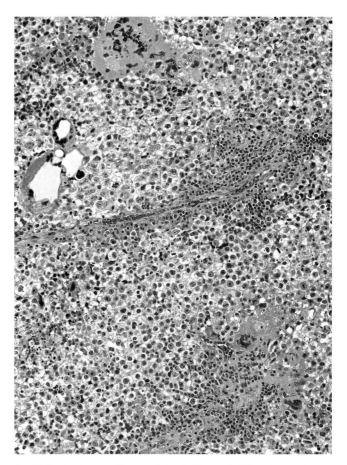

Fig. 13.32 Seminoma with syncytiotrophoblast cells. Intracytoplasmic lacunae are present in some of the syncytiotrophoblast cells.

Radiotherapy for seminoma is associated with a slight (hazard ratio 1.36) increased risk for second malignant neoplasms.[480] Most recurrences arise outside of the radiated field, in the mediastinum, cervical lymph nodes, or lungs.[472,481]

With the increasingly chosen option of surveillance for clinical stage I patients, 13% to 20% of patients will undergo relapse.[482-484] Nevertheless, chemotherapy salvages virtually all relapses, and therefore 5-year disease-specific survival for surveillance management approaches 100%.[484] About 92% of relapses are within the first 3 years, and 87% are detected by computed tomography (CT) (as opposed to tumor markers).[484]

Chemotherapy is recommended for patients with bulky retroperitoneal involvement or in more advanced stages. ("Bulky" is defined variously in different studies as metastases greater than 5 cm, 6 cm, or 10 cm in diameter.) There is an 87% progression-free survival for advanced-stage seminoma patients who are initially treated with chemotherapy, whereas such patients who are initially irradiated and then treated with chemotherapy for persistent disease have a 3-year progression-free survival of 69%.[485] A four-cycle etoposide and platinum regimen has been evaluated to attempt to limit bleomycin toxicity in patients with germ cell tumors and retroperitoneal disease, but these patients are four times more likely to have active cancer in the retroperitoneal specimen when compared with the standard three-cycle bleomycin, etoposide, and platinum treatment.[486]

A prominent lymphocytic reaction has been associated with improved prognosis.[487,488] Elevation of serum hCG levels may

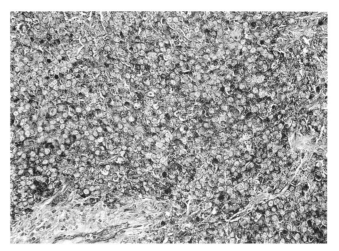

Fig. 13.33 Periodic acid-Schiff positivity in a seminoma, indicating abundant glycogen.

indicate a poorer prognosis, although there are contradictory results in the literature.[223,359,363,365,367,368,489,490] In one study, primary tumor size (>4 cm), testicular vascular invasion, rete testis invasion, tunica albuginea penetration, spermatic cord invasion, epididymis invasion, and vascular invasion of the cord were predictive of metastasis in univariate analysis, but only tumor size (>6 cm) and rete testis invasion were independently predictive in multivariate analysis.[491] Rete testis involvement was not

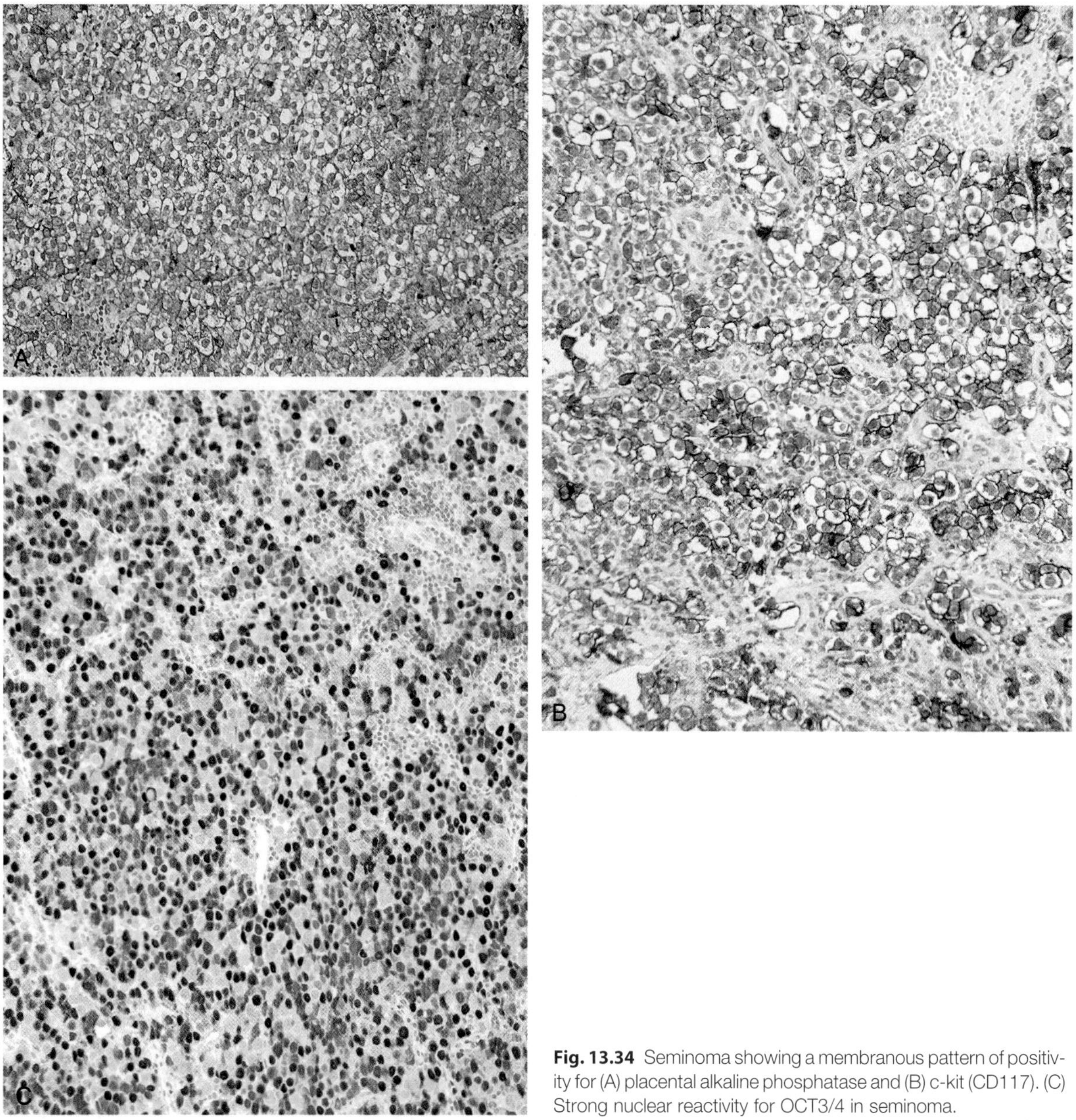

Fig. 13.34 Seminoma showing a membranous pattern of positivity for (A) placental alkaline phosphatase and (B) c-kit (CD117). (C) Strong nuclear reactivity for OCT3/4 in seminoma.

independently predictive of relapse of stage in other studies.[479,492] In a series of 1954 stage I seminoma patients in Denmark followed on a surveillance program, size, vascular invasion, and epididymis involvement were significant predictors of relapse.[493] Lymphovascular invasion, however, is often overdiagnosed in seminoma, with the rate of apparent lymphovascular invasion dependent on the handling of the gross specimen.[494] Immunohistochemical expression of p53, Ki67, CD30, and loss of CD117/c-kit expression in a group of 62 seminomas did not correlate with metastasis or other histopathologic risk factors for metastasis, unlike a different study.[399,495] In a mixed group of testicular germ cell tumors, high-level microsatellite instability by molecular analysis was significantly predictive of poorer prognosis, and a similarly significant but lower-magnitude difference was observed with loss of mismatch repair protein (MLH1) expression by immunohistochemistry.[496] In germ cell tumor patients undergoing postchemotherapy retroperitoneal lymph node dissection, the number of lymph nodes removed has prognostic significance with a calculated 2-year relapse-free probability of 90% when 10 lymph nodes are removed

compared with 97% when 50 lymph nodes are removed.[497] Patients with viable seminoma in postchemotherapy retroperitoneal lymph node dissection specimens have decreased 5-year survival, 54% in a recent series.[498]

Prognostic factors in patients with clinical stage I seminoma have been reviewed.[499,500] Rete testis invasion was associated with relapse in some studies, but lymphovascular invasion, young age, and preoperative hCG level were not associated with recurrence. It seems likely that the nonsignificance of lymphovascular invasion stems from the difficulty in judging true versus pseudoinvasion.[494] It would be useful to identify a subset of seminoma patients with a poor prognosis at an early stage, because it is likely that initial treatment with chemotherapy would improve the outcome in such a group. It is likely that the poor prognosis relates to the tendency of such cases to transform to nonseminomatous tumors, given the high frequency of nonseminomatous tumors at autopsy in patients who died after resection of pure testicular seminoma.[20,54]

Testis-sparing surgery, not typically considered appropriate for germ cell tumors, has been performed for small (20 mm or

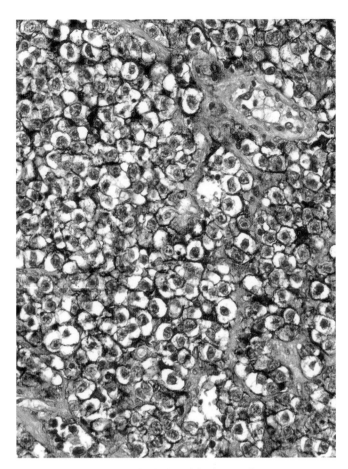

Fig. 13.35 Membranous podoplanin staining in a seminoma.

smaller), clinical stage I, synchronous or metachronous bilateral germ cell tumors to attempt to allow preservation of fertility.[501] Although testosterone production is consistently maintained, almost one-third of patients develop local recurrence, and only one-sixth achieve conception.[501] Frequent local recurrences are expected, as, in addition to the frequent presence of GCNIS in these patients, about one-fourth of germ cell tumors are multifocal, and multifocality can be present even in small tumors.[502]

Embryonal Carcinoma

Although very common in mixed germ cell tumors (occurring in 87% of nonseminomatous germ cell tumors,) embryonal carcinoma is less frequent as a pure testicular tumor, comprising only 2.3% of cases in a referral practice and about 10% of testicular tumors in two general series.[39,345,503] A decline in the reported proportion of pure embryonal carcinoma among testicular germ cell tumors is largely attributable to the recognition of foci of yolk sac tumor in such cases, leading to their categorization as mixed germ cell tumors. This finding reflects the capacity of embryonal carcinoma to differentiate into other forms of testicular neoplasia, as verified by experimental observations including tissue culture.[504-508] Embryonal carcinoma expresses the stage-specific embryonic antigen (SSEA) indicative of a primitive, undifferentiated stage of development, SSEA-3, but not SSEA-1, which indicates a more mature phenotype.[509]

Clinical Features

The peak incidence occurs at about 30 years of age, and embryonal carcinoma is distinctly rare in prepubertal children and likely

limited to those with a disorder of sexual development.[39,510-513] It usually presents as a testicular mass, with gynecomastia or symptoms of metastases each occurring in about 10% of cases.[514] Rare cases may present with sudden death caused by massive tumor thromboemboli to the lungs.[515,516] However, metastases are clinically or radiographically evident in about 40% of patients at presentation, and two-thirds of patients who are pathologically staged have metastases.[514] As in seminoma, limbic encephalopathy may be a rare form of presentation.[355]

Serum AFP elevation in embryonal carcinoma is usually the result of misclassification of mixed germ cell tumor (embryonal carcinoma and yolk sac tumor), and it is uncommon for morphologically pure embryonal carcinoma to be associated with serum AFP elevation.[503,517] Many embryonal carcinomas are associated with syncytiotrophoblast cells, accounting for serum hCG elevation in 60% of cases.[517] PLAP, LDH, and CA19-9 levels may also be elevated.[518,519]

Pathologic Features

Grossly, embryonal carcinoma is usually poorly circumscribed and gray-white to pale yellow or tan with prominent areas of hemorrhage and necrosis (Fig. 13.36). Microscopically, there are three major patterns, solid, glandular, and papillary, all of which consist of cohesive groups of primitive, anaplastic epithelial cells. In the solid pattern, the cells are arranged in diffuse sheets (Fig. 13.37).[448] In the tubular or glandular pattern, well-defined, glandlike or tubule-like structures are formed by epithelium varying from cuboidal to columnar (Fig. 13.38). Anastomosing (Fig. 13.39) or sievelike (Fig. 13.40) patterns may be seen. The luminal spaces are cleftlike or round. In the papillary pattern, the papillae may or may not have stromal cores (Fig. 13.41). When vascular stromal cores are cut transversely, a radial arrangement of tumor cells at their periphery resembles the endodermal sinus-like structures of yolk sac tumor ("pseudoendodermal sinuses"; Figs. 13.42 and 13.43). Uncommon patterns include nested, micropapillary, pseudopapillary, and blastocyst-like (Fig. 13.44).[376,448] A "double-layered" pattern of embryonal carcinoma has also been described in which a papillary arrangement of embryonal carcinoma is accompanied by a parallel layer of flattened neoplastic epithelium (Fig. 13.45).[520] This pattern, however, is more accurately classified as embryonal carcinoma with yolk sac tumor and should therefore be regarded as a mixed germ cell tumor.

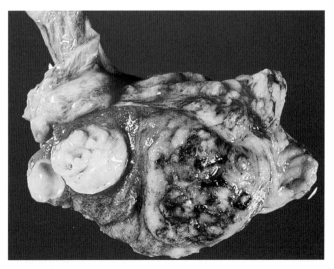

Fig. 13.36 The large yellow-tan nodule is embryonal carcinoma, showing areas of hemorrhage and necrosis.

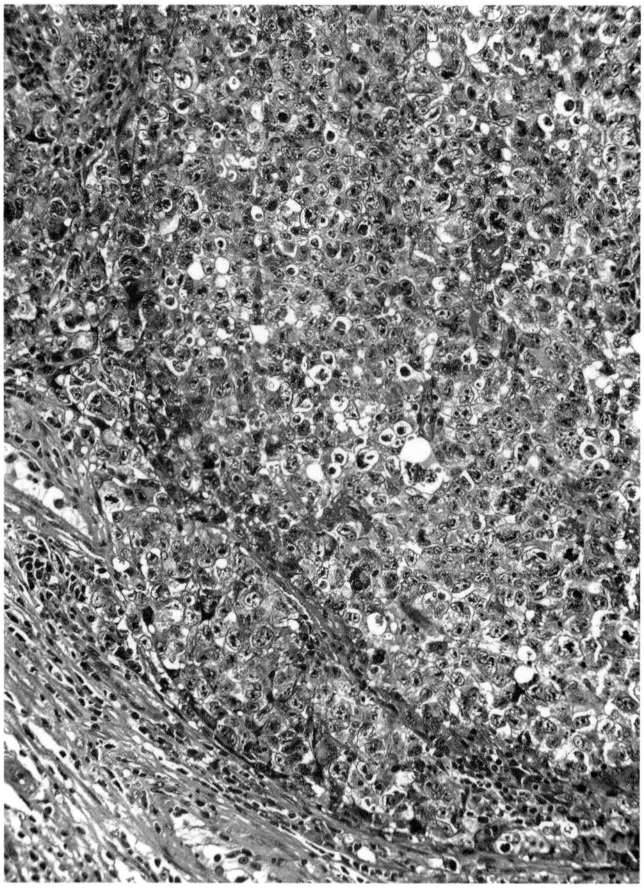

Fig. 13.37 Embryonal carcinoma with a solid pattern.

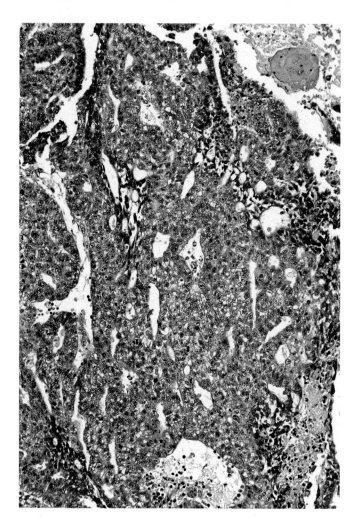

Fig. 13.38 Embryonal carcinoma with a glandular pattern.

At high magnification, the cells have variable staining, abundant cytoplasm, and large, vesicular, irregular nuclei with prominent macronucleoli (Fig. 13.46). The cell borders are characteristically ill defined, unlike seminoma, and the nuclei are often crowded, appearing to abut or overlap. Karyorrhectic fragments are frequent in the background, and the mitotic rate is high. Potentially deceptive histologic features occur in some cases, including foci of cells with clear cytoplasm and well-defined cytoplasmic borders, possibly causing concern for seminoma (Fig. 13.47). Glands lined by tall, columnar cells may be mistaken for teratoma (Fig. 13.48). In both circumstances, the pleomorphic nature of the nuclei supports embryonal carcinoma.[448,521] Occasionally, the tumor cells may have clear cytoplasmic vacuoles giving the tumor a "lipoid" appearance (Fig. 13.49).

Prominent foci of eosinophilic, coagulative necrosis are common in all forms of embryonal carcinoma. Cells with smudged, hyperchromatic nuclei are distinctive but nonspecific (Fig. 13.50). These commonly appear "applied" to the periphery of tumor nests ("appliqué" appearance).[448] Such cells are considered to be degenerate embryonal carcinoma cells, but they may be misinterpreted as syncytiotrophoblast cells, thereby leading to a misdiagnosis of choriocarcinoma. Unlike syncytiotrophoblast cells, however, these degenerate embryonal carcinoma cells lack hCG and are not usually associated with hemorrhage.

The capacity of embryonal carcinoma to generate a minor amount of undifferentiated neoplastic stroma (Fig. 13.51) is widely recognized.[25,375] The stroma may either be reactive, fibrous, and nonneoplastic or a neoplastic derivative of the tumor with atypia and mitotic activity.[448] Although some regard neoplastic stroma within the spectrum of embryonal carcinoma, rationalizing that it is part and parcel of a primitive neoplasm recapitulating an early phase of embryonic development, we believe that neoplastic stroma should be considered a teratoma component. Based on the experience of the BTTP, no significant prognostic difference was noted in embryonal carcinoma with or without a stromal component, but these data were obtained in an era before effective chemotherapy.[24] Because teratoma components in the testis are associated with an increased risk for persistent tumor in metastatic sites after chemotherapy, those BTTP data should have no bearing on current classification.

In about one-fourth of cases, embryonal carcinoma is associated with an intratubular embryonal carcinoma component, which is typically extensively necrotic, having a comedocarcinoma-like appearance (Figs. 13.52 and 13.53).[448] Such necrotic foci may undergo dystrophic calcification leading to the formation of so-called "hematoxylin-staining bodies."[522] Such coarse intratubular calcifications in scarred areas are excellent evidence of a regressed germ cell tumor.[522,523]

The identification of vascular invasion in nonseminomatous germ cell tumors (including embryonal carcinoma) may be helpful in deciding whether patients with clinical stage I tumors are appropriate candidates for "surveillance only" management and is a key

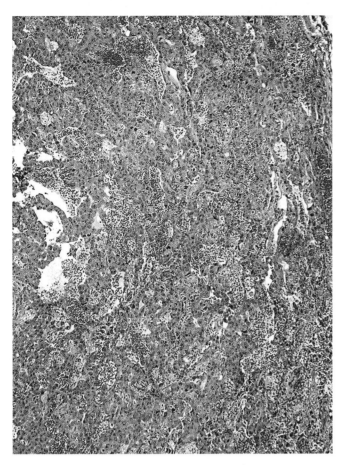

Fig. 13.39 Embryonal carcinoma with an anastomosing pattern.

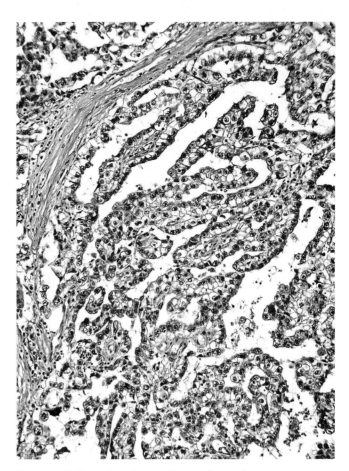

Fig. 13.41 Embryonal carcinoma with a papillary pattern.

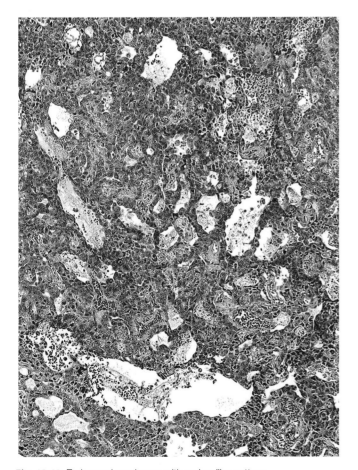

Fig. 13.40 Embryonal carcinoma with a sievelike pattern.

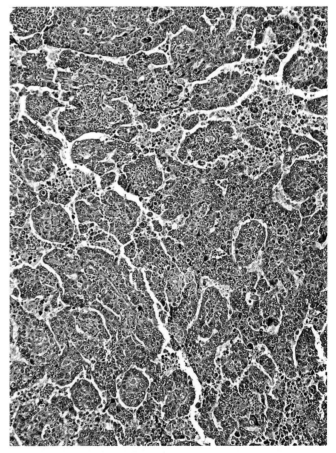

Fig. 13.42 Embryonal carcinoma with papillary structures with central blood vessels resembling the endodermal sinus pattern of a yolk sac tumor.

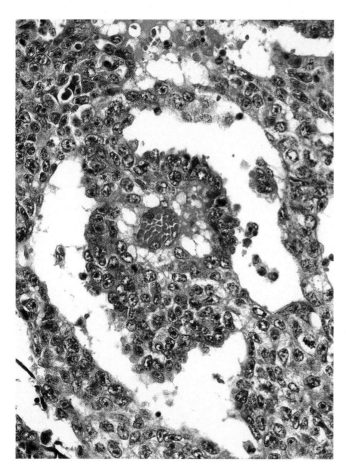

Fig. 13.43 Embryonal carcinoma with an endodermal sinuslike pattern at high magnification. The arrangement of tumor cells around the blood vessels resembles a Schiller-Duval body.

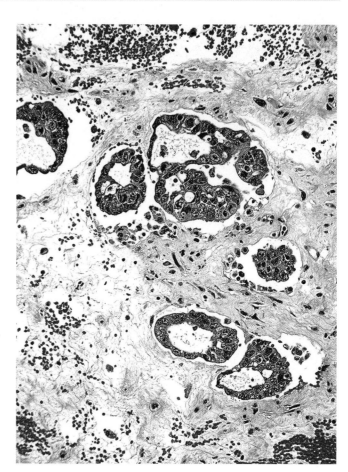

Fig. 13.44 Embryonal carcinoma with a blastocyst-like pattern with tumor cell nests with a central vesicle-like space.

feature in tumor staging. Embryonal carcinoma is the angioinvasive element in most cases when such invasion is present. There are some pitfalls in deciding if vascular invasion is present. First, intratubular neoplasm may closely resemble intravascular neoplasm. The presence of residual Sertoli cells in a possible "vessel" is good evidence that it is a tubule (Fig. 13.54). Additionally, intratubular tumors are often extensively necrotic, and the tubules are nonbranching and of relatively similar caliber, whereas intravascular tumors do not typically show extensive necrosis and may occur in branched vessels of different sizes (Fig. 13.55). Second, stringent criteria must be applied such that invaded tissue spaces are clearly lined by endothelial cells before regarding them as vessels. Third, germ cell tumors, and especially embryonal carcinoma and seminoma, are quite cellular and friable, leading to artifactual, knife-implantation of tumor cells into vascular spaces. Such implants, however, are loosely cohesive and unassociated with vascular thrombosis (Fig. 13.56), whereas legitimate vascular invasion is characterized by neoplasm conforming to the shape of the vessel, which may also show evidence of thrombosis. Commonly, artifactual vascular implants are also associated with implants on the surfaces of tissues. It is usually easiest to appreciate vascular invasion a short distance away from the periphery of the neoplasm.

Special Studies

Only a small percentage of cases of pure embryonal carcinoma demonstrate AFP immunoreactivity, but such positivity is more common in the embryonal carcinoma component of a mixed germ

cell tumor, a fact that likely represents early biochemical transformation to a yolk sac tumor component in cases of mixed germ cell tumor before morphologic differentiation.[524,525] PLAP positivity occurs in 86% to 97% of cases, but is usually patchy and weaker than in seminoma.[41,288,526] Several different cytokeratin classes are present in embryonal carcinoma, most prominently cytokeratins 8 and 18, but also cytokeratin 19, and occasionally cytokeratins 4 and 17.[527] Most authors therefore report strong and diffuse positivity for cytokeratins in the majority of embryonal carcinomas, including routinely processed cases.[41,528] Immunostains for CD30 (Ber-H2, Ki-1) are positive in 84% of cases (Fig. 13.57), whereas EMA is negative in almost all embryonal carcinomas.[41,529,530] CD117 and podoplanin (D2-40), in contrast with seminoma, are negative or only focally positive in embryonal carcinoma. OCT3/4, a nuclear transcription factor, is highly sensitive and mostly specific for embryonal carcinoma (Fig. 13.58), seminoma, and GCNIS, with no staining observed in other germ cell tumor types or sex cord–stromal tumors, and only very rare positivity seen in lung and renal cell carcinomas and in large B-cell lymphomas.[44,404] More recently, SOX2 has emerged as a valuable marker for embryonal carcinoma, with negativity in the other germ cell tumors except for immature teratoma.[49,50,283,300,301] GATA3 is negative or only very focally positive (as opposed to consistent staining in choriocarcinoma).[531] There is therefore a characteristic immunohistochemical profile: positivity for cytokeratin, PLAP, OCT3/4, SOX2, and CD30 and negativity for EMA, CD117, and podoplanin. This profile can be of great value in distinguishing embryonal carcinoma in an extragonadal site (either a metastasis or

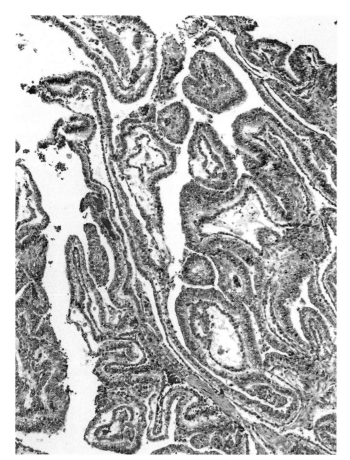

Fig. 13.45 The "double-layered" pattern of embryonal carcinoma, consisting of ribbons of embryonal carcinoma with a parallel layer of flattened cells. This is classified as mixed germ cell tumor, sometimes termed *diffuse embryoma,* and consists of embryonal carcinoma and yolk sac tumor (the flattened layer).

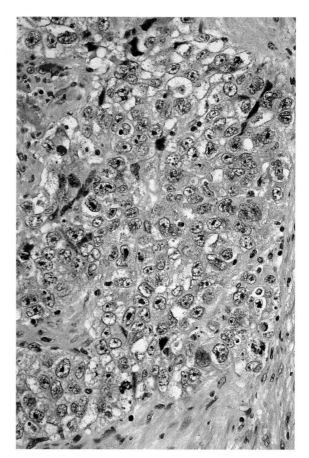

Fig. 13.46 Embryonal carcinoma. Note the ill-defined cell borders and large, crowded, vesicular nuclei with large nucleoli.

an extratesticular primary) from a poorly differentiated carcinoma of nongerm cell origin (typically, cytokeratin and EMA positive, PLAP variable [but most commonly negative], and negative for CD30 and OCT3/4).[413] The presence of CD30 in embryonal carcinoma indicates the necessity for caution and additional supportive evidence before accepting a CD30-positive, poorly differentiated malignant neoplasm as an anaplastic large cell lymphoma. Occasionally, embryonal carcinoma will also stain for α-1-antitrypsin, Leu-7, vimentin, LDH, human placental lactogen (hPL), and ferritin.[41,414,524,532] The product of the *TP53* tumor suppressor gene is often identifiable in embryonal carcinoma, although the absence of mutations with molecular biologic techniques support that this is the result of nonmutated overexpression.[243-246]

Ultrastructurally, embryonal carcinoma usually resembles a poorly differentiated, primitive adenocarcinoma with ill-defined lumens in solid areas and well-defined, large lumens in glandular areas.[60] The lumens are bordered by cells having well-defined junctional complexes with characteristically long tight junctions.[533] Short microvilli project into the luminal spaces, and the cytoplasm contains ribosomes, a prominent Golgi body, rough endoplasmic reticulum, teleolysosomes, mitochondria, glycogen, and occasional lipid droplets. The nuclei are large, deeply indented, often contain cytoplasmic inclusions, and have large nucleoli with complex nucleolonema.[60]

Embryonal carcinoma has a DNA index ranging from 1.4 to 1.6 times normal, which is significantly less than that of seminoma.[51,62] Embryonal carcinoma often contains isochromosome 12p, and increased copy numbers of i(12p) have correlated with a more aggressive clinical course.[424] The presence of i(12p) or other 12p amplifications in a poorly differentiated carcinoma, either metastatic or a primary neoplasm of an extragonadal site, may be a useful means of separating embryonal carcinoma from other poorly differentiated neoplasms.[534,535] The detection of 12p abnormalities can be accomplished in interphase cells obtained from fresh biopsy samples or in paraffin-embedded tumor by the fluorescence in situ hybridization (FISH) technique.[536,537]

Differential Diagnosis

The distinction of embryonal carcinoma from seminoma was discussed earlier in this chapter. The distinction of embryonal carcinoma from yolk sac tumor depends on the presence, in yolk sac tumor, of one of several distinctive patterns, and the larger and more pleomorphic nature of the neoplastic cells in embryonal carcinoma. Yolk sac tumor often contains hyaline globules and intercellular basement membrane, which are usually lacking in embryonal carcinoma, and AFP is much more likely to be present in yolk sac tumor than in embryonal carcinoma.[538] CD30 positivity is characteristic of embryonal carcinoma and is not usually present in yolk sac tumor.[283,529] OCT3/4 and SOX2 are positive in embryonal carcinoma and negative in yolk sac tumor.[45,282,283] Glypican-3, an immunohistochemical marker for yolk sac tumor,

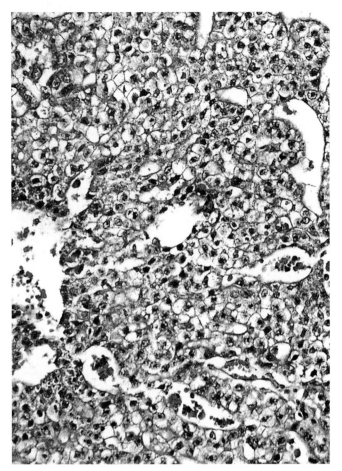

Fig. 13.47 Embryonal carcinoma with seminoma-like cells.

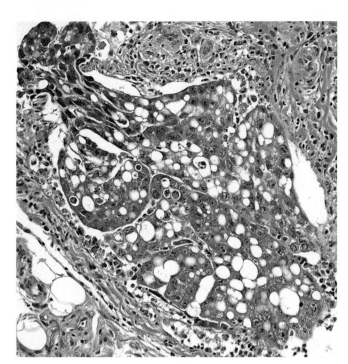

Fig. 13.49 Embryonal carcinoma with prominent cytoplasmic vacuolization (lipoid appearance).

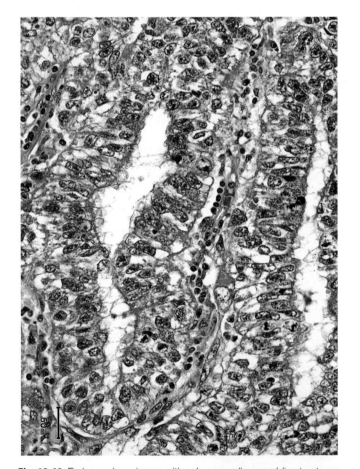

Fig. 13.48 Embryonal carcinoma with columnar cells resembling teratoma.

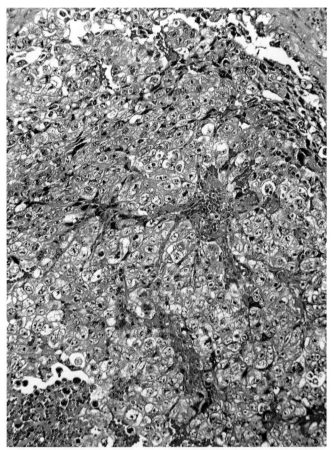

Fig. 13.50 Solid pattern of embryonal carcinoma with degenerate, smudged cells (appliqué pattern) and focal necrosis.

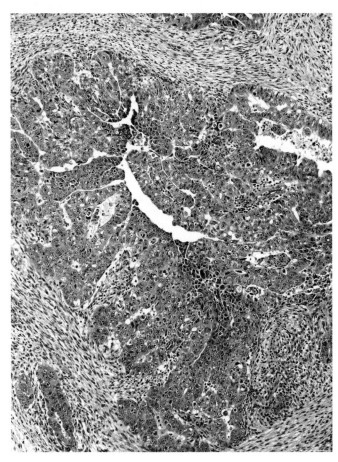

Fig. 13.51 Neoplastic stroma in an embryonal carcinoma. Classification as embryonal carcinoma and teratoma is recommended, although some regard the neoplastic stroma within the spectrum of embryonal carcinoma.

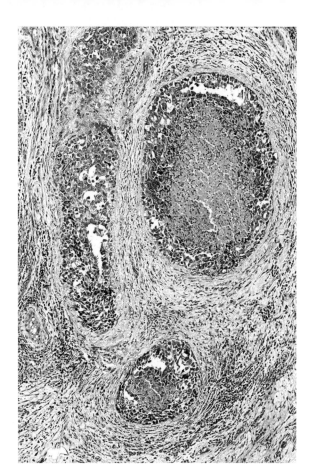

Fig. 13.53 Intratubular embryonal carcinoma with characteristic abundant necrosis.

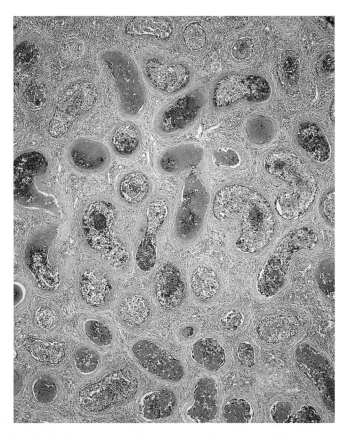

Fig. 13.52 Extensive intratubular embryonal carcinoma with prominent necrosis.

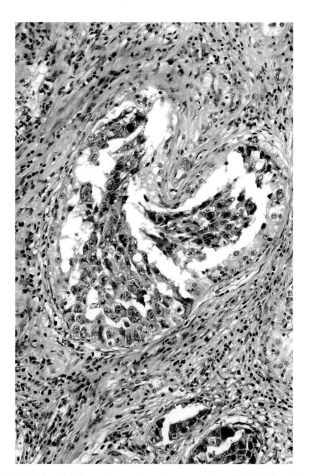

Fig. 13.54 Intratubular embryonal carcinoma can be reliably distinguished from vascular invasion if there are residual Sertoli cells.

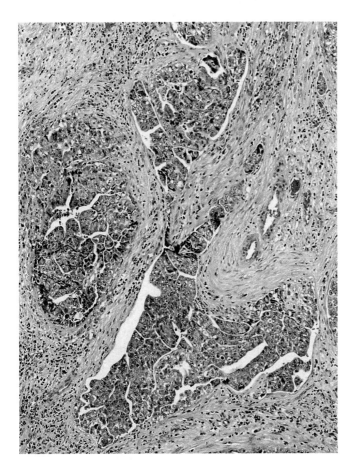

Fig. 13.55 Vascular invasion that was peripheral to embryonal carcinoma. Note the branching pattern.

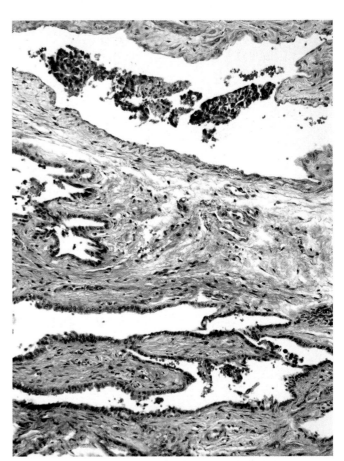

Fig. 13.56 Artifactual "knife implantation" of tumor groups into vascular spaces. Note the loose tumor cell groups unassociated with vascular thrombosis.

is negative in seminoma and positive in 0% to 8% of embryonal carcinoma.[455,456] Because embryonal carcinoma may transform into yolk sac tumor, there are foci where the distinction is arbitrary. Such cases, however, invariably show areas of both neoplastic types. The smudged, degenerate cells common in embryonal carcinoma may be misinterpreted as syncytiotrophoblast cells, causing a misdiagnosis of choriocarcinoma. These cells, however, lack hCG, and the background is usually not hemorrhagic, unlike true choriocarcinoma. Large cell lymphoma usually occurs in older patients, lacks the epithelial patterns usually identified in embryonal carcinoma, has an interstitial growth pattern, is not associated with GCNIS, is PLAP negative, only rarely OCT3/4 positive, cytokeratin negative, and LCA positive, features contrasting with those of embryonal carcinoma.[413] The differential with "anaplastic" spermatocytic tumor is discussed on the Spermatocytic Tumor section later in this chapter.

Treatment and Prognosis

The treatment of nonseminomatous germ cell tumors, including embryonal carcinoma, depends on the clinical stage of the patient. Most patients with clinical stage I tumor receive surveillance management after orchiectomy, although patients at risk for occult metastases of chemoresistant elements (somatic-type malignancies, see the Teratoma with Somatic-Type Malignancy section later in this chapter) are often recommended for nerve-sparing retroperitoneal lymph node dissection (RPLND) tailored to excise the commonly involved nodal groups ipsilateral to the affected testis. From

20% to 30% of clinical stage I patients with nonseminomatous germ cell tumors relapse on surveillance management protocols.[484,539–541] These are almost entirely caused by nondetected retroperitoneal involvement. As evidence for this conclusion, in one series of clinical stage I patients, RPLND confirmed pathologic stage II disease in 28%.[542] Adjuvant chemotherapy (two courses of cisplatin, etoposide, and bleomycin) without RPLND for clinical stage I patients has also been evaluated in a prospective trial.[543] A recent study of 382 patients with clinical stage I nonseminomatous germ cell tumor randomized to RPLND or one course of chemotherapy (bleomycin, etoposide, and cisplatin) found equivalent quality of life outcomes.[544]

With surveillance management, relapse can often be detected early by serum marker elevation, allowing almost all relapsing patients to be salvaged by standard chemotherapy. Surveillance thus avoids unnecessary RPLND in the 69% to 81% of clinical stage I patients who are cured by orchiectomy alone.[484,542,545,546] A review of 560 clinical stage I patients managed by "surveillance only" found that 97% were tumor-free and that 72% required no therapy after orchiectomy.[547] About 90% of patients who relapse do so within 2 years.[484] Only 1.6% of patients who relapse do so after 5 years or more.[546] Relapse is detected by abdominal CT scan or by serum tumor markers in an approximately equal number of cases.[484] With treatment, patients have an excellent prognosis even with relapse, with the 5-year disease-specific survival approaching 100% for the entire group of surveillance-managed clinical stage I nonseminoma patients.[484]

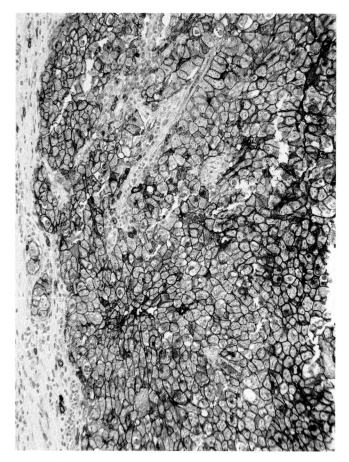

Fig. 13.57 Immunostaining for CD30 in embryonal carcinoma with strong membrane reactivity.

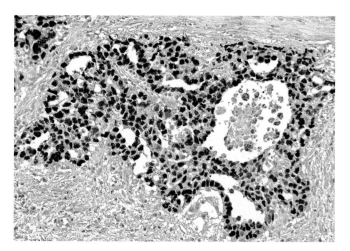

Fig. 13.58 Immunostaining for OCT3/4 in embryonal carcinoma showing strong nuclear positivity.

The proportion of clinical stage IA (clinical T1, N0, M0) patients managed by surveillance increased from 65% between 2004 and 2005 to 74% between 2012 and 2013.[548] Some clinical stage I patients at high risk for relapse may be less suitable candidates for "surveillance only" and may be identified by a careful, multifactorial analysis of the orchiectomy specimen. Factors that correlate with relapse or occult retroperitoneal metastases include: lymphovascular invasion, large proportion or volume of embryonal

carcinoma, pure embryonal carcinoma, absence of a yolk sac tumor component, embryonal carcinoma in the absence of teratoma, less than 50% teratoma, the presence of choriocarcinoma, rete testis invasion, high S or G_2M+S phase values as determined by flow cytometry, a high proportion of proliferating tumor cells, and highly aneuploid tumor stemlines.[514,546,547,549-567] In a recent study of nonseminomatous germ cell tumors, only vascular invasion, rete testis invasion, and hilar soft tissue invasion were predictive of advanced clinical stage in multivariate analysis.[568] Embryonal carcinomas with a high Ki-67 labeling index, low apoptosis, and low p53 expression have a better overall survival.[569] A pre-orchiectomy AFP value exceeding 80 ng/mL and an abnormally slow decline in AFP values after orchiectomy have also correlated with relapse.[554,557] In Europe, lymphovascular invasion has been used as a sole risk factor to recommend one cycle of chemotherapy (if lymphovascular invasion is present) or the choice between chemotherapy and surveillance (if absent).[477]

Patients having clinically apparent, nonbulky retroperitoneal involvement (clinical stage II) may be managed by RPLND with either close follow-up or a limited course of adjuvant therapy or with initial chemotherapy. Survival in excess of 95% is expected.[570,571] For patients with bulky clinical stage II or more advanced tumor, treatment is combination chemotherapy followed by surgical resection of residual masses if the serum markers have normalized. Survival of 70% to 80% is expected.[17,572] Specimens resected after chemotherapy must be carefully evaluated pathologically to determine the need for additional chemotherapy.[573] Total lymph node count of 28 or more is associated with a slightly decreased risk for relapse after RPLND compared with patients with fewer lymph nodes identified.[574] It should be noted that even in the absence of viable tumor in a postchemotherapy RPLND specimen, recurrence may be seen in approximately 18% of patients.[575]

Several different studies have been conducted to identify prognostic factors in patients with nonseminomatous testicular germ cell tumors. The most important factors are tumor stage, the extent of serum marker elevation, the age of the patient (older being worse), the presence of choriocarcinoma, and the proliferative fraction by flow cytometry.[572,576-579] HER2 overexpression was prognostically significant for mixed germ cell tumors in one study but not in another.[580,581] Epidermal growth factor receptor (EGFR) immunohistochemical overexpression has been reported in 43% of cases of chemorefractory metastatic embryonal carcinoma, suggesting that anti-EGFR targeted therapy could be a possibility for this group.[582] Most of these tumors (71%) have polysomy for chromosome 7 rather than amplification of the *EGFR* gene.[582] Treatment-resistant germ cell tumors are also more likely to have *BRAF* mutations, lack expression of the mismatch repair proteins MLH1 or MSH6, and demonstrate microsatellite instability on molecular analysis.[583] The association with *BRAF* mutation in particular is of interest because of the possibility of tyrosine kinase inhibitor treatment in patients with relapse after initial chemotherapy.[583]

A consensus classification of germ cell tumors into good, intermediate, and poor prognosis categories was published in 2013 and reproduced in the recent WHO Classification.[23,584] Nonseminomatous germ cell tumors of gonadal or retroperitoneal location, low serum tumor markers (AFP less than 1000 ng/mL, hCG less than 500 U/L, LDH less than 1.5 times the upper limit of normal), and no extrapulmonary visceral metastases are in the favorable prognosis category. Those with intermediate-level serum tumor marker elevation are in the intermediate prognosis category. Those with high-level tumor marker elevation (AFP over 10,000 ng/mL, hCG over 50,000 U/L, LDH greater than 10 times the upper limit of normal) or extrapulmonary visceral metastases are in the poor prognosis category.

Late recurrences are seen in a small percentage of patients (1% to 6%), can occur 30 years or more after initial treatment, and are likely to be treatment resistant.[585] Somatic-type malignancies are seen in approximately 23% of late recurrences.[586] Up-front surgical resection should be considered for late recurrences.[587]

Yolk Sac Tumor, Postpubertal-Type

Yolk sac tumor is the most recently recognized among the five major categories of testicular germ cell tumor. For years, ovarian yolk sac tumor was misclassified, along with ovarian clear cell carcinoma, as "mesonephroma." Teilum recognized the identity between testicular and ovarian yolk sac tumor and the frequent admixture of the testicular lesion with other forms of germ cell tumor.[588] This observation permitted the classification of yolk sac tumor as a form of germ cell neoplasm and removal of the ovarian lesion from the "mesonephroma" category.[589] Subsequently, Teilum recognized the resemblance of the mesenchyme of yolk sac tumor to the extraembryonic mesenchyme of development and its glomeruloid structures to the endodermal sinuses of the rat placenta.[590,591]

Clinical Features

Postpubertal patients with yolk sac tumor fall within the usual age spectrum for nonseminomatous testicular germ cell tumor, ranging from 15 to 45 years and averaging 25 to 30 years; rare cases have been reported in elderly patients.[592] Prospective studies of nonseminomatous germ cell tumors have shown yolk sac tumor elements in 44% of cases.[593]

Adults with yolk sac tumor in a mixed germ cell tumor are more likely to have lower-stage disease than those without a yolk sac tumor component, and the absence of a yolk sac tumor component in a mixed germ cell tumor may be a positive predictor of occult metastases in clinical stage I tumors.[558] Almost all patients with yolk sac tumor have significant elevation of serum AFP, typically ranging from hundreds to thousands of ng/mL.[59,594] Embryonal carcinoma or enteric elements of teratoma may cause minor elevation of serum AFP, but this is unusual.[503,594]

Pathologic Features

The appearance is usually heterogeneous, with frequent areas of hemorrhage, necrosis, and cystic change (Fig. 13.59). Numerous microscopic patterns are seen in yolk sac tumor and commonly include hybrid, incomplete, and transitional forms. The patterns, modified from Talerman, include: (1) microcystic (honeycomb, reticular, vacuolated); (2) endodermal sinus (perivascular); (3) papillary; (4) solid; (5) glandular/alveolar; (6) myxomatous; (7) sarcomatoid; (8) macrocystic; (9) polyvesicular vitelline; (10) hepatoid; and (11) parietal.[595]

The microcystic pattern is most common and is characterized by intracellular vacuoles creating attenuated lengths of cytoplasm connected in a spiderweb-like array (Fig. 13.60). The cells often resemble lipoblasts, with vacuoles compressing the nuclei, although they do not contain lipid. In some cases, the cells are arranged in cords and surround extracellular spaces, creating a reticular arrangement (Fig. 13.61). The microcystic pattern is often seen with a myxoid stroma and blends with the myxomatous pattern (Fig. 13.62). The solid pattern is also commonly intermingled with the microcystic (Fig. 13.63).

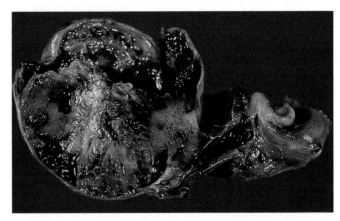

Fig. 13.59 Yolk sac tumor, postpubertal-type, showing hemorrhage, cystic degeneration, and myxoid change. (From Sternberg SS. *Diagnostic Surgical Pathology*. Raven Press, New York, NY; 1989:1885–1947, with permission of Raven Press.)

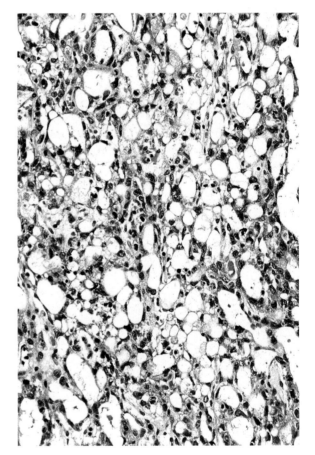

Fig. 13.60 Microcystic pattern of a yolk sac tumor resulting from intracellular vacuoles.

The endodermal sinus pattern consists of a central vessel rimmed by fibrous tissue that is surrounded by malignant epithelium. This structure is set in a cystic space that is often lined by flattened tumor cells (Figs. 13.64 and 13.65). Oblique cuts of these structures result in fibrovascular cores of tissue that are "draped" or "festooned" by malignant cells with an accompanying complex ("labyrinthine") arrangement of anastomosing extracellular spaces (Fig. 13.66). This pattern is also designated as a "perivascular" or

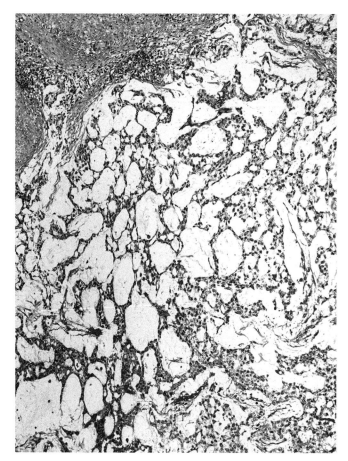

Fig. 13.61 Microcystic pattern of a yolk sac tumor created by cords of cells surrounding extracellular space (also referred to as reticular pattern).

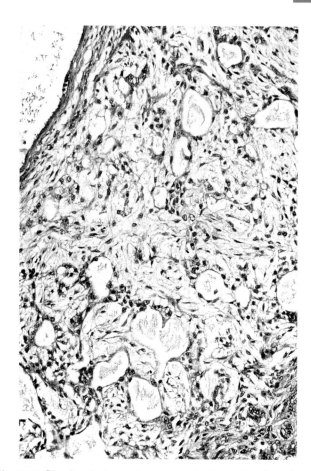

Fig. 13.62 Blending of microcystic and myxoid patterns of a yolk sac tumor. Neoplastic cells appear to "bud" from microcystic structures and blend into a myxoid stroma.

"festoon" pattern, and the endodermal sinus-like structure is termed a *glomeruloid* or *Schiller-Duval body*.[591]

The papillary pattern has papillae, with or without fibrovascular cores, which project into cystic spaces (Fig. 13.67). The cells are often cuboidal to low columnar and may have a "hobnail" configuration secondary to apical protrusion of the nucleus. Exfoliated clusters of neoplastic cells may be present in the cystic spaces. The papillary pattern may blend with the endodermal sinus pattern.

The solid pattern is quite common and may resemble seminoma, consisting of sheets of relatively uniform cells with lightly staining to clear cytoplasm and well-defined borders (Fig. 13.68).[454] However, the lymphoid component and fibrous septa of seminoma are usually absent, and the cells are more pleomorphic than those of seminoma. Some areas of solid pattern tumor have prominent thin-walled blood vessels, and focal microcysts may also be seen in an otherwise solid pattern (Fig. 13.63). In some cases, the solid pattern has small cells with scant cytoplasm resembling blastema (Fig. 13.69); such foci are intimately intermingled with classic patterns of yolk sac tumor (Fig. 13.70).

Well-defined glands, often with enteric features, are common in yolk sac tumor (Fig. 13.71), present in 34% of cases in one series.[538] The glands may be contiguous with vesicles typical of the polyvesicular vitelline pattern, or may appear in a background of myxomatous, microcystic, or solid patterns. Usually the glands are simple, round, and tubular, but may show an elaborate branching pattern or become quite intricate and complex (Fig. 13.72). Unlike the glands of teratoma, those of yolk sac tumor are not

associated with other teratomatous components and lack circumferential smooth muscle that is common but not invariable in teratoma.[596] The nuclei of the glands are often more bland than those of the surrounding yolk sac tumor and may show subnuclear vacuolation, reminiscent of early secretory pattern endometrium. As a consequence, predominantly glandular ovarian yolk sac tumor has been termed *endometrioid-like*.[597] Purely or predominantly glandular testicular yolk sac tumor is more rare than in the ovary, but may be associated with a high serum AFP.[269] Purely glandular yolk sac tumor is more common after chemotherapy and is therefore usually found in metastases; it is particularly more frequent in late recurrences.[586]

The myxomatous pattern is common, consisting of neoplastic epithelioid to spindle cells dispersed in a stroma that is rich in mucopolysaccharide, staining only lightly with hematoxylin and eosin (Fig. 13.73). A prominent vascular network is common, and Teilum described this pattern as "angioblastic mesenchyme" that he felt was homologous with the extraembryonic mesenchyme (the "magma reticulare") of development.[598] Myxomatous foci commonly merge with other patterns, and hybrids of microcystic and myxomatous patterns are more the rule than the exception (Fig. 13.62). By light microscopy, the spindle cells appear to arise from solid or microcystic foci by budding from them and blending into the surrounding myxoid stroma (Fig. 13.74). Intense cytokeratin immunoreactivity within these cells supports derivation from the epithelial component of yolk sac tumor.[599] These cells are, in fact, pluripotent cells with the capacity to form differentiated

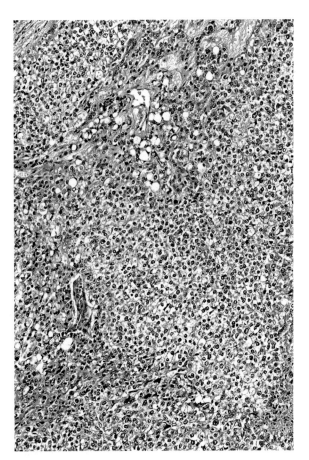

Fig. 13.63 Mixture of solid and microcystic patterns of a yolk sac tumor.

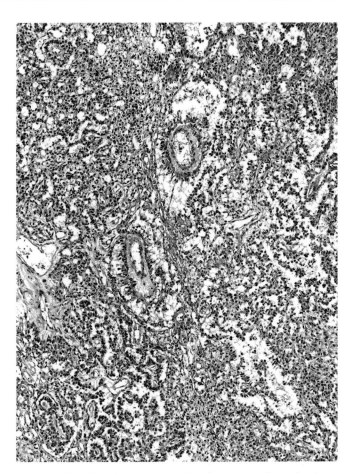

Fig. 13.64 Endodermal sinus pattern of a yolk sac tumor. Several endodermal sinuslike structures are present in this field.

mesenchymal tissue such as skeletal muscle, cartilage, and bone, thus blurring the distinction between yolk sac tumor and teratoma (Fig. 13.74).[599] Classification of such elements as yolk sac tumor is justified by the recognition that the surrounding tissues are typical yolk sac tumor.

The uncommon sarcomatoid pattern consists of a cellular proliferation of spindle, and usually also epithelioid, cells (Fig. 13.75) in continuity with other yolk sac tumor patterns, most commonly microcystic. It is distinguished from the solid pattern by the spindle cell nature of the component cells and the myxomatous pattern by its greater size as a single pattern. Despite the sarcomatoid appearance, the spindle cells express cytokeratin and glypican-3 and may also react for SALL4 but not AFP. It is likely that some embryonal rhabdomyosarcomas arising in testicular germ cell tumors derive from differentiation of sarcomatoid spindle cells to rhabdomyoblastic cells.[600] The occasional intimate admixture of embryonal rhabdomyosarcoma with yolk sac tumor supports this hypothesis. Spindle cell patterns in yolk sac tumor have also been reported in primary mediastinal examples.[601]

The macrocystic pattern appears to arise from coalescence of microcystic spaces to form large, round to irregular cysts (Fig. 13.76), and the surrounding pattern is often microcystic.

In the uncommon polyvesicular vitelline pattern, vesicle-like structures are lined by flattened, innocuous-appearing epithelium, in a myxoid to fibrous stroma (Fig. 13.77). Sometimes the vesicles have a central constriction, resembling a dumbbell or a figure 8. Teilum compared these vesicles to the embryonic subdivision of the primary yolk sac into the secondary yolk sac.[602] At the point of constriction, the epithelium may change from flattened to

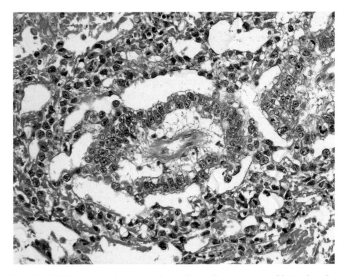

Fig. 13.65 Endodermal sinus pattern of a yolk sac tumor. Note also the basement membrane deposits in the peripheral tumor.

cuboidal or columnar; the latter often has enteric features, including an apical brush border. AFP is often present in the epithelium of the vesicles, and hyaline globules are occasionally seen within them. In some cases, a transition from a microcystic to polyvesicular vitelline pattern can be identified. The bland cytologic appearance of the polyvesicular vitelline pattern may falsely suggest a

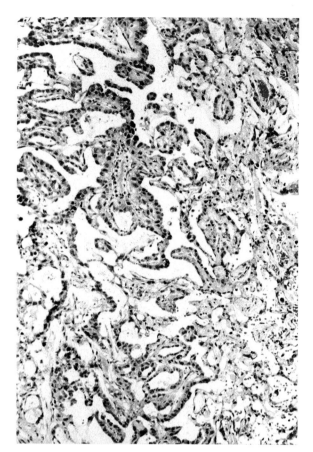

Fig. 13.66 Oblique sections of endodermal sinuslike structures result in geographic configurations with festoons of malignant epithelium at the periphery and a complex, labyrinthine pattern of interconnecting, extracellular spaces.

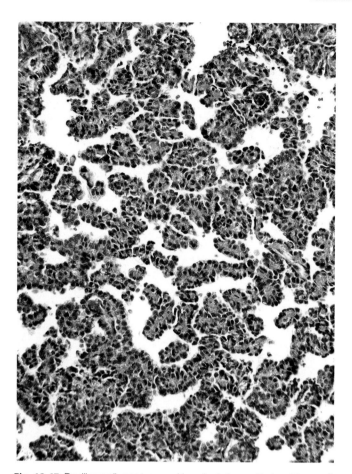

Fig. 13.67 Papillary yolk sac tumor with a single layer of hobnail-type cells on fibrovascular cores.

benign neoplasm, but the presence of other patterns should prevent this pitfall. The polyvesicular pattern is less frequent in testicular yolk sac tumor than in its ovarian counterpart, where it may rarely occur in pure form.[603]

A hepatoid pattern also occurs in about 20% of yolk sac tumors and consists of small clusters of polygonal, eosinophilic cells arranged in sheets, nests, or trabeculae (Fig. 13.78).[538,604] The cells have round, vesicular nuclei with prominent nucleoli and contain abundant AFP; hyaline globules are common in hepatoid foci as are bile canaliculi, although bile is a rare finding.[376,605] Hepatoid foci are scattered randomly in yolk sac tumor and usually are minor components; rarely, a more diffuse hepatoid pattern may be seen, although a prominent hepatoid pattern is more common in ovarian tumors and in late recurrences of testicular tumors.[586,606,607]

The parietal pattern has extensive deposits of extracellular basement membrane, with only scattered neoplastic cells in an abundant, eosinophilic matrix (Fig. 13.79). It is considered the extreme end of parietal differentiation (see later) in which basement membrane is deposited in the extracellular space in a variety of yolk sac tumor patterns. In a true parietal pattern yolk sac tumor, the basement membrane deposits efface the underlying yolk sac tumor pattern. This is a rare pattern, most often seen after chemotherapy, particularly in late recurrences.[586,608] There is some overlap with the sarcomatoid pattern when the tumor cells are spindled, and we have seen some cases that, in postchemotherapy resections, mimicked osteosarcoma.

The frequency of the different patterns of yolk sac tumor is difficult to determine because of lack of uniformity in classification. The microcystic, solid, and myxomatous patterns are most common, with glandular, macrocystic, endodermal sinus, hepatoid, and papillary patterns also occurring frequently. The polyvesicular vitelline pattern is less common, and sarcomatoid and parietal patterns are unusual. If only four patterns are employed for classification, the frequency of the patterns diminishes from reticular to solid to endodermal sinus to polyvesicular vitelline. Jacobsen noted a "vacuolated network" in 91% of yolk sac tumors, microcystic pattern in 67%, myxomatous pattern in 51%, macrocystic pattern in 44%, solid pattern in 27%, hepatoid areas in 23%, labyrinthine formations in 17%, and endodermal sinus-like structures in 9%.[520]

A common feature of yolk sac tumor is the deposition of extracellular basement membrane, identified in 92% of cases.[538] These deposits generally are irregularly shaped, eosinophilic bands between the neoplastic cells (Fig. 13.80) and have been referred to as parietal differentiation because of their homology to the parietal layer of the embryonic yolk sac of the rodent, which rests on a thick basement membrane (known as Reichert membrane).[538,602] Such intercellular basement membrane, although not specific for yolk sac tumor, is characteristic and can be helpful in diagnosis, particularly in small biopsy samples taken from extratesticular tumors. Another characteristic but nonspecific feature in most yolk sac tumors is the presence of intracellular, round, hyaline globules

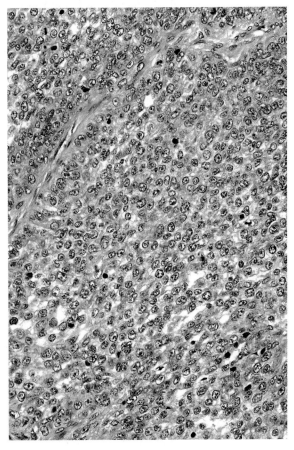

Fig. 13.68 Solid pattern of a yolk sac tumor.

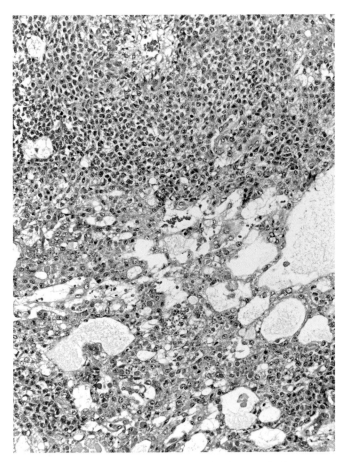

Fig. 13.70 Solid pattern of a yolk sac tumor with blastema-like focus next to more typical patterns of yolk sac tumor.

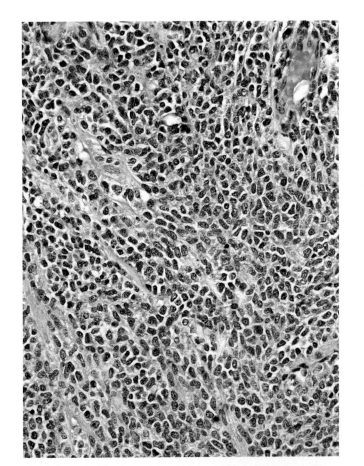

Fig. 13.69 Solid areas in a yolk sac tumor composed of small, blastema-like cells.

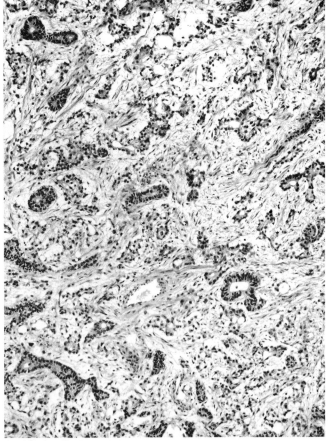

Fig. 13.71 Glandular structures in a microcystic (reticular) pattern of a yolk sac tumor.

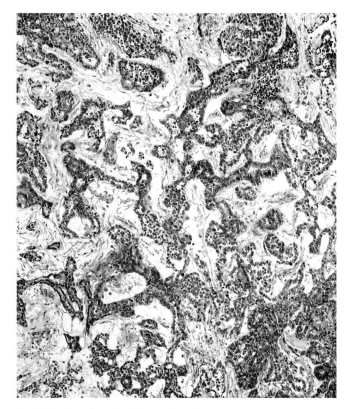

Fig. 13.72 Complex glands in a yolk sac tumor.

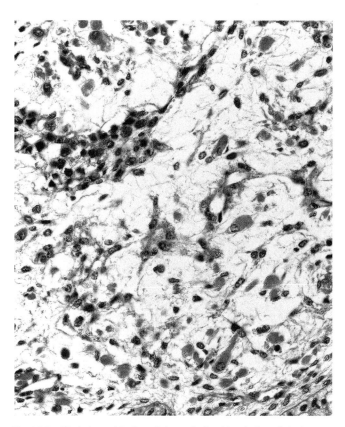

Fig. 13.74 Rhabdomyoblastic cells intermingle with spindle cells in the myxomatous portion of a yolk sac tumor.

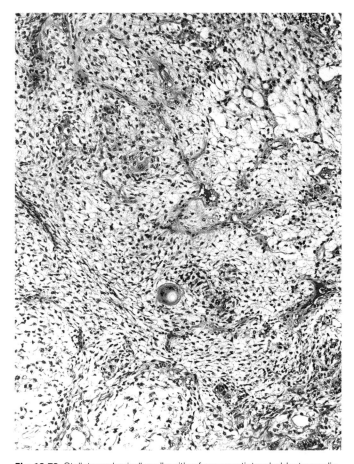

Fig. 13.73 Stellate and spindle cells with a few syncytiotrophoblasts are dispersed in a myxoid stroma in the myxomatous pattern of a yolk sac tumor. Overgrowth of this pattern justifies a diagnosis of sarcomatoid yolk sac tumor.

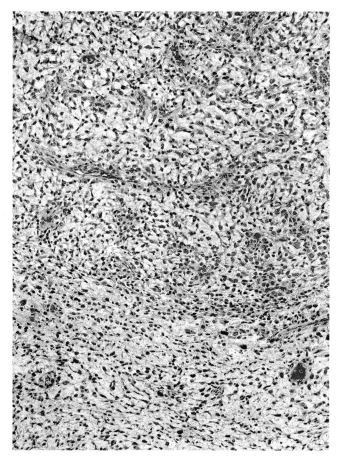

Fig. 13.75 Sarcomatoid yolk sac tumor with a myxoid background.

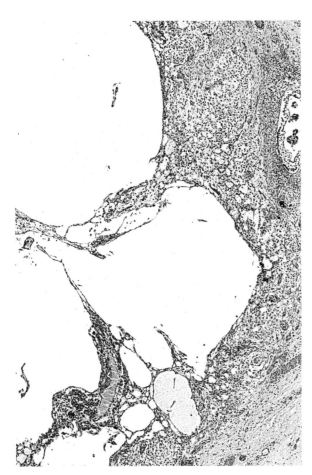

Fig. 13.76 Macrocystic pattern of a yolk sac tumor. Note the adjacent microcystic pattern.

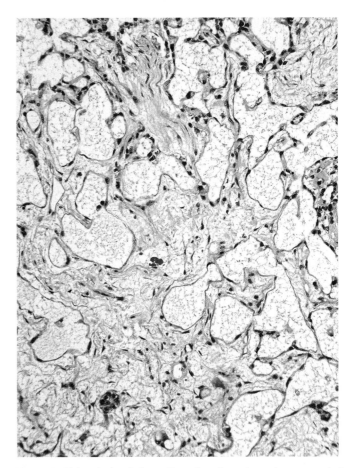

Fig. 13.77 Polyvesicular vitelline pattern of a yolk sac tumor is composed of irregular, often constricted, vesicle-like structures lined by flattened epithelium in loose stroma.

of variable size (from 1 to more than 50 μm in diameter) (Fig. 13.81). These globules are PAS-positive and diastase-resistant and may be present in the extracellular space after cell necrosis. Occasionally these globules may stain positively for AFP, but most do not; hence the staining is considered nonspecific. The hyaline globules and basement membrane deposits of yolk sac tumor are separate and distinct findings, although they have sometimes been confused in the literature.

Hematopoietic elements, usually erythroblasts, are present in a minority of testicular yolk sac tumors, usually in vascular spaces or myxomatous tissues.

Special Studies

Most yolk sac tumors show cytoplasmic AFP positivity on immunostaining; the frequency varies from 50% to 100% depending on the technique employed and the number of blocks examined.[41,59,454,524,609] Positivity is characteristically patchy (Fig. 13.82); intense staining is usually present in hepatoid foci. Postpubertal-type yolk sac tumor stains more frequently for AFP than prepubertal-type.[524] Glypican-3, a proteoglycan that plays a role in embryonic growth, is positive in yolk sac tumor and is much less commonly expressed in most other forms of testicular germ cell tumor (Fig. 13.83).[455,456,610] Glypican-3 is more sensitive for yolk sac tumor than AFP, staining 100% of cases in one study compared with 58% for AFP.[457] Staining was seen in all patterns of all cases evaluated, except the solid pattern of a single case.[457] Glypican-3 staining has been reported in some tumors

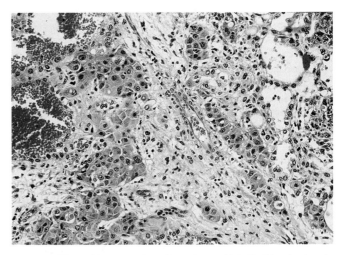

Fig. 13.78 Hepatoid pattern of a yolk sac tumor. Note the islands of eosinophilic cells with round nuclei and prominent nucleoli adjacent to microcystic (reticular) pattern.

other than yolk sac tumor and hepatocellular carcinoma, however, including cholangiocarcinoma, hepatoblastoma, immature teratoma, melanoma, and pulmonary squamous cell carcinoma, so caution is necessary if these tumors are in the differential diagnosis.[611] Among other primary testicular tumors, focal staining may

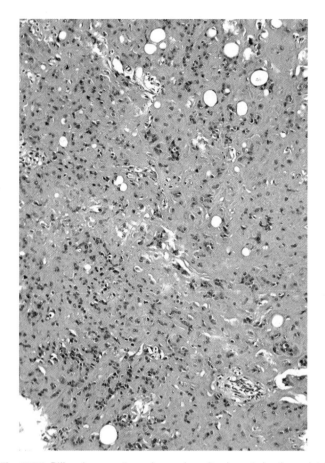

Fig. 13.79 Diffuse basement membrane deposits characterize the parietal pattern of a yolk sac tumor.

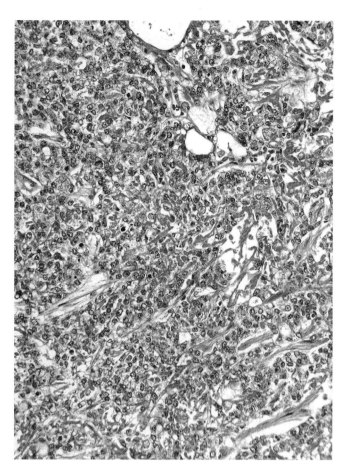

Fig. 13.80 Bands and irregularly shaped deposits of basement membrane constitute parietal differentiation in a yolk sac tumor.

be seen in some embryonal carcinomas, teratomas, and spermatocytic tumors.[612] Positivity for α-1-antitrypsin occurs in about 50% of yolk sac tumors, and the enteric glands may stain for carcinoembryonic antigen and villin, which also highlight the purely glandular tumors.[41,59,532,538]

SALL4, a regulator of OCT3/4, is a nuclear marker that is expressed in essentially all cases of GCNIS, seminoma, spermatocytic tumor, embryonal carcinoma, and pre- and postpubertal type yolk sac tumors.[409,613] This marker is consistently negative in testicular tumors other than germ cell tumors (including stromal tumors), so it is useful to identify germ cell tumors as a group.[409] It is also useful to identify metastatic germ cell tumors, such as in the setting of a metastatic yolk sac tumor with glandular or solid pattern and absent AFP expression, although occasional somatic malignancies including esophageal, gastric, and colonic adenocarcinomas may show weak staining.[614] Among somatic malignancies, ovarian serous carcinoma has the highest (29%) frequency of SALL4 staining, but urothelial and gastric carcinomas stain in almost one-fourth of cases, and other tumors stain in single-digit percentages.[613] SALL4 tends to be more diffusely positive in yolk sac tumor (Fig. 13.84) than glypican-3. Cytokeratin is present in virtually all cases, although cytokeratin 7 is characteristically absent.[41,454,615] Positivity with HEA 125, an epithelial marker, occurs in most cases.[616] Albumin, ferritin, neuron-specific enolase, and Leu-7 are present in a variable number of cases.[41,532] Chromogranin reactivity is unusual.[616] From 39% to 85% of yolk sac tumors are reported as positive for PLAP, and EMA is usually negative, as is CD99.[41,281,288,616] p53 may

be identified in yolk sac tumor, and laminin and type IV collagen are present in areas of parietal differentiation.[245,538] We have noted reactivity of hepatoid foci for hepatocyte-specific antigen (HepPar1; clone OCH1E5) (unpublished observations, 2001) and others have reported HepPar1 positivity in occasional yolk sac tumors in the absence of light microscopically evident hepatoid features.[617] In addition to HepPar1, other endodermal lineage markers such as TTF1 (2 of 15 cases) and CDX2 (6 of 15 cases) may show intermediate- to high-level expression in some testicular yolk sac tumors.[618] The growth differentiation factor 3 (GDF3) antibody is immunoreactive with yolk sac tumors and a GDF3+/OCT3/4–/CD30– immunophenotype is supportive of the diagnosis in morphologically difficult cases.[283] GATA3 is expressed by yolk sac tumor, but choriocarcinomas are also positive; focal staining may be seen in some embryonal carcinomas, and staining is seen in carcinomas of many somatic sites, limiting its usefulness.[531]

Ultrastructurally, yolk sac tumor shows clusters of epithelial cells joined by junctional complexes. Glands have microvilli with glycocalyceal bodies and long anchoring rootlets.[538] Basement membrane material can be identified in the extracellular space, and flocculent material is present within dilated cisternae of endoplasmic reticulum, often with a central lucent zone.[60,538,619,620] Cytoplasmic glycogen may be conspicuous.[619,621] The nuclei are usually irregular, with complex nucleolonema. Densely osmiophilic, cytoplasmic, nonmembrane bound, round bodies correspond to the hyaline globules observed at the light microscopic level.

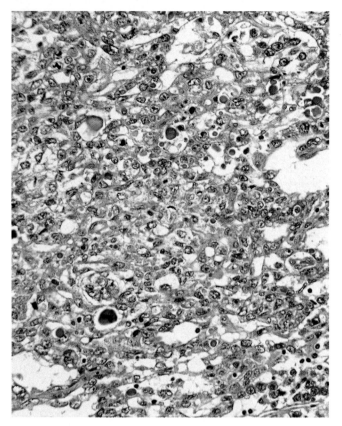

Fig. 13.81 Solid and microcystic patterns of a yolk sac tumor with eosinophilic, hyaline globules.

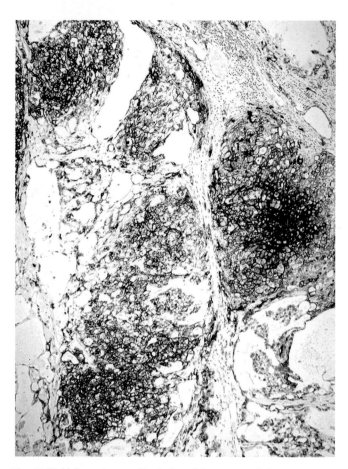

Fig. 13.83 Yolk sac tumor with glypican-3 immunoreactivity.

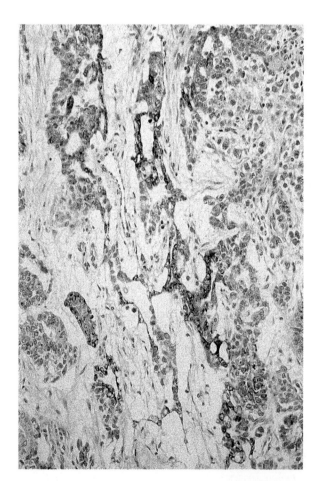

Fig. 13.82 Patchy immunoreactivity for alpha-fetoprotein in a yolk sac tumor.

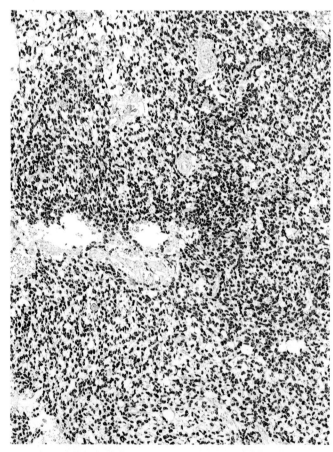

Fig. 13.84 Yolk sac tumor with SALL4 diffuse nuclear immunoreactivity.

Differential Diagnosis

Solid pattern yolk sac tumor must be distinguished from seminoma, an issue that has been addressed in the Seminoma section earlier in this chapter. The distinction of yolk sac tumor from embryonal carcinoma has less clinical significance but is based on the distinctive patterns of yolk sac tumor and the less pleomorphic, less atypical nature of the neoplastic cells. CD30, OCT3/4, AFP, and glypican-3 stains are helpful; the first two are positive in embryonal carcinoma but not yolk sac tumor, and the latter two are positive in many yolk sac tumors and usually negative in embryonal carcinomas. Embryonal carcinoma probably transforms to yolk sac tumor, so there are transitional forms that are difficult to categorize.[622] A hyperplastic reaction of the rete testis with hyaline globules may be induced by invasion of the rete by a neoplasm, thus simulating yolk sac tumor (Fig. 13.85).[623] The arborizing pattern of the rete testis and the bland nature of the hyperplastic cells should prevent this misinterpretation, although immunostains can also be used if doubt persists.[623]

Treatment and Prognosis

Adult patients with yolk sac tumor are treated in a fashion similar to that outlined previously, although the presence of a yolk sac tumor component in a patient with clinical stage I tumor has been associated with a decreased likelihood of occult metastases.[558,624] Patients with metastatic yolk sac tumor do not respond as well to chemotherapy as do patients with other forms of metastatic nonteratomatous testicular germ cell tumor, and therefore seem to have a poorer prognosis.[625] The greater chemoresistance of yolk sac tumor in adult patients compared with other forms of germ cell tumor is reflected in a higher frequency of yolk sac tumor metastases at autopsy in the chemotherapeutic era compared with the prechemotherapeutic era.[626]

Choriocarcinoma and Other Trophoblastic Neoplasms

Clinical Features

Choriocarcinoma is an uncommon component of mixed germ cell tumors (present in 15% of cases), and pure choriocarcinoma is quite rare, representing only 0.3% of testicular tumors in a registry of 6000 cases and 0.6% of cases in a recent large series.[375,593] Most patients with choriocarcinoma present with symptoms secondary to metastases, unlike other testicular tumors in which a palpable mass is the usual presenting complaint. Often the testicular tumor remains occult even after the diagnosis of metastatic choriocarcinoma. Typically, metastases are in a hematogenous distribution, often affecting the lungs, brain, and gastrointestinal tract, although retroperitoneal lymph node involvement may occur. In rare instances, patients may present with cutaneous or pancreatic metastases.[627,628] Most patients are in the second and third decades, and choriocarcinoma has not been reported before puberty outside of a disorder of sex development.[510] Serum levels of hCG may be highly elevated, resulting in secondary hormonal manifestations such as gynecomastia and thyrotoxicosis caused by similar stimulating effects of hCG, luteinizing hormone, and thyroid-stimulating hormone, because of their shared α-subunits.[488,598,629]

Pathologic Features

Grossly, the testis may be externally normal; the cut surface usually shows a hemorrhagic and necrotic nodule (Fig. 13.86), although in some instances regression of the primary lesion has occurred, with residual scar as the only evidence of prior neoplasm. Classically, choriocarcinoma consists of a random mixture of mononucleated trophoblast cells with clear to lightly staining cytoplasm (cytotrophoblasts and intermediate trophoblasts) and multinucleated syncytiotrophoblast cells, the latter often with smudged or degenerate-appearing nuclei and densely eosinophilic cytoplasm (Fig. 13.87). Cells of intermediate size with eosinophilic cytoplasm are also common. The syncytiotrophoblast cells may have intracytoplasmic lacunae containing an eosinophilic precipitate or

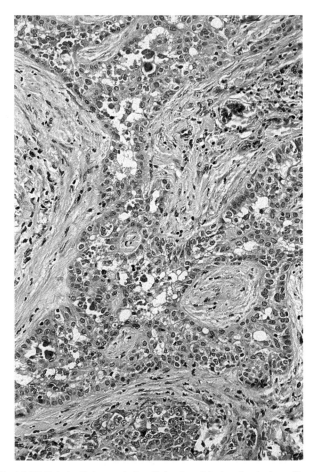

Fig. 13.85 Rete testis hyperplasia with hyaline globules. Confusion with yolk sac tumor is possible.

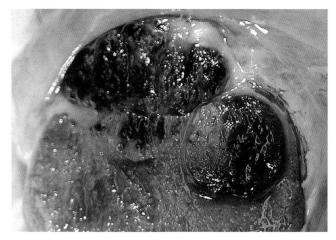

Fig. 13.86 Choriocarcinoma of the testis. Note the hemorrhagic nodules.

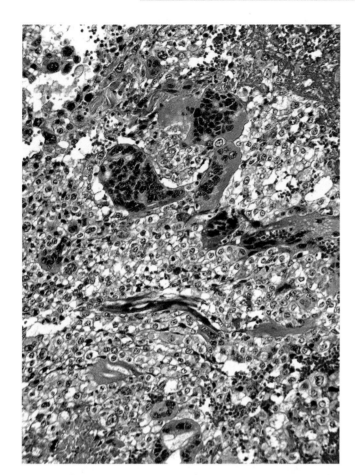

Fig. 13.87 Characteristic mixture of syncytiotrophoblast cells and mononucleated trophoblast cells in choriocarcinoma. The background is hemorrhagic.

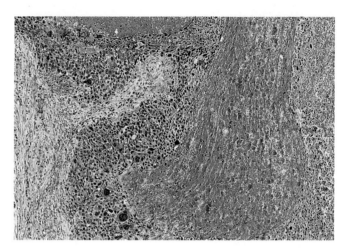

Fig. 13.88 Viable choriocarcinoma forms a rim around pools of blood and fibrin.

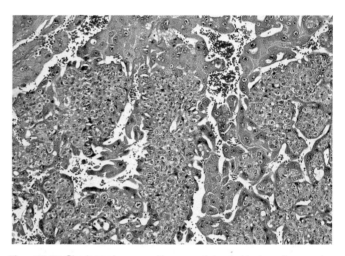

Fig. 13.89 Choriocarcinoma with syncytiotrophoblast cells capping cytotrophoblast cells in a villuslike fashion.

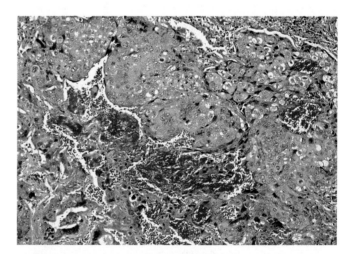

Fig. 13.90 Choriocarcinoma in which the syncytiotrophoblast cells are subtle, appearing as intermingled, smudged cells. Note the hemorrhage and typical syncytiotrophoblast cells at the bottom.

erythrocytes. The area surrounding a choriocarcinoma is almost always hemorrhagic, and the central portions of the neoplasm are typically hemorrhagic and necrotic. Extensive sampling of such tumors may therefore be necessary to demonstrate the diagnostic cell types, usually at the periphery (Fig. 13.88). In the best-organized examples, the syncytiotrophoblast cells appear to surround or "cap" masses of mononucleated trophoblast cells, like the arrangement in immature placental villi (Fig. 13.89). However, in some cases the syncytiotrophoblast cells are inconspicuous, having relatively scant cytoplasm and a degenerate appearance (Fig. 13.90). In other cases, descriptively characterized as "monophasic choriocarcinoma," a biphasic pattern of intermingled syncytiotrophoblast and mononucleated trophoblast cells is absent; instead, there occurs a proliferation of atypical trophoblastic cells of varying size.[630] These are usually mononucleated and occasionally binucleated trophoblast cells, and the background typically remains hemorrhagic (Fig. 13.91). Lymphovascular invasion is a consistent finding in choriocarcinoma.[631]

Special Studies

Immunostains for hCG are useful in establishing the diagnosis of a trophoblastic proliferation, including choriocarcinoma. Positivity for hCG is strongest in syncytiotrophoblast cells and in large mononucleated trophoblast cells that may represent transitional forms between cytotrophoblast cells and syncytiotrophoblast cells (Fig. 13.92).[41,59,632] Cytotrophoblast cells generally have only weak or absent staining for hCG. Similarly, pregnancy-specific

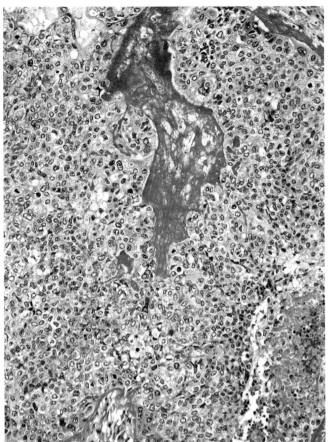

Fig. 13.91 "Monophasic" choriocarcinoma. There is a diffuse pattern of mostly mononucleated trophoblast cells in a hemorrhagic background.

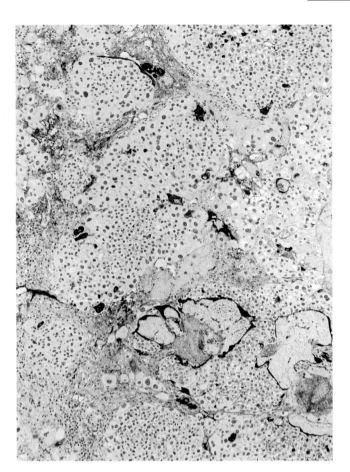

Fig. 13.92 Choriocarcinoma with strongest positivity for hCG in syncytiotrophoblast cells and large mononucleated trophoblast cells.

β-1-glycoprotein and human placental lactogen (hPL) may be identified in syncytiotrophoblast cells and intermediate-sized trophoblast cells but are not seen in the cytotrophoblast population.[632] Inhibin-α is positive in syncytiotrophoblast cells.[616,633,634] About one-half of choriocarcinomas stain for PLAP, and carcinoembryonic antigen (CEA) can be identified in both syncytiotrophoblast cells and cytotrophoblast cells in about 25% of cases.[41,635] Cytokeratin is readily identifiable in both the syncytiotrophoblastic and cytotrophoblastic components of choriocarcinoma, including cytokeratins 7, 8, 18, and 19.[41,376,636] EMA positivity is noted in about one-half of choriocarcinomas, usually within syncytiotrophoblast cells, whereas most other nonteratomatous germ cell tumors of the testis do not express EMA. SALL4 reactivity occurs in the mononucleated trophoblast cells.[41,409] Choriocarcinomas are positive for p63 and hPL, with cytotrophoblasts showing p63 staining (Fig. 13.93) and absence of hPL staining, and intermediate trophoblasts are p63 negative and weak or negative for hPL.[631] hPL is strongly positive in syncytiotrophoblasts.[631] GATA3 is positive in most testicular choriocarcinomas, and GATA3 is also expressed in gestational choriocarcinoma, suggesting that GATA3 is a useful and sensitive trophoblastic marker.[637]

Ultrastructurally, the multinucleated syncytiotrophoblast cells have prominent cisternae of rough endoplasmic reticulum, which often contain electron dense material, and show interdigitating microvilli on the cell surface.[60,638] Cytotrophoblast cells lack the prominent rough endoplasmic reticulum but have numerous free cytoplasmic ribosomes. Desmosomes are identified in all cell types.

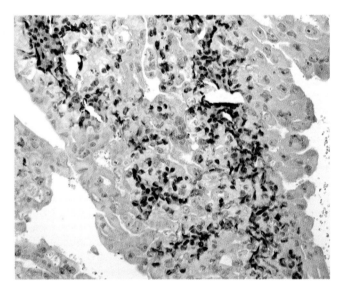

Fig. 13.93 Choriocarcinoma with p63 immunoreactivity in cytotrophoblast cells.

Differential Diagnosis

Other types of germ cell tumor may contain trophoblast cells, but they are scattered as individual cells or small nests and lack the biphasic pattern of choriocarcinoma. For example, the syncytiotrophoblast cells that occur in many seminomas are randomly distributed as separate cells and small islands without accompanying mononucleated trophoblast cells. Neither is there a distinct nodule of trophoblast cells of varying sizes as may be seen in some cases of choriocarcinoma. Embryonal carcinoma may show degenerate cells that mimic choriocarcinoma with a poorly defined syncytiotrophoblastic component. The lack of hemorrhage and hCG reactivity and the presence of OCT3/4 reactivity in such cases distinguish them from choriocarcinoma. Rare cases of embryonal carcinoma may show transformation to choriocarcinoma[639]; if the background is hemorrhagic and the admixed multinucleated cells are positive for hCG but not OCT3/4, choriocarcinoma should be diagnosed rather than embryonal carcinoma. "Monophasic" variants of choriocarcinoma should be distinguished from seminoma and solid-pattern yolk sac tumor.[630] Diffuse hCG reactivity is helpful in this regard, as is the absence of AFP and OCT3/4 staining and a greater degree of pleomorphism compared with seminoma. The placental site trophoblastic tumor and epithelioid trophoblastic tumor may be distinguished from choriocarcinoma based on the absence of a biphasic pattern and their strong and diffuse reactivity for hPL and p63, respectively. GATA3 is consistently expressed by choriocarcinoma and may in some situations be a useful marker, but it should be remembered that yolk sac tumors are also positive, focal staining may be seen in embryonal carcinoma, and staining is seen in many somatic carcinomas.[531]

Treatment and Prognosis

Choriocarcinoma tends to metastasize before detection of the primary lesion, and most patients have an advanced-stage tumor at the time of diagnosis.[631] It often shows a less orderly pattern of metastasis than other germ cell tumors, frequently skipping the retroperitoneum and metastasizing in a hematogenous pattern to the lungs, liver, central nervous system, and other sites.[375,640] The prognosis is therefore overall poorer than for other germ cell tumors.[631] The prognosis for mixed germ cell tumors with a predominant component of choriocarcinoma is also poorer than that of other germ cell tumors, although a recent study failed to find a negative prognostic impact when the amount of choriocarcinoma was less than 5%.[631,641a] The aggressive nature of choriocarcinoma is supported by several studies demonstrating a poorer prognosis in patients with nonseminomatous germ cell tumors who had elevated serum hCG levels, and in those with choriocarcinoma in mixed germ cell tumors.[488,641-644]

Nonchoriocarcinomatous Trophoblastic Tumors

There are other trophoblastic tumors in the testis apart from choriocarcinoma. These include placental site trophoblastic tumor, epithelioid trophoblastic tumor, and cystic trophoblastic tumor. Placental site trophoblastic tumor resembles the uterine tumor of the same name (Fig. 13.94).[630] It consists of a nodular proliferation of "intermediate" trophoblast cells that stain positively for human placental lactogen and is mostly negative for p63. There is lack of the biphasic pattern of choriocarcinoma. This tumor has been described in a 16-month-old boy who had no evidence of disease at 8 years follow-up after orchiectomy in the absence of any adjuvant therapy.[630] Additional cases have been described in a 24-year-old man that was associated with teratoma, had GCNIS and 12p amplification by FISH, and had a favorable outcome with orchiectomy alone, and in a 39-year-old man in association with retroperitoneal teratoma after orchiectomy and chemotherapy for testicular germ cell tumor.[645,646]

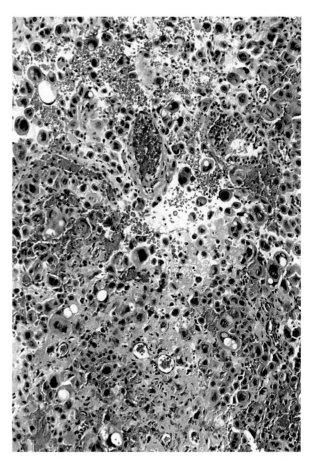

Fig. 13.94 Placental site trophoblastic tumor. There is a sheetlike arrangement of intermediate trophoblast cells with densely eosinophilic cytoplasm in a hemorrhagic background. The tumor cells were strongly and diffusely reactive for human placental lactogen.

Microscopically, discohesive cells and clusters of cells with large nuclei and abundant eosinophilic cytoplasm are seen in a fibrous background, and vascular wall infiltration is characteristic.[646] Prognosis is thought to be better than in choriocarcinoma, although experience is limited.[646]

Epithelioid trophoblastic tumor (Fig. 13.95) consists of mononucleated squamoid chorionic-type intermediate trophoblast cells with pleomorphic, hyperchromatic nuclei, abundant eosinophilic cytoplasm, and prominent cell membranes.[646] Apoptotic bodies and fibrinoid necrosis are often admixed. The cells are positive for p63, but hPL is negative or focal.[646,647] Inhibin, GATA3, and PLAP are also positive, and staining for hCG is variable.[646] Five cases, two testicular and three in resections after chemotherapy, have been reported.[646,647] The patients were 19 to 43 years of age, and four of the five tumors were associated with teratoma. As with placental site trophoblastic tumor, the prognosis is thought to be more favorable than in choriocarcinoma.[646]

Cystic trophoblastic tumors may occur as a spontaneous testicular tumor or after chemotherapy in metastatic sites.[648-650] Rarely it may be seen in metastases in patients not previously treated with chemotherapy.[651] It consists of mostly mononucleated trophoblast cells that line cysts that may contain fibrinoid material, pink-staining fluid, or appear mostly empty (Fig. 13.96). The trophoblasts show variable cytoplasmic vacuoles and only rare mitotic figures.[648] In testicular specimens, it is usually a minor (10% or less)

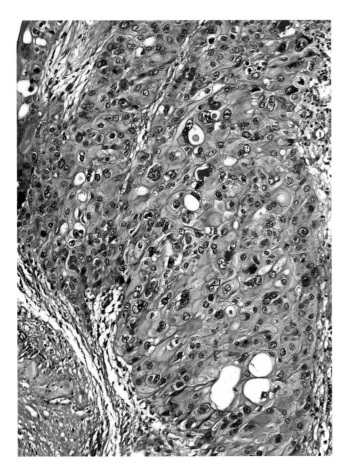

Fig. 13.95 Epithelioid trophoblastic tumor consisting of mononucleate chorionic-type intermediate trophoblast cells. Note admixed, eosinophilic apoptotic bodies.

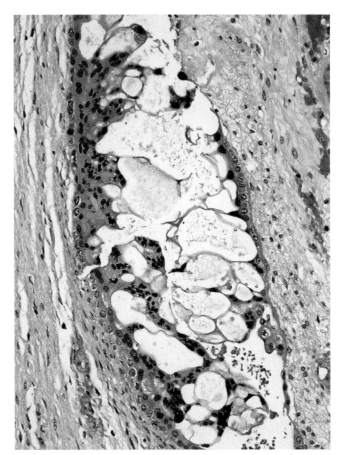

Fig. 13.96 Cystic trophoblastic tumor showing prominently vacuolated trophoblastic cells lining a space.

component of a germ cell tumor with other components.[649,650] Inhibin and hCG are focally positive, and p63 is variable.[649,650] Only about 15% of patients with cystic trophoblastic tumor in retroperitoneal lymph node specimens have had choriocarcinoma in the preceding orchiectomy.[649,650] The prognosis in retroperitoneal lymph node dissection specimens is similar to teratoma, and no further treatment is required if other components are absent.[648]

Teratoma, Postpubertal-Type

Clinical Features

Teratoma, postpubertal-type, usually occurs in adults as a component of a mixed germ cell tumor and is present in more than one-half of all mixed germ cell tumors and in approximately 25% of all nonseminomatous germ cell tumors.[345,640] In contrast with teratoma, prepubertal-type, it carries a definite risk for metastases even when present in pure form. Hence, there are reports of "pure mature teratoma" metastasizing as "pure mature teratoma" and also pure mature teratoma associated with metastases of nonteratomatous type, such as embryonal carcinoma.[652-658] The explanation for these observations is that postpubertal patients with pure teratoma develop teratoma from GCNIS through an intermediary of invasive, nonteratomatous malignant germ cell tumor.[659] This is supported by the frequent identification of GCNIS in seminiferous tubules adjacent to pure teratoma of the testis in postpubertal patients.[78] Nonteratomatous malignant elements are initially a component of a teratoma-containing mixed germ cell tumor, but transformation of the nonteratomatous elements to teratoma

(and/or their regression) occurs before orchiectomy. Metastasis of nonteratomatous elements with subsequent transformation at the metastatic site to teratomatous elements explains the phenomenon of mature teratoma metastasizing as mature teratoma; failure to transform at the site of metastasis explains mature teratoma of the testis associated with metastases of nonteratomatous type. It is of paramount importance to recognize that almost all pure, mature teratomas in postpubertal patients are malignant, although there is now evidence of rare benign cases (analogous to the benign pediatric teratomas).[29]

Most patients with testicular teratoma present with a testicular mass, although patients may have symptoms secondary to metastases. Serum marker elevation may occur because of admixed yolk sac tumor or syncytiotrophoblast cells either in the primary tumor or in metastases; in addition, mild AFP elevation may occur in patients with pure teratoma secondary to synthesis of AFP by endodermal glandular structures of teratomatous type.[57,59,532]

Pathologic Features

Grossly, teratoma has a variable appearance. Mature teratoma often contains multiple cysts, generally less than 1 cm in diameter, which contain watery to mucoid fluid (Fig. 13.97). Semi-translucent nodules of gray-white cartilage may be present, and a fibromuscular stroma may be seen among the cartilaginous and cystic structures. In other areas, the tumor may be solid (Fig. 13.98). Fleshy, encephaloid, and hemorrhagic areas usually correspond to foci of immaturity, which, if extensive, may justify a diagnosis of teratoma

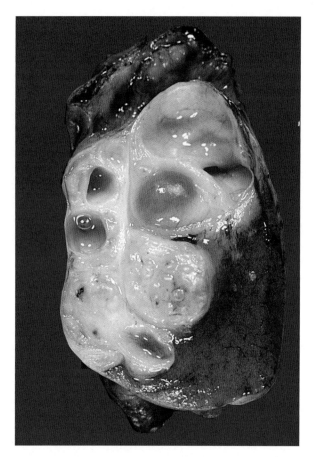

Fig. 13.97 Teratoma with several cysts and cartilage.

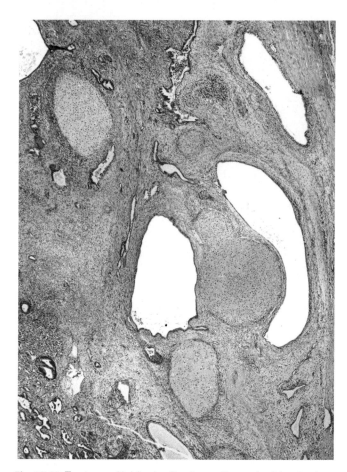

Fig. 13.99 Teratoma with islands of hyaline cartilage, glandular structures lined by enteric-type epithelium, and fibromuscular stroma.

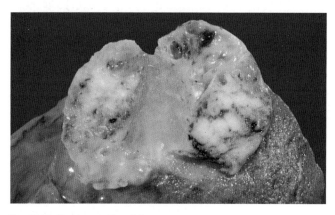

Fig. 13.98 Teratoma with solid appearance.

with a secondary malignant component. Such foci may also represent intermixed nonteratomatous elements.

Microscopically, mature teratoma consists of a variety of somatic-type tissues (Fig. 13.99), commonly including cartilage, smooth and skeletal muscle, neuroglia, enteric-type glands (Fig. 13.100), squamous epithelial islands and cysts, respiratory epithelium, and urothelial islands. Less commonly, bone and pigmented choroidal epithelium, and rarely kidney, liver, meninges, choroid plexus, or prostatic tissues, are present. These tissues are considered mature, but it is quite common to find significant cytologic atypia (Figs. 13.101 and 13.102). This atypia correlates with

the presence of aneuploidy in mature testicular teratoma, reflecting their derivation (see earlier discussion).[660] There is no evidence that the grading of the degree of atypia, based on qualitative assessment of nuclear enlargement, hyperchromasia, and mitotic rate, has any prognostic significance. The testicular parenchyma adjacent to postpubertal-type teratomas has GCNIS in about 90% of the cases and usually shows tubular atrophy and sclerosis with hypospermatogenesis.[77] Microlithiasis also may be seen.

Immature elements are common in postpubertal-type teratoma but are not known to have any prognostic significance. This was recognized in the 2004 WHO classification, which no longer drew a distinction between mature and immature testicular teratomas and is also the case in the current classification.[23,661] Such elements are easily recognized when they consist of highly immature tissues such as neuroectoderm, blastema, or embryonic tubules. Neuroectoderm consists of small, hyperchromatic cells arranged in tubules and rosettes (Fig. 13.103). Blastema consists of nodular collections of oval cells with scant cytoplasm and hyperchromatic nuclei (Fig. 13.104); such blastematous elements may be mixed with embryonic tubules lined by cuboidal cells with scant, inconspicuous cytoplasm. When intermixed, these two components resemble a primitive blastomatous neoplasm such as nephroblastoma or pulmonary blastoma (Fig. 13.104). Lower-grade "immature" elements are common, including a hypercellular or a myxomatous, hypocellular mesenchyme (Fig. 13.105). Such stroma likely represents a precursor to smooth muscle, as it is often arranged concentrically around islands of epithelium in a manner similar to

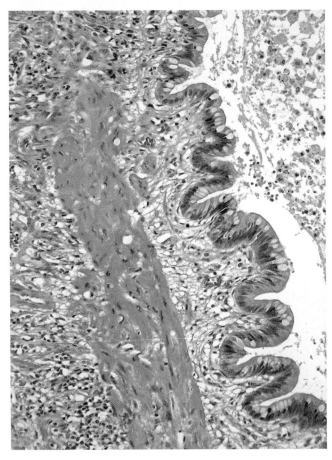

Fig. 13.100 Mature enteric-type epithelium in a teratoma with associated smooth muscle.

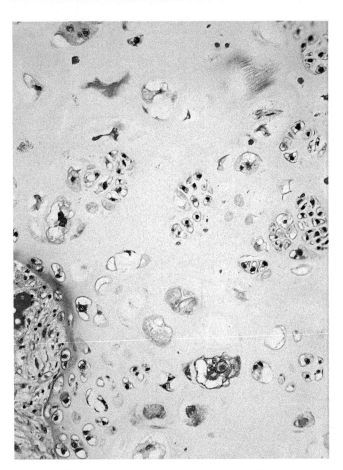

Fig. 13.102 Cytologic atypia of hyaline cartilage in a teratoma.

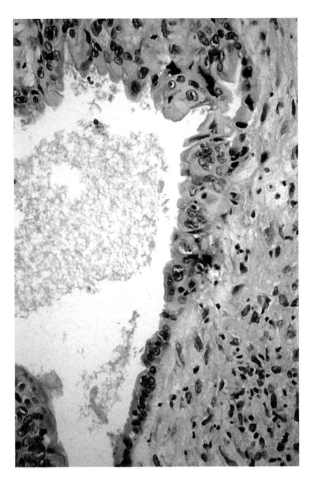

Fig. 13.101 Cytologic atypia of glandular epithelium in a teratoma.

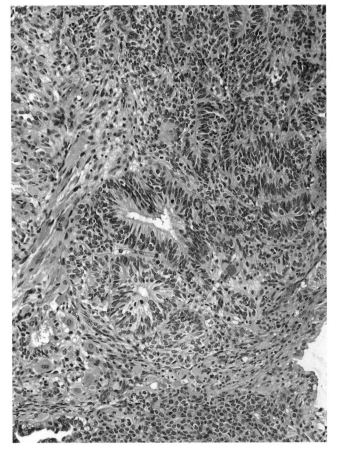

Fig. 13.103 Embryonic-type neuroectoderm in a teratoma.

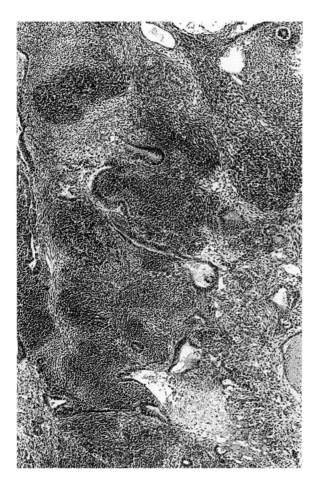

Fig. 13.104 Cellular nodules of blastema with glands in a teratoma.

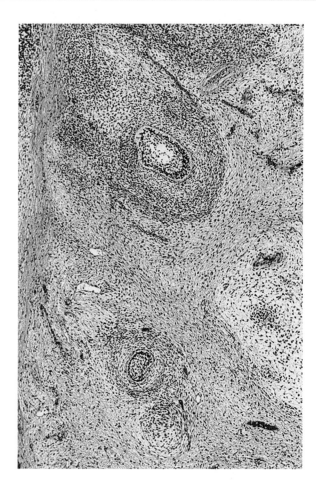

Fig. 13.105 A lower degree of immaturity in this teratoma, compared with Fig. 13.104, with modestly cellular stroma around islands of epithelium.

muscularis propria of the gastrointestinal or respiratory system (Fig. 13.105).

Special Studies

Immunohistochemical staining of teratomatous elements yields results expected for the nature of the particular tissue.[615,616,662] AFP may be present within glands of enteric or respiratory type, as well as within liver-like tissue[57,59,532]; therefore pure teratoma may be associated, theoretically, with modestly elevated serum AFP, although this rarely is manifest. Alpha-1-antitrypsin, CEA, and ferritin may also be produced by teratomatous epithelium, and PLAP-positivity may be expressed in glands of a minority of teratomas.[281,288,402,532] Focal SALL4 reactivity occurs in some postpubertal-type teratomas.[409] IMP3, an oncofetal protein expressed in many malignancies, is expressed in testicular teratoma and in other testicular germ cell tumor components, but not in ovarian teratoma, supporting the malignant nature of testicular postpubertal-type teratoma.[663]

Mature postpubertal-type teratoma usually has aneuploid DNA content, frequently in the hypotriploid range.[664-666] The i(12p) marker chromosome is also found in most postpubertal-type teratomas.[424,666,667] These data support the derivation of postpubertal-type teratoma from GCNIS. As mentioned previously, the karyotype of the prepubertal teratomas is normal. The fibrous stroma of postpubertal-type teratoma has isochromosome 12p or other overrepresentation of 12p similar to the epithelial and other components, supporting its neoplastic nature and common origin with the epithelial components.[667]

Differential Diagnosis

It is important to distinguish postpubertal-type and prepubertal-type teratomas because of the benign nature of the latter.[29,375,668-672] Dermoid cyst, now considered a subtype of prepubertal-type teratoma, often has grossly evident hair within a largely cystic lesion, unlike postpubertal-type teratoma.[661] On microscopic examination, it has an organotypical arrangement of hair and adnexal structures to an epidermal surface, a feature rarely encountered in postpubertal-type teratoma. Although it shares with postpubertal-type teratoma the presence of diverse tissue types, including intestinal mucosa, cartilage, bone, and others, these lack the cytologic atypia that may be seen in postpubertal-type teratoma. Most importantly, dermoid cyst is not associated with GCNIS.[670] Similar comments pertain to the nondermoid postpubertal-type teratomas; although these lack the organoid cutaneous-like component, they often show organoid bronchus-like or, less commonly, enteric-type structures. Moreover, even when organoid arrangements are less apparent, prepubertal-type teratomas frequently show prominence of ciliated and squamous epithelium and smooth muscle. Absence of "dysgenetic" tubular changes and GCNIS is also helpful in recognizing them, as is their cytologically bland appearance. Epidermoid cyst, now considered a subtype of prepubertal-type teratoma, is lined with keratinizing squamous epithelium but lacks associated adnexal structures. Unlike postpubertal-type teratoma, epidermoid cysts do not display cytologic atypia, and there is absence of GCNIS.[78,673] Although squamous predominant postpubertal-type teratomas are infrequently encountered, close inspection almost always discloses nonsquamous elements. Furthermore, the squamous epithelium is typically arranged as multiple nests of different sizes rather than as a single cystic lesion. If additional assurance is needed to make the distinction of postpubertal-type from prepubertal-type teratoma, FISH study of the teratoma can be done for chromosome 12p amplification, which is present in the former but not in the latter.

Treatment and Prognosis

Postpubertal-type teratomas have a guarded prognosis. In two referral series of adult patients with "pure mature teratoma," the frequency of metastases was over 40%, to some extent reflecting referral bias.[657,658] Johnson et al. performed orchiectomy and RPLND in 18 patients with "mature teratoma," some of whom also had a seminomatous component, and reported 100% 5-year survival.[674] Conversely, 2 of 12 adult patients with pure teratoma reported by the British Testicular Tumor Panel died of nonteratomatous metastases.[656] Dixon and Moore reported 70% 5-year survival for patients with teratoma, with or without seminoma. The prepubertal-type teratomas (including epidermoid and dermoid cyst) are cured by orchiectomy.[675]

Teratoma With Somatic-Type Malignancy

Somatic-type malignancies may occur in association with teratoma, usually in posttreatment specimens but occasionally in the untreated testis. Somatic-type malignant components are encountered most frequently in metastases to the lung or retroperitoneal lymph nodes, but also at other sites.[676] These tumors share 12p amplification and loss of heterozygosity, supporting origin from the same progenitor cell.[584] They have also been referred to as "teratoma with malignant transformation," an unfortunate consequence of borrowing terminology that was used for ovarian teratomas, which are mostly of different pathogenetic nature. This term, however, incorrectly suggests that postpubertal-type teratoma in the absence of such transformation is not malignant. Also, somatic-type malignancies may occur after testicular germ cell tumors lacking a teratoma component (30% of cases), and some of these originating tumors express AFP or glypican-3, suggesting that the somatic-type malignancy may be of yolk sac tumor derivation.[677,678]

A somatic-type malignancy in a teratoma may have either a mature or immature appearance. Carcinoma of somatic type, representing the destructive growth of epithelium with a mature phenotype, is recognized by its invasive features. It forms masses of cytologically malignant epithelium or irregularly configured, infiltrating cords or nests associated with a desmoplastic reaction. Carcinomas showing glandular (Fig. 13.106), squamous, or neuroendocrine differentiation or lacking differentiation may occur. Glandular tumors with glypican-3 and AFP expression and scant to absent keratin 7 and EMA expression may, however, represent glandular pattern yolk sac tumor.[677] Glandular pattern yolk sac tumor has a poor prognosis, similar to or poorer than somatic-type adenocarcinoma arising in germ cell tumor.[677] SALL4 may be a useful marker for these tumors when seen at distant sites, although it is more consistently positive in glandular pattern yolk sac tumor (71% of cases) than in adenocarcinoma arising from a germ cell tumor (36% of cases).[677] It is notable that CDX2 expression is frequent in glandular pattern yolk sac tumors (83% of cases) and adenocarcinomas arising in germ cell tumors (63% of cases).[677]

Sarcoma may occur either as a specific histologic type (e.g., chondrosarcoma, leiomyosarcoma, well-differentiated

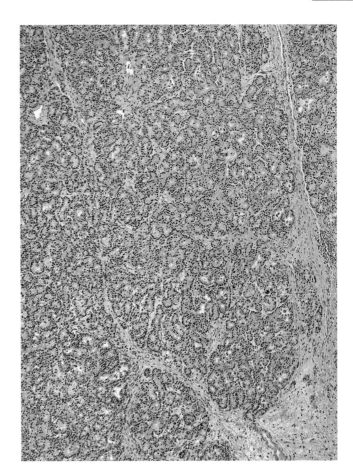

Fig. 13.106 Carcinoma with glandular differentiation showing confluent growth in a teratoma.

liposarcoma) or as a spindle cell sarcoma with no apparent specific differentiation.[676] Because invasion of mesenchymal elements is not easily distinguished from atypical mesenchyme that remains an integral component of a teratoma, we require that sarcomas manifest independent growth by producing a pure proliferation of a single type of highly atypical mesenchyme of at least a $4 \times$ field (5-mm diameter).[679] Overgrowth of embryonic-type neuroectoderm or nephroblastic tissue results in primitive neuroectodermal tumors or Wilms tumors, respectively.[680-683] Embryonal rhabdomyosarcoma represents a pure overgrowth of mitotically active primitive rhabdomyoblastic cells (Fig. 13.107). Because identical primitive elements may occur in teratoma, there is need to find a "pure" proliferation of such elements before concluding that one of these types of somatic-type malignancy is present. Sarcomatoid tumors lacking differentiation to a specific tumor type and with expression of keratin AE1/AE3 and glypican-3 may represent sarcomatoid yolk sac tumor (Fig. 13.75 and the discussion of postchemotherapy resections later in this chapter), with prognosis similar to or poorer than sarcoma arising in a germ cell tumor.[677,678] SALL4 may be a useful marker to support germ cell origin for sarcomatoid yolk sac tumor at distant sites (positive in about 60% of cases), but expression has not been reported in sarcomas arising from germ cell tumors (0% of cases).[677] Sarcomatoid yolk sac tumor may show myxoid tumor "ringlets," intercellular basement membrane deposits (parietal differentiation), and have variable nuclear atypia.[678] Grading using the French Federation of Cancer Centers Sarcoma group system is prognostic for sarcomatoid tumors arising in testicular germ cell tumors.[677,684]

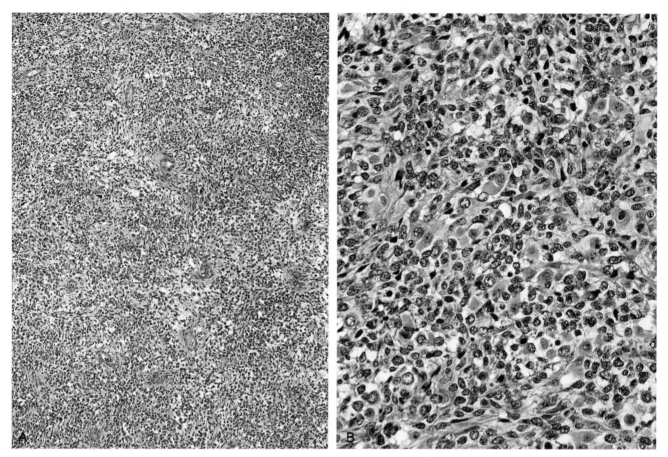

Fig. 13.107 Embryonal rhabdomyosarcoma in a teratoma. (A) Low magnification shows tumor overgrowth. (B) High magnification shows primitive cells with differentiated rhabdomyoblasts.

Disseminated somatic-type malignancies do not respond well to the usually effective chemotherapy for metastatic germ cell tumors, so aggressive surgical resection is the crucial component of treatment.[676,685] Compared with patients with other metastatic germ cell tumors, the prognosis is worse for these patients, especially when the somatic component is primitive neuroectodermal tumor or rhabdomyosarcoma.[679,680,686-688] The secondary malignancies in such cases have been shown to have the abnormalities of chromosome 12p.[685,689]

The clinical significance of teratoma with a secondary malignant component in the testis in the absence of known metastatic disease is not clear. Patients with such tumors probably more commonly develop chemoresistant "nongerm cell" neoplasms after chemotherapy.[679,690] Ahmed et al. with 5 patients and Colecchia et al. with 12 patients did not document a poor prognosis in germ cell tumors with somatic-type malignant components that were clinically confined to the testis.[676,687]

Primitive Neuroectodermal Tumor

This neoplasm results from overgrowth of embryonic-type neuroectodermal elements that are a common component of immature testicular teratoma. It is best to reserve the term "primitive neuroectodermal tumor" of the testis for those rare cases that are a pure proliferation of such elements, and to diagnose cases with residual teratomatous or other germ cell tumor elements as having areas of primitive neuroectodermal tumor with other germ cell tumor components.[34,691-693] The distinction of such cases from teratoma depends on overgrowth of a primitive neural component, as previously described.

These cases occur in the typical age range for adult-type germ cell tumors, but may rarely occur in children.[694] Gray-white, partially necrotic tumors are identified. Microscopically, the tumors contain small, hyperchromatic, poorly differentiated neural-type cells arranged in rosettes, tubules, or diffusely (Fig. 13.108).[691,693] The tumors most commonly resemble medulloepithelioma of the central nervous system, and may show glial differentiation that is reflected by immunoreactivity for glial fibrillary acidic protein and sometimes by features that are of overtly malignant glial type (Fig. 13.109).[680,695] Similar to central nervous system primitive neuroectodermal tumors, most germ cell tumor–derived cases lack the t(11;22) translocation typical of peripheral primitive neuroectodermal tumor.[695] Very rare cases of peripheral primitive neuroectodermal tumor of the testis, however, may have chromosome 22 rearrangement detectable by FISH.[696] Neurosecretory granules may be identified ultrastructurally.[693] Immunohistochemical studies utilizing neural markers, including chromogranin, synaptophysin, and CD99, may be useful if positive, but neuroendocrine markers other than CD57 are frequently negative.[680,695] Other small cell tumors in the differential diagnosis include teratoma with embryonic-type neuroectodermal elements, metastatic small cell carcinoma, malignant lymphoma, and nephroblastoma. As discussed earlier, the distinction from teratoma is based on the amount of primitive neural tissue. Small cell carcinoma does not form the well-defined tubules

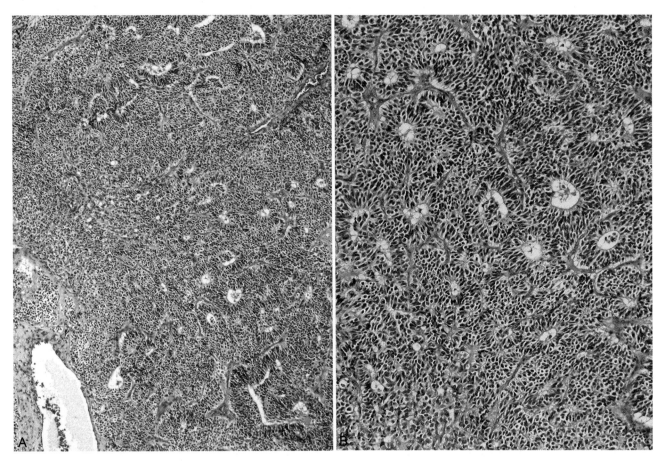

Fig. 13.108 (A) Primitive neuroectodermal tumor with neural-type cells arranged in rosettes, tubules, and diffusely. (B) Stratified, hyperchromatic tumor cells line tubules.

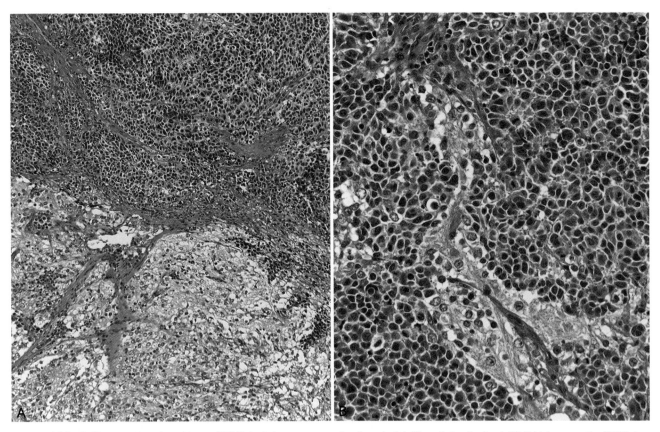

Fig. 13.109 (A) A primitive neuroectodermal tumor (PNET, *top*) shows an area of malignant glial differentiation *(bottom).* (B) At high power, the PNET shows a small focus *(bottom)* with glial differentiation.

and rosettes that occur in most primitive neuroectodermal tumors and usually shows more intense and widespread cytokeratin reactivity that contrasts with the focal, weak, or absent reactivity in primitive neuroectodermal tumor. The absence of GCNIS in small cell carcinoma metastatic to the testis contrasts with its usual presence in testicular primitive neuroectodermal tumor. Additionally, small cell carcinoma tends to occur in older patients who often have a history of lung cancer or cancer at another appropriate primary site.[693] The absence of GCNIS, tubules, and rosettes and the tendency for interstitial growth help in the differential with lymphoma, although immunohistochemistry offers a powerful method for distinction. Overgrowth of blastema and epithelium in a teratoma can produce a tumor resembling a nephroblastoma that is easily confused with a primitive neuroectodermal tumor (Fig. 13.110).[683] Distinction may require immunohistochemistry for neural markers, which are negative in nephroblastoma-like tumors, and WT1. Ultrastructural or immunohistochemical studies permit separation of the other alternative diagnoses.

Testicular germ cell tumors with primitive neuroectodermal tumor behave more aggressively than germ cell tumors lacking it as a component. Seven of 15 clinical stage I patients with a component of testicular primitive neuroectodermal tumor either had metastases or relapsed on surveillance management.[681] Of the 23 patients who presented with metastatic primitive neuroectodermal tumor and received chemotherapy, only three had a complete response.[681] The mainstay of treatment therefore is complete surgical excision of metastatic lesions.[685]

Mixed Germ Cell Tumor

Mixed germ cell tumors have more than one type of germ cell tumor component, including one or more nonseminomatous elements, and are thus classified as nonseminomatous tumors, even if seminoma is the chief neoplastic type. Mixed germ cell tumors are common, accounting for about one-third of germ cell tumors and 69% of all nonseminomatous germ cell tumors of the testis.[39] Virtually any combination of elements may be present. Frequent combinations include: embryonal carcinoma and teratoma; embryonal carcinoma and seminoma; embryonal carcinoma, yolk sac tumor, and teratoma; embryonal carcinoma, teratoma, and choriocarcinoma; embryonal carcinoma, teratoma, and seminoma; and teratoma and seminoma.[39] Although seminoma with syncytiotrophoblast cells is histopathologically a mixed germ cell tumor, it is classified as a variant of seminoma rather than a mixed, nonseminomatous neoplasm because the natural history and treatment are similar to seminoma.

Clinical Features

Patients with mixed germ cell tumor have the same clinical features as those with nonseminomatous germ cell tumor, and most present with a testicular mass. Those with a predominance of embryonal carcinoma average 28 years of age, whereas patients with a predominance of seminoma average 33 years.[697] AFP and hCG elevation occurs in about 60% and 55% of patients with mixed germ cell tumor, respectively.[358]

Pathologic Features. Grossly, mixed germ cell tumors are often variegated because of their different components (Fig. 13.111). Foci of hemorrhage and necrosis are common. The microscopic features are like those of the individual components described elsewhere in this chapter. It is common for foci of yolk sac tumor with microcystic or vacuolated patterns to be contiguous with areas of embryonal carcinoma, and such foci are easily overlooked (Fig. 13.112). A "double-layered" pattern of embryonal carcinoma has been described in which ribbons of columnar embryonal carcinoma cells are accompanied by a parallel ribbons of flattened tumor cells (Fig. 13.45); the intense AFP immunoreactivity of this flattened cell layer, together with its morphology, indicates yolk sac

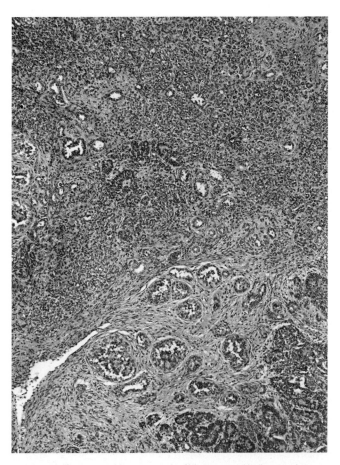

Fig. 13.110 Teratoma with overgrowth of blastema, epithelium, and stroma resembling nephroblastoma.

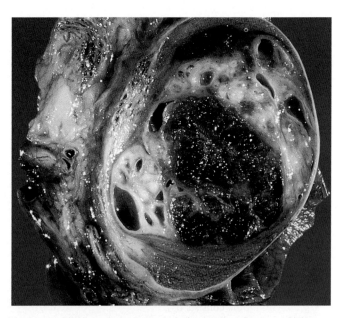

Fig. 13.111 Variegated appearance of mixed germ cell tumor, with hemorrhagic, cystic, and fleshy areas.

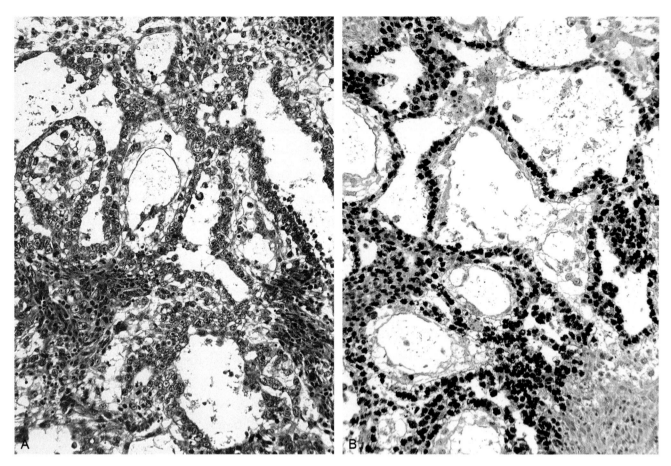

Fig. 13.112 (A) Luminal spaces lined by embryonal carcinoma cells with yolk sac tumor cells on the adluminal aspect. (B) OCT3/4 highlights the nuclei of the embryonal carcinoma but spares those of the yolk sac tumor.

tumor differentiation, and this pattern should therefore be classified as a form of mixed germ cell tumor (embryonal carcinoma and yolk sac tumor).[520,698] This pattern has sometimes been described as "necklace-like" or "diffuse embryoma" (see later).

Polyembryoma and Diffuse Embryoma

Polyembryoma is a distinct form of mixed germ cell tumor that recapitulates the embryo at approximately 13 to 18 days of gestation and is very rare as a dominant pattern.[699,700] The embryoid body consists of a central core of cuboidal to columnar, sometimes stratified, embryonal carcinoma cells, a "ventral" yolk sac tumor component forming a yolk sac–like vesicle, and a "dorsal" space similar to that of the amniotic sac and lined by flattened epithelium (Fig. 13.113).[701,702] The embryoid body is surrounded by loose, myxomatous, richly vascular tissue, similar to extraembryonic mesenchyme, which is also commonly identified in yolk sac tumor (Fig. 13.113). Because of the yolk sac tumor component, patients with polyembryoma may have substantial AFP elevation.[701] In some cases, intestinal and squamous differentiation of the "amniotic" epithelium is present, as well as hepatic differentiation in the yolk sac–like zone.[701] Imperfectly formed embryoid bodies are occasionally seen in mixed germ cell tumors, consisting of small nodular collections of embryonal carcinoma admixed with yolk sac tumor, surrounded by a myxomatous to fibrous stroma (Fig. 13.114).

Diffuse embryoma consists of a sheetlike admixture of embryonal carcinoma and yolk sac tumor in approximately equal proportions (Fig. 13.115), with the two components retaining their expected immunohistochemical reactivities.[703,704] The "double-layered" tumor pattern (Fig. 13.45) may also be considered "diffuse embryoma." The behavior and treatment of polyembryoma and diffuse embryoma is similar to other mixed germ cell tumors with these components.

Treatment and Prognosis

Patients with mixed germ cell tumors are managed like patients with nonseminomatous tumors. Tumors consisting of embryonal carcinoma and teratoma are less likely to metastasize than tumors having the same volume of embryonal carcinoma but lacking a teratomatous component, suggesting that the ability of embryonal carcinoma to differentiate is associated with a decrease in metastatic potential.[705] A similar observation has been made for cases having a yolk sac tumor component, with a decrease in metastatic potential.[558] However, improved prognosis with a yolk sac tumor component has not always been observed, as in a recent series of 615 patients, where yolk sac tumor in the primary tumor was associated with a poor prognosis, with coexisting yolk sac tumor and seminoma having the poorest outcome.[706] This seems likely related to the poorer chemosensitivity of yolk sac tumor when metastatic.

Germ Cell Tumors of Unknown Type

Regressed Germ Cell Tumors

Some patients with extragonadal germ cell tumor lack clinical evidence of a primary testicular tumor.[707-710] Some have primary extragonadal germ cell tumor, especially those with tumor confined to the mediastinum or pineal region without retroperitoneal

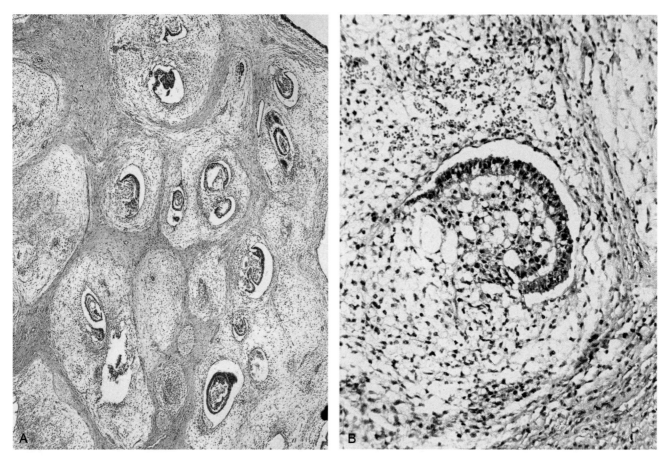

Fig. 13.113 (A) Polyembryoma consists of embryoid bodies in a myxoid stroma. (B) Embryoid body composed of a central core of embryonal carcinoma, a "ventral" yolk sac tumor component, and a "dorsal" amnion.

involvement. Current evidence suggests that retroperitoneal tumor, frequently thought in the past to be a common site of primary extragonadal germ cell tumor, is often caused by metastasis with regression of a primary testicular tumor.[336,710] Such cases are treated as testicular primary tumors.[711] Examination of the testis in cases with retroperitoneal germ cell tumor often demonstrates foci of testicular scarring and, less frequently, GCNIS.[336] This phenomenon of primary testicular tumor regression in the presence of metastases is documented in autopsy studies in which almost 10% of patients who die of metastatic testicular germ cell tumor show "burnt-out" primary tumors.[712] In our experience, essentially all types of germ cell tumor are susceptible to regression and, not unexpectedly, regressed seminoma composes the single greatest proportion of cases, given the large fraction of testicular germ cell tumors that seminoma represents.[523] It is also clear that many (possibly all) cases of "pure" postpubertal-type teratoma of the testis represent what were originally mixed germ cell tumors that had regression of the nonteratomatous components.[713]

Regression can be recognized from a constellation of findings (Figs. 13.116 to 13.118). All cases have scarred areas that may have either nodular or stellate configurations. These scars often contain a variably intense lymphoplasmacytic infiltrate and have prominent curvilinear blood vessels. They usually also have "ghost" remnants of hyalinized seminiferous tubules, which therefore do not represent evidence for a nonneoplastic process causing scarring.[185,523] Coarse intratubular calcifications in the scar provide very good evidence for a regressed germ cell tumor that had an intratubular embryonal carcinoma component, because these commonly undergo comedonecrosis in the tubules with dystrophic calcification. Peripheral to the scar, there invariably is tubular atrophy and sclerosis with impaired spermatogenesis, reflecting the usual testicular background on which postpubertal-type germ cell tumors develop. Additional findings include GCNIS in about one-half of cases, tubular microliths in about one-third, and prominent clusters of Leydig cells in about 40%.[523] We consider intratubular coarse calcifications within expanded tubular outlines in a scar or GCNIS peripheral to a scar to be diagnostic of a regressed germ cell tumor, whereas the other features are supportive but not entirely specific.

Postchemotherapy Specimens

Chemotherapy in patients with metastatic testicular germ cell tumor often results in a marked decrease in tumor size, although large masses may persist. Persistent masses are often surgically excised, and the pathologic findings are of prime importance in determining the future treatment for these patients.[573,714]

Following chemotherapeutic cytoreduction, residual masses may consist of necrosis (often associated with a xanthomatous reaction), fibrosis, and viable-appearing germ cell tumor histologically similar to the original tumor or with an altered morphology. Additionally, malignant neoplasms resembling non–germ cell tumors (e.g., sarcoma, primitive neuroectodermal tumor, and carcinoma) may occur.[573,679,686] Patients with teratoma in postchemotherapy retroperitoneal lymph node specimens have a significantly more favorable prognosis than patients with nonteratomatous components.[715] Patients with necrosis, fibrosis, and mature (although

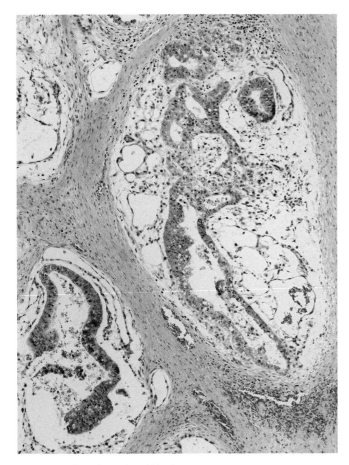

Fig. 13.114 Complex embryoid body.

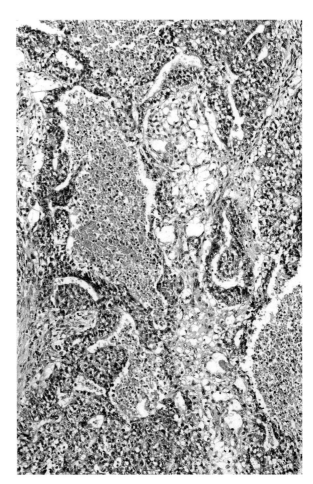

Fig. 13.115 Diffuse embryoma consists of an approximately equal mixture of embryonal carcinoma and yolk sac tumor.

often atypical-appearing) teratomatous lesions after chemotherapy are not usually treated with additional chemotherapy; conversely, those who have persistent embryonal carcinoma, yolk sac tumor, choriocarcinoma, or seminoma are candidates for second-line ("salvage") chemotherapy, sometimes with bone marrow transplantation. The treatment of postchemotherapy sarcoma, primitive neuroectodermal tumor, and carcinoma is problematic and often ineffective, but is usually primarily by surgical resection.[681,685,686] In one study of 101 patients with advanced, nonseminomatous germ cell tumor treated with cisplatin-based chemotherapy and resection of residual masses, 51% had necrosis or fibrosis; 37% had residual mature teratoma; and 12% had residual malignant, nonteratomatous germ cell tumor.[716]

Necrotic foci in postchemotherapy resections often appear as tan, granular nodules surrounded by a thin yellow rim (Fig. 13.119). Microscopically, there is central, coagulative necrosis consisting of eosinophilic debris with ghostlike outlines of necrotic tumor cells, typically lacking prominent karyorrhectic debris. Macrophages with abundant, foamy cytoplasm surround the areas of necrosis (Figs. 13.120 and 13.121), accounting for the grossly visible yellow rim. The nuclei of these cells may be mildly atypical, which, in conjunction with the clear cytoplasm, can lead to misinterpretation as seminoma (Fig. 13.121).[573] The absence of significant atypia and inconspicuous mitotic activity are usually sufficient to permit separation without resorting to special stains for glycogen, placental alkaline phosphatase, OCT3/4, and macrophage markers. If immunohistochemical staining is necessary, OCT3/4 immunohistochemistry is a sensitive and specific

marker for metastatic seminoma and embryonal carcinoma.[717] An active fibroblastic proliferation may be intermingled with the foamy macrophages, creating a fibroxanthomatous reaction.

Grossly, fibrosis in postchemotherapy resections is firm and white and, microscopically, consists of scattered spindle cells set in dense collagenous tissue. Some spindle cells may be enlarged and cytologically atypical but do not form fascicles and are scattered randomly, creating a hypocellular appearance (Fig. 13.122). Some of the apparent fibrous lesions may represent postchemotherapy persistence of the hypocellular, spindled cell component of yolk sac tumor, based on the identification of this yolk sac tumor pattern in the orchiectomy specimen and the intense cytokeratin reactivity of the spindle cells.[600] It is probably best, however, to consider the hypocellular, collagenous lesions as "fibrosis" rather than creating clinical confusion by characterizing it as persistence of a yolk sac tumor component, because it does not merit additional chemotherapy.

Some spindle cell lesions after chemotherapy display increased cellularity and mitotic activity in a more myxomatous background.[600] They have a fibrous (Fig. 13.123) to myxoid stroma (Fig. 13.124) and variable cellularity (Figs. 13.123 and 13.124) and often have a component of epithelioid cells. Tumor cell "ringlets" showing an empty space with surrounding tumor cells occur in a minority (Fig. 13.124). Based on their reactivity for cytokeratins, glypican-3, and SALL4, as well as their "magma reticulare"–like appearance, they should be classified as sarcomatoid yolk sac

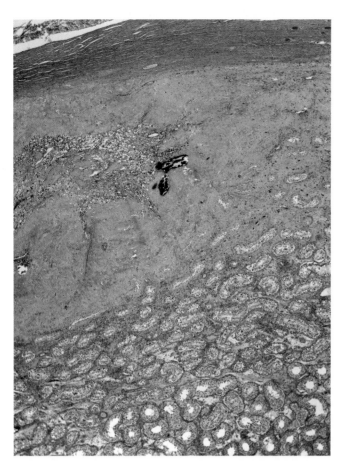

Fig. 13.116 Regressed germ cell tumor consisting of a discrete scar containing dystrophic, intratubular, coarse calcifications—a pathognomonic finding.

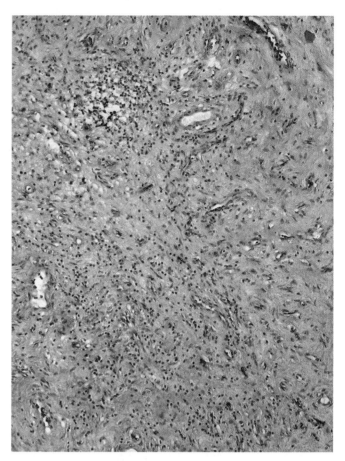

Fig. 13.117 Regressed germ cell tumor with scarring, lymphocytes, and prominent vessels.

tumors.[677,718] AFP positivity is usually absent in these lesions, as it is in the spindle cell component of the primary lesion.[600] Their cellularity and mitotic activity distinguishes them from the similarly derived examples of "fibrosis" discussed in the preceding paragraph. We have seen some of these sarcomatoid proliferations eventually evolve to embryonal rhabdomyosarcoma after multiple recurrences characterized by gradually increasing cellularity (Fig. 13.125). The prognosis of patients with high-grade spindle cell lesions in postchemotherapy resections is guarded.[600,677]

Teratomatous lesions after chemotherapy are common, and are readily diagnosed by those aware that metastatic teratoma may be seen after orchiectomy for germ cell tumors in which it is absent.[715,719] Metastatic teratoma usually appears as a multicystic mass with intervening fibrous or muscular tissue (Fig. 13.126); the cysts typically contain clear, serous fluid, but mucoid or hemorrhagic cyst contents may also be seen. Microscopically, there are often glands, squamous nests, islands of cartilage, smooth and striated muscle, and intervening fibromuscular stroma. Significant cytologic atypia can be identified in these tumors.[8,698,720] Glandular epithelium, although confined to round, noninvasive glands, may be stratified with enlarged, hyperchromatic, and mitotically-active nuclei, which raise a concern for embryonal carcinoma (Fig. 13.127). However, the primitive, vesicular nuclei and macronucleoli of embryonal carcinoma are absent. These glands often have intestinal differentiation, with goblet cells and eosinophilic absorptive-type cells. Squamous nests and cartilage may also display cytologic atypia. Stromal invasion by highly atypical

elements indicates a diagnosis of carcinoma or sarcoma; criteria for invasion are the same as in primary teratoma with a secondary malignant component.

Metastatic teratoma may be life threatening. Mature teratoma may undergo progressive enlargement and impinge on vital structures, especially in the mediastinum. This has been described as the "growing teratoma syndrome" and is one reason for complete excision of metastatic teratomatous tumor whenever feasible.[721-724] Although often diagnosed as mature teratoma, these tumors contain cells with a malignant genotype (as well as phenotype) based on karyotypic and ploidy studies.[660,725,726] Consequently, such lesions should be surgically excised before evolution of more aggressive clones of cells results in overgrowth with a malignancy of teratomatous origin.[665,726,727] Despite the cytologic atypia that occurs in metastatic teratomatous lesions after polychemotherapy, such atypia, in the absence of evolution to an invasive malignant neoplasm, does not have known prognostic significance.[720]

A variety of malignancies resembling tumors of non–germ cell origin ("somatic-type" malignancies) may be identified in postchemotherapy resections. Tumors with both yolk sac tumor and seminoma are most likely to undergo somatic transformation, and pure seminoma only rarely does so.[706,728] These consist of fleshy or necrotic areas among fibrous tissue and cysts. Embryonal rhabdomyosarcoma and primitive neuroectodermal tumor are the most common tumors of this type; others include malignant glioma, adenocarcinoma, undifferentiated carcinoma, and undifferentiated sarcoma.[679] One report describes a case with two distinct somatic-

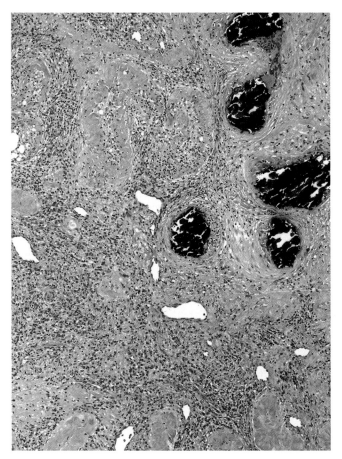

Fig. 13.118 Regressed germ cell tumor showing lymphocytes, coarse intratubular calcifications in expanded tubular profiles, and hyalinized tubules within a scar.

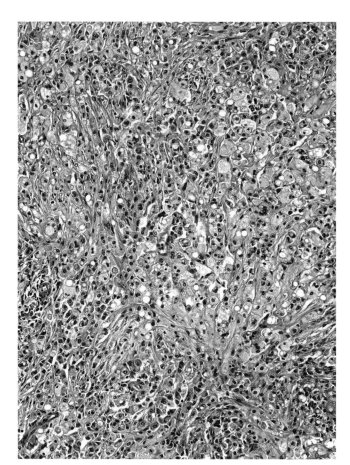

Fig. 13.120 The fibroxanthomatous reaction that often surrounds foci of tumor necrosis induced by chemotherapy may be highly cellular.

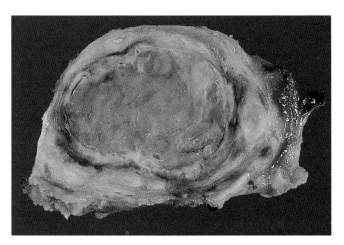

Fig. 13.119 Tumor necrosis after chemotherapy. A tan, granular nodule is surrounded by a yellow rim with peripheral fibrosis.

type malignancies, adenocarcinoma and leiomyosarcoma.[729] About one-fourth of sarcomatoid neoplasms in the postchemotherapy setting show glypican-3 and keratin AE1/AE3 reactivity and can be considered sarcomatoid yolk sac tumors (Figs. 13.123 and 13.124), which share the poor prognosis of the somatic-type malignancies.[728] The prognosis of germ cell tumors with somatic-type malignancies is guarded, with 5-year cancer-specific survival of approximately 64%.[685,728] For germ cell tumors with sarcoma or sarcomatoid yolk sac tumor, grading with the French sarcoma grading system may have prognostic value.[684,728]

The morphology of persistent, postchemotherapy, nonteratomatous germ cell tumor is usually like that of primary testicular neoplasms. However, exceptions to this rule occur, particularly with trophoblastic proliferations. Unlike the biphasic proliferation of syncytiotrophoblast and cytotrophoblast cells in classic choriocarcinoma, the trophoblastic proliferations in postchemotherapy resections often lack definite syncytiotrophoblast cells. Instead, mononucleated trophoblast cells may be identified in the absence of a syncytiotrophoblast component. Mazur described this pattern in patients treated for gestational choriocarcinoma as "atypical choriocarcinoma," but we prefer "monophasic" choriocarcinoma (Fig. 13.91).[730] In some cases, the trophoblast cells are exclusively mononuclear and form the epithelial lining of cysts, closely mimicking teratomatous cysts composed of atypical squamous epithelium (Fig. 13.128) but having focal hCG and/or inhibin reactivity.[731] The distinction between these cystic trophoblastic tumors and teratoma does not appear to be clinically important if there is no evidence of stromal invasion. We found no difference in outcome when such cystic trophoblastic tumors were identified with teratoma in postchemotherapy resections compared with historical outcomes for teratoma alone in the same setting.[648] They may, however, be associated with minor elevation in serum hCG. Solid, monophasic proliferations of trophoblastic cells, in contrast, merit additional chemotherapy, when feasible. Additionally, we have found that the appearance of yolk sac tumor may be different in postchemotherapy resections, especially in the context

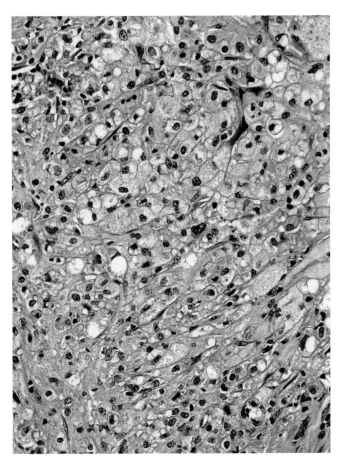

Fig. 13.121 The histiocytes in the fibroxanthomatous reaction adjacent to a necrotic tumor may show mild cytologic atypia.

of late recurrence. There tends to be a predominance of glandular (Fig. 13.129A), hepatoid (Fig. 13.129B), and parietal patterns in this setting, often to the extent that the clinical history of late recurrence can be predicted from the morphology.[586]

A potential pitfall in the interpretation of postchemotherapy retroperitoneal resections is the presence of paraganglionic tissue. The pale cytoplasm in these structures and diffuse to nested arrangement may lead to misinterpretation as persistent metastatic seminoma (Fig. 13.130). They are not, however, present in nodal tissue; the cytoplasm shows a subtle basophilic granularity; they are associated with small nerves; and the nuclear features are bland. If doubt remains, immunostains are diagnostic.

The outcome of patients undergoing excision of persistent masses after chemotherapy for metastatic testicular germ cell tumor varies depending on the pathologic findings. Eighty-eight percent of patients with only necrosis in retroperitoneal lymph node dissections were well on follow-up.[732] Similarly, only 1 of 25 patients (4%) with "fibrosis" relapsed on follow-up.[733] Residual mature teratoma is also associated with a favorable prognosis; a combination of three series reported benign follow-up in 90% of 42 cumulative patients.[733-735] Conversely, 24 of 30 patients (80%) with malignant, somatic-type neoplasms developed recurrent tumor after resection, and another series reported a 5-year survival of 51%.[686,720,736] For patients with persistent, apparently viable germ cell tumor other than teratoma in postchemotherapy resections, the prognosis is also guarded. Those who do well include patients who have complete surgical excision of persistent tumor, who have received only primary chemotherapy before resection, and who also receive postresection chemotherapy; patients with retroperitoneal tumor who meet these criteria have a 70% disease-free survival.[737] Patients who have persistent retroperitoneal germ cell tumor other than teratoma after salvage therapy and who are completely resected have a 40% disease-free survival.[737] Inability to completely resect

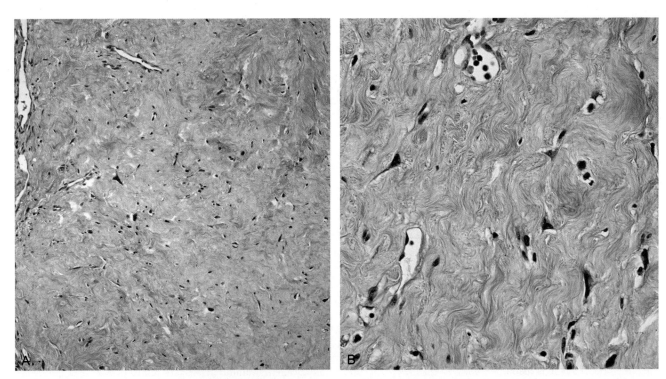

Fig. 13.122 (A) Fibrous lesion after chemotherapy contains widely scattered spindle and stellate cells. (B) High power shows mild cytologic atypia.

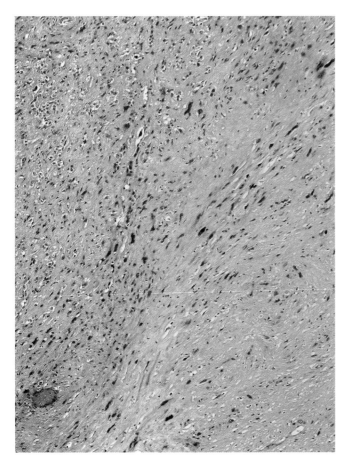

Fig. 13.123 Increased cellularity, especially at left, in conjunction with supporting immunoreactivity, justifies classification as sarcomatoid yolk sac tumor.

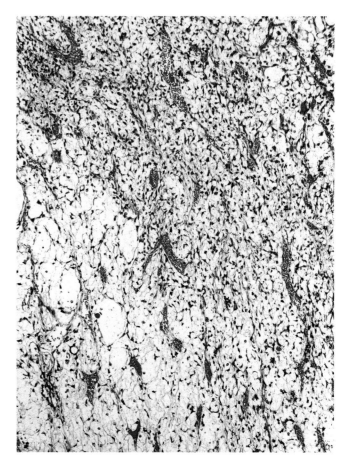

Fig. 13.124 Myxoid sarcomatoid yolk sac tumor.

viable germ cell tumor other than teratoma after primary or salvage chemotherapy carries a poor prognosis, with only 9% remaining clinically tumor free.[737] Additionally, only about one-third of patients with late recurrence of nonteratomatous germ cell tumor remain disease free after resection.[586]

Germ Cell Tumors Not Derived From Germ Cell Neoplasia in Situ

Spermatocytic Tumor

Clinical Features

Historically this tumor, known previously as "spermatocytic seminoma," was considered a variant of seminoma. Today it is recognized as a unique clinicopathologic entity with morphology, clinical features, and pathogenesis distinct from seminoma and other postpubertal germ cell tumors.[738] Originally described by Masson in 1946, spermatocytic tumor is an unusual neoplasm that represents only 1% to 2% of testicular germ cell tumors and occurs with about one-twentieth the frequency of seminoma.[39,739,740] Unlike other types of germ cell tumor, it occurs only in the testis (or, in one unique case, a dysgenetic gonad), slightly more frequently on the right side.[741-744] Also, unlike almost all other germ cell tumors that occur in postpubertal patients, spermatocytic tumor is not associated with cryptorchidism, GCNIS, or other types of germ cell tumor.[329,740] It occurs as a pure lesion, except in rare cases in which it is associated with a sarcoma.[743,745-747] Spermatocytic tumor is bilateral in up to 9% of cases, about four

times as frequently as seminoma, and there does not appear to have been a definite increase in incidence over time.[86,740,748]

Most patients with spermatocytic tumor are older than those with other types of testicular germ cell tumor. In various case series, the average age varied from 52 to 59 years, compared with an average of 40 years for patients with seminoma.[39,743,748-750] Nonetheless, 30% are in the fourth decade.[748] Most are white, but occurrence in African Americans and Asians has been reported.[743] Most patients present with painless, often long-standing, testicular enlargement.[740,743] Serum marker studies (AFP, hCG, and LDH) are negative.

Pathologic Features

Grossly, spermatocytic tumor usually ranges 3 to 15 cm in diameter and has a variable appearance, with zones of fleshy, white to tan tissue, mucoid or gelatinous change, friability, hemorrhage, and cystic degeneration (Fig. 13.131).[740] Necrosis, however, is uncommon. A multinodular appearance is frequent (Fig. 13.131), and paratesticular extension is infrequent.[743,751] Several patterns may be identified, often including a diffuse, sheet-like pattern that may be interrupted by follicle-like (Fig. 13.132) or irregular spaces (Fig. 13.133) caused by edema, which is present in up to 90% of cases. Multiple, cellular tumor nodules that are separated by an edematous stroma are also characteristic (Fig. 13.134). A partial surrounding rim of fibrin may occur at the periphery of some nodules (Fig. 13.135).[748] In about 20% of cases, intricate anastomosing tumor islands are seen (Fig. 13.136).[748] Corded growth occurs in a minority (20%) of cases, usually at the tumor

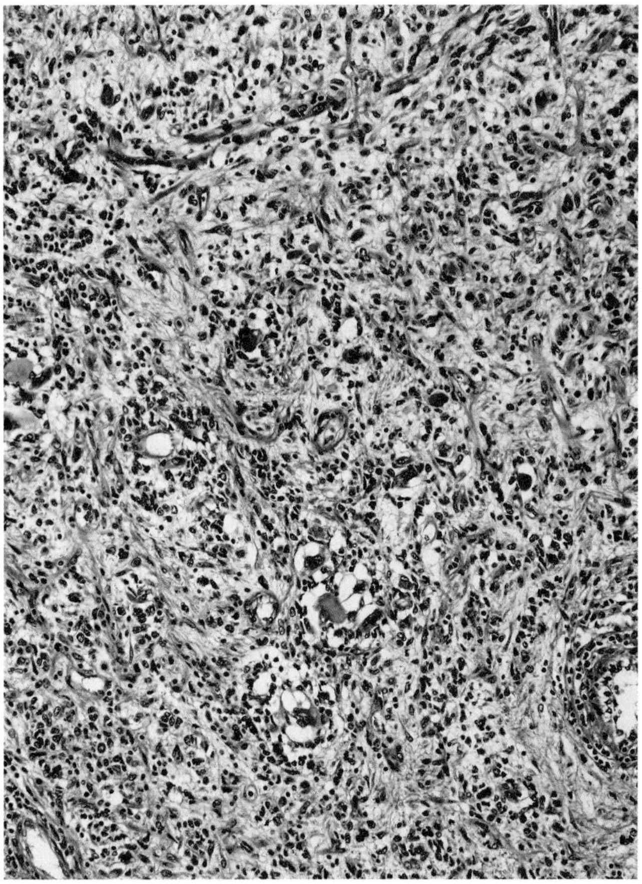

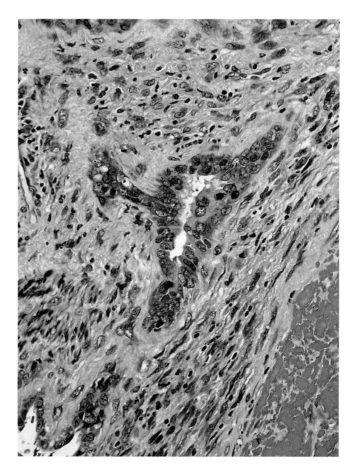

Fig. 13.125 Embryonal rhabdomyosarcoma after chemotherapy.

Fig. 13.127 High-grade epithelial atypia in a teratomatous gland embedded in atypical stroma.

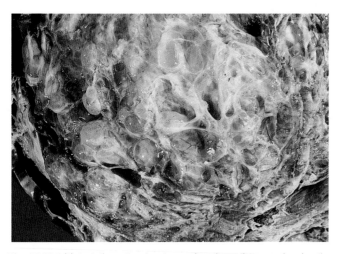

Fig. 13.126 Metastatic mature teratoma after chemotherapy, showing the characteristic multicystic appearance.

periphery. A prominent infiltrate of lymphocytes is uncommon (8% of cases), although rare clusters are present in about 40% (Fig. 13.137).[748] Granulomatous reactions are virtually never encountered, unlike seminoma. Apoptosis is almost always present and may be prominent, with many clusters of apoptotic cells (Fig. 13.138). The microscopic hallmark of spermatocytic tumor is a polymorphous population of cells (Fig. 13.139) that consists of three major types: a small, lymphocyte-like cell 6 to 8 μm in

diameter; an intermediate-sized cell averaging 15 to 20 μm in diameter; and giant cells, some of which may be multinucleated (Fig. 13.139), averaging 50 to 100 μm in diameter. The smallest cell has smudged, degenerate-appearing chromatin and scant eosinophilic to basophilic cytoplasm. The intermediate-sized cell has a round nucleus, usually with granular chromatin and scant cytoplasm. The nucleoli in the intermediate and giant cells are variably prominent. In some intermediate-sized and giant cells, the chromatin has a distinctive filamentous appearance that is like the chromatin of meiotic-phase, nonneoplastic spermatocytes ("spireme" chromatin). The borders between the cells, in contrast with seminoma, are generally indistinct. Intratubular growth is common (Fig. 13.140), and probably gives rise to separate invasive foci that cause the common multinodular or lobulated pattern of the tumor.[752]

An "anaplastic" variant of spermatocytic tumor was described in 1996, and isolated cases have been reported since then.[753] These tumors have conventional areas but, additionally, large areas with a uniform population of cells with vesicular nuclei and prominent nucleoli (Fig. 13.141) that may resemble either usual seminoma or embryonal carcinoma. Nonetheless, the immunohistochemical features are those of spermatocytic tumor (see later), including negativity for PLAP, OCT3/4, and cytokeratins. Because there is, yet, no clear evidence that these tumors behave more aggressively than other spermatocytic tumors, we discourage the use of this terminology, which is not recognized in the current WHO Classification.

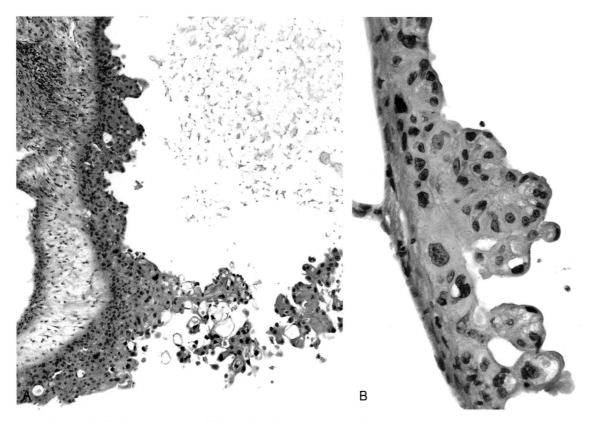

Fig. 13.128 Cystic trophoblastic tumor showing (A) intracystic proliferation of stratified trophoblast cells, some of which have cytoplasmic lacunae. (B) High power of the trophoblast cells lining the cyst.

Special Studies

In contrast with seminoma, spermatocytic tumor lacks glycogen. Most immunohistochemical markers are negative, including OCT3/4, vimentin, actin, desmin, AFP, hCG, NSE, carcinoembryonic antigen, and leukocyte common antigen.[282,404,407,742,743,753,754] Stains for placental alkaline phosphatase are also generally negative, although rare, focal positivity for PLAP may occur in isolated clusters of cells.[743,754] Cytokeratin stains are also usually negative, although perinuclear, dotlike positivity for cytokeratin 18 can be seen infrequently.[411,742] CD117, in contrast, is frequently positive in spermatocytic tumor, and such reactivity represents a potential pitfall in mistaking spermatocytic tumor for seminoma.[407,755] More recently, spermatocytic tumor has been found to be reactive for SALL4, a general germ cell tumor marker.[614] Spermatocytic tumor also expresses a variety of proteins, known as cancer testis antigens, that are characteristic of spermatogonia and spermatocytes (synaptonemal complex protein 1, synovial sarcoma on X chromosome, and xeroderma pigmentosa type A), indicating a more "mature" form of tumor differentiation than classic seminoma.[446,756] Several cancer testis antigens, GAGE7, NY-ESO-1, MAGE-A4, and NUT (nuclear protein in testis), may be used as diagnostic markers with high specificity if only diffuse strong staining is considered a positive result.[23,757] Differential expression of OCT2 and SSX family member 2-4 protein may divide spermatocytic tumor into subtypes resembling different stages of spermatogonial maturation.[752] Spermatocytic tumors show a characteristic amplification of a portion of chromosome 9 that encompasses the *DMRT1* gene; hence immunostains for DMRT1 protein are also positive.

Ultrastructurally, spermatocytic tumor may show intercellular bridges similar to those described in spermatocytes, as well as leptotene stage-type chromosomes (filamentous chromosomes with lateral fibrils).[758,759] These features suggest meiotic phase differentiation, but their presence and specificity are disputed.[760] Adjacent cells occasionally show macula adherens type junctions, and a Golgi body is a variably prominent feature. Other features include scattered mitochondria, occasional profiles of rough endoplasmic reticulum, nuclei with prominent nucleoli, and a thin basement membrane surrounding nests of tumor cells.[758,760] One ultrastructural feature of spermatocytic tumor is the presence of "nuage," cytoplasmic electron-dense deposits that lack a membrane and may be free in the cytoplasm or appear to bind mitochondria together ("intermitochondrial cement").[761] The presence of both nonmitochondria-associated nuage and intermitochondrial cement is characteristic of, and relatively specific for, normal male and female germ cells, but it is not seen in usual seminoma.[761] This observation may provide further support for the concept that spermatocytic tumor represents a more differentiated phenotype than usual seminoma.[761]

Flow-cytometric studies have demonstrated variable DNA content, including hyperdiploidy, peritriploidy, diploidy, peridiploidy, tetraploidy, and aneuploidy.[329,407,754,760] No haploid population has ever been found, arguing against spermatocytic tumor being postmeiotic. These variable results probably reflect the heterogeneous population of these neoplasms, because static cytophotometry of spermatocytic tumor has demonstrated a diploid or near-diploid DNA content in the small cell component, and a DNA content ranging up to 42C in the giant cell population, with intermediate values in the intermediate-sized cells.[762] One study suggested that the cells of spermatocytic tumor arise after cycles of polyploidization, refuting the notion of a meiotic phase tumor.[763] A karyotypic and differential gene profiling study (versus usual seminoma) found that spermatocytic tumor

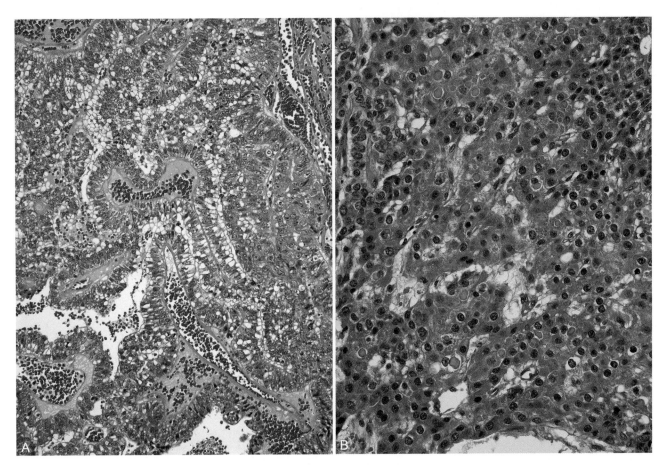

Fig. 13.129 Glandular (A) and hepatoid (B) patterns in postchemotherapy yolk sac tumor.

showed consistent gain in chromosome 9, failed to express the stem cell–associated genes typical of usual seminoma, and expressed genes associated with prophase of meiosis I.[764] These data support the derivation of spermatocytic tumor from the primary spermatocyte. Either *HRAS* or fibroblast growth factor receptor *(FGFR3)* gene mutations are seen in approximately 20% of cases.[752]

Treatment and Prognosis

There are only four cases of metastasizing spermatocytic tumor in which there was histologic documentation of the metastatic tumor.[765-768] Three of these cases had known lymphovascular invasion, which is ordinarily identified in only about 10% of cases.[748] At least some reported cases of metastatic spermatocytic tumor represent misinterpretations of lymphoma.[744] Because several hundred cases of spermatocytic tumor have been reported in the literature, the frequency of malignant behavior is well under 1%. Therefore orchiectomy alone is adequate treatment; adjuvant therapy is not indicated and may be harmful.[740,750]

Differential Diagnosis

The major differential diagnosis of spermatocytic tumor is seminoma. A summary of features helpful in this distinction is listed in Table 13.4. For the "anaplastic" variant, embryonal carcinoma is a consideration. The presence of the usual triphasic appearance of spermatocytic tumor, at least in foci, is quite helpful in such cases, as is the round nuclear contour that contrasts with the much more irregularly shaped nuclei of embryonal carcinoma. Absence

of GCNIS supports spermatocytic tumor, although some examples of intratubular spermatocytic tumor may mimic GCNIS (Fig. 13.142). Strong cytokeratin, OCT3/4 (nuclear), and CD30 (membranous) reactivity is expected for embryonal carcinoma but absent in spermatocytic tumor.[769] Positive markers for spermatic tumor are now available and include NUT, GAGE7, MAGE-A4, NY-ESO-1, and DMRT1.[757,764] Nuclear immunoreactivity should be strong and diffuse to be considered supportive of spermatocytic tumor, and a scoring system has been presented.[757] CD117 positivity is supportive of spermatocytic tumor but may be negative in valid cases (and is, of course, also expected in seminoma).

Spermatocytic Tumor With Sarcoma

Several cases of spermatocytic tumor associated with sarcoma have been reported.[743,745-748] Some of the patients gave histories of stable testicular masses that underwent rapid enlargement or became painful.[745,746] Some patients had symptoms secondary to metastases.[745] Grossly, many of the tumors were hemorrhagic, necrotic, and had a whorled appearance on cut surface.[745,746] Microscopically, the sarcoma was often admixed with the spermatocytic tumor (Fig. 13.143A) and usually described as an undifferentiated spindle cell sarcoma (Fig. 13.143B) or embryonal rhabdomyosarcoma, although chondrosarcomatous differentiation is also possible.[743,745-748,770] In contrast with pure spermatocytic tumor, over one-half of the reported cases of spermatocytic tumor with sarcoma metastasized, frequently with a fatal outcome.[745-747] The metastases were in a hematogenous distribution, with the lung being the most common metastatic site, and consisted solely of sarcoma.

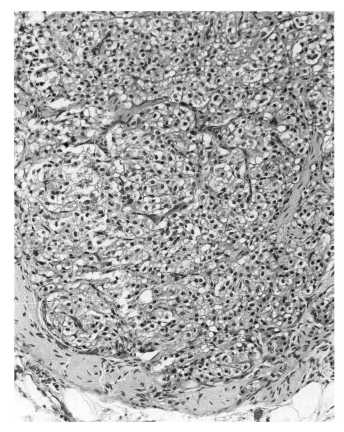

Fig. 13.130 Paraganglionic tissue in a retroperitoneal resection associated with small nerves.

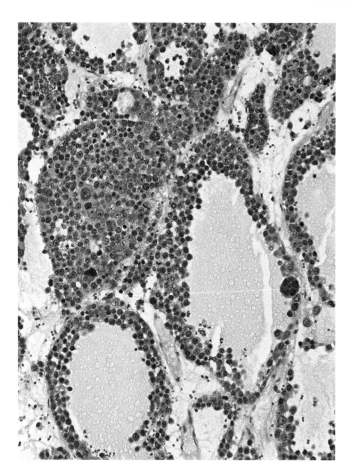

Fig. 13.132 Follicle-like spaces in an edematous spermatocytic tumor. Note the multinucleated tumor giant cell.

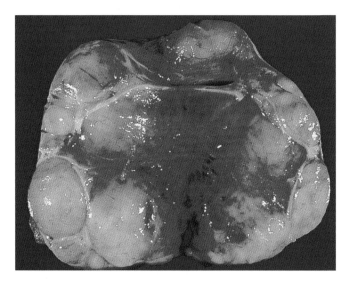

Fig. 13.131 Cut surface of spermatocytic tumor showing a multinodular, tan-yellow tumor with a central zone of hemorrhage. (Courtesy of RH Young, MD, Harvard Medical School, Boston, MA).

Teratoma, Prepubertal-Type

Teratoma is the second (after yolk sac tumor) most common form of testicular germ cell tumor (14% to 18% of cases) in children according to some registry series, but is a higher proportion (48%) in the combined experience in four pediatric centers.[510,771,772] In a recent single hospital series of pediatric testicular lesions, teratoma was more common than yolk sac tumor,

suggesting that the previous series finding that yolk sac tumor was more common may have been subject to referral bias.[773] Prepubertal-type teratoma occurs mostly as a pure neoplasm, at a median age of 13 months, and is commonly found during routine physical examination or by a parent.[771] Prepubertal-type teratoma in patients older than 4 years of age is unusual, but is now recognized to rarely occur in adult patients.[29,771] The pathogenesis of prepubertal-type teratomas is fundamentally different from postpubertal-type teratomas, a supposition supported by the absence of GCNIS in prepubertal-type teratomas.[76,78] These tumors do not develop from an invasive malignant germ cell (as is the case with postpubertal-type teratoma) but derive from a benign germ cell through an unknown mechanism. This viewpoint is supported by the normal karyotype of prepubertal-type teratomas, their benign outcome, differences in their patterns of genomic imprinting compared with postpubertal-type germ cell tumors, and absence of 12p amplification.[29,79,80,82,656,774-776]

Prepubertal-type teratomas have a different appearance than postpubertal-type teratomas. Those that are of dermoid type (see later), which are now considered a subtype of this group, may show the grossly evident hair and keratinous material commonly seen in the ovarian examples. The nondermoid prepubertal-type teratomas are not necessarily distinguishable from their postpubertal counterparts but frequently show cysts, keratinous material, a mucoid quality (Fig. 13.144), and no necrosis. They have a more organoid arrangement of elements that contrasts with the more frequently random arrangements of the postpubertal-type (Fig. 13.145). Ciliated respiratory-type epithelium is often prominent and invested

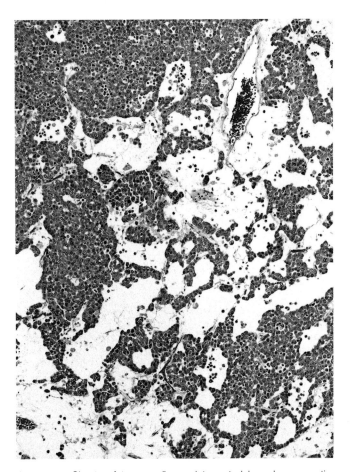

Fig. 13.133 Sheets of tumor cells are interrupted by edema, creating irregular spaces and cords in a spermatocytic tumor.

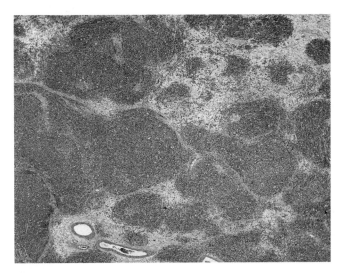

Fig. 13.134 Highly cellular tumor nodules in a spermatocytic tumor.

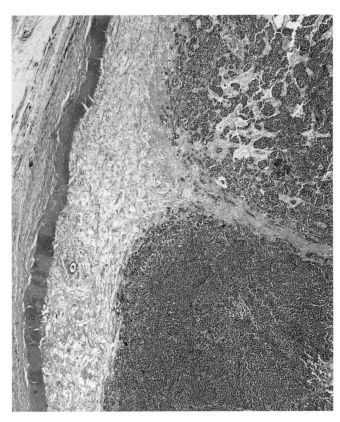

Fig. 13.135 A rim of fibrin surrounds tumor cell nodules in some spermatocytic tumors.

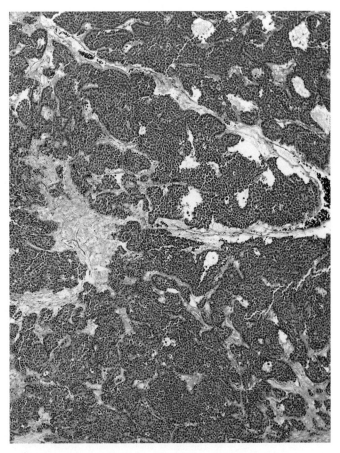

Fig. 13.136 Anastomosing tumor islands in a spermatocytic tumor.

by thick bundles of smooth muscle and with associated seromucinous acini, thus resembling bronchus (Fig. 13.145). Other teratomatous elements, including cysts lined by squamous or intestinal-type epithelium, intestinal type mucosa with accompanying muscularis mucosa, gastric pyloric-type epithelium, thyroid, pancreas,

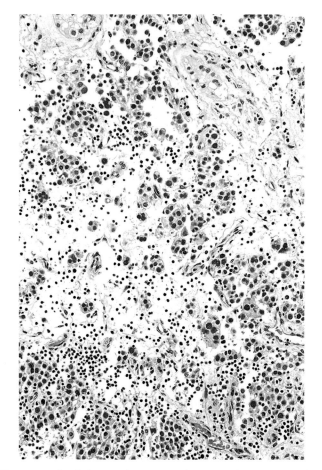

Fig. 13.137 Small clusters of spermatocytic tumor cells are separated by edematous stroma. Note the admixed lymphocytes, an unusual feature.

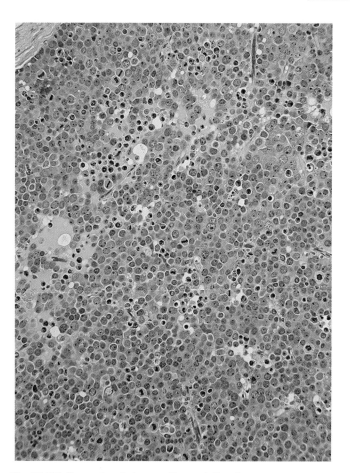

Fig. 13.138 Spermatocytic tumor with apoptotic cells.

salivary gland, cartilage, smooth muscle, adipose tissue, and bone may also be seen.[29,375,668-670,777-779]

Prepubertal-type teratoma must be diagnosed with caution in adults because of its differing prognosis and treatment (versus postpubertal-type teratoma). Careful evaluation for GCNIS, absence of "dysgenetic" testicular changes (i.e., tubular atrophy, peritubular sclerosis, impaired spermatogenesis, microlithiasis), absence of cytologic atypia, and FISH evaluation for isochromosome 12p/12p amplification are important to exclude postpubertal-type teratoma.[29,779]

In contrast with postpubertal-type teratomas, immaturity may be germane in prepubertal-type teratomas. Although immaturity does not have prognostic significance in the postpubertal setting, it is much more commonly seen in this group and was therefore described with postpubertal-type teratomas.

Prepubertal-type teratomas are almost invariably cured by orchiectomy, with only a single report of metastasis in a 6-month-old infant who had an 11-cm "immature" teratoma in an intraabdominal testis resected 3 months previously.[780] Testis-sparing surgery has been used successfully for prepubertal boys with pure teratoma.[781-783]

Dermoid Cyst

Dermoid cysts are considered a subset of prepubertal-type teratoma. They are cystic masses filled with friable, keratinous debris and hair. Analogous to the common ovarian counterpart, the wall of the cyst is composed of epidermis and dermis with hair follicles, sebaceous glands, and apocrine and eccrine sweat glands (Fig. 13.146), and a mural protuberance may also be present.[668,784] Other teratomatous elements, similar to those of the nondermoid prepubertal-type teratomas, may also be seen.[785,786] A helpful finding is a lipogranulomatous reaction in the adjacent parenchyma caused by leakage of sebaceous/keratinous cyst contents (Fig. 13.147). Patients ranged in age from 14 to 42 years in two series totaling fifteen cases.[670] GCNIS is absent, as is 12p amplification.[29,670] These tumors are benign, and testis-sparing surgery has been successful.[670,787]

Epidermoid Cyst

This lesion is now classified as a subtype of prepubertal-type teratoma like dermoid cyst and the nondermoid prepubertal-type teratomas; it is not associated with GCNIS, and it is uniformly benign.[78,672,673] It characteristically occurs in patients in the second to fourth decades of life.[671,788] The ultrasonographic appearance may be characteristic, with most cases having an "onion ring"–like laminated appearance.[788] Grossly, an epidermoid cyst usually is 2 to 3 cm in diameter, typically located at the periphery of the testis close to the tunica albuginea, and filled with white to yellow, friable, often pungent keratinous material (Fig. 13.148).[789] Microscopically, there is a single cyst lined by squamous epithelium with a granular cell layer and a fibrous wall of variable thickness (Fig. 13.149). The lining is often compressed to just a few flattened layers of cells. Unlike dermoid cyst, there are no adnexal structures in the wall of the cyst. It is crucial to examine the surrounding testis for GCNIS, which is an indication of postpubertal-type teratoma. Epidermoid cysts lack

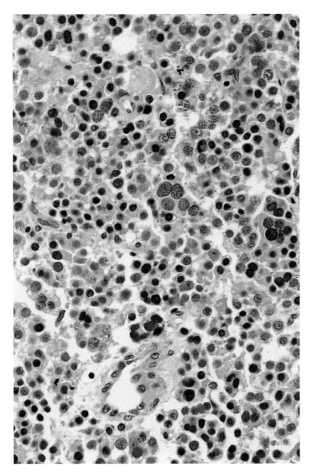

Fig. 13.139 The characteristic polymorphous cell population of a spermatocytic tumor. Several cells have granular to filamentous chromatin.

isochromosome 12p and 12p overrepresentation, in contrast with postpubertal-type teratoma, so FISH studies may be helpful in problematic cases.[790]

The epidermoid cyst requires no additional therapy after orchiectomy.[671,672] In cases in which testicular preservation is considered essential, it may be justifiable to locally excise the cyst and a rim of surrounding testis, with frozen section examination to determine the presence of GCNIS or other forms of germ cell tumor.[778,791] Testis-sparing surgery has been used successfully in pediatric patients, and follow-up in conservatively managed patients has been uneventful, but it is important to sample enough of the testicular parenchyma to confidently exclude GCNIS.[673,781,783,792]

Well-Differentiated Neuroendocrine Tumor (Monodermal Teratoma)

Well-differentiated neuroendocrine tumor, formerly termed *carcinoid tumor,* of the testis is considered a monodermal form of teratoma; and in support of this concept, 15% to 28% of testicular carcinoid tumors are associated with other teratomatous elements.[793-796] These rare tumors constituted 0.17% of testicular tumors in the files at the Armed Forces Institute of Pathology.[794] They have been said to occur more frequently than other germ cell tumors in older patients, with a median age of 45 to 50 years, with some cases in elderly men, although some occur in the typical age range of most germ cell tumors, and the mean age in a recent series of 29 cases was 36 years.[793-798] Rare cases are in children.[799] Most

patients present with a testicular mass; carcinoid syndrome is uncommon (occurring in 7% to 12% of cases) but correlates with increased metastatic potential.[795,796] It is more common to identify serotonin in tissue or serum, or its metabolites in urine, than for clinical carcinoid syndrome to occur.[795] AFP and hCG levels are normal (except for a single case associated with yolk sac tumor that had AFP elevation).[796] If metastases occur (16% of cases), they are usually in a hematogenous distribution, affecting liver, lung, bone, soft tissue, heart, and skin.[799]

Grossly, testicular well-differentiated neuroendocrine tumors are solid, yellow to tan, and well-circumscribed, varying from 0.3 to 8 cm in diameter (Fig. 13.150).[793,795,796] Associated cystic spaces may represent a teratomatous component; calcification occurs in about 10% of cases.[795] Microscopically, a pattern of mid-gut carcinoid tumor is the usual finding, with solid nests and acini of cells in a fibrous to hyalinized stroma that tends to retract from the epithelium (Fig. 13.151). The cells have eosinophilic, granular cytoplasm and round nuclei with a punctate or "salt-and-pepper" chromatin pattern. Vascular invasion or extratesticular extension occur in about 20% of testicular carcinoids, but they do not correlate with clinical malignancy in most instances.[795,798] Argyrophil and argentaffin stains are typically positive, and luminal mucin can be identified in some cases. Rarely a pure trabecular pattern or spindle cell pattern may occur.[796,797] Serotonin, substance P, chromogranin, synaptophysin, neuron specific enolase, gastrin, vasoactive intestinal polypeptide, neurofilament protein, and cytokeratin have been identified in these tumors, and one would expect to find positivity for other substances typical of mid-gut type carcinoid tumors in many cases.[795,800-803] Immunohistochemical stains for OCT3/4, CD30, c-kit, TTF-1, and CDX-2 are negative.[804] Ultrastructurally, the tumor cells contain pleomorphic neurosecretory granules typical of mid-gut carcinoid tumor.[793,795,800] Flow cytometry has demonstrated aneuploid or tetraploid DNA values and variable S-phase fractions.[795,798] Despite the relationship of well-differentiated neuroendocrine tumor to teratoma, the cases we and others have seen have lacked GCNIS, including the 29 cases in a recent report, although there are contradictory reports suggesting the possibility of a dual genetic pathogenesis.[796,802,804-807] Similarly there are conflicting data on the presence of isochromosome 12p, with some reports of absence and others of its presence.[796,804]

It is prognostically important to differentiate primary well-differentiated neuroendocrine tumor from metastasis to the testis. The occurrence of other teratomatous elements in some testicular well-differentiated neuroendocrine tumors is an indication of their primary nature. The occurrence of bilateral involvement, multifocal tumor, vascular invasion, or extratesticular spread favor well-differentiated neuroendocrine tumor metastatic to the testis rather than a primary testicular tumor. Primary well-differentiated neuroendocrine tumor is a low-grade malignancy; in their comprehensive review, Stroosma and Delaere found a metastatic rate of 16%; in a paper that postdates that of Stroosma and Delaere, Wang et al. identified malignant behavior in only 1 of the 23 cases with follow-up.[796,799] Large size (average diameter of metastasizing tumors = 7.3 cm versus average diameter of nonmetastasizing tumors = 2.9 cm) and the carcinoid syndrome were the strongest predictors of metastasis in one study.[795] Features of atypical carcinoid/grade 2 neuroendocrine tumor (≥2 mitoses/10 high-power fields and/or necrosis) may be the best indicator of malignant potential; Wang et al. in their review found no convincing evidence of metastasis from classic carcinoid tumor of the testis and argued that all metastatic cases were atypical carcinoids.[796] Most cases are

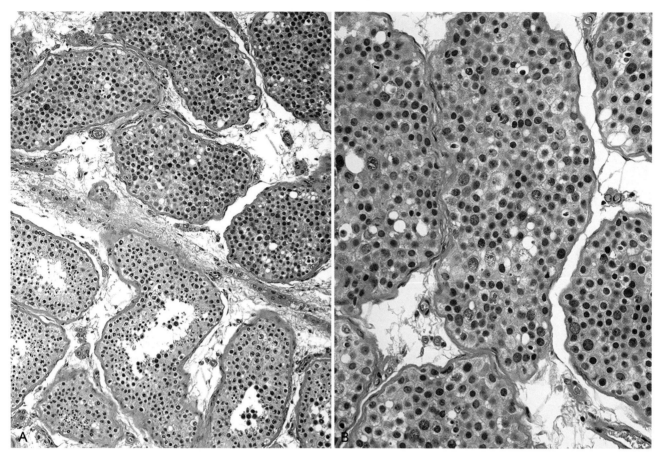

Fig. 13.140 (A) Intratubular spermatocytic tumor. (B) High magnification shows cells with variable nuclear size, including some large nuclei with granular to filamentous chromatin.

cured by orchiectomy. The course of patients with metastases is often indolent, and the utility of retroperitoneal lymph node dissection is unknown.

Very rare tumors (other than well-differentiated neuroendocrine tumors; see the Teratoma, Prepubertal-Type section earlier in this chapter) have been considered monodermal teratomas. Monodermal teratomas such as well-differentiated neuroendocrine tumor (carcinoid tumor) are now considered to belong in the prepubertal-type teratoma category. However, identification of coexisting GCINS in a tumor composed of one tissue type is supportive of germ cell origin and potential for malignant behavior. Additionally, one published case of pure cartilaginous teratoma (with retroperitoneal metastasis) lacked morphologic evidence of GCNIS, but showed chromosome 12p overrepresentation by FISH.[808]

Mixed Teratoma and Yolk Sac Tumor, Prepubertal-Type

Mixed teratoma and yolk sac tumor, prepubertal-type, is composed of a combination of prepubertal-type teratoma and yolk sac tumor and occurs about one-tenth as frequently as prepubertal-type yolk sac tumor.[23] In one pediatric case, an apparently pure prepubertal-type teratoma was associated with an elevated AFP and recurred as a retroperitoneal metastasis composed of yolk sac tumor.[809] Mixed teratoma and yolk sac tumor of prepubertal-type should be treated as would prepubertal-type yolk sac tumor.[810]

Mixed teratoma and yolk sac tumor of prepubertal type, lacking GCNIS and 12p overrepresentation, may also rarely occur in adulthood, as in two cases in the recently reported series of Oosterhuis et al., one of which was primarily teratoma and one of which was primarily yolk sac tumor.[30] Behavior was favorable without treatment other than orchiectomy.

Yolk Sac Tumor, Prepubertal-Type

In registry series of prepubertal testicular tumors, yolk sac tumor is the most common neoplasm, accounting for 82% of testicular germ cell tumors and the majority of all testicular neoplasms.[510] This dominance, however, is questioned as secondary to reporting bias because yolk sac tumors represented only 15% of the cases in the combined experience at four centers with testicular tumors in patients younger than 12 years of age.[772] In a recent single-hospital study, yolk sac tumors were 20% of pediatric germ cell tumors.[773] They occur in children from birth to 9 years of age, with a median age of 17 to 18 months.[771,811,812] They are rare after 3.5 years of age.[813] Unlike postpubertal-type yolk sac tumors, those of prepuberta type are usually pure without other germ cell tumor components; when another element is present, it is invariably teratoma. The usual epidemiologic associations of testicular germ cell tumor do not apply to prepubertal type yolk sac tumor. There is no association with cryptorchidism, and the predilection for whites more than other races is lacking.[814] Additionally, unlike the postpubertal-type tumors, whose incidence steadily increased during the twentieth century, the pediatric germ cell tumors showed a stable rate.

Children with yolk sac tumor almost always present with a painless testicular mass; clinical evidence of metastasis is rare at presentation, occurring in only 6% of cases.[811,815]

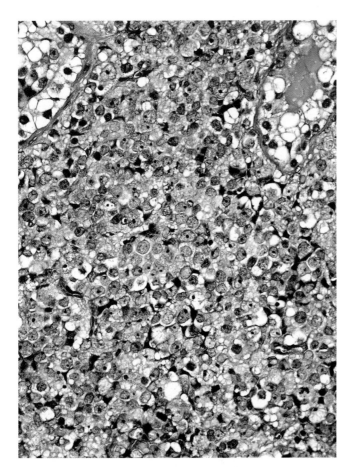

Fig. 13.141 "Anaplastic" spermatocytic tumor. There is a predominance of intermediate-sized cells with prominent nucleoli.

TABLE 13.4	Comparison of the Clinical and Pathologic Features of Spermatocytic Tumor and Typical Seminoma	
	Spermatocytic Tumor	**Seminoma**
Mean age	55 years	40 years
Proportion of germ cell tumors	~1%	40%-50%
Sites	Testis only	Testis, ovary (dysgerminoma), mediastinum, pineal, RP
Associated with cryptorchidism	No	Yes
Association with GCNIS	No	Yes
Association with sarcoma	Rare	No
Composition	Three cell types, with denser cytoplasm, round nuclei	One cell type, often clear cytoplasm, "boxy" nuclei
Intercellular edema	Common	Less common
Stroma	Scanty	Prominent
Lymphoid reaction	Rare to absent	Prominent
Granulomas	Virtually never	Often prominent
Glycogen	Absent to scant	Abundant
PLAP staining	Absent to scant	Prominent
OCT3/4 staining	Absent	Prominent
hCG staining	Absent	Present in 10%
Metastases	Rare	Common

GCNIS, Germ cell neoplasia in situ; *hCG*, human chorionic gonadotropin; *PLAP*, placental-like alkaline phosphatase; *RP*, retroperitoneum.
Modified from Murphy WM. Urological Pathology. WB Saunders, Philadelphia, PA; 1989:314–379; and Scully RE. Spermatocytic seminoma of the testis. A report of 3 cases and review of the literature. Cancer. 1961;14:788–794.

In a series of pediatric testicular tumors, serum AFP differed significantly between yolk sac tumor patients (mean: 4600 ng/mL) and patients with teratoma (mean: 20 ng/mL).[781] It is possible that rare yolk sac tumors of the pediatric type (type I, lacking GCNIS and excess i12p by in situ hybridization) may present in early adulthood.[30]

Grossly, prepubertal-type yolk sac tumor appears as solid, gray/white to tan, relatively homogeneous nodules with myxoid or gelatinous cut surfaces (Fig. 13.152); cystic change may be present. The microscopic features are not distinguishable from the postpubertal form. The most common histologic pattern is reticular-microcystic, but macrocystic, papillary, endodermal sinus (with Schiller-Duval bodies), myxomatous, labyrinthine, glandular, and solid patterns can also be seen.[812] Immunohistochemical features are largely similar to those of yolk sac tumor, postpubertal-type, but yolk sac tumor, prepubertal-type stains less frequently for AFP than postpubertal-type.[524] These cases lack i(12p) on karyotypic analysis, although very rare cases may have gains of 12p by FISH.[79,81,727] About 30% of prepubertal-type yolk sac tumors are diploid, with peritetraploid values in the remainder, whereas postpubertal-type tumors are almost invariably nondiploid.[61] Hypermethylation of the promoter of a probable tumor suppressor gene, *RUNX3*, and loss of heterozygosity at 1p36.1 are typical of prepubertal-type yolk sac tumor but not postpubertal-type.[816]

Juvenile granulosa cell tumor may mimic yolk sac tumor; both may be seen in very young children, but juvenile granulosa cell tumor usually (90% of cases) is seen in children younger than 6 months of age, whereas yolk sac tumor tends to occur in older children, the peak being at 17 to 18 months of age.[771,811,817,818] Histologically both tumors may show microcystic, macrocystic, and solid patterns, as well as high mitotic rates and cellular atypia. Follicles lined by multiple layers of tumor cells and a lobular arrangement are key to the recognition of juvenile granulosa cell tumor. The presence of other characteristic patterns is helpful in recognizing yolk sac tumor; intracellular AFP, glypican-3, PLAP, and nuclear SALL4 do not occur in juvenile granulosa cell tumor but are usually seen in pediatric yolk sac tumor.[34,616] Positivity for inhibin-α and CD99 occur in juvenile granulosa cell tumor but not in yolk sac tumor.[616] Serum AFP levels may be physiologically "elevated" in infants younger than 6 months of age, and should not be overinterpreted to support the diagnosis of yolk sac tumor rather than juvenile granulosa cell tumor.[819]

Eighty to 90% of prepubertal-type yolk sac tumors are pathologic stage I, and most with clinical stage I tumors (including postorchiectomy AFP levels) receive surveillance management rather than RPLND.[811,815,820,821] Prepubertal-type yolk sac tumor has an increased frequency of hematogenous metastases to the lung (relative to postpubertal-type one), and the reported frequency of retroperitoneal involvement is 0% to 14% of cases, significantly less than the postpubertal-type tumor. RPLND is usually no longer thought to be indicated in children without persistent retroperitoneal disease after chemotherapy, persistently elevated AFP after

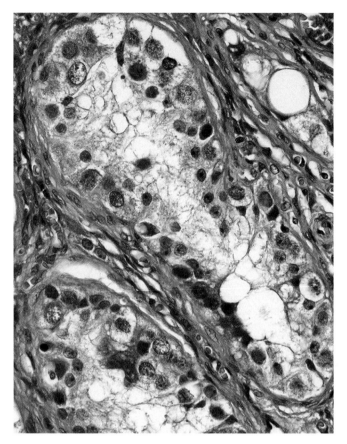

Fig. 13.142 A single layer of tumor cells in intratubular spermatocytic tumor, a mimic of GCNIS.

chemotherapy without apparent tumor on imaging, or normal or unknown AFP level before chemotherapy (making AFP unreliable as a tumor marker).[812,820,822]

The prognosis of childhood yolk sac tumor is good, with a 5-year survival of more than 90%.[512,823] Differences in prognosis with respect to age in children are no longer identified, perhaps as a result of contemporary therapies.[512,771,811] Presence of two or more risk factors (tumor size >4.5 cm, rete testis and/or epididymis invasion, and necrosis) in stage I cases has been associated

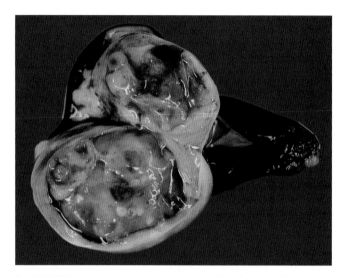

Fig. 13.144 Teratoma, prepubertal-type consists of a myxoid, lobulated, and variegated tumor with focal hemorrhage.

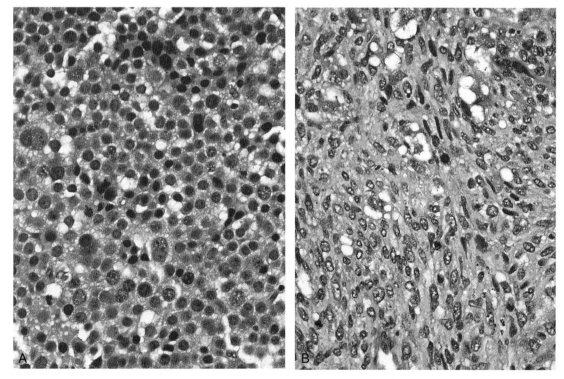

Fig. 13.143 A spermatocytic tumor (A) with a spindle cell sarcoma component (B).

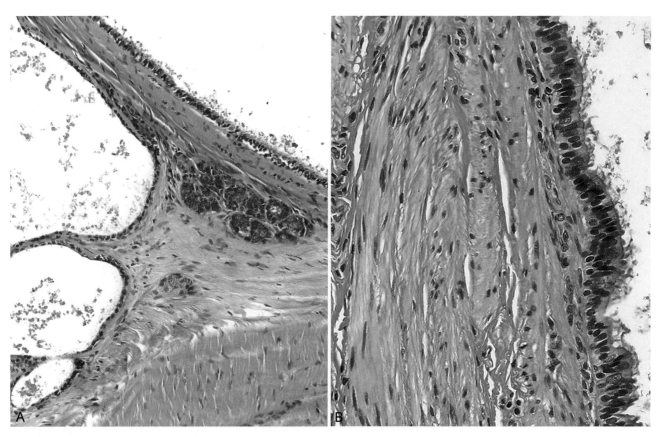

Fig. 13.145 Prepubertal-type teratoma with serous acini and ciliated epithelium with surrounding smooth muscle.

with poorer outcome, but in this study none of the 24 patients diagnosed after 1956 with follow-up died of yolk sac tumor.[812]

Sex Cord–Stromal Tumors

Sex cord–stromal tumors make up only about 4% of testicular neoplasms.[170,789] These include Leydig cell tumor, Sertoli cell tumor, granulosa cell tumor, and sex cord–stromal tumors of mixed and unclassified (indeterminate) types. Many authors also include within the sex cord–stromal tumor category those hyperplastic or hamartomatous lesions of the testis in patients with the adrenogenital syndrome, Nelson syndrome, and the AIS, which are derived from interstitial cells and Sertoli cells, although those occurring with the adrenogenital syndrome and Nelson syndrome are almost always hyperplasias induced by high levels of adrenocorticotrophic hormone. These lesions are discussed with the neoplasm that they most closely resemble: Leydig cell tumor (for the adrenogenital syndrome and Nelson syndrome) and Sertoli cell tumor (for the androgen insensitivity syndrome).

Leydig Cell Tumor

Clinical Features

Leydig cell tumor accounts for about 3% of testicular neoplasms.[824] It has two age peaks, with about 20% of cases occurring in children (most commonly between 5 and 10 years of age and exceptionally rare in infants younger than 2 years of age) and 80% occurring in adults (most commonly between 20 and 60 years with an average of 47 years).[824-829] Children usually present with significantly smaller tumors because of the early clinical detection

of androgen production manifest by isosexual pseudoprecocity, the presenting feature in virtually all pediatric cases.[824] Such patients may not have palpable tumors, and testicular ultrasound or differential testicular vein sampling for androgens may be required for clinical diagnosis. About 10% of children have gynecomastia superimposed upon virilization.[826] Adults, in whom neoplastic androgen production is much less evident than in children, most commonly present with a testicular mass, with about 30% of patients developing gynecomastia.[824] Bilateral involvement occurs in about 3% of cases.[824] Leydig cell tumors share some of the epidemiologic features of testicular germ cell tumors, occurring more commonly in patients with cryptorchidism, testicular atrophy, and infertility, but the predominant sparing of African Americans that occurs in the germ cell tumors (3% of cases) is absent in Leydig cell tumors (24% of cases).[317,829] Familial occurrence is described, and Leydig cell tumors may be seen, along with hereditary leiomyomatosis and renal cell carcinoma, in association with germline fumarate hydratase mutations.[830,831] Additionally, some of the Leydig cell tumors in children have been found to have acquired activating mutations in the luteinizing hormone receptor.[832-834]

Pathologic Features

Most Leydig cell tumors appear as yellow, brown, or tan, solid, sometimes lobulated, intratesticular nodules, infrequently with areas of necrosis or hemorrhage (Fig. 13.153). The majority are 2 to 5 cm in diameter, but some exceed 10 cm; children more often have Leydig cell tumors less than 1 cm in diameter. Extratesticular extension occurs in about 10% of cases.[824] A variety of light microscopic patterns may be seen; the solid, sheetlike pattern is most common (Figs. 13.154 and 13.155), but pseudoglandular

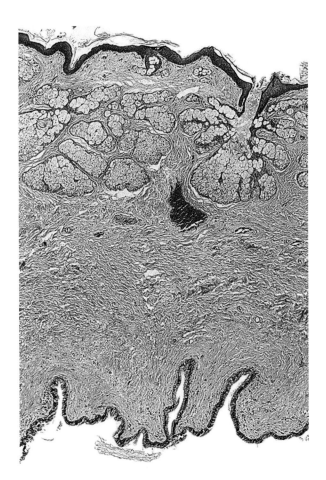

Fig. 13.146 Dermoid cyst. Note the skinlike arrangement of adnexal structures and the additional glandular cyst *(bottom).*

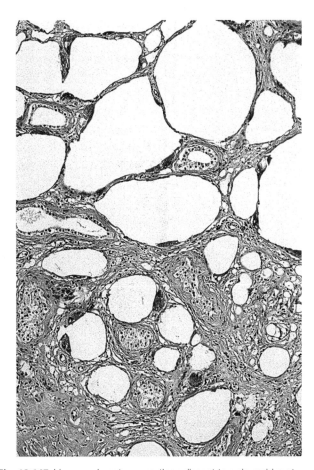

Fig. 13.147 Lipogranulomatous reaction adjacent to a dermoid cyst.

(Fig. 13.156), cordlike (trabecular), and compact nested patterns may also be present, often in the same neoplasm. Rare tumors may have a microcystic pattern, potentially causing confusion with yolk sac tumor (Fig. 13.157), and also rare are cases in which the tumor cells are spindle-shaped, either focally or as the predominant pattern (Fig. 13.158).[835,836] It is frequent for nodular aggregates of tumor cells to be separated by edematous or fibrous stroma (Fig. 13.159). The cells are polygonal, with abundant, eosinophilic cytoplasm, round, variably sized nuclei, and conspicuous, central nucleoli (Figs. 13.155 and 13.160). Finely granular lipofuscin pigment is present in the cytoplasm of some tumors from postpubertal patients (Fig. 13.160) (usually giving a tan to brown gross appearance), and careful search allows the identification of rod-shaped, intracytoplasmic crystals of Reinke in up to 40% of cases (Fig. 13.155).[789] Eosinophilic cytoplasmic globules may correspond to precursors of these crystals (Fig. 13.161). Cytoplasmic accumulation of lipid imparts a clear, finely vacuolated appearance resembling the zona fasciculata of the adrenal cortex in some cases and, in rare tumors, the cells may have optically clear cytoplasm (Fig. 13.162). Infrequently, fat cells are seen as a component of Leydig cell tumors (Fig. 13.163) either deriving from lipid accumulation within tumor cells or from differentiation of stromal cells.[836,837] Rarely, calcifications and ossification may be seen, apparently more frequently in tumors with fatty metaplasia.[836,838,839] Mitotic figures are usually infrequent, and a rate of 3 or more per 10 high-power fields is a feature that suggests

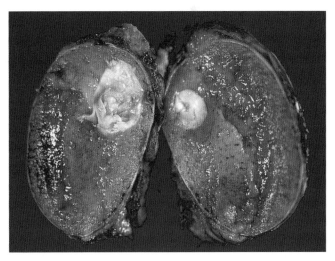

Fig. 13.148 Epidermoid cyst containing friable, yellow-white keratinous material. Note the proximity to tunica albuginea.

malignancy (see later). The nuclei may have a ground-glass appearance (Fig. 13.164).

Immunohistochemistry can assist with the diagnosis of Leydig cell tumor. Inhibin-α is positive in almost all Leydig cell tumors, as are stains for Melan-A (MART1) and calretinin.[616,840-843] The steroidogenic factor 1 (SF1) immunohistochemical stain appears to be the most sensitive marker for sex cord–stromal tumors as a group.[844] CD99 is detected in about two-thirds of cases.[616] p53

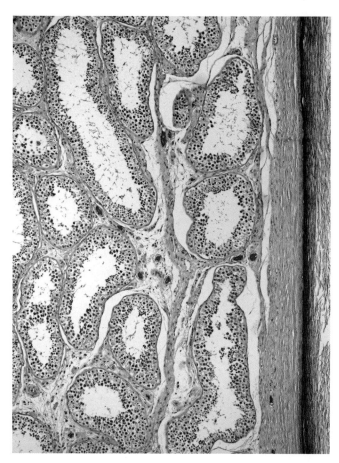

Fig. 13.149 Epidermoid cyst showing a thin, compressed layer of stratified squamous epithelium *(right)* lining a space filled with keratin. The surrounding seminiferous tubules show intact spermatogenesis with no evidence of GCNIS.

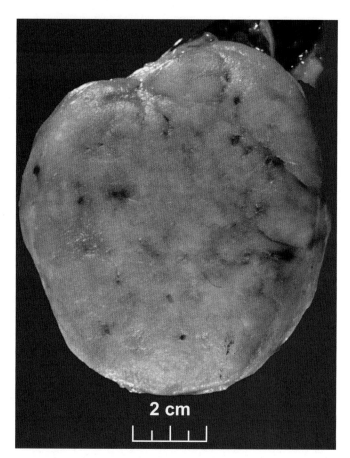

Fig. 13.150 Testicular well-differentiated neuroendocrine tumor (carcinoid tumor) with a solid, tan appearance. (Courtesy of RH Young, MD, Massachusetts General Hospital, Boston, MA).

is detected in some malignant cases and may be helpful in recognizing malignant examples.[845,846] Infrequently, Leydig cell tumors may stain for placental alkaline phosphatase.[616] Vimentin is the dominant cytoplasmic intermediate filament, although cytokeratin reactivity may also be seen.[847] One case with enkephalin immunoreactivity has been described.[848] Ultrastructurally, Leydig cell tumors have features of steroid hormone–synthesizing cells, including abundant lipid droplets, prominent cisternae of smooth endoplasmic reticulum, and mitochondria with tubular cristae.[849,850] Reinke crystals appear as sharply demarcated geometric shapes, such as hexagons, rectangles, and rhomboids, which have a lattice-like substructure.[851] A specific activating mutation of the luteinizing hormone receptor gene *(D578H)* has been observed in Leydig cell tumors, but can also be present in Leydig cell hyperplasia.[852]

Treatment and Prognosis

The frequency of malignant behavior in Leydig cell tumors has historically been described as approximately 10%, but it has been suggested that this may currently be an overestimate, perhaps because tumors now present at smaller size (40% less than 2 cm).[829,853] This viewpoint is supported by a review of Leydig cell tumors from the Surveillance, Epidemiology, and End Results (SEER) program, which found a cancer-specific mortality of 6.6%.[829] In the patients who ultimately died, the median survival was 12 months. Some

clinical features correlate with the natural history of Leydig cell tumors, including that older patients are more likely to have malignant tumors, that malignant behavior has not been reported before puberty (although there is a reported case of a histologically malignant Leydig cell tumor in a 13-month-old without documented metastasis), and that gynecomastia is more common with benign cases.[824,825,828,854,855] Malignant behavior also correlates with a number of pathologic features (Fig. 13.165), including: larger tumors (>5 cm), higher mitotic rates (>3 to 5 mitotic figures per 10 high-power fields), atypical mitotic figures, vascular space invasion, significant nuclear atypia, necrosis, infiltrative borders, invasion of the rete testis or beyond, DNA aneuploidy, high proliferative activity (>5%) as assessed by staining with the MIB-1 antibody, and increased expression of p53 protein by the tumor cells.[824,845,846,856,857] In a study by Kim et al. that included as risk factors size ≥5 cm, infiltrative margins, lymphovascular invasion, necrosis, a mitotic index of >3 per 10 high-power fields, and grade 2 or 3 cytologic atypia, 5 of 5 clinically malignant cases had ≥4 criteria, whereas 12 of 14 clinically benign cases had none, 1 had one, and 1 had three.[824] In a recent series of testicular sex cord–stromal tumors, 37 patients with either no (34 patients) or one (3 patients) high-risk factor underwent surveillance, and none recurred.[858] Among patients in this series with RPLND performed for pathologic risk factors in the absence of radiographic evidence of retroperitoneal disease, only 1 of 6 had involvement in the RPLND specimen.[858] None of the malignant/high-risk features, however, is pathognomonic of malignancy, and, indeed, malignant

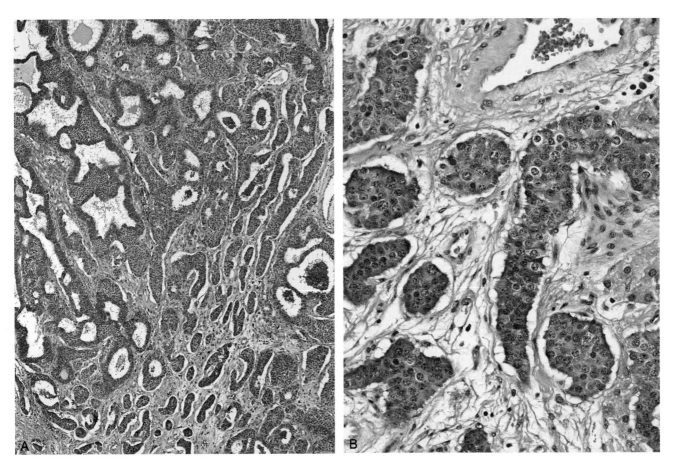

Fig. 13.151 (A) Insular, glandular, and trabecular patterns in testicular well-differentiated neuroendocrine tumor. (B) Note the punctate chromatin and cytoplasmic granules.

behavior has been found in 0.9% of cases of "testicular stromal tumors" (that included 70% Leydig cell tumors) where no risk factor was found.[859]

Orchiectomy is the standard treatment, but testis-sparing surgery has been employed in patients with bilateral tumors and has gained acceptance for single tumors in the pediatric group as well as being discussed in clinical stage I adult patients.[36,860,861] Small (<2.5 cm) lesions with negative tumor markers have been treated

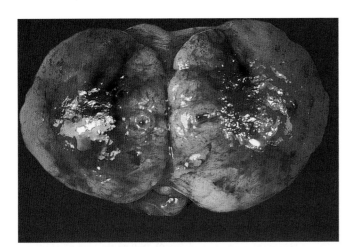

Fig. 13.152 Yolk sac tumor, prepubertal-type. Solid, tan-yellow, focally hemorrhagic nodule with a myxoid quality.

by testis-sparing surgery with favorable results.[792,853,862-864] In a recent series of 31 testicular sex cord–stromal tumors (27 Leydig cell tumors and 4 Sertoli cell tumors) with a median size of 0.7 cm there were no metastases, although there was one local recurrence requiring orchiectomy, and in another series of 22 patients there were no local recurrences or metastases.[863,865]

Radiation and chemotherapy are not effective in the treatment of malignant Leydig cell tumor.[865] Retroperitoneal lymphadenectomy may be curative in patients with clinical stage II disease.[865] It may also be performed in clinical stage I tumors with malignant features/recurrence risk factors, but the role of this intervention remains unclear.[865,866] Late metastases are infrequent but may develop more than a decade after orchiectomy.

Differential Diagnosis

Several entities should be considered in the differential diagnosis of Leydig cell tumor.[789] Leydig cell hyperplasia, although usually diffuse, may form nodules that mimic Leydig cell tumor. However, this is an interstitial, nondestructive process that preserves many seminiferous tubules.[867] It may be seen in patients with elevated gonadotropin levels, including those with elevated hCG levels. Apparent Leydig cell hyperplasia occurs in many cases of testicular atrophy because of a normal population of Leydig cells in a reduced testicular volume. It is seen in Klinefelter syndrome where other pathologic features of that disorder are present and help with the diagnosis. Patients who have the adrenogenital syndrome or Nelson syndrome (Cushing syndrome associated with occult pituitary adenoma that becomes clinically evident with high levels of

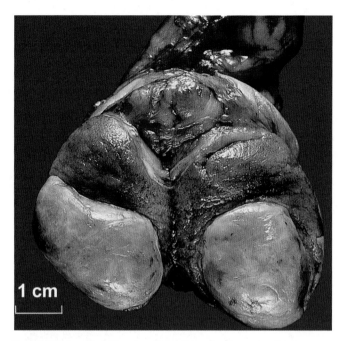

Fig. 13.153 Leydig cell tumor with a solid, yellow-tan cut surface.

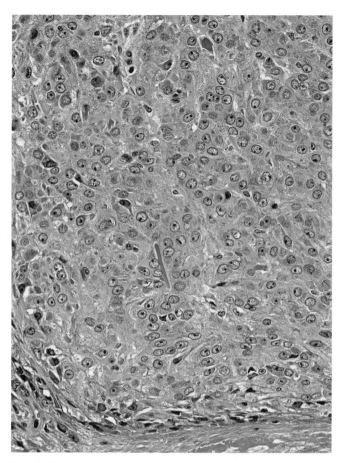

Fig. 13.155 Prominent Reinke crystals in a Leydig cell tumor. Note the uniform nuclei with single, conspicuous nuclei.

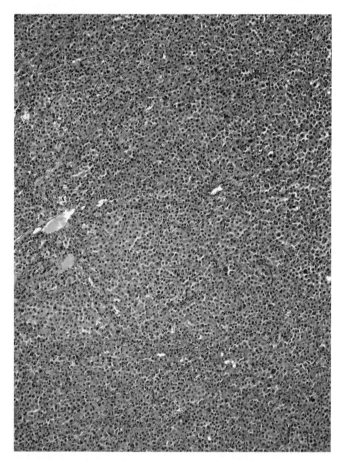

Fig. 13.154 Sheets of eosinophilic cells in a Leydig cell tumor.

adrenocorticotrophin after bilateral adrenalectomy) may develop testicular nodules that closely resemble Leydig cell tumors.[868-872] These nodules appear to be hyperplastic and are usually distinguished from Leydig cell tumors by their multifocality, bilaterality,

uniform absence of Reinke crystals, frequent fibrous bands (Fig. 13.166), tendency for prominent lipofuscin deposits, and clinical history, although some patients present in the absence of known adrenogenital syndrome.[789] An additional helpful feature is the occurrence of small basophilic cytoplasmic granules in the cytoplasm of some of the adrenogenital syndrome–associated nodules that are not a feature of Leydig cell tumor (Fig. 13.167). Although both may be reactive for synaptophysin, the testicular tumor of the adrenogenital syndrome (TTAGS) shows stronger, more widespread reactivity. The TTAGS also shows greater reactivity for CD56 than Leydig cell tumors, and is negative for androgen receptor, in contrast with Leydig cell tumors.[870] Other markers of adrenal and testicular steroidogenesis have been evaluated, and a DLK1+/INSL3– immunophenotype supports TTAGS, with the opposite pattern typical of Leydig cell tumors.[871] TTAGS often regresses when treated with glucocorticoid to suppress adrenocorticotrophin levels. Clinical history is of value in such cases. It is hypothesized that the TTAGS derives from nodular steroid cell nests that are normally located near the testicular hilum (Fig. 13.168). These, by themselves, may cause some concern for Leydig cell tumor, but they are less than 3 mm in size, occur in the absence of a history of endocrine disorder, and often have a trabecular architecture and sinusoidal vasculature.[873]

Large cell calcifying Sertoli cell tumor, an entity that is associated with Carney complex, may resemble Leydig cell tumors because the neoplastic cells are usually polygonal with abundant eosinophilic cytoplasm.[2,4,874,875] Unlike Leydig cell tumors, large cell calcifying Sertoli cell tumors may be bilateral and multifocal (when Carney

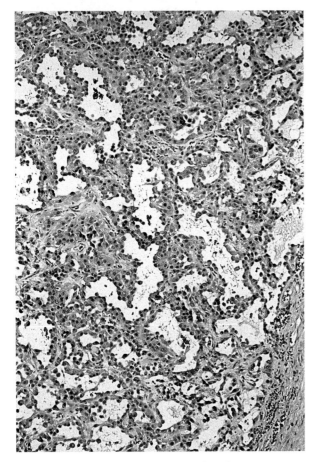

Fig. 13.156 Pseudoglandular pattern in a Leydig cell tumor.

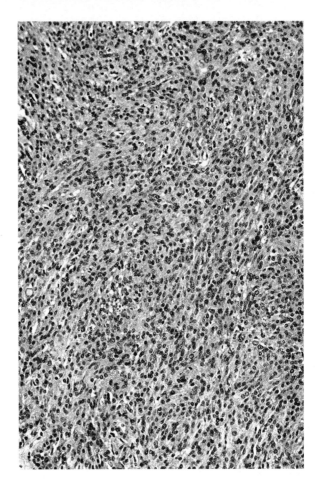

Fig. 13.158 Leydig cell tumor with a vaguely fascicular arrangement of spindle cells.

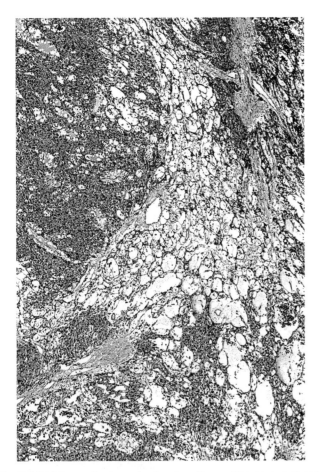

Fig. 13.157 Microcystic change in a Leydig cell tumor. The more usual, solid pattern is also present.

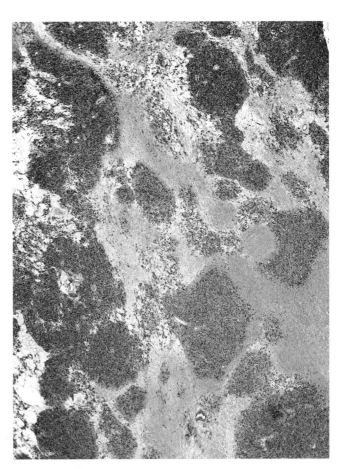

Fig. 13.159 Nodular pattern in a Leydig cell tumor.

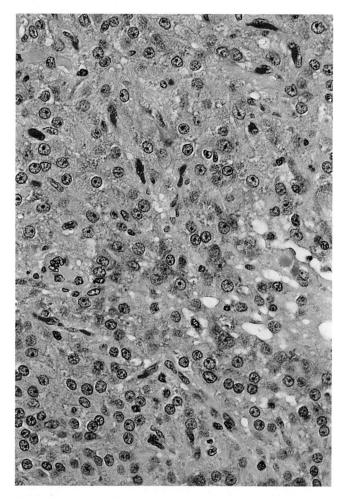

Fig. 13.160 Leydig cell tumor with intracytoplasmic lipofuscin. Note the eosinophilic cytoplasm and round nuclei with moderate-sized nucleoli.

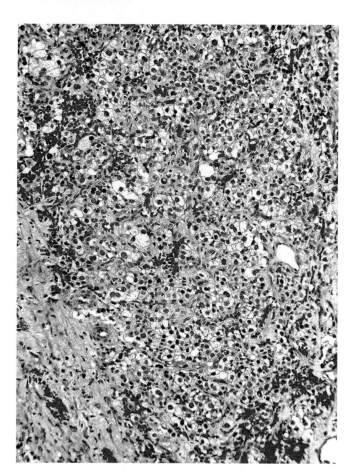

Fig. 13.162 Leydig cell tumor with clear cytoplasm.

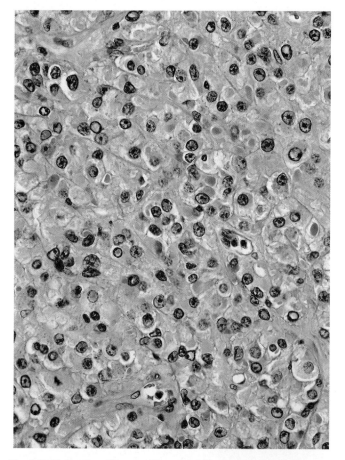

Fig. 13.161 Leydig cell tumor with eosinophilic cytoplasmic globules.

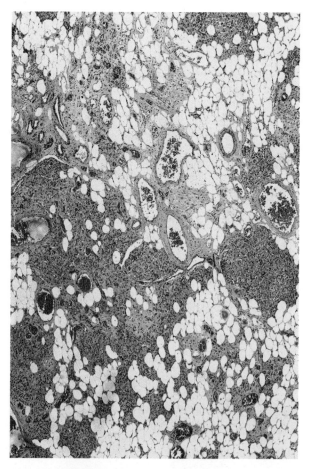

Fig. 13.163 Leydig cell tumor with fatty metaplasia.

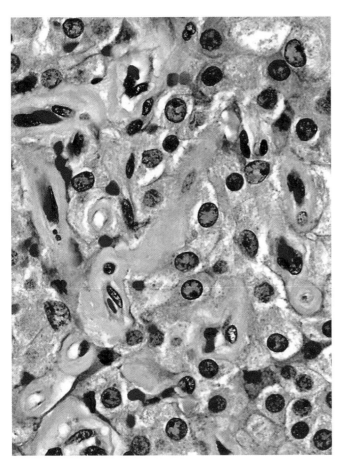

Fig. 13.164 Leydig cell tumor with ground glass nuclei.

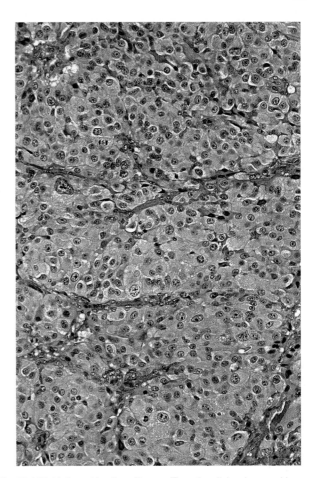

Fig. 13.165 Malignant leydig cell tumor. There is cellular pleomorphism and an elevated mitotic rate.

complex associated), lack Reinke crystals, are more consistently associated with calcifications (and sometimes ossification), may show intratubular growth, and tend to have a more myxoid stroma, often with a neutrophilic infiltrate.[4,789] There is significant overlap in the immunostaining patterns of these two neoplasms, although it has been claimed that patchy (as opposed to diffuse) positivity for Melan-A and CD10, as well as reactivity for S100 protein-β, favor large cell calcifying Sertoli cell tumor.[432,876]

Young and Talerman reported metastatic prostate carcinoma to the testis mimicking Leydig cell tumor, but immunostains against prostate specific antigen and prostatic acid phosphatase were positive, resolving the differential diagnosis.[789] Leydig cell tumor with prominent cytoplasmic clarity may be misinterpreted as seminoma, but the clarity is caused by lipids, often yielding a finely vacuolated appearance, rather than glycogen, as in seminoma, which causes a "water-clear" appearance. Additionally, there is no association with GCNIS, and the characteristic lymphoid infiltrate and granulomatous reaction of seminoma are absent. Malakoplakia may resemble Leydig cell tumor but has intratubular infiltrates of eosinophilic histiocytes and cytoplasmic calcifications (Michaelis-Gutmann bodies) that are not seen in Leydig cell tumors.

Sertoli Cell Tumor, Not Otherwise Specified

Clinical Features

Sertoli cell tumor, not otherwise specified (NOS) is infrequent but, in our experience, probably not as rare as the commonly cited 1% of testicular neoplasms for children and adults.[877] A review of

SEER data found it was about 40% as frequent as Leydig cell tumor.[829] Like Leydig cell tumors, it does not show the marked proclivity of the germ cell tumors to occur in white men.[829] It can occur at virtually any age but is most common in middle age, with a median age of 39 years.[829] Most patients present with a testicular mass, but estrogen production by the tumor can cause gynecomastia or impotence, which can be the presenting complaints.[826,878] Isolated gynecomastia may be the initial manifestation of Sertoli cell tumor in a child; children with Leydig cell tumor, in contrast, do not develop gynecomastia without virilization.[826] Patients with Peutz-Jeghers syndrome have been reported with testicular Sertoli cell tumor, but most of these appear to represent a different neoplastic process that is intratubular.[3,6]

Pathologic Features

Grossly, Sertoli cell tumor typically is a solid, gray, white, tan, or yellow nodule, usually under 4 cm in diameter, although larger tumors may occur but should raise concern for malignancy (Fig. 13.169).[879] Occasional tumors have cystic change. On microscopic examination, the hallmark is tubule formation.[468] These may be either hollow or solid, usually in a fibrous (often hyalinized) to myxoid stroma (Fig. 13.170). Sheetlike arrays of tumor cells (Fig. 13.171), solid nests (Fig. 13.172), trabeculae, and cords may also occur but are not diagnostic alone. Rarely a retiform pattern may be seen (Fig. 13.173). A combination of solid, tubular, and nested patterns is not uncommon (Fig. 13.174). The tumor cells typically have scant to moderate amounts of pale to clear

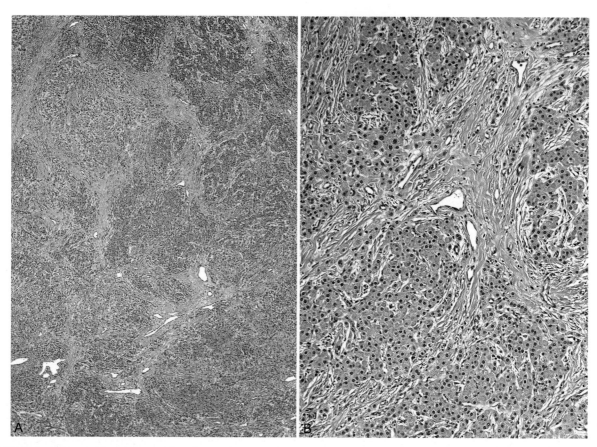

Fig. 13.166 Testicular tumor of the adrenogenital syndrome with nodules of hyperplastic Leydig cells that are characteristically multifocal, bilateral, lack Reinke crystals, and are segregated by fibrous bands.

cytoplasm (Fig. 13.172), but it may also be eosinophilic (Fig. 13.175). Prominent cytoplasmic vacuolization may create a microcystic pattern or signet ring-like appearance (Figs. 13.174 and 13.176), and some have considered tumors where this was a prominent feature a separate lesion, a viewpoint we disagree with.[880,881] The nuclei are round to oval, relatively uniform, and usually lack large nucleoli. The cytoplasmic clarity is caused by abundant cellular lipid, which may be demonstrable on fresh tissue with special stains. Zones of fibrosis with sclerotic blood vessels and elastic fibers encrusted by calcium and hemosiderin deposits may be seen in some cases. One case of a Sertoli cell tumor with a heterologous sarcomatous component has been reported.[882]

The so-called "sclerosing Sertoli cell tumor" is now considered a morphologic variant of Sertoli cell tumor rather than a separate entity. It has been found in patients with an average age of 35 to 37 years and a range of 18 to 80 years, and has clinical features similar to the nonsclerotic cases.[883,884] The gross features only differ by a firmer consistency, reflected by a stromal predominance. Because the hypocellular stroma comprises at least 50% of the lesion, the tumor cells are often compressed to cords or trabeculae, although small nests and tubules also may be seen (Fig. 13.177).[884] Mitotic activity and cytologic atypia are infrequent.[883] Frequent *CTNNB1* gene mutations and nuclear positivity for β-catenin are typical of sclerosing Sertoli cell tumors, as they are of Sertoli cell tumors, NOS.[883-889]

On immunohistochemical study, 30% to 90% of Sertoli cell tumors are inhibin-α reactive, 60% to 80% are positive for cytokeratin, 90% to 100% are positive for vimentin, 30% to 64% are positive for S100, 0% to 82% are positive for chromogranin,

45% are reactive for synaptophysin, and they are usually negative for EMA, although in our experience with malignant examples, EMA reactivity occurred in most.[469,616,840,890-892] About one-half of Sertoli cell tumors, NOS, in our experience, stain for calretinin, although such positivity may be quite focal. NSE positivity has been described in several cases, and very focal reactivity for anti-müllerian hormone has been reported.[879,893] Newer immunohistochemical markers such as SF1, SOX9, and FOXL2 appear to be more sensitive than inhibin and calretinin, but are not especially useful in the distinction from other sex cord–stromal tumors.[844] Nuclear β-catenin immunoreactivity is seen in 64% of Sertoli cell tumors, NOS and correlate with mutation in the *CTNNB1* gene.[885,894] Only membranous and cytoplasmic β-catenin staining is seen in other sex cord–stromal tumors such as Leydig cell tumors, large cell calcifying Sertoli cell tumors, adult and juvenile granulosa cell tumors, and sex cord–stromal tumors, unclassified.[894] Features of steroid synthesizing cells are identified ultrastructurally, including abundant cisternae of smooth endoplasmic reticulum and numerous intracytoplasmic lipid droplets. Adjacent cells are connected by desmosomes.[895] Charcot-Böttcher filaments (perinuclear arrays of filaments) are considered pathognomonic of Sertoli cell differentiation. They have been identified in ovarian Sertoli cell tumor and in large cell calcifying Sertoli cell tumor, but most reports of testicular Sertoli cell tumor, NOS have not mentioned their presence.[875,896-898]

A higher proportion of Sertoli cell tumors are clinically malignant as compared with Leydig cell tumors. Although about 10% of Sertoli cell tumors were considered malignant in some studies, review of the SEER database for 2004 to 2012 showed that

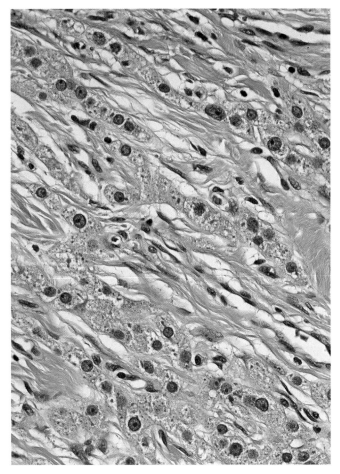

Fig. 13.167 Testicular tumor of the adrenogenital syndrome may also have small basophilic cytoplasmic granules in some cells, a feature not seen in Leydig cell tumors.

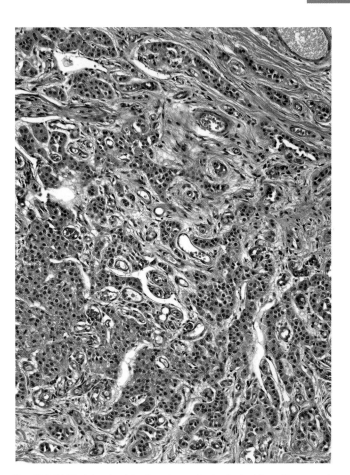

Fig. 13.168 Nodular steroid cell nest near the testicular hilum. These nests are less than 3 mm in size and typically have a trabecular and sinusoidal architecture; they are hypothesized to be the source of the adrenogenital syndrome "tumors."

35% of cases presented with advanced-stage disease.[829] In contrast with Leydig cell tumor, malignant cases may occur in children.[164,469,878,879,899] Gynecomastia appears to be more common in malignant tumors than in benign ones.[879] As in Leydig cell tumors, malignant behavior in Sertoli cell tumors, NOS may be difficult to predict from pathologic features alone. Features that correlate with an increased likelihood of malignancy include: size of 5 cm or more, significant cytologic atypia and pleomorphism, invasive borders, mitotic activity in excess of 5 mitotic figures per 10 high-power fields, vascular invasion, and necrosis (Fig. 13.178).[879,900-902] In the study by Young et al., which did not include invasive borders as a criterion, the malignant cases had at least two of these features.[468] MIB1 proliferation index greater than 30% correlates with malignant behavior, and we noted malignant behavior in a group of Sertoli cell tumors with a predominance of a diffuse growth pattern.[469,891]

The sclerosing variant appears to have a better overall prognosis, with only 1 of 31 reported cases having a malignant course, and this tumor had both an invasive growth pattern and lymphovascular involvement.[884,903]

Differential Diagnosis

Sertoli cell tumor must be distinguished from the rare seminoma with a tubular pattern, a differential diagnosis discussed in the Seminoma section earlier in this chapter.[380] Patients with the

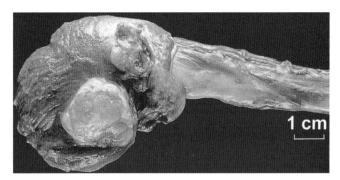

Fig. 13.169 Sertoli cell tumor with a gray-white cut surface.

AIS (also known as the testicular feminization syndrome) may develop multiple hamartomatous testicular nodules composed of closely spaced tubules lined by Sertoli cells, but, in contrast with true Sertoli cell tumors, these lesions also have intervening Leydig cells within the interstitium (Fig. 13.179).[253,262] About 25% of patients with AIS also develop multifocal, bilateral Sertoli cell adenomas composed of pure proliferations of Sertoli cell–lined tubules (Fig. 13.180).[262] These lesions may be indistinguishable from well-differentiated Sertoli cell tumors, and it is uncertain if they are neoplastic or hamartomatous. Some have a prominent component of globular basement membrane deposits. Malignant

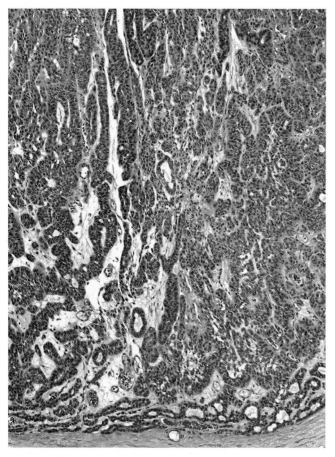

Fig. 13.170 Sertoli cell tumor composed of mostly solid tubules.

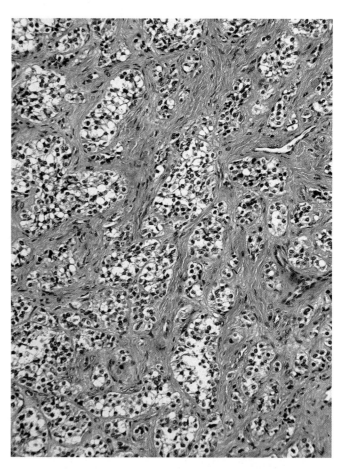

Fig. 13.172 Solid nests and focal tubules in a Sertoli cell tumor.

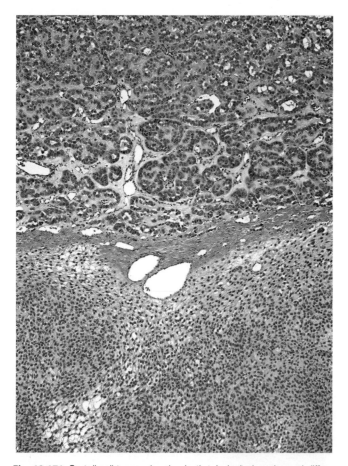

Fig. 13.171 Sertoli cell tumor showing both tubular/trabecular and diffuse patterns.

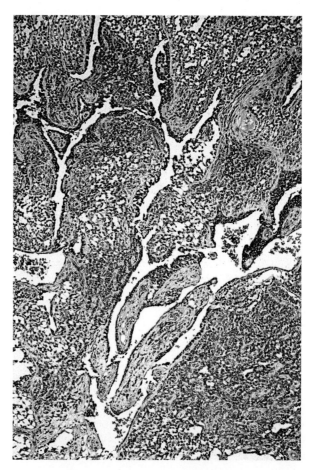

Fig. 13.173 Retiform pattern in a sertoli celltumor.

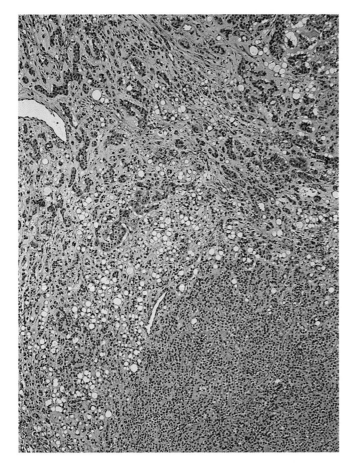

Fig. 13.174 Sertoli cell tumor with multiple patterns including tubular, signet ring cells, and solid/diffuse.

In patients with germ cell tumors, they may be colonized by GCNIS, simulating gonadoblastoma (Fig. 13.184).

Sertoli cell tumors may show large areas of sheetlike arrangement and, furthermore, have an associated lymphocytic infiltrate and prominence of clear or pale cytoplasm (Fig. 13.185). These features mimic seminoma and can be a source of serious diagnostic error.[469] Features of assistance include, in Sertoli cell tumor, the absence of GCNIS, foci with typical tubules, less-atypical-appearing nuclei, and lower mitotic rates. Immunohistochemistry is helpful as well, with OCT3/4, SALL4, and PLAP being negative in Sertoli cell tumors and positive in seminomas.[469]

The distinction of a Sertoli cell tumor from a Leydig cell tumor depends on the formation of tubules, at least focally, in the former. Additionally, the eosinophilic cytoplasm of most Leydig cell tumors contrasts with the less conspicuous and lighter-staining cytoplasm of most Sertoli cell tumors, although exceptions may be seen. Leydig cell tumors may show Reinke crystalloids, unlike Sertoli cell tumors. Inhibin-α is less consistently expressed in Sertoli cell tumors than in Leydig cell tumors, being positive in 30% to 80% of Sertoli cell tumors but in virtually all Leydig cell tumors.[616,891] CD99 is also more commonly expressed in Leydig cell tumors than in Sertoli cell tumors.[616] About two-thirds of Sertoli cell tumors express nuclear β-catenin, but not Leydig cell tumors.[894]

Treatment and Prognosis

Standard treatment for primary tumors is orchiectomy (and is, of course, required for diagnosis in most cases), but for small (less than 2 cm) lesions, testis-sparing surgery has been used with favorable results.[862,865]

Metastatic Sertoli cell tumors do not usually respond to radiation and chemotherapy. Retroperitoneal lymphadenectomy therefore remains an important option if the tumor has not disseminated beyond the scope of the dissection.

Large Cell Calcifying Sertoli Cell Tumor

Large cell calcifying Sertoli cell tumor is a variant that has some unique clinical associations.[7,908-910] Some are a component of the Carney complex characterized by lentigines of the face; myxomas of the heart, skin, soft tissue, and elsewhere; myxoid fibroadenomas of the breast; blue nevi of the skin; pigmented nodules of the adrenal cortex associated with Cushing syndrome; growth hormone–producing adenomas of the pituitary gland; and psammomatous melanotic schwannomas.[2,7,875,911-914] Many of these patients have a germline mutation in the *PRKAR1A* gene on the long arm of chromosome 17. Some sporadic tumors may have acquired *PRKAR1A* mutations.[915] About 40% of large cell calcifying Sertoli cell tumors are associated with the Carney complex, so its diagnosis should prompt consideration of this association because of the potential life-threatening complications of cardiac myxomas and, rarely, adrenocortical carcinoma.[916] Typically the patients with Carney complex are found in childhood or adolescence with small, bilateral, and multifocal testicular tumors, whereas those with sporadic tumors have solitary lesions and are older.[4,889] A testicular mass is the usual presenting complaint, but gynecomastia and isosexual pseudoprecocity may also occur, especially in those cases that are syndrome associated.[897,917] The hormones responsible for these manifestations may be produced by the neoplasm or by associated nodules of hyperplastic Leydig cells.

Grossly, large cell calcifying Sertoli cell tumor is usually tan or yellow with associated "gritty" calcification and may be multifocal, with a 40% frequency of bilaterality.[874,911] Microscopically,

behavior in pure Sertoli cell proliferations in patients with AIS have not been reported; thus the term *Sertoli cell adenoma* is appropriate even though it connotes a neoplastic process.[253,262] A unique case of a malignant sex cord–stromal tumor in a patient with AIS did not have the features of a typical Sertoli cell adenoma and more closely resembled juvenile granulosa cell tumor, although ultrastructure supported Sertoli cell differentiation.[904]

The cordlike pattern of the sclerosing variant may be misinterpreted as trabecular carcinoid tumor, but most primary well-differentiated neuroendocrine tumors have an insular pattern, and they may be associated with teratomatous elements. The presence of a cordlike or tubular pattern with vacuolated cells may also suggest an adenomatoid tumor, but the primarily paratesticular location of adenomatoid tumors and immunohistochemical negativity for inhibin and strong reactivity for EMA and mesothelial markers are helpful differential features.

Mostly microscopic, nonencapsulated nodules composed of small tubules lined by immature-appearing Sertoli cells are common incidental findings in orchiectomy specimens, and may be more common in cryptorchid testes (Fig. 13.181).[202,203,905] Rarely, they are sufficiently large to be clinically detectable (Fig. 13.182).[906] These "Sertoli cell nodules" often contain central accumulations of basement membrane that can be seen in continuity with thickened peripheral basement membrane surrounding the tubules. In contrast with true Sertoli cell tumors, these are almost always incidental microscopic findings, although rarely they may be up to 1 cm or more, and sometimes have admixed spermatogonia (Fig. 13.183), unlike Sertoli cell tumors, NOS.[905-907]

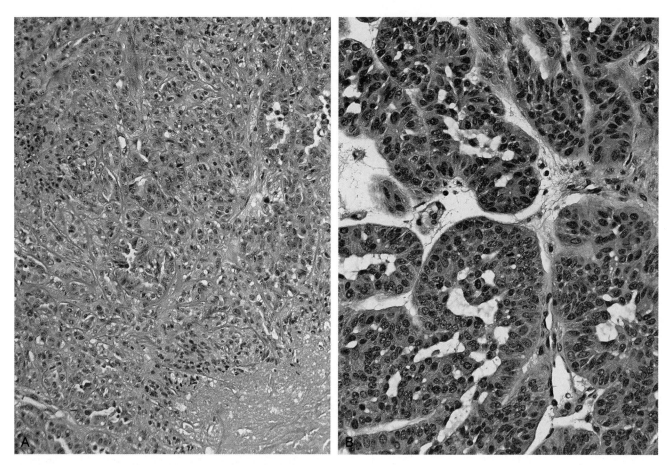

Fig. 13.175 Metastasizing Sertoli cell tumor showing (A) foci of necrosis *(bottom right)* and (B) cytologic atypia and mitotic figures.

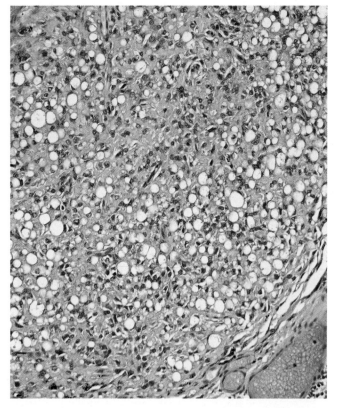

Fig. 13.176 Sertoli cell tumor with prominent cytoplasmic vacuolization creating a signet ring-like appearance.

there are nests and cords of cells with abundant, eosinophilic cytoplasm in a myxoid to collagenous stroma that is calcified or even ossified in about one-half of cases (Fig. 13.186). A neutrophilic stromal infiltrate is characteristic. Intratubular neoplasm and calcifications are common. Nuclei are usually round and may have prominent nucleoli, but mitotic figures are typically rare. Malignant cases do occur but are uncommon.[4,874,918] They usually develop on a sporadic basis in patients older than 25 years of age rather than in association with Carney complex; hence malignant tumors are solitary and can mostly be recognized as having metastatic potential on the basis of size greater than 4 cm, extratesticular growth, tumor cell necrosis, high-grade atypia, vascular space invasion, or mitotic rate in excess of 3 mitotic figures per 10 high-power fields.[4,889,918] Malignant cases typically exhibit at least two of these features, and benign tumors typically lack all of them.[4] Immunohistochemical study has shown vimentin, inhibin, calretinin, SF1, S100, NSE, desmin, EMA, and focal cytokeratin reactivity.[4,841,844,909,919,920] Ultrastructural studies have demonstrated Charcot-Böttcher filaments and other features of Sertoli cells.[875,897] The main differential diagnostic problem posed by a large cell calcifying Sertoli cell tumor is separation from a Leydig cell tumor, which was previously discussed.

Intratubular Large Cell Hyalinizing Sertoli Cell Neoplasia

Patients with the Peutz-Jeghers syndrome develop multifocal, bilateral intratubular proliferations of Sertoli cells having abundant

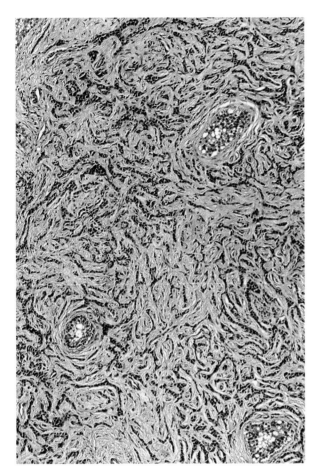

Fig. 13.177 "Sclerosing Sertoli cell tumor," now considered a morphologic variant of Sertoli cell tumor, not otherwise specified, with cordlike growth and densely collagenous stroma.

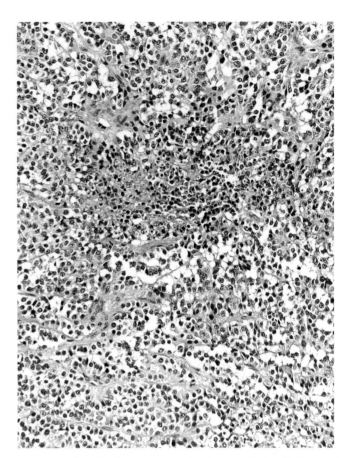

Fig. 13.178 Sertoli cell tumor, not otherwise specified, with focus of necrosis.

eosinophilic cytoplasm, similar to those seen in the large cell calcifying Sertoli cell tumor.[5,6,921] Descriptively termed *large cell hyalinizing Sertoli cell neoplasia,* these intratubular lesions occur in conjunction with thickened, peritubular basement membrane that is internalized into the expanded tubules and infrequently calcified (Fig. 13.187).[6] These expanded tubules occur in lobular clusters throughout the parenchyma. Most of the patients present in childhood with gynecomastia, which is the result of tumor-produced aromatase converting endogenous androgens to estrogens. Occasional invasive tumors are seen in association with the intratubular tumor, and these may be very similar in appearance to the large cell calcifying Sertoli cell tumor, but they more commonly do not have calcifications or the prominent fibromyxoid stroma with neutrophils.[6] Patients may have a mutation of the *STK11* gene on the short arm of chromosome 19, different from the mutation associated with the large cell calcifying Sertoli cell tumor. Conservative management of patients with aromatase inhibitors who have no evidence of an invasive tumor (the majority) by ultrasonographic follow-up permits testicular preservation in many patients, although the development of a distinct mass or hormonal complications may necessitate orchiectomy. Malignant behavior has not been reported.[5,6]

The differential diagnosis includes the large cell calcifying Sertoli cell tumor, which, in contrast with the Peutz-Jeghers lesion, is dominated by invasive tumor. Furthermore, the intratubular component in these cases does not show as great a degree of tubular expansion or as prominent basement membrane deposits and often displays conspicuous calcifications. Despite these differences in morphology and genetics, and abundant literature has considered the Peutz-Jeghers tumors to be large cell calcifying Sertoli cell tumors, a viewpoint we disagree with. Sertoli cell nodules may also be confused with the Peutz-Jeghers lesion because of their clustered seminiferous tubules with basement membrane deposits, but they have small fetal-type Sertoli cells and may contain spermatogonia.

Granulosa Cell Tumor

Adult Granulosa Cell Tumor

There are two major types of granulosa cell tumor of the testis: adult and juvenile. The adult type is rare, occurring in patients from 14 to 87 years of age.[789,922-929] These tumors have been associated with hyperestrogenism, and were described as often causing gynecomastia in previous reports.[926] However, a recent large series reported endocrine symptoms in none of 32 patients, so this appears to be an uncommon presentation.[929] Grossly, the tumor may be solid, cystic, or both, and is typically yellow to gray.[789,924,929] Gross hemorrhage and necrosis may correlate with malignant behavior.[927] Microscopically, the patterns of the more common granulosa cell tumor of the ovary may be identified, including microfollicular, macrofollicular, trabecular, gyriform, insular, and diffuse (Fig. 13.188). Call-Exner bodies are characteristic of the microfollicular pattern. The cells have scant, lightly staining cytoplasm, and the nuclei are pale, angulated to oval, and frequently grooved. Mitotic figures are usually infrequent but there may rarely be up to 6 to 18 per 10 high-power

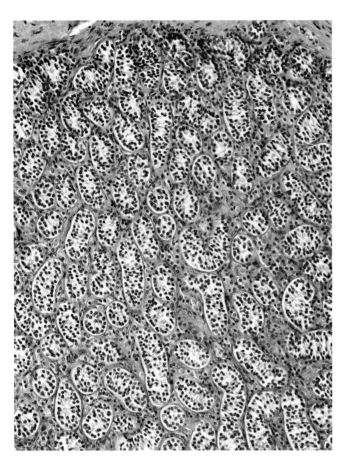

Fig. 13.179 Nodule of seminiferous tubules lined by small, immature-appearing Sertoli cells with intertubular Leydig cells in a patient with the androgen insensitivity syndrome. Such lesions are considered hamartomas.

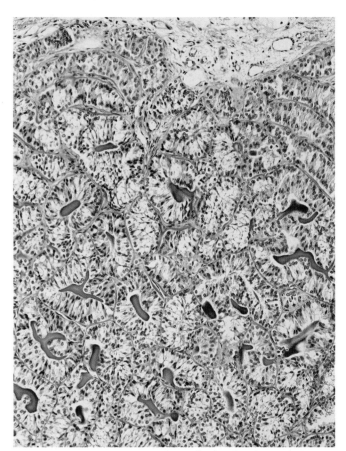

Fig. 13.180 Sertoli cell adenoma in a patient with the androgen insensitivity syndrome. There is a circumscribed proliferation of closely packed tubules lined by immature Sertoli cells. Basement membrane deposits are prominent.

fields.[927,929] Positivity for inhibin, calretinin, vimentin, cytokeratins 8 and 18, smooth muscle actin, S100, and CD99 has been reported, although one study reported an absence of cytokeratin reactivity in five of five cases.[922,925,927-931] EMA is negative.[922,925,927,930] FOXL2 and SF1 immunohistochemical stains are consistently positive but not specific, as staining is also seen in other sex cord–stromal tumors.[844] Ultrastructural studies have shown results similar to ovarian granulosa cell tumor.[923,925] FOXL2 (forkhead box L2) 402C→G mutation, consistently seen in ovarian adult granulosa cell tumors, is seen in a minority of testicular adult granulosa cell tumors.[932]

Most reported cases have been benign, but malignant behavior is a possibility.[926,927] A recent series with review of previous studies estimates a metastatic frequency of 16%.[929] Large tumor size (>7 cm), vascular invasion, hemorrhage, and necrosis have been considered useful in identifying cases with the greatest risk for malignant behavior, but a recent literature review found only tumor size (>5 cm) to be statistically associated with malignancy.[927,933]

Juvenile Granulosa Cell Tumor

Juvenile granulosa cell tumor of the testis is similar in appearance to its ovarian counterpart but occurs in a more restricted age range, with most patients younger than 5 months of age.[817,818,934-938] There are a few cases of this tumor presenting later in childhood in 4- to 10-year-old boys and a single report in a 27-year-old man.[818,939,940] There are no well-established risk factors, although

a disproportionate number occur in patients with either gonadal dysgenesis or anomalies of sex chromosomes, including patients with X/XY mosaicism.[255,818,941,942] A testicular mass is invariably the presenting feature. Grossly, it consists of a solid to cystic, gray to yellow nodule (Fig. 13.189).[817] The cystic foci are filled with mucoid to watery fluid. Microscopically, juvenile granulosa cell tumor has solid, cellular zones admixed with follicle-like, cystic structures filled with watery, eosinophilic to basophilic, faintly mucicarminophilic fluid (Fig. 13.190). Often the follicles are lined by several layers of stratified tumor cells and surrounded by a spindle cell stroma (Fig. 13.190A). The "solid" areas may display small inconspicuous (Fig. 13.190B) to absent follicles (Fig. 13.191), although even in the latter there typically is seen a lobular arrangement (either follicular or solid), with an intervening hypocellular fibromuscular stroma (Figs. 13.190 and 13.191). Columnar cells lining spaces create gland-like structures in about one-fourth of the cases.[818] Many neoplastic cells have abundant pale to eosinophilic cytoplasm with round, hyperchromatic nuclei and identifiable nucleoli (Fig. 13.190B).[789,817] Mitoses and cellular apoptosis may be prominent (Fig. 13.190B), but malignant behavior has not been reported, another feature that differs from ovarian juvenile granulosa cell tumor.[817,892,943,944] A recent large series described intratubular growth in 43% of cases.[818] Immunohistochemical studies reveal inhibin, vimentin, CD99, and focal cytokeratin, smooth muscle actin, and desmin reactivity.[892,937,943,945] FOXL2 and SF1 are the most sensitive markers and are consistently

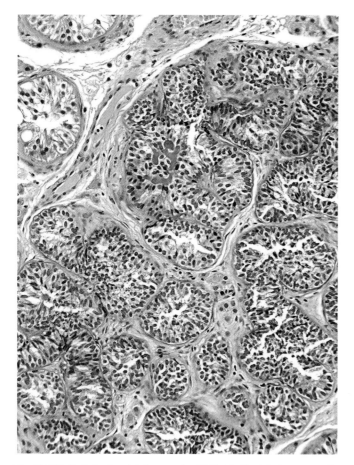

Fig. 13.181 Sertoli cell nodule in a cryptorchid testis. The tubules are smaller than the surrounding seminiferous tubules, are lined only by fetal-type Sertoli cells, and have focal central accumulations of basement membrane.

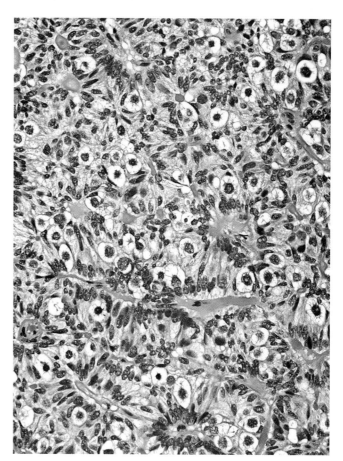

Fig. 13.183 Sertoli cell nodule with admixed spermatogonia.

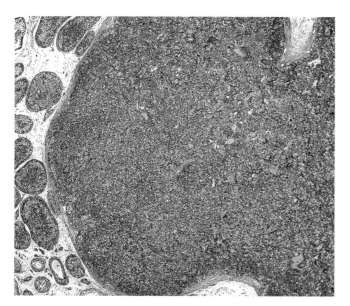

Fig. 13.182 Macroscopic sertoli cell nodule.

expressed.[818] AFP and SALL4 are negative. The histogenesis of this tumor is unknown; intratubular growth may indicate Sertoli cell derivation that exhibits aberrant differentiation based on FOXL2

expression, which is not seen in the normal testis but is characteristic of granulosa cell differentiation, even if not specific.[844,946] Because of the exclusive occurrence in infants and young children; the solid, cystic, and reticular patterns; and (physiologically) elevated serum AFP in some cases, juvenile granulosa cell tumor may be confused with testicular yolk sac tumor.[818] (This differential diagnosis was discussed previously.) Behavior has been uniformly benign.[818] Testis-sparing enucleation has been suggested for suspected juvenile granulosa cell tumors in infants with serum AFP in the normal range for age.[938,944]

Tumors in the Fibroma-Thecoma Group

Testicular tumors resembling ovarian fibroma or thecoma are rare; some reported examples likely represent unclassified sex cord–stromal tumors with a predominance of spindle cells. Cases have been reported in men over a wide age range (16 to 69 years) with a mean age of 44 years.[947] Patients present with palpable masses.[947,948] They are circumscribed, solid, yellow-white to tan tumors that lack necrosis. On microscopic examination, there is moderate to dense cellularity and short fascicles or storiform arrangements of uniform spindle to ovoid cells (Fig. 13.192). Acellular, hyaline plaques of collagen may be seen (Fig. 13.192), as well as prominent interstitial deposits of collagen. Mitotic activity is usually less than 5 mitotic figures per 10 high-power fields, but may be up to 10 per 10 high-power fields without known adverse prognosis.[947] Inhibin, calretinin, vimentin, actin, desmin, SF1, FOXL2, and SOX9 are frequently positive on immunohistochemical study.[844,947,948] Behavior is benign.[947]

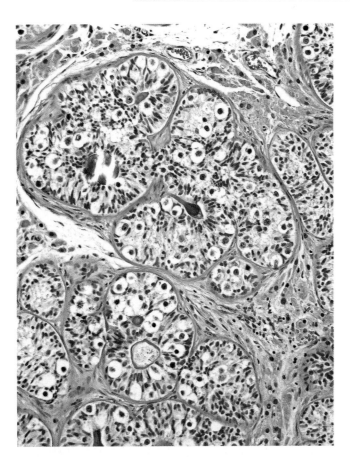

Fig. 13.184 Sertoli cell nodule partially populated by GCNIS cells.

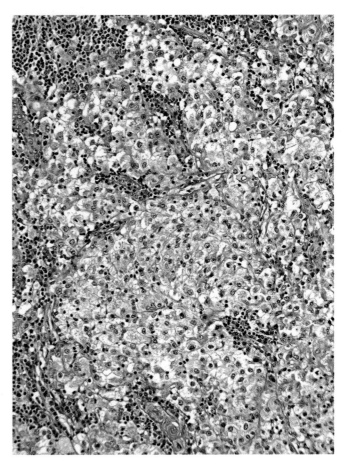

Fig. 13.185 This malignant Sertoli cell tumor has a sheetlike pattern of pale cells and a prominent inflammatory reaction that mimic seminoma.

Myoid Gonadal Stromal Tumor

Some of the purely spindled unclassified "sex cord–stromal tumors" represent myoid gonadal stromal tumors that express both S100 protein and smooth muscle markers similar to the peritubular myoid cells.[949-952] Because they lack a sex cord component, they should be considered a pure gonadal stromal neoplasm. These very rare tumors are composed of fascicles of fusiform to elongated spindled cells (Fig. 13.193), occur at a mean age of 37 years, and are not associated with hormonal symptoms.[952] In addition to S100 and SMA expression that is required for diagnosis, SF1 and FOXL2 expression is typical and focal inhibin staining is common.[844] Behavior has been benign in the small number of reported cases.[952]

Tumors may also have a combination of spindled and sex cord components with S100 and smooth muscle actin expression in the spindled component, and CD99 and inhibin reactivity occurring in the sex cord component, but these tumors should be placed in the unclassified sex cord–stromal tumor category.[952-955] In other cases, the presence of myofilaments in spindled stromal tumors suggests origin from myofibroblastic cells of the testicular interstitium.[950,951,956] Such cases should probably be classified as pure mesenchymal tumors rather than unclassified sex cord–stromal tumors.

Mixed and Unclassified Sex Cord–Stromal Tumors

A sizable group of sex cord–stromal neoplasms of the testis show admixtures of various forms of differentiation or incomplete differentiation. Such cases are classified as mixed or unclassified sex cord–stromal tumors, respectively. An example of a mixed sex cord–stromal tumor is adult granulosa cell tumor with tubules lined by Sertoli cells. Unclassified sex cord–stromal tumors consist of proliferations of incompletely differentiated sex cord or stromal elements that cannot be further characterized at the light microscopic level. These neoplasms are heterogeneous and have been grouped into a "wastebasket" category. Mixed and unclassified sex cord–stromal tumors occur at all ages, with 50% of cases occurring in children.[957] They usually present as a testicular mass, and 15% of cases are associated with gynecomastia.[789] Most consist of gray, tan, or yellow solid nodules of variable size. Both epithelial (sex cord) and stromal differentiation may be apparent at the light microscopic level (Fig. 13.194), and reticulum stains may enhance the different elements, surrounding groups of sex cord–like cells and individual stromal cells. In some tumors, sex cord elements of nonspecific type may compose most or the entire tumor. In other cases, the stromal component may be dominant, consisting of a relatively pure spindle cell proliferation.[953,955,958] Many of those cases are small (1 to 2 cm), occur close to the rete testis, and have benign features.[954] Occasional cases are overtly sarcomatoid, sometimes having "heterologous" mesenchymal differentiation.[959] Inhibin is often scant in the stromal cells and more impressive in the sex cord cells. SF1 and FOXL2 are more consistently expressed.[844] The demonstration of epithelial features by electron microscopy and immunohistochemistry suggests that some of these "stromal" tumors are spindled forms of epithelial (sex cord) origin.[955,960]

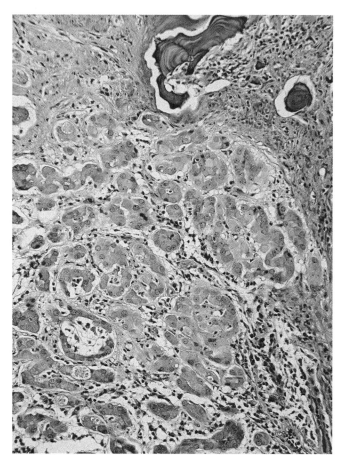

Fig. 13.186 Large cell calcifying sertoli cell tumor. Note the focal calcification and neutrophilic infiltrate.

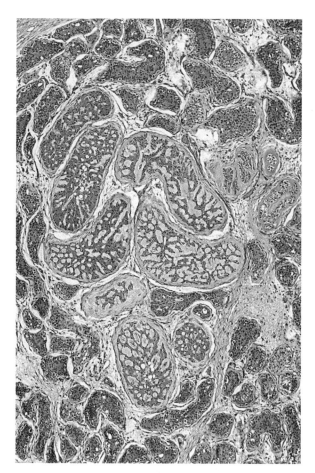

Fig. 13.187 Cluster of expanded seminiferous tubules containing proliferations of large Sertoli cells with abundant, eosinophilic cytoplasm and prominent basement membrane deposits in a patient with Peutz-Jeghers syndrome.

Mixed and unclassified sex cord–stromal tumors have thus far behaved in a benign fashion in children younger than 10 years of age, but metastases develop in 20% of older patients.[943,957,961] The presence of cellular atypia and pleomorphism, a high mitotic rate, necrosis, vascular invasion, invasive margins, and large tumor size are features that identify patients at risk for metastases. These tumors are usually managed by radical orchiectomy, with retroperitoneal lymph node dissection reserved for patients with clinical evidence of metastatic involvement or "high-risk" pathologic features.

Tumors Containing Both Germ Cell and Sex Cord–Stromal Elements

Gonadoblastoma

Clinical Features

Gonadal pathology in individuals with disorders of sex development has been recently reviewed.[962] Gonadal dysgenesis, a disorder of sex development resulting from a mutation or deletion of a gene upstream from *SOX9* (a transcription factor essential in Sertoli cell development) in the presence of a Y chromosome (or that portion of the Y chromosome including the *TSPY* locus), is associated with a distinctive tumor known as gonadoblastoma.[962] Gonadoblastoma is composed of a mixture of seminoma-like cells, immature germ cells, spermatogonia-like cells, and sex cord cells having some features of both granulosa cells (with strong nuclear FOXL2 nuclear reactivity) and Sertoli cells (with weaker SOX9 reactivity

and Charcot-Böttcher filaments in the cytoplasm).[963-966] Among patients with gonadoblastoma, 80% are phenotypically female and 20% are phenotypically male, but ambiguous genitalia occur in many cases.[967] Phenotypically male patients present in childhood or early adolescence with cryptorchidism, hypospadias, or other anomalies of the external genitalia and gynecomastia. Surgical exploration of the cryptorchid testes often demonstrates persistence of female-type internal genital structures stemming from failure of involution of the müllerian ductal system.[265] Bilateral involvement by gonadoblastoma occurs in about one-third of cases.[967] Karyotypic analysis of the patients, regardless of sexual phenotype, almost always reveals a Y-chromosome, with 46,XY and 45,X/46,XY occurring most commonly.[265] In patients with 45,X or 46,XX peripheral karyotypes, it is most likely that there is mosaicism with the gonads harboring nondeleted Y-chromosomal material. In children with 45,X/46,XY mosaicism, germ cell tumor risk varies by observed external masculinization, with highest risk among those with ambiguous phenotype, intermediate risk among boys with mild undervirilization, and lowest risk among girls with female (Turner syndrome) phenotype.[968]

Pathologic Features

Grossly, gonadoblastoma usually forms solid, yellow and tan nodules with gritty calcifications (Fig. 13.195). Microscopically, the nodules usually consist of well-defined, rounded nests of large, pale

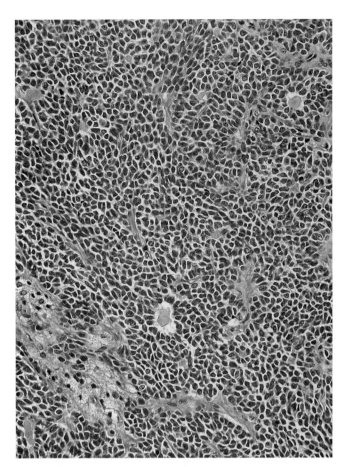

Fig. 13.188 Testicular granulosa cell tumor of the adult type showing a mostly diffuse pattern with occasional Call-Exner bodies.

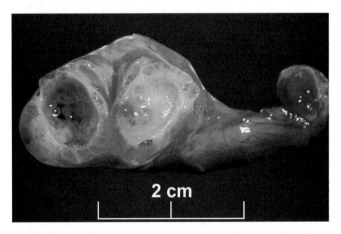

2 cm

Fig. 13.189 Juvenile granulosa cell tumor has a solid and cystic, yellow to tan cut surface. (Courtesy of Carlos Galliani, MD, Fort Worth, TX).

seminoma-like cells admixed with small, dark, angular, sex cord cells that may form a peripheral palisade around the cellular nests (Fig. 13.196). Close inspection also discloses that some of the germ cells lack a seminoma-like morphology and appear more like spermatogonia or primitive gonocytes, in keeping with molecular data.[286,295] Foci of hyalinized basement membrane can be seen in the center of these nests and at the periphery. Calcifications appear initially on this basement membrane, and may become

quite prominent, sometimes assuming a "mulberry-like" profile. In the stroma adjacent to gonadoblastoma, collections of Leydig-like cells lacking Reinke crystals may be seen in about two-thirds of cases.[253,967] In many classic gonadoblastomas, a trabecular growth pattern of seminoma-like cells and frequently inconspicuous sex cord cells may occur in tandem (Fig. 13.197). This pattern, which has been termed *dissecting gonadoblastoma of Scully* because of Dr. R.E. Scully's use of this nomenclature, appears to represent the same variation in gonadoblastoma morphologically as "undifferentiated gonadal tissue."[969] Biopsies of such tissue, however, may be difficult to recognize because the germ cells and sex cord cells are frequently relatively inconspicuous within a dominant nonneoplastic stroma. If the sex cord component is overlooked, it may be misinterpreted as a corded pattern of germinoma. An additional "dissecting" variant that mimics germinoma is represented by "expansile" confluent nests of gonadoblastoma that, however, retain the germ cell heterogeneity, sex cord cells, and basement membrane deposits (Fig. 13.198).

Special Studies

Many of the germ cells of gonadoblastoma have the immunohistochemical reactivities seen in GCNIS.[295] Some appear to be germ cells with delayed maturation that also express fetal-type germ cell markers.[286] The sex cord component stains for inhibin and the Wilms tumor gene protein (WT1).[970] The morphologically ambiguous sex cord cells of gonadoblastoma coexpress SOX9 (a transcription factor involved in Sertoli cell development) and, more strongly, FOXL2 (a transcription involved in granulosa cell tumor development), supporting that the cells are incompletely differentiated.[966] FISH in patients with gonadoblastoma and 45,X/46,XY mosaicism has demonstrated disproportionate representation of the Y chromosome in the gonadoblastoma cells, implicating it in tumor genesis.[971] Mapping studies have defined a susceptibility region on the Y chromosome that encompasses five candidate genes.[972–974] Accumulation of OCT3/4-positive germ cells and loss of expression of testis-specific protein on the Y chromosome (TSPY) has been observed by immunohistochemistry in the progression from gonadoblastoma to invasive germ cell tumor.[975]

Treatment and Prognosis

Gonadoblastoma is a premalignant lesion from which invasive germ cell tumors can develop; most are seminomas, but any nonseminomatous germ cell tumor may occur.[967] Excision of a gonad with gonadoblastoma before development of an invasive lesion is curative. Bilateral gonadectomy is indicated because of the dysgenetic nature of the gonads and the high frequency of bilaterality of gonadoblastoma.

Differential Diagnosis

Sertoli cell nodules colonized by GCNIS may be misinterpreted as gonadoblastoma (Fig. 13.184). However, this lesion is mostly microscopic rather than macroscopic, and the associated gonad is not dysgenetic, nor does the patient have somatosexual ambiguity. In some cases, the colonization by GCNIS is focal, and the seminoma-like cells are not uniformly distributed throughout the Sertoli cell nodule, whereas gonadoblastoma contains seminoma-like cells that are an integral and diffusely distributed component. Additionally, the constituent cells of these lesions contain both X and Y chromosomes by FISH, unlike gonadoblastoma.[976] This distinction is important because the diagnosis of gonadoblastoma implies an underlying dysgenetic gonad and much higher risk for bilateral

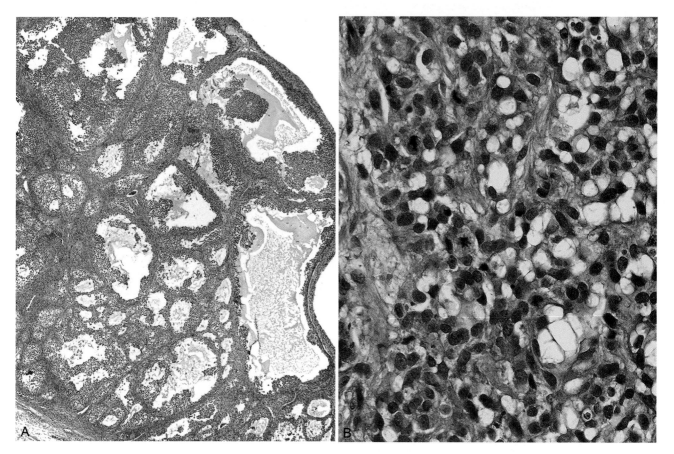

Fig. 13.190 Juvenile granulosa cell tumor with (A) follicle-like structures lined by multiple layers of tumor cells and containing watery to mucoid secretion and (B) solid foci with mitotic figures and apoptosis.

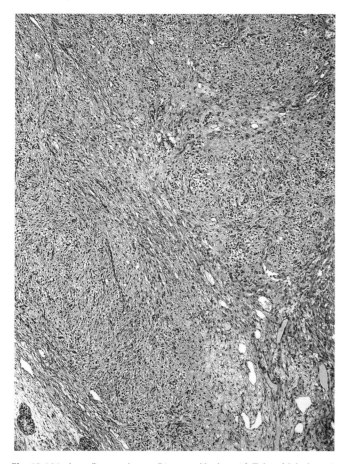

Fig. 13.191 Juvenile granulosa cell tumor with absent follicles. A lobular pattern with intervening fibromuscular stroma is appreciable.

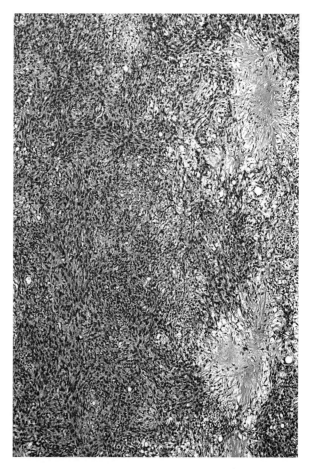

Fig. 13.192 Cellular fibroma. Note the plaques of hyalinized collagen.

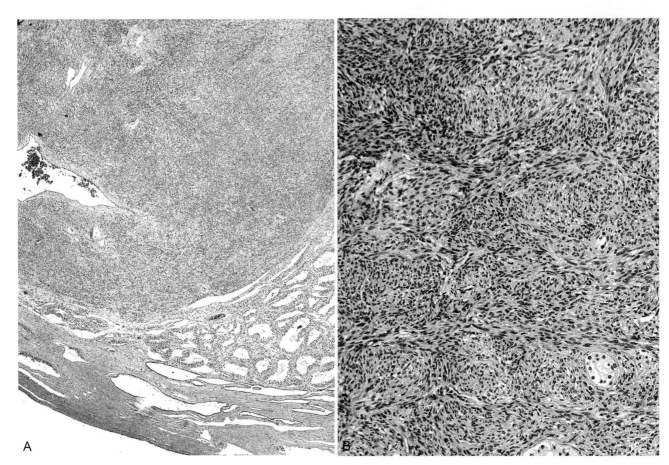

Fig. 13.193 Myoid gonadal stromal tumor with circumscribed profile (A) and fascicles of fusiform to elongated spindled cells (B).

gonadal involvement by a premalignant lesion. In contrast, a patient with a Sertoli cell nodule with GCNIS probably has a risk for bilateral involvement like that of any patient with GCNIS in one testis, approximately 1% to 5% of cases. SOX9 expression is greater and FOXL2 staining is absent in Sertoli cell nodule with GCNIS as compared with gonadoblastoma (where less intense SOX9 staining and positive FOXL2 staining are seen).[966]

The dissecting patterns of gonadoblastoma require distinction from a germinoma. This can be accomplished by appreciation of their sex cord components, usual basement membrane deposits, and frequent heterogenous nature of their germ cells. Immunostains can assist with this recognition if necessary.

An additional consideration is sex cord–stromal tumor with entrapped, nonneoplastic germ cells.[977] It, however, does not have a discretely nested arrangement of the lesional cells, nor do the germ cells show reactivity for GCNIS markers but retain features of spermatogonia (Fig. 13.199).

Miscellaneous Tumors of the Testis and Paratesticular Tissue

Ovarian-Type Epithelial Tumors

Tumors that resemble the surface epithelial tumors of the ovary may occur in and near the testis. More commonly they occur in the paratestis, involving the surface of the testis or structures such as the epididymis, and these are discussed in chapter 14.

Occasionally, however, they are found within the parenchyma and therefore merit a few comments here.

Borderline tumors of serous or mucinous types may occur in the testis, as may mucinous cystadenomas, serous cystadenofibromas, benign or malignant Brenner tumors, serous carcinomas, endometrioid adenocarcinomas, and mucinous adenocarcinomas.[978-990] They occur over a wide age range and typically present as palpable masses or as a hydrocele. These are usually cystic lesions, in keeping with their frequently borderline nature. The histologic appearances are like those seen in the much more common ovarian examples. In our experience, the serous tumors are the most common (Fig. 13.200). In the mucinous tumors, several of the cases we have seen were associated with mucin extravasation into the parenchyma with consequent fibrosis and dystrophic calcifications (Fig. 13.201). Some of the cases had marked cytologic atypia in the absence of stromal invasion, so-called "intraepithelial carcinoma."[981]

The distinctive appearance of the serous borderline tumors readily permits their diagnosis, although this diagnosis in the paratestis is complicated by the differential with papillary mesothelioma.[991-993] Mucinous tumors and Brenner tumors are potentially subject to confusion with teratoma. The absence of other teratomatous elements, cytologic atypia (usually), and of GCNIS assists with this differential, which may be facilitated by an older patient age, although there is overlap in the age range with patients having teratomas.[994] Additionally, at least in younger patients, the absence of "dysgenetic" parenchymal changes (i.e., tubular atrophy, peritubular sclerosis, tubular hyalinization, Sertoli cell–only tubules, microlithiasis) can

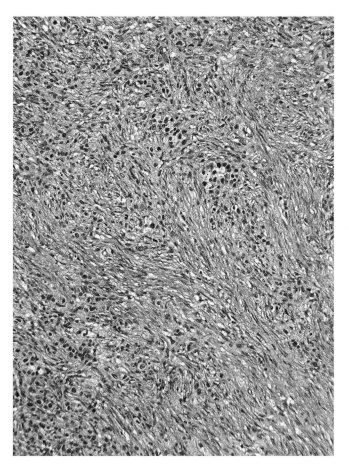

Fig. 13.194 Unclassified sex cord–stromal tumor has clusters of sex cord cells admixed with spindle cells.

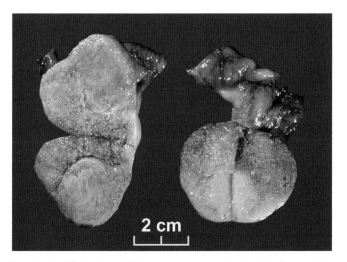

Fig. 13.195 Bilateral gonadoblastomas composed of solid, yellow and tan nodules with a gritty consistency. There are associated pink and white germinomas. (Photograph courtesy of RH Young, MD, Boston, MA).

assist in the differential diagnosis with postpubertal-type teratoma. Endometrioid tumors may be positive on estrogen and progesterone receptor protein immunohistochemical staining.[989] Rare cases of paratesticular endometriosis have been reported in men with prostate cancer treated with estrogen hormonal therapy and may represent metaplasia of the stromal cells of the tunica vaginalis, thus

providing the basis for endometrioid tumors.[995] Orchiectomy appears to be curative for tumors lacking stromal invasion.

Miscellaneous Lesions

Juvenile Xanthogranuloma

In infants, juvenile xanthogranuloma, including a series of three cases, has been described as a solitary testis mass.[996] These tumors are composed of an interstitial infiltrate of round and spindled mononuclear cells (Fig. 13.202) that are positive for CD68, vimentin, and factor XIIIa and negative for S100 protein and CD1a.[996] Touton giant cells, although characteristic, may be sparse to absent.

Hemangioma

Testicular hemangioma (including epithelioid hemangioma) has been reported in isolated reports.[997-1004] In a recent series of 8 cases, patient age ranged from 9 to 54 years (mean, 32 years), mean tumor size was 1.7 cm, and 3 of the 8 were recognized as hypervascular lesions by ultrasound preoperatively.[1005] Hemangiomas commonly have an infiltrative appearance and may extend between seminiferous tubules; they may show capillary, cavernous, or epithelioid morphology and always lack endothelial nuclear atypia or atypical mitoses.[1005] Several of them have anastomosing architecture ("anastomosing hemangioma"; Fig. 13.203).[1005] These, however, lack the cellular stratification and hyperchromasia of angiosarcoma. Vascular markers such as CD31, CD34, ERG, and factor VIII–related protein are positive.[1005,1006] Behavior has been benign, including in a case with up to 5 mitoses per high-power field.[1005,1006]

Testicular hemangioendothelioma has also been reported and, along with angiosarcoma, would be considered for a vascular tumor with nuclear atypia and/or atypical mitoses.[1007-1009] Angiosarcoma in the testis is usually a teratoma-associated somatic-type malignancy, so associated germ cell tumor would need to be carefully excluded. Very rare primary testicular angiosarcomas in the absence of germ cell tumor may occur in elderly men with chronic hydrocele.[1010] The possibility of angiosarcoma metastatic to the testis should also be considered.

Other Soft Tissue Tumors

Numerous other soft tissue tumors of the testis may rarely be seen, and some can be difficult to separate from unclassified sex cord–stromal tumors, but this distinction should be based on the absence of recognizable sex cord or epithelial differentiation and, possibly, lack of inhibin reactivity. Thus neurofibroma, fibroma of gonadal stromal origin, leiomyoma, inflammatory myofibroblastic tumor, osteosarcoma, chondrosarcoma, leiomyosarcoma, fibrosarcoma, rhabdomyosarcoma, and unclassified sarcoma of the testis have been reported.[997,1011-1025] Some of these may represent overgrowth of teratomatous elements of a germ cell tumor; we have seen several cases of pure testicular embryonal rhabdomyosarcoma associated with GCNIS, and one other case has been reported in the literature, suggesting that some testicular sarcomas are of teratomatous origin.[1026] Because patients who have testicular sarcoma developing from germ cell tumor may have conventional germ cell tumor elements at metastatic sites (which would be amenable to chemotherapy), the distinction of primary sarcoma versus sarcoma of germ cell tumor origin is important. The occurrence of testicular sarcoma in younger adult

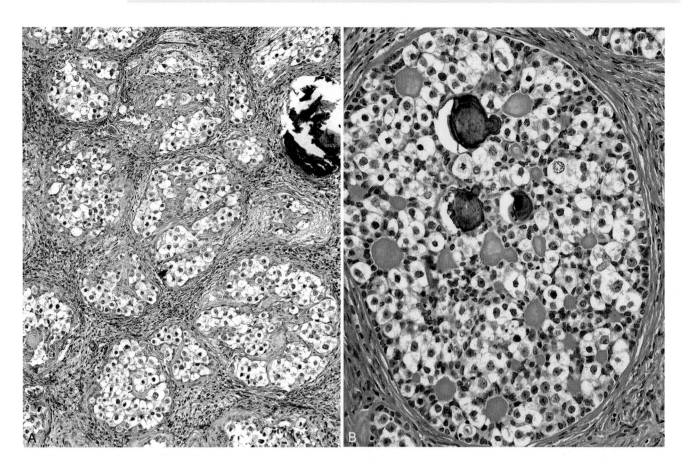

Fig. 13.196 Gonadoblastoma. (A) There are multiple, circumscribed, discrete nests. (B) The nests contain germ cells (some with a seminoma-like appearance and others resembling spermatogonia), sex cord cells, and round deposits of basement membrane, some with calcification.

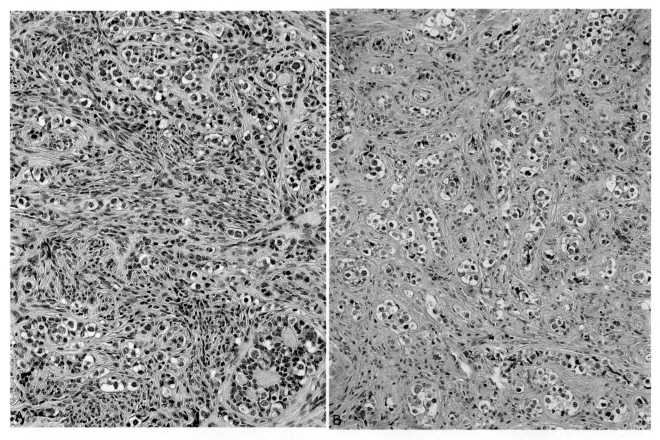

Fig. 13.197 Gonadoblastomas (A and B) with a trabecular growth pattern of seminoma-like cells and frequently inconspicuous sex cord cells, a pattern that has been termed *dissecting gonadoblastoma of Scully.*

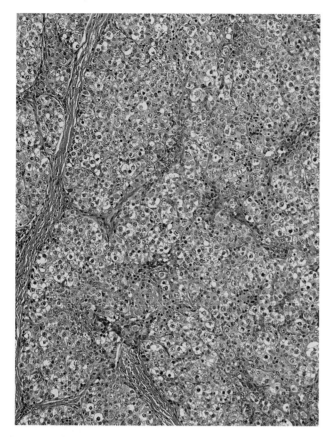

Fig. 13.198 An additional "dissecting" variant mimicking germinoma with confluent nests of gonadoblastoma that retain sex cord cells and basement membrane deposits.

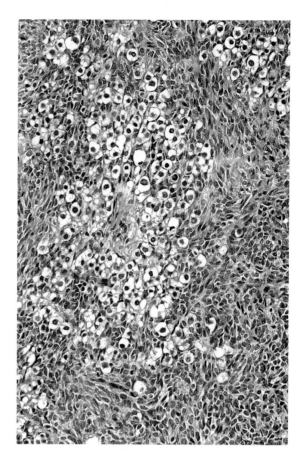

Fig. 13.199 Sex cord–stromal tumor with entrapped, nonneoplastic germ cells may mimic gonadoblastoma. It does not have a discretely nested arrangement of the lesional cells or germ cells reactivity for GCNIS markers.

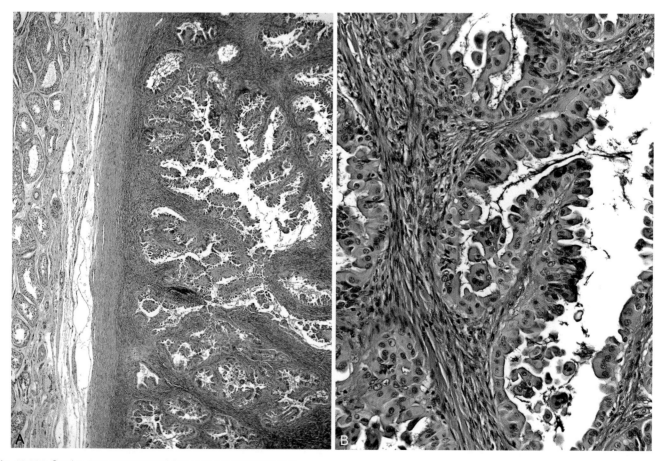

Fig. 13.200 Ovarian-type tumor resembling serous borderline tumor.

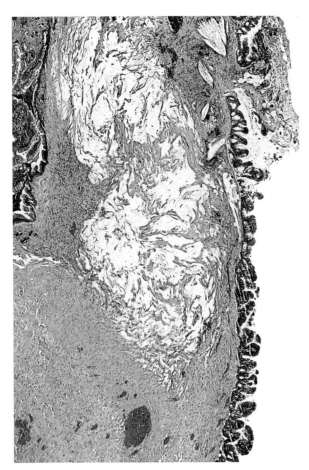

Fig. 13.201 Borderline mucinous tumor with extravasated mucin. Note the characteristic filigree pattern of the lining epithelium.

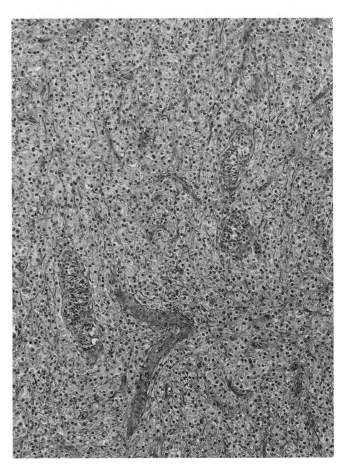

Fig. 13.202 Juvenile xanthogranuloma composed of an interstitial infiltrate of round and spindled mononuclear cells. Occasional seminiferous tubules remain.

patients is a suspicious finding for sarcoma in the context of germ cell tumor. The identification of chromosome 12p amplification also indicates that a testicular sarcoma is derived from germ cell neoplasia. Additionally, some sarcomas may occur as a "dedifferentiation" phenomenon in Leydig cell tumors and spermatocytic tumors.[745,746,836]

Hematolymphoid Tumors

Lymphoma

Lymphoma in the testis usually represents secondary spread from lymph nodes, although there are occasional cases that meet the criteria for primary testicular lymphoma.[412,414,461,463,467,1027] These criteria include principal involvement of the testis and absence of nodal involvement after careful staging.[461] However, these restrictions may be inadequate for recognizing lymphoma originating in the testis. The tendency of apparently primary testicular lymphoma to progress rapidly after excision, with high rates of recurrence, supports the belief that many originated elsewhere but spread to the testis and became clinically evident.[461,463,464,1028,1029] Consistent clonal rearrangements of the immunoglobulin light-chain genes in synchronous, bilateral testicular lymphoma likely indicates occult dissemination of lymphoma with seeding of the testes, and argues against primary bilateral testicular lymphoma.[1030] The unfavorable survival of patients with bilateral lymphoma provides

additional support for this view.[1027] In many studies of testicular lymphoma, it is not clear if the tumor is primary extranodal lymphoma or lymphoma that originated elsewhere and subsequently spread to the testis, making interpretation of this literature difficult.

Clinical Features

Patients with testicular lymphoma are usually older than those with germ cell tumors, with a mean age of about 60 years[458-463,1027]; 50% of testicular neoplasms occurring in patients older than 60 years of age are lymphomas.[789] Although most patients present secondary to a testicular mass, systemic symptoms such as fever, sweats, and weight loss also occur.[461] Bilateral testicular involvement occurs in about 20% of cases and is usually metachronous but may also be synchronous.[459,461-463,1031,1032]

Pathologic Features

Grossly, testicular lymphoma forms a fleshy, white-gray to pink mass that often diffusely replaces the testicular parenchyma (Fig. 13.204). Foci of necrosis may be conspicuous. It may be difficult to distinguish grossly from seminoma, although extension into the paratesticular structures suggests lymphoma rather than seminoma.[467,1027] Microscopically, lymphoma often has an interstitial pattern, with neoplastic cells surrounding but not replacing seminiferous tubules deep within the tumor

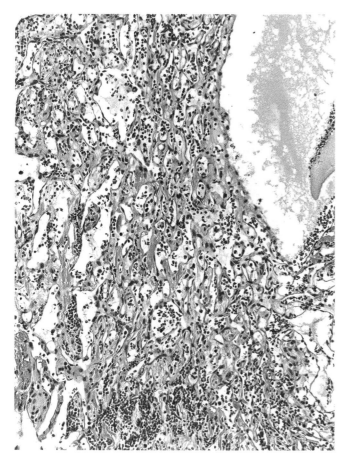

Fig. 13.203 "Anastomosing hemangioma" with interconnecting vascular channels. Note the lack of cellular stratification and hyperchromasia.

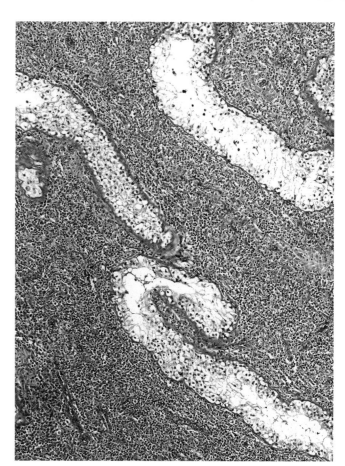

Fig. 13.205 Typical interstitial pattern of lymphoma, with preservation of several seminiferous tubules.

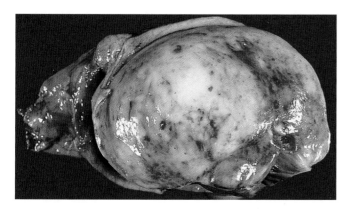

Fig. 13.204 Lymphoma in the testis. Note the fleshy, pink to cream-colored tumor.

(Fig. 13.205). Transtubular migration of the neoplastic cells may occur, and there may rarely be conspicuous intratubular involvement (Fig. 13.206).[1033] Despite interstitial growth, the seminiferous tubules may eventually be destroyed and replaced by tumor, so the absence of an interstitial pattern does not exclude lymphoma. Most testicular lymphomas in adults are diffuse large cell type of B-cell immunophenotype.[387,458, 460-462,1027,1029,1034-1036] They are furthermore mostly of the nongerminal center cell type of B-cell lymphoma, a type associated with a more aggressive course.[1037] They are generally not

associated with Epstein-Barr virus or human herpes virus 8.[1034] Many express bcl-2 protein in the absence of a 14:18 chromosomal translocation.[1038] In children, Burkitt lymphoma is the most common one in the testis, and shows the characteristic features, including small, mitotically active cells with round nuclei having several small nucleoli intermixed with macrophages containing phagocytosed nuclear debris.[1031] Rare cases of Burkitt lymphoma of the testis have occurred in adults.[1039] Hodgkin lymphoma involving the testis was not seen in a large testicular lymphoma case series, although a single case has been reported.[1027,1031,1040,1041] Infrequent cases of pediatric testicular follicular lymphoma have been reported, with very favorable outcomes.[1042,1043] Several additional types have been described in the testis: anaplastic large cell lymphoma (sometimes showing conspicuous intratubular involvement), nasal-type T/natural killer cell lymphoma, follicular lymphoma, low-grade T-helper cell lymphoma, B-lymphoblastic lymphoma, and histiocytic sarcoma.[1033,1043-1056] A discussion of the features of these lymphomas is beyond the scope of this chapter.

Prognosis

The stage of testicular lymphoma is the most important prognostic factor. In patients with stage I disease, there is a 60% 5-year tumor-free survival, whereas patients with more advanced stage disease have only a 17% 5-year tumor-free survival.[1027] Histologic classification is also prognostically useful; in a multivariate analysis, lymphoma with sclerosis had a significantly more favorable outcome,

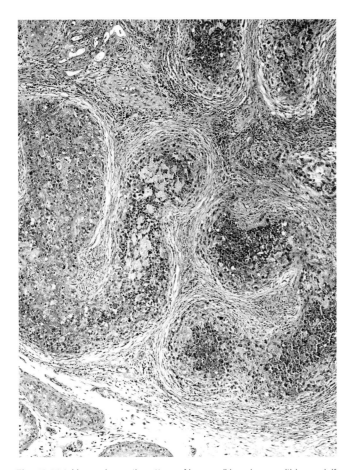

Fig. 13.206 Unusual growth pattern of large cell lymphoma within seminiferous tubules. Note the comedo-like tumor necrosis.

and, for unclear reasons, so did right-sided testicular lymphoma.[462,1027] A recent series of 43 primary testicular lymphomas found Eastern Cooperative Oncology Group (ECOG) performance status, infiltration of adjacent tissues (such as epididymis or spermatic cord), and bulky disease (>9 cm) were independently prognostically significant factors and also predicted benefit from rituximab treatment (with only the low-risk patients showing benefit).[1057]

Differential Diagnosis

A major differential diagnostic consideration in testicular lymphoma is seminoma, which is addressed in the Seminoma section earlier in this chapter. Anaplastic large cell lymphoma with intratubular growth may be confused with embryonal carcinoma. Both are CD30 reactive and may show prominent comedo-type necrosis of the intratubular component, but the strong cytokeratin and OCT3/4 reactivity of embryonal carcinoma and its negativity for lymphoid markers serve to assist in the distinction, as does the absence of GCNIS in lymphoma. A potential pitfall in this differential diagnosis, however, is the uncommon occurrence of OCT3/4 reactivity in large cell lymphomas (Tickoo, S.K., 2013, personal communication), illustrating the benefit of a panel of immunostains. Chronic orchitis may also be confused with lymphoma but contains a heterogeneous cell population, consisting of lymphocytes, polyclonal plasma cells, and neutrophils without atypia. Reactive lymphoid hyperplasia within the testis is a rare

condition and has been described as testicular "pseudolymphoma"; its distinction from lymphoma is based on the same criteria used at other sites.[1058]

Plasmacytoma

Plasmacytoma of the testis is rare and usually occurs in older patients with an established or concurrent diagnosis of multiple myeloma.[1059-1063] Some of these patients may have bilateral involvement, either synchronous or asynchronous.[1062,1063] Even more rarely, however, testicular plasmacytoma may be an apparently isolated finding, and, in such cases the patient must be carefully worked up and followed for multiple myeloma, although some have not progressed.[1061,1062,1064,1065] The testis may be the site of relapse of treated multiple myeloma, suggesting that the blood–testis barrier may make the testis a sanctuary site, as in acute lymphoblastic leukemia.[1066] Autopsy studies of patients with multiple myeloma demonstrate an approximately 2% frequency of testicular involvement, but the majority of such involvement remains clinically inapparent.[789] Grossly, plasmacytoma often appears as a soft, fleshy, gray-white and hemorrhagic intratesticular mass. Microscopically, sheets of variably differentiated neoplastic plasma cells are identified, often with an interstitial pattern of involvement (Fig. 13.207). Unlike chronic orchitis, a polymorphic cell population is absent and there is light chain restriction. In the poorly differentiated examples, misinterpretation as seminoma, lymphoma, or metastatic melanoma is possible.[1062]

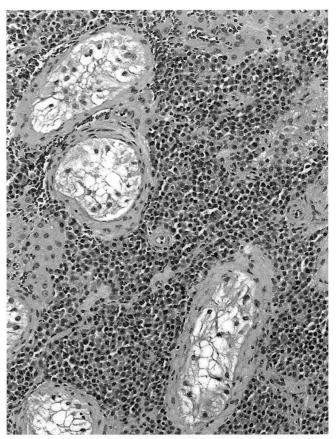

Fig. 13.207 Plasmacytoma with sheets of neoplastic plasma cells in an interstitial pattern.

Immunostains for light chain restriction, CD138, CD79a, and with monoclonal antibody VS38 are often helpful in identifying plasmacytoma.

Leukemia, Including Myeloid Sarcoma

Leukemic infiltrates occur commonly in the testis, with frequency rates at autopsy of 40% to 65% of patients with acute leukemia and 20% to 35% of patients with chronic leukemia.[1040,1067] Leukemia is the most common neoplasm to involve the testis in children.[773] Acute lymphoblastic leukemia is especially prone to testicular involvement, and the testis may be a "sanctuary" site for leukemic cells such that testicular biopsy may detect leukemic infiltrates during periods of otherwise complete remission. The detection of leukemia in the testis in such cases occurs in 5% to 10% of patients and is predictive of subsequent systemic relapse.[1068-1070] The probability of a second remission from non–B-cell childhood leukemia is higher for patients with isolated testicular relapse than those with relapse at other sites.[1071] The leukemic testis is usually not enlarged, and the diagnosis is established by biopsy of patients at risk. Occasionally, diffuse testicular enlargement, induration, or a testicular mass may be observed.[1070] Bilateral involvement is common. Exceptionally, leukemia may initially present as testicular enlargement.[789,1072] Microscopically, leukemia usually shows an interstitial pattern of infiltration, similar to lymphoma. The neoplastic cells are characteristic of the leukemia. It may not be possible to morphologically distinguish between some types of lymphoma and leukemia, and clinical information regarding peripheral blood involvement and bone marrow studies are required. The distinction between neoplastic monocytic and myelocytic infiltrates and lymphoid neoplasia may require histochemical and immunohistochemical studies.

Rarely, myeloid sarcoma occurs in the absence of leukemia; typically, subsequent leukemia is found, although one patient who was treated for lymphoma because of pathologic misinterpretation survived for 12 years without evidence of leukemia.[1073-1076] In one case of myeloid sarcoma presenting in the testis of an infant, cerebrospinal fluid was involved at presentation but bone marrow involvement was not histopathologically identified.[1077] Myeloid sarcoma, because of its frequent paratesticular involvement and overlapping morphology, is prone to misinterpretation as lymphoma or plasmacytoma.[1075,1076] If eosinophilic myelocytes are present, the correct diagnosis is greatly facilitated. CD45 may be positive and therefore may not discriminate between myeloid sarcoma and lymphoma.[1076] More helpful are stains directed against myeloperoxidase and lysozyme, as well as chloroacetate esterase stains.[1076]

Rosai-Dorfman Disease

Testicular Rosai-Dorfman disease (sinus histiocytosis with massive lymphadenopathy) may occur over a wide age range but is most common in middle-age adults.[1078,1079] These lesions are composed of a mixed inflammatory infiltrate with lymphocytes, plasma cells, and large histiocytes with emperipolesis. The disorder is an abnormal proliferation of S100-positive histiocytic cells with characteristic phagocytosis of lymphocytes.[1078,1079] The differential diagnosis could include germ cell tumors, hematolymphoid tumors, metastatic tumors such as melanoma, and granulomatous orchitis. Occasional patients have had a history of previous lymphoproliferative disease.[1078]

Tumors of Collecting Duct and Rete Testis

Adenoma

Adenoma of the rete testis is rare, consisting of papillary or glandular proliferations of cytologically bland cells.[1080-1082] Four adenomas were reported in patients from 21 to 79 years of age.[1083] They ranged from 1.5 to 3.6 cm in diameter and were composed of cysts lined by bland, sometimes stratified or tufted epithelium, with prominent intervening fibrous stroma.

About 25 cases of Sertoliform cystadenoma of the rete testis have now been reported since the original elaboration of its features by Jones et al.[1083-1085] In the largest series of 15 cases, the patients were 1 to 84 years of age, and all presented with masses except for one that was incidental in an orchiectomy specimen.[1085] These cystic and solid lesions are centered in the testicular hilum and have an appearance similar to that of a Sertoli cell tumor, although most of the proliferation occurs within the dilated channels of the rete testis (Fig. 13.208). They form hollow and solid tubules, cords, and nests in a hyalinized to myxoid stroma and, less commonly, solid sheets, festoons, individual cells, and papillae.[1085] The lesional cells are cuboidal to columnar and have bland cytologic features with few (0 to 2 per 10 high-power fields) mitotic figures.[1085] They usually express SF1 and inhibin.[1085] Follow-up has been benign.

Cystadenomas, adenofibromas, and a complex multilocular cystic lesion of the rete testis with smooth muscle hyperplasia have also been reported.[1083,1086,1087] Approximately 54% of men with von

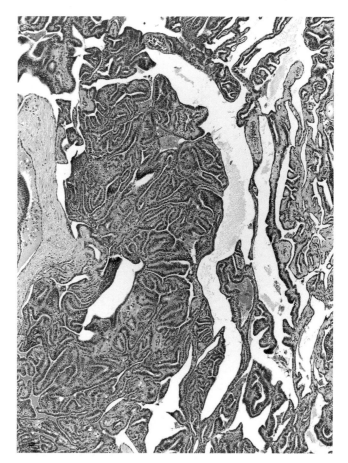

Fig. 13.208 Sertoliform cystadenoma of the rete testis with a tubular and papillary proliferation of epithelium within dilated channels of the rete testis.

Hippel–Lindau disease have enlargement of the epididymis compatible with epididymal cystadenoma.[1088]

Hartwick et al. described adenomatous hyperplasia of the rete testis in a series of nine cases in patients ranging from 30 to 74 years of age; in three cases, the hyperplasia produced grossly evident, solid, and cystic masses in the testicular hilum.[1089] Nistal et al. reported 20 cases in patients ranging from 2 months to 74 years of age, 11 associated with cryptorchidism and 4 with a germ cell tumor.[1090] Microscopically, these lesions are tubulopapillary proliferations of bland cells within distended rete testis. Whether these cases are distinct from adenoma is unclear; they do not appear to be similar to the hyperplastic reaction of the rete testis typically seen in cases of germ cell tumor (Fig. 13.85).[623] Conservative surgical treatment (excision rather than orchiectomy) for small lesions has been recommended.[1091]

Cystic Dysplasia

Scattered case reports describe cystic dysplasia of the rete testis associated with absence or dysplasia of the ipsilateral kidney.[1092,1093] These lesions mostly present in children and young adults as a painless scrotal swelling with a multicystic appearance on ultrasound and negative tumor markers.[1094] Rarely the lesion may present as a painful and solid mass.[1095] There is often prominent dilatation of the rete testis with compression of residual testicular parenchyma.

Adenocarcinoma

Adenocarcinoma of the rete testis is very rare, occurring in patients from 20 to 91 years of age.[1083,1096,1097] Most patients are older than 60 years of age.[1083] Many present with symptoms of testicular pain and swelling. The initial clinical impression is often epididymitis or hydrocele, and hydrocele is found associated with the tumor in 25%.[1096] Because of the posterior location of the tumor, a mass may be difficult to palpate. Some patients present with metastatic scrotal or perineal nodules. Grossly, there is a white to tan, yellow, or brown, ill-defined mass near the testicular hilum, often with extension into paratesticular structures. Some degree of cystic change may be present but is usually not prominent. Microscopically the tumor displays solid, papillary, and glandular patterns. The tumor often has an intraluminal component, which distends the spaces of the rete, as well as a component that infiltrates the supporting stroma of the rete (Fig. 13.209). There may be associated rete testis hyperplasia, and, ideally, a transition from benign to malignant epithelium is seen in the lining of the rete (Fig. 13.209B), but this finding may not be demonstrable and may furthermore be mimicked by metastatic carcinomas that involve the rete testis and undermine its epithelial lining.[1096,1098,1099] The solid pattern is often punctuated by slitlike lumens, and a spindle cell pattern rarely occurs.[1100] The papillae may have hyalinized fibrous cores and project into cysts. The tumor cells typically have round to oval nuclei, sometimes with grooves, and scant cytoplasm. Immunohistochemical studies typically yield

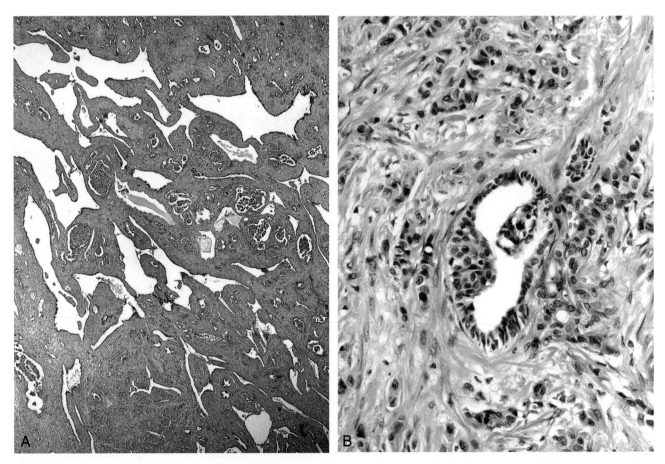

Fig. 13.209 Adenocarcinoma of the rete testis with (A) an intraluminal component and infiltrating component in the supporting stroma of the rete. (B) In the central tubule there is transition from cytologically bland rete epithelium to dysplastic epithelium.

positive reactions for cytokeratins and EMA and less consistent reactivity for CEA. Lymphatic metastases occur most commonly and initially involve retroperitoneal lymph nodes; sometimes there is involvement of the skin of the scrotum or perineum.[1101] The prognosis is poor, with only 36% of patients being tumor-free on follow-up.[1096] The differential diagnosis includes carcinomas and borderline tumors of ovarian epithelial type; these occur more commonly in the paratesticular area, probably from metaplasia of the mesothelium or müllerian remnants, but also rarely occur within the testis, perhaps from metaplasia of mesothelial inclusions. It is likely that some cases of papillary serous borderline tumor have been reported as adenocarcinoma of the rete testis, thus leading to an overly optimistic prognosis for rete testis carcinoma.[1096] Psammoma bodies, squamous metaplasia, or mucinous cell type should raise the question of müllerian-type neoplasms. The differential is probably not of great importance except when it involves the distinction of a borderline tumor from an invasive carcinoma. Mesothelioma, which in some cases is associated with a history of asbestos exposure, should also be considered, and immunohistochemical studies to distinguish between adenocarcinoma and mesothelioma may help in difficult cases.[1102] Malignant mesothelioma of the tunica vaginalis consistently expresses calretinin, WT-1 (nuclear), and EMA, and thrombomodulin, cytokeratin 7, and cytokeratin 5/6 reactivity is also seen in most cases, although many of these may also occur in rete adenocarcinoma.[993,1102,1103] More helpful are positivity in rete adenocarcinoma for PAX8 and with antibodies BerEp4 and MOC31. Prostatic carcinoma may involve the rete testis, but the clinical history and immunostains for prostate-specific antigen should allow its identification.

Metastatic Tumors

Metastases to the testis are most commonly identified in patients with known malignancies, and the most common sites of origin (excluding leukemia and lymphoma) are the prostate, stomach, lung, skin (melanoma), colon/rectum, kidney, urinary bladder, and elsewhere.[786,1104-1115] It is likely that the predominance of the prostate in this ranking represents at least a partial selection bias resulting from examination of therapeutic orchiectomy specimens from patients with metastatic prostatic carcinoma.[1116] In children, there is a predominance of neuroblastoma and rhabdomyosarcoma, but metastatic rhabdomyosarcoma may also involve the testis in adults.[1107,1117-1121] Rarely metastases to the testis may present as apparent primary testicular tumors, including those originating in the prostate, lung, kidney, gastrointestinal tract (stomach and colon), urinary bladder, skin (melanoma), thyroid gland (medullary carcinoma), pancreas, and liver, and well-differentiated neuroendocrine tumor.[786,789,1109,1112,1122-1124] One case of occult gastric signet ring carcinoma presented as a spermatic cord and testis mass (and was considered a "Krukenberg tumor in a male patient").[1125] Although bilateral involvement may be seen in some cases, often the tumors are unilateral and solitary masses, complicating the distinction from primary tumors.[786,1107,1109,1125] A proclivity to involve the right testis has been identified in several studies.[786,1107,1109] Misinterpretation of metastatic carcinoma or melanoma as embryonal carcinoma, Leydig cell tumor, or Sertoli cell tumor may occur, or metastatic well-differentiated neuroendocrine tumor may be misinterpreted as primary testicular well-differentiated neuroendocrine tumor.[786,794,1109,1112] We have seen several metastatic prostate carcinomas that had a prominent intratubular component (Fig. 13.210) or that prominently involved the rete testis (Fig. 13.211), potentially causing confusion

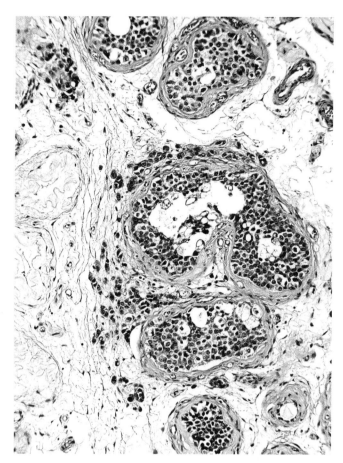

Fig. 13.210 Metastatic prostate carcinoma to the testis with a prominent intratubular component.

with primary testicular neoplasms, especially for the latter, Sertoliform cystadenoma of the rete testis or rete testis carcinoma. The nested and tubular pattern of metastatic renal cell carcinoma of clear cell type is prone to misinterpretation as Sertoli cell tumor.[786] Some metastatic melanomas may show prominent foamy tumor cells, overlapping with an appearance that may be seen in Leydig cell tumors.[1109] Additionally melanomas may have relatively scant cytoplasm and display prominent intertubular growth, features that are readily confused with lymphoma (Fig. 13.212). The presence of an extensive interstitial pattern, prominent microvascular involvement, multifocality, and bilaterality are features that favor metastasis rather than primary testicular tumor, but they are not always present.[1112,1116,1126] The clinical history may also be of value because patients with metastatic lesions to the testis are, on average, older (mean age, 57 years) than patients with a germ cell tumor such as embryonal carcinoma (mean age, 30 years). However, patients with metastatic stomach and small intestinal cancer may fall within the usual age range of those with testicular germ cell tumor.[1127] Serum AFP and hCG levels are much more likely to be elevated in patients with germ cell tumor. The absence of GCNIS in the surrounding seminiferous tubules increases the probability of a metastatic tumor over germ cell tumor, as do EMA positivity and PLAP, SALL4, and OCT3/4 negativity.[413,1126] Other immunohistochemical studies may prove useful, including prostate-specific antigen, renal cell carcinoma and melanoma markers, and inhibin stains.

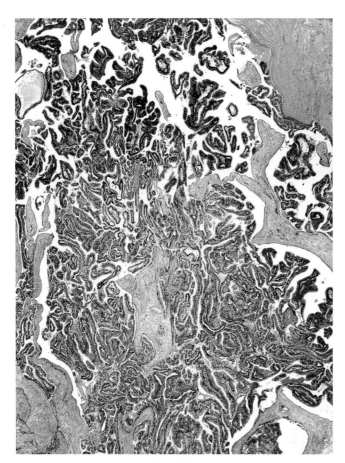

Fig. 13.211 Metastatic prostate carcinoma with prominent intrarete growth. The pattern is similar to sertoliform cystadenoma of the rete (Fig. 13.208), although the cytologic features and immunoreactivity are distinctly different.

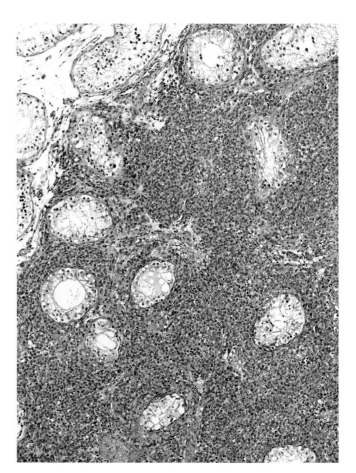

Fig. 13.212 Metastatic melanoma. The tumor cells show prominent interstitial growth, mimicking the low-power appearance of lymphoma.

Diagnostic Approach to Testicular Tumors

From the preceding information, it is apparent that several recurring morphologic patterns are observed in testicular tumors. The differential diagnostic considerations for tumors with certain patterns may include tumors of germ cell origin, tumors of sex cord–stromal origin, and secondary tumors. In most cases, careful attention to the morphologic features, along with the clinical history, will allow establishment of the correct diagnosis, and the most important differential diagnostic considerations have been discussed earlier and elsewhere.[8,10,284,1128-1132] In some of these cases, immunohistochemical staining provides crucial supportive evidence.[13]

Some of the common patterns include solid tumors composed of cells with pale cytoplasm; tumors with a glandular and/or tubular pattern; tumors with a microcystic pattern; oxyphilic tumors with a predominant solid pattern; and tumors with spindle cell morphology.[1128]

Solid tumors composed of cells with pale cytoplasm may include seminoma, spermatocytic tumor, solid-pattern embryonal carcinoma, solid-pattern yolk sac tumor, metastatic adenocarcinoma, Sertoli cell tumor, Leydig cell tumor, and lymphoma. Several light microscopic features and immunohistochemical reactions assist the separation of these entities (Fig. 13.213). These may be distinguished based on the presence of associated GCNIS, the presence of focal glandular architecture, the presence of a predominantly interstitial growth pattern, and the immunohistochemical

staining pattern for OCT3/4, SALL4, PLAP, CD30, AFP, inhibin, SF1, and LCA (Fig. 13.213).

Tumors with a glandular or tubular pattern include embryonal carcinoma, yolk sac tumor, tubular pattern seminoma, rete testis neoplasm, metastatic adenocarcinoma, and Sertoli cell tumor (Fig. 13.214). These may be distinguished based on the presence of associated GCNIS, nuclear features and the presence of elongated glandular spaces, the presence of hyaline globules and other patterns of yolk sac tumor, the presence of intertubular growth pattern or solid tubules, and OCT3/4, SALL4, PLAP, CD30, AFP, keratin, and inhibin staining patterns (Fig. 13.214).

Tumors that may have a microcystic pattern include yolk sac tumor, seminoma, Sertoli cell tumor, Leydig cell tumor, juvenile granulosa cell tumor, and adenomatoid tumor (Fig. 13.215). Features helpful in distinguishing these tumors include patient age, the presence of GCNIS, nuclear features such as nuclear size variability and flattened cellular profiles within the cysts, the presence of cords of tumor cells and lipid-rich cells, and staining for keratin, OCT3/4, AFP, SALL4, PLAP, inhibin, and calretinin (Fig. 13.215).

Oxyphilic tumors with a predominantly solid pattern include Leydig cell tumor, large cell calcifying Sertoli cell tumor, hepatoid pattern yolk sac tumor, well-differentiated neuroendocrine tumor, metastatic adenocarcinoma, melanoma, plasmacytoma, and adenomatoid tumor (Fig. 13.216). Cytoplasmic lipofuscin or Reinke crystals, the presence of associated fibromyxoid stroma, the presence of GCNIS, the presence of insular and trabecular patterns or teratomatous elements, the presence of overtly malignant nuclear features and intratubular growth, and staining patterns

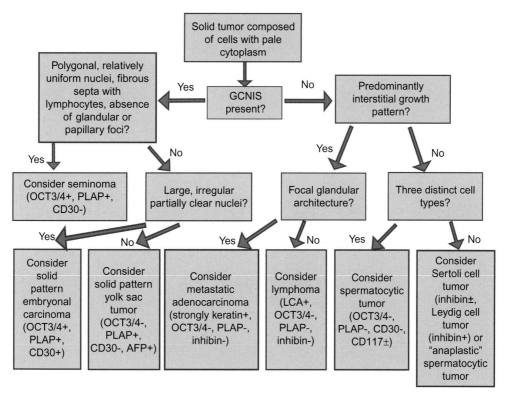

Fig. 13.213 A general approach for the diagnosis of tumors with a diffuse arrangement of pale to clear cells. (Modified from Emerson RE, Ulbright TM. Morphological approach to tumours of the testis and paratestis. *J Clin Pathol*. 2007;60:866–880.)

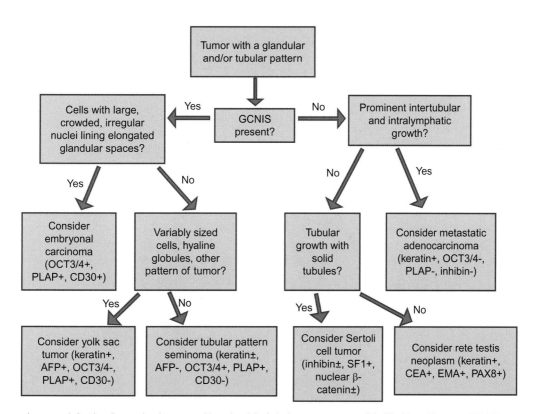

Fig. 13.214 A general approach for the diagnosis of tumors with a glandular/tubular arrangement. (Modified from Emerson RE, Ulbright TM. Morphological approach to tumours of the testis and paratestis. *J Clin Pathol*. 2007;60:866–880.)

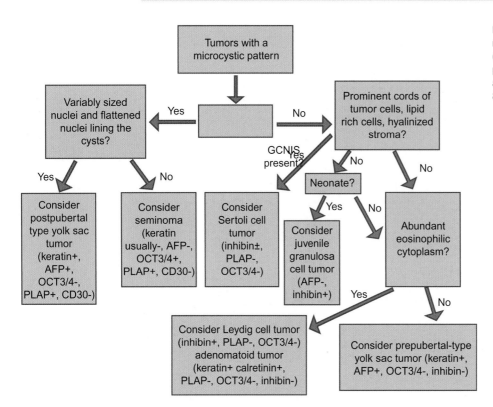

Fig. 13.215 A general approach for the diagnosis of tumors with a microcystic pattern. (Modified from Emerson RE, Ulbright TM. Morphological approach to tumours of the testis and paratestis. *J Clin Pathol.* 2007;60: 866–880.)

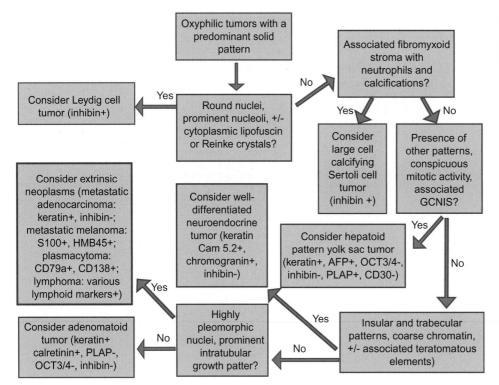

Fig. 13.216 A general approach for the diagnosis of tumors composed mostly of oxyphilic cells. (Modified from Emerson RE, Ulbright TM. Morphological approach to tumours of the testis and paratestis. *J Clin Pathol.* 2007;60:866–880.)

with keratin, inhibin, SALL4, PLAP, calretinin, and markers specific for extrinsic neoplasms can be useful in differentiating these tumors (Fig. 13.216).

Tumors with a largely or entirely spindle cell pattern may include Leydig cell tumor, unclassified sex cord–stromal tumor, sarcomatoid carcinoma, mesothelioma, some benign mesenchymal lesions such as testicular tunic fibroma, and a variety of sarcomas (Fig. 13.217).

These may be distinguished based on the presence of foci of recognizable oxyphilic Leydig cells, nuclear cytology and mitotic activity, and immunohistochemical staining pattern for actin, desmin, CD34, keratin, inhibin, and S100 protein (Fig. 13.217).

References are available at expertconsult.com

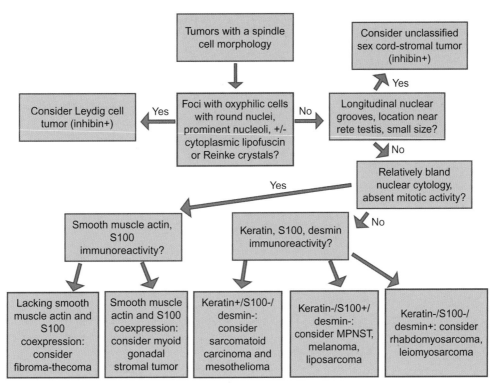

Fig. 13.217 A general approach for the diagnosis of tumors composed mostly of spindle cells. (Modified from Emerson RE, Ulbright TM. Morphological approach to tumours of the testis and paratestis. *J Clin Pathol.* 2007;60:866–880.)

14

Spermatic Cord and Testicular Adnexa

DAVID G. BOSTWICK AND JUN MA

Introduction

The paratesticular region includes the testicular tunics, efferent ductules, epididymis, spermatic cord, and vas deferens. Most studies of paratesticular region pathology include the rete testis despite its intratesticular location.[1] Numerous rare and interesting lesions arise in this region, including cysts, "celes," inflammatory diseases, embryonic remnants, neoplasms, and neoplasm-like proliferations (Table 14.1). In children, one of the common neoplasms is paratesticular rhabdomyosarcoma. In adults the most common pathologic conditions, in order of frequency and excluding "celes," are epididymitis, lipoma of the spermatic cord, adenomatoid tumor of the epididymis, and sarcoma of the spermatic cord.[2]

It is often difficult to diagnose paratesticular masses before or during surgery due to their varied morphologic appearance and rarity. An inguinal surgical approach is usually indicated when there is a suspicion of malignancy. The pathologist should document the anatomic site of origin, histologic classification, and extent of spread of the lesion.

Embryology and Normal Anatomy

The paratesticular region contains numerous anatomically complex epithelial and mesenchymal structures, often within embryonic remnants (Fig. 14.1). The rete testis of the mediastinum of the testis, the first element of the wolffian collecting system, connects the seminiferous tubules and efferent ductules.

The most common abnormalities of the paratesticular region are benign, including hydrocele, lipoma, and inflammatory conditions such as epididymitis, but a variety of cystic and proliferative lesions also occur and are diagnostically challenging.

Embryology

The embryology of the testis and its adnexa is described in Chapter 12; herein is a brief summary of significant events in the development of paratesticular tissues. The testis and head of the epididymis arise from the genital ridge. The wolffian ducts, the male genital ducts, are paired tubes that are associated with the developing gonads and degenerating mesonephric tubules.[3] The body and tail of the epididymis, the vas deferens, and the ejaculatory duct arise from the mesonephric tubules; other degenerating tubules often persist as embryonic remnants including the appendix epididymis, paradidymis, and cranial and caudal aberrant ductules (Fig. 14.1). The paired vasa deferentia connect to the ejaculatory ducts within the prostate that, in turn, have their outlets in the prostatic urethra adjacent to the müllerian tubercle. Blind diverticula of the distal vas deferens form the seminal vesicles. The müllerian duct, or paramesonephros, regresses in men but may persist as embryonic remnants such as the appendix testis and prostatic utricle.

Anatomy

Scrotum and Testicular Tunics

The sac of the scrotum is divided by a partial median septum into two compartments, each of which contains a testis and epididymis and the lower portion of the spermatic cord. The scrotal wall consists of six layers, from the inside outward: the tunica vaginalis, the internal spermatic fascia, the cremasteric muscle, the external spermatic fascia, the dartos muscle, and the skin. The tunica vaginalis is a thin mesothelium-covered layer of the parietal peritoneum that

TABLE 14.1	Paratesticular Tumors and Cysts in the Ccanadian Reference Center for Cancer Pathology, 1949 to 1986

Diagnosis	No. of Cases
Cysts	
Mesothelial cyst	4
Epididymal cyst	1
Benign Neoplasms and Pseudotumors	
Adenomatoid tumor	23
Nodular and diffuse fibrous proliferation	6
Leiomyoma	6
Cystadenoma of epididymis	3
Hamartoma of rete testis	1
Adenomatous hyperplasia of epididymis	1
Adenomatous hyperplasia of rete testis	1
Mixed gonadal stromal tumor	1
Adrenal cortical heterotopia	1
Rhabdomyoma	1
Miscellaneous soft tissue tumors	8
Malignant Neoplasms	
Primary	
Rhabdomyosarcoma	14
Liposarcoma	9
Leiomyosarcoma	7
Malignant mesothelioma	7
Malignant fibrous histiocytoma	3
Malignant mesenchymoma	1
Plasmacytoma	1
Papillary serous cystadenocarcinoma of low malignant potential	1
Sarcoma, not otherwise specified	3
Secondary	
Metastatic carcinoma	4
Metastatic carcinoid tumor	2
Metastatic non-Hodgkin lymphoma	2

From Srigley JR, Hartwick RWH. Tumors and cysts of the paratesticular region. *Pathol Annu* 1990:25(Pt 2):51–108 (review), with permission.

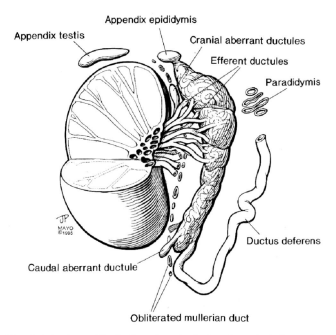

Fig. 14.1 Anatomy of the testis and paratesticular adnexa, including embryonic remnants.

testis, eventually merging into 12 to 20 ducts (the efferent ductules, or ductuli efferentes that perforate the tunica vaginalis and form the head of the epididymis at the upper pole of the testis). After puberty, elastic fibers are present in the muscular coat of the ductules, epididymis, and vas deferens.

Epididymis

The epididymis is a highly convoluted tubule that is attached to the dorsomedial portion of the testis, connecting the efferent ductules of the rete testis with the vas deferens. It is about 6 m long. The head consists of a series of conical masses, the lobules, each of which contain a single duct measuring 15 to 20 cm long; it is lined by tall columnar epithelium and invested with a thick layer of smooth muscle. The body of the epididymis is a single highly convoluted tube that increases in diameter distally to form the tail. The tail distally merges with the vas deferens.

Development of the efferent ducts and ductus epididymis follows a biphasic pattern. Progressive development occurs from the fetal period to infancy between 2 and 4 months of age, but this development is transient and regresses during later infancy. At childhood, definitive development is initiated and finishes at puberty. These changes are probably related to the androgen dependence of the epididymis, the different stages of testicular maturation, and the steroidogenic activity of the Leydig cells.[5] The epididymis plays a critical role in maturation and viability of spermatozoa; SED1 facilitates epididymal cell adhesion, and its loss leads to breakdown of the epididymal epithelium and consequent development of spermatic granulomas.[6]

A variety of morphologic variations occur in the epididymal columnar cells and vas deferens including cribriform hyperplasia (42% of patients), patchy or diffuse eosinophilic granular cell change (Paneth cell–like metaplasia) (8.3%), intranuclear eosinophilic inclusions, nuclear atypia with "monstrous" cells (14%), adenomatous hyperplasia, prostatic-type glands, epithelial luminal pitting, multiple diverticula in the cauda epididymis in the elderly, and accumulation of lipofuscin pigment.[7-18]

also covers the white fibrous tunica albuginea of the testis and epididymis; it is initially in contact with the peritoneal cavity from which it arises but becomes isolated with regression of the processus vaginalis. A common stimulus such as androgens is likely required for obliteration of the processus vaginalis and epididymal development, a hypothesis supported by the common coexistence of epididymal anomalies and patency of the processus vaginalis.[4]

The internal spermatic fascia is a continuation of the transversalis fascia, and the external fascia is a continuation of the external oblique aponeurosis. The cremasteric muscle consists of incomplete slips of muscle, usually in the upper part of the scrotal wall. The dartos muscle consists of smooth muscle embedded in loose areolar tissue. The scrotum is supplied by the external and internal pudendal, cremasteric, and testicular arteries. Lymphatics drain to the superficial inguinal lymph nodes.

Rete Testis

The rete testis is formed by the convergence of the seminiferous tubules (see Chapter 12). The tubules follow a cranial and dorsal course through the fibrous connective tissue of the mediastinum

Vas Deferens (Ductus Deferens) and Spermatic Cord

The vas deferens is about 46 cm long, traversing the spermatic cord and inguinal canal to connect the tail of the epididymis with the ejaculatory ducts. In the spermatic cord, it is invested with a thick, muscular coat that includes the internal spermatic, cremasteric, and external spermatic fasciae; other structures of the spermatic cord include the pampiniform plexus, the testicular artery, lymphatics, and nerves. Upon exiting the spermatic cord, the vas deferens passes extraperitoneally upward, and laterally in the pelvis, then medial to the distal ureter and the posterior wall of the bladder, and terminates at an acute angle in a dilated ampulla that, with the duct of the seminal vesicle, forms the ejaculatory duct. The vas deferens is supplied by its own artery, the artery of the vas deferens, which is usually a branch of the internal iliac or umbilical artery.

The vas deferens is lined by columnar epithelium in low folds, with morphologic variations like those in the epididymis (see earlier). The wall of the vas deferens consists of three layers of smooth muscle: the inner longitudinal, middle circular, and outer longitudinal layers. Elastic fibers appear in the muscular wall after puberty.

Congenital Anomalies

Abnormal development of the paratesticular region may result in a variety of anomalies, including embryonic remnants, agenesis, atresia, ectopia, and cysts. There is an increased frequency of anomalies in boys with cryptorchidism and congenital rubella. Bilateral anomalies result in sterility.

Agenesis and atresia of the testis, epididymis, and vas deferens result from failure of development of the genital ridge, often with anomalies of other wolffian derivatives and renal ectopia, agenesis, or dysplasia. Congenital absence of the vas deferens may be autosomal recessive, partial or complete, unilateral or bilateral, and is often associated with cystic fibrosis (see later). Testicular biopsies in patients with congenital absence of the vas deferens reveal normal spermatogenesis or hypospermatogenesis in up to 45% of cases, and clinical investigation should include semen analysis, renal ultrasound, and genetic cystic fibrosis screening.[19,20] Congenital unilateral absence of the vas deferens is more commonly associated with renal agenesis than bilateral absence (74% versus 12%, respectively).[19]

Duplications may involve any structure of the adnexa, but they are rare. Ectopic insertion of the ureteric bud in the epididymis, vas deferens, or seminal vesicles also may occur. Congenital or developmental cysts of the epididymis are rare and may be associated with intrauterine exposure to diethylstilbestrol.[21] The cysts are usually solitary but may be multiple and bilateral. Ectopic epididymis may be found anterior to the testis, in the retroperitoneum, and within the kidney. Epididymal abnormalities are commonly associated with ectopic or cryptorchid testes (72% of cases), ranging from simple elongation of the epididymis (33%) to more complex changes such as complete disruption (39%).[22]

Splenogonadal Fusion

Splenogonadal fusion is a rare congenital anomaly in which there is fusion of the splenic and gonadal anlage.[23] About 100 cases have been reported, usually on the left side (98%) in men (95%). Patients may present with nontender scrotal mass or intestinal obstruction, but most cases are discovered incidentally at autopsy

or surgery for cryptorchidism or inguinal hernia. About 57% are associated with other congenital anomalies, including peromelia, micrognathia, and cardiac anomalies. Hepatogonadal fusion has also been reported.[24]

There are two types of splenogonadal fusion. The continuous type is characterized by connection of the spleen and the splenogonad by a fibrous cord. The cord usually arises in the upper pole of the spleen and may be retroperitoneal or anterior to the small bowel or colon. Splenic tissue may be present at both ends of the cord or stud the cord throughout its length. The discontinuous type of splenogonadal fusion has no connection between the spleen and splenogonad. The splenic tissue appears within the tunica albuginea or scrotum, or along the vascular pedicle.

Splenogonadal fusion probably results from early fusion of the spleen and gonad during embryonic development, perhaps as the result of inflammation or adhesions. The spleen develops during the fourth and fifth weeks of gestation, and rotates into proximity with the urogenital fold and developing gonadal mesoderm. During the eighth to tenth weeks, the gonads migrate caudally, probably accompanied by a portion of the spleen in cases of splenogonadal fusion. The limb buds and mandible are developing at the same time, accounting for the close association of splenogonadal fusion with peromelia and micrognathia.

Preoperative diagnosis of splenogonadal fusion by splenic scan may avoid unnecessary orchiectomy. Splenogonadal fusion and accessory spleen are important to consider when splenic ablation is needed.

Adrenal Heterotopia and Renal Ectopia

Adrenal cortical tissue may be present anywhere along the route of descent of the testis from the abdomen to the scrotum.[25] It is usually an incidental finding at inguinal herniorrhaphy or epididymoorchiectomy, present in 1% to 3% of children undergoing such operations.[26-28] Adrenal cortical tissue has been identified in inguinal hernia sac, spermatic cord (Fig. 14.2), epididymis, and rete testis.[29] It may present as a palpable tumor, and appears as small, round-to-oval, 1 to 5 mm in diameter, yellow-orange nodules, usually near the inguinal ring. The lesions almost always consist of adrenal cortical tissue resembling zona glomerulosa and fasciculata. Rarely they contain medullary tissue. Involution during childhood is the rule, but exceptional cases persist and become functional, rarely harboring neoplasms or developing into "tumors" in the adrenogenital syndrome and Nelson syndrome; rare cases occur in adults.[29] Removal of functional rests may result

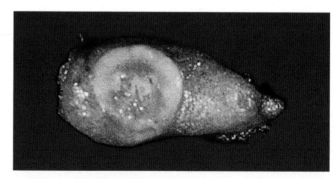

Fig. 14.2 Heterotopic adrenal cortical tissue in the left spermatic cord forming a discrete yellow-orange nodule.

in adrenal insufficiency. Ectopic renal tissue has rarely been observed in the scrotum, consisting of tubules and immature glomeruli.

Wolffian and Müllerian Remnants

Numerous embryonic remnants are found in the paratesticular area, including the appendix testis (hydatid of Morgagni), appendix epididymis, paradidymis, and vasa aberrantia. Precise classification of cystic remnants may be challenging.[30,31]

Appendix Testis (Hydatid of Morgagni)

The appendix testis is attached to the surface of more than 90% of testes at autopsy; ultrasound examination found an incidence rate of 44%.[32] This structure is located at the superior pole of the testis adjacent to the epididymis. Grossly it varies from 2 to 4 mm, appearing as a polypoid or sessile nodular excrescence. Microscopically it consists of a fibrovascular core of loose connective tissue covered by simple cuboidal or low columnar müllerian-type epithelium that is in continuity with the tunica vaginalis at the base. The fibrovascular core may contain tubular inclusions lined by similar cuboidal epithelium. Torsion of the appendix testis may be painful and mimic testicular torsion, and is the most common cause of acute scrotum in children.[33,34]

The severity of the acute inflammatory cell infiltrates is associated with longer duration of symptoms and clinical evidence of torsion of the testicular appendages.[35] No other association was detected between the pattern or degree of acute inflammatory cell infiltrate and any other clinicopathologic variable that may indicate pyogenic infection. No bacteria or fungal elements were identified. Marked lymphatic dilation may be the only histologic finding to indicate the presence of early torsion in cases of scrotal pain secondary to torsion of the appendix testis.

Appendix Epididymis (Vestigial Caudal Mesonephric Collecting Tubule)

The appendix epididymis is present in about 35% of testicles examined at autopsy; ultrasound examination found an incidence rate of 18%.[32] Grossly it is a pedunculated spherical cystic or elongate structure arising from the anterosuperior pole of the head of the epididymis. Microscopically it is lined by cuboidal to low columnar epithelium that may be ciliated and show secretory activity. The wall consists of loose connective tissue and is covered by flattened mesothelial cells that are continuous with the visceral tunica vaginalis. The appendix epididymis may become dilated by serous fluid and, when enlarged, may mimic a tumor. Torsion may occur, sometimes in cryptorchidism.

Paradidymis (Organ of Giraldes)

This wolffian duct embryonic remnant consists of clusters of tubules lined by cuboidal to low columnar epithelium within the connective tissue of the spermatic cord, superior to the head of the epididymis.[36]

Vasa Aberrantia (Organ of Haller)

Vasa aberrantia are wolffian duct remnants that appear as clusters of tubules that are histologically similar to the paradidymis. They arise within the groove between the testis and epididymis. Torsion of the vas aberrans is rare.[37]

Other Lesions Associated With the Epididymis

Other rare epididymal lesions have been described, including epididymal cyst, duplication, and ectopic epididymal tissue associated with inguinal hernia. Cyst and duplication may arise from the caudal vasa aberrantia.

Walthard Rest

The remnant Walthard rest, probably of müllerian origin, consists of solid and cystic nests of uniform epithelial cells with ovoid nuclei and characteristic longitudinal grooves.

Hernia Sac Specimens: Glandular Inclusions Versus Vas Deferens or Epididymis

Herniorrhaphy in children is surgically challenging, particularly in strangulated hernia sac, accounting for the vulnerability of the epididymis and vas deferens that may be inadvertently transected during the procedure. This problem is compounded by the diagnostic difficulty in classifying glandular inclusions in hernia sacs; a challenging problem in young children is separating these structures and embryonic remnants before puberty. Benign glandular inclusions in inguinal herniorrhaphy specimens may represent Müllerian remnants, wolffian remnants, transected vas deferens, or transected epididymis. It is critical to make this distinction due to the potential impact on reproductive function and medicolegal issues.[38-41] Disruption of one vas deferens may generate antisperm antibodies.

Classification of glandular inclusions is often subjective; in one study, interobserver agreement was reported in only 44% to 52% of cases.[39] Epididymis typically has a well-formed concentric muscular coat, whereas embryonic remnants lack a muscular coat but have a mantle of fibrous tissue. Some have advocated the use of Masson trichrome stain and muscle-specific actin to make this distinction, but this has been refuted by others as inconclusive.[39] Comparative analysis reveals that the combination of glandular diameter (with special attention to patient age, recognizing possible changes with advancing development) and histochemical and immunohistochemical stains (trichrome, muscle-specific actin, and CD10) should allow distinction in most cases (Table 14.2). Reliance on light microscopic features alone may be misleading.[38]

Should inguinal hernia repair specimens be routinely submitted for histopathologic examination? One study of 456 specimens from 371 patients younger than 20 years revealed four unexpected cases with epididymal tissue (1%), leading the authors to conclude that pathologic study was an unnecessary expense.[42] In a study of almost 1500 inguinal herniorrhaphies, the authors found vas deferens in 0.13% of cases (Table 14.2).[43] Another report of more than 7000 consecutive pediatric herniorrhaphies found incidence rates of 0.23% vas deferens, 0.3% epididymis, and 0.41% embryonal rests.[39] Inguinal hernia characteristically shows cremasteric muscle fiber hypertrophy that accounts for the palpable thickening of the spermatic cord (see later Hamartoma [Smooth Muscle Hyperplasia] section).[44]

Cystic Fibrosis

Cystic fibrosis is a genetic abnormality that often affects the testicular adnexa, resulting in infertility due to agenesis or atresia of mesonephric structures or anomalies of the testes (see Chapter 12). Patients with congenital bilateral absence of vas

TABLE 14.2 Glandular Inclusions in Herniorrhaphies: Comparative Features

	Incidence in Herniorrhaphies (%)	Mean Diameter (mm)	Immunophenotype
Embryonic remnants	1.5[40] 2.6[282] 2.9[39] 6.0[41]	0.17[40] 0.20[282]	Muscle-specific actin negative; CD10 negative[-38]
Vas deferens	0.16[40] 0.23[39]	0.6[38] 1.2-1.4 (age, 4 months)[40]	Muscle-specific actin positive in wall; CD10 positive[+38]
Epididymis	0.16[40] 0.30[39] 0.88[42]	0.20[282]	Muscle-specific actin positive in wall; CD10 positive[+] in epithelium[38]

deferens often have cystic fibrosis, although this finding may occur in patients without cystic fibrosis.

Nonneoplastic Diseases of the Spermatic Cord and Testicular Adnexa

"Celes" and Cysts

Hydrocele

This mesothelial-lined cyst results from accumulation of serous fluid between the parietal and visceral tunica vaginalis of the testis (Fig. 14.3). There are two variations of spermatic cord hydrocele: the "encysted" variety that does not communicate with the peritoneal cavity, caused by defective closure at both proximal and distal ends of processus vaginalis; and the "funicular" variety that does communicate with the peritoneal cavity, caused by defective closure of only the distal end of tunica vaginalis. The encysted type can be confused with an inguinal mass (lymphadenopathy, hernia) and a primary tumor of the cord.[45,46]

Congenital hydrocele occurs when a patent processus vaginalis within the spermatic cord communicates with the peritoneal cavity. The prevalence of congenital hydrocele is about 6% at birth and 1% in adulthood. Most cases of hydrocele are idiopathic, but they may be associated with inguinal hernia, scrotal trauma, epididymoorchitis, or tumors of the testis or paratesticular region. Possible causes of idiopathic hydrocele include excessive secretion within the testicular tunics by parietal mesothelial cells, decreased reabsorption, and congenital absence of efferent lymphatics.

Hydrocele is lined by a single layer of cuboidal or flattened mesothelial cells, sometimes with prominent atypia, with underlying connective tissue stroma. The luminal fluid is usually clear and serous unless complicated by infection or hemorrhage. The surface is often covered by fibrinous adhesions and inflammation, and subepithelial chronic inflammation and fibrosis may be present. In some cases progressive fibrosis narrows or obliterates the cyst lumen, creating adhesions and multiple cysts. Spermatocele may rupture into the hydrocele sac.

Contralateral hydrocele, commonly seen in cases of neonatal testicular torsion, is of minimal clinical significance and does not warrant formal inguinal exploration for treatment, thereby minimizing the potential of contralateral spermatic cord injury in the neonate.[47]

Hematocele (Hematoma)

Hematocele refers to the accumulation of blood in the space between the parietal and visceral tunica vaginalis, often in association with hydrocele (Fig. 14.3). Long-standing hematocele becomes calcified and fibrotic, with numerous hemosiderin-laden macrophages. The causes of hematocele are like those for hydrocele. Idiopathic hematoma arising in the spermatic cord or epididymis may be mistaken for neoplasm.[48]

Varicocele

Varicocele is a mass of dilated tortuous veins of the internal testicular vein and pampiniform venous plexus of the spermatic cord that occurs posterior and superior to the testis, sometimes extending into the inguinal ring (Fig. 14.3). The venous plexus normally empties into the internal spermatic vein near the internal inguinal ring; poor drainage and progressive dilatation and elongation result from incompetent valves of the left internal spermatic vein that empties into the renal vein. The right internal spermatic vein is less likely to be involved with varicocele because it drains directly into the inferior vena cava and has a lower probability of having incompetent valves.

Varicocele results from many conditions, but most cases are idiopathic. Unilateral varicocele in older men may indicate the presence of a renal tumor that has invaded the renal vein and occluded the spermatic vein drainage. Varicocele is associated with maternal exposure to diethylstilbestrol. Patients with varicocele sometimes present with testicular pain associated with sexual activity. Long-standing varicocele may result in testicular damage in some males, causing testicular atrophy with impaired sperm production and decreased Leydig cell function, whereas in others the varicocele may seemingly cause no ill effects. In adult men, varicocele is frequently present and surgically correctable, yet the measurable benefits of surgical repair are slight.[49] Although occurring more commonly in infertile men than fertile men, only 20% of those with varicocele will suffer from fertility problems. Most varicoceles found in adolescents are detected during routine medical examination, and it is difficult to predict which adolescent presenting with a varicocele will ultimately show diminished testicular function in adolescence or adulthood. As in adults, the mainstay of treatment for varicocele in adolescents is surgical correction. Treatment consists of ligation of the internal spermatic vein at the level of the internal inguinal ring and does not usually yield a pathologic specimen for analysis.

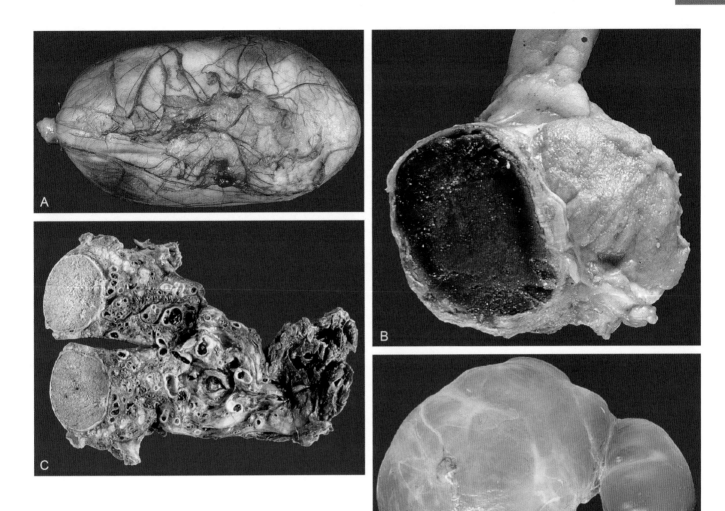

Fig. 14.3 (A) Hydrocele. (B) Encapsulated hematocele. (C) Varicocele. (D) Spermatocele.

Microscopic changes in the pampiniform plexus with varicocele include vascular wall thickening, segmental obliteration, medial hypertrophy of longitudinal smooth muscle fibers, fragmentation of the internal elastic lamina, and occasional occlusive thrombi.[50,51] Compared with control group without varicocele, affected patients have significant thickening of the tunica adventitia and tunica media of the spermatic veins (control versus varicocele: tunica adventitia 0.22 ± 0.10 mm versus 0.35 ± 0.08 mm, respectively; tunica media: 0.09 ± 0.04 mm versus 0.25 ± 0.05 mm, respectively).[52]

Spermatocele (Acquired Epididymal Cyst)

Spermatocele is a dilatation of an efferent ductule in the region of the rete testis or caput epididymis.[53] The inner lining consists of a single layer of cuboidal to flattened epithelial cells that are often ciliated. The wall is composed of fibromuscular soft tissue, often with chronic inflammation, and the cyst may be unilocular or multilocular (Fig. 14.3).[54] Spermatocele is distinguished from hydrocele by the presence of spermatozoa within the cyst fluid (Fig. 14.4), a distinction that can be made by aspiration cytology. Torsion is a rare complication of spermatocele.[55,56]

Benign papilloma may arise within the epithelial lining of spermatocele. The papillae contain fibrovascular cores lined by a single layer of columnar epithelium with vacuolated cytoplasm. The epithelium appears cytologically benign, and there is no evidence of subepithelial invasion.

Mesothelial Cyst

Mesothelial cyst arises within the tunica vaginalis, tunica albuginea, or, less commonly, the epididymis and spermatic cord. The cyst may be single or multiple, measuring up to 2.5 cm in diameter, and lined by a single layer of uniform cuboidal to flattened attenuated mesothelial cells.

Mesothelial cyst of the tunica vaginalis arises from the connective tissue of the tunica. There may be nodular or diffuse proliferation of mesothelial cells, sometimes with squamous metaplasia. This cyst is probably an embryonic remnant or an inclusion of vaginalis mesothelium resulting from inflammation, trauma, or neoplasm, similar to mesothelial cyst of the tunica albuginea.

Mesothelial cyst of the tunica albuginea most often occurs in men older than 40 years, but all ages are affected. It is usually located anterior and lateral to the testis, measuring up to 4 cm in diameter. The cyst is filled with clear or blood-tinged serous fluid, and the lining consists of typical mesothelial cells with a wall composed of hyalinized fibrous tissue. Unilocular and multilocular mesothelial cyst of the spermatic cord is rare and probably arises

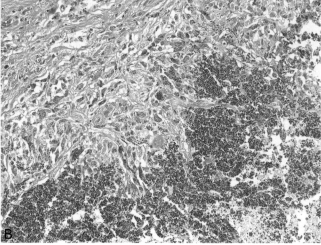

Fig. 14.4 Spermatocele with sperm granuloma. (A) Caput epididymis with dilated efferent ductules filled with abundant spermatozoa. (B) Abundant extravasation of sperm *(lower right)* rimmed by macrophages *(upper left)*.

from embryonic mesothelial remnants such as the processus vaginalis.[57]

Epidermoid Cyst (Epidermal Cyst)

Epidermoid cyst is common in the testis, comprising about 1% of testicular tumors, but may also rarely arise in the paratesticular area and epididymis.[58] Epidermoid cyst consists of a lining of benign keratinizing squamous epithelium and a wall composed of fibrous connective tissue, often with inflammation. Diligent search is required to exclude the presence of adnexal structures or teratomatous elements. Paratesticular epidermoid cyst may arise from squamous metaplasia of wolffian duct structures, displacement of squamous epithelium from the scrotal skin to paratesticular structures during embryogenesis, squamous metaplasia of mesothelial cyst, or monomorphic epidermal development of a teratoma. Epidermoid cyst in the paratesticular area does not recur after surgical excision. Some consider this tumor to be a cholesteatoma when it arises in the epididymis.

Dermoid Cyst (Mature Teratoma)

Dermoid cyst most often involves the testis and paratesticular structures, but may occur in the spermatic cord and, rarely, in the testicular tunics.[59] This cyst measures up to 4 cm in diameter and contains soft, cheesy, yellow-white amorphous material with or without hair and calcifications. The cyst is lined by keratinized squamous epithelium, and the wall contains typical dermal adnexal structures such as pilosebaceous units, although these may be difficult to identify without thorough sectioning. Dermoid cyst does not recur or metastasize after excision.

Simple Cyst and Cystic Dysplasia of the Rete Testis

Simple cyst of the rete testis is rare and is typically unilocular, up to 1 cm in diameter, lined by normal rete testis tubular epithelium, and bulges into the testis proper. When multilocular, it is often associated with epididymal cysts.[60]

Cystic dysplasia of the rete testis is a benign congenital lesion of newborns and young boys that is frequently associated with ipsilateral renal agenesis and dysplasia.[61] It clinically mimics testicular cancer. Long-term follow-up for possible recurrence is recommended.

Cystic transformation of the rete testis and epididymis is common in men undergoing dialysis for chronic renal insufficiency. Histologic changes include columnar transformation of the epithelium, accumulation of calcium oxalate crystals, fibrosis, and giant cell reaction.[62-64] Other causes of cystic transformation include mechanical obstruction of the epididymis by tumor or trauma, ischemia, hormonal alterations such as those in cirrhosis, or cryptorchidism.[65]

Patients with cryptorchidism display changes in the rete testis referred to in one report as dysgenetic rete testis; changes included metaplastic epithelium with columnar or large cuboidal cells, rete testis hypoplasia, combined hypoplasia and cystic dysplasia, or adenomatous hyperplasia.[10,66] These findings may result from a primary abnormality of the rete testis or incomplete pubertal maturation. A rare case was reported of a 35-year-old with a seminal vesicle cyst that extended through the inguinal canal.[67]

Inflammatory and Reactive Diseases

Epididymitis

Epididymitis may be acute or chronic, depending on the inciting agent and the duration of infection.[68] It usually occurs in association with orchitis or after trauma but rarely is an isolated finding. Most cases result from retrograde spread by vesicoepididymal urine reflux, but hematogenous and lymphatic spread account for some. Congenital anomalies such as ureteral ectopia may cause epididymitis in infants. The surgical pathologist rarely receives specimens of these diseases. Urethral and epididymal smears and cultures are useful in identifying the causative infectious agent.

Acute Epididymitis

Patients with acute epididymitis usually present with unilateral painful enlargement of the epididymis, more commonly on the right side, often involving the testicle (50% of cases have epididymoorchitis) and vas deferens (Fig. 14.5). The epididymis is thickened, congested, and edematous, with white fibrinopurulent exudate in the tubules and stroma. Microabscesses and fistulae may occur, but rupture is uncommon. The tubules may be damaged or destroyed by the inflammation, sometimes with squamous metaplasia and regenerative changes.

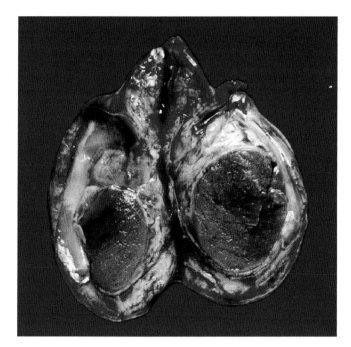

Fig. 14.5 Acute Epididymitis With Associated Testicular Infarction.

TABLE 14.3	Comparison of Bacterial and Chlamydial Epididymitis	
	Bacterial Epididymitis[a]	Chlamydial Epididymitis
Clinical Features		
Patient age (range), y	59.8 (39-79)	42.8 (22-74)
Pain	Yes	Infrequent
Laboratory Features		
Pyuria	Frequent	Infrequent
Elevated erythrocytic sedimentation rate	Yes	No
Elevated C-reactive protein	Yes	No
Pathologic Features		
Tissue destruction	Yes	Minimal
Xanthogranuloma	Yes	Minimal
Abscess and necrosis	Yes	Minimal
Cytoplasmic location of antigens	Histiocytes	Epithelial cells

[a]Usually *Escherichia coli.*

Modified from Hori S, Tsutsumi Y. Histologic differentiation and bacterial epididymitis: nondestructive and proliferative versus destructive and abscess forming—immunohistochemical and clinicopathologic findings. *Hum Pathol* 1995;26:402–407.

Acute epididymitis is commonly caused by bacteria. Coliforms account for most cases in children, whereas *Neisseria gonorrhoeae* and *Chlamydia trachomatis* are most frequent in young men, and *Escherichia coli* and *Pseudomonas* predominate in older men.[69] Other bacteria that may cause acute epididymitis include *Klebsiella, Staphylococcus, Streptococcus pneumoniae, Neisseria meningitidis, Aerobacter aerogenes,* and *Haemophilus influenzae.* The epididymis is a reservoir for *N. gonorrhoeae,* and although infection may be asymptomatic, microabscesses and edema are common, usually without extensive necrosis. The round cytoplasmic inclusions of *C. trachomatis* are difficult to identify in routinely stained sections, and immunohistochemical stains, culture, or genotypic studies are usually required for diagnosis.

Clinical and histopathologic findings allow separation of some cases of chlamydial and bacterial epididymitis (Table 14.3).[70] *C. trachomatis*–positive cases are clinically indolent, with minimally destructive periductal and intraepithelial inflammation and epithelial regeneration.[71] Lymphoepithelial complexes and squamous metaplasia are sometimes present. *E. coli*–positive cases are characterized by scrotal pain, pyuria, leukocytosis, and highly destructive epididymitis with abscesses and xanthogranulomas.

Viral causes of acute epididymitis include mumps and cytomegalovirus, like those causing orchitis (see Chapter 12). Mumps epididymitis, present in 85% of cases of mumps orchitis, occurs before testicular involvement, usually appearing as unilateral scrotal swelling after parotiditis. The epididymis shows vascular congestion, edema, and interstitial lymphocytic inflammation; neutrophils are usually not a prominent feature. Cytomegaloviral epididymitis may occur in patients with AIDS or those receiving immunosuppression for transplantation.[72,73]

In endemic areas such as India, parasitic infection by *Wuchereria bancrofti* preferentially involves intrascrotal juxtatesticular lymphatic vessels, with nests of microfilaria with a mean diameter of 0.3 cm^2 observable by ultrasonography.[74,75] These infections form epididymal and spermatic cord nodules that contain larvae (microfilariae), eggs, and adult worms, visible in cytologic smears. Early diagnosis and treatment prevents the more severe manifestation of the disease, lymphatic filariasis. Traumatic acute epididymitis is characterized by vascular congestion, petechial hemorrhages, and hematocele. Drugs such as amiodarone may also cause epididymitis.[76]

Chronic Epididymitis

Although many cases of acute epididymitis resolve, some become chronic. The epididymis in chronic epididymitis is indurated and scarred, with cystically dilated tubules, marked fibrosis, chronic inflammation, and sperm granulomas; similar changes may account for the "late vasectomy syndrome" in which patients report pain many months or years after vasectomy.[77] The epithelium shows reactive or metaplastic changes, often with cytoplasmic vacuolization and lumenal hyaline aggregates. Epididymitis nodosa, a proliferative lesion of the epididymis, may result from chronic inflammation or trauma, reminiscent of vasitis nodosa.[78] Coarse granular cytoplasmic changes appear in the epididymis in the setting of ductal obstruction. Calcification is common in chronic epididymitis, and there may be a foreign body giant cell reaction. Xanthogranulomatous epididymitis may also occur. Special stains for bacteria and fungi may be of value.

Specific causes of chronic epididymitis include tuberculosis, leprosy, malakoplakia, sarcoidosis, and sperm granuloma. The epididymis is the reservoir for tuberculous involvement in the male genital tract, with secondary testicular involvement and other local sites of involvement in about 80% of cases; 40% of cases of renal tuberculosis are accompanied by epididymal infection. Patients usually present with painless scrotal swelling, but other signs and symptoms include unilateral or bilateral mass, infertility, and scrotal fistula.[79,80] Caseating granulomatous inflammation is prominent, with fibrous thickening and enlargement of the epididymis and adjacent structures (Fig. 14.6). Rarely miliary tuberculosis causes small punctate white lesions. One case of bilateral tuberculous epididymoorchitis followed intravesical bacillus Calmette–Guérin therapy for urothelial carcinoma of the

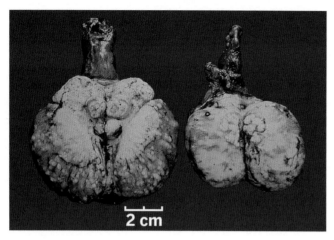

Fig. 14.6 Tuberculosis of the Epididymis and Testis.

bladder.[81] The auramine-rhodamine stain is preferred over the Ziehl–Neelsen stain because of its greater sensitivity (60% positive in aspiration smears).[82] Fine needle aspiration cytology was diagnostic in 67% of patients with tubercular epididymitis or epididymoorchitis, with epithelioid cell granulomas with caseation.[82]

Lepromatous leprosy frequently involves the epididymis, usually after testicular involvement, but rarely spreads to the vas deferens. Patients report painful scrotal swelling, and the epididymis and testis are thickened and enlarged. The inflammation consists chiefly of perivascular and perineural lymphocytic infiltrates, often with sheets of macrophages that contain acid-fast bacilli set in a dense sclerotic stroma. Sterility results from testicular azoospermia rather than epididymal blockage. The dartos muscle of the testicular tunics shows a predilection for lepromatous myositis.

Malakoplakia of the epididymis is uncommon, usually occurring with testicular involvement.[83] Patients are asymptomatic or present with painful scrotal swelling or hydrocele. The histologic findings are similar to malakoplakia at other sites.

Sarcoidosis involves the genital tract in about 5% of cases at autopsy but is rarely symptomatic. The epididymis is the most common site of genital involvement.[84-86] Patients present with painful or painless scrotal swelling that is bilateral in about 33% of cases. Nonnecrotizing granulomatous inflammation is typical, similar to involvement at other sites. The main differential diagnostic consideration is sperm granuloma, but extravasated sperm are absent in sarcoidosis.

Epididymitis may also result from other fungi,[12] bacteria, parasites, and viruses. *Candida albicans* epididymoorchitis with candiduria is rare, usually after instrumentation of the urinary tract.[87] *Histoplasma capsulatum* creates necrotizing inflammation and abscesses that mimic sperm granuloma; typical silver-stained 2- to 4-μm fungal spores are usually present.[88] *Coccidioides immitis* produces necrotizing and nonnecrotizing granulomas of the epididymis and prostate; silver-stained fungal spherules measuring about 100 μm in diameter contain numerous endospores. Systemic *Blastomyces dermatitidis* involves the epididymis in up to 30% of systemic cases, producing microabscesses that contain silver-stained budding fungal spores up to 15 μm in diameter with thick refractile capsules.[89] Other causes of epididymitis include *Paracoccidioides brasiliensis*, *Actinomyces*, *Sporothrix schenckii*, *Schistosoma haematobium*, *Treponema pallidum*, typhoid, brucellosis, rickettsia, and hydatid cyst. The degenerating worms of *W. bancrofti* filariasis produce granulomas, often with prominent tissue and blood

eosinophilia; scrotal and penile elephantiasis results from lymphatic obstruction.[90] Human papillomavirus was identified by polymerase chain reaction in dysplastic squamous metaplastic epithelium of the epididymis in a 39-year-old man.[91] Young syndrome is characterized by the association of sinobronchial disease and azoospermia resulting from bilateral epididymitis-associated obstruction in the distal ductuli efferentes.[92,93]

Idiopathic granulomatous epididymitis is a rare but significant finding at autopsy or during surgery (less than 1% incidence rate), arising in the caput epididymis.[94] This lesion contains zonal necrosis of efferent ducts with epithelial damage and regeneration. Macrophages are plentiful, as are cholesterol crystals, foreign body–type giant cells, and spermatozoa.

Sperm Granuloma

Sperm granuloma is an exuberant foreign body giant cell reaction to extravasated sperm and occurs in up to 42% of patients after vasectomy and 2.5% of routine autopsies.[95] Patients may have no symptoms but often present with a history of pain and swelling of the upper pole of the epididymis, spermatic cord, and, rarely, testis. Others have a history of trauma, epididymitis, and orchitis. In some cases sperm granuloma mimics testicular or spermatic cord tumor.

Sperm granuloma appears as a solitary yellow nodule or multiple small indurated nodules measuring up to 3 cm in diameter. Foreign body–type granulomas are present, with necrosis in the early stages and progressive fibrosis in late stages (Fig. 14.4). Extravasated sperm are often present in large numbers, but are quickly engulfed by macrophages (referred to as *spermiophages*) and eventually disappear. Yellow-brown ceroid pigment, a lipid degradation product of sperm, may persist. Vasitis nodosa occurs in about one-third of cases of sperm granuloma.

Disruption of the tubules and extravasation of sperm results in sperm granuloma, but isolated sperm may be present in the interstitium without significant inflammation. Ligation vasectomy accounts for most cases of sperm granuloma, whereas cauterization vasectomy rarely results in granuloma. Secondary oxalosis with crystal deposition from chronic renal failure may be accompanied by sperm granuloma.[63] Experimental injection of ceroid pigment produces granulomatous inflammation, suggesting that destruction of sperm initiates the process. An autoimmune process has been proposed but is not favored.

Vasitis and Vasitis Nodosa

Inflammation of the vas deferens (vasitis, or deferentitis) usually occurs in association with epididymitis or posterior urethritis.[96] Vasitis nodosa is a benign ductular proliferation that produces nodular and fusiform enlargement of the vas deferens, often after vasectomy. It resembles salpingitis isthmica nodosa and clinically mimics sperm granuloma.

In vasitis nodosa the vas deferens may be more than 1 cm in diameter, with diffuse enlargement or rounded indurated masses punctuated by small lumens. The ductular proliferation is prominent and may be mistaken for metastatic prostatic adenocarcinoma. Chronic inflammation and fibrosis are always observed, although in variable amounts, and are sometimes accompanied by muscular hyperplasia of the wall. The ductules vary from discrete, round, acinar structures to plexiform masses of irregular acini. The cells are cuboidal or low columnar, with a moderate amount of pale granular cytoplasm, central large nuclei with uniform chromatin, and single enlarged nucleoli. Cilia may be present. Perineural invasion is common and often extensive, and may be mistaken for malignancy; benign vascular invasion may also occur. Sperm granulomas are present in about 50% of cases, and sperm are often present in the acinar lumens of vasitis nodosa. As the number of sperm granulomas declines, the amount of ceroid pigment increases, resulting from lipid breakdown products of spermatozoa. A histologically similar process may occur in the epididymis (epididymitis nodosa).

Vasitis nodosa is a benign reactive process. Trauma or surgery results in epithelial rupture with release of sperm into the soft tissues of the vas deferens, invariably invoking a prominent fibroinflammatory response. However, some cases have no history of trauma and are idiopathic.

Funiculitis (Inflammation of the Spermatic Cord)

Inflammation of the spermatic cord, or funiculitis, often accompanies vasitis, usually as the result of direct extension from the vas deferens, but isolated involvement may occur by hematogenous spread from other sites of inflammation.[97,98] Funiculitis appears as painful enlargement of the spermatic cord. Tuberculous funiculitis is rare, presenting as multiple large, discrete masses or diffuse thickening with typical necrotizing granulomatous inflammation.[99] Perforation of an incarcerated hernia may cause extravasation of fecal contents and vegetable fibers, resulting in an exuberant foreign body giant cell reaction in the cord. Sclerosing endophlebitis and thrombosis of the pampiniform plexus may accompany funiculitis, resulting in necrosis and gangrene. Recent reports described diabetes-associated, *Actinomyces*-infected xanthogranulomatous funiculitis and *Dirofilaria repens*–induced chronic funiculitis and epididymitis.[69,100] *S. haematobium*–induced funiculitis can be diagnosed by semen analysis in infected men.[101] An unusual incidental finding during hernia repair in a 70-year-old was incarcerated colonic diverticulum with fecalith that was "parasitized" onto the spermatic cord.[102]

Meconium-Induced Inflammation

Prenatal or antenatal perforation of the colon may cause meconium leakage through the patent processus vaginalis into the scrotum, resulting in foreign body giant cell reaction, chronic inflammation, and scarring; this is referred to as meconium periorchitis, meconium granuloma, or meconium vaginalitis.[103] Fewer than 30 cases have been reported, rarely in association with cystic fibrosis. Grossly the tunica vaginalis contains a single mass or is studded with numerous orange or green nodules composed of chronically inflamed myxoid stroma, sometimes containing bile, cholesterol, or lanugo hairs within histiocytes. Hydrocele is often present.

Vasculitis

Vasculitis may be part of systemic vasculitis or may exist as single-organ/isolated vasculitis; the distinction is important because in other forms of single-organ vasculitis, surgical therapy alone may be curative. Isolated epididymal or spermatic cord vasculitis is rare and usually occurs in men presenting with a mass in the absence of systemic symptoms and normal laboratory results.[104,105] In most patients with isolated vasculitis, neoplasm is initially suspected, and vasculitis is an unexpected finding. After surgical removal, isolated vasculitis does not require systemic therapy.

Systemic vasculitides may affect the epididymal and testicular vessels, sometimes resulting in hydrocele or swelling of the affected structures.[106] Polyarteritis nodosa is observed in these vessels at autopsy in 80% of affected patients, although clinical involvement is rare.[107,108] There are no histopathologic differences between systemic vasculitis and most forms of isolated necrotizing vasculitis of testicular and epididymal tissue.[105]

Other Nonneoplastic Diseases

Torsion of the Spermatic Cord and Embryonic Remnants

Torsion of the spermatic cord results in hemorrhagic infarction of the testis (see Chapter 12), as well as thrombosed veins surrounded by fat necrosis with cystic cavities bounded by wavy hyaline membranes.[109-111] Torsion of embryonic remnants is a much rarer event that may clinically mimic torsion of the cord. Torsion of a hernia sac is rare, presenting as acute scrotum in children.[112]

Torsion is a common abnormality of the appendix testis. Patients report acute scrotal pain, often after vigorous exercise. About 90% of patients are boys between 10 and 12 years of age, accounting for the most common cause of acute scrotum in children, but men of all ages are affected. Typical histologic features of torsion are present, including severe congestion, edema, and hemorrhagic infarction. Severe acute inflammation is associated with longer duration of symptoms.[35] Bilateral involvement is rare.[113]

Torsion of the appendix epididymis is much less common than of the appendix testis, and the histologic findings are similar. Torsion of the vasa aberrantia is rare, with fewer than 10 reported cases.

Calculi and Calcification

Acute and chronic epididymitis and vasitis predispose to calculus formation usually in the epididymis, vas deferens, and scrotum (Fig. 14.7). The calculi are brown and composed of phosphates and carbonates, measuring up to 1 cm in diameter. Their occurrence in varicocele veins has been referred to as "varicolithiasis."[114]

Idiopathic mural calcification of the vas deferens occurs in up to 15% of males with diabetes. These deposits in the smooth muscle are focal and variable in appearance, rarely with osseous metaplasia. Inflammation-induced calcifications are scattered throughout the smooth muscle, usually associated with chronic inflammation and fibrosis.

Myositis ossificans has also been reported forming a spermatic cord tumor, as has heterotopic ossification.[115,116] Osseous metaplasia of the epididymis occurs sporadically of in association with fibrous pseudotumor, sometimes forming a mass that may be mistaken for a neoplasm. Microscopically it consists of trabecular bone set in connective tissue stroma.

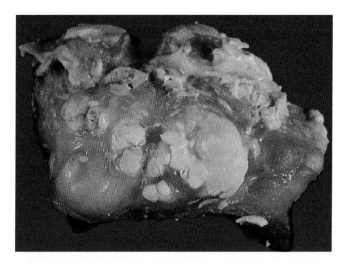

Fig. 14.7 Idiopathic scrotal and epididymal calcinosis in an otherwise healthy 37-year-old man forming a multinodular mass measuring 3 cm in greatest dimension.

Neoplasms

Benign Neoplasms and Pseudotumors

A variety of unusual tumors and tumor-like proliferations arise in the paratesticular region, often of uncertain histogenesis. Because of the rarity of many of these benign tumors, they may be erroneously considered malignant.

Lipoma

Lipoma is the most common paratesticular tumor, accounting for up to 90% of spermatic cord tumors (Fig. 14.8).[117] Lipoma usually occurs in adults, but may be seen at all ages. Grossly it is a circumscribed, unencapsulated mass of lobulated yellow adipose tissue, measuring up to 30 cm in diameter and weighing as much as 3.2 kg.[118] The microscopic appearance is similar to lipoma at other sites, consisting of mature adipose tissue. Variants include angiolipoma, hibernoma, fibrolipoma, fibromyxolipoma, myxolipoma, and myxoid myolipoma (Fig. 14.9).

Lipoma was identified in 23% of hernia repairs; of these, 51% were associated with indirect hernia, 17% with direct hernia, 1% with pantaloon and femoral hernia, and 31% without hernia.[119] Autopsy study with careful inguinal dissection revealed 75% with discrete masses of adipose tissue within the inguinal canal, and the majority of lipomas measured more than 4 cm in length with pedunculation and a bulbous distal tip.[120]

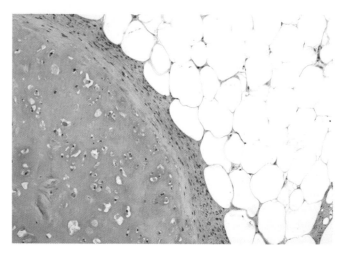

Fig. 14.9 Chondrolipoma of the paratestis arising in a 53-year-old. The mass was 3 cm in diameter, circumscribed, and composed chiefly of mature fat and cartilage with scant fibrous connective tissue.

Adenomatous Hyperplasia

Adenomatous hyperplasia of the rete testis and epididymis consists of a poorly circumscribed tubular or tubulopapillary proliferation of uniform benign cuboidal to low columnar epithelial cells with back-to-back crowding; there is no stromal invasion or other features of malignancy. This lesion is a frequent finding in the undescended testis and is considered benign.[121]

Adenomatoid Tumor (Benign Nonpapillary Mesothelioma)

Adenomatoid tumor is the most common tumor of the epididymis and cord, and second in frequency only to lipoma in the paratesticular area; it accounts for about one-third of nonlipoma paratesticular tumors.[122,123] It also arises in the tunica vaginalis or tunica albuginea, and may be present in association with hydrocele.

Adenomatoid tumor is usually seen in men between 20 and 50 years of age, but has been reported in those as old as 79 years; rare cases occur in childhood.[124] Patients often present with a painless scrotal mass, but some lesions are found incidentally at epididymoorchiectomy or autopsy. Adenomatoid tumor consists of a firm, circumscribed, solid mass, measuring up to 2 cm in greatest dimension, and usually arising in the head of the epididymis or rarely in the lower pole of the epididymis, testicular tunics, or spermatic cord. The cut surface is homogeneous and white-gray. The characteristic microscopic findings are irregular tubules, cell nests, and solid trabeculae of cuboidal to flattened epithelioid or endothelioid cells (Fig. 14.10).[125] The tumor cells are eosinophilic, with variably sized cytoplasmic vacuoles. In some cases excessive vacuolization creates thin strands of cytoplasm spanning lumina; alternatively, it creates a signet ring cell pattern. Nuclei are small and vesicular with inconspicuous nucleoli. The stroma contains fibroblasts, blood vessels, and smooth muscle. Focal stromal hyalinization may be present, and the tumor may infiltrate the testis. Adenomatoid leiomyoma consists of adenomatoid tumor in association with prominent smooth muscle.

Tumor cell cytoplasm contains hyaluronidase-sensitive acid mucopolysaccharides, similar to mesothelioma. Immunohistochemistry reveals cytoplasmic staining for cytokeratin in most cases, focal luminal surface staining for epithelial membrane antigen in some cases, and negative staining for carcinoembryonic antigen, vimentin, factor VIII–related antigen, and *Ulex europaeus*

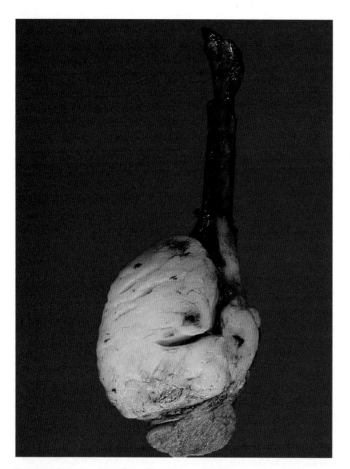

Fig. 14.8 Lipoma of the Cord Dwarfing the Testis.

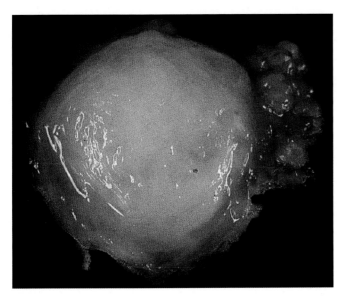

Fig. 14.10 Adenomatoid Tumor of the Epididymis. (A) Grossly the tumor was a firm white-gray mass. (B) Anastomosing tubules lined by cells with small nuclei and punctuated by thin-walled vessels.

agglutinin 1, although focal staining for factor VIII has been occasionally reported. Proliferative activity by MIB1 staining is less than 1%, and the tumor is diploid.[126] Ultrastructural studies reveal mesothelial differentiation including slender microvilli, intermediate filaments adjacent to the nuclei, intracellular canaliculi, desmosomes, basal lamina, and transition forms with features of both typical mesothelial cells and stromal spindle cells. Mesothelial origin is likely for adenomatoid tumor because of the anatomic continuity between the surface mesothelium of the tunica vaginalis and tumor cells in some cases, as well as identification of rare cases of adenomatoid tumor in the retroperitoneum. The mesothelial theory of histogenesis has displaced earlier theories, including endothelial origin, mesonephric origin, and müllerian origin.

Despite the potential for local invasion, adenomatoid tumor is benign, with no metastatic potential. Intraoperative frozen section diagnosis allows local resection with preservation of the epididymis and testis. This tumor may recur if incompletely excised but does not recur after complete excision.

Hamartoma (Smooth Muscle Hyperplasia)

Separation of smooth muscle hamartoma (tumor-like overgrowth of normal tissue) and hyperplasia may be difficult and perhaps arbitrary, according to a study of 16 cases in which there was predominantly concentric periductal, perivascular, or interstitial proliferation of muscle fascicles.[127] Hamartoma of the spermatic cord may be composed chiefly of smooth muscle or fibrous connective tissue. One case of hamartoma of the rete testis arose as a testicular mass in a 2-year-old. The tumor consisted of a disorganized cluster of tubules embedded in a loose connective tissue stroma. The tubules were lined by cells that were cytologically similar to normal rete testis. Another case of smooth muscle hyperplasia of the rete testis arose in association with multilocular cyst and myxoid stroma with scattered Leydig cells mimicking Leydig cell tumor.[128]

Reactive Mesothelial Hyperplasia

Reactive mesothelial hyperplasia appears as a small solid nodule of mesothelial cells that is usually microscopic and clinically asymptomatic. It probably arises as a result of mechanical irritation or inflammation. Reactive mesothelial hyperplasia has also been described in association with hydrocele, hematocele, inguinal hernia sac, and fibrous pseudotumor. Reactive hyperplasia consists of solid nests, tubules, simple papillae, or small cysts of cytologically benign mesothelium set in a fibrous stroma, often appearing beneath the surface mesothelium. Mild cytologic atypia may be present, and squamous metaplasia is rarely seen. Histologic mimics include benign papillary mesothelioma, malignant mesothelioma, and metastatic adenocarcinoma. Benign papillary mesothelioma has more complex papillary architecture. Malignant mesothelioma is also architecturally complex, often with nuclear atypia, increased mitotic activity, and stromal infiltration. Metastatic adenocarcinoma usually shows severe nuclear abnormalities that stand in contrast with the adjacent surface mesothelium; stains for neutral or hyaluronidase-resistant mucin may also be of value, with negative staining suggesting adenocarcinoma rather than mesothelioma.

Benign Papillary Mesothelioma

Benign papillary mesothelioma is a rare tumor of the tunica vaginalis that usually appears in young men.[129,130] Grossly it consists of a hydrocele sac with papillary or adenomatous excrescences and cystic or solid areas. Microscopically there are complex papillae covered by cuboidal, columnar, or flattened mesothelial cells with large vesicular nuclei and glassy eosinophilic cytoplasm (Fig. 14.11). There is no significant nuclear atypia. Psammoma bodies are often present. Careful search should be made to determine whether the papillary lining of the tumor is in continuity with the mesothelium of the adjacent tunica vaginalis. The tumor contains hyaluronidase-sensitive mucin, and ultrastructural study reveals mesothelial differentiation. Multicystic mesothelioma rarely arises in the spermatic cord.[131]

Papillary Cystadenoma of the Epididymis

Papillary cystadenoma of the epididymis is a benign tumor that accounts for about one-third of all primary epididymal tumors; one case was located in the spermatic cord.[132] It occurs in men between 16 and 81 years of age (mean, 36 years). More than 50 cases have been reported.[133] About two-thirds of cases of papillary cystadenoma of the epididymis occurs in patients with von Hippel-Lindau syndrome, and are more frequently bilateral in this syndrome.[134] Other manifestations of von Hippel-Lindau syndrome include hemangioblastoma of the cerebellum, cerebrum, spinal cord, retina, pancreas, and urinary bladder; meningioma; syringomyelia; paraganglioma; renal cell carcinoma; pheochromocytoma; islet cell tumor; adrenal cortical adenoma; and a variety of cysts of the liver, kidney, adrenal, and pancreas. Somatic von Hippel–Lindau mutations are present in some, but not all, cases.[135]

About 40% of cases of papillary cystadenoma of the epididymis are bilateral, and these appear as cystic masses in the head of the epididymis that measure up to 6 cm in diameter. The cut surface is gray-brown with yellow foci, and the tumor often contains cyst fluid that varies from clear and colorless to yellow, green, or blood-tinged (Fig. 14.11).

Microscopically, papillary cystadenoma consists of dilated ducts lined by papillae with a single or double layer of cuboidal to low columnar epithelium (Fig. 14.11).[136] The cells have characteristic clear glycogen-filled cytoplasm with secretory droplets and cilia at the surface. The papillary cores and cyst walls consist of fibrous connective tissue that may be hyalinized or inflamed. This appearance may be mistaken for metastatic renal cell carcinoma.[135]

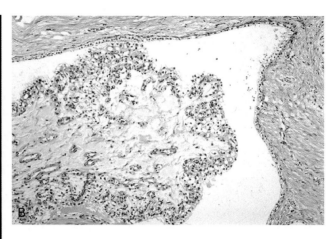

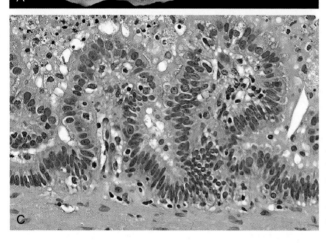

Fig. 14.11 Papillary Cystadenoma of the Epididymis. (A) Grossly the tumor consisted of a papillary mass. (B) Cystic space containing well-formed papillae. This 35-year-old man had a history of von Hippel-Lindau syndrome, including bilateral renal cell carcinoma and cerebellar and retinal hemangioblastomas. (C) Another case of papillary cystadenoma from a patient without a history of von Hippel-Lindau syndrome. *(A and B, courtesy Dr. Bernd Scheithauer, Rochester, Minnesota.)*

The cells stain with soybean agglutinin lectin and are immunoreactive for low- and intermediate-weight cytokeratins CAM5.2 and AE1/AE3, epithelial membrane antigen, α_1-antitrypsin, α_1-antichymotrypsin, and vimentin.[135,137]

Rare cases of mucinous subtype of papillary cystadenoma have been reported, including one case with intestinal-type goblet cells.[138] There was no significant cytologic atypia, and the neoplastic cells displayed immunoreactivity for carcinoembryonic antigen, cytokeratin 20, CDX2, epithelial membrane antigen, and CD15; they were negative for PAX8 and Wilms tumor 1 protein.[138]

Fibrous Pseudotumor (Nodular and Diffuse Fibrous Proliferation)

Fibrous pseudotumor encompasses a wide variety of fibroproliferative lesions of the testicular tunics, epididymis, and spermatic cord.[139-141] This lesion has been referred to as chronic periorchitis, proliferative funiculitis, fibrous proliferation of the tunics, fibroma, nonspecific paratesticular fibrosis, nodular fibrous periorchitis, nodular fibropseudotumor, inflammatory pseudotumor, reactive periorchitis, and pseudofibromatous periorchitis.[142,143] Early cases of spermatic cord and epididymal fibroma were probably fibrous pseudotumors. This nonneoplastic fibroinflammatory reactive lesion clinically mimics testicular and paratesticular neoplasm, especially when it encases the testis and manifests grossly as indurated testis. Patients are typically in the third decade of life, but age ranges from 7 to 95 years. It usually involves the tunics and may be associated with hydrocele, hematocele, or both. Less commonly the epididymis or spermatic cord are involved. A history of epididymoorchitis, trauma, or inflamed hydrocele is often elicited.[144]

Fibrous pseudotumor is a nodular or diffuse thickening of firm white tissue, measuring up to 9.5 cm in diameter, often with focal yellow calcifications (Fig. 14.12). Histologically it consists of granulation tissue with chronic inflammation, but long-standing tumors contain only paucicellular hyalinized fibrous connective tissue with calcification and ossification. Sclerosing lipogranuloma-like changes may be present.

The condition is considered reactive. Resection of the tumor, perhaps with the tunica vaginalis, is curative, but it is frequently difficult

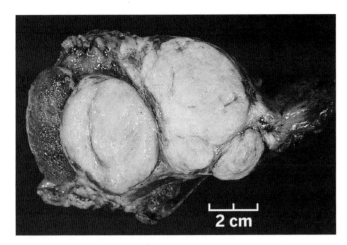

Fig. 14.12 Fibrous Pseudotumor of the Testicular Tunics.

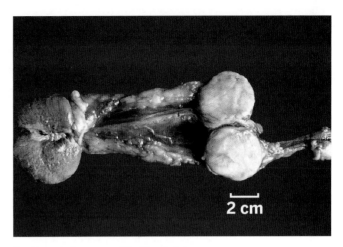

Fig. 14.13 Leiomyoma of the Vas Deferens.

to confirm the benign nature of the process preoperatively, and orchiectomy is often used.[144] One case was associated with lipoma and diffuse mast cell infiltration of unknown significance.[145]

Based on similarities to other fibroinflammatory disorders characterized by infiltrates of IgG4-expressing plasma cells and included under the heading of IgG4-mediated diseases, Bosmuller and colleagues investigated the plasma cell distribution and immunoglobulin isotypes in paratesticular fibrous pseudotumor.[146] They found that all three of their cases contained a high number of IgG4-positive plasma cells, with an IgG4/IgG ratio of 44% to 48%, suggesting that paratesticular fibrous pseudotumor belongs to the growing list of IgG4-related diseases, including retroperitoneal fibrosis, sclerosing pancreatitis and cholangitis, Riedel thyroiditis, and sclerosing sialadenitis. The differential diagnosis includes solitary fibrous tumor, idiopathic fibromatosis, neurofibroma, and leiomyoma.

Leiomyoma

Reports of the relative frequency of leiomyoma to adenomatoid tumor of the epididymis vary from 1:1 to 1:9.[147,148] Men with genital leiomyoma range in age from 25 to 81 years (mean, 48 years).[149] Hydroceles or hernia sacs are identified in up to 21% of cases, and up to 39% of cases of leiomyoma are bilateral.[150,151] Leiomyoma appears as a round, firm, gray-white mass, measuring up to 8 cm in diameter; the cut surface is homogeneous and whorled and bulges from the adjacent soft tissues (Fig. 14.13). It has typical microscopic features of leiomyoma, including interlacing fascicles of spindled smooth muscle cells with few or no mitotic figures. Tumor cells are immunoreactive for vimentin, desmin, and smooth muscle actin.[152] Rare cases of leiomyoma with bizarre nuclei have been described.[153] Angioleiomyoma has also been reported.[154] Spermatic cord leiomyoma may clinically mimic irreducible inguinal hernia without scrotal involvement.[155] Surgical excision of epididymal leiomyoma is curative.

Differential diagnostic considerations include smooth muscle hyperplasia, low-grade leiomyosarcoma, and solitary fibrous tumor. The number of mitotic figures is the most reliable criterion for making this separation, but quantitative reporting in smooth muscle tumor of the epididymis and spermatic cord has not been validated. Leiomyoma is less common in the spermatic cord than the epididymis, with fewer than 20 reported cases. Patient age is similar.

Melanotic Neuroectodermal Tumor of Infancy (Progonoma; Retinal Anlage Tumor)

Rare cases of melanotic neuroectodermal tumor of infancy have arisen in the head of the epididymis and paratestis.[156-159] Patients range in age from newborn to 24 months (mean, ∼7 months). The tumor is a solitary, circumscribed, solid blue-brown or black mass, measuring up to 3 cm in diameter. Microscopically it consists of cells with uniform round nuclei and abundant melanin granules lining small cystic spaces of variable size. Smaller round cells with hyperchromatic nuclei, prominent nucleoli, and minimal cytoplasm are observed within lumen spaces and the stroma. Tumor cells resemble neuroblasts and may form glomeruloid bodies, sometimes surrounded by a fibrous matrix set in a collagenous stroma.

Melanotic neuroectodermal tumor of infancy may replace the epididymis, but there are no reports of testicular or spermatic cord invasion. No recurrences of metastases have been identified at this site, but the number of cases is small, and the length of follow-up is limited; some speculate that this tumor has the potential for local recurrence and lymph node involvement.

Brenner Tumor

Brenner tumor of the testicular tunics is rare, occurring in men between 37 and 61 years of age. The tumors are small, usually less than 3 cm in diameter, and appear as solid masses with smooth external surfaces and typical histologic features of Brenner tumors elsewhere. Brenner tumor may share a common histogenesis with adenomatoid tumor or Walthard cell rest.

Gonadal Stromal Tumor

Gonadal stromal tumor accounts for up to 3% of testicular tumors, and rare extratesticular examples have been reported. Embryogenesis of the testis can account for extratesticular nests of germ cells and stromal cells. Microscopic foci of gonadal interstitial cells are occasionally observed in extratesticular sites such as the spermatic cord and epididymis in orchiectomy specimens removed for other reasons, and these may account for gonadal stromal tumor at such sites.

Other Benign Tumors

Other rare benign paratesticular tumors and tumor-like conditions include mucinous adenoid tumor, pleomorphic adenoma, desmoid, neurofibroma, pheochromocytoma/paraganglioma, blue nevus, and hemangioma of the testicular tunics.[160-168] Lymphangiectasia,

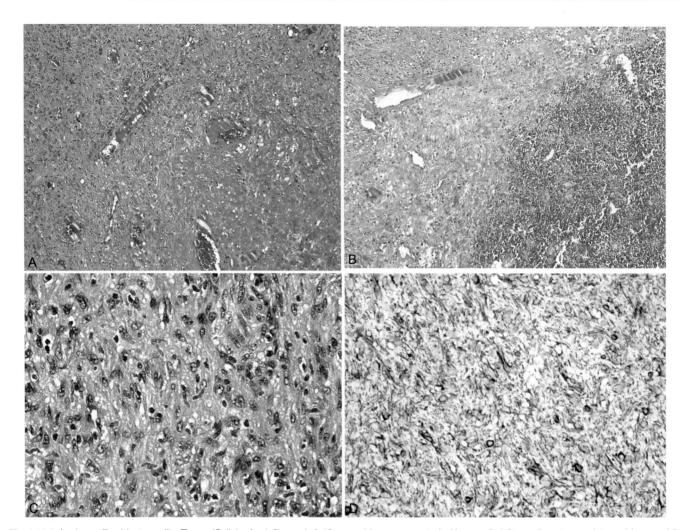

Fig. 14.14 Angiomyofibroblastoma-like Tumor (Cellular Angiofibroma). A 48-year-old man presented with a small, 1.2-cm-diameter, oval, tan rubbery mobile mass near the left epididymis. The tumor is a variably cellular proliferation of tapered uniform spindled cells containing numerous small- to medium-sized irregularly ectatic vessels, patchy red cell extravasation, and fine collagenous stroma (A to C). Scattered epithelioid-appearing stromal cells are seen, but no necrosis or mitotic activity is observed. (D) Tumor cells exhibit immunoreactivity for vimentin, muscle-specific actin (shown), and smooth muscle actin; negative immunostains include progesterone receptors, estrogen receptors, CD34, desmin, and S100 protein.

arteriovenous malformation, lymphangioma, hemangioma, angiomyolipoma, angiomyofibroblastoma, angiomyofibroblastoma-like tumor (cellular angiofibroma) (Fig. 14.14), and neurofibroma may arise in the spermatic cord or epididymis.[169-177] There have been rare case reports of granular cell tumor, paratesticular myxoma, carcinoid, solitary fibrous tumor, extratesticular Leydig cell tumor, and rhabdomyoma of the spermatic cord and epididymis.[178-187] Aggressive angiomyxoma of the spermatic cord was reported in two 13-year-old boys, appearing as a benign myxoid tumor immunoreactive for vimentin and smooth muscle actin.[188-190] Another case arose in an 82-year-old that was also positive for vimentin but negative for actin, desmin, and CD34.[191] Four cases of aggressive angiomyxoma contained estrogen and progesterone immunoreactivity in the majority, similar to cases in women.[192] Fibrous hamartoma of infancy occasionally arises in the scrotum or spermatic cord, and usually requires surgical excision for diagnosis.[193]

Malignant Neoplasms

Spermatic cord sarcoma accounts for 2% of all urologic tumors; it is usually treated initially with surgery and has a poor prognosis.[194]

The most common histologic types are liposarcoma (46%), leiomyosarcoma (20%), malignant fibrous histiocytoma (13%), and rhabdomyosarcoma (9%). The median age of diagnosis for rhabdomyosarcomas was 26.3 years, whereas for others it was 64.7 years.[195] According to Rodriguez et al., worse outcome was observed with undifferentiated tumor grade, distant disease, positive lymph nodes, and leiomyosarcoma or malignant fibrous histiocytoma cell histology.[195] Other reports described the following adverse outcome variables: patient age, performance status, size, grade depth of invasion, and surgical margin status.[196,197]

Liposarcoma

The most common sarcoma of the paratesticular region in adults is spermatic cord liposarcoma.[198-201] Mean patient age is about 63 years (range, 16 to 90 years).[202] Grossly liposarcoma is a lobulated mass of yellow tissue ranging from 3 to 50 cm (mean, 12 cm) that often resembles lipoma (Fig. 14.15).[202,203] Microscopically the most common pattern is well-differentiated liposarcoma (lipoma-like liposarcoma), often with prominent sclerosis or abundant myxoid stroma.[204,205] Myxoid/round cell liposarcoma and dedifferentiated/pleomorphic liposarcoma may also occur.[202,206-210]

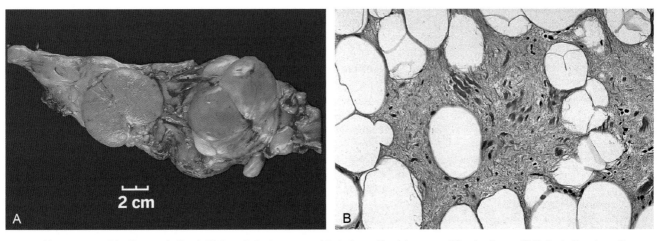

Fig. 14.15 Liposarcoma of the Spermatic Cord. (A) Grossly the tumor consisted of a multinodular mass of firm tan tissue. (B) Delicate fibrosis and increased cellularity were observed within adipose tissue.

Well-differentiated liposarcoma displayed immunoreactivity for MDM2 in 95% of cases and CDK4 in 78%.[200,205] Cytogenetics in 13 cases showed ring and giant marker chromosomes; fluorescence in situ hybridization revealed amplification of 12q13 to 12q15 in all cases evaluated.[205,211]

Paratesticular liposarcoma is treated by radical orchiectomy with high ligation of the spermatic cord.[199] Hemiscrotectomy may be required in cases with inadequate surgical resection margins to avoid local recurrence. Lymphadenectomy is usually not indicated, especially with well-differentiated and myxoid liposarcoma. The role of radiation therapy and chemotherapy is uncertain, but they are commonly employed. The majority of patients with paratesticular liposarcoma treated by resection with negative surgical margins are clinically free of tumor, and those with well-differentiated liposarcoma have a prolonged course, sometimes with late recurrence.[202] In a surgical series, Bachmann et al. reported 100% disease-free survival rate at 3 years after radical resection and 64% overall survival at 4.5 years.[212] However, 23% of patients with liposarcoma experience local recurrence and less than 10% experience development of metastases, invariably in those with dedifferentiated or high-grade liposarcoma.

Dedifferentiated liposarcoma (DDL) may be pure low grade (14% of cases) or pure or mixed high grade (86%).[213] Mixed patterns are common and may coexist with osteosarcoma and leiomyosarcoma. Low-grade DDL may have fibrosarcoma, myxofibrosarcoma, or inflammatory-like patterns, whereas high-grade DDL may display undifferentiated pleomorphic sarcoma-like, myxofibrosarcoma, fibrosarcoma, and myxofibrosarcoma-like patterns. Osseous metaplasia may also occur.[214] DDL occurs at a median age of 71 years (range, 43 to 90 years) and has a median size of 10.9 cm (range, 3 to 30 cm). Most are high grade, with occasional cases mixed with osteosarcoma or leiomyosarcoma. Recurrence is common, developing at a median of 24 months (range, 2 to 180 months). Size, grade, and margin status are not predictive of recurrence. Fluorescence in situ hybridization reveals amplification of MDM2 in the majority of cases.[215]

The differential diagnosis of well-differentiated liposarcoma includes sclerosing lipogranuloma and lipoma. Myxoid liposarcoma should be distinguished from rhabdomyosarcoma and myxoid malignant fibrous histiocytoma. Pleomorphic liposarcoma may be difficult to distinguish from other types of high-grade sarcoma.

A rare case of DDL and contralateral angiolipoma has been described in a 60-year-old man.[216]

Rhabdomyosarcoma

Paratesticular rhabdomyosarcoma may arise in the testicular tunics, epididymis, or spermatic cord. When the tumor is large or locally invasive, the exact site of origin cannot be determined. Rhabdomyosarcoma is the most common sarcoma of the paratesticular area in children, with a peak incidence at about 9 years, although it may occur at any age.[217-220]

Grossly, rhabdomyosarcoma is an encapsulated white-gray mass with focal hemorrhage and cystic degeneration that measures up to 20 cm in diameter. Most are embryonal rhabdomyosarcoma, consisting of small, round cells with dark nuclei, scant cytoplasm, and variable numbers of cells showing myoblastic differentiation. The connective tissue stroma may be myxoid. Alveolar, botryoid, and pleomorphic patterns have rarely been observed at this site.[218]

Rhabdomyosarcoma usually spreads to retroperitoneal lymph nodes, and patients without distant metastases are treated by radical inguinal orchiectomy with high ligation of the spermatic cord and ipsilateral or bilateral retroperitoneal or pelvic lymphadenectomy. Retroperitoneal lymphadenectomy can be avoided after radical inguinal orchiectomy when radiologic studies such as computerized tomography are negative. The extent of lymphadenectomy determines the likelihood of postoperative fertility. Locally invasive rhabdomyosarcoma that involves the skin or arises with clinically suspicious inguinal lymph nodes is treated by orchiectomy, scrotectomy, and inguinal lymphadenectomy. Long-term survival rates of greater than 80% are observed in patients receiving adjuvant radiation therapy and combination chemotherapy.

Leiomyosarcoma

Leiomyosarcoma is more common in the spermatic cord than in the epididymis, with more than 125 reported cases.[221-224] It arises in patients of all ages, with a peak in the sixth and seventh decades of life; more than 80% of patients are older than 40 years.[202,225,226]

Grossly, leiomyosarcoma is a solid gray-tan, 2 to 9 cm in diameter mass involving the intrascrotal portion of the spermatic cord, scrotal subcutis and dartos muscle, epididymis, or testicular tunics.[227] It consists of a spindle cell proliferation with typical features of leiomyosarcoma at other sites. Features that conclusively separate low-grade leiomyosarcoma and leiomyoma are lacking, although the presence of necrosis, a high number of mitotic figures, nuclear pleomorphism, and marked cellularity suggest malignancy. Most cases are high grade at diagnosis, although this has been refuted.[227]

Paratesticular leiomyosarcoma is treated by radical inguinal orchiectomy. The role of retroperitoneal lymphadenectomy is uncertain and is usually not recommended because of the propensity of leiomyosarcoma for hematogenous spread rather than lymphatic spread. Adjuvant radiation therapy and chemotherapy are considered palliative. Leiomyosarcoma may recur locally and metastasize, and about one-third of patients die of metastases. Survival rates after treatment are 75% and 50% at 5 and 10 years, respectively.[228] Enucleation was undertaken in one patient with good long-term results.[229]

Malignant Mesothelioma

Paratesticular malignant mesothelioma is uncommon, with fewer than 300 reported cases. Most occur in the tunica vaginalis, with very few in the spermatic cord and epididymis.[230-233] Mean patient age is about 55 years and ranges from 12 to 84 years. Primary peritoneal malignant mesothelioma may present as a mass in an inguinal hernia. The most common presenting symptom is either hydrocele of unknown origin or intrascrotal mass.

Malignant mesothelioma of the tunica vaginalis may appear in pipe fitters after asbestos exposure, raising the possibility of asbestos as a contributory factor, similar to pleural and peritoneal mesothelioma, and may account for an estimated 30% to 40% of cases.[231] Bilateral mesothelioma of the tunica vaginalis occurs rarely.

Grossly, malignant mesothelioma appears as multiple friable cystic and solid masses and small nodules studding the lining of a hydrocele sac, hernia sac, or the peritoneum (Fig. 14.16). Continuity between the tumor and adjacent mesothelium of the tunica vaginalis may be apparent, and there may be invasion of adjacent structures.

Histologically paratesticular malignant mesothelioma is similar to mesothelioma at other sites and may be epithelial, spindle cell, or biphasic, with a wide morphologic spectrum (Fig. 14.16). The epithelial pattern is most common, accounting for about 75% of cases, and may be mixed with papillary, tubular, and solid areas. Spindle cells predominate in the sarcomatous pattern and may merge perceptively with solid epithelioid nests. Tumor cells are cuboidal or flattened, with variable amounts of eosinophilic cytoplasm and atypical vesicular nuclei, often with prominent nucleoli. Mitotic figures are usually present. One case mimicked adenomatoid tumor because of the presence of small tubular and microcystic glands lined by flattened epithelioid cells and vague signet ring cells set in a myxofibrous stroma.[234] The combination of calretinin, cytokeratin 5/6, and thrombomodulin appears to be useful in separating epithelioid mesothelioma from metastatic carcinoma; these markers are also positive in benign and reactive mesothelium.[235] Few cases have been identified or suspected preoperatively on cytologic examination.

Malignant mesothelioma is aggressive, with potential for late recurrence or metastasis. It recurs locally along the vas deferens or in the pelvis, and usually spreads by lymphatic routes to pelvic, retroperitoneal, or distant lymph nodes. Radical inguinal orchiectomy is recommended with high ligation of the spermatic cord at the internal inguinal ring. Hemiscrotectomy or hemiscrotal irradiation may be useful to avoid local recurrence when transscrotal incision is made. Primary retroperitoneal lymphadenectomy is often used in patients with clinical or radiologic evidence of lymphatic metastases or in those without distant metastases. The utility of adjuvant chemotherapy is uncertain. About one-half of patients remain free of tumor up to 18 years after treatment.

The predominance of the epithelial or spindle cell component determines the differential diagnostic considerations. Epithelial malignant mesothelioma may be mistaken for reactive mesothelial hyperplasia, adenomatoid tumor, benign papillary mesothelioma, adenocarcinoma of the epididymis, paratesticular müllerian serous tumor, and metastatic adenocarcinoma. Paratesticular mesothelioma

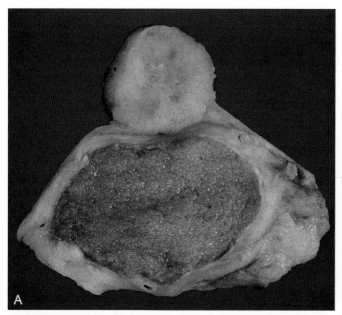
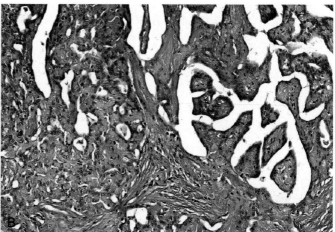

Fig. 14.16 Malignant Mesothelioma of the Tunica Vaginalis. (A) Grossly the tumor consisted of a large exophytic papillary mass. (B) Micropapillations are lined by flattened to cuboidal tumor cells. *(Courtesy Dr. Jan Kennedy, Atlanta, Georgia.)*

should be suspected in cases with in situ mesothelioma in the adjacent tunics, typical tubulopapillary architecture, and a lack of extrascrotal involvement. Spindle cell malignant mesothelioma should be distinguished from the variety of soft tissue sarcomas that arise at this site. Biphasic mesothelioma may be confused with stromal fibrosis, synovial sarcoma, and carcinosarcoma.

Papillary Serous Tumor of Müllerian Epithelium (Benign and Malignant)

Rarely müllerian epithelial tumors (also referred to as ovarian-type epithelial tumors) arise in the testis and paratesticular structures, perhaps from embryonic remnants such as the appendix testis.[156,236] One case arose in the torsed appendix testis of a young boy.[237] Some early reports of adenocarcinoma of the testicular appendages apparently represent papillary serous tumor of müllerian epithelium or malignant mesothelioma.

Papillary serous tumor of low malignant potential may occur in the tunica vaginalis, testis, spermatic cord, and epididymis and is grossly, microscopically, and immunohistochemically identical to its ovarian counterpart.[126,238] Patients range in age from 6 to 77 years (mean, 56 years) and present with an apparent testicular tumor. Proliferative activity by MIB1 staining ranges from 1% to 10% (mean, 5.5%), and most are diploid. Radical orchiectomy is the treatment of choice, and the tumor does not recur or metastasize after complete resection.[126]

Papillary serous carcinoma typically consists of invasive papillae lined by serous cuboidal or columnar cells with eosinophilic cytoplasm, frank nuclear anaplasia, and abundant psammoma bodies.[239] Cancer cells display immunoreactivity for broad-spectrum keratin AE1/AE3, S100 protein, epithelial membrane antigen, and Ber-EP4; variable positive staining is seen with Leu M1, B72.3, CEA, PLAP, and vimentin. Serum concentration of CA-125 is elevated in some patients. Cancer tends to recur within 5 to 7 years.

The differential diagnosis of serous tumor of müllerian epithelium includes papillary cystadenoma of the epididymis, benign papillary mesothelioma, malignant mesothelioma, adenocarcinoma of the rete testis or epididymis, and metastatic adenocarcinoma.

Adenocarcinoma of the Epididymis

Fewer than 30 cases of epididymal adenocarcinoma have been reported.[8,240-243] Mean patient age is 44 years (range, 5 to 78 years). The tumors measure up to 9 cm in diameter and may be multicystic or solid. About one-half are associated with hydrocele.

Microscopically there are typical features of adenocarcinoma including papillary, glandular, mucinous, and solid undifferentiated patterns; clear cells often predominate.[244] Squamous cell carcinoma may also be admixed. The main differential diagnostic consideration is metastatic renal cell carcinoma.[245]

Nearly one-half of reported patients experience development of metastases. Treatment is uncertain, but surgery and chemotherapy are most often used. Palliative radiation therapy has no apparent durable effect on cancer progression.[246]

Malignant Fibrous Histiocytoma

Fewer than 40 reported cases of malignant fibrous histiocytoma involving the spermatic cord and paratesticular area have been reported.[247-250] Most cases occur in patients older than 50 years. Grossly the tumor is solid gray or yellow-white, has a whorled cut surface, and measures up to 10 cm in diameter. Histologic patterns include myxoid, inflammatory, and pleomorphic malignant fibrous histiocytoma; the storiform-pleomorphic pattern accounted for more than 80% of reported cases.[248]

About one-third of patients with malignant fibrous histiocytoma experience local recurrence or distant metastases. The treatment of choice is radical inguinal orchiectomy with high ligation of the spermatic cord. The value of adjuvant therapy is unknown, although one patient was cancer-free 6 years after adjuvant radiation therapy.[251] Tumor size did not predict outcome.[248]

Other Sarcomas and Malignancies

More than 60 cases of spermatic cord and epididymal fibrosarcoma have been described, but some of these probably represent other forms of sarcoma.[252] Most occur in adults, but all ages may be affected. The gross and microscopic appearances of fibrosarcoma of the paratesticular area are similar to other sites. More than one-half of patients die of locally recurrent or metastatic tumor.

Most types of sarcoma have been described in the paratesticular area including primary neuroblastoma, neurofibrosarcoma, angiosarcoma, chondrosarcoma, myxofibrosarcoma, and undifferentiated sarcoma (Fig. 14.17).[253,254] Peripheral neuroectodermal tumor (extraskeletal Ewing sarcoma) also has been reported.[255] Carcinosarcoma of the tunica vaginalis occurred after radiation therapy for prostate cancer.[256] Paraganglioma with malignant features was recently described.[257]

Germ Cell Tumor

A variety of germ cell tumors have been described in the paratesticular area including seminoma, embryonal carcinoma, and teratoma; rare cases may be burned out and pose a diagnostic challenge.[258] The epididymis is more commonly involved than the spermatic cord, but germ cell tumor at either site is rare. The demographic and pathologic features of paratesticular germ cell tumor are like those of the testis. These tumors probably arise from misplaced germinal elements. Contiguous subepithelial spread of seminoma along the vas deferens was reported in a 56-year-old man.[259]

Malignant Lymphoma and Hematopoietic Neoplasms

Malignant lymphoma is the most common tumor of the testis in men older than 50 years, yet paratesticular lymphoma is uncommon.[260] Rare cases of primary epididymal or spermatic cord lymphoma have been described.[260-264] Secondary lymphoma has been described in all sites of the paratesticular area, invariably in association with testicular involvement. Occlusion of spermatic cord vessels by lymphoma may result in testicular ischemia.[265] Plasmacytoma of the epididymis and spermatic cord has also been reported.[266]

Metastases

Metastases to the paratesticular area are rare, and usually arise from the prostate, kidney, lung, and stomach, and other sites.[267-273] Renal primary should always be considered in clear cell carcinoma at this site; misdiagnoses include Sertoli cell tumor, Sertoli-Leydig cell tumor, and clear cell cystadenoma of the epididymis.[274] Rare cases have originated from colonic adenocarcinoma (Fig. 14.18), pancreatic adenocarcinoma, esophageal squamous cell carcinoma, urothelial carcinoma, ileal carcinoid, Wilms tumor, and malignant melanoma.[275-281] Patients with paratesticular metastases usually have a poor outcome.

References are available at expertconsult.com

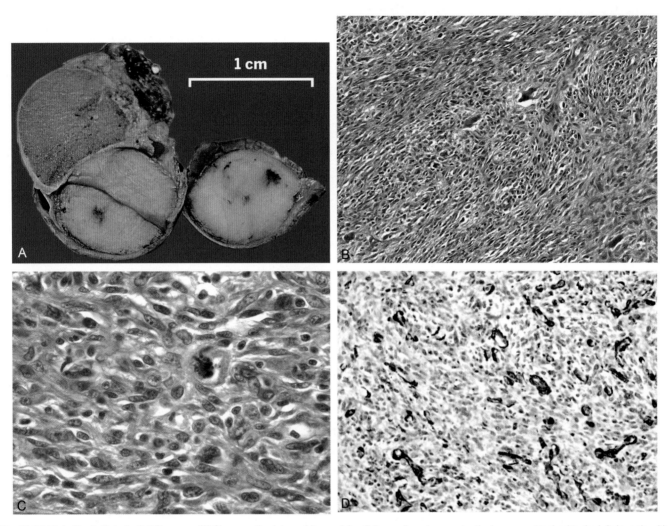

Fig. 14.17 High-Grade Spindle Cell Sarcoma. (A) Circumscribed, tan-white, nodular, 2.5-cm-diameter, paratesticular mass attached to the inferior pole without invasion. (B) The fascicular pattern is composed of plump spindle cells with pleomorphic nuclei and tumor giant cells. (C) There is brisk mitotic activity with rare abnormal mitotic figures. (D) Tumor cells display diffuse intense cytoplasmic immunoreactivity for vimentin, myo-D1 (shown), and myoglobulin; focal staining for calponin, smooth muscle actin, and muscle-specific actin; and negative staining for pankeratin, CD34, CD68, CD99, S100 protein, caldesmon, and desmin.

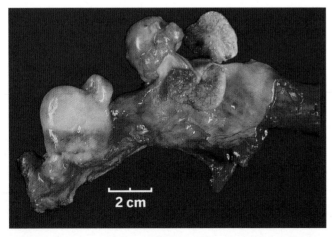

Fig. 14.18 Hernia Sac Containing Multiple Nodules of Metastatic Colonic Adenocarcinoma.

15
Penis and Scrotum

JAE Y. RO, MUKUL K. DIVATIA, KYU-RAE KIM, MAHUL B. AMIN AND ALBERTO G. AYALA

CHAPTER OUTLINE

Penis

Normal Anatomy and Histology

The penis consists of three portions: the root, the body, and the glans. The root lies in the superficial perineal pouch and provides fixation and stability. The body constitutes the major part of the penis and is composed of three cylinders of spongy erectile tissues: the paired corpora cavernosa and the single corpus spongiosum. The two cavernous bodies lie on the dorsum of the penis and are surrounded by a double layer of dense fibrous connective tissue called *Buck fascia* and *tunica albuginea*. The corpus spongiosum lies in the ventral aspect of the penis and surrounds the urethra in its center. The glans is the distal expansion of the corpus spongiosum; it is conical and normally ensheathed by the loose skin of the prepuce. In uncircumcised males, five to six layers of stratified nonkeratinizing squamous epithelium line the mucosal surface of the glans and become keratinized after circumcision.

The foreskin, or prepuce, of the penis is remarkably thin, dark, and loosely connected to the tunica albuginea. It has features of true skin but is devoid of subcutaneous adipose tissue. Sebaceous glands (Tyson glands) without associated hair follicles and sweat glands are present in the superficial dermis.

Histologically, the foreskin comprises five layers: epidermis, dermis, dartos muscle, lamina propria, and squamous mucosa. The squamous mucosa of the foreskin is a prolongation of that of the glans and balanopreputial sulcus. Langerhans cells are present in the mucosal epithelium of the foreskin and are more numerous in the foreskin than those identified in the female cervical tissue.[1] The foreskin is highly vascular. Most of its blood supply arises from the internal pudendal artery, which has three main branches: the deep artery, the bulbar artery, and the urethral artery. The venous return is through three channels: the cavernous veins, the deep veins, and the superficial dorsal veins. The lymphatic drainage is through the superficial and deep inguinal lymph nodes that drain to the external and common iliac nodes.

The glans is composed of epithelium, lamina propria, corpus spongiosum, tunica albuginea, and corpora cavernosa. The epithelium of the glans is keratinized or nonkeratinized squamous epithelium, depending on the status of circumcision. The lamina propria consists of a 1- to 3-mm-thick loose connective tissue layer containing small vessels, lymphatics, nerves, and occasional Vater-Pacini corpuscles.

The corpus spongiosum is the main structure of the glans; it consists of an 8- to 10-mm-thick layer of highly vascularized erectile tissue with varying-sized vessels, smooth muscle fibers, and peripheral nerves. The transition between the lamina propria and corpus spongiosum is usually not well delineated and often difficult to determine (Fig. 15.1). The corpora cavernosa form the main component of the shaft of penis and extend into the glans to a variable degree among males. The corpus spongiosum is separated from the corpora cavernosa by a dense, white, fibroelastic membrane—tunica albuginea (Fig. 15.2). It is 1 to 2 mm thick in the flaccid state but becomes thinner during erection and serves as an important barrier to the spread of cancer to the corpora cavernosa.

The coronal sulcus between the glans and the shaft is a narrow and circumferential cul-de-sac located just below the corona of the penis. The sulcus is composed of squamous mucosa, lamina propria, dartos muscle, and Buck fascia, and is a common site for recurrence of carcinoma or a positive margin in cases of primary foreskin carcinoma.[2]

The body or shaft of the penis is composed of: (1) a thin, wrinkled, pigmented epidermis with few adnexal structures; (2) dermis; (3) dartos muscle; (4) adipose tissue; (5) Buck fascia with numerous vessels and nerves; (6) tunica albuginea; and (7) erectile tissue of corpora cavernosa and corpus spongiosum, the latter encasing the urethra (Fig. 15.3). Histogenetically, the penis has two separate origins for its three erectile bodies. The corpora cavernosa are derived from the genital tubercles, whereas the urethra and corpus spongiosum are formed from the urogenital sinus and the urogenital folds. A comprehensive list of penile lesions is included in Table 15.1.

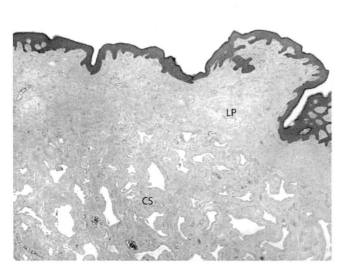

Fig. 15.1 Glans penis with lamina propria *(LP)* and corpus spongiosum *(CS)* showing venous channels with fibromuscular stroma.

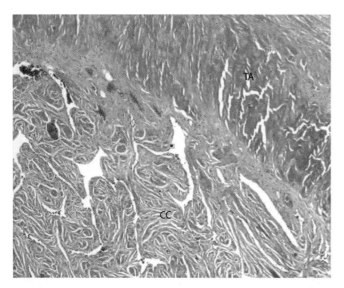

Fig. 15.2 Tunica albuginea *(TA)* and corpus cavernosum *(CC)* showing erectile tissue similar to corpus spongiosum, with a more muscular appearance.

Congenital Anomalies

Congenital absence of the upper wall of the urethra is known as *epispadias.* In this anomaly, the urethral opening is situated on the dorsum of the penis as a groove or cleft. The incidence of epispadias is 1 in 80,000 male births.[3,4] According to the location, the three types of epispadias are penopubic, penile, and glanular, with penopubic being most frequent.[3] Urinary incontinence is frequently observed with penopubic epispadias and occasionally with penile type, but it is not associated with glanular epispadias.[4] Buried penis and epispadias are usually isolated congenital anomalies, although they can also be seen in association with each other. An underlying penile anomaly may be seen in children with buried penises and unretractable foreskin. This warrants careful examination of the dorsum of the glans through the foreskin, because a dorsal cleft might indicate an associated epispadiac urethra. Associated congenital anomalies include diastasis of the pubic

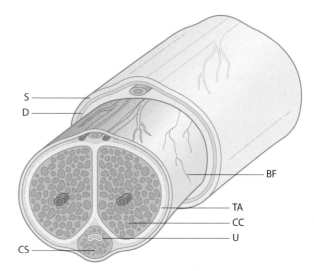

Fig. 15.3 Anatomy of penile shaft: skin *(S)*, dartos *(D)*, Buck fascia *(BF)*, tunica albuginea *(TA)*, corpus cavernosum *(CC)*, corpus spongiosum *(CS)*, and urethra *(U)*.

symphysis, bladder exstrophy, renal agenesis, and ectopic pelvic kidney.[4-12]

Hypospadias is a developmental anomaly in which the urethra opens on the underside of the penile shaft or on the perineum (Fig. 15.4).[13-15] Hypospadias is frequently associated with chordee (Fig. 15.5) but also seen as an independent finding. Hypospadias is classified based on the location of the meatus (glanular, subcoronal, distal penile, midshaft, proximal penile, penoscrotal, scrotal, or perineal) (Fig. 15.6).[13,14] The incidence of hypospadias is 1 per 300 live male births.[14,16] Associated anomalies include cryptorchidism and inguinal hernia. Association with anomalies of the upper urinary tract is uncommon unless other anomalies are present in other organ systems. Delayed surgery may be detrimental for patients because factors related to age may influence the rate of complications. Many surgical techniques are described based on the following three commonly assessed parameters: penile straightening, urethroplasty, and reconstruction of the ventral side of penis. The two main complications are fistulae and stenosis.[14-18]

Micropenis is diagnosed based on correct measurement of length. If stretched penile length is below the value corresponding to -2.5 standard deviations of the mean in a patient with normal internal and external male genitalia, a diagnosis of micropenis may be considered. It can be caused by a variety of factors including structural or hormonal defects of the hypothalamic-pituitary-gonadal axis and can also be a component of many congenital syndromes. Endocrinologic tests are important to establish the causative factor. The ratio of the length of the penile shaft to its circumference is normal (Fig. 15.7). The corpora cavernosa may be severely hypoplastic. The scrotum is generally fused but often diminutive, and the testes usually are small and frequently cryptorchid. A webbed or concealed penis often resembles a micropenis, but the penile shaft is of normal length. The three most common causes of micropenis are hypogonadotropic hypogonadism, hypergonadotropic hypogonadism (primary testicular failure), and idiopathic.[19-21]

Concealed penis is a normally developed penis that becomes buried in a suprapubic fat pad (Fig. 15.8). This anomaly may be congenital or idiopathic after circumcision. A concealed penis may be visualized by retracting skin lateral to the penile shaft.

TABLE 15.1 Diseases of the Penis

Congenital abnormalities

Inflammation
Phimosis and paraphimosis
Fibroepithelial polyp
Balanoposthitis
Plasma cell balanitis (Zoon balanitis)
Balanitis xerotica obliterans (lichen sclerosus et atrophicus)
Reiter syndrome
Peyronie disease
Os penis
Penile prosthesis
Priapism

Infections
Gonorrhea
Syphilis
Herpes simplex
Lymphogranuloma venereum
Granuloma inguinale
Chancroid (soft chancre)
Candidiasis
Scabies
Pediculosis pubis
Molluscum contagiosum
Erythrasma
Penile lesions in AIDS

Tumor-like lesions
Condyloma
Pearly penile papules
Penile cysts
Pseudoepitheliomatous keratotic and micaceous balanitis
Verruciform xanthoma
Lipogranulomas
Tancho nodules
Fournier gangrene: Corbus disease
Wegener granulomatosis
Other (includes sarcoidosis, Crohn disease, amyloidosis, sebaceous hyperplasia, inflammatory pseudotumor)

Tumors

Benign tumors
Papilloma
Hemangioma
Neurofibroma, schwannoma
Leiomyoma
Glomus tumor
Fibrous histiocytoma
Granular cell tumor
Myointimoma

Premalignant conditions
Penile intraepithelial neoplasia
  Differentiated
  Undifferentiated
    Warty
    Basaloid
    Warty-basaloid

Malignant epithelial tumors
Squamous cell carcinoma, non-HPV related
  Usual type
  Acantholytic (pseudoglandular or adenoid)
  Verrucous
  Papillary, not otherwise specified
  Carcinoma cuniculatum
  Pseudohyperplastic nonverruciform carcinoma
  Sarcomatoid (spindle cell) carcinoma[a]
  Mixed (hybrid) carcinomas
  Adenosquamous carcinoma
Squamous cell carcinoma, HPV related
  Basaloid, including papillary variant
  Warty (condylomatous)
  Warty-basaloid
  Clear cell
  Medullary
Basal cell carcinoma
Paget disease (see Scrotum section)

Melanocytic tumors
Nevi and other benign melanocytic proliferations
Malignant melanoma

Malignant mesenchymal tumors
Kaposi sarcoma
Angiosarcoma
Leiomyosarcoma
Rhabdomyosarcoma
Epithelioid sarcoma
Others

Hematopoietic tumors
Malignant lymphoma

Secondary (metastatic) tumors

HPV, *Human papillomavirus.*
[a]*Carcinosarcoma is included with sarcomatoid carcinoma for the purposes of this work. These tumors are also designated metaplastic carcinoma by some authors.*

Affected patients have poor sexual function, urinary dribbling with subsequent skin breakdown, and balanitis xerotica obliterans with subsequent urethral stricture. Limited surgical repairs can lead to reburying of the penis and a progression of urethral disease. Escutcheonectomy (surgical removal of suprapubic fat pad), scrotoplasty, and split-thickness skin grafting have proved to be beneficial in limited series with intermediate-term outcomes.[22] Penoplasty alone or penoplasty with liposuction of prominent prepubic fat pad used to correct concealed penis alleviates the initial complaint and provides good cosmetic and functional results with greater satisfaction in older patients.[23]

Aphallia (penile agenesis) results from failure of the genital tubercle to develop. The incidence is 1 in 10,000,000 live male births; less than 100 cases have been reported.[24-26] The usual appearance is that of a well-developed scrotum with descended testes but no penile shaft. In most cases the urethra opens at the anal verge adjacent to a small skin tag or, in other cases, opens into the rectum. Gender reassignment is of prime significance in such cases, necessitating immediate clinical assessment. Associated malformations include cryptorchidism, vesicoureteral reflux, horseshoe kidney, renal agenesis, imperforate anus, and musculoskeletal and cardiopulmonary abnormalities.[24-27]

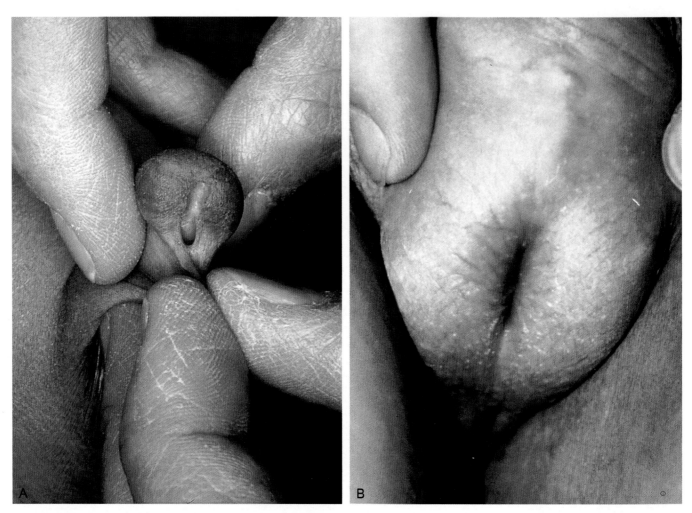

Fig. 15.4 (A) Distal hypospadias with the urethral meatus at the junction of the glans and penile shaft. (B) Proximal hypospadias with the urethral meatus at the base of the scrotum. *(Courtesy of Dr. Hyun Yul Rhew, Kosin University, Busan, Korea.)*

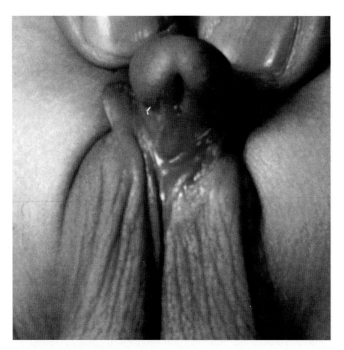

Fig. 15.5 Hypospadias with chordee. *(Courtesy of Dr. Hyun Yul Rhew, Kosin University, Busan, Korea.)*

Diphallus, or duplication of the penis, is a rare anomaly that ranges from a small accessory penis to complete duplication (Fig. 15.9).[28,29] It has an estimated frequency of 1 per 5,000,000 neonates. Approximately 100 cases have been reported to date. The embryologic causes for diphallia have not been fully elucidated, but it is believed that the various entities in this spectrum represent different embryopathies. True penile duplications are considered a part of caudal duplication defects, and hemiphalluses represent a part of the exstrophy-epispadias complex. Most patients present with true duplications (two penises, each with two corpora, a urethra, and spongiosum) or pseudoduplications (accessory rudimentary nonfunctional penises). Glans duplication is the rarest form of diphallia. The patients usually present with esthetic/sexual complaints or an abnormal voiding pattern. Associated anomalies include hypospadias, bifid scrotum, duplication of the bladder, renal agenesis or ectopia, and diastasis of the pubic symphysis. Anal and cardiac anomalies are also common.[28-30]

Chordee, a congenital or acquired bend of the penis, is caused by decreased elasticity in one or more of the fascial layers of the penis, leading to shortness of one corpus cavernosum when erection occurs. The bend may be ventral, dorsal, lateral, or complex. Chordee is most frequently associated developmentally with hypospadias when the mesenchyme distal to the meatus ceases to differentiate, creating a fan-shaped band of dysgenetic fascia.[31,32]

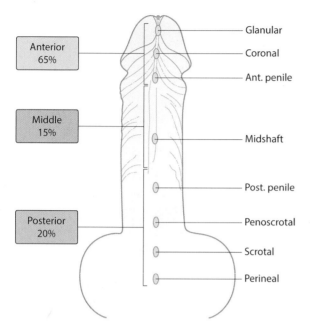

Fig. 15.6 Location of hypospadias. *Ant,* Anterior; *Post,* posterior. *(From Mr. Subhendu Chakraborty, Houston Methodist Hospital, Houston, Texas.)*

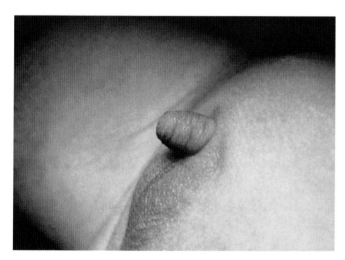

Fig. 15.7 Micropenis. *(Courtesy of Dr. Hyun Yul Rhew, Kosin University, Busan, Korea.)*

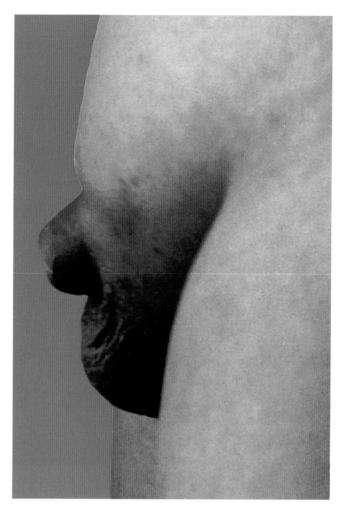

Fig. 15.8 Concealed penis. *(Courtesy of Dr. Hyun Yul Rhew, Kosin University, Busan, Korea.)*

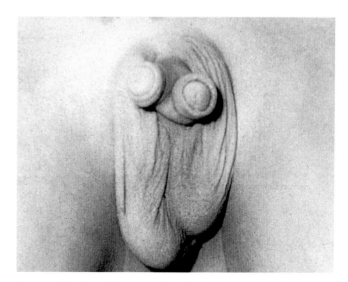

Fig. 15.9 Diphallus. *(Courtesy of Dr. Hyun Yul Rhew, Kosin University, Busan, Korea.)*

Acquired chordee may result from trauma or Peyronie disease.[33] Congenital chordee and penile torsion are commonly observed in the presence of hypospadias, but can also be seen with the meatus in its orthotopic position. Varying degrees of penile curvature are observed in 4% to 10% of males in the absence of hypospadias. Penile torsion can be observed at birth or in older boys who were circumcised at birth. The most widely used surgical techniques include penile degloving and dorsal plication.[32]

Scrotal engulfment (penoscrotal transposition) results from incomplete migration of the inferomedial labioscrotal swelling (Fig. 15.10). This has been termed *bifid scrotum, doughnut scrotum, prepenile scrotum,* and *shawl scrotum.* Frequently it occurs in conjunction with perineal, scrotal, or penoscrotal hypospadias with chordee.[34]

Ectopic scrotum is rare and refers to the anomalous position of one hemiscrotum along the inguinal canal, most commonly the suprainguinal canal, although it may be within the infrainguinal canal or the perineum. It is theorized that a defect in the gubernacular development leads to ectopic scrotum. Associated anomalies include cryptorchidism, inguinal hernia, exstrophy, renal agenesis,

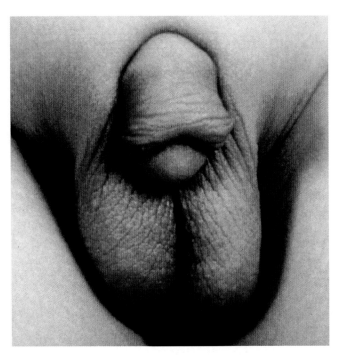

Fig. 15.10 Scrotal engulfment. *(Courtesy of Dr. Hyun Yul Rhew, Kosin University, Busan, Korea.)*

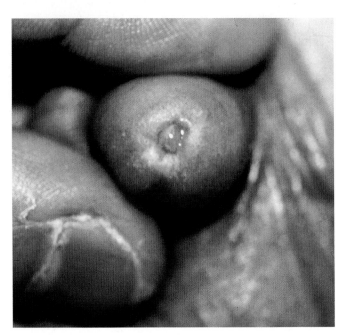

Fig. 15.11 Phimosis. *(Courtesy of Dr. Hyun Yul Rhew, Kosin University, Busan, Korea.)*

renal dysplasia, and ectopic urethra.[35] Magnetic resonance imaging (MRI) renders excellent anatomic interpretation of complex genital anomalies and associated abnormal pelvic tissues, thereby assisting surgeons in conceptualizing the anomalous structures and contributing to management.[36] After surgical correction of anomalies, long-term follow-up studies have shown that adulthood satisfaction with voiding and sexual function is achieved in approximately two-thirds of patients and some degree of dissatisfaction in one-third. Epispadias repair is a much more complicated procedure, and long-term results are seldom reported. Nevertheless, good results are achieved with respect to continence (~80% success) and sexual function.[37]

Nonneoplastic Diseases

Inflammation

Phimosis and Paraphimosis

Phimosis is a condition in which the foreskin cannot be retracted behind the glans penis (Fig. 15.11). In adolescents and adults the foreskin can normally be retracted beyond the corona with relative ease, but it is important to note that in children younger than 5 years the foreskin is not retractable.[38] Phimosis may arise in uncircumcised men at any age.

Phimosis may be congenital or acquired. Congenital phimosis is much rarer and is secondary to a small preputial orifice or an abnormally long foreskin. Secondary phimosis usually results from an accumulation of smegma, which is due to poor hygiene and can lead to chronic inflammation, edema, and fibrosis. Balanoposthitis (inflammation of the glans and prepuce) and balanitis xerotica obliterans may cause phimosis. Balanitis is the most common inflammatory disease of the penis. The accumulation of yeasts and other microorganisms under the foreskin contributes to

inflammation of the surrounding penile tissue. The clinical presentation of inflammatory penile conditions includes itching, tenderness, and pain. Penile inflammation is responsible for significant morbidity, including acquired phimosis, balanoposthitis, and balanitis xerotica obliterans.[38,39]

Circumcision is the treatment for phimosis, regardless of causative factor. Surgical specimens from men should be carefully examined for areas of induration that might indicate dysplastic or neoplastic lesions.[38] Microscopically, phimotic prepuces may be histologically normal or show varying degrees of inflammation, fibrosis, edema, and vascular congestion. Lymphocytes and plasma cells are the predominant inflammatory components.[40] Patients with phimosis often report irritation, but significant pain is uncommon unless ballooning of the foreskin occurs as a result of urinary obstruction.

Paraphimosis is a condition in which the foreskin has been retracted behind the glans penis and cannot be advanced back over the glans.[38] Constriction of the glans causes pain from vascular engorgement and edema. Paraphimosis is often iatrogenic, occurring after examination of the penis or after urinary tract instrumentation. Rarer reported causes include *Plasmodium falciparum* malaria and carcinoma metastatic to the penis.[41-43] Paraphimosis requires circumcision or emergency dorsal slit surgery.[38]

Phimosis often coexists with penile carcinoma and is a risk factor for it (see later discussion).[44,45] Difficulty in foreskin retraction and phimosis are risk factors for penile carcinoma that may be related to the anatomically variable length of the foreskin. Velazquez et al. compared foreskin length and status in the general population and patients with penile cancer, and found that 77% of men without cancer had a long foreskin and only 7% had phimosis.[46] Seventy-eight percent of patients with cancer had a long foreskin, and phimosis was significantly increased in frequency (52%).

Coexistence of a long foreskin and phimosis may explain the high incidence of penile cancer in some geographic regions. Because phimosis appears to be a major factor, the presence of a long foreskin may be a necessary, but not a sufficient, condition for cancer development. For these reasons Velazquez et al. supported preventive circumcision in patients with long and phimotic foreskins who are living in high-risk areas.[46]

Fibroepithelial (Lymphedematous) Polyp

Fibroepithelial polyp is rare in the penis and usually manifests as a polypoid or cauliflower-like mass or masses involving the glans penis or prepuce.[47-50] It ranges from less than 1 cm to greater than 7.5 cm in greatest dimension and is strongly associated with long-term condom catheter use, or rarely it may develop in association with phimosis. These lesions are characterized by their large size, and histopathologic examination demonstrates loose, edematous, cellular stroma containing numerous small vessels with luminal dilatation and occasional multinucleated mesenchymal cells; the term *lymphedematous fibroepithelial polyp* has been assigned to this entity. The age of the patients ranges from 4 to 58 years (median, 40 years) at the time of initial surgical resection, and the preoperative duration varies from 6 months to 10 years. The majority of fibroepithelial polyps affect the ventral surface of the glans near the urethral meatus.

Clinically, the differential diagnosis includes cutaneous fibroepithelial polyp (acrochordon), condyloma acuminatum, and even squamous or urothelial carcinoma. Lymphedematous fibroepithelial polyps of the penis are histologically and clinically distinct from the standard acrochordons that are commonly encountered in dermatopathology practice. In contrast with the cutaneous fibroepithelial polyps, lymphedematous fibroepithelial polyps of the penis are typically larger; show stromal hypercellularity with occasional multinucleated cells, increased mast cells, and stromal edema; and have a prominent vascular pattern with dilatation and thickening of vessels. In addition, lymphedematous fibroepithelial polyps have been described occurring only on the penis, whereas the typical locations for cutaneous fibroepithelial polyps are the neck, axilla, eyelid, and inframammary folds. The location and clinical appearance raise the clinical impression of condyloma acuminatum; however, no features such as papillomatosis or koilocytosis are seen to suggest this diagnosis. These polyps do not demonstrate any features of a cutaneous or mucosal carcinoma, such as invasion of normal structures, cytologic atypia, or mitoses. The stromal hypercellularity and occasional multinucleation may appear worrisome on low power; however, high-power examination shows bland cytologic morphology. Immunohistochemically, the stromal cells of lymphedematous fibroepithelial polyp demonstrate limited immunoreactivity for muscle-specific actin, α-smooth muscle actin (SMA), and desmin, and show no reactivity for S100 protein or CD34.[47-50]

The precise pathogenesis of these lesions is not known; however, considering the strong association with condom catheter use, they are likely reactive. Treatment with local excision has been successful in all reported cases. Although fibroepithelial polyp may recur, recurrences are also managed in a similar fashion.[47] This rare entity may be currently underrecognized or underreported by pathologists or dermatopathologists. In cases in which clinical information regarding the use of a condom catheter may not be readily available, recognizing the distinct histologic features of this lesion with edematous, hypercellular stroma with occasional multinucleated cells and prominent vasculature is important for a correct diagnosis, because they will likely be the dermatopathologists' only diagnostic clues.

Balanoposthitis (inflammation of the glans penis and prepuce) and balanitis (inflammation of the glans penis) occur most commonly in uncircumcised men.[51-53] The usual cause of balanoposthitis is poor hygiene. Failure to regularly retract and clean the foreskin leads to accumulation of smegma (desquamated epithelial cells and debris), which incites an inflammatory response, and may subsequently result in phimosis.

Balanoposthitis also can result from specific dermatologic lesions or infectious agents (Table 15.2). Various bacterial species and yeasts under the foreskin have the potential to cause penile inflammatory conditions. *Candida albicans* is the most frequent fungal isolate from the penis. Bacteria, especially *Streptococcus* spp., by themselves are the second most common cause of infectious balanitis. Less common are *Haemophilus parainfluenzae, Klebsiella* spp., *Staphylococcus epidermidis, Enterococcus, Proteus* spp., *Morganella* spp., and *Escherichia coli. Chlamydia trachomatis*, genital mycoplasmas, and bacterial sexually transmitted infections (STIs) such as *Neisseria gonorrhoeae, Haemophilus ducreyi*, and others can be associated with balanitis and balanoposthitis. *Gardnerella vaginalis* is responsible for symptomatic anaerobic-related balanitis in men. Other causes of balanitis and balanoposthitis include viral STIs, such as high-risk human papillomavirus (HPV) types, and parasitic infections such as *Trichomonas vaginalis* and protozoa, all more common in uncircumcised men.[52,54,55] Balanoposthitis caused by *Pseudomonas aeruginosa* coproducing metallo-β-lactamase and 16S rRNA methylase in children with hematologic malignancies has been reported, although it is rare.[54] Candidal balanoposthitis is discussed later in this chapter (see Infections). Discussion of papulosquamous and vesiculobullous diseases is beyond the scope of this text.

Plasma Cell Balanitis (Zoon Balanitis)

Plasma cell balanitis (Zoon balanitis or balanitis circumscripta plasmacellularis) is a disorder that was first described in 1952 by Zoon.[56] The disease is not rare and is important because it clinically resembles squamous cell carcinoma (SCC) in situ of the glans penis.[57,58] Plasma cell balanitis is a benign disorder of unknown etiology that is thought to represent a reaction to a multitude of diverse stimuli. Houser et al. reported a case of Zoon balanitis

TABLE 15.2	Balanoposthitis: Inflammation of Glans Penis and Prepuce	
Balanoposthitis, not otherwise specified	Balanitis circinata of Reiter syndrome
Candidal balanitis	Contact dermatitis
Plasma cell balanitis (Zoon balanitis)	Allergic
	Irritant
Balanitis xerotica obliterans (lichen sclerosus)	Vesiculobullous diseases: may simulate balanitis clinically
Papulosquamous diseases	Cicatricial pemphigoid
Lichen planus	Fixed drug eruption
Psoriasis	

in an African American man with HIV. Plasma cell balanitis affects only uncircumcised males.[59,60] It is similar clinically and histologically to its vulvar counterpart, vulvitis circumscripta plasmacellularis. It usually manifests as a single, large (≥2 cm), bright red, moist patch on the glans or inner prepuce (Fig. 15.12). Rarely, multiple patches may be present, and in severe cases it may consist of extensive visibly eroded lesions. The clinical appearance of the lesion overlaps with that of candidal balanitis and SCC in situ, so biopsy is mandatory. Cases of combined dysplastic conditions such as erythroplasia of Queyrat with Zoon balanitis have been reported, and this combination can create a diagnostic dilemma.[61] A case of plasma cell balanitis has been reported in a 57-year-old Hispanic man with a remote history of syphilis who presented with a 6-month nonhealing, granulating ulcer of the foreskin and glans penis that had been repeatedly mistaken for syphilis and treated unsuccessfully with circumcision. Biopsy of the glans penis

demonstrated denuded chronic granulation tissue showing a fibrotic stroma with numerous blood vessels and a mixed inflammatory infiltrate including scattered plasma cells. It is important to differentiate plasma cell balanitis from a syphilitic chancre in a patient presenting with a nonhealing penile lesion. This case report demonstrates that these entities may be seen in the same patient at different times.[62]

Histologically, the hallmark of plasma cell balanitis is a distinct upper dermal bandlike infiltrate containing numerous plasma cells (Fig. 15.13).[60-65] In some cases the number of plasma cells may be scant or moderate, and the histologic findings must be correlated with the clinical observations. The dermis also contains numerous dilated capillaries adjacent to extravasated erythrocytes or hemosiderin deposits. The overlying epidermis is thin and may occasionally be absent or partially separated from the dermis. The most distinctive feature within the epidermis is the presence of flattened or diamond- or rhomboid-shaped keratinocytes that are separated by uniform intercellular edema. Aggarwal et al., in their study of 17 cases, demonstrated that 35.3% demonstrated ≥50 IgG4-positive plasma cells per high-power field, with an IgG4/IgG ratio greater than 40%, at least focally, in two of these cases.[65] The plasma cells were polytypic in 12 of 15 cases, with an increased proportion of κ-positive plasma cells in three cases. Thus plasma cell balanitis should be considered in the expanding list of inflammatory disorders that can have significantly increased IgG4 plasma cells, but that do not represent IgG4-related sclerosing disease and that can have increased κ-positive plasma cells in the absence of malignant lymphoma.

Mucinous metaplasia of the penis is an uncommon lesion that occurs usually in elderly patients and appears to be a metaplastic change associated with severe chronic inflammation, especially with Zoon balanitis. Mucinous metaplasia may affect the glans penis and the mucosal surface of the foreskin.[66,67] Mucin deposition is seen in superficial epithelial layers ranging from numerous large goblet cells to subtle deposits. The epithelium exhibits polygonal (squamoid) or cuboidal differentiation, whereas columnar differentiation is not always identified. A bandlike inflammatory infiltrate is consistently present. Metaplastic epithelium consistently expresses cytokeratin 7 (CK7), carcinoembryonic antigen (CEA), and epithelial membrane antigen (EMA) either in the entire epithelium or in a superficial band, whereas CK14,

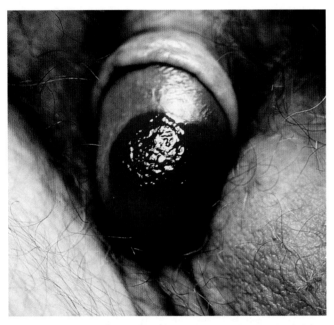

Fig. 15.12 Zoon balanitis. *(Courtesy of Dr. Hans Stricker, Henry Ford Hospital, Detroit, Michigan.)*

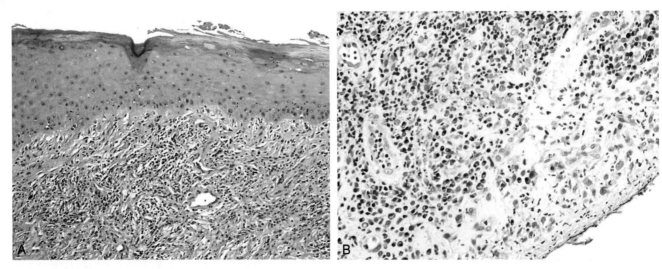

Fig. 15.13 (A) Zoon balanitis with reactive epithelial changes in the epidermis and a dermal inflammatory infiltrate accompanied by edema (low power). (B) Zoon balanitis with abundant plasma cells in the inflammatory infiltrate (high power).

CK10, GCDFP-15, and lysozyme are mostly negative, and staining for CK20 and S100 is also negative. Comparison with Paget disease demonstrates similar staining characteristics, but in a scattered pattern of mucinous cells within preserved squamous epithelium and not in a bandlike pattern as in mucinous metaplasia. Nuclear pleomorphism and Ki67[+] mucinous cells in superficial epithelial layers are seen in Paget disease, but not mucinous metaplasia. No evidence of HPV-specific DNA has been found in cases of mucinous metaplasia.[66]

Currently, the treatment of choice for Zoon balanitis is circumcision, but application of topical calcineurin inhibitors, mupirocin ointment, photodynamic therapy, and topical tacrolimus therapy has been used with variable success.[57,58,64,68-70]

Balanitis Xerotica Obliterans (Penile Lichen Sclerosus)

Balanitis xerotica obliterans is a chronic atrophic mucocutaneous condition that affects the epidermis and dermal connective tissue that most commonly involves the genital and perianal skin of both males and females.[71] Extragenital lesions may accompany genital lesions, although they also may occur alone.[71] *Balanitis xerotica obliterans* is a term used as a synonym for *lichen sclerosus of the glans penis and prepuce*.[72] This lesion is associated with penile carcinoma, and it has been postulated to be a preneoplastic condition for at least some types of penile cancer, particularly non-HPV variants of SCC.[73-85]

Balanitis xerotica obliterans is commonly encountered in preputial resections for phimosis in older men. In contrast, the prepubertal incidence rate in a series of 117 patients was only 4%.[86] The idiopathic form of balanitis xerotica obliterans is not associated with phimosis and manifests with classic clinical and pathologic features. The cause of this classic form of balanitis xerotica obliterans is unknown, but an autoimmune mechanism has been suggested.[72,87-90] Patients with balanitis xerotica obliterans may have increased organ-specific antibodies (thyroid microsomal and parietal cell antibodies in women and smooth muscle and parietal cell antibodies in men).[87-90] Association with autoimmune diseases, including vitiligo and alopecia areata, further supports the premise that autoimmune pathogenetic mechanisms may play an important role in this disease.

Clinically, balanitis xerotica obliterans manifests as a well-defined and marginated white patch on the glans penis or prepuce that envelops or involves the urethral meatus, the navicularis, and the penile urethra, but not the bulbar urethra, resulting in urethral strictures (Fig. 15.14).[88] It also may manifest as a lichenoid scale with a roughened surface. In long-standing cases, the lesion is firm because of the underlying fibrosis, which may cause phimosis in uncircumcised men.[91,92] Most lesions occur on the glans penis or prepuce, but the shaft is occasionally involved. Urethral involvement may cause stricture.[93] Pruritus, pain, and dyspareunia are common in vulvar lichen sclerosus et atrophicus, but balanitis xerotica obliterans is usually asymptomatic.

Histologically, active lesions of balanitis xerotica obliterans show pronounced orthokeratotic hyperkeratosis accompanied by striking atrophy of the epidermis, a distinctive combination of features. Basal cell vacuolation and clefting of the dermoepidermal junction also may occur; in rare instances, bullae may be seen. Orthokeratotic plugging of cutaneous follicles, a feature of lichen sclerosus et atrophicus, is not seen in balanitis xerotica obliterans because of the absence of follicles in this area.[76,77] The upper dermis is markedly edematous, and the collagen forms a homogenized band, beneath which a lymphoplasmacytic infiltrate may be present (Fig. 15.15).

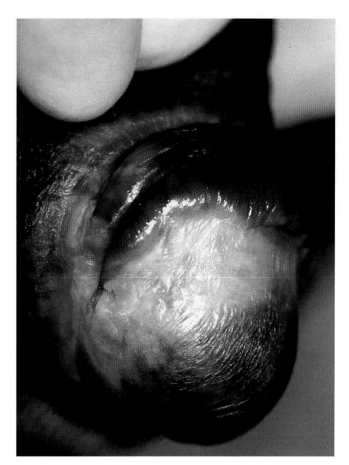

Fig. 15.14 Balanitis xerotica obliterans.

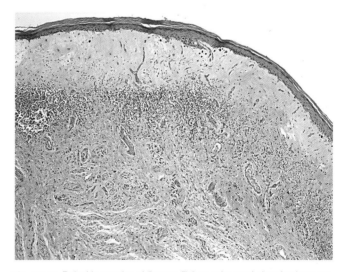

Fig. 15.15 Balanitis xerotica obliterans (lichen sclerosus) showing homogeneous collagen in upper dermis with a band of chronic inflammation just below.

Over time, four principal changes occur: the basal layer of the epidermis becomes mature; the upper dermis is gradually replaced by sclerotic collagen; the inflammation in the middermis becomes patchy or absent and is seen in the superficial dermis; and areas of epithelial hyperplasia may alternate with areas of atrophy. In rare cases, frank atypia may be evident. Small capillaries in the upper dermis and papillary dermis may be widely patent because of retraction by the sclerotic collagen. The chief differential diagnostic considerations are lupus erythematosus, morphea, and lichen planus.

The treatment of balanitis xerotica obliterans is often difficult. Circumcision, laser therapy, and topical administration of steroids, antifungal agents, and retinoids have been used with variable results. A recent report stated that after successful treatment of balanitis xerotica obliterans with long-term corticosteroids, purple to red asymptomatic angiomatoid nodules resembling the clinical features of Kaposi sarcoma developed.[94]

Balanitis xerotica obliterans may precede, coexist with, or arise after the development of carcinoma. Balanitis xerotica obliterans is preferentially associated with non-HPV variants of SCC. When balanitis xerotica obliterans is associated with malignancy, it often shows, in addition to hyperplastic epithelium, the presence of a low-grade squamous intraepithelial lesion (LSIL). These findings suggest that balanitis xerotica obliterans may represent a preneoplastic condition for at least some types of penile cancer, those not related to HPV.[83,95]

Whether balanitis xerotica obliterans represents a premalignant process remains a matter of some debate. Barbagli et al. retrospectively reviewed the histology of 130 patients with balanitis xerotica obliterans and reported premalignant or malignant features in 11 (8.4%).[88] In the largest series to date, SCC was found in 2.3% of 522 patients diagnosed with balanitis xerotica obliterans.[91] Nasca et al. reported on a series of 86 patients with balanitis xerotica obliterans in which SCC was subsequently found in only 5.8%.[90] In all cases, epithelial dysplasia and balanitis xerotica obliterans were found adjacent to tumor foci, indicating possible histologic progression from chronic inflammation to dysplasia and eventually to malignant transformation. Although European guidelines consider balanitis xerotica obliterans to be a premalignant condition, no consensus has been reached on the follow-up of these patients.[92]

Reiter Syndrome

In 1916 Reiter described a patient who experienced systemic illness with polyarthritis, conjunctivitis, and nongonococcal urethritis after an episode of bloody diarrhea. Although this was not the first reported case, the syndrome characterized by the triad of arthritis, urethritis, and conjunctivitis is now commonly referred to as *Reiter syndrome*. More than two-thirds of patients have associated mucocutaneous lesions, supporting the argument that Reiter syndrome is better defined by a tetrad of symptoms that includes mucocutaneous lesions.[96] More than 90% of patients are males, with onset of symptoms in the third and fourth decades of life.[97] Epidemic (enteric) and endemic (urogenital) modes of presentation have been described, with the latter being much more common.[97-99] Patients frequently report a history of recent sexual contact with a new partner that is followed by the development of urethritis. The less common epidemic form is secondary to enteric infection and occurs in children. Urethritis occurs in 90% of the postdysenteric or enteric form of the disease, so it should not be assumed that urethritis and Reiter syndrome are always transmitted sexually.

C. trachomatis probably is the most common cause for the sexually acquired form of Reiter syndrome, although *Ureaplasma urealyticum, Shigella flexneri, Salmonella* species, *Campylobacter* species, *Yersinia enterocolitica*, and *N. gonorrhoeae* also have been implicated.[96-101] Genetic susceptibility plays an important role; 60% to 80% of patients are positive for human leukocyte antigen (HLA)-B27. It is postulated that HLA-B27, either as a result of

molecular mimicry or by virtue of its relation to antigens linked to genes controlling immune responses to certain infectious agents, produces an exaggerated or abnormal immune response to specific microbiologic agents that culminates in the inflammatory manifestations of the disease.[102]

Genital involvement occurs as part of the mucocutaneous manifestations of Reiter syndrome and is common in the sexually acquired form of the disease. The lesions take two forms: balanitis circinata and keratoderma blennorrhagica. Balanitis circinata is the more common form and occurs in up to 85% of men with the sexually acquired form of the syndrome.[103-105] It consists of a painless lesion that begins as small red papules that enlarge centrifugally to form a circular or ringlike configuration. In circumcised men the lesion is hyperkeratotic and resembles the second lesion, keratoderma blennorrhagica. Keratoderma blennorrhagica is predominantly a cutaneous lesion, most commonly affecting the palms and soles. It begins as erythematous macules that enlarge to form hyperkeratotic papules with red halos. This form is clinically and histologically similar to psoriasis, and some cases of Reiter syndrome progress to become indistinguishable from psoriatic arthritis.[105] Histologically, the early lesions are indistinguishable from psoriasis vulgaris or pustular psoriasis, and they demonstrate psoriasiform hyperplasia, hyperkeratosis, parakeratosis, and neutrophilic exocytosis within the stratum corneum, with formation of spongiform pustules.[106] The spongiform pustules seen in the upper epidermis are the most characteristic histologic feature of Reiter syndrome. The papillary dermis is thickened by edema and may contain a neutrophilic perivascular infiltrate. In later stages the pustules are absent, and the epidermis shows nonspecific findings, including acanthosis, hyperkeratosis, and focal parakeratosis. Reliable distinction of Reiter syndrome from pustular psoriasis and psoriasis vulgaris may be difficult and requires clinicopathologic correlation.

Various therapies used in the management of Reiter syndrome are nonsteroidal antiinflammatory drugs, antibiotics, and disease-modifying antirheumatic drugs such as sulfasalazine or methotrexate. Successful treatment of Reiter syndrome with tumor necrosis factor-α blockers has been reported.[107]

Peyronie Disease

Peyronie disease (also called *plastic induration, fibrous sclerosis*, and *fibrous cavernositis*) manifests with painful erection accompanied by distortion, bending, or constriction of the erect penis.[108-111] Observations resembling Peyronie disease were made in 1561 by the Italian anatomist, Fallopius, but the first detailed description was by de la Peyronie, in a series of patients with deformities of the erect penis.

Peyronie disease affects men between the ages of 20 and 80 years (median, 53 years) but is uncommon in men younger than 40 years. The prevalence rate of patients younger than 40 years at diagnosis is only 1.5%.[112,113] Peyronie disease is more prevalent in patients with diabetes and urolithiasis.[114] In addition, genetic predisposition, trauma of the penis, systemic vascular diseases, smoking, and alcohol consumption are other possible causative factors in the development of the disease.[115] More than 66% of patients report painful erection. In contrast, in patients without pain, the manifesting symptom is penile bending (Fig. 15.16), which varies in duration from an overnight appearance to a few months or, in some instances, a few years. Patients concerned about the presence of tumor may seek attention after feeling a plaque. These lesions often are palpable as firm nodules or plaques on

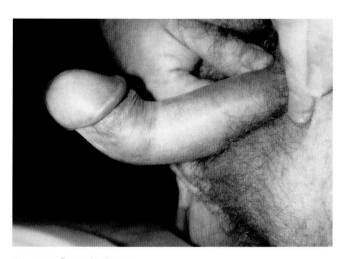

Fig. 15.16 Peyronie disease.

the dorsal surface of the erect penis. Examination of the flaccid penis may be unremarkable. Rarely, multiple plaques may be present. Some suggest Peyronie disease may be related to fibromatosis because of its association with Dupuytren contractures or palmar or plantar fibromatosis, seen in 10% to 20% of patients.[116] Others have suggested that it may be an inflammatory fibrotic reaction secondary to urethritis. Peyronie disease also appears to be related to coital trauma and urethral instrumentation, and has been associated with use of β-blockers, hypertension, diabetes, and immune reactions.[117-121] It is not associated with antigens of certain HLA systems.[122] Although some earlier studies suggested a relationship between specific HLA types and Peyronie disease, further studies failed to corroborate this association.[123] In addition, Hauck et al. failed to demonstrate the occurrence in Peyronie disease of 16S rDNA, which is a highly sensitive marker for the presence of bacteria in inflammatory processes.[124] The results of this study argue against an association between Peyronie disease and bacterial infection. Bivens et al. reported six patients with Peyronie disease and carcinoid syndrome, and suggested a causal role for elevated serum serotonin levels.[125] Guerneri et al. found chromosomal aberrations in 9 of 14 patients.[126]

Hauck et al. found an increased frequency of the homozygous genotype of the single nucleotide polymorphism G915C in patients with Peyronie disease in contrast with healthy control subjects (89.2% versus 79%).[127] However, no significant differences in allelic frequencies of the single nucleotide polymorphism T869C were found. These results indicate that the homozygous wild type of the G915C single nucleotide polymorphism in the coding region of the *TGFB1* gene, which was associated with elevated transforming growth factor-β1 production and pulmonary fibrosis, may influence the predisposition to Peyronie disease. However, it does not represent a major genetic risk factor.[127] The expression levels of transforming growth factor-β1 and pro-fibrotic and antifibrotic gene products, as well as the nitric oxide/reactive oxygen species ratio in the tunica albuginea, appear to be essential for the formation and progression of the Peyronie disease plaque and affect the expression of multiple genes. This can be assessed with recently developed DNA-based chip arrays, and results with the Peyronie disease plaque have been encouraging. OSF1 (osteoblast recruitment), MCP1 (macrophage recruitment), procollagenase IV (collagenase degradation), and other profibrotic genes have been identified as possible candidate regulatory genes. Gene-based therapy for the treatment of Peyronie disease is being investigated and may eventually reduce the need for surgical intervention.[128]

Although the chief pathologic finding in Peyronie disease is fibrosis of the tunica albuginea, it does not affect the erectile tissue of the corpora cavernosa. Calcification and ossification may occur in the fibrous plaques. Histologically, Peyronie disease begins with perivascular inflammation in the loose connective tissue between the tunica albuginea and the sinusoids of the corpora cavernosa. Deposition of fibrin in the tunica albuginea may be the primary event, followed by inflammation, fibrosis, and collagenization. In surgical specimens the histologic features are less dramatic than the clinical presentation, often consisting only of a cellular proliferation resembling fibromatosis or merely fibrosis (Fig. 15.17). Studies have shown excessive amounts of type III collagen in the plaques.[129] Ultrasonography of the penis is a helpful tool to the urologist, providing anatomic detail of soft tissue structures, and recently it has been used in the assessment of Peyronie disease.[130,131] Smith et al. studied ultrasonography in Peyronie disease and demonstrated tunica thickening,

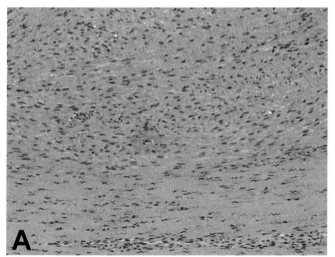
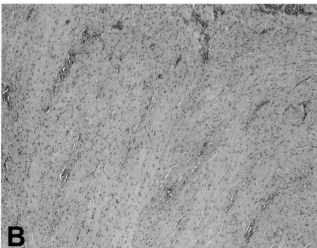

Fig. 15.17 (A) Peyronie disease, cellular region. (B) Peyronie disease, densely collagenous region.

calcifications, septal fibrosis, and intracavernosal fibrosis in 50%, 31%, 20%, and 15% of men, respectively.[131] Men 40 to 59 years of age were more likely to have subtunica calcifications relative to men younger than 40 years. Men with septal fibrosis had fewer chronic medical conditions such as diabetes, hypertension, and coronary artery disease, and presented within 1 year of disease onset. Men with septal fibrosis were less likely to have lost penile length and more likely to be able to have intercourse. Men with intracavernosal fibrosis were less likely to have penile pain but more likely to have penetration difficulty during intercourse, an additional penile deformity, or rapid onset of disease. Tunica thickening was associated with decreased ability to have intercourse.[130]

The clinical course is variable. The disease resolves spontaneously in fewer than one-third of the patients, progresses in up to 40%, and remains stable in the rest.[132] Treatment has included surgical excision of the plaques, intracavernosal plaque excision, radiotherapy, intralesional injection of interferon, steroid injections, and extracorporeal shock wave therapy.[122-137] Surgical approach with tunica excision in patients with palpable lesions and penile curvature can result in impotence and decreased penile sensation. Eisenberg et al. and Bella et al. described a novel method of excision of such lesions with preservation of the tunica that maintained potency and penile sensation.[138,139] Collagenase clostridium histolyticum (Xiaflex) has recently become the mainstay and gold standard of minimally invasive management of Peyronie disease.[140] Other treatment options include stem cell therapy and different types of surgery using a host of grafting materials.[141,142]

The combination of colchicine and vitamin E (which has antifibrotic, antimitotic, and antiinflammatory effects) in modifying the early stages of Peyronie disease has been used in one study and was an effective and well-tolerated way to stabilize the disease, but more extensive studies are needed, comparing these results with other oral therapies.[143] Prostheses may be required to restore potency.[144]

Heterotopic penile bone (os penis) is occasionally found in the plaques of Peyronie disease, particularly in elderly men.[145] In children, the presence of os penis is considered a congenital anomaly related to the normal occurrence of penile bone in numerous carnivorous animals, a feature lost in humans.[146] The bone is usually deposited just beneath the tunica albuginea.

Cutaneous Horn and Leukoplakia

Cutaneous horn is a rare exophytic, conical, keratotic mass that arises in areas of chronic inflammation. Little is known about its pathogenesis, but long-standing preputial inflammation and phimosis are known to play an important role.[147] It has a risk for malignant transformation into low-grade verrucous or keratinizing SCC, reported in approximately 30% of patients.[148]

Leukoplakia of penis is rare and consists of white verrucous plaques that can arise on mucosal surfaces. Genital lesions occur primarily on the glans or prepuce and can clinically resemble areas of balanitis xerotica obliterans. They occur more commonly in patients with diabetes, probably related to recurrent and chronic infection. Dysplastic changes have been reported in 10% to 20% of patients.[149,150]

Penile Prosthesis

Penile prostheses are surgically implanted devices that aid in erection by providing penile rigidity.[151] Since their introduction in the early 1970s the technology has greatly advanced, chiefly because of

better understanding of erectile physiology and pathophysiology. These developments have resulted in widespread patient and physician acceptance of these devices, as well as a substantial reduction in complications.

The indications for prosthetic implantation are organic and psychogenic impotence. Organic causes include diabetes, paraplegia, quadriplegia, and Peyronie disease. Therapeutic advances in vascular surgery and pharmacotherapy are leading to decreased use of penile prostheses in patients with organic causes, because other modalities offer better results.[151]

The two general categories of penile prosthesis are malleable devices and inflatable devices. These differ from one another in their construction and operation.[151-153] Malleable devices provide simplicity of implantation and have no mechanical parts that may fail. They require very little manual dexterity because they merely need to be bent upward before use. They are disadvantageous because neither the size nor the rigidity of the penis changes. Inflatable devices are based on hydraulic principles that allow inflation for sexual intercourse with deflation in the detumescent phase. These devices are more difficult to implant and have limited life span because of eventual mechanical failure.

Complications of penile prostheses may occur during surgery (usually crural or corporal perforation), postoperatively (mainly infection or component failure), or later because of device erosion. More than 90% of patients report satisfaction; the reoperative rate has significantly improved with new designs and surgical advances.[154-156]

Besides penile erection, endourethral prostheses for urethral stricture have been used in clinical practice with variable success.[157]

Priapism

Priapism is one of the most common urologic emergencies. Priapism is defined as a prolonged and persistent penile erection that is unrelated to sexual interest or stimulation and lasts longer than 4 hours. Three main types of priapism have been defined: ischemic (low flow), nonischemic (high flow), and stuttering (recurrent). Ischemic priapism is a persistent erection marked by rigidity of the corpora cavernosa and by little or no cavernous arterial inflow. Arterial (high-flow) priapism is a persistent erection caused by unregulated cavernous arterial inflow. Stuttering priapism, also termed intermittent or recurrent priapism, is a distinct condition characterized by repetitive, painful episodes of prolonged erections. Ischemic priapism is the most common form of priapism, accounting for more than 95% of all priapism episodes. Ischemic priapism is identified as idiopathic in most patients; sickle cell anemia is the most common cause in childhood.[158]

Priapism may be primary, secondary, or idiopathic. Secondary causes include genital trauma, thromboembolism, hemostasis, and leukostasis (fat embolism, sickle cell anemia, leukemia), neurologic defects (anesthetic agents, spinal cord injury, and autonomic dysfunction), infiltration by cancer (predominantly from urinary bladder, prostate, rectum), pharmacologic effects (alcohol, drugs acting on the central nervous system, total parenteral nutrition), and intracavernous injections for diagnostic procedures (papaverine hydrochloride, prostaglandin E, and phentolamine).[158,159] In a review of 230 cases, more than 33% were idiopathic, 21% were reactions to drugs and alcoholism, 12% were caused by trauma, 11% were caused by sickle cell anemia (an important cause of priapism in children), and less than 1% were due to neoplasms.[160] Priapism can be caused by hematologic malignancy with hypercoagulation or metastatic disease involving the corpora cavernosa with thrombosis of the venous outflow from the penis.[161]

Data on pathologic findings in priapism are extremely limited. The corporeal tissue may be edematous, indurated, and ultimately sclerotic. Ultrastructural examination reveals interstitial edema within 12 hours, destruction of sinusoidal endothelium and exposure of basement membrane with adherence of platelets by the end of 24 hours, and, finally, vascular thrombi associated with ischemic necrosis of smooth muscle tissue at 48 hours.[162]

Besides control of the precipitating factors, treatment includes conservative therapy with analgesics, sedatives, and fluids; control of pain with penile block; aspiration and injection of anesthetic agent, injection of α-adrenergic receptor agonists, intracavernosal injection of thrombolytic medications, and surgery for cavernosal shunt.[163,164]

Infections

Gonorrhea

Gonorrhea is caused by *N. gonorrhoeae*, a gram-negative, nonmotile, non–spore-forming, biscuit-shaped diplococcus. The term *gonorrhea* was coined by Galen in the second century and means "flow of semen," referring to the exudate of gonorrheal urethritis. The disease was recorded before the common era in descriptions by Hippocrates and Celsius. Gonorrhea is a global disease that infects approximately 60 million people annually. In the United States there are approximately 300,000 cases each year, with an incidence of approximately 100 cases per 100,000 population.[165,166]

The gonococcus infects a diverse array of mucosal surfaces, some of which include the urethra, endocervix, pharynx, conjunctiva, and rectum. In men, gonorrhea typically produces urethritis with urethral discharge, which may be profuse, purulent, or scant, and burning micturition. This disease is sexually acquired, and the risk for infection increases as the number of sexual partners increases. The penis is involved only as a complication of the disease, with cutaneous lesions, infection of the median raphe, penile abscess, and gonococcal tysonitis (inflammation of the preputial glands).[167,168] The chief complication is urethral stricture. Laboratory tests are essential because the disease is frequently mimicked by, and coexists with, chlamydial infection.[169] Standard diagnostic procedures include Gram stain, culture, and microbial susceptibility testing.[165,166] The Centers for Disease Control and Prevention (CDC) has given guidelines for its treatment, consisting primarily of antibiotic therapy.[170] Treatments for uncomplicated urogenital, anorectal, or pharyngeal gonococcal infections include cephalosporins and macrolides. Fluoroquinolones should not be used in patients who live in or may have contracted gonorrhea in Asia, the Pacific islands, or California, or in men who have sex with men. Gonorrhea infection should prompt physicians to test for other sexually transmitted diseases, including HIV.[171,172]

Syphilis

"Know syphilis in all its manifestations and relations, and all other things clinical will be added unto you."
—SIR WILLIAM OSLER, 1897

Syphilis is one of the most fascinating diseases affecting humans and has been investigated and described by clinical scholars, playwrights, and poets, including Fracastoro, who in 1530 wrote in his poem about the suffering shepherd Syphilis.[173] Although the disease was thought to be declining in incidence, it seems to have made a comeback in recent years.[174-176] Syphilis is produced by *Treponema pallidum*, a microaerophilic gram-negative spirochete, after a 9- to 90-day incubation period. In its classic form, untreated syphilis occurs in three stages: primary, secondary, and tertiary.

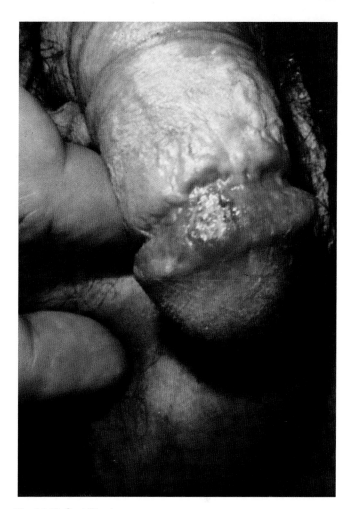

Fig. 15.18 Syphilitic chancre.

In the primary stage, penile involvement commences as a tiny papule, usually at the site of genital trauma on the glans penis, coronal sulcus, prepuce, frenulum, or shaft. In homosexual men the lesion may occur in the anal canal or rectum. The lesion progresses through the papular phase into an ulcerated chancre. The classic chancre is a single round, painless ulcer with sharp margins and a clean, indurated base (Fig. 15.18). Lymphadenopathy develops within a week, and the nodes are typically painless, rubbery, and nonsuppurative. With or without therapy, the primary ulcer heals within 6 to 8 weeks.[173,174]

Dark-field microscopy is the mainstay of diagnosis during this phase of the disease, because the antibody response lags.[174] Biopsy is usually not necessary but may be performed if the diagnosis of syphilis is not suspected. Histopathologic features include epidermal ulceration with acanthosis at the margins. The submucosa or dermis contains an inflammatory infiltrate of lymphocytes and plasma cells that is mostly diffuse but may be concentrated around blood vessels and associated with pronounced proliferation of endothelial cells (Fig. 15.19).[173,177] The Warthin-Starry or Levaditi stain reveals spirochetes in the epidermis or in the dermis around capillaries. The organisms typically have 8 to 12 convolutions, but reticulin fibers may mimic them and interpretation must be cautious.[177] The lymph nodes exhibit follicular hyperplasia, with many plasma cells and endothelial proliferation. Special stains may show numerous spirochetes in lymph nodes.

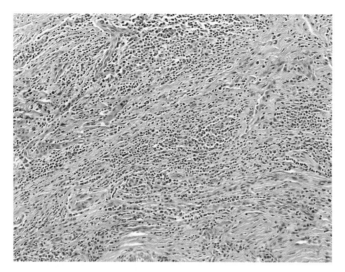

Fig. 15.19 Syphilis. Dense chronic inflammatory infiltrate with predominantly plasma cells and endothelial cell hyperplasia.

In secondary syphilis, penile involvement is usually part of the systemic mucocutaneous manifestations of this stage. The *T. pallidum* organisms circulate in the blood and lymphatic systems for 6 weeks to 6 months after the primary stage, producing symmetric skin lesions and generalized lymphadenopathy. The skin lesions are maculopapular, annular, and usually hyperpigmented. Secondary syphilis may manifest with nodular lesions.[178,179] Condyloma latum and mucous patches are included in the constellation of mucocutaneous lesions. Smears from these lesions should be examined by dark-field microscopy for organisms. A biopsy may yield variable histologic features and by itself is nonspecific, because in up to 25% of patients the plasma cell infiltrate and capillary endothelial proliferation typical of syphilis are absent.[180] The lesions that lack plasma cells and endothelial proliferation may mimic other cutaneous diseases such as lichen planus or psoriasis. A pronounced lymphocytic response may also be mistaken for mycosis fungoides.[181] The epidermal changes include parakeratotic scales, acanthosis, ulceration, spongiosis, exocytosis, dyskeratosis, and basal vacuolation. Condyloma latum shows prominent epithelial hyperplasia that may become pseudoepitheliomatous with ulceration and exocytosis with neutrophils.[182]

The third stage (tertiary syphilis) is characterized by granulomas referred to as *gummata*. These lesions may be nodular or gummatous—that is, accompanied by central necrosis. Nodular lesions lack tissue necrosis and are composed of hard granulomas accompanied by endothelial proliferation and perivascular inflammation. Central caseous necrosis heralds the gummatous phase, which has an intense inflammatory infiltrate in addition to the granulomas.

Until recently, syphilis was considered a major cause of penile cancer, but the possible role of syphilis was discarded without much debate with the acceptance of certain HPVs primarily involved as causative agents. A recent study with logistic regression showed that patients with penile cancer did not have a syphilis history significantly more often than control patients with colon and stomach cancers.[183]

Therapy is stage dependent, consists predominantly of antimicrobial drugs, and is successful if timely. The CDC recommends counseling all patients for risks and testing for HIV infection, which also reactivates syphilis.

Herpes Simplex and Zoster

Herpes (from Greek, meaning "to creep") simplex virus (HSV) infection involving the genital system is an important sexually transmitted disease that may have a causal role in cervical carcinoma and has high morbidity and mortality in infants. The virus is a double-stranded DNA virus that has two subtypes. HSV type 1 produces oral lesions, whereas HSV type 2 predominantly affects the genitalia; only 10% to 25% of HSV type 2 infections produce oral lesions.[184,185] Herpes genitalis and infections caused by HPV are increasingly common, particularly in young, sexually active people. However, HSV infection remains the most common infectious cause of genital ulceration, with evidence that many infections are asymptomatic.[185,186]

Clinical manifestations are more severe and fulminant in the first episode than in recurrent disease.[187,188] Initial episodes often have systemic symptoms (fever, malaise, and headache) and affect multiple extragenital and genital sites. Pain, itching, urethral discharge, dysuria, and tender lymphadenopathy are the most common local symptoms. The genital lesions appear as multiple vesicles with erythematous bases that may coalesce, rupture, form pustules, and eventually become encrusted (Fig. 15.20A). Asymptomatic viral shedding may occur for a prolonged period.[189] The clinical diagnosis may be confirmed by scraping the lesion and

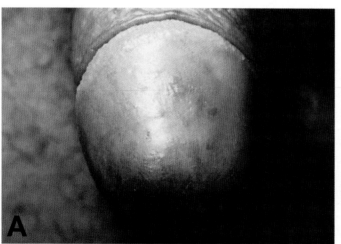

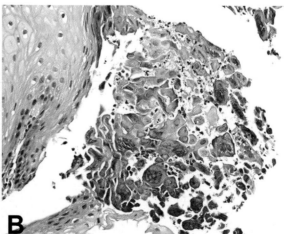

Fig. 15.20 (A) Herpes simplex. (B) Herpes simplex vesicle with 3M (multinucleation, nuclear molding, and margination).

obtaining a Tzanck smear (stained with Wright-Giemsa, toluidine blue, or Papanicolaou procedures), which reveals large multinucleated giant cells with ballooning degeneration and characteristic intranuclear inclusions. However, this method cannot differentiate between HSV and varicella zoster virus (VZV) infection. The diagnosis of HSV and VZV infection is often made clinically; however, laboratory confirmation is required in some cases. Viral culture has been considered the gold standard test, although molecular methods have been shown to be more rapid and sensitive, resulting in increased use of these techniques. Currently, most laboratories perform real-time polymerase chain reaction (PCR) for the detection of HSV and VZV. Multiplex assays offer the potential to detect multiple pathogens in a single test, which may reduce the amount of sample required, the hands-on time, and turnaround time for results.[190]

Histologically, HSV and VZV lesions are identical, characterized by unilocular or multilocular intraepidermal vesicles produced by profound acantholysis (Fig. 15.20B).[191] The vesicles contain proteinaceous material and are surrounded by epidermal cells with reticular and ballooning degeneration, features that are hallmarks of herpes infection but absent in other vesiculobullous diseases that may enter into the differential diagnosis. Cytopathic changes may be evident in adnexal and pilosebaceous structures, endothelial cells, and fibroblasts, but are typically seen in the epidermal cells, which exhibit chromatin margination and inclusion bodies (ranging from small, demarcated acidophilic bodies to large, homogeneous, ground-glass acidophilic to basophilic bodies) surrounded by halos.

Atypical clinical manifestations of HSV may occur in HIV-positive immunocompromised patients presenting with tumor-like nodules or condylomatous or hypertrophic lesions, rather than classic ulcer. Such unusual presentations raise the risk for misdiagnosis and a delay in appropriate treatment. Therefore it is important to be aware of these unusual presentations to provide a correct diagnosis and prompt, effective treatment for HSV. Several studies suggest that aggressive treatment of HSV in combination with highly active antiretroviral therapy provides a significant survival benefit. Pathobiology mechanisms of unusual and exaggerated tumor-like inflammatory response are not completely elucidated.[192] Complications of herpes include neonatal complications; nervous system abnormalities (aseptic meningitis, encephalitis, radiculopathies); extragenital lesions on buttocks, groin, thighs, or other sites; disseminated infection resulting in arthritis, hepatitis, or hematologic disorders; superinfections; intractable nonhealing ulcers in patients with AIDS; and possibly cervical cancer in women.[193] Treatment options are limited. Acyclovir is effective in decreasing the intensity and duration of both primary and recurrent episodes but is not curative. For adults and adolescents with a recurrent clinical episode of genital HSV infection the World Health Organization (WHO) STI guideline suggests the use of acyclovir over valaciclovir or famciclovir.

Herpes zoster is a common dermatologic infection and predominantly affects the trunk in up to 50% to 60% of patients, followed by the head region (10% to 20%), with sacral dermatomes involved in only up to 5% of patients. Penile zoster is neither commonly seen by dermatologists nor reported in dermatologic journals.[194] The diagnosis of herpes zoster is made clinically; however, laboratory confirmation is necessary in a subset of cases and is readily established with the aid of molecular techniques.[190] Patients with penile herpes zoster present with vesicular rash involving S2 to S4 dermatomes. Postherpetic neuralgia is the most frequently reported complication, and risk factors include older age, more severe acute pain, and greater rash severity. Bladder dysfunction and urinary retention have been reported in patients with herpes zoster, and penile herpes zoster should not be overlooked in patients with unilateral vesicular rash.

Lymphogranuloma Venereum

Lymphogranuloma venereum is a sexually transmitted disease caused by *C. trachomatis* subtypes L1, L2, and L3. It was established in 1913 by Durand, Nicolas, and Favre as a clinicopathologic entity separate from other venereal diseases.[195] Lymphogranuloma venereum is sporadic in the United States and most European countries, but it is highly prevalent in Africa, Asia, and South America. Rarely it is associated with HIV infection.[196]

Like syphilis, lymphogranuloma venereum has three stages: primary genital stage; secondary inguinal stage characterized by acute lymphadenitis with bubo formation; and a rare chronic tertiary stage with genital ulcers, fistulas, elephantiasis, and rectal strictures.[197,198] After an incubation period of 3 days to 6 weeks, the lesion begins as a papule, which transforms into a pustule and heals without treatment; therefore in 50% of patients, the penile lesion is not clinically examined. The pathognomonic clinical sign is inguinal lymphadenopathy, commonly known as *bubo*. It is painful, usually unilateral (66%), and may enlarge to form an abscess and rupture (33%).[197-199]

The histologic features are nonspecific and nondiagnostic. The ulcer is coated with exudate and neutrophils; the base is composed of granulation tissue, with a mixed inflammatory infiltrate containing large mononuclear cells with occasional granulomas.[200] Giemsa stains may demonstrate purple chlamydial inclusions in the macrophages, but this procedure lacks specificity and sensitivity. The lymph nodes show follicular hyperplasia and elongate stellate abscesses like those of cat scratch disease, tularemia, and fungal and atypical mycobacterial infections.

Culture of the organisms by aspirating the lymph nodes is a useful method of detection but is technically difficult and costly. The Frei test is no longer used, but serologic tests have gained wide acceptance for diagnosis of lymphogranuloma venereum.[201] Genetic testing is now widely available and is rapid and specific. Lymphogranuloma venereum can be confirmed by the detection of lymphogranuloma venereum–specific DNA from specimens such as bubo aspirates, ulcer swabs, urethral swabs, first voided urine, and rectal biopsy material. The real-time polymerase chain reaction assay simultaneously detects and differentiates lymphogranuloma venereum (LGV) from non-LGV strains using swab specimens. This assay offers a relatively rapid and sensitive alternative for the diagnosis of LGV infection and is a useful tool for screening and for outbreak investigations.[202] Antibiotics are effective if the diagnosis is made in a timely fashion.

Granuloma Inguinale (Donovanosis)

Granuloma inguinale is a chronic, progressive, sexually transmitted disease caused by *Calymmatobacterium granulomatis*, a nonmotile, gram-negative, pleomorphic intracellular bacillus of uncertain classification. Although rare in the United States, it is more prevalent in areas of Australia, India, the Caribbean, and Africa.[203,204]

Granuloma inguinale is only mildly contagious and affects the penis, anal region, and vulva. The incubation period varies from 8 to 80 days. The lesion starts as single or multiple small papules that subsequently form ulcers that bleed readily and have abundant beefy-red granulation tissue at their bases.[203-206] Ulcers are the hallmark of the disease and are typically nontender, indurated, and firm. A verrucous form occurs in the perianal region and may simulate carcinoma.[207-209] Severe ulcerative genital diseases can cause destruction of the prepuce, glans, or sometimes the entire penis (phagedena). Partial destruction of the prepuce from donovanosis has been reported.[209]

Histologically, granuloma inguinale consists of a central ulcer bordered by acanthotic epidermis with features of pseudoepitheliomatous hyperplasia.[207,208] The dermis below the ulcer contains granulation tissue with vascular ectasia and endothelial proliferation, microabscesses with neutrophils, and large histiocytes (25 to 90 μm). These histiocytes have cytoplasmic vacuoles that contain dark particulate inclusions (Donovan bodies), seen best with Giemsa or Warthin-Starry stains.[210] Donovan bodies are often easier to see in smears than in histologic sections. Mimicking granuloma inguinale, organisms may be evident within histiocytes in rhinoscleroma, histoplasmosis, coccidioidomycosis, and leishmaniasis, but the small size (1 to 2 μm) of *C. granulomatis* is an important distinguishing feature for granuloma inguinale.[211] The diagnosis must be established by microscopy because the bacilli are not readily cultured.[212] Serologic testing using indirect immunofluorescence is available in some laboratories.[213] Azithromycin has emerged from practical experience as the agent of choice per the major treatment guidelines. Surgical intervention may be needed in severe cases, especially those with pseudoelephantiasis.[214]

Chancroid (Soft Chancre)

Chancroid is a sexually transmitted disease caused by the gram-negative, facultatively anaerobic, biochemically relatively inert bacteria *Haemophilus ducreyi.* It is characterized by necrotizing genital ulceration that may be accompanied by inguinal lymphadenitis or bubo formation in 50% of cases. First described by Ricord in France in 1838, chancroid is a major cause of genital ulceration in Africa, with a recent increase in prevalence in the United States.[215,216]

The ulcer develops after a 4- to 7-day incubation period, beginning as a tender erythematous papule that erodes, ulcerates, and becomes pustular. The ulcer is not indurated, but has undermined edges and is covered by grayish yellow exudate. The lymphadenitis is unilateral, and the lymph nodes may enlarge and rupture spontaneously.[216]

Histologically, the cutaneous findings are relatively distinctive, forming three zones: a surface zone containing exudate, fibrin, neutrophils, and debris at the base of the ulcer; a wide intermediate zone in which prominent vascular proliferation and ectasia with focal thrombosis are seen; and a deep zone containing a dense infiltrate of lymphocytes and plasma cells.[217] The adjacent epidermis may show acanthosis, spongiosis, and a neutrophilic infiltrate. The presumptive diagnosis based on the recognition of these typical zonal histologic features may be confirmed by demonstrating the bacteria by Giemsa, Gram, or methylene blue stain. The bacteria are more easily seen in smears than in histologic sections.[217] In smears, the organisms have a "railroad track" or "school of fish" pattern of alignment of short rods.[218] The organisms may be cultured on a selective agar medium and directly detected by PCR DNA amplification.[219,220]

Evidence indicates that chancroid is a risk factor for heterosexual spread of HIV.[221-223] Cell-mediated immunity in the host response to *H. ducreyi* infection may play a more critical role in the transmission of HIV than humoral immunity.[224] Antibiotic therapy is usually curative, although cases associated with HIV infection do not respond as well.

Candidiasis and Other Fungal Infections

Candidiasis of the penis mimics balanitis or balanoposthitis, visible clinically as bright red patches, numerous minute pustules, and erosions. It is common in uncircumcised men in whom heat and retained moisture within the preputial sac create a favorable environment.[225,226] Diabetes mellitus, lengthy antibiotic treatment, and immunosuppression are other predisposing factors.[227] *C. albicans* is the most common species and may be identified in the curd-white exudate that often overlies the lesions. Microscopy of a wet-mount preparation with potassium hydroxide is sufficient for diagnosis. Conversely, positive culture alone is not diagnostic, because fungi may colonize other forms of balanitis. Therapy consists of eliminating environmental factors predisposing to the infection, improving local hygiene, and application of topical antifungal agents. If local treatment fails, circumcision may be necessary. Patients may have concurrent candidal intertrigo. Other penile fungal infections include penile pityriasis versicolor and tinea genitalis caused by dermatophyte fungi.[55,228] Penoscrotal histoplasmosis is rarely reported. A case with penoscrotal histoplasmosis has been reported after bladder carcinoma that had been treated with intravesical bacille Calmette–Guérin therapy. The patient presented with multiple ulcers on the penis and scrotum that coalesced, followed by the appearance of cutaneous lesions. The condition responded well to itraconazole.[229] Severe life-threatening *Candida* infections with formation of emphysematous lesions are rare.[230]

Scabies

Believed to be the first human disease with a known causative agent, scabies was discovered in 1687 and found to be caused by the bite of the human itch mite (*Sarcoptes scabiei*).[231] Prolonged personal contact is required for transmission, and affliction of several members of a family or infection of sexual partners is likely.[232,233] Scabies also may be an undetected contributor to recurrent staphylococcal or streptococcal infections. A recent report described a patient with AIDS and Norwegian scabies who presented with a single, crusted plaque localized to the glans penis.[233]

Scabies is clinically characterized by severe pruritus that is more pronounced at night and may be severe enough to provoke profound excoriation. In addition to the genitalia, the palms, wrists, feet, and elbows may be involved. Burrowing by female mites produces scaly red patches that may be papular, nodular, or excoriated. Vesicles may be visible at the ends of burrows.[186,232]

The diagnosis may be made by teasing the mite out from the burrow with a needle or scraping the skin with a sharp scalpel and examining the fragments with a microscope. Definitive histopathologic diagnosis requires demonstration of the mite or its products. The burrow is housed within the horny layer, where the female mite, approximately 400 μm long, resides (Fig. 15.21).[234-237] In the absence of the mite, eggs that contain larvae or egg shells (chitin walls with marked eosinophilia and periodic acid–Schiff [PAS] positivity) are diagnostic of scabies. Epidermal spongiosis and dermal eosinophilia are clues aiding recognition. Treatment consists of antipruritic agents and antiscabietic drugs, which also should be administered to family members and sexual partners.[238,239]

Pediculosis Pubis

Pediculosis pubis, or phthiriasis, is caused by infection with *Phthirus pubis,* the crab louse that, along with the head louse, account for nearly 3 million cases annually in the United States. History, physical examination, and a high index of suspicion are necessary to make the correct diagnosis.[186,240] Pediculosis should be suspected when itching occurs in hair-bearing regions of the

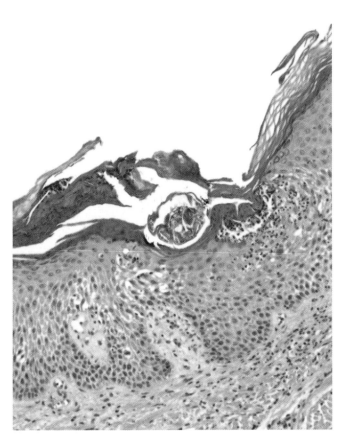

Fig. 15.21 Scabies burrow in the epidermis.

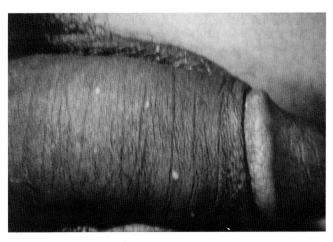

Fig. 15.22 Molluscum contagiosum.

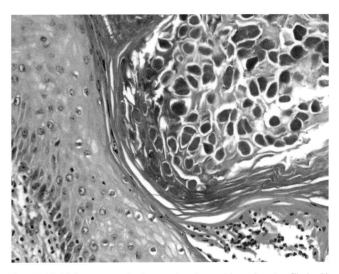

Fig. 15.23 Molluscum contagiosum showing epidermal crater filled with molluscum bodies.

groin, scrotum, and thighs. Penile lesions may be evident as blue spots. Transmission occurs with physical contact and contamination of clothing.[241,242] The lice and mites may be seen in the pubic hair with a magnifying lens. Treatment, essential for the patient, sexual partners, and close family members, consists of mechanical measures, such as combing, topical insecticide in cream or shampoo form, and antibiotics, if necessary, for secondary infection.[243-245]

Molluscum Contagiosum

Molluscum contagiosum is a fairly common viral mucocutaneous disorder caused by the large, brick-shaped DNA pox virus.[246] The lesion was named in 1817 by Bateman for its pedunculated gross appearance and contagious nature. Lymphangioma circumscriptum of the penis may clinically mimic molluscum contagiosum.[247]

The incubation period is 2 to 7 weeks, and lesions appear as multiple, discrete, dome-shaped, 3- to 6-mm papules (Fig. 15.22) with small central umbilications through which milky-white contents may be extruded under pressure.[248] Molluscum contagiosum occurs in children, adolescents, young adults, and immunocompromised patients (including AIDS patients). In immunocompromised patients, hundreds of lesions may fail to involute.

Histologically, the characteristic low-power picture is a cup-shaped invagination of acanthotic epidermis into the dermis (Fig. 15.23).[249,250] The basal layer is uninvolved, but the cells of the stratum malpighii acquire cytoplasmic inclusions that progressively enlarge as they reach the surface. The inclusions, known as *molluscum bodies* (Henderson-Paterson bodies), contain viral particles. The inclusions initially are eosinophilic but gradually acquire basophilia and granularity as they enlarge and displace the nuclei. The stratum corneum ultimately ruptures, releasing the molluscum bodies through a central crater. The underlying dermis usually lacks significant inflammation unless the molluscum bodies and epidermal contents rupture into it.[251]

Most lesions regress spontaneously within 6 to 12 months, but treatment is necessary to prevent autoinoculation and transmission to others. Treatment consists of curettage with application of podophyllin or silver nitrate or laser vaporization. Imiquimod and cryotherapy have been used to treat molluscum contagiosum.[252]

Erythrasma

Erythrasma is a superficial, asymptomatic, noninflammatory disease caused by the diphtheroid organism *Corynebacterium minutissimum*.[253] The lesions are often overlooked, appearing as sharply delineated, round-to-oval patches or plaques with fine scales in intertriginous areas (the genitocrural form). Examination with a Wood light (ultraviolet light in the ultraviolet A range) reveals characteristic coral-red fluorescence. The histologic abnormalities are limited to the stratum corneum, where hyperkeratosis and small gram-positive bacilli are seen.[254,255] The basal epidermis and dermis lack specific histologic changes. The disease is more common in tropical and subtropical climates. Treatment with antibiotics is effective.

Penile Lesions in AIDS

Almost all sexually transmitted diseases are common in patients with AIDS. These include gonorrhea, syphilis, herpes, candidiasis, chancroid, molluscum contagiosum, HPV, scabies, Reiter syndrome, and others.[256-260] In patients with AIDS, these diseases are generally more severe, of longer duration, and less responsive to therapy than in other patients.

Kaposi sarcoma, multiple squamous carcinomas, and multifocal carcinoma in situ are malignancies of penile skin associated with AIDS.[31,261-263] Condyloma acuminata and anal intraepithelial neoplasia arise in the perianal region of homosexual males. Screening methods presently employed for anal intraepithelial neoplasia, a precursor for anal cancer, combine anal Papanicolaou cytology and high-resolution anoscopy with biopsy of suspicious lesions. Significant barriers to establishing anal cancer screening programs include the small number of healthcare professionals who perform high-resolution anoscopy and the lack of data showing that anal cancer screening can reduce morbidity and mortality related to anal carcinoma. The rising incidence of this disease in some groups supports routine screening programs in high-risk populations, especially in HIV-positive men who have sex with men. Currently, it is recognized that there is an HPV-related and an HPV-independent pathway to developing SCCs in the anus and vulva. Most precursor lesions and SCCs in the anus and vulva are high-risk HPV (HR-HPV) associated, with HPV16 the most common type. Given the morphologic overlap and biologic equivalence of HPV-related preinvasive squamous lesions of the lower anogenital tract, a unified, two-tiered histopathologic nomenclature is now recommended. In contrast, mutations in the *TP53* gene have been associated with HPV-independent vulvar and anal SCCs. Apart from squamous and melanocytic lesions, the differential diagnosis includes extramammary Paget disease, a nonsquamous intraepithelial lesion of the vulva and anus that may be a primary epidermotropic apocrine neoplasm or may represent secondary involvement by a synchronous/metachronous adenocarcinoma.[264]

Tumor-like Conditions

Condyloma Acuminatum

HPV causes substantial disease in men, including benign and malignant lesions of the external genitalia. Condyloma, or genital wart, is a common clinical manifestation of nononcogenic genital HPV infection. These benign epithelial lesions are highly infectious and occur most frequently among men 25 to 29 years of age. It has been consistently shown that nononcogenic mucosal HPV types 6/11 are detected in 75% to 100% of condylomas, and that one-half are coinfected with oncogenic mucosal HPV types, particularly HPV16.[265-270]

Most condylomas are transmitted sexually. Men whose sexual partners have HPV-related cervical lesions have an increased (50% to 85%) incidence of penile condyloma.[270] When genital condyloma occurs in children, sexual abuse should be suspected.[271] After the initial infection, autoinfection is common. The incubation period for penile condyloma varies from several weeks to months or even years.[272] Condyloma is most often located on the corona of the glans, the penile meatus, or the fossa navicularis

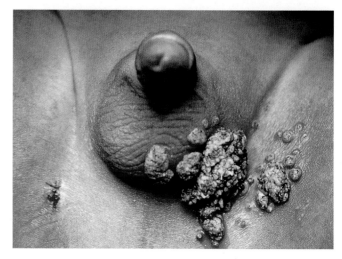

Fig. 15.24 Condylomata acuminata. *(Courtesy of Dr. Julian Wan, State University of New York, Buffalo, New York)*

urethrae, but it also occurs on the scrotal skin and perineum (Fig. 15.24).[272] Condyloma may be flat, delicately papillary, or warty and cauliflower-like. Histologically it consists of a proliferation of squamous epithelium with an acanthotic and papillomatous architecture, showing orderly epithelial maturation (Fig. 15.25A). Hyperkeratosis, parakeratosis, and koilocytic atypia are common (Fig. 15.25B).[273] Although cytologic atypia is usually minimal in penile condyloma and mitotic figures are confined to the basal layer, treatment with podophyllin or lasers may cause bizarre cytologic changes that mimic malignancy.[274] To avoid an erroneous diagnosis of carcinoma, information should be obtained regarding treatment. HPV can be demonstrated in condyloma by in situ hybridization or immunohistochemistry.[275-278] HPVs 6 and 11 are common in typical condyloma without dysplasia, whereas HPVs 16, 18, 31, and 33 are common in dysplastic condyloma.[265-267,269,270,275-279] Less invasive methods such as swabbing the surface of a genital lesion to obtain a sample for HPV DNA testing have been investigated but may not represent HPV types present in lesional tissue. Anic et al. examined the concordance of HPV types detected in swab and biopsy samples from 165 genital lesions in men between the ages of 18 and 70 years.[276] Lesions included 90 condyloma, 10 penile intraepithelial neoplasia (PeIN), 23 noncondyloma with a known histology, and 42 lesions with an undetermined histology. Both sampling methods showed high agreement for HPV DNA detection in condyloma (87.8%) and PeIN (100%). There was also high concordance for detection of HR-HPV genotypes 16 and 18 in PeIN; however, agreement was low to moderate for detecting low-risk HPV (LR-HPV) genotypes 6 and 11 in condyloma. Low to moderate agreement was also observed between sampling methods for detecting individual HPV types in the noncondyloma and lesions with an indefinite histology. These findings indicate that obtaining a biopsy in addition to swabbing the surface of a lesion provides additional significant data about specific HVP types associated with male genital lesions.

Although condyloma may regress spontaneously, it persists in approximately 50% of patients. The lesion is usually treated with topical podophyllin or laser and, in most cases, responds to treatment. The excision of HPV-induced anogenital lesions using carbon dioxide laser remains an efficient treatment, even if it needs to be repeated because lesions recur or persist.[280] The relationship of HPV infection to carcinogenesis is discussed later in this chapter.

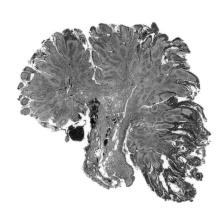
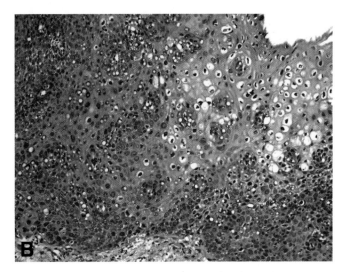

Fig. 15.25 (A) Condyloma acuminatum with marked papillomatosis and hyperkeratosis. (B) Condyloma acuminatum with koilocytic atypia.

Videodermatoscopy (VD) is a noninvasive technique that has greatly improved the diagnostic accuracy for pigmented and non-pigmented skin disorders. Micali and Lacarrubba studied selected cases of penile growths to identify specific VD patterns.[281] Pearly penile papules, Fordyce spots, genital warts, molluscum contagiosum, angiokeratoma of Fordyce, and median raphe penile cysts showed specific VD features. VD may enhance diagnostic accuracy and aids in the differential diagnosis of selected infectious and non-infectious penile growths. In single or clinically nonspecific lesions, VD allows noninvasive recognition of specific patterns and features to make a more definitive diagnosis and rule out clinically similar growths, thus avoiding biopsy and other invasive measures in some cases.[281]

Pearly Penile Papules

Pearly penile papules, also called *hirsutoid papillomas*, are common penile lesions without clinical significance that are present in approximately 10% to 20% of males.[282] These lesions are thought to be embryologic remnants of an organ that is well developed in other mammals. Pearly penile papules are typically 1 to 3 mm in diameter. They appear as yellow-white papules on the corona or, rarely, on the frenulum of the penis.[283] The individual lesions are domelike and are usually arranged in rows. Histologically, they show epithelial thickening covering a central fibrovascular core resembling angiofibroma, and lack they glandular elements. The differential diagnosis includes condyloma acuminata, Tyson glands, or molluscum contagiosum. These lesions do not demonstrate the presence of HPV, and there is no association between condyloma and the presence of pearly penile papules. Unlike Tyson glands, which are modified sebaceous glands in a parafrenular distribution, these papules are not predominantly parafrenular and have no glandular component. Molluscum contagiosum lesions can be distinguished clinically from pearly penile papules based on their umbilicated appearance, their larger size, and their characteristic inclusion bodies.[283] Two cases of sebaceous gland hyperplasia of foreskin manifested as penile papular lesions with centrally umbilicated features resembling molluscum contagiosum.[284]

These lesions can cause psychological issues that may warrant treatment. Current treatment options include cryotherapy, electro-dessication, and curettage. However, these modalities may have considerable adverse cosmetic effects, including scarring, pain, and pigmentary changes. Laser treatment offers an advantage for improved cosmetic outcome in treatment but is not routinely used.[285]

Penile Cysts

Epidermal cyst is the most common cystic lesion of the penis and usually occurs on the penile shaft. It varies in size from 0.1 to 1 cm in diameter.[286,287] A penile epidermal inclusion cyst in adult men is rare. It can develop after an inadequate procedure for penile girth enhancement and should be treated by complete resection.[288]

Mucoid cyst of the penis arises from ectopic urethral mucosa.[289,290] It is lined by stratified columnar epithelium with mucous cells and is filled with mucoid material. Usually located on the prepuce or the glans, most are unilocular and range from 0.2 to 2 cm in diameter. Median raphe cyst arises during embryogenesis from incomplete closure of the genital fold. This cyst is lined by pseudostratified columnar epithelium and may be unilocular or multilocular.[286,291-293]

Pseudoepitheliomatous Keratotic and Micaceous Balanitis

The rare lesion pseudoepitheliomatous keratotic and micaceous balanitis primarily affects elderly, uncircumcised men. The foreskin often becomes phimotic, and a solitary, well-circumscribed, hyperkeratotic lesion develop on the glans with a laminated (micaceous) appearance.[294] It was first described by Lortat-Jacob and Civatte as a rare scaling, raised lesion of the glans penis characterized by acanthosis, hyperkeratosis, and pseudoepitheliomatous hyperplasia.[295] Pseudoepitheliomatous keratotic and micaceous balanitis often recurs and may be a precursor of verrucous carcinoma.

Verruciform Xanthoma

Verruciform xanthoma is a warty lesion characterized by acanthosis, hyperkeratosis, parakeratosis, and long rete ridges associated with a neutrophilic infiltrate. A variable (often prominent) xanthomatous infiltrate occupies the dermis between the rete ridges (Fig. 15.26). This lesion is usually solitary and arises in the oral cavity; only a few genital lesions have been described (scrotal, penile, and vulvar areas). Despite the architectural resemblance of verruciform xanthoma to other verruciform mucocutaneous lesions of the penis related to HPV infection, this lesion is most likely not an

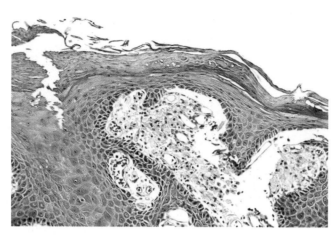

Fig. 15.26 Verruciform xanthoma with infiltrate of foamy histiocytes in dermal papillae.

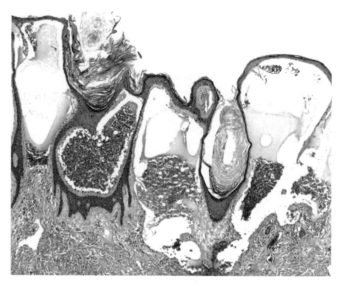

Fig. 15.27 Angiokeratoma with dilated vascular channels.

HPV-associated penile lesion.[296] Furthermore, it can simulate a HPV viral lesion such as condyloma and malignant neoplasia such as verrucous SCC. Therefore an accurate diagnosis is important to avoid overtreatment, considering it is a benign lesion that does not require any radical treatment.[297] The xanthoma cells have been reported to be weakly and focally positive for CK, CD68, and factor XIIIa but negative for S100 protein and HPV immunostains. Mohsin et al. postulated that the xanthoma (foam) cells, a histologic hallmark of the lesion, are possibly derived from dermal dendritic cells.[298]

A recent case report documents the occurrence of multiple, coexisting verruciform xanthomas of the anogenital region in the setting of cutaneous trauma. The etiology and pathogenesis of verruciform xanthoma have yet to be determined; however, recent literature reported that multifocal cutaneous verruciform xanthomas are frequently associated with preexisting inflammatory processes. A significant number of verruciform xanthomas of the skin coexist with cutaneous disorders, including graft-versus-host disease, discoid lupus erythematosus, pemphigus vulgaris, and recessive dystrophic epidermolysis bullosa. Therefore Cumberland et al. speculate that severe cutaneous trauma and chronic inflammation may induce epithelial keratinocytes to respond aberrantly, leading to epidermal hyperplasia and foamy cell formation characterizing the verruciform xanthoma lesion.[299]

Neoplastic Diseases

Benign Neoplasms

Benign tumors of epithelial origin are rare, and squamous papilloma and syringoma have been described.[300,301] Among the benign soft tissue tumors of the glans penis, tumors of vascular origin, including capillary or cavernous hemangioma, pyogenic granuloma (lobular hemangioma), epithelioid hemangioma, and lymphangioma, are the most common.[302-306] These are followed by neurofibroma, traumatic neuroma, schwannoma, leiomyoma, glomus tumor, multiple glomangiomas, fibrous histiocytoma, neurothekeoma, myofibroma, and granular cell tumor.[288,302-314] Epithelioid hemangioma can demonstrate exuberant proliferation and is often confused with epithelioid hemangioendothelioma and epithelioid angiosarcoma.[315] Several cases of juvenile xanthogranuloma have been reported. Awareness of these lesions in the differential diagnosis of penile masses presenting in early childhood is important to avoid

potentially unnecessary ablative genital surgery. Careful assessment also should be made for any systemic involvement and for associated pathologies.[316]

Benign soft tissue tumors are more often located on the distal part, whereas malignant lesions are more common on the proximal shaft. Angiokeratoma is a distinctive, asymptomatic, well-circumscribed, benign vascular lesion with red or blue papules but is not considered to be a true neoplasm.[317,318] This lesion characteristically involves the scrotum, but it may involve the penis. Morphologically, this lesion reveals superficial vascular ectasia with overlying warty epidermal changes (Fig. 15.27). The four clinical types are: (1) angiokeratoma corporis diffusum in association with Fabry disease, in which multiple angiokeratomas appear late in childhood; (2) angiokeratoma of Mibelli, in which bilateral angiokeratomas are found on the dorsum of fingers and toes; (3) angiokeratoma of Fordyce, in which angiokeratoma characteristically occurs on the scrotum, with rare occurrence on the shaft or glans penis (one recent case report documented the occurrence of angiokeratoma of Fordyce after penile carcinoma and thus raising a differential diagnosis of recurrent squamous carcinoma); and (4) solitary angiokeratoma.[319,320]

Another recently described lesion, myointimoma (myointimal proliferation), involves the corpus spongiosum of the glans penis.[321,322] Patients range in age from 2 to 61 years (mean age, 29 years) and present with a mass that varies in size from 0.5 to 1.9 cm in greatest dimension. The lesion is present from 4 days to more than 6 months before surgical intervention. Microscopically, a prominent, often occlusive, fibrointimal proliferation is seen, with plexiform architecture involving the vasculature of the corpus spongiosum. The proliferation consists of stellate-shaped and spindled cells embedded in abundant fibromyxoid matrix. Occasional lesional cells have well-developed myoid characteristics with moderately abundant eosinophilic cytoplasm, blunt-ended nuclei, and juxtanuclear vacuoles. Foci with degenerative changes, including ghost cell morphology, are also present. The myointimal process is extensively immunoreactive for SMA, muscle-specific actin (HHF-35), and calponin, but it is minimally reactive for desmin. The myointimal cells are nonreactive for CD34, S100 protein, and keratin. Factor VIII antigen, CD31, and CD34 highlight intact endothelial cells lining suboccluded vessels, scattered capillaries that penetrate the proliferation, and normal uninvolved vasculature. The lesion is benign without evidence of metastasis.

Myofibroma, late-stage intravascular (nodular) fasciitis, vascular leiomyoma, and plexiform fibrohistiocytic tumor are potential differential diagnoses.

Benign melanocytic lesions such as melanocytic nevi, melanosis, and lentiginous melanosis also occur on the penis.[323] These lesions preexist or coexist with penile melanoma.

Premalignant Lesions of the Penis

Premalignant lesions of the penis can be difficult to distinguish from other benign dermatoses and have an uncertain natural history. A tendency for delayed presentation, often with a history of long-term self-management or unsuccessful treatment, can result in progression to invasive carcinoma, requiring more extensive surgery. Accurate early diagnosis and treatment before invasion provides the best approach to the management of these lesions. One of the major areas of confusion in the nomenclature of penile lesions is the terminology of premalignant epithelial proliferations. The terms *erythroplasia of Queyrat*, *Bowen disease*, and *bowenoid papulosis* were used in the past to describe lesions that are histologically similar but may have different clinical presentations and biologic behaviors (Table 15.3).[93,324,325] A series of studies have consistently provided data that support replacement of these older terms by newer terminologies such as PeIN or carcinoma in situ.[326-332] Over the past two decades, the studies of Cubilla et al. and Chaux and associates have established that there are two groups of precancerous and invasive carcinomas (typical squamous carcinoma and the warty-basaloid carcinoma), consistent with the bimodal hypothesis of the existence of non–HPV-related (typical squamous), differentiated PeINs and HPV-related (warty, basaloid, and mixed warty-basaloid), undifferentiated PeINs.[326,330]

Premalignant penile lesions can be broadly divided into those related to HPV infection and those not HPV related but caused by chronic inflammation. HPV-related lesions include Bowen disease, erythroplasia of Queyrat, and bowenoid papulosis, which are associated with HR-HPV types 16 and 18. LR-HPV types 6 and 11 are associated with other premalignant lesions, such as giant condylomata Buschke-Lowenstein tumors. Another report stated that HPVs 6 and 11 are the most prevalent genotypes for penile HPV-associated lesions, with HR-HPV types in high-grade PeIN and LR-HPV types in low-grade PeIN.[331]

Non–HPV-related lesions are primarily linked to genital lichen sclerosus and lichen planus. However, they are also associated with rarer chronic inflammatory conditions such as penile cutaneous horn, leukoplakia, and pseudoepitheliomatous hyperplasia, keratotic, and micaceous balanitis. Unlike HPV-related tumors, progression of these premalignant lesions is largely to keratinizing or verrucous SCCs.[332]

A heterogeneous spectrum of epithelial alterations and atypical lesions affecting the squamous epithelium of penile mucosal anatomic compartments was documented in 2004.[326] It was reported that squamous hyperplasia was more commonly associated with usual squamous, papillary, and verrucous carcinomas than with warty and basaloid invasive carcinomas (Fig. 15.28). LSIL was associated with all types of SCCs but was rarely present adjacent to basaloid or verrucous tumors. High-grade squamous intraepithelial lesion (HSIL) was present in two-thirds of invasive warty, basaloid, and mixed warty-basaloid tumors, in about one-half of usual SCCs, and was absent in papillary and verrucous carcinomas. There was definitive correlation of special types of invasive carcinomas with subtypes of dysplasia (squamous intraepithelial lesion) based on the morphologic correspondence of invasive tumor and the associated intraepithelial lesion. LSIL was preferentially associated with verrucous, papillary, and usual

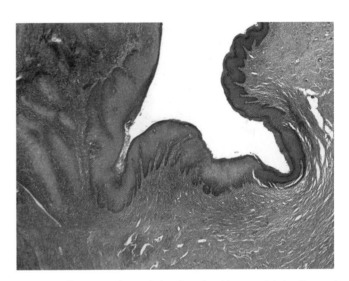

Fig. 15.28 Squamous hyperplasia of penile skin associated with usual invasive squamous cell carcinoma (on the left).

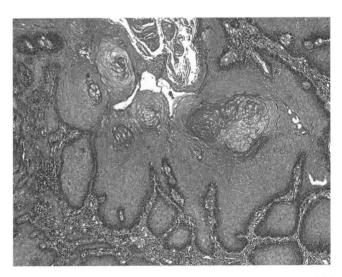

Fig. 15.29 Low-grade squamous intraepithelial lesion with superficial koilocytic changes associated with usual squamous cell carcinoma.

TABLE 15.3	Histologic Risk Groups for Penile Cancers		
Low-Risk Group	**Intermediate-Risk Group**	**High-Risk Group**	
Usual, grade I	Usual, grade II	Usual, grade III	
Verrucous carcinoma	Warty (condylomatous)	Basaloid	
Papillary, not otherwise specified	Mixed	Warty-basaloid	
Pseudohyperplastic		Papillary-basaloid	
Cuniculatum		Sarcomatoid carcinoma	

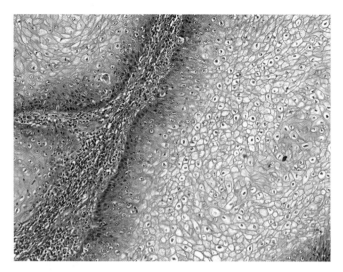

Fig. 15.30 Warty low-grade squamous intraepithelial lesion with prominent koilocytic features usually seen in association with warty or warty-basaloid carcinomas of the penis.

SCCs (Fig. 15.29), and warty LSIL with invasive warty and mixed warty-basaloid carcinomas (Fig. 15.30). Differentiated HSIL was frequently found in SCCs of usual type but was rarely present with warty or basaloid carcinomas (Fig. 15.31A). Basaloid HSIL was associated with basaloid carcinoma (Fig. 15.31B), and HSIL of warty type with either warty or mixed warty-basaloid carcinomas.

Chaux et al. also described and classified precursor conditions as PeIN, and these lesions were classified into two major groups: differentiated and undifferentiated (Fig. 15.32).[333] The latter was further divided in warty, basaloid, and warty-basaloid subtypes. Among 121 patients, 95 were associated with invasive SCCs. Differentiated lesions predominated (68%), followed by warty-basaloid (14%), basaloid (11%), and warty (7%) subtypes. Multifocality was found in 15% of the patients. Differentiated lesions were preferentially located in the foreskin, whereas warty and basaloid subtypes were more prevalent in the glans. The former lesions were preferentially seen in association with keratinizing

variants of SCC, whereas the latter subtypes were found mostly in conjunction with invasive warty, basaloid, and warty-basaloid carcinomas. Balanitis xerotica obliterans was present in 51% of differentiated lesions and absent in warty and basaloid subtypes. The authors stated that the proper pathologic characterization of these lesions may provide important clues to the understanding of the pathogenesis and natural history of penile cancer. In addition, they reported that p16, Ki67, and p53 immunostains are useful to identify differentiated PeIN versus undifferentiated PeIN or squamous hyperplasia, with squamous hyperplasia being negative for p16 and p53 and having variable Ki67 positivity; differentiated PeIN being negative for p16 and positive for Ki67, with variable p53 positivity; and undifferentiated (basaloid and warty) PeIN being consistently positive for p16 and Ki67, with variable p53 positivity.[334]

Cubilla et al. reported that p16^{INK4a} overexpression was found to be a reliable marker for HR-HPV and a helpful tool in the differential diagnosis of low-grade verruciform and high-grade solid penile tumors.[335] SCC variants depicting basaloid features were more likely to be positive for HPV and p16^{INK4a} than low-grade, keratinizing lesions. They also observed a tendency toward HPV positivity in high-grade nonbasaloid tumors. Chaux et al.,[336] in their study of 141 cases, reported a sensitivity rate of 82% p16 positivity for discriminating types of PeIN, with a specificity of 100% and an accuracy of 95%. Balanitis xerotica obliterans was identified in 42 cases, and their epithelial component was p16$^-$ in all cases. These studies convincingly elucidated that p16 overexpression is a valuable tool for discriminating differentiated from warty, basaloid, and warty-basaloid PeINs. Their results indicated concordance between HPV and p16^{INK4a} status, and this observation may have diagnostic and prognostic implications.[335,336]

There appears to be a distinctive distribution of penile precursor lesions depending on the geographic region in consideration. PeIN with warty and/or basaloid features predominated in low-incidence areas, whereas differentiated PeIN was more prevalent in regions endemic for penile cancers.[337] Similar results have been reported from the study of various precancerous and cancerous lesions exclusively affecting the foreskin in a region of high penile cancer incidence. The frequent coexistence of balanitis xerotica obliterans, squamous hyperplasia, differentiated PeIN, and low-grade SCC suggests a common non–HPV-related

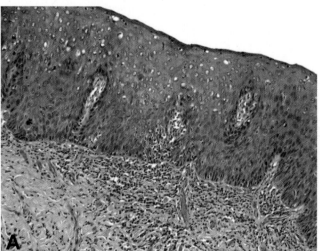

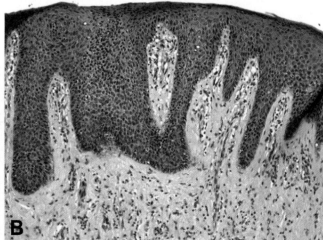

Fig. 15.31 (A) High-grade squamous intraepithelial lesion (HSIL) with surface koilocytosis, increased mitotic activity, and significant nuclear atypia seen adjacent to usual invasive squamous cell carcinoma. (B) Basaloid HSIL with characteristic morphology encountered frequently in cases of invasive basaloid penile carcinomas.

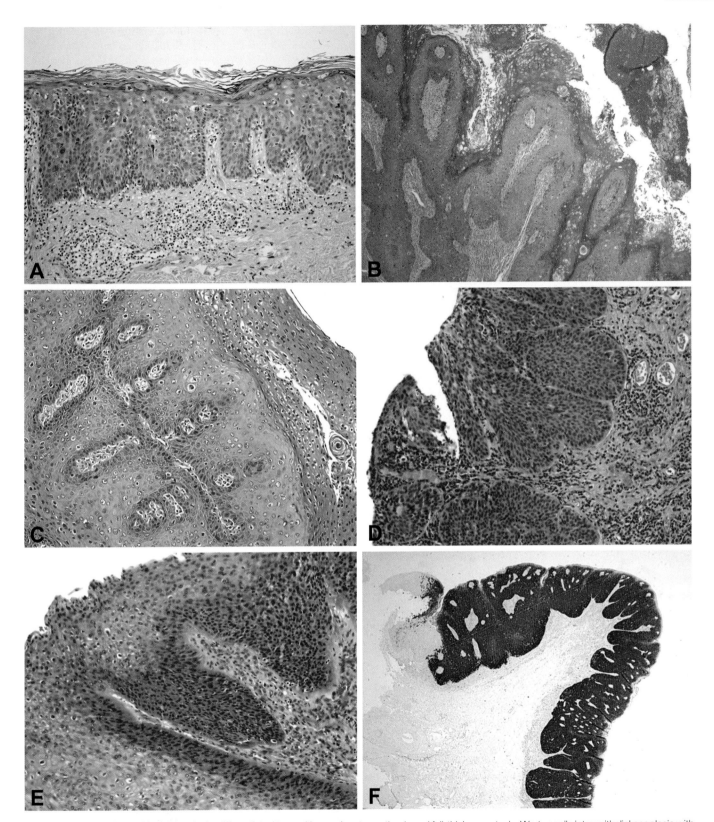

Fig. 15.32 (A) Penile intraepithelial neoplasia, differentiated type with prominent acanthosis and full-thickness atypia. Warty penile intraepithelial neoplasia with parakeratosis and koilocytic changes in the papillomatous epithelium (B and C). (D) Basaloid penile intraepithelial neoplasia with a monotonous population of amphophilic or basophilic epithelial cells with scant cytoplasm. (E) Warty-basaloid penile intraepithelial neoplasia lined by hyperchromatic basaloid-type cells in the basal and parabasal layers, with clear, koilocytic-type cells on the surface. (F) Strong and diffuse block positivity pattern of p16 immunohistochemical staining in basaloid penile intraepithelial neoplasia.

pathogenic pathway for preputial lesions and highlights the importance of circumcision in symptomatic patients for the prevention of penile cancer.[338]

Many different options and treatment modalities are available for premalignant penile lesions. The choice of treatment should be tailored to the type and site of the lesion, considering patient preference and likely compliance with treatment regimens and the need for close follow-up with the more minimally invasive techniques. Available treatment modalities include: (1) topical chemotherapy and immunotherapy (5-fluorouracil and imiquimod); (2) laser (carbon dioxide or neodymium-doped yttrium aluminum garnet [Nd:YAG]); (3) cryotherapy; (4) photodynamic therapy; and (5) surgical excision with glans resurfacing (partial or total), circumcision, or Mohs micrographic surgery.[331,339] The precise follow-up procedure after treatment for premalignant penile lesions is unclear. Although it largely depends on the type of lesion and treatment modality used, a logical and standardized protocol for follow-up should be used, especially given the uncertain natural history, the risk for malignant transformation in up to 30% of patients, and the risk for recurrence in up to 30% after certain treatment modalities. Patients should be seen every 3 months for the first 2 years, reducing to every 6 months for at least 5 years of follow-up, although lifelong follow-up would give a better insight into the natural course of this rare condition.[331]

Malignant Neoplasms

Cancer of the penis is uncommon, affecting approximately 1 in 100,000 men and accounting for less than 0.5% of all neoplasms in men in North America and Europe.[340,341] As per the American Cancer Society, it is estimated that 2320 patients would experience development of penile cancer in 2018, leading to 380 deaths caused by this disease.[342] The total number of penile cancers globally has been estimated to be 26,000 cases per year.[341] The incidence is much higher in some areas of Asia, Africa, and South America compared with Western Europe and North America, partly due to differences in socioeconomic conditions and religious practices. The highest incidence rate of penile cancer is reported from Brazil, where an epidemiologic study reported an incidence between 2.9 and 6.8 per 100,000, predominantly affecting low-income and uncircumcised men. Uganda has the second highest reported incidence of penile cancer in the world. In the United States, the incidence of penile cancer between the years 1993 and 2002 has been estimated at 0.58 per 100,000, with Hispanics having the highest incidence, followed by Alaskan Native Americans and African Americans. In recent years the incidence of penile cancer has been steadily decreasing because of several factors, including improved hygiene, neonatal circumcision, increased condom use, smoking cessation, and expanding HPV vaccination programs for both sexes.[343-346] Worldwide, more than 95% of cases of penile cancer are SCC, with sarcoma accounting for most of the remaining 4% to 5%. Rarely, other cancers such as melanoma and basal cell carcinoma arise in the penis. Urothelial carcinoma usually arises in the penile urethra (see Chapter 9).

Squamous Cell Carcinoma

Risk factors for SCC of the penis include HPV status, lack of circumcision, poor hygiene, phimosis, tobacco use, penile trauma, and psoralen and ultraviolet A radiation therapy.[73,74,83-85,340,341,344,347-350] SCC is extremely unusual among individuals who were circumcised in infancy; for example, it is rare among Jews

and Nigerians who practice circumcision shortly after birth.[349,351] Circumcision in late childhood or adolescence seems to confer partial protection.[352-354] Although the data indicate that circumcision at birth provides excellent protection, it appears that equally low incidence rates can be achieved in uncircumcised males who practice good hygiene. The very low rate of penile carcinoma in Northern European countries, where males are not circumcised but where good hygiene is practiced, supports this conclusion.[355] Almost 50% of patients with penile carcinoma also have phimosis.[356]

Like head and neck and lower anogenital tract cancers, penile carcinomas are considered to develop through two carcinogenic pathways: a non–HPV-related pathway and an HPV-related pathway. The overall prevalence rate of HPV in penile cancer ranges from 33% to 63%, with HPV being more prevalent in developed countries.[357-366] It has been proposed that there are two separate pathways of penile carcinogenesis that exhibit differing histologic features.[327,328] The current WHO histologic classification of penile carcinoma supports this dual-pathway theory and separates invasive neoplasia into HPV related and non-HPV related.[367,368] In the HPV-associated group, tumors with warty or basaloid morphology predominate, and the non–HPV-associated group is composed of more differentiated keratinizing variants of SCCs and sarcomatoid carcinomas. Sanchez et al. evaluated data from several studies and found that there was a correlation between tumor types and incidence of nodal metastasis and survival.[367] They further classified these penile tumors according to their behavior into three groups—low, intermediate, and high—with differing risks for regional tumor spread and mortality risk. The various subtypes are categorized as listed in Table 15.3. PeIN is often found adjacent to invasive carcinomas and often demonstrates similar morphology in both the in situ and invasive components. The nomenclature of PeIN, subclassified into differentiated and warty-basaloid subtypes, has been adopted in the WHO classification of urologic malignancies.[329,368,369]

Currently, there are relatively fewer reports of HPV in penile precancerous lesions, and they do not address the subtypes of PeIN.[279,331,360,370-374] There are also some lesions that can be found in association with penile cancer where a causal relation is not well defined, like squamous hyperplasia and condylomas, and information regarding HPV status is limited. Penile neoplastic lesions are often complex with multiple lesional areas and different histologic patterns. Alemany et al. reported that HPV-related and non–HPV-related lesions can be found in the same case, and multiple HPV genotypes are found in 18% and 9% of whole-tissue sections of precancerous and cancerous lesions, respectively.[363] When HPV detection is based on the presence of HPV DNA or RNA in whole-tissue sections, it is impossible to decide the true association of individual lesions with HPV. p16[INK4a] has been used as a marker for HR-HPV genotypes 18 and 19 and generally supports the idea of multiple pathways, but its expression is not specific for HPV carcinogenesis and is positive only in HR-HPV and absent in neoplasia associated with LR-HPV.

In a recently published study, Fernandez-Nestosa and colleagues reported the use of laser capture microdissection-polymerase chain reaction (LCM-PCR) supported by p16[INK4a] staining to demonstrate HPV DNA in penile lesions, including squamous hyperplasia, flat lesions, condylomas, PeIN, and invasive SCCs.[364] HPV was detected in both whole-tissue sections and LCM-PCR. LCM was demonstrated as a more precise technique than whole-tissue section analysis in assigning individual genotypes to specific lesions. HPV was negative or very infrequently detected in squamous hyperplasia, differentiated PeIN, and low-grade keratinizing variants of squamous carcinomas. HPV positivity was strongly associated with condylomas, warty-basaloid PeIN, adjacent flat lesions, and warty-basaloid carcinomas. A single HPV genotype was found in each lesion. Some condylomas and flat lesions, especially those with atypia, were preferentially associated with HR-HPV. Eighteen HPV genotypes were detected in PeIN, usually HPV 16 in basaloid PeIN, but marked HPV heterogeneity in warty PeIN with 11 different genotypes. Variable and multiple HPV genotypes were identified in multicentric PeIN, whereas unifocal PeIN was usually associated with a single genotype. There was a correspondence among HPV genotypes in invasive carcinoma and associated PeIN. p16^{INK4a} was positive in most HPV-positive lesions except condylomas containing LR-HPV. p16 staining was usually negative in squamous hyperplasia, differentiated PeIN, and low-grade keratinizing variants of SCCs. The heterogeneity of HPV genotypes in PeIN and the differential association of HPV genotypes with subtypes of PeIN were notably highlighted in this study. The presence of atypia and HR-HPV in condylomas and adjacent flat lesions implies a precursor role, and the correspondence of HPV genotypes in invasive carcinomas and associated PeIN indicates a causal relationship with HPV.

Balanitis xerotica obliterans, porokeratosis, and lichen planus are appreciated as possible risk factors for penile carcinoma in HPV-negative SCC.[372,375] In addition, ultraviolet radiation also may contribute to SCC of the penis and scrotum, according to studies of patients with psoriasis who have been treated with oral 8-methoxy-psoralen and ultraviolet A phototherapy or ultraviolet B.[376]

Penile carcinoma usually occurs in older men.[248,347,371,377,378] Patient age at diagnosis ranges from 20 to 90 years, but it rarely affects men younger than 40 years.[378,379] This may be changing, however. In a 1992 study from the United States, 22% of the patients were younger than 40 years, and 7% were younger than 30 years.[378]

Patients usually have an exophytic or ulcerated mass. Penile pain, discharge, difficulty in voiding, and lymphadenopathy are manifesting symptoms.[340-342,344,347-349] Autoamputation of the penis has been reported, even in this era of advanced medical care, as signs and symptoms are ignored resulting in autoamputation.[380] The majority arise in the glans or the prepuce, and primarily involve the penile shaft and urethral meatus (Table 15.4).[340-342,344,347-349,371,377-379]

The two main types of penile carcinoma are the fungating or exophytic type and the ulcerating or infiltrating type (Figs. 15.33 and 15.34). No unique grading system exists for penile SCC; the grading system for cutaneous SCC is used. In the modified Broders grading system (Table 15.5), the degree of keratinization is the most important feature.[381] Most SCCs are

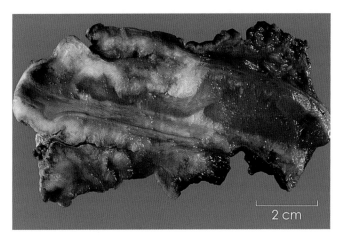

Fig. 15.33 Squamous cell carcinoma of penis. The glans and prepuce are eroded and replaced by a fungating mass, which invades the corpus cavernosum (sagittal section in plane of urethra).

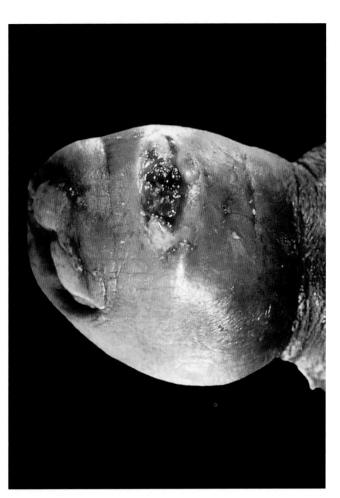

Fig. 15.34 Squamous cell carcinoma of the penis has eroded through the foreskin of this uncircumcised penis.

TABLE 15.4	Primary Sites of Squamous Carcinoma of the Penis	
Site(s)	Frequency (%)
Glans	48
Prepuce	21
Glans, prepuce, and shaft	14
Glans and prepuce	9
Coronal sulcus	6
Shaft	2

low grade at the time of biopsy. Well-differentiated SCC consists of finger-like downward projections of atypical squamous cells that originate from a thickened, hyperkeratotic, papillomatous epidermis (Fig. 15.35). These projections often resemble nests of cells within the dermis. Concentrically arranged masses of cells often surround accumulations of anucleated keratin known as *keratin*

TABLE 15.5 Grading of Squamous Carcinoma (Modified Broders System)

Grade	Differentiation	Histologic Features
1	Well	Prominent intercellular bridges Prominent keratin pearl formation Minimal cytologic atypia Rare mitotic figures
2/3	Moderately	Occasional intercellular bridges Fewer keratin pearls Increased mitotic activity Moderate nuclear atypia
4	Poorly	Marked nuclear pleomorphism Numerous mitotic figures Necrosis No keratin pearls

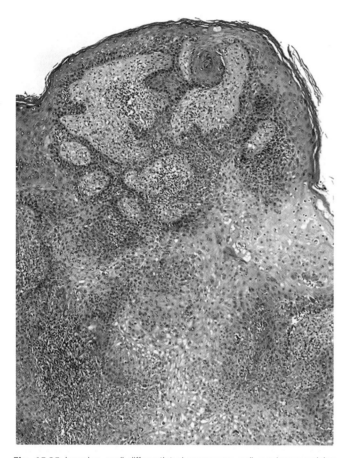

Fig. 15.35 Invasive, well-differentiated squamous cell carcinoma arising from downward projections of atypical squamous cells from a thickened, hyperkeratotic, papillomatous epidermis.

pearls (Fig. 15.36A). These represent a disorganized attempt by the malignant cells to undergo differentiation. Intercellular bridges often are prominent (Fig. 15.36B). Well-differentiated (grade 1) cancer has limited atypia, consisting of nuclear enlargement and pleomorphism and the presence of one or more large nucleoli. Mitotic figures usually can be found but are rare. Individual cells may be dyskeratotic with deeply eosinophilic cytoplasm. The dermis along the tumor margin usually contains a dense lymphocytic

or mixed inflammatory infiltrate. Poorly differentiated SCC (grade 3) lacks evidence of keratinization and forms few or no keratin pearls (Fig. 15.37), but it has marked nuclear pleomorphism and hyperchromasia and may have areas of necrosis and superinfection. Mitotic figures are usually numerous, and the cancer is deeply invasive (Fig. 15.38). Moderately differentiated carcinoma (grade 2) shows histologic differentiation intermediate between grades 1 and 3, with moderate nuclear atypia, more mitotic activity, and evidence of keratinization and fewer keratin pearls than grade 1.

Maiche et al. proposed a scoring system for grading SCC of the penis on the basis of four criteria: the degree of keratinization, the number of mitotic figures per high-power field (×400), the degree of nuclear atypia, and the presence of inflammatory cells (Table 15.6).[382] They reported that this grading system was practical and showed a correlation between histologic grade and stage.[382] In their series, stage I and II cancers were grades 1 and 2 more frequently than stage III and IV cancers. The highest proportion of poorly differentiated grade 4 cancer was found in patients with stage IV disease. These authors also found that histologic grade was a valuable prognostic factor. The 5- and 10-year relative survival rates are highest for patients with grade 1 tumors and lowest for those with grade 4 cancers. No significant difference was seen in the survival rates between patients with grade 2 and 3 cancers.[382]

A prognostic index was described for penile cancer based on histologic grade and location. Cancer was categorized as low (scores 1 to 3), intermediate (score 4), and high prognostic index (scores 5 and 6) (Table 15.7). Velazquez et al. demonstrated in their study that tumor grade and perineural invasion are better predictors for lymph node metastases than tumor thickness in penile SCC invading 5 to 10 mm.[383]

Penile cancer spreads superficially through the epithelial mucosal compartment, following the penile fascia, following spaces formed by feeding vessels in the tunica albuginea, by direct vertical invasion, or along the urethral epithelium.[2,384] The urethra and periurethral tissues, including the penile fascia, are common sites of involvement, followed by the corpus spongiosum and corpora cavernosa (Fig. 15.39), and fistula formation may occur.[384] Despite the rich vascularity of the corpus cavernosum, hematogenous spread is uncommon. Infrequent involvement of the corpora cavernosa probably reflects the barrier function of the tunica albuginea.[384] Distant metastasis usually occurs through lymphatics, and the inguinal lymph nodes are generally the first involved. The lymphatics of the penis consist of richly anastomosing channels that cross the midline along the shaft and at the penile base. Therefore metastasis may be to either side or both sides. The number of lymph nodes containing metastases correlates with prognosis.[385] Lymphovascular invasion (LVI) is a strong predictor of lymph node metastasis and subsequent prognosis. It is characterized by the presence of tumor emboli seen within endothelium-lined spaces separated from the primary tumor by at least one high-power field. The presence or absence of LVI is vastly important in prognosis and is therefore listed as a defining criterion for distinguishing category T1b versus T1a primary tumors of the penis, respectively.[386]

Infection of the primary tumor can cause inguinal lymph node enlargement without metastases; therefore sentinel node biopsy is commonly performed to stage the tumor accurately. Because most patients present with clinical stage I or II, controversy exists regarding the role of prophylactic bilateral inguinal node dissection.[387-392] Palpation of the inguinal lymph nodes is 70% to

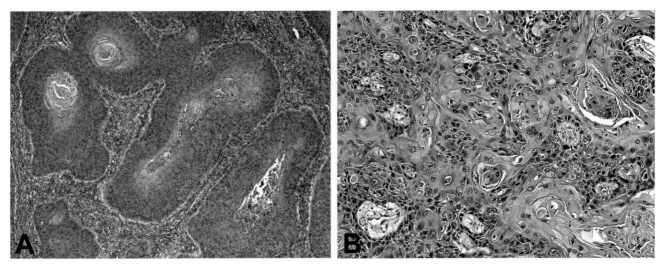

Fig. 15.36 (A) Squamous cell carcinoma forming keratin pearls. (B) Squamous cell carcinoma of penis showing glassy cytoplasm of keratinizing cells.

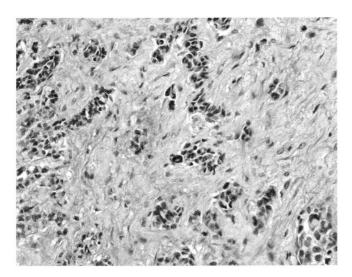

Fig. 15.37 Squamous cell carcinoma infiltrating the penis as small nests of cells.

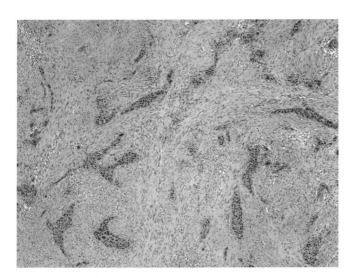

Fig. 15.38 Deeply Invasive poorly differentiated squamous cell carcinoma.

TABLE 15.6	**Histologic Scoring System for Squamous Cell Carcinoma of Penis**

Degree of Keratinization

Points

0	No keratin pearls. Keratin in <25% of cells
1	No keratin pearls. Keratin in 25%-50% of cells
2	Keratin pearls incomplete or keratin in 50%-75% of cells
3	Keratin pearls complete or keratin in >75% of cells

Mitotic Activity

Points

0	≥10 mitotic cells/field
1	6-9 mitotic cells/field
2	3-5 mitotic cells/field
3	0-2 mitotic cells/field

Cellular Atypia

Points

0	All cells atypical
1	Many atypical cells/field
2	Moderate number of atypical cells/field
3	Few atypical cells/field

Inflammatory Cells

Points

| 0 | No inflammatory cells present |
| 1 | Inflammatory cells (lymphocytes) present |

Grading

Grade 1	8-10 points
Grade 2	5-7 points
Grade 3	3-4 points
Grade 4	0-2 points

From Maiche AG, Pyrhonen S, Karkinen M. Histological grading of squamous cell carcinoma of the penis: a grading system. Br J Urol 1991;67:522-526.

85% sensitive and 50% specific for detection of metastases. If clinical evaluation of the groin lymph nodes is delayed several weeks after excision of the primary tumor, the false-positive rate drops to approximately 15%. Bilateral inguinal lymph node dissection (ILND) carries a significant risk for morbidity and mortality; thus many surgeons advocate that inguinal node dissection be performed

TABLE 15.7	Prognostic Index for Squamous Carcinoma of Penis	
NUMERICAL VALUES OF HISTOLOGIC GRADE		
Grade	Value	
I	1	
II	2	
III	3	
NUMERICAL VALUES OF ANATOMIC LEVELS OF INVASION		
Site	Level	Value
Glans	Epithelium	0
	Lamina propria	1
	Corpus spongiosum	2
	Corpora cavernosa	3
Foreskin	Epithelium	0
	Lamina propria	1
	Dartos	2
	Skin	3
Coronal sulcus	Epithelium	0
	Lamina propria	1
	Dartos	2
	Buck fascia	3

From Young RH, Srigley JR, Amin MB, et al. The penis and scrotum. In: Young RH, Srigley JR, Amin MB, Ulbright TM, et al., eds. *Tumors of the prostate gland, seminal vesicles, male urethra, and penis: atlas of tumor pathology.* Washington, DC: Armed Forces Institute of Pathology, 2000.

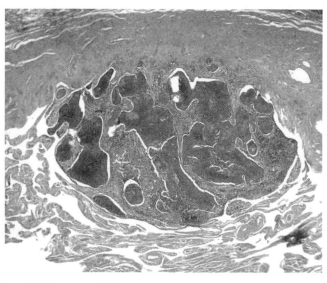

Fig. 15.39 Tumor emboli in corpus cavernosum.

only for patients with palpable lymph nodes several weeks after primary surgery to allow the inflammatory reaction in the nodes to subside. Minimally invasive lymph node staging with accurate localization is significantly helpful in the surgical management of penile SCC. In patients with clinically node-negative disease, there is evidence supporting the employment of sentinel lymph node biopsies. Dynamic sentinel lymph node biopsy confers a minimal risk to the patient and provides enhanced sensitivity and specificity compared with alternate nodal staging techniques. Improvements in inguinal or pelvic lymphadenectomy in the presence of locoregional

disease have notably decreased morbidity rates and improved oncologic outcomes. A multimodality-based treatment approach of chemotherapy and surgery has demonstrated a survival benefit for patients with advanced disease. More robust long-term data on multicenter patient cohorts are required to determine the optimal management of lymph nodes in penile cancer.[388-393] A recent study from the Netherlands on prophylactic pelvic lymph node dissection in penile cancer included 79 chemotherapy-naive patients without preoperative evidence of pelvic disease who were treated with prophylactic pelvic lymph node dissection. Pelvic nodes were positive in 24% of the patients. Inguinal extranodal extension or two or more tumor-positive nodes were predictive of tumor-positive pelvic nodes. The 5-year disease-specific survival rate in patients with pelvic lymph node involvement was 17%.[394]

[18]F-fluorodeoxyglucose positron emission tomography (PET) computed tomography (CT) is a useful staging examination for invasive penile cancer. Souillac et al. assessed inguinal lymph node status in patients with penile cancer using PET scan. In 22 cN0 cases (total of 44 inguinal lymph node basins analyzed), PET had 75% sensitivity and 87.5% specificity.[395] Positive and negative predictive values were 37.5% and 97.2%, respectively. In the eight cN[+] cases (a total of 16 inguinal lymph node basins analyzed), this type of imaging had 100% sensitivity, specificity, and positive predictive value. In three cases staged clinically as cN1, PET imaging revealed several metabolically active lesions on the same side, which was confirmed by histologic examination, upstaging these cases to pN2. These data confirm that PET detects clinical and subclinical inguinal lymph node metastasis.

Cubilla et al. classified penile carcinoma as superficially spreading SCC; vertical growth SCC; verruciform carcinoma (including warty or condylomatous carcinoma); verrucous carcinoma; papillary carcinoma, not otherwise specified; and multicentric carcinoma.[396] Superficially spreading carcinoma occurred most frequently. Inguinal lymph node metastases were found in 82% of patients with vertical growth carcinoma, 42% with superficially spreading carcinoma, and 33% with multicentric carcinoma. Superficial spreading carcinoma usually involves more than one compartment (glans, foreskin, or coronal sulcus), but occasionally is confined to either the glans or foreskin. When vertical growth occurs, invasion of the corpora or skin of the prepuce may occur. Approximately 20% of cases of penile carcinoma display vertical growth, which is characterized by a large, fungating, often ulcerated, whitish gray or hemorrhagic mass.

Exophytic penile carcinoma forms a large polypoid mass. Histologically, most are well-differentiated SCCs, with extensive keratinization and finger-like projections invading the stroma. Ulcerating carcinoma tends to originate on the glans penis, grows invasively, and is usually moderately to poorly differentiated, with a higher incidence of lymph node metastases than the exophytic type. Lesions adjacent to the invasive carcinoma show undifferentiated (or bowenoid) PeIN, defined by full-thickness atypia throughout the epithelium, and differentiated PeIN, characterized by atypia confined to the lower third of the epithelium. Undifferentiated PeIN is always associated with warty (condylomatous), basaloid, or mixed SCC, and differentiated PeIN and squamous hyperplasia are associated with underlying balanitis xerotica obliterans and usual or verrucous SCC.[397]

A high prevalence of cervical cancer–associated high-risk types of HPV has been demonstrated in premalignant and invasive squamous cell lesions of the penis, but large studies correlating histologic characteristics with HPV status are few. Krustrup et al. studied tumor tissues from 145 patients with invasive ($n = 116$) or in situ ($n = 29$) penile SCC by systematic histologic evaluation and PCR tested for 14 HR-HPV types and 23 LR-HPV types.[398] They found approximately 52% of invasive and 90% of in situ lesions were positive for HR-HPV type, of which HPV 16 was by far the predominant type (91% of HR-HPV–positive lesions). In relation to histologic characteristics, HR-HPV positivity was statistically significantly more common in high-grade tumors, lesions dominated by small tumor cells, lesions with a high number of multinucleated cells and mitoses, and lesions with a small amount of parakeratosis.

The extent of penile shaft involvement of SCC, the growth pattern, mean depth of invasion, and LVI correlate with the frequency of lymph node metastases.[399] Patients with tumors of the shaft and those with ulcerating growth have a greater likelihood of metastasis. Inguinal lymph node metastases are frequent in cases with vertical growth and skin involvement.[384] The size of the primary tumor, the grade, and the length of the delay in diagnosis do not correlate with the incidence of lymph node metastasis.[378,385,399] Limitations exist in interpretation of biopsies in patients with penile SCC. Therefore important pathologic prognostic factors cannot depend on biopsy information alone, because this may be insufficient to make a decision whether to perform a groin dissection or to predict those patients in whom other treatment modalities should be considered.[400]

With a diagnosis of SCC of the penis, a significant need still exists to define the tumor criteria that allow the disease to be stratified according to the risk for development of lymph node metastases. To answer this question, the histopathology of the primary tumor in 72 consecutive patients with resected SCC of the penis was reviewed by Alkatout et al. Tumor tissue was reviewed for histologic grade, invasion pattern, tumor stage, proportion of poorly differentiated tumor cells, invasion depth, proportion of tumor necrosis, LVI, histologic classification, number of lesions, growth pattern, number of mitoses, degree of keratinization, and clinical groin status.[401] They found that the presence of inguinal lymph node metastases correlated in descending order of frequency with grade G2 or G3, clinically positive groin status, reticular invasion, stage pT2 or T3, more than 50% poorly differentiated tumor cells, depth of invasion, and comedo-like tumor necrosis. These results revealed that the risk for inguinal lymph node metastasis in penile carcinoma can be predicted on the basis of three major factors: histologic grade, pattern of invasion, and clinical groin status.[401] A similar result was reported from Chinese patients, with histopathologic classification, pathologic tumor stage, and depth of invasion of the primary lesion being significant predictors of regional lymph node metastasis.[402]

Protzel et al. reported that all patients with decreased or negative expression of metastasis suppressor protein KAI1 (kang ai 1)/cluster of differentiation 82 (KAI1/CD82) in penile carcinoma had lymph node metastases.[403] In contrast, patients with positive KAI1/CD82 expression showed better survival. The presence of HPV DNA was associated with decreased or negative KAI1/CD82 expression. Absent or decreased expression of metastasis suppressor gene KAI1/CD82 appears to be a prognostic parameter for the occurrence of lymph node metastases in penile cancers.

D2-40 (podoplanin) immunohistochemical expression was investigated by Minardi et al. in tissue specimens from 39 patients with SCC of the penis who underwent partial or total penectomy between 1987 and 2008.[404] They found that intratumoral lymphatic vessel density greater than 2.0 units had 83.3% sensitivity and 78% specificity in predicting lymph node metastasis. Analysis of cell immunoreactivity showed cytoplasmic D2-40 positivity in intratumoral and normal tissue in 89.7% and 65.5% of patients,

respectively. A strong correlation emerged between grade of cell differentiation and D2-40 immunoreactivity in intratumoral tissue; 88.9% of tumors with weak podoplanin expression were G1, whereas strong cellular immunoreactivity was detected in 83.3% of patients with G3. A significant correlation was also noted between pattern of reactivity and tumor grade because the basal layer was positive in patients with undifferentiated tumors (100% of G3) and in 72.2% of G1 tumors.

Palpable inguinal lymphadenopathy is present at diagnosis in 58% of patients.[393,394] Of these, less than 50% have metastases; the others have inflammatory lymphadenopathy resulting from infection of the primary tumor. Approximately 20% of patients with nonpalpable lymph nodes have metastases.[393] In patients with SCC of the penis, the presence and extent of metastases involving the inguinal nodes are the most important predictors of survival. Favorable prognostic indicators of survival in surgically treated patients in whom metastases develop include minimal nodal disease, unilateral involvement, no evidence of extranodal extension of cancer, and absence of pelvic nodal metastases. Therefore prophylactic lymphadenectomy in selected patients at high risk for metastases seems reasonable.[394,405] Dynamic sentinel node biopsy is now recommended for the patients with clinically node-negative penile cancer to reduce the morbidity of radical inguinal lymphadenectomy.[406-409] Perdona et al. reported that this procedure is minimally invasive and easy to perform, with results similar to those of radical inguinal lymphadenectomy and with lower morbidity.[406] Kroon et al. compared the clinical outcome of early and delayed excision of lymph node metastases in patients with penile SCC and found that cancer-specific 3-year survival of patients with positive lymph nodes detected during surveillance was 35%, whereas those who underwent early resection of occult inguinal metastases detected on dynamic sentinel biopsy had an 85% survival rate.[410] However, Izawa et al. reported that dynamic sentinel node biopsy using intraoperative lymphatic mapping is a promising technique but requires further testing for penile cancer among high-volume centers.[411] Contemporary superficial and modified inguinal dissection techniques with intraoperative frozen section remain the gold standard for identifying microscopic metastases. Tabatabaei et al. evaluated lymphotropic nanoparticle-enhanced MRI with ferumoxtran-10 to determine the presence of regional lymph node metastases in patients with penile cancer.[412] They found that lymphotropic nanoparticle-enhanced MRI had sensitivity, specificity, and positive and negative predictive values of 100%, 97%, 81.2%, and 100%, respectively. Venous or lymphatic embolization predicted lymph node involvement and could be used to determine which patients with clinically negative lymph nodes should undergo immediate lymphadenectomy.[413] Among the pathologically node-positive patients, factors adversely influencing survival in multivariate analysis were bilateral nodal metastases, number of positive inguinal nodes, pelvic nodal metastases, and extranodal extension.[414] Presentation with distant metastases is rare in the absence of regional lymph node metastasis. Hematogenous dissemination is rare; less than 2% of patients with penile carcinoma have distant visceral metastases at the time of diagnosis. However, hepatic, pulmonary, osseous, and, rarely, cutaneous metastases can occur in untreated cases.[415-417] In some studies, it has been shown that the presence of HPV does not influence prognosis.[417] However, other studies have reported different results.[402]

Sanchez et al. evaluated data from several studies and found that there was a correlation between tumor type and incidence of nodal metastasis and survival.[418] They further classified these penile tumors into three groups—low, intermediate, and high—according to their behavior, with differing risks for regional tumor spread and mortality risk. The low-risk group tumors were usually grossly large, replaced more than one anatomic compartment, but were histologically low-grade, noninvasive, or superficially invasive (verrucous, cuniculatum, and pseudohyperplastic carcinomas), or in some cases deeply invasive (papillary carcinoma). However,

the outcome in these cases was excellent, with a significantly low mortality rate. Tumors in the high-risk category were the usual poorly differentiated carcinoma, basaloid, warty-basaloid, papillary basaloid, and sarcomatoid carcinomas. Most of these neoplasms were large and locally destructive with high-grade histology, perineural and vascular invasion, and deep invasion of corpora cavernosa, resulting in frequent nodal metastasis and poor outcomes with increased mortality. The third category was that of intermediate-risk tumors, comprising about one-half of penile carcinomas. To this group belonged the usual moderately differentiated carcinoma, warty and mixed carcinomas. Typically, these neoplasms were grade 2 carcinoma and invaded up to penile corpus spongiosum, with low rates of perineural or vascular invasion. Regional metastasis and outcome were intermediate or low, more like the low-risk tumors and significantly different from high-risk tumors.

The most widely used clinical staging systems for penile cancer are the Jackson system (Table 15.8) and the American Joint Committee on Cancer system (Table 15.9).[386,419] Grade and stage are the most reliable prognostic factors for penile carcinoma, although stage is dominant. Survival is shortened when spread occurs to

---

TABLE 15.8	Jackson Staging System for Squamous Cell Carcinoma of the Penis

Stage	Description
I	Confined to glans, prepuce, or both
II	Extending onto penile shaft or corpora
III	Operable inguinal lymph node metastases
IV	Inoperable inguinal lymph node metastases, adjacent structure involvement, and/or distant metastases

From Jackson SM. The treatment of carcinoma of the penis. *Br J Surg* 1966;53:33-35.

TABLE 15.9	TNM: The Staging System of the American Joint Committee on Cancer

TNM Classification

T—Primary Tumor

TX	Primary tumor cannot be assessed
T0	No evidence of primary tumor
Tis	Carcinoma in situ (penile intraepithelial neoplasia)
Ta	Noninvasive localized squamous cell carcinoma
T1	Glans: tumor invades lamina propria
	Foreskin: tumor invades dermis, lamina propria, or dartos fascia
	Shaft: tumor invades connective tissue between epidermis and corpora regardless of location
T1a	Tumor is without lymphovascular invasion or perineural invasion and is not high grade (i.e., grade 3 or sarcomatoid)
T1b	Tumor exhibits lymphovascular invasion and/or perineural invasion and is high grade (i.e., grade 3 or sarcomatoid)
T2	Tumor invades corpus spongiosum (either glans or ventral shaft) with or without urethral invasion
T3	Tumor invades into corpora cavernosa (including tunica albuginea) with or without urethral invasion
T4	Tumor invades into adjacent structures (i.e., scrotum, prostate, pubic bone)

N—Regional Lymph Nodes (Pathologic Stage Definition)

pNX	Regional lymph nodes cannot be assessed
pN0	No regional lymph node metastasis
pN1	$\leq$2 unilateral inguinal metastases, no extranodal extension
pN2	$\geq$3 unilateral inguinal metastases or bilateral metastases
pN3	Extranodal extension of lymph node metastases or pelvic lymph node metastases

M—Distant Metastasis

M0	No distant metastasis
M1	Distant metastasis present

Anatomic Stage/Prognostic Groups

Stage 0	Tis	N0	M0
	Ta	N0	M0
Stage I	T1a	N0	M0
Stage IIA	T1b	N0	M0
	T2	N0	M0
Stage IIB	T3	N0	M0
Stage IIIA	T1-3	N1	M0
Stage IIIB	T1-3	N2	M0
Stage IV	T4	Any N	M0
	Any T	N3	M0
	Any T	Any N	M1

M, Metastasis; *N*, node; *T*, tumor.
Adapted with permission from Amin MB, Edge S, Greene F, et al. *AJCC Cancer Staging Manual.* 8th ed. New York, NY: Springer; 2017.

inguinal or iliac lymph nodes, or when distant metastases occur.[420] Histologic grade correlates well with the clinical stage. Patients with low-grade cancer have a favorable prognosis, and more than 80% are long-term survivors. Patients with high-grade cancer tend to have advanced stage at presentation and a poor prognosis. Approximately 50% of cancers appearing on the shaft are high grade in contrast with only 10% arising in the prepuce.[421]

DNA flow cytometric analysis also may be a useful prognostic factor in penile cancer.[38,422-424] Yu et al. reported that patients with diploid cancer had longer survival than those with aneuploid cancer, and low S-phase fraction was associated with favorable outcome.[422] The incidence of aneuploidy rises with increasing stage. Yu et al. also reported that all patients who appeared cured had diploid tumors, whereas 80% of patients dying of cancer had aneuploid tumors.[422] Gustafsson et al. reported similar results; they found that low-grade cancer was predominantly diploid and high-grade cancer was not.[423] Death from cancer occurred in only 1 of 14 patients with diploid cancer, but it occurred in 4 of 12 patients with nondiploid cancer.[423] Ki67 antibody and cyclin D1 overexpression have been reported to be high in high-grade tumors and seem to parallel each other, supporting the concept that cyclin D1 and Ki67 serve as cell-cycle activators and their overexpression may be used as a prognostic factor of poor outcome in penile carcinoma.[425,426]

Gunia et al. reported a multi-institutional study on invasive penile carcinoma for the prognostic value of p16^{INK4a} in conjunction with other prognostic parameters.[427] Multivariate analysis identified koilocytosis, p16^{INK4a} expression, and histologic stage and grade as independent prognostic factors for cancer-specific survival.[427]

PD-L1 (programmed death ligand 1) inhibits T-cell function and prevents tumor eradication. This is facilitated by PD-L1–positive tumor cells and PD-L1–positive immune cells, and can be prevented by anti–PD-1 (programmed death 1)/PD-L1 immunotherapy. In advanced penile cancer there is a need for new therapeutic strategies. Ottenhof et al. investigated PD-L1 expression in penile cancers and compared PD-L1 expression with disease-specific survival, lymph node metastases at diagnosis, and HR-HPV status in a large patient cohort, and reported that PD-L1 was expressed in 48% of penile carcinomas and mainly in HR-HPV–negative tumors.[428] The pattern of expression was a prognostic factor because marginal expression was associated with absence of lymph node metastases and diffuse expression was associated with poor survival.

Treatment of choice for penile cancer is surgical resection with inguinal lymphadenectomy, with few therapeutic advances in the past two decades. Major progress includes methods for less disfiguring treatment of the primary lesion for some patients, improved survival by altering the timing of groin dissection for those at risk for metastases, and multimodal therapy (radiotherapy and chemotherapy) for treating metastases.[429,430] Assessment of penile cancer based on clinical findings alone often results in inaccurate staging and suboptimal treatment. Imaging of primary site and metastases optimizes treatment planning. MRI, both T1- and T2-weighted, is the most accurate imaging modality in the assessment of primary penile cancer and metastases.[431] ^{18}F-fluorodeoxyglucose PET or PET/CT may be used in SCC of the penis for detection of metastases and for therapeutic strategy planning for which invasive procedures, such as total bilateral inguinal lymphadenectomy, that have a high morbidity may be avoided.[432]

Resection margin control is critical for cancer control, but the traditional 2-cm free resection margin is unnecessary. Minhas et al.

reported that excision margins of only a few millimeters offered excellent control.[433] The role of sentinel lymph node biopsy, lymphatic mapping, prophylactic lymphadenectomy, and the template for lymph node dissection will be better defined in the future.[434]

In patients with penile SCCs, lymphadenectomy can be curative and should be considered in cases deemed high risk for metastatic spread to regional lymph nodes. However, management of patients without palpable lymphadenopathy remains controversial, and current guidelines for T1 penile SCCs based on previous studies have suggested that moderately differentiated tumors are at low risk for metastatic disease and recommend surveillance without lymph node removal. Malhotra et al. reported a total of 34 patients with SCC, of which 10 were stage T1, with 7 having moderately differentiated carcinoma without vascular invasion on pathologic evaluation.[435] Metastatic disease was present in one patient at the time of diagnosis and subsequently developed in three of the remaining six patients during follow-up. Thus 57% of the patients experienced metastatic disease. Our experience suggests that patients in this category are at higher risk for metastatic disease and may be offered early groin dissection in place of expectant management.

Patients receiving inguinal lymphadenectomy involving eight or more lymph nodes experienced improved overall 5-year survival than lymphadenectomy involving fewer than eight lymph nodes. Guidelines should not only be given more emphasis but possibly also should be updated to reflect the benefit of extensive lymph node dissection in patients with high-risk penile cancer (grade 3 and pT2 to pT4 disease).[435] Some of the potential strategies for the prevention of penile cancer could include circumcision, reducing the risk for transmission of penile HPV infection with male vaccination, early treatment of phimosis, smoking cessation, and hygienic measures. Implementing some of these measures would require extensive cost-benefit analysis, with significant changes in the global health policy.[436]

Variants of Squamous Cell Carcinoma (Human Papillomavirus Related)

Basaloid Carcinoma, Including Papillary Variant. Basaloid carcinoma is an unusual but distinctive variant of SCC, frequently associated with HPV, with deeper invasion and higher mortality rate than typical SCC, not otherwise specified (Table 15.10).[437] It is similar to basaloid cancer occurring at other sites, such as the vulva, and it may coexist with other types of SCC such as typical carcinoma, warty, pseudoglandular, anaplastic, and spindle types (Fig. 15.40A).[437] The tumor usually appears as a mass in the glans and perimeatus but may extend to the coronal sulcus, skin of the penile shaft, and urethra, and it may infiltrate deeply into the corpus cavernosum, corpus spongiosum, Buck fascia, dartos muscle, skin, and the urethra. Grossly it manifests with a white-gray, flat or elevated, irregular, firm mass with necrotic foci. Microscopically, downward proliferation of closely packed solid nests with focal or central comedonecrosis is often seen (Fig. 15.40B). The cells have basaloid features with uniform, small, basophilic nuclei with inconspicuous nucleoli and numerous mitotic figures. Individual cell necrosis occasionally forms a "starry sky" appearance. Strong en bloc positivity for p16, a surrogate marker for HPV, is seen these tumors (Fig. 15.40C). Differential diagnosis includes typical SCC, urothelial carcinoma, basal cell carcinoma, small cell (neuroendocrine) carcinoma, and metastatic carcinoma.

The papillary variant of basaloid carcinoma, which has an exophytic configuration, is a distinct variant of basaloid carcinoma that

TABLE 15.10	Variants of Squamous Cell Carcinoma				
	Basaloid	Warty	Verrucous	Papillary Carcinoma, Not Otherwise Specified	Sarcomatoid
Human papillomavirus	+	+	-	-	-
Age (mean), y	55	61	50	60	60
Incidence, %	10	6	3	10	1
Size, cm	>4	4	3	≤14	5-7
Koilocytosis	Absent	Prominent	Absent	Absent	Absent
Fibrovascular core	Rare	Present	Rare	Present	Absent
Base	Irregular and infiltrative	Rounded or irregular	Regular, pushing	Irregular, jagged	Irregular, jagged
Metastasis	Yes	Rare	No	Yes	Yes
Prognosis	Poor	Good	Excellent	Fair	Poor

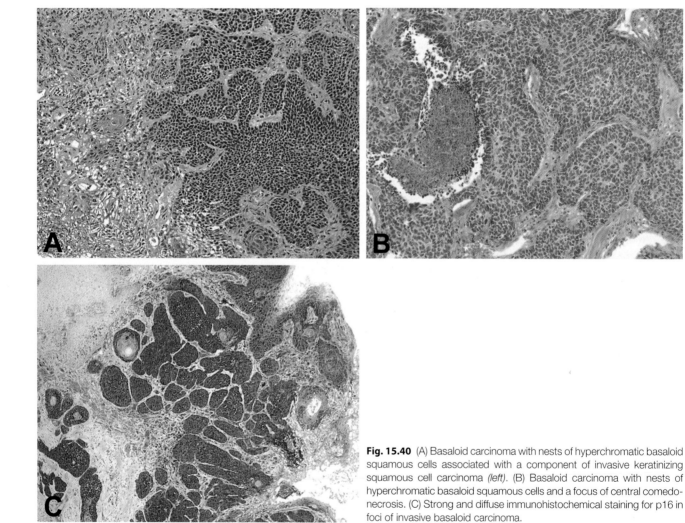

Fig. 15.40 (A) Basaloid carcinoma with nests of hyperchromatic basaloid squamous cells associated with a component of invasive keratinizing squamous cell carcinoma *(left)*. (B) Basaloid carcinoma with nests of hyperchromatic basaloid squamous cells and a focus of central comedonecrosis. (C) Strong and diffuse immunohistochemical staining for p16 in foci of invasive basaloid carcinoma.

is similar to urothelial carcinomas and composed of papillae with central fibrovascular cores covered by poorly differentiated uniform cells like those of basaloid penile carcinomas.[438] This papillary small cell pattern may superficially be part of basaloid or warty-basaloid invasive carcinomas. Parakeratosis and focal koilocytosis at the surface may be present. This tumor, despite its papillomatous pattern, is a distinctive HPV-related neoplasm of the family

of basaloid carcinomas and should not be classified in the group of highly keratinized papillary not otherwise specified carcinomas.[326] The differential diagnosis includes warty, warty-basaloid, basaloid, papillary not otherwise specified, and urothelial carcinomas. Warty and warty-basaloid carcinomas are condylomatous tumors with papillomatosis and highly keratinized squamous cells and pleomorphic koilocytic features not present in the papillary variant of basaloid carcinomas where few koilocytes may be observed on the papillae surface. Papillary not otherwise specified carcinomas are also composed of large, low-grade keratinizing squamous cells, distinguishing them from features seen in the papillary basaloid variant. The distinction from urothelial papillary carcinomas may be challenging, but immunohistochemical stains including GATA3 and uroplakin II are helpful in establishing the diagnosis of urothelial carcinoma.

Warty (Condylomatous) Carcinoma. Warty carcinoma is a morphologically distinct verruciform neoplasm that is like its counterpart in the vulva. The cancer may involve single or multiple anatomic sites such as the glans, coronal sulcus, and foreskin.[439]

Grossly, warty cancer forms exophytic, cauliflower-like, white-gray firm masses that are mainly papillomatous, with acanthosis, hyperkeratosis, and horny cysts (Table 15.10). The papillae contain prominent fibrovascular cores, and the epithelium has large, wrinkled, hyperchromatic, often binucleated nuclei and clear cytoplasm. The epithelial-stromal border is infiltrative, pushing, or mixed (Fig. 15.41).[365] HPV DNA is present in up to 45% of cases, more than with typical SCC.[327,365] The differential diagnosis includes other verruciform neoplasms such as verrucous carcinoma, giant condyloma, and papillary SCC, not otherwise specified.

It is difficult to identify the early cases of warty carcinoma in the literature because of the diverse nomenclature used in the past for the verruciform lesions, including giant condyloma Buschke-Lowenstein tumor, verrucous carcinoma, and papillary SCC. A useful feature is its preferential association with HPV in contrast with other types of penile cancer, and it may be a malignant counterpart of giant condyloma.[327,365] Giant condylomas are a rare sexually transmitted disease usually caused by HPV subtypes 6 and 11, but also by 16 and 18, among others. They are expansive, cauliflower-like, destructive lesions that most frequently affect the anogenital region. Approximately 30% of giant condylomas progress to warty condylomatous SCC.[327] The tumor has a definite risk for regional lymph node metastasis, although this is less frequent than with typical SCC.[327,365] Therefore it is important to distinguish this tumor from verrucous carcinoma and other verruciform tumors.[364,365]

Warty-Basaloid Carcinoma. This HPV-related tumor demonstrates a combined morphology of warty and basaloid carcinomas, and should be diagnosed after exclusion of both of these morphologic subtypes. It is seen in older patients and usually involves the glans.[440] Most tumors are exophytic, but exoendophytic growth can occur. These are large tumors with an irregular or papillomatous surface. Microscopic examination shows areas of warty and basaloid carcinoma admixed in varying proportions. The warty component is frequently present over the surface, and the basaloid component is identified in deeper invasive areas such as corpora cavernosa. Both morphologic patterns may also be present in the same tumor nest with central koilocytic areas and a peripheral basaloid appearance.[440] The tumor can also be almost entirely composed of papillae with small basaloid cells and clear, koilocytic cells. The differential diagnosis includes not only pure warty or basaloid carcinomas but also the papillary variant of basaloid carcinoma.[440]

Clear Cell Carcinoma. Liegl and Regauer described five cases of penile clear cell carcinoma presenting in middle-aged men on the inner side of the foreskin.[441] The tumors were large, exophytic, partly ulcerated, and widely invasive, with sharp demarcation from the adjacent benign skin and mucosa. Histologically, these clear cell carcinomas were composed of large clear cells with intracytoplasmic diastase-resistant, PAS-positive material, and extensive lymphatic and blood vessel invasion (Fig. 15.42). Intense cytoplasmic immunoreactivity for MUC1, EMA, and CEA was seen. All carcinomas contained HPV16, although only one displayed HPV-related cytologic cell changes. All patients had extensive, partly cystic inguinal lymph node metastases with striking clear cell differentiation and focal dense sclerotic basement membrane material, either at diagnosis or within several months. Two patients were alive after 7 and 10 years, one patient died after 9 months with widespread cancer, and two other patients were alive at 7 and 17 months with widespread lymphatic and hematogenous metastases despite adjuvant chemotherapy and radiation therapy. In contrast with SCC, penile clear cell carcinoma showed extensive vascular and lymphatic invasion, and early metastases to regional lymph nodes. Clear cell carcinomas are aggressive HPV-related tumors that arise in the penile mucosa, involve the glans or foreskin, and demonstrate a clear cell morphology.[441,442] They exhibit a typically nested growth pattern with confluent nests in

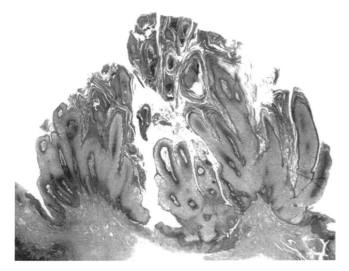

Fig. 15.41 Warty carcinoma. This well-differentiated variant of squamous carcinoma shows marked surface keratinization with broad bulbous rete downgrowths pushing into the stroma.

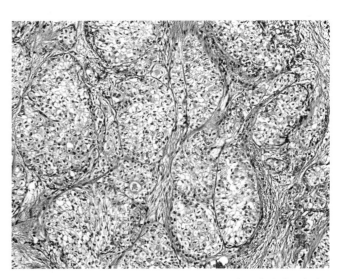

Fig. 15.42 Penile clear cell carcinoma composed exclusively of clear tumor cells.

some cases and prominent geographic as well as comedo-type necrosis. The nests contain PAS-positive material amid clear cells that show strong p16 positivity on immunohistochemical staining. The differential diagnosis includes warty carcinoma, cutaneous adnexal sweat gland tumors, and metastatic neoplasms with a clear cell morphology. Features that aid in establishing a diagnosis of penile clear cell carcinoma include a nonverruciform growth pattern and presence of solid tumor nests in contrast with warty carcinomas.[441,442] Immunohistochemical stains are significantly helpful in ruling out metastatic tumors such as clear cell renal cell carcinoma (PAX8 positive) or cutaneous adnexal sweat gland tumors.

Medullary Carcinoma of the Penis. Recently Canete-Portillo et al. reported a series of 12 cases of a novel penile tumor associated with HPV.[443] The patients' ages ranged from 42 to 92 years (average, 71 years), and most tumors arose in the glans. A characteristic microscopic finding of this tumor is the presence of a moderate to dense tumor-associated inflammatory cell infiltrate composed of neutrophils, lymphocytes, plasma cells, or eosinophils. The tumor cells are arranged in large solid sheets, nests, or trabeculae. These tumors are composed of large and poorly differentiated or anaplastic cells with enlarged nuclei and prominent nucleoli. Keratinization is minimal or absent. Conspicuous mitotic activity is seen, and tumor necrosis is commonly present. Tumor-associated inflammatory cells, especially neutrophils and eosinophils, are an important component of this tumor. The inflammatory cells can be present at the periphery of the tumor, akin to medullary carcinomas of breast, or more commonly located within the tumor itself.[443]

Deep invasion of the corpora cavernosa is frequently seen, implying more aggressive behavior. In the published series, p16[INK4a] and HPV-DNA were positive in all cases tested, whereas mRNA detection was positive in nine cases only. En bloc p16 positivity with diffuse nuclear and cytoplasmic staining was seen. The prevalent genotype was HPV16 (nine cases, 75%). Other genotypes identified were HPV genotypes 58, 33, and 66.[443]

The differential diagnoses include sarcomatoid, basaloid, and lymphoepithelioma like SCCs. In non–HPV-related, poorly differentiated SCC, there are more recognizable features of cell maturation, keratinization, and desmoplastic stromal reaction. Sarcomatoid carcinomas may exhibit pleomorphic or anaplastic cells, like those described in medullary carcinomas, but spindle cells predominate. Basaloid carcinomas may show a solid pattern in some cases, but a nesting pattern with comedonecrosis is usually present, in addition to basaloid cytomorphology. Lymphoepithelioma-like carcinoma is characterized by proliferation of noncohesive, poorly differentiated epithelial cells with a lymphocytic predominant stroma. In medullary carcinomas, cells are more cohesive with a solid pattern, and neutrophils and eosinophils are more commonly encountered than lymphocytes.[443]

Variants of Squamous Cell Carcinoma: Non–Human Papillomavirus Related

Verrucous Carcinoma. Since its first description in the oral cavity, verrucous carcinoma has been identified in numerous organs, including the larynx, vulva, vagina, anus, and penis (Table 15.10). Verrucous carcinoma of the penis accounts for 5% to 16% of penile malignancies.[444] It is commonly seen in middle-aged men.[444-450] Typically, it appears as a large, fungating, frequently ulcerated warty lesion that burrows through the normal tissues (Fig. 15.43). Most arise on the coronal sulcus and spread to the glans and preputial skin. Microscopically, verrucous carcinoma is a very well-differentiated SCC with exophytic and endophytic papillary growth (Fig. 15.44). Central fibrovascular cores are not prominent. Characteristically, the tumor shows a broad-based "pushing" pattern of infiltration (Fig. 15.45). Cytologic atypia is minimal, and mitotic figures are rare and usually confined to the deeper aspect of the tumor. No cytoplasmic clearing or koilocytotic nuclear atypia of HPV-related tumors is seen (Table 15.11).[449]

Verrucous carcinoma tends to grow locally and does not metastasize. If inadequately treated, multiple recurrences may appear. The main differential diagnosis includes condyloma acuminatum, warty carcinoma, and the usual type of keratinizing SCC. When the lesion is large, giant condyloma Buschke-Lowenstein tumor enters the differential diagnosis. Whether verrucous carcinoma and giant condyloma Buschke-Lowenstein tumor are the same or different entities remains controversial. The consistent absence of HPV genotypes 6, 11, 16, 18, and 31 in verrucous carcinoma suggests a fundamental difference between verrucous carcinoma and giant condyloma.[449,450] Masih et al. reported the uniform absence of the common genital HPV in their cases of verrucous

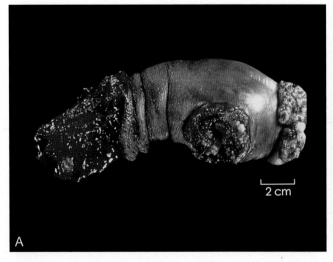
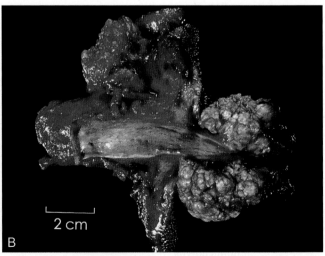

Fig. 15.43 (A) Verrucous carcinoma has grown out of the preputial orifice and eroded through the prepuce. (B) Dissection reveals that verrucous carcinoma has grown extensively in the glans and prepuce, obliterating the preputial space. (From Fletcher CDM. Diagnostic histopathology of tumors. Edinburgh: Churchill Livingstone, 1995.)

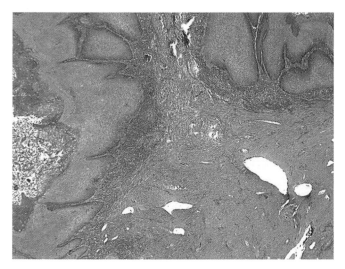

Fig. 15.44 Verrucous carcinoma with marked hyperkeratosis and a regular but pushing border with the dermis.

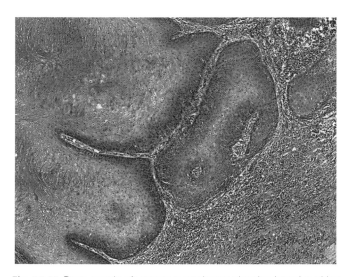

Fig. 15.45 Deep margin of verrucous carcinoma showing broad pushing invasion with lack of irregular infiltration. Note the lack of nuclear atypia.

TABLE 15.11	Histopathologic Features of Verrucous Carcinoma
Morphologic Features	**Frequency**
Club-shaped, hyperplastic rete ridges	+++
Pushing deep margins	+++
Well-differentiated squamous epithelium	+++
Polygonal squamous cells with glassy cytoplasm	+++
Intercellular bridges	+++
Centrally located vesicular nuclei	+++
Central single nucleolus	+++
Well-formed intercellular edema	+++
Individual cell necrosis	+++
Hyperkeratosis	+++
Parakeratosis	+++
Keratin-filled clefts	+++
Cystic degeneration of rete ridges	+++
Heavy subepithelial inflammatory cell infiltrates	++
Intact basement membrane	++
Crust formation	++
Epithelial abscesses	++
Koilocyte-like cells	++
Superficial fibrovascular cores	++
Keratohyaline granules	+
Dermal abscesses	+
Anaplastic foci (hybrid verrucous and regular)	+
True koilocytes	+
True fibrovascular cores	+

carcinoma and concluded that verrucous carcinoma is a distinct clinicopathologic entity that does not have a place in the morphologic spectrum of condyloma acuminatum and giant condyloma (penile giant condyloma of Buschke-Lowenstein has the same human HPV subtypes as condyloma acuminatum, with similar frequency).[449] Conversely, some authors found HPV genotypes 6 and 11, as well as preexisting condyloma acuminatum, in some cases of verrucous carcinoma, suggesting a viral causative agent.[448,450] The lack of cytologic atypia, mitotic figures, and infiltrative growth pattern are helpful features in differentiating verrucous carcinoma from the usual type of SCC. According to Saeed et al., the mean BCL2/BAX ratio was significantly lower in verrucous carcinoma in contrast with typical SCC.[451] BAX expression was comparable in verrucous carcinoma and low-grade SCC, but BCL2 expression was significantly higher in high-grade SCC. These findings indicate that penile verrucous carcinoma and typical SCC are immunophenotypically distinct.

Stankiewicz et al. studied HPV infection and immunochemical detection of cell-cycle markers in verrucous carcinoma of the penis.[452] They found p16^{INK4a} and Ki67 expression were significantly lower in verrucous carcinoma than in the usual SCC type. HPV detection was seen in only 3 of 13 verrucous carcinoma cases. Based on these findings, they report that penile verrucous carcinoma pathogenesis is unrelated to HPV infection.[452]

Clinical outcome for patients with verrucous carcinoma varies according to the type of treatment. Partial or radical penectomy reduces the recurrence rate to 33%, in contrast with 80% recurrence in patients treated with local excision.[444,449,450] Therefore partial or total penectomy is recommended. Intraaortic infusion chemotherapy has recently been used to treat penile verrucous carcinoma with the uniqueness of preserving the anatomic structure and sexual function in complete responders. For penile verrucous carcinoma, especially in younger patients, intraaortic infusion chemotherapy may be considered organ-sparing treatment before penectomy.[453] Radiation therapy is contraindicated because it induces dedifferentiation of verrucous carcinoma.[444,449,450]

Papillary Carcinoma, Not Otherwise Specified. Papillary carcinoma, not otherwise specified is an exophytic SCC lined by atypical cells without HPV-related features and with infiltrative borders (Fig. 15.46; Table 15.10). This variant occurs commonly in the fifth and sixth decades of life. Glans alone is the most commonly involved site (51%), followed by glans, coronal sulcus, and foreskin in 37%, glans and sulcus in 9%, and foreskin in 3%.[454] Microscopically, it is a well-differentiated, hyperkeratotic carcinoma with irregular, complex papillae, with or without fibrovascular cores (Fig. 15.47). Unlike verrucous carcinoma, the interface with the underlying stroma is infiltrative and irregular. Although papillary carcinoma, not otherwise specified can invade the corpus spongiosum or cavernosum, regional lymph node metastases are exceptional, and therefore the prognosis is excellent. In warty SCC, as in papillary carcinomas, the interface of tumor and stroma is irregular, but the prominent condylomatous papillae and conspicuous

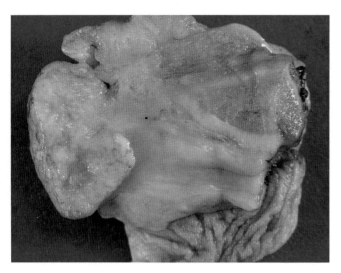

Fig. 15.46 Papillary squamous cell carcinoma, not otherwise specified, of the penis. Gross picture of a penectomy specimen with an exophytic papillomatous tumor extending through the glans and coronal sulcus, and involving the urethra.

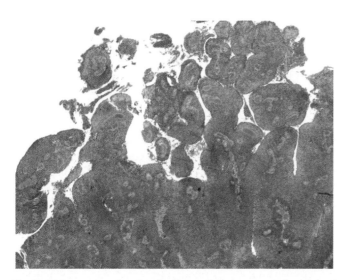

Fig. 15.47 Low-power view showing the papillomatous exophytic pattern of growth of papillary carcinoma of the penis. Variability in size and shape of papillae with irregular fibrovascular cores is noted.

pleomorphic koilocytosis, hallmarks of warty tumors, are absent in papillary SCC. In some cases, immunohistochemistry for p16^{INK4a} or HPV identification and genotypification may be required for the distinction, with negative HPV in papillary SCC. Although morphologically quite different, the papillary variant of basaloid carcinoma, given its exophytic configuration, also should be considered in the differential diagnosis. This unusual tumor is like urothelial carcinoma and composed of papillae with central fibrovascular cores lined by poorly differentiated and uniform cells like those of basaloid penile carcinomas (Fig. 15.48). This papillary small cell pattern may superficially be part of basaloid or warty-basaloid invasive carcinomas. Parakeratosis and focal koilocytosis at the surface may be present. As stated earlier, papillary SCC is typically negative for HPV and p16^{INK4a}. This tumor, despite its papillomatous pattern, is a distinctive HPV-related neoplasm of the family of basaloid carcinomas and should not be classified in the group of highly keratinized papillary SCCs, not otherwise specified. In a study by

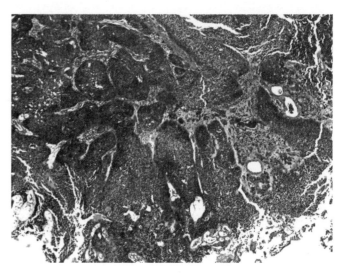

Fig. 15.48 Basaloid squamous cell carcinoma with papillary features showing papillae with conspicuous fibrovascular cores and lined by tumor cells with basaloid features.

Cubilla and colleagues of 12 cases of basaloid SCC with papillary features, the tumors were either exophytic or exoendophytic.[334] Microscopically, a papillomatous pattern of growth with a central fibrovascular core and small basophilic cells lining the papillae was seen. Positivity for HPV was present in 11 of 12 tumors (92%). Single genotypes found were HPV16 in nine tumors and HPV51 in one tumor. Multiple genotypes (HPV16 and HPV45) were present in another case. Overexpression of p16 was observed in all cases. Uroplakin III was negative in all cases. The differential diagnosis included basaloid, warty-basaloid, warty, and papillary SCC, as well as urothelial carcinomas. Local excision (four cases), circumcision (three cases), and partial penectomy (five cases) were preferred treatment choices. Tumor thickness ranged from 1 to 15 mm (average, 7 mm). Two patients with tumors invading 11 and 15 mm into the corpus spongiosum experienced inguinal nodal metastasis. Of the 11 patients followed (median, 48 months), 7 were alive with no evidence of metastatic disease, 3 died of causes other than penile cancer, and another died postoperatively. Unlike in typical basaloid carcinomas, the overall prognosis was excellent. However, deeply invasive tumors were associated with regional nodal metastasis, indicating a potential for tumor-related death. Sometimes a low-grade usual SCC may superficially resemble papillary carcinoma, but the former usually does not exhibit a verruciform pattern of growth, and papillomatosis is not a prominent feature. Finally, pseudohyperplastic carcinoma may exhibit a focal papillary growth.[334]

Carcinoma Cuniculatum. Carcinoma cuniculatum, a low-grade SCC of plantar skin, was first described in 1954 by Aird et al. and manifests with ulcerated, fungating masses with fine papillary architecture.[455] Microscopic examination of the tumors reveals bulbous acanthosis, parakeratosis, and a well-defined lower border circumscribed by chronic inflammatory cells. This variant of SCC has been described as a variant of penile SCC characterized by its peculiar deeply penetrating and burrowing pattern of growth (Fig. 15.49). This low-grade, verruciform penile neoplasm is like plantar carcinoma cuniculatum. Barreto et al. described clinical and pathologic features of seven patients.[456] Seven partial penectomies and four bilateral inguinal node dissections were performed. The mean patient age was 77 years. Grossly the tumors were white to gray, exoendophytic, and papillomatous, with a

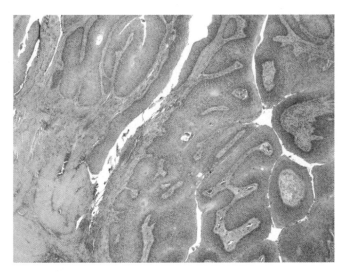

Fig. 15.49 Carcinoma cuniculatum of the penis characterized by a labyrinthine exoendophytic growth and a penetrating tumor tract.

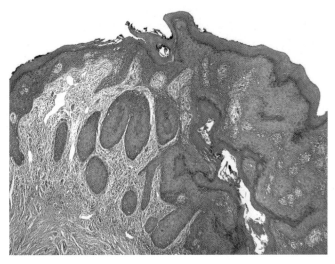

Fig. 15.50 Pseudohyperplastic nonverruciform squamous cell carcinoma with superficially infiltrating, well-differentiated carcinoma composed of nests of variable sizes and minimal atypia surrounded by fibrous stroma.

cobblestone or spiky appearance. All cases affected the glans and extended to coronal sulcus and foreskin (average size, 6.3 cm). The hallmark of the lesion was noted on the cut surface, where deep tumoral invaginations formed irregular, narrow, and elongated neoplastic sinus tracts connecting the surface of the neoplasm to deep anatomic structures. The neoplasm invaded through lamina propria and corpus spongiosum, and grew along the loose connective tissue of Buck fascia to involve the tunica albuginea and corpora cavernosa (average depth, 32 mm). Deeply invasive keratin-filled cysts or crypts, on serial sections, were shown to be connected to the surface tumor. Fistulization to the skin also was noted. Microscopically, the lesions corresponded to well-differentiated carcinomas with a bulbous front of invasion. Focal areas of higher histologic grade and more infiltrative and jagged borders were seen in four cases. Inguinal nodes were negative in four patients in which groin dissection was performed. Carcinoma cuniculatum is a variant of penile SCC with distinctive growth pattern and should be distinguished from other verruciform tumors such as verrucous, papillary, and warty carcinomas. Unlike most subtypes of penile SCCs and despite the deep invasion, none of the tumors showed groin or systemic dissemination at the time of diagnosis.

Pseudohyperplastic Nonverruciform Squamous Cell Carcinoma. The pseudohyperplastic nonverruciform SCC variant of penile carcinoma was recently described by Cubilla et al. as well-differentiated SCC with pseudohyperplastic features.[95] Most low-grade penile cancers are verruciform, either verrucous or papillary carcinoma, not otherwise specified subtypes. At presentation, the median age is 69 years. Most are multicentric and preferentially involve the inner mucosal surface of the foreskin. Grossly, pseudohyperplastic carcinoma is typically flat or slightly elevated, white and granular, and measures approximately 2 cm in diameter. Characteristic histologic features include keratinizing nests of squamous cells with minimal atypia surrounded by a reactive fibrous stroma (Fig. 15.50). In biopsies or select foci of resected specimens, separation from pseudoepitheliomatous hyperplasia is very difficult, but samples of sufficient size contain obvious evidence of infiltration. The adjacent squamous epithelium typically shows changes often associated with SCC, including squamous hyperplasia and low-grade or high-grade squamous intraepithelial neoplasia. Well-developed balanitis xerotica obliterans is invariably present.

Patients are treated by circumcision or partial penectomy, and they are cured with rare exceptions.

Spindle Cell (Sarcomatoid) Squamous Cell Carcinoma. Although spindle cell SCC is common in the oral cavity, upper respiratory tract, and esophagus, only a few cases have been reported in the penis (Table 15.10).[457,458] This variant also has been reported as a carcinosarcoma.[459] Two recent series reported that the incidence rate of spindle cell carcinoma is 1.4% to 4%.[460,461] The cancer tends to form polypoid masses on the glans penis and deeply invades corpora cavernosa. Histologically, it is composed of spindle cell sarcomatoid and squamous carcinoma components (Fig. 15.51A) or exclusively spindle cell malignant component, mimicking a sarcoma (Fig. 15.51B). Marked nuclear pleomorphism and numerous mitotic figures are common in the spindle cell component.[460] HPV is negative, and high-molecular-weight CK (34βE12) and p63 appear to be more specific and sensitive markers than other epithelial markers to confirm epithelial derivation.[460] Most cases are very aggressive, with early lymph node metastasis and distant metastases, including to the lung, skin, bone, pericardium, and pleura.[457-461]

Mixed Carcinoma. Approximately 25% of cases of penile verrucous carcinoma contain microscopic foci of cellular anaplasia, higher mitotic activity, and ruptured basement membranes.[444,449] These tumors are referred to as *hybrid squamous-verrucous carcinoma*, similar to their counterpart in the oral cavity.[462] Hybrid squamous-verrucous carcinoma and verrucous carcinoma have multiple similarities, including patient age, location, and outcome after treatment, although the data on hybrid squamous-verrucous carcinoma are limited.[444,449] DNA ploidy and cell-cycle studies by Masih et al. showed that both verrucous carcinoma and hybrid squamous-verrucous carcinoma are diploid and have similar proliferative indices.[449] Foci of invasive SCC have been found in up to 30% of verrucous carcinoma. Verrucous carcinoma should be recognized as a unique subtype of carcinomas.[463] Other mixed carcinomas include warty-basaloid carcinoma, adenocarcinoma-basaloid carcinoma (adenobasaloid carcinoma), and squamous carcinoma–neuroendocrine carcinoma (Fig. 15.52).

Adenosquamous Carcinoma. Adenosquamous carcinoma of the penis is a rare, biphasic malignant tumor with SCC and adenocarcinoma components. Reports indicate that the squamous

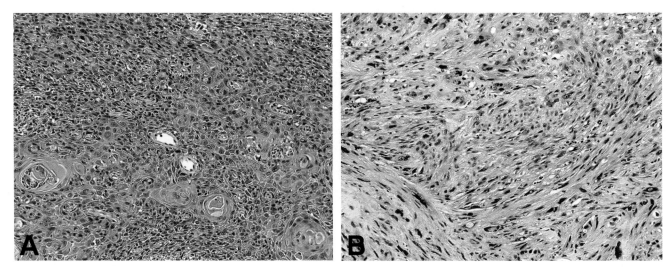

Fig. 15.51 (A) Spindle cell squamous cell carcinoma *(top)* with an adjacent area of keratinizing squamous cell carcinoma *(bottom)*. (B) Spindle cell squamous cell carcinoma with an exclusively spindled growth pattern resembling a primary sarcoma.

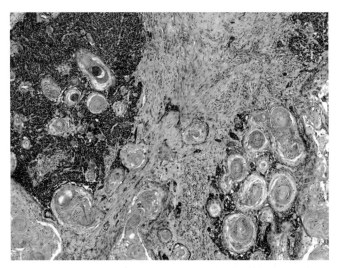

Fig. 15.52 Combined small cell neuroendocrine carcinoma *(left)* intermixed with areas of keratinizing squamous cell carcinoma *(right)*.

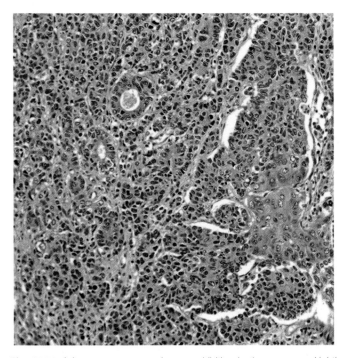

Fig. 15.53 Adenosquamous carcinoma exhibiting both squamous *(right)* and glandular *(left)* differentiation.

component is either the warty or usual type of SCC, or the adenocarcinomatous component is mucin secreting.[464] To make a diagnosis of adenosquamous carcinoma, we recommend that the adenocarcinoma component should be truly glandular with either definite gland formation or mucin production (Fig. 15.53). Acantholysis of the squamous component (acantholytic SCC, adenoid SCC) with pseudogland formation should not be included as adenosquamous carcinoma.[465] HPV positivity has also been reported in primary penile adenosquamous carcinoma arising from the skin.[466] Adenosquamous carcinoma can metastasize, but very limited follow-up data are available.[464,466] Cases of mucoepidermoid carcinoma arising in the glans penis have been reported, some of which have exhibited more aggressive behavior than original descriptions implied.[467,468]

Acantholytic Squamous Cell Carcinoma. Acantholytic SCC also may be referred to as *adenoid squamous cell carcinoma* or *pseudoglandular squamous cell carcinoma*. This variant was initially described in 1947 as a tumor composed of both solid and glandlike epithelial proliferations extending into the dermis and labeled

adenoacanthoma of sweat glands. Most authors now regard acantholytic SCC as a variant of SCC rather than a sweat gland tumor.[469] It usually has a typical SCC pattern in combination with glandular formations, dyskeratotic cells, and acantholysis.

Clinically, this tumor is most often seen in the sun-exposed areas of the head and neck of elderly patients, and most likely arises from acantholytic actinic keratoses. Cases have been reported, however, of this tumor occurring in sun-protected areas such as the dorsum of the foot and penis.[465] A striking male predominance is seen. Fewer than 10 cases of acantholytic SCC of the penis have been reported. Acantholytic SCC may appear as a flesh-colored, pink, red, or brown nodule. Crusting, scaling, or ulceration may be present.

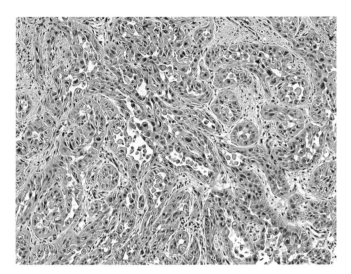

Fig. 15.54 Acantholytic squamous cell carcinoma showing formation of pseudoglandular spaces lined by atypical cells with squamous differentiation.

Histologically, the tumor is composed of strands and islands of atypical epithelial cells extending into the dermis. Connection to the overlying epidermis is seen in most cases, which may show hyperkeratosis and parakeratosis. However, this connection may be only focal or, in some cases, absent. Many of the tumor strands may show tubular and alveolar formations, referred to as *pseudoglandular appendages*. These spaces contain acantholytic cells that result from loss of cohesion of the tumor cells (Fig. 15.54). These acantholytic cells may appear extremely bizarre, large, or multinucleated. Mitotic figures are variably present.

Acantholytic SCC may be mistaken for adenosquamous carcinomas, metastatic adenocarcinomas, or epithelioid angiosarcomas. In adenosquamous carcinomas the glandular spaces are lined with PAS⁺ cells, whereas in acantholytic SCC the cells are negative for PAS. Also, acantholytic SCC lacks the production of CEA, S100 protein, and amylase, which can be seen in true glandular malignancies. In epithelioid angiosarcoma, the vascular spaces contain red blood cells, as opposed to the atypical keratinocytes seen in acantholytic SCC. Acantholytic SCC also may contain red blood cells within the pseudoglandular spaces. In these cases immunohistochemical stains may be required. Angiosarcomas are typically positive for vimentin, CD31, CD34, and FLI1, whereas acantholytic SCC is positive for CK and EMA. Clinically, acantholytic SCC of the penis is a highly aggressive type of SCC and is probably not related to HPV. Pathologists should be familiar with this entity because it shows distinct clinical features and prognosis, and by histologic examination it can mimic other penile tumors.[470,471]

Penile carcinoma is rare in the United States and Europe but is an important cause of morbidity and mortality in many other countries. Therefore it is important to implement preventive measures to decrease the incidence of disease and improve quality of life.[472] Early detection plays a vital role in disease control, and the proper diagnostic modalities must be used to accurately identify the cancer and its progression. The use of imaging in combination with biopsy is an effective means to determine disease stage and grade.[473]

Partial amputation is the most traditional procedure and is indicated for invasive distal lesions (stages T2 to T4) or large T1. Local recurrences after radiotherapy or brachytherapy are usually salvaged by partial penectomy. Partial penectomy is recognized as an effective procedure for local disease control, with low local recurrence rates. During partial amputation, it is mandatory to maintain a residual penile shaft with at least 4 cm of length, which allows for standing micturition and intercourse. Therefore it is essential to have free surgical margins. Intraoperative frozen section assessment is very helpful in this regard.

Disadvantages of partial penile amputations include penile shortening or its distal contour deformations, and are associated with both physical and psychological issues. Recently partial or total glans resections have been strongly advocated for selected cases of distal glans lesions (stage Ta/T1 or T2). These techniques preserve the corporal tips maintaining the penile length, and the shape is almost unchanged. For small lesions, Tis, Ta/T1, and selected T2 (and not involving the urethra), a partial glansectomy with resection until exposure of tunica albuginea of the corpora is performed. Total glansectomy with neoglans reconstruction with cavernous rotation and free-skin grafting technique was proposed for the treatment of balanitis xerotica obliterans and has become popular for treating penile cancer. The whole glans resection achieves satisfactory cosmetic and oncological results (<4% local relapses), but loss of graft, meatal stenosis, and phimosis can occur after surgery.[474]

Micrographic Mohs surgery achieves its best results for small and low-grade superficial or in situ lesions. Laser ablation for penile cancer plays a role in superficial (Ta/T1) and Tis lesions, with benefits of early local control, minimal scars, and preservation of adjacent uninvolved areas. The most commonly used are low-penetration lasers such as CO_2 or Nd:YAG (neodymium-yttrium-garnet), but with the latter it is not possible to procure specimens for pathologic examination. Patients with preputial Tis or small Ta-1 foreskin lesions can be treated with wide local excision or circumcision. If there are diffuse Tis or associated phimosis, a circumcision is mandatory. For distal preputial lesions, an extended circumcision is required.

ILND should be undertaken after proper assessment for metastatic spread to the nodes via dynamic sentinel lymph node biopsy in combination with fine needle aspiration cytology. The use of lymph node MRI has shown promise as a new tool for detecting lymph node metastasis and is a possible standard future approach to the evaluation of inguinal lymph nodes. The degree of ILND depends greatly on the extent of lymph node involvement and grade. Video endoscopic inguinal lymphadenectomy has proved to be an effective treatment option for ILND, with a superior complication rate to open nodal dissection. Further data regarding its use and the different approaches to metastatic lymph node disease management are essential and would greatly benefit the advancement of penile cancer care.[473]

Advanced penile cancer holds a poor prognosis and must be approached via a multimodal treatment regimen that includes neoadjuvant chemotherapy followed by surgical resection. In select cases the use of radiotherapy has been shown to be effective in the reduction of bulky nonresectable disease to allow for surgical removal. The chemotherapy combination that has so far been shown to be the most effective and well tolerated is paclitaxel, ifosfamide, and cisplatin. However, large randomized trials are lacking in this area and would shed light as to the best therapy for advanced penile cancer.[473,475]

Molecular Pathology of Penile Squamous Carcinoma

Recent studies have demonstrated clinical benefits with epidermal growth factor receptor (EGFR)-targeted therapy in patients with penile carcinoma, although there is no test that provides accurate patient selection. Silva Amancio et al. recently evaluated the prognostic value of *EGFR* gene and protein status in tumor samples from patients with primary penile SCC.[476] They assessed the expression of wild-type and two mutant EGFR isoforms (delA746-E750 and mL858R) by immunohistochemistry in 139 samples, of which 49 were also evaluated for EGFR copy number by fluorescence in situ hybridization (FISH). Positive immunohistochemical staining of wild-type and mutant EGFR was evidenced by complete and strong membranous staining. For FISH analysis, cases were considered unaltered, polysomic, or amplified, as determined by signals of the *EGFR* gene and chromosome 7. An independent cohort of 107 penile carcinoma samples was evaluated for mutations in *EGFR*, *KRAS*, and *BRAF*. Protein overexpression was noted in nearly half of the cases and was associated with cancer recurrence and perineural invasion. Expression of the two mutated EGFR isoforms was not observed. The FISH status was not associated with protein expression. Altered FISH (polysomy and gene amplification) was an independent risk factor for mortality due to penile cancer. Only 1 of 107 patients showed presence of KRAS mutations, and no mutations of EGFR or BRAF were observed.[476]

Despite aggressive multimodal therapy, locally advanced or metastatic penile SCC is associated with significant morbidity and mortality, indicating a need for new therapeutic options. Given the emerging clinical utility of immunotherapeutics, Udager et al. sought to assess the incidence and potential clinical significance of PD-L1 expression in penile squamous carcinomas.[477] They found that the majority of primary penile SCCs express PD-L1, which is associated with high-risk clinicopathologic features and poor clinical outcome. These data provide a rational basis for further investigation of anti–PD-1 and anti–PD-L1 immunotherapeutics in patients with advanced penile SCC. Anti–PD-1/PD-L1 immunotherapy is another treatment modality to treat penile cancer.[428]

The rarity of penile carcinoma, together with the technical difficulties inherent in this tumor because of the presence of inflammation, necrosis, and poor growth in cell culture, have led to few results and reviews about molecular alterations of penile carcinoma.[478]

Molecular alterations include alterations in the number of the DNA copies; HPV infection and p53 expression; gene overexpression, underexpression, and mutations; imbalanced protein expression; and DNA hypermethylation in the promoter region of the gene. Molecular alterations in penile carcinoma include copy number gains of 8q24, 16 p11 to 16 p12; deletions of 13q21 to 13q22 and 4q21 to 4q32; aneuploidy; TP53 overexpression and mutations; PIK3CA, KRAS, and HRAS mutations; BCL2 overexpression; and DNA hypermethylation in the promoter region of p16INK4A, RUNX3, FHIT, and MGMT.[478]

Other Malignant Tumors (Nonsquamous Neoplasms)
Basal Cell Carcinoma
Basal cell carcinoma is the most common malignant skin tumor elsewhere on the body, but it is rare in penile or scrotal skin.[479-483] It may involve any portion of the penis but most often involves the shaft (56%), the glans (30%), and the prepuce (14%).[481,482] Rarely, it may arise from the inner surface of the foreskin.[484] Patients range in age from 37 to 79 years.[481,482] Most patients are white, although one Japanese patient was reported.[482] Grossly, basal cell carcinoma manifests as a small, irregular, ulcerated mass. Histologically, it contains nests of small, uniform basaloid cells with peripheral palisading (Fig. 15.55). The cells tend to form nests with bulbous finger-like invaginations from the epidermis. The

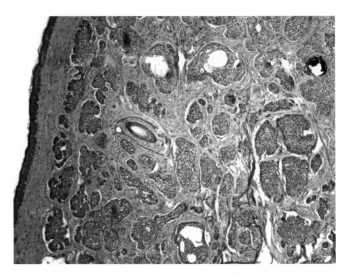

Fig. 15.55 Basal cell carcinoma. Nests of hyperchromatic basaloid tumor cells with characteristic retraction artifact.

cells lack intercellular bridges, and the nuclei display little variation in size, shape, or intensity of staining. The stroma adjacent to the tumor often shows a proliferation of young fibroblasts; alternatively, it may appear mucinous. Frequently the stroma retracts around the islands of basal cell carcinoma, resulting in peritumoral lacunae or cleftlike spaces. The clinical course tends to be indolent, and local excision is usually curative.

Malignant Melanoma
Approximately 100 cases of malignant melanoma of the penis have been reported, including melanoma in situ, accounting for less than 1% of all penile cancers.[405,485-493] Most occur in white men in their fifth and sixth decades of life, a decade older than is typical for most cutaneous melanomas.[494] In contrast with SCC, penile malignant melanoma is rare in men of African ancestry. In most cases it arises on the glans (Fig. 15.56).[81,405,491,492,495]

Patients present with a black, brown, or blue variegated papule or ulcerated plaque. The histologic findings are identical to those in other mucosal or cutaneous sites (Fig. 15.57).[81] Variants of

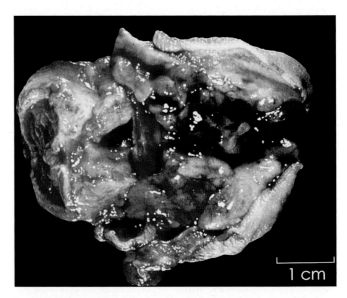

Fig. 15.56 Malignant melanoma arising in the glans penis.

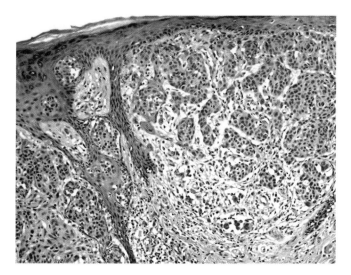

Fig. 15.57 Nests of malignant melanoma cells undermine the epidermis.

primary penile malignant melanoma include nodular, superficial spreading, acral lentiginous, and desmoplastic types.[405,489-494,496]

Stage I melanoma is confined to the penis, stage II melanoma is metastatic to regional lymph nodes, and stage III melanoma has distant metastases. The prognosis depends on the depth of invasion and the stage. Penile melanoma with a thickness ≤0.75 mm has an excellent prognosis, whereas a depth of invasion of ≥1.5 mm carries an extremely poor prognosis because of the high frequency of metastases.[81,405] Overall, 50% of patients have lymph node metastases at the time of diagnosis.[81] Prophylactic superficial lymph node dissection is recommended as an adjunct to penectomy for stage I penile malignant melanoma more than 1.5 mm thick. Bilateral ILND is standard treatment for stage II melanoma.[405]

Malignant melanoma of soft parts (clear cell sarcoma) is an uncommon neoplasm occurring most frequently in the tendons and aponeuroses of the extremities and rarely arising in the penis.[497]

Sarcoma and Other Tumors

Sarcoma is the second most common type of penile cancer, accounting for less than 5% of penile malignancies. Sarcomas arise in men of all ages, with a typical peak occurrence in the fifth and sixth decades of life; exceptions include rhabdomyosarcoma (young children) and epithelioid sarcoma (young adults).[498,499] With the exception of Kaposi sarcoma, which most commonly arises on the glans penis, sarcoma is most frequently located on the shaft.[499]

Vascular sarcomas, including Kaposi sarcoma, epithelioid hemangioendothelioma, and angiosarcoma, are the most common type of penile sarcoma. Sarcoma of myogenic, neurogenic, and fibrous origin also occurs.[302,500] The histologic features of these lesions are like those of their counterparts arising at other locations. Penile pseudomyogenic hemangioendothelioma/epithelioid sarcoma-like hemangioendothelioma, an intermediate-grade malignant tumor composed of spindle- to oval-shaped atypical cells with variably prominent nucleoli, has also been documented.[501] The lesional cells are positive for endothelial markers, such as ERG, FLI1, and CD31. They can also exhibit nuclear and cytoplasmic FOSB positivity, which is not expressed in epithelioid hemangioendothelioma or epithelioid sarcoma. Chromosome

banding analysis, FISH, mRNA sequencing, reverse transcriptase PCR, and quantitative real-time PCR have shown that these tumors are characterized by a balanced translocation t(7;19) (q22;q13), resulting in the fusion of the *SERPINE1* and *FOSB* genes. The role of *SERPINE1*, which is highly expressed in vascular cells, in this gene fusion is probably to provide a strong promoter for FOSB. FOSB encodes a transcription factor belonging to the FOS family of proteins, which together with members of the JUN family of transcription factors are major components of the activating protein 1 complex.

AIDS-related Kaposi sarcoma of the penis is a well-established entity.[502,503] Approximately 20% of male patients with AIDS with Kaposi sarcoma have lesions on the penis, and as many as 3% initially present with penile Kaposi sarcoma (Fig. 15.58). The penis is rarely the first site of involvement of Kaposi sarcoma, and occurrence is usually associated with systemic lesions.[504] The tumor typically involves the skin of the shaft or the glans. When it involves the glans or corpus spongiosum, Kaposi sarcoma may cause urethral obstruction. Clinically, it manifests with violaceous papules, plaques, or nodules because of the vascular nature of the lesions, but rarely with yellow-green penile plaques in black men.[505] Spindle-shaped tumor cells stain for vascular markers CD34, ERG, and human herpesvirus 8 (HHV8) (Fig. 15.59). HHV8 is detected in tumor tissue and peripheral blood mononuclear cells. Kaposi sarcoma may arise in HIV⁻ patients.[506-508] Local excision is effective for small localized lesions, as is radiation therapy.[509,510] Although Kaposi sarcoma is rare in HIV⁻ patients, cases have been reported, and also in association with HHV8 infection.[511-513]

Rarely, vascular sarcoma arises in the corpora cavernosa; approximately 35 cases have been reported.[514] The majority are hemangioendothelioma and tend to be indolent. Epithelioid hemangioendothelioma is composed of anastomosing networks of irregularly shaped vascular spaces lined by plump, often piled-up endothelial cells with low-grade morphology.[515-517] High-grade tumors with solid masses of anaplastic tumor cells, hemorrhage, and necrosis have also been reported. These may metastasize to

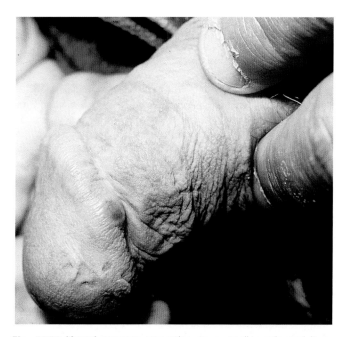

Fig. 15.58 Kaposi sarcoma presenting as a small purple nodule on the corona of the glans penis. (*Courtesy of Dr. A. Hood, Indiana University, Indianapolis, Indiana.*)

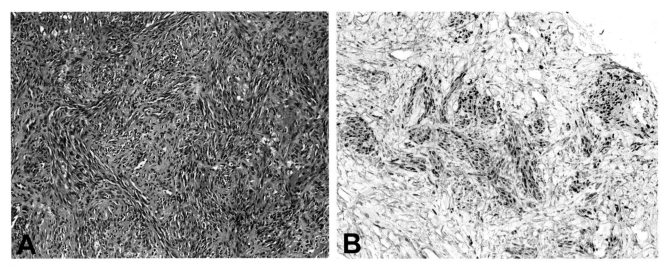

Fig. 15.59 (A) Kaposi sarcoma showing monomorphic spindle cells arranged in ill-defined fascicles with slitlike vessels and extravasated red blood cells. (B) Human herpesvirus 8 immunostain demonstrated strong immunoreactivity in lesional spindle cells.

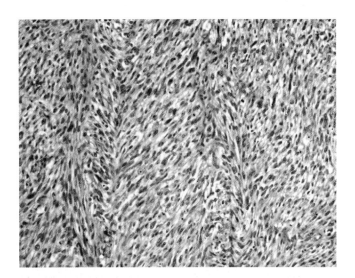

Fig. 15.60 Leiomyosarcoma of the penile shaft comprising intersecting fascicles of hyperchromatic spindle cells with moderate pleomorphism.

lymph nodes or hematogenously to distant sites such as lung, liver, and bone.

Leiomyosarcoma of the penis is rare, with fewer than 30 reported cases. It usually occurs in the fifth to seventh decades of life and involves the prepuce, distal shaft, circumcision scar line, or base of the penis.[518,519] Superficial leiomyosarcoma is thought to arise from the smooth muscle of the glans, frenulum, or the dermis of the shaft, and usually forms subcutaneous nodules.[520] Patients with superficial leiomyosarcoma tend to do well with local excision, but the tumor may recur locally. Deep leiomyosarcoma (Fig. 15.60) is less common, arising from the smooth muscle of the corpora cavernosa and tending to invade the urethra and metastasize early. Tumor depth and size are currently the best predictors of outcome for primary leiomyosarcoma. Small (≤2 cm diameter) superficial tumors are best managed by wide local excision, but large (>5 cm), deep-seated sarcomas have a poor prognosis because of their tendency for widespread metastases despite aggressive surgical intervention.[516,521] Radiation and chemotherapy are unproven as primary treatments for penile leiomyosarcoma.

Fibrosarcoma can be superficial or deep and usually manifests as a slow-growing, firm, nontender mass on the dorsum of the shaft or glans. It shares many clinical and gross features with leiomyosarcoma.[522,523] Immunohistochemical stains (CK, SMA, desmin, and vimentin) and the absence of overlying in situ carcinoma are useful to confirm soft tissue derivation and rule out spindle cell–SCC.

Malignant fibrous histiocytoma is rare in the penis, with only two cases reported in the literature, including one case of inflammatory malignant fibrous histiocytoma.[524,525]

Rhabdomyosarcoma in the penis arises on the shaft near the root. Most reported cases appeared in children and were embryonal rhabdomyosarcoma.[526,527]

Fewer than 20 cases of epithelioid sarcoma of the penis have been reported.[499,528-530] Patients ranged in age from 23 to 43 years (mean, 32 years). The sarcoma manifested as single or multiple, firm, slow-growing, painless subcutaneous nodules. The masses may produce surface ulceration, resulting in erectile pain or dysuria. Therefore epithelioid sarcoma may mimic Peyronie disease, urethral stricture, or ulcerating squamous carcinoma. Radical excision is the preferred method of treatment, although local excision combined with radiation therapy has been used with success. Epithelioid sarcoma is a slow-growing but aggressive tumor in the penis, as it is elsewhere in the body. Regardless of therapy, up to 80% recur locally. Metastases to the lung have been reported in two cases, but most reports lack long-term follow-up. The so-called proximal type of epithelioid sarcoma has been reported in the penis.[499]

Other soft tissue sarcomas, including hemangiopericytoma, malignant schwannoma, and extraskeletal osteosarcoma with malignant fibrous histiocytoma-like component, may arise in the penis.[531]

Lymphoma

Primary lymphoma of the penis is rare, with fewer than 40 reported cases. Most are high-grade, diffuse, large B-cell lymphoma, but other subtypes include T-cell lymphoma, mucosa-associated lymphoid tissue lymphoma, and Hodgkin disease.[532-535] Penile lymphoma at presentation may mimic Peyronie disease, may form a penoscrotal mass, may present with priapism or paraphimosis, or may present with skin thickening or inflammatory skin ulcers. When clinical disease primarily involves penile skin, primary cutaneous lymphoma must be distinguished from lymphoma with secondary skin involvement.[535] Patients commonly describe painless, progressive swelling or ulceration of the shaft or glans penis and foreskin.[536] All circumcision specimens in adults should be submitted for pathologic examination for proper evaluation of penile lesions.

Tissue examination, ideally in concert with flow cytometer, is essential to achieve the correct diagnosis, and histologic analysis must include immunohistochemical tests to differentiate lymphoma from undifferentiated sarcoma or carcinoma, as well as to distinguish between B-cell and T-cell lymphoma. The absence of lymphoid tissue in the penis suggests that penile lymphoma is a manifestation of occult nodal disease or part of a systemic process; this is the rationale for combined treatment modalities (chemotherapy, radiation therapy, or surgery). Primary lymphoma appears to have a good prognosis, and treatment options are the same as for systemic lymphoma.[532,533]

Germ Cell Tumors
Pediatric extragonadal yolk sac tumors have been documented to originate in the anterior mediastinum, cranium (pineal body and optic chiasm), retroperitoneum, or sacrum. A case of extragonadal germ cell tumor (yolk sac tumor) was recently reported in the penis.[537]

Metastases to the Penis
Although the penis has a rich and complex vascular circulation interconnected to the pelvic organs, metastases are rare and usually represent a late manifestation of systemic metastasis.[538-541] In all reported series the most common primary sites were the prostate gland and urinary bladder, followed by the rectosigmoid colon and kidney (Fig. 15.61).[43,538-549] Less common primary sites include the testes, ureters, and nonpelvic organs such as the lung, pancreas, nasopharynx, larynx, thyroid, and bone.[75,159,538-556]

The most common site for metastatic deposits is the corpus cavernosum.[538-543] Clinically, metastases usually manifest as multiple, palpable, painless nodules that involve the skin and ulcerate, mimicking syphilitic chancre. In 25% of patients, diffuse involvement of the corpus cavernosum causes priapism.[543] Hematuria and

dysuria also may occur. In most cases penile metastases occur in the terminal stage of known cancer and pose no diagnostic difficulty, although rarely they may be the primary presentation of an occult cancer.[75,553] Metastases to the penis should be suspected in any patient with known cancer who has an onset of priapism or an unusual penile lesion. MRI can be accepted as a reliable noninvasive method for the evaluation of the extent of penile metastases and involvement of tunica albuginea or urethra.[554]

The prognosis is poor for patients with metastases to the penis. In a study of 17 patients, the time interval between primary tumor and penile metastasis ranged from 3 to 60 months (mean, 19 months) and between diagnosis of penile metastasis and death ranged from 0.25 to 18 months (mean, 6 months).[543] Similarly, another study reported that 71% of patients died within 6 months of diagnosis and suggested that total penectomy may be indicated for relief of pain or severe urinary symptoms if metastases are confined to the penis without extension to the pelvis or pelvic diaphragm.[556] Palliative local resection or radiation treatment can relieve pain and improve the quality of life.[541]

Scrotum

Normal Anatomy and Histology

The scrotum consists of skin, dartos muscle, and external spermatic, cremasteric, and internal spermatic fasciae. The internal fascia is loosely attached to the parietal layer of the tunica vaginalis. The epidermis covers the dermis, and the deepest layer of the dermis merges with the smooth muscle bundles of the dartos tunic. Although scattered fat cells are present, there is no subcutaneous adipose tissue layer. The dermis contains hair follicles and apocrine, eccrine, and sebaceous glands.

The scrotum contains the testes and the lower parts of the spermatic cords. The surface of the scrotum is divided into right and left halves by a cutaneous raphe that continues ventrally to the inferior penile surface and dorsally along the midline of the perineum to the anus. The left side of the scrotum is usually lower because of the greater length of the left spermatic cord.

Embryologically, the scrotum originates from the genital swellings that meet ventral to the anus and unite to form the two scrotal sacs. A median raphe of fibrovascular connective tissue separates both halves. Median raphe cysts of the perineum are uncommon congenital lesions of the male genitalia. They can be found from the distal penis and scrotum to the perineum in a midline position. They are considered congenital alterations in embryologic development. It is important that adult and pediatric urologists recognize these lesions and their management to provide the appropriate information to the parents.[557]

The scrotum derives its blood supply from the external and internal pudendal arteries, and additional blood comes to it from the cremasteric and testicular arteries that traverse the spermatic cords. Lymphatic drainage of the scrotum is to the superficial inguinal nodes.

Nonneoplastic Diseases

Fournier Gangrene
Fournier gangrene is an idiopathic form of necrotizing fasciitis of the subcutaneous tissue and skeletal muscle of the genitals and perineum, particularly that of the scrotum.[558,559] It begins as reddish plaques with necrosis (Fig. 15.62) and is accompanied by severe systemic symptoms, including pain and fever. The lesions progress

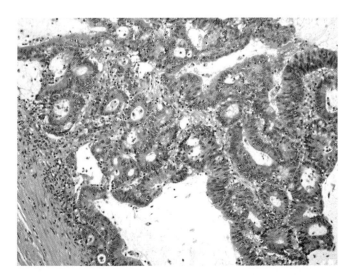

Fig. 15.61 Metastatic colonic adenocarcinoma with malignant enteric-type glands invading the corpus cavernosum.

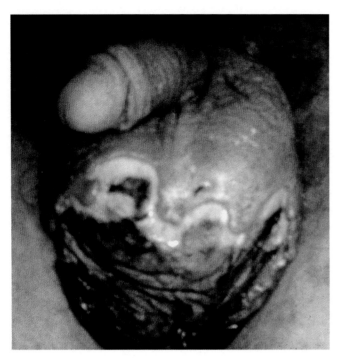

Fig. 15.62 Fournier gangrene. *(Courtesy of Dr. Hans Stricker, Henry Ford Hospital, Detroit, Michigan.)*

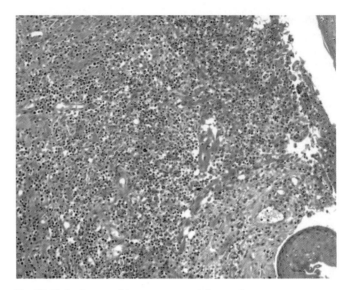

Fig. 15.63 Acute necrotizing gangrenous inflammation.

to develop localized edema, become insensitive, and form blisters that overlie an area of cellulitis. Most cases have accompanying scrotal emphysema. Without prompt diagnosis and aggressive treatment, ulceration and gangrene ensue.

Fournier gangrene probably results from infection by staphylococcal or streptococcal species, which may be pure or, more commonly, are mixed with other gram-negative bacilli and anaerobic bacteria. Diabetes, alcoholism, immunosuppression, recent surgical intervention, trauma, and morbid obesity are predisposing factors but are not necessary for development of Fournier gangrene.[559] Fournier gangrene is a serious, life-threatening condition that requires vigorous and prompt therapy.[558-560] Clinically, the infection resembles clostridial gas gangrene, and in the past, frozen sections were performed to detect gas bubbles. Today most believe that this does not yield clinically significant information and is unnecessary. Definitive treatment includes wide debridement, intravenous broad-spectrum antibiotics, and skin grafting.[560-562] SCC may develop in the scar of Fournier gangrene after a long delay, which differentiates it from other scar carcinomas or Marjolin ulcer.[563]

A necrotizing inflammatory process that is clinically like Fournier gangrene but involves the glans penis is called *Corbus disease* or *gangrenous balanitis*.[564-566] This condition is caused by anaerobic bacteria and can cause total necrosis of the glans penis (Fig. 15.63). Gangrene of the penis also may be caused by constricting bands from external urinary drainage devices and other constricting injuries.[567,568]

Hidradenitis Suppurativa

Hidradenitis suppurativa is a chronic, suppurative inflammatory disease that is part of the follicular occlusion triad—hidradenitis suppurativa, acne conglobata, and perifollicular capitis.[569] First described by Verneuil in 1854, hidradenitis suppurativa is included with other lesions of the triad because of histologic and pathogenetic similarities.[570]

The term *hidradenitis suppurativa* is a misnomer because it is an inflammatory process of apocrine and eccrine glands that are obstructed by follicular hyperkeratosis.[571] Thus follicular hyperkeratosis is the root cause of the rupture of dilated pilosebaceous structures that extrude keratin, apocrine and eccrine products, and commensal bacteria into the dermis, inciting the acute necrotizing and granulomatous reaction with abscess formation that extends into the deep connective tissue and upward onto the epidermis as sinus tracts in the lesions typically seen by surgical pathologists.

The cause of the obstructing follicular hyperkeratosis is not fully understood but may include genetic, hormonal, mechanical, and environmental factors.[572,573] Women with androgenic disturbances, obese patients, and those with intertrigo are especially predisposed to hidradenitis suppurativa. Puberty is also a risk factor. Cultures are often negative, but superinfection is usually due to staphylococci, streptococci, or a mixture of bacteria, including anaerobes and *Actinomyces* species.[574]

Clinically, hidradenitis suppurativa begins as tender erythematous papules and progresses to form fluctuant nodules that may have draining sinuses. Coalescence of adjacent involved follicles forms large plaques. The axilla is the most common site, but it also occurs in the skin of the groin, perianal, areolar, and periumbilical regions. Genitoperineal hidradenitis suppurativa is a debilitating and disfiguring disease that results in the need for repeated abscess drainage operations, chronically painful skin boils, and chronic foul-smelling infectious discharge. It can be associated with lymphedema of surrounding tissues, requiring removal of tissues not originally affected by the disease. Debridement with complete surgical resection and reconstruction with skin flaps and grafts provides a viable treatment option for these patients.[575]

Idiopathic Scrotal Calcinosis

Scrotal calcinosis occurs in two settings: calcification of preexisting epidermal or pilar cysts and calcification of dermal connective tissue in the absence of cysts (idiopathic scrotal calcinosis).[576,577] The hypothesis for the latter form favors origin from eccrine duct milia because of immunoreactivity for CEA, a marker for eccrine sweat glands.[578] A recent study indicated that the idiopathic form may be related to trauma.[579]

Approximately 123 cases of scrotal calcinosis have been described.[580] Saladi et al. classified scrotal calcinosis according to the proposed causal mechanisms: calcific degeneration of epidermoid cysts (34 cases), dystrophic calcification of dartos muscle (3 cases), calcification of eccrine sweat ducts (4 cases), and idiopathic/undetermined (82 cases).[581]

Patients are usually young men, but children and older men also have been affected.[582,583] They usually have multiple (up to 50), long-standing, firm to hard nodules varying in size from a few millimeters up to 3 cm. The overlying skin is usually intact but may ulcerate, releasing cheesy material. Occasionally, a single hard nodule may be present.[584]

Histologically, scrotal calcinosis lies within the dermis and contains granules and globules of hematoxylinophilic calcific material. It may or may not be accompanied by giant cell granulomatous inflammation and recognizable cyst wall fragments (Fig. 15.64). It is plausible that idiopathic scrotal calcinosis represents an end-stage phenomenon of numerous "old" epidermal cysts that over time have lost their cyst walls.[585-587] Treatment may be unnecessary for asymptomatic lesions, but surgery is indicated for infected, recurrent, or extensive lesions.

Lipogranuloma

Lipogranuloma (also known as *paraffinoma*, *sclerosing lipogranuloma*, and *Tancho nodules*) may involve the penile or scrotal skin. Penile lipogranuloma is usually due to hypodermic injection of substances such as paraffin, silicone, oil, or wax into the penis for penile enlargement or sexual gratification.[588-591] In the scrotum, trauma, cold weather, and topical application of ointment (suggesting percutaneous absorption) also have been implicated.[588,592] Most lipogranulomas arise in men younger than 40 years who report a localized plaque or mass that may be tender and indurated, and as large as several centimeters in diameter. Biopsy is necessary, especially in the absence of clinical history of injection of exogenous material. The importance of lipogranuloma lies in differentiating it from malignancy to avoid extensive surgery. It is normally treated with total or partial excision. However, a recent report stated that surgery should be reserved for recurrent or refractory cases when steroids have failed as first-line treatment.[593]

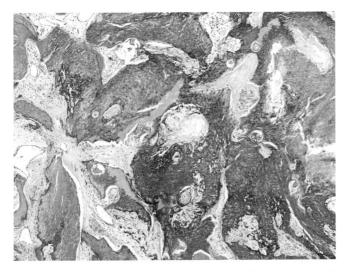

Fig. 15.64 Scrotal calcinosis with deposition of basophilic calcified material in the dermis.

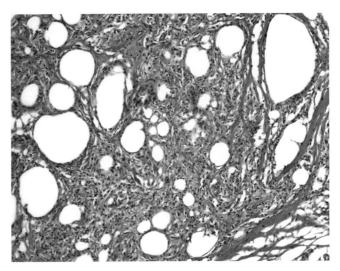

Fig. 15.65 Scrotal lipogranuloma. Lipid vacuoles with marked size variation are seen along with a histiocytic infiltrate, fibrosis, and hyalinization.

Microscopically, lipogranuloma consists of lipid vacuoles embedded in a sclerotic stroma, usually accompanied by a histiocytic or foreign body granulomatous infiltrate with or without eosinophils (Fig. 15.65).[592] CD68 staining is strongly positive in multinucleated giant cells and epithelioid histiocytic cells. Most of the lymphocytes infiltrating the lesions are T cells associated with some S100-positive dendritic cells. T-cell–mediated immune reaction appears to be important in the histogenesis of lipogranuloma. The histogenesis is generally considered to be a foreign body reaction to degenerated or damaged fatty tissue or lipids, but no apparent causative factors can be identified in some reported cases.[594] The differential diagnosis includes signet ring cell carcinoma and malakoplakia. The diagnosis of lipogranuloma may be confirmed by histochemical stains for lipid, but light microscopy is usually sufficient.

Epidermal Cyst

Epidermal cyst (keratinous cyst) is common in the scrotum.[81,595-597] It manifests as single or multiple rubbery-firm subdermal or intradermal nodules. Typically, it contains gray-white cheesy material resulting from exfoliation of the keratinizing squamous epithelium.[595] Hoomayoon et al. reported epidermal cysts in children, and none had a history of exposures to diethylstilbestrol, cryptorchidism, cystic fibrosis, or von Hippel–Lindau disease.[596] Only one patient required surgical excision as a result of persistent pain, and the epidermal cysts resolved in other patients who completed follow-up. Dechev et al. reported a case of epidermoid cyst with signs of malignancy.[598] Because of this feature a histologic study should be a must after surgical removal of the cyst; it is the only method to prove beyond doubt the presence or absence of malignant transformation of the epithelium.[598]

Fat Necrosis

Fat necrosis of the scrotum usually occurs in children and adolescents, appearing as firm nodules in the lower portion of the scrotal wall.[599] Two-thirds of patients have bilateral nodules.[599] The lesion may develop when scrotal fat crystallizes after exposure to cold. Because scrotal fat necrosis has specific imaging features, ultrasound appearance combined with the characteristic clinical presentation can confirm the diagnosis of scrotal fat necrosis.[600]

Neoplastic Diseases

A hamartomatous lesion with angioleiomyomatous features (angioleiomyomatous hyperplasia) rarely occurs in the scrotum and may occasionally simulate malignancy. This lesion is probably underrecognized and has been poorly described in the literature, labeled with various terms, including *hamartoma, muscular hyperplasia, leiomyoma,* and *vascular leiomyoma.*[601-603] Van Kooten et al. reported that chronic scrotal lymphedema may induce hyperplasia of the dartos muscle, resulting in the histologic appearance of scrotal hamartoma.[602]

Benign and malignant neoplasms of the scrotum are rare, and most arise from the skin and adnexal structures.[81,604-607] Melanoma of the scrotum is uncommon with few cases in the reported literature.[405] Hemangioma, lymphangioma, leiomyoma, bizarre leiomyoma, fibrous hamartoma, cellular angiofibroma, neurofibroma, ancient schwannoma, and angiokeratoma are the most common benign scrotal neoplasms.[81,608-620] Atypical fibrous histiocytoma, lipoblastoma, ganglioneuroma, and granular cell tumor also have been reported.[621-624] SCC is the most common scrotal cancer.[625-631] Merkel cell carcinoma and basal cell carcinoma also arise in the scrotum.[632,633] Mucinous cystadenoma, large cell neuroendocrine carcinoma, and apocrine carcinoma have been reported.[634-636] Cases of metastatic carcinoma to the scrotum have been reported.[637,638] Cases of aggressive angiomyxoma and angiomyofibroblastoma also were reported at this site.[639-643]

Squamous Cell Carcinoma

Scrotal SCC was the first cancer linked to occupational exposure to a carcinogen. In the eighteenth century men exposed to soot and dust (e.g., chimney sweeps and cotton factory workers) had an increased incidence of scrotal SCC. Pott described this association, and the tumor was subsequently referred to as *Pott cancer* or *chimney sweep cancer.*[644] SCC of the scrotum also occurs in men with other occupations, including tar workers, paraffin and shale oil workers, machine operators in the engineering industry, petroleum wax pressmen, workers in the screw-making industry, and automatic lathe operators.[626] Seabra et al. reported an interesting observation that three of six patients with scrotal cancer were truck drivers, raising the hypothesis that being a member of this profession with contact with the diesel exhaust expelled by the engine or engaging in sexual promiscuity would imply a larger risk for development of scrotal cancer.[645] Later, 3'4'-benzpyrene was discovered to be the causative agent.[646] Other risk factors include psoriasis treated with coal tar, mineral oil, arsenic, or ultraviolet therapy; condyloma acuminatum; HPV; and multiple cutaneous epitheliomas.[626,646-648] Abhyankar et al. described scrotal carcinoma arising in a 45-year-old man with a history of chronic scrotal and penile lymphedema of filarial origin, and Shifrin et al. reported a case of scrotal carcinoma in a radiation technologist.[649,650]

The incidence of SCC of the scrotum is much lower than that of penile carcinoma.[625-631] To date, approximately 500 cases have been reported.[630] The overall incidence rate varied at approximately 1.5 to 10 per 1,000,000 persons/year. The overall 5-year relative survival rate was 82%, with 77% and 95% for patients with squamous and basal cell carcinoma, respectively. In all, 18% of the patients were diagnosed with a second primary tumor.[630,631]

SCC usually manifests as a solitary slow-growing pimple, wart, or nodule, usually on the anterolateral aspect of the scrotum. It later ulcerates and forms raised, rolled edges with variable amounts of seropurulent discharge. Invasion of the scrotal contents or the penis may occur in patients with advanced cancer. Some authors

suggest that scrotal cancer is uncommon among black men; however, the relatively small number of cases in each reported series limits current understanding of the racial distribution.[627]

SCC of the scrotum occurs primarily in the sixth and seventh decades of life.[626,627] The left scrotum is more frequently affected than the right, and this predominance seems to reflect the site of exposure to carcinogens.[626,627] When occupational exposure is excluded, the sides are equally frequently affected. Ipsilateral inguinal lymphadenopathy is observed at the time of initial presentation in 50% of patients.[626]

Microscopically, SCC of the scrotum is like that of the penis. It is usually well differentiated or moderately differentiated, and keratinization is common. The adjacent epidermis shows hyperkeratosis, acanthosis, and dyskeratosis. A strong correlation exists between stage and survival, but grade does not appear to add prognostic information, although most studies are limited by small sample size.

The full spectrum of subtypes of HR-HPV involved in scrotal SCC has not been elucidated. Matoso et al. recently published their finding in a series of 27 cases of scrotal SCC assessed for viral loads of all 15 subtypes of HR-HPV using multiplex real-time PCR.[651] The results were correlated with histopathologic features, p16 expression, and in situ hybridization for HR-HPV. HR-HPV was identified in two-thirds of the cases. In situ carcinomas had higher viral loads than invasive tumors. The average age of HPV+ and HPV- cases was overall similar. The highest proportion of HR-HPV positivity was seen in basaloid and warty types (100%), followed by usual type (44%); findings akin to vulvar or penile tumors. Additionally, 70% of HR-HPV16/18–positive cases were also reported to be coinfected with other subtypes. The authors of this study stratified SCC of the scrotum into two major groups: groups 1 and 2. Group 1, positive for p16 and elevated Ki67, is associated with HPV infection and displays predominantly a basaloid or warty morphology, although many them are of usual type. Group 2 tumors are negative for p16 with variable Ki67 expression and display predominantly usual-type morphology. SCC of the scrotum in the United States currently affects primarily white-collar professionals. The majority present with in situ lesions, and the high rate of positive margins at first excision indicates that these tumors are clinically ill-defined lesions. Occupational exposures to carcinogens do not comprise the major causative agents of scrotal SCC in the developed world. Currently, common risk factors include HPV infection, immunocompromised states, and chronic scrotal inflammatory conditions.[651] Pigmented SCC was reported in the scrotum in a 70-year-old man, like its counterpart in the oral cavity and conjunctiva. Microscopically, the tumor had typical features, including keratinization, intercellular bridges, and colonization by plump dendritic melanocytes with marked pigmentation. The tumor cells were positive for high-molecular-weight CK and the colonizing melanocytes for HMB45. Because the tumor was associated with a lentiginous lesion, melanocytes entrapped from the lentigo may have been activated during cancer enlargement, resulting in melanocytic colonization.[652]

The differential diagnosis of scrotal SCC includes a wide variety of lesions, including nevus, epidermal cyst, eczema, psoriasis, folliculitis, syphilis, tuberculous epididymitis, and periurethral abscess, as well as benign and malignant neoplasms such as hemangioma, lymphangioma, basal cell carcinoma, malignant melanoma, Paget disease, and sarcoma.[653]

The staging system for scrotal cancer was proposed by Lowe (Table 15.12) and is not included in the current American Joint

TABLE 15.12	Staging System for Scrotal Carcinoma
Stage	**Description**
A1	Localized to scrotal wall
A2	Locally extensive tumor invading adjacent structure (testis, spermatic cord, penis, pubis, perineum)
B	Metastatic disease involving inguinal lymph nodes
C	Metastatic disease involving pelvic lymph nodes without evidence of distant spread
D	Metastatic disease beyond the pelvic lymph nodes involving distant organs

From Lowe FC. Squamous cell carcinoma of the scrotum. *J Urol* 1983;130:423–427.

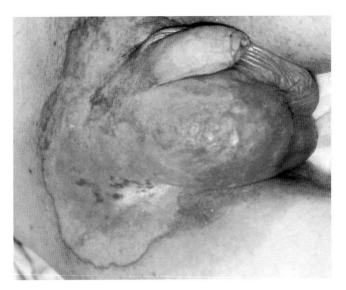

Fig. 15.66 Extramammary Paget disease.

Committee on Cancer staging classification.[386,653] The prognosis is poor for those with SCC; the 5-year survival rate is 30% to 52%. Ray and Whitmore reported a 5-year survival rate of 70% for patients with stage A carcinoma and 44% for patients with stage B carcinoma.[654] Patients with stage C or stage D cancer have little chance for long-term survival. The use of sentinel lymph node biopsy in SCC of the scrotum has been advocated as a safe method of limiting the morbidity associated with bilateral ilioinguinal dissections.[629,655]

Basal Cell Carcinoma

Basal cell carcinoma of the scrotum is rare, accounting for less than 10% of scrotal malignancies.[625,656-660] Mean patient age is 65 years (range, 42 to 82 years).[658] Clinically, it manifests as painless plaques or ulcerated nodules or rarely with a polypoid appearance.[661] Nonulcerative basal cell carcinoma also may occur, clinically mimicking angiokeratoma or seborrheic keratosis.[662] A predilection is seen for the left side of the scrotum.[657] Unlike in SCC, no occupational risk factor or carcinogen has been identified. HPV infection does not appear to play a role.[663] A case of basal cell carcinoma associated with Langerhans cell histiocytosis was reported in a patient with occupational exposure to coal tar and dust.[664] Other causative factors such as chronic skin irritation, previous trauma, exposure to ionizing radiation and other carcinogens, or immunosuppressive drugs may be responsible for the development of the tumors at non–sun-exposed areas such as the scrotum.[665] It has been reported that basal cell carcinoma of the scrotum is more aggressive and likely to metastasize than basal cell carcinoma arising at other sites.[633,658,666,667] Therefore these patients should be kept under surveillance for metastasis for 2 to 5 years after excision of the tumor.[665]

Paget Disease

Extramammary Paget disease rarely involves the penile or scrotal skin.[668-672] Most cases arise in apocrine gland–bearing skin, most commonly the vulva, followed by the perianal region, although other sites have been reported less commonly, including the male genitalia. Unlike mammary Paget disease, most cases of extramammary Paget disease do not arise in association with an underlying malignancy, but occasional cases are associated with underlying carcinoma (either adnexal or visceral), including cancers of the urinary bladder, prostate, rectum, urethra, and sweat glands.[672-678] Penile and scrotal Paget disease most often occur during the sixth and seventh decades of life, usually manifesting as a scaly, eczematous lesion (Fig. 15.66). Microscopically, extramammary Paget

disease consists of an intraepithelial proliferation of atypical cells with vacuolated cytoplasm and large vesicular nuclei (Fig. 15.67). The atypical cells tend to cluster at the tips of the rete ridges. Shiomi et al. recently defined six patterns of extramammary Paget disease: (1) glandular, (2) acantholysis-like, (3) upper nest, (4) tall nest, (5) budding, and (6) sheetlike.[679] The frequencies of the different proliferation patterns they reported were glandular, 36.8%; acantholysis-like, 73.7%; upper nest, 68.4%; tall nest, 28.9%; budding, 47.4%; and sheetlike, 23.7%. The upper nest pattern and presence of more than three patterns were significantly more frequent in invasive extramammary Paget disease than in in situ extramammary Paget disease ($P < 0.05$). They identified the histopathologic patterns of Paget cell proliferation in the epidermis in extramammary Paget disease and suggested that the characteristic patterns and the diversity of patterns could be associated with progression and dermal invasion in extramammary Paget disease. Hyperkeratosis, parakeratosis, and papillomatosis are common. The intraepithelial neoplastic cells contain intracytoplasmic neutral and acidic mucopolysaccharides that can be demonstrated by PAS, mucicarmine, Alcian blue, and aldehyde fuchsin stains. Primary scrotal involvement may rarely coexist with Bowen disease alone or HPV31+ Bowen disease and HPV6+ condyloma acuminatum.[672,677]

The differential diagnosis of extramammary Paget disease includes SCC in situ and malignant melanoma. Intracytoplasmic mucin is not a feature of melanoma or squamous carcinoma in situ, so mucin stain is helpful in establishing the diagnosis. Immunohistochemical stains for CEA, S100 protein, and HMB45 also may be helpful because the cells of Paget disease often contain CEA, whereas melanoma cells are negative, and melanoma cells usually are positive for either S100 protein or HMB45, whereas the cells of Paget disease are negative for these reactions.[675] Paget cells in cases of extramammary disease express a uniform phenotype of mucin (MUC1+ MUC2- MUC5AC+) that is different from that of mammary Paget disease (MUC1+ MUC2- MUC5AC-).[676] The differential diagnosis of pagetoid Bowen disease includes primarily Paget disease, malignant melanoma in situ, and other less common entities. Williamson et al. reported two cases of pagetoid Bowen disease, one in a 65-year-old man with a thigh lesion and the other in a 25-year-old man with a lesion in the penile and scrotal region.[680] Neither patient had clinical

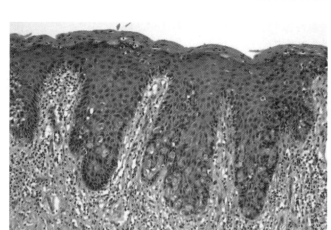
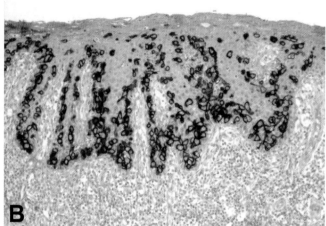

Fig. 15.67 Extramammary Paget disease. (A) Large atypical cells with vacuolated cytoplasm, mainly located at the basal layer of the epidermis. (B) Cytokeratin 7 demonstrates immunoreactivity of tumor cells.

evidence of an internal malignant neoplasm. In both cases the neoplastic cells were positive for CK7/19 and were negative for CK18/20, CEA, gross cystic disease fluid protein 15 (GCDFP15), HER2, S100 protein, and HMB45. Others have shown that CK7 is an almost invariable marker of Paget disease. These two cases illustrated that CK7 can be expressed by pagetoid Bowen disease and should not be a cause of confusion in the differential diagnosis.[680] Cutaneous extramammary Paget disease is characteristically positive for CK7, negative for CK20, and positive for GCDFP15, whereas endodermal extramammary Paget disease shows a CK7/20+ GCDFP15- phenotype. MUC1 and HER2 are also positive in cutaneous extramammary Paget disease, whereas the endodermal subtype is frequently associated with internal malignancy and positive MUC2 and CDX2.[681] HER2 expression in extramammary Paget disease was reported to be higher than in breast Paget disease (31.9%), but scrotal Paget disease was negative for HER2.[682]

Uncommonly, primary extramammary Paget disease is a manifestation of an underlying primary adenocarcinoma of a skin appendage, and the presence of an underlying adnexal carcinoma is thought to be a strong predictor of poor survival in most series. Zhu et al. reported that two of three patients with concomitant sweat gland carcinoma had lymph metastases and eventually died of cancer.[678] Chanda[683] reviewed 197 cases of extramammary Paget disease and reported deaths in 46% patients with underlying adnexal adenocarcinoma. Thus a biopsy diagnosis of extramammary Paget disease with cutaneous sweat gland carcinoma is an indication for curative surgical excision and routine evaluation of regional lymph nodes. A thorough investigation for internal malignancies is also recommended when extramammary Paget disease is diagnosed. The incidence of internal malignancies is low (<10%) in penoscrotal Paget disease.[679,684] Moreover the incidence of coexisting cancer in Asians seems to be lower than that in Caucasians.[679,684,685]

Choi et al. found that the best predictors of late recurrence for extramammary Paget disease were LVI and surgical margin involvement.[685] Yang et al. reported that patients with positive surgical margins developed local recurrence at a median of 8 months; therefore the authors recommended local excision with

intraoperative frozen biopsy analysis.[684] Hegarty et al. reported 20 cases of extramammary Paget disease of the scrotum or penis; 8 had invasive adenocarcinoma, 2 of whom died of the disease, and 3 of whom had residual or recurrent cancers at 5, 7, and 40 months of follow-up and were undergoing multimodal therapy.[686] No patient (12 cases) whose disease was exclusively intraepidermal died of the disease. The prognosis for primary extramammary Paget disease confined to the epidermis is excellent. However, patients with extramammary Paget disease with dermal invasion are at risk for nodal or systemic progression of cancers.

Tsutsumida et al. found a significantly higher risk for lymph node metastases in extramammary Paget disease with reticular dermis or subcutaneous tissue invasion.[687] In their series, 8 of 12 patients with deeper invasion had obvious lymph node metastases. Hatta et al. evaluated sentinel lymph node biopsies in 13 patients with extramammary Paget disease and found that 4 had positive lymph nodes.[688] Of the four patients with positive nodes, dermal invasion was present in three cases, and microdermal invasion was noted in one.[688] The two reports showed a dismal outcome in patients with lymph node metastasis. By contrast, lymph node metastasis was rare in other reports.[678,685] Because inguinal lymphadenectomy is associated with significant morbidity in older patients, sentinel lymph node biopsy might be an appropriate procedure in those cases with dermal invasion. However, the survival benefit of early lymphadenectomy needs further evaluation.

Shan et al. recently reported that overexpression of survivin and human telomerase reverse transcriptase correlated strongly with recurrence and local invasion in extramammary Paget disease lesions.[689]

Sarcoma

Sarcoma of the scrotum, excluding extension of sarcoma from the spermatic cord, is extremely rare.[690] The most common type is leiomyosarcoma, which arises from the dartos muscle; fewer than 20 cases have been reported.[691-696] The age at presentation ranges from 35 to 89 years. A case of radiation-induced leiomyosarcoma was reported in the scrotum.[691] Only five patients had long-term follow-up, and four had distant metastases.[690] Scrotal leiomyosarcoma appears to behave similarly to subcutaneous leiomyosarcoma

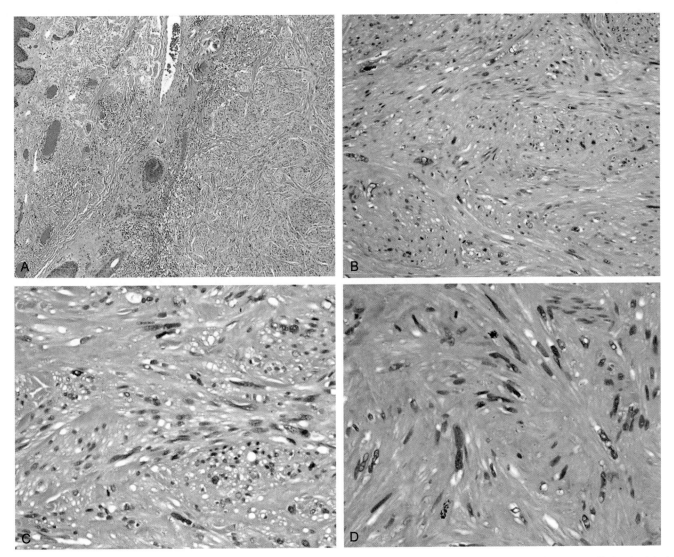

Fig. 15.68 Leiomyosarcoma of the scrotum (A to D). Leiomyosarcoma arising from dartos muscle showing fascicular growth patterns with focal cytologic atypia and mitotic figures.

(Fig. 15.68). Scrotal leiomyosarcoma comprises a proliferation of spindled tumor cells with cigar-shaped nuclei and eosinophilic cytoplasm. A rim of uninvolved overlying dermis may be identified (Fig. 15.68A). Cellular pleomorphism with bizarre or giant tumor cells have been reported as features present in this tumor (Fig. 15.68B to D). The mitotic count may be variable (Fig. 15.68D). Lymphatic metastases are rare, but long-term follow-up is necessary because of the possibility of late visceral metastases or recurrence. Recently a case with combined features of liposarcoma and leiomyosarcoma was reported in the scrotum.[697] Cases of liposarcoma, malignant fibrous histiocytoma, epithelioid sarcoma, embryonal rhabdomyosarcoma, and synovial sarcoma arising from the scrotal wall also have been reported.[698-704] Other malignant tumors are rare and include malignant lymphoma and melanoma, both of which may manifest as a large exophytic mass.[705] Froehner et al. reported a case of gastrointestinal stromal tumor extending through the right inguinal canal that presented as a scrotal mass. Scrotal posttraumatic spindle cell nodule may mimic sarcoma.[706,707] To avoid misdiagnosis, clinicopathologic evaluation is required.

References are available at expertconsult.com

16
Adrenal Glands

ERNEST E. LACK AND EDINA PAAL

CHAPTER OUTLINE

Embryology and Normal Gross Anatomy

Adrenal Cortex

The primordium of the adrenal cortex becomes evident at Carnegie stage 14 (~5 to 7 mm and 32 days), just lateral to the base of the dorsal mesentery near the cranial end of the mesonephros.[1,2] The adrenal cortical primordia are of mesodermal origin and, during development in the late embryo and fetus, the portion of the developing cortex that occupies the greatest volume is referred to as the *fetal* or *provisional cortex*. This layer of cortex makes up approximately 80% of the newborn adrenal gland and undergoes marked regression in the first weeks of life; this is shown graphically in Fig. 16.1, in which the combined weight of the adrenal glands decreases by almost 50% by the 9th to 14th week after birth.[3] The adult, or definitive, cortex forms a much thinner outer zone beneath the adrenal capsule and ultimately becomes the trilayered adrenal cortex of the adult. Convincing evidence exists for centripetal migration or displacement of adrenal cortical cells in experimental animals, thus supporting the original cell migration theory of Gottschau that proposed that migrating adrenal cortical cells can produce all the major adrenal cortical steroids.[3]

On gross examination, the late fetal or neonatal adrenal gland is relatively soft, and, in transverse sections, the fetal zone may have rather dark coloration, which at this stage is quite broad. This dark appearance, shown in Fig. 16.2, may be misinterpreted as adrenal hemorrhage or apoplexy. The adrenal glands in newborns have smoother external surfaces than in adults. In the adult, the right adrenal gland is roughly pyramidal and the left is more elongated (Fig. 16.3). Inspection of the intact capsular surface of the gland after removal of periadrenal connective tissue and fat may reveal small capsular extrusions of cortex; some of these are directly connected with the underlying cortex, but others seem to lie free on the

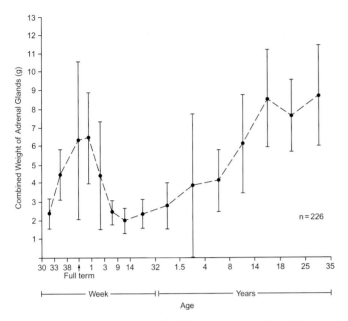

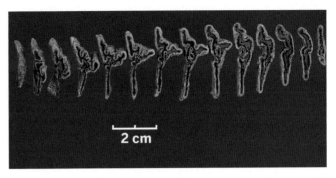

Fig. 16.4 Normal adrenal gland from an adult. An incomplete cuff of cortical cells is present around a central adrenal vein in the medulla. The adrenal vein is present on the ventral surface toward the head of the gland. The dorsal ridge (crista) is flanked by lateral and medial extensions (alae). Medullary tissue is concentrated in the body and head and appears gray-white, in contrast with the bright-yellow cortex.

Fig. 16.1 Average combined weight of the adrenal glands from 226 autopsies by age. Note the marked reduction in combined weight in the first few weeks of life caused by regression of the fetal (provisional) cortex. (From Lack EE, Kozakewich HPW. Embryology, developmental anatomy, and selected aspects of nonneoplastic pathology. In: Lack EE, ed. Pathology of the Adrenal Glands. New York: Churchill Livingstone; 1990:1–74.)

capsular surface or unattached in periadrenal fat. Transverse sections of adrenal gland in the adult reveal a bright yellow, relatively uniform cortex with a gray-white medulla that is concentrated in the head and body of the gland (Fig. 16.4). A cuff of cortical cells may be noted partially or entirely surrounding larger tributaries of the adrenal vein. The dorsal surface of the adrenal gland has a longitudinal ridge or crista flanked by medial and lateral extensions or alae (wings). The anterior (or ventral) surface of the adrenal gland is relatively smooth, and it is from this surface of the gland that the adrenal veins exit and drain into the inferior vena cava on the right side and the renal vein on the left. The orientation of the adrenal gland in vivo differs from that depicted in gross photographs of specimens in surgical or autopsy material. As seen in Fig. 16.5, the glands are oriented in a more vertical axis, with the ridge (or crista) projecting posteriorly and flanked by medial and lateral alae. The thickness of the adult cortex is approximately 2 mm or more throughout most of the gland, although some variability may be seen from area to area, and cortical nodularity may complicate the morphology.[3]

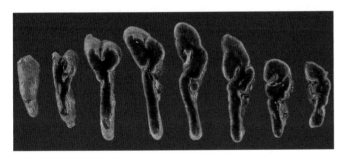

Fig. 16.2 Adrenal gland from a newborn infant. Note the dark congested fetal (provisional) cortex and thin rim of pale adult (definitive) cortex. Cortical extrusion is also present centrally.

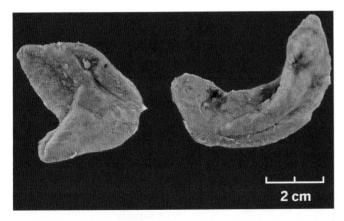

Fig. 16.3 Normal adrenal glands from an adult. The right is roughly pyramidal (*left side of photo*), whereas the left is elongated (*right side of photo*). The longitudinal ridge (crista) is flanked by lateral extensions (alae).

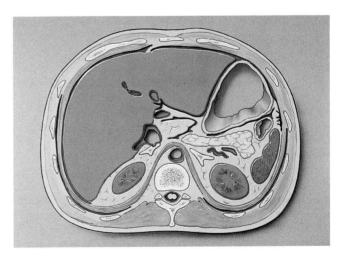

Fig. 16.5 Diagram of transverse cut of abdomen in an adult showing orientation of the adrenal glands and relation with the kidneys. The ventral aspect of both glands is relatively flat, and the dorsal surface has a longitudinal ridge (crista). Lateral extensions (alae) are often referred to as *medial and lateral limbs* on CT scans.

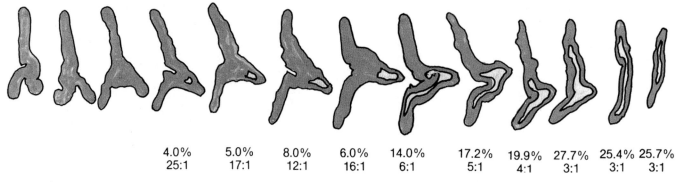

	4.0%	5.0%	8.0%	6.0%	14.0%	17.2%	19.9%	27.7%	25.4%	25.7%
	25:1	17:1	12:1	16:1	6:1	5:1	4:1	3:1	3:1	3:1

Fig. 16.6 Schematic drawing of transverse sections of adrenal gland from an adult. Chromaffin tissue is concentrated in the body and head. Figures indicate the percentage of cross-sectional area occupied by medulla (*top row*) and ratio of areas of cortex to medulla (*bottom row*).

Adrenal Medulla

Chromaffin tissue of the adrenal medulla in the fetal and newborn adrenal gland is inconspicuous on gross examination of transverse sections of the gland. In the adult, however, chromaffin tissue is concentrated in the body and head of the gland, with the latter regions being directed inferomedially in vivo.[3,4] As seen in Fig. 16.6, the ratio of area occupied by cortex relative to that of medulla decreases considerably from the tail to the body and head of the gland. The normal overall ratio of cortex to medulla is approximately 10:1. The distribution and amount of chromaffin tissue within the gland, as well as other factors, such as adrenal weight, may be important in determining whether adrenal medullary hyperplasia (AMH) is present.[4] Another consideration is morphologic abnormalities of the adrenal cortex, such as adrenal cortical atrophy, which can affect the overall ratio. The adrenal medulla is composed of chromaffin cells derived from primitive sympathicoblasts of neural crest origin that migrate into the dorsomedial aspect of the adrenal primordium and become apparent at Carnegie stages 16 and 17 (~11 to 14 mm and 41 days).[1,2] Most of the developing chromaffin tissue in fetal life is extraadrenal, with the largest collections of cells in the paraaortic region, near the origin of the superior mesenteric and renal arteries down to the aortic bifurcation; these chromaffin structures were first characterized in the human fetus by Zuckerkandl in 1901, who referred to them as *aortic bodies.*[5]

Microscopic Anatomy

At birth, the thin rim of adult (definitive) cortex blends imperceptibly into cells of the fetal (provisional) cortex. The definitive cortex apparently begins to grow soon after birth, with zonation into the zona glomerulosa and zona fasciculata first appearing at 2 to 4 weeks.[6] According to some investigators, the zona reticularis appears at approximately 4 years, but others contend that it appears before 1 year.[6,7] The zona glomerulosa contains cells with dark round nuclei and relatively scant cytoplasm arranged in interlacing cords and spherules; this zone is normally thin and ill defined, and it may appear discontinuous in the normal adult gland (Fig. 16.7). This layer blends imperceptibly into the zona fasciculata, which constitutes most of the adult cortex, and consists of long columns of larger cells with pale, finely vacuolated cytoplasm in the unstressed gland. The transition between the innermost zona fasciculata and the zona reticularis contains cells with more compact eosinophilic cytoplasm separated by thin-walled sinusoids and irregular short cords of cells. Reticularis cells may contain prominent granular

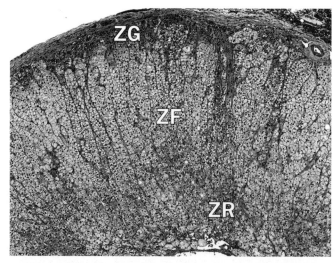

Fig. 16.7 Normal adult adrenal cortex. Zona glomerulosa (*ZG*) is at the top of the field beneath the adrenal capsule and forms a thin, discontinuous layer of cells. Most of the cortex is occupied by radial interconnecting cords of zona fasciculata (*ZF*), which contain cells with pale-staining, lipid-rich cytoplasm. The zona reticularis (*ZR*) has interconnecting short cords of cells with compact, eosinophilic cytoplasm and congested microvasculature.

pigment representing lipofuscin. Chromaffin cells of the adrenal medulla are polyhedral and arranged in short anastomosing cords or nests with a prominent vascular network, or a more solid or diffuse arrangement of cells may be seen. Adrenal chromaffin cells secrete predominantly epinephrine, with lesser amounts of norepinephrine.[4] In the fetal and neonatal adrenal gland, small nests of primitive neuroblastic cells may be encountered (Fig. 16.8), which may be a part of normal developmental anatomy (see the In Situ Neuroblastoma section later in this chapter).[3,4]

The zona glomerulosa is the site of aldosterone production and is responsive to stimulation by angiotensin and adrenocorticotropic hormone (ACTH). The zona fasciculata produces corticosteroids such as cortisol, whereas the zona reticularis is responsible for sex steroid production. Longitudinal pillars of smooth muscle are found predominantly in the head of the adrenal gland around tributaries of the adrenal vein and are thought to act as "sluice gates" that retard the flow of blood from the medullary venous sinuses and plexus reticularis during muscle contraction.[8] The muscular bundles may help regulate medullary blood flow and influence the degree of congestion in the zona reticularis and zona fasciculata of the adjacent cortex.

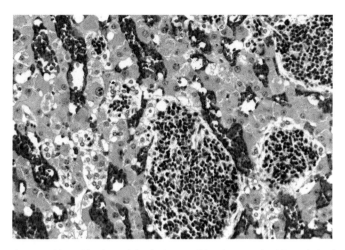

Fig. 16.8 Neuroblastic nodules in the provisional zone of a 16-week fetal adrenal gland.

Examination of the Adrenal Glands

Examination of the intact adrenal gland is best accomplished by careful removal of as much investing connective tissue and fat as possible to obtain an accurate weight. The weight of the cleanly dissected gland may provide valuable information regarding adrenal cortical or medullary pathology. In the study by Stoner et al., the average combined weight of the adrenal glands at birth was 10 g (range, 2 to 17 g), whereas the average weight was 6 g at 7 days of age and 5 g at 2 weeks of age.[6] Quinan and Berger studied the adult adrenal gland, concentrating on ostensibly healthy subjects who had died suddenly, and found that the average weight of each gland was 4.15 g, with no significant difference between the right and left sides.[9] Studzinski et al. examined surgically removed adrenal glands from women with breast cancer and reported an average weight of 4 g, with little variation (standard deviation, 0.8 g).[10] Adrenal glands obtained at autopsy from individuals who had not died suddenly or unexpectedly tended to be heavier, with an average individual weight of 6 g; this difference was attributed to the stress of illness and the trophic influence of endogenous ACTH.[10] Using these data, each normal adrenal gland should weigh less than 6 g, provided excess periadrenal fat and connective tissue are carefully removed.

Congenital and Other Abnormalities

Congenital Adrenal Aplasia and Hypoplasia

Congenital adrenal aplasia or agenesis is rare. Unilateral adrenal aplasia has been reported in about 10% of patients with unilateral renal agenesis.[11] Complete bilateral adrenal aplasia is also rare and may occur in a familial setting.[12] The diagnosis should be viewed with caution because there may be small amounts of residual adrenal tissue present in the suprarenal fat pad that can be missed on sensitive abdominal imaging or routine autopsy.[13] Bilateral congenital adrenal aplasia has nonetheless been documented at careful autopsy examination.[14] Congenital adrenal hypoplasia refers to distinct clinical conditions characterized by underdevelopment or hypoplasia of the adrenal cortex, and based on its physiopathology can be broadly classified as primary or secondary.[15] The causes of adrenal cortical insufficiency in general are complex, even in the congenital category, and can have varied phenotypic

manifestations. DAX-1 (dosage-sensitive sex reversal-adrenal hypoplasia congenita critical region on the X-chromosome) and steroidogenic factor-1 (SF-1) are two important transcription factors that belong to the nuclear receptor superfamily.[16] These play an important role in human adrenal and reproductive development. Alterations in the genes encoding these factors (e.g., deletions, mutations) are associated with an ever-expanding range of phenotypic adrenal and reproductive abnormalities. Adrenal hypoplasia congenital (AHC) is not to be confused with the much more common disorder congenital adrenal hyperplasia (CAH). *NROB1* is the gene encoding DAX-1 and is the key gene in which alterations are known to cause X-linked AHC with infantile-onset acute primary adrenal insufficiency. This severe adrenoprival disorder in male infants can manifest as vomiting, difficulty feeding, dehydration, and shock caused by salt wasting. If unrecognized or left untreated, acute adrenal insufficiency can be rapidly fatal with hyperkalemia, acidosis, and shock. At autopsy, combined adrenal weights can be markedly decreased (e.g., 0.5 g in the first week of life). In X-linked AHC, several histologic patterns of cortical atrophy have been described. The miniature adult form has small amounts of cortical tissue resembling the adult or definitive cortex, and the cytomegalic form has enlarged cells with abundant cytoplasm and absence or near absence of the adult or definitive cortex.

Phenotypic variation can occur with X-linked form of AHC with delayed onset into adult life or variation in manifestation of hypogonadotropic hypogonadism. Other forms of AHC exist, with some having autosomal inheritance and even presentation in females. SF-1 is also a nuclear receptor with encoding gene *NR5A1* located on the long arm of chromosome 9. This is a pivotal factor in initiation and fetal maturation of the adrenal cortex. In the absence of SF-1 expression, the adrenal gland does not form as shown by adrenal aplasia in SF-1 knockout mice.[16] Alterations in SF-1 are rarely associated with adrenal cortical insufficiency, but a range of reproductive phenotypic abnormalities are more common including 46XY disorders such as gonadal dysgenesis, hypospadias, and anorchia; in 46XX females, alterations in SF-1 are associated with primary ovarian insufficiency.[17]

Adrenal Heterotopia

During embryologic development, the adrenal primordium is in close proximity to the urogenital ridge, accounting for the accessory and heterotopic adrenal tissue that may occur in sites in the upper abdomen and along lines of descent of the gonads.[3] Heterotopic adrenal tissue has been described in up to 32% of patients in the region of the celiac axis, and, at this site, approximately one-half of the lesions contained both cortex and medulla.[18] Accessory adrenal tissue in sites further removed from the upper abdomen usually consists of cortical tissue alone, without the distinctive zonation of the normal adult adrenal gland. Other sites of heterotopia include the broad ligament near the ovary (23%), the liver, the kidney (6%, usually subcapsular), along the spermatic cord (3.8% to 9.3%; a higher incidence was observed for males undergoing surgery for an undescended testis), the testicular adnexa (7.5%), and other rarely described sites that defy ready embryologic explanation such as the placenta, lung, mediastinum, and an intracranial intradural location.[19-29] Only rarely have intratesticular or intraovarian cortical rests occurred within the substance of the gonads.[30,31] Cases have been reported of hyperplastic cortical nodules arising from accessory adrenal tissue along the spermatic cord and the broad ligament, and adrenal cortical neoplasms have been reported, rarely, in hepatic parenchyma and the spinal canal.[32-36] Intraadrenal bile ductules have been reported in association with adrenohepatic fusion; heterotopic intraadrenal liver has also been reported.[37,38]

Union and Adhesion

Union or adhesion of the adrenal gland to kidney or liver has been reported, the distinction being whether a continuous connective tissue capsule separates the two organs.[39] Adrenal fusion is a rare anomaly in which the adrenal glands are fused in the midline and may be associated with other congenital midline defects such as spinal dysraphism or indeterminate visceral situs.[3] Abnormal adrenal shape has been reported in some cases of renal agenesis, in which the glands may be ovoid with smoother contours.[3]

Adrenal Cytomegaly

Congenital adrenal cytomegaly is usually an incidental finding in an adrenal gland that otherwise appears grossly normal. It has been reported in approximately 3% of newborn autopsies and 6.5% of premature stillborns.[40] The cytomegaly affects cells of the fetal (provisional) cortex and may be bilateral or unilateral, focal or diffuse. The cytomegalic cell has an enlarged hyperchromatic nucleus and increased volume of cytoplasm. Nuclei may be markedly pleomorphic and occasionally contain intranuclear pseudoinclusions, which are indentations of the nucleus with invagination of cytoplasm. Despite the marked nuclear abnormalities, mitotic figures are characteristically absent.

Adrenal cytomegaly is a characteristic component of the Beckwith-Wiedemann syndrome (Fig. 16.9), sometimes called the *EMG syndrome,* which refers to a major triad of findings—exomphalos, macroglossia, and gigantism.[3,41-43] The estimated frequency of this disorder is 1 in 13,000 births; most reported cases are sporadic, although some seem to have a mendelian pattern of inheritance.[3] The disorder is caused by dysregulation of growth-regulatory genes within the 11p15 region, resulting in loss of normal growth control and increased incidence of certain cancers.[44,45] The adrenal glands in this disorder are enlarged, with combined weights as high as 16g. The adrenal cytomegaly is usually marked and is typically bilateral and diffuse. Curiously, adrenal chromaffin

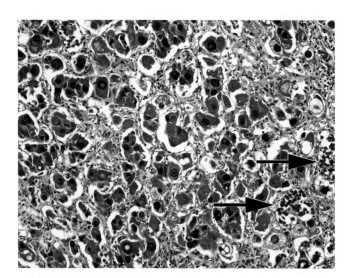

Fig. 16.9 Adrenal gland in Beckwith-Wiedemann syndrome. Provisional zone of the fetal adrenal gland shows prominent cytomegaly with cells having greatly enlarged hyperchromatic nuclei. Small nests of neuroblastic cells are also evident (*arrows*).

tissue may be hyperplastic or inappropriately mature.[4,43] Visceromegaly may be present, affecting the kidneys and pancreas, and some infants develop severe neonatal hypoglycemia that may prove fatal. An increased incidence of malignant tumors is seen in this disorder, usually Wilms tumor or adrenal cortical carcinoma (ACC), but other neoplasms have been reported including neuroblastoma, pancreatoblastoma, and hepatoblastoma.[3,46-49] The presence of hemihypertrophy in children predicts a greater risk for the development of a malignant neoplasm. Adrenal cytomegaly has also been associated with fetal hydrops resulting from Rh incompatibility or hemoglobin Bart.[50]

Adrenoleukodystrophy

Adrenoleukodystrophy (ALD) is a clinically heterogeneous disease and occurs in multiple forms. Most cases of ALD are X-linked. The molecular basis of X-linked ALD is mutation of the gene (*ABCD1*) encoding a peroxisomal membrane protein (ALDP), resulting in an increase in very-long-chain fatty acids and reduced oxidation thereof in the peroxisomes.[51-54] The lipid material accumulates in tissue as cholesterol esters that may exert a toxic effect on cells, with crystallization of lamellae and disruption of cell membranes.[3] This mechanism may account for the pathogenesis of adrenal cortical insufficiency and degeneration of white matter, particularly involving the posterior cerebrum, cerebellum, and descending corticospinal tracts. Three main forms of X-linked ALD are known: (1) the childhood form, which is a progressive central demyelination leading to total disability within 2 years of onset; (2) the adult form, also known as *adrenomyeloneuropathy,* in which a slowly progressive spastic paraparesis and distal polyneuropathy occur, with onset usually in the second or third decade of life; and (3) a variant that has a primary presentation of adrenal insufficiency.[3] ALD or adrenomyeloneuropathy should be considered in the differential diagnosis of boys or young men who present with unexplained adrenal cortical insufficiency, because neurologic symptoms may not be evident at the time of presentation.[51-54] A rare fourth neonatal form usually has an autosomal recessive inheritance.[3]

The adrenal glands in ALD are often quite small. Thinning of the adrenal cortex occurs, with characteristic enlargement of cortical cells having abundant ground-glass or waxy cytoplasm; these cells have been called *balloon cells* and may have a fibrillar or striated appearance caused by lipid material being extracted during routine processing.[55] On ultrastructural examination, bilamellar and lamellar lipid inclusions can be seen, which are virtually pathognomonic for the disorder. The adrenal cortical insufficiency in this disorder is primary and not caused by pituitary or hypothalamic dysfunction. The recent molecular advances regarding the X-linked form of this disease have major implications for the possibility of gene-based therapy.[51,54,56] A comprehensive review of the pathophysiology of X-linked ALD has recently been published.[57]

Congenital Adrenal Hyperplasia

CAH, also known as adrenogenital syndrome, is a rare autosomal recessive disorder usually caused by a deficiency of one of five different enzymes in the steroid biosynthetic pathway of the adrenal cortex (Fig. 16.10).[3,58] The first description of a case of CAH was in 1865 by the Italian anatomist de Crecchio, who dissected the cadaver of an apparent male of approximately 40 years of age who had bilateral cryptorchidism and partial hypospadias; however, further examination revealed a vagina, uterus, fallopian tubes, ovaries, and very large adrenal glands.[59] The subject was also said to

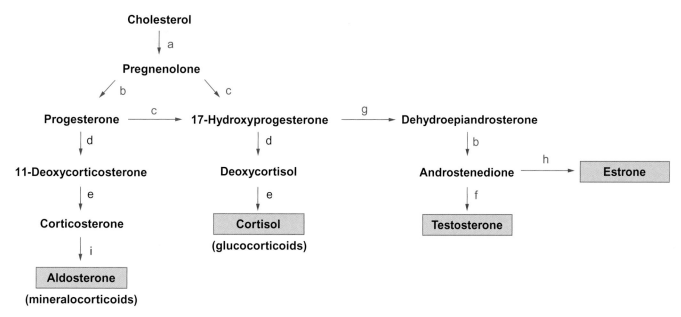

Fig. 16.10 Normal biosynthetic pathway of adrenal cortical steroid synthesis. *a* = 20,22 hydroxylase and 20,22 desmolase; *b* = 3β-hydroxysteroid dehydrogenase; *c* = 17-hydroxylase; *d* = 21-hydroxylase; *e* = 11β-hydroxylase; *f* = 17-ketosteroid reductase; *g* = 17,20 desmolase; *h* = P450 aromatase; *i* = 18-hydroxylase and 18-aldehyde synthetase.

have had frequent diarrhea and vomiting and in his final days had extreme weakness and exhaustion, which almost certainly represented an addisonian crisis.

The most common cause of CAH is 21-hydroxylase deficiency, which accounts for approximately 90% to 95% of cases.[58,60] This deficiency has been divided into a classic form, with an incidence of 1 in 5000 to 15,000 live births in most white populations; a nonclassic form, which is among the most frequent of autosomal recessive disorders in the white population; and a cryptic form in which patients are asymptomatic despite having the same biochemical abnormality.[58,60] Mutations in the encoding gene have been confirmed as the basis of endocrine disease in all adrenal steroidogenic enzymes required for the synthesis of cortisol. In 21-hydroxylase deficiency, insufficient production of cortisol occurs, resulting in a lack of negative feedback at the hypothalamic-pituitary level and secondary trophic stimulation of the adrenal glands by increased ACTH levels. In approximately two-thirds of cases of the classic disorder, biosynthesis of aldosterone is also affected, leading to salt wasting; if unrecognized or severe enough, this may result in death in the first few weeks of life.[3] The remaining one-third of cases have simple virilizing disease, without significant impairment of aldosterone biosynthesis. Because of the enzymatic block, precursor steroids accumulate and spill over into the sex steroid pathway with increased androgen production. The development of external genitalia is under the control of androgens in utero, and, because of this, affected females usually have ambiguous genitalia with clitoromegaly and fusion of the labioscrotal folds, although the internal female organs develop normally. In females, the ambiguous genitalia may be so extreme that the child is incorrectly assumed to be male. Affected males usually appear normal at birth. For this reason, males with the disorder may not be diagnosed until they present with more severe symptoms, often related to a potentially fatal salt-wasting crisis. The identification of mutations in the *CYP21* gene, which encodes the 21-hydroxylase enzyme, has led to advances in DNA diagnosis, including prenatal and newborn screening programs.

Approximately 5% to 8% of cases of CAH are caused by the classic form of 11β-hydroxylase deficiency because of mutations in the *CYP11B1* gene.[61] Other enzymatic defects causing CAH include deficiency of 3β-hydroxysteroid dehydrogenase, 17α-hydroxylase, and the rare mutation in the gene encoding steroidogenic acute regulatory protein (StAR), which seriously interferes with adrenal and gonadal steroidogenesis by a defect in the conversion of cholesterol to pregnenolone.[62] The latter defect causes *congenital lipoid hyperplasia.*

Pathology of Adrenal Glands in Congenital Adrenal Hyperplasia

Today it is very uncommon to examine the adrenal glands of patients who died of unrecognized or untreated CAH. Grossly, the adrenal glands are enlarged, often with a convoluted or cerebriform surface with excess cortical plications and folding. The glands frequently have a light-brown color reminiscent of the zona reticularis, resulting from the sustained trophic effect of ACTH and the conversion of lipid-rich, pale-staining cells to cortical cells with lipid-depleted compact eosinophilic cytoplasm (Fig. 16.11). In children, the weight of each adrenal gland may be 10 to 15 g, whereas in older individuals each gland may weigh 30 to 35 g.[3] *Congenital lipoid hyperplasia* is the most fatal form of CAH in which there is accumulation of cholesterol and cholesterol esters giving the adrenal glands a bright-yellow or white appearance on cross-section.[62]

Testicular Adrenal Rest Tumors in Congenital Adrenal Hyperplasia

Male patients with CAH—particularly but not exclusively the salt-wasting form of 21-hydroxylase deficiency—may develop one or more testicular adrenal rest tumors (TARTs). In a study of 244 patients with CAH, the prevalence of TART on ultrasound examination was 33% in boys and 44% in men.[63] The tumors are often bilateral (83%) and may cause testicular pain and tenderness.[64] Several reports in the literature clearly document that the tumors

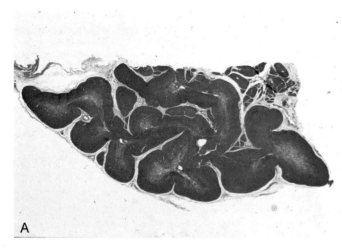
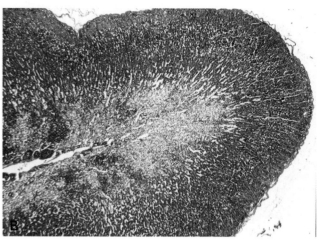

Fig. 16.11 Adrenal gland in congenital adrenal hyperplasia. (A) Note the convoluted or cerebriform surface of the gland in this whole-mount section. (B) Microscopically, the adrenal cortical cells have a compact eosinophilic cytoplasm with depletion of the normal lipid content.

are ACTH dependent, as evidenced by reduction in testicular size and associated symptoms with suppressive doses of dexamethasone and recrudescence of testicular enlargement with ACTH stimulation. Laboratory testing also has demonstrated ACTH-dependent steroidogenesis by the tumors.[65]

The tumors may be 2 to 10 cm in diameter in older patients. Most of the smaller tumors appear to be in the hilum of the testis, but with larger tumors the precise site of origin is difficult to determine.[64] Rete testis–associated nodular steroid cell nests have been reported with immunoreactivity for melan A, inhibin, and calretinin, and may represent the putative histogenetic cell for TART.[66] On cross-section, TARTs often have a lobulated appearance with bulging, tan to dark-brown nodules. The histologic appearance resembles that of a Leydig cell tumor; however, some features may distinguish these two tumors. Nuclei are usually round to oval with a single prominent nucleolus, which may be central or somewhat eccentric. Cells have granular, pink cytoplasm with relatively distinct cell borders. The cells are usually arranged in sheets or small nests with intersecting fibrous bands, and reticulum stain often demonstrates an intimate pattern of isolation of individual and small clusters of cells. As opposed to Leydig cell tumors, TARTs lack Reinke crystalloids, exhibit more extensive fibrosis, and may contain lymphoid aggregates. Nuclear pleomorphism is reportedly prominent in contrast with Leydig cell tumors, and mitotic activity is rare. Most TARTs are strongly positive for synaptophysin, whereas only rare Leydig cell tumors are immunoreactive with synaptophysin.[67]

Virtually identical testicular tumors of this type have been reported in males with Nelson syndrome (pituitary adenoma after bilateral adrenalectomy); rarely, a female with Nelson syndrome may develop similar adrenal rest tumors in the region of the ovaries, where heterotopic adrenal cortical tissue occasionally is found.[68] Rare examples of histologically similar tumors have been reported in the ovary of women with CAH.[69,70] It is unclear whether TARTs are true neoplasms or hyperplastic nodules. In favor of hyperplasia are their ACTH dependence and bilaterality.

Other Tumors Associated With Congenital Adrenal Hyperplasia

Rare cases of adrenal cortical adenoma (ACA) and ACC have been reported in patients with CAH.[3,71,72] It has been suggested that persistent ACTH stimulation may result in neoplastic transformation of some adrenal cortical cells, but this is unproved.

Other tumors have been reported in association with CAH, including bilateral adrenal myelolipomas, osteosarcoma, and Ewing sarcoma, but their relationship with CAH and the underlying biochemical abnormality is unclear.[73,74]

Stress-Related Changes of the Adrenal Gland

One of the most common histologic changes observed in the adrenal gland of patients under stress is the conversion of lipid-rich, pale-staining cortical cells of the zona fasciculata to cells with compact, lipid-depleted eosinophilic cytoplasm. This is particularly common in acquired immunodeficiency syndrome (AIDS) (Fig. 16.12). Another abnormality reported in stress-related conditions is degeneration of the outer zona fasciculata, initially described as *tubular degeneration;* this abnormality appears with scattered necrosis of cortical cells, shedding of vacuolated cytoplasm, and exudation of fluid into cords of cortical cells in the outer zona fasciculata.[75] A peculiar vacuolization of the fetal adrenal cortex has been described in infants with erythroblastosis fetalis, and nearly identical changes have been observed in thalassemia major.[3] A relationship with intrauterine stress and hypoxia has been

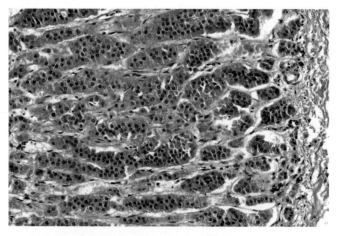

Fig. 16.12 Adrenal gland of an adult who died of acquired immunodeficiency syndrome. The cortex showed severe lipid depletion, characterized by numerous cells with compact eosinophilic cytoplasm. The capsule of the adrenal gland is present on the *far right.*

suggested. A pattern of focal lipid depletion has been reported as lipid reversion, which suggests recovery from stress and replenishment of lipid in cells of the inner zona fasciculata. In areas of lipid reversion, the outer aspect of the adrenal cortex contains little or no lipid, although lipid is prominent in the inner zona fasciculata.[7]

Other Abnormalities

Conspicuous iron accumulation occurs in the form of hemosiderin in cells of the outer cortex, particularly the zona glomerulosa, in conditions such as primary hemochromatosis and transfusion hemosiderosis.[3] In some cases, associated hypothalamic-pituitary dysfunction is caused by excess iron deposition, which may result in endocrine insufficiency of the gonads, thyroid gland, and adrenal glands. A variety of drugs and cytotoxic agents have direct antiadrenal activity; examples include dichlorodiphenyltrichloroethane (DDT) and its derivative o,p'DDD, which has been used for palliative treatment of patients with ACC because of its adrenolytic effect on normal and neoplastic cortical cells. Another agent with antiadrenal activity is ketoconazole, a broad-spectrum antifungal drug that blocks adrenal steroid synthesis.[3] Linear hyaline fibrosis has also been reported in the zona reticularis after radiation, probably because of structural damage of the vascular plexus in this zone.[76]

Anencephaly is a severe developmental defect of anterior neural tube structures with agenesis of much of the brain and cranial vault. The pituitary gland is difficult to find grossly but is often identified in histologic sections, albeit reduced in amount. The adrenal glands are often extremely small in this disorder, with an average combined weight in one study of 1.8 g, but a significant number weighed less than 1 g.[77] The fetal cortex is often normal in size and structure until approximately 20 weeks of gestation, after which it progressively involutes, like changes that normally occur after birth; chromaffin tissue may appear relatively prominent.

Nonneoplastic Diseases

Chronic Adrenal Cortical Insufficiency (Addison Disease)

Idiopathic or Autoimmune Addison Disease

In developed countries, 80% to 90% of cases of primary adrenal insufficiency are caused by autoimmune adrenalitis that can be isolated (40%) or part of an autoimmune polyendocrine syndrome (APS; 60%).[78] The most common type of Addison disease is idiopathic or autoimmune and is regarded as an organ-specific autoimmune form of adrenalitis. It has been suggested that Addison disease has a strong genetic component, including APS and, more often there is expression of disease susceptibility with alleles associated with organ-specific autoimmunity (MHC, CTLA4, PTPN22), and those that encode proteins of innate immune response.[79] It has been shown that presence of autoantibodies directed against the enzymes of steroid hormone production, predominantly 21-hydroxylase, and their detection may be helpful in predicting the risk for developing the disease.[79,80] A recent detailed review summarizes adrenal insufficiency including epidemiology and pathophysiology.[78] The frequency of the causes of primary adrenal insufficiency in children differs substantially from that in the adult population. Genetic forms are more common, with the most frequent cause of primary adrenal insufficiency being CAH (72%) with other genetic causes accounting for another 6%; autoimmune Addison disease was diagnosed in only 13%.[81]

The adrenal gland in this disorder may be greatly reduced in size and volume, making gross identification difficult at autopsy unless numerous tissue blocks from the suprarenal bed are examined. The adrenal cortex has a large endocrine reserve, and it is estimated that up to 90% or more of the cortex must be ablated before functional impairment is apparent.[3] In some cases, intercurrent illness, infection, or surgery may precipitate an addisonian crisis. The residual cortex is often thin and discontinuous, with scattered islands of cortical cells (Fig. 16.13) admixed with lymphocytes, plasma cells, and occasional lymphoid follicles, sometimes with reactive germinal centers. Cortical cells may be enlarged, with ample compact, eosinophilic cytoplasm and occasional nuclear alteration, including pseudoinclusions. On occasion, residual cortex may be difficult to identify, and little or no inflammation may be present. Adrenal medulla may appear relatively prominent.

APS is characterized by the association of two or more organ-specific disorders and has been divided into two forms: APS type 1, also known as autoimmune polyendocrinopathy–candidiasis–ectodermal dystrophy (APECED) and APS type 2. APS type 1 is a rare autosomal recessive disorder with endocrine insufficiency involving various organs, including the adrenal cortex. Numerous mutations in the gene responsible for the disease, AIRE (autoimmune regulator), have been identified. The gene is located on

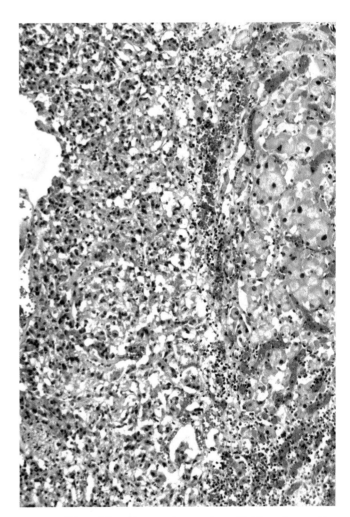

Fig. 16.13 Primary idiopathic or autoimmune form of Addison disease. Atrophic adrenal cortex (*right side*) contains cells with compact, eosinophilic cytoplasm. The medulla is present on the *left*.

chromosome 21 (21q22) and encodes a protein involved in transcriptional regulation.[82-85] This disorder has a variety of manifestations including Addison disease.[86] APS type 2 is defined by the occurrence of Addison disease, thyroid autoimmune disease, or type 1 diabetes mellitus. The combination of nontuberculous Addison disease and thyroid insufficiency is sometimes referred to as *Schmidt syndrome.*[87]

Adrenal Tuberculosis

Adrenal tuberculosis once was the leading cause of Addison disease.[88] According to the review by Guttman of cases between 1900 and 1929, 70% resulted from tuberculosis, and 19% were caused by primary or idiopathic atrophy.[89] The endemic nature of bovine tuberculosis in the early decades of the twentieth century is reflected in the comment by Dunlop, who characterized cream on top of the milk in those days as often being composed of "tuberculous pus."[90] The tuberculous adrenal gland is often enlarged, with extensive areas of caseous necrosis. A classic granulomatous reaction with numerous epithelioid histiocytes is present typically in extraadrenal sites but not the adrenal, suggesting that the locally high levels of adrenal corticosteroids dampen the host inflammatory response.[3]

Histoplasmosis and Other Fungal Infections

Disseminated histoplasmosis is a recognized cause of Addison disease and typically involves the glands bilaterally. In a study of almost 100 cases, 7% of patients had chronic adrenal cortical insufficiency.[91] Similar to tuberculosis, extensive caseous necrosis is a common finding, although a granulomatous response is the exception rather than the rule. Perivasculitis involving extracapsular adrenal vessels may lead to extensive infarction and caseous necrosis, resulting in loss of adrenal parenchyma and development of Addison disease. Other mycotic infections causing Addison disease are less frequent, including North American blastomycosis, South American blastomycosis, coccidioidomycosis, and paracoccidioidomycosis.[3,92] On microscopic examination, the organisms are often found clustered within the cytoplasm of macrophages (Fig. 16.14). They are spherical to oval and typically have single buds attached by a relatively narrow base.

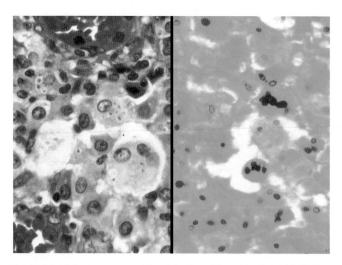

Fig. 16.14 *Histoplasma capsulatum* infection of the adrenal gland (*left*). Fungal organisms present within macrophages are highlighted by Gomori methenamine silver stain (*right*).

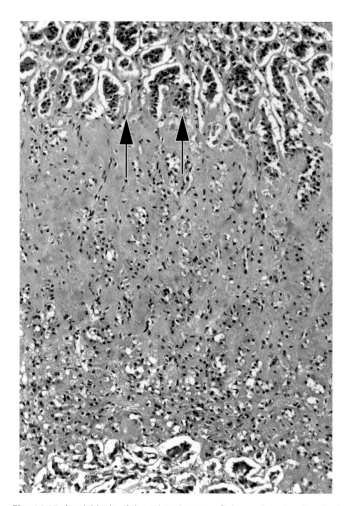

Fig. 16.15 Amyloidosis of the adrenal cortex. Only small nests of cortical cells remain (*arrows*).

Amyloidosis

The adrenal gland may be involved in primary and secondary forms of amyloidosis. In primary amyloidosis, involvement of arterioles tends to occur; whereas, in the secondary form, there is usually extensive involvement of the cortex by the characteristic homogeneous eosinophilic material, resulting in severe atrophy and distortion of cells in the zona fasciculata and zona reticularis (Fig. 16.15). In advanced cases, cortical function can be impaired.[93] A historical review of amyloidosis is provided elsewhere.[94]

Acute Adrenal Cortical Insufficiency

Acute adrenal cortical insufficiency can occur in the setting of systemic infection with Waterhouse-Friderichsen syndrome but is seldom documented by laboratory or biochemical studies. Waterhouse-Friderichsen syndrome is seen classically in meningococcemia, but occasionally other bacteria, such as *Streptococcus* species, staphylococci, *Rickettsiae, Ehrlichia, Clostridium* species, *Klebsiella* species, *Legionella* species, *Bacillus anthracis,* and *Treponema pallidum,* are responsible.[95] The course of the disease is usually fulminant, with a fatal outcome within 48 hours of onset, and accompanied by mucocutaneous petechial hemorrhages and vascular collapse. The adrenal gland is usually intensely hemorrhagic, with confluent areas of coagulative necrosis, often associated with small fibrin deposits within sinusoids; occasionally more extensive hemorrhage occurs, with expansion of the gland and periadrenal hemorrhage (Fig. 16.16).

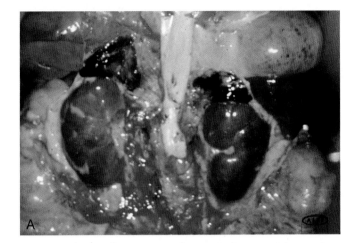

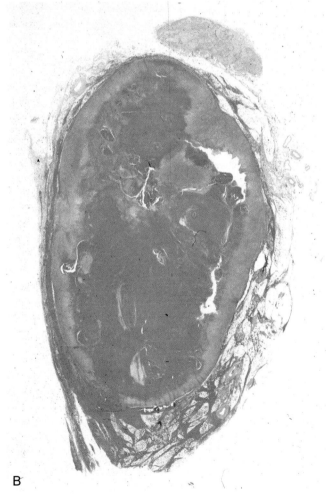

Fig. 16.16 Adrenal glands in Waterhouse Friderichsen syndrome. (A) In situ photograph showing bilateral hemorrhagic adrenal glands in a suprarenal location (autopsy specimen, from files of Armed Forces Institute of Pathology, Washington, DC). (B) Extensive necrosis and hemorrhage are seen in this adrenal gland and extend into periadrenal connective tissue. (From Lack EE, Kozakewich HPW. Pathology. In: Javadpour N, ed. Principles and Management of Adrenal Cancer. Berlin: Springer-Verlag; 1987:19–55).

Inflammation and Other Infections

Nonspecific Adrenalitis

Focal chronic adrenalitis is common and has been found in up to 48% of autopsies, appearing as small aggregates of lymphocytes admixed with plasma cells adjacent to veins or venules in the corticomedullary junction.[96] Focal chronic adrenalitis of this type is not considered to be a primary adrenal disorder but may represent a nonspecific inflammatory reaction, possibly related to inflammation in neighboring organs, such as chronic pyelonephritis. Autoantibodies may be directed against adrenal medullary or chromaffin cells in type 1 (insulin-dependent) diabetes mellitus, and this organ-specific autoimmunity might be related to diabetic autonomic neuropathy.[4]

Herpetic Adrenalitis

Members of the herpes virus group may infect the adrenal gland, including herpes simplex virus, cytomegalovirus (CMV), and varicella-zoster virus. A characteristic pattern of herpetic adrenalitis occurs with disseminated herpes simplex infection in newborns, referred to as *neonatal hepatoadrenal necrosis* and first described by Hass in 1935. The foci of herpes simplex or varicella-zoster infections tend to be small, circumscribed, punched-out areas of coagulative necrosis, with scant inflammation.[97] The necrosis within the cortex may become widespread and confluent.[3] Eosinophilic Cowdry type A intranuclear inclusions are the diagnostic hallmark, usually occurring in cells bordering the zones of necrosis (Fig. 16.17A). It may not be possible to distinguish varicella-zoster infection from herpes simplex by routine light microscopy.

Disseminated CMV infection in newborns involves a wide variety of organs and tissues, including the adrenal gland. Some infants may have multiple mobile blue-gray subcutaneous nodules caused by dermal erythropoiesis. The appearance of the pigmented nodules may be striking, giving the infant an appearance described as a "blueberry muffin."[3] The viral cytopathic effect in CMV adrenalitis is virtually pathognomonic, with sharply defined large amphophilic intranuclear inclusions having characteristic halos and small, basophilic granules within the cytoplasm (Fig. 16.17B). CMV adrenalitis was relatively common in patients with AIDS; death is attributed in part in some cases to adrenal cortical insufficiency. In one study, approximately 50% of patients with AIDS had evidence of CMV infection at autopsy, and the adrenal glands were most commonly involved (75%) with cortical or medullary necrosis.[98] Necrosis of the medulla caused by CMV infection may be greater than that of the cortex, but it is useful to note that there is no deficiency syndrome caused by destruction of the adrenal medulla. CMV infection of the adrenal gland in AIDS may result in latent or overt adrenal cortical insufficiency, requiring prophylactic treatment with corticosteroids.[99]

Rare Infections

Rarely, the adrenal gland is involved by other infectious agents, such as *Pneumocystis jiroveci* (Fig. 16.18), the most common opportunistic infection in patients with AIDS that rarely occurs in immunocompetent individuals.[100,101] Malakoplakia of the adrenal gland has been reported.[102,103] Echinococcal cyst of the adrenal gland is usually an incidental autopsy finding.[104] A review of adrenal infections by Paolo and Nosanchuk is available.[105]

Adrenal Cortical Hyperplasia

Nodular Adrenal Gland

Cortical nodularity in the adrenal gland can pose significant diagnostic problems for the pathologist at the autopsy table and in

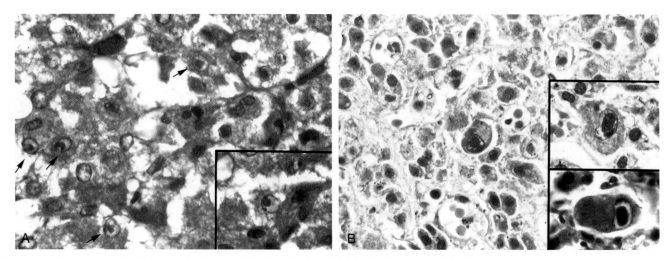

Fig. 16.17 Herpetic adrenalitis. (A) Herpes simplex virus infection. Note the multiple intranuclear eosinophilic Cowdry type A inclusions (*arrows*) with peripheral displacement of nuclear chromatin (*inset*). (B) Cytomegalovirus infection. The adrenal cortical cells infected by the virus show the characteristic cytomegalic changes. *Insets* highlight the large, amphophilic intranuclear inclusions with peripheral halo.

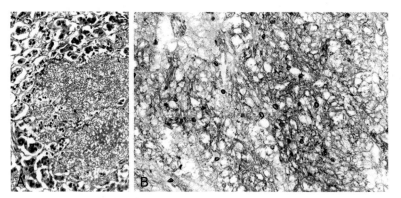

Fig. 16.18 (A) Adrenal gland extensively involved by *Pneumocystis jiroveci* infection in a patient with acquired immunodeficiency syndrome. Note the characteristic foamy exudate in the cortex. (B) Gomori methenamine silver stain shows several *P. jiroveci* organisms (*arrow*); some organisms have cup-shaped indentations when viewed in profile.

surgical material. Nodularity usually occurs in individuals without biochemical or clinical signs or symptoms of adrenal cortical hyperfunction. By definition, *hyperplasia* refers to an increase in the number of cells in tissue or in an organ, which may result in *hypertrophy*. In the adrenal cortex, the changes may be diffuse unilateral or bilateral with or without formation of cortical nodules (Fig. 16.19). The morphologic spectrum of diffuse and nodular adrenal cortical hyperplasia is broad. The incidence of cortical nodularity with eucorticalism can be analyzed from material obtained at autopsy or in patients who are discovered to have incidental cortical nodules in vivo.

Incidental Cortical Nodule/Adenoma at Autopsy

Early studies of incidental adrenal cortical nodularity at autopsy considered any solitary adrenal cortical nodule greater than 3 to 5 mm in diameter to be a nonfunctional adenoma.[3] Several autopsy studies have shown that the incidence of cortical nodularity increases with age and may be associated with hypertension and diabetes mellitus.[106,107] The early study by Spain and Weinsaft identified solitary ACA in 29% of elderly women.[108] Another autopsy study reported a cortical adenoma 1.5 cm or larger in up to 20% of hypertensive individuals in contrast with only 1.8% of normotensive patients.[109] In two of the largest autopsy studies of ACA (study population over 16,000), lesions were detected in 1.5% to 2.9% of cases.[110,111] More recent data indicate a prevalence of an incidental adrenal mass to occur in approximately 3% to 7% of the adult

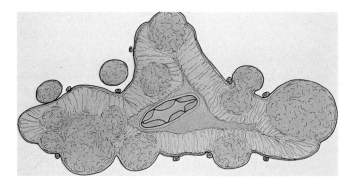

Fig. 16.19 Schematic view of nodular adrenal gland in transverse section. Accessory nodules of cortical cells may be seen lying free within periadrenal fat, on the capsular surface, or attached to the underlying cortex (capsular extrusion). A dominant macronodule within the cortex can simulate a neoplasm. Multiple small capsular arterioles are present on the surface of the gland. The central adrenal vein in the medullary compartment has discontinuous bundles of smooth muscle, allowing close contact of chromaffin cells or cortical cells with vascular lumina. Occasionally a mushroom-like intravascular protrusion by cortical or medullary cells can be seen.

population.[112] The average size of the incidental adrenal cortical nodule/adenoma in one study was 2.8 cm, but some reached 5 cm in diameter. The autopsy study by Dobbie showed that incidental adrenal cortical nodules may be present in virtually every region of the cortex, with the degree of nodularity varying widely from gland to gland.[106] Adrenal nodularity was almost always bilateral, and, in some cases, there was significant disparity in the weights of the glands from an individual patient. Some nodules were as large as 3 cm in size and may display lipomatous or myelolipomatous metaplasia. Although no specific size criteria have been developed for distinguishing cortical nodules and adenomas, most cortical nodules are less than 1 cm in size. Some cortical nodules seemed to be related to capsular arteriopathy which, in turn, is related to aging, and one theory in pathogenesis of cortical nodules was localized ischemia with secondary regenerative change.[106] Based on this theory, most cortical nodules could be regarded as secondary to hypertension rather than a cause of it. Other investigators have logically questioned the validity of this theory.

Incidental Adrenal Mass Discovered in Vivo

With increasing use of high-resolution abdominal imaging, an adrenal mass may be detected as an incidental finding that is often referred to as an adrenal "incidentaloma," but the significance in most cases is unclear.[112-114] Fortunately, the prevalence of malignant tumors among incidentaloma is relatively low. In a study from the Mayo Clinic, there were a large number of patients with an adrenal mass detected by computed tomography (CT) scan and following exclusion of patients with known malignancy, tumors previously documented by biochemical study, and adrenal nodules less than 1 cm in size, there were 342 patients remaining with an adrenal tumor. Histologic proof of diagnosis was obtained in 55 patients at the time of adrenalectomy; 5 patients had a malignant tumor (1.4%), 4 had an ACC, and 1 had a metastatic carcinoma of unknown primary site. Interestingly, the smallest malignant tumor was 5 cm in size, and of the benign, incidentally discovered lesions, only 6% were 5 cm or larger.[115] Another study showed that the likelihood of malignancy doubles to 10% with tumors 4 cm or larger and there is more than a ninefold increase in the likelihood of malignancy in tumors 8 cm or larger.[116]

Magnetic resonance imaging (MRI) may provide some information on tissue characterization of adrenal masses; T_2-weighted pulse sequences provide some specificity in separating nonhyperfunctioning cortical adenomas, which have low signal intensity, from metastases with intermediate signal intensity and pheochromocytomas, which tend to have high signal intensity.[117] Pheochromocytomas, however, are not always "light bulb bright" on T_2-weighted MRI. This imaging modality does not allow for clear distinction between functional and nonfunctional (or nonhyperfunctional) ACA or small ACC that lack necrosis and other secondary changes. Adrenal cortical scintigraphy with a radioiodinated cholesterol precursor often showed tracer uptake, indicating cortical steroid synthesis.[118,119] Various enzymes involved in cortical steroid synthesis are present, based on immunohistochemical staining, indicating that the nodules have the capacity for corticosteroidogenesis, although not in sufficient amounts to elicit signs or symptoms of endocrine hyperfunction or abnormal biochemical findings to alter the hypothalamic-pituitary-adrenal axis.[120] Many incidental cortical nodules (or adenomas) are therefore considered nonhyperfunctional rather than nonfunctional, without excess production of adrenal cortical steroids. Cortical nodularity in this setting has been compared with nodular euthyroid (nontoxic) goiter.

Incidental Pigmented Cortical Nodule

Incidental pigmented nodules of adrenal cortex usually vary from 0.1 to 1.5 cm in size and are usually located in or straddle the zona

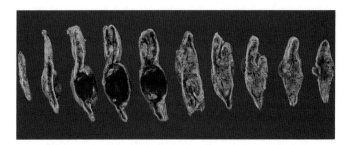

Fig. 16.20 Incidental pigmented adrenal cortical nodule. The adjacent cortex contained numerous small pale-yellow nodules.

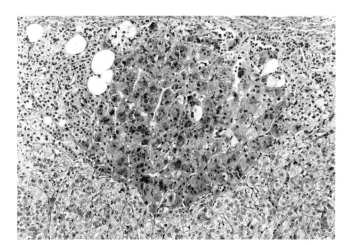

Fig. 16.21 Incidental pigmented adrenal cortical nodule. Cells contain abundant granular lipofuscin pigment. Nuclei are uniform, and many contain a small central to eccentric nucleolus.

reticularis, often with expansion and distortion of the adjacent cortex or medulla (Fig. 16.20). The frequency of grossly identifiable pigmented nodules at autopsy varies according to the method of adrenal sectioning, the number of sections examined, and the level of interest of the pathologist in specifically searching for the lesions. Retrospective studies of autopsy material reported pigmented adrenal cortical nodules in 2.2% to 10.4% of cases.[121,122] When the glands were thinly sectioned in a prospective study, pigmented nodules were detected in 37% of cases.[121] Pigmented nodules are usually solitary but may be multiple, and in 11% of cases are bilateral. Histologically, the cells have compact eosinophilic cytoplasm with variable amounts of intracellular granular brown pigment, which has staining characteristics like those of lipofuscin (Fig. 16.21). One study suggested the presence of neuromelanin.[122]

Management of the Incidental Adrenal Mass Discovered in Vivo

There have been a number of recommendations over the past few decades addressing the strategy or algorithm in the workup of patients with an incidentaloma.[113,114,123,124] According to the National Institutes of Health consensus panel (Table 16.1), all patients with incidentaloma should undergo a 1-mg dexamethasone suppression test and measurement of plasma-free metanephrines. Patients with hypertension should undergo measurement of serum potassium and plasma aldosterone concentration–plasma renin activity ratio. Patients with biochemical evidence of pheochromocytoma, patients with tumors larger than 6 cm, and patients with tumors larger than 4 cm who meet other criteria should undergo

TABLE 16.1 National Institutes of Health Consensus Conference on Adrenal Incidentalomas

- All patients with an incidentaloma should have a 1-mg dexamethasone suppression test and measurement of plasma free metanephrines.
- Patients with hypertension should also undergo measurement of serum potassium and plasma aldosterone concentration–plasma renin activity ratio.
- A homogenous mass with a low attenuation value (<10 Hounsfield units) on computed tomography is probably a benign adenoma.
- Surgery should be considered in all patients with functional adrenal cortical tumors that are clinically apparent.
- All patients with biochemical evidence of pheochromocytoma should undergo surgery.
- Data are insufficient to indicate the superiority of a surgical or non-surgical approach to manage patients with subclinical hyperfunctioning adrenal cortical adenomas.
- Recommendations for surgery based on tumor size are derived from studies not standardized for inclusion criteria, length of follow-up, or methods of estimating the risk for carcinoma. Nevertheless, patients with tumors >6 cm usually are treated surgically, and those with tumors <4 cm are generally monitored. In patients with tumors between 4 and 6 cm, criteria in addition to size should be considered in the decision to monitor or proceed to adrenalectomy.
- The literature on adrenal incidentaloma has proliferated in the past several years. Unfortunately, the lack of controlled studies makes formulating diagnostic and treatment strategies difficult. Because of the complexity of the problem, the management of patients with adrenal incidentalomas will be optimized by a multidisciplinary team approach involving physicians with expertise in endocrinology, radiology, surgery, and pathology. The paucity of evidence-based data highlights the need for well-designed prospective studies.
- Open or laparoscopic adrenalectomy is an acceptable procedure for resection of an adrenal mass. The procedure choice will depend on the likelihood of an invasive adrenal cortical carcinoma, technical issues, and the experience of the surgical team.
- In patients with tumors that remain stable on two imaging studies done at least 6 months apart and do not exhibit hormonal hypersecretion over 4 years, further follow-up may not be warranted.

Data from Anonymous. NIH state-of-the-science statement on management of the clinically inapparent adrenal mass ("incidentaloma"). NIH Consens State Sci Statements. 2002; 19:1–25; and Grua JR, Nelson DH. ACTH-producing pituitary tumors. Endocrinol Metab Clin N Am. 1991;20:319–362.

surgical resection. Incidentaloma smaller than 4 cm should be followed by imaging. These masses may grow over time. If the growth is rapid, surgical resection is considered. It is estimated that up to 20% of patients with incidentalomas have abnormal cortisol production and could be classified as having subclinical Cushing syndrome.[125] In general, all functional incidentalomas should be surgically resected. A detailed flowchart for incidentalomas detected on CT or MRI was developed by the Incidental Findings Committee of the American College of Radiology and provides useful guidelines for these patients.[112]

Fine-needle aspiration under CT or ultrasound guidance may provide valuable information, particularly when it is not possible to reliably distinguish a metastasis from an adrenal cortical nodule or neoplasm (Fig. 16.22). The distinction between ACA and ACC is not always reliable by fine-needle aspiration. Occasionally, aspiration yields cells with bare nuclei stripped of cytoplasm, which might be confused with a small cell malignancy. Correlation of cytologic findings with imaging results, clinical findings, and endocrinologic data is essential.

Adrenal Cortical Hyperplasia With Hypercortisolism

Cushing syndrome has several basic endogenous or noniatrogenic causes (Fig. 16.23). A more detailed tabulation of causes of endogenous Cushing syndrome is given in Table 16.2.[126] The three most common causes of Cushing syndrome are pituitary-dependent ACTH overproduction, commonly referred to as *Cushing disease,* which accounts for approximately 60% to 70% of cases in adults; adrenal cortical neoplasm with autonomous overproduction of cortisol: ACA 10% to 22% and ACC 5% to 7% of cases in adults; and ectopic production of ACTH (5% to 10% of cases); or, very rarely, ectopic production of corticotropin-releasing hormone. In childhood, Cushing syndrome is most often caused by a cortisol-producing cortical neoplasm, particularly in the very young, whereas older children are more likely to have an ACTH-dependent form of hypercortisolism (Cushing disease).[127] Most patients with an ACTH-dependent form caused by ACTH overproduction have a pituitary microadenoma or macroadenoma. In some cases, no pituitary tumor is detected, and the disease may result from hyperplasia of ACTH-producing corticotrophs or abnormal hypothalamic regulation with secondary ACTH hypersecretion by corticotrophs, which has been referred to as tertiary hypercortisolism.

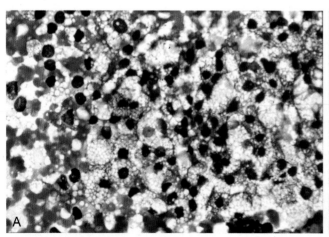
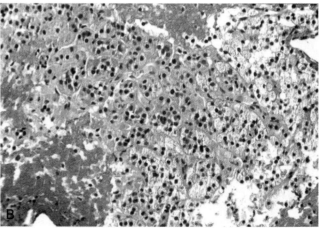

Fig. 16.22 Adrenal incidentaloma. (A) Fine-needle aspiration (Diff-Quik stain) of adrenal cortical adenoma showing clusters of adrenal cortical cells with microvesiculated cytoplasm and eccentrically placed, round to oval nuclei. (B) The corresponding cell block preparation (hematoxylin and eosin stain) shows a proliferation of adrenal cortical cells, some with microvesiculated, lipid-filled cytoplasm (*right*) interspersed by cells with a more compact eosinophilic cytoplasm (*left*).

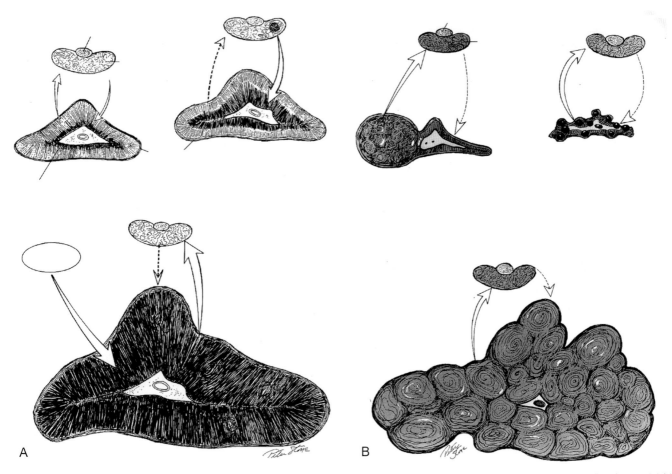

Fig. 16.23 (A) Normal hypothalamic-pituitary-adrenal axis (*upper left*). Pituitary (or adrenocorticotropic hormone)-dependent hypercortisolism (*upper right*) is characteristic of Cushing disease. Ectopic adrenocorticotropic hormone syndrome (*lower half*) with enlarged, dark adrenal gland caused by trophic influence of adrenocorticotropic hormone with predominance of cells with compact, lipid-depleted cytoplasm. (B) Noniatrogenic causes of Cushing syndrome. Cortisol-secreting cortical neoplasm (*upper left*) with autonomous hyperfunction and feedback inhibition of adrenocorticotropic hormone release from adenohypophysis. Rare examples of Cushing syndrome are caused by primary pigmented nodular adrenal cortical disease (*upper right*) and macronodular hyperplasia with marked adrenal enlargement (*lower half*).

Pituitary or Adenocorticotropic Hormone–Dependent Hypercortisolism (Cushing Disease)

Diffuse and Micronodular Adrenal Cortical Hyperplasia

With the high success rate of transsphenoidal adenomectomy for ACTH-producing pituitary neoplasms, the pathologist rarely has the opportunity to examine adrenal glands in this disorder. Bilateral adrenalectomy is usually done only after failed resection of a pituitary adenoma or when the primary (ectopic) ACTH-secreting neoplasm cannot be identified or removed. Bilateral laparoscopic adrenalectomy has gained an increasing role as a safe and effective therapeutic option.[128] The pathologic alterations in the resected adrenal gland(s) may be so subtle that the gland might be regarded as normal if the alterations are not correlated with clinical and biochemical data.[3,71] The size and weight of the mildly stimulated gland may be only slightly increased—usually between 6 and 12 g; the average weight in the study by Smals et al. was 8.2 g.[129]

On transverse sectioning, the adrenal gland may have a somewhat rounded contour, and the larger glands may demonstrate a mild degree of nodularity (Fig. 16.24) with nodules up to 3 mm in diameter randomly distributed throughout the cortex. Capsular extrusions may appear accentuated, as well as the cuff of cortical cells around tributaries of the central adrenal vein. The microscopic

hallmark of ACTH stimulation in Cushing disease is conversion of lipid-rich, pale-staining cortical cells in the inner one-third to one-half of the cortex into cells with compact eosinophilic cytoplasm, like those in the zona reticularis (Fig. 16.25). The net effect is what appears to be a greatly expanded zona reticularis except for the absence of lipochrome pigment in the outer part, which is zona fasciculata.[3,71] The extent to which vacuolated, lipid-rich cells are converted into compact, lipid-depleted cells is variable and may be influenced by a variety of physiologic factors.[3] The zona glomerulosa may be even more difficult to identify because of expansion of the zona fasciculata. Some cortical cells may extend irregularly into periadrenal adipose tissue or intermingle in irregular nests with chromaffin cells. Some of these changes may be subtle, particularly in mildly stimulated glands, and correlation with clinical and biochemical data is crucial.[3,71]

Macronodular Hyperplasia

Macronodular hyperplasia is present in approximately 20% of cases of hyperplasia with Cushing disease, but this is variable.[3,130,131] The morphology may be more confusing than that of diffuse or micronodular hyperplasia. Nodules up to 2 cm in diameter or

TABLE 16.2 Causes of Endogenous Cushing Syndrome

	Proportion (%)	Age (peak)	Female:male	Features
ACTH-dependent	70–80	..	..	..
Cushing disease	60–70	..	..	..
Corticotroph adenoma	60–70	3rd–4th decades	3–5:1	Roughly 50% non-visible on MRI
Corticotroph hyperplasia	Very rare	..	..	..
Ectopic ACTH*	5–10	..	..	..
Malignant neuroendocrine tumours	About 4	5th–6th decades	0·6–1:1	Might have very high ACTH
Benign neuroendocrine tumours	About 6	3rd–4th decades	..	Might respond to dexamethasone, CRH, desmopressin
Occult neuroendocrine tumours	About 2	..	..	..
Ectopic CRH	Very rare	..	..	Causes pituitary corticotroph hyperplasia
ACTH-independent	20–30	..	..	..
Unilateral adrenal	..	..	..	..
Adenoma	10–22	4th–5th decades	4–8:1	Most pure cortisol secretion
Carcinoma	5–7	1st, 5th–6th decades	1·5–3:1	Mixed cortisol and androgen frequent
Bilateral adrenal	1–2	..	..	..
Bilateral macronodular adrenal hyperplasia†	<2	5th–6th decades	2–3:1	Modest cortisol secretion compared with size; raised steroid precursors; might have combined androgen and mineralocorticoid cosecretion
Aberrant G-protein-coupled receptors	..	..	..	..
Autocrine ACTH production	..	..	..	..
Sporadic or familial (*ARMC5*)	..	..	..	..
Bilateral micronodular adrenal hyperplasias	<2	..	..	Adrenal size often normal
Primary pigmented nodular adrenocortical disease	Rare	1st–3rd decades	0·5:1 <12 years / 2:1 >12 years	Frequent paradoxical increase of urine free cortisol with Liddle's oral dexamethasone suppression test
Isolated or familial with Carney complex	Rare	1st–3rd decades	..	..
Isolated micronodular adrenocortical disease	Very rare	Infants	..	Non-pigmented adrenal micronodules
Primary bimorphic adrenocortical disease	Very rare	Infants	..	..
McCune-Albright syndrome	Rare	Infants (<6 months)	1:1	Internodular adrenal atrophy
Bilateral adenomas or carcinomas	Rare	4th–5th decades	2–4:1	..

ACTH=adrenocorticotropic hormone. CRH=corticotropin-releasing hormone. *Most frequent sources of ectopic ACTH syndromes are small cell lung carcinoma and neuroendocrine tumours of lung, thymus, and pancreas. Less frequent causes include medullary thyroid carcinoma, gastrinoma, phaeochromocytoma, prostate carcinoma, and several others. †In bilateral macronodular adrenal hyperplasia tissues, autocrine and paracrine ACTH might be produced and contribute to cortisol secretion. If confirmed by in-vivo studies, the ACTH-independent classification will need to be modified in the future.
From Lacroix A, Feelders RA, Stratakis CA, Nieman LK. Cushing's syndrome. *Lancet.* 2015;386:913–927.

larger (Fig. 16.26) protrude from one or more sides of the gland; they also may be situated deep within the adrenal gland, identifiable only when the gland is sectioned in the transverse plane. Smals et al. used the designation macronodular hyperplasia for grossly visible nodules 0.5 cm or more in diameter, with some nodules up to 5 cm in size.[129] Separation of micronodular and macronodular hyperplasia is difficult, and a morphologic continuum exists between the two processes, making this distinction arbitrary.

Macronodular hyperplasia is often characterized by disparity in size and weight between the adrenal glands. In the study by Smals et al., the female-to-male ratio for macronodular hyperplasia was 5:1, identical to that for diffuse and micronodular hyperplasia.[129] However, there were several important differences between micronodular and macronodular hyperplasia. The average age of patients with macronodular hyperplasia (44 years) is considerably older than those with diffuse and micronodular hyperplasia (31 years), and disease duration is longer with macronodular hyperplasia (8 years versus 2 years). The average adrenal gland in macronodular

hyperplasia weighed 16 g, nearly twice the observed weight in diffuse and micronodular hyperplasia.[129] As noted by Cohen et al., the medullary compartment may be compressed by the prominent cortical nodules and, in many sections, it may be difficult to recognize (Fig. 16.27).[131] Foci of lipomatous or myelolipomatous metaplasia may be present.

Ectopic Adrenocorticotropin Hormone Syndrome With Secondary Hypercortisolism

Approximately 5% to 10% of cases of Cushing syndrome in adults result from ectopic production of ACTH by neoplasms such as bronchial carcinoid tumor, bronchogenic small cell carcinoma, pancreatic endocrine neoplasm, medullary thyroid carcinoma, pheochromocytoma, or other rare tumors.[132,133] Ectopic production of corticotropin-releasing hormone may occur, very rarely, and be accompanied by orthotopic ACTH secretion by the pituitary gland (tertiary hypercortisolism).[3,71] Nearly all normal tissues are capable of producing small amounts of the inactive precursor of

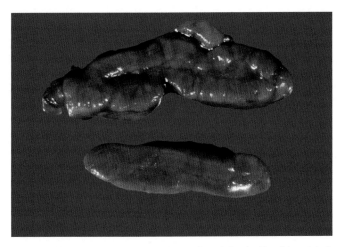

Fig. 16.24 Transverse sections of a 3.5 g adrenal gland with mild nodularity surgically resected from an 8-year-old boy with Cushing disease. Patient underwent several attempts at transsphenoidal pituitary resection. The patient was also treated with radiation (4800 cGy), but the tumor recurred on several occasions. Nelson syndrome subsequently developed, with radiologically detectable changes in the sella.

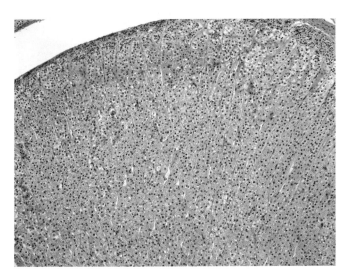

Fig. 16.25 Adrenal gland in Cushing disease caused by an adrenocorticotropic hormone–producing pituitary adenoma. The cortex is hyperplastic, with conversion of many cells throughout the zona fasciculata into reticularis-type cells with compact, eosinophilic cytoplasm caused by lipid depletion.

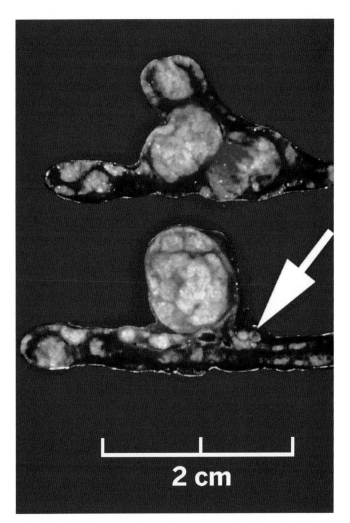

Fig. 16.26 Macronodular adrenal cortical hyperplasia in a patient with multiple endocrine neoplasia, type 1, who developed Cushing syndrome caused by a presumed adrenocorticotropic hormone–producing pituitary adenoma. Multiple pale cortical nodules range up to 1.5 cm in diameter, including small capsular extrusions (*arrow*). (Modified from Lack EE, Travis WD, Oertel JE. Adrenal cortical nodules, hyperplasia, and hyperfunction. In: Lack EE, ed. Pathology of the Adrenal Glands. New York: Churchill Livingstone; 1990:75–113.)

ACTH, probably proopiomelanocortin. Cancers may overproduce this substance, although few convert it into ACTH; in this regard, ectopic ACTH production may not be ectopic.[134] Correct identification of the source of ACTH secretion is essential to avoid unnecessary pituitary surgery.[135] In ectopic ACTH syndrome, serum levels of ACTH are usually quite elevated, sometimes greater than 250 pg/mL, whereas in Cushing disease ACTH levels are rarely over 200 pg/mL and are commonly in the upper range of normal or only slightly elevated.[71] Inferior petrosal sinus sampling can identify a pituitary source of ACTH via central (petrosal sinus) to peripheral blood concentration gradient with a high degree of accuracy.[136] Some patients with aggressive, fast-growing tumors, such as bronchogenic small cell carcinoma, lack signs and symptoms of Cushing syndrome, with the clinical findings dominated by electrolyte disturbances and cachexia. Some slowly growing neoplasms, such as bronchial carcinoid tumor, may be associated with marked changes of Cushing syndrome, although the primary tumor remains occult, sometimes for years.[137]

On gross examination, the adrenal glands are often symmetrically enlarged with rounded contours and frequently weigh 10 to 15 g each; occasionally, the individual adrenal gland may weigh more than 20 g or, rarely, 30 g.[3,71] In this setting, the adrenal glands are under intense and persistent trophic stimulation by ACTH and on transverse sectioning may be tan to brown because of the conversion of lipid-rich, pale-staining cortical cells to cells with more compact eosinophilic cytoplasm (Fig. 16.28). The cortex is hyperplastic, being 0.3 to 0.4 cm thick, but, in some cases, may be even thicker. Typically, diffuse cortical hyperplasia is present, but sometimes vague nodularity may be seen (Fig. 16.29).

Primary Pigmented Nodular Adrenal Cortical Disease

Primary pigmented nodular adrenal cortical disease (PPNAD) is a rare form of pituitary or ACTH-independent hypercortisolism

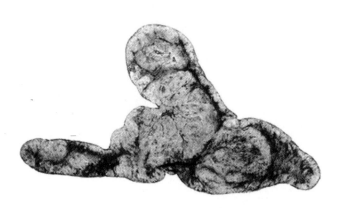

Fig. 16.27 Pituitary-dependent macronodular adrenal cortical hyperplasia (same as in Fig. 16.26). Irregular expansile cortical nodules blend with adjacent hyperplastic cortex. The adrenal medulla was difficult to identify in random transverse sections of the gland. (From Lack EE. Tumors of the Adrenal Glands and Extraadrenal Paraganglia. Atlas of Tumor Pathology, Series 4. Washington, DC: Armed Forces Institute of Pathology; 2007:75.)

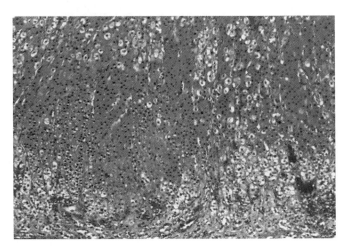

Fig. 16.29 Ectopic adrenocorticotropic hormone syndrome. The adrenal cortex is markedly hyperplastic, with columns and cords of lipid-depleted cells. Faint nodularity was evident in some areas.

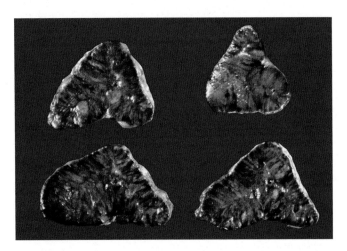

Fig. 16.28 Ectopic adrenocorticotropic hormone syndrome caused by a bronchial carcinoid tumor that was occult for several years. The right adrenal gland weighed 12 g and the left 11 g. The dark appearance on cross-section is caused by intense stimulation by adrenocorticotropic hormone with conversion of lipid-rich cortical cells to lipid-depleted cells with compact, eosinophilic cytoplasm. (From Lack EE. Tumors of the Adrenal Glands and Extraadrenal Paraganglia. Atlas of Tumor Pathology, Series 4. Washington, DC: Armed Forces Institute of Pathology; 2007:90.)

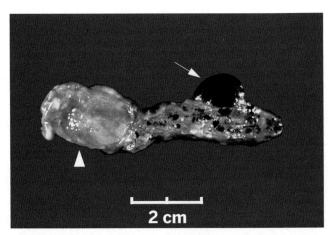

Fig. 16.30 Primary pigmented nodular adrenal cortical disease. Transverse section of the adrenal gland shows numerous dark-pigmented nodules, one nearly 1 cm in diameter (*arrow*). Another nodule (*arrowhead*) is pale-yellow and has small foci of necrosis. The patient was a member of a family with the complex of myxomas, spotty pigmentation, and endocrine overactivity. (From Lack EE. Tumors of the Adrenal Glands and Extraadrenal Paraganglia. Atlas of Tumor Pathology, Series 4. Washington, DC: Armed Forces Institute of Pathology; 2007:86.)

typically seen in young individuals, with a predilection for females. It is a benign, bilateral adrenal cortical hyperplasia that can be seen as an isolated/sporadic process, but most are characteristic components of Carney complex (see later discussion).[138-142] The associated Cushing syndrome may be severe, with bone pain and pathologic fractures.[138] A variety of endocrinologic studies, including dynamic endocrine testing, indicate a primary adrenal source for the hypercortisolism. Imaging studies of the sella and pituitary fossa reveal no abnormalities, and selective venous sinus sampling of the inferior petrosal sinus excludes a pituitary origin for PPNAD.

The adrenal glands in PPNAD are usually normal on CT scan, but unilateral or bilateral nodularity may be present, including macronodules greater than 1 cm in diameter.[71] The weight of each gland varies from 0.9 to 13.4 g, with an average combined weight of 9.6 g; the gland is usually normal in size.[138] Small pigmented micronodules, 1 to 3 mm in diameter, may be seen through the intact capsular surface of the gland, but transverse sections usually reveal the pigmented nodules to better advantage (Fig. 16.30). Complete removal of the investing connective tissue and fat may be impeded by these small nodules when they protrude through the capsule or extend into the periadrenal fat. The pigmented nodules are light gray, gray-brown, dark brown, or jet black. The term *micronodular* is somewhat arbitrary because many of the intensely pigmented nodules are grossly apparent, even when they are less than 1 mm in size.

The gross pathology of the pigmented nodules is often much more striking than the histologic features (Fig. 16.31). The pigmented nodules are usually round to oval and are present within the zona reticularis or interface with the adjacent medulla. Their configuration varies from hourglass and strings of beads to links

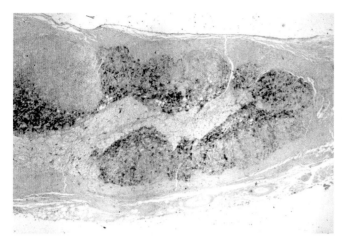

Fig. 16.31 Pigmented nodules contain cells that are argentaffin positive, causing them to stand out in contrast with the remaining gland. Some areas show marked atrophy of the internodular cortex.

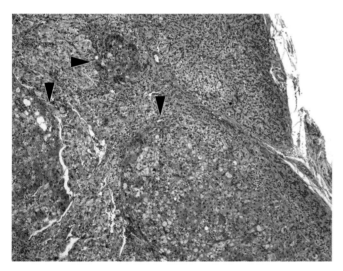

Fig. 16.32 Several pigmented micronodules in primary pigmented nodular adrenal cortical disease (*arrowheads*) are located in the inner aspect of the cortex and impinge on the medulla.

of sausages. The pigmented nodules are typically unencapsulated but have expansile borders and may cause distortion or compression of adjacent uninvolved cells (Fig. 16.32). Occasionally, intraluminal projection of a small pigmented nodule into tributaries of the central adrenal vein at sites with interrupted bundles of smooth muscle may be seen. In most nodules, the cells contain compact eosinophilic cytoplasm with variable amounts of coarse granular pigment, which usually has the staining characteristics of lipofuscin. Some nodules contain cells with pale-staining, lipid-rich cytoplasm; occasionally, cells may be large with a ballooned appearance. Sparse lymphocytic infiltrates have been noted, rarely, around vessels or within the nodules, and, occasionally, a lipomatous or even myelolipomatous metaplastic component may be seen.[71]

Regardless of whether familial or isolated/sporadic, PPNAD is linked to mutation of PRKAR1A, a gene encoding the regulatory subunit of a cyclic adenosine monophosphate (cAMP)-dependent protein kinase that is located on chromosome 17 (17q22–24). Studies of families with Carney complex raise the possibility of a second locus affected in the disease on chromosome 2 (2p16).[141]

The exact pathogenesis of PPNAD is unknown, but several theories have been proposed such as hamartomatous malformation or dysplasia of the cortex; primary abnormality of the zona reticularis; occult adrenocorticotropic hormone–producing pituitary adenoma with adrenal cortical nodules becoming functionally autonomous; embryonic developmental error in the cortex at the adrenarche; block in evolution of zona fasciculata cells into cells of the zona reticularis, with accumulation of autonomous cells at the interface; and an organ-specific autoimmune hypercortisolism (Cushing syndrome).

The autoimmune theory of hypercortisolism is based on reports of circulating adrenal-stimulating immunoglobulin in this disorder; the adrenal-stimulating immunoglobulin is presumably directed against ACTH receptors or receptor-binding sites.[143] Further study should determine whether PPNAD is an autoimmune disorder or one in which the circulating adrenal-stimulating immunoglobulin is merely an epiphenomenon. An immunohistochemical study of PPNAD revealed the nodules to be strongly reactive for synaptophysin, whereas the extranodular or internodular cortex was nonreactive.[144] This immunohistochemical differential may be helpful in the detection of small nodules in apparently unaffected cortex and suggest a possible neuroendocrine role for the genes involved. A previous report revealed intense immunoreactivity for all enzymes involved in steroidogenesis in cells of the cortical nodules, particularly those with abundant eosinophilic cytoplasm, unlike cells of the internodular cortex.[145]

The treatment of choice for PPNAD is bilateral adrenalectomy, with the removal of both adrenal glands even if they appear normal or small.[146] In some cases, subtotal resection may be possible, although approximately one-third of patients initially treated by unilateral or subtotal adrenalectomy require completion or total adrenalectomy because of persistence or recurrence of Cushing syndrome.[146] It is important to note that Nelson syndrome has not been reported after bilateral adrenalectomy in patients with PPNAD. Recently the original four cases of PPNAD were revisited after 30 years, and none of the patients' primary relatives had Cushing syndrome or Carney complex; these original four patients also had an isolated form of PPNAD without stigmata of Carney complex.[147]

Complex of Myxomas, Spotty Pigmentation, and Endocrine Overactivity: Carney Complex

This is a complex array of diverse abnormalities that, in the review by Carney et al., included cardiac myxoma (72%); spotty mucocutaneous pigmentation (65%); testicular tumors, particularly large cell calcifying Sertoli cell tumor (56% of males); PPNAD (45%); cutaneous myxoma (45%); mammary myxoid fibroadenoma (30% of females); and other abnormalities such as growth hormone–secreting pituitary tumor and psammomatous melanotic schwannoma.[3,71,148] Carney et al. reported four cases of unusual congenital bone tumors associated with Carney complex that they have provisionally named *osteochondromyxoma of bone*.[149] Carney complex has an autosomal dominant inheritance. Two chromosomal loci, 17q22–24 and 2p16, have been identified that are believed to harbor the genes for PPNAD and/or Carney complex.[140,141] Germline inactivating mutations (PRKAR1A) have been observed in both Carney complex and PPNAD.[150-153] Cardiac myxomas have a significant risk for morbidity and mortality, especially in the setting of Cushing syndrome. Therefore, if a patient has two or more elements of this complex, particularly PPNAD, bilateral large cell calcifying Sertoli cell tumor of the testis, or mucocutaneous pigmentation, investigation for cardiac myxoma (which may be multiple) is recommended for early detection and treatment. Recently, 37 cases of Carney complex were studied at the Mayo Clinic with 29 having clinical, pathologic, or laboratory evidence of an adrenal cortical disorder; 17 were found to have classic Cushing syndrome, 15 had PPNAD proven by total or subtotal adrenalectomy, and 2 patients were left untreated.[154]

Macronodular Hyperplasia With Marked Adrenal Enlargement

Macronodular hyperplasia with marked adrenal enlargement (MHMAE) is a rare primary autonomous form of adrenal hypercortisolism that is ACTH and pituitary independent.[3,71] It is a heterogenous disorder in which cortisol secretion can be mediated by hormones other than ACTH because of the aberrant or ectopic expression of various hormone receptors. Ectopic receptors for gastric inhibitory polypeptide, β-adrenergic receptor agonists, vasopressin, and 5-hydroxytryptamine have been identified, which can act as cortisol secretagogues.[155-157] Careful endocrinologic investigation, including dynamic endocrine testing, usually reveals elevated plasma cortisol levels, depressed or undetectable ACTH levels, and loss of diurnal rhythmicity, suggesting a primary adrenal cortical neoplasm. Paradoxically, radiographic imaging reveals bilateral adrenal gland enlargement, with no detectable abnormality of the sella or pituitary fossa, including in one patient who was reinvestigated almost 26 years later.[158] An unusual case of ACTH-independent MHMAE occurred in a male patient who presented with feminization and Cushing syndrome; the combined adrenal glands weighed 86 g.[71] Another reported case describes massive adrenal gland enlargement, with the left gland weighing 199 g and the right gland weighing 93 g.[159] The average patient age is approximately 50 years, with a slight male preponderance (although one series reports a 3:1 female preponderance), and the duration of Cushing syndrome ranges from approximately 1 to 10 years.[160]

The adrenal glands in MHMAE are significantly enlarged and can simulate an adrenal neoplasm.[71] Typically, the combined weight ranges from 60 to 180 g, with an extraordinary degree of nodular cortical hyperplasia; the nodules in one study ranged in size from 0.2 to 3.8 cm (Fig. 16.33).[161] The nodules are yellow or golden-yellow, typically unencapsulated, and blend imperceptibly with the hyperplastic cortex. The medullary compartment may be distorted and difficult to recognize in random sections of the gland, similar to macronodular hyperplasia. Cortical cells have a variable amount of finely vacuolated, lipid-rich, pale-staining cytoplasm (Fig. 16.34). Scattered cells with compact eosinophilic cytoplasm may be seen. Rarely, cells with large ballooned vacuolated cytoplasm are present, and occasionally there is a small component of lipomatous or myelolipomatous metaplasia. Weak

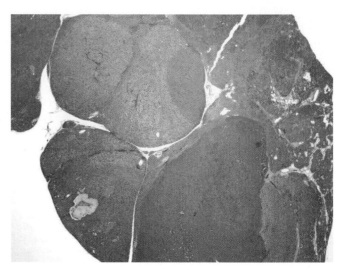

Fig. 16.34 Macronodular adrenal cortical hyperplasia with marked adrenal enlargement. Note the multiple irregular nodules of hyperplastic adrenal cortex. Most hyperplastic cells had lipid-rich, pale-staining cytoplasm.

immunoreactivity in MHMAE is seen for 3β-hydroxysteroid dehydrogenase and other enzymes involved in steroidogenesis, whereas strong staining is noted in ACA and PPNAD.[145,162] In situ hybridization study of P-450c17 has been used to localize the site of steroidogenesis, and results suggest that the degree of corticosteroidogenesis by individual cortical cells is low and that a significant increase in cell numbers is necessary before excessive cortisol production causes Cushing syndrome.[162]

As indicated in Fig. 16.35, some had questioned a possible relationship between MHMAE and macronodular hyperplasia of Cushing disease, but current evidence does not support this. Recently the genetic basis of a significant number of cases of MHMAE has been elucidated and found to be associated with germline mutations in armadillo repeat containing 5 (*ARMC5*) and may coexist with somatic second hit mutations of ARMC5 in MHMAE.[156,157] Recently, it has been shown that in addition to cortisol secretion being controlled by aberrant receptors within MHMAE, ACTH is also produced within the adrenal cortical tissue, which may act as a local amplifier for the action of these receptors through some autocrine mechanism(s).[155] Some cases, therefore, may not be entirely ACTH independent. The treatment proposed for this rare disorder is bilateral adrenalectomy. As in macronodular hyperplasia in Cushing disease, the clinical, imaging, and biochemical features may be misleading and suggest an underlying adrenal cortical neoplasm.

Multiple Endocrine Neoplasia Type 1

Multiple endocrine neoplasia (MEN) type 1 (Wermer syndrome) occurs as an autosomal dominant trait with somewhat variable expression or affects family members in whom manifestations are detectable only after close scrutiny.[163] The genetic defect is located on chromosome 11q13.[164] In a review by Ballard et al., adrenal findings at autopsy included cortical adenoma, miliary adenoma, hyperplasia, multiple adenomas, and nodular hyperplasia, but only 1 in 31 patients had clinical hypercortisolism.[165] Cushing disease may occur in MEN1, but it is rare (Figs. 16.26 and 16.27).[166] There is a study reporting 12 malignant endocrine neoplasms in 42 cases of MEN1, 2 of which were ACC; thus, although malignancies tend to play a lesser role in MEN1 than in the other

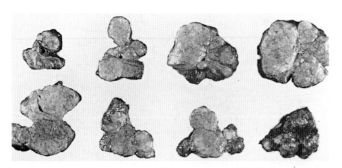

Fig. 16.33 Macronodular adrenal cortical hyperplasia with marked adrenal enlargement. Transverse sections of one adrenal gland are displayed. The combined weight of both glands was approximately 90 g.

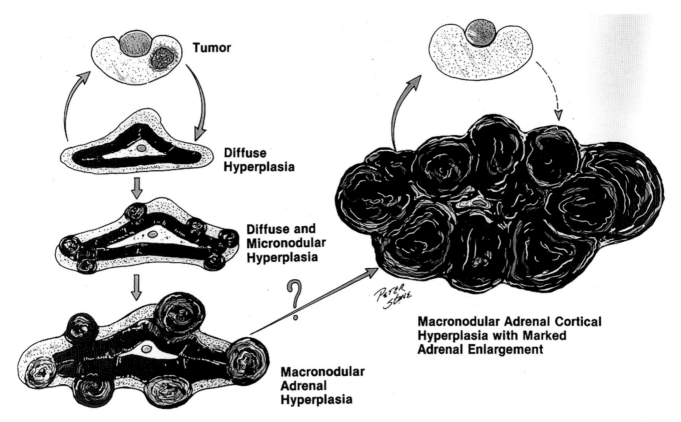

Fig. 16.35 Schematic diagram of progression of pituitary (or adrenocorticotropic hormone)-dependent Cushing disease into micronodular and macronodular adrenal cortical hyperplasia. Macronodular adrenal cortical hyperplasia with marked adrenal enlargement appears to be a primary form of adrenal hypercortisolism (Cushing syndrome) by sensitive imaging and biochemical studies. The relationship with macronodular adrenal hyperplasia (*lower left*) is uncertain.

MEN syndromes, patients still need to be examined and followed with this possibility in mind.[167]

Other Rare Causes of Cushing Syndrome

Cushing syndrome has several other rare causes. One of these is McCune-Albright syndrome (triad of polyostotic fibrous dysplasia, café au lait spots, and precocious puberty), with hyperfunction of various endocrine glands, including adrenal hypercortisolism resulting from a somatic mutation of the *GNAS1* gene (a stimulatory gene of the G-protein family) and activation of a signal transduction pathway generating cAMP.[168,169] Histologically, the predominant finding is an alternating pattern of nodular cortical hyperplasia and distinct pattern of cortical atrophy thus constituting a bimorphic cortical pathology.[170]

Adrenal Cortical Hyperplasia With Hyperaldosteronism

Endocrine causes of secondary hypertension include primary hyperaldosteronism (5% to 10% of hypertensive patients) and much less commonly (<1%) Cushing syndrome, pheochromocytoma, hyperparathyroidism, and hypo- and hyperthyroidism.[171,172] The most common form of primary hyperaldosteronism is idiopathic, with bilateral hyperplasia of the zona glomerulosa accounting for 60% to 70% of cases (Table 16.3).[172] Patients are usually managed medically; adrenalectomy is reserved for patients with unilateral disease, most frequently an aldosterone-producing adenoma, because of a more predictable response in terms of amelioration or normalization

TABLE 16.3	Causes of Primary Hyperaldosteronism	
Cause	**Proportion**
Idiopathic bilateral hyperplasia	60%-70%
Aldosterone-producing adenoma	30%-35%
Familial hyperaldosteronism (FH)	<1%
• FH Type 1 (glucocorticoid remediable)	
• FH Type 2 (linked to chromosome 7p22 mutation)	
• FH Type 3 (linked to KCNJ5 potassium channel mutation)	
Adrenal cortical carcinoma	<1%

Modified from Velasco A, Vongpatanasin W. The evaluation and treatment of endocrine forms of hypertension. Curr Cardiol Rep. 2014;16:528.

of systemic hypertension.[173,174] Recent reports identify 14% to 17% of unilateral adrenal disease to be unilateral hyperplasia.[175]

Adrenal Cortical Hyperplasia With Excess Sex Steroid Secretion

Adrenal cortical hyperplasia with excess sex steroid secretion is essentially limited to cases of CAH.

Adrenal Medullary Hyperplasia

AMH has been reported in a sporadic setting as a distinct entity.[176] AMH had been reported as a precursor lesion for pheochromocytoma in MEN2a and MEN2b, where it could be diffuse or nodular and is often multicentric and bilateral.[177-180] A cutoff of 1 cm in size was proposed for the diagnosis of pheochromocytoma, because this was the smallest tumor in the publication by Karsner.[178,181] AMH in this familiar setting is now regarded as a small or micropheochromocytoma because it shows the same genetic abnormalities.[182]

Sporadic AMH has been reported in patients with symptoms of pheochromocytoma including paroxysmal or sustained hypertension, headache, palpitations, and diaphoresis; surgical exploration fails to reveal a catecholamine-secreting tumor. AMH in this setting may be unilateral and enters into the differential diagnosis of pseudopheochromocytoma. AMH also has been reported in patients with cystic fibrosis and Beckwith-Wiedemann syndrome.[4,43,71]

Adrenal Cyst

Nonneoplastic adrenal cysts are uncommon, usually occurring in the fifth and sixth decades of life, although cases have been reported from birth to 76 years.[183] A predilection for women is seen, with a female-to-male ratio of approximately 3:1.[184] Adrenal cysts may be small and discovered incidentally at autopsy. Rarely, they may be extremely large, containing several liters of fluid and compressing the abdominal contents. Adrenal cysts have been classified as parasitic (7% of cases, usually echinococcal), epithelial (9%), endothelial (45%), and pseudocyst (39%).[183,185] Epithelial cysts are subdivided into three categories: true glandular or retention cysts; embryonal cysts lined by cylindrical epithelium derived from displaced urogenital tissue that has undergone cystic transformation; and cystic change within an adrenal adenoma, carcinoma, or pheochromocytoma.[186] It has also been proposed that an epithelial-lined adrenal cyst rarely may develop from entrapped mesothelium.[187,188]

Adrenal pseudocysts are the most common type of adrenal cyst seen at surgery and often appear as a large unilocular cyst with an irregular lining, containing red-brown bloody fluid (Fig. 16.36). Some adrenal pseudocysts probably arise by hemorrhage into normal or pathologic adrenal glands; a small number result from hemorrhage into an underlying tumor.[183,186,189] Immunohistochemical studies show a vascular endothelial lining in some adrenal pseudocysts.[190-192] Some hemorrhagic cysts may arise when hemorrhage occurs in an existing vascular malformation.[191] Entrapment of nests of cortical cells by extravasated blood may occur, and this

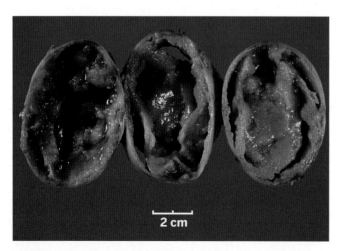

Fig. 16.36 Adrenal pseudocyst on cross-section contains grumous, soft, pale-tan debris. Dystrophic calcification was present in the cyst wall.

hemorrhagic cyst should be distinguished from a necrotic adrenal cortical neoplasm. Breast carcinoma has initially manifested as metastasis to an adrenal cyst, and mature adipose tissue and myelolipomatous metaplasia have been described within adrenal pseudocysts.[193]

Microscopic cysts are a frequent histologic finding in the permanent cortex of fetal and premature adrenal glands, being reported in up to 62% of stillbirths under 35 weeks gestational age.[194] A significant correlation with short gestation and short survival after birth has been reported.[195] Three possible pathogenetic mechanisms have been proposed: an intrinsic developmental process, infection, and a generalized reaction to stress.

Adrenal Hemorrhage

Adrenal hemorrhage can complicate cardiac disease, thromboembolic disease, sepsis, postoperative or postpartum state, or coagulopathy (e.g., heparin administration).[3] A recent autopsy study found that 61% of individuals dying of bacterial sepsis develop some degree of adrenal hemorrhage.[95] Patients may become symptomatic with abdominal or lower chest pain and fever. Newborn infants may present with manifestations of adrenal hemorrhage or hematoma formation.[3] Occasionally, adrenal hemorrhage is bilateral and massive.[196] Unfortunately, the diagnosis is made only infrequently during life. A high index of suspicion is required because of the nonspecific clinical presentation and the frequent comorbidity of other factors. Imaging techniques are useful in establishing a timely diagnosis so that appropriate intervention can prevent a poor outcome.[197]

Adrenal Neoplasms

Adrenal Cortical Neoplasms

Adrenal Cortical Adenoma With Cushing Syndrome

ACA is usually small, weighing less than 50 g. In one series, the tumors had an average weight of 36 g (range, 12.5 to 126 g).[198] On transverse section, it usually appears as a sharply circumscribed or encapsulated mass.[71,199] Almost all tumors are unilateral and solitary, although rare exceptions have been noted.[200,201] Adenomas may be yellow or golden-yellow throughout or have irregular mottling or diffuse dark brown areas (Fig. 16.37). The color of the tumor depends on many factors, including the presence of congestion or hemorrhage and the content of neutral lipid and lipofuscin.[71,199,202]

Although many tumors appear grossly encapsulated, histologic study may reveal a relatively smooth expansile border, in some cases with formation of a pseudocapsule. Compression of adjacent adrenal parenchyma and connective tissue, including the expanded adrenal capsule itself, contributes to the encapsulation of the ACA. Adenomas usually consist of cells with relatively abundant pale, lipid-rich cytoplasm resembling the zona fasciculata, but cells with more compact eosinophilic cytoplasm may be seen. Architecturally, the cells are arranged in short trabeculae, blunt cords, or a nesting or alveolar pattern (Fig. 16.38). Nuclei are usually vesicular, with a single, small nucleolus. Nuclear enlargement and pleomorphism may occur, but it is usually focal and mild to moderate in degree (Fig. 16.39). Also, foci of lipomatous or myelolipomatous metaplasia may be found. Endocrinologic data and clinical information are often essential to distinguish an adrenal cortical neoplasm associated with Cushing syndrome from an incidental nonhyperfunctioning adenoma or one associated with a different endocrine syndrome.[71,199] An important clue to the presence of

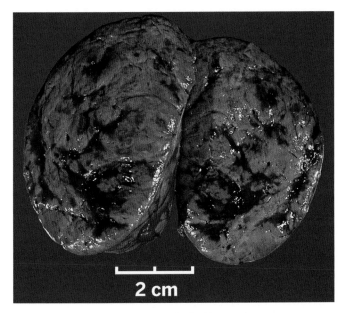

Fig. 16.37 Adrenal cortical adenoma in Cushing syndrome.

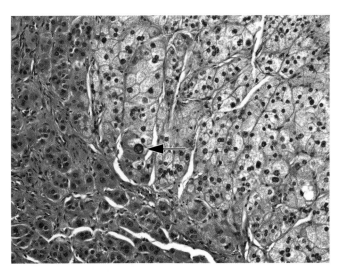

Fig. 16.39 Adrenal cortical adenoma in Cushing syndrome. Note the focal variability in nuclear size and hyperchromasia. Many cells in this field have compact, eosinophilic cytoplasm, and some have nuclear pseudoinclusions (*arrow*).

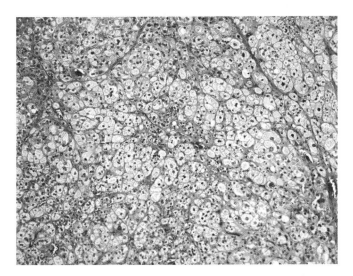

Fig. 16.38 Adrenal cortical adenoma in Cushing syndrome. Cells are arranged in alveoli or short cords.

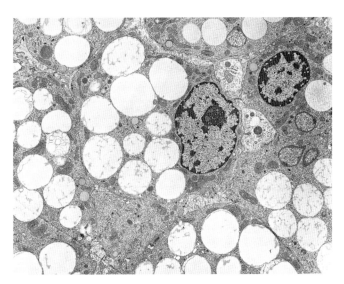

Fig. 16.40 Adrenal cortical adenoma in Cushing syndrome. Cells contain large lipid globules and prominent smooth endoplasmic reticulum (×3500). (From Lack EE, Travis WD, Oertel JE. Adrenal cortical neoplasms. In: Lack EE, ed. Pathology of the Adrenal Glands. New York: Churchill Livingstone; 1990:115–171.)

Cushing syndrome is cortical atrophy in the attached adrenal or the contralateral gland. In most cases, ultrastructural study reveals abundant intracytoplasmic lipid (Fig. 16.40). Mitochondria may have tubulovesicular cristae, similar to normal cells of zona fasciculata, or lamellar cristae characteristic of the zona reticularis. Smooth endoplasmic reticulum is usually abundant.

The Carney triad was described in 1977 and currently is composed of gastric stromal sarcoma, pulmonary chondroma, and extraadrenal paraganglioma. ACA has recently been recognized as the fourth component of the Carney triad, and has been associated with subclinical Cushing syndrome.[203] Incidentalomas, as previously noted, have become increasingly common as more abdominal imaging is performed, and the most common secretory syndrome is subclinical Cushing syndrome, also referred to as adrenal mild hypercortisolism.[204] Duan et al. provide a detailed overview of clinicopathologic correlates of adrenal Cushing syndrome including an in-depth discussion of molecular and genetic abnormalities.[205]

Adrenal Cortical Adenoma With Primary Hyperaldosteronism (Conn Syndrome)

An estimated 30% to 35% of cases of primary hyperaldosteronism are caused by an aldosterone-secreting ACA (Table 16.3).[172] Recent data indicate that idiopathic bilateral hyperplasia is a more frequent cause, particularly if mild examples are included. Three types of familial primary hyperaldosteronism have been identified, all inherited in an autosomal dominant manner and together account for less than 1% of primary hyperaldosteronism.[172,206] A variety of genetic abnormalities have been reported in primary hyperaldosteronism and are addressed elsewhere in recent publications.[207,208]

The aldosterone-secreting ACA is an important surgical lesion because it may be a curable form of systemic hypertension. Adrenal vein sampling is a widely accepted method for localizing aldosterone-secreting ACA and is useful in distinguishing adenomas from hyperplasias.[209] The prevalence of an aldosterone-secreting adenoma in the hypertensive population ranges from 0.5% to 8%, although Conn suggested that primary hyperaldosteronism may be the cause of up to 20% of all cases of essential hypertension based on the incidence of a solitary adenoma 1.5 cm or more in diameter reported in hypertensive individuals at autopsy (20%).[109,199,210] However, incidental cortical nodules are relatively common in patients 50 to 80 years of age and those with hypertension.[106] It is unclear whether hypertension results from the incidental nodule or adenoma or is a cause of it, perhaps in some cases related to capsular arteriopathy. This controversy can forever be rekindled, however, because it can be postulated that, over time, conversion may occur of glomerulosa-type cells within these incidental nodules to cells having different functional characteristics. When the incidental adenoma is discovered, the patient may already have established systemic hypertension without the expected biochemical profile of an aldosterone-secreting adenoma.[199]

Aldosterone-secreting ACA (aldosteronoma) is usually solitary, small, and measures only a few centimeters in diameter; many are smaller than 2 cm, although most are large enough to be visible on abdominal CT.[199] Grossly, the tumor may project from one portion of the gland, although it may be difficult to appreciate in the intact gland without transverse sectioning. It is often homogeneous, diffusely bright yellow-orange, and may be sharply demarcated from the adjacent cortex, simulating encapsulation (Fig. 16.41). Architectural patterns include alveolar or nesting arrangement, short cords, or trabeculae of cells (Fig. 16.42).

Four types of cells have been described by light microscopy, often with multiple types in the same tumor.[7,211] The most common cell type is large, with pale-staining, lipid-rich cytoplasm resembling cells of the zona fasciculata. This cell type has been associated with the genetic mutation KCNJ5.[207] A second cell type appears as clusters of smaller cells resembling those of the zona glomerulosa, with a high nuclear-to-cytoplasmic ratio and a small amount of vacuolated cytoplasm. The third type consists of scattered cells with compact eosinophilic cytoplasm similar to cells of the zona reticularis. The fourth cell type, hybrid cell, has morphologic features intermediate between those of zona glomerulosa–type and zona fasciculata–type cells. The attached or contralateral adrenal gland may show hyperplasia of the zona glomerulosa, with a broad focal or discontinuous zone beneath the capsule

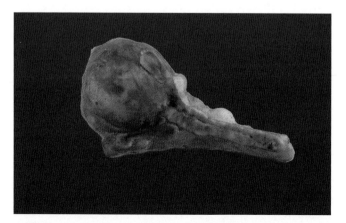

Fig. 16.41 Aldosterone-secreting adrenal cortical adenoma. The tumor was 1 cm in diameter and yellow-orange on cross-section.

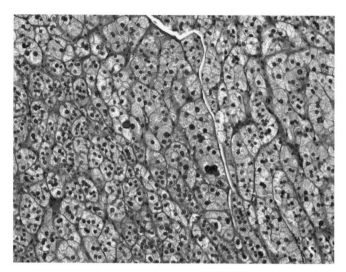

Fig. 16.42 Aldosterone-producing adrenal cortical adenoma. Most cells have lipid-rich, finely vacuolated cytoplasm.

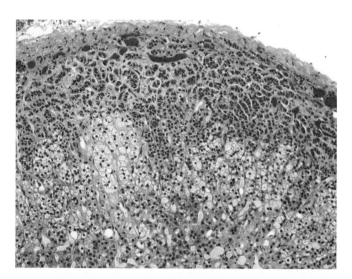

Fig. 16.43 Hyperplasia of the zona glomerulosa is apparent as a continuous band of cells beneath the capsule. Numerous foci such as this may be present in the cortex adjacent to aldosterone-secreting adenomas.

(Fig. 16.43), sometimes with small tongues of glomerulosa-type cells extending inward from the capsule.[7,211] The term *hybrid* refers to the capacity of the cell to synthesize cortical steroids, which are normally produced by the zona glomerulosa (aldosterone) or the zona fasciculata (cortisol). Aldosterone-secreting adenomas may originate from hybrid cells or zona fasciculata–type cells. This would account for the functional behavior of tumor cells in vivo, as evidenced by modulation of aldosterone secretion by ACTH, lack of responsiveness to angiotensin II (the dominant secretagogue and trophic hormone for the glomerulosa-type cells under normal conditions), secretion of the hybrid steroids in large quantities, and the ability of the cells to produce cortisol in vitro and sometimes in large quantities in vivo.[212] Ultrastructurally, these cells show morphologic heterogeneity, including round to elongated mitochondria with cristae that are short and tubular, vesicular, or lamellar, typical of zona glomerulosa–type cells.[71,213]

Spironolactone bodies are lightly eosinophilic, scroll-like intracytoplasmic inclusions that have been described in the zona glomerulosa of the nonneoplastic cortex in patients treated with the aldosterone antagonist spironolactone (Aldactone) (Fig. 16.44).[214] Occasionally, these inclusions can be seen within the tumor cells.[71,199] Ultrastructural study suggests origin from tightly packed tubules of endoplasmic reticulum.[215] The spironolactone bodies typically range in size from 2 to 12 μm, but most are equal in size or slightly larger than the adjacent nucleus. These structures may be highlighted with Luxol fast blue stain because of their rich phospholipid content.[71,199] Although the specificity of these inclusions has been questioned, they are generally regarded as rather specific markers for spironolactone administration. In one study, the number of spironolactone bodies within cells of the aldosterone-secreting adenoma correlated positively with the proportion of glomerulosa-type cells.[216]

Functional Pigmented (Black) Adrenal Cortical Adenoma

Pigmented (black) ACA is characterized by diffuse black pigmentation on cross-section (Fig. 16.45), although some areas may be dark brown or yellow-brown.[217] Pigmented ACA is usually diagnosed in the third to the fifth decades of life, with a distinct predilection for females.[199] This tumor is most often associated with

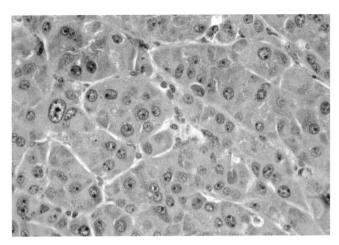

Fig. 16.46 Pigmented (black) adenoma causing Cushing syndrome. Tumor cells form nests and short cords and have abundant intracytoplasmic granular lipofuscin pigment.

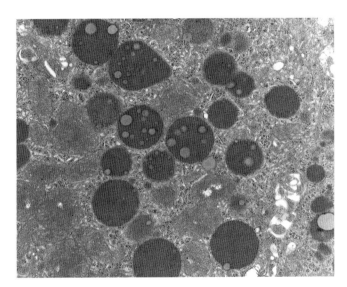

Fig. 16.47 Black adenoma of adrenal gland from a patient with Cushing syndrome. Note the numerous electron-dense structures, some containing small lipid droplets. (×17,000).

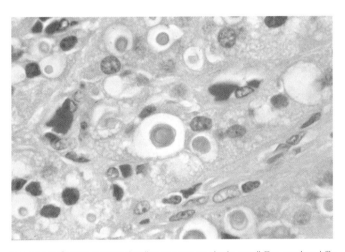

Fig. 16.44 Spironolactone bodies appear as single scroll-like, eosinophilic inclusions within zona glomerulosa cells. Many are surrounded by a clear space.

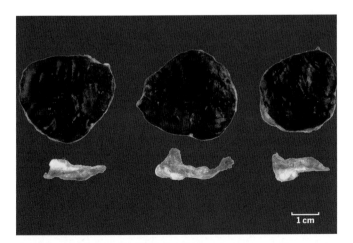

Fig. 16.45 Pigmented (black) adrenal cortical adenoma with Cushing syndrome. The tumor is 3.5 cm in diameter. Sectioned surfaces of tumor are diffusely black, with vague lobulation. Residual adrenal gland (*lower row*) shows marked cortical atrophy.

Cushing syndrome, although it also has been reported with primary hyperaldosteronism.[71,199] Microscopically, the architectural patterns are similar to those of other adenomas. The histologic hallmark is the conspicuous brown or golden-brown granular pigment in the cytoplasm (Fig. 16.46), which has the staining characteristics of lipofuscin. One study, however, suggested that some of the pigment may be neuromelanin.[122] As with other adenomas, areas of lipomatous or myelolipomatous metaplasia may be present.[71] Ultrastructurally, the cells contain relatively few lipid globules but have a variable number of electron-dense structures that are often associated with small lipid vacuoles (Fig. 16.47) characteristic of lipofuscin.[71,199] No melanosomes or premelanosomes are seen.

Adrenal Cortical Neoplasms With Virilization or Feminization

Adrenal cortical neoplasms associated with virilization or feminization are clinically important because of the potential for malignant behavior. Many have unfavorable gross or microscopic findings such as large size and areas of necrosis. A review of women with virilizing adrenal cortical tumors found that at least 17% were clinically malignant; an even greater proportion of feminizing adrenal cortical neoplasms were malignant.[218,219] Histologically, a predominance of cells with compact eosinophilic cytoplasm is often seen, but this histologic pattern is not specific. Virilization has been reported with tumors classified as Leydig cell adenoma of the adrenal gland, which contain Reinke crystalloids, a pathognomonic feature of Leydig (or hilus) cells.[220] Rarely, Leydig cells have been reported in the adrenal cortex, probably because of the close embryologic relation between developing adrenal primordia and gonads.[221] Virilization is present with many of the childhood adrenal cortical tumors and may be part of a mixed endocrine along with Cushing syndrome.

Oncocytic Adrenal Cortical Neoplasms (Adrenal Oncocytoma)

Rarely, adrenal cortical neoplasms are composed of cells with abundant, finely granular, eosinophilic cytoplasm typical of oncocytoma (Fig. 16.48).[222-225] Eosinophilic cytoplasmic inclusions have been described in some of these tumors that are thought to be a mitochondria-associated degenerative change and not specific for the adrenal cortex or its products.[226] The vast majority of these tumors are clinically nonfunctional, but some may exhibit low levels of enzyme activity in cortical steroidogenesis.[223] Although most adrenal cortical oncocytic neoplasms are benign, cases of oncocytic carcinomas have been reported.[227-231] It has been suggested that oncocytic carcinomas represent low-grade ACC.

Adrenal Cortical Carcinoma

ACC is rare, occurring annually in approximately 0.7 to 2 cases per million population in the United States.[232] Many large series of ACC have been reported in the last few decades, mainly in adults. A slight female preponderance is seen. The age distribution is bimodal, with peak incidence in the fifth to seventh decades of life with a second peak in childhood.[233] Presenting signs and symptoms include abdominal pain, a palpable mass, fatigue, weight loss, and, in 10% to 20% of patients, intermittent low-grade fever that may be caused by tumor necrosis.[71,199] Regional or distant metastases occur in 25% or more of patients.[71,199,234,235] Because ACCs are usually inefficient producers of steroids, clinical evidence of excess hormone secretion usually does not become apparent until the tumor is large. Some tumors are therefore classified clinically as nonfunctional or functionally inactive. When adrenal cortical neoplasms are functional, they most commonly produce cortisol, but in some cases the patient may present with a mixed endocrine syndrome (e.g., Cushing syndrome and virilization). Purely virilizing ACC is uncommon in adults, and feminizing ACC is rare. Primary hyperaldosteronism caused by ACC is also relatively uncommon.[71,199] A study reported five adrenal cortical neoplasms clinically mimicking pheochromocytoma with biochemical evidence of elevated catecholamine secretion in serum or urine; two were ACC and three were ACA.[236]

ACC is usually large, and careful gross examination often may suggest malignancy, with areas of necrosis, hemorrhage, and cystic change.[71,199] On cross-section, the tumors are often variegated in color, ranging from yellow, yellow-orange, to tan-brown. Larger tumors are often coarsely lobulated with intersecting fibrous bands (Fig. 16.49). The average recorded weight in several series ranged from 705 to 1210 g.[71] Tang and Gray reported that all adrenal cortical tumors over 95 g were malignant, whereas those weighing less than 50 g were benign.[237] However, weight alone is not entirely reliable as a distinguishing characteristic, because some small ACCs have metastasized, including tumors weighing 40 g or less.[71,191,238] Also, some adrenal cortical neoplasms weighing more than 1000 g may prove to be clinically benign after prolonged follow-up. Size has also been reported to be an important indicator of malignancy. The clear majority of ACCs are greater than 6 cm in diameter, but several cases of small ACC measuring less than 5 cm have been reported.[239] The reverse is also true. ACA may be quite large—more than 5 cm—sometimes because of central degeneration, hemorrhage, or calcification and fibrosis.[240] A study of the Surveillance Epidemiology and End Results (SEER) database indicated that for adrenal cortical neoplasms 4 cm or larger the likelihood of malignancy essentially doubles to approximately 10% and increases more than ninefold in tumors 8 cm or larger.[116]

ACC has a variety of architectural patterns, including trabecular, alveolar (nesting), and solid (diffuse). The most characteristic pattern is a trabecular arrangement of cells with broad anastomosing columns separated by delicate elongated vascular spaces (Fig. 16.50). Some of the trabeculae, when cut in cross-section or oblique planes, appear as free-floating islands of tumor cells.

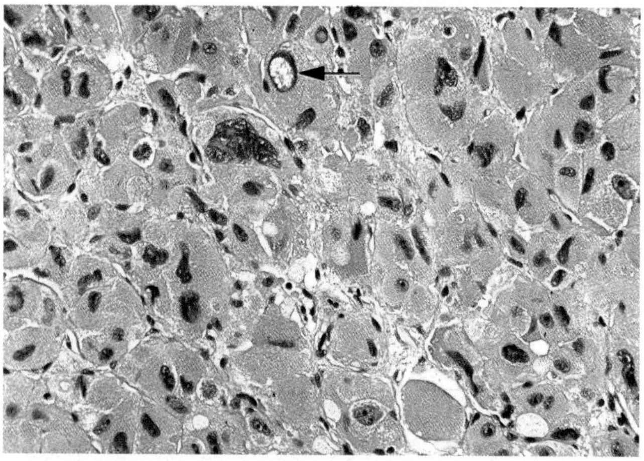

Fig. 16.48 Incidental nonhyperfunctional adrenal cortical adenoma is composed of cells with abundant, granular eosinophilic cytoplasm (oncocytoma). Nuclei are moderately pleomorphic and hyperchromatic, with occasional nuclear pseudoinclusions (*arrow*). The tumor weighed less than 15 g.

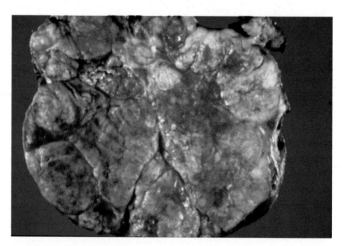

Fig. 16.49 Adrenal cortical carcinoma. Note the coarsely nodular cut surface.

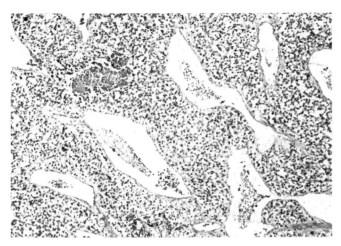

Fig. 16.50 Adrenal cortical carcinoma. The tumor has broad anastomosing trabeculae and gaping sinusoids with delicate endothelium. Tumor cells have compact, eosinophilic cytoplasm and small, uniform nuclei. The patient died of metastases within 1 year of diagnosis and at autopsy had massive invasion of the inferior vena cava.

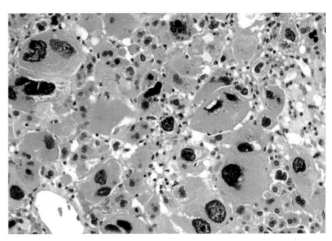

Fig. 16.51 Adrenal cortical neoplasm that proved to be benign and hence atypical adenoma. Tumor cells have marked nuclear pleomorphism and hyperchromasia. The tumor was found incidentally on computed tomography and weighed 99 g. The patient was alive and well 11 years later.

Rarely, a pseudoglandular arrangement of cells may be seen, or the tumor may have a myxoid appearance.[71,199] Most tumor cells in ACC have compact, eosinophilic cytoplasm that is lipid poor. Foci of vascular invasion when present usually appear as unattached plugs of tumor within vascular spaces. Nuclear pleomorphism and hyperchromasia can be spectacular in ACC, but nuclear atypia alone is not a reliable indicator of malignancy and can also be seen in ACA (Fig. 16.51).[71,199] Mitotic figures may be numerous in ACC and are rare in ACA and adrenal hyperplasia (Fig. 16.52). In the study by Weiss, only two nonmetastasizing adrenal cortical tumors contained fewer than 3 mitotic figures per 50 high-power fields (hpf), whereas 78% of ACCs contained more than 5 mitotic figures per 50 hpf, and 17% had more than 50 per 50 hpf.[241] In addition to mitotic activity, tumor necrosis is more frequent in ACC than in ACA.[235,242-246] One investigation of 56 cases reported no necrosis in 8 of the ACA reviewed, whereas 45 of the 48 ACCs displayed variable amounts of necrosis.[235] An unusual feature of ACC (and some adenomas) is the presence of intracytoplasmic hyaline globules, similar to those commonly seen in pheochromocytoma (Fig. 16.53).[71] An ACC or ACA with an alveolar growth pattern and cells with compact, eosinophilic cytoplasm along with intracytoplasmic globules may be mistaken for a pheochromocytoma. Another pitfall in the diagnosis of adrenal cortical neoplasms is immunoreactivity for synaptophysin or neuron-specific enolase, markers that are used for documenting neuroendocrine differentiation.[247,248] Ultrastructurally, intracytoplasmic lipid vacuoles are often sparse or absent and cellular organelles may be moderate or few in number.[249] Flattened cisternae of rough endoplasmic reticulum in stacks or short parallel lamellae may be seen. Smooth endoplasmic reticulum may form an intricate anastomosing network.

Many studies have proposed histologic criteria to predict malignant behavior. Hough et al. reported that the strongest predictors were broad fibrous bands, a diffuse growth pattern, and vascular invasion.[242] Weiss et al. analyzed the predictive value of nine histologic parameters and found that recurrence or metastasis occurred only in tumors with a mitotic rate greater than 5 per 50 hpf, atypical mitotic figures, and invasion of venous structures.[245] Van Slooten et al. used a histologic index based on seven histologic

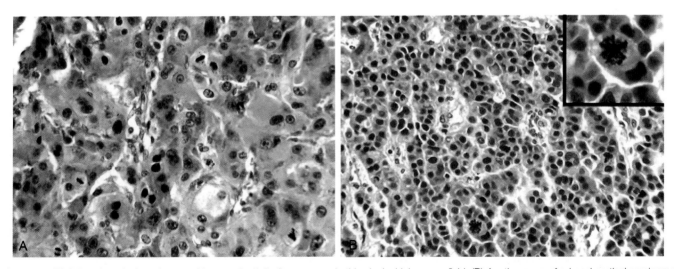

Fig. 16.52 (A) Adrenal cortical carcinoma with several mitotic figures seen in this single, high-power field. (B) Another case of adrenal cortical carcinoma composed of cells with dense, compact eosinophilic cytoplasm arranged in a trabecular growth pattern; an atypical mitotic figure is highlighted (*inset*).

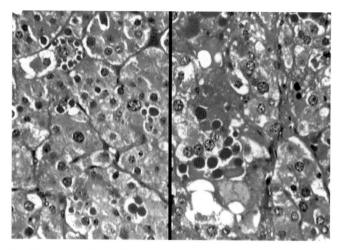

Fig. 16.53 Adrenal cortical adenoma with intracytoplasmic globules, similar to what is more commonly encountered in pheochromocytoma. *Right,* High-power image of globules.

parameters to predict outcome.[243] Volante et al. introduced an algorithmic approach to evaluate adrenal cortical neoplasms that may be useful in borderline cases.[244] This approach incorporates evaluation of the reticulin network with the modified Weiss criteria. Based on this approach, all adrenal cortical tumors with a disrupted reticulin network qualify for carcinoma as do those with maintained reticulin pattern and any one of the following: mitoses greater than 5 per 50 hpf, necrosis, or venous invasion. Despite these findings, it is clear that a small but significant number of adrenal cortical neoplasms have unpredictable biologic behavior, and long-term follow-up in some of these troublesome cases is the final arbiter in diagnosis.[234] Mitotic rate has been used to separate low-grade and high-grade ACC; the median survival for patients with low-grade ACC (≤20 mitotic figures per 50 hpf) was 58 months in contrast with 14 months for high-grade tumors (>20 mitotic figures per 50 hpf).[245] Immunohistochemistry for cell cycle regulatory proteins has been applied to ACC; with Ki-67, there was a 5% cutoff, and none of the 33 ACA reached this cutoff value; more than 75% of ACCs in this study had 6 or more mitoses per 50 hpf.[250] A large international study has recently concluded that current practices in Ki-67 scoring assessment vary greatly, and novel digital microscopy-enabled methods could provide critical aid in improving reproducibility and reliability in the clinical setting.[251] DNA ploidy analysis has been used to predict outcome, but the results have been controversial.[71,252-256] According to some investigators, the greatest value of DNA ploidy analysis in predicting outcome is in patients undergoing potentially curative surgical resection.[256]

More recently, molecular studies have revealed multiple chromosomal aberrations that may be related to ACC.[257,258] Some chromosomal loci correlate with abnormal familial syndromes including Li-Fraumeni syndrome (p53, 17p13), MEN1 (11q13), Beckwith-Wiedemann syndrome (11p15.5 associated with IGFII overexpression), and Carney complex (2p16). Additionally, loss of heterozygosity on chromosomes 11p, 13q, and 17p has been reported in ACC, whereas these chromosomal changes have not been seen in ACA or hyperplasia. Numerous other studies on chromosomal and immunohistochemical associations with malignancy in adrenal cortical tumors have been reported in recent years, the results of which are beyond the scope of this chapter.[257,258] Suffice it to say, as our understanding of the molecular pathogenesis of these neoplasms progresses, improved diagnostic and treatment strategies may become available.

The pattern of metastasis of ACC reflects both lymphatic and hematogenous dissemination. The sites of metastases in patients dying of ACC include liver (92%), lung (78%), retroperitoneum (48%), intraabdominal lymph nodes (32%), intrathoracic lymph nodes (26%), and other sites such as bone.[199] On rare occasion, the tumor can extend into the inferior vena cava with occlusion of this vessel and even extend into the right atrium.[71,259]

Percutaneous fine-needle aspiration may be helpful in the preoperative diagnosis of ACC, but extreme caution must be exercised in trying to differentiate ACC from a benign adrenal cortical neoplasm on cytologic features alone.[71,199] A major drawback to the cytologic differentiation of ACC versus adenoma is sampling error. If a good specimen with obvious cytologic features of carcinoma is obtained, the diagnosis can be made with a fair amount of certainty.[71] However, if the specimen has only minor cytologic abnormalities that could be seen in ACA, to definitively rule out the possibility of carcinoma on a fine-needle aspiration specimen would not be prudent. Careful correlation with clinical and endocrinologic data is needed, combined with knowledge of other features such as tumor size and imaging characteristics.[71] The same can be said for core needle biopsy specimens.

The differential diagnosis of ACC may be aided by special studies, including immunohistochemistry. Typically, adrenal cortical neoplasms are positive for vimentin and negative for epithelial markers such as cytokeratin, CAM5.2, and epithelial membrane antigen; however, occasionally, adrenal cortical neoplasms may express keratin reactivity, especially with low-molecular-weight cytokeratins.[260] Antibodies to the α subunit of inhibin have been found to be expressed by adrenal cortical tissue, both normal and neoplastic (Fig. 16.54); additionally, the majority of adrenal cortical neoplasms are immunoreactive with calretinin and melan A.[260] Another antibody that shows sensitive and specific reactivity is SF-1.[261] Immunohistochemistry is quite useful in differentiating adrenal cortical neoplasms from other neoplasms such as pheochromocytoma and metastatic tumors, especially renal cell carcinoma.[261,262]

Disease-free and overall survival rates have been strongly correlated with ACC stage. Most patients have relatively advanced disease at the time of diagnosis; only approximately 30% of patients have tumor confined to the adrenal gland (Table 16.4).[71,263] ACCs have been stratified to three risk groups: the low-risk group includes stage I to II disease with a mitotic rate of 9 or fewer per 50 hpf; the intermediate-risk group includes stage I to II disease with mitoses

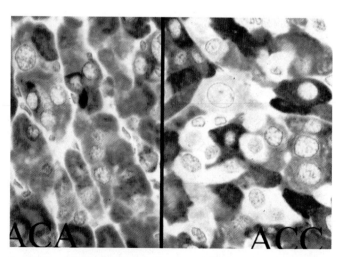

Fig. 16.54 Adrenal cortical adenoma (*ACA*) and adrenal cortical carcinoma (*ACC*), both showing strong cytoplasmic staining with antibodies to the α subunit of inhibin.

TABLE 16.4	Staging of Adrenal Cortical Carcinoma			
%	Stage	TNM		Staging Criteria
2.8	I	$T_1N_0M_0$	T_1	Tumor ≤5 cm, no extraadrenal invasion
29	II	$T_2N_0M_0$	T_2	Tumor >5 cm, no extraadrenal invasion
19.3	III	$T_1N_1M_0$	T_3	Tumor of any size, locally invasive but not involving adjacent organs
		$T_2N_1M_0$		
		T_3 Any N M_0	T_4	Tumor of any size, with invasion of adjacent organs or large blood vessels
48.9	IV	Any T, any N, M_1	N_0	Negative regional lymph nodes
		T_3, N_1	N_1	Positive regional lymph nodes
		T_4	M_0	No distant metastases
			M_1	Distant metastases

Used with permission of the American College of Surgeons, Chicago, Illinois. The original source for this information is the AJCC Cancer Staging Manual, Eighth Edition (2017) published by Springer International Publishing.

greater than 9 per 50 hpf or stage III to IV disease and a mitotic count of 9 or fewer per 50 hpf; and the high-risk group includes stage III to IV disease with a mitotic count greater than 9 per 50 hpf.[263]

Adrenal cortical neoplasms in children remain somewhat of an enigma for pathologists. Their clinical and biologic behavior can be quite distinct from that of histologically similar counterparts in adults. Attempts to identify pathologic criteria of malignancy have been made, with some success, but further studies are required for a better understanding of adrenal cortical neoplasms in children.[246,264,265] A big factor in the difficulty of assessing these lesions is the rarity with which ACC occurs in this population.

Other Adrenal Cortical Neoplasms

Several examples of adrenal carcinosarcoma have been reported in adults, consisting of mixtures of sarcomatous elements and ACC.[266-269] An example of virilizing adrenal cortical blastoma was reported in an infant who had an elevated serum level of α-fetoprotein.[270]

Pheochromocytoma

Pheochromocytoma is a catecholamine-secreting tumor arising from neural crest–derived chromaffin cells of the sympathoadrenal system. It is relatively uncommon in surgical pathology practice, with an estimated average annual incidence of 8 per 1 million person-years (excluding familial cases).[271] It has been suggested that for every pheochromocytoma diagnosed during life, two remain undiscovered, but recent data show more of them diagnosed during life, probably reflecting increased clinical awareness, heightened diagnostic acumen, and more sensitive laboratory testing. The peak age at diagnosis is in the fifth decade, but pheochromocytoma can affect any age group. Most clinical series report a roughly equal sex incidence.

Hereditary Pheochromocytoma–Paraganglioma

Pheochromocytoma has been referred to as the "10% tumor"—10% familial, 10% malignant and 10% extraadrenal, and 10% occurring in childhood—but this may no longer apply given the advances in identifying genetic markers for increased susceptibility for hereditary/familial pheochromocytoma/paraganglioma.[272] There have been at least 14 susceptibility genes identified since 1990, and 10 have been validated in large studies (Table 16.5).[273] Additional genes will probably be tested and

TABLE 16.5	Detected Germline Mutations in 3694 Pheochromocytoma/Paraganglioma Patients
Mutation	Frequency
SDHB (paraganglioma 4)	10.3%
SDHD (paraganglioma 1)	8.9%
VHL	7.3%
RET	6.3%
NF-1	3.3%
SDHC (paraganglioma 3)	1.0%
SDHA (paraganglioma 5)	<2%
SDHAF2 (paraganglioma 2)	<2%
TMEM 127	<2%
MAX	<2%

From Lenders JW, Duh QY, Eisenhofer G, et al. Pheochromocytoma and paraganglioma: an endocrine society clinical practice guideline. J Clin Endocrinol Metab. 2014;99:1915–1942.

validated in future studies.[274] In lieu of the "10% tumor," some have proposed the "10-gene tumor." Pheochromocytoma/paraganglioma is a significant heritable form of neoplasia in humans with about 40% of cases associated with familial syndromes having autosomal dominant traits.[273] These include neurofibromatosis type 1, MEN2a and MEN2b, von Hippel-Lindau disease, renal cell carcinoma with SDHB mutation, Carney triad, and Carney-Stratakis dyad (paraganglioma and gastric stromal tumor).[275,276] The profile for possible hereditary/familial pheochromocytoma/paraganglioma includes a family history of such tumors (or the presence of syndromic features) or the presence of tumors with some of the following: (1) multiple tumors (e.g., >1 paraganglioma or pheochromocytoma including bilateral pheochromocytoma); (2) multifocal tumors, synchronous or metachronous, in different anatomic sites; (3) malignant tumors; and (4) early onset (e.g., <45 years).[273] It is notable that germline mutations have been found in 24% of patients who presented with nonsyndromic apparently sporadic pheochromocytoma, and the following features were significantly associated with mutations: younger age, multifocal tumors, and extraadrenal tumors (paraganglioma).[277]

Eight studies, each having more than 200 patients, have been involved with genotyping of the main pheochromocytoma-paraganglioma susceptibility genes (SDHB, SDHD, VHL, and RET), with the total cohort of patients being 3694; of these, 1250 individuals harbored germline mutations (33.8%), indicating that at least one-third of all patients with pheochromocytoma-paraganglioma have disease-associated genetic mutations.[273] Genotypic/phenotypic correlations have been identified in pheochromocytoma-paraganglioma syndromes with at least 40% or more of tumors with SDHB mutations exhibiting malignant behavior.[273,278,279] In addition, tumors having any of the *SDH* mutations tend to be more often extraadrenal, whereas those with a *RET* mutation are usually confined to the adrenal or immediate area. Five of the susceptibility genes in Table 16.5 were found in 2% or fewer of cases studied including two of the more recently reported genes, *TMEM127* and *MAX* (MYC-associated factor X).[273,280,281]

A task force organized to formulate clinical practice guidelines for pheochromocytoma-paraganglioma has recommended that genetic testing should be *considered* in each patient, but this does not mean to imply that genetic testing should be *done* on each patient. Genetic testing has limited incremental value in patients with unilateral pheochromocytoma, no syndromic or malignant features, and absence of positive family history.[273] Evidence available in the literature apparently justifies SDHB genetic testing in patients with malignant pheochromocytoma-paraganglioma.

Pathology of Pheochromocytoma

Sporadic pheochromocytoma usually forms a unicentric spherical or ovoid mass that is often sharply circumscribed and may appear encapsulated. Histologic sections taken at the periphery of the tumor often show a fibrous pseudocapsule or, at times, no capsule at all. Most pheochromocytomas are 3 to 5 cm in diameter, with an average weight in several large series ranging from 73 to 156.5 g.[4,71,272] The average weight of clinically malignant tumors tends to be greater than that of benign tumors. Pheochromocytoma is usually resiliently firm, with a glistening gray-white surface (Fig. 16.55), which may be altered by degenerative change such as congestion, hemorrhage, or necrosis, and some tumors undergo cystic change that may be marked. Rarely, pheochromocytoma grows into the inferior vena cava and may extend into the right atrium, mimicking renal cell carcinoma.[4,71,272]

Pheochromocytoma usually has an anastomosing cell cord pattern (Fig. 16.56), or sometimes an alveolar or zellballen architectural growth pattern in which the neoplastic cells form rounded to oval nests that are surrounded by a delicate fibrovascular network of supporting cells, the most characteristic cell being the sustentacular cell. Sustentacular cells typically are not apparent on routine stained sections. Occasionally, tumor cells are arranged in a predominantly solid or diffuse pattern (Fig. 16.57). A compressed fibrous pseudocapsule may be present between the

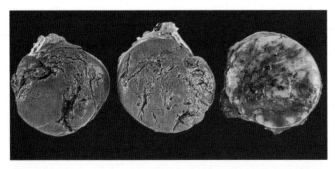

Fig. 16.55 Pheochromocytoma. Cross-section of a 3.5-cm tumor on the *right* is fleshy and pale tan, with mottled areas of congestion. Two other portions of the same tumor fixed in Zenker solution show a positive chromaffin reaction with a mahogany brown color.

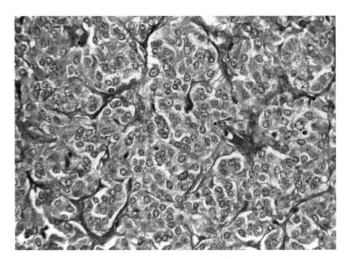

Fig. 16.56 Pheochromocytoma with an anastomosing cell cord pattern. The cells have a finely granular, basophilic cytoplasm with round to oval, eccentrically placed nuclei.

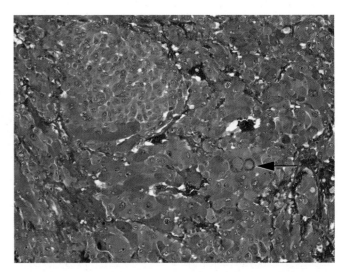

Fig. 16.57 Pheochromocytoma with a solid or diffuse growth pattern. Cells have abundant amphophilic cytoplasm. Note the marked nuclear pleomorphism and hyperchromasia and nuclear pseudoinclusions (*arrow*).

pheochromocytoma and the adjacent cortex, but sometimes no intervening fibrous connective tissue is present (Fig. 16.58), and there may be intermingling with nonneoplastic cortical cells at the periphery. Alterations in the supporting stroma, including sclerosis, edema, and changes in the vasculature, which could create diagnostic confusion, also may be present. One study reported amyloid deposition in 14 of 20 pheochromocytomas (70%), but no electron microscopic illustrations were provided.[282] Another study identified amyloid deposition in only 2 of 22 cases (9.1%) examined with supporting special stains, immunohistochemical stains, and electron microscopy.[283]

The pheochromocytoma cells, or pheochromocytes, are typically polygonal in shape with a finely granular cytoplasm that is basophilic to lightly eosinophilic. Nuclear pseudoinclusions have been reported in approximately one-third of pheochromocytomas, typically appearing as sharply defined round to oval structures that contain cytoplasm having the same staining intensity as the remainder of the cell, although they sometimes appear pale or empty (Fig. 16.59).[4,272] Some tumors contain cells with prominent nuclear hyperchromasia and pleomorphism, but these

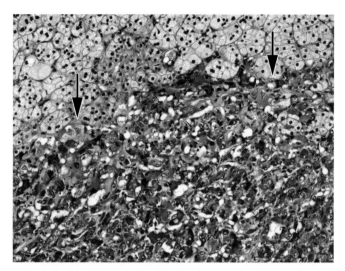

Fig. 16.58 Pheochromocytoma with a vague alveolar or nesting pattern. Section taken through the periphery of the tumor shows junction with the residual cortex (*arrows*) and lack of encapsulation.

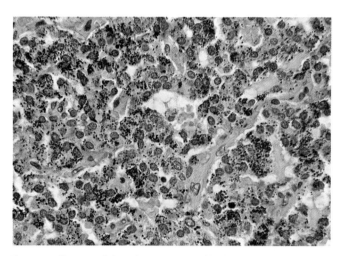

Fig. 16.60 Pigmented pheochromocytoma with abundant granular pigment that is consistent with lipofuscin. Ultrastructural study revealed no melanosomes or premelanosomes. A heavily pigmented tumor such as this may be mistaken for a pigmented black adenoma or malignant melanoma.

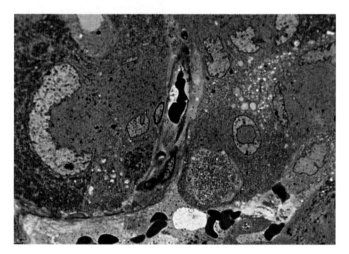

Fig. 16.59 Pheochromocytoma. A nuclear pseudoinclusion is present on the *right side* of the field viewed en face. The nucleus of the tumor cell on the *left side* shows a deep indentation with a jagged border that represents a pseudoinclusion viewed in profile (toluidine blue stain, ×1000.)

features alone are not useful in predicting biologic behavior. Cytoplasmic hyaline globules can be found in some pheochromocytomas and are characteristically positive for periodic acid–Schiff stain and resistant to diastase predigestion. The globules are slightly refractile and identical to those that may be found in the normal medullary chromaffin cells. These globules are detected in almost 50% of cases of sympathoadrenal paragangliomas and are possibly related to secretory activity.[284] Rarely, in some tumors, the cytoplasm is deeply eosinophilic and copious representing oncocytic change. Lipid degeneration gives the cytoplasm a clear, vacuolated appearance that can mimic an adrenal cortical neoplasm.[285,286] Some pheochromocytomas contain scattered cells resembling neuronal or ganglion cells with tapering cytoplasmic processes and peripheral aggregation of basophilic material resembling Nissl substance. Periadrenal brown fat may be associated with pheochromocytoma, but its incidence and functional importance are unclear.[287,288] Pigmented pheochromocytomas and extraadrenal paragangliomas are extremely rare.[71,289,290] These tumors may

have a jet-black gross appearance caused by an abundance of intracytoplasmic granules of lipofuscin (Fig. 16.60). The differential diagnosis of pigmented (black) adrenal neoplasms includes cortical adenoma, pheochromocytoma, and malignant melanoma (primary or secondary).

Pheochromocytoma in Multiple Endocrine Neoplasia Type 2

MEN2a (Sipple syndrome) is an autosomal dominant disorder with a high degree of penetrance, including various combinations of pheochromocytoma, medullary thyroid carcinoma, and parathyroid hyperplasia.[291] MEN2b also has an autosomal dominant mode of inheritance, but some patients appear to have the isolated or sporadic form of the disorder. The molecular background of MEN2a and MEN2b syndromes is activating mutations of the RET protooncogene.[292] It is possible that clinically aggressive medullary thyroid carcinoma that occurs in the setting of MEN2b causes death at an early age without the patient being able to pass the genetic syndrome on to a future generation.[4] Some cases may be truly sporadic as a result of gene mutations. The pheochromocytoma in MEN2a and MEN2b are frequently multicentric (Fig. 16.61) and bilateral (Fig. 16.62), and in some cases in which residual chromaffin tissue is recognizable, extratumoral medullary hyperplasia may be seen.[293] Gross morphologic features may be sufficiently distinctive that the surgical pathologist may be alerted to the possibility of the associated syndrome.[4,293]

In older literature, AMH in MEN2 was considered to be the precursor of pheochromocytoma.[176,177] AMH in this setting is now regarded as a small or early pheochromocytoma because they share the same genetic abnormality.[182] In MEN2a and MEN2b, one of the earliest manifestations of early pheochromocytoma is an elevated ratio of epinephrine to norepinephrine in the urine.[176] One suggested treatment for such patients is bilateral total adrenalectomy. Others suggest good long-term results with conservative unilateral adrenalectomy, with removal of the larger gland. Involvement of the adrenal glands may be symmetric or asymmetric. Carney et al. had adopted a cutoff point of 1 cm in size to diagnose pheochromocytoma, but even smaller nodules can be regarded as tumors in the setting of MEN2.[178] This size was chosen because it was the lower limit in size range for pheochromocytoma reported in the first series

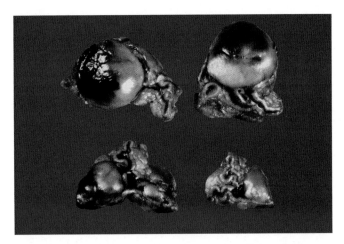

Fig. 16.61 Multifocal early pheochromocytomas in multiple endocrine neoplasia 2a (Sipple syndrome). The adrenal glands had a similar gross appearance. Transverse sections of the left adrenal gland show multiple nodules expanding the medullary compartment, with the largest nodule 1.5 cm in diameter.

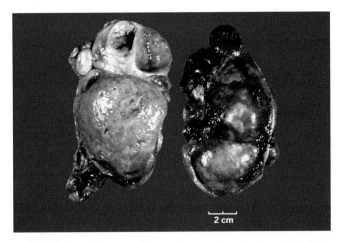

Fig. 16.62 Bilateral pheochromocytoma in multiple endocrine neoplasia 2a. The tumors weighed 168 and 220 g. One gland is depicted here; the outer surface is on the *right,* and the cut surface is on the *left.*

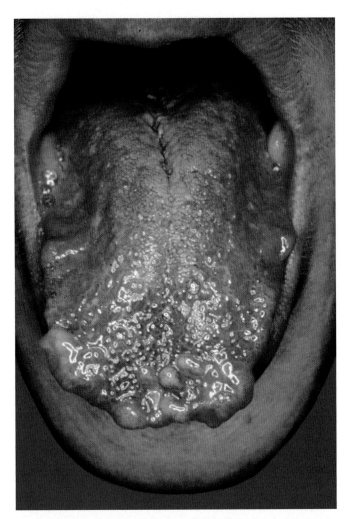

Fig. 16.63 Patient with multiple endocrine neoplasia 2b. The tongue is studded with neuromatous nodules, particularly along the lateral borders and the tip. (From Lack EE. Tumors of the Adrenal Glands and Extraadrenal Paraganglia. Atlas of Tumor Pathology, Series 4. Washington, DC: Armed Forces Institute of Pathology; 2007:245.)

fascicle from the Armed Forces Institute of Pathology dealing with tumors of the adrenal gland.[181] A recent study showed identical molecular changes in these lesions and pheochromocytoma from patients with MEN2 and concluded that these are not hyperplastic but instead neoplastic (i.e., a small pheochromocytoma).[182] Histologically, the lesions consist of expansile nodular growth of the medulla with distortion of the adjacent cortex or adjacent normal-appearing medulla. There may be numerous extensively vacuolated cells, as well as intracytoplasmic hyaline globules, some of which appear to be present in the extracellular space. Mitotic figures may be present but usually are not numerous, and some nuclear pleomorphism may be seen. In a study of MEN2 and pheochromocytoma, DNA content was found to be diploid or euploid in normal and hyperplastic glands, whereas 87% of clinically benign pheochromocytoma and all malignant pheochromocytoma had nondiploid or aneuploid DNA histograms.[180]

The phenotypic expression of MEN2b is very distinctive. Medullary thyroid carcinoma in this syndrome is usually aggressive, and recurrence and metastasis are its most pernicious components.[4,272]

Pheochromocytoma is often preceded by what used to be called AMH.[176,177]

In MEN2b, there is a low incidence of clinical and biochemical hyperfunction of the parathyroid glands, in contrast with that in MEN2a.[4,272] Characteristic mucosal neuromatous proliferation involves the lips, tongue (Fig. 16.63), oral mucosa, and conjunctivae; ganglioneuromatosis may involve the upper aerodigestive and lower gastrointestinal tracts. This may lead to a variety of intestinal manifestations, including motility disorders and megacolon mimicking Hirschsprung disease.[4,272] Other findings include ocular abnormalities such as thickened corneal nerves, conjunctival and eyelid neuromatous lesions, and, rarely, failing vision. Various neuromuscular abnormalities have been described, such as marfanoid habitus, elongated facies, dolichocephaly, laxity of joints, lordosis, kyphosis, pes cavus, and coxa valga. The gastrointestinal manifestations in MEN2b are important to recognize because they may form a prominent component of the syndrome, often antedating the endocrine neoplasms.[294]

Composite Pheochromocytoma

The term *composite pheochromocytoma* refers to a pheochromocytoma in which a component resembles neuroblastoma,

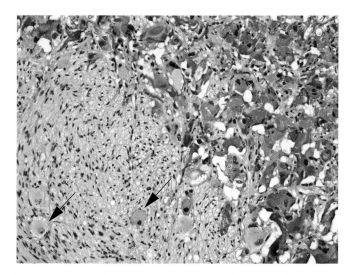

Fig. 16.64 Composite pheochromocytoma-ganglioneuroma. Mature ganglion cells within the ganglioneuroma component (*left*), marked by *arrows*.

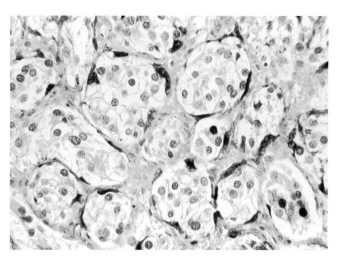

Fig. 16.65 Pheochromocytoma. Sustentacular cells are demonstrated by immunostaining for S100 protein, which highlights nuclei and slender cytoplasmic extensions. These cells are located at the periphery of nests and cords of pheochromocytoma cells.

ganglioneuroblastoma, ganglioneuroma (Fig. 16.64), or malignant peripheral nerve sheath tumor (malignant schwannoma).[4,71] A few have secreted vasoactive intestinal peptide (VIP), causing the watery diarrhea syndrome. The capacity for synthesis and secretion of VIP has been associated with a neuronal or ganglionic phenotype, but this is not always apparent. Neoplastic chromaffin cells in vitro may exhibit intense neuritic outgrowth of cell processes, indicative of one of several neuronal characteristics. The existence of composite pheochromocytoma with neural and endocrine features in vivo is ample testimony to the close morphologic and functional kinship of the nervous system and the endocrine system.[4] An example of composite pheochromocytoma-ganglioneuroma of the adrenal gland has been reported in a patient with MEN2a.[295]

Pseudopheochromocytoma

The term *pseudopheochromocytoma* refers to the unusual circumstance in which a patient has signs or symptoms of a pheochromocytoma, but no neoplasm is found on surgical exploration. Reported examples include AMH, adrenal myelolipoma, renal cyst, coarctation of the abdominal aorta, and astrocytoma.[4,272] Rarely, patients may develop signs and symptoms suggesting pheochromocytoma after surreptitious administration of epinephrine or other agents that produce provocative clinical manifestations.[4] Rarely adrenal cortical tumor has been reported mimicking pheochromocytoma.[236]

Immunohistochemistry and Other Features

The catecholamine-synthesizing enzymes tyrosine hydroxylase, dopamine β-hydroxylase, and phenylethanolamine N-methyltransferase have been identified in pheochromocytoma and correlate with the functional capacity of this tumor to produce norepinephrine and epinephrine.[4] The ratio of epinephrine to norepinephrine in the normal adrenal medulla is approximately 4:1, whereas norepinephrine predominates in pheochromocytoma.[4] The immunohistochemical profile of pheochromocytoma is quite broad; it typically expresses neuron-specific enolase and other neuroendocrine markers such as chromogranin A, synaptophysin, and CD56.[286] Pheochromocytoma also can express a broad array of other regulatory peptides and hormones, including enkephalins, somatostatin, VIP, substance P, ACTH, and calcitonin.[296] Rare

cases are associated with a paraneoplastic syndrome caused by the secretion of one of the neuropeptides, such as VIP, with watery diarrhea syndrome and ACTH with Cushing syndrome.[4] Sustentacular cells are the supporting cells in pheochromocytoma, appearing as S100 protein immunoreactive cells at the periphery of cords and clusters of neoplastic chromaffin cells (Fig. 16.65). Cytokeratin reactivity has been reported in an oncocytic pheochromocytoma.[297] However, another report fails to support keratin reactivity in more traditional pheochromocytoma, but immunopositive staining for keratin (CAM5.2 and AE1/3) was noted in a few extraadrenal paragangliomas.[298]

The ultrastructural hallmark of pheochromocytoma is the presence of dense-core neurosecretory-type granules, which have variable distribution and density within neoplastic cells.[299] Sparse numbers of these granules in some cells may help explain a low to equivocal intensity of immunostaining for neuroendocrine markers such as chromogranin A in some cases. Tannenbaum found that granule morphology correlated with catecholamine content as determined biochemically.[300] Two distinct types of granules were recognized. Those associated with norepinephrine storage had a distinctly prominent, eccentric halo or electron lucent space adjacent to the dense core; and those associated with epinephrine storage were more uniform (Fig. 16.66). Given the wide array of neuropeptides and hormones that may be detected in pheochromocytoma, the distinction based solely on granule morphology is no longer tenable.[4,272] Some granules, in fact, may be quite pleomorphic, and some could conceivably contain more than one peptide.

Fine-needle aspiration of pheochromocytoma may create problems in cytologic interpretation, and a malignant diagnosis rendered solely on the basis of cytologic and nuclear atypia may be erroneous.[4] Occasional complications also have been reported, including catecholamine crisis with a marked alteration in blood pressure and sometimes with uncontrollable intraabdominal hemorrhage.[4] In smear and imprint preparations of pheochromocytoma, nuclei may appear suspended in a syncytium of ill-defined cytoplasm, and considerable variations in nuclear size and shape may be seen (Fig. 16.67). Other cytologic features include intranuclear pseudoinclusions and enlarged hyperchromatic nuclei, sometimes stripped of cell cytoplasm.[4]

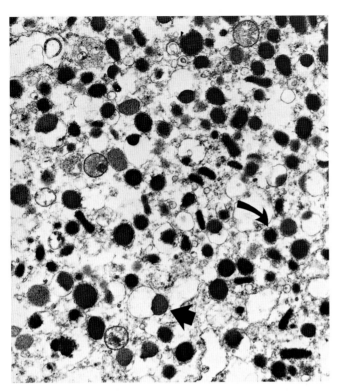

Fig. 16.66 Pheochromocytoma. Electron micrograph shows numerous dense-core neurosecretory granules; some have an investing membrane with a uniform thin halo (*curved arrow*), whereas others have an eccentric dense core with a wide asymmetric halo (*straight arrow*). Other neurosecretory granules are pleomorphic. (×15,000.)

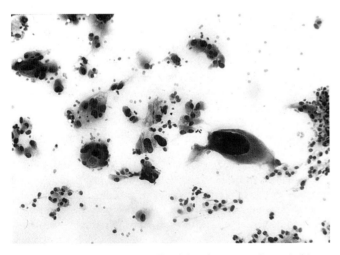

Fig. 16.67 Pheochromocytoma. Touch imprint smear of resected tumor shows marked variation in nuclear size, which might lead to a presumptive diagnosis of malignancy (Diff-Quik stain).

Malignant Pheochromocytoma

The incidence of clinically malignant pheochromocytoma is relatively low, and it is important to consider these separately from intraabdominal extraadrenal paragangliomas, which tend to have a significantly higher incidence of malignant behavior.[4] Early reviews cite a frequency of malignant behavior in pheochromocytoma of 2.4% to 2.8% in adults, whereas in children 2.4% were malignant.[301-303] A study from 2006 reports a relatively high incidence (47%) of malignancy in 30 children with

pheochromocytoma and extraadrenal paraganglioma.[304] In this study, however, 18 of the children had extraadrenal paraganglioma and only 12 had pheochromocytoma (defined as tumors arising from the adrenal medulla), which may account for the higher incidence. Overall, recent studies show an incidence of malignancy ranging from 7% to 14%.[4] It is notoriously difficult on gross and histologic evaluation to predict which tumors will prove to be malignant. The histology of benign and malignant pheochromocytoma overlaps to such an extent that the most important criterion acceptable for malignancy is the presence of metastases to sites where nonneoplastic chromaffin tissue is not normally found.[305] However, some histologic features have been noted to be more frequently associated with malignant behavior.[306] In the study by Thompson, the following features were more frequent in malignant pheochromocytoma: loss of the small alveolar or nesting pattern, to be replaced by larger cell nests lacking the well-formed fibrovascular supporting network; a diffuse growth pattern; tumor cell spindling; confluent tumor necrosis; increased mitotic rate (>3 per 10 hpf); and the presence of atypical mitotic figures.[307] Based on these findings, a scoring system (pheochromocytoma of the adrenal gland scaled score [PASS]) for pheochromocytoma was proposed to separate benign from malignant tumors. Selected features were weighed to come up with a single score, with a total score of 4 or more suggesting malignancy. Another scoring system that was proposed for both pheochromocytomas and extraadrenal paragangliomas is the grading system for adrenal pheochromocytoma and paraganglioma (GAPP).[308] There is no universal agreement on the applicability and reproducibility of PASS, and probably the same may apply to the GAPP system.[274]

In some studies, DNA quantification has suggested that ploidy may be an independent prognostic factor, because there were fewer deaths of patients with diploid pheochromocytoma.[309,310] Aneuploid histograms have been reported, however, in pheochromocytomas that are clinically benign or cured by surgery. A low proportion (or absence) of S100 protein immunoreactive cells has been correlated with malignant behavior of paragangliomas, but this may not be a reliable discriminator in the evaluation of individual cases.[311-313] Other markers recently investigated as possible predictors of high risk for malignant/recurrent pheochromocytoma include Ki-67 labeling greater than 4% and absence of S100 positive sustentacular cells.[314] Cell cycle and apoptosis markers, including p53, Bcl-2, mdm-2, cyclin D1, p21, and p27, seem to play no significant role in predicting malignant behavior.[315]

Surgical resection has been the mainstay of treatment for pheochromocytoma. Laparoscopic adrenalectomy may be a less invasive procedure for patients, but, for suspected malignant pheochromocytoma, conversion to open surgery may be indicated. A case has been reported of local spillage of tumor during laparoscopic manipulation resulting in iatrogenic pheochromocytomatosis.[316]

Peripheral Neuroblastic Tumors: Neuroblastoma, Ganglioneuroblastoma, and Ganglioneuroma

Peripheral neuroblastic tumors are defined as embryonal tumors of the sympathetic nervous system derived from the neural crest and arise in anatomic sites paralleling the distribution of the sympathoadrenal neuroendocrine system. Peripheral neuroblastic tumors include a spectrum of tumors ranging from neuroblastoma and ganglioneuroblastoma to fully mature ganglioneuroma. The

TABLE 16.6	Peripheral Neuroblastic Tumor Classification Recommended by the International Neuroblastoma Pathology Committee	
Category		**Subtype**
Neuroblastoma (schwannian stroma-poor)		• Undifferentiated • Poorly differentiated • Differentiating
Ganglioneuroblastoma, intermixed (schwannian stroma-rich) Ganglioneuroblastoma, nodular[a] Ganglioneuroma (schwannian stroma-dominant)		• Maturing • Mature

[a]Ganglioneuromatous component may be stroma-rich or stroma-dominant, and nodule(s) may be composed of undifferentiated, poorly differentiated, or differentiating neuroblastoma.
Modified from Shimada H, Ambros IM, Dehner LP, Hata J, Joshi VV, Roald B. Terminology and morphologic criteria of neuroblastic tumors: recommendations by the International Neuroblastoma Pathology Committee. Cancer. 1999;86:349–363.

current terminology for peripheral neuroblastic tumors is shown in Table 16.6, which is adopted by the International Neuroblastoma Pathology Committee and based on a modification of the earlier Shimada age-linked classification.[317-320] This classification defines the various categories of peripheral neuroblastic tumors. Subtypes of neuroblastoma are undifferentiated, poorly differentiated, and differentiating. Subtypes of ganglioneuroblastoma are intermixed and nodular. The amount of spindle cell schwannian stroma delineates neuroblastomas from ganglioneuroblastomas and ganglioneuromas because in neuroblastomas the amount of schwannian stroma is less than 50% of the total surface area of the tumor in representative histologic sections.

In Situ Neuroblastoma

The concept of in situ neuroblastoma was introduced in 1963 and refers to a small adrenal tumor similar histologically to classic childhood neuroblastoma but without gross or microscopic evidence of tumor elsewhere in the body.[321] In situ neuroblastoma has been detected in about 1 in 200 autopsies on infants up to 3 months of age. The lesions consist of poorly differentiated neuroblasts. Apoptotic figures and microcysts may be present, but mitoses are infrequent. In situ neuroblastoma is much more frequent than clinical neuroblastoma, and if truly neoplastic then the clear majority must be assumed to undergo spontaneous regression or maturation. It should be noted that neuroblastic foci are an integral part of normal development of the adrenal gland and may linger until early infancy, and their distinction from in situ neuroblastoma may be problematic.

Peripheral Neuroblastic Tumors

Neuroblastoma ranks fourth in frequency of malignant tumors in patients younger than 15 years of age, exceeded only by leukemia, brain tumors, and malignant lymphoma.[322] The incidence of neuroblastoma and ganglioneuroblastoma is estimated at 9.1 per million. Age is a strong factor bearing on incidence, with neuroblastoma predominating in children younger than 5 years of age and making up most tumors arising during infancy.[322] A

slightly increased incidence of neuroblastoma is seen in males (9.8 per million) in contrast with females (9.2 per million). In a series of 118 patients from Boston Children's Hospital, 88% were 5 years of age or younger at diagnosis, with a median age of 21 months.[323] Neuroblastomas and ganglioneuroblastomas are rare in the second decade of life and exceedingly rare in adults.[324] When these tumors do arise in adolescents or adults, they appear to have different biologic characteristics from their pediatric counterparts and have a poor prognosis regardless of stage.[324] Occasionally, neuroblastoma appears in several members of a family, and some data suggest an autosomal dominant pattern of inheritance. However, obvious difficulties exist in determining the incidence and penetrance of an inherited susceptibility because of the capacity for regression or spontaneous maturation, as well as early death and long-term treatment complications that prevent reproduction and the evaluation of multiple pedigrees.[325,326] Neuroblastomas and ganglioneuroblastomas may have some unusual associations: watery diarrhea syndrome resulting from VIP production, Cushing syndrome, opsoclonus/myoclonus, and alopecia. Horner syndrome and heterochromia iridis have been reported because of involvement of cervical sympathetic ganglia.[4,327] Occasional tumors are associated with Beckwith-Wiedemann syndrome, neurofibromatosis types 1 and 2, Hirschsprung disease, central hypoventilation syndrome (Ondine's curse) secondary to *PHOX2B* mutation, and other syndromes and congenital malformations.

The first screening for neuroblastoma began in Japan in 1974, and other studies have followed.[4,328,329] Screening in Japan has resulted in an increased annual detection rate for these tumors (93 per million) in contrast with the baseline rate of 13.3 per million. Children are screened at 6 months of age with a qualitative vanillylmandelic acid spot test. The prognosis for children with neuroblastoma detected by screening is favorable because of low clinical stage and early age at diagnosis, both important independent prognostic factors.[4,327] Most infants are considered to be in a low-risk subgroup with potential for spontaneous regression, and although screening programs do increase the number of newly diagnosed cases, they do not appear to reduce population-based mortality in infants, nor do they result in a decreased incidence of advanced-stage disease in older children.[330-333] Screening infants could potentially result in overdiagnosis and lead to unnecessary diagnostic and therapeutic procedures with possible physical and psychological harm.

The anatomic location of peripheral neuroblastic tumors parallels that of the sympathoadrenal neuroendocrine system with tumors arising in any location from the neck to the pelvis. The anatomic distribution of primary tumors in the series of 118 patients from Boston Children's Hospital was as follows: intraabdominal (67.8%), with most arising in the adrenal glands (38.1%) and 29.7% being nonadrenal; intrathoracic (20.3%); cervical (3.4%); and pelvic (3.4%); in 5.1%, the precise anatomic origin was undetermined.[323] Patients with neuroblastoma and ganglioneuroblastoma may have spinal cord compression caused by an extradural intraspinal ("dumbbell") configuration of the tumor; similar spinal cord compression may occasionally be seen with ganglioneuroma.[4,327]

Neuroblastoma and ganglioneuroblastoma usually present as a solitary spherical or ovoid mass, and tumors can be quite large, measuring up to 10 cm or more.[4,327] On cross-section, they are variable in appearance and consistency depending on the amount of immature neuroblastic component present. Neuroblastomas of the undifferentiated or poorly differentiated subtypes may be soft and friable with areas of hemorrhage (Fig. 16.68). The tumors may have coarse lobulations. Yellow flecks of calcification or pale foci of

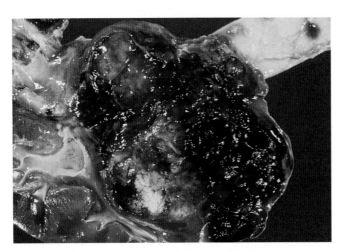

Fig. 16.68 At autopsy, neuroblastoma virtually replaces the entire adrenal gland and compresses the adjacent kidney. The cut surface of the tumor has coarse lobulations and is hemorrhagic.

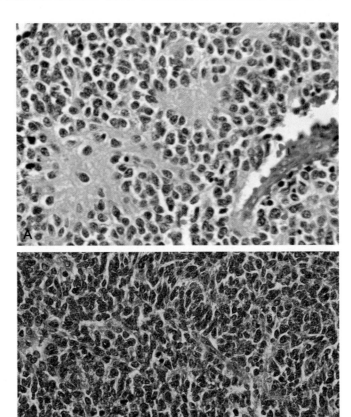

Fig. 16.69 Neuroblastoma. (A) Stroma-poor in the Shimada classification. The cells are closely packed, with indistinct cellular borders. Note the Homer Wright rosettes. (B) Undifferentiated neuroblastoma. Sheets of small blue cells with elongated nuclei and indistinct cellular borders. Nuclear chromatin is stippled (salt and pepper). Neuropil is absent.

necrosis may be present. With increasing differentiation, the cut surface may be tan-yellow and less friable.

Undifferentiated and poorly differentiated neuroblastoma is the prototypical "small, blue cell tumor" of childhood, and often has an ill-defined lobular or nesting growth pattern with delicate incomplete fibrovascular septa.[334] Some tumors have a more diffuse or solid pattern. Typical Homer Wright rosettes can be found in some tumors (Fig. 16.69A), with the center consisting of a pale-staining tangled skein of neuritic cell processes.[335] This neurofibrillary matrix has been likened to neuropil of the central nervous system and may form the center of rosettes or form broad mats with irregular contour. Rarely, rosettes may have a rhythmic or palisaded configuration. In undifferentiated neuroblastoma (Fig. 16.69B), the neurofibrillary matrix is absent or equivocally present, and the tumor may require ancillary techniques (e.g., immunohistochemistry or electron microscopy) to establish a correct diagnosis. In differentiating neuroblastoma, the tumor cells are transitioning to ganglion cells and show synchronous enlargement of nucleus and cytoplasm. The diameter of the cell should be two times the diameter of the nucleus to qualify as a differentiating neuroblast, and at least 5% of the cells should have this appearance for a tumor to be designated as a differentiating neuroblastoma. Nucleoli are inconspicuous, and chromatin may be finely dispersed with a "salt-and-pepper" pattern (Fig. 16.70).

Morphologic evidence of ganglion cell differentiation includes nuclear enlargement, increased amount of eosinophilic cytoplasm, distinct cell borders, prominent nucleolus, and peripheral granular material within the cytoplasm that represents Nissl substance (Fig. 16.71). The degree of ganglion cell differentiation varies from tumor to tumor and within different areas of the same tumor. Some peripheral neuroblastic tumors have unusual histopathologic features such as a sclerosing pattern, spindle-shaped neuroblasts, and a dense lymphoplasmacytic component, and the latter may be related to tumor regression in some cases. Anaplastic neuroblastoma has marked cellular and nuclear pleomorphism, but this finding has no apparent impact on survival after controlling for disease stage.[336,337] Cystic neuroblastoma is uncommon and may simulate an adrenal cyst or hematoma.[338] Pigmented ganglioneuroblastoma is very rare with cytoplasmic pigment thought to be neuromelanin.[339]

Ganglioneuroblastoma is classified as a schwannian stroma-rich tumor with schwannian matrix accounting for at least 50% of the surface area in representative histologic sections. There may be

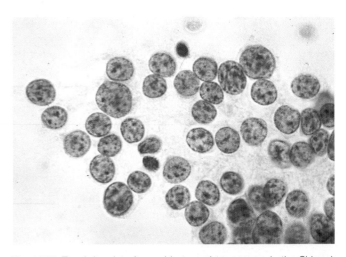

Fig. 16.70 Touch imprint of neuroblastoma (stroma-poor in the Shimada classification). Nuclei have dispersed chromatin (salt-and-pepper nuclei), and are separated by pale pink cytoplasm with indistinct borders.

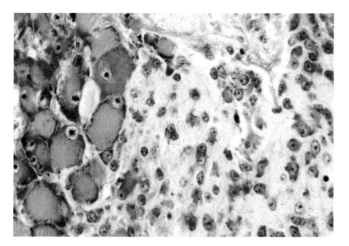

Fig. 16.71 Ganglioneuroblastoma with well-developed ganglion cells that have Nissl substance in peripheral cytoplasm and prominent nucleoli (toluidine blue).

clusters of neuroblasts accompanied by neurofibrillary matrix and showing cytodifferentiation into recognizable ganglion cells or their immediate precursors. Two types of ganglioneuroblastoma are recognized: ganglioneuroblastoma intermixed and ganglioneuroblastoma nodular.[320,340,341] Ganglioneuroblastoma intermixed has microscopic nests of neuroblasts with differentiating neuroblasts or immature ganglion cells predominating. Poorly differentiated neuroblasts are less conspicuous or absent. On gross

Fig. 16.72 (A) Stroma-rich neuroblastoma according to the Shimada age-linked classification of neuroblastoma proposed in 1984. Survival data are indicated for the favorable and unfavorable groups. (B) Stroma-poor neuroblastoma according to the Shimada age-linked classification. Favorable and unfavorable prognosis groups are indicated along with survival data. *MKI*, Mitosis-karyorrhexis index; *y/o*, years old. (From Lack EE, ed. Pathology of adrenal and extraadrenal paraganglia. In: Major Problems in Pathology. Vol 29. Philadelphia: Saunders; 1994:315–370.) Newer revised classification of neuroblastic tumors is shown in Tables 16.6 and 16.7.

examination, the cut surface of ganglioneuroblastoma intermixed is yellow to tan, rubbery, and less friable. In ganglioneuroblastoma nodular, there are one or more *grossly visible* neuroblastic nodules usually sharply demarcated and often hemorrhagic in a tumor that elsewhere conforms to ganglioneuroblastoma intermixed or ganglioneuroma. In some examples of ganglioneuroblastoma nodular, the neuroblastic nodule(s) may be poorly delimited or overwhelm the schwannian-rich or schwannian-dominant component with only a narrow rim of ganglioneuroblastoma intermixed or ganglioneuroma identified. Another variation of ganglioneuroblastoma nodular occurs when a small neuroblastic nodule may be overlooked in a ganglioneuroblastoma intermixed or ganglioneuroma, but there is metastatic neuroblastoma in another site.

Original Age-Linked Classification of Neuroblastoma

In 1984, Shimada et al. introduced an age-linked classification of neuroblastoma, based on the patient's age at diagnosis, degree of maturation or percentage of differentiating elements, and the mitosis-karyorrhexis index (MKI).[317,342] The stroma-rich category showed extensive growth of schwannian and other supporting elements, with three groups (Fig. 16.72A): the well-differentiated and intermixed groups had a favorable prognosis (92% to 100% survival), and the nodular group had a poor prognosis (18% survival). The stroma-poor category had two groups (Fig. 16.72B): the favorable group had a survival of 84%, and the unfavorable group had a survival of 4.5%.

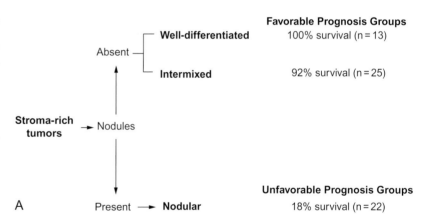

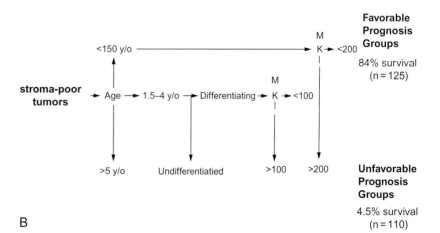

International Neuroblastoma Pathology Classification

The morphologic classification of peripheral neuroblastic tumors incorporating age at diagnosis as just noted was initially proposed in 1984, established a few years later, and revised in 2003; this classification was recently summarized in an updated WHO classification on tumors of endocrine organs.[320] Basically, tumors are classified as favorable histology or unfavorable histology (Table 16.7) based on the following: (1) the amount of spindle cell schwannian stroma (stroma-poor, stroma-rich, and stroma-dominant); (2) the degree of neuroblastic differentiation (undifferentiated, poorly differentiated, and differentiating); (3) the MKI score (low, intermediate, or high); and (4) the age of the patient at diagnosis.[320] The MKI is defined as the number of mitotic figures and karyorrhectic cells per 5000 neuroblastic cells, and one of three scores is reported: (1) low: less than 2% (<100/5000); (2) intermediate: 2% to 4% (100 to 200/5000); and high: greater than 4% (>200/5000). Hyperchromatic nuclei that are not fragmented are not included in the MKI. The microscopic fields selected for the MKI should be representative of the tumor with avoidance of necrotic zones. A Ki-67 index has recently been proposed as a surrogate marker for the MKI.[343]

As shown in Table 16.7, favorable histology tumors include poorly differentiated or differentiating neuroblastoma (schwannian stroma-poor) with low or intermediate MKI until 1.5 years (18 months) of age; differentiating neuroblastoma (schwannian stroma-poor) with a low MKI 1.5 to 5 years (18 to 60 months) of age; and ganglioneuroblastoma intermixed (schwannian stroma-rich) and ganglioneuroma (schwannian stroma-dominant) of either subtype, mature or maturing at any age. Unfavorable histology tumors include undifferentiated neuroblastoma (schwannian stroma-poor) at any age and neuroblastoma of any subtype with a high MKI at any age; poorly differentiated neuroblastoma (schwannian stroma-poor) and differentiating neuroblastoma (schwannian stroma-poor) with an intermediate MKI at 1.5 to 5 years (18 to 60 months) of age; and neuroblastoma (schwannian stroma-poor) of any subtype over 5 years of age. With ganglioneuroblastoma nodular, placement into the favorable or unfavorable histology categories is dependent on the histology or character of the neuroblastic (schwannian stroma-poor) component described previously. For this distinction, the same age-dependent evaluation criteria for grade (or subtype) of neuroblastic differentiation and MKI are applied to the neuroblastomatous components as are used in the neuroblastoma (schwannian stroma-poor) category.[320]

TABLE 16.7	Histopathologic Age-Linked Prognostic Indicators According to the International Neuroblastoma Pathology Classification
Favorable Histology	**Unfavorable Histology**
Less Than 1.5 Years (18 Months)	
• Neuroblastoma (schwannian stroma-poor) poorly differentiated with low/intermediate MKI • Neuroblastoma (schwannian stroma-poor), differentiating with low/intermediate MKI	
1.5–5 Years (18-60 Months)	
• Neuroblastoma (schwannian stroma-poor), differentiating with low MKI	• Neuroblastoma (schwannian stroma-poor), poorly differentiated • Neuroblastoma (schwannian stroma-poor), differentiating with intermediate MKI
More Than 5 Years (60 Months)	
	• Neuroblastoma (schwannian stroma-poor), of any subtype
Any Age	
• Ganglioneuroblastoma, intermixed (schwannian stroma-rich) • Ganglioneuroma (schwannian stroma-dominant), maturing or mature	• Neuroblastoma, (schwannian stroma-poor), undifferentiated • Neuroblastoma, (schwannian stroma-poor), any subtype with high MKI

Ganglioneuroblastoma, nodular (composite, schwannian stroma-rich/dominant and schwannian stroma-poor) is classified in either the favorable or unfavorable histology group depending on the characteristics of its neuroblastomatous nodules. For this distinction, the same age-dependent evaluation criteria for grade of neuroblastic differentiation and MKI are applied to the neuroblastomatous components as are used in the neuroblastoma (schwannian stroma-poor) category.

Modified from Shimada H, DeLellis RA, Tissier F. Neuroblastic tumors of the adrenal gland. In: Lloyd RV, Osamura RY, Klöppel G, Rosai J, World Health Organization, International Agency for Research on Cancer, eds. WHO Classification of Tumours of Endocrine Organs. Lyon, France: International Agency for Research on Cancer (IARC); 2017:196–203.

Ancillary Techniques

Neuroblastomas are characteristically immunoreactive for a variety of neural markers such as chromogranin, synaptophysin, PGP 9.5, CD 57, neurofilament protein, and PHOX2B.[320,344] Immunostaining for S100 protein highlights slender dendritic cells near fibrovascular septa, which represent Schwann cells. Large numbers of S100 protein immunoreactive cells in undifferentiated neuroblastoma have been associated with a more favorable prognosis.[345] Conversely, large numbers of ferritin-positive cells have been associated with a poor prognosis.[4,327] Undifferentiated neuroblastomas are immunoreactive for PHOX2B and PGP 9.5 and are sometimes positive for tyrosine hydroxylase; these tumors are usually negative for other neural markers.[346] Ultrastructural characteristics of neuroblastoma and ganglioneuroblastoma include neuritic extensions with neurofilaments, neurotubules, and dense-core neurosecretory granules, which are usually few (Fig. 16.73).[334]

Molecular Genetics in Neuroblastomas

A variety of molecular and genetic changes are present in neuroblastomas involving mutations, as well as gains and losses of whole chromosomes and segmental chromosome alterations.[320,341,347-350] MYCN amplification occurs in about 20% of neuroblastomas and produces an excess of Myc-N protein that prevents cellular differentiation and promotes cellular proliferation and apoptosis; it is an ab initio finding in a subset of aggressive tumors.[320,341,349,351] Thus tumors with MYCN amplification are usually undifferentiated or poorly differentiated subtypes of neuroblastoma with increased mitotic rate and karyorrhectic cells—that is, high MKI. MYCN amplification is an important oncogenic driver, and the presence of more than 10 copies is associated with a poor prognosis.

Another important oncogenic driver is an activating mutation of the *ALK* gene, which is found in 8% to 10% of neuroblastomas, or amplification of a wild-type *ALK* gene in another 2% to 4% of

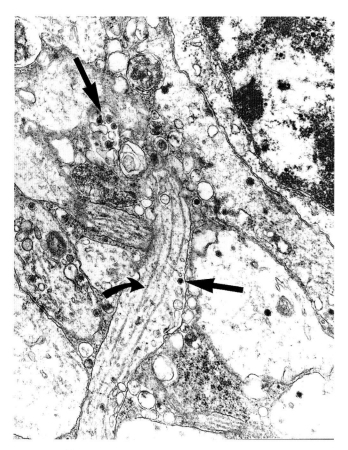

Fig. 16.73 Neuroblastoma. Neuritic processes contain microtubules (*curved arrow*) and sparse numbers of dense-core neurosecretory granules (*straight arrows*) (×27,000).

neuroblastomas.[352-355] Mutations in genes involved in chromatin remodeling are found in neuroblastomas including *ATRX, ARID1A, ARID1B,* and *DAXX*.[356-358] *ATRX* in particular is mutated in a high

proportion of metastatic neuroblastomas, mainly in children and adolescents with a chronic but progressive clinical course. *ARID1A* and *ARID1B* are mutated in about 2% to 3% of neuroblastomas and are found in a subset of highest-risk neuroblastomas.[357] Other mutations have recently been reported in clinically aggressive neuroblastomas, including *CHD9, TERT, PTK2, NAV1, NAV3,* and *FZD1*.[350,359] Various chromosomal abnormalities are common in neuroblastomas. An unbalanced gain of 17q is found in more than one-half of neuroblastomas, often as part of an unbalanced translocation between chromosomes 1 and 17, and is associated with more aggressive neuroblastomas.[360] Deletion of 1p indicates a poor prognosis and is observed in most tumors with MYCN amplification.[361] DNA ploidy analysis has shown that near-diploid tumors have a poor prognosis, whereas near-triploid ones tend to manifest at a lower stage and thus have a more favorable prognosis.[362-364] There are other molecular and genetic abnormalities in peripheral neuroblastic tumors that cannot be covered in the limited space herein.

Staging of Neuroblastoma and Ganglioneuroblastoma

The staging classification proposed by Evans et al. has been popular for decades.[365,366] In 1992, an interim working staging system was also proposed, with incidence and survival data based on stage of tumor at diagnosis (Table 16.8).[367] Of patients with neuroblastoma and ganglioneuroblastoma, 60% to 70% have metastases at the time of presentation (stages IV and IV-S) and 30% to 40% have localized disease (stages I, II, and III).[4] Children with a tumor primary in the cervical, intrathoracic, or pelvic areas have a more favorable prognosis stage than do patients with intraabdominal primaries, but a disproportionate number may have a low-stage tumor or be younger than 2 years of age and frequently younger than 1 year of age at diagnosis.[4] Revisions of the International Neuroblastoma Staging System have been reported (Table 16.9) and vary slightly from those in Table 16.8.[368] More recent is the International Neuroblastoma Risk Group Staging System, which incorporates overall staging based on the extent of disease

TABLE 16.8	Staging System Proposed by the International Staging System Working Party with Incidence and Survival According to Stage of Tumor and Diagnosis		
	Staging Criteria	Incidence (%)	Survival at 5 years (%)
Stage I	Localized tumor confined to the area of origin, complete gross excision, with or without microscopic residual disease; identifiable ipsilateral and contralateral lymph nodes negative microscopically	5	≥90
Stage IIa	Unilateral tumor with incomplete gross excision; identifiable ipsilateral and contralateral lymph nodes negative microscopically	10	70-80
Stage IIb	Unilateral tumor with complete or incomplete gross excision; with positive ipsilateral regional lymph nodes; identifiable contralateral lymph nodes negative microscopically		
Stage III	Tumor infiltrating across the midline with or without regional lymph node involvement; or midline tumor with bilateral regional lymph node involvement	25	40-70 (depending on completeness of surgical resection)
Stage IV	Dissemination of the tumor to distant lymph nodes, bone, bone marrow, liver, and/or other organs (except as defined in stage IV-S)	60	>60 if age at diagnosis is younger than 1 year; 20 if age at diagnosis is older than 1 year and younger than 2 years; 10 if age at diagnosis is older than 2 years
Stage IV-S	Localized primary tumor as defined for stage I or II with dissemination limited to liver, skin, and/or bone marrow	5	>80

From Philip T. Overview of current treatment of neuroblastoma. Am J Pediatr Hematol Oncol. 1992;14:97–102.

TABLE 16.9 International Neuroblastoma Risk Group Staging System

Stage	Definition
L1	Localized tumor, not involving vital structures as defined by the list of image-defined risk factors and confined to one body compartment
L2	Locoregional tumor with the presence of one or more image-defined risk factors
M	Distant metastatic disease (except stage MS)
MS	Metastatic disease in children younger than 18 months of age with metastases confined to the skin, liver, and/or bone marrow (<10% of all nucleated cells)

Modified from Louis CU, Shohet JM. Neuroblastoma: molecular pathogenesis and therapy. Annu Rev Med. 2015;66:49–63.

and preoperative, radiographic, and image-defined risk factors used to assess resectability (Table 16.9).[369] The recently proposed International Neuroblastoma Risk Group Consensus Pretreatment Classification Schema protocol currently incorporates stage, age, histology, ploidy, MYCN status, and the presence or absence of 11q aberrations into risk stratification and treatment protocols.[348]

Stage IV-S Neuroblastoma and Patterns of Spread by Peripheral Neuroblastic Tumors

Stage IV-S (S = special) neuroblastoma refers to a distinctive group of patients with disseminated neuroblastoma involving liver, skin, or bone marrow without radiologic or other evidence of bone metastases and limited to age younger than 1 year (median, ~3 months).[4,327,367,368] These children usually have a small adrenal primary, but, in a minority of cases, no primary can be identified. Overall the prognosis is favorable, with survival rates of 80% or more, and many of the tumors undergo spontaneous regression. There is a small subset of children with stage IV-S neuroblastoma, usually in the first 6 weeks of life, who have marked abdominal distention because of massive liver involvement by the tumor. The outlook for these patients is less favorable, because massive hepatomegaly may cause secondary complications such as compromise in cardiorespiratory function.[370] Some investigators speculate that stage IV-S neuroblastoma is a mass of hyperplastic nodules of mutated cells that lack the genetic events for transformation into an overtly malignant tumor.[371]

A fascinating aspect of neuroblastoma and ganglioneuroblastoma is the occasional spontaneous regression or maturation into fully mature ganglioneuroma.[4,327,372] The concept of Collins law has been applied to children with neuroblastoma and gives a rough approximation of the doubling time of a tumor measured as a period of risk that is equal to the patient's age at diagnosis plus 9 months.[373] According to this concept, a child with neuroblastoma who has not been cured of the tumor will relapse within this time span; theoretically, older children must therefore be followed for a much longer time because of the expanded period of risk. Two syndromes of metastatic neuroblastoma can be found in the early literature, the Pepper syndrome with prominent hepatic metastases and the Hutchison syndrome with skull metastases manifesting at a somewhat later age.[374] The cases described by Pepper in 1901 probably correspond to stage IV-S neuroblastoma.[4,327] Because no correlation exists between the laterality of the adrenal tumor and the pattern of metastases, the concept of these syndromes is obsolete. Metastatic spread of neuroblastoma and ganglioneuroblastoma occurs by both hematogenous and lymphatic routes, with involvement of sites such as bone and lymph nodes. Cranial involvement by metastatic neuroblastoma is usually confined to calvarial bone, leptomeninges, and dura, with intrinsic involvement of brain parenchyma being rare.[4,327]

Ganglioneuroma

Ganglioneuroma consists of mature or mildly dysmorphic ganglion cells set in an abundant mixture of mature Schwann cells.[4,327] Most patients with ganglioneuroma are older than 10 years of age at diagnosis, and the tumor is usually located in the posterior mediastinum; it also may be seen in the retroperitoneum but is relatively uncommon in the adrenal gland.[4,327] Other, more unusual locations include cervical and parapharyngeal area, urinary bladder, prostate, pancreas, orbit, and appendix. Ganglioneuroma typically manifests as a circumscribed tumor that is firm, rubbery, and gray-white to tan-yellow (Fig. 16.74). Grossly, the cut surface of ganglioneuroma may have a trabecular or whorled appearance reminiscent of leiomyoma. Larger tumors may have degenerative features such as hemorrhage and cystic change. Histologically, considerable variation is often seen in the distribution and density of ganglion cells (Fig. 16.75); areas with a paucity or absence of ganglion cells may be mistaken for a neurofibroma or schwannoma. Ganglion cells may be exceedingly well differentiated with Nissl substance and a complete or partial collarette of satellite cells, and some ganglion cells may contain granular tan to brown pigment resembling lipofuscin or neuromelanin; red granules may be present possibly representing megamitochondria.

In the International Neuroblastoma Pathology Committee scheme, ganglioneuroma is in the category ganglioneuroma (schwannian stroma-dominant) *mature* subtype, and should not be confused with ganglioneuroma (schwannian stroma-dominant) *maturing* subtype, where, in the latter, dispersed individual differentiating neuroblasts and maturing ganglion cells are seen.

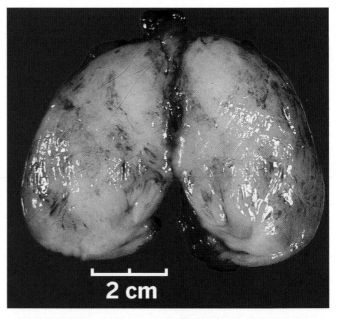

Fig. 16.74 Ganglioneuroma is homogeneous pale tan on cross-section. The tumor measured 7 × 5 × 4 cm.

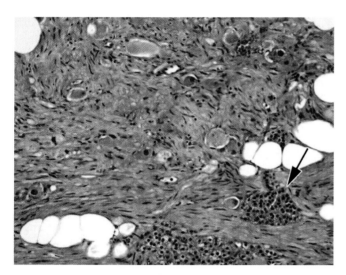

Fig. 16.75 Ganglioneuroma. A tumor with ganglion cells mingling with Schwann cells replacing much of the cortex. Small islands of residual adrenal cortex are noted (*arrow*).

Diagnosis of mature ganglioneuroma requires the absence of any neuroblastomatous component. Thus when making a diagnosis of mature ganglioneuroma, it is imperative that one examines the tumor thoroughly to be certain that no areas of immature neuroblastic tissue exist, even in small amounts.

Whether ganglioneuroma arises de novo or by maturation (differentiation) of a preexisting neuroblastoma or ganglioneuroblastoma remains controversial. Transformation of ganglioneuroma to malignant peripheral nerve sheath tumor (malignant schwannoma) has been rarely observed.[4,71] In some cases, malignant schwannoma has arisen de novo without any history of chemotherapy, radiation treatment, or von Recklinghausen disease, but other cases have developed after radiotherapy. A few examples have been reported of adrenal ganglioneuroma with hilus or Leydig cells containing typical crystalloids of Reinke; the tumor reported by Aguirre and Scully was associated with masculinization.[375,376]

Other Adrenal Tumors

Myelolipoma

Adrenal myelolipoma is a benign tumefactive lesion consisting of mature adipose tissue admixed with a variable amount of hematopoietic elements. This lesion occurs most frequently in the adrenal gland, although it also occurs in extraadrenal sites, including the retroperitoneum, stomach, liver, mediastinum, pleura, spleen, nasal cavity, and presacral region.[186,377-383] The pathogenesis is unknown, although some data suggest that it arises under hormonal influence by metaplasia of adrenal cortical or stromal cells.[186] Intraadrenal fat and hematopoietic tissue have been induced experimentally by injecting crude pituitary ACTH extract into adrenal glands, and myelolipomatous foci may be seen in patients with excess cortical activity, such as a hyperfunctioning ACA or adrenal cortical hyperplasia.[71,384] Others suggest that myelolipoma derives from emboli from the bone marrow or from embryonic rests of hematopoietic tissue.[186] A recent study suggests a clonal origin for myelolipoma, as supported by nonrandom X chromosome inactivation.[385]

The incidence of adrenal myelolipoma at autopsy is 0.01% to 0.2%, and it is most common in individuals older than 40 years of age, with a roughly equal gender predilection.[386] Most patients are asymptomatic, and most cases are discovered incidentally. When patients are symptomatic, it is usually because of the large size of the myelolipoma, resulting in abdominal or flank pain, dysuria, hematuria, or, rarely, catastrophic spontaneous retroperitoneal hemorrhage.[387] It may occur in patients with concurrent endocrinologic disorders such as Cushing disease, Cushing syndrome, Conn syndrome, Addison disease, and CAH.[71,388-390] A case of subclinical Cushing syndrome caused by adrenal myelolipoma has been reported.[391]

Grossly, myelolipoma forms a soft, well-circumscribed mass that is variegated yellow to red-brown (Fig. 16.76). It ranges in size from a few millimeters to 34 cm. Microscopically, hematopoietic tissue contains various combinations of the three cell lines, with an admixture of mature adipose tissue (Fig. 16.77). Bony trabeculae, hemorrhage, and fibrosis are occasionally seen. Myelolipoma is detected more frequently with the advent of CT and MRI. Fine-needle aspiration biopsy has proved useful in preoperative diagnosis. Treatment varies from radiographic surveillance for small

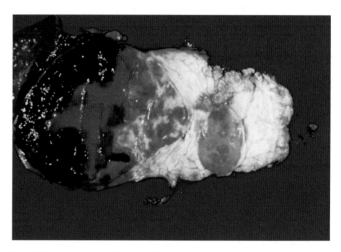

Fig. 16.76 Adrenal myelolipoma. The tumor is well circumscribed with a thin fibrous capsule. On cross-section, it is red-brown because of abundant hematopoietic elements with a focal area of hemorrhage. The lesion appears quite large and is enveloped by abundant adipose tissue.

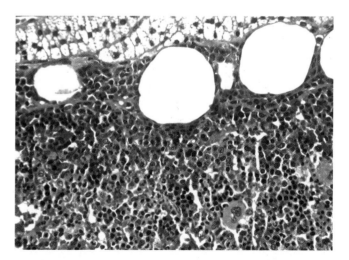

Fig. 16.77 Myelolipoma consists of fat mixed with hematopoietic elements, including megakaryocytes. Note the rim of compressed adrenal cortical tissue (*top*).

lesions in asymptomatic patients to surgical excision of large or symptomatic lesions.

Adenomatoid Tumor

Although rare, adenomatoid tumors have been described in extra-genital sites, including the adrenal gland.[392-397] Adenomatoid tumors of the adrenal gland are benign tumors of mesothelial origin, with the characteristic histomorphology of adenomatoid tumors more commonly seen in or near the genital tract. The tumor may have an infiltrative border and typically has a sievelike appearance. It is composed of epithelioid cells with uniform nuclei and intracytoplasmic vacuoles forming tubular or glandlike spaces (Fig. 16.78). Recently a cystic adrenal adenomatoid tumor was reported resembling a cystic lymphangioma.[398] Immunohistochemical evaluation shows strong immunoreactivity for cytokeratin and vimentin, weak reactivity for epithelial membrane antigen, and negative immunostaining for carcinoembryonic antigen, factor VIII–related antigen, and CD34. Strong staining for calretinin also is seen (Fig. 16.79). Electron microscopy reveals desmosomes,

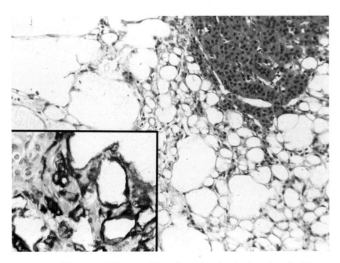

Fig. 16.78 Adenomatoid tumor. Note the uninvolved adrenal cortical tissue (*upper right*) intimately adjacent to the tumor cells, forming cystic, tubular, and glandlike spaces. The *inset* demonstrates strong staining of the tumor cells with antibodies to cytokeratin (AE1/AE3).

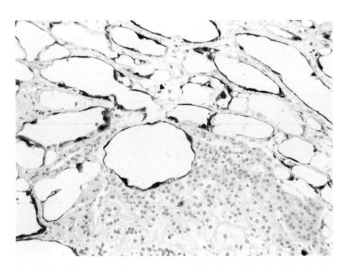

Fig. 16.79 Adenomatoid tumor. Immunohistochemical stain showing the tumor cells immunoreactive for calretinin.

tonofilaments, and long "bushy" cytoplasmic microvilli typical of mesothelial cells.

Malignant Lymphoma

Malignant lymphoma secondarily involving the adrenal gland usually occurs in the setting of widespread or advanced-stage tumor, with an incidence in fatal cases of 18% to 25%.[4,186] Bilateral adrenal involvement has been reported in 9% of cases of Hodgkin disease and 18% of non-Hodgkin malignant lymphoma.[186] Malignant lymphoma rarely manifests primarily in the adrenal gland without detectable extraadrenal involvement, although several cases have been reported.[399,400] Rarely, Addison disease may result from massive involvement of the adrenal glands by malignant lymphoma, and the adrenal cortical insufficiency may resolve after treatment with combination chemotherapy.[71,186,401] Adrenal cortical insufficiency also has been reported with a form of malignant lymphoma having prominent vascular involvement and intravascular lymphomatosis, previously referred to as *malignant angioendotheliomatosis.* Plasmacytoma manifesting primarily in the adrenal gland is extremely unusual and may represent an early stage of malignant lymphoma with plasmacytoid features.[186,402] A study suggesting a possible association between Epstein-Barr virus infection and the development of adrenal lymphoma has been reported.[403]

Mesenchymal Tumors

Primary vasoformative neoplasms of the adrenal glands are extremely unusual. Adrenal hemangioma may be found incidentally at autopsy, but several cases have been detected during life as a surgical lesion.[404] A case has also been reported in association with subclinical Cushing syndrome.[405] At times, a cortical adenoma may show hemorrhage with extensive degenerative change with vascular organization that may mimic hemangioma (Fig. 16.80). Visceral hemangioma also may occur in the setting of hereditary hemorrhagic telangiectasia (Rendu-Osler-Weber syndrome), but adrenal involvement is very rare.[186] Adrenal hemangioma is usually of the cavernous type, although capillary hemangioma has been reported. Adrenal angiosarcoma has been reported rarely and may have epithelioid features that include

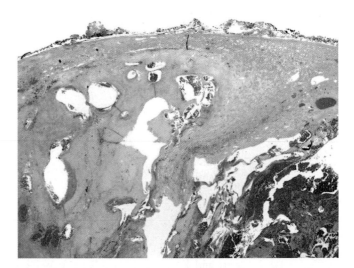

Fig. 16.80 Adrenal cortical adenoma with hemorrhage showing organization. This pattern may be mistaken for hemangioma. Note the residual cortical adenoma at the periphery.

the presence of epithelial-specific immunohistochemical markers such as cytokeratin.[406-408] Both leiomyoma and leiomyosarcoma occur, rarely, in the adrenal gland, with histologic features similar to smooth muscle neoplasms occurring in other sites.[71,409-411] A case of adrenal leiomyosarcoma has been reported in association with AIDS.[412] Adrenal lipoma and even liposarcoma have rarely been reported.[413]

Neurilemoma and neurofibroma arising in the adrenal gland are extremely unusual.[71,414,415] Malignant peripheral nerve sheath tumor (malignant schwannoma) has been reported and in one case was part of a composite pheochromocytoma.[416,417]

Malignant Melanoma

Primary malignant melanoma of the adrenal gland is extremely rare and highly malignant, usually occurring in middle-aged individuals.[71,418-420] Origin of a malignant melanoma within the adrenal gland is reasonable given the common embryogenesis of adrenal chromaffin cells and melanocytes from the neural crest. Melanin pigment is typically present in varying amounts, but the tumor may be amelanotic. There may be a nesting pattern or a biphasic growth pattern consisting of epithelioid and spindle cells. Rarely, a meningothelial-like growth pattern may be seen. Immunohistochemical studies are important in confirming the diagnosis. The neoplastic cells of an adrenal melanoma, like those of other melanomas, typically show strong reactivity with S100, HMB45, and tyrosinase. Immunostain for melan A (MART-1) is positive, but there also may be staining of an adrenal cortical neoplasm that might enter into the differential diagnosis of melanoma. It may be very difficult to exclude the possibility of primary mucocutaneous malignant melanoma that has metastasized to the adrenal gland.

Other Unusual Tumors and Tumor-like Lesions

Ovarian thecal metaplasia is an incidental microscopic lesion composed of bland spindle cells. It is typically wedge-shaped and attached to the adrenal capsule, and may contain small nests of cortical cells.[3,71] Foci measure up to 2 mm and may be multiple.[421] Most cases occur in females, but rare cases have been seen in males. Rarely, such lesions may arise in association with ectopic adrenal cortical tissue.[71] A recent case was reported in association with Beckwith-Wiedemann syndrome.[422] Some regard the lesion as a radial scarlike spindle cell nodule composed of myofibroblasts.[423] Macroscopic tumefactive spindle cell lesions of the adrenal glands have been described in two individuals, one male and one female, and S100 protein immunoreactivity suggested an origin from Schwann cells.[424] A case of granulosa cell tumor of the adrenal gland also has been reported.[425] Leydig cells have been described in the adrenal gland as an incidental finding, a component of adrenal ganglioneuroma, or, rarely, a pure adrenal Leydig cell tumor. Other rare adrenal tumors include solitary fibrous tumor, inflammatory myofibroblastic tumor, calcifying fibrous tumor, Ewing sarcoma/primitive neuroectodermal tumor, and malignant perivascular epithelioid cell tumor.[426-430]

Tumors Metastatic to the Adrenal Glands

The adrenal gland is the fourth most common site of metastatic cancer after lung, liver, and bone; per unit weight, it is more

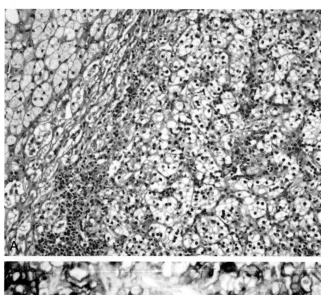
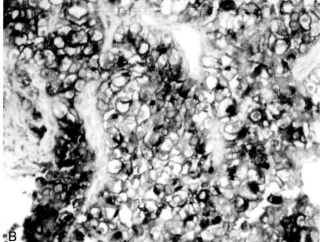

Fig. 16.81 Metastatic renal cell carcinoma. (A) The tumor cells have optically clear cytoplasm in contrast with the adrenal cortex (*upper-left corner*) showing pale staining, finely vacuolated lipid-rich cytoplasm. (B) CD10 immunostain is strongly positive.

frequently involved than the other sites, probably because the adrenal vascular supply has a high flow volume and a sinusoidal vascular pattern.[71,186] Metastases to the adrenal gland most commonly originate in the lung and breast, but other primary sites include the kidney (Fig. 16.81), stomach, pancreas, and skin (malignant melanoma). Rarely, metastases to the adrenal gland are massive, resulting in adrenal cortical insufficiency (Addison disease).[71,186] CT-guided or ultrasound-guided fine-needle aspiration biopsy may be useful in documenting the presence of adrenal metastases. Metastatic carcinoma to the adrenal gland can simulate poorly differentiated ACC.

The views expressed in this chapter are those of the authors and do not reflect the official policy of the Department of Army/Navy/Air Force, Department of Defense, Department of Veterans Affairs, or US government.

References are available at expertconsult.com

Note: Page numbers followed by *f* indicate figures, *t* indicate tables, *b* indicate boxes and fn indicate foot notes.